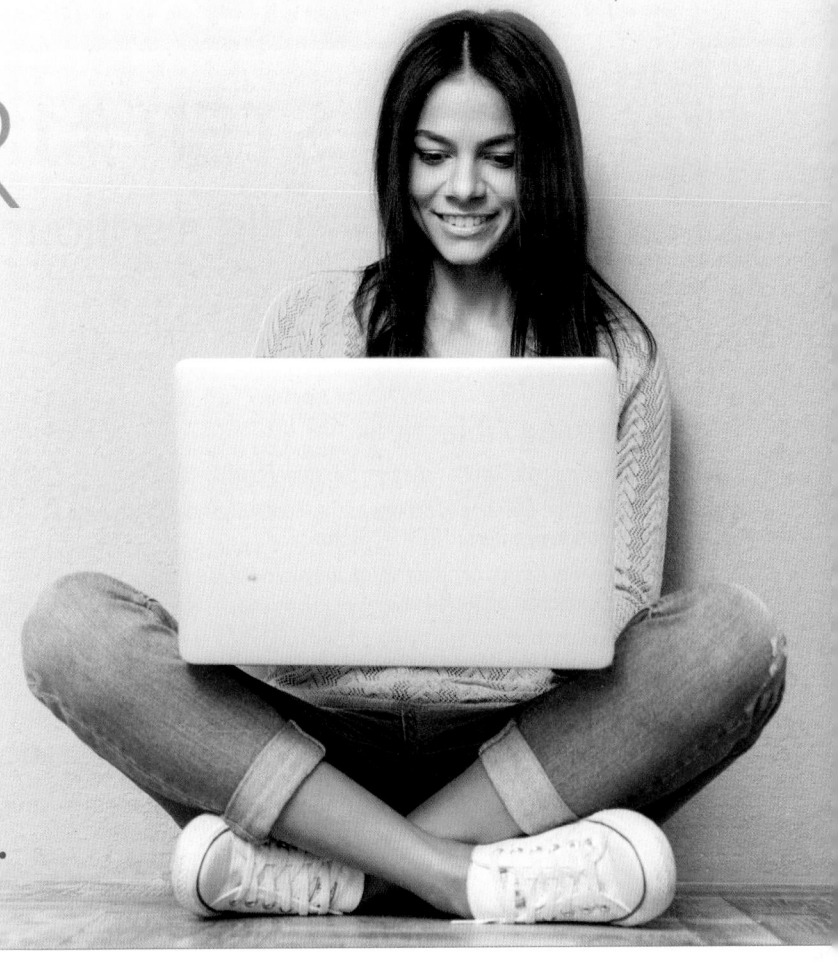
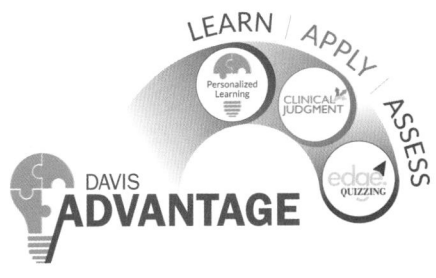

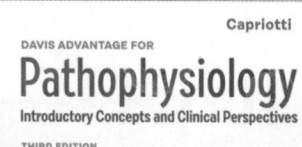

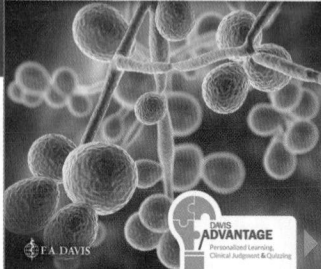

DAVIS ADVANTAGE FOR

Pathophysiology
Introductory Concepts and Clinical Perspectives

Capriotti

THIRD EDITION

TEXT

STEP #1
Build a solid foundation.

Learning Objectives

After completion of this chapter, the student will be able to:

- Describe the various actions of the kidney and how these actions are affected in renal dysfunction.
- Identify causes of prerenal, intrarenal, and postrenal dysfunction of the kidney.
- Explain the signs and symptoms of major causes of kidney dysfunction.

- Recognize assessment modalities and laboratory tests used to diagnose kidney dysfunction.
- Differentiate between acute kidney injury and chronic kidney disease.
- Discuss pharmacological and nonpharmacological treatment modalities used in renal dysfunction.

Learning Objectives at the beginning of each chapter guide your reading and highlight the information you'll need to know.

Clinical Concept boxes explain how key information applies to clinical practice.

 CLINICAL CONCEPT

Individuals who have chronic hypoxia, such as those with chronic obstructive lung disease, often have higher-than-normal hemoglobin and hematocrit levels because of constant secretion of erythropoietin. Conversely, patients with renal failure have lower hemoglobin and hematocrit levels because of deficient erythropoietin.

ALERT! Respiratory acidosis can occur with severe asthma despite the patient having tachypnea. The breathing rate is increased, but the breaths are very shallow and do not eliminate CO_2. CO_2 accumulates, causing increased production of acids in the bloodstream.

 Alerts, highlighted in red, warn you of potential problems or complications that can arise in patients based on the underlying pathophysiology.

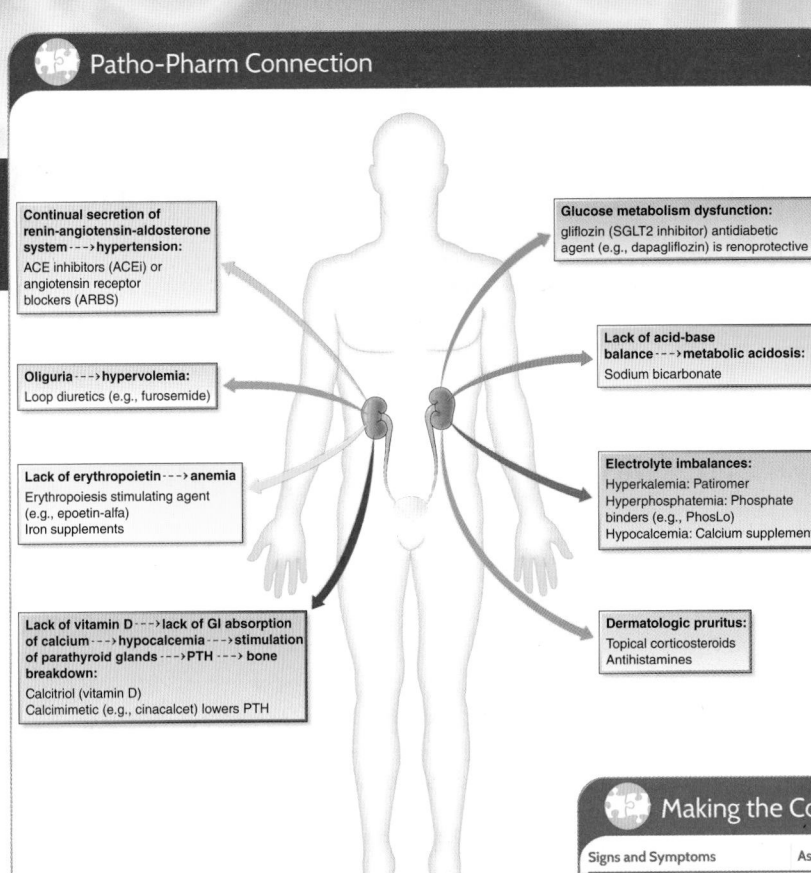

Patho-Pharm Connection

Continual secretion of renin-angiotensin-aldosterone system - - -> hypertension:
ACE inhibitors (ACEi) or angiotensin receptor blockers (ARBS)

Oliguria - - -> hypervolemia:
Loop diuretics (e.g., furosemide)

Lack of erythropoietin - - -> anemia
Erythropoiesis stimulating agent (e.g., epoetin-alfa)
Iron supplements

Lack of vitamin D - - ->lack of GI absorption of calcium - - -> hypocalcemia - - ->stimulation of parathyroid glands - - ->PTH - - -> bone breakdown:
Calcitriol (vitamin D)
Calcimimetic (e.g., cinacalcet) lowers PTH

Glucose metabolism dysfunction:
gliflozin (SGLT2 inhibitor) antidiabetic agent (e.g., dapagliflozin) is renoprotective

Lack of acid-base balance - - -> metabolic acidosis:
Sodium bicarbonate

Electrolyte imbalances:
Hyperkalemia: Patiromer
Hyperphosphatemia: Phosphate binders (e.g., PhosLo)
Hypocalcemia: Calcium supplement

Dermatologic pruritus:
Topical corticosteroids
Antihistamines

NEW! Patho-Pharm Connection boxes highlight how pathophysiology relates to disease processes and their treatment.

Renal failure causes multiple systemic complications. Pharmacological agents are used to counteract the potential adverse effects. With the kidneys not functioning, fluid balance is disturbed and hypervolemia can occur. Loop diuretics can enhance water loss from the body. The failing kidney does not secrete erythropoietin; therefore, epoetin-alfa (synthetic erythropoietin) is administered. This stimulates RBC production, which requires iron supplementation. Blood pressure (BP) is not controlled when the kidneys fail; HTN occurs due to constant secretion of renin. Therefore, antihypertensive medications such as ACE inhibitors or angiotensin receptor blockers are commonly used to control BP. Vitamin D is not produced when the kidneys fail; therefore, Calcitriol (vitamin D supplement) is

necessary. There is c[...]
glands in kidney fail[...]
tions can decrease [...]
metabolism is disru[...]
glifozin-type antidia[...]
turbances occur such[...]
hyperphosphatemia. [...]
level, phosphate bin[...]
ments can be given. [...]
when the kidneys [...]
Sodium bicarbonate[...]
endings become hyp[...]
bloodstream causing[...]
roids and antihistam[...]

Chapter Summary

- Between 1990 and 2015, the prevalence of ESRD has increased almost 100% within the population. Aging of the population and increased prevalence of DM and HTN are reasons for increased kidney disease in the United States.
- As of 2021, one in seven adults in the United States have chronic kidney disease (CKD). Also, as many as 9 in 10 adults with CKD do not know they have this disorder.
- African Americans have the greatest incidence of kidney disease.
- The renal blood filtered per unit of time is known as the GFR. Normal GFR is 90 to 120 mL/min.
- To calculate accurate GFR, clinicians need to use a specific formula that involves age and sex of the patient and serum creatinine.
- The GFR decreases as a physiological change of aging. Because older adults take the greatest number of prescription drugs, decreased GFR raises risk of medication toxicity.

Chapter Summaries make it easy for you to review the most important concepts.

Making the Connections

Signs and Symptoms	Assessment Findings	Diagnostic Tests	Treatment
Nephrotic Syndrome | Any disorder that causes glomerular injury. When glomeruli are injured, they become highly permeable and allow proteins to filter out of blood. Albumin leaves the blood and is excreted in the urine, called proteinuria or albuminuria. Hypoalbuminemia causes edema. Glomerulonephritis caused by infection and immunological inflammatory disease is a cause of nephrotic syndrome.			
Edema, especially of periorbital region and face.	Edema of the face is common, especially in the periorbital region. HTN. With severe albumin loss, edema of lower extremities, pleural effusion, and ascites can develop.	Albuminuria. Hypoalbuminemia. Hematuria. Hyperlipidemia. Hypertriglyceridemia. Elevated serum creatinine and BUN. 24-hour urine collection shows more than 3 grams of protein /dL. ANAs may be positive if etiology is an autoimmune disease.	Diet low in sodium. Adequate protein and fluid. ACE inhibitors or ARBs may be used.
Nephrolithiasis | The formation of calculi in the kidney, which can cause obstructive uropathy. Calculi are commonly composed of calcium.			
Severe back pain with radiation into the groin. Severe abdominal pain. Chills.	CVA tenderness. Hematuria. Crystalluria.	Blood may show high calcium, uric acid, or purines, depending on the etiology of nephrolithiasis. Elevated blood pressure and tachycardia are caused by pain. Urinalysis shows RBCs and crystals. Abdominal x-ray, CT, or ultrasound can show calculi.	IV fluid. Analgesics. Strain urine. Urinalysis needed. Increase oral fluid intake to more than 3 liters/day. Lithotripsy. Ureterocystoscopic surgery.
Pyelonephritis | Infection of the upper urinary tract, commonly caused by an ascending lower UTI.			
Back pain. Fever. Malaise. Chills. Dysuria. Frequency.	CVA tenderness. Fever.	Elevated WBC count. Microscopic hematuria. Pyuria. Bacteriuria. Proteinuria.	Antibiotics. Antipyretics and analgesics may be necessary.
Polycystic Kidney Disease | Disease causing multiple cysts in the kidneys and dysfunction caused by genetic mutation at			
Back pain. Fever (if infection).	CVA tenderness, if infection.	Hematuria. Crystalluria. Bacteriuria. Ultrasound or CT scan can show cysts within kidneys.	Supportive treatment: low-sodium diet, physical activity, smoking cessation, and normal body weight maintenance. Tolvaptan. ACE inhibitors or ARBs to treat HTN. Prevention and treatment of UTIs. Hemodialysis if necessary. Renal transplant.

Making the Connections boxes relate pathophysiology to the clinical manifestations, assessment, and management of key disorders.

Personalized Learning

LEARN

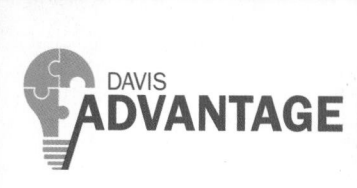

DAVIS ADVANTAGE

STEP #2
Make the connections to key topics.

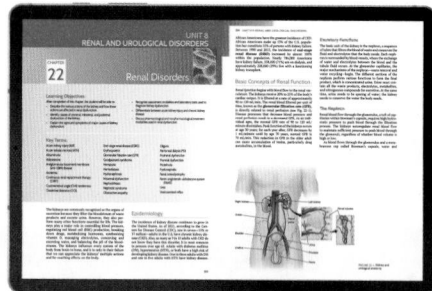

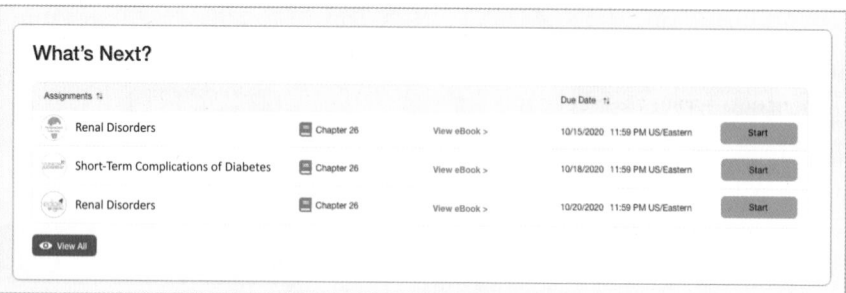

Assignments in Davis Advantage correspond to key topics in your book. Begin by reading from your printed text or click the ebook button to be taken to the **FREE, integrated ebook.**

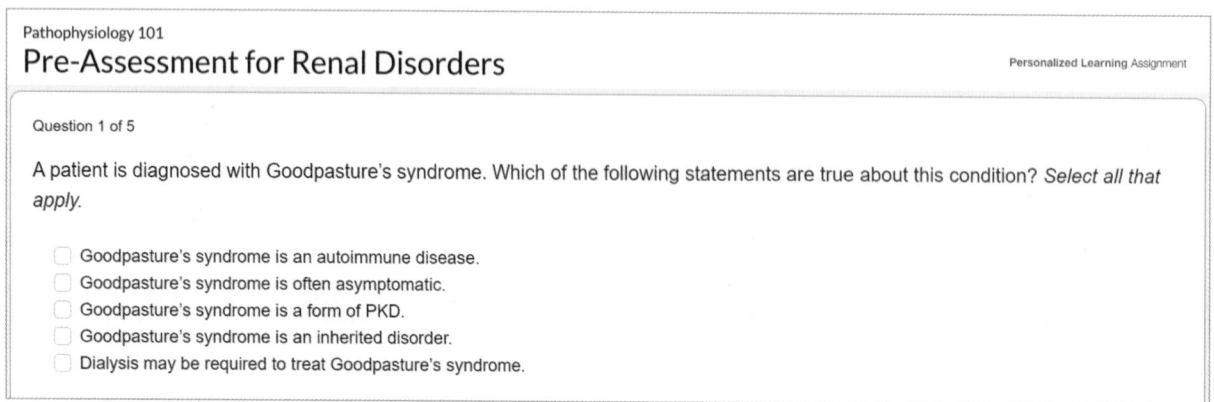

Pathophysiology 101
Pre-Assessment for Renal Disorders

Personalized Learning Assignment

Question 1 of 5

A patient is diagnosed with Goodpasture's syndrome. Which of the following statements are true about this condition? *Select all that apply.*

- [ ] Goodpasture's syndrome is an autoimmune disease.
- [ ] Goodpasture's syndrome is often asymptomatic.
- [ ] Goodpasture's syndrome is a form of PKD.
- [ ] Goodpasture's syndrome is an inherited disorder.
- [ ] Dialysis may be required to treat Goodpasture's syndrome.

Following your reading, take a **Pre-Assessment** to evaluate your understanding of the content. Questions feature single answer, multiple-choice, and select-all-that-apply formats.

Immediate feedback identifies your strengths and weaknesses using a thumbs up, thumbs down approach. *Thumbs up* indicates competency, while *thumbs down* signals an area of weakness that requires further study.

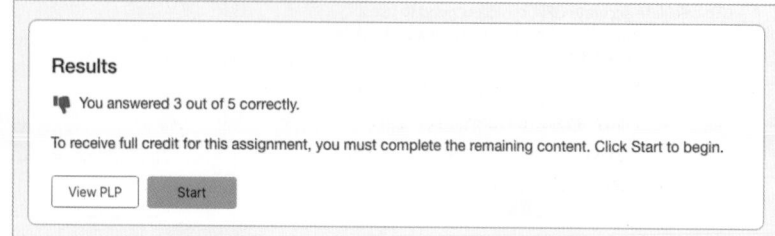

Results

👎 You answered 3 out of 5 correctly.

To receive full credit for this assignment, you must complete the remaining content. Click Start to begin.

View PLP   Start

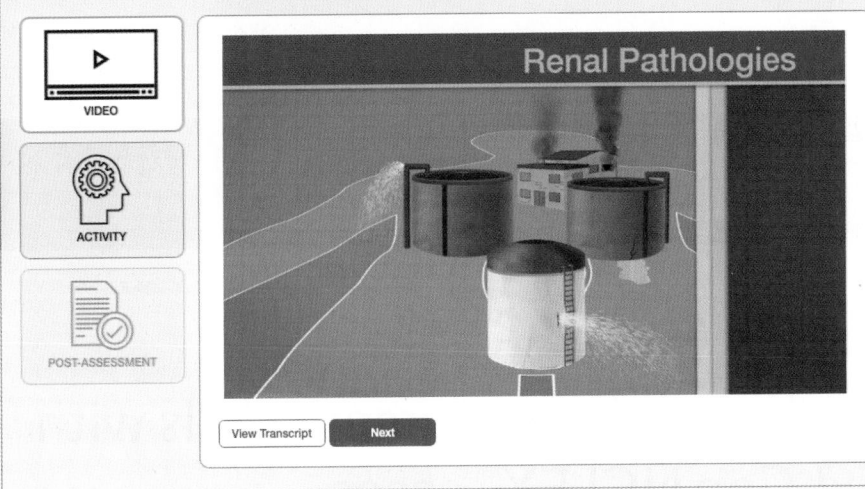

After working through the video and activity, a **Post-Assessment** tests your mastery.

Mini-lecture videos make key concepts easier to understand, while **interactive learning activities** allow you to expand your knowledge and make the connections to important topics.

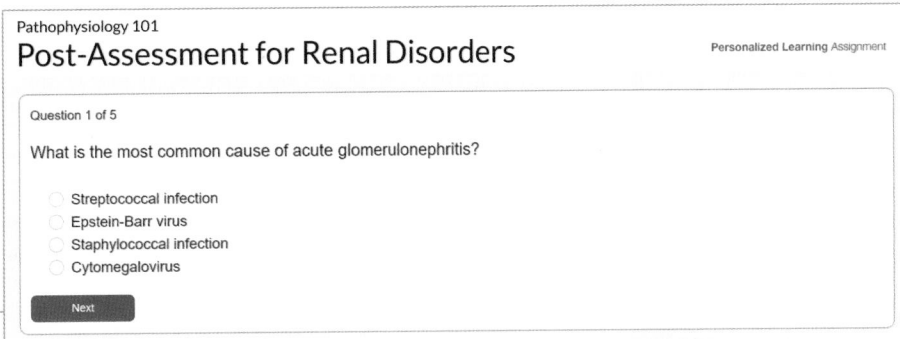

Pathophysiology 101
Post-Assessment for Renal Disorders

Personalized Learning Assignment

Question 1 of 5

What is the most common cause of acute glomerulonephritis?

- Streptococcal infection
- Epstein-Barr virus
- Staphylococcal infection
- Cytomegalovirus

Next

Personalized Learning at a Glance

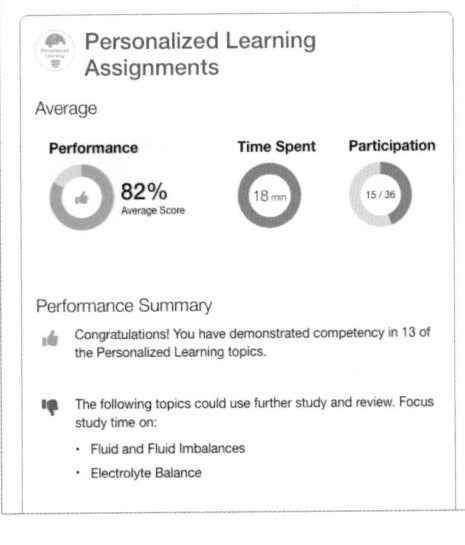

Personalized Learning Assignments

Average

Performance	Time Spent	Participation
82% Average Score	18 min	15 / 36

Performance Summary

Congratulations! You have demonstrated competency in 13 of the Personalized Learning topics.

The following topics could use further study and review. Focus study time on:
- Fluid and Fluid Imbalances
- Electrolyte Balance

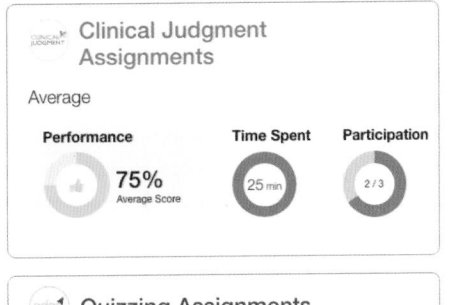

Clinical Judgment Assignments

Average

Performance	Time Spent	Participation
75% Average Score	25 min	2 / 3

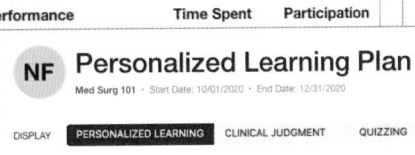

Quizzing Assignments

Average

Performance	Time Spent	Participation

Your **Dashboard** provides an at-a-glance snapshot of your performance as you work through your assignments.

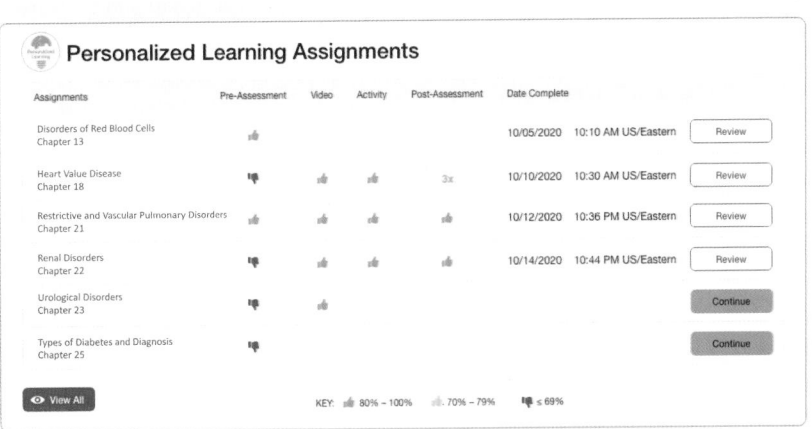

Your **Personalized Learning Plan** is tailored to your individual needs and tracks your progress **across all your assignments**, helping you to identify the specific areas that require additional study.

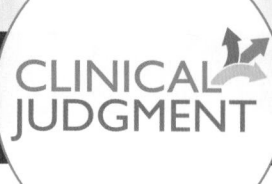

CLINICAL JUDGMENT

APPLY

STEP #3
Develop clinical judgment skills with Next Gen NCLEX® cases.

Short-term Complications of Diabetes

Clinical Judgment **Assignment**

Short-term Complications of Diabetes

Twenty-two-year-old female college student presents in emergency department with suspected diabetic ketoacidosis.

This case consists of six clinical judgment questions. Read each question carefully and select the best answer(s). Use the chart to help answer the question. The chart is dynamic and may change as the case progresses.

Next

Real-world cases mirror the complex clinical challenges you will encounter in a variety of health care settings. Each **case study** begins with a patient photograph and a brief introduction to the scenario.

Scenario

Twenty-two-year-old female college student presents in emergency department with suspected diabetic ketoacidosis. Use the chart to answer the questions. *The chart may update as the scenario progresses.*

History and Physical Assessment	**Nurses' Notes**	**Vital Signs**	**Laboratory Results**

Medical/Surgical history: Patient diagnosed with type 1 diabetes mellitus at age 11. Patient admitted to hospital with diabetic ketoacidosis at age 14 and age 16. Anterior cruciate ligament repair (L knee) 2 years ago.

Social history: Senior in college, business major. Sorority member. Volunteers in after school youth program. Denies use of tobacco and recreational drugs. Seldom uses alcohol. (Often serves as designated driver for friends.)

Family history: Uncle (father's brother) diagnosed with type 1 diabetes mellitus at age 10. Father in good health. Mother diagnosed with ulcerative colitis last year (age 46). One older sibling, suffers from depression.

Physical Assessment: Patient is distressed. Patient breathing is heavy

The **Patient Chart** displays tabs for History and Physical Assessment, Nurses' Notes, Vital Signs, and Laboratory Results. As you progress through the case, the chart expands and populates with additional data.

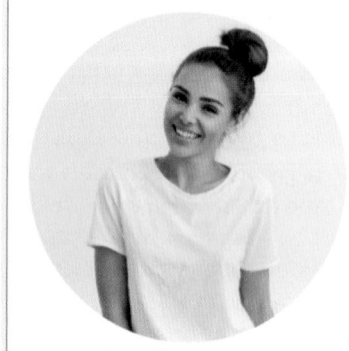

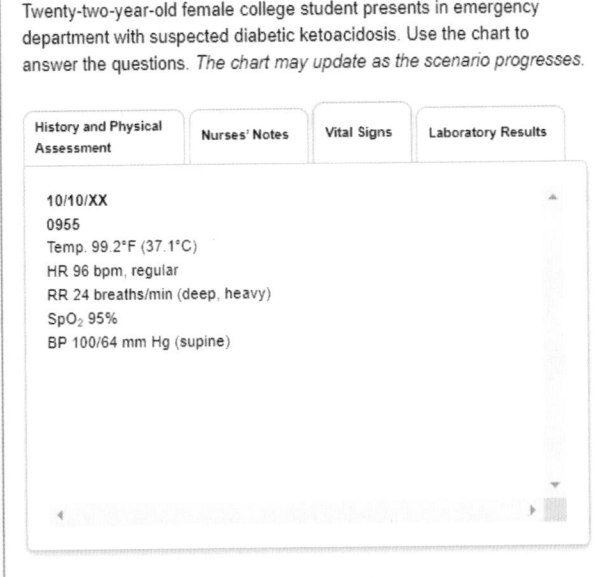

Twenty-two-year-old female college student presents in emergency department with suspected diabetic ketoacidosis. Use the chart to answer the questions. *The chart may update as the scenario progresses.*

History and Physical Assessment	Nurses' Notes	Vital Signs	Laboratory Results

10/10/XX
0955
Temp. 99.2°F (37.1°C)
HR 96 bpm, regular
RR 24 breaths/min (deep, heavy)
SpO_2 95%
BP 100/64 mm Hg (supine)

Question 4 of 6

If diabetic ketoacidosis has developed in the patient, indicate for each laboratory value listed whether it will likely be "elevated" or "decreased" in the patient. *Select one option in each row.*

	Elevated	Decreased
Blood pH	●	○
$PaCO_2$	●	○
Acetone	○	●
Blood K^+	○	●
Anion gap	●	○
Blood glucose	○	●
HCO_3-	○	●

Previous

Next

Short-term Complications of Diabetes

Clinical Judgment Assignment

Results

You answered 2 out of 6 questions correctly

Review the questions, answers and rationales below to improve your understanding. Identify which questions you answered correctly (indicated by a green check mark) and incorrectly (identified by a red x). Remember, you must choose all correct options and only the correct options to get a question correct. Expand the questions to review your individual answer choices, the correct answers (indicated by green shading), and complete rationales.

Hide All Details ▲   Return to Assignments

❌ Question 4 of 6   Hide ▲

If diabetic ketoacidosis has developed in the patient, indicate for each laboratory value listed whether it will likely be "elevated" or "decreased" in the patient. *Select one option in each row.*

	Elevated	Decreased
Blood pH	●	○
$PaCO_2$	●	○
Acetone	○	●
Blood K^+	○	●
Anion gap	●	○
Blood glucose	○	●
HCO_3-	○	●

Rationale

If the patient has developed diabetic ketoacidosis, ketones, which are acidic, will be elevated. The acidic ketones will lower blood pH and to compensate for the reduced pH, ventilation will increase, reducing carbon dioxide levels. Bicarbonate ion levels will be lower than normal, as bicarbonate is a base that buffers the elevated acidic levels.

Blood K^+ levels will increase as in metabolic acidosis, H^+ ions shift into cells, while K^+ ions leave the cells and enter the blood. The anion gap will also be elevated, as bicarbonate levels are lower than normal.

If insulin is lacking, blood glucose will be elevated.

Clinical Judgment Cognitive Skill: Analyze Cues, Prioritize Hypotheses   Page Reference: P. 605

💬 Test-Taking Tip   Memorizing values is not enough. Be able to justify your answer to yourself. For example, for "Blood K+," be able to provide an explanation such as "K+ levels may elevate in the blood because during acidosis, H+ ions enter the cells, and K+ ions leave the cell. This results in higher K+ levels in the blood." By justifying your answer, you prevent mistakes and "guessing."

NGN-format questions that align with the cognitive areas of the **NCSBN Clinical Judgment Measurement Model** require careful analysis, synthesis of the data, and multi-step thinking.

Immediate feedback with **detailed rationales** identifies the cognitive skills practiced according to the NCSBN Clinical Judgment Measurement Model and includes page references to the text for further remediation.

Test-taking tips provide important context and strategies for how to consider the structure of each question type when answering.

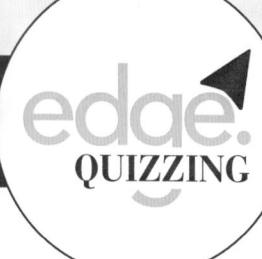

STEP #4
Improve scores and build confidence with NCLEX®-style questions.

High-quality questions, including **Next Gen NCLEX® bowtie and trend questions**, test your knowledge and challenge you to think critically.

Renal Disorders
Quizzing: Assignment

Question 14 of 15

For which of the following would antibiotics be appropriate as the primary treatment? Select all that apply.

- ☐ Group A beta-hemolytic streptococci (GABHS) glomerulonephritis
- ☐ Nephrotic syndrome
- ☐ Pyelonephritis
- ☐ Goodpasture's syndrome
- ☐ Polycystic kidney disease

Feedback

👍 **You answered 9 out of 10 correctly.**
Review the questions, answers and rationales below.

[Hide All Details ▲]   [Return to Assignments]

✓ Question 13 of 15

For which of the following would antibiotics be appropriate as the primary treatment? Select all that apply.

- ☑ Group A beta-hemolytic streptococci (GABHS) glomerulonephritis
  Rationale: GABHS glomerulonephritis is a disorder caused by streptococcal bacteria.

- ☐ Nephrotic syndrome
  Rationale: Nephrotic syndrome is not due to a bacterial infection.

- ☑ Pyelonephritis
  Rationale: Pyelonephritis is an infection of the renal pelvis.

- ☐ Goodpasture's syndrome
  Rationale: Goodpasture's syndrome is an autoimmune disorder.

- ☐ Polycystic kidney disease
  Rationale: Polycystic kidney disease is a genetic disorder.

💬 Test-Taking Tip   The question stem is essentially asking which of the... infection.

Question ID:
PATHO2-RDDFE-12

Course Topic:
Renal Disorders

Concept:
Urinary Elimination

Cognitive:
Evaluation [Evaluating]

Immediate feedback with **comprehensive rationales** explains why your responses are correct or incorrect. **Page-specific references** direct you to the relevant content in your text, while **test-taking tips** improve your test-taking skills.

Practice Quizzes
[Create Practice Quiz]

You may generate their own practice quizzes (NCLEX®-style assessments) to test or expand your understanding of topics).

Assignments		Competency	Percent Correct	Date Complete	
Renal Disorders	15 Questions	👍	85%	09/11/2020 10:40 PM US/Eastern	[Review]
Types of Diabetes and Diagnosis	15 Questions	👍	79%	09/25/2020 10:45 PM US/Eastern	[Review]

👁 View All

KEY: 👍 80% – 100%   👍 70% – 79%   👎 ≤ 69%

Create your own **practice quizzes** to focus on topic areas where you are struggling, or to use as a study tool to review for an upcoming exam.

GET STARTED TODAY!
Use the access code on the inside front cover to unlock
Davis Advantage for Pathophysiology!

DAVIS ADVANTAGE FOR

Pathophysiology
Introductory Concepts and Clinical Perspectives

THIRD EDITION

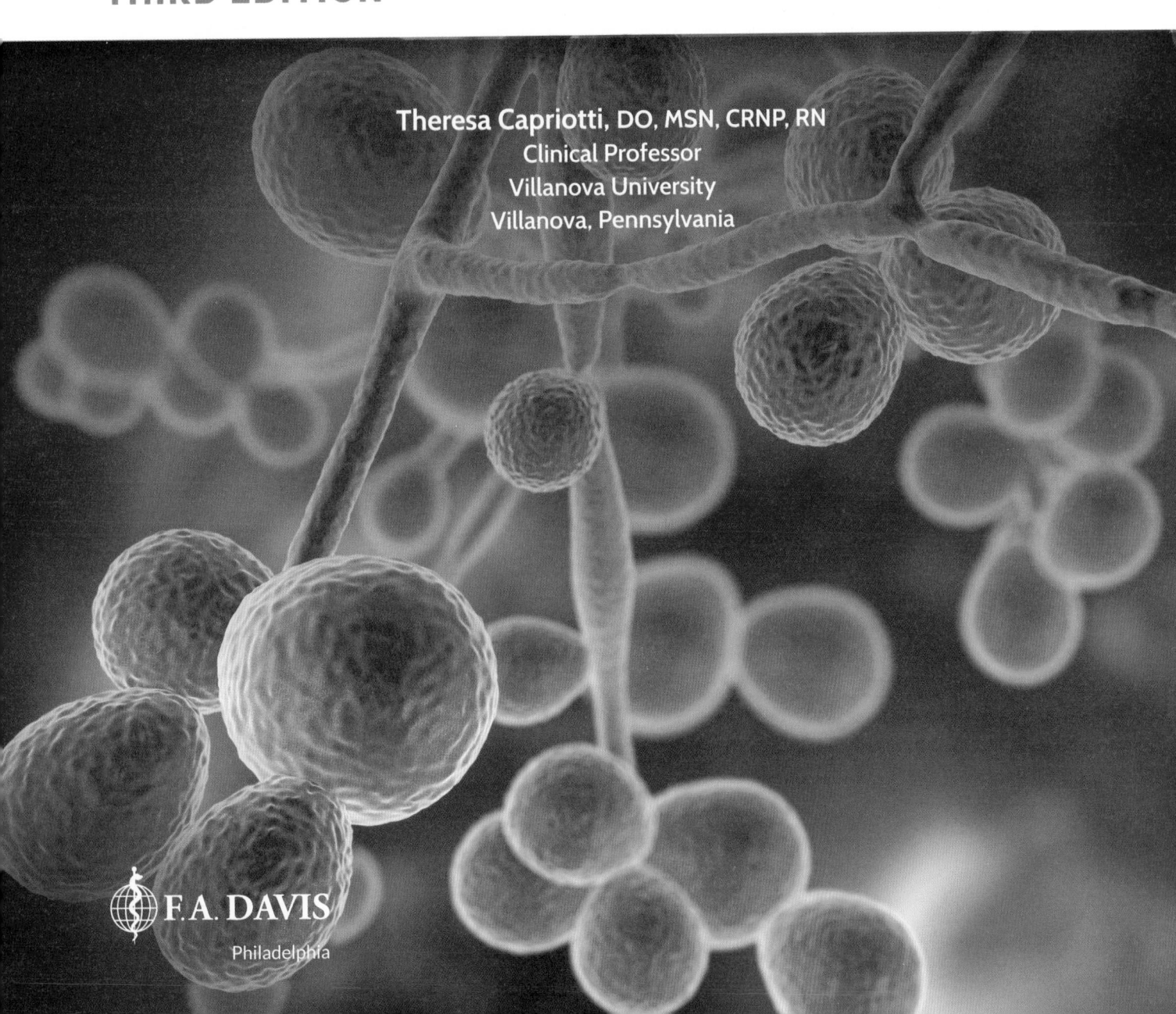

Theresa Capriotti, DO, MSN, CRNP, RN
Clinical Professor
Villanova University
Villanova, Pennsylvania

F.A. DAVIS
Philadelphia

F. A. Davis Company
1915 Arch Street
Philadelphia, PA 19103
www.fadavis.com

Copyright © 2024 by F. A. Davis Company

Printed in the United States of America

Last digit indicates print number: 10 9 8 7 6 5 4 3 2 1

Publisher, Nursing: Suzanne Czehut Toppy
Senior Content Project Manager: Amy M. Romano
Design and Illustration Manager: Carolyn O'Brien

As new scientific information becomes available through basic and clinical research, recommended treatments and drug therapies undergo changes. The author(s) and publisher have done everything possible to make this book accurate, up-to-date, and in accord with accepted standards at the time of publication. The author(s), editors, and publisher are not responsible for errors or omissions or for consequences from application of the book, and make no warranty, expressed or implied, in regard to the contents of the book. Any practice described in this book should be applied by the reader in accordance with professional standards of care used in regard to the unique circumstances that may apply in each situation. The reader is advised always to check product information (package inserts) for changes and new information regarding dose and contraindications before administering any drug. Caution is especially urged when using new or infrequently ordered drugs.

Library of Congress Cataloging-in-Publication Data

Names: Capriotti, Theresa, author.
Title: Davis advantage for pathophysiology : introductory concepts and
  clinical perspectives / Theresa Capriotti.
Other titles: Pathophysiology | Advantage for pathophysiology
Description: Third edition. | Philadelphia, PA : F.A. Davis Company, [2024]
  | Includes bibliographical references and index.
Identifiers: LCCN 2023013768 (print) | LCCN 2023013769 (ebook) | ISBN
  9781719648592 (hardcover) | ISBN 9781719650533 (ebook)
Subjects: MESH: Disease | Pathologic Processes—nursing | Nurses
  Instruction
Classification: LCC RB113 (print) | LCC RB113 (ebook) | NLM QZ 140 | DDC
  616.07—dc23/eng/20230726
LC record available at https://lccn.loc.gov/2023013768
LC ebook record available at https://lccn.loc.gov/2023013769

I think it is very important for students, particularly those studying the health-care sciences, to remember that this book is really about people. Diseases affect people. Pathophysiology is essentially the study of suffering. If you are studying to become a health-care provider, please remember that you are treating people, not diseases—people who have aspirations, loved ones, and responsibilities that are turned upside down by disease. I hope that this book will help you understand the challenges of people affected by diseases and disorders.

I want to thank those who have inspired me—my mother, Johanna Capriotti, and my father, Vincent Capriotti, for making me laugh, even now after they are gone; my three sons, David, Michael, and Peter Wolinsky, who have grown to be men that I am so proud of; my niece, Erica Plower, who has been like a daughter to me; my grandsons, Ethan and Caleb Wolinsky, who are brand new to this world; and my best friends, Rocco, Gianna, and Bambino, who waited patiently to go out while I typed each word in this book.

–Teri Capriotti

CONTRIBUTORS
(to this edition or the first edition)

Elise M. Alverson, DNP, RN, FNP-BC, CNE
Professor Emerita
Valparaiso University
Valparaiso, Indiana

Kenya Beard, EdD, CNE, AGACNP-BC, ANEF, FAAN
Dean, Nursing & Health Sciences
Nassau Community College
Garden City, New York

Linda Brandon
Heart Failure Care Manager
New England Quality Care Alliance
Braintree, Massachusetts

Erin Caroulis, MPH, RD, LDN, CDE, CPT
Diabetes Educator
Diabetes Center at Children's Hospital of Philadelphia
Philadelphia, Pennsylvania

Dona Rinaldi Carpenter, RN, EdD
Undergraduate Program Director
Scranton University
Scranton, Pennsylvania

Linda A. Carrick, PhD, RN, CNAA
Adjunct Assistant Professor of Nursing
University of Pennsylvania, School of Nursing
Philadelphia, Pennsylvania

Deborah W. Chapa, PhD, ACNP-BC
Assistant Professor, Director, Doctor of Nursing Practice
George Washington University, School of Nursing
Washington, D.C.

Michael Clinton, RN, PhD
Professor
American University of Beirut, Hariri School of Nursing
Beirut, Lebanon

Ferne M. Cohen, EdD, CRNA
Assistant Chair, Nurse Anesthesia Program
Drexel University
Philadelphia, Pennsylvania

Denise Coppa, PhD, RNP
Associate Professor
University of Rhode Island, School of Nursing
Kingston, Rhode Island

Darleen Crisileo, RN
Staff RN, Post-Anesthesia Care Unit
Massachusetts General Hospital
Canton, Massachusetts

Renee Crossman, BN, RN, MHS
Lecturer
Memorial University School of Nursing
St. John's, Newfoundland
Canada

Angela J. Daniel, MSN, MBA, RN
Atlanta, Georgia

Stephanie Denninghoff, MSN, CNOR
Faculty
School of Nursing
Purdue University Global, Inc.

Elaine K. Diegmann, CNM, ND, FACNM
Program Director, Nurse Midwifery
University of Medicine and Dentistry of New Jersey, School of Nursing
Newark, New Jersey

Sr. Rosemary Donley, PhD, APRN, FAAN
Professor, Jacques Laval Chair for Social Justice
Duquesne University School of Nursing
Pittsburgh, Pennsylvania

Patricia A. Dunn, PhD, RNC
Associate Professor
Holy Family University
Philadelphia, Pennsylvania

Claire Faust, MSN, APN
Nursing Program Coordinator, College of Nursing & Allied Health
Burlington County College
Pemberton, New Jersey

Cynthia M. Finn, RN, BS, CCRN
Staff RN, Cardiac Surgical ICU
Massachusetts General Hospital
Boston, Massachusetts

Elizabeth Galik, PhD, CRNP
Associate Professor
University of Maryland School of Nursing
Baltimore, Maryland

Diane M. Gay, RN
Boston, Massachusetts

Catherine A. Griffith, PhD, RN, ACNP-BC
Clinical Research Nurse
Harvard Catalyst Clinical & Translational Science Center at Massachusetts General Hospital
MGH Clinical Research Center
Boston, Massachusetts

Kathie Judy Guth, MS, RN
Baltimore, Maryland

Kimberly Harding, PhD
Professor, Department of Science
Colorado Mountain College
Glenwood Springs, Colorado

Patricia Hindin, PhD, CNM
Assistant Professor
Rutgers, The State University of New Jersey
Newark, New Jersey

Janice J. Hoffman, PhD, RN, ANEF
Associate Professor, Assistant Dean of the Baccalaureate Nursing Program
University of Maryland School of Nursing
Baltimore, Maryland

Joanna F. Hofmann, NP
New York, New York

Susan H. Jones, RN, BSN, MS, EdD
Associate Professor, Nursing (Retired)
Hampton University School of Nursing
Hampton, Virginia

Emily Karwacki Sheff, PhD, MS, RN, FNP
Partnership Liaison, Project REEP
Rivier University
Nashua, New Hampshire

Julie A. Koch, DNP, RN, FNP-BC
Assistant Professor, FNP Program Coordinator
Valparaiso University College of Nursing and Health Professions
Valparaiso, Indiana

Marianne Kraemer, RN, EdM, MPA, CCRN
Chief Nursing Officer
Kennedy Health System
Stratford, New Jersey

Ginette Lange, PhD, CNM, RN
Associate Professor
University of Medicine and Dentistry of New Jersey, School of Nursing
Newark, New Jersey

Ciara Levine, MSN, RN
Assistant Professor of Nursing
La Salle University
Philadelphia, Pennsylvania

Claude Lieber, MD, FACS
Clinical Associate Professor of Surgery, Thomas Jefferson Medical College, Philadelphia, Retired
Chief of Surgery, Wilmington VA Medical Center, Retired
Adjunct, Department of Nursing, Florida Gulf Coast University, Retired

Sandra MacDonald, RN, BN, MN, PhD
Professor
Memorial University of Newfoundland School of Nursing
St. John's, Newfoundland
Canada

Carol Isaac MacKusick, AGNP-C, CNE
Adult Gerontology Nurse Practitioner
Doctors Making Housecalls
Arden, North Carolina

April Manuel, PhD, BN
Assistant Professor
Memorial University School of Nursing
St. John's, Newfoundland
Canada

James Mendez, PhD, RN
Clinical Associate Professor
Villanova University
Villanova, Pennsylvania

Kimberly Meyer, MSN, CNRN, ACNP-BC
Neurosurgery Nurse Practitioner
University of Louisville Medical Center Trauma Institute
Louisville, Kentucky

Helen Miley, RN, PhD, CCRN, AG-ACNP
Specialty Director, Adult Geriatric Acute Care Nurse Practitioner Program
Rutgers University
Newark, New Jersey

Judy I. Murphy, PhD, RN, CNE, CHSE
Simulation Coordinator, Nurse Researcher
Rhode Island College School of Nursing
Assistant Professor of Clinical Medicine
Alpert Medical School Brown University
Providence, Rhode Island

Kathleen O'Rourke Vito, PhD, PHCNS-BC, RN
Associate Professor of Nursing
Felician College
Lodi, New Jersey

Joan Parker Frizzell, PhD, CRNP, ANP-BC
Associate Professor
School of Nursing & Health Sciences
La Salle University
Philadelphia, Pennsylvania
Nurse Practitioner
Roxborough Memorial Hospital
Philadelphia, Pennsylvania

Margie Pierce, MS, RRT, CPFT
Director of Respiratory and Neurophysiology Services
Pennsylvania Hospital
Philadelphia, Pennsylvania

Susan Padham Porterfield, PhD, FNP-c
Assistant Dean for Graduate Programs, College of Nursing
Florida State University
Tallahassee, Florida

AliceMarie S. Poyss, PhD, CNL, APRN-BC
Associate Clinical Professor, CNL Track Director
Drexel University College of Nursing and Health Professions
Philadelphia, Pennsylvania

Ingrid Pretzer-Aboff, PhD, RN
Associate Professor, Co-Director of The Nurse Managed Health Center, Parkinson's Clinic
University of Delaware
Newark, Delaware

Francia I. Reed, MS, RN, FNP-C
Clinical Assistant Professor
State University of New York, Institute of Technology
Utica, New York

Kimberly D. Ryan-Nicholls, RPN, RN, BScN, MDE
Associate Professor, Psychiatric Nursing
Brandon University, School of Health Studies
Brandon, Manitoba
Canada

Mary Clare A. Schafer, MS, RN, ONC, CRRN
Orthopaedic Day Rehabilitation Coordinator
Magee Rehabilitation Hospital
Philadelphia, Pennsylvania

Deborah Schiavone, PhD, PMHCNS-BC, CNE
Program Director
Stratford University
Woodbridge, Virginia

Susan K. Smith, DNP, RN, CEN, CCRN
SK Smith Consulting
Warriors Mark, Pennsylvania

Julia Spinolo, DNP
Owner
Centered Self, LLC
Atlanta, Georgia

Angela Starkweather, PhD, MSN, CCRN, CNRN, PhD, RN, ANCP-BC, CNRN, FAAN
Associate Dean
Professor, Academic Affairs
University of Connecticut, School of Nursing
Storrs, Connecticut

Kimberly Subasic, PhD, MS, BSN
Assistant Professor
University of Scranton
Scranton, Pennsylvania

Patricia A. Thompson, BSN, MSN, FNP-BC
Family Nurse Practitioner
Hattiesburg Clinic, Wiggins Clinic
Hattiesburg, Mississippi

Ann B. Tritak, EdD, RN
Associate Dean Department of Graduate Nursing
Felician University
Division of Nursing and Health Management
Lodi, New Jersey

Diane M. Wieland, PhD, MSN, RN, PMHCNS-BC, CNE
Associate Professor
La Salle University, School of Nursing and Health Sciences
Philadelphia, Pennsylvania

Mary Wilby, PhD, MSN, RN
Assistant Professor of Nursing
La Salle University
Philadelphia, Pennsylvania

Joyce S. Willens, PhD, RN, BC
Assistant Professor
Villanova University
Villanova, Pennsylvania

Tamara L. Zurakowski, PhD, GNP-BC
Clinical Associate Professor
Concentration Coordinator, Adult-Gerontology Primary Care Nurse Practitioner Program
Virginia Commonwealth University
Richmond, Virginia

Erica Allen, DNP, MBA, RN
Associate Professor, Program
  Coordinator
Chicago State University
Chicago, Illinois

Charita L. Barlow-Walls, DNP, MSN, RN
Faculty Professor–Lecturer
Chicago State University
Chicago, Illinois

Rhonda L. Bishop, EdD, MSN, RN, CNE
Associate Professor
Ferris State University
Big Rapids, Michigan

Maria Brosnan, MSN, APRN, ACNP-BC, CNE, CHSE
Associate Professor
Carroll College
Helena, Montana

Edward Campbell, EdD, RN, CNE
Instructor
The University of Alabama at
  Birmingham
Birmingham, Alabama

Rachel Choudhury, MSN, MS, RN, CNE
Dean of Nursing
Arizona College of Nursing
Ontario, California

Aaron Cyr, MSN, RN
Director of Assessment and
  Evaluation
Arizona College of Nursing
Phoenix, Arizona

Amy J. Edmison, DNP, RN
Associate Dean of Undergraduate
  Programs
King University
Bristol, Tennessee

Jami England, DNP, FNP-BC
Assistant Professor of Nursing
Lincoln Memorial University
Harrogate, Tennessee

Anita Fitzgerald, PhD, RN, APRN, CNE
Assistant Professor
California State University, Long
  Beach
Long Beach, California

Becka Foerster, MS, RN, CNE
Lecturer
South Dakota State University
Brookings, South Dakota

Kitty M. Garrett, RN, MSN, CCRN-K
Assistant Professor, Department of
  Physiological and Technological
  Nursing
Augusta University
Augusta, Georgia

Bonnie Gary, MSN, RN, CNE
Senior Lecturer
Georgia Southwestern State
  University
Americus, Georgia

Masoud Ghaffari, PhD, MSN/RN, MEd, MT (ASCP)
Associate Professor
Benedictine University
Lisle, Illinois

Alisa L. Hearl, MSN, RN, CDCES
Instructor
King University
Bristol, Tennessee

Jamie Hunsicker, DNP, MS, RN
Associate Professor of Nursing
Ohio Northern University
Ada, Ohio

Robin F. Johns, PhD, RN
Associate Professor
Augusta University, Athens Campus
Athens, Georgia

Amber Kool, DNP, RN
Associate Provost
Arizona College of Nursing
Phoenix, Arizona

Lilian Nyindodo, PhD, MPH
Chair and Associate Professor
  Biomedical Sciences
Baptist Health Sciences University
Memphis, Tennessee

Michael Perlow, DNS, RN
Professor of Nursing
Murray State University
Murray, Kentucky

Tara Price, RNC, DNP, WHNP-BC, CNS
Assistant Professor
University of Mississippi Medical
  Center, School of Nursing
Jackson, Mississippi

Rhonda R. Reid, RN, BSN, MSN-LHCM, MSN-ED
Simulation and Lab Skills Instructor
Arizona College of Nursing
Tempe, Arizona

Bedelia H. Russell, RN, PhD, CPNP-PC, CNE
Associate Professor and Interim
  Associate Provost
Tennessee Tech University, Whitson-
  Hester School of Nursing
Cookeville, Tennessee

Laurie J. Singel, PhD, MSN, RN, MEDSURG-BC
Nurse Educator
Ascend Learning Inc.
San Antonio, Texas

Lisa B. Soontupe, EdD, RN, CNE
Professor
Nova Southeastern University, Ron
  and Kathy Assaf College of Nursing
Fort Lauderdale, Florida

Nancy L. Stark, RN, DNP
Associate Professor
University of South Carolina Aiken
Aiken, South Carolina

Michael W. Thompson, PhD
Instructor, Department of Biology
Indiana State University
Terre Haute, Indiana

**Theresa Turick-Gibson, EdD
  candidate, MA, PPCNP-BC,
  RN-BC**
Professor Emerita, Curriculum
  Chair–Department of Nursing
Hartwick College
Oneonta, New York

Elizabeth A. VandeWaa, PhD
Professor
University of South Alabama College
  of Nursing
Mobile, Alabama

Barbara Voshall, DNP, MN, RN
Professor of Nursing
Graceland University
Independence, Missouri

Denyce Watties-Daniels, DNP, RN
Associate Professor, Director
  Simulation and Learning Resource
  Centers
Coppin State University, College of
  Health Professions
Baltimore, Maryland

**Melissa L. Weir, PhD, RN, CNE,
  CPEN, CEN**
Assistant Professor
Howard University
Washington, D.C.

**Mary B. Winton, PhD, RN,
  ACANP-BC**
Associate Professor
Tarleton State University
Stephenville, Texas

Pricilla Wyatt, DNP, MSN, RN
Faculty Instructor
Abilene Christian University
Abilene, Texas

Pathophysiology, in its simplest definition, is the study of the altered processes of the body as a result of a disease or disorder. A solid understanding of pathophysiology builds a strong foundation for later nursing and health sciences courses. It provides the key to understanding core components of care, such as why certain drugs are chosen, how to assess clinical manifestations, and how to choose interventions and prioritize care.

The subtitle of this book is "Introductory Concepts and Clinical Perspectives." It highlights how this text intends to approach the learning of this important subject matter. There are many pathophysiology texts and resources; however, all too often, they focus on "the science" alone. This book and its digital components strive to keep pathophysiology oriented in the clinical context, never forgetting the patient. The content of the text, the pedagogical features, and the online components are firmly tied to patient care, providing the framework for a solid understanding of pathophysiology and its applications and, thus, fostering clinical judgment skills.

Organization

The text begins with a general description of the basic unit of the body—the cell—and fundamental genetic concepts. It then covers important body processes that affect overall health and functioning. From there, the rest of the units follow a systems approach to explain aspects of pathophysiology. Each chapter begins with an overview of concepts regarding the normal anatomy and physiology of the system under study. The chapter then covers pathophysiological concepts and ties them to clinical application.

Pedagogical Features

- Each chapter begins with **Learning Objectives** to help focus students' reading of the chapter.
- Throughout each chapter, important **Clinical Concepts** are pulled out in a special design, helping readers connect important concepts to patient care.
- **Alerts** highlight information critical to providing safe and effective patient care.
- At the end of each chapter, the **Chapter Summary** provides key points, and the **Making the Connections** box helps students synthesize pathophysiology with the clinical manifestations,

assessment, and management of key diseases and disorders.
- Select chapters contain a feature new to the third edition called **Patho-Pharm Connection,** which are illustrations that highlight the drug classes typically prescribed for a complex clinical disorder and demonstrate how the drugs act to treat the condition. Pathophysiology and pharmacology are interwoven, and this feature helps students understand pathophysiology not only as it relates to the disease process, but also how it relates to treatment.

The Teaching and Learning Package

How students learn is evolving. In this digital age, we consume information in new ways. The possibilities to interact and connect with content in new, dynamic ways are enhancing students' understanding and retention of complex concepts.

In order to meet the needs of today's learners, how faculty teaches is also evolving. Classroom (traditional or online) time is valuable for active learning. This approach makes students responsible for the key concepts, allowing faculty to focus on clinical application. Relying on the textbook alone to support an active classroom leaves a gap. *Davis Advantage* is designed to fill that gap and help students and faculty succeed in core courses. It comprises the following:

- **A Strong Core Textbook** that sets out to explain critical aspects of the most common clinical disorders affecting patients in the health-care setting. Readers' understanding is enhanced by the approachable writing style and detailed art program, which helps students visualize important processes and concepts.
- **An Online Solution** that provides resources for each step of the learning cycle: learn, apply, assess.
- **Personalized Learning** assignments are the core of the product and are designed to prepare students for classroom (live or online) discussion. They provide directed learning based on needs. After completing text reading assignments, students take a pre-assessment for each *topic*. Their results feed into their *Personalized Learning Plan*. If students do not pass the pre-assessment, they are required to complete further work within the topic: watch

an animated mini-lecture, work through an activity, and take the post-assessment.

The personalized learning content is designed to connect students with the foundational information about a given topic or concept. It provides the gateway to helping make the content accessible to all students and complements different learning styles.

- **Clinical Judgment** assignments are case-based and build off key Personalized Learning topics. These cases help students develop clinical judgment skills through exploratory learning. Students will link their knowledge base (developed through the text and personalized learning) to new data and patient situations. Cases include dynamic charts that expand as the case progresses and use complex question types that require students to analyze data, synthesize conclusions, and make judgments. Each case will end with comprehensive feedback, which provides detailed rationales for the correct and incorrect answers.
- **Quizzing** assignments build off Personalized Learning Topics (and are included for every topic) and help assess students' understanding of the broader scope and increased depth of that topic. The quizzes use NCLEX®– and Next Generation NCLEX®–style questions to assess understanding and synthesis of content. Quiz results include comprehensive feedback for correct and incorrect answers to help students understand why their answer choices were right or wrong.
- **Online Instructor Resources** are aimed at creating a dynamic learning experience that relies heavily on interactive participation and is tailored to students' needs. Results from the post-assessments are available to faculty, in aggregate or by student, and inform a **Personalized Teaching Plan** that faculty can use to deliver a targeted classroom experience. Faculty will know students' strengths and weaknesses before they come to class and can spend class time focusing on where students are struggling. Suggested in-class activities are provided to help create an interactive, hands-on learning environment that helps students connect more deeply with the content. NCLEX®– and Next Generation NCLEX®–style questions from the **Instructor Test Bank** and **PowerPoint slides** that correspond to the textbook chapters are referenced in the Personalized Teaching Plans. Also included are NGN-style questions to help familiarize students with the alternative style questions on the Next Generation NCLEX®.

CONTENTS

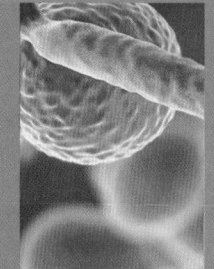

CHAPTER

1

The Cell in Health and Illness

Learning Objectives

After completion of this chapter, the student will be able to:

- Recognize the major organelles and their functions within the cell.
- Describe the functions of the nucleus and consequences of DNA damage.
- Distinguish between the components that make up DNA versus RNA.
- Compare and contrast the processes of transcription and translation.
- Discuss the difference between aerobic and anaerobic metabolism.

Key Terms

Aerobic metabolism
Anaerobic metabolism
Autolysis
Cellular dehydration
Cellular edema
Cellular hypoxia
Codon
Deoxyribonucleic acid (DNA)

Free radicals
Glycoproteins
Heterolysis
Homeostasis
Lysosomes
Mitochondria
Na⁺/K⁺ pump
Nucleotides

Organelles
Plasma membrane
Purine bases
Pyrimidine bases
Ribosomes
Transcription
Translation

All forms of disease start with disruptions of normal cellular structure and function, which is why tissues and their cellular components need to be examined when studying illness. Biochemical diagnostic studies provide insight into these physiological changes. Because disease is initiated at the cellular level, it is first necessary to understand the cell's basic internal microenvironment.

Cell Structure and Function

All body tissues and organs are composed of cells—the basic unit in which all structural, functional, and environmental alterations occur in disease processes. Each cell performs internal processes vital for the body's normal physiological function. Specialized intracellular structures, called **organelles,** carry out specific activities to sustain life. At the same time, cells sense and respond to their external environment while freely exchanging materials and energy with their surroundings. Through these actions, cells ensure **homeostasis,** regulating the internal environment to maintain balance and equilibrium in response to internal and external changes. When these responses are compromised, illness occurs. In other words, an illness of the whole organism is the macroscopic presentation of what is occurring at a microscopic level within the cell.

The cell is bounded by a **plasma membrane** and composed of cytoplasm, organelles, and a nucleus. Cytoplasm is a colloidal internal fluid environment that contains water, ions, proteins, carbohydrates, and lipids; it is a gel-like substance that suspends the cellular organelles within it (see Fig. 1-1). The nucleus contains genetic material, **deoxyribonucleic acid (DNA),** that ultimately regulates cellular activity.

Normal cell function, including the cell's major functions of growth, energy production and metabolism,

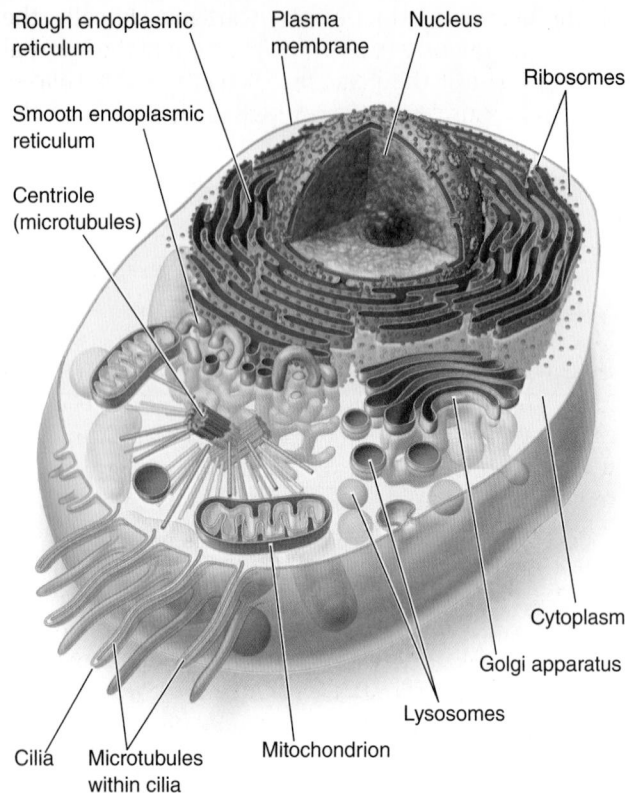

Rough endoplasmic reticulum

Plasma membrane

Nucleus

Ribosomes

Smooth endoplasmic reticulum

Centriole (microtubules)

Cilia   Microtubules within cilia   Mitochondrion

Lysosomes

Golgi apparatus

Cytoplasm

FIGURE 1-1. The cell is the body's basic structural unit. It contains a nucleus, which houses the DNA. It also contains organelles, which are surrounded by cytoplasm.

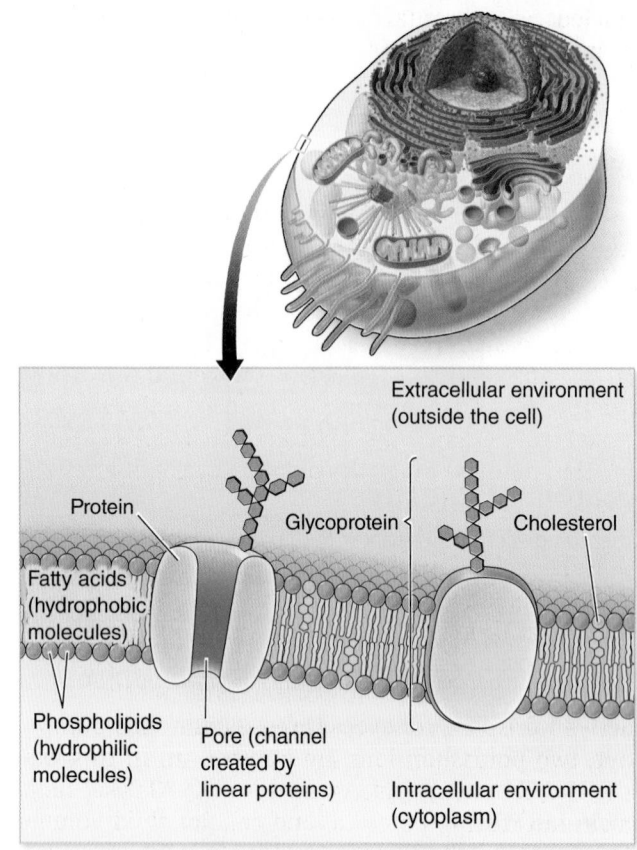

Extracellular environment (outside the cell)

Protein

Glycoprotein

Cholesterol

Fatty acids (hydrophobic molecules)

Phospholipids (hydrophilic molecules)

Pore (channel created by linear proteins)

Intracellular environment (cytoplasm)

FIGURE 1-2. The plasma membrane consists mainly of lipids and proteins. The membrane's fundamental structure is the phospholipid bilayer, which forms a stable barrier between the extracellular compartment, which is the outside of the cell, and the intracellular compartment, which is the inside of the cell. Proteins embedded within the phospholipid bilayer carry out the specific functions of the plasma membrane, which include active transport of molecules.

replication, and protein synthesis, requires synchronized organelle function, biochemical processes, and specific environmental conditions. Disease arises most commonly from dysfunction of one or more of the cellular organelles, proteins, or biochemical processes. This chapter will review concepts regarding the structure and function of the major cellular organelles and clinical consequences of their dysfunction from a clinical perspective.

The Plasma Membrane

The plasma membrane acts as a barrier to the cell's external environment and protects the internal organelles from injury. The cell's outside layer separates the intracellular and extracellular environments (see Fig. 1-1). Its major component is a phospholipid bilayer that contains proteins and cholesterol. The protein structures have varied functions, some of which include ion channels for exchange with the extracellular environment (see Fig. 1-2). The plasma membrane is semipermeable, which means it selectively allows substances in or out.

Extracellular and intracellular fluid, ions, and other molecules can diffuse back and forth through the pores of the semipermeable plasma membrane. The core lipid region remains impermeable to water and water-soluble substances, while at the same time allowing lipid-soluble substances such as oxygen and carbon dioxide to diffuse across. When disease alters the plasma membrane's

configuration, excess fluid can enter the cell's internal environment, causing swelling, referred to as **cellular edema.** Conversely, intracellular fluid can leak out of the cell through the pores, causing cell shrinkage, termed **cellular dehydration.** Either cellular edema or dehydration can disrupt organelle function.

On the plasma membrane's outer surface, carbohydrates attach to cell surface protein molecules; these structures are called **glycoproteins** (see Fig. 1-2). Glycoproteins are surface markers, also called *antigens,* that identify cells as part of the individual's own tissues. For example, a red blood cell contains glycoprotein surface markers that identify the individual's blood type as A, B, O, or AB. When any of these cellular surface markers are altered, the immune system will recognize them as foreign and provoke an attack on the cell. Identifying "self" from "non-self" substances is a major function of the immune system. The provocation of the immune system is the basis for allergies, autoimmune disorders, transplant rejection, and transfusion reactions.

Damage to the plasma membrane causes a breach in the security of the cell's interior environment. A damaged plasma membrane leaves all organelles open to injurious agents. It is particularly dangerous to the nucleus, which contains the DNA, leaving it vulnerable to injury.

The Sodium–Potassium Pump (Na⁺/K⁺ Pump)

For optimal cell function, it is necessary for potassium (K^+) ions to be at a higher concentration inside the cell compartment and for sodium (Na^+) to be at higher concentration outside the cell. The plasma membrane is more soluble to K^+ ions and less soluble to Na^+ ions, so K^+ ions tend to leak out of the cell and Na^+ ions are retained. Also, because of osmosis, water tends to travel from outside the cell to inside it. This causes a gradient of more positivity outside the cell than inside the cell.

The maintenance of the cellular movement of Na^+ outside and K^+ inside requires energy. The sodium–potassium pump uses adenosine triphosphate (ATP) to constantly move these two ions in opposite directions across the plasma membrane (see Fig. 1-3). The mechanism is called *active transport* by Na^+/K^+. In active transport, for every three sodium ions pumped out, two potassium ions are pumped in. In this way, the **Na^+/K^+ pump** (also termed Na^+/K^+ ATPase) helps maintain resting potential and cellular fluid volume. For most animal cells, the Na^+/K^+ pump is responsible for one-third of the cell's energy expenditure. For neurons, the Na^+/K^+ pump is responsible for two-thirds of the cell's energy expenditure.

The Na^+/K^+ pump can be pharmacologically altered through the administration of certain drugs. For instance, the Na^+/K^+ pump found in the membrane of heart cells is an important target for cardiac glycosides, which are drugs used to improve the force of the heart's contraction. In heart muscle cells, the Na^+/K^+ pump works to pump calcium out of the internal environment of the heart muscle cells, which relaxes the heart muscle. Pharmacological slowdown of the Na^+/K^+ pump keeps more calcium inside the heart muscle cell, strengthening its force of contraction.

Mitochondria

Mitochondria are the cell's energy producers. Cell types differ in their number of mitochondria according to their energy needs. For example, muscle cells have abundant numbers of mitochondria because they require a high amount of energy to function, whereas bone cells have fewer mitochondria. The mitochondria's primary function is to convert organic nutrients into cell energy in the form of ATP. Mitochondria accomplish this through the process of **aerobic metabolism,** which requires oxygen. When no oxygen is available for cells, a situation called **cellular hypoxia,** the cell converts to another form of metabolism: **anaerobic metabolism.** Anaerobic metabolism, also referred to as *glycolysis,* occurs outside the mitochondria. In anaerobic metabolism, glucose is used to create energy.

Energy Metabolism

Aerobic metabolism requires oxygen and provides the maximum amount of energy for cellular function: a net yield of 34 ATP. When oxygen is not available, anaerobic metabolism produces significantly less cellular energy: a net yield of 2 ATP, as well as pyruvic acid.

Pyruvic acid is converted into acetyl-coenzyme A, which triggers a series of reactions known as the *Krebs cycle,* also called the *citric acid cycle.* With the use of oxygen, mitochondria produce a net yield of 34 ATP from the Krebs cycle (see Fig. 1-4). However, in cellular hypoxia, pyruvic acid is converted to lactic acid, which is noxious to cells, causing muscle pain and biochemical alterations such as acidosis.

Mitochondrial DNA

Mitochondria are unique because they are the only cellular organelles that have their own distinctive DNA. Cell biologists speculate that mitochondria were self-sustaining, independent-living, bacteria-like organisms that, over the course of evolution, became incorporated into human cells. However, because they contain their own DNA, they are also able to reproduce within the cell whenever there is an increased need for ATP formation. For example, exercise stimulates the formation of increased numbers of mitochondria in a muscle cell. Because of this, the muscle uses more oxygen and yields more energy.

During human fertilization, the sperm provides minimal mitochondria, which results in almost all the mitochondrial DNA being derived maternally. Because

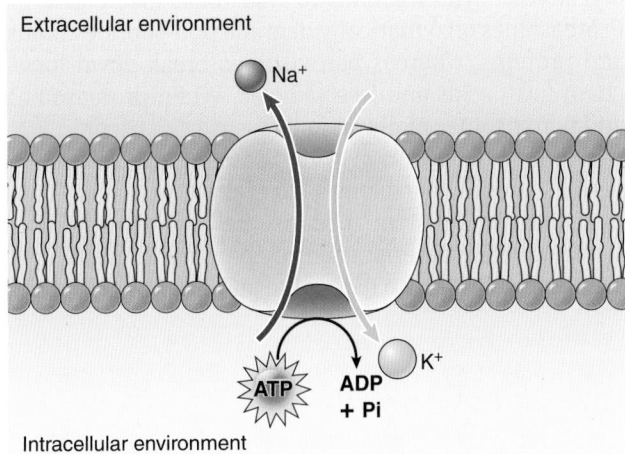

Extracellular environment

Na⁺

ADP + Pi

ATP

K⁺

Intracellular environment

FIGURE 1-3. The sodium–potassium (Na⁺/K⁺) pump uses energy to actively transport sodium out of the cell and bring potassium into the cell. The pump is located in the plasma membrane of all cells. Active transport is responsible for the intracellular compartment containing relatively high concentrations of potassium ions but low concentrations of sodium ions. The pump moves these two ions in opposite directions across the plasma membrane. For every three sodium ions pumped out, two potassium ions are pumped in.

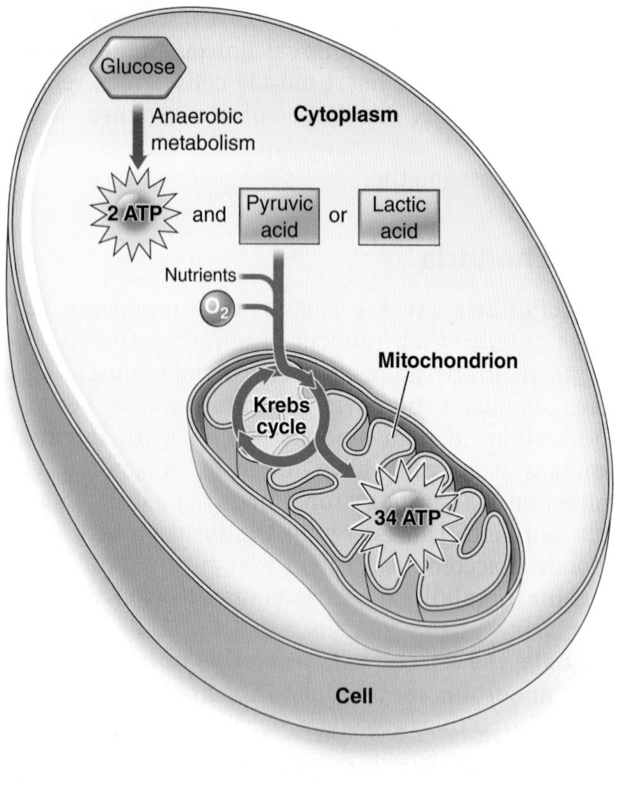

FIGURE 1-4. Cellular energy production. The mitochondrion uses oxygen to produce a net yield of 34 ATP through the process of aerobic metabolism. When no oxygen is available, the cell enters anaerobic metabolism to convert glucose to 2 ATP and pyruvic acid, which occurs outside the mitochondria in the cytoplasm. If oxygen is present, pyruvic acid is converted into acetyl coenzyme A, which triggers the Krebs cycle (citric acid cycle). In cellular hypoxia, pyruvic acid is converted to lactic acid, which is noxious and causes muscle pain and biochemical alterations.

of this unique characteristic of mitochondrial DNA, geneticists use it to study an individual's maternal hereditary lineage.

Mitochondrial DNA is subject to mutation by oxygen-derived **free radicals,** also called *reactive oxygen species.* It is theorized that in aging and disorders such as diabetes, cancer, and heart failure, mitochondrial DNA undergoes mutations, and the mitochondrial damage is partly responsible for the cellular impairment observed in the diseases. There are also diseases that target mitochondria specifically. Injury of mitochondria can occur in the cells of different organs, and mitochondrial disease causes a wide array of problems, including energy depletion and severe muscle weakness (see Chapter 3: Genetic Basis of Disease).

CLINICAL CONCEPT

Mitochondrial diseases present with significant symptoms when the defective mitochondria are present in the muscles, cerebrum, or nerves, because these cells use more energy than most other cells in the body.

Lysosomes

Lysosomes are small, membrane-enclosed organelles with a more acidic internal environment than the rest of the cell. They contain digestive enzymes such as lysozyme, proteases, and lipases (see Fig. 1-1). These enzymes degrade ingested foreign substances and cellular debris. Whenever a cell dies, lysosomes release digestive enzymes to destroy the cell parts in a process called **autolysis.**

Lysosomal Heterolysis
Macrophages, major defensive white blood cells of the body, contain a large number of lysosomes. Because macrophages constantly engulf and ingest foreign substances that invade the body, they rely on lysosomal enzymes to digest the material. When lysosomes are used to digest foreign matter ingested by a macrophage, the process is called **heterolysis.**

Lack of Lysosomal Enzymes and Disease
Lysosomes play an important part in cellular metabolic processes. Lysosomal enzymes constantly degrade waste products, cellular debris, and foreign matter. Lack of lysosomal enzymes can cause a harmful accumulation of a nondegraded substance. For example, Tay-Sachs disease is a lipid storage disease resulting from a deficiency in a lysosomal enzyme. This causes the accumulation of ganglioside, a specific type of lipid found in the central nervous system. Ganglioside then accumulates in the cells of the liver, heart, nervous system, retina, and spleen, causing organ dysfunction and widespread systemic illness.

Proteasomes and Peroxisomes

Proteasomes and peroxisomes are organelles with digestive enzymes similar to lysosomes (see Fig. 1-1). Proteasomes enzymatically degrade polypeptide chains and proteins, whereas peroxisomes break down long-chain fatty acids and free radicals. When proteasomes and peroxisomes malfunction, disease can occur.

Adrenoleukodystrophy is a disorder of dysfunctional peroxisomes in which long-chain fatty acids accumulate in the nervous system. The disease evolves over time, slowly causing deterioration of the nervous system; it can eventually lead to dementia, paralysis, and death.

CLINICAL CONCEPT

Accelerated cellular proteasome activity occurs in cachexia (wasting of body mass) associated with cancer.

Endoplasmic Reticulum

The endoplasmic reticulum (ER) is a network of tubules within the cell that act as a transport system. There are two main types of ER: smooth and rough. The smooth

ER is the location for lipid production, which includes corticosteroids, oils, and phospholipids. The rough ER is a tubular network with attached ribosomes that synthesize proteins. During ER stress, proteins cannot travel to their proper intracellular locations and are rapidly degraded. Increasing numbers of studies suggest that ER stress is involved in the pathogenesis of a number of diseases, including neurodegenerative diseases, cancer, obesity, diabetes, and atherosclerosis.

Ribosomes

Ribosomes are small, spherical organelles composed of ribosomal ribonucleic acid (rRNA). Some are freestanding within the cytoplasm, and some are attached to rough ER. Ribosomes can be likened to cellular "protein factories" (see Fig. 1-1). Proteins manufactured by ribosomes are destined to become parts of the cell, enzymes, or exported protein secretions. Different types of cells manufacture different proteins. For example, ribosomes in pancreatic beta islet cells synthesize the proteins that make up insulin, whereas thyroid cell ribosomes manufacture proteins that build thyroxine. In all cells, protein synthesis by the ribosomes is directed by specific information received from the nucleus. Messenger RNA (mRNA) from the nucleus acts as a blueprint for the construction of proteins. Transfer RNA (tRNA) plays a key role in the assembly of proteins. During severe hypoxic states, ribosomal protein synthesis ceases.

 CLINICAL CONCEPT

Some antibiotics interfere with the function of bacterial ribosomes, thereby inhibiting bacterial protein synthesis.

Golgi Apparatus

Once protein synthesis has been completed by ribosomes, the proteins are transported via the ER to the Golgi apparatus to be processed, packaged, and secreted (see Fig. 1-1).

An example of this process is seen in the formation of hormones such as insulin and adrenocorticotropic hormone (ACTH). The initial protein is manufactured in the ribosome and referred to as a *preprohormone*. The preprohormone contains a signal peptide that directs its transfer to the ER. As the preprohormone is transferred from the ribosome to the ER, the signal peptide is removed. At this point, it is referred to as a *prohormone* and is transported to the Golgi apparatus. Within the Golgi apparatus, further processing converts the prohormone into the actual hormone that will be secreted by the endocrine gland's cells. This processing may include dividing the prohormone into smaller units or the addition of carbohydrate units. The completed hormone is stored in a secretory granule within the Golgi apparatus until it leaves the cell to be secreted by the gland.

Secretory Vesicles

Secretory vesicles, which are formed by the ER–Golgi apparatus system, store substances that are secreted by cells before their release. Secretory vesicles move to the cell's periphery, waiting for the release of their contents into the extracellular space.

Microtubules and Microfilaments

Microtubules are hollow filaments composed of protein subunits called *tubulin*. They have a dynamic structure, meaning that they are constantly being formed, broken down, and reformed. Microtubules comprise structures involved in cell division such as centrioles and the mitotic spindle. They also provide a pathway for transporting secretory vesicles to the cell's perimeter. For example, microtubules form tunnel-like pathways for the movement of neurotransmitters down the axon of a neuron to the synapse.

Cilia are cellular projections that contain microtubules. The movement of cilia propels substances along the outside of the cells. An example of this is seen in the mucociliary apparatus of the respiratory tract. The ciliated respiratory epithelial cells propel mucus and inhaled debris out of the lung through a sweeping motion.

Microfilaments are solid, flexible fibers, sometimes referred to as *actin filaments*. Microfilaments help the cell change shape, as seen in the amoeboid movements of macrophages and the contraction of muscles. Actin and myosin are the key proteins in the contractile units of muscle cells. During contraction, one end of the actin filament elongates while the other end contracts.

The Nucleus

The nucleus is the cell's mastermind. It contains the body's genetic material, DNA, which regulates all cell structure and function. DNA consists of extremely long, double-stranded helical chains containing variable sequences of **nucleotides,** known as the *DNA double helix.* The DNA nucleotides consist of nitrogenous bases and a phosphate bound to a pentose (five-carbon sugar) called *deoxyribose.* The nitrogenous bases are either **purine bases,** consisting of adenine and guanine, or **pyrimidine bases,** consisting of thymine and cytosine. The DNA molecule resembles a twisted ladder with a phosphate–pentose backbone and the purine–pyrimidine base pairs represented by the individual steps on the ladder (see Fig. 1-5). These uniquely sequenced base pairs form the individual's genetic code.

Within the helical structure of DNA, there is a precise pairing of purine and pyrimidine bases: adenine always binds with thymine and guanine always binds with cytosine. This precise pairing of the nitrogenous bases provides DNA with the unique molecular ability to replicate.

DNA Replication

When DNA reproduces or replicates itself, both strands are duplicated, resulting in two identical DNA helices. However, as a result of the replication process, each

Chromatin is DNA folded upon itself within the nucleus.

Each "step" in the ladder is made up of purine–pyrimidine base pairs; adenosine (A), thymine (T), cytosine (C), guanine (G). These uniquely matched base pairs form the genetic code of each individual.

Nucleus

Deoxyribose sugar and phosphate

DNA helix untwists and separates into 2 strands.

One strand acts as a TEMPLATE for the synthesis of a new structure called RNA.

DNA strand acting as a template.

New strand of RNA synthesized from the DNA template.

rRNA (ribosomal RNA) section

tRNA (transfer RNA) section

mRNA (messenger RNA) section

FIGURE 1-5. Within the nucleus, DNA is folded in on itself and is known as *chromatin.* When DNA is stretched out, it forms a double helix that resembles a twisted ladder with purine–pyrimidine nitrogenous base pairs represented by the individual steps on the ladder. The purine–pyrimidine nitrogenous base pairs consist of the amino acids adenosine, cytosine, thymine, and guanine. These are matched in a unique sequence to form an individual's distinctive genetic code.

DNA helix contains one original strand and one newly formed daughter strand.

Specific enzymes called *DNA polymerase* are involved in the process of DNA replication. First, the DNA strand uncoils and begins to split into two separate strands. Each strand becomes a template, and the new nucleotides begin to pair up in an orderly fashion with the DNA template strands. As the purine bases pair up with the pyrimidine bases, hydrogen bonds are formed. This bonding enables the newly created daughter strand to be formed alongside the original strand. At the completion of the process, there are two identical strands of DNA.

Transcription and Translation

Protein synthesis is a requirement for normal physiological function. DNA directs the cell to carry out

protein synthesis through a two-step process known as **transcription,** which occurs in the nucleus, and **translation,** which occurs in the ribosome.

During transcription, the two strands of the helical DNA structure uncoil and separate. One of the strands acts as a template for the synthesis of RNA.

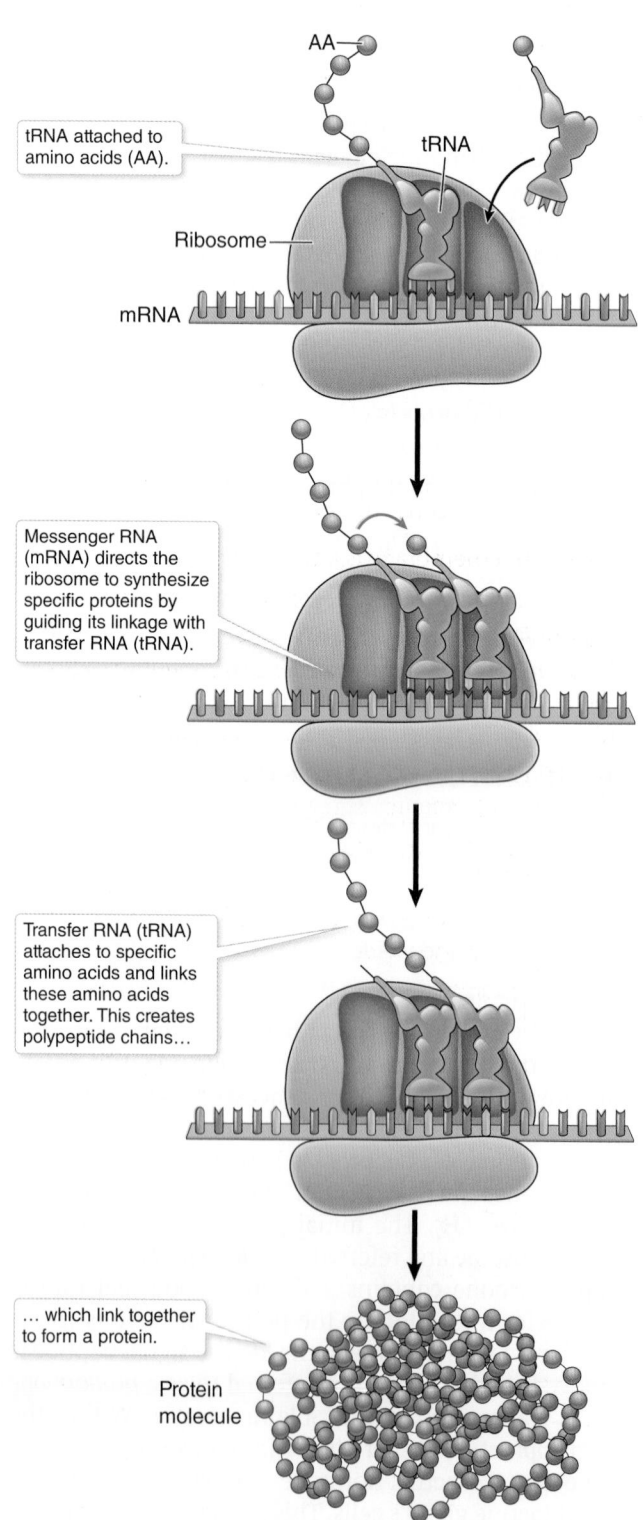

AA

tRNA attached to amino acids (AA).

tRNA

Ribosome

mRNA

Messenger RNA (mRNA) directs the ribosome to synthesize specific proteins by guiding its linkage with transfer RNA (tRNA).

Transfer RNA (tRNA) attaches to specific amino acids and links these amino acids together. This creates polypeptide chains…

… which link together to form a protein.

Protein molecule

FIGURE 1-6. Translation. After the process of transcription, the process of translation occurs at the ribosome. This is how RNA transfers genetic information to the ribosome for the synthesis of specific cellular proteins.

RNA differs from DNA in some important ways; for example, it is single stranded and can travel to sites outside of the nucleus. The pentose sugar in RNA is ribose, and the pyrimidine base thymine is replaced with uracil.

The RNA molecule copies genetic information from the main DNA molecule and then leaves the nucleus. The RNA molecule is composed of three types of RNA (see Fig. 1-6):

1. mRNA (messenger RNA)
2. tRNA (transfer RNA)
3. rRNA (ribosomal RNA)

Protein Synthesis

The single RNA strand transports the genetic information for protein synthesis from the nuclear DNA to the ribosomes. At the ribosomes, RNA begins the next process, called *translation*. During translation, ribosomes interpret the message from mRNA in order to manufacture proteins. tRNA gathers and joins the exact amino acids that will form the protein designated by mRNA (see Fig. 1-6). rRNA is mainly involved in the formation of the ribosome itself.

There is specificity within the combination of nitrogenous bases that enables selection of the correct sequence of amino acids to form the desired protein. Three nitrogenous bases form a **codon** that is interpreted by the ribosome. Each codon has a specific link to an exact amino acid. One codon signals the start of protein synthesis, other codons link to specific amino acids, and another codon signals the end of the protein synthesis. By interpreting the codons, specific proteins are formed to meet the cell's needs.

Chapter Summary

- The plasma membrane is a semipermeable barrier.
- A defect in the plasma membrane's integrity makes organelles vulnerable to injury.
- Glycoproteins are surface markers that identify cells as part of the individual's own tissues.
- The sodium–potassium pump (Na^+/K^+ pump), which maintains the cellular movement of Na^+ outside and K^+ inside the cell, requires energy.
- Aerobic metabolism occurs at the mitochondria and yields 34 ATP.
- Anaerobic metabolism occurs outside the mitochondria within the cell and yields 2 ATP, as well as lactic acid.
- The mitochondria have their own DNA that is solely inherited from the individual's mother.
- Lysosomes are small, spherical organelles that contain digestive enzymes and perform autolysis or heterolysis.
- Proteasomes break down proteins, and peroxisomes break down lipids.
- Ribosomes can be likened to cellular protein factories.
- In the nucleus, RNA is formed from DNA in the process called transcription.
- At the ribosomes, mRNA provides the direction for specific protein synthesis.
- DNA is composed of purine bases, consisting of adenine and guanine, and pyrimidine bases, consisting of thymine and cytosine.
- RNA is composed of purine bases, consisting of adenine and guanine, and pyrimidine bases, consisting of uracil and cytosine.

Bibliography

Available online at fadavis.com

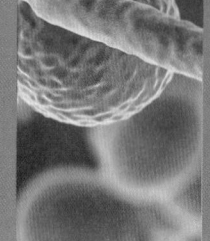

Cellular Injury, Adaptations, and Maladaptive Changes

Learning Objectives

After completion of this chapter, the student will be able to:

- Identify etiologic factors that can cause cellular adaptive and maladaptive changes.
- List common cellular adaptations and maladaptations that occur in the body.
- Explain endothelial injury, ischemic tissue damage, and infarction of tissue.
- Compare and contrast characteristics of malignant cancer cells versus normal, healthy cells.
- Discuss therapeutic interventions to repair cell injury and cell death.
- Distinguish between the processes of therapeutic cloning versus reproductive cloning.

Key Terms

Aneurysm
Angiogenesis
Apoptosis
Atherogenesis
Atrophy
Benign
Biopsy
Dysplasia
Endothelin
Etiology

Free radicals
Gangrene
Histology
Hyperplasia
Hypertrophy
Hypoxia
Infarction
Ischemia
Malignant
Metaplasia

Necrosis
Neoplasia
Oncogenes
Oxidative stress
Pathognomonic changes
Pathological hypertrophy
Physiological hypertrophy
Pluripotent stem cells
Vascular endothelial growth factor (VEGF)

The human body's intricate processes are vulnerable to many kinds of insults and stresses that can cause cells to take on distinctive changes and put the body's normal function and structure at risk for either temporary or permanent injury.

Injurious agents are also known as *etiologic agents*; an **etiology** is the original cause of a cellular alteration or disease. For example, the etiology of a sore throat is commonly streptococcus, a bacterial organism. On microscopic examination, cells infected with streptococcus demonstrate distinctive alterations associated with the infection, including inflammation and swelling.

In general, cells exhibit characteristic changes associated with specific etiologic agents or changes in their environment. Different etiologic agents create distinctive cellular changes, for example:

- Exposure to extreme cold temperatures will cause localized frostbite and tissue necrosis.
- Exposure to electrical current can burn tissue and cause cardiac rhythm disturbances.
- Alcohol abuse can cause the liver to take on characteristic fatty changes.

Cells are capable of maintaining homeostasis in the face of temporary stressors, insults, or changes in their environment. However, prolonged or severe insults can cause homeostasis to be disrupted. Therefore, under the influence of different etiologic agents, cells can do one of two things:

1. Develop adaptive, compensatory changes in an attempt to maintain homeostasis
2. Develop maladaptive changes, which are derangements of structure or function

In circumstances of overwhelming insult, cell injury or cell death can occur. Cell injury can be reversible,

 CLINICAL CONCEPT

The point at which cells can no longer achieve reversible changes varies according to the type of cell. For example, brain cells cannot withstand low oxygen delivery, referred to as **hypoxia,** for more than 6 minutes, whereas skeletal muscle can tolerate hypoxia for prolonged periods.

but if the injurious agent is persistent or severe enough, cell injury can lead to cell death.

Basic Concepts of Cellular Adaptations and Maladaptive Changes

Cellular adaptations and maladaptive changes occur as a result of specific disease processes, altered cell function, or environmental influences. Cells that undergo these changes develop distinctive structural or functional characteristics. The study of specific cell alterations can assist clinicians in identifying the etiology and predicting the consequences of cell changes.

Histology is the microscopic study of tissues and cells, and it yields important diagnostic information for the clinician. A **biopsy** extracts a cell sample from an organ or mass of tissue to allow for histological examination. Identifiable histological findings can assist clinicians in identifying the etiology of cellular changes. Unique histological findings that represent distinct disease processes are referred to as **pathognomonic changes.** For example, an inflamed, craterlike breach in the gastrointestinal mucosa, as seen on an endoscopic examination of the stomach and duodenum, is pathognomonic for peptic ulcer disease.

Histological changes are also examined on autopsy specimens. An autopsy is an examination of the tissues and organs of a deceased individual that allows for a study of the cause of death. Clinicians can learn significant details about cellular adaptations, maladaptations, cell injury, and cell death from autopsy specimens. The following sections detail the most common adaptive and maladaptive cellular changes encountered in patients in the clinical setting.

Atrophy

Atrophy is a cellular adaptation in which cells revert to a smaller size in response to changes in metabolic requirements or their environment. Atrophy occurs when a cell's environment cannot support its metabolic requirements. The cell's smaller size allows for less metabolic demand and more efficient functioning that is compatible with survival.

Atrophy is best exemplified by the shrinking of skeletal muscle cells in an individual with upper extremity paralysis (see Fig. 2-1). Paralysis causes lack of muscle contraction, loss of nerve stimulation, and decreased workload of the muscles. Gradually, the size of skeletal muscle cells decreases and they undergo diminished metabolic activity. Causes of cellular atrophy include:

- Disuse or diminished workload
- Lack of nerve stimulation (paralysis)
- Loss of hormonal stimulation
- Inadequate nutrition

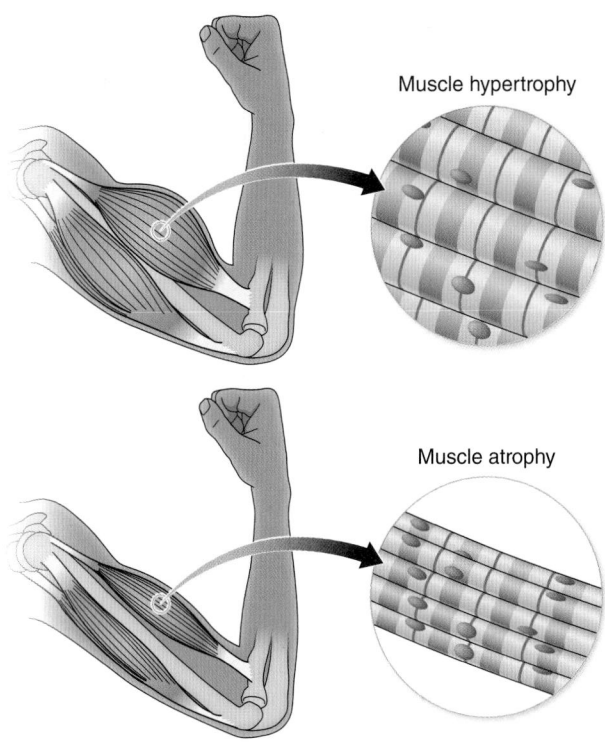

Muscle hypertrophy

Muscle atrophy

FIGURE 2-1. Skeletal muscle cell atrophy versus hypertrophy. Atrophy of the arm muscle occurs when skeletal muscle cells revert to a smaller size in response to changes in their environment, such as lack of circulation, diminished workload (disuse), or decreased neural stimulation. Conversely, hypertrophy of the arm muscle occurs when skeletal muscle cells enlarge in size in response to increased workload.

- Decreased blood flow (ischemia)
- Aging

Hypertrophy

Hypertrophy is an increase in individual cell size that results in an enlargement of functioning tissue mass (see Fig. 2-1). In hypertrophy, each individual cell becomes larger. Hypertrophy increases the cell's functional components, which leads to greater metabolic demand and energy needs.

Physiological Hypertrophy vs. Pathological Hypertrophy

Hypertrophy can occur as a result of normal physiological stimuli or abnormal pathological conditions. Normal physiological stimuli include exercise, which increases muscle mass. Exercise stimulates physiological hypertrophy of muscle cells, enhances the functional components of each cell, and increases the number of blood vessels that perfuse the enlarged muscle. Exercise stimulates **angiogenesis,** the growth of new blood vessel branches. Exercise also increases the number of mitochondria in each muscle cell, which in turn increases energy production. For example, a weightlifter who wants to develop stronger biceps lifts weights to increase workload on the biceps muscles. The increased workload stimulates increased size of each skeletal muscle cell within each biceps muscle. The stimulus for hypertrophy increases the muscle cell's actin and myosin filaments, enzymes, mitochondria, blood vessel growth, and adenosine triphosphate (ATP) production.

In **physiological hypertrophy,** the enlarged muscle is adequately perfused and supplied with blood flow, oxygen, and nutrients because of angiogenesis. In well-trained athletes, the heart physiologically hypertrophies because of the enlargement of each individual myocardial cell. There is a proportional increase in myocardial cell size and enhancement of coronary blood supply of the myocardial cells. Therefore, the enlarged heart in an athlete is supplied with abundant coronary artery blood flow, which delivers large amounts of oxygen and nutrients (see Fig. 2-2).

Pathological hypertrophy occurs when there is an increase in cellular size without an increase in the supportive structures necessary for the enlarged cell's increased metabolic needs. Pathological hypertrophy of cells can occur in disease processes or may be a compensatory maladaptation to changed environmental conditions. For example, in hypertension, blood pressure within the aorta and systemic arterial circulation is elevated. High aortic blood pressure creates a higher workload for the left ventricle; in response, each cardiac muscle cell undergoes pathological hypertrophy. Although each cardiac muscle cell increases in size, in pathological hypertrophy there is no corresponding increase in blood vessel growth to supply these muscle cells. As each cardiac muscle cell in the left ventricle undergoes hypertrophy, the whole left ventricle eventually hypertrophies. This resulting enlarged left ventricular muscle mass has an increased need for oxygen and blood flow; however, without concurrent growth of blood vessels, it outgrows its supply of coronary

blood flow and is susceptible to effects of inadequate blood flow, also called **ischemia**.

CLINICAL CONCEPT

As a result of hypertension, the left ventricle undergoes pathological hypertrophy. During cardiovascular physical assessment, left chest palpation locates the point of maximal impulse (PMI). The PMI's location correlates with the location of the heart's apex, which is usually located just under the left nipple. However, with left ventricular hypertrophy, the PMI is displaced to the left.

Hyperplasia

Hyperplasia is the increase in the number of cells in a tissue or organ. It occurs only in tissues with cells that are capable of mitotic division, such as the epithelium and glandular tissue. Hyperplasia is stimulated by hormonal or compensatory cellular mechanisms. An example of hormonal stimulation of hyperplasia occurs in pregnancy, when estrogen stimulation results in mitotic division of breast gland cells. Hyperplasia can also occur as a maladaptive mechanism when overcompensation causes the cell mass necessary for regeneration to be exceeded. Excessive numbers of cells in a specific tissue or organ can have detrimental effects. For example, a keloid is a maladaptive hyperplastic accumulation of epithelial cells and connective tissue that can occur in wound healing. It creates an elevated, disfiguring scar that requires cosmetic surgery (see Fig. 2-3).

It was generally thought that stable cells, which include cardiac, nerve, skeletal muscle, and brain cells, do not divide and do not have the capacity for regeneration. However, new research suggests that cardiac muscle cells may be able to divide and regenerate. According

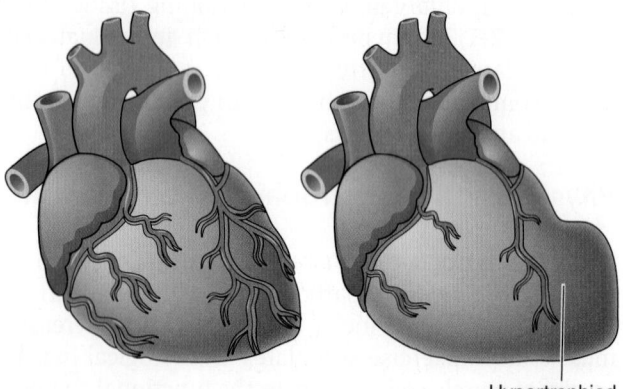

Hypertrophied left ventricle

FIGURE 2-2. Physiological versus pathological hypertrophy of heart muscle. (A) In physiological hypertrophy, the heart muscle is proportionately enlarged and significant coronary blood vessel growth occurs, allowing for sufficient coronary blood flow. (B) In this figure, there is disproportionate enlargement of the left ventricle compared with the remainder of the heart muscle. This is pathological hypertrophy of the left ventricle, which occurs in long-standing hypertension. In pathological hypertrophy, there is lack of growth of coronary vasculature to supply the enlarged cardiac muscle.

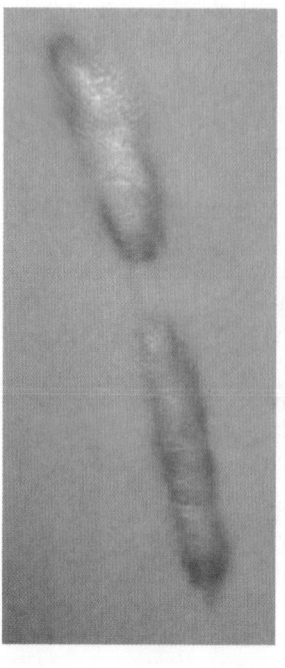

FIGURE 2-3. Keloid.

to Haubner, et al. (2018), in response to hypoxic conditions, the neonatal heart is capable of regenerating lost myocardium, and the adult heart is capable of modest self-renewal. It is believed that human organs contain limited populations of self-renewing cells, called *stem cells*. Stem cell research is demonstrating the regenerative power of stable cells and has the potential to change previously held theory (see the section "Regenerative Medicine Using Stem Cells"). At this time, the theory that stable cells cannot undergo mitosis or regeneration is still generally accepted.

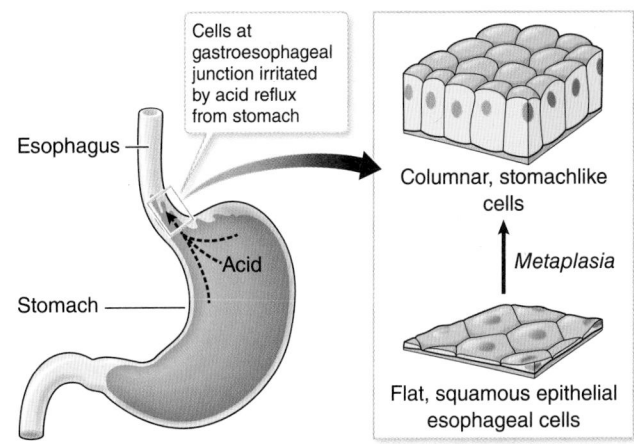

FIGURE 2-4. Metaplasia can occur in gastroesophageal reflux disease (GERD). In GERD, cells in the gastroesophageal junction are chronically irritated because of exposure to stomach acid. Lower esophageal squamous epithelial cells can undergo a metaplastic change into columnar stomachlike cells. When this condition develops, it is called Barrett's esophagus.

 CLINICAL CONCEPT

Hyperplasia caused by hormonal stimulation occurs in older adult males. As males age, prostate gland cells increase in number because of testosterone stimulation. As a result, a condition known as *benign prostatic hyperplasia (BPH)* occurs.

Metaplasia

Metaplasia is the replacement of one cell type by another cell type. It is likely a result of the cell's genetic reprogramming in response to a change in environmental conditions. Commonly, metaplasia occurs in response to chronic inflammation, and the substitution of cells enables the tissue's survival.

 CLINICAL CONCEPT

One of the best examples of metaplasia can occur in gastroesophageal reflux disease (GERD). In GERD, the lower esophageal sphincter is weakened and allows stomach acid to reflux into the lower esophagus. The acid irritates the lower esophageal cells, causing inflammation of the esophagus. Without treatment, and if prolonged, these lower esophageal cells, which are normally squamous epithelium–type cells, transform into columnar stomach-like cells. The stomach-like cells have greater tolerance for the acid reflux (see Fig. 2-4).

ALERT! The metaplastic change that occurs in GERD is a condition referred to as *Barrett's esophagus*, which requires periodic examination and aggressive treatment because it can deteriorate into cancer of the esophagus (see Fig. 2-5).

Dysplasia

Dysplasia is deranged cellular growth within a specific tissue, often as a result of chronic inflammation or a

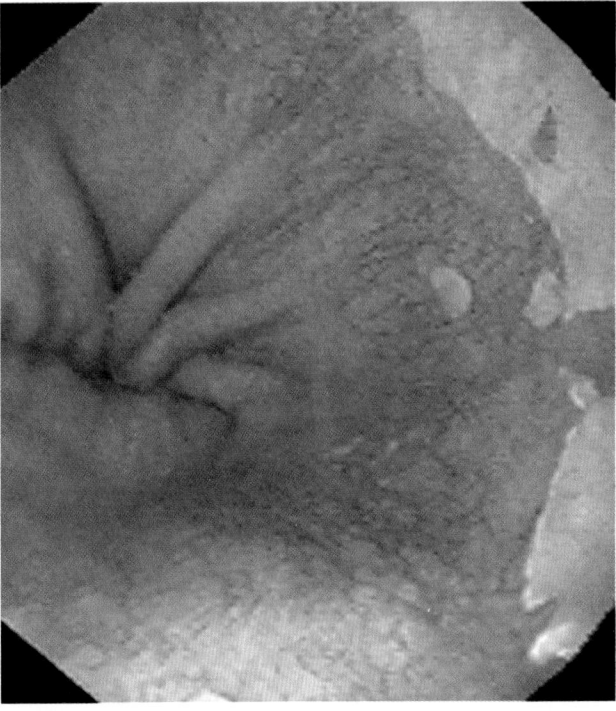

FIGURE 2-5. Metaplastic lower esophageal cells visualized on endoscopic examination. Lower esophageal cells, which are normal squamous epithelium-type cells, as shown in pale pink, change into cells that are columnar stomach-like cells in response to acid reflux, as shown in dark pink. This condition is called Barrett's esophagus. *(Courtesy of H. Worth Boyce, MD.)*

precancerous condition. On histological examination, dysplastic cells vary in size, shape, and architectural organization compared with healthy cells. Cervical dysplasia, often detected on a Papanicolaou (Pap) test, is a common example of this cellular change (see Fig. 2-6). When discovered, frequent examinations are necessary because dysplasia is the classic precursor to cancer of the cervix.

Normal cervix

Normal cervical cells

Cervical dysplasia

Dysplastic cervical cells
(precancerous)

FIGURE 2-6. Normal cervix and cervical cells versus cervical dysplasia and dysplastic cells.

Neoplasia

Neoplasia means *new growth* and usually refers to disorganized, uncoordinated, uncontrolled proliferative cell growth that is cancerous. The words *tumor* and *neoplasm* are often used interchangeably, and both indicate new cells growing within a specific tissue or organ.

Neoplasms can be classified as **benign** or **malignant,** depending on an important cell characteristic called differentiation (see Box 2-1). Differentiation is the process whereby newly growing cells acquire the

---

BOX 2-1. Cellular Differentiation: Benign and Malignant Neoplasms

Cellular differentiation is a characteristic used to designate a neoplasm as benign or malignant. Neoplastic cells that resemble the normal, healthy cells within the tissue where they are found are termed *well differentiated.* Benign neoplasms contain well-differentiated cells, or cells that resemble the healthy cells of the tissue of origin. Another characteristic of benign neoplasms is that the cells do not metastasize or break loose from the tissue of origin.

Conversely, neoplastic cells can appear very different from the healthy cells within their tissue of origin, in which case the cells are termed *poorly differentiated.* Malignant neoplasms contain poorly differentiated cells, which have a tendency to break away, enter the lymphatic or circulatory systems, and metastasize to distant sites to form secondary neoplasms.

---

specialized structure and function of the cells they replace. For example, skin cells that are sloughed daily are replaced by normally differentiated epithelial cells. The new epithelial cells are structurally and functionally exact copies of the sloughed cells. However, in cases of malignant melanoma (skin cancer), poorly differentiated, neoplastic epithelial cells, which do not look or act like normal skin cells, replace normal epithelial cells. Additionally, the cells are arranged in a disorganized fashion so that when viewed with a microscope, the normal cellular arrangement or tissue architecture is altered (see Fig. 2-7).

Basic Concepts of Cellular Injury

Cell injury occurs when cells are exposed to a severe stress that no longer allows them to maintain homeostasis, resulting in structural and functional changes. The basic changes of cell injury include dysfunction of the sodium–potassium pump (Na^+/K^+ pump), loss of plasma membrane integrity, mitochondrial dysfunction, defects in protein synthesis, intracellular accumulations, cellular swelling, and DNA damage. If the damaging stimulus is removed, cellular injury may be reversible. If the stress is prolonged, the cells may reach a critical point when recovery is not possible, which is variable for different cells, resulting in organelle disruption and irreversible cell injury.

Dysfunction of the Na^+/K^+ Pump

When the cell is unable to produce sufficient ATP, a high-energy compound, cellular physiological functions are reduced. Lack of sufficient ATP contributes to failure of active transport mechanisms such as the Na^+/K^+ pump.

Under normal, healthy circumstances, the Na^+/K^+ pump expels three sodium ions from the intracellular environment and pumps in two potassium ions. This contributes to the development of membrane polarity in excitable tissues such as muscle cells and neurons. It also maintains the normal osmotic relationships between ions, with sodium being the major extracellular ion and potassium the major intracellular ion.

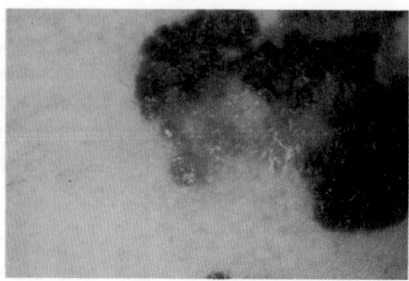

FIGURE 2-7. Normal skin vs. malignant melanoma. In normal skin, skin cells are lined up in an orderly fashion. In malignant melanoma, skin cells are numerous and disorderly in architecture.

However, when this active transport system is not functioning, the normal osmotic balance is altered. The intracellular sodium ion concentration is increased because it is not being adequately pumped out of the cell. This increase in intracellular sodium draws in water, leading to cellular swelling.

Dysfunction of the Calcium Pump

With a lack of ATP, an energy-dependent calcium pump—which maintains intracellular calcium at extremely low levels—also becomes dysfunctional. As a result, calcium accumulates within the cell and disrupts numerous biochemical processes. Calcium also activates a number of enzymes that further deplete ATP, damage the plasma membrane, disrupt DNA, and induce cell degeneration. Pathological calcification, the deposition of calcium and other minerals within tissues, occurs in a variety of conditions. Calcifications often accumulate in areas of cell injury and cell death (see Box 2-2).

 CLINICAL CONCEPT

On mammography, microcalcifications often indicate that the tissue has cancerous changes.

Loss of Plasma Membrane Integrity

The plasma membrane surrounds the whole perimeter of the cell and acts as a guardian of internal organelles. With a breach of membrane integrity, injurious agents can affect any of the organelles. In addition, water can enter the intracellular compartment, causing cellular swelling. The mitochondria can be damaged, which would halt the cell's ability to produce energy. Organelles can swell and deteriorate. The nucleus,

which contains the DNA, would be left vulnerable to injury, and the cell will be left without the ability to regenerate.

Defects in Protein Synthesis Ability

When the cell is low in energy because of hypoxia or mitochondrial dysfunction, there is a decrease in ATP. With dwindling ATP availability, the critical cellular process of protein synthesis begins to fail. The cells cannot manufacture proteins, which are crucial constituents for their own regeneration and many different kinds of body processes. Lack of protein synthesis can begin the process of cell degeneration or cell death.

Intracellular Accumulations

Cells can accumulate excessive amounts of various substances, such as cellular constituents, environmentally acquired substances, or cell breakdown products, because of abnormal metabolic function, exposure to high amounts of environmental material, or aging. Accumulated substances may be harmless or toxic to the cell and can be transient or permanently embedded in the cell.

If the accumulation is caused by a problem that can be brought under control, the cellular accumulation may be reversible. However, if accumulation is progressive and continual, cellular injury can occur. For example, intracellular accumulation can occur in the liver when exposed to excessive amounts of alcohol. Hepatocytes, which are integrally involved in lipid metabolism, can sustain toxic injury from alcohol and accumulate large quantities of intracellular fat. Fatty liver is a distinctive histological change associated with alcoholism that causes the liver to enlarge and become dysfunctional (see Fig. 2-8).

Another intracellular accumulation occurs in familial hypercholesterolemia, a condition that causes defective cholesterol metabolism. Xanthomas and xanthelasma are yellow, raised skin lesions that develop

---

BOX 2-2. Conditions That Cause Pathological Calcification

- In arteriosclerosis, calcifications accumulate within long-standing plaque. Calcified plaque is hardened, fragile, and likely to break apart into small pieces that can travel in the bloodstream.
- Aortic sclerosis, a common disorder in older individuals, involves a calcified aortic heart valve. Calcification causes thickening and narrowing of the heart valve with consequent blood disruption.
- On mammography, a breast lesion containing microcalcifications is often indicative of a malignancy. Calcium deposits are seen within the nutrient-deprived cells of a malignant tumor in the breast.

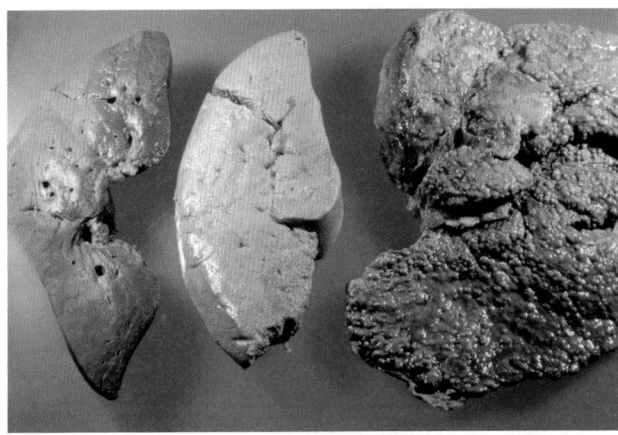

FIGURE 2-8. Normal liver versus fatty liver. *(From Arthur Glauberman/ Photo Researchers, Inc. Enhancement by: Mary Martin/Science Source.)*

because of intracellular accumulation of excess choles-terol within epithelial cells (see Fig. 2-9).

An example of an environmentally derived cellular accumulation occurs in anthracosis, otherwise known as coal miner's lung disease. Individuals who chronically inhale coal dust demonstrate accumulations of this substance within respiratory tract epithelial cells, which leads to blackening of the lung tissues (see Fig. 2-10).

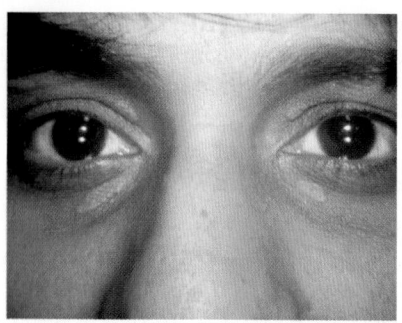

FIGURE 2-9. Xanthelasma is an intracellular accumulation of cholesterol within skin cells around the eyelids. This condition is seen in individuals with familial hypercholesterolemia. *(Courtesy of Wills Eye Hospital, Philadelphia, PA.)*

 CLINICAL CONCEPT

An accumulation of bilirubin in the bloodstream causes jaundice. Bilirubin, a yellow pigmented substance, is a breakdown product of hemoglobin. It is also a constituent of bile, which is synthesized by the liver. If excess RBC breakdown or liver dysfunction occurs, bilirubin accumulates in the bloodstream. Bilirubin has high affinity for elastin, a component of the skin and sclera of the eye, causing a yellow hue (see Fig. 2-11). Jaundice, the yellow hue of the skin and sclera, diminishes when bilirubin levels are reduced.

Genetic Damage

Injury to the cell's DNA can cause mutations, which, in turn, initiate changes in cell structure and function. Mutated DNA will be transcribed in the nucleus to produce mutated RNA. The abnormal RNA will, in turn, direct the cell's ribosomes to produce abnormal proteins. The abnormal proteins then rebuild the cell in an abnormal fashion and manufacture abnormal secretions.

Changes in the cell's structure and function often will be incompatible with life. Commonly, changes in the cell's DNA will initiate changes that bring about genetically programmed cell degeneration, also called **apoptosis**.

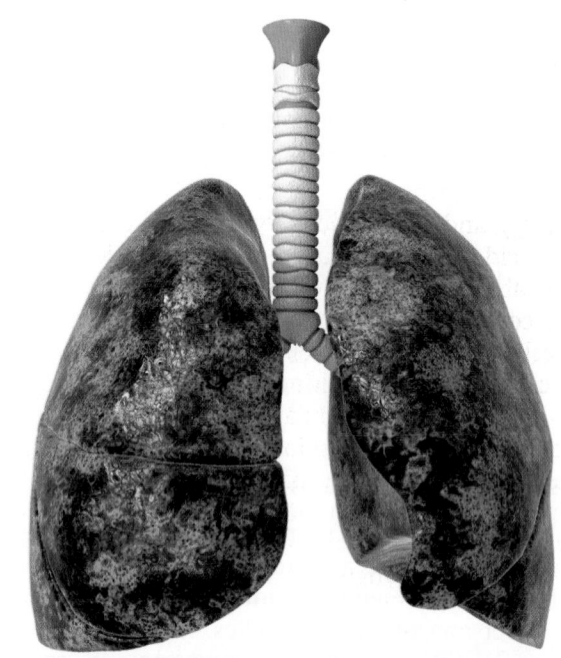

FIGURE 2-10. Anthracosis, also known as coal miner's lung and black lung. *(From David Mack/Science Source.)*

 CLINICAL CONCEPT

DNA mutations are common with exposure to high doses of radiation. With radiation damage, genes can mutate into **oncogenes,** which trigger cancerous cell changes. The cancerous cells manufacture cancerous proteins, also called *oncoproteins*.

Causes of Cell Injury

Many stressors and injurious agents can cause cellular injury. Causes of cell injury can be categorized as follows:

• Hypoxic cell injury
• Free radical injury (oxidative stress)
• Physical agents of injury
• Chemical injury

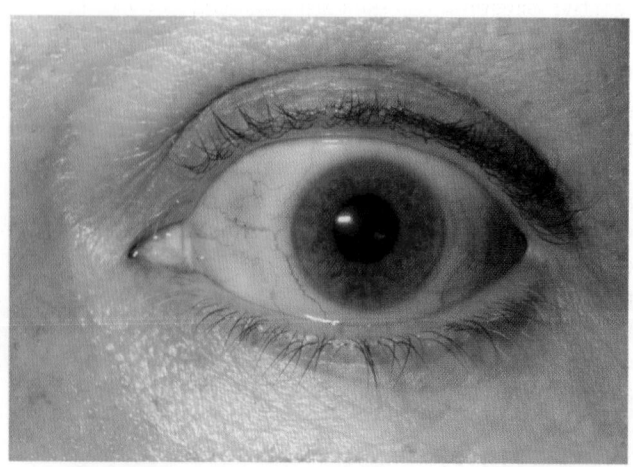

FIGURE 2-11. Jaundice of the sclera. Jaundice is caused by bilirubin, a yellow pigment that can accumulate in the sclera and skin in liver disease and other disorders. *(From Dr. P. Marazzi/ Science Source.)*

- Infectious agent injury
- Injurious immunological reactions
- Genetic defects
- Nutritional imbalances

Hypoxic Cell Injury

Hypoxia is the most common cause of cell injury. Cellular hypoxia commonly results when the blood cannot deliver enough oxygen to the cells. The most common cause of cellular hypoxia is ischemia, or diminished circulation. Ischemia occurs most often because of obstruction of arterial blood flow. The obstruction is commonly atherosclerotic plaque and clot formation, which blocks circulation downstream from the clot.

Another cause of cellular hypoxia is anemia. In anemia, the blood lacks sufficient hemoglobin (Hgb), which is the molecule in the red blood cell that carries oxygen. Inadequate Hgb results in insufficient oxygen carried by the blood, which, in turn, results in the cells not receiving fully oxygenated blood. This results in hypoxia.

Hypoxia causes the cell to enter anaerobic metabolism, during which it generates 2 ATP, a low amount of energy, and pyruvic acid. Pyruvic acid changes into lactic acid. The inadequate cell energy slows down all metabolic functions of the cell, and the lactic acid alters cellular biochemical activity. Lactic acid is particularly irritating to muscle cells. Anaerobic metabolism cannot sustain cell life for a prolonged time.

Other causes of hypoxia include exposure to low concentrations of oxygen in the environment, such as occurs at high altitudes; inadequate oxygen diffusion at the alveoli, as in pneumonia; suffocation injury; or airway obstruction caused by a foreign body or inflammation of oropharyngeal tissues.

Free Radical Injury

Cells generate energy in the mitochondria through a process called *oxidative phosphorylation*. During this process, often described as a respiratory burst, small amounts of reactive oxygen molecules are produced as by-products. These reactive oxygen molecules are referred to as **free radicals** or *reactive oxygen species*. Free radicals are also present in many environmental substances such as cigarette smoke, pesticides, and other toxins.

Free radicals have a single unpaired electron in an outer orbit that creates instability and reactivity with adjacent molecules; they react with constituents of the cell's plasma membrane and organelle membranes, causing oxidative degradation. Free radicals are oxidizing agents with the ability to penetrate the cell's plasma membrane, disrupt internal organelles, and damage the nucleus and its DNA.

Cells have multiple mechanisms to remove free radicals and thereby minimize injury. These mechanisms involve a series of enzymes referred to as *superoxide dismutases*. However, free radical generation can overwhelm the mechanisms of removal, in which case, a form of cell injury known as **oxidative stress** occurs.

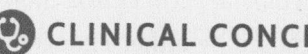

CLINICAL CONCEPT

Individuals can counteract free radical injury through consumption of antioxidants such as vitamins A, E, and C, and beta-carotene.

Oxidative stress commonly occurs in cells that undergo transient ischemia and subsequent resumption of circulation, also known as *ischemic-reperfusion injury*. Depending on the ischemic insult's intensity and duration, variable numbers of cells may proceed to die after blood flow is restored to tissues. This is because new damaging forces are activated by reactive free radicals during the reperfusion phase, causing the death of cells that might have recovered otherwise.

CLINICAL CONCEPT

In the clinical setting, heart disease commonly involves ischemic-reperfusion injury, which often occurs when a blood clot that obstructs a coronary artery causes cardiac muscle ischemia. After this occurs, the region undergoes reperfusion with clot dissolution. The mitochondria in the region undergo interrupted oxidative phosphorylation because of the temporary hypoxia and release of free radicals as by-products, which cause injury to surrounding tissue.

Physical Agents of Injury

There are many different physical agents of cell injury. Mechanical trauma from an external force such as a laceration, gunshot wound, or fall are obvious causes of physical cell injury. Temperature extremes, which can result in such injuries as burns and frostbite; radiation; electrical shock; and extreme changes in environmental pressure can also cause cell injury. Sunburn, brought upon by excessive exposure to sunlight, is an observable example of cell injury caused by a physical agent. Excessive noise is considered a mechanical stressor of the inner ear's delicate organs.

In addition to direct trauma to the cells and tissues, physiological responses to trauma often include the initiation of the inflammatory response, which can lead to healing or further cell damage (see Chapter 9: Inflammation and Dysfunctional Wound Healing).

CLINICAL CONCEPT

Hypertension, high pressure within the arteries, acts as a physical force against the endothelial lining of the vasculature. The constant stress of the pulsatile force of blood flow against the arterial endothelium causes a shearing injury. Endothelial injury caused by the forces of hypertension initiates the development of atherosclerosis throughout the arterial system.

Chemical Injury

Chemical injury can be caused by either endogenous biological substances or exogenous synthetic substances that influence the cell. Chemical agents commonly injure the plasma membrane and gain access to the cell's interior to cause dysfunction of organelles.

Imbalances of the body's biological chemical constituents, such as electrolytes, can cause cell injury. For example, high sodium levels in the bloodstream, termed *hypernatremia,* cause intracellular fluid depletion (cellular dehydration) and reversible cell shrinkage. The symptoms associated with this include lethargy, weakness, irritability, and confusion (see Chapter 7: Fluid and Electrolyte Imbalances).

In uncontrolled diabetes mellitus (DM), high glucose levels in the bloodstream, termed *hyperglycemia,* cause chemical injury of the endothelial cells that line the arteries. High levels of blood glucose react with endothelial membrane constituents to yield substances called *advanced glycation end products,* which can damage the coronary and cerebral arteries, the arteries of the kidneys, the vessels of the lower extremity, and the retinas of the eyes. The endothelial injury associated with uncontrolled DM initiates the process of atherosclerosis. Consequently, individuals with chronically uncontrolled diabetes are susceptible to diseases associated with atherosclerosis: coronary artery disease, peripheral arterial disease, and cerebrovascular disease (see Chapter 25: Diabetes Mellitus and the Metabolic Syndrome).

Alternatively, exogenous chemical substances such as drugs, environmental pollutants, or poisons can cause cellular injury in various ways. Many drugs, such as nonsteroidal anti-inflammatory drugs (NSAIDs) and antibiotics such as aminoglycosides, can have nephrotoxic side effects. Nephrotoxic drugs have chemically damaging effects on the cells of the kidney's nephron tubules.

🔍 CLINICAL CONCEPT

Carbon monoxide (CO) binds very tightly to the hemoglobin molecule, decreasing its oxygen-carrying capacity. Thus the amount of oxygen delivered to the tissues is decreased in CO poisoning.

Infectious Agents of Injury

A wide variety of microorganisms, including bacteria, viruses, fungi, and parasites, can cause cellular injury. Each type of microorganism carries out injurious cell processes in a distinctive manner. An example is the human papillomavirus (HPV), a sexually transmitted infectious agent that can cause cancerous cell changes within the cervix. Another example is *Helicobacter pylori,* which causes peptic ulcer disease. *H. pylori* is a bacterium that erodes the gastrointestinal mucosal lining and allows gastric acids to penetrate and damage underlying cells (see Fig. 2-12). The constant acid

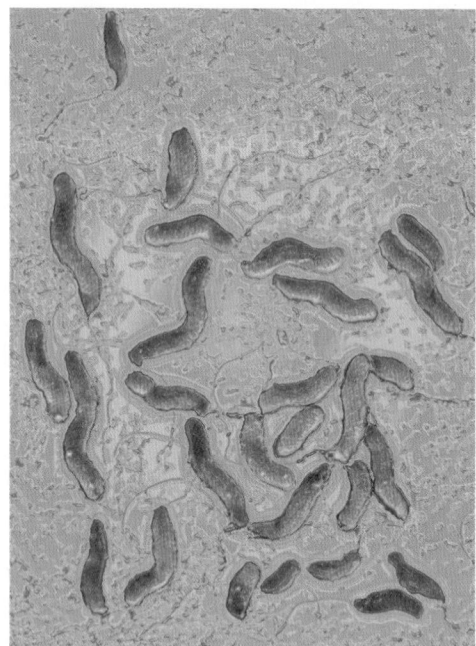

FIGURE 2-12. Histological view of *Helicobacter pylori,* which is a bacterial organism that erodes the gastric mucosa to cause peptic ulcer disease. *(From James Cavallini/Science Source.)*

irritation leads to ulceration of the gastrointestinal cells, also termed *peptic ulcer* (see Chapter 29: Esophagus, Stomach, and Small Intestine Disorders).

Injurious Immunological Reactions

The immune system is the body's major defense mechanism against infectious agents. In some instances, however, the immune system can overreact and attack the body's own cells, causing cell injury and creating disease. For example, allergies are adverse immune reactions in response to contact with an environmental substance known as an *antigen.* In allergy, the immune system is triggered to synthesize antibodies that cause inflammatory changes in the body.

Another example of immunological cell injury occurs in autoimmune diseases such as rheumatoid arthritis, where immune system cells such as T cells and B cells are triggered by an unknown antigen to attack the body's own joints.

Genetic Defects

Genetic disorders can damage and mutate DNA, resulting in the initiation of events that can cause cell injury. Damaged DNA is transcribed as defective RNA, which transmits flawed instructions to the ribosomes. At the ribosomes, the defective RNA causes synthesis of abnormal cellular proteins, which can initiate disease.

Nutritional Imbalances

Undernutrition, overnutrition, and malnutrition are all capable of causing cell injury. Starvation can cause inadequate supply of the nutrients necessary for proper cell function. Without sufficient proteins, carbohydrates, vitamins, and minerals, cell dysfunction can occur. An example of the effects of protein starvation can be seen in disorders such as marasmus and kwashiorkor, which are conditions seen in individuals suffering from severe protein starvation.

CLINICAL CONCEPT

Protein starvation causes low levels of albumin in the bloodstream, which leads to fluid shifting from the blood into the interstitial spaces. Excess fluid accumulation within the peritoneal cavity is most apparent in these starving individuals. The individuals demonstrate wasting of the trunk, bony extremities, and protuberant abdominal swelling.

Obesity, or excessive nutrition, can also cause cell injury. Excessive fat stores can place stress on the heart and pancreas, resulting in heart disease and diabetes. Excess body weight increases the heart's workload because of the obese body's increased metabolic requirements. Excess body weight also places strain on joints, which predisposes to arthritis.

Malnutrition, the inadequate daily intake of carbohydrates, fats, protein, vitamins, and minerals, can also adversely affect cell function. Optimal cellular function requires daily ingestion of sufficient quantities of essential amino acids, glucose, fats, vitamins, and trace amounts of minerals for enzymatic reactions. Carbohydrates are needed for all cellular functions, particularly brain cell metabolism. Fat is necessary in the diet for the storage of fat-soluble vitamins A, D, E, and K; synthesis of hormones; and formation of all cell membranes. Proteins are the basic building blocks of all cells in the body.

Many persons have difficulty obtaining the daily requirement of vitamins, minerals, and nutrients from diet alone. For this reason, many nutritionists recommend adding a daily multivitamin to the diet.

Significance of Endothelial Cell Injury

The arterial blood vessels are lined by a continuous layer of endothelium that plays a key role in vascular function. Endothelial cells constitute a large area of responsive and secretory tissue that is influenced by blood flow changes, shear stress forces, inflammatory mediators, and various circulating substances. One of the substances secreted by endothelium is angiogenesis growth factor, also called **vascular endothelial growth factor (VEGF),** which stimulates the synthesis of collateral blood vessel branches. The endothelial cells also secrete vasodilating substances, such as nitric oxide (NO), and vasoconstricting substances, such as **endothelin.** Blood constituents such as glucose, lipids, platelets, norepinephrine, epinephrine, acetylcholine, vasopressin, natriuretic peptides, and angiotensin II act on the endothelium. Each constituent affects the vasculature's function differently and may have detrimental effects, such as endothelial injury.

> **ALERT!** The endothelium can be considered the body's largest organ because of its vast area. When it is injured, there are widespread effects. Recognition that the arterial endothelium is an extensive, body-wide, active tissue that is highly vulnerable to injury is key to understanding cardiovascular disease.

Endothelial cell injury acts as an initiator of arteriosclerosis and is the fundamental cell change that causes cardiovascular disease. The most significant injurious agents of the endothelial cells are hypertension, diabetic hyperglycemia, free radicals, persistent secretion of angiotensin II, and low-density lipoprotein cholesterol (LDL-C). These are the most common insults that lay the foundation for cardiovascular disease. It is important for clinicians to understand all the etiologies of endothelial injury because cardiovascular disease is currently the most common disease among Americans.

Hypertension

Hypertension exerts a shearing force against the endothelial cell membranes, creating multiple areas of injury on the interior walls of arteries. The high blood pressure force of hypertension can also weaken the integrity of the smooth muscle within the arterial walls. A weakened area in an arterial wall is called an **aneurysm.** After the formation of an aneurysm, the persistent, pulsatile force of hypertension can further weaken its wall, causing rupture and hemorrhage. For example, a berry aneurysm is an example of a cerebral aneurysm located on the arterial network known as the *circle of Willis* within the brain (see Fig. 2-13). A surge in blood pressure can rupture a cerebral aneurysm and cause a fatal cerebral hemorrhage.

Diabetic Hyperglycemia

In uncontrolled diabetes, high blood glucose levels chemically injure the membranes of endothelial cells. Glucose reacts with the constituents of the endothelial membrane and creates advanced glycation end products, which further undermine the endothelial cells' integrity. High-circulating glucose also stimulates the endothelium to secrete endothelin, a potent vasoconstrictor, thereby causing arterial narrowing. Diabetes provokes the combined effects of endothelial injury and vasoconstriction, which stimulates arterial vessel narrowing and accelerates the development of arteriosclerosis throughout the body. The endothelial injury and vasoconstriction are particularly apparent in the lower extremities, which develop peripheral arterial disease. This arterial disease can lead to ischemia of the lower extremities, leading to cellular necrosis and gangrene and resulting in amputation.

FIGURE 2-13. A weakening in an arterial wall is referred to as an aneurysm. An aneurysm of a cerebral artery is often called a berry aneurysm because of its resemblance to a berry hanging from a vine. *(From Living Art Enterprises/Science Source.)*

Free Radicals

Free radicals are highly reactive oxidizing molecules found within the environment and generated by certain cellular processes in the body. Cigarette smoke is a major source of free radicals, which injure the arterial endothelial cells and initiate arteriosclerosis. Cigarettes also contain nicotine, which provokes arterial vasoconstriction. Endothelial injury in combination with vasoconstriction results in widespread cardiovascular disease.

Persistent Secretion of Angiotensin II

Angiotensin II, a product of the renin–angiotensin–aldosterone cascade, acts as a potent arterial vasoconstrictor. In heart disease, constant secretion of angiotensin II is a persistent stimulus for arterial vasoconstriction, which narrows arteries and raises blood pressure. High blood pressure and arterial vasoconstriction create detrimental resistance and a high workload for the heart. Persistent secretion of angiotensin II leads to heart disease. For this reason, angiotensin-converting enzyme (ACE) inhibitors and angiotensin II receptor blockers (ARBs) are the antihypertensive medications commonly prescribed in heart disease.

LDL Cholesterol

Atherogenesis is the gradual and progressive development of atherosclerotic plaque within the arteries that is initiated by endothelial injury. Areas of endothelial injury undergo inflammation, which attracts white blood cells and platelets to the region. These inflammatory changes cause diminished vasodilatory capacity of the artery and set up conditions for the

LDL-C deposition and clot formation. LDL-C accumulates within macrophages to form foam cells, which form the foundation for large spans of atherosclerotic plaque along the artery walls.

Also, during the formation of atherosclerosis, endothelial cell nitric oxide (NO) is depleted, which inhibits the ability of coronary arteries to vasodilate. Vasodilation ability is crucial to sustain enough coronary artery blood flow to the heart muscle, particularly during exercise. Therefore, depletion of NO, which inhibits vasodilation, in addition to the inflammatory changes of the endothelium and LDL deposition, create arterial narrowing and atherosclerosis—a highly detrimental combination for coronary arteries (see Fig. 2-14).

Cell Degeneration and Death

Apoptosis and necrosis are the two major forms of cell death. In apoptosis, cells degenerate at a specific time with no adverse effects on the body. Cellular necrosis, however, is cell death caused by injury. The cell is overcome by an insult, cannot maintain homeostasis, becomes severely dysfunctional, and may adversely affect neighboring tissues or the organ as a whole.

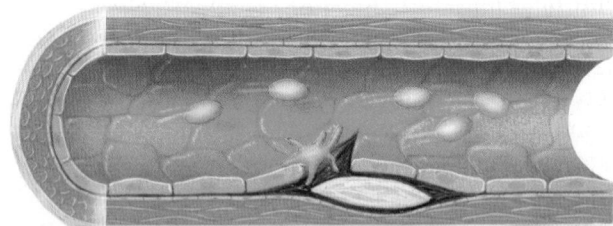

A Endothelial injury with LDL cholesterol settling into arterial wall.

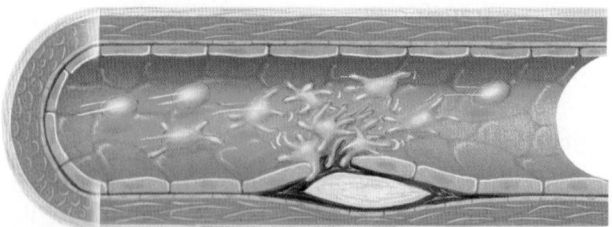

B Inflammation pulls macrophages into area and macrophages engulf lipid. Also, arterial vasoconstriction occurs due to depletion of nitric oxide.

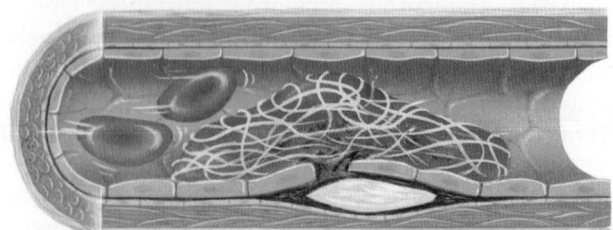

C LDL cholesterol, inflammation, and platelet accumulation form arteriosclerotic plaque with concurrent vasoconstriction that obstructs blood flow.

FIGURE 2-14. Endothelial injury and development of atherosclerosis. *(From BSIP/Science Source.)*

Apoptosis

Apoptosis is a genetically programmed degenerative change that results in cell death. It is an organized process that eliminates unwanted, unnecessary, or damaged cells without inflammation or any adverse effects on surrounding tissue (see Fig. 2-15). It can occur as a normal physiological process or may be involved in a disease process.

An example of physiological apoptosis occurs during the hand's embryonic development, which originates as a paddle-shaped structure. Apoptosis of select cells occurs within the paddle-shaped hand plate to form indentations to shape the individual fingers. The apoptotic cells disintegrate in a stepwise manner without disrupting other cells.

Physiological apoptosis also occurs in female adult ovaries during menopause. During this time, the ovaries become dysfunctional and degenerate according to a genetically determined life span. Cells that have completed their function and need elimination also undergo apoptosis. For example, white blood cells that become exhausted after participation in immune reactions undergo apoptosis.

Some disorders are associated with the dysfunction of cellular apoptosis; as a consequence, cellular life span is prolonged. In these disorders, cells have an abnormally long survival, accumulate, and become disadvantageous to the body. Cells that fail to undergo apoptosis can give rise to certain cancers, tumors, and detrimental hyperplastic cell changes. Prostate cancer is theorized to arise from cells that lose their apoptotic function. In older males, the prostate gland enlarges because apoptosis fails and cells continually multiply. Some of the prostate cells that fail to experience apoptotic cell death undergo cancerous transformation.

Alternatively, some disorders are associated with increased cellular apoptosis, which results in excessive cell death rates. Certain degenerative neurological diseases, such as spinal muscular atrophy, are thought to arise from nerve cells that undergo increased apoptotic rates and consequently die prematurely. In another example, accelerated apoptosis of thyroid epithelial cells results in thyroid gland dysfunction. Hashimoto's thyroiditis is a common autoimmune disease that causes gradual failure of the thyroid gland because of increased apoptotic cell death.

Cell Necrosis

Necrosis occurs when cells die when stressors or insults overwhelm their ability to survive. Necrosis is an irreversible process whereby the cell undergoes a series of changes, including membrane disintegration, chromatin fragmentation, lysosomal activation, and lysis. With cell necrosis, lysosomes break open and release digestive enzymes, initiating autolysis. The body initiates an inflammatory reaction against the necrotic cells, and necrotic cell bodies are left as remnants (see Fig. 2-16). The enzymes and other cellular chemicals that are released from the dead cells enter the systemic circulation and can be measured as indicators of cell death.

Infarction, also called *ischemic necrosis,* is the death of tissue as a consequence of prolonged ischemia. For example, when there is a lack of sufficient coronary artery blood supply to the myocardial muscle, ischemia occurs. If ischemia is prolonged without resumption of circulation to the region of myocardial muscle, infarction occurs. When infarction occurs, lysosomal enzymes and proteins from dead cardiac cells are released into the bloodstream. In myocardial infarction, blood levels of the lysosomal enzyme CPKmb and the cardiac protein troponin are measured to confirm death of myocardial tissue (see Fig. 2-17).

Any tissue that sustains prolonged ischemia is susceptible to infarction, but individual cell types have different tolerance levels. For example, in ischemic conditions, brain and myocardial cells undergo infarction and cell death within minutes, whereas skeletal muscle cells can tolerate lack of circulation for hours.

Gangrene

After cells die, tissue necrosis develops. Dead tissue is a medium for certain types of bacteria, a condition known as **gangrene.** Gangrene can occur when tissues endure prolonged ischemia, undergo infarction and necrosis, and then are exposed to bacteria that thrive on the decaying tissue. *Clostridium perfringens* is an anaerobic bacterium that proliferates in exposed necrotic tissue and emits a gas identifiable as a foul odor associated with gangrene. In clinical settings, gangrene is most often seen in patients with peripheral arterial disease (PAD) of the lower extremities. PAD can cause prolonged ischemia of the lower extremities that leads to infarction, followed by necrosis of tissue and superimposed gangrenous infection (see Fig. 2-18).

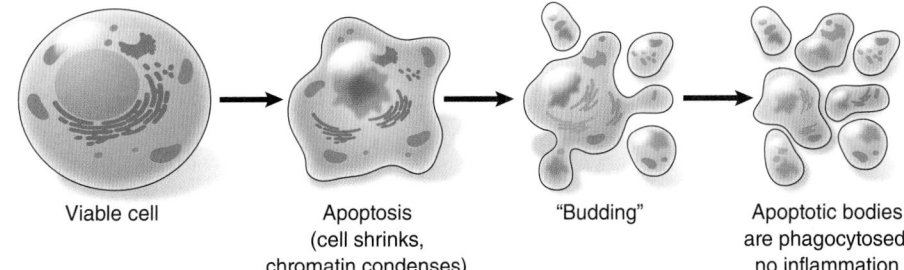

FIGURE 2-15. Apoptosis is a genetically programmed, step-by-step, involutional cellular process. The cell shrinks, DNA undergoes orderly fragmentation, and organelles degenerate. The degenerated cells are phagocytosed by white blood cells, do not stimulate inflammation, and do not have adverse effects on the body.

Viable cell

Apoptosis (cell shrinks, chromatin condenses)

"Budding"

Apoptotic bodies are phagocytosed; no inflammation

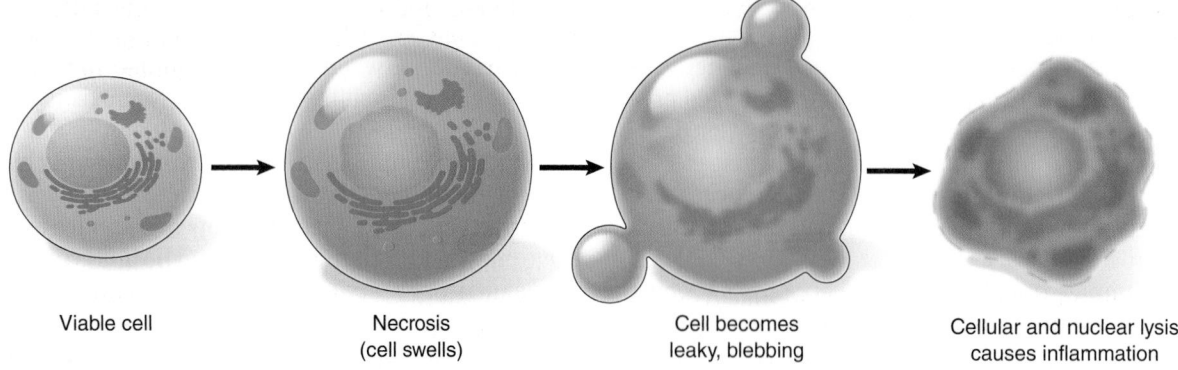

Viable cell

Necrosis
(cell swells)

Cell becomes
leaky, blebbing

Cellular and nuclear lysis
causes inflammation

FIGURE 2-16. The stages of cellular necrosis. In cellular necrosis, the cell swells, loses cellular integrity, and stimulates inflammation.

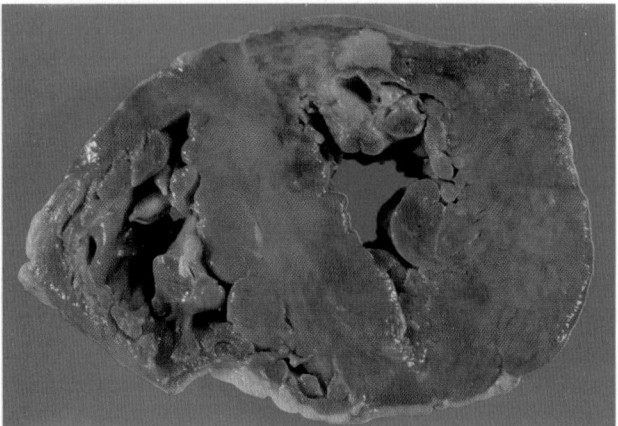

FIGURE 2-17. Cross section of the heart showing an enlarged left ventricle with myocardial infarction. *(From Dr. E. Walker/Science Source.)*

Clinical Interventions to Reverse Cell Injury

Clinical interventions can reverse the effects of cell injury and death through various medical and surgical treatment modalities. In some cases, injured cells can be treated to reverse the damage so that cellular regeneration can take place. Different types of cellular changes require specific types of therapy.

Removal of injurious stimuli can reverse muscle atrophy. If the atrophy is caused by lack of circulation or nerve stimulation, restoration of these processes can allow for rehabilitation of normal cell size. With hyperplasia, metaplasia, and hypertrophy, the eradication of injurious stimuli can allow for the resumption of normal growth patterns in some cases.

 CLINICAL CONCEPT

Hyperplasia of the uterine endometrium can resolve with appropriate hormone therapy that counteracts the effects of excessive estrogen. Acid suppression treatment can resolve the metaplasia of Barrett's esophagus. Treatment of hypertension can cause some regression of left ventricular hypertrophy.

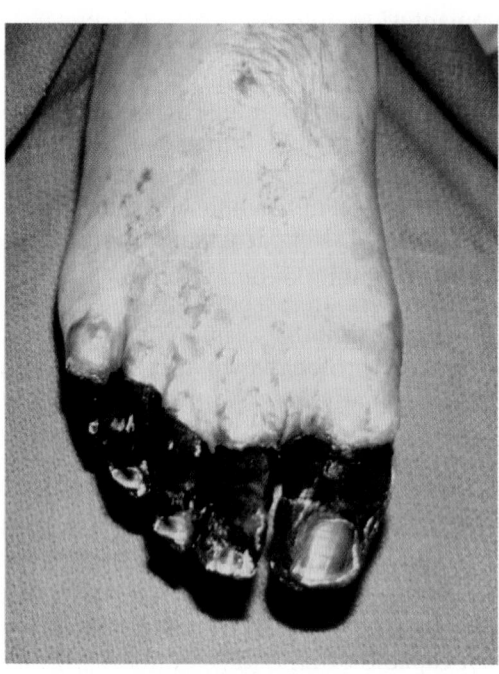

FIGURE 2-18. Gangrene. *(Courtesy of CDC/William Archibald.)*

Neoplastic growths usually require surgical removal. If the neoplasia is malignant, more intense treatment modalities, such as radiation and chemotherapy, may need to be employed to completely eliminate all tumor cells.

Intracellular accumulations can usually be eradicated by resolving the etiology of the metabolic derangement. If the etiology is irreversible, then only palliative or supportive treatments for the disease's effects are available.

Interventions to Treat Permanent Cell Injury

Treatments to reverse permanent cell injury are limited. For example, in myocardial infarction, the heart muscle cells die and are assumed to be permanently dysfunctional. This dead myocardium leaves a segment of the heart muscle as a noncontracting unit, which weakens the heart pump overall. If a large region of cardiac muscle is damaged, heart failure is inevitable. Interventions to treat permanent cell injury include organ and tissue transplantation, regenerative medicine using stem cells, and therapeutic cloning.

Transplantation

Transplantation, a surgical intervention that replaces irreversibly injured cells, tissues, and organs with viable donor tissue, has historically proven successful for many patients. The field of transplantation is complex and involves the solicitation of donors, harvesting of organs, matching of donor organs and recipients, surgical implantation, and interventions to prevent organ rejection. It has proven successful for resolution of many conditions, such as kidney failure, heart failure, and pancreatic and liver disease. Bone marrow transplants have also demonstrated success for different types of cancers and hematologic disorders.

Transplantation therapy, however, is associated with many obstacles: Short supplies of donor organs, exact tissue matching of donor and recipient organs, and transplant rejection are just some of the obstacles within this form of therapy. Researchers are continuing to search for better methods to restore depleted cells, dead tissues, and dysfunctional organs.

Regenerative Medicine Using Stem Cells

Cell biologists have been studying regeneration of cells previously thought incapable of mitosis, such as brain, neuron, and heart muscle cells. It was believed that other than through transplantation, these cells were not capable of functional restoration; therefore cell biologists are developing procedures to regenerate these kinds of cells.

Research in biotechnology and genetic engineering has introduced new modalities of cellular regeneration involving pluripotential cells, called *embryonic stem cells*. Embryonic stem cells are derived from fertilized eggs in the blastocyst stage, a phase of primitive cell division occurring shortly after fertilization. The primitive cells are at an undifferentiated stage and are capable of developing into any specialized tissue or organ. Investigators have found that they could use human embryonic stem cells for tissue repair and cell regeneration. However, human embryonic stem cell research has raised ethical issues about destroying a potential human life. Human embryonic stem cells are obtained from human in-vitro fertilization (IVF) embryos that cannot be used for the couple's infertility treatment. Single cells biopsied from eight-cell stage embryos can be used to develop organs (Damdimopoulou et al., 2016).

Due to the controversy of using embryos and a limited supply, several other methods of deriving pluripotential stem cells have been developed. Umbilical cord blood (UCB) is a rich source of mesenchymal stem cells and can be supplied by placentae, which were previously discarded after childbirth. The value of UCB has prompted the establishment of UCB banks throughout the world. After a woman gives birth, there is an option to store and bank the umbilical cord blood for future use.

Human umbilical cord–mesenchymal stem cells (HUC-MSCs) have remarkable potential to differentiate and proliferate, and have low immunogenicity. Currently, HUC-MSCs are used to treat more than 10 types of diseases, and more major therapeutic breakthroughs are expected. It has been shown that HUC-MSCs injected intravenously into diabetic animals can home to pancreatic islets and differentiate into functional islet-like cells that secrete insulin. In animals, HUC-MSCs improve control of blood glucose and reverse some complications due to diabetes. Diabetic retinopathy, ulcerative foot disease, and renal disease due to diabetes have shown improvement using these cells (Xie et al., 2020).

In persons with liver disease, HUC-MSCs significantly improve hepatocellular necrosis and inflammation without triggering adverse reactions (Zhang et al., 2017). HUC-MSCs also have immunoregulatory function and have improved cases of severe and refractory systemic lupus erythematosus that had failed to respond to pharmacological therapy (Wang et al., 2018). HUC-MSCs have been shown to effectively treat osteoarthritis by differentiating into osteoblasts, inhibiting the proliferation of cytotoxic T cells and inflammatory cytokines, and suppressing inflammation (Dhillon et al., 2022). In brain injury and cerebrovascular disease, HUC-MSCs are found to reduce neuronal degeneration by increasing the expression of glial cell-derived neurotrophic factor, which has a neuroprotective effect (Thomi et al., 2019).

HUC-MSCs have also been shown to treat and relieve various cardiovascular diseases, including myocardial infarction, heart failure, myocardial ischemia, and myocarditis. These cells promote cardiac tissue regeneration and angiogenesis, inhibit inflammation, and significantly reduce infarct size and mortality (Ni et al., 2019). HUC-MSCs are also being used in the treatment of patients with spinal cord injury (SCI). Treated patients have improved sensation, movement, and self-care ability, as indicated by higher American Spinal Injury Association scores and daily life activity scores. Several studies have documented that timely transplantation of HUC-MSCs effectively treats SCI by promoting the recovery of nerve function (Wu et al., 2020).

HUC-MSCs also have clinical applicability in viral infections, cancers, and respiratory diseases such as COPD and asthma. HUC-MSCs are revolutionizing the field of regenerative medicine. Further research and clinical applications hold promise for curative treatment of many chronic diseases. There is an unlimited supply of UCB, and its use is not limited by moral and ethical restrictions. UCB may become the pluripotent stem cell source with the best prospects for broad clinical applications of the future (Xie et al., 2020).

Therapeutic Cloning

At present, cloning technology and stem cell research are under investigation for the creation of transplant organs. The combination of these technologies is called *therapeutic cloning*. This procedure has the potential to develop new organs using human somatic cells (body cells) without any use of a human embryo. Therapeutic cloning is also referred to as *somatic cell nuclear transfer (SCNT)*. The following procedure is used:

- A scientist extracts the nucleus from a donated unfertilized ovum.
- The ovum nucleus holds DNA, which is removed, resulting in an empty ovum.
- The scientist then takes a somatic cell from a patient, which is any body cell other than an ovum or sperm, and extracts the nucleus from this somatic cell.
- The nucleus that is extracted from the somatic cell is then inserted into the unfertilized ovum, which had its nucleus previously removed.
- The ovum then contains the patient's nucleus with the patient's DNA.
- The ovum containing the patient's DNA is now a new cell with a complete set of DNA.
- Scientists then stimulate this new cell to divide.
- Shortly thereafter, the new cell forms a cluster of cells known as a *blastocyst*.

The newly generated blastocyst has an inner layer of cells that is rich in **pluripotent stem cells** containing the same DNA as the patient. These blastocyst cells are undifferentiated. Scientists can harvest these cells and induce them to develop into any organ. This procedure is in early experimental stages but has potential for creating organs for transplant. The newly generated organs would contain the same DNA as the patient, making a perfect match.

Researchers have also found that some adult organs contain small populations of stem cells. Adult stem cells have been found in the brain, bone marrow, peripheral blood, blood vessels, skeletal muscle, skin, teeth, heart, gut, liver, ovarian epithelium, and testis. They are thought to reside in a specific area of each tissue called a *stem cell niche*. Adult stem cells have the potential to develop into mature cells of the organ through an induction process. In this way, they have the potential to serve as an internal repair system that can regenerate new tissue. There is a very small number of stem cells in each tissue, and once removed from the body, their capacity to divide is limited, making generation of large quantities of stem cells difficult. Scientists in many laboratories are trying to find better ways to grow large quantities of adult stem cells in cell culture and to manipulate them to generate specific cell types so they can be used to treat injury or disease.

Research into the curative properties of stem cells is being investigated in many different diseases. For example, in Parkinson's disease, specific dopamine-producing brain cells undergo degeneration and progressively die, causing the patient to endure gradual, progressive neurological deterioration. Current stem cell research in Parkinson's disease is showing promise. Investigators have successfully implanted stem cells into the damaged area of the brain in monkeys with Parkinson's disease. The stem cells replace the diseased cells and regenerate that area of brain tissue (Kikuchi et al., 2017). This has not yet been attempted in humans. Currently, human adult stem cells harvested from many different organs, including cardiac muscle tissue, are under investigation for their potential to regenerate new tissue and treat diseases.

Reproductive Cloning

Research into the therapeutic use of embryonic stem cells has coincided with another field of investigation called *reproductive cloning*. Reproductive cloning is a new and controversial biotechnological field that involves genetic engineering, or manipulation of genetic material. In 1996, a group of scientists in Edinburgh, Scotland, experimented with a process termed *nuclear transfer* for reproductive cloning. After many attempts, the scientists accomplished a nuclear transfer procedure that succeeded. They extracted the nucleus of a mammary cell from an adult sheep and placed it in a donated unfertilized egg, which had its nucleus removed. They then implanted the egg containing the new nucleus into the uterus of a "foster mother" sheep. After the appropriate period of development within the uterus, the foster mother sheep gave birth to a lamb named Dolly, the first cloned sheep. Dolly was an identical newborn version of the original donor sheep. After reaching adulthood, breeders successfully enabled Dolly to give birth to offspring of her own. Unfortunately, after 6 years of adulthood, Dolly died an early death caused by multiple health problems, a common occurrence in animal clones.

Since the 1980s, scientists have been experimenting with the reproductive cloning of farm animals with varying success rates. Published data show that, on average, 1% to 3% of cloned embryos lead to live births. Many cloned offspring die late in pregnancy or soon after birth, and investigations demonstrate that clones that live into adulthood commonly have abnormalities. Currently, reproductive cloning is performed among livestock, such as cattle, pigs, and goats. Clones of rabbits, mice, rats, mules, and cats have also been created.

Presently there is an international debate regarding the scientific use of reproductive cloning technology, as there are many ethical issues surrounding its use. However, breakthroughs in research continue to occur and cannot be rescinded. The debate regarding the use of this biotechnology will likely continue for quite some time.

Chapter Summary

- Cells are vulnerable to many kinds of injurious agents that can cause adaptations, maladaptive changes, and reversible or irreversible damage.

- Physical trauma, temperature extremes, electrical injury, radiation, free radicals, high circulating glucose in diabetes, and high blood pressure can all damage the plasma membrane and leave cellular organelles vulnerable to injury.

- Atrophy is the diminished size and growth of tissue, whereas hypertrophy is an increase in the size of each individual cell of an organ or tissue.

- The most common organ damaged by injurious agents is the endothelium. Endothelial injury initiates arteriosclerosis, which leads to circulatory obstruction.

- Hypertension, high cholesterol levels, hyperglycemia, and free radicals are major injurious agents of the endothelium.

- Ischemia is the lack of adequate blood flow to tissues. Ischemia leads to cellular hypoxia, the most common form of cell injury. Prolonged ischemia leads to infarction or death of tissue.

- Apoptosis is the cell's genetically programmed degeneration.

- Transplantation may not be the only remedy for non-regenerative organs. Stem cell research offers a future alternative to transplant.

- Cellular regeneration of nonmitotic cells, such as brain and cardiac muscle tissue cells, is under investigation; somatic cell transfer procedures are under intense scrutiny.

Bibliography

Available online at fadavis.com

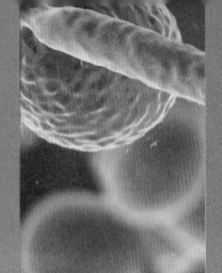

Genetic Basis of Disease

Learning Objectives

Upon completion of this chapter, the student will be able to:

- Describe the major components that make up the double helix of human DNA.
- Define gene mutation and single nucleotide polymorphism and how these can lead to human disease.
- Identify how specific genes can be labeled according to a gene locus.

- Differentiate between Mendelian, sex-linked, and complex multifactorial inheritance patterns.
- Recognize procedures involved in the analysis of DNA, isolation of individual genes, and prenatal diagnosis.
- Discuss common disorders caused by chromosomal abnormalities and genetic mutations.

Key Terms

3-prime end	Gene	Oncogene
5-prime end	Gene locus	Oncoproteins
Allele	Genetics	Pedigree
Aneuploidy	Genogram	Pharmacogenomics
Autosomal	Genome	Phenotype
Autosomes	Genomics	Recessive
Carrier	Genotype	Single nucleotide polymorphisms (SNP)
Centromere	Heterozygous	Transcription
Codon	Homozygous	Translation
CRISPR-Cas9	Intron	Translocation
Dominant	Karyotype	Tumor suppressor gene
Epigenetics	Mutation	
Exons	Nucleotide	

Many disease processes are the result of abnormal cellular activity that occurs from alterations in the cell's genetic control (see Chapter 1: The Cell in Health and Illness). When there is a change in the sequence of DNA nucleotides, there may be changes in cellular physiology. Many changes in nucleotide sequence are not related to diseases at all, but are simply common variations. Other changes are linked to specific diseases, and clinicians can often identify precise changes in DNA that are related to specific diseases. Also, because DNA is passed on to subsequent generations, specific inheritance patterns can often be identified. These changes in DNA, inheritance patterns, and their associated illnesses compose the genetic basis of disease. At the same time, there are also changes in protein production that are not related to changes in the DNA nucleotide sequence. Epigenetic changes are alterations in gene expression that arise due to stressors in the environment, behaviors, or lifestyle. These

changes switch genes on and off within DNA, which affects the individual. Because epigenetic changes can be inherited, offspring can be affected as well.

The fundamental unit of DNA is the **gene,** which is located on a chromosome. The **genome** refers to the collection of all of an organism's genes. The Human Genome Project was established by the National Institutes of Health and other research organizations to determine the sequence of DNA in the human genome. It was a major 13-year research study conducted from 1990 through 2003, and its results have enabled researchers to identify tens of thousands of genes linked to specific disorders and traits. The project revolutionized our understanding of DNA and continues to provide increasing knowledge regarding gene mapping and disease predisposition. Having the human genome sequenced provided the foundation to study gene function in health, disease, and responses to medications **(pharmacogenomics).**

Basic Concepts of Genetics

It is important to distinguish between genetics and genomics. **Genetics** is the study of inherited traits and patterns of inheritance. **Genomics** is the study of the interactions of all the nucleotide sequences (not just genes) within an organism. This includes both those areas that code for proteins and those that do not.

DNA Components

DNA is a double helical structure that can be broken down into nucleotides. A **nucleotide** is a combination of a pentose sugar molecule, phosphate, and a purine or pyrimidine nitrogen base. The nitrogen bases are adenine (A), thymine (T), guanine (G), and cytosine (C) (see Fig. 3-1). The nitrogenous base pairs combine in specific ways in DNA: adenine and thymine (A)–(T) or guanine and cytosine (G)–(C). In ribonucleic acid (RNA), there is one different nitrogen base called uracil that replaces thymine. As a result, RNA base pairs combine as adenine and uracil (A)–(U) or guanine and cytosine (G)–(C).

Genes

Each DNA molecule contains many genes—the basic units of heredity. A gene is a specific arrangement of nucleotide bases, which carry a code for constructing proteins. The human genome is estimated to be composed of between 20,000 and 25,000 genes. Human genes vary widely in length, often extending over thousands of bases, but only about 10% of the genome is known to include the protein-coding sequences called **exons.** Interspersed within genes are **intron** sequences, which do not provide coding information for protein synthesis.

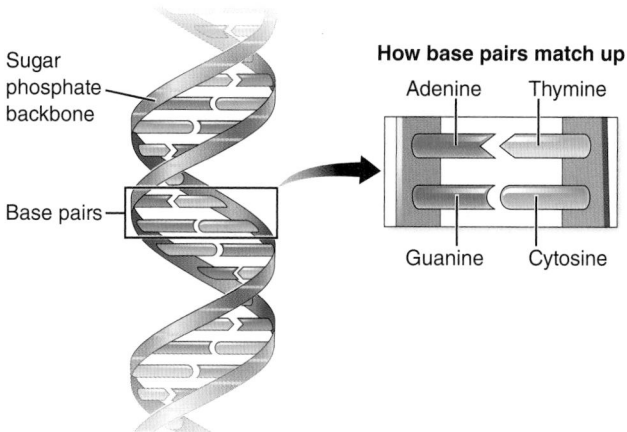

Sugar phosphate backbone

Base pairs

How base pairs match up

Adenine   Thymine

Guanine   Cytosine

FIGURE 3-1. The nitrogenous bases of DNA. When DNA is stretched out, it forms a double helix that resembles a twisted ladder with purine–pyrimidine nitrogenous pairs represented by individual steps on the ladder. The purine–pyrimidine nitrogenous pairs consist of the amino acids adenosine, cytosine, thymine, and guanine. These are matched in a unique sequence to form an individual's genetic code.

Within a gene, an arrangement of three specific DNA bases is called a **codon.** Codons contain a code that is complementary to a specific amino acid; for example, the base sequence ATG codes for the amino acid methionine. An average-sized gene is made of 3,000 nitrogenous base pairs. Because three bases code for one amino acid, an average gene can code for 1,000 amino acids. These amino acids link together to form the proteins synthesized by the cell; this means that the genetic code is a series of codons that specify which amino acids are required to make up specific proteins. In addition, there are codons that signal that protein production should begin or should stop.

Mutations

Mutations are changes in DNA or RNA sequence. Some of these changes can cause disease, but most do not. Common changes in DNA sequence are called polymorphisms. A **mutation** occurs when a gene is damaged or changed in such a way that it alters the genetic code carried by that gene. A mutation can be inherited from parents or can occur spontaneously because of environmental influences. Gametes, also referred to as germ cells, include the sperm and the ovum. Mutations that affect the gamete genes, otherwise known as germ cell mutations, can be passed down to future offspring. Mutations that arise in body cells, also called somatic cells, can contain mutations, but these are not passed down to offspring.

Mutations can occur at a single point in the DNA sequence. These are called point mutations and can be the result of a change in one nucleotide for another (substitution). Point mutations often result in coding for a different amino acid, which then causes a change in the synthesized protein. Removal of a single nucleotide (deletion) or addition of an extra nucleotide (insertion) are termed *frameshift mutations*. Frameshift mutations cause shifts in the reading frame during the translation process. These mutations result in more harmful consequences in coded proteins than do single-point mutations. Such mutations and errors most often result in nonfunctional proteins when all the subsequent codons in the coding sequence are changed. Gene variations can also occur in larger portions of gene sequences or even whole chromosomes.

Gene Nomenclature

As researchers have discovered the various genes in the human genome, each has been given a label. Some genes have been given names that are acronyms of diseases or names that identify their effect. For example, one gene that is associated with breast cancer is called the *BRCA1* gene, and the gene that is associated with retinoblastoma is the *Rb* gene. We all have these genes, but when they are damaged, they can cause diseases.

Not all genes, however, have specific names. To identify any gene, a specific type of nomenclature is followed. All genes can be identified according to their **gene locus,** or their location on a chromosome (see Fig. 3-2).

Understanding a gene locus requires knowledge of chromosomal structure. Each chromosome is divided into two sections, based on a point of narrowing of the linear chromosome, called the **centromere.** The shorter segment, relative to the centromere, is known as the "p" arm, while the longer segment is known as the "q" arm.

Chromosomes are further divided into zones called regions, bands, and sub-bands.

When indicating a specific gene locus, the chromosome number, arm, and region are designated. For example, the gene linked to Duchenne's muscular dystrophy has been located at Xp21.2, the short arm ("p") of the X chromosome in the 21.2 region. Cystic fibrosis (CF) is caused by a variety of different defects at the gene locus 7q31.2. This indicates that the gene is located on the long arm ("q") of the seventh chromosome in a region designated as 31.2.

Some genes have specific names, but others are identified only by their location; for example, one gene that can cause breast cancer when damaged can be referred to as the *BRCA1* gene or 17q21. This indicates that the *BRCA* gene is located on the 17th chromosome's long arm in the 21st region. Another gene that can cause breast cancer when damaged is *BRCA2*. Its locus is 13q12-q13, indicating that it is on the long arm of chromosome 13. Breast cancer only becomes likely when these genes are damaged. Table 3-1 identifies the gene locus for different genetic diseases.

The Human Karyotype

A **karyotype** is an organized arrangement of all the chromosomes within a cell. The human karyotype

TABLE 3-1. Genetic Diseases and Their Gene Locus

Disease	Gene Locus
Huntington's disease	4p16
Cystic fibrosis	7q31
Hemophilia type A	Xq28
Marfan's syndrome	15q15–15q21
Sickle cell anemia	11p15
Breast cancer *BRCA1*	17q21
Breast cancer *BRCA2*	13q
Fragile X syndrome	Xq27
Phenylketonuria	12q21
Duchenne's muscular dystrophy	Xp21
Retinoblastoma	13q14
Hemochromatosis	6p21
Familial hypercholesterolemia	19p13
Polycystic kidney disease	16p4
Alpha 1 antitrypsin deficiency	14q31 and 14q32
Familial Alzheimer's disease	21q11
Cleft palate	Xq13
Tay Sachs disease	15q22
Familial adenomatous polyposis	5q21 and 5q22
Neurofibromatosis type 1	17q11

contains 23 pairs of chromosomes (see Fig. 3-3). Although the human karyotype can be assembled from any human cell with a nucleus, karyotype testing is commonly performed on an individual's white blood cells (WBCs) or buccal mucosal cheek cells. During the metaphase portion of cell division, the chromosomes are stretched out and easier to identify. During this stage, geneticists can study individual chromosomes and genes by obtaining a picture of the 23 chromosome pairs (the karyotype). Each individual has a unique karyotype—a distinct picture of their 23 pairs of chromosomes. A karyotype can be used to identify an individual, similar to how fingerprints are used.

Of the 23 chromosome pairs, 22 pairs carry genes related to body traits, called **autosomes.** The 23rd pair is the sex chromosomes. Most females possess the XX sex chromosome pair, and most males possess the XY pair. The Y chromosome is much smaller than the X and contains the sex-determining region. Both sex chromosomes carry genes for other traits not related to sex, but because the X chromosome is so much larger

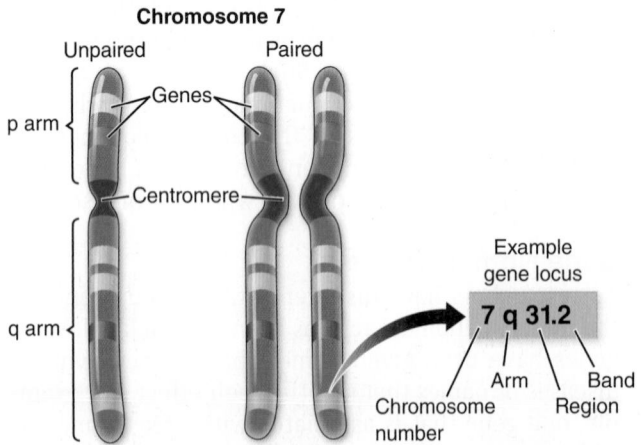

Chromosome 7

FIGURE 3-2. A gene locus is the gene's location on the chromosome. The central region of a pair of chromosomes is called the centromere, which divides the chromosome into a short arm (p) and a long arm (q). A gene is named by listing the chromosome number, followed by the arm it sits on: p or q. The numbered region on the p or q arm is listed and can be further broken down into band and sub-band, for example: 7q31.2.

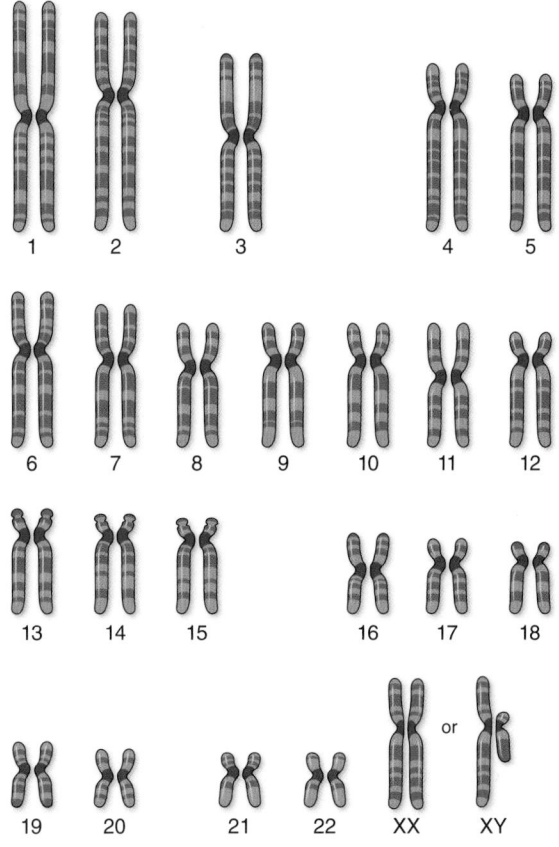

FIGURE 3-3. The human karyotype is a picture of the 23 pairs of chromosomes. Each pair of chromosomes is numbered 1 to 23. The 23rd pair contains the sex chromosomes. The 1st to 22nd pairs are called autosomes, which determine the body's genetic characteristics. Each person has a unique karyotype, which is why a karyotype can be used to identify a specific individual.

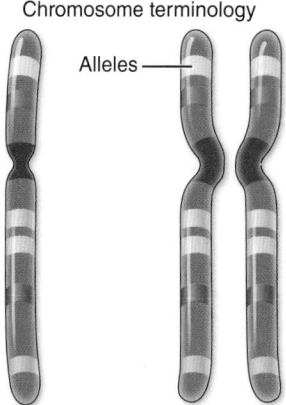

Chromosome terminology

Alleles

FIGURE 3-4. On every pair of chromosomes there are genes that determine the same characteristic. Each individual gene is called an allele. They occupy the same position on each chromosome. One allele is inherited from the mother, and the other allele is inherited from the father.

than the Y, it carries far more genes. Every chromosome has genes that contain traits of inheritance that transmit information from one generation to another (see Fig. 3-4).

> ### 🔬 CLINICAL CONCEPT
>
> The normal human karyotype contains 22 pairs of autosomal chromosomes and 1 pair of sex chromosomes. The most common female karyotypes are 46,XX and males are 46,XY.

Regulation of Gene Expression

Daily cellular function involves the production of proteins and other substances that are responsible for maintaining physiological homeostasis. DNA is transcribed into messenger RNA (mRNA) in the nucleus in a process known as **transcription.** After the strand of mRNA is created, it leaves the nucleus and travels to the ribosomes. At the ribosomes the process called **translation** occurs, which is the manufacture of specific proteins according to the directions provided by mRNA.

Transcription

The process of transcription within the nucleus begins when the enzyme RNA polymerase, along with the help of transcription factors, binds to a promoter region on the DNA molecule. During transcription, the double helix of DNA unwinds and separates into two distinct strands. One strand acts as a template for the production of a complementary strand of RNA. An enzyme RNA polymerase acts on the DNA template to create the strand of mRNA. The promoter region serves as a "start" signal for gene transcription. The RNA polymerase then helps unwind and separate the DNA strand, exposing the base pairs to be transcribed. Transcription occurs in sections of DNA, moving in a specific direction from the DNA template to create mRNA. A DNA template fragment has two opposite ends, termed prime ends. The RNA polymerase reads the exposed DNA template starting from the **3-prime end** and moving toward the **5-prime end.** From the 3-prime end to the 5-prime end, nucleotides that bind in complementary fashion are added to the exposed base pairs on the DNA strand to create mRNA. The complementary base pairing for DNA and mRNA are the same, except that the thymine of DNA molecules is replaced with uracil in mRNA. Thus a DNA strand that reads ACTGA is transcribed into UGACU on the mRNA strand.

Several RNA polymerases can be used to transcribe a section of DNA, and these initial transcripts undergo further modification before leaving the nucleus. When DNA is first transcribed, the transcript contains introns, which are intervening sequences that do not encode for proteins. Introns are removed as part of mRNA processing. The portions of the transcript that encode for protein—exons—will remain in the transcript. The process of intron removal is carried out by spliceosomes—large enzymatic molecules that precisely splice out specific sections of mRNA. Introns are excised so that exons can be joined together in a specific manner to create the precise mRNA molecule that can create proteins later in the process during translation.

The processing of an mRNA transcript is not the only way genetic regulation occurs. All cells contain the same genes. However, cells carry out different functions; thus not all cells express the same genes, nor do all cells maintain the same levels of gene expression. Controlling gene expression at the level of transcription is crucial for each cell. This level of genetic control can be seen in the use of enhancers and silencers of transcription. Enhancers and silencers are transcription factor binding sites located on the DNA. As their names imply, enhancers are areas where, when transcription factors bind, the transcription rate of a given gene is enhanced or increased. On the other end of the spectrum, silencers are transcription factor binding areas that reduce or inhibit genetic transcription. The use of enhancers and silencers is one mechanism used by the cell to regulate its genetic expression.

Translation

Once the processed mRNA leaves the nucleus, the mRNA transcript will serve as the template for protein formation in the process of translation. The translation process occurs in the ribosomes, located in the cytoplasm. Ribosomes are composed of structural proteins, enzymes, and ribosomal RNA (rRNA). The mRNA transcript binds to a portion of the rRNA on the ribosome. The "reading" process of the mRNA transcript during translation engages three nucleotides at a time that act as a code for a specific amino acid. The mRNA nucleotides are aligned with specific amino acids by transfer RNA (tRNA). The link between the nucleotides on the mRNA and specific amino acid is coordinated by tRNA.

On one end of the tRNA is a three-sequence nucleotide that binds with complementary base pairs to the sequence on the mRNA. The other end of the tRNA carries the corresponding amino acid associated with the three-nucleotide sequence. As the mRNA transcript is read and each tRNA delivers a specific amino acid encoded by the transcript, the amino acids are linked together by peptide bonds in the proper sequence to form a growing peptide chain. Peptide chains connect to each other. The lengthening chain of peptides is assembled into a specific protein that will be secreted by the cell.

Although every cell in the body contains identical DNA with its accompanying genetic information, not all the genes are active. Some genes are silenced. The active genes are only those necessary for the particular tissue's function. For example, each pancreatic beta cell contains the whole human genome (all of the individual's DNA). However, because the pancreatic beta cells need to produce insulin, those genes required for synthesis of insulin are turned on and the genes for synthesis of other hormones are turned off. Regulatory regions, usually just outside of a gene coding sequence, determine whether a gene is active or inactive. Also, specific transcription factors interact with these regulatory regions in turning protein synthesis on or off.

Inheritance Patterns

The transmission of genetic information from parents to children begins with the formation of the gametes (sperm and ova). During the process of meiosis, gametes are formed that contain DNA derived from both parents. When the gametes fuse to form a zygote, chromosome pairs are formed. One chromosome of each pair comes from the mother, and the other chromosome comes from the father. Each chromosome carries with it the genes for certain traits, so except for those genes located on the sex chromosomes, everyone has two copies of each gene. Each individual gene is an **allele** that is inherited from each parent. The two alleles may be the same or different, and their combination determines inheritance of a certain trait. A person may be either heterozygous or homozygous for a certain trait, which has implications for how the trait will be manifested in the individual. If a person is **heterozygous** for a certain allele, it means that the gene from their mother is different from the gene from their father. If a person is **homozygous** for a particular trait, it means that they inherited the same gene variation from their mother and their father.

A **genotype** is the set of genes inherited from the individual's mother and father, which are responsible for a certain trait. Depending on their inheritance from parents, an individual can have a genotype that is heterozygous or homozygous. A **phenotype** is defined as how genes are manifested in the individual; it is the actual physical or somatic expression of the genotype.

Alleles can be either **dominant** or **recessive** (see Fig. 3-5). If an allele is dominant, it will be expressed even if the person has only one copy (one allele from the mother and a different allele variation from the father). The dominant allele will be the one expressed. For example, the trait polydactyly (having more than five fingers on one hand) is a heterozygous trait. If a baby has one copy of the gene that causes polydactyly inherited from their mother and a normal copy of the gene from their father, the baby will have polydactyly. If an allele is recessive, a person will need to have identical alleles from their mother and father for the trait to be expressed. CF is a disease caused by a recessive trait. For a baby to have this condition, they must inherit a CF gene from both their mother and father.

When letters are used to diagram the genetic trait, capital letters are used for dominant characteristics. Lowercase letters represent recessive characteristics. For example, polydactyly is determined by the alleles inherited from both parents. P represents a dominant gene, so if present, the individual will have polydactyly; p represents a recessive gene, which represents the trait for five fingers. A person can be heterozygous,

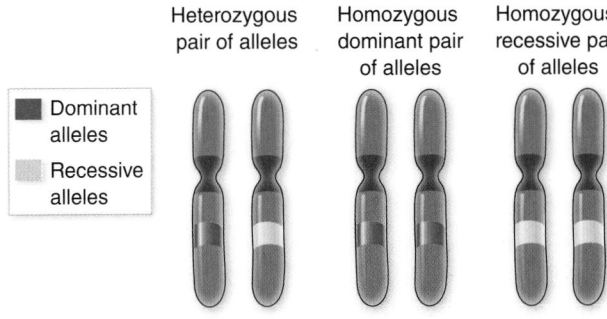

Heterozygous pair of alleles   Homozygous dominant pair of alleles   Homozygous recessive pair of alleles

■ Dominant alleles
▫ Recessive alleles

FIGURE 3-5. Genetic traits can be either dominant or recessive, with the dominant trait usually being expressed over the recessive genetic trait. Individuals can be homozygous or heterozygous with regard to genetic traits. Homozygous individuals have both alleles expressing the same trait. Heterozygous individuals have both alleles expressing different traits.

where their genotype is Pp, or homozygous, where their genotype is PP or pp. If a person has the homozygous genotype PP, which are two dominant genes, they will have the phenotype of polydactyly. If the person has the heterozygous genotype Pp, their phenotype is also polydactyly because P is dominant. If a person has a homozygous genotype with a p from their mother and a p from their father, their genotype is pp, and their phenotype is five fingers.

As seen in the previous example, a dominant trait is usually expressed if corresponding alleles are homozygous or heterozygous. In a heterozygous state, the dominant allele silences the recessive allele. A **carrier** is a person who is heterozygous for a recessive trait and does not manifest it; in other words, a carrier possesses a recessive allele, but the dominant allele silences it. The carrier does not externally demonstrate the recessive trait, but can pass it on to their offspring. CF is caused by a recessive trait. An individual can carry the trait for CF but not have the disease themselves. Their genotype consists of one CF gene and one healthy gene (Pp). The CF gene is recessive, and the healthy gene is dominant. Therefore they have the genotype that makes them a carrier of CF but a phenotype of no disease. They would not be affected but would be able to pass on the disease to their children if they mated with another carrier. A person who has CF (recessive) would have a genotype of pp.

The inheritance of some genetic traits is sex linked. As stated earlier, the female genotype is usually XX, whereas the male genotype is usually XY. Because the Y chromosome is smaller than the X chromosome, it does not have comparable alleles for many of the X chromosome traits. Therefore genetic traits on the X chromosome are dominant in males. However, they may be either dominant or recessive in females. Traits that are not sex linked are referred to as **autosomal** traits.

Mendelian Inheritance
The basic concepts of genetics were initially developed through the work of Gregor Mendel, a 19th-century Augustinian monk. As a high school science teacher, he began to study inheritance patterns by examining the characteristics of pea plants in his garden. His descriptions of inheritance patterns of dominant and recessive traits have been used to introduce the concepts of heredity. However, some genetic traits and illnesses are inherited in more complicated ways and do not follow Mendelian inheritance patterns.

In Mendelian inheritance, the Punnett Square is used to depict the chance of dominant versus recessive traits being expressed. This method is used to configure possible combinations of gene traits in offspring. The allelic traits of each parent are used to configure all possible combinations. The alleles contributed by one parent are placed across the top of the square, and the alleles contributed by the other parent are placed on the left of the square.

Autosomal Inheritance
If a mother and a father are heterozygous for the gene variants that cause polydactyly (Pp) and they want to know the chances of their offspring having polydactyly, the Punnett Square method can be used (see Fig. 3-6). The results of the Punnett Square depicted in Fig. 3-6 demonstrate that there is a 25% chance that the offspring will be homozygous for the gene causing polydactyly (PP), a 50% chance that the offspring will be heterozygous for polydactyly (Pp), and a 25% chance that the offspring will be homozygous (pp). Because the allele causing polydactyly is dominant, any offspring that has at least one P will show the traits. The P gene is dominant and silences the p gene, which is recessive.

Parents who possess the sickle cell anemia trait often need information about the chances that their offspring will have sickle cell anemia. Sickle cell anemia is considered an autosomal-recessive disorder. The sickle cell trait is carried by more than 100 million people worldwide. An individual with sickle cell trait is heterozygous for sickle cell anemia. People with sickle cell trait are carriers for the disease; they can pass the disease

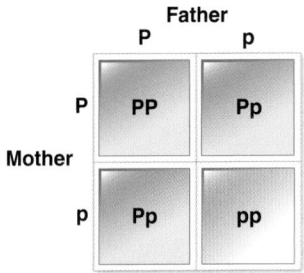

FIGURE 3-6. Using a Punnett Square to determine the chance of having offspring with polydactyly. In this Punnett Square, the mother is Pp genotype heterozygous for polydactyly. The father is Pp genotype also. There is a 25% chance of the child being homozygous with genotype PP and a 25% chance of the child being homozygous with genotype pp. The chance of an offspring that will be heterozygous for polydactyly like their parents (Pp) will be 50%.

on to their children if they mate with another carrier. But they may also experience some disease symptoms when they are dehydrated or exercise at high intensity. A Punnett Square can be used to configure the possible genetic combinations of offspring (see Fig. 3-7).

The results of the Punnett Square in Fig. 3-7 demonstrate that there is a 25% chance that each of this couple's offspring will be homozygous for sickle cell anemia (Hgb S–Hgb S), a 50% chance that their offspring will be heterozygous for sickle cell anemia (Hgb S–Hgb normal), and a 25% chance that their offspring will not have sickle cell anemia (Hgb normal–Hgb normal). Therefore there is a 25% chance that the parents with sickle cell trait will have an offspring who will suffer from sickle cell anemia and a 50% chance that each offspring will be a carrier.

Sex-Linked Inheritance

If the gene is located on the X chromosome, the inheritance pattern is sex linked, or X-linked. Because the X chromosome has no corresponding allele on the Y chromosome, the X allele is dominant. The X alleles will dominate over the lack of Y alleles. Therefore the X allele will always be expressed in male offspring. However, for female offspring, it will follow a similar pattern to autosomal dominant or recessive. Because there are few non–sex-related genes on the Y chromosome, there are very few Y-linked diseases. The Y chromosome contains only about 2% of all the DNA within the cell.

An example of the X-linked disease inheritance pattern can be seen in hemophilia. The gene responsible for hemophilia is carried on the X chromosome. There is no corresponding allele on the Y chromosome. Females can have one X chromosome with the hemophilia allele and one normal X chromosome. The normal X chromosome allele silences the allele with hemophilia. Therefore females can be carriers of hemophilia but not express the disease. Because the allelic trait is on the X chromosome in the male and the male Y chromosome has no corresponding allele, hemophilia is expressed in the male. There is no Y allele to silence the hemophilia allele on the X chromosome. Therefore males express the allele on the X chromosome and suffer from the disease (see Fig. 3-8).

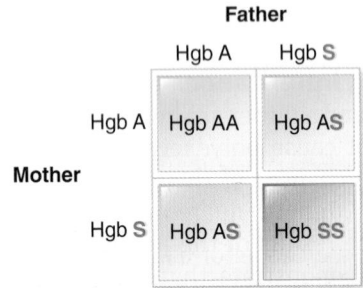

FIGURE 3-7. Using a Punnett Square to determine sickle cell disease. In this Punnett Square, the mother is heterozygous and the father is heterozygous. The mother and father, who are both carriers of sickle cell anemia, have a 25% chance of having a child with full sickle cell disease, a 25% chance of having a child with no trait at all, and a 50% chance of having a heterozygous child.

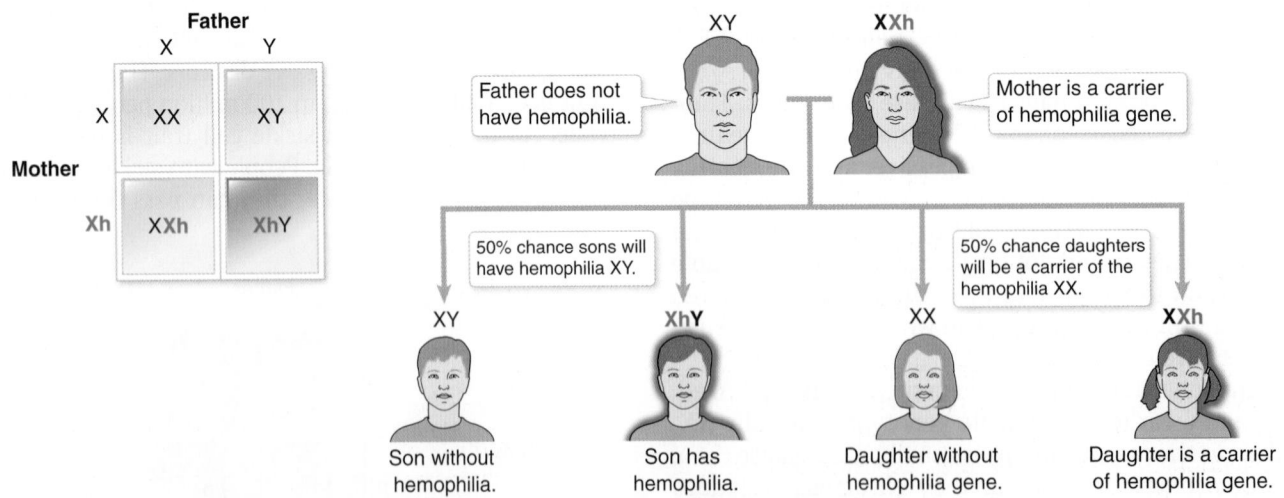

FIGURE 3-8. The following Punnett Square and pedigree show how hemophilia, which is an X-linked genetic disorder, is inherited. The X chromosome, which is dominant over the Y chromosome, determines the trait's heredity in an X-linked disorder. The X chromosome is a full chromosome, whereas the Y chromosome is a piece of chromosomal material. In this genogram, the mother is a carrier of hemophilia; therefore her genotype is XXh. The father does not have hemophilia, and his genotype is XY. A Punnett Square can be used to determine the chances of the child having hemophilia or carrying the trait. There is a 25% chance that the parents will have a daughter who is a carrier of hemophilia, a 25% chance of having a son with hemophilia, a 25% chance of having a son without the disorder, and a 25% chance of having a daughter who is not a carrier.

Penetrance and Variable Expressivity

Sometimes when two individuals have the same genotype, their phenotype is different. One person may have a disease, whereas another with the same disease-causing genotype will not. This difference is the result of varying penetrance of the genetic characteristic. Penetrance refers to what percentage of people with the genotype will show the phenotype. For example, if everyone with a particular genotype has the phenotype, the trait is considered to be fully penetrant. If 50% of people with the genotype have the phenotype, the trait is considered to be roughly 50% penetrant, or incompletely penetrant. For example, women who inherit the *BRCA1* or *BRCA2* gene have an increased risk of developing breast cancer. Thus the penetrance of these genes is based on the likelihood or lifetime risk of developing cancer. In women who inherit *BRCA1*, the penetrance is about 85%; for *BRCA2*, it is about 20%. This is important information that must be considered in deciding whether to be tested for the presence of the *BRCA1* and *BRCA2* genes.

Sometimes in heterozygous-dominant disease, a person who has a damaged gene copy from both parents will have a more severe form of the disease. Variable expressivity means that people with the same disease-causing genotype have varying levels of disease severity. This can be seen in Marfan's syndrome, a connective tissue disorder that results in affected people being tall with elongated limbs and cardiovascular complications. Marfan's syndrome is caused by a mutation in the gene *FBN1*. But even though people with Marfan's syndrome carry a mutation of the same gene, the severity of symptoms they experience varies. Some are just tall and have long thin limbs, whereas others are severely affected with heart and blood vessel problems that can cause sudden death.

Complex (Multifactorial) Inheritance

Single-gene inherited disorders or single mutations are quite rare. The majority of diseases are the result of multifactorial genetic influences. Diseases such as hypertension, heart disease, diabetes mellitus (DM), and most cancers are caused by a combination of genetics and environment or a combination of several defective genes working, or not working, together. In these diseases, an individual inherits one or more gene defects that predispose them to a disorder, and then environmental or behavioral triggers such as diet, exposure to toxins, or sedentary lifestyle contribute to disease development. For example, multifactorial inheritance factors are involved in the development of type 1 and type 2 DM:

- The exact cause of type 1 DM (T1DM) is unknown. However, gene variations within the immune system, particularly the human leukocyte antigen (HLA) complex, are implicated, and T1DM is considered an autoimmune disease. In this case, the person's own immune system attacks the beta cells of the pancreas, causing them to stop making insulin. But HLA variations are responsible for only about 40% of cases, and researchers believe that some HLA variants may actually be protective.
- In type 2 DM (T2DM), obesity, sedentary lifestyle, and increased abdominal fat distribution patterns are associated with insulin resistance, which characterizes the disorder. There is also a strong family history of T2DM in affected individuals. Over 150 variations in DNA have been associated with T2DM. A combination of genetics, environment, and behavior appears to cause the disease.

An interesting aspect of complex inheritance relates to common variations in genes. A type of these variations is known as **single nucleotide polymorphisms (SNPs).** In an SNP, one nucleotide is substituted for another. For example, in the sequence ATCGTA, the C may be replaced with a T, leading to the nucleotide sequence ATTGTA (see Fig. 3-9). Although a single nucleotide substitution may seem minor when considering the entire human genome, SNPs can have profound effects on health and disease, as a single base substitution may code for a different amino acid. The substituted amino acid may disrupt the functionality of the peptide formed. In addition, SNPs may lead to disease development and affect responses to environmental factors such as drugs or chemicals. SNPs can affect genetic functioning even if found in noncoding areas of the DNA, as SNPs may disrupt the binding of transcription factors and other signals used to regulate gene expression.

Sickle cell anemia is an example of a disease caused by an SNP. Other diseases may manifest from the interplay of several SNPs, but in the case of sickle cell anemia, a single nucleotide change is involved. An alteration in the nucleotide sequence for the beta chain of hemoglobin results in an amino acid substitution that

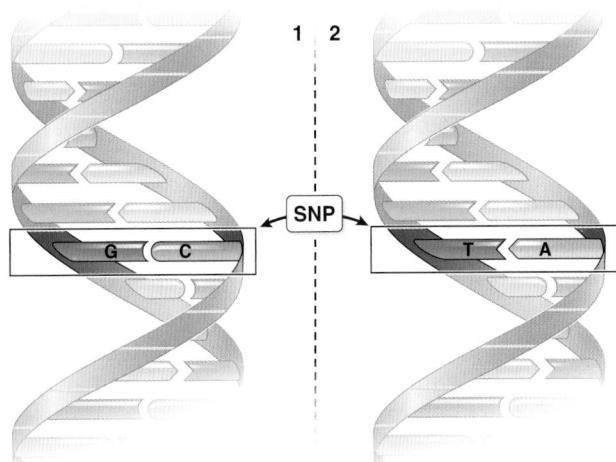

FIGURE 3-9. A single-nucleotide polymorphism is a variation in a DNA sequence occurring when a single nucleotide—A, T, C, or G—in the genome differs between a pair of chromosomes.

disrupts the normal polypeptide chain for hemoglobin. In normal hemoglobin, a portion of the DNA sequence is GAG, encoding for the amino acid glutamate. However, in the case of sickle cell anemia, the DNA sequence has an SNP, resulting in the nucleotide sequence of GTG, which encodes for valine. This simple nucleotide substitution and subsequent amino acid alteration change the function and shape of the beta hemoglobin chain, resulting in the disease characteristics associated with sickle cell anemia.

Mitochondria and Inherited Diseases

Mitochondria are the cell's powerhouses, producing energy through a series of complex biochemical reactions. Their activity is required for supplying energy for all physiological functions. Additionally, mitochondria are the only cellular organelles that have their own distinctive ribosomes and DNA. Mitochondrial DNA is a double-stranded, circular single chromosome responsible for the formation of the key components of energy production. Cell biologists speculate that mitochondria were self-sustaining, independent-living, bacteria-like organisms that over the course of evolution became incorporated into human cells.

During human fertilization, the ovum destroys the sperm's mitochondria, which results in virtually all mitochondrial DNA being derived from the mother. Because mitochondrial DNA is unique, geneticists can use it to study an individual's maternal hereditary lineage.

Alterations in nutrient delivery to the cell can damage mitochondria. In addition, mitochondrial DNA can be subject to impairment or mutation by free radicals. Although there is a repair process for DNA within the cell's nucleus, this does not usually happen for mitochondrial DNA. Cumulative damage of mitochondrial DNA has been implicated in the aging process and in diseases such as diabetes, cancer, and heart failure.

Not all mitochondrial disease is due to damage to the DNA in the mitochondria. Some genes that produce proteins needed for the mitochondria to function are located on nuclear chromosomes.

Inherited mitochondrial disorders include neurogenerative disorders, hypertrophic cardiomyopathy, ophthalmoplegia, and maternally inherited deafness. This inheritance pattern is passed on from the mother to all offspring. Other inherited mitochondrial diseases include disorders of balance and sensation, classified as ataxia–neuropathy syndromes. It is theorized that the cellular damage and symptoms are related to the progressive decrease in cellular mitochondrial activity. The symptoms are more evident when the altered mitochondrial function affects the muscles and the nerves.

Biomedical and genetic technological procedures have made it possible to edit defective mitochondrial DNA. Biotechnologists can remove defective mitochondrial DNA from the ovum of a female with mitochondrial disease. The defective mitochondrial DNA can be replaced with normal mitochondrial DNA from a healthy female donor that is implanted into the female parent's ovum. The edited ovum then contains the donor mitochondrial DNA, making it a healthy ovum. However, the edited ovum is composed of DNA from two different females; mitochondrial DNA from the donor female and nuclear DNA from the parent female. This has posed an ethical dilemma because the donor becomes a kind of "third" parent involved in the process of conception when the edited ovum and sperm unite.

In addition to editing mitochondrial DNA, scientists are now able to edit whole genes in the early stages of embryonic development. In 2019, a highly controversial procedure termed clustered regularly interspaced short palindromic repeats (CRISPR) was performed on humans in China, which edited the genes of twin females in their early embryonic stages. The editing procedure changed the females' genes that coded for specific surface antigens on their cells. The editing procedure was able to imbue the embryos with specific surface antigens that endowed cellular resistance to HIV infection. Investigations that use the CRISPR procedure to eradicate genetic mutations that cause disease are emerging. CRISPR is a highly controversial procedure in the scientific community, with many ethical issues surrounding this technological process.

 CLINICAL CONCEPT

Mitochondrial DNA is maternally inherited, which enables researchers to trace maternal lineage far back in time.

Pharmacogenomics

Individuals differ in their response to medications. Genetic variations that alter drug response most commonly alter drug metabolism, but there can also be genetic changes in drug absorption, drug transport, and drug receptors. One example of a variation in drug response involves the enzyme *N*-acetyltransferase enzyme (NAT). There are two common variations in the gene that codes for this metabolic enzyme. About half the population are "slow acetylators." They process drugs that are metabolized by NAT more slowly, leading to higher blood levels and longer activity. Those who are "fast acetylators" metabolize drugs that require NAT quickly, leading to lower blood levels. Some drugs that require acetylation include sulfamethoxazole, hydralazine, procainamide, and caffeine.

Pharmacogenomics has also provided more understanding of individual responses to warfarin (Coumadin), which is used to decrease the formation of blood clots in patients. However, individual responses to this medication are variable. Some people obtain therapeutic effects quickly, whereas others require higher dosages to achieve the same effects. Some persons are at high risk for bleeding because their blood levels of the drug are much higher than expected and they remain higher longer. This variability in response has been linked to variations in primarily two genes. One is a gene affecting metabolism (*CYP2C9*), and the other is a warfarin target gene. The Food and Drug Administration (FDA) requires that precautions be placed on warfarin labels informing health-care providers that people with certain genetic variations may require lower starting doses.

Pharmacogenomics has also provided more understanding of individual responses to many other drugs. The FDA now places warnings on several drugs regarding variable responses among patients based on their genetic variations. Clinicians are beginning to be able to personalize drug therapy for individuals based on their genetics, which affects the patient's expected response to the pharmacological agents.

An example of how genomics influences pharmacological therapy is in the management of hypertension in people of African descent. Uncontrolled hypertension (HTN) is particularly prevalent and devastating among Black individuals, who disproportionately suffer the complications of this condition compared with persons in other racial/ethnic groups. Research demonstrates that angiotensin-converting enzyme inhibitors (ACEi), angiotensin receptor blocker (ARBs), and beta 1 adrenergic blockers are ineffective at controlling HTN among hypertensive patients of African ancestry. Recent studies have now identified novel genetic variants unique to people of African ancestry that influence the effect of certain pharmacological agents in control of blood pressure (Liang et al., 2018). Based on pharmacogenomic studies that link genetic variations with specific medications, it is now known that calcium channel blockers and diuretics are most effective to manage HTN in people of African ancestry (Brewster et al., 2016). Findings such as these will likely lead to other discoveries of genetic variations within sectors of the population that influence pharmacological treatment. The study of pharmacogenomics is still in its infancy; however, discoveries of specific genetic influences on pharmacological treatment are increasingly becoming part of precision medicine. Precision medicine is a new approach in health care that customizes medical treatment so that it is appropriate for a patient's unique genetic makeup, specific metabolic processes, and life circumstances.

Alterations in DNA

The DNA within the nucleus must be protected because it contains the vital information for heredity and all cellular activity in the body. DNA is vulnerable to damage if a breach occurs in the nuclear membrane or an injurious agent penetrates the nucleus. However, there are internal repair processes that attempt to restore DNA to its normal state. If the change in DNA

involves an altered nitrogenous base sequence in one strand of the DNA, its complementary strand can act as a template for repair. The mismatched base sequence is removed from the altered strand. The DNA replication process then uses the complementary strand to match up the appropriate bases, completing the repair process.

Genetic mutations are referred to as either hereditary or acquired, also called *sporadic*. A hereditary alteration would be evident in prior and present generations, whereas an acquired alteration would be seen in the individual and possibly in their offspring. If the DNA is damaged in a germ cell (egg or sperm), it will be passed on to the next generation even if the parents' genome does not carry this mutation.

In cases of DNA injury, damaged genes are defective and, in turn, transcribed as defective mRNA. Defective mRNA will then carry defective directions to the ribosomes, which in turn manufacture defective proteins. Defective proteins synthesized by the cell can be the cause of a disease process.

DNA alterations or mutations are changes in nucleotide sequences, deletions, or insertions of nucleotides. These changes can represent the change of base sequences in a codon, leading to a change in the protein structure. For example, a nucleotide base substitution results in a different amino acid being included in hemoglobin formation, leading to the development of sickle cell anemia. The normal nucleotide base sequence is GAG (guanine–adenine–guanine), which codes for glutamic acid. In sickle cell disease, the sequence is GTG (guanine–thymine–guanine), which codes for valine. This change in amino acid alters the hemoglobin structure, forming the sickle cell HgbS.

Deletion of a nucleotide may cause its specific gene to be nonfunctional. This is the case with individuals with phenylketonuria (PKU). Affected individuals are unable to produce a specific enzyme, phenylalanine hydroxylase, which converts phenylalanine to tyrosine. Lack of phenylalanine hydroxylase leads to a buildup of phenylalanine in the systemic circulation. The accumulation of phenylalanine can cause PKU, a disease that includes growth inhibition, hypopigmentation, and intellectual disability.

 CLINICAL CONCEPT

Most newborns in developed countries are screened for PKU soon after birth. A sign of PKU is a musty odor of the urine and sweat.

Oncogenes and Tumor Suppressor Genes

An individual can possess a genetic mutation called an activated **oncogene**, which increases risk of cancer. Proto-oncogenes are normal genes that control cell proliferation. Mutation of proto-oncogenes leads to activated oncogenes. This mutation causes uncontrolled cellular proliferation or insuppressible cancerous growth.

Activated oncogenes can be inherited or acquired. When the cell that possesses this activated oncogene undergoes transcription, the RNA will carry the defective message of the activated oncogene onto the ribosomes. The ribosomes, in turn, will synthesize defective proteins called **oncoproteins.** These oncoproteins will direct the cell to undergo uncontrolled proliferation, persistent mitotic divisions, or persistent cancerous growth, which is why activated oncogenes can be considered cancer-causing genes.

Another genetic defect associated with cancer involves **tumor suppressor genes,** which are genes that inhibit uncontrolled cellular mitosis and persistent proliferation. An example is the p53 tumor suppressor gene, which stops the mitotic cell division cycle. When defective, tumor suppressor genes do not suppress cancerous transformation of cells, and cancer growth occurs uninhibited.

Another way that cancer occurs is through viral insertion of an oncogene. For example, the human papilloma virus (HPV) inserts its DNA into the DNA of tissue cells. When activated, this DNA stimulates the abnormal growth cycle associated with cancer cells. Additionally, it inhibits the action of p53, a tumor suppressor gene. This is the mechanism for the development of cervical, anal, and oropharyngeal cancer from HPV infection.

There is also the multistage theory of cancer development. According to this theory, there must be an initial exposure to a carcinogen that mutates the gene. The next step involves continued exposure to that carcinogen or another carcinogen with similar effects. Finally, the alterations lead to tumor development. Small cell lung cancer in smokers is believed to develop in this way.

 CLINICAL CONCEPT

An activated oncogene can lead to formation of oncoproteins and a cancerous change in the cell. A defective tumor suppressor gene can also lead to a cancerous change in the cell.

Knudson's "Two-Hit" Hypothesis

Pairs of alleles make up an individual's genotype. If one of the pair's alleles becomes damaged or mutated, in most cases, the normal corresponding allele can counteract the effect. In 1971, Alfred Knudson proposed the "two-hit" hypothesis to explain the genetic mechanisms in the initiation of certain cancers. He was studying retinoblastoma, a cancer of the retina, which can occur spontaneously or as a hereditary disorder.

It had been observed that retinoblastoma occurred in a younger age in patients with a hereditary predisposition for the cancer than in patients without a hereditary predisposition. Additionally, children with retinoblastoma were more likely to develop the cancer in both eyes than those adults who developed it spontaneously. Knudson tried to understand why cancer developed in only some persons with hereditary predisposition and not others with the same hereditary risk. He studied individuals born with a genetic mutation in one allele for retinoblastoma. For actual cancer to develop, Knudson noted that a mutation of one allele was not sufficient because the normal allele counteracted the effect. He termed the initial allelic mutation the "first hit" in his theory. In his investigations, he noted that cancer developed only in persons who acquired a second allelic mutation. Persons who developed cancer possessed a hereditary mutation on one allele and acquired a second mutation on their normal allele sometime in the course of their lifetime. Therefore he hypothesized that for many cancers to develop, both corresponding alleles on a chromosome must be mutated. Hence, Knudson called this the "two-hit" hypothesis, which has been found to hold true as the required initiating events for many diseases, as well as many types of cancer.

For example, if an individual discovers they have inherited a disease-causing mutation in the *BRCA1* or *BRCA2* gene, this does not mean that the individual is 100% likely to develop cancer. The individual has a heightened risk of cancer because of the allelic mutation, but this is not the only factor involved in the development of cancer. A second allelic mutation would need to be acquired, perhaps through carcinogen exposure, for the disease to develop.

Many tumors are examined to determine whether one mutation is accompanied by a second mutation. This information has been helpful in cancer research. In terms of hereditary cancer syndromes, it is important to note that an additional mutation is often needed for tumor development.

This model of the "two-hit hypothesis" has been applied to the development of other illnesses as well. For example, the tendency to develop schizophrenia can be linked to specific genes related to neurological development. Once the "at-risk" gene has been transmitted to offspring (first hit), an environmental factor during the nervous system's development (second hit) alters the formation of neural networks, leading to the development of schizophrenia.

As Knudson proposed, in many diseases both alleles must be mutated for a disease to manifest in an individual. This holds true unless a disease is notably autosomal dominant, meaning only one allele needs to be mutated for the disease to come to fruition. Hereditary familial adenomatous polyposis (FAP) is an autosomal-dominant disorder, and in these individuals only one allele needs to be mutated for the disease to manifest.

Chromosomal Alterations

Genetic disorders also occur because of changes in the number or structure of chromosomes. Alterations in chromosome division during meiosis can result in a different number of chromosomes. This condition is known as **aneuploidy.** This usually occurs when a chromosomal pair does not separate in the anaphase stage of meiosis, a condition known as nondisjunction and anaphase lag. The gamete will have one additional or one fewer chromosome. Other chromosomal alterations can occur when a piece of one chromosome breaks off and joins another. This is referred to as **translocation.** A chromosome can also break and lose a portion of genetic material; this is called a chromosomal deletion.

The most common chromosomal alteration is Down syndrome, a major cause of intellectual disability. About 95% of individuals with Down syndrome have a trisomy of chromosome 21. They have three copies of chromosome 21 instead of two, giving them a total of 47 chromosomes. Some individuals have a translocation of chromosomal material from chromosome 21 to either chromosome 22 or 14; this is another form of Down syndrome.

Turner's syndrome, a disorder that affects females, causes hypogonadism and physical characteristics such as a webbed neck, broad chest, and short stature. Instead of 46 chromosomes, females with Turner's syndrome have 45 chromosomes—and instead of two X chromosomes, they have only one, giving them a designation of 45,X or 45,XO. Some women with Turner's syndrome have a portion of the second X chromosome.

Errors of the mitosis of cells in early embryonic development can give rise to a condition known as mosaicism. Mosaicism occurs when there are cells with different numbers of chromosomes within the same individual. Mosaicism that affects the sex chromosomes is fairly common. In the division of a fertilized ovum, an error can develop where one cell has 45,X and another cell has 47,XXX. All descendent cells from these abnormal cells will have either 45,X or 47,XXX. The individual will exhibit a variation of Turner's syndrome. Some people with Down syndrome are mosaic, which means that some of their cells contain three copies of chromosome 21 and others contain only two copies.

Many more structural and numerical errors of chromosomes can occur that result in abnormal karyotypes. Those discussed here are major types of chromosomal errors. It is estimated that 7.5% of all conceived embryos have a chromosomal abnormality. Often these types of chromosomal abnormalities are not compatible with life, resulting in fetal or embryonic death. Causes of abnormalities in chromosome number and structure include advanced maternal age and environmental factors.

Epigenetics

Epigenetics is the study of how behaviors, lifestyle, and environmental factors can influence genes and the way they are expressed. Epigenetic changes do not change your DNA sequence, but change the way your body reads the DNA sequence. They are reversible changes and work by either turning genes "on" or "off." Epigenetic changes affect gene expression in the following ways (CDC, 2020):

- DNA methylation: In DNA methylation, a chemical group is added to the DNA, which can "turn on" or "turn off" a gene.
- Histone modification: Histones are proteins that can wrap around genes and turn them on or off.
- Non-coding RNA: Non-coding RNA is not used to make proteins; it influences how ribosomes read the RNA to make proteins.

Epigenetic changes can be caused by various environmental agents and conditions. For example, exposure to opioids causes long-term changes to brain regions involved in reward processing and motivation. Opioid use can lead vulnerable individuals to engage in pathological drug seeking and drug taking for a lifetime. The persistence of these neuroadaptations is mediated in part by epigenetic remodeling of gene expression in specific brain regions. Current evidence shows that chronic use of opioids promotes histone modification and DNA methylation in brain cell DNA sequences involved in reward circuitry (Browne et al., 2020).

Genetic Assessment

When dealing with heritable disorders, assessment includes a family history with multigenerational patterns of illness, as well as ethnic, cultural, and social practices. The multigenerational history should include, at a minimum, three generations of a family. This information is then displayed in a **pedigree** (also called a **genogram)** (see Fig. 3-10).

Gathering assessment data may require a tactful approach from the health-care professional because some families are reluctant to divulge all this information during an initial visit. Certain illness patterns are seen in specific ethnic groups, so it is important to gather this information. For example, Tay Sachs disease is more common among people of Ashkenazi Jewish ancestry. Thalassemia anemia is more prevalent in people of Mediterranean or East Asian descent. People of African or Asian descent have a G6PD deficiency more often than people without this ancestry. Cultural practices and shared dietary patterns may increase the risk of developing multifactorial disorders such T2DM and cardiovascular disease. This aspect of history taking can provide important clues in evaluating the risk of developing certain heritable disorders.

Family History by Genogram

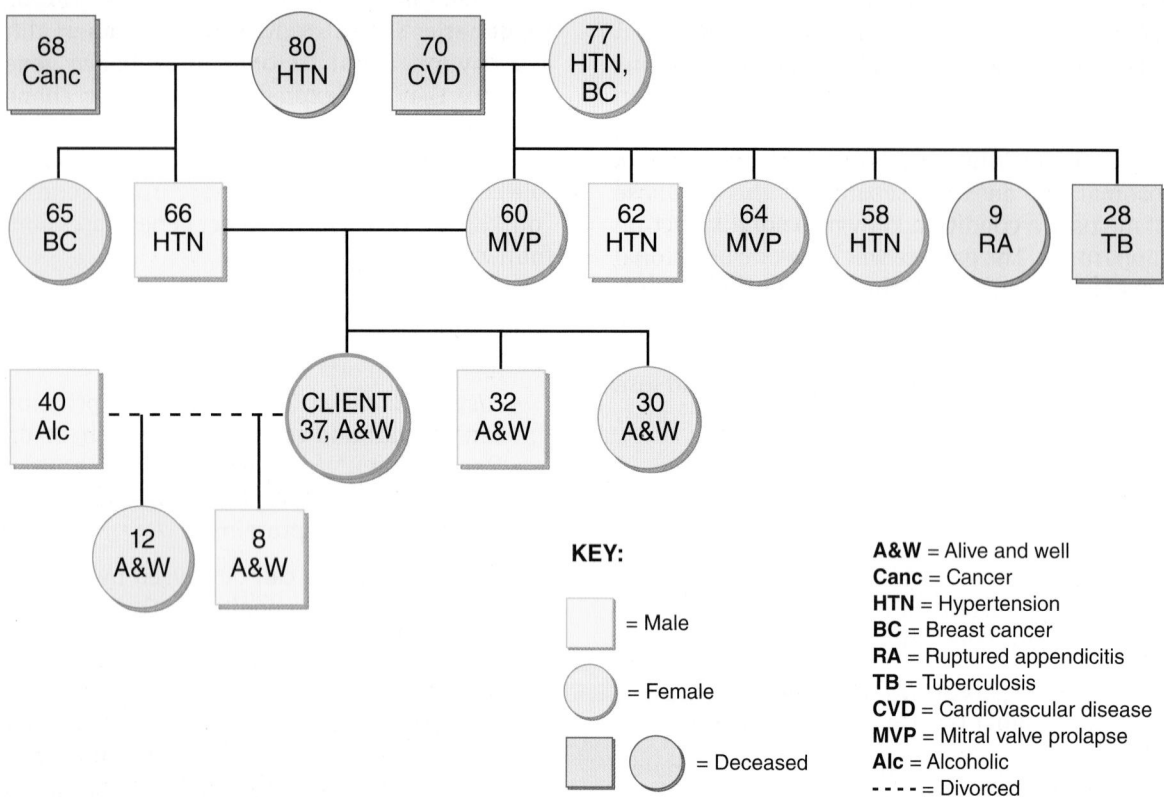

FIGURE 3-10. Example of a pedigree.

KEY:

☐ = Male

◯ = Female

☐ ◯ = Deceased

A&W = Alive and well
Canc = Cancer
HTN = Hypertension
BC = Breast cancer
RA = Ruptured appendicitis
TB = Tuberculosis
CVD = Cardiovascular disease
MVP = Mitral valve prolapse
Alc = Alcoholic
- - - - = Divorced

Molecular Analysis of Genetic Disorders

It is possible to identify mutations at the DNA level, and clinicians can now offer diagnostic tests for an increasing number of genetic disorders. Acquired or inherited genetic alterations can be detected using molecular analysis techniques such as polymerase chain reaction (PCR) and fluorescence in situ hybridization (FISH).

Karyotyping

A karyotype analysis involves staining the condensed chromosomes of mitotic cells with Giemsa dye. It provides an overall picture of an individual's chromosome pairs. The dye stains regions of chromosomes that are rich in the base pairs adenine (A) and thymine (T), producing a dark band. A common misconception is that bands represent single genes, but in fact, the thinnest bands contain over a million base pairs and potentially hundreds of genes. The analysis allows for comparisons of chromosomes for their numbers, structure, placement of centromeres, and location and sizes of bands.

Polymerase Chain Reaction

PCR is a procedure that produces multiple copies of a short segment of DNA and amplifies the segment for further study in the laboratory. The PCR procedure can be applied to a very small sample of DNA and be used for diagnostic testing. It does not require mitotic cells, as does karyotyping. It is commonly used for genetic analysis in cancer and infectious disease detection, forensics, and research.

Fluorescence In Situ Hybridization

FISH is a procedure used to map the genetic material in an individual's cells. It has been used for detection of numeric abnormalities of chromosomes, subtle chromosomal microdeletions, and translocations not detectable by routine karyotyping. It does not require mitotic cells, as does karyotyping.

Southern Blotting

Southern blotting is a molecular genetic testing technique used to detect DNA fragments, which can vary because of various types of mutations; these include gene insertions, gene deletions, expanded trinucleotide repeats, and single nitrogenous base changes. For example, Southern blotting could be used to locate a particular gene or DNA fragment within an entire genome.

Prenatal Diagnosis of Genetic Disorders

Prenatal diagnosis or prenatal screening is used for early detection of birth defects and genetic diseases in a fetus or embryo in utero. This diagnosis can identify disorders such as neural tube defects, Down syndrome, chromosome abnormalities, spina bifida, cleft palate, Tay Sachs disease, sickle cell anemia, thalassemia, CF, and fragile X syndrome. Screening can also be used for prenatal sex discernment. Common testing procedures include chorionic villus sampling (CVS), amniocentesis, and percutaneous umbilical cord blood sampling (PUBS). In general, genetic testing is offered to couples or individuals identified as being at risk for a particular genetic problem. Some of the risk factors that health-care providers consider in deciding who should be offered testing include family history, medical history, and ethnicity. Examples include:

- Women 35 years or older who are pregnant or are planning to become pregnant
- Abnormal ultrasound findings
- Couples who are close blood relatives, such as first cousins
- Women who have a condition, such as diabetes, that can be associated with an increased risk of fetal problems
- Ethnicity—two parents of Ashkenazi heritage would be at higher risk for a number of autosomal-recessive conditions than two parents of non-Ashkenazi heritage
- Unexplained or multiple miscarriages
- Family history of an inherited condition, intellectual disability, or birth defects

Maternal Serum Screening

Maternal serum screening refers to tests performed on a pregnant woman's blood for the purpose of determining if her developing fetus may have an increased risk of having an open neural tube defect (ONTD), Down syndrome, or trisomy 18. Proteins that are produced by the developing placenta and fetus enter the mother's blood. The most commonly tested proteins are alpha-fetoprotein (AFP), human chorionic gonadotropin (hCG), unconjugated estriol (uE3), and dimeric inhibin A (DIA). Cell-free DNA from the placenta can also be tested and provides a higher level of accuracy than many other prenatal blood tests. If a maternal serum screening test is positive, it indicates an increased chance for a fetal problem. In this case, additional, more specific diagnostic testing is done.

Chorionic Villus Sampling

CVS is a diagnostic procedure performed during pregnancy to diagnose chromosome abnormalities, some inherited disorders, and certain birth defects in a fetus. CVS is most commonly offered when a woman is at an advanced maternal age (35 years and older at the time of delivery) because of the increased chance of a fetal chromosome problem. CVS may also be offered if an inherited genetic problem is identified in the family. CVS is performed between 10 and 12 weeks of pregnancy. Under the visualization of ultrasound, a thin

needle is either inserted through the abdomen or a specially designed catheter is passed through the vagina and a small sample of placenta is removed. The placenta contains cells generated by the fetus. Approximately 99% of fetal chromosome abnormalities can be diagnosed from CVS.

ALERT! CVS is contraindicated in pregnant women with vaginal bleeding, uterine fibroids, retroverted uterus, and those carrying twins.

Amniocentesis

Amniocentesis is a test primarily used to diagnose fetal chromosome problems. It can also help diagnose fetal defects, such as spina bifida, abdominal wall defects, and some inherited disorders. Amniocentesis is performed on amniotic fluid, usually between 16 and 18 weeks of pregnancy. As the fetus grows and sheds cells, those cells can be found in the amniotic fluid and used to study the fetal chromosomes.

Amniocentesis detects about 99% of fetal chromosome abnormalities. A thin needle is inserted through the mother's abdomen (under ultrasound guidance) into the amniotic sac, and a small amount of amniotic fluid is removed.

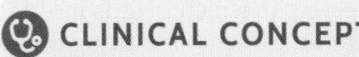

CLINICAL CONCEPT

Amniocentesis, commonly done between 16 and 18 weeks, is recommended for pregnant women older than 35 years.

Percutaneous Umbilical Cord Blood Sampling

PUBS, also called cordocentesis, is a diagnostic genetic test that examines blood from the fetal umbilical cord to detect fetal abnormalities. It provides a means of rapid chromosome analysis and is useful when information cannot be obtained through amniocentesis, CVS, or ultrasound. This test carries a significant risk of complication and is typically reserved for pregnancies determined to be at high risk for genetic defects.

Gene Therapy: Reversing and Preventing Disease

Gene therapy is the prevention and treatment of a disease through transferring genetic material into the cells of patients. Gene therapy is revolutionizing the treatment of several diseases and utilizes different strategies to achieve its therapeutic goal. Initial gene therapy strategies used ex vivo gene delivery strategy. Researchers collected and cultured the patient's genetically defective cells, modified the genetic defect, and then readministered the corrected cells back to the patient. Retroviruses were used as vectors to deliver a normal copy of a specific defective gene into the genome of the corrected cells. Ex vivo gene delivery has been successfully applied in the treatment of severe combined immunodeficiencies, β-thalassemia, and large B-cell lymphoma (Tang & Xu, 2020).

Another strategy, termed in vivo gene therapy, directly delivers a normal copy of a specific defective gene into the target cells through local delivery or systemic delivery. Adenoviruses are used as vectors to deliver the genetic material. The adenovirus can facilitate insertion of genetic material into target cells for a limited time. They are not permanent genetic changes. This type of gene therapy has shown some success in treatment of cystic fibrosis (CF), a disease that causes mucus-obstructed airways. Vector-assisted, in vivo gene therapy, allows for delivery of a corrected gene to the respiratory mucosal cells in CF. Patients demonstrate significant ventilatory improvement for as long as 10 weeks after treatment (Guggino & Ceboratu, 2017).

In traditional gene therapy, a normal copy of a specific defective gene is delivered into the target cells and restores the function of the defective gene temporarily. However, a recent breakthrough in genome editing technology, termed CRISPR-Cas9, has opened up the possibility of removal or correction of defective genes in a genome permanently. Genome editing is a type of genetic engineering in which DNA is inserted, deleted, or replaced in the genome of a living organism. Scientists first observed this kind of genomic editing performed by bacteria in the natural environment. They then experimented for many years to attempt to mimic the process in the laboratory with animal cells. The result, CRISPR technology, is revolutionizing gene therapy (NIH, 2019).

To edit the genome of an organism, scientists have to break a specific DNA sequence at a precise location within the double helix of DNA. To achieve this precise DNA break, researchers have developed the **CRISPR-Cas9** (clustered regularly interspaced short palindromic repeats and CRISPR-associated protein 9) system. With CRISPR-Cas9, researchers create a short RNA template, termed *guide RNA*, which matches a target DNA sequence in the genome. Strands of RNA and DNA bind to each other when they have matching sequences. The RNA guide portion of the CRISPR technology directs the Cas9 enzyme to the targeted DNA sequence. The Cas9 enzyme is a laboratory-created nuclease that cuts the genome at the specific location to make the edit. The cell then uses its own DNA repair machinery to proceed with making the change in the genome (Komor et al., 2017).

There are two different categories of gene therapies: germline therapy and somatic therapy. Germline gene therapy changes DNA in reproductive cells: sperm and ova. Changes to the DNA of reproductive cells can be passed down from generation to generation. Somatic gene therapy makes changes in nonreproductive body cells. These changes affect only the person who receives the gene therapy. There are ethical concerns with germline gene editing as it requires experimentation on embryos. The NIH, for example, does not fund research to edit human embryos (Swartjes et al., 2020).

Recently, a combination of ex vivo gene therapy and genetic editing, termed chimeric antigen receptor (CAR-T) gene therapy, has become one of the most promising therapies for treatment of cancer. Instead of delivering a normal copy of a specific defective gene to a patient, it extracts some of the patient's T cells and then modifies and fortifies them to target cancer cells. A patient with cancer has some T cells extracted, cultured, and modified genetically. The T cells are modified so that their genome includes a gene that codes for development of a specific receptor that targets the patient's cancer cells. The T cells with this newly developed receptor are then re-administered to the patient and are able to target and annihilate the patient's specific cancer cells. CAR-T gene therapy has been successful in treatment of large B-cell lymphoma and B-cell precursor acute lymphoblastic leukemia (Tang & Xu, 2020).

Gene therapy and genome editing are revolutionizing prevention and treatment of numerous diseases. These technologies are not widely used clinically for patients yet. The efficacy and safety of gene therapy and gene editing requires thorough investigation before it is widely used clinically. However, it is exciting research and holds great promise for millions of patients suffering from presently incurable and untreatable diseases.

Ethical Concerns

Health-care professionals are sometimes asked to counsel patients about what the results of genetic testing mean for them. Genetics professionals are skilled at this type of counseling, and it is important that people at high genetic risk and those considering genetic testing receive counseling by certified genetic counselors. Patients need to know what their genetic testing results actually mean and all available treatment options. Because this is a relatively new area of health care, health-care professionals are exploring the best approaches to use in each instance of testing for inheritable disorders. This area needs further research.

Pathophysiology of Selected Genetic and Chromosomal Disorders

Familial Hypercholesterolemia

Familial hypercholesterolemia (FH) is an autosomal-dominant disorder that causes severe elevations in total cholesterol and low-density lipoprotein (LDL) cholesterol. Although hypercholesterolemia is a common finding in many individuals, heterozygous FH occurs in approximately 1 per 500 persons in the United States. Homozygous FH, which is a more severe disease than the heterozygous form, occurs in approximately 1 in 1 million individuals in the United States. FH is a disorder of absent or dysfunctional LDL receptors. The LDL receptor gene is located on the short arm of chromosome 19.

In FH, the liver, which normally processes cholesterol, lacks effective receptors for LDL cholesterol, preventing the liver from taking it up. This increases blood LDL levels. Normally, the uptake of LDL by the hepatocytes will suppress the liver's synthesis of cholesterol. However, when LDL is not taken up by hepatocytes, hepatic synthesis of cholesterol is not suppressed. This leads to further cholesterol production despite high levels of circulating cholesterol. The total cholesterol levels of infants and children with homozygous FH are higher than 600 mg/dL. In patients with heterozygous FH, half the LDL receptors are normal and half are rendered ineffective by the mutation. These patients' total cholesterol and LDL cholesterol levels are twice as high as the recommended level of LDL (less than 100 mg/dL). LDL cholesterol levels of 200 to 400 mg/dL are common in heterozygous FH.

In homozygous FH, severe and widespread atherosclerosis occurs early in life. Children are at risk for early acute myocardial infarction. In heterozygous FH, early adulthood coronary artery disease is the most serious clinical manifestation. Untreated men are likely to develop symptoms by the fourth decade of life, and women in the fifth decade. Early manifestations include xanthomas and xanthelasma, which are deposits of cholesterol under the skin. Xanthelasma specifically occurs in the skin around the eyes. Corneal arcus is a light-colored ring that is within the periphery of the cornea of the eye. Cholesterol-lowering drugs, a low-fat diet, and daily exercise are the treatment recommendations.

 CLINICAL CONCEPT

A family history of early cardiovascular disease, such as myocardial infarction in a first-degree relative younger than age 55 years, is suggestive of FH.

Familial Adenomatous Polyposis

FAP is usually inherited in an autosomal-dominant fashion. It is characterized by the early onset of hundreds to thousands of adenomatous polyps throughout the colon. If left untreated, patients with this syndrome develop colon cancer by age 40 years. In addition, an increased risk exists for the development of other malignancies.

FAP is caused by a mutated gene at 5q21 called the *APC* gene. Under normal conditions, the *APC* gene is a tumor suppressor gene that triggers apoptosis in colon cells. The mutation of this gene prevents its function as a tumor suppressor and allows uncontrolled growth of colonic tumors called polyps. The polyps have a high likelihood of becoming malignant tumors, and colorectal cancer can develop.

In the autosomal-dominant disorder, every colonic cell in patients with FAP has one mutated APC allele. Inactivation of the other normal allele of the APC gene removes the tumor-suppressive function of APC, thus allowing uncontrolled growth of adenomatous polyps. There is also an autosomal-recessive form of the disease involving mutation of the *MUTYH* gene, which is involved in DNA repair.

Incidence varies from 1 case in 6,850 persons to 1 case in 31,250 persons worldwide. The cause of death is colorectal cancer, which develops in all patients unless they prevent the disease. The mean age at which colorectal cancer develops in patients with classic FAP is 39 years. Patients can be asymptomatic until cancer has already metastasized. In patients with FAP, 75% to 80% have a family history of polyps or colorectal cancer at age 40 years or younger. Symptoms, if present, include unexplained rectal bleeding (hematochezia), diarrhea, or abdominal pain. To detect disease, patients with a family history should have a colonoscopy every 1 to 2 years beginning at age 10 to 12 years.

Surgical treatment to excise and biopsy polyps is necessary. The patient may require removal of the colon (colectomy). The patient with FAP is also susceptible to other types of cancer, such as thyroid, liver, adrenal, pancreatic, or gastric cancer, as well as medulloblastoma.

Marfan's Syndrome

As discussed earlier, Marfan's syndrome is an inherited connective tissue disorder transmitted as an autosomal-dominant trait. It affects about 1 in 10,000 individuals and perhaps as many as 1 in 3,000 to 5,000. About 75% of affected individuals have an affected parent. Sporadic mutation accounts for the remaining 25%.

Marfan's syndrome results from mutations in the fibrillin-1 (*FBN1*) gene on chromosome 15, which contains the code for the glycoprotein fibrillin. Fibrillin is a major building block of microfibrils, which constitute the structural components of the aorta and other heart valves, airways of the lung, suspensory ligament of the lens, dura mater of the spinal cord, and other connective tissues of the body. The mitral, tricuspid, and aortic heart valves are commonly affected. Cardiovascular disease, mainly aortic dilation and dissection, is the major cause of morbidity and mortality. Death after infancy usually involves ascending aortic dissection and chronic aortic regurgitation. Dissection generally occurs at the aortic root and is uncommon in childhood and adolescence.

If untreated, Marfan's syndrome can be highly lethal; the average age at death is 30 to 40 years. There are many clinical signs and symptoms, such as:

- Tall stature with elongated arms and fingers
- Kyphoscoliosis
- Ligament hypermobility of the hips, knees, ankles, arches, wrists, and fingers
- Heart murmur from aortic regurgitation or mitral prolapse
- Dysrhythmia
- Abrupt onset of thoracic pain, which occurs in more than 90% of patients with aortic dissection
- Syncope
- Shock
- Pallor
- Pulselessness
- Paresthesia or paralysis in the extremities
- Low back pain near the tailbone
- Burning sensation and numbness or weakness in the legs caused by dura mater defects
- Joint pain (adult patients)
- Dyspnea, severe palpitations, and substernal pain in severe pectus excavatum (concave sternum)
- Breathlessness, often with chest pain, in spontaneous pneumothorax
- Visual problems, including loss of vision, from lens dislocation or retinal detachment

CLINICAL CONCEPT

In Marfan's syndrome, sudden onset of hypotension may indicate aortic rupture.

Physicians experienced in connective tissue disorders can make the clinical diagnosis. Common tests used to help with clinical diagnosis are chest x-ray, aortic angiogram, echocardiogram, CT, and magnetic resonance imaging (MRI). Genetic testing is used to confirm or rule out a diagnosis in persons with a family history of Marfan's syndrome or those with uncertain clinical findings.

Heart valve problems are a priority in treatment. Preventive procedures for cardiovascular disease are necessary, such as valve replacement and medications to prevent dysrhythmias. Scoliosis may require orthopedic surgery. Pneumothorax needs to be treated with a chest tube to suction. Pectus excavatum may require surgery. Ophthalmological consultation is needed as well. Genetic counseling is important to inform patients and families and to assist with family planning and reproductive decisions.

CLINICAL CONCEPT

Individuals with Marfan's syndrome are at increased risk of spontaneous pneumothorax, aortic dissection, and heart valve abnormalities.

Neurofibromatosis

Neurofibromatosis (NF) is a genetic disorder with cutaneous, neurological, and orthopedic manifestations. There are primarily two types of disease: NF type 1 (*NF1*) and NF type 2 (*NF2*). *NF1* is more common than *NF2*, and there is less cutaneous involvement in *NF2* compared with *NF1*. The manifestations of *NF1* result from a mutation in the *NF1* gene, which is a tumor-suppressor gene that codes for the protein neurofibromin. Decreased production of this protein results in various clinical features. The *NF1* gene has been localized to the long arm of chromosome 17. The estimated incidence of *NF1* is 1 in 3,000. *NF1* and *NF2* are autosomal-dominant conditions, but approximately half of the cases are caused by a new, sporadic genetic mutation.

Schwannomatosis is often considered a third type of NF. It results in benign tumors associated with chronic pain. Most cases of schwannomatosis are sporadic and not inherited. Only about 20% of cases run in families.

The *NF2* gene is located on the long arm of chromosome 22. The *NF2* gene protein product, known as merlin, serves as a tumor suppressor; decreased production of this protein results in a predisposition to develop tumors of the central and peripheral nervous systems. The estimated incidence of *NF2* is 1 in 37,000 per year. Although the genetic change causing *NF2* is present at conception, as with *NF1*, the clinical manifestations occur over the course of many years. The typical age of onset of symptoms is in the late teens to early 20s. Many of the problems associated with NF do not appear until adolescence; therefore, the diagnosis is often delayed. The clinical criteria used to diagnose NF are as follows:

- Six or more café-au-lait spots (hyperpigmented macules)
- Axillary or inguinal freckles
- Two or more typical neurofibromas or one large neurofibroma
- Optic nerve tumor
- Two or more tumors in the iris (Lisch's nodules), often only identified by an ophthalmologist
- Long-bone abnormalities
- First-degree relative (e.g., mother, father, sister, brother) with the *NF1* mutation

The earliest clinical findings in childhood are café-au-lait spots. These are darkly pigmented, flat macules. Cutaneous neurofibromas, which are irregularly shaped, darkly pigmented, raised lesions, appear over time in older children, adolescents, and adults. Other signs include optic and acoustic nerve tumors, scoliosis, bowing of the legs, tumors of the meninges and spinal cord, and macrocephaly. NF is a great example of variable expressivity. Some people have only café-au-lait spots, whereas others have many large tumors even though they carry the same mutation. Tumors in NF are typically benign, but transformation to malignant peripheral nerve sheath tumors can occur. Diagnosis requires genetic testing, CT, MRI, neurological evaluation, and acoustic and ophthalmological examinations. Periodic neurological examination is needed throughout life. Surgical treatment of tumors with radiation or chemotherapy is common, but the goal is to relieve pain, as there is no cure. Genetic counseling is important to inform patients and families and to assist with family planning and reproductive decisions.

Ehlers-Danlos Syndrome

Ehlers-Danlos syndrome (EDS) is a group of disorders that characteristically involve diminished strength and integrity of the skin, joints, and other connective tissues. The patient's skin is highly elastic, and joints are hypermobile. EDS is caused by abnormalities in the synthesis of collagen and other connective tissue proteins. Collagen is the most abundant protein in the body. A minimum of 29 genes contribute to the collagen protein structure, and the genes are located on 15 of the 23 pairs of human chromosomes. The classic form of EDS occurs because of a mutation on the 9q34.2 and 9q34.3 loci, which is the location of the *COL3A1* and *COL3A2* genes.

The prevalence of EDS has been reported as 1 in 5,000 to 10,000 persons, but the exact figure is unknown. The clinical manifestations include skin hyperelasticity, hypermobility of joints, easy bruising, and poor wound healing. Affected persons may also have mitral valve prolapse (MVP), arterial aneurysms, dissections, and occlusions. Genetic testing, MRI, CT, and echocardiogram are used in diagnosis. Skin biopsy is inconclusive.

The patient should not place undue stress on joints, as they can dislocate. Periodic cardiovascular examination may be necessary for those with MVP, aneurysm, or aortic dissection. Treatment is symptomatic, as there is no cure. Patients are usually prescribed over-the-counter pain relievers and are monitored carefully for complications.

Cystic Fibrosis

CF is the most common lethal inherited disease in persons of European ancestry. The incidence of CF varies according to ethnicity. The incidence is 1 in 3,500 in European Americans, 1 per 9,500 in Hispanic Americans, 1 per 15,000 in African Americans, and 1 in 31,000 among Asian Americans.

CF is an autosomal-recessive disease caused by defects in the CF transmembrane conductance regulator (*CFTR*) gene, which encodes for a protein that functions as a chloride channel and regulates the flow of other ions across the surface of epithelial cells. The *CFTR* gene locus is 7q31.

CF involves multiple organ systems, but chiefly the respiratory system and pancreas. Pancreatic enzyme insufficiency with associated complications occurs. The water content of secretions is reduced, which causes thick mucus plugging of the pancreas's ductules. The clogged ducts prevent pancreatic enzymes from reaching the intestine. This often causes malabsorption and failure to thrive in infants. Pancreatitis, cholelithiasis, and cirrhosis of the liver occur in many patients. Pulmonary involvement occurs in 90% of patients. The respiratory epithelium produces excess amounts of thick mucus that blocks airways and causes a high susceptibility to pulmonary infection for the patient's lifetime. CF also affects the pancreas, causing reduced digestive enzymes leading to steatorrhea and vitamin malabsorption. Signs and symptoms include pulmonary wheezes, rhonchi, excess mucus in sputum, sinusitis, nasal polyps, diarrhea, malabsorption, abdominal pain caused by pancreatitis and cholecystitis, cirrhosis of the liver, and rectal prolapse.

A patient is usually diagnosed by age 1 year. Newborn screening for CF is universally required in the United States. Diagnostic testing involves screening for immunoreactive trypsinogen (IRT), a pancreatic protein typically elevated in infants with CF. If that test is positive, repeat IRT testing and DNA testing are done. A sweat test called the quantitative pilocarpine iontophoresis test (QPIT) is used to collect sweat and analyze its chloride content. However, the sweat test is not always reliable. Chest x-ray, abdominal x-ray, chest CT, and abdominal ultrasound are used in the diagnosis as well. Genetic testing (carrier testing) is recommended for individuals with a positive family history who are planning a pregnancy. Treatment for affected individuals includes pancreatic enzyme supplements, bronchodilators, mucolytics, nebulizer treatments, antibiotics, and anti-inflammatory medications. Patients may require nutritional supplements and insulin.

Ivacaftor (Kalydeco) was approved by the FDA in January 2012 to treat people with certain mutations (about 4% to 5% of patients with CF). Ivacaftor is a *CFTR* potentiator. Since 2012, additional CFTR potentiators have been created to treat CF. End-stage lung disease is the principal cause of death in many individuals, and lung transplant is sometimes considered. With treatment, an individual with CF born in the United States today is expected to survive longer than 40 years.

Lysosomal Storage Disease

Lysosomes are cellular organelles that contain digestive enzymes used to break down cellular debris. Lysosomal storage diseases are rare inherited disorders characterized by the failure of lysosomal function. In these diseases there is an accumulation of undigested or partially digested molecules, which ultimately cause cellular dysfunction. Organomegaly, connective tissue problems, ocular pathology, and central nervous system (CNS) dysfunction are known to occur in these disorders.

More than 50 lysosomal storage diseases have been identified. Some of the more common lysosomal storage diseases are Tay Sachs disease, Niemann-Pick disease, and Gaucher disease. Lysosomal storage diseases are classified according to the accumulated substances, which include the sphingolipidoses, oligosaccharidoses, mucolipidoses, mucopolysaccharidoses (MPSs), lipoprotein storage disorders, lysosomal transport defects, and others. Each lysosomal storage disease presents differently according to the undigested substance that accumulates within the cells and according to which major organ is affected.

Tay Sachs Disease

Tay Sachs disease is a lysosomal storage disease that results from a mutation on chromosome 15. The lysosomal enzyme, hexosaminidase A, is severely deficient. The disease is prevalent among Ashkenazi Jews in whom a carrier rate of 1 in 30 persons has been found. The enzyme that is deficient ordinarily breaks down ganglioside, which is abundant in many organs, including the heart, liver, spleen, and brain. Ganglioside accumulates in the cells, particularly the CNS. The accumulation of ganglioside causes progressive destruction of neurons and brain cells. The cerebellum, basal ganglia, brainstem, spinal cord, and autonomic nervous system are notably affected.

Infants born with Tay Sachs appear normal until approximately age 6 months. As the infant matures, motor incoordination, lethargy, muscle flaccidity, and increasing cognitive impairment become apparent. A sign that is diagnostic of Tay Sachs is a "cherry red spot" seen on the retina on ophthalmological examination. The nervous system becomes increasingly impaired throughout the first year of life. Death usually occurs by age 3 years. Prenatal diagnosis and carrier detection of Tay Sachs disease are possible. Genetic counseling is important to inform patients and families and to assist with family planning and reproductive decisions.

Niemann-Pick Disease

Niemann-Pick disease is a group of autosomal-recessive disorders that result from a defect at gene 11p15.4. This defect causes a deficiency of the lysosomal enzyme sphingomyelinase. Sphingomyelin is a lipid that is a normal component of cell membranes. However, due to the enzyme deficiency, sphingomyelin accumulates abnormally within the brain, spleen, liver, lymph nodes, bone marrow, GI tract, and lungs. There are four main types of the disease: type A, type B, type C1, and type C2. The classifications are based on variations in the symptoms and the genetic causes. Type A is a severe deficiency that causes widespread neurological involvement and visceral accumulation of sphingomyelin. Type B is similar except for the lack of CNS involvement. Individuals affected by type A usually die by age 3, whereas those with type B live into adulthood. Types C1 and C2 have similar symptoms and typically childhood onset, but they have different genetic causes.

As with Tay Sachs disease, Niemann-Pick disease occurs largely in Ashkenazi Jews. Clinical manifestations in type A are apparent by age 6 months. A protuberant abdomen, progressive GI problems, fever, enlarged spleen, and generalized lymphadenopathy are present. The infant exhibits progressive motor dysfunction. The diagnosis is made by biochemical assays for sphingomyelinase in a biopsy of the liver or bone marrow. Carriers can be detected by DNA testing. Genetic counseling is important to inform patients and families and to assist with family planning and reproductive decisions.

Gaucher Disease

Gaucher disease is an autosomal-recessive disorder caused by a mutation in the gene 1q21 that codes for the enzyme glucocerebrosidase. This disease is the most common lysosomal storage disease. As a result of the missing enzyme, the glycolipid glucocerebroside accumulates in macrophages and the CNS. Gaucher disease type 1 occurs most commonly in Ashkenazi Jews. Types 2 and 3 are not more common among Ashkenazi Jews than in the general population. In Ashkenazi Jews, the frequency of the genetic mutation is 1 in 15 persons and the disease frequency is as high as 1 in 450. In contrast, the incidence in the non-Jewish general population is 1 to 2 per 100,000. There are several types of disease, but type 1 Gaucher disease is present in 99% of affected individuals.

More than 150 gene mutations can cause Gaucher disease, and it is not possible to diagnose the disease based on one single genetic test. Type 1 disease affects the CNS, spleen, skeleton, and WBCs. Type 2 Gaucher disease affects neurons and is apparent in infants. Progressive CNS involvement occurs, with death coming at an early age.

In the cellular analysis of Gaucher disease, cells that have accumulated glucocerebroside are called Gaucher cells. They are found throughout the body in the spleen, liver, bone marrow, lymph nodes, tonsils, thymus, and Peyer's patches in the GI tract.

Type 1 Gaucher disease may not become apparent until adulthood. Symptoms are related to splenomegaly or bone marrow involvement. Thrombocytopenia and bone fractures can occur. Replacement enzyme therapy is possible, and so a fairly long life expectancy is seen. Bone marrow transplantation is also done.

Wilson Disease

Wilson disease is a rare, autosomal-recessive, inherited disorder of copper metabolism. The condition is characterized by excessive deposition of copper in the liver, brain, and other tissues. The major physiological problem is excessive absorption of copper from the small intestine and decreased excretion of copper by the liver. The genetic defect is at 13q14, which is the copper-transporting adenosine triphosphatase gene (*ATP7B*) in the liver. The predominant route of copper excretion (approximately 95%) in the body is in the bile synthesized by the liver. However, in Wilson disease excretion of excess copper into bile is impaired. Initially, the excess copper accumulates in the liver, leading to damage to hepatocytes. Eventually, as liver copper levels increase, it increases in the circulation and is deposited in other organs. Current research indicates that a normal variation in the *PRNP* gene may change the progression of the disease, resulting in later onset but more neurological problems.

The prevalence of Wilson disease is 1 per 30,000 individuals in the United States. It commonly presents as hepatic dysfunction in more than half of patients, with the most common initial presentation being cirrhosis. Another common presenting symptom is tremor, occurring in approximately half of individuals. Characteristic corneal Kayser-Fleischer rings are seen in the eyes of at least 98% of patients. Frequent early symptoms include difficulty speaking, excessive salivation, ataxia, mask-like facies, clumsiness with the hands, and personality changes. Late manifestations include dystonia, spasticity, grand mal seizures, rigidity, and flexion contractures. Psychiatric symptoms may be present. Skeletal involvement is a common feature of Wilson disease, with more than half of patients exhibiting osteopenia on radiological examination and an arthropathy that is similar to osteoarthritis. The arthropathy generally involves the spine and large appendicular joints, such as knees, wrists, and hips. Hemolytic anemia is a rare (10% to 15%) complication of the disease. Urolithiasis, hematuria, nephrocalcinosis, and proteinuria are common signs of kidney involvement.

Diagnosis is made by both biological and clinical findings. Serum ceruloplasmin levels and urine copper levels can be measured and liver biopsy done. CT and MRI scans can show lesions in the brain. The main treatment for Wilson disease is pharmacological therapy with chelating agents. Liver transplantation may be necessary.

G6PD Deficiency

Glucose-6-phosphate dehydrogenase (G6PD) deficiency is the most common enzyme disorder in humans. Inherited as a recessive X-linked disorder, G6PD deficiency affects 400 million people worldwide. Over 200 mutations have been found in the *G6PD* gene. Like sickle cell anemia, G6PD deficiency is common in areas where malaria is present. It has been suggested that the trait results in protection against malaria, but this is unconfirmed.

G6PD deficiency is an X-linked inherited disease that primarily affects men. The highest prevalence rates of 5% to 25% occur in Africa, the Middle East, Asia, and the Mediterranean. All mutations that cause G6PD deficiency are found at the gene locus Xq28.

The disorder is characterized by abnormally low levels of G6PD, a metabolic enzyme involved in the pentose phosphate pathway that produces nicotinamide adenine dinucleotide phosphate (NADPH), which is especially important in red blood cell (RBC) metabolism. NADPH protects the RBCs against oxidative stresses that can destroy them. People deficient in G6PD have RBCs that undergo hemolysis under stresses such as infection or exposure to certain medications or chemicals. Interestingly, individuals with G6PD deficiency can undergo hemolysis in response to ingestion of fava beans; because of this, some refer to this disorder as favism. Individuals can have a mild case of G6PD deficiency, in which they are asymptomatic, or a severe case of the disorder, in which they often exhibit hemolysis. Hemolysis most often is exhibited as jaundice: yellowing of the skin and sclera. Symptomatic patients can present at birth with neonatal jaundice and acute hemolytic anemia.

G6PD deficiency is typically identified during newborn screening, but symptoms may appear at any time. Diagnostic tests include testing blood levels of G6PD. Other tests include bilirubin level, complete blood count, measuring hemoglobin in the urine, haptoglobin level, lactate dehydrogenase (LDH) test, methemoglobin reduction test, and reticulocyte count.

Prevention of acute hemolytic anemia is the most important measure in G6PD deficiency. Patients should avoid drugs and foods that cause hemolysis. If hemolysis is severe, blood transfusions may be necessary. Transfused RBCs are not G6PD deficient and will live a normal life span in the recipient's circulation. Some patients require removal of the spleen because this is a site of RBC destruction. Folic acid should be given because the body is in a state of high RBC synthesis.

Klinefelter's Syndrome

Klinefelter's syndrome is one of the most common male chromosomal genetic disorders. Approximately 1 in 500 to 1,000 males is born with this disorder, and approximately 250,000 men in the United States are affected. Males with Klinefelter's syndrome commonly have a 47,XXY karyotype; however, an extra X or Y can be present in some variants of the disorder. The error occurs in the separation of chromosomes during meiosis. The X chromosome carries genes that code for testes function, brain development, and growth. The addition of more than one extra X or Y chromosome to a male karyotype results in variable physical and cognitive abnormalities. However, not all affected individuals are cognitively impaired.

The consequences of an extra sex chromosome are numerous. Lack of development of the testes, gynecomastia, and skeletal and cardiovascular abnormalities are common. Mental ability diminishes with extra chromosomes. All major areas of cognitive development, including expressive and receptive language, are affected by extra X chromosome material. Testosterone deficiency causes tall, lanky body proportions; sparse or absent facial, axillary, and pubic hair; decreased muscle mass and strength; feminine distribution of adipose tissue; decreased physical endurance; and osteoporosis. These patients are at a higher risk of autoimmune diseases, DM, MVP, osteopenia and osteoporosis, breast and testicular tumors, SLE, and RA.

Klinefelter's syndrome can be diagnosed prenatally by amniocentesis; however, it may not be suspected until adolescence or much later. Many men with Klinefelter's syndrome are not diagnosed until they seek treatment for infertility.

Genetic testing and hormone analysis can be done to confirm the diagnosis. Echocardiogram and bone density testing should be done with diagnosis because of the high prevalence of MVP and osteoporosis.

Testosterone replacement should begin at puberty, around age 12 years, and the dose should increase until it is sufficient to raise all sex hormones to normal levels. Psychoeducational evaluation and support are necessary. Physical therapy may be needed to build and tone muscles. Infertility treatment is possible because not all patients are completely sterile. Microsurgical sperm extraction for in-vitro fertilization is possible in some cases.

 CLINICAL CONCEPT

In Klinefelter's syndrome, XXY males commonly have weaker muscles and reduced strength. As they grow older, they tend to become taller than average and lack changes associated with puberty.

Turner's Syndrome

Turner's syndrome, discussed earlier, results from a complete or partially missing X chromosome in the female, so that karyotype is 45,X or 45,XO. It affects 1 in 2,000 births. As many as 15% of spontaneous abortions, also referred to as miscarriages, have a 45,X karyotype. There are many variations of the abnormal karyotype that makes this disease more severe in some than in others. Some affected individuals have a mosaic chromosome pattern. At birth, the infant commonly has lymphedema of the feet and neck. The lymphedema subsides, leaving an elastic skin of the neck, later referred to as webbed neck. More than 95% of adult women with Turner's syndrome exhibit short stature and infertility. Lack of breast development and amenorrhea at puberty occur in many of those affected, though pubic hair distribution is often normal. An abundance of pigmented nevi, a broad shield-shaped chest, and small hips are common.

Cardiovascular problems include hypertension, coarctation of the aorta, aortic valve abnormalities, and an underdeveloped left side of the heart. Scoliosis may be present, and the arms may have a deformity called cubitus valgus, which is a skeletal abnormality of the arm's carrying angle. Hypothyroidism is common, as are visual problems such as strabismus, cataract, and amblyopia. The patient presents with ovarian failure at puberty, and the oocytes are often degenerated.

Patients with suspected Turner's syndrome require genetic testing and hormone level evaluation. Echocardiogram, bone density, and bone age testing are necessary. Treatment involves estrogen therapy and growth hormone administration. The patient should be treated symptomatically for all other effects of the disease.

Fragile X Syndrome

Fragile X syndrome, also termed Martin-Bell syndrome, is the most common cause of inherited cognitive impairment and is the second most common cause of genetically associated mental disabilities after trisomy 21. It is a disorder of the X chromosome at Xq27.3, characterized by long repeating sequences of the three nucleotides cytosine (C), guanine (G), and guanine (G). The Xq27.3 gene is also called the familial mental retardation 1 gene (FMR1). The altered gene turns off production of the fragile X mental retardation protein, and this results in the symptoms. The incidence is 1 in 4,000 for males and 1 in 8,000 for females. Problems include mild-to-moderate autistic-like behavior (most notably, hand flapping and avoidance of eye contact), shyness, sensory integration difficulties, attention deficits, hyperactivity, impulsivity, depressed affect, anxiety, mathematical learning disabilities, aggressive tendencies, deficiency in abstract thinking, developmental delays particularly in language, and decreasing IQ with increasing age.

In addition to the cognitive, behavioral, and neuropsychological findings, the organ systems most frequently involved include the craniofacial, genital, and musculoskeletal systems. Males have a long face with large mandible, large everted ears, and large testicles. Hypermobile joints, high arched palate, scoliosis, and MVP are also common.

The standard diagnostic test involves molecular genetic techniques. The exact number of CGG triplet repeats can be determined by Southern blot and PCR. Treatment is symptomatic according to the patient's various health problems. Genetic counseling is important to inform patients and families and to assist with family planning and reproductive decisions.

Down Syndrome

Down syndrome, discussed earlier, is the most common chromosomal disorder in humans and the most common cause of intellectual disability. It is characterized by cognitive impairment, dysmorphic facial features, congenital heart defects, and other distinctive traits. Down syndrome is primarily caused by trisomy of chromosome 21: three chromosomes of chromosome number 21. Trisomy 21 causes multiple systemic complications, but not all defects occur in each patient, as there is a wide variation in the severity of the disorder.

The frequency is about 1 case in 800 live births. Each year, approximately 6,000 children are born with Down syndrome. It can be diagnosed prenatally with amniocentesis, PUBS, CVS, and extraction of fetal cells from the maternal circulation. It is often diagnosed shortly after birth by recognition of the characteristic features, though they are most obvious in children older than age 1 year.

The disorder's occurrence is strongly dependent on maternal age. It varies from an incidence of 1 in 1,500 births in a mother aged 15 to 29 years to an incidence of 1 in 50 births to mothers older than 45 years. As a woman's eggs age, their ability to correctly undergo meiosis can be impaired.

The clinical features of Down syndrome include flat facial profile, oblique palpebral fissures, and epicanthic folds around the eyes. Approximately 80% of children have an IQ of 25 to 50. The remaining 20% have average or near-average intelligence. Approximately 40% of children with Down syndrome have congenital heart disease and esophageal and intestinal malformations. Children have a 10- to 20-fold increased risk of developing leukemia. The immune system is weak, which makes children with Down syndrome susceptible to infection.

Currently, technological advances in medicine have lengthened the lives of adults with Down syndrome to an average of 47 years. Many affected adults can become employed and lead normal lives with assistance. Almost all long-living adults with Down syndrome eventually develop a dementia that is similar to Alzheimer's disease.

Prader-Willi Syndrome

Prader-Willi syndrome (PWS) occurs with a frequency of 1 in 10,000 to 30,000 people. The mutation usually occurs on the paternal chromosome of pair number 15. Recall that there are two copies of each gene, one inherited from the mother and one from the father. In the majority of cases of PWS, a gene on chromosome 15 (commonly gene locus 15q.11–q.13) inherited from the father is missing or defective. In some cases, the whole chromosome 15 from the father is missing. The gene inherited from the mother is normal, but both genes are required for healthy functioning. In PWS, only one gene is normal, causing a lack of protein synthesis in the hypothalamus.

The defect results in abnormal function of the hypothalamus. Consequently, multiple body systems are involved. Commonly associated characteristics include severe obesity, hypotonia, low IQ, short stature, hypogonadotropic hypogonadism, strabismus, small hands and feet, ataxic gait, behavioral problems, and seizures. Persons with PWS overeat and do not have the normal sensation of satiety. The person endures constant hunger because of dysfunction of the hypothalamus. Individuals need monitoring for development of morbid obesity, diabetes, and thyroid problems.

Complications from hypogonadism, such as osteoporosis and fracture, behavioral issues such as psychoses, T2DM, and heart failure may shorten life expectancy. PWS causes many lifelong multisystem problems, although patients frequently reach adulthood and are able to function in a group home setting.

Angelman's Syndrome

Angelman's syndrome is caused by a similar defect in the same gene that causes PWS. However, the defective gene is on the mother's chromosome 15 in the same location of q.11–q.13. For a child to be born with Angelman's syndrome, the defective gene is inherited from the mother and the gene inherited from the father is normal. Angelman's syndrome is rare, with a frequency of 1 in 12,000 to 20,000 people. Children with Angelman's syndrome have primarily neurological problems. They tend to have intellectual disability, seizures, and movement disorders such as ataxia. They tend to be excitable but are usually smiling and laughing, sometimes with hand-flapping movements.

Huntington's Disease

Huntington's disease (HD) is an adult-onset, autosomal-dominant inherited disorder associated with degeneration of specific neurons in the basal ganglia and cortex. The frequency of HD is between 3 and 7 per 100,000 people of European ancestry. The disorder appears to be less common in other populations, including people of Japanese, Chinese, and African descent. The average age of onset of HD ranges from 35 to 44 years, whereas the average age of death of an individual with HD ranges from 51 to 57 years. Most patients survive between 10 and 25 years after the onset of illness.

HD is caused by a trinucleotide repeat in the gene that codes for huntingtin protein (*HTT*). When the CAG codon is repeated again and again, it causes a problem in the ability of the gene to code for the protein. The repeats tend to increase with each generation. People who have 27 to 35 repeats of CAG do not show any signs of HD, but they can pass the disease on to their children. When the repeats get up to 36 or more, the child will develop HD at some point in their life.

There are two forms of HD. The most common is adult onset; persons with this form usually develop symptoms in their mid-30s and 40s. This disease is considered to have age-related penetrance. A rare early-onset form of HD begins in childhood or adolescence.

The clinical presentation of HD includes a movement disorder, a cognitive disorder, and a behavioral disorder. Patients may present with one or all disorders in varying degrees. Chorea is the most common movement disorder seen in HD. Initially, mild chorea causes dance-like movements or tics. Severe chorea occurs later and can cause uncontrollable flailing of the extremities, termed ballism. As the disease progresses, chorea is replaced by parkinsonian features, such as slowed movements, muscle rigidity, and postural instability. In advanced disease, patients develop an akinetic-rigid syndrome, without movement at all. Other late features are spasticity, dysarthria (the inability to speak), and dysphagia, which is difficulty swallowing. Slowed cognition to dementia occurs gradually. Severe depression, mental decline, and suicidal ideation are common.

No specific imaging study can be used to diagnose HD. Patients who have the condition and predominant features of bradykinesia and rigidity may benefit from Parkinson-type treatment of levodopa or dopamine agonists. Antidepressants, antipsychotic medications, and anticonvulsants may be necessary. Genetic testing can show the defect of HD, and family members need genetic counseling. More research is needed for treatments of this disease. At this point, there is no cure.

Chapter Summary

- A genome refers to the collection of all of an organism's genes.
- A nucleotide is a combination of a pentose sugar molecule, phosphate, and purine or pyrimidine nitrogen base. The nitrogen bases in DNA are adenine (A), thymine (T), guanine (G), and cytosine (C), or ATGC. In RNA, uracil replaces thymine as the nitrogen base, so the bases in RNA are adenine, uracil, guanine, and cytosine, or AUGC.
- Transcription is the synthesis of mRNA from DNA in the nucleus, and translation is the synthesis of proteins from mRNA at the ribosomes.
- SNPs are changes in one nucleotide of a gene sequence that occur with some frequency within a population.
- SNPs can also be called genetic variations. For example, if the majority of persons in the population have the DNA nitrogen base sequence ACTG that codes for a specific protein, an example of an SNP would be ATTG, which would code for a different protein.
- A gene locus is the gene's position on a specific chromosome.
- The two chromosomes in a pair are joined at their central point, called the centromere, creating two arms. The upper arm of a chromosome is the "p" arm, and the lower arm is called the "q" arm.
- A karyotype is an overall picture of all an individual's chromosome pairs. The dye stains regions of chromosomes that are rich in the base pairs adenine (A) and thymine (T), producing a dark band.
- A genotype is the technical allelic makeup of a trait. A phenotype is the physical expression of the genotype.
- An individual can possess allelic traits that are homozygous or heterozygous.

- A Punnett Square can be used to predict single-gene inheritance patterns.
- A carrier is a person who is heterozygous for a recessive trait but does not manifest it; the dominant allele silences it.
- If a gene is located on the X chromosome, the inheritance pattern is considered to be sex linked, or X-linked.
- Genetic mutations are hereditary or acquired (also called sporadic).
- Activated oncogenes and defective tumor-suppressor genes are involved in carcinogenesis.
- Mitochondria have their own DNA, which is maternally inherited. The ovum's mitochondria drive the developing embryo, and the sperm's mitochondria are deactivated.
- The severity of a genetic disorder may vary from one individual to another based on penetrance and expressivity.
- In an individual with a mosaic genetic pattern, some cells contain the gene or chromosome variation and some do not.
- Aneuploidy refers to a disorder related to chromosome number. Sections of chromosomes can be translocated from one chromosome to another or lost.
- Epigenetics is the study of how cellular environments can cause changes in the expression of genes. Unlike genetic changes, epigenetic changes are reversible and do not change the DNA sequence, but they can change how the body reads a DNA sequence.
- PCR and FISH are molecular techniques for identifying genes.
- CVS and amniocentesis are common procedures used for prenatal diagnosis.

- CRISPR-Cas9, which is short for clustered regularly interspaced short palindromic repeats and CRISPR-associated protein 9, is a technology that allows for genome editing. Genetic material is added, removed, or altered at particular locations in the genome.

- Gene therapy is an experimental technique that uses genes to treat or prevent disease.
- There are many genetic and chromosomal disorders. They range in severity from asymptomatic to being incompatible with life.

Making the Connections

Signs and Symptoms	Physical Assessment Findings	Diagnostic Testing	Treatment
Familial Hypercholesterolemia | Most commonly caused by a defect in the LDL receptor gene that codes for the LDL receptor in the liver; liver processing of cholesterol cannot occur; liver produces excessive cholesterol.			
Premature arteriosclerosis. Premature coronary artery disease. Premature myocardial infarction.	Cholesterol deposits under the skin called xanthoma and xanthelasma.	Extremely high serum cholesterol and LDL. Genetic testing.	Anti-lipidemia medications.
Familial Adenomatous Polyposis | Mutation at gene locus 5p21, the *APC* gene, which causes numerous intestinal polyps and susceptibility to colon cancer.			
Melena, diarrhea, hematochezia, abdominal pain, and malabsorption.	None.	Colonoscopy reveals hundreds of polyps. Biopsies needed to rule out colon cancer. Genetic testing.	Removal of the colon may be necessary.
Marfan's Syndrome | Mutation in the fibrillin-1 gene on chromosome 15, which contains the code for the glycoprotein fibrillin. Fibrillin is normally found in heart valves, airways, and other tissue. Fibrillin is deficient in Marfan's syndrome.			
Sudden dyspnea with pneumothorax. Sudden chest pain with aortic dissection. Lower back pain in tailbone with spinal dura involvement.	Tall, lanky appearance. Elongated arms and fingers. Heart murmur, pectus excavatum, ligament hypermobility, and kyphoscoliosis.	Genetic testing. Echocardiogram, chest X-ray, aortic angiogram, and others that diagnose various conditions associated with genetic defects.	Treatment is for symptoms and multiple conditions that result from the genetic defect.
Neurofibromatosis | Mutation in the *NF1* or *NF2* gene. The *NF* gene is a tumor-suppressor gene that codes for the protein neurofibromin; decreased production of this protein results in tumors of various organs.			
Vision and hearing defects. Back pain caused by scoliosis and spinal cord tumors.	Characteristic café-au-lait spots. Scoliosis; bowing of the legs; tumors of the meninges, spinal cord, and skin. Macrocephaly.	Genetic testing. CT, MRI, neurological evaluation, acoustic and ophthalmological examinations because of various tumors.	Treatment is for symptoms and multiple conditions that result from the genetic defect.
Ehlers-Danlos Syndrome | Mutation of the *COL3A1* and *COL3A2* genes that code for collagen. Results in collagen deficiency.			
Easy bruising and poor wound healing.	Skin hyperelasticity. Joint hypermobility. Heart murmur of MVP.	Genetic testing, MRI, CT, angiograms, and echocardiograms are used in diagnosis.	Treatment is for symptoms and multiple conditions that result from the genetic defect.

Continued

Making the Connections—cont'd

Signs and Symptoms	Physical Assessment Findings	Diagnostic Testing	Treatment
Cystic Fibrosis | Defects in the *CFTR* gene, which encodes for a protein that functions as a chloride channel and regulates the flow of other ions across the surface of epithelial cells. The *CFTR* gene locus is 7q31. Chiefly affected organs are the respiratory system and pancreas. Excessive mucus and thickened secretions form plugs.			
Chronic cough, upper respiratory infections, and GI disturbances caused by pancreatitis, cirrhosis of liver, and gallstones.	Pulmonary wheezes, rhonchi, and excess mucus in sputum. Sinusitis, nasal polyps, abdominal pain caused by pancreatitis and cholecystitis, and cirrhosis of the liver. Rectal prolapse.	Genetic testing. IRT, a pancreatic protein typically elevated in infants with CF. A sweat test called QPIT is used to collect sweat and analyze its chloride content. Chest X-ray, abdominal X-ray, chest CT, and abdominal ultrasound.	Pancreatic enzyme supplements, bronchodilators, mucolytics, nebulizer treatments, antibiotics, and anti-inflammatory medications.
Tay Sachs Disease | Mutation on chromosome 15. The lysosomal enzyme, hexosaminidase A, is severely deficient, which allows ganglioside to accumulate in tissues, particularly the brain and spinal cord.			
Lethargy and cognitive impairment.	Muscle flaccidity, poor suck reflex in infant. Lack of completing developmental milestones.	Genetic testing. A characteristic "cherry red spot" is seen on the retina on ophthalmological examination.	Treatment is for symptoms and multiple conditions that result from the genetic defect.
Niemann-Pick Disease | Defect at gene at 11p15.4 that causes deficiency of the lysosomal enzyme sphingomyelinase. Cells of various organs such as the brain, spleen, lymph nodes, lungs, and liver accumulate sphingomyelin.			
Gastrointestinal problems, enlarged abdomen, generalized lymphadenopathy, and motor dysfunction.	Splenomegaly, protuberant abdomen, fever, and generalized lymphadenopathy are present. The infant exhibits progressive motor dysfunction.	The diagnosis is made by biochemical assays for sphingomyelinase in a biopsy of the liver or bone marrow. Carriers can be detected by DNA testing.	Treatment is for symptoms and multiple conditions that result from the genetic defect.
Gaucher's Disease | An autosomal-recessive disorder caused by a mutation in the gene 1q21 that codes for the enzyme glucocerebrosidase. Accumulation of glucocerebroside protein in the CNS, spleen, skeleton, and WBCs.			
Enlarged spleen and liver. Bone lesions that may be painful. Weakness, numbness, and paresthesias. Easy bruising. Susceptibility to infection.	Splenomegaly and hepatomegaly. Weakness of extremities. Lymphadenopathy, arthropathy, and distended abdomen. Brownish tint to the skin. Yellow fatty deposits on the sclera. Distended abdomen. Swelling of lymph nodes and adjacent joints.	Cellular analysis of Gaucher's disease: cells that have accumulated glucocerebroside are called Gaucher's cells. They are found throughout the body in the spleen, liver, bone marrow, lymph nodes, tonsils, thymus, and Peyer's patches in the GI tract.	Replacement enzyme therapy is possible, and so a fairly long life expectancy is seen. Bone marrow transplantation is also done.
Wilson's Disease | Autosomal-recessive inherited disorder of copper metabolism. Genetic defect is at 13q14, which is the copper-transporting adenosine triphosphatase gene (*ATP7B*) in the liver, causing excessive deposition of copper in the liver, brain, and other tissues.			
Jaundice caused by liver dysfunction. Grand mal seizures.	Jaundice. Difficulty speaking.	Kayser-Fleischer rings in the eye. Liver enzymes may be elevated. Osteopenia on	Chelating agents that bind copper. Liver transplantation.

Making the Connections—cont'd

Signs and Symptoms	Physical Assessment Findings	Diagnostic Testing	Treatment
Psychiatric symptoms. Joint pain and abdominal pain caused by kidney stones.	Excessive salivation. Ataxia, mask-like facies, clumsiness, muscle spasticity, rigidity, and flexion contractures. Joint pain of spine and large appendicular joints, such as knees, wrists, and hips.	radiological examination. Urolithiasis, hematuria, nephrocalcinosis, and proteinuria are common signs of kidney involvement. Serum ceruloplasmin levels and urine copper levels elevated, and liver biopsy shows copper. CT and MRI scans can show lesions in the brain.	

G6PD Deficiency | All mutations that cause G6PD deficiency are found at the gene locus Xq28. A metabolic enzyme involved in RBC metabolism. Some of the RBCs undergo hemolysis when the body is under stress.

Jaundice with stresses to the body.	Hemolysis that presents as jaundice.	Blood levels of G6PD, bilirubin level, complete blood count, measuring hemoglobin in the urine, haptoglobin level, LDH test, methemoglobin reduction test, and reticulocyte count.	Periods of hemolysis and jaundice do not require treatment and resolve on their own. Avoid drugs and foods that cause hemolysis. Blood transfusions may be necessary for severe hemolysis. Possibly removal of the spleen. Folic acid should be given because the body is in a state of high RBC synthesis.

Klinefelter's Syndrome | Males commonly have a 47,XXY karyotype; however, an extra X or Y can be present in some variants of the disease.

Decreased physical endurance. Osteoporosis. High risk of autoimmune disease. DM, MVP, osteopenia and osteoporosis, breast and testicular tumors, SLE, and RA.	Tall, lanky body proportions. Sparse or absent facial, axillary, and pubic hair. Decreased muscle mass and strength. Feminine distribution of adipose tissue.	Genetic testing and hormone analysis can be done to confirm the diagnosis. Echocardiogram and bone density testing should be done with diagnosis caused by high prevalence of MVP and osteoporosis.	Testosterone therapy and other treatment for symptoms and multiple conditions that result from the genetic defect.

Turner's Syndrome | A combination of disorders that results from a complete or partially missing X chromosome in the female so that the karyotype is 45,X or 45,XO.

Amenorrhea. Infertility. Hypothyroidism. Hypertension, coarctation of the aorta, and aortic valve abnormalities. Vision problems. Lack of energy and fatigue caused by hypothyroidism.	Short stature. Webbed neck. Possible cyanosis or dyspnea related to heart problems. Lack of breast development. Abundance of pigmented nevi. Broad shield-shaped chest. Obesity. Small hips. Scoliosis. Cubitus valgus. Strabismus. Cataract. Amblyopia. Lymphedema at birth.	Genetic testing and hormone level evaluation. Echocardiogram, bone density, and bone age testing.	Estrogen therapy and growth hormone administration. Surgery may be necessary for cardiac defects. Patient should be treated symptomatically for all other effects of the disease.

Continued

Making the Connections–cont'd

Signs and Symptoms	Physical Assessment Findings	Diagnostic Testing	Treatment
Down Syndrome | Chromosomal abnormality that usually involves three copies of chromosome 21; this abnormality causes multiple organ system problems.			
Delay in developmental milestones. Congenital heart defects are common: dyspnea, cyanosis, and syncope (fainting) can result. Esophageal and intestinal complications are also common, which can cause problems with swallowing and malabsorption.	Infant has facial features that are distinctive for Down syndrome. Flat facial profile. Oblique palpebral fissures and epicanthic folds around the eyes. Heart murmur. Cyanosis. Dyspnea. Approximately 80% of children have IQ of 25 to 50. The remaining 20% have normal or near-normal intelligence.	Genetic testing. Echocardiogram, electrocardiogram, and chest and abdominal X-rays to test for common problems with the heart, lungs, and intestine.	Treatment is for symptoms and multiple conditions that result from the genetic defect.
Fragile X Syndrome | Disorder of the X chromosome at Xq27.3, characterized by long repeating sequences of the three nucleotides: cytosine (C), guanine (G), and guanine (G).			
Mild-to-moderate autistic-like behavior (most notably, hand flapping and avoidance of eye contact). Shyness. Attention deficits. Hyperactivity. Impulsivity. Anxiety. Cognitive difficulties. MVP.	Males have a long face with large mandible, large everted ears, and large testicles. Hypermobile joints. High arched palate. Scoliosis.	Genetic testing. The exact number of CGG triplet repeats can be determined by Southern blot and PCR.	Treatment is for symptoms and multiple conditions that result from the genetic defect.
Prader-Willi Syndrome | Loss of function of certain genes in the proximal arm of chromosome 15. The mutation usually occurs on the paternal chromosome of pair number 15.			
Seizures. Behavioral problems such as stubbornness and temper outbursts. Sleep abnormalities.	Excessive hunger and obesity. Hypotonia. Mild to moderate intellectual disability. Short stature. Hypogonadotropic hypogonadism. Strabismus. Small hands and feet. Ataxic gait.	Genetic testing. A number of diagnostic tests, depending on disease manifestations.	Treatment is for symptoms and multiple conditions that result from the genetic defect.
Angelman's Syndrome | Loss of function of specific genes on the proximal arm of chromosome 15. The mutation usually occurs on the maternal chromosome of pair number 15.			
Delayed development. Seizures. Ataxia.	Small head size (microcephaly). Poor speech. Intellectual disability. Movement and balance problems. Happy demeanor. Hand flapping movements. Hyperactivity.	Genetic testing. A number of diagnostic tests, depending on disease manifestations.	Treatment is for symptoms and multiple conditions that result from the genetic defect.

Making the Connections—cont'd

Signs and Symptoms	Physical Assessment Findings	Diagnostic Testing	Treatment
Huntington's Disease | Genetic defect at 4p16.3, called the huntingtin gene. The gene defect causes a part of DNA called a CAG repeat sequence to repeat many more times than it should and form the huntingtin protein. Autosomal-dominant inherited disorder associated with degeneration of specific neurons in the basal ganglia and cortex.			
Lack of control of movements called chorea. Cognitive decline. Depression and psychosis possible. Dementia late in course of disease.	Muscle spasticity. Difficulty with speech and swallowing. Subtle, tic-like movements may progress to flailing-type movements. Lack of movement, blank facies, tremor, and rigidity. Eventually akinesia or lack of any movement occurs.	No imaging studies can show deterioration well. Genetic testing, inheritance pattern, and clinical picture make diagnosis.	May benefit from Parkinson-type treatment of levodopa or dopamine agonists. Antidepressants, antipsychotic medications, and anticonvulsants may be necessary. Genetic testing can show the defect of HD, and family members need counseling.

Bibliography

Available online at fadavis.com

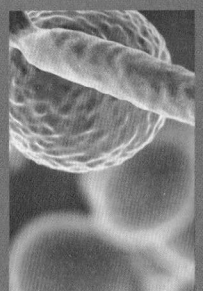

Stress, Exercise, and Immobility

Learning Objectives

Upon completion of this chapter, the student will be able to:

- Understand how chronic stress can lead to physical and psychological dysfunction according to the theories of Selye, Cannon, and McEwen.

- Recognize risk factors that can lead to stress-related illnesses and understand recommended techniques to manage and reduce stress.

- Identify the benefits of exercise and specific disorders that are counteracted by regular physical activity.

- List the various systemic complications of sedentary behavior and immobility.

- Discuss the clinical interventions needed to prevent complications of immobility.

Key Terms

Adaptive ability
Allostasis
Allostatic load
Allostatic overload
Contractures
Distress
Eustress

Fight-or-flight reaction
General adaptation syndrome
Homeostasis
Immunosuppression
Natriuresis
Negative nitrogen balance
Orthostatic hypotension

Pathological fracture
Pressure injury
Polysomnography
REM sleep
Trabecular bones

Stress can be a physical or psychological experience that disturbs comfort, threatens safety, or imperils life. It can develop because of physical injury, such as fracture of a bone, or because of feelings related to work, school, social, or family issues.

A certain amount of psychological stress is advantageous in that it can motivate an individual. **Eustress** describes stress that stimulates a person positively, such as a job promotion that provokes positive feelings and reactions. However, **distress** describes stress that evokes negative feelings and adverse reactions. For many in society, psychological stress can rise to overwhelming levels, which can lead to disruption of normal functioning and major health problems.

Any type of stress triggers a primal physical response from the body. This response can be useful in that it excites the nervous, endocrine, and musculoskeletal systems and allows one to quickly react to an emergent situation. During acute stress, the body automatically initiates a set of involuntary responses; the heart rate speeds up and myocardial contractile function strengthens. The bronchioles dilate, allowing more air to enter the lungs. Chemical mediators provoke stress hormones that are released into the bloodstream, priming the body to be alert. Concentration becomes more focused, reaction time is faster, and strength and agility increase. When the stressful situation ends, hormonal signals switch off the stress response and the body returns to normal. Primitive man depended on this stress response for survival. In prehistoric times, stress was an intermittent experience, and its intensity varied according to environmental factors. The stress response was evoked infrequently and ended after the threat was avoided.

However, in our modern society, stress is often a frequent, constant, or long-term experience. Electronic forms of communication have created a sense of urgency in personal interactions, employer–employee relationships are less permanent than in the past, relocation for employment is expected, social support is often lacking for individuals, many persons lack time for leisure activities, citizens are asked to be vigilant about threats of terrorism on a daily basis, and acts of violence have become commonplace in U.S. society. Stress has become part of our daily culture, and coping with stressors has become necessary in today's society.

This constant stress puts great strain on the body. Frequent or long-term stressors cause stress hormones to continually pulse through the system at high levels, causing them to never leave the blood and tissues. Research shows that such long-term activation of the stress response can have a hazardous effect on the body, diminishing immunity and increasing the risk of autoimmune disease, cancer, heart disease, depression, and a variety of other illnesses. Chronic stress in childhood has also been linked to the secretion of excess free radicals that cause oxidative cellular changes. Mitochondrial dysfunction and telomere shortening, which are markers of biological aging, are found in young children exposed to early childhood stressful events. It is further speculated that these cellular changes due to early childhood stress and trauma may be transmitted to future generations.

The Effects of Stress

There is a human mind–body connection that significantly affects the individual's total well-being. Emotions and psychological conditions can cause biological responses that can lead to physical illness. This is seen when an anxious individual develops physical symptoms of chest pain, hyperventilation, tachycardia, and diaphoresis; this individual feels physically ill despite the emotional etiology of the condition.

Conversely, physiological disorders can influence a person's state of mind and cause emotional consequences: an individual enduring the chest pain of myocardial infarction commonly experiences anxiety, a psychological reaction to the physical disturbance.

The mind–body connection has provoked many investigations into stress and stress-related illnesses. The body's reaction to an acute stress has been well researched; less is known about the cumulative effects of prolonged stress. At present, theories devised by physiologists Hans Selye, Walter Cannon, and Bruce McEwen are well-accepted explanations of the effects of stress on the body.

Selye's Stress Response Theory

Hans Selye, a scientist who studied physiological reactions to stress in the 1930s and 1940s, first described the body's reaction to acute stress. According to Selye, a stressor is a challenging demand on the body that arouses a response from multiple organ systems. Stressors can be positive or negative experiences for the individual and have the potential to cause adverse health effects. Fear, bereavement, promotion, new role assumption,

home relocation, trauma of any type, infection, surgery, debilitating illness, and exposure to intense heat or cold are examples of stressful experiences.

In addition to the stressor, the individual's adaptive ability is an important element in the body's stress reaction. **Adaptive ability** is the way in which the individual manages the stress and reduces the stressor's effect on their life. Effective adaptive ability allows an individual to maintain homeostasis. **Homeostasis** is a condition of equilibrium when various physiological parameters such as blood pressure, respirations, heart rate, oxygen tension, blood pH, blood glucose, body temperature, and white blood cell (WBC) count are within narrow normal ranges.

An individual's adaptive ability depends on coping mechanisms and conditioning factors. Coping mechanisms are the emotional and behavioral responses used to manage threats to physiological and psychological homeostasis. How a person copes with stressful events depends on how they perceive and interpret the event. For example, an individual can perceive an employment promotion as a positive new challenge or a negative added burden. The mind's interpretation of the stressful event influences the stressor's physiological effects.

An individual's reaction to a stressor is also influenced by conditioning factors, such as age, gender, genetic predisposition, preexisting health conditions, life experiences, developmental level, educational level, and social support. For example, how an individual copes with a diagnosis of cancer is greatly influenced by their past experiences with the disease. An individual may fear the diagnosis if they observed the suffering of another with the same diagnosis. Alternatively, the individual may not fear the diagnosis if they are encouraged by others who conquered and survived the disease.

 CLINICAL CONCEPT

A major surgical procedure is a physical and psychological stressor for a patient. Health-care providers can enhance the patient's adaptive ability and coping mechanisms by encouraging a supportive family member or friend to stay with the patient in the preoperative setting and during recovery.

Neuroendocrine and Immune Responses

The physiological reaction to stress can have protective, restorative effects or damaging, injurious consequences on the body. In the short term, there is a protective activation of the neurological, endocrine, and immune systems, the major organ systems affected by stress, as the body increases its defenses to cope with the acute threat. However, prolonged exposure to stress and long-term activation of the neuroendocrine and immune systems eventually has a negative effect on the body.

According to Selye, regardless of the source, stress is a threat to homeostasis that provokes a coordinated, adaptive reaction called the **general adaptation syndrome.** Selye developed this theory as an attempt to scientifically analyze the body's reaction to stress. In 1936, his research involved exposing animals to unpleasant or harmful stimuli such as physical trauma and extreme cold and examining the physiological responses. He found that all animals showed a similar set of reactions that involved three stages:

1. Alarm
2. Resistance
3. Exhaustion

Alarm Stage. The alarm stage is a state of arousal characterized by the central nervous system, sympathetic nervous system (SNS), and adrenal gland stimulation. The SNS, also known as the adrenergic nervous system, releases the catecholamine norepinephrine, which increases alertness and stimulates cardiorespiratory and vascular responses. Norepinephrine also causes vasoconstriction of the arterial blood vessels that bring blood to the heart muscle, lungs, and skeletal muscles. Heart and respiratory rate increase as peripheral circulation decreases in the extremities. Decreased circulation of the hands and feet creates cold, clammy extremities. Sweat gland activity increases to disperse excess heat generated by a surge in energy. The pupils dilate, which increases visual acuity, and the bronchioles dilate to enhance respiratory capacity. Blood flow to the gastrointestinal (GI) and genitourinary systems diminishes, which slows activity in these areas.

Discharge of the SNS provides the temporary ability to endure a stressor. This neurological discharge also occurs in the **fight-or-flight reaction,** first described by Walter B. Cannon in the 1920s. The fight-or-flight reaction is a basic survival response to an acute, severe stressor that incites involuntary neuroendocrine physiological changes. The effects of the alarm stage in Selye's theory of stress are the same as those described in Cannon's fight-or-flight reaction theory (see Fig. 4-1).

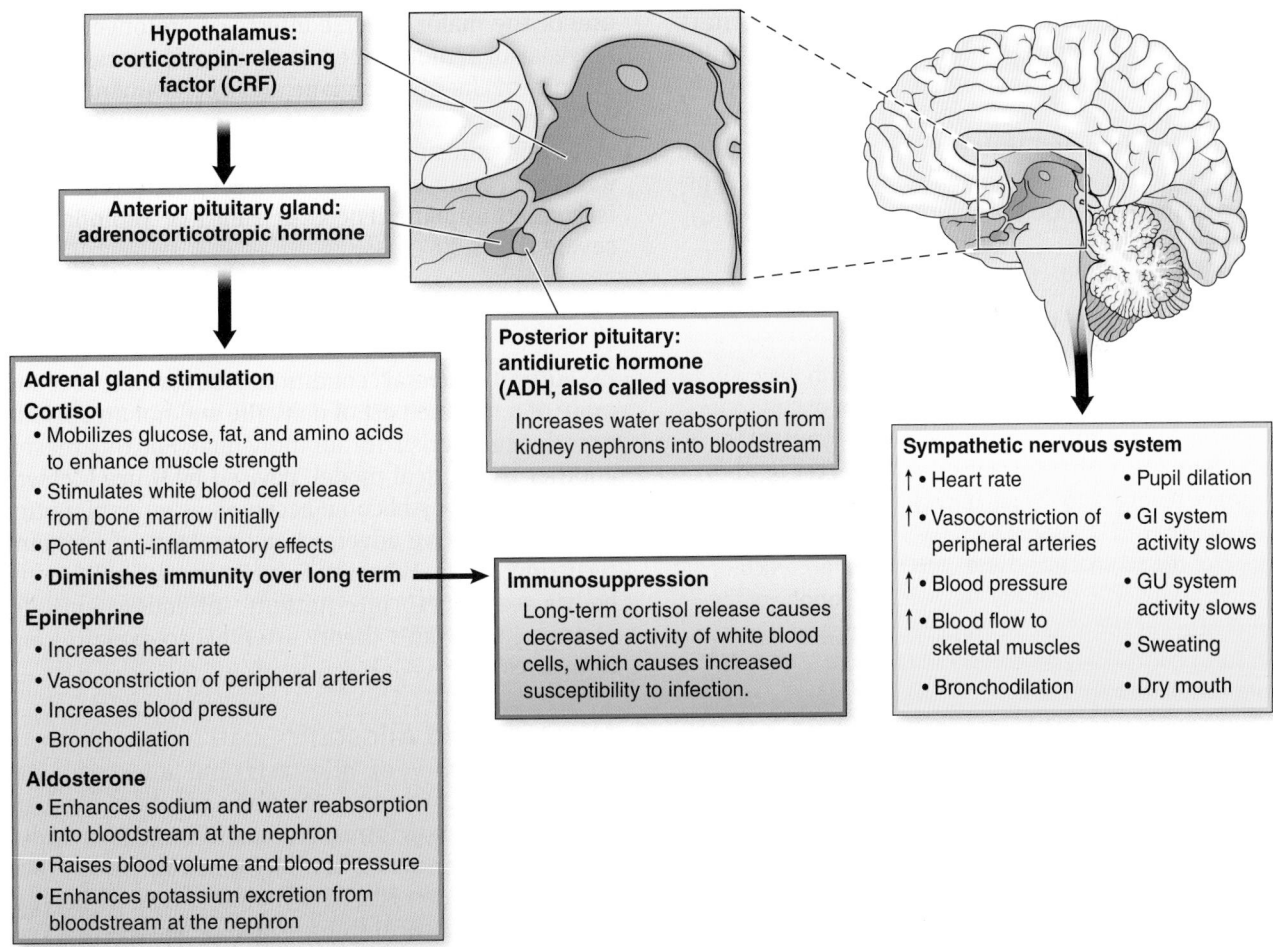

FIGURE 4-1. The fight-or-flight reaction is a basic survival response to an acute, severe stressor that incites involuntary neuroendocrine physiological changes. The fight-or-flight reaction causes the same effects as those described in the alarm stage of Selye's theory of stress. During severe stress, the hypothalamus of the brain releases corticotropin-releasing factor, which in turn stimulates the anterior pituitary to secrete ACTH. ACTH stimulates the adrenal gland to secrete cortisol, epinephrine, and aldosterone. Concurrently, the posterior pituitary secretes antidiuretic hormone, also called vasopressin. Long-term stimulation of cortisol causes diminished activity of WBCs, which causes immunosuppression.

Also during the alarm stage of Selye's stress response, the hypothalamus of the brain releases corticotropin-releasing factor, which stimulates the anterior pituitary gland to secrete adrenocorticotropic hormone (ACTH). ACTH acts on the adrenal cortex to secrete the glucocorticoid cortisol, which raises blood glucose levels, enhances muscle strength, and potentiates sympathetic activity. Cortisol powerfully enhances the body's ability to resist stress by mobilizing glucose, amino acids, and fat stores for cellular energy production (see Fig. 4-1).

In acute stress, cortisol also causes an increase in WBC response and counteracts inflammation. Immunity is enhanced for the initial 3 to 5 days, but if stress is prolonged, cortisol will cause **immunosuppression.** Long-term, elevated cortisol levels diminish the activity of WBCs.

The adrenal medulla is also stimulated to secrete the catecholamine epinephrine and the mineralocorticoid aldosterone. Epinephrine potentiates the sympathetic reaction, and aldosterone acts at the kidney's nephrons to increase sodium and water reabsorption into the bloodstream. Concurrently, the posterior pituitary gland secretes antidiuretic hormone (ADH), also called vasopressin, which further enhances water reabsorption from the kidney nephrons into the bloodstream. The extra sodium and water in the bloodstream and vasoconstrictive effects of norepinephrine and epinephrine increase blood pressure (see Fig. 4-1).

CLINICAL CONCEPT

A potent anti-inflammatory effect occurs with the administration of the pharmacological form of cortisone, also called prednisone or dexamethasone. However, long-term use of pharmacological cortisone will send negative feedback to the pituitary gland and shut off secretion of ACTH. Lack of ACTH will decrease stimulation of the adrenal gland and reduce natural corticosteroid secretion. Eventually, this leads to atrophy of the adrenal gland and resultant immunosuppression. For this reason, pharmacological cortisone should be used only for short-term treatment.

CLINICAL CONCEPT

Some studies show that stress-induced cortisol secretion may contribute to central fat accumulation.

Resistance Stage. Selye termed the second phase of the general adaptation syndrome the resistance stage. During this stage, the body attempts to stave off the effects of stress through continual hormone and catecholamine secretion. However, this is a time-limited stage; if the stress subsides, then the SNS and adrenal stimulation abate, and the parasympathetic nervous system (PSNS) responses resume a state of relaxation. Activation of the PSNS, also known as the cholinergic nervous system, causes the opposite effects of the SNS. The PSNS slows heart rate, constricts the bronchioles, decreases pupil size, and enhances GI and genitourinary activity (see Table 4-1). Under the influence of the PSNS, the body is in a relaxed, quiet state.

Exhaustion Stage. If the stressor does not subside and the stress is prolonged, the high levels of hormone and catecholamine secretion cannot be sustained and the exhaustion stage ensues. During this stage, stress overwhelms the body's ability to defend itself. The body's resources are depleted and signs of systemic dysfunction occur. During this stage, an individual commonly feels run-down, unable to cope, depressed, anxious, and physically ill.

Chronic stress can have a cumulative, negative effect on physical health and mental well-being. Long-term secretion of cortisol suppresses immunity, and WBC responses become sluggish and less efficient—one of the major adverse effects of prolonged stress. Selye also demonstrated that chronic stress causes atrophy of the thymus gland and a consequent decline in T lymphocytes, another cause of immunosuppression. Immunosuppression predisposes the individual to infection and other diseases; therefore, illness is commonly experienced at times of prolonged or severe stress.

McEwen's Stress Response Theory

In current societal conditions, stress has become more of a routine part of daily life and not an episodic experience or crisis for an individual. For this reason, another theoretical model, devised by Bruce McEwen in the 1990s, has become accepted as an explanation of the cumulative adverse health effects of frequent, recurring stress. Whereas Selye's theory explains the body's reaction to intermittent, infrequent episodes of stress, McEwen's theory attempts to explain long-term stress.

Allostasis and Allostatic Load

McEwen's theory of allostasis and allostatic load attempts to explain how the body adapts to frequent stressors and how stressors can change the body's set points of homeostasis. McEwen coined the term **allostasis** to describe a dynamic state of balance that changes according to exposure to stressors (see Fig. 4-2). In contrast, homeostasis is a set state of balance with strict, unchanging parameters or set points. According to past stress theory, the body's reactions to stress occur with the intent to reestablish homeostasis with definite set points of normal. McEwen theorizes that frequent stressors change the body's physiological balance and create new set points. For example, individuals exposed to job stress on a daily

TABLE 4-1. Effects of the Autonomic Nervous System

	Sympathetic Nervous System (Adrenergic)	Parasympathetic Nervous System (Cholinergic)
Neurotransmitter	Norepinephrine	Acetylcholine
Heart	Increased heart rate	Decreased heart rate
Vascular	Vasoconstriction of peripheral arteries Increased blood pressure	Vasodilation of peripheral arteries Decreased blood pressure
Lungs	Bronchodilation	Bronchoconstriction
Pupils	Pupil dilation (mydriasis)	Pupil constriction (miosis)
Gastrointestinal system	Decreased blood flow to GI system slows activity	Increased blood flow to GI system normalizes activity
Genitourinary system	Decreased blood flow to GU system slows activity	Increased blood flow to GU system normalizes activity
Other	Sweating (diaphoresis) Dry mouth Feelings of nervousness Tremors possible	Feeling of relaxation

GI, gastrointestinal; GU, genitourinary.

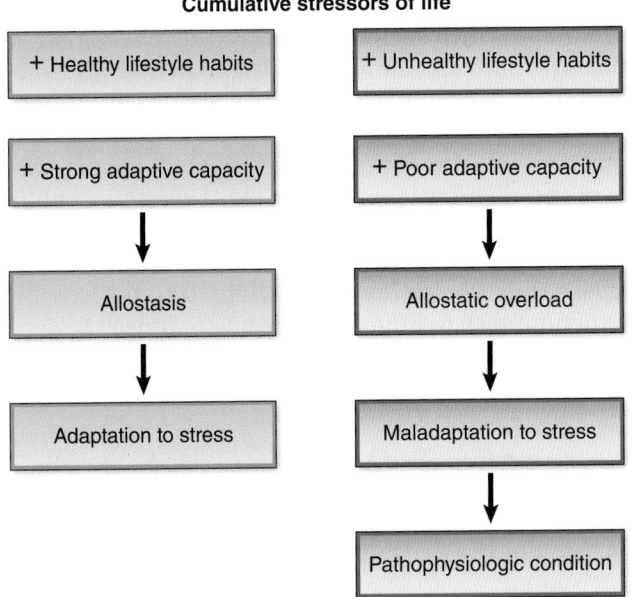

FIGURE 4-2. McEwen's theory of allostasis and allostatic load. Frequent, cumulative stressors exert an allostatic load. The individual's lifestyle and adaptive capacity influence the reaction to the cumulative stress. An individual with a healthy lifestyle and strong adaptive capability will be able to balance and adapt successfully to stressors, a state called allostasis. An individual with an unhealthy lifestyle and poor adaptive capability will experience allostatic overload, which results in a pathophysiological state.

basis may develop high blood pressure while in the work environment. If this stress becomes chronic, it can drive the individual's physiological blood pressure to high levels that persist in and out of the work environment.

CLINICAL CONCEPT

Long-term high blood pressure causes endothelial damage and accelerates the development of atherosclerosis over time; in this way, atherosclerosis caused by hypertension is a stress-related disease.

Allostatic load can be defined as the wear and tear on body systems caused by stress reactions. In prolonged stress, hormones and catecholamines have a cumulative, noxious effect and are part of the allostatic load on the body (see Fig. 4-2). For example, chronic secretion of the hormone epinephrine causes arterial vasoconstriction and raises blood pressure. Chronic cortisol secretion causes immunosuppression and sleep disruption.

According to McEwen, allostatic load can accumulate because of any of the following four mechanisms:

1. **Repeated stressful experiences:** This mechanism of allostatic load can occur when, for example, a person experiences multiple stresses consecutively or simultaneously. Death of a loved one, illness, moving to another home, and divorce are common types of stresses for an individual. If a person has to deal with all of these at once, the neuroendocrine stress reaction is provoked multiple times and the body isn't given sufficient time to recover and reestablish homeostasis.

2. **Inability of the individual to adapt to stress:** Every individual differs in their adaptive ability

to deal with stress. Some have fewer coping mechanisms than others or insufficient social support. For example, those who relocate to live in a new region that is unfamiliar to them may experience diminished adaptive ability to handle stress because of lack of support from friends and family.

3. **Prolonged reaction to a stressor:** This mechanism of allostatic load occurs when an individual has an inappropriately prolonged reaction to a stressor. When a person is called upon to take an examination, they experience the neuroendocrine stress response before and during the examination. Many individuals also experience the stress for a lengthy time after the termination of the experience. For such persons, the stress reaction begins before the stressful event and does not shut down in a timely manner, creating an inappropriately detrimental, lengthened exposure to the stress hormones and catecholamines. Interestingly, studies show that with aging, stress-induced hormones and catecholamines return to baseline values more slowly after the conclusion of a stressful event. For example, with exertion, an older person's heart rate increases more slowly and returns to normal more gradually than in the younger adult.

4. **Inadequate response to a stressor:** Lastly, allostatic load can result from an inadequate neuroendocrine response to a stressful experience. Some individuals have a faulty stress response that causes imbalanced neuroendocrine activity and lack of feedback mechanisms to shut off the reaction. The individual has inappropriate hypoactivity and hyperactivity of different systems involved in the stress response. Laboratory animals that secrete inadequate amounts of cortisol during stress demonstrate inadequate shutdown of localized inflammatory mediators. These laboratory animals, in turn, demonstrate more autoimmune and inflammatory diseases. These studies have led to theories that many autoimmune and inflammatory diseases are stress-related in etiology.

According to McEwen, allostatic load is not only determined by the stressor but also by how well the individual adapts to the stressor. The individual's adaptive ability is influenced by genetic makeup, cognitive ability, developmental level, socioeconomic status, lifestyle choices, diet, exercise, preexisting conditions, past life experiences, and support of others. When stress exceeds the body's ability to adapt, **allostatic overload** results, initiating pathophysiological disorders (see Fig. 4-2). For example, an obese, sedentary individual who overeats has a high risk of developing insulin resistance and type 2 diabetes. The excess fat and insulin resistance are stressors to the body, and the individual's adaptive ability is hindered by sedentary behavior and poor eating habits. The

stressors and lack of adaptive ability contribute to the allostatic load. In the individual who develops insulin resistance and type 2 diabetes, the allostatic load overwhelms the individual's ability to return the body to homeostasis and causes a state of pathological imbalance. The body can resume an allostatic state of stability with treatment for diabetes and reduce allostatic load through exercise and weight loss. If allostatic load is reduced significantly, the body may be able to reestablish homeostasis and diabetes can subside.

Stress is an increasingly significant consideration in the diagnosis and treatment of many common illnesses (see Box 4-1). Clinicians frequently recommend stress management, weight reduction, smoking cessation, and exercise in addition to medical, pharmacological, and surgical treatments. These recommendations aim to lessen lifestyle-related stressors on the body, thereby reducing allostatic load. Stress reduction can boost immunity and reverse many of the negative effects of illness.

There is an emerging field of research that asserts certain societal pressures exist that cause discordant, unavoidable, deeply ingrained stress for certain segments of the population. A phenomenon termed structural racism is increasingly being investigated as it relates to health disparities among certain sectors of the population. Structural racism refers to the totality of ways in which societies foster racial discrimination through mutually reinforcing systems of housing, education, employment, earnings, benefits, credit, media, health care, and criminal justice. These patterns and practices in turn reinforce discriminatory beliefs, values, and distribution of resources. Experts in public health, such as the American Heart Association, are beginning to recognize the influence of these societal-level stressors and assert that our future focus on structural racism offers a promising approach toward advancing health equity and improving population health (Bailey et al., 2017; Churchwell et al., 2020).

BOX 4-1. Common Stress-Related Disorders

- Asthma
- Atherosclerosis
- Autoimmune diseases
- Cardiac rhythm disturbances
- Cerebrovascular disease
- Coronary artery disease
- Diabetes
- General anxiety disorder
- Hypertension
- Irritable bowel disease
- Migraine headache
- Peptic ulcer disease
- Skin disorders such as urticaria (hives)
- Substance abuse

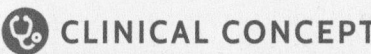

CLINICAL CONCEPT

Older individuals have less resilience against stress, as the body requires more time for recovery from a stressful event.

Treatment of Stress

Overwhelming stress or allostatic overload occurs when the individual's adaptive ability is exceeded. Symptoms such as nervousness, irritability, headaches, lack of ability to concentrate, insomnia, changes in appetite, depression, and panic attacks are often the result of allostatic overload. When stress interferes with normal daily functioning, many persons seek treatment from clinicians or counselors. Lifestyle modifications, stress-management programs, psychotherapy, alternative medical practices, and pharmacological treatments are often recommended for excessive stress.

Lifestyle Practices

Many lifestyle factors affect how the body deals with stress. Adequate sleep, exercise, and nutrition are necessary elements for resilience against stress.

Reducing Caffeine Intake

Caffeine is a stimulant contained in coffee, tea, cola, chocolate, and many appetite suppressants. Nine out of 10 Americans consume some type of caffeine regularly. For most people, moderate doses of caffeine (200 to 300 mg, or about two to three cups of brewed coffee a day) aren't harmful.

Caffeine readily crosses the blood–brain barrier and acts as an antagonist of adenosine receptors found in the brain. The reduction in adenosine activity results in increased activity of the neurotransmitter dopamine, which causes mental alertness. Caffeine can also increase levels of epinephrine and serotonin. Epinephrine stimulates the SNS, leading to increased heart rate, blood pressure, and blood flow to muscles and vasoconstriction of arterioles, which perfuse the skin and inner organs. Biochemically, it stimulates glycogenolysis, inhibits glycolysis, and stimulates gluconeogenesis to produce more glucose for the muscles and release of glucose into the bloodstream from the liver. Also, caffeine stimulates serotonin in the brain, which produces positive changes in mood.

Side effects of excessive caffeine intake include nervousness, tremulousness, and increased heart rate and blood pressure. Many studies have been done to investigate an association between caffeine, coffee drinking, and coronary artery disease. Caffeine can stimulate occasional premature atrial contractions in the heart, which can be perceived as palpitations by an individual. However, research studies have not established a link between caffeine and development of coronary artery disease.

CLINICAL CONCEPT

In individuals experiencing a high level of stress, even moderate coffee-drinking can cause increased jitteriness, nervousness, insomnia, and heart palpitations. These individuals should either decrease or eliminate their caffeine intake.

CLINICAL CONCEPT

Caffeine tolerance develops very quickly, especially among heavy coffee drinkers. Caffeine-habituated individuals can experience caffeine withdrawal 12 to 24 hours after the last dose of caffeine. It resolves within 24 to 48 hours. The most prominent symptoms are headache, irritability, anxiety, fatigue, and drowsiness.

Ensuring Restorative Sleep

For the body to cope with daily stress, restorative sleep is necessary. Studies show that restorative sleep is a heightened anabolic state, when there is growth and rejuvenation of the immune, nervous, skeletal, and muscular systems. Restorative sleep requires a sufficient length of time devoted to sleep so that the body can enter the five different stages of sleep that begin after the body is relaxed and preparing for sleep (see Box 4-2).

CLINICAL CONCEPT

To examine sleep patterns, a diagnostic test called **polysomnography** is performed. Sensors are placed on the patient to monitor electrical activity of the brain, eye movement, muscle contraction, and cardiac and respiratory function during sleep.

Lack of Sufficient Sleep. Generally, sleep disorders affect the quality, duration, and onset of sleep. Sleep deprivation, a frequently changing sleep schedule, stress, and environment all affect the progression of the sleep cycle.

CLINICAL CONCEPT

Various studies worldwide have shown the prevalence of insomnia in 10% to 30% of the population, some even as high as 50% to 60%. It is common in older adults, females, and people with medical and mental health disorders and is often a problem that goes unrecognized by primary care clinicians.

BOX 4-2. The Five Stages of Sleep

STAGE 1
Stage 1 sleep, or drowsiness, is first in the sequence. On polysomnography, brain waves show a 50% reduction in activity between wakefulness and stage 1 sleep. The eyes are closed. This stage usually lasts between 5 and 10 minutes.

STAGE 2
Stage 2 is a period of light sleep during which polysomnographic readings show spontaneous periods of muscle tone mixed with periods of muscle relaxation. The heart rate slows, and body temperature decreases. At this point, the body prepares to enter deep sleep.

STAGE 3 AND STAGE 4
In stage 3, slow brain waves called *delta waves* begin to appear, interspersed with smaller, faster waves. By stage 4, the brain produces delta waves almost exclusively. It is very difficult to wake someone during stages 3 and 4, which together are called deep sleep. There is no eye movement or muscle activity. People awakened during deep sleep do not adjust immediately and often feel groggy and disoriented for several minutes after they wake up.

STAGE 5
Stage 5 is referred to as **REM sleep** because rapid eye movement (REM) occurs during this stage. Although REM sleep is not completely understood, some physiological changes are distinguishable during this stage. Breathing becomes more rapid, irregular, and shallow, and the eyes jerk rapidly in various directions. There is a decrease in the activity of monoamine neurotransmitters, such as norepinephrine, in the brain. Muscles of the extremities become temporarily paralyzed, heart rate increases, and blood pressure rises. Uniquely, dreaming occurs during REM sleep.

Although REM sleep is not well understood, many theories exist about its function and significance. Theories have stated REM sleep is important because it:
- Allows for consolidation of procedural and spatial memories
- Helps the monoamine receptors in the brain recover to regain full sensitivity
- Provides the neurological stimulation needed to form mature neural connections for proper central nervous system development in newborns

Experts agree that there seem to be no ill effects from lack of REM sleep, but it appears to be necessary for restorative sleep. Researchers have found that suppressing REM sleep greatly increases the number of attempts an individual will make to enter REM sleep. Also, once the suppression ceases, the proportion of time spent in REM sleep will increase significantly, an event known as REM rebound.

THE SLEEP CYCLE
When people sleep, they cycle through the stages of sleep in a repetitive manner. A complete sleep cycle takes approximately 90 to 110 minutes and is composed of stages 1 through 5, with stage 2 and 3 repeated before stage 5. A normal sleep cycle has the following pattern: restful wakefulness; stage 1, 2, 3, and 4; repeat of stage 3; repeat of stage 2; and then stage 5 REM sleep. A person may complete five cycles in a typical night's sleep.

Irritability and moodiness are the first symptoms a person experiences from lack of sleep. Sleep deprivation can cause apathy, slowed speech, flattened emotional responses, impaired memory, poor judgment, and an inability to multitask. Extreme sleep deprivation causes a person to fall into microsleeps (5 to 10 seconds) that result in lapses of attention and possible hallucinations.

Individual sleep needs vary. In general, most healthy adults function best with 8 to 10 hours of sleep a night. However, some individuals are able to function without sleepiness or drowsiness after as little as 6 hours of sleep. The need for sleep doesn't decline with age; however, the ability to sleep for 6 to 8 hours at one time may be reduced.

CLINICAL CONCEPT
Obstructive sleep apnea (OSA) is a common cause of nonrestorative sleep. OSA is caused by the relaxation of pharyngeal soft tissue that collapses over the airways during sleep. The hallmark symptom of OSA is excessive daytime sleepiness; the patient may also report snoring and repetitive pauses in breathing.

Improving Nutrition
Stress can affect eating patterns and the nutritional status of an individual. Conversely, nutritional status can affect the ability to deal with stress. Individual eating patterns vary in response to stress. Many persons report that they eat excessively when under stress; others complain of a loss of appetite because of stress. Eating six small nutritious meals instead of three large meals is often recommended as a strategy for those under stress. Also, slowing down, taking a seated position, and relaxing while eating are recommended.

Persons under stress commonly skip meals, which is an unhealthy practice. Skipping meals can lead to hypoglycemia, which causes dizziness, tachycardia, diaphoresis, poor ability to concentrate, possible syncope, and poor intake of daily recommended vitamins and minerals. Conversely, some persons under stress overeat or increase their intake of fast food. These are unhealthy practices that can lead to obesity, sluggishness, and indigestion.

Many persons under stress endure indigestion, heartburn, constipation, diarrhea, nausea, and vomiting. Conditions such as inflammatory bowel disease and irritable bowel syndrome are exacerbated by stress. Considerable research has been done that confirms a brain–gut axis, which is a neurological connection between the central nervous system, autonomic nervous system, and GI tract.

The Role of Serotonin and Tryptophan. Research is focusing on the role of serotonin in GI disorders. Serotonin is an important neurotransmitter found in both the brain and GI tract. In the GI system, cells of the small intestine, called enterochromaffin cells, release serotonin, which stimulates peristaltic, secretory, vasodilatory, and parasympathetic activity. Serotonin allows for full, complete, and relaxed function of the GI system. During stress there is a deficit of serotonin, causing decreased GI function and higher susceptibility to indigestion.

It is theorized that serotonin levels in the brain also become depleted during stress. Studies with humans and animals show that serotonin in the brain promotes feelings of calm, personal security, relaxation, confidence, and concentration, whereas lack of serotonin in the brain causes a lack of feelings of well-being.

Tryptophan, one of the essential amino acids obtained from dietary sources, is the precursor to serotonin. Some dietary sources of tryptophan include meats, soy products, some kinds of cheese, milk, brown rice, and peanuts. Many protein sources contain the essential amino acids, with a small percentage in the form of tryptophan. In order to form serotonin, tryptophan must cross the blood–brain barrier and compete with the other ingested amino acids. Insulin is a carrier molecule that facilitates the transport of glucose, some amino acids, and fatty acids into muscle and liver cells. In the presence of insulin, most competing amino acids are absorbed into muscle cells, whereas tryptophan remains behind in the circulation. By facilitating absorption of competing amino acids into muscle, insulin frees tryptophan so that it can enter the brain.

Ingestion of carbohydrates is the greatest dietary stimulus for the release of insulin; carbohydrates, which stimulate insulin, enhance the uptake of competing amino acids into muscle and allow the brain to absorb tryptophan. Once inside the brain, tryptophan is converted into serotonin. At the pineal gland, located within the brain, some serotonin is converted to melatonin, an enhancer of sleep, which is why tryptophan has earned a reputation as having calming, relaxing effects on individuals. Anecdotally, many persons claim that some carbohydrate-rich foods are comforting; these individuals report increased intake of carbohydrates when under stress. Occasional indulgence in this type of food is probably useful to relieve anxiety in the short term, but habitually consuming foods rich in carbohydrates is likely to cause obesity.

Balancing Work and Leisure Activities

Working persons need to balance their lives with sufficient time for recreation and leisure. Initially, increased stress produces increased performance. However, after a certain point prolonged stress results in decreased performance, as efforts to work harder become either unproductive or even counterproductive.

One of the first symptoms of distress is fatigue and irritability. These symptoms are signals that the individual's adaptive ability is reaching its threshold and stress relief is necessary, or exhaustion can result.

Utilizing Social Support

Persons under stress often need to talk about their problems with a supportive, active listener. Social support from friends, coworkers, or relatives can provide some relief of stress. Supportive others can offer feedback, validation, encouragement, and advice. Many times, simply allowing the individual to voice their feelings enables stress relief.

 CLINICAL CONCEPT

Journaling is another form of expression that can be useful for relieving stress. Although not a social medium, writing affords the person a private place to express feelings, work out problems, and organize thoughts about specific issues, much as they would with a supportive listener.

Using Humor

Humor can be used as a coping mechanism to reduce stress and promote general wellness. Studies show that among cancer patients, various types of humorous material lessened anxiety and discomfort and provoked open discussion of concerns and fears. Researchers also found that humor has a positive effect on the immune system. Humor is associated with an increased pain threshold and enhanced function of specific WBCs called natural killer cells. In addition, research shows that patients demonstrate specific neuroendocrine changes associated with improved physical stress responses and increased feelings of well-being after humorous interventions.

Exercising

Exercise can reduce stress, alleviate depression and anxiety, enhance coping mechanisms, and boost self-confidence. It stimulates blood flow to the brain, which enhances secretion of the neurotransmitters serotonin, norepinephrine, and dopamine, which counteract depression and anxiety.

Over the long term, exercise reduces the effect of neuroendocrine excitation that is provoked by stress. The long-term effect of regular exercise is likened to meditation, in that it can activate the PSNS and endow the individual with a relaxation effect.

Utilizing Psychotherapy

Individual psychotherapy involves regularly scheduled counseling sessions between the patient and a mental health professional such as a psychologist, psychiatrist, social worker, or psychiatric clinician. The sessions may focus on current or past problems; sources of anxiety; and current thoughts, feelings, or relationships. Sharing these experiences with an objective mental health professional allows a patient to ventilate and come to understand how to manage stress and anxiety.

Cognitive-behavioral therapy and interpersonal psychotherapy are the major types of psychotherapeutic techniques used. Cognitive-behavioral therapy explores the patient's beliefs; expectations; and cognitive appraisals of self, the world, and the nature of personal problems. The therapist attempts to explore the patient's sources of anxiety and give recommendations regarding coping behaviors to manage the stress. In interpersonal therapy, the therapist attempts to enhance the patient's insight into their problems, identify sources of stress, and facilitate the recognition of the patient's own coping abilities or disabilities.

Stress-Management Programs

Stress-management programs assist an individual in coping with various types of stress through education, counseling, and support group interaction. These types of programs are commonly available within hospitals or other clinical settings. Usually directed by a psychologist or psychiatrist, patients are able to verbalize their problems and anxieties, explore their sources of stress, and receive advice for coping from others in the support group and a mental health professional.

Alternative Practices to Reduce Stress

Individuals who want natural remedies for disorders have been increasingly using alternative medical practices and complementary therapies. Research studies have shown that meditation and yoga are techniques that can reduce stress.

Meditation

Meditation is a state of concentrated attention. It involves turning the attention inward to a single point of reference. Different meditative disciplines encompass a wide range of spiritual and psychophysical practices that can emphasize development of either a high degree of mental concentration or mental quiescence.

Many persons who meditate retreat to a quiet area and focus intently on one word or concept for a daily prearranged period with the body in a resting state in order to free the mind. Research demonstrates that daily periods devoted to quiet, restful meditation can alleviate stress.

Yoga

Yoga is an exercise technique that uses different poses to induce relaxation, body alignment, muscle strength, stamina, flexibility, and stress reduction. The person's own body weight provides the resistance needed to strengthen muscles from head to toe.

Yoga enables a person to stretch tight muscles, increase range of motion, enhance balance, and improve alignment. It also boosts energy; calms the person; and enhances awareness, focus, and patience. Research shows that a set period devoted to yoga in a quiet environment combined with meditation relieves stress.

Pharmacological Treatments to Reduce Stress

Some pharmacological agents can be prescribed for stress, including sedatives, sleep aids, and antidepressants. Keep in mind that pharmacological agents should be used in combination with professional counseling or psychotherapy.

Sedatives

Stress can cause insomnia, and patients may require sleep aids or substances to help them sleep. A sedative is a substance that depresses the central nervous system, resulting in relaxation, anxiety relief, drowsiness, and slowed breathing. A sedative can also cause slurred speech, unstable gait, poor judgment, and slowed reflexes. Sedatives may be referred to as tranquilizers, depressants, anxiolytics, soporifics, sleeping pills, "downers" (slang), or sedative-hypnotics. When a patient experiences extreme stress or an anxiety attack, sedatives are most often the prescribed medication for rapid relief. There are several types of prescribed sleep medications, but the most utilized is the over-the-counter sleep aid diphenhydramine (Benadryl).

However, sedatives can be abused to produce an overly calming effect; alcohol is the most common sedating substance used within the population. At high doses or when abused, many of these drugs can cause unconsciousness and death.

Antidepressants

Antidepressants are often the treatment of choice for adults with moderate or severe depression and anxiety. Sadness, anxiety, depression-related sleep and appetite disorders, concentration, and energy levels all can improve with antidepressant medications. They achieve their effect by modulating the neurotransmitters in the brain—serotonin, norepinephrine, or dopamine. Dozens of antidepressants are available, and each affects brain neurotransmitters in a different way. Patients often must try different medications to find the particular one that is effective and suitable for them.

> ## 🩺 CLINICAL CONCEPT
> Antidepressants usually require at least 3 weeks to reach therapeutic blood levels.

Sleep Hygiene

It is recommended that a person develop a sleep routine using natural techniques such as quiet time, reading, warm milk, or chamomile tea to induce sleep. It is advisable to avoid caffeine, alcohol, and any stimulant medications such as phenylephrine or pseudoephedrine, as these can interfere with sleep. It is also advisable to turn off the screens of electronic devices close to bedtime.

The Beneficial Effects of Exercise

Daily physical activity is a necessary component of health promotion and disease prevention. Regular exercise is associated with cardiovascular health, respiratory fitness, decreased risk of chronic disease, bone strengthening, regulation of blood sugar, emotional well-being, and greater longevity (see Box 4-3).

In general, most people can participate in some form of exercise. As a rule, persons younger than age 35 years in good health do not need a medical examination before starting an exercise program. However, individuals with cardiovascular disease, chronic respiratory illnesses, diabetes, or disabling conditions should consult a physician before beginning an exercise regimen.

The basic types of exercise include those that facilitate stretching and flexibility, aerobic fitness, muscular strength, and endurance. In general, the public health recommendation is moderate-intensity physical activity for 40 minutes 3 to 4 days per week. It is suggested that persons alternate between flexibility, aerobic, and isometric exercise in order to target all muscle groups.

Weight

Physical activity is important to prevent obesity, a significant public health problem in the United States.

Obesity is defined as excess body fat resulting from consumption of calories in excess of those expended. Exercise requires energy and expends the calories consumed by the individual. As one exercises, energy is derived from the breakdown of glycogen and fat stores; this process can decrease obesity.

Heredity, sociocultural factors, and environmental influences also play a role in the development of obesity. Obesity is associated with multiple disease processes, including cancers (see Box 4-4).

Cardiovascular System

There is an inverse relationship between the level of physical activity and the incidence of cardiovascular disease. Individuals who exercise regularly demonstrate less atherosclerosis and coronary artery disease and fewer acute cardiac events. Exercise improves coronary blood flow and vascular endothelial function. The vascular endothelium or lining of arterial blood vessels responds to exercise by producing vasodilator compounds such as prostacyclin and nitric oxide. These vasodilator compounds widen the arterial blood vessels, allowing more blood flow to various regions of the body. Specifically, nitric oxide–dependent vasodilation of the coronary arteries increases myocardial perfusion and prevents endothelial inflammation, platelet activation, and thrombus formation.

Individuals who exercise are found to have lower levels of fibrinogen, an indicator of active clot formation, and C-reactive protein, an inflammatory mediator. For this reason, it is theorized that exercise has an antiatherogenic effect on the endothelium, which prevents endothelial injury and arteriosclerotic plaque and clot formation.

In addition, exercise stimulates angiogenesis, which is the growth of collateral blood vessels. Physical activity stimulates vascular endothelial growth factor secretion, which provokes synthesis of new blood vessels by the endothelial cells. Within the heart muscle, the growth of collateral coronary artery branches provides extra circulatory routes for blood flow to the myocardium. Within the extremities, growth of

---

BOX 4-3. Therapeutic Effects of Exercise

- Increases number of mitochondria in muscle cells
- Raises HDL-C
- Stimulates angiogenesis
- Enhances glucose entry into muscle cells
- Improves cardiovascular conditioning: increases perfusion of myocardium and cardiac output, enhances vascular dilation capacity, increases venous return, increases efficiency of heart, decreases blood pressure and pulse rate over long term
- Stimulates osteoblastic activity
- Decreases body fat
- Builds muscle mass
- Creates positive psychological effects on mood and stress relief

---

BOX 4-4. Obesity-Related Disorders

- Cardiovascular disease
- Deep vein thrombosis
- Degenerative joint disease
- Diabetes mellitus
- Gallbladder disease
- Higher risk for breast, prostate, colon, and uterine cancer
- Poor wound healing
- Sleep apnea
- Venous insufficiency

collateral arterial blood vessels provides new routes of blood flow to the leg muscles. For this reason, walking is recommended to counteract peripheral arterial occlusive disease. Walking stimulates the development of new vascular branches off existing arterial vessels, which, in turn, increases routes of circulation in the extremities.

Regular exercise also lowers blood pressure and pulse rate over time. It enhances the heart's efficiency by increasing cardiac muscle mass and growth of coronary vessel branches. A muscular, well-perfused heart contracts more efficiently and requires fewer contractions to yield cardiac output. The efficient heart beats at a slower pace and has adequate time for cardiac filling during diastole. The athletic heart can beat at a slower pace to eject sufficient blood from the ventricles for the body's metabolic requirements. Exercise also stimulates peripheral arterial vasodilation, which opens blood vessels throughout the body, diminishes resistance, and decreases resting systemic blood pressure. Peripheral vasodilation decreases the aortic resistance against the left ventricle and eases the heart's workload.

Venous return is greatly enhanced during aerobic exercise. Contraction of the large leg muscles, in particular, creates a pumping action to facilitate upward flow of venous blood back to the heart. The contractile muscle action and blood flow counteracts venous stasis and clot formation in the legs. Increased amounts of venous blood return to the right side of the heart, lungs, and left side of the heart. Greater venous return raises stroke volume and cardiac output in the healthy heart.

Exercise also increases the formation of high-density lipoprotein cholesterol (HDL-C). The total cholesterol in the body is derived from foods and synthesized by the liver. Total cholesterol is composed of low-density lipoprotein (LDL-C) and HDL-C. The body metabolizes cholesterol to yield either form. LDL-C is deposited within the endothelium to become atherosclerotic plaque, and the HDL-C component is excreted. It is advantageous for more of the total cholesterol in the body to become HDL-C versus LDL-C. Exercise stimulates the body to form more HDL-C than LDL-C. Persons who exercise demonstrate lower total cholesterol levels and higher levels of HDL-C compared with sedentary individuals.

Current research data suggest that epigenetic modifications occur with performance of continual aerobic and resistance exercise. Genetic changes are seen in cells of the brain, blood, skeletal and cardiac muscle, and adipose tissue. Six months of aerobic exercise alters whole-genome DNA methylation in skeletal muscle and adipose tissue and directly influences lipogenesis, which enhances lean body mass. Research in the field of exercise epigenomics is increasingly delineating mechanisms by which exercise confers a healthier phenotype and improves performance (Denham et al., 2014).

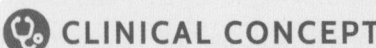

CLINICAL CONCEPT

Exercise stimulates angiogenesis, increases the number of mitochondria in the muscles, and raises HDL-C.

Cardiac Exercise Stress Testing

Exercise stress testing is used to evaluate the cardiovascular status of patients by measuring their energy expenditure and physiological responses while walking or running on a treadmill. Changing the speed and incline of the treadmill can vary the exercise workload on the body. The patient's heart rate, blood pressure, and electrocardiogram are continuously monitored during the stress test. The patient is challenged to exercise at various levels until maximal heart rate is reached, which is estimated by age.

As a general rule, the predicted maximal heart rate can be estimated by subtracting age from 220. For example, the target heart rate for a 70-year-old person would be 220 − 70, or 150 beats/minute. For optimal exercise effects, persons are encouraged to reach at least 85% of their maximal heart rate.

Exercise capacity assessed by a cardiac stress test is a strong predictor of risk of death from cardiovascular disease. During a stress test, the patient is gradually challenged to exercise to peak capacity on a treadmill so clinicians can assess cardiovascular status. Along with physiological monitoring, the individual's feelings during exertion are monitored as the treadmill speed and incline increase. Research shows that as an individual's exercise capacity increases, risk of death from cardiovascular disease decreases. Research also shows that less fit or less active persons can improve their survival if they increase their level of physical activity. A program of regular exercise can improve fitness by 15% to 30% within 3 to 6 months. Exercise levels must be maintained or else the benefits wane with discontinued activity.

Pulmonary System

Exercise increases the depth and rate of breathing, ventilatory capacity of the lungs, and oxygen and carbon dioxide diffusion at the alveolar–capillary membranes. Enhanced cardiac output creates a greater volume of blood delivered to the pulmonary vasculature, and pulmonary perfusion increases. Greater depth and rate of breathing increase the blood's oxygenation.

As exercise continues and a person tires, increased levels of carbon dioxide, decreased levels of oxygen, and decreased blood pH stimulate chemoreceptors in the medulla, aorta, and carotid arteries to increase breathing rate. How long a person is able to exercise depends on the ability of the cardiovascular system and lungs to deliver oxygenated blood to the contracting muscles.

Muscles work most efficiently when using oxygen to perform aerobic metabolism. Muscles that do not receive adequate oxygen eventually enter into anaerobic metabolism, which can only support the exercising body for a short period.

Musculoskeletal System

Isometric exercise can build muscle strength; it enlarges muscle size by contracting muscles against increasing levels of workload. Weightlifters typically perform isometric exercises to build muscle mass. Aerobic exercise is both an endurance and isometric type of activity. Walking and running are aerobic exercises that increase efficiency of the muscles, build muscle mass, increase the number of mitochondria, and enhance blood supply.

With isometric exercise, muscles can hypertrophy and double in size. Muscle fibers enlarge, the number of mitochondrial enzymes increases substantially, and there is an increase in stored glycogen and triglycerides. Increased glycogen and triglycerides enhance the potential for anaerobic metabolic activity in the muscles, whereas the increase in mitochondrial enzymes augments the aerobic metabolic capacity of the muscles.

Both aerobic and isometric types of exercise can increase metabolic rate, or the amount of energy used by the body during rest. Metabolic rate is directly proportional to lean body mass; the more muscle mass, the greater the metabolic rate. Muscles expend more calories than fat. For example, a pound of muscle can burn up to 50 more calories a day than a pound of fat. Therefore an exercise program that combines aerobic and isometric activities appears to be the best approach for increasing muscle efficiency, raising metabolic rate, and controlling body weight.

Bone
Bone is a dynamic organ continually undergoing remodeling by osteoblastic and osteoclastic activity. Osteoblasts continually deposit new bone, and osteoclasts actively absorb bone. Normally, except in growing bones, the rates of bone deposition and absorption are equal to each other so that total mass of bone remains constant. Bone is deposited according to compressional loads and remodels according to load stress patterns.

Physical activity stimulates increases in bone diameter and strength throughout the life span. Exercise-stimulated bone strengthening and remodeling diminish the risk of fracture by counteracting the development of osteoporosis.

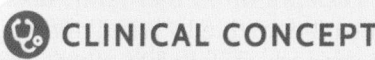 **CLINICAL CONCEPT**
Weight-bearing exercises stimulate osteoblastic activity and calcification of bone.

Glucose Tolerance

Exercise enhances cellular glucose uptake and reduces glucose intolerance. For reasons not clearly understood, muscle cells become more permeable to glucose during the process of contraction even in the absence of insulin. For persons with diabetes, exercise is recommended as an adjunct to dietary restrictions and weight control, as these therapies combined can often reverse the disease process.

ALERT! Persons with diabetes mellitus must be vigilant for hypoglycemia during periods of intense exercise.

Gastrointestinal System

During intense exercise, blood is shunted away from the GI tract toward active skeletal muscles and the cardiorespiratory system. However, over the long term, regular exercise is known to assist peristaltic activity; counteract constipation; and reduce risk of colon cancer, diverticulosis, and inflammatory bowel disease.

Psychological Effects

Regular exercise increases oxygen delivery to the brain and stimulates neurotransmitters such as dopamine, serotonin, and norepinephrine, which can elevate mood. There is also evidence that endorphins, which are natural pain relievers, increase in the bloodstream after exercise. High endorphin levels in the brain endow an individual with a feeling of well-being. Lastly, exercise is hypothesized to have a detoxification effect on the body, as it may increase metabolism sufficiently to allow the body to excrete stress hormones more rapidly.

The Harmful Effects of Physical Inactivity and Immobility

Lack of physical activity has become a public health problem in the United States. Immobility may be a consequence of severe neuromuscular injury, as experienced by paralyzed individuals; a prerequisite for healing, as in stabilization of a fractured bone; or it can be a lifestyle choice. Regardless of the cause, immobility is a risk factor for obesity, cardiovascular deconditioning, muscular atrophy, osteoporosis, and other disease processes (see Box 4-5).

Lack of regular physical activity causes a characteristic pattern of suboptimal systemic function. It reduces stimulation of the cardiovascular, pulmonary, GI, genitourinary, and musculoskeletal systems.

BOX 4-5. Effects of Immobility

- Atelectasis
- Bone demineralization
- Deconditioning of the heart and muscles
- Decreased pulmonary ventilation, including vital capacity, tidal volume, and functional residual capacity
- Pressure ulcers (pressure injury)
- Depression
- Diminished peristalsis and constipation
- Disorientation
- Gait and balance disturbance
- Gastroesophageal reflux
- Increased susceptibility to aspiration
- Increased susceptibility to orthostatic hypotension
- Joint contractures
- Kidney stones
- Loss of appetite
- Muscle atrophy
- Reduced cough effectiveness
- Stasis of pulmonary secretions and increased risk of pneumonia
- Urinary stasis
- Urinary tract infection
- Venous stasis
- Venous thromboembolism

Prolonged inactivity can cause electrolyte imbalances, glucose intolerance, circulatory dysfunction, skin breakdown, and altered sensory perception.

Circulatory System Changes

With immobility, changes occur in the arteries and veins. Veins are weak-walled structures with valves that often fail to direct blood flow upward to the heart. Arteries, although muscular structures, do not vasoconstrict rapidly with position changes, causing a condition called orthostatic hypotension.

Venous Stasis

When walking, the leg muscles contract against the force of gravity and exert a positive pressure force on the veins of the legs. The gastrocnemius muscle of the lower leg, in particular, keeps blood pumping up toward the heart. In the supine position, the body cannot counteract the forces of gravity. With immobility, there is stagnation of venous blood in the lower extremities—a condition called venous stasis. The stasis of venous blood increases hydrostatic pressure within the veins of the legs, which is then transmitted into the capillaries. With this increase in pressure, fluid is displaced from the blood into the interstitial tissue, forming edema. Ankle edema is common in persons with venous insufficiency.

Because the blood is stagnant in venous stasis, it is susceptible to clotting. A clot that forms in the venous circulation of the legs is called deep vein thrombosis (DVT).

Pulmonary Embolism

The risk of pulmonary embolism (PE) increases with immobility and venous insufficiency. A venous clot can form in the stagnant blood of a deep vein of the lower extremity. The venous clot then can travel into the inferior vena cava and into the right side of the heart. When a clot travels, it is referred to as an embolism. From the right ventricle the clot is pumped into the pulmonary artery and can lodge and obstruct pulmonary circulation. The clot is then referred to as a PE—a potentially fatal condition because it blocks the perfusion of lung tissue.

 CLINICAL CONCEPT

Patients on bedrest can develop venous stasis, which can lead to DVT and, eventually, PE. A PE can be fatal, and prevention is the most effective strategy. Thrombo-embolic dressing (TED) stockings, sequential pneumatic compression devices, and anticoagulant medications are often used to decrease the risk of DVT in patients on bedrest.

Orthostatic Hypotension

Orthostatic hypotension occurs when a patient attempts to resume the upright position after a prolonged period of bedrest. After an extended period in the supine position, an individual's arterial baroreceptors (pressure sensors that stimulate the SNS to vasoconstrict the arterial blood vessels) require time to readjust to the upright position. Under normal conditions, as a person changes from the lying to standing position, the arterial blood vessels experience a drop in blood pressure that stimulates the baroreceptors inside the walls of the arteries. The baroreceptors then stimulate the SNS to vasoconstrict arteries and increase heart rate in response to the drop in blood pressure. Blood pressure then readjusts to ensure cerebral perfusion.

When the patient with orthostatic hypotension attempts to rise to a standing position, they commonly experience a delay in arterial vasoconstriction, and the patient's blood pressure temporarily falls as they stand. During this episode, the patient experiences a temporary interval of inadequate cerebral perfusion. Patients often feel faint, dizzy, or weak; they may also be unable to stand and may experience syncope, or loss of consciousness. This transient episode of inadequate cerebral perfusion lasts until arterial vasoconstriction occurs to raise blood pressure.

> **ALERT!** A supine patient who attempts to assume the standing position quickly can experience symptoms of orthostatic hypotension. These symptoms include dizziness, tachycardia, diaphoresis, and possibly syncope. Clinicians need to be vigilant for this syndrome to prevent falls in patients and should assist patients in assuming a sitting position for a short time before standing.

> **ALERT!** Older individuals and individuals on antihypertensive medications have increased susceptibility to orthostatic hypotension.

Natriuresis

In the first few days of bedrest, body fluid volume redistribution causes a temporary natural diuretic effect called **natriuresis,** which is water loss from the body. Initially, when the body assumes the supine position, heightened centralized blood volume, which inhibits ADH and aldosterone, suppresses the baroreceptors. The suppression of ADH and aldosterone inhibits water reabsorption from the nephron tubules into the bloodstream and enhances natriuresis. Plasma volume becomes more concentrated with the initial water loss, but after a few days, fluid volume stabilizes.

Cardiovascular System Changes

With prolonged inactivity or immobility, the cardiovascular system becomes deconditioned and the heart must work harder and beat faster in order to eject sufficient ventricular blood to supply the organs with adequate circulation. Cardiac output initially increases in the supine position because of the redistribution of blood volume to the centralized region of the body. With extended periods of bedrest, however, venous return decreases, which diminishes cardiac filling. Left ventricular end diastolic volume decreases, stroke volume decreases, and reduced cardiac output results. To compensate for the decreased cardiac output, heart rate increases. A rapid heart rate compromises the amount of diastolic filling time in the ventricles.

Pulmonary System Changes

Bedrest and immobility cause pulmonary changes in lung volumes and breathing mechanics because the supine position is not conducive to full ventilation and lung expansion. In the upright position, breathing is facilitated by the rib cage, intercostal muscles, and diaphragm. In the supine condition, the abdominal muscles cannot optimally facilitate pulmonary expansion.

CLINICAL CONCEPT

Individuals must exert more energy to breathe in the supine position, and because of this, they tend to have shallow ventilations. Clinicians must recognize that the ideal position to facilitate the patient's breathing is in the upright, seated position.

Patients on bedrest have diminished ability to expand the lungs, decreased strength of cough, and consequent susceptibility to atelectasis, or collapse of the alveoli. Atelectasis causes areas of submaximal oxygenation within the lungs and consequent hypoxemia, or low oxygen in the bloodstream. Because of the lack of strength of the cough reflex and shallow ventilation, pulmonary secretions tend to accumulate and pool. Pooled pulmonary secretions create conditions conducive to pneumonia.

Bedridden patients are commonly at risk for aspiration or choking. Aspiration occurs when gastric contents or food particles are swallowed into the lungs versus the esophagus. Because of weakened muscles, pulmonary inefficiency, weakened cough, and possibly a weak gag reflex, the patient may not be able to adequately coordinate swallowing to prevent choking. The bedridden patient may also be at increased risk of gastroesophageal reflux, which can cause gastric contents to enter the lungs and lead to aspiration pneumonia.

Musculoskeletal System Changes

To function efficiently, muscles need periodic contraction and relaxation. The sliding actin and myosin subunits within a muscle require activation. Similarly, bones require weight-bearing conditions to stimulate their growth and remodeling. With immobility, muscle and bone experience negative effects.

Effects on Muscle

Unstimulated, noncontracting muscle fibers have fewer metabolic requirements and adapt by decreasing in size, which is why muscles undergo disuse atrophy when an individual is immobilized or on bedrest.

Muscles also weaken in strength and shorten in length with disuse. **Contractures** occur when muscles shorten over joints that are inactive for prolonged periods. An inactive joint contracts and constricts and becomes increasingly limited in terms of range of motion. The connective tissue around inactive joints also undergoes shortening and degeneration, which contributes to the contracture. This is most apparent in paralyzed individuals who do not receive range-of-motion exercises.

CLINICAL CONCEPT

Without activity, the joints naturally assume positions of flexion contractures—fingers clench and wrists flex inward, arms flex at the elbows, hips and legs flex toward the medial aspect of the body, and the neck flexes forward to bring the chin to the chest. The immobilized, inactive body will assume a fetal position if joints are allowed to develop contractures (see Fig. 4-3). For this reason, clinicians need to ensure proper body alignment, turn immobile patients, and perform daily passive range-of-motion exercises on those with limited mobility.

Effects on Bone

Bone also begins to degenerate with lack of weight-bearing activity or exercises. **Trabecular bones,** which have a nonsolid, latticelike interior, are the first to undergo degeneration because of inactivity. Cortical bone, which has a solid interior, degenerates slower.

The hip joint (femur head and neck), wrist, and vertebrae are areas that contain a high amount of trabecular bone. In individuals with osteoporosis, fracture is common in these areas. Vertebral compression fractures are also a major cause of disability in older adults. These fractures are often subtle, painful, and lead to the spinal deformities that cause the patient to assume a hunched posture.

ALERT! Hip fracture is a major cause of morbidity, disability, and mortality among older adults. Between 25% and 75% of older individuals who suffer hip fracture can neither walk independently nor achieve their previous level of independent living within 1 year after their fracture. Between 18% and 33% of older hip fracture patients die within 1 year of their fracture.

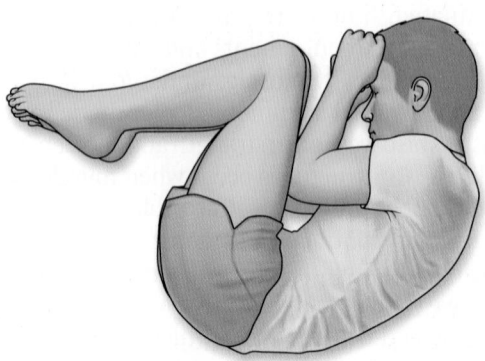

FIGURE 4-3. The fetal position.

Bone metabolism is a function of the opposing actions of the osteoblasts and osteoclasts. With lack of physical activity, osteoblasts are not sufficiently stimulated to keep producing bone; osteoclasts, however, continue to absorb bone unopposed. Osteoclastic activity overtakes osteoblastic activity, causing bone demineralization and osteoporosis.

When bones demineralize, calcium and phosphorus leach out into the bloodstream and then into the urine. The urinary calcium can increase susceptibility to kidney stone formation, particularly if the patient is dehydrated. In immobile patients, replacement of calcium without weight-bearing exercise is of no value and adds to the calcium excreted in the urine.

Osteoporosis from inactivity can weaken bones to the point of pathological fracture. A **pathological fracture** is a break in the bone's integrity caused by extreme stress from a nontraumatic etiology. The bone is internally weakened by a preexisting condition and fractures easily without trauma or with only slight trauma. Osteoporosis, neoplasms or cancerous tumors within bone, and metabolic conditions that internally weaken bones can cause pathological fracture.

CLINICAL CONCEPT

Osteoporosis often causes pathological fracture of the hip or vertebrae because these are composed of trabecular, nonsolid bone that undergoes deterioration earlier than cortical, solid bone.

Renal and Urological System Changes

The renal system functions optimally when gravitational forces assist urine to flow downward from the kidneys, into the ureters and bladder, and then into the urethra. The supine position does not facilitate urine drainage as efficiently as the upright position. Because of this, urinary stasis, or pooling of urine in the bladder, is more common when the patient is in the supine position.

CLINICAL CONCEPT

Urinary stasis, which occurs with prolonged immobility, predisposes to urinary tract infections because urine is a medium for bacteria.

ALERT! Prolonged bedrest places the individual at greater risk for kidney stone formation, as the excess protein and calcium from the deterioration of muscle and bone are excreted in the urine.

Gastrointestinal System Changes

The supine position is not conducive to efficient digestive processes and peristaltic activity. Peristaltic-wave activity significantly diminishes, and the lack of physical activity inhibits movement of intestinal contents and gas. Patients on bedrest also tend to have diminished appetite, slowed peristalsis, and decreased rate of intestinal absorption. The muscle atrophy that occurs also causes diminished strength of the diaphragm and abdominal and pelvic muscles, which are needed for defecation. Constipation is a frequent consequence of physical inactivity. In addition, the supine position increases susceptibility to gastroesophageal reflux.

 CLINICAL CONCEPT

In the upright position, gravitational forces pull gastric contents downward and oppose the regurgitation of fluids or food particles into the esophagus and pharynx. Elevation of the head and chest of the patient on bedrest can counteract the risk of reflux and possible aspiration.

Metabolic and Endocrine System Changes

Inactive people have lower energy requirements than those who exercise, but they also have lower metabolic rates. Lack of physical activity leads to muscle protein breakdown, catabolic activity, and negative nitrogen balance. Catabolism is the breakdown of cells and production of waste products from the degeneration. During catabolism, proteins derived from different body tissues break down into amino acids. Amino acids are nitrogen-rich compounds that keep the body supplied with a source of nitrogen. As proteins break down, amino acids released into the bloodstream are then excreted in the urine. The loss of amino acids diminishes the amount of nitrogen in the body, a state referred to as **negative nitrogen balance.**

Carbohydrate or glucose intolerance also begins to develop with prolonged physical inactivity. After 2 weeks of bedrest, peripheral cellular glucose uptake decreases by 50% and blood glucose levels rise. Pancreatic insulin secretion is forced to increase to maintain normal blood glucose levels.

Parathyroid hormone levels increase in response to immobility, which stimulates osteoclastic activity and bone degeneration and facilitates the leaching of calcium from bones. Calcium then increases in the bloodstream and enters the kidney. In the kidney an excess of calcium can precipitate in the urine and form kidney stones.

Thyroid hormone, growth hormone, and epinephrine levels change with immobility as well. Circadian rhythm peak and trough levels of these hormones change, which may be why persons on bedrest experience changes in appetite, sleep, and mood.

Integumentary System Changes

During bedrest, a large surface area of the skin is in contact with the bed and under constant pressure; this pressure is particularly transmitted to skin that lies over bony prominences, including the occiput of the skull, shoulders, elbows, sacrum, ankles, and heels. The constant pressure irritates the epithelium; impairs blood flow to the area under pressure; and interferes with tissue–blood exchange of nutrients, oxygen, and waste products. Also, body moisture and shear force from bed linens contribute to skin breakdown.

Pressure Ulcer/Pressure Injury

Skin breakdown and tissue ischemia can lead to the development of pressure injuries, previously called pressure ulcers, decubitus ulcers, or bedsores. There are four stages of **pressure injury.** These stages are categorized according to the depth of tissue involvement (see Fig. 4-4):

- **Stage I:** Skin exhibits persistent redness and irritation.
- **Stage II:** There is loss of skin in the epidermal or dermal layers.
- **Stage III:** Ulcers show deterioration of epidermis, dermis, and deeper layers of subcutaneous tissue.
- **Stage IV:** There is loss of full thickness of tissue down into the fascia, muscle, and bone.

 CLINICAL CONCEPT

Clinicians need to frequently reposition immobilized patients in bed and keep skin dry and free from irritation to prevent pressure injuries. Once pressure injuries form, extensive measures of wound care are necessary. Common sites for pressure injury are shown in Figure 4-5.

ALERT! Pressure injuries are vulnerable to bacterial contamination and infection; these can extend into the bloodstream and cause septicemia, which is a bloodstream infection.

Psychosocial Changes

Inactivity and prolonged bedrest can alter an individual's mood, orientation, and cognitive ability. Social isolation and sensory deprivation may also occur with prolonged inactivity and bedrest. Research shows that individuals exhibit heightened anxiety, depression,

Four stages of pressure injuries

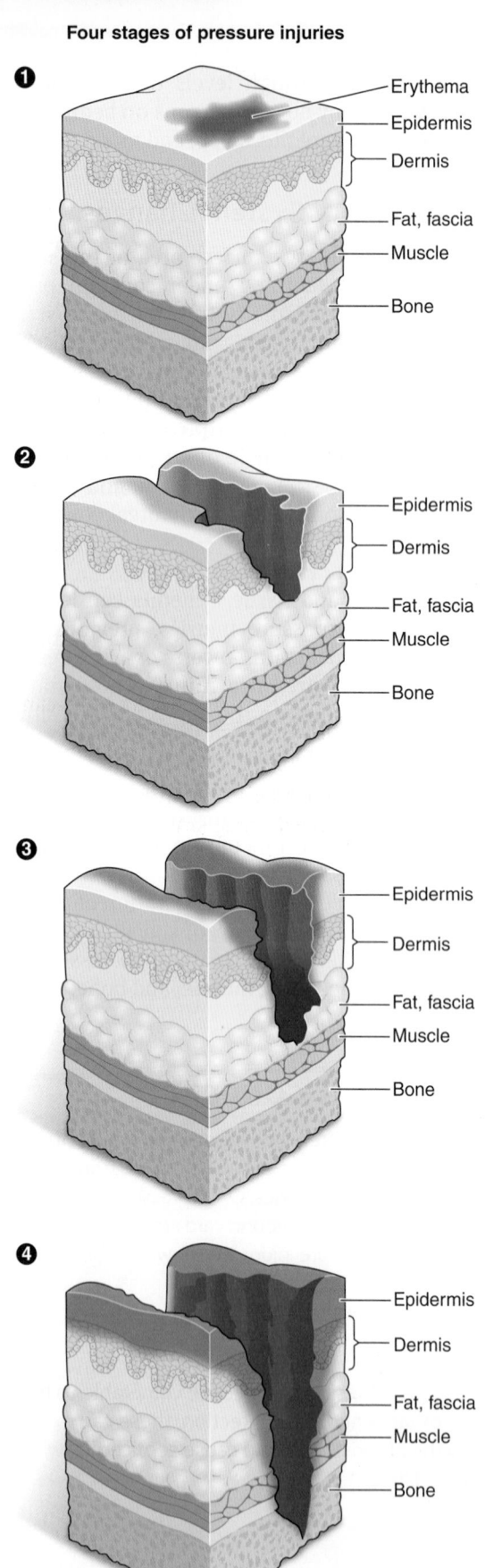

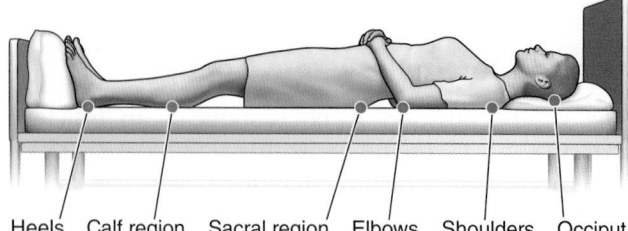

FIGURE 4-5. Sites at risk for pressure injuries for patients in the supine position.

Heels   Calf region   Sacral region   Elbows   Shoulders   Occiput

FIGURE 4-4. The four stages of pressure injury. Stage I: Epidermis has an area of persistent erythema over the region of skin subjected to pressure. Stage II: Area of skin loss and ulceration or blistering through epidermis and dermis. Stage III: Area of deep ulceration through dermis down through fat to fascia. Stage IV: Area of extensive destruction of tissue down through fascia, muscle, tendons, and exposing bones.

restlessness, fear, and mood swings when enduring isolation. Individuals can also experience decreased levels of concentration, decreased problem-solving ability, disorientation, hallucinations, vivid dreams, ineffective thought processes, and altered tactile responses. Older adults who are subjected to prolonged bedrest and social isolation commonly exhibit episodes of acute delirium, clinical depression, and cognitive decline.

Interventions to Counteract Effects of Immobility

Rehabilitative interventions are necessary to counteract the many systemic consequences of inactivity and prolonged bedrest. Active and passive range-of-motion exercises and early mobilization of hospitalized patients are necessary measures to prevent complications of inactivity. Isometric and aerobic exercise regimens can rebuild muscle, improve cardiac and pulmonary function, enhance GI activity, strengthen bones, and counteract venous stasis. Regular exercise is recommended to counteract depression and relieve mental stress.

To prevent skin breakdown and pressure injuries, patients on bedrest should assume positional changes at least every 2 hours, or more frequently, depending on the presence of other associated conditions. Immobile patients need to be turned onto their sides periodically. In general, the prone position is avoided because it hinders chest excursion for optimal respiratory function. When possible, patients should be seated in a chair for part of the day and ambulate small distances. Areas of the body where bony prominences irritate skin should be cushioned to relieve pressure. Special mattresses and padding are available for this purpose. Health-care providers should assess the patient's skin for areas of erythema and irritation periodically to prevent development of pressure injuries. Dependent areas, particularly the sacral region, need to be assessed frequently. TED stockings are used to facilitate venous return from the distal areas of the limbs upward.

Chapter Summary

- A stressor is a challenging demand on the body that arouses a response from multiple organ systems.

- Eustress is stress that results in a positive response.

- Adaptive ability is the way in which the individual manages the stress and reduces the effect of the stressor on their life.

- Selye's general adaptation syndrome of stress consists of three stages: alarm, resistance, and exhaustion.

- Stimulation of the SNS causes a fight-or-flight reaction.

- Cortisol powerfully enhances the body's ability to resist stress by mobilizing glucose, amino acids, and fat stores for cellular energy production.

- Long-term secretion of cortisol or prolonged use of pharmacological cortisone causes immunosuppression.

- According to McEwen, allostatic load can be defined as the wear and tear on body systems caused by stress reactions. In prolonged stress, hormones and catecholamines have a cumulative, noxious effect and are part of the allostatic load on the body.

- When stress exceeds the body's ability to adapt, allostatic overload results, which initiates pathophysiological disorders.

- There are five stages of sleep that begin after the body is relaxed and preparing for sleep. Stage 5, REM sleep, is necessary for restorative sleep.

- Exercise stimulates blood flow to the brain; this enhances secretion of the neurotransmitters serotonin, norepinephrine, and dopamine, which counteract depression and anxiety.

- Exercise has many systemwide therapeutic effects, including stimulation of vascular endothelial growth factor, elevation of HDL-C, and stimulation of osteoblastic activity.

- Immobility has widespread negative effects on the body, including susceptibility to skin breakdown, pulmonary infection, muscle atrophy, contractures, orthostatic hypotension, urolithiasis, osteoporosis, DVT, and PE.

- Skin breakdown in the form of pressure injury can occur over the bony prominences of the body when in the supine position for long intervals.

- Infection of pressure injuries is common and can lead to septicemia (systemwide infection).

Bibliography

Available online at fadavis.com

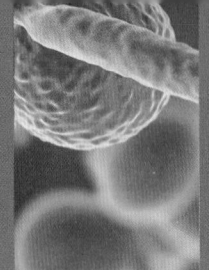

Obesity and Nutritional Imbalances

Learning Objectives

Upon completion of this chapter, the student will be able to:

- Identify the risk factors involved in the development of obesity.
- Describe the pathophysiological mechanisms involved in obesity.

- Recognize the methods of diagnosis in obesity.
- Discuss treatment measures for obesity.
- Give examples of vitamin and mineral imbalances.
- Recognize the signs and symptoms of eating disorders.

Key Terms

Adipokine

Adiponectin

Adiposity

Anorexia nervosa

Bariatric surgery

Basal metabolic rate (BMR)

Binge eating

Body mass index (BMI)

Bulimia nervosa

Dumping syndrome

Gastric banding

Ghrelin

Intragastric balloon therapy

Laparoscopic gastric sleeve surgery (LGS)

Leptin

Lipolysis

Night eating syndrome (NES)

Purging disorder

Resistin

Roux-en-Y gastric bypass (RYGB)

Few issues affect individuals as comprehensively as their weight. Many people in the United States and other industrialized nations struggle to maintain their weight within normal parameters. Once individuals exceed their ideal weight by 20%, they are considered overweight. When that level rises to 30%, they meet the criteria of obesity, which is defined as increased body weight related to excess fat accumulation. Obesity is particularly problematic because it predisposes an individual to multiple conditions, including cardiovascular disease, arthritis, diabetes, nonalcoholic fatty liver disease, and hyperlipidemia. It also exerts an effect on the whole body, including psychological well-being.

Epidemiology

There are a disproportionate number of obese individuals in the United States compared with the rest of the world. According to the latest reports from the National Institute of Diabetes and Digestive and Kidney Diseases, more than 65% of Americans are overweight or obese; in addition, 1 in 20 adults is morbidly obese. The National Heart, Lung, and Blood Institute rates obesity at epidemic proportions, and the problem is steadily worsening.

The United States doesn't stand alone when dealing with this health issue. Most industrialized nations have seen a tremendous increase in the rate of obese individuals. Over the last 20 years, the percentage of overweight adults worldwide has increased by 300%. In the United States, obesity prevalence rates have progressively risen, from 19.4% in 1997 to 42% in 2018.

Age

Once thought of as a problem of aging caused by increasingly sedentary lifestyles, obesity is becoming a greater problem among younger individuals. Recent studies have shown that more than 20% of children between the ages of 6 and 11 years old are obese. Childhood obesity, already at levels that are alarmingly high, continues to rise.

> **ALERT!** Childhood obesity is a direct contributor to adult obesity and predisposes to an earlier onset of myriad health problems.

Gender

According to the Centers for Disease Control and Prevention, 42.4% of the adult population in the United States is obese. In terms of gender, 37.9% of men and 41.1% of women are considered to be obese. If you combine the two categories of overweight and obesity, the prevalence estimates are 73.7% for men and 69% for women. Therefore, more than two-thirds of the U.S. population requires intervention for weight loss and management.

Race

There are large disparities in obesity prevalence by race-ethnic group. According to the CDC, 2021, non-Hispanic Black adults have the highest age-adjusted prevalence of obesity at 49.6%, followed by Hispanic adults at 44.8%, non-Hispanic White adults at 42.2%, and non-Hispanic Asian adults at 17.4%.

Socioeconomic Status

Obesity is linked to both affluence and poverty. Affluent individuals may overindulge and take in excessive calories—and in some developing nations, being overweight or obese may be viewed as a status symbol and a public representation of a person's wealth. By contrast, in the United States, obesity is associated with poverty and lack of appropriate food choices. Many people who live in lower socioeconomic areas have little or no access to nutrient-rich, low-calorie foods or fresh produce. Many in the lower socioeconomic areas rely on fast food, which is inexpensive and commonly rich in fat, sodium, and sugar.

Etiology

Obesity results when energy intake exceeds energy expenditure. If the body doesn't expend all the energy it takes in, it stores this energy as fat. However, individuals vary widely in their propensity to gain weight and accrue fat mass. People differ in their susceptibility to gain weight, even at identical levels of caloric input and activity. This indicates that factors other than excess food intake and inadequate activity are involved in the accumulation of excess body fat. A science of obesity is emerging and current research is broadening our understanding, but there are still many unanswered questions.

Obesity is a metabolic disorder caused by changes in cellular insulin sensitivity, glucose utilization, fat accumulation, hepatic glucose production, and fluid balance. Fat cells, also called *adipocytes,* are considered endocrine cells. They secrete **adipokines,** which are hormones and proteins that affect body metabolism. Adipocytes can increase in number and each cell can hypertrophy to cause fat mass.

The subcutaneous tissue and the omentum, the membranous covering over the intestine, are major areas of fat storage in the body. Visceral fat can be found surrounding organs as well. Adipokines affect cellular insulin sensitivity, fat breakdown, blood lipid levels, and hepatic glucose production. They also influence appetite, hunger, and satiety. The more adipose tissue in the body, the greater the influence of adipokines. Obesity itself increases susceptibility to additional accumulation of adipose tissue.

Genetics is another etiological factor of obesity, though the link between genetics and obesity is not well understood. Only a small number of genetic disorders are known to cause obesity. Data suggest that 5% of children who are obese have mutations at 2p23 and 18q21.3. Persons who lack the leptin gene or have leptin receptor gene mutations at 7q31 are found to be obese. Some patients with enzyme alterations caused by a mutation at 5q15-21 have significant obesity. Severe obesity is seen in individuals with a mutation in an adipocyte transcription factor gene at 3p25. Many different gene loci are being investigated as potential "obesity genes."

It is currently thought that a combination of genes and environmental influences is the cause of obesity. In addition, familial influences, traditions, and culture significantly contribute to the way individual eating habits develop.

Various disorders cause obesity as a secondary effect. Hypothyroidism, Cushing's syndrome, and polycystic ovarian syndrome are three diseases that cause body fat accumulation, but there are many others. When the primary disorder is remedied, obesity may no longer be a problem.

Pathophysiology

Adipose tissue provides insulation, warmth, and cushioning for body organs and serves as a storage depot for excess energy. However, fat is not simply a repository of triglycerides that break down into fatty acids. Adipocytes are metabolically active and secrete a wide variety of repetitive adipokines (see Fig. 5-1). Adipokines include the inflammatory mediators, tumor necrosis factor alpha (TNF-alpha), and interleukin-6 (IL-6), as well as the vascular activators angiotensinogen (AGT) and plasminogen activator inhibitor (PAI). Other adipokines, called *adiponectin, leptin,* and *resistin,* are "good" adipokines that regulate glucose, insulin, and lipid metabolism, respectively. Therefore, adipose tissue influences many metabolic processes in the body.

Adipokines

Adiponectin is a plasma protein that enhances cellular sensitivity to insulin, exerts anti-inflammatory effects, and protects against the formation of arteriosclerosis; it has an inverse relationship with the fat content, or **adiposity,** of the body. The lower the adiposity, the greater amount of adiponectin produced. The greater the adiposity, the less adiponectin produced.

High adiposity with resulting lower adiponectin decreases cellular sensitivity to insulin, which, in turn,

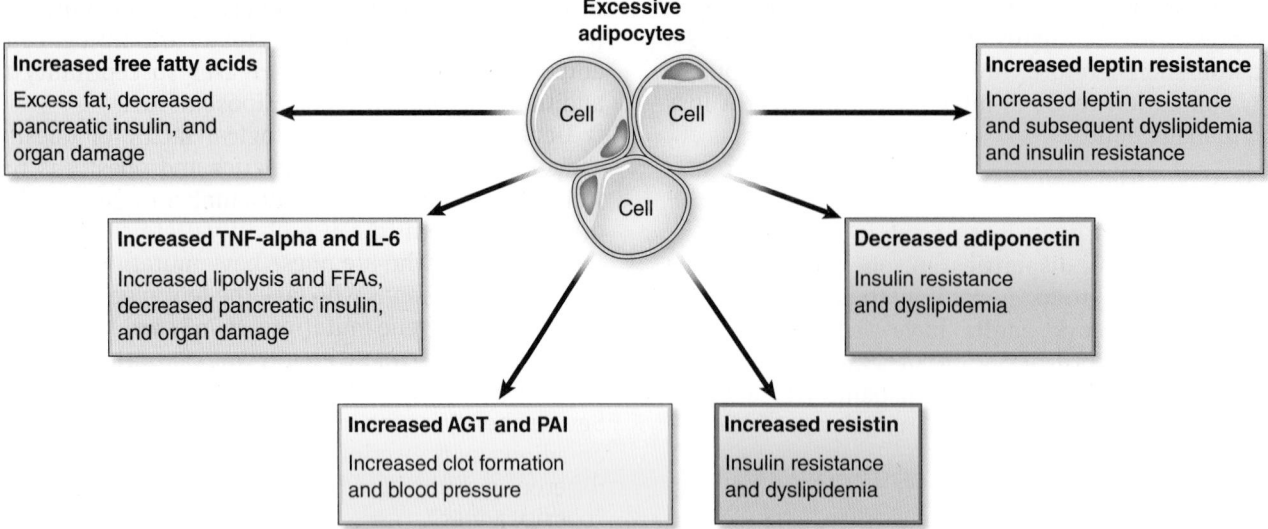

FIGURE 5-1. Adipocytes and released adipokines and their effects.

leads to glucose intolerance and subsequent elevations in blood glucose levels; this situation is also correlated with low high-density lipoprotein (HDL) levels and high triglyceride levels. Because of the beneficial effects, some researchers have referred to adiponectin as a "good" adipokine. However, obese individuals produce less adiponectin and cannot reap the benefits.

Leptin, another "good" adipokine, is a hormone produced by adipocytes that affects body weight, appetite, and energy expenditure. As the amount of fat stored in adipocytes rises, leptin is released into the blood and sends signals to the brain that the body has had enough to eat. Research shows that obese individuals have high levels of leptin but are resistant to its effects, resulting in leptin desensitization. This results in the individual not receiving a feeling of satiety after a meal. Leptin also works with adiponectin to enhance cellular sensitivity to insulin, reduce triglyceride levels, and inhibit fat accumulation.

Resistin is another adipokine that is found in the blood of individuals with obesity. It is known to interfere with the actions of insulin, causing insulin resistance in mice. Resistin also enhances hepatic glucose production, raises triglyceride levels, reduces HDL levels, and causes endothelial dysfunction that predisposes to early arteriosclerotic lesion formation. Whether resistin activity in mice can be ascribed to a similar role in humans is controversial. However, because of its actions, resistin has been called a "bad" adipokine.

Vascular Mediators as Adipokines

AGT is a precursor to angiotensin II, a major vasoconstrictor that raises blood pressure. Adipocytes release AGT, which has led to an association between excess adipose tissue and increased vascular tone. Studies have shown a correlation between high circulating levels of AGT, hypertension, and preliminary vascular changes of arteriosclerosis.

Tissue plasminogen activator (tPA) is one of the body's natural fibrinolytic substances that dissolves clots. PAI, a product of adipocytes, blocks the action of tPA. Because obesity produces PAI and blocks fibrinolysis, obesity increases susceptibility to clot formation. The combination of AGT and PAI is associated with clot formation, hypertension, and arteriosclerosis; therefore, these are "bad" adipokines. The larger the number of fat cells, the greater the risk of cardiovascular disease because of adipose tissue secretion of adipokines, AGT, and PAI.

Inflammatory Mediators as Adipokines

TNF-alpha and IL-6 are inflammatory mediators that reduce cellular insulin sensitivity, blunt the beneficial effect of adiponectin, and promote lipolysis. **Lipolysis** causes formation of free fatty acids (FFAs), which have negative effects on the body.

FFAs are highly destructive to tissues, causing damage to intracellular membranes through lipid oxidation and injury to mitochondria. Excess FFAs in the bloodstream are deposited in various organs, causing organ dysfunction. An excess of FFA overwhelms the pancreas, leading to reduced secretion of insulin and resulting glucose intolerance. Excess FFAs are also deposited in the liver, causing nonalcoholic steatohepatitis (NASH) (also called nonalcoholic fatty liver disease [NAFLD]) , which leads to cirrhosis. The myocardium is also affected by excess FFAs, decreasing the efficiency of the heart muscle. Therefore, excess adipose tissue, which secretes inflammatory mediators and indirectly stimulates formation of FFAs, can lead to pancreatic, liver, and myocardial dysfunction.

Intestinal Peptides and Food Intake

Food intake is influenced by hunger and satiety, which are regulated by the hypothalamus. Low blood glucose triggers the hunger center of the hypothalamus. The empty stomach also generates impulses interpreted as hunger pangs that transmit signals to the hypothalamus. **Ghrelin** is a peptide secreted in the stomach that stimulates hunger and regulates short-term food intake; it is also theorized to regulate long-term body weight and adiposity because it stimulates secretion of growth hormone.

Appetite is distinguished from hunger in that it is primarily the result of visual, olfactory, and emotional triggers. The appetite center is in a slightly different location of the hypothalamus than the hunger center. Variations in appetite are also influenced by culture, environment, and social and economic factors. Satiety, or a sense of fullness, usually occurs after consumption of a meal. Gut distention causes the release of peptides, cholecystokinin, and glucagon-like peptide in the gastrointestinal (GI) tract that gives the body a feeling of satiety and signals the brain to stop eating. Increased levels of circulating leptin also trigger the brain to stop eating.

Risk Factors

Each individual needs a certain number of calories to meet the needs of daily energy expenditure. Approximately 70% of required calories are utilized for energy by the body at rest. About 10% of caloric expenditure is used for the metabolic processing of food. The remaining 20% of calories are used for energy required for activity and exercise. As discussed earlier, weight gain occurs when caloric intake exceeds caloric expenditure, which is why risk factors for obesity include excess calorie ingestion and sedentary behavior. Other risk factors include poverty, female gender, age, smoking cessation, disorders that cause obesity as a secondary effect, and genetic susceptibility.

- **Excess calorie ingestion:** Poor food choices, such as fast foods that are high caloric and nutrient poor, put individuals at risk for obesity. Unlike home-cooked meals, fast food and restaurant meals are typically large in portion size and high in calories, salt, and fat.
- **Sedentary behavior:** Lack of physical activity is a major risk factor for obesity. Activity stimulates the use of glucose by the muscles and subsequent activation of fat stores.
- **Poverty:** Poverty is a risk factor because people living in impoverished communities usually have fewer healthy food choices and fewer recreational areas for exercise. Many urban and rural areas in the United States do not have supermarkets or grocery stores that provide fresh produce and healthy food choices; these are referred to as food deserts.
- **Female gender:** On average, men have more muscle than women. Because muscle burns more calories than other types of tissue, men use more calories than women, even at rest, which is why women are more likely than men to gain weight with the same calorie intake. Pregnancy is also a risk factor for obesity. Women tend to weigh an average of 4 to 6 pounds more after a pregnancy than before the pregnancy. Weight gain often compounds with each pregnancy, and this weight gain contributes to obesity in women.
- **Age:** People tend to lose muscle and gain fat as they age, and they also experience a slowing of their metabolic rate. These consequences of aging lower calorie requirements; if older individuals don't change their eating habits or increase their activity level, they will then put on weight.
- **Smoking cessation:** When used habitually, cigarettes can act as an appetite suppressant. Habitual cigarette smokers generally have lower body weight than comparably aged nonsmokers. In addition, habitual smokers who abstain from smoking often have an increase in body weight. Both psychological and physiological explanations have been suggested to account for this phenomenon. Research studies show that nicotine administration and cigarette smoking are accompanied by a decreased consumption of sweet-tasting, high-caloric foods. These findings may help explain the changes in body weight that accompany smoking cessation. Persons who stop smoking report an average weight gain of 10 pounds.
- **Disorders that cause obesity as a secondary effect:** Many disorders cause obesity as a secondary effect (see Box 5-1). For example, persons affected by hypothyroidism are susceptible to obesity because of a lack of thyroid hormone. Cushing's syndrome, caused by the overactivity of the adrenal gland, also causes weight gain. Many disorders increase the risk of obesity; usually, if the major pathological condition is remedied, the accumulation of fat can be alleviated.

BOX 5-1. Disorders and Conditions That Cause Obesity

Cushing's syndrome
Prader-Willi syndrome
Growth hormone deficiency
Hypogonadism
Hypothalamic obesity
Hypothyroidism
Insulinoma
Polycystic ovarian syndrome
Pregnancy
Pseudohypoparathyroidism
Tube-feeding–related obesity

- **Genetic susceptibility:** Genetic susceptibility to obesity is a subject that requires more research. Only a few genetic disorders are known to directly cause obesity, but there is a wide spectrum of ways in which genes can favor fat accumulation in a given environment.

Genes can influence the body in the following ways:

- Drive to overeat
- Tendency to be sedentary
- Diminished ability to use dietary fats as fuel
- Enlarged, easily stimulated capacity to store body fat

Not all people living in industrialized countries with abundant food and reduced physical activity become obese, nor do all obese people have the same body fat distribution or suffer the same health issues. This diversity occurs among groups of the same racial or ethnic background and even within families living in the same environment. The variation in how people respond to the same environmental conditions is an additional indication that genes play a role in the development of obesity.

Clinical Manifestations

Body weight consists of lean body mass and fat. Obese individuals have an excess amount of fat on their bodies. Overweight individuals have a body weight that is approximately 20% over ideal weight. Obesity occurs when a patient's body weight is approximately 30% over the ideal. Morbid obesity is diagnosed when an individual's body weight is 40% or more greater than ideal.

The location of fat accumulation on an individual's body often can be categorized as apple shaped or pear shaped. Apple-shaped, or central, obesity is characterized by fat accumulation around the abdomen. Pear-shaped obesity is characterized by fat accumulation around the hips and buttocks. Central obesity has a higher associated risk of health problems.

In obese persons, fat accumulation is not limited to the subcutaneous region. On autopsy, it is apparent that organs are covered in visceral fat, and the heart and arteries collect fat within both the interior and outer walls. Researchers find that there is high cardiometabolic disease risk from excess visceral adipose tissue—excess fat accumulation in liver, heart, and lean muscle tissue.

> ### CLINICAL CONCEPT
> Central obesity is associated with cardiovascular disease risk. A waist measurement that exceeds 35 inches in women or 40 inches in men is considered a cardiovascular risk factor.

Diagnosis

Two key factors in determining obesity are amount and location of body fat. Typically, the amount of body fat is difficult to measure. The main techniques used for this purpose are categorized as follows:

- **Density-based:** Hydrodensitometry and air displacement plethysmography
- **Scanning:** Computed tomography (CT), magnetic resonance imaging, and dual-energy x-ray absorptiometry
- **Bioelectrical impedance and anthropometric:** Skinfold, waist circumference, and waist-to-hip ratio

The majority of these methods are not practical for patient use and are limited to research settings. Anthropometric measures using skinfold calipers are most commonly used to estimate an individual's percentage of body fat. It is recommended that three specific sites be measured on the body:

- **Men:** Chest, abdomen, and thigh
- **Women:** Triceps, suprailiac, and thigh

It is recommended that the three sites be measured three times each to get as near an accurate result as possible. Mathematical equations have been developed to yield percentage of body fat based on skinfold measurements (see Box 5-2).

Lean body mass is determined by multiplying body fat percentage by weight; the result is an estimate of how many pounds of fat make up the body. Subtract that number from weight, and this yields lean body mass. It is generally recommended that females have no more than 30% and males have no more than 25% body fat.

The most common method used to compare a patient's body weight to the ideal standard is the calculation of **body mass index (BMI).** BMI makes a comparison of height to weight and gives a score in relationship to ranges (see Box 5-3). The formula for BMI is:

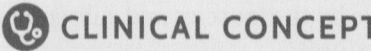

$$\text{Weight in pounds} \times 703 \,/\, \text{height in inches} \,/\, \text{height in inches}$$

Weight in pounds × 703 divided by height in inches and then divided by height in inches again.

> ### CLINICAL CONCEPT
> BMI may not be accurate in individuals with high muscle mass.

> ### CLINICAL CONCEPT
> Weight cycling, also known as yo-yo dieting, has been associated with increased cardiovascular disease in some research studies. Weight fluctuation is also a risk factor for gallbladder disease.

BOX 5-2. Calculating Percentage of Body Fat

The formula for men is:

%Fat = 495 / (1.0324 – 0.19077(log(waist – neck)) + 0.15456(log(height))) – 450

The formula for women is:

%Fat = 495 / (1.29579 – 0.35004(log(waist + hip – neck)) + 0.22100(log(height))) – 450

The American Council on Exercise uses the following categories based on percentage of body fat:

	Women	Men
Essential fat	10% to 12%	2% to 4%
Athletes	14% to 20%	6% to 13%
Fitness	21% to 24%	14% to 17%
Acceptable	25% to 31%	18% to 25%
Obese	32% or more	26% or more

LEAN BODY MASS OR FAT-FREE MASS. This is derived by subtracting the calculated value of body fat from the total weight.

Lean Body Mass = Weight × (100 – % Body Fat)

BOX 5-3. Body Mass Index Values

- Underweight: <18.5
- Normal weight: 18.5–24.9
- Overweight: 25–29.9
- Obesity: ≥30
- Morbid obesity: ≥40

Treatment

Diet

Nutrient balance is achieved by consuming foods from each of the three major categories: carbohydrates, proteins, and lipids, as well as vitamins and minerals. The U.S. Department of Agriculture (USDA) provides guidelines for nutritional intake on the Web site choosemyplate.gov, which aims to guide consumers in healthy food choices by detailing approximately the amount of different food types that should appear on a plate of food (see Fig. 5-2). In addition, the USDA

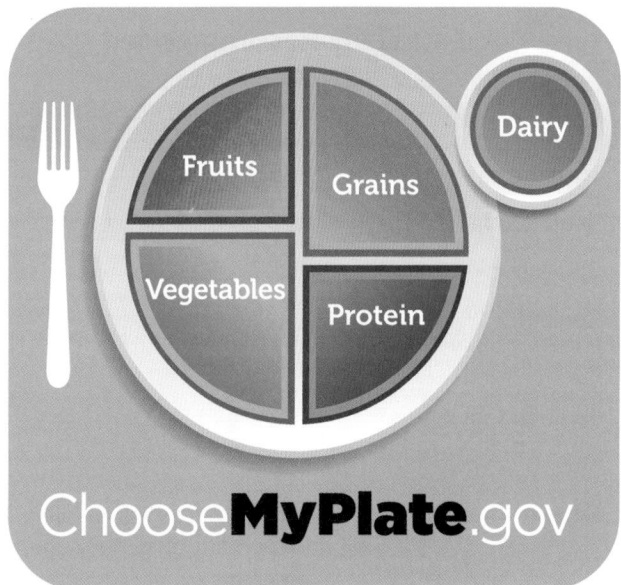

FIGURE 5-2. USDA MyPlate. *(Courtesy of the USDA's Center for Nutrition Policy and Promotion.)*

publishes recommended daily allowances for all nutrients (see Table 5-1).

Dietary approaches to treating obesity involve calorie restriction. Adjustments made to the diet must create a negative caloric balance. Total calories consumed daily must be fewer than calories expended. The recommended method begins by calculating an individual's **basal metabolic rate (BMR),** the minimum caloric requirement needed to sustain metabolic processes in a resting state (see Box 5-4). This calculation is based on age, sex, and size. BMR is responsible for burning up to 70% of total calories expended per day. The remaining 30% of calories are used for activity.

According to exercise physiologists McArdle and Katch, the average maintenance level for women in the United States is 2000 to 2100 calories per day and the average for men is 2700 to 2900 per day. These are only averages; caloric expenditure varies widely among individuals and is higher for athletes and lower for sedentary individuals.

Based on an average intake of 2000 calories per day, a low-calorie diet creates a caloric deficit of 500 to 1000 cal/day, which will yield a weight loss of 1 to 2 pounds per week. These diets, which allow approximately 1000 to 1500 cal/day, may be balanced in nutrient intake or may be restrictive of certain food groups. These diets are best used for individuals with a BMI of 35 or greater.

Very low-calorie diets allow 800 calories or fewer per day and are reserved for people with a BMI greater than 30 who need to achieve rapid weight loss. Individuals can lose about 3 to 5 pounds per week. Long-term results may not be any more effective than those achieved with less-restrictive plans. This diet regimen should be used only under the supervision of a healthcare provider.

TABLE 5-1. Daily Recommended Allowances*

Nutrient	Daily Values
Total fat	<65 g
Saturated fat	<20 g
Cholesterol	<300 mg
Sodium	<2,400 mg
Potassium	3,500 mg
Total carbohydrates	<300 g
Fiber	25 g
Protein	approximately 45 g–60 g (depending on gender, age, pregnancy)
VITAMINS	
Calcium	1,000 mg
Folate	400 mcg
Iron	18 mg
Niacin	20 mg
Riboflavin	1.7 mg
Thiamin	1.5 mg
Vitamin A	5,000 IU
Vitamin B_6	2.0 mg
Vitamin B_{12}	6.0 mcg
Vitamin C	60 mg
Vitamin D	400 IU
Vitamin E	30 IU
Vitamin K	80 mcg

*Based on a 2000-calorie intake; for adults and children 4 or more years of age. (Courtesy of the U.S. Food and Drug Administration.)
<, less than

CLINICAL CONCEPT

Benefits of weight loss, such as decreased blood pressure in hypertension and improved glycemic control in diabetes, are seen with even a small reduction in weight.

Activity

Activity is related to weight management by causing caloric expenditures. Moderate levels of physical activity help maintain the balance of caloric intake and expenditure, and therefore weight. Increases in

BOX 5-4. Calculating Basal Metabolic Rate

To calculate BMR, use the following formulas. Keep in mind that 1 inch equals 2.54 centimeters and 1 kilogram equals 2.2 pounds.
- **Men:** BMR = 66 + (13.7 × wt in kg) + (5 × ht in cm) – (6.8 × age in years)
- **Women:** BMR = 655 + (9.6 × wt in kg) + (1.8 × ht in cm) – (4.7 × age in years)
- **Example:** You are a 30-year-old woman who is 5′6″ (167.6 cm) tall and weighs 120 lb (54.5 kg). Your BMR = 655 + (9.6 × 54.5) + (1.8 × 167.6) – (4.7 × 30) = 655 + 523 + 302 – 141 = 1,339 calories/day.

Now that you know your BMR, you can calculate total daily energy expenditure by multiplying your BMR by your activity multiplier:
- **Sedentary:** BMR × 1.2 (little or no exercise)
- **Lightly active:** BMR × 1.375 (light exercise/sports 1–3 days/wk)
- **Moderately active:** BMR × 1.55 (moderate exercise/ sports 3–5 days/wk)
- **Very active:** BMR × 1.725 (hard exercise/sports 6–7 days/wk)
- **Extra active:** BMR × 1.9 (hard daily exercise/sports, a physical job, or twice-a-day training [i.e., marathon, contest])
- **Example:** Your BMR is 1,339 calories per day. You work out three to four times per week, so your activity level is moderately active. Your activity factor is 1.55. Your total daily energy expenditure = 1.55 × 1,339 = 2,075 calories/day.

physical activity, especially aerobic activity, stimulates the use of glucose and subsequent activation of glycogen stores. After utilization of glycogen stores, fat becomes mobilized and reduced. Walking is a simple activity recommended by most clinicians. Different kinds of physical activity allow for different amounts of calorie expenditure (see Table 5-2).

Pharmacology

Pharmacological agents are possible adjunctive treatments when combined with lifestyle changes. Weight loss results are modest and medications are usually effective for only as long as the medication is taken.

According to the NIH, pharmaceutical interventions should be reserved for individuals who have increased medical risks related to obesity. Medications such as appetite suppressants are only for short-term use and require health-care provider prescription. Appetite suppressants commonly do not facilitate long-term maintenance of weight reduction. Individuals need to also employ behavior modifications and dietary adjustments and engage in some physical activity along with appetite suppressants.

TABLE 5-2. Exercise and Calorie Expenditure

A 154-pound man who is 5'10" will use up (burn) about the number of calories listed doing each activity here. **Those who weigh more will use more calories; those who weigh less will use fewer calories.** The calorie values listed include both calories used by the activity and the calories used for normal body functioning during the activity time.

	Approximate calories used (burned) by a 154–pound man	
MODERATE physical activities	In 1 hour	In 30 minutes
Hiking	370	185
Light gardening/yard work	330	165
Dancing	330	165
Golf (walking and carrying clubs)	330	165
Bicycling (less than 10 mph)	290	145
Walking (3.5 mph)	280	140
Weight training (general light workout)	220	110
Stretching	180	90
VIGOROUS physical activities	In 1 hour	In 30 minutes
Running/jogging (5 mph)	590	295
Bicycling (more than 10 mph)	590	295
Swimming (slow freestyle laps)	510	255
Aerobics	480	240
Walking (4.5 mph)	460	230
Heavy yard work (chopping wood)	440	220
Weight lifting (vigorous effort)	440	220
Basketball (vigorous)	440	220

From USDA. ChooseMyPlate.gov. Retrieved from https://www.choosemyplate.gov/physical-activity-calories-burn.

Over-the-counter appetite suppressants are generally not recommended because of their sympathomimetic side effects.

Semaglutide (Ozempic, Rybelsus), a glucagon-like peptide-1 (GLP-1) receptor agonist, is used to treat type 2 diabetes and has shown efficacy in facilitating weight loss. This agent stimulates insulin release and inhibits glucagon secretion, slows gastric emptying, and increases satiety after eating. It is labeled as an adjunct to diet and exercise for weight management in overweight or obese adults. Studies show patients can lose from 10 to 13 lbs on average when continually taking this medication combined with diet and exercise. Semiglutide improves cardiometabolic markers such as blood pressure, waist circumference, body mass index, and A1c. However, long-term maintenance of these improvements remains uncertain (Wilding, 2021).

 CLINICAL CONCEPT

Antiobesity pharmacological agents are indicated for individuals with a BMI of 30 or more or a BMI of 27 or more with concurrent obesity-related medical problems. Individuals should be under a health-care provider's care while on the agent.

Surgical Options

Liposuction is considered a minor procedure that focuses on fat reduction in a specific site. For individuals with severe obesity, bariatric surgery is recommended. The two categories of bariatric surgery are gastric bypass and gastric restrictive procedures.

Liposuction

Liposuction is the most commonly performed cosmetic procedure in the United States. The ideal candidate is physically fit and eats well-balanced meals but is unable to reduce a fatty deposit that is well localized. Liposuction does not remove visceral fat (fat around organs). Small-volume liposuction is commonly performed on an outpatient basis under local anesthesia. Large-volume liposuction may require general anesthesia. A small incision and tunnel are formed at the site of subcutaneous fat accumulation. A suction catheter is used to remove fat. Compression garments and absorptive pads are applied for the immediate postoperative period. Return to physical activities may occur within a few days depending on the patient's comfort. Complications are minimal, with the most significant complications attributed to anesthesia or fluid shifts secondary to large-volume liposuction. To maintain weight loss, individuals must adhere to behavior modification guidelines.

ALERT! Liposuction performed in one session for persons who are morbidly obese is associated with high risk of mortality from fluid shifts.

Bariatric Surgery

Surgical therapy to decrease obesity is termed **bariatric surgery.** This is appropriate for persons with a BMI of 40 or greater and individuals with a BMI of between 35 and 40 who have medical problems related to their obesity. Successful bariatric surgery has been shown to reduce weight and provide beneficial physiological changes in the patient. After weight reduction, patients often experience resolution of hypertension, diabetes, sleep apnea, NASH (NAFLD), hyperlipidemia, and other complications of obesity.

To determine eligibility for surgical procedures, patients must undergo a thorough assessment. Two general categories of the procedures are gastric bypass and gastric restrictive procedures.

Intragastric Balloon Therapy. **Intragastric balloon (IGB) therapy** is the insertion of a space-occupying device into the stomach by endoscopy. This space-occupying device gives the patient the sensation of gastric fullness, which in turn impedes overeating. Patients with intragastric balloons can eat less during a meal and feel satiated. Studies show significant weight loss in patients after 6 months of therapy. However, long-term maintenance of weight reduction requires patient continuance of lifestyle and diet modifications. Studies show avoidance of obesity-related comorbidities such as new-onset diabetes mellitus for up to 5 years. However, studies also show that some patients require repeat IGB therapy to achieve goals after 6 months and some patients use this procedure as a bridge to major bariatric surgery (Chan et al., 2021).

Laparoscopic Roux-en-Y Gastric Bypass. **Roux-en-Y gastric bypass (RYGB)** is done by surgically restructuring the upper portion of the stomach to leave an extremely small pouch available for food digestion. The surgeon then connects the stomach to the jejunum portion of the small intestine, bypassing the duodenum and leaving it as a blind pouch.

The procedure promotes weight loss in two ways. First, it limits the volume of food consumed to $\frac{1}{2}$ to 1 ounce and the individual experiences satiety sooner. Second, it alters the ability of the stomach and small bowel to absorb calories and nutrients, while simultaneously preserving the health of the remaining distal portion of the stomach. RYGB alters hormonal responses by bypassing the duodenum and excluding the fundus of the stomach. Ghrelin levels are lower and leptin levels higher after RYGB, which results in decreased hunger and increased satiety.

RYGB usually results in significant weight loss in a short period. At 2 years postsurgery, the expected weight loss from an RYGB is approximately 70% to 75% of that in excess of a patient's ideal body weight. For example, a patient who is 6 feet tall and weighs 400 pounds is approximately 200 pounds overweight. This patient can expect to lose 150 pounds after the surgery. To maintain weight loss, individuals must adhere to behavior modification guidelines.

Along with weight loss, RYGB has been shown to decrease lipid levels, reduce the incidence of diabetes, improve blood pressure, reduce sleep apnea, and reduce gastroesophageal reflux disease (GERD). However, multiple potential complications exist. Malabsorption and dumping syndrome commonly occur, and nutritional supplements are necessary. It is particularly important to include calcium and vitamin D in the diet or supplement, as lack of these nutrients can lead to osteopenia or osteoporosis. Postoperative GI leak, stomal stenosis, jejunal ulceration, gastric fistula, small bowel obstruction, and intestinal hernia are possible complications.

Gastric Banding. **Gastric banding,** such as vertical banding and lap-band procedures, are done by surgically separating a smaller upper portion of the stomach from the lower portion, while maintaining a small opening between the two sections. The banding process keeps the opening from enlarging. The anatomical attachment of the duodenum to the distal portion of the stomach is undisturbed. The gastric band consists of a soft, locking silicone ring connected to an infusion port placed in the subcutaneous tissue. The port may be accessed using a syringe and needle. Injection of saline into the port leads to reduction in the band diameter, resulting in an increased degree of restriction. This procedure promotes weight loss by limiting the amount of food that can be consumed and producing early satiety. The goal of gastric banding is to give the patient a restriction of approximately 1 cup of dried food and satiety for at least 1.5 to 2 hours after a meal.

Laparoscopic Sleeve Gastrectomy. In **laparoscopic sleeve gastrectomy (LSG),** a large portion of the stomach along the greater curvature is removed; approximately 70% to 80% is surgically excised (see Fig. 5-3). This decreases the size of the stomach and the patient's capacity for food ingestion. There are also some anorexic effects after LSG due to changes in hormonal control of appetite. Ghrelin, an appetite stimulant, is normally secreted by glands in the fundus of the stomach. LSG removes this region of the stomach so the patient feels appetite satiety early in the course of eating a meal. Glucagon-like peptide (GLP-1) is increased after LSG, and it is theorized that increased levels of GLP-1 contribute to weight loss by improving glucose metabolism, reducing hunger, and increasing satiety.

After sleeve gastrectomy, the patient does not endure side effects of malabsorption. Patients should consume a high-protein, low-fat diet and supplement with multivitamins, iron, and calcium, usually on a twice-daily basis. Ursodiol may be given to minimize the risk of developing gallstones during the period of acute weight loss. Patients must modify their eating habits by avoiding chewy meats and other foods that may inhibit normal emptying of their stomach pouch. Metabolic blood tests should be performed on a frequent basis: at 6 months after surgery, 12 months after surgery, and then annually thereafter. At 5 years after LSG, the average patient loses 60.5% of excess body weight and achieves a BMI of 30. Besides weight loss, LSG has also been shown to result in improvement or resolution of a number of comorbid medical conditions such as diabetes. Postoperative bleeding after LSG has been seen in up to 15% of cases. It can occur within the lumen of the stomach, intra-abdominally, or at the incision sites. LSG can also be complicated by staple line leak along the stomach or development of stricture within the stomach. Surgical reintervention may be required if complications develop. Portomesenteric vein thrombosis has been reported in up to 1% of patients undergoing LSG. Epigastric pain is the most common symptom. Diagnosis is usually made on CT scan of the abdomen. Stable patients with nonocclusive disease can be treated with anticoagulation for 3 to 6 months. Patients with occlusive disease require thrombolysis and/or operative thrombectomy and subsequent anticoagulation.

Surgical Complications

Although the procedures described can be performed by laparoscopy, they carry all of the typical operative risks such as vascular injury, bowel perforation, wound infection, fascial dehiscence, or complications of pneumoperitoneum. In addition to those risks, gastric procedures may cause vitamin and mineral deficiencies, especially of B_{12}, calcium, and iron. Herniation of the proximal stomach pouch, rupture of the suture line, and vomiting may also occur.

Dumping syndrome, also called *rapid gastric emptying,* is another possible postoperative complication. It occurs when the undigested contents of the stomach are transported, or "dumped," into the small intestine too rapidly. Dumping syndrome causes malabsorption of important nutrients, vitamins, and minerals. Symptoms that occur shortly after eating include abdominal cramps, nausea, and diarrhea. Diarrhea, sweating, tachycardia, and severe hypotension can occur hours after eating. Some people also experience hypoglycemia related to excessive levels of insulin delivered to the bloodstream as part of the syndrome. Most cases of dumping syndrome improve as the digestive system adjusts and the patient learns to modify eating habits by eating smaller meals a few times a day; avoiding fluids with meals; eating high-protein, high-fiber meals; and limiting high-sugar foods and fluids. Alternatively, clinicians can prescribe medications such as acarbose or octreotide that slow the passage of food out of the stomach.

Nutritional Imbalances

Nutritional imbalances include vitamin and mineral deficiencies and excesses. Both types of disorders have serious adverse effects on the body.

Vitamin and Mineral Deficiencies

Vitamin deficiencies can have serious effects on overall health (see Table 5-3). B vitamins and vitamin C are water soluble and are not stored in the body. Deficiencies of B vitamins are related to beriberi (thiamine), pellagra (niacin), irritability and depression (B_6), and

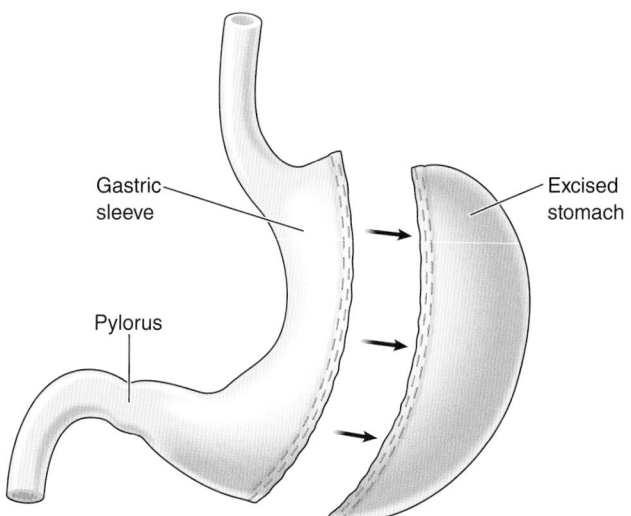

Gastric sleeve

Excised stomach

Pylorus

FIGURE 5-3. Laparoscopic gastric sleeve surgery.

TABLE 5-3. Vitamin and Mineral Deficiencies

Vitamin/Mineral	Clinical Disorder Related to Deficiency
Folate	Megaloblastic anemia
Niacin	Pellagra: pigmented rash on sun-exposed areas
Riboflavin	Cheilosis: fissures and irritation at edges of mouth
Thiamine	Beriberi: neuropathy, muscle weakness, and wasting
Vitamin A	Night blindness
Vitamin B_6	Neuropathy, depression, microcytic anemia
Vitamin B_{12}	Megaloblastic anemia
Vitamin C	Scurvy: petechiae, ecchymosis, inflamed and bleeding gums
Vitamin D	Rickets: skeletal deformities, osteomalacia
Vitamin E	Peripheral neuropathy, retinopathy, skeletal muscle atrophy
Vitamin K	Bleeding, elevated prothrombin time

megaloblastic anemia (folic acid and B_{12}). Insufficient vitamin C leads to scurvy.

Fat-soluble vitamins—A, D, E, and K—can be stored in the liver and fat tissue; as such, they are less likely to be related to deficits. Although labeled a vitamin, vitamin D is a hormone produced in the body as a result of exposure to sunshine. Vitamin D works in close correlation with parathyroid hormones to regulate the absorption of calcium. Individuals with little opportunity for sun exposure, such as homebound persons or those living in northern climates, may need to take vitamin D supplements.

Minerals are as essential as vitamins in maintaining normal physiological functioning. Mineral deficits can be reflected in diminished capacity to maintain water balance, conduct nerve impulses, and contract muscle fibers. For example:

- Calcium deficit is related to decreased bone formation and altered nerve conduction.
- Iron deficit is related to fatigue and anemia.
- Potassium deficit is related to muscle weakness, especially of cardiac muscle.
- Sodium deficit can be associated with weakness and GI disturbances.
- Zinc deficits are related to inadequate growth, especially secondary sex characteristics.

Vitamin and Mineral Excesses

Vitamin and mineral excesses, which occur when an individual consumes large quantities of vitamins and minerals over short periods, can lead to toxicity. Medical problems triggered by excess vitamins, or hypervitaminosis, are as serious as those caused by vitamin deficits. Overdoses of fat-soluble vitamins are more dangerous than those of water-soluble vitamins. For example, extremely large doses of vitamin A may cause nausea, vomiting, abdominal pain, hair loss, and headaches. Excess vitamin D can lead to nausea, vomiting, loss of appetite, and confusion. Among water-soluble vitamins, excesses of vitamin C can cause diarrhea and nausea. Excess vitamin B_6 is related to irreversible nerve damage.

 CLINICAL CONCEPT

Excessive amounts of vitamins are generally defined as 10 times the recommended level.

Eating Disorders

Eating disorders include anorexia nervosa, bulimia nervosa, and binge eating. Some persons with eating disorders also engage in purging. Purging includes self-induced vomiting, laxative abuse, inappropriate diuretic use, and excessive exercising.

Anorexia Nervosa

Anorexia nervosa is an eating disorder characterized by an individual who refuses to maintain body weight within minimal normal standards. Although individual weights may vary, weights that fall below the 85th percentile, or a BMI of less than 17.5, may indicate anorexia nervosa.

The term *anorexia* is a bit of a misnomer: by pure definition, it actually describes a loss of appetite. The individual with anorexia nervosa does not lose appetite; instead, he or she intentionally undertakes starvation practices. Individuals often have a disturbed body image, imagining their body as fat. The individual achieves weight loss by a number of means such as severely restricting diet, binging and purging, misusing laxatives and diuretics, and exercising excessively.

Patients with anorexia nervosa often display other personality traits such as a desire for perfection, academic success, and a denial of hunger in the face of starvation. Psychiatric characteristics include excessive dependency needs, developmental immaturity, social isolation, obsessive-compulsive behavior, and constriction of affect. Many patients also have comorbid mood disorders, with depression being most prevalent.

In the United States, prevalence of anorexia nervosa is 0.3% to 1%; however, some studies have shown rates as high as 4% among women. The rates among men are estimated at 0.1%. It is difficult to estimate prevalence, as many individuals do not admit to eating disorders. As much as 13% of adolescent girls exhibit symptoms of anorexia but do not meet full diagnostic criteria. Anorexia nervosa is found in all developed countries and in all socioeconomic classes. Eighty-five percent of patients have onset between the ages of 13 and 18.

In any eating disorder, malnutrition can lead to protein deficiency, hypoglycemia, anemia, and vitamin deficiencies. Thyroid function can become suppressed, and electrolyte disturbances are common. Delayed puberty, amenorrhea, anovulation, low estrogen states, increased growth hormone, decreased antidiuretic hormone, hypercarotenemia, and hypothermia can occur. Decreased gonadotropin levels and hypogonadism may occur among males who are affected.

Prolonged starvation can affect many body systems. Cardiovascular effects include mitral valve prolapse, supraventricular and ventricular dysrhythmias, long QT syndrome, bradycardia, orthostatic hypotension, and congestive heart failure. Renal disturbances include decreased glomerular filtration rate, elevated blood urea nitrogen (BUN), edema, acidosis with dehydration, hypokalemia, hypochloremic alkalosis with vomiting, hypoalbuminemia, and hyperaldosteronism. GI findings include constipation, delayed gastric emptying, and gastric dilation and rupture when binge eating. Patients who induce vomiting develop dental enamel erosion, palatal trauma, enlarged parotids, esophagitis, Mallory-Weiss lesions, and elevated liver enzymes.

Studies show that with psychiatric treatment, 47% of patients with anorexia show complete recovery, 33% show some improvement, and 20% of patients develop chronic, relapsing anorexia. Mortality rates are from 4% to 18%, and suicide is a common cause of death.

Bulimia Nervosa

Bulimia nervosa is an eating disorder characterized by two key features:

1. An individual eats a very large quantity of food in a short period. This is considered binging and usually takes place in a specified amount of time, often in minutes and usually less than 2 hours. For diagnostic purposes, these binges must occur at least twice weekly for 3 months or longer. Generally, the type of food consumed is high in calories and sugar. This binging is usually associated with a sense of loss of control perceived by the individual.

2. The individual will rid himself or herself of the food just eaten to avoid any associated weight gain. The individual may utilize similar inappropriate behaviors as the anorexic, including vomiting, laxative abuse, or excessive exercise. The person who suffers from bulimia is usually within the normal weight range, or may be slightly higher or lower than his or her expected weight. This disorder is also associated with increased symptoms of depression or mood disorders.

Bulimia nervosa is thought to be significantly underrecognized because most persons do not report it. In the United States, the prevalence of bulimia nervosa is estimated at 1%. From those who report the syndrome, lifetime prevalence is 0.5% for males and 1.5% for females. Approximately 65.3% of patients with bulimia have a normal BMI between 18.5 and 29.9 and only 3.5% have a BMI less than 18.5. Bulimia nervosa is prevalent in all ethnic, racial, and socioeconomic groups. It is mainly a disease of young women, with average age of onset at 19 years old. It is estimated to be prevalent in as much as 20% of certain male population groups that require maintenance of body weight, such as competitive athletes.

Signs and symptoms are related to the activities an individual uses to avoid weight gain, such as vomiting or the use of laxatives. Typical problems include electrolyte imbalances, sore throat, lymph node enlargement, worn tooth enamel, tooth decay, GERD, severe dehydration, and renal complications related to diuretic abuse. Diagnostic studies include electrolyte levels, liver enzymes, serum albumin, BUN, electrocardiogram (ECG), and serum creatinine. With malnutrition and if weight drops to severely low levels, there are similar metabolic consequences as in anorexia nervosa.

Binge Eating

Binge eating is a disorder that resembles bulimia. A person with this disorder either will eat a large quantity of food in a small period or may eat continuously for the entire day. The eating is not triggered by hunger and is not discontinued with signs of satiety. The individual may continue to eat despite the fact that he or she is physically uncomfortable from being full.

Outwardly, these individuals may show no signs of having problems, except that some may be obese or overweight. In addition to the previously noted symptoms, these individuals may hoard food, frequently eat alone, make repeated unsuccessful attempts at dieting, and may feel depressed about their size. Unlike people suffering from bulimia, binge-eaters do not engage in inappropriate compensatory behaviors to prevent weight gain or promote weight loss. Severe obesity is a common consequence of binge eating.

Complications are similar to those experienced by obese individuals, such as cardiovascular issues, including hypertension. Additionally, binge eating is closely linked to psychiatric disorders of anxiety and depression.

Purging Disorders

Individuals with **purging disorder** regularly use self-induced vomiting, laxatives, diuretics, or other extreme methods to control their weight or shape. Some engage in excessive bouts of exercise. Usually the individual is not significantly underweight or overweight; however, they are commonly obsessed about weight control. Individuals with purging disorder usually do not have large, out-of-control binge-eating episodes. They do not engage in restricted eating. They eat normal meals but have certain times when they feel obliged to purge in order to control weight. Individuals who purge, like those with anorexia or bulimia, have significant body image disturbances and high incidence of anxiety and depression. If weight drops to severely low levels,

there are similar metabolic consequences as those found in anorexia nervosa.

Night Eating Syndrome

Night eating syndrome (NES), also known as *nocturnal eating syndrome,* is an eating disorder characterized by a persistent pattern of late-night binge eating. Affected individuals claim to be unaware of eating while asleep. The diagnosis is controversial. It affects between 1% and 2% of the population and can affect all ages and both sexes. However, most cases are not reported. NES is commonly associated with depression. It has been proposed that individuals have low nocturnal levels of the hormones melatonin and leptin.

 CLINICAL CONCEPT

A combination of psychotherapy, behavior modification, and treatment of underlying mental health disorders is necessary for successful treatment of eating disorders.

Chapter Summary

- Over the last 20 years, the percentage of overweight adults worldwide has increased by 300%.
- Obesity results when energy intake exceeds energy expenditure; fat is a form of stored energy. Individuals vary widely in their propensity to gain weight and accrue fat mass, even at identical levels of caloric input and activity.
- BMI is the current method used to measure body weight; however, it doesn't accurately reflect adiposity, and it is inaccurate in highly muscular individuals.
- Adipose tissue is an endocrine organ that secretes adipokines such as adiponectin, leptin, and resistin.
- Adipokines are hormones, thrombogenic substances, inflammatory mediators, and proteins that exert influence on glucose and lipid metabolism, hunger, and satiety.
- Adiponectin enhances cellular sensitivity to insulin, exerts anti-inflammatory effects, and is protective against the formation of arteriosclerosis; it has an inverse relationship with the fat content, or adiposity, of the body.

- As the amount of fat stored in adipocytes rises, leptin is released into the blood and sends signals to the brain that the body has had enough to eat. Obese individuals have high levels of leptin but are resistant to its effects, resulting in leptin desensitization.
- Disorders associated with obesity include cardiovascular disease, diabetes mellitus, osteoarthritis, sleep apnea, and gallbladder and liver disease.
- Diet and exercise are the recommended treatment for excess body fat.
- Bariatric surgery, in addition to causing weight loss in persons with severe obesity, can resolve diabetes, hypertension, hyperlipidemia, NAFLD, sleep apnea, and other obesity-related disorders.
- Vitamin and mineral deficiencies often occur in individuals with poor diet.
- Food intake can be an emotional issue that is involved in mental health problems such as anorexia, bulimia, and purging.

Making the Connections

Signs and Symptoms	Physical Assessment Findings	Diagnostic Testing	Treatment
Obesity | A metabolic disorder that involves excess fat accumulation caused by lack of sufficient activity and excess caloric intake. Obesity is a metabolic disorder that involves changes in cellular insulin sensitivity, satiety, glucose utilization, fat accumulation, hepatic glucose production, and fluid balance.			
Lethargy. Indigestion caused by GERD. Osteoarthritis caused by excessive weight on knees and hips.	Apple-shaped or pear-shaped excess fat accumulation. Waist circumference in males >40 inches; in females >35 inches.	BMI ≥30. Skinfold fat measurement >25% in males, >30% in females. Dyslipidemia: low HDL, high LDL, high triglycerides. Elevated blood glucose. Elevated blood pressure.	Diet. Exercise. Pharmacological agents: appetite suppressors. Liposuction. Bariatric surgery.
Anorexia Nervosa | Intentional self-restriction of food, causing severe weight loss.			
Patient usually denies any problems. Individual sees self as overweight and is obsessed with taking off body weight through not eating or purging. Disturbed self/body image. Refusal to put on weight.	BMI <17.5. Multiple system disturbances; lack of body fat, hair loss, cold intolerance, delayed puberty, orthostatic hypotension, amenorrhea, heart murmur of mitral valve prolapse. Abnormal heart rhythm. Edema.	Electrolyte imbalances such as hypokalemia. Complete blood count abnormalities showing anemia. Increased BUN showing dehydration. ECG abnormalities. Elevated liver enzymes. Low thyroid function. B_{12} deficiency. Low estrogen.	Psychiatric treatment. Nasogastric tube feedings. Rehydration and correction of any complications.
Bulimia Nervosa | An illness in which a person binges on food or has regular episodes of overeating and feels a loss of control. The person then uses different methods—such as self-induced vomiting or laxative abuse—to prevent weight gain. Some with bulimia also have anorexia nervosa.			
Patient usually denies problems.	Patient may be of normal body weight. Typical problems include electrolyte imbalances, sore throat, lymph node enlargement, worn tooth enamel, tooth decay, GERD, severe dehydration, and renal complications related to diuretic abuse.	Diagnostic studies for electrolyte levels, liver enzymes, serum albumin, BUN, ECG, and serum creatinine.	Psychiatric treatment. Correction of any side effects.
Binge Eating | Eating a large quantity of food in a small period, or eating continuously for the entire day. The eating is not triggered by hunger and is not discontinued with signs of satiety or feeling uncomfortably full.			
Patient usually denies problems.	Obesity is common. Patient may hoard food, eat alone, or try numerous diets.	None.	Psychiatric treatment. Treatment for obesity, including diet and activity.

Continued

Making the Connections—cont'd

Signs and Symptoms	Physical Assessment Findings	Diagnostic Testing	Treatment
Purging Disorder | Individuals with purging disorder regularly use self-induced vomiting, laxatives, diuretics, or other extreme methods to control their weight or shape. Some engage in excessive bouts of exercise. Usually the individual is not significantly underweight or overweight but is commonly obsessed with weight control.			
Patient usually denies problems.	Normal weight is common.	None.	Psychiatric treatment.
Night Eating Syndrome | Characterized by a persistent pattern of late-night binge eating. Affected individuals claim to be unaware of eating while asleep.			
Obesity.	Obesity.	None.	Psychiatric treatment.

Bibliography

Available online at fadavis.com

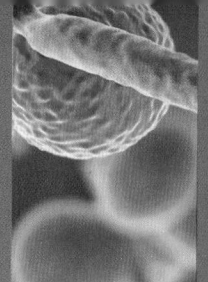

Learning Objectives

After completion of this chapter, the student will be able to:

- Describe the gate control and neuromatrix theories of pain.
- List common neurotransmitters involved in pain transmission.
- Discuss how to comprehensively assess a patient's pain.
- Describe the WHO step ladder approach for prescribing opioid, nonopioid, and adjuvant medications.
- Identify nonpharmacological treatments for pain.
- Distinguish among abuse, tolerance, physical dependence, and withdrawal of opioid drugs.
- Recognize specific types of pain syndromes.

Key Terms

Addiction
Afferent neuron
Catastrophize
Colic
Controlled substance
Dermatomes
Efferent neuron
Gate control theory

Modulation
Neuromatrix theory
Neuropathic pain
Nociceptors
OLDCART
Paresthesia
Perception
Phantom limb pain

Referred pain
Schedule
Simple reflex arc
Tolerance
Transduction
Transmission
Withdrawal

Pain has been recognized as a source of human suffering since ancient times, when our ancestors believed evil spirits and sin to be its cause. Later, pain was associated with apparent tissue damage, whereas pain without apparent cause was thought to be unreal, psychosomatic, or caused by patient malingering. In the last decade, there have been changes in the assessment and treatment of pain. Clinicians have given the patient's perception of pain greater credibility than in the past and now ask patients to describe and quantify their pain, regardless of evident pathology, with the knowledge that pain is a subjective experience. The International Association for the Study of Pain defines pain as an unpleasant sensory and emotional experience associated with actual or potential tissue damage.

Although unpleasant, it is important to remember that pain is a protective mechanism; it allows the body to detect injury while also enabling the body to protect itself from more serious injury.

Epidemiology

Numerous research studies have identified the detrimental effects of uncontrolled pain on morbidity and mortality, quality of life, and health-care costs. Optimal pain management is associated with a quicker rate of recovery, better functioning, and fewer postoperative complications. Pain is the most common symptom that prompts people to seek medical attention, accounting for over 70 million office visits per year in the United States. It is also the second leading reason for work absenteeism, resulting in over 50 million lost workdays per year and an estimated $3 billion in lost wages. Pain costs employers an estimated $80 billion per year because of lost productivity, health-care costs, and compensation.

Basic Concepts Related to Pain

An understanding of how pain sensation is interpreted by the body involves the spinal cord and brain. At times, pain triggers an immediate response without interpretation by the brain through a simple reflex. At other times, pain signals travel from the periphery to an ascending tract in the spinal cord up to the brain for interpretation.

Nociceptors, which are specialized pain nerve fibers, and neurotransmitters, which work to transmit impulses from one neuron to another, are involved in the travel of pain sensation in the spinal cord. The brain can inhibit the experience of pain through natural neurochemicals called endogenous opioids. Endorphins are examples of these natural opioids. The assessment of pain requires knowledge of areas on the body represented by sensory and motor nerves called dermatomes and myotomes. Localizing pain to specific dermatomes or myotomes can give clinicians diagnostic clues regarding the source of pain.

The Central Nervous System and Pain

The brain and spinal cord are integral components in the experience of pain perception. Within the center of the spinal cord there is an H-shaped region called the substantia gelatinosa. Spinal nerves enter the spinal cord at the posterior region of the substantia gelatinosa called the dorsal horn. The neurons that enter the dorsal horn are called afferent neurons. **Afferent neurons** are sensory nerves that carry pain, temperature, touch, proprioception, vibration, and pressure sensations into the spinal cord. **Efferent neurons** are motor nerves; these neurons exit the spinal cord through the ventral horn and extend to the muscles of the body.

The afferent neurons that carry information for pain are categorized as A-delta and C fibers. A-delta fibers are larger in diameter than C fibers, and are myelinated. These fibers conduct impulses rapidly and cause the first, short-lived acute experience of pain, such as occurs when a finger senses a burn and pulls away from the heat source. C fibers are smaller in diameter and unmyelinated. These fibers conduct impulses slowly and cause longer-lasting, persistent, dull pain, such as the pain that occurs after a burn has taken place.

Simple Reflex Arc

A simple reflex occurs in the body without need for interpretation by the brain. In a **simple reflex arc**, an afferent neuron carries sensory impulses into the dorsal horn of the spinal cord. The afferent neuron connects with an interneuron in the substantia gelatinosa. The interneuron connects to an efferent neuron that exits via the ventral horn and enacts motor activity.

The simple reflex is protective: It allows for immediate action by the body without requiring time for interpretation by the brain. For example, when touching a hot stove, the finger senses the heat, and afferent neurons bring the sensory impulses into the spinal cord via the dorsal horn. It connects with an interneuron, which connects with an efferent neuron that enacts the motor activity of pulling the finger away immediately. A protective response is elicited before the brain has a chance to interpret the event (see Fig. 6-1).

A simple reflex arc is also seen when a clinician tests a patient for deep tendon reflexes. For example,

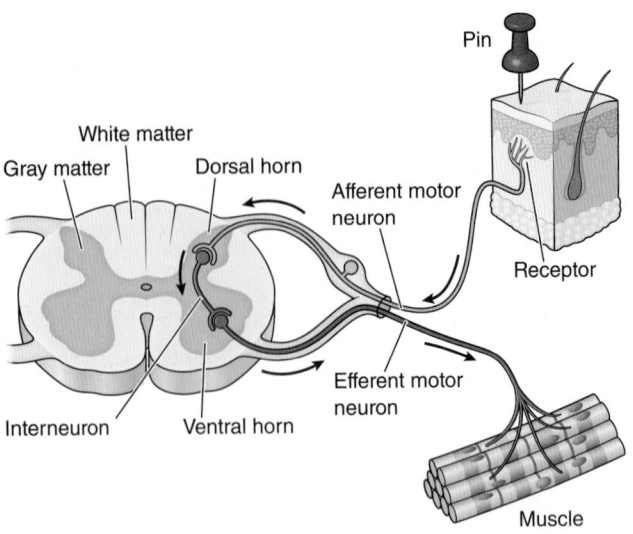

FIGURE 6-1. In a simple reflex arc, a sensation is felt and transmitted via a nerve impulse that travels via the afferent neuron into the dorsal horn of the spinal cord. It connects with an interneuron located in the spinal cord, which connects with an efferent neuron that travels out the ventral horn of the spinal cord and stimulates a motor activity. A simple reflex arc enables a quick action response before the brain has a chance to interpret the event.

the clinician tests the patellar reflex when tapping the tendon of the quadriceps muscle at the knee with a reflex hammer. Afferent neurons carry the signal into the spinal cord, where they connect with interneurons. An interneuron then connects to an efferent motor neuron, and the reflexive kick motion of the quadriceps muscle occurs.

The brain can also interpret pain in the pain sensory experience. The afferent neuron carries sensory information from the periphery into the dorsal horn of the spinal cord, where it synapses with an interneuron in the substantia gelatinosa. The interneuron then synapses with another neuron that is within an ascending tract called the spinothalamic tract. The spinothalamic tract directs sensory neuronal impulses from the spinal cord up through the brainstem to the hypothalamus and upper regions of the brain cortex. The axons of the spinothalamic tract cross over to the other side of the spinal cord before their arrival in the brain. From the sensorimotor portion of the brain, motor neurons descend downward in the spinal cord and cross over at the medulla to control the opposite side of the body. These motor neurons, known as the corticospinal tract, exit via the ventral horn of the spinal cord to control muscles of the body (see Fig. 6-2).

Nociception

Nociception is the response of the nervous system to painful stimuli. Afferent nerve fibers that respond to noxious stimuli are termed **nociceptors.** Nociceptors are found in the skin; muscle; connective tissue; bone; circulatory system; and abdominal, pelvic, and thoracic viscera. Although not all afferent neurons are nociceptors, all nociceptors are afferent neurons.

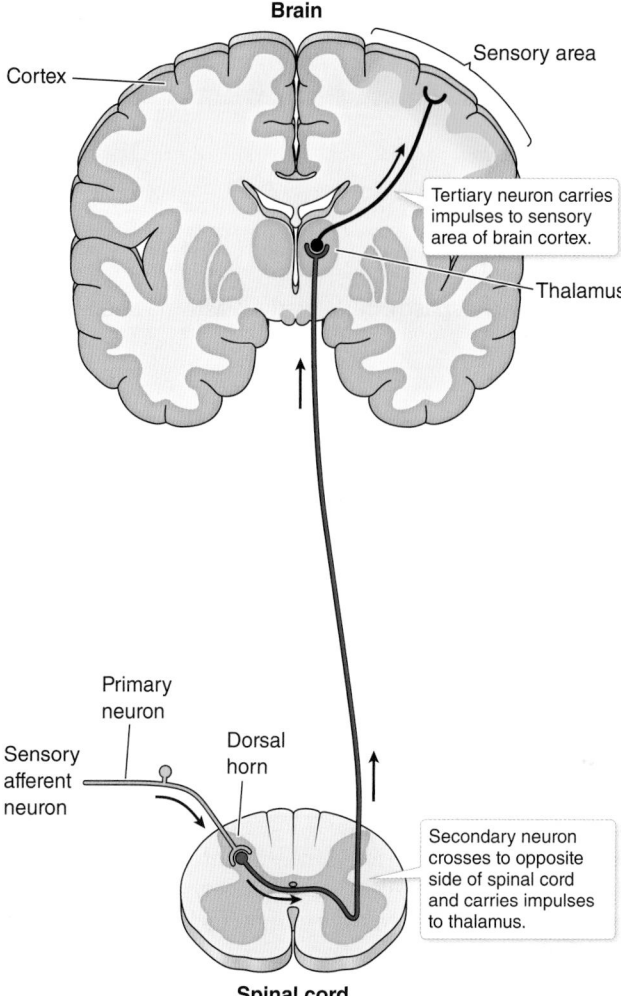

FIGURE 6-2a. The spinothalamic tract directs afferent sensory impulses from the periphery into the dorsal horn of the spinal cord (primary neuron). It connects with an interneuron in the spinal cord that crosses over to the opposite side of the spinal cord (secondary neuron) to the thalamus. The interneuron then connects with another neuron (tertiary neuron) that directs impulses to the upper regions of the brain sensorimotor cortex (sensory area).

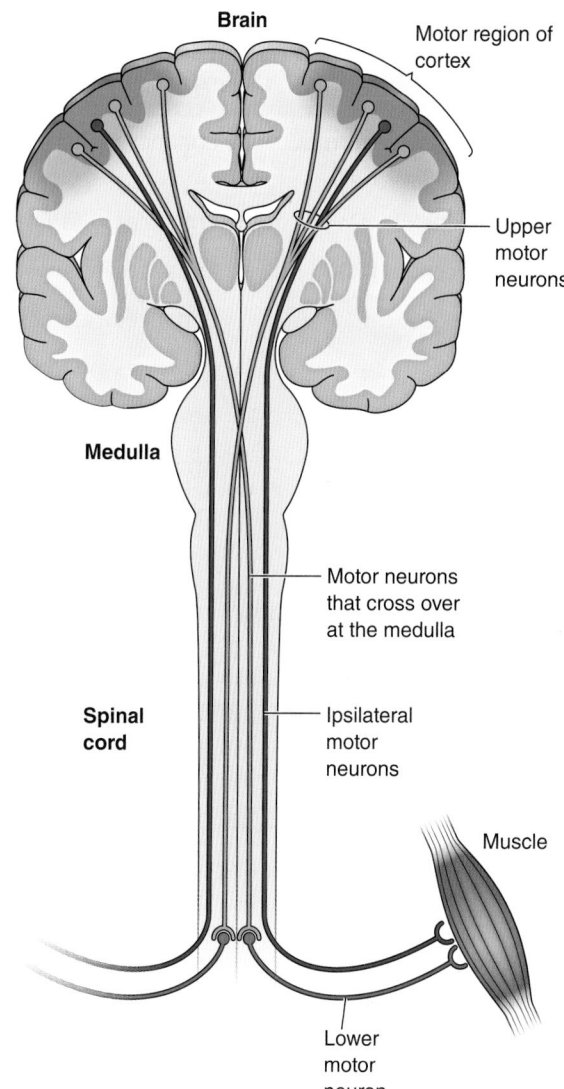

FIGURE 6-2b. From the sensorimotor region of the brain, corticospinal tract neurons descend down into the medulla, where the majority of neurons cross over to the opposite side of the spinal cord. The area of crossover in the medulla is called the area of decussation. Some corticospinal tract neurons do not cross over and remain ipsilateral. The motor neurons descend via the spinal cord and exit via the ventral horn of the spinal cord, then connect to a lower motor neuron to stimulate muscle activity.

Neurotransmitters

Neurotransmitters are excitatory or inhibitory chemical mediators that are released from one neuron to stimulate another (see Table 6-1). There are approximately 50 neurotransmitters, including acetylcholine, norepinephrine, dopamine, serotonin, and gamma-aminobutyric acid (GABA). Acetylcholine and norepinephrine are excitatory neurotransmitters, whereas dopamine, serotonin, and GABA are inhibitory. A nerve impulse travels down a neuron from dendrites to the cell body into the axon and eventually the presynaptic membrane, which contains vesicles that release neurotransmitters into a synaptic cleft. In the postsynaptic membrane, receptors on the adjoining neuron pick up freely flowing neurotransmitters. Once the neurotransmitter is picked up by receptors in the postsynaptic membrane, the molecule is internalized in the neuron and the impulse continues. Within the dorsal horn of the spinal cord and brain, communication

of nociceptive information between various neurons occurs via neurotransmitters. Knowledge about the mechanisms of neurotransmitters means that they can be manipulated for pharmacological management of pain. For example, the neurotransmitter serotonin is stimulated by the pharmacological agent sumatriptan as a remedy for migraine headache.

Endogenous Opioids

Endogenous opioids are natural analgesic neurochemicals that inhibit pain sensation and are similar to neurotransmitters. Endogenous opioids include endorphins, enkephalins, and dynorphins. Major areas of the midbrain and brainstem, called the periaqueductal gray matter (PAG) and nucleus raphe magnus

TABLE 6-1. Influence of Neurochemicals and Neurotransmitters on Pain

Neurochemicals	Action
Prostaglandins (from COX-1 enzymatic pathway)	Enhances inflammation, pain, edema
Interleukins	Enhances inflammation, pain, edema
Tumor necrosis factor	Enhances inflammation, edema, and pain and decreases appetite
Leukotrienes	Enhances inflammation, edema, and bronchospasm, particularly in asthma and allergy
Bradykinins	Enhances inflammation
Glutamate	Amplifies pain signal
Substance P	Amplifies pain signal
Enkephalins, endorphins	Inhibitory influence on pain; natural opioid
Acetylcholine	Inhibitory action on pain in the spinal cord
Gamma-aminobutyric acid	Inhibitory action on pain in the spinal cord and brain
Norepinephrine	Inhibitory action on pain in the spinal cord
Dopamine	Inhibitory action on pain in the spinal cord and brain
Serotonin	Conveys analgesic signals from the PAG area to the NRM of the brain (serotonin is diminished in migraine headache)

(NRM), are particularly influential in pain inhibition (see Fig. 6-3). Stimulation of the PAG activates enkephalin-releasing neurons that project to the NRM in the brainstem.

From the NRM, serotonin-releasing neurons descend to the dorsal horn of the spinal cord, where there is a connection with interneurons in the spinal cord that release endogenous opioids. The natural opioids bind to and inhibit receptors in the axons of incoming C and A-delta fibers, which carry pain signals of nociceptors from the periphery.

The NRM is also specifically involved in migraine headaches, which are theorized to evolve from a serotonin deficiency that causes abnormal cerebral vasodilation and vasoconstriction. Migraine medications work by stimulating NRM neurons to release serotonin, which, in turn, stimulates interneurons to release endogenous opioids.

Sensitization

The pain mechanism may be altered in some individuals, as well as in some diseases and conditions. For instance, some neurons may increase the rate or intensity of firing at the level of the dorsal root ganglion. Repeated or excessive stimulation of C fibers, a process known as wind-up, sensitizes the afferent neurons so that even mild stimulation may be perceived as painful. Sensitization exaggerates excitement of nerve fibers and impairs inhibitory

(analgesic) interneuron influences at the level of the dorsal horn, brainstem, or both. An example of sensitization occurs when an individual lightly rubs a certain area of skin over and over. At first this is sensed as slight tactile contact. However, with continual light rubbing the skin becomes hypersensitive. The afferent neurons are repeatedly stimulated until eventually they become extremely sensitive to any kind of tactile contact.

Dermatomes and Myotomes

Spinal nerves contain both motor fibers and sensory fibers. The motor fibers innervate certain muscles, whereas the sensory fibers innervate certain areas of skin. A **dermatome** is a skin area innervated by the sensory fibers of a single nerve root; a myotome is a group of muscles primarily innervated by the motor fibers of a single nerve root. Dermatome and myotome patterns of distribution are relatively consistent from person to person (see Fig. 6-4). Dermatomes are named according to the spinal nerve roots that supply them and can be correlated with spinal nerve dysfunction. For example, with impingement of the fifth cervical spinal nerve (C5), the patient complains of pain in the area of the C5 dermatome, which encompasses the shoulder and upper arm. A clinician can correlate the dermatome of the patient's pain with the specific spinal nerve that is involved in the disorder.

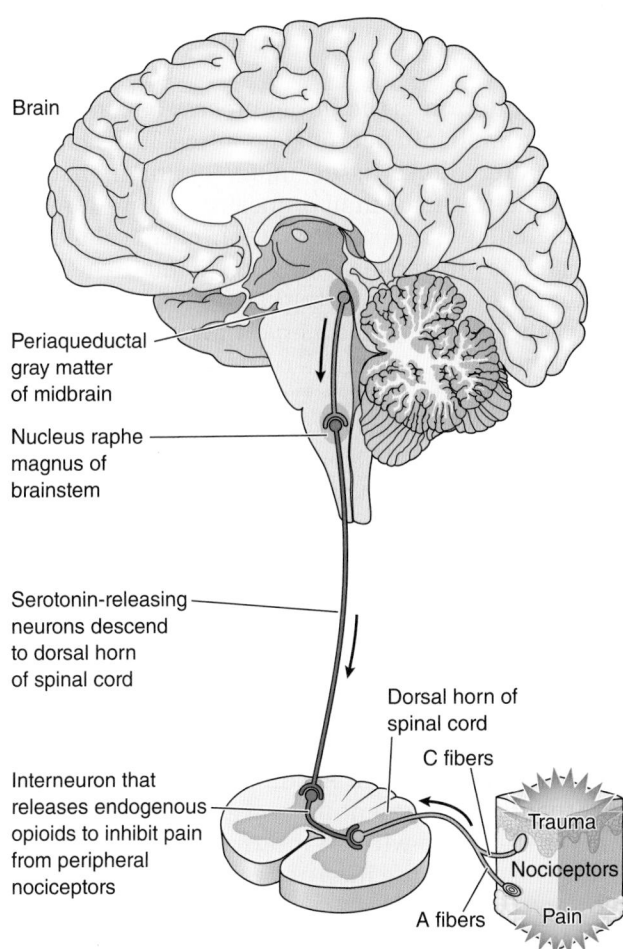

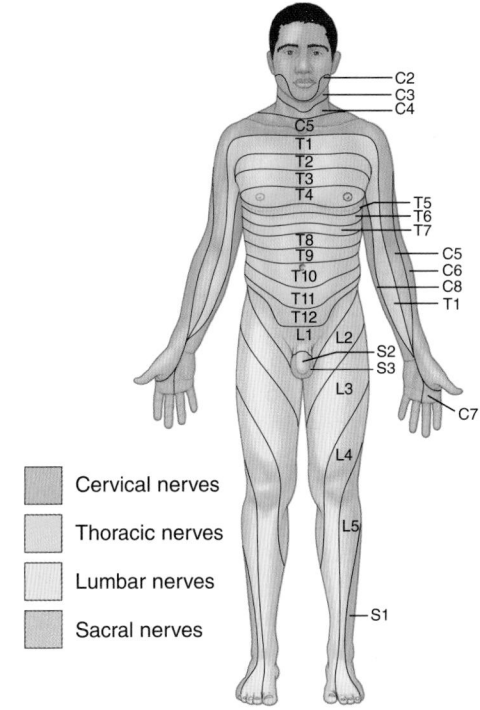

FIGURE 6-4. Sensory dermatomes. A dermatome is the area of skin supplied by nerves originated from a spinal nerve.

FIGURE 6-3. Pain inhibition by natural opioids. Stimulation of the PAG matter of the midbrain activates enkephalin-releasing neurons that project to the NRM in the brainstem. Serotonin released from the NRM descends to the dorsal horn of the spinal cord, where it forms connections with inhibitory interneurons that release endogenous opioids. The endogenous opioids bind to opioid receptors in the axons of incoming C and A-delta fibers carrying pain signals from nociceptors activated in the periphery.

CLINICAL CONCEPT

Sciatica, a cause of low back pain, is a common reason for individuals to seek primary health care. The pain arises from sciatic nerve impingement. The patient complains of pain in the region of the dermatome, which originates in the L4–S1 region of the back and radiates down the posterior leg.

Basic Pathophysiological Concepts Related to Pain

The mechanism of pain is complex, and several theories have provided a framework for our understanding. Pain diminishes the quality of life, and patients look to the clinician for relief. In order to implement interventions that can alleviate pain, the source and process need to be understood.

Pain Theories

In 1965, researchers Melzack and Wall developed the landmark **gate control theory,** which revolutionized our understanding of pain and changed how clinicians treat pain. According to this theory, there are two major points:

1. Pain is not necessarily proportional to the amount of tissue injury.
2. Sensation travels both to and from the brain.

Before the development of this theory, only the central nervous system (CNS), spinal cord, and brain were recognized as integral parts of the pain experience. The gate control theory proposed that tissue injury and inflammation stimulate specific pain fibers in peripheral nerves and send signals to the spinal cord. In the spinal cord, the neural signals are influenced by other neurons, where the pain signal can become dampened or amplified. The signals then continue up to the brain, where interpretation occurs. Signals can also come down from the brain to the neurons in the spinal cord and modulate the pain.

Further research, however, demonstrated that the gate control theory was not a complete explanation of the pain experience, as it did not explain chronic pain syndromes, phantom limb pain, and other types of pain without an obvious cause. This prompted Melzack to develop the **neuromatrix theory** of pain, which emphasizes the brain's influence in experiences of pain. According to this theory, pain is not simply a sensory experience but one that involves our thoughts, past experiences, emotions, and stress. Our understanding of pain now involves both of these theories—and there is still further research needed.

Gate Control Theory

The gate control theory involves impulse conduction of pain through a three-neuron chain. The first neuron is an afferent neuron, which is stimulated by pain in the periphery, sending an impulse into the spinal cord. The second neuron is an interneuron that is influenced by descending nerve tracts from the brain or ascending nerve tracts from the spinal cord. The third neuron's impulse projects upward into the brain (see Fig. 6-5).

According to the gate control theory, to produce pain, A-delta and C fiber afferent nociceptive nerve impulses within the three-neuron chain go through four processes:

1. Transduction
2. Transmission
3. Modulation
4. Perception

Transduction is the initial process of converting painful stimuli into neuronal impulses. Transduction occurs after direct tissue injury or inflammation. In traumatic tissue injury, nociceptors are directly stimulated. In tissue inflammation, chemical mediators such as prostaglandins (PGs) stimulate the nociceptor. After the nociceptor is stimulated, impulses are produced along the nerve's axon to enter the dorsal horn of the spinal cord. The travel of the impulse along the axon is **transmission.** In the dorsal horn of the spinal cord, synaptic connections occur between the incoming afferent neuron and an interneuron, which can be influenced by ascending and descending nerve tracts from the brain. The influence on the afferent neuron by other neurons in the spinal cord is **modulation.** The spinothalamic tract, which travels from the spinal cord up to the brain, is the most prominent nociceptive pathway in the spinal cord.

Modulation is the effect of the interneuron on the afferent neuron; the effect can be amplification or dampening of pain. According to the gate control theory, the afferent neuron encounters a "gate" when it connects with an interneuron in the spinal cord. The gate is the interneuron's influence on the afferent neuron, which can be negative or positive. The interneuron can be influenced by descending pathways from the brain or ascending pathways from the spinal cord. If the gate is opened, pain is amplified; if the gate is closed, pain may be dampened. Neurotransmitters released by the interneuron are involved in the gate's amplification or dampening of pain. Examples of pain modulation can be seen when an individual experiences an obvious painful stimulus from the environment but does not feel the pain.

For example, neurotransmitters called endorphins are negative influences that dampen an afferent neuron's pain stimulus. Long-distance runners, who do not experience pain when running to the point of exhaustion, often report a pleasant feeling due to the effect of endorphin modulation on the pain stimulus. Pain modulation can also be seen when a person walks on hot coals without experiencing pain. The afferent neuron brings the signal of pain from the feet into the spinal cord, but the influence of an interneuron modulates the pain signal, in essence closing the gate. The interneuron is influenced by descending nerve pathways from the brain that conduct impulses from thoughts that distract the person from feeling the pain.

Conversely, a person can experience a minor pain stimulus but perceive it as extremely painful. In this case, the afferent nociceptive stimulus is minor, but the interneuron is open to the influence of descending pathways from the brain that augment the experience of pain. The person cognitively perceives the pain is

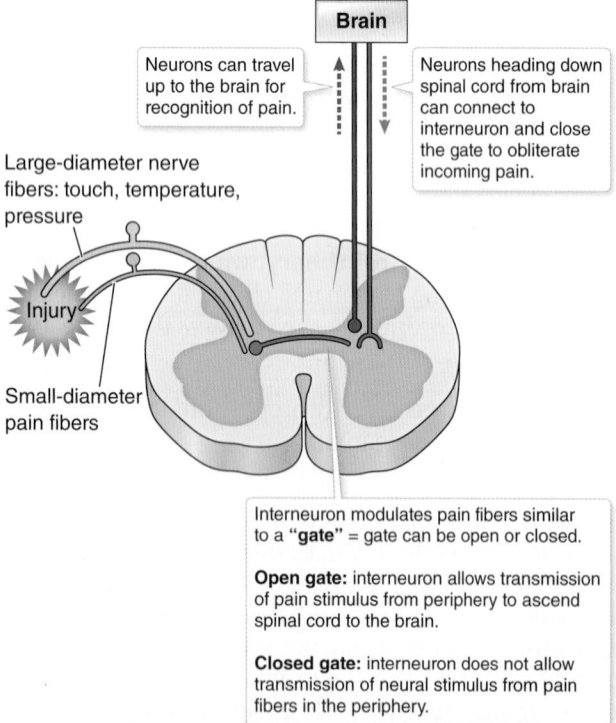

Neurons can travel up to the brain for recognition of pain.

Brain

Neurons heading down spinal cord from brain can connect to interneuron and close the gate to obliterate incoming pain.

Large-diameter nerve fibers: touch, temperature, pressure

Injury

Small-diameter pain fibers

Interneuron modulates pain fibers similar to a **"gate"** = gate can be open or closed.

Open gate: interneuron allows transmission of pain stimulus from periphery to ascend spinal cord to the brain.

Closed gate: interneuron does not allow transmission of neural stimulus from pain fibers in the periphery.

FIGURE 6-5. Gate control mechanism. When large nerve fibers from the periphery are stimulated, small-diameter pain fibers cannot get through the interneuron gate. The gate is closed. Therefore when injury occurs, rubbing, cold treatment, or shaking off pain can dull or obliterate the pain. When pain nerve fibers from the periphery are stimulated and the interneuron gate is open, the neural stimulus is transmitted up the spinal cord to the brain for recognition. Pain can also be influenced by descending spinal nerves from the brain down into the spinal cord to the interneuron. The descending neural pathway can close the interneuron gate. This is how distraction and endorphins can obliterate pain.

extreme, and this influences the pain experience. This often occurs in persons who overreact when receiving an intramuscular injection. The injection in reality is a minor pinching sensation; however, many persons perceive it as severe because of cognitive influences on the experience.

Perception of pain is the conscious awareness of the experience of pain. Perception results from impulse transmission up to the thalamus, limbic system, midbrain, cerebral cortex, and reticular system. This is where the individual interprets the pain. An individual's perception of pain is influenced by a multitude of factors, including developmental level, memory, past experiences, attention, distraction, fatigue, fear, stress, and mood states such as anxiety and depression.

The Neuromatrix Theory

The neuromatrix theory of pain developed by Melzack in 1990 highlights the brain's role in pain sensation. Melzack developed the theory mainly because the gate control theory cannot explain pain experienced with no apparent pathological source. For example, **phantom limb pain** commonly occurs after a patient undergoes an amputation—burning, cramping, and shooting pains are experienced by 70% of amputees long after the amputation has occurred. Patients experience pain in the absent extremity as though the extremity is still part of the body, and the pain is often intractable with no effective treatment. Phantom limb pain particularly illustrates the complex role of the brain in modulating the body's sensation of pain.

The neuromatrix theory proposes that pain is a multidimensional experience produced from characteristic neurosignature patterns arising from nerve impulses generated by a widely distributed neural network, called the body-self neuromatrix, located in the brain. Similar to the gate control theory, the brain can be triggered by sensory input from nociceptors in the periphery, but according to the neuromatrix theory, the brain can also generate painful sensations independently. Nociceptive stimulation is not a prerequisite for pain sensation.

The neuromatrix is genetically determined and shaped by sensory input during the individual's life. The neuromatrix is the brain's perception of the body. It consists of complex neural networks that are built into the brain from birth and develop throughout life. With time, all sensory input from the body undergoes repeated processing so that characteristic patterns of input, known as a neurosignature, are impressed on the brain.

With these principles in mind, phantom limb pain can be understood. The absence of sensory input does not stop the brain from generating messages about missing body parts. The body's extremities are part of the neurosignature impressed upon the neuromatrix. Well-developed neurological pathways involving the extremities have been present in the brain since before birth. The extremities are part of the neurosignature, and the brain still perceives the extremities and their pain.

Types of Pain

The major types of pain include acute, chronic, and neuropathic. Acute pain is experienced immediately after tissue injury. Chronic pain is a prolonged pain sensation that may or may not be related to tissue injury. Neuropathic pain is often difficult for the patient to describe; it is a feeling of pain perpetuated by dysfunctional neurons. Neuropathic pain is reported by the patient in many different ways, from numbness to sharp, piercing pain.

Acute Pain

Acute pain results from new onset of tissue injury or inflammation. Acute pain is sudden, lasts hours to days, and resolves with healing of the disorder. Acute pain plays a biologically protective role because it facilitates tissue repair and healing by making the injured area and surrounding tissue hypersensitive to all kinds of stimuli. This, in turn, makes the injured individual avoid exposing the area to external stimuli, thereby allowing for an undisturbed healing process. Acute pain occurs after surgery and in disorders such as myocardial infarction, fracture, and appendicitis.

Chronic Pain

Chronic pain persists beyond the expected time for a given disease process or injury and is defined as having a duration greater than 6 months. Chronic pain may arise as a result of sustained noxious stimuli such as persistent inflammation. Cancer, osteoarthritis, and rheumatological diseases such as rheumatoid arthritis commonly cause chronic pain. Unlike acute pain, chronic pain is debilitating and does not serve any biological or protective function. It is pain that initially occurred because of a pathological condition; however, it does not subside when the condition no longer exists. In chronic pain, the pain itself eventually becomes the patient's focus. For example, fibromyalgia is a syndrome of chronic musculoskeletal pain with no readily apparent pathological tissue, yet it is defined as a condition of chronic pain.

In some cases of chronic pain, the neuromatrix theory is well illustrated. Chronic pain can begin as acute pain caused by acute pathology. After the acute pathology resolves, chronic pain can persist and continue to be perceived by the brain. This is a complex condition that is difficult to treat but can be explained by the neuromatrix theory. The pain continues because its neural network evolves into a neurosignature that becomes imprinted onto the brain. There is no pathological condition, yet the pain is still perceived. Commonly, chronic pain does not respond to conventional analgesic treatments.

Neuropathic Pain

Neuropathic pain is caused by injury or malfunction of the spinal cord and/or peripheral nerves. Neuropathic pain is typically a burning, tingling, shooting, stinging, or pins-and-needles sensation, often referred to as **paresthesia.** Some people also complain of a stabbing, piercing, cutting, and drilling pain.

Neuropathic pain is a unique kind of pain because it cannot be described as either acute or chronic. It can occur within days, weeks, or months of an injury and tends to occur in waves of frequency and intensity. Neuropathic pain is diffuse and occurs either at the level or below the level of injury, most often in the legs, back, feet, thighs, and toes, although it can also occur in the upper body. Some disorders that cause neuropathic pain include postherpetic neuralgias, spinal nerve radiculopathy, diabetic polyneuropathy, postsurgical pain syndromes, and complex regional pain syndrome (CRPS). Neuropathic pain is very difficult to treat. Often alternative therapies, such as transcutaneous electrical neural stimulation (TENS), antidepressants, anticonvulsants, or acupuncture, are needed to provide relief.

Sources of Pain

There are various sources of pain; some sources are obvious, such as traumatic body injury. However, some sources of pain may not be readily apparent, yet they are clearly perceived by the brain. Pain from areas rich in nociceptors is easy to locate. However, some areas of the body can be painful because of damage to an internal organ that sends neural impulses far from the origin of injury; this is called referred pain.

Cutaneous Pain

Injury to the skin or superficial tissues causes cutaneous pain. Cutaneous nociceptors terminate just below the skin, where a high concentration of nerve endings exists. Cutaneous nerve endings produce a well-defined, localized pain of short duration. Examples of injuries that produce cutaneous pain include minor cuts and bruises, first-degree burns, and lacerations.

Deep Somatic Pain

Deep somatic pain originates from ligaments, tendons, bones, blood vessels, and nerves themselves. These areas contain small numbers of somatic nociceptors. The scarcity of pain receptors in these areas produces a dull, poorly localized pain of longer duration than cutaneous pain; examples include sprains and broken bones. Myofascial pain is a type of somatic pain that is usually caused by tender points in muscles, tendons, and fascia; it may be localized or referred.

Visceral Pain

Visceral pain is defined as pain emanating from deep organs, usually resulting from disease processes. It is very different from cutaneous nociception because of the small number of nociceptors. Visceral pain can be vague and not well localized and is usually described as pressure-like, deep squeezing, dull, colicky, or diffuse. Most visceral pain occurs because of distention of hollow, muscular-walled organs, such as the gastrointestinal tract, genitourinary tract, and gallbladder. The nerves within an organ are distended, and this signal is interpreted as pain by the brain.

Inflammation, as in cystitis or pancreatitis, is also a cause of visceral pain. This type of visceral pain commonly occurs because of PGs and other inflammatory mediators that are produced by tissues in inflammation. PGs cause edema, pain, and fever, as well as continually stimulate inflammation. Visceral pain can also be associated with systemic symptoms, such as malaise, weakness, and nausea.

Referred Pain

Referred pain occurs when the pain response occurs at a distance from the actual pathology. It is a hallmark of visceral pain (see Fig. 6-6) but occurs in other conditions as well. Referred pain occurs when nerve fibers from regions of high sensory input, such as the skin, and nerve fibers from regions of normally low sensory input, such as the internal organs, converge on the same levels of the spinal cord.

The best-known example of referred pain is pain experienced during myocardial infarction. Nerves from damaged heart tissue convey pain signals to spinal cord levels C4–T4 on the left side, which happen to be the same levels that receive sensation from the left side of the chest and part of the left arm. The brain doesn't have a strong neurosignature of the heart, but it does have a strong impression from the adjoining thoracic skin and muscles, so it interprets the signals from the heart as pain in the chest and left arm.

Referred pain often occurs at the shoulder from irritation of the diaphragm muscle. A ruptured organ beneath the diaphragm gives off escaped air that stays beneath the diaphragm and acts as an irritant. An inflamed organ can enlarge and also irritate the diaphragm. There is not a strong neurosignature of the diaphragm muscle in the brain. If the diaphragm is irritated, the patient feels shoulder pain. This occurs because the diaphragm is innervated by the sensory

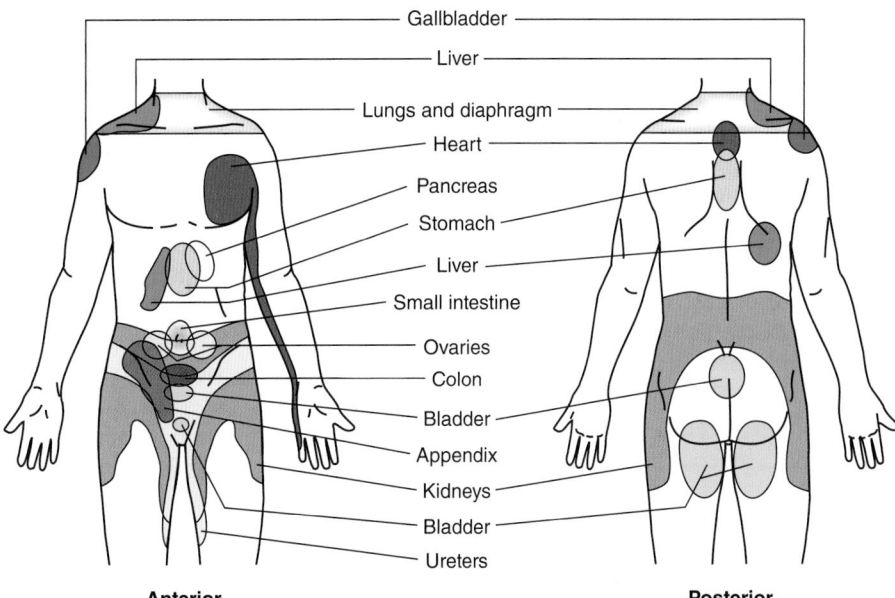

FIGURE 6-6. Sites of referred pain.   **Anterior**   **Posterior**

fibers of the cervical spinal nerves C3 through C5. These nerves also innervate the shoulder muscles and skin. When there are pain signals from C3 through C5, the brain interprets the signals as coming from the shoulder because it has a better neurosignature of the shoulder muscles and skin compared with the diaphragm.

Phantom Pain

Phantom pain is the sensation of pain originating in an amputated part of the body. Patients describe a burning, stinging, or cramping pain, or they may describe a feeling that the missing body part is positioned awkwardly or painfully. Phantom pain is constant and is most intense right after the amputation. The pain usually develops within the first month after amputation and most often develops in patients who had a high degree of pain preamputation. The pain becomes intermittent and resolves with time, although some patients still experience phantom pain years after the amputation. Phantom pain is usually worse at night, after the extremity has been in a dependent position, and it can be worsened by anxiety and stress. The neuromatrix theory explains the reason for phantom limb pain best. The body's extremities are part of the neurosignature impressed upon the neuromatrix since birth. Well-developed neurological pathways are part of the neurosignature, and the brain still perceives the extremities despite their amputation.

Pain Assessment

Pain is referred to as the fifth vital sign because its assessment is so important to the patient's health. It is important for the clinician to listen to the patient's complaint of pain, including its quality, duration, associated features, and alleviating factors. A thorough history is necessary, as is careful physical assessment. The clinician should allow the patient to point to the area of pain before the physical examination; this area should always be examined last.

Clinical Presentation

Pain is subjective, and pain behaviors differ from person to person. Some patients are stoic and suppressed in their expression, whereas others can exaggerate their pain. Nonverbal and behavioral expressions are not consistent or reliable indicators of pain intensity or quality, and they should not be used to determine the presence or absence of pain. However, because pain is a subjective feeling, the clinician cannot assume the patient is inaccurate in their description, which is why assessment relies heavily on the patient report.

Pain is often accompanied by symptoms and physiological conditions that offer diagnostic clues of the complete clinical picture, including tachycardia, hypertension, tachypnea, mydriasis, diaphoresis, hypervigilance, anxiety, and increased muscle tone. To assess the pain and accompanying symptoms, the initial history can be obtained by using the **OLDCART** (onset, location, duration, characteristics, aggravating or relieving factors and associated symptoms, and treatment) mnemonic, which prompts essential questions (see Box 6-1).

If a patient cannot find words to describe the character of pain, the clinician should prompt the patient by asking if the pain is throbbing, aching, stabbing, crushing, or piercing. It is common for the clinician to

---

BOX 6-1. OLDCART

Use the OLDCART mnemonic to assess pain, its features, and its treatment.
- **O**nset: When did the pain begin?
- **L**ocation: Where does it hurt? Can you point to where it hurts?
- **D**uration: How long does it last?
- **C**haracteristics: What does it feel like?
- **A**ggravating factors: Does anything make it worse?
- **R**elieving factors: Does anything make it better?
- **T**reatment: Did anything make it better (pain medication, ice, heat)?

---

use a 0 to 10 scale and ask the patient for a number that describes the pain's severity, with 1 being mild to 10 being the worst pain ever experienced. The clinician should also ask about associated symptoms, such as depression, anxiety, anorexia, nausea, and insomnia, which may affect the treatment plan.

Distinguishing Features of Pain

Pain can have certain characteristics and associated symptoms. When seeking a diagnosis, it is necessary to obtain a complete clinical picture of the problem by searching for additional distinguishing features of the pain. For example, myocardial pain can present like the epigastric pain of esophagitis. However, distinguishing features that characterize the pain as cardiac include associated dyspnea, pallor, and diaphoresis. These associated features enable the clinician to make the specific diagnosis of cardiac chest pain (see Table 6-2).

Another example is colicky pain. **Colic** is a pain that occurs in waves; it builds to a peak and then declines. Spasmodic pain within hollow organs, such as the hyperperistalsis of gastroenteritis, can cause colicky pain. If the hollow organ is the intestine, its muscular walls can spasm to cause colicky pain. Other abdominal organs can also cause colicky pain, particularly the gallbladder in cholecystitis. A gallstone can develop in cholelithiasis. The muscular walls of the gallbladder or cystic duct can spasm around the gallstone, causing colicky pain.

Cholecystitis, appendicitis, pancreatitis, and diverticulitis are often referred to as disorders of the acute abdomen. The pain of the acute abdomen is unique because organs of the gastrointestinal tract that lie within the peritoneal cavity can cause inflammation of the peritoneal membrane. Peritoneal inflammation is intense and exhibited by abdominal muscle rigidity, a phenomenon called guarding. Rebound tenderness also occurs in peritoneal inflammation; pain occurs when the examiner palpates and lifts the hand from the abdomen. The patient with peritoneal inflammation usually cannot tolerate movement because it aggravates the peritoneal membrane. With this in mind, asking the patient to jump or cough usually makes the pain worse.

Interestingly, when there is rupture of an organ beneath the diaphragm, free air can escape from the organ and irritate the diaphragm. The diaphragm's irritation refers pain to the shoulder; it is necessary that the clinician recognize patterns of referred pain (see Fig. 6-6).

Some people who suffer from chronic pain conditions **catastrophize,** which is defined as an exaggerated negative orientation toward actual or anticipated pain experiences. These misinterpretations of pain can lead to a cycle of avoidance of activity, disuse, and disability.

In the face of continuing pain, people may have pain-related anxiety and feel they have no control over the pain. Depression is also common in patients with chronic pain. Prolonged pain is difficult to endure and, as a result, people undergo major affective and behavior changes, including increased or decreased appetite, restricted activity levels, social withdrawal, life role changes, poor sleep, chronic fatigue, and decreased concentration.

Physical Assessment

Following the history, a thorough examination should be conducted to detect sensory, motor, and coordination abnormalities. Patients with pain may have changes in the way they respond to touch. The motor examination may reveal increased or decreased muscle tone, weakened muscles, tremor, paralysis, hyporeflexia, or hyperreflexia. The patient's gait should be observed; abnormalities may be seen with musculoskeletal pathology, altered balance, or incoordination. Some types of pain, such as peritoneal irritation, decrease when the patient is stationary. When observing the patient, the examiner should note whether a position change lessens or worsens the pain. Other types of pain, such as pain associated with peristalsis, gallstones, and kidney stones, decrease when the patient moves.

The physical examination will also provide clues as to the amount of physical disability the patient experiences because of the pain. The clinician should be aware of sensory dermatomes and myotomes, as these can assist in the localization of pain.

Diagnosis

Pain severity may be assessed by one of several reliable and valid tools for measuring pain, such as the McGill Pain Scale, which assesses the quality and severity of the patient's pain, and the visual analog scale (VAS), which assesses pain on a sliding scale. Clinicians commonly use the VAS by asking the patient to quantify their pain on a scale of 0 to 10, with 0 being no pain

TABLE 6-2. Distinguishing Features of Pain in Common Disorders

Disorder	Pain	Associated Features
Myocardial infarction	Squeezing, crushing chest pain	Radiation into left arm Radiation possibly up into jaw Radiation to back Dyspnea Diaphoresis Pallor Hypotension Levine's sign (fist to chest)
Peripheral arterial disease	Intermittent claudication of lower extremity	Cramping in the leg that occurs with a similar distance each time it is sensed Associated with pallor, paresthesias, cooler leg temperature Caused by lack of sufficient arterial flow
Pleuritis/pneumonia/pleurisy	Chest pain with coughing or deep breathing	Pleural friction rub heard on auscultation with stethoscope; squeaking or grating sounds of the pleural linings rubbing together that can be described as the sound made by treading on fresh snow
Cholecystitis/cholelithiasis (inflammation of gall-bladder with gallstone)	Biliary colic; intense pain comes on in waves	Nausea Vomiting Eructation (belching) Full feeling of stomach Tenderness of the right upper quadrant of the abdomen with palpation; called Murphy's sign
Appendicitis	Pain starts in the umbilical area then gradually becomes localized to right lower quadrant of abdomen; called McBurney's point	Extreme tenderness of right lower quadrant Signs of peritoneal inflammation include: • Patient wanting to remain stationary • Jumping, coughing that hurts abdomen • Psoas sign • Rebound tenderness • Guarding • Rovsing's sign • Rectal pain
Nephrolithiasis (kidney stone)	Colicky pain from costovertebral region around body into the groin	Patient cannot find a comfortable position; intense pain and hematuria
Uterine/ovarian/fallopian disorders	Pelvic or abdominal pain radiates down leg to inner thigh obturator nerve	Air can collect under the diaphragm, causing referred shoulder pain
Stomach/duodenum peptic ulcer	Gnawing, burning pain	Pain occurs between meals; food soothes pain
Ruptured peptic ulcer/pancreatitis	Pain in umbilical area straight into the back	Tachycardia Nausea Vomiting Anxiety
Aortic aneurysm/aortic dissection	Tearing, midthoracic pain	Pallor Hypotension Anxiety

and 10 being most severe pain (see Fig. 6-7). The Wong-Baker FACES scale, which is commonly used for children and adults with cognitive impairment, is a variation of the VAS that is also valid and reliable (see Fig. 6-8). In comatose or noncommunicative patients, the Critical Care Pain Observation Tool (CPOT) or the Faces, Legs, Activity, Cry, and Consolability Tool (FLACC) can be used.

Diagnostic tests may be employed based on clinical findings, patient disorders, or to guide treatment approaches. Various imaging techniques or nerve studies may also be helpful (see Box 6-2).

> ### 🩺 CLINICAL CONCEPT
>
> Normal results on studies should not deter the clinician from diagnosing and treating the patient if the clinical examination is consistent with a certain type of pain. In fact, allowing the pain to continue without treatment may be associated with the initiation of chronic pain pathways.

Treatment

The World Health Organization's (WHO) Step Analgesic Ladder provides an approach to the pharmacological management of pain. Although initially created to treat cancer pain, this tool has been proposed as an excellent model for all types of pain (see Fig. 6-9). Some researchers have recently recommended modifications regarding the inclusion of a fourth step that describes procedures for intractable pain. The modification also adds opioids—tramadol, oxycodone, hydromorphone, and buprenorphine—and new ways of administering them, such as patient-controlled analgesia, epidural administration, and transdermal patch.

There are three major classes of pharmacological pain relievers: opioid, nonopioid, and adjuvant medications. The analgesic ladder proposes that treatment of pain should begin with a nonopioid medication, such as an NSAID. If the pain is not properly controlled, a weak opioid should be introduced. If the use of this medication is insufficient to treat the pain, a more powerful opioid can be used instead. Two products belonging to the same category should not be used simultaneously, as they would not offer any different pain control while also increasing risk of adverse effects. When using multiple pain relievers, each drug should have a different mode of action. The WHO analgesic ladder

---

BOX 6-2. Diagnostic Studies for Pain

There is a wide variety of diagnostic studies for pain because of the many different possible causes. The etiology of pain influences the manner of treatment.

- **Blood tests:** Detect diabetes; vitamin deficiencies; and liver, kidney, or immune problems.
- **Nerve conduction study:** Shows how fast nerves are able to transmit impulses, as well as the strength of those signals. Can determine whether muscle function is a problem or whether other neurological conditions such as multiple sclerosis are present.
- **Electromyography:** Measures the electrical activity of one or more muscles while being flexed. Shows how well muscles are receiving impulses from nerves.
- **Nerve injection:** Injection of the nerve with lidocaine or bupivacaine (Marcaine) just above the site of involvement can be the most valuable diagnostic tool. The patient can define the extent of relief obtained from such an injection, which can be helpful in defining the zone of injury and expected relief from surgical release or excision.
- **Myelogram:** Contrast medium is injected into the subarachnoid space to visualize the spinal cord.
- **Ultrasound, computed tomography scan, or magnetic resonance imaging:** Checks whether cysts, tumors, blood vessels, or bones are compressing nerves.

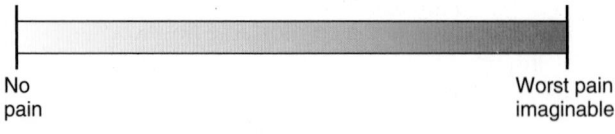

No pain   Worst pain imaginable

FIGURE 6-7. Visual analog scale.

Wong-Baker FACES® Pain Rating Scale

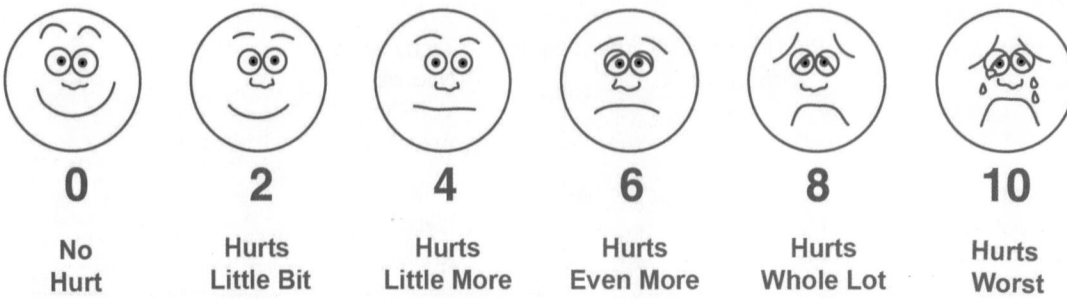

0	2	4	6	8	10
No Hurt	Hurts Little Bit	Hurts Little More	Hurts Even More	Hurts Whole Lot	Hurts Worst

FIGURE 6-8. Wong-Baker FACES Pain Rating Scale. (*www.wongbakerFACES.org. © 1983. Wong-Baker FACES Foundation. Used with permission.*)

WHO analgesic (pain relief) ladder

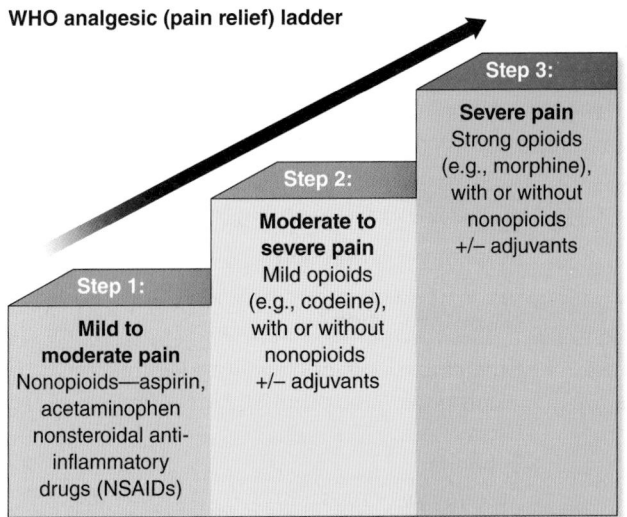

Step 1:
Mild to moderate pain
Nonopioids—aspirin, acetaminophen nonsteroidal anti-inflammatory drugs (NSAIDs)

Step 2:
Moderate to severe pain
Mild opioids (e.g., codeine), with or without nonopioids +/– adjuvants

Step 3:
Severe pain
Strong opioids (e.g., morphine), with or without nonopioids +/– adjuvants

FIGURE 6-9. WHO step ladder approach to analgesic treatment. The "pain ladder" is a term coined by the WHO to describe its guidelines for the use of drugs in pain management. Originally applied to the management of cancer pain, it is now widely used for the management of all types of pain. The general principle is to start with first-step drugs and then to climb the ladder if pain is still present. The medications range from over-the-counter drugs with minimal side effects at the lowest rung to more powerful opioids at the highest rung. *(Adapted from WHO, https://www.ncbi.nlm.nih.gov/books/NBK554435)*

recommends the use of adjuvant treatments, such as antidepressants for neuropathic pain or for unrelieved pain associated with cancer.

The analgesic ladder can be used in a bidirectional fashion: the slower upward pathway for chronic pain and cancer pain and the faster downward direction for intense acute pain and uncontrolled chronic pain. The ladder can be used to ascend slowly one step at a time

in the case of chronic pain and, if necessary, increase the rate of climb according to the intensity of the pain. Once pain is controlled, the WHO recommends that the patient "step down" on the ladder.

Modifications to the WHO analgesic ladder have been recommended (see Fig. 6-10), expanding it to include nonpharmacological modalities of pain management, such as physiotherapy, acupuncture, occupational therapy, and psychological counseling. Nonpharmacological measures are discussed later in this chapter.

Opioids

Opioids are powerful medications that may be used alone or in conjunction with other analgesics. Opioids, also referred to as opiates or narcotics, are derived from the opium poppy plant. They are considered controlled substances by the Federal Drug Administration (FDA). A **controlled substance** is a drug or chemical whose manufacture, possession, or use is regulated by the federal government. According to the FDA, controlled substances have abuse potential and can cause physical dependence. Mishandling, abusing, or dispensing controlled substances without a license can lead to criminal prosecution. Controlled substances are further categorized according to a **schedule,** ranging from Schedule I through Schedule V. The abuse rate and potential for dependence are determining factors in the scheduling of a drug. Schedule I drugs have a high potential for abuse and the potential to create severe psychological and/or physical dependence. As the drug schedule number increases, the abuse and dependence potential decreases; Schedule V drugs represent the least potential for abuse. A listing of drugs and their schedule were designated by the Controlled Substance Act (CSA). Table 6-3 displays

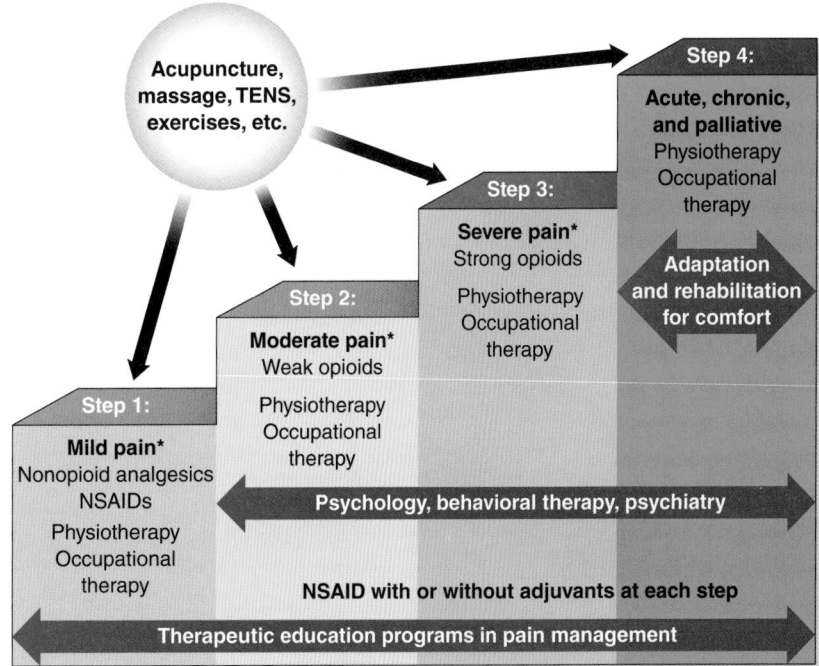

Acupuncture, massage, TENS, exercises, etc.

Step 1:
Mild pain*
Nonopioid analgesics
NSAIDs
Physiotherapy
Occupational therapy

Step 2:
Moderate pain*
Weak opioids
Physiotherapy
Occupational therapy

Step 3:
Severe pain*
Strong opioids
Physiotherapy
Occupational therapy

Step 4:
Acute, chronic, and palliative
Physiotherapy
Occupational therapy

Adaptation and rehabilitation for comfort

Psychology, behavioral therapy, psychiatry

NSAID with or without adjuvants at each step

Therapeutic education programs in pain management

FIGURE 6-10. Modified WHO ladder that includes nonpharmacological modalities of pain management. *(From Grisell Vargas-Schaffer, G., & Cogan, J. [2014]. Patient therapeutic education. Canadian Family Physician, 60(3), 235–241. Copyright © The College of Family Physicians of Canada.)*

NSAID—nonsteroidal anti-inflammatory drug, TENS—transcutaneous electrical nerve stimulation.
*Acute and chronic pain

TABLE 6-3. Commonly Used Opioid Analgesics

Drug	Indication	Side Effects
SCHEDULE II		
Morphine (MS Contin, Roxanol)	Severe pain Prototypical opioid medication	Drowsiness Euphoria Respiratory depression Constipation Nausea/vomiting
Hydrocodone (Vicodin)	Moderate pain 10% of people lack the enzyme needed to make codeine active (CYP2D6)	Greater amounts of nausea and vomiting compared with other opioids Drowsiness Euphoria Respiratory depression
Hydromorphone (Dilaudid)	Severe pain Duration of action is slightly less than morphine	Drowsiness Euphoria Respiratory depression
Meperidine (Demerol)	Severe pain	Repeated dosing not recommended, as accumulation of meperidine metabolites can cause central nervous system excitation and high risk of seizures
Methadone (Dolophine, Methadose)	Severe pain Can be used to wean off opioids in a detoxification program	Drowsiness or insomnia Dizziness Nausea Vomiting Hypotension Constipation
Oxycodone (Oxycontin, Percocet, Endocet, Roxicodone, Roxicet)	Severe pain	Drowsiness Euphoria Respiratory depression Constipation
Fentanyl (Duragesic, Oralet, Actiq, Sublimaze, Innovar)	Severe pain May be administered via intravenous (IV), subcutaneous (SQ), transmucosal, epidural, and intrathecal route Short duration of action compared with morphine	Diarrhea Drowsiness Urinary retention Weakness Dyspnea Indigestion Dry mouth
Tapentadol	Opioid + norepinephrine/serotonin reuptake inhibitor Moderate to severe chronic pain	Dizziness Constipation Nausea, vomiting
SCHEDULE III		
Buprenorphine (Suboxone, Subutex)	Moderate to severe pain Can be used to wean off opioids in detoxification	Drowsiness Dizziness Nausea Vomiting Constipation Numbness

TABLE 6-3. Commonly Used Opioid Analgesics–cont'd		
Drug	**Indication**	**Side Effects**
SCHEDULE IV		
Tramadol	Moderately severe pain Oral and extended-release	Seizures Dizziness Somnolence Constipation Nausea

the names and uses of some of the most commonly prescribed opioids and their schedule.

Side effects of opioids include diminished concentration ability, nausea, vomiting, feeling of bodily warmth, heaviness of the extremities, dry mouth, pruritus, and respiratory depression. Constipation often occurs with opioid use, and stool softeners can be given to counteract this effect. Miosis (constriction of pupils) will be found on physical assessment. Opioids can also suppress a cough.

Morphine is the prototypical opioid and can be administered in many forms. It is effective against pain from skeletal muscles, joints, viscera, and skin structures. It can produce analgesia, euphoria, and sedation.

Morphine is most effective when given before the painful stimulus; this approach plays a protective role by preventing central sensitization. Central sensitization occurs when neurons involved in pain become more sensitive to pain-causing stimuli. The pain then occurs with less provocation, eventually leading to chronic pain. In general, controlled-release opioids given on a scheduled basis are recommended for patients with persistent or continuous pain to promote constant levels of analgesia, prevent fluctuations in blood levels, and avoid adverse events associated with high peak opioid levels.

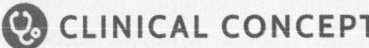

ALERT! Opioids have high abuse potential. Tolerance, physical dependence, and addiction can occur.

CLINICAL CONCEPT

Morphine can cause respiratory depression, particularly in patients with lung disease.

Complications of Opioid Use

Complications of opioid use include substance abuse, tolerance, withdrawal, and physical dependence. For this reason, opioids should be used sparingly in the lowest dose that can alleviate the pain.

Substance Abuse. Substance abuse refers to the dysfunctional use of a substance in amounts or methods not condoned by health-care professionals. Patients with problems of substance abuse may suffer from pain, but many abusers feign the amount of pain they are experiencing. In fact, some abusers may not have any pain at all.

Predictors of substance abuse among patients with chronic pain include a familial or personal history of substance abuse; history of legal problems or criminal activity; regular contact with high-risk people; problems with past employers, family, or friends; medication craving; risk-taking or thrill-seeking behavior; heavy tobacco use; and history of severe depression or anxiety. Many psychosocial and behavioral factors are involved in substance abuse, and patients require a consultation with an addiction specialist who can provide ongoing care.

CLINICAL CONCEPT

Patients who are prescribed opioid medications have the potential for abuse. Appropriate screening should take place with the Screener Opioid Assessment for Patients with Pain before initiating drug therapy.

Tolerance, Physical Dependence, and Opioid Withdrawal. **Tolerance** is a state of adaptation in which chronic exposure to a drug causes gradual decreasing results over time. As a person takes an opioid for an extended period, receptors in the brain become less sensitive, and higher dosages are required to achieve the same effect. When the body can no longer make enough natural opioids to satisfy the less sensitive receptors, the body becomes dependent on the external source. This is physical dependence, a state of adaptation that is manifested by a drug withdrawal syndrome that can be produced by abrupt cessation, rapid dose reduction, decreasing blood level of the drug, or administration of an antagonist.

For patients who have been on long-term opioid treatment such as morphine, there is a normal physiological tolerance to the drug. The patient becomes habituated to a certain dosage of opioid and reliant on the drug. Opioid **withdrawal** occurs when the patient develops systemic symptoms in response to a lack of adequate opioid dosage needed by the body. Symptoms of withdrawal can be seen within hours of missing a regular dose and include nausea, vomiting, tachycardia, sweating, restlessness, irritability, insomnia, lacrimation, and rhinorrhea. The extent of symptoms will depend on the drug dose and how long it has been taken. Tapering the medication slowly over several weeks can help minimize the intensity of symptoms. Clonidine may also be used to treat withdrawal.

Addiction to opioids is a common disorder developed after frequent use of the drugs. **Addiction** is a primary, chronic, neurological disease with genetic, psychosocial, and environmental factors influencing its development and manifestations. It is characterized by behavior that includes one or more of the following:

- Impaired control over drug use
- Compulsive use of drug
- Continued use despite harm from using the drug
- Craving of the drug

CLINICAL CONCEPT

Patients with opioid addiction require a multidisciplinary approach to rehabilitation. Methadone, a synthetic opioid, is commonly administered to prevent the symptoms of opioid withdrawal. Methadone does not have the euphoric effects of opioids such as heroin. It is commonly administered in decreasing dosages to slowly wean the patient off opioids and diminish the effects of withdrawal.

Buprenorphine is a newer medication used as opioid replacement therapy to wean patients from opioids. It is a partial opiate receptor agonist that causes less analgesia and euphoria than methadone but ameliorates withdrawal symptoms. As a partial agonist, buprenorphine has a "ceiling effect"; that is, after a certain point, taking more will not increase any of the effects of the drug. It is not a respiratory depressant, which adds to its safety in accidental or intentional overdose. In addition, buprenorphine has a high affinity for the mu (μ) opioid receptor, which means that it reduces the effects of additional opioid use.

Opioid Overdose and Naloxone. Persons addicted to opioids are at risk for overdose. Naloxone is a drug that helps counter the effects of opiate overdose because it has an extremely high affinity for opioid receptors in the CNS. Naloxone is a competitive antagonist that blocks opioid attachment to neural receptors. It is specifically used to counteract life-threatening depression of the CNS and respiratory system. High-dose intranasal naloxone is available for emergency opioid overdose.

ALERT! Naloxone will cause rapid onset of withdrawal symptoms in patients who are physically dependent on opioids.

ALERT! According to the CDC, there were an estimated 100,306 drug overdose deaths in the United States during 2021, which is an increase of 28.5% from 2020. Illicitly manufactured fentanyl (and analogues) are the drugs most responsible for this rise in opioid deaths.

Nonopioid Analgesics

Nonopioid analgesics include acetaminophen (Tylenol) and NSAIDs such as aspirin, ibuprofen, naproxen sodium, and celecoxib. All of these agents except for acetaminophen work by blocking cyclo-oxygenase enzymes (COX-1 and -2) that prevent the release of PGs from white blood cells and inflammatory tissue. PGs are chemical mediators involved in physiological processes and the inflammation reaction. Some PGs are necessary for gastric mucus production, renal perfusion, and thrombus formation; these PGs utilize the COX-1 enzyme pathway. Other PGs cause edema, pain, inflammation, and dysmenorrheal uterine contractions; these PGs utilize the COX-2 enzyme pathway (see Fig. 6-11). Most NSAIDs are nonselective cyclo-oxygenase pathway inhibitors that block both COX-1 and -2 enzymes. Because NSAIDs are nonselective, they can cause some adverse physiological effects, including diminished gastric mucus and ulceration, decreased renal perfusion, and diminished clotting. Patients who routinely use NSAIDs should be counseled about the side effects of gastric irritation, clotting deficit, and renal insufficiency (see Fig. 6-11).

Celecoxib (Celebrex) is a selective COX-2 enzyme inhibitor. Specific inhibition of the COX-2 enzyme pathway blocks PGs that cause edema, inflammation, and pain. COX-2 inhibitors were developed so that the selectivity of the drug would avoid the adverse side effects of the nonselective NSAIDs. However, recent research and clinical experience have shown that those who used the COX-2 inhibitor rofecoxib (Vioxx) had an increased risk of myocardial infarction, strokes, and deep vein thrombosis. Rofecoxib was taken off the market, but celecoxib is still available and prescribed.

Acetaminophen is an antipyretic and analgesic agent, but it does not inhibit inflammation. Its mechanism is not fully understood; however, it blocks prostaglandin synthesis, activates serotonin receptors, and inhibits endocannabinoid reuptake in the CNS.

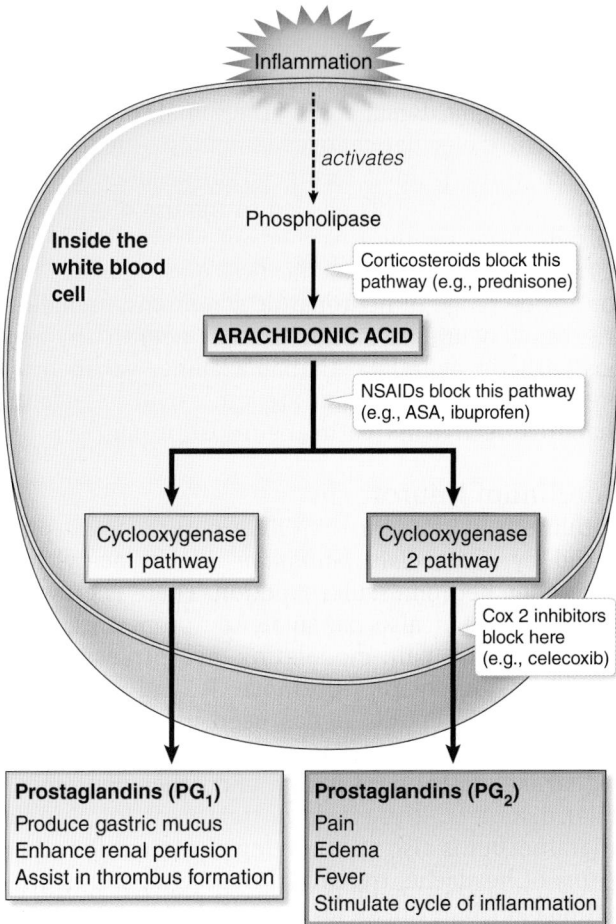

FIGURE 6-11. Inflammation pathways of PGs and sites of anti-inflammatory drug action. After inflammation stimulates the inflammatory reaction, white blood cells produce PGs via the cyclo-oxygenase pathways. The COX-1 pathway produces prostaglandins (PG1s) that assist the body in performing significant functions. The COX-2 pathway produces prostaglandins (PG2s) that cause uncomfortable side effects of inflammation. Anti-inflammatory drugs block the formation of PGs at the sites shown. Corticosteroids and NSAIDs block the formation of both types of PGs. Therefore corticosteroids and NSAIDs block gastric mucus production, decrease renal perfusion, and inhibit thrombus formation. COX-2 inhibitors can specifically block the PG2s that cause the uncomfortable side effects of inflammation.

Adjuvant Medications

Adjuvant medications are used to amplify the analgesic effect of pain medication. Commonly, acetaminophen can be added to an analgesic agent to boost its effect. An example is oxycodone plus acetaminophen (Percocet). However, it is important to warn patients that many over-the-counter (OTC) drugs contain acetaminophen, and it is important to read labels so as not to overdose on acetaminophen. For example, Theraflu is a common OTC medication used to relieve cold symptoms. It contains 650 mg of acetaminophen per tablet. This isn't apparent by the name of the drug, and a person may take it with additional acetaminophen, not recognizing the high dosage already contained in the drug.

ALERT! An average OTC combination drug contains up to 500 mg of acetaminophen. The FDA has recommended a limit of 4000 mg of acetaminophen per day. Acetaminophen toxicity can cause liver failure.

Other adjuvant medications include antidepressants and anticonvulsants, particularly used for neuropathic pain. Local anesthetic agents and corticosteroids can also assist in pain relief. Injection of these medications into joints for musculoskeletal pain is common.

With the increasing acceptance of cannabis as a medicinal drug, cannabinoids (CBDs) can be added to the group of adjuvant medications. They have demonstrated efficacy in the palliative care of cancer patients, patients affected by AIDS, and in some neuropathic pain disorders.

Antidepressants

Antidepressants can increase synaptic serotonin, norepinephrine, and dopamine levels. They also have been found to enhance the effect of analgesics in some types of neuropathic pain. Tricyclic antidepressants (TCAs), however, have many unpleasant and potentially dangerous side effects, limiting their use in some patients. Older adults, for example, are prone to toxic effects from TCAs.

ALERT! Overdose of TCAs is often fatal.

Serotonin-norepinephrine reuptake inhibitors have also proven to be effective for treating some types of neuropathic pain. They are safer to use than TCAs and are a better option for patients with cardiac disease. The relative risk for withdrawal because of side effects is low, and there is no need for drug-level monitoring. Side effects include sedation, confusion, hypertension, nausea, vomiting, constipation, loss of appetite, and weakness.

Local Anesthetics

Local anesthetics produce anesthesia by inhibiting excitation of nerve endings or by blocking conduction in peripheral nerves. This is achieved by anesthetics reversibly binding to and inactivating sodium channels. Sodium influx through these channels is necessary for the depolarization of nerve cell membranes and subsequent propagation of impulses along the course of the nerve. When a nerve loses depolarization and capacity to propagate an impulse, the individual loses sensation in the area supplied by the nerve. Commonly used agents include lidocaine, mepivacaine, prilocaine, procaine, and benzocaine.

Peripheral Nerve Blockade

Peripheral nerve blocks (PNBs) are mainly used for postoperative pain management, most commonly after orthopedic surgery. Analgesic and anesthetic agents can be administered as a single injection or continuous infusion via a perineural catheter. A continuous infusion provides a longer duration of pain management. PNB is often used in combination with systemic analgesia (e.g., opioids).

Injected Corticosteroids

Steroids are the most potent anti-inflammatory agents available and are used to reduce inflammation of the tissue compressing the affected nerves, as well as to reduce neuronal edema. Corticosteroids can be injected into joints to treat musculoskeletal disorders, as well as into the epidural space to reduce spinal nerve root impingement from spinal degenerative conditions such as disc herniation. Prolotherapy, an injection of lidocaine and a corticosteroid into affected muscles and joints, can be used to treat mechanical low back pain and fibromyalgia.

Topical Pain Relievers

Topical analgesics are effective and alternative means to systemic therapy, often minimizing the adverse drug effects and complications of systemic analgesic use. They are most effective with localized nociceptive pain, as in osteoarthritis, localized tissue injury, or some neuropathic pain. Topical or transdermal capsaicin can be applied at the region of pain. Capsaicin depletes a chemical (substance P) responsible for transmitting painful impulses from peripheral sites to the CNS and thus provides analgesia in some disorders. Topical lidocaine has limited systemic absorption when applied to intact skin and exerts its analgesic effects through the blockage of sodium channels on afferent nerves. Available topical NSAIDs include diclofenac in a patch, gel, or solution, which are indicated for minor strains, sprains, and contusions (patch) and osteoarthritis (gel and solution). In osteoarthritis of the knee, topical diclofenac has shown equal efficacy compared with oral diclofenac in terms of pain reduction (Ling et al., 2020).

 CLINICAL CONCEPT

Epidural administration of local anesthetic and corticosteroid is often used for intractable back pain.

Anticonvulsants

Neuropathic pain, whether of peripheral or central origin, is characterized by a neuronal hyperexcitability in damaged areas of the nervous system. In peripheral neuropathic pain, damaged nerve endings exhibit abnormal changes at neural sodium and calcium channels, glutamate receptors, and GABA inhibition. The peripheral hyperexcitability is due to molecular changes at the level of the peripheral nociceptor, dorsal root ganglia, dorsal horn of the spinal cord, and the brain. The molecular changes in neuropathic pain are similar to the cellular changes that occur in certain forms of epilepsy. This has led to the use of anticonvulsant drugs for the treatment of neuropathic pain. A trial of antiepileptic medication may be beneficial for a wide range of neuropathic symptoms, including trigeminal neuralgia, painful diabetic neuropathy, and postherpetic neuralgia. Carbamazepine, gabapentin, pregabalin, and lamotrigine are anticonvulsant agents that are effective in treating neuropathic pain.

Botulinum Neurotoxin

Botulinum neurotoxin (BoNT), a natural toxin produced by *Clostridium botulinum,* blocks acetylcholine at the neuromuscular junction. There is growing evidence that it also has analgesic properties, as it blocks various pain-modulating neurotransmitters, including glutamate, substance P, and calcitonin gene–related peptide. It has been used extensively for relief of painful muscle spasm in multiple sclerosis, stroke, spinal cord injury, and other neuromuscular disorders. It is effective treatment for chronic migraine, but is also an emerging treatment for other forms of headache, trigeminal neuralgia, and neuropathic pain. BoNT has a favorable safety profile, and a single injection can provide long-lasting relief. More research is needed to explore BoNT as an analgesic and investigate the best routes of administration and optimal dosages.

Potential of Cannabinoids

Cannabinoids are natural endogenous substances, plant-based substances (marijuana), and synthetic pharmacological agents (Dronabinol, Epidiolex). The endogenous endocannabinoid system (ECS) is active throughout the CNS and peripheral nervous system (PNS) in modulating pain. The ECS alleviates pain through a variety of receptor and nonreceptor mechanisms, including direct analgesic and anti-inflammatory effects, modulatory actions on neurotransmitters, and interactions with endogenous and administered opioids. Endocannabinoids are naturally produced in the CNS to dampen sensitivity to pain.

The use of plant-based cannabinoids (marijuana) has been found to relieve pain in some disorders. However, the use of marijuana for medicinal purposes is a controversial subject with evidential studies that both support and deny the efficacy of the agents in various disorders. Part of the controversy involves cannabis (marijuana) being designated as a Schedule I controlled substance by the FDA. Schedule I drugs are considered to have the highest potential for abuse and physical/psychological dependence.

Studies have shown that cannabinoids can reduce pain in neuropathic disorders, multiple sclerosis, fibromyalgia, rheumatoid arthritis, and cancer. The study of the role of cannabinoids in pain management is evolving. More studies are needed to support the analgesic benefit of cannabinoids, as well as determine optimal routes of administration, effective dosages, adverse effects, and drug interactions.

A significant mechanism of cannabis is stimulation of natural endorphins by the ingredient tetrahydrocannabinol (THC). This effect on endorphins has shown that cannabinoids used with opioids can be opiate sparing; less opioid drug can be used to achieve a high level of pain relief. The use of cannabinoids in conjunction with opioid drugs has been shown to prevent opioid tolerance, overuse, and withdrawal (Campbell et al., 2018; Nielsen et al., 2017). In the future, adjunctive treatments that combine opioids with cannabinoids may enhance the analgesic effect of both agents. Such strategies may permit use of lower doses of opioid analgesics for therapeutic benefit, minimize adverse side effects, and decrease potential for opioid abuse and overdose. More research is needed to replicate studies that demonstrate this opioid-sparing benefit.

Nonpharmacological Pain Management

Nonpharmacological methods of pain management may be used alone or in conjunction with pharmacological agents for pain relief. Integrative medicine is a branch of medicine that emphasizes nonpharmacological therapies and attends to the patient's physical, psychological, emotional, and social experience of pain. These methods include complementary and alternative therapies that offer nontraditional approaches to lessen pain and enhance function and quality of life. This is a new paradigm based on evidence-based methods that are effective in the management of both acute and chronic pain. Many treatments are effective because they activate the body's own endorphins and enkephalins. Therapies include healing touch, physiotherapy, imagery, yoga, cognitive-behavioral therapy (CBT), acupuncture, and others.

Nursing Interventions
Nursing interventions have been shown to diminish pain severity and normalize vital signs in patients across different clinical settings. Dialogue, proper body positioning, and splinting the postsurgical site are pain-relieving nursing interventions. Healing touch, commonly used by nurses, reduces anxiety, facilitates relaxation, and decreases pain in patients. In patients with dementia, hand-holding and stroking the forehead or shoulder have been shown to decrease patient distress. Neonates who are closely held in skin-to-skin contact, swaddled, and rocked by nurses during painful procedures are noted to demonstrate less agitation and lower heart rate. Patient education provided by nurses has also been shown to lessen patient stress levels.

Physiotherapy
Physiotherapy consists of function-oriented exercises and manual treatments that aim to optimize patient strength, flexibility, and aerobic capacity. Physiotherapy is often a component of pain management after surgery or in conjunction with pharmacotherapy. It is most effective with musculoskeletal pain, such as complex regional pain syndrome (CRPS), chronic headache, fibromyalgia, whiplash injury, lower back pain, and osteoarthritis. Physiotherapy begins with physical assessment of the patient's specific limitations and sensitive areas, followed by an individualized treatment plan of supervised exercise and hands-on manual therapies. Manual therapies include soft tissue manipulation, heat and cold therapy, ultrasound, joint mobilization, trigger point massage, iontophoresis, spinal manipulation, and other modalities. Treatment plans include counseling regarding self-management of pain.

Occupational Therapy
Occupational therapy teaches patients how to live and function with their disability. Patients learn how to perform activities of daily living without discomfort and using the least amount of energy. Occupational therapists perform a complete evaluation of the patient's abilities and disabilities and plan goals for rehabilitation. Occupational therapy services include assessment of the patient's home and other environments (e.g., workplace, school), recommendations for adaptive equipment, and education for family members and caregivers.

Acupuncture
Acupuncture is an ancient Chinese medical intervention that involves the stimulation of the body using thin, solid metallic needles that are inserted by hand. The aim of the procedure is to improve levels of qi (pronounced *chi*), which practitioners believe is the energy force behind all life, and to restore balance in the opposing forces of yin and yang. The needles are placed along specific, invisible energy channels called meridians that run along the length of the body.

Research studies have shown acupuncture can help relieve neuropathic pain associated with spinal cord injury, chronic pelvic pain, hot flashes associated with menopause, breathlessness associated with chronic obstructive pulmonary disease, and postchemotherapy fatigue. More research is needed to investigate acupuncture's benefits for other disorders.

Guided Imagery
Guided imagery is a program of directed thoughts and suggestions that guide the imagination toward a relaxed, focused state. Instructors, videos, or scripts assist the patient through this process. Guided imagery is based on the concept that the body and mind are connected. Using all the senses, the body can respond as though the imagined scenario is real. Guided

imagery promotes relaxation, which can lower blood pressure and reduce other problems related to stress. It has been used for weight loss, smoking cessation, and pain management.

Virtual Reality

Virtual reality (VR) is a computer-generated environment that immerses the user in an interactive artificial world. This ability to distract from reality has been utilized for the purposes of providing pain relief from noxious stimuli. As technology rapidly matures, there is potential for anaesthetists and pain physicians to incorporate virtual reality devices as nonpharmacological therapy in a multimodal pain management strategy. Some studies demonstrate that VR is an effective adjunct modality for pain management in intraoperative settings, labor and delivery, painful wound dressing changes, and chronic pain conditions (Chuan et al., 2021).

Transcutaneous Electrical Nerve Stimulation

TENS is the use of low-voltage electrical current to help relieve pain. A small, battery-operated device delivers electrical current through the skin via electrodes placed near the source of pain. It is theorized that the electricity stimulates nerves in the affected area and sends signals to the brain that scramble normal pain perception. TENS has been shown to be helpful to relieve pain of diabetic neuropathy, degenerative disc disease, and dysmenorrhea.

Ultrasound-Guided Peripheral Nerve Stimulation

Peripheral nerve stimulation using electrical current is a commonly used modality for postoperative orthopedic surgery. Electrical stimulation activates large-diameter myelinated afferent peripheral nerve fibers, which in turn inhibit pain signals from the small-diameter pain fibers to the central nervous system.

Peripheral Nerve Cryoanalgesia

Cryoanalgesia is the application of extremely cold temperatures to peripheral nerves involved in the pain propagation. The cold temperature ablates the nerve fibers and provides analgesia in the distribution of the nerve until the nerve regenerates, often for up to several months. This modality is mainly employed to blunt chronic pain.

Intradiscal Electrothermal Therapy

Intradiscal electrothermal therapy (IDET) uses heat to modify the nerve fibers of a spinal disc and to destroy pain receptors in the area. In this procedure, a wire called an electrothermal catheter is placed through an incision in the disc. An electrical current passes through the catheter, heating a small outer portion of the disc to a temperature of 194°F. IDET is performed as an outpatient procedure while the patient is awake and under local anesthesia. Early studies indicate that some patients may have continued pain relief for up to 6 months or longer. The long-term effects of this procedure on the disc have not been determined.

Psychological Counseling for Chronic Pain

Chronic pain, typically defined as persistent pain that has continued for longer than 3 to 6 months, is a complex biopsychosocial condition, requiring a multimodal approach to management. Evidence supports the effectiveness of various cognitive-behavioral interventions for reducing pain intensity and improving a patient's coping skills. The most common interventions include acceptance and commitment therapy (ACT) and traditional CBT. Both ACT and CBT interventions decrease pain intensity, disability, and pain interference. Both increase patient readiness to create changes in coping with chronic pain, depression, or anxiety. The methods used within CBT include managing moods, attention, thoughts, and activity. Relaxation and physical exercise techniques are used to alter negative thoughts, increase control, and create positive goals. ACT is similar to CBT but it incorporates mindfulness-based treatment methods. Mindfulness is a time of meditation that focuses the person on a particular object, thought, or activity to achieve a mentally clear and emotionally calm state. Mindfulness has been shown to decrease blood pressure, slow heart rate, and alleviate anxiety.

Selected Clinical Pain Syndromes

Some disorders have specific patterns and characteristics of pain. The clinician needs to recognize the manifestations of these specific pain syndromes. Recognizing specific pain patterns and qualities can assist in the diagnosis and treatment of these disorders.

Cancer Pain

One out of every three persons suffering from cancer endures pain. Cancer pain can be dull, aching, or sharp. It can be intermittent or constant and result from the cancerous lesion or the treatment.

Tumors can cause pain by putting pressure on or destroying adjacent tissue. Cancer cells secrete enzymes and inflammatory mediators that penetrate and irritate tissues. Enzymatic destruction of adjoining tissues is also common in cancer. Pain can come from the primary tumor itself or from other areas in the body where the cancer has metastasized. Tumors secrete chemical mediators such as endothelin-1, which is a strong vasoconstrictor that decreases circulation to certain areas. Tumors also secrete PGs and substance P, which can cause pain, edema, and constant inflammation.

Some cancer treatments, such as chemotherapy, can cause painful side effects such as mouth sores, diarrhea, and nerve damage. Radiation treatment in cancer can leave a burning sensation in the radiated region. Surgery can leave painful scars along with a burning sensation.

Bone pain is a debilitating form of pain that is often caused by the metastasis of cancer. The outer periosteal layer of bone tissue is highly pain sensitive and a frequent source of pain. Tumors within the center of bone involve the endosteal and haversian nerve supply. Interior tumors secrete enzymes and inflammatory mediators that stimulate nociceptors and produce dull, diffuse pain. When the cancer cells have established themselves within bone, the mechanical dynamics of the bone matrix become weaker as skeletal strength decreases. This leads to several other complications throughout the body, including pain, that decrease the patient's quality of life.

Spinal Nerve Radiculopathy

Spinal nerve radiculopathy, also called radiculitis, is spinal nerve impingement. It is a common cause of low back pain when the sciatic nerve is entrapped by a herniated vertebral disc. Often this is caused by a traumatic twisting of the lower back or from cumulative trauma on the vertebrae. The pain of sciatic nerve radiculopathy, commonly called sciatica, occurs at the lumbosacral region with radiation down the leg. The patient may also report numbness and tingling in the foot and may have decreased motion and weight-bearing ability in the leg.

Cervical radiculopathy is another common site of spinal nerve impingement. This is often caused by herniation of a cervical disc that places pressure on the spinal cord. There is pain in the neck that radiates down the arm. The patient may report numbness in the hand or fingers and may have weakness in the extremity.

Diabetic Peripheral Neuropathy

Diabetic peripheral neuropathy affects both sensory and motor nerves in the extremities. In uncontrolled diabetes, hyperglycemia causes increased levels of intracellular glucose in nerves. This leads to biochemical changes that cause impaired axonal transport and structural breakdown of nerves. The deleterious effects cause abnormal action potential propagation in both sensory and motor nerves. The individual loses sensation in the feet and suffers from imbalance because of a lack of motor control.

The reaction of excess glucose with nerve cell membranes results in advanced glycation end (ACE) products that disrupt neuronal integrity. ACE products also cause endothelial injury, predisposing the individual to arteriosclerotic plaque accumulation in arterial blood vessels. Arteriosclerosis in the small vessels of the lower extremities causes diminished circulation. The lack of neural sensation, decreased motor control, and diminished circulation in the lower extremities increases susceptibility to trauma and wound formation. The individual with diabetes often loses sensation in the feet and cannot perceive injury of the foot. In a numb foot, a minor injury can become severe. Without a pain stimulus to warn the individual of the injury, the injury often worsens and becomes infected. Poor wound healing because of dysfunction of white blood cells in diabetes increases susceptibility to infection and pain. Together, all the conditions in uncontrolled diabetes increase the risk of lower extremity amputation.

Complex Regional Pain Syndrome

CRPS is a chronic, progressive disorder characterized by severe pain, edema, discoloration, and changes in the skin. Its cause is currently unknown. Precipitating factors include injury and surgery, although there are cases that have no injury associated with the site of pain. CRPS often affects an arm or a leg and may spread to another part of the body. It is associated with dysfunction of the autonomic nervous system, resulting in impairment and disability. Treatment is often unsatisfactory, but early multidisciplinary therapy such as combined physical therapy, pain medications, and occupational therapy can bring improvement in some patients. There are two types of CRPS:

1. Type I CRPS has been formerly called many different names, including reflex sympathetic dystrophy, Sudeck's atrophy, reflex neurovascular dystrophy, and algoneurodystrophy. In Type I CRPS, there is no demonstrable nerve lesion.
2. Type II CRPS, formerly known as causalgia, has evidence of obvious nerve damage.

Postherpetic Neuralgia

Varicella zoster is a viral infection that presents in childhood as chicken pox. The virus produces a characteristic pruritic, vesicular rash that often starts on the trunk and spreads out to the extremities, face, and head. After the acute phase, the virus enters the sensory nervous system, where it remains dormant within the dorsal root of the spinal nerves throughout adulthood. When dormant, there are no symptoms. With advancing age or immunocompromised states, the virus reactivates along a nerve and an eruption called shingles occurs.

Shingles is the reactivation of varicella zoster, but it is renamed herpes zoster when it develops in the adult. Even though the rash might appear the same, shingles does not have the same effect on the body as chicken pox. It is commonly an acute, vesicular, and linear rash along a nerve dermatome that causes excruciating pain. The pain develops as the acute rash subsides; sharp pain can persist in shingles-affected areas for months. This is a common pain syndrome known as postherpetic neuralgia. Studies show that postherpetic neuralgia is difficult to treat, and fewer than 50% of sufferers attain pain relief. Oral TCAs, pregabalin, and the lidocaine 5% patch are recommended as first-line therapies. Gabapentin has also been used with some success. Some clinicians combine gabapentin and pregabalin despite a lack of compelling evidence to support this tactic. Capsaicin preparations, in patch and cream formulations, may also be used.

Fibromyalgia

Fibromyalgia is a common syndrome in which people experience long-term, body-wide pain, as well as pain in joints, muscles, tendons, and other soft tissues. The disorder has also been linked to fatigue, sleep problems, headaches, depression, anxiety, and other symptoms. Its cause is unknown. Men and women of all ages can contract fibromyalgia, but the disorder is most common among women aged 20 to 50 years.

The primary symptom of fibromyalgia is pain, and the exact locations of the pain are called tender points. Tender points are found in the soft tissue on the back of the neck, shoulders, sternum, lower back, hips, shins, elbows, and knees and can include fibrous tissue or muscles of specific body areas (see Fig. 6-12). The pain, which is described as deep-aching, radiating, gnawing, shooting, or burning, spreads out from these areas and ranges from mild to severe. The joints are not affected, although the pain may feel like it is coming from them.

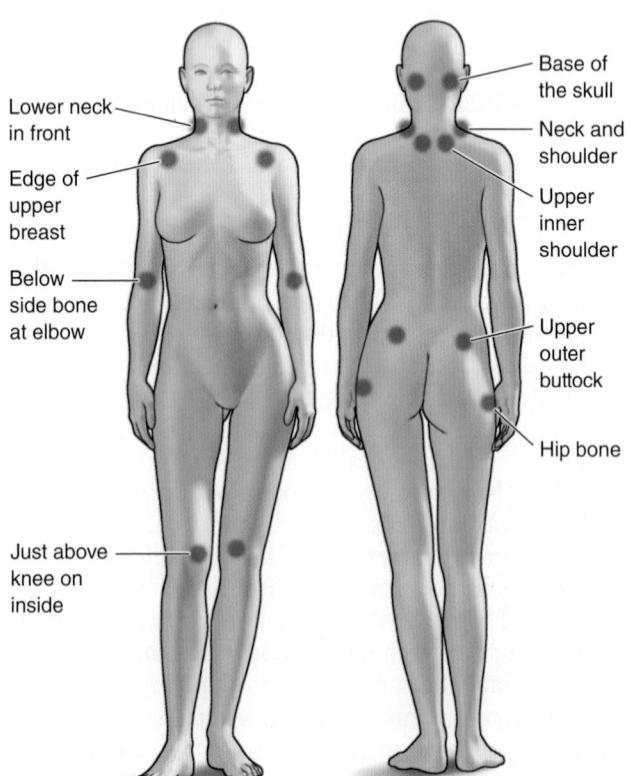

Lower neck in front
Edge of upper breast
Below side bone at elbow
Just above knee on inside

Base of the skull
Neck and shoulder
Upper inner shoulder
Upper outer buttock
Hip bone

FIGURE 6-12. Trigger points, or tender points, are used to diagnose fibromyalgia. Individuals who have fibromyalgia experience abnormal sensitivity when light pressure is applied to the areas delineated in the diagram.

People with fibromyalgia tend to wake up with body aches and stiffness. For some patients, pain improves during the day and increases again during the evening, though many patients have day-long, nonstop pain. Pain can increase with activity, cold or damp weather, anxiety, and stress. Fatigue and problems with sleep are seen in almost all patients with fibromyalgia.

Diagnosis requires a history of at least 3 months of widespread pain, and pain and tenderness in at least 11 of 18 tender-point sites (see Fig. 6-12). Sometimes, laboratory tests and x-rays are done to help confirm the diagnosis by ruling out other conditions that may have similar symptoms. Treatment should focus on not only relieving symptoms but also on helping patients learn how to cope with their symptoms. Studies show that some individuals achieve moderate symptom management with pregabalin, a GABA analog that inhibits calcium channels in neurons within the CNS. There is evidence that gabapentin (an anticonvulsant) may relieve symptoms in fibromyalgia. A study has shown that gabapentin in combination with osteopathic manipulative therapy has provided pain relief. If these methods fail to improve symptoms, an antidepressant or muscle relaxant is often tried to relieve symptoms. Pharmacotherapy should be accompanied by physical therapy, exercise, and methods for reducing stress.

Trigeminal Neuralgia

Trigeminal neuralgia, also called tic douloureux, is a nerve disorder that causes a stabbing or electric shock–like pain in parts of the face. The pain arises from the trigeminal nerve, cranial nerve V, which carries pain and sensation to the face. It can affect part or all of the face, as well as the surface of the eye. The condition usually affects older adults. Often, no specific cause is found, though pressure on the trigeminal nerve from a swollen blood vessel or tumor or multiple sclerosis may be a cause. The patient feels very painful, sharp, electric-like spasms that usually last a few seconds or minutes but can become constant. Pain is usually only on one side of the face, often around the eye, cheek, and lower part of the face. It can be triggered by touch, sounds, or common activities, such as brushing teeth, chewing, drinking, eating, or shaving. Diagnosis includes a neurological examination, which is usually normal. Tests performed to look for the problem's cause include blood tests, magnetic resonance imaging of the head, and trigeminal reflex testing.

Certain medications such as anticonvulsants, muscle relaxers, and TCAs can help reduce the pain and the rate of attacks. Botulinum toxin type A injections have provided effective pain relief. Patients may need surgery to relieve pressure on the nerve.

Postoperative Pain

An estimated 25 million inpatient surgeries and an additional 35 million ambulatory surgeries are performed annually in the United States. More than 80% of surgical patients experience postoperative pain, and 39% experience "severe" to "extreme" postoperative pain. Pain has adverse effects on postoperative recovery, including prolonging recuperation time and hospital stay. Also, the use of postoperative opioids results in adverse effects, such as sedation, constipation, dizziness, somnolence, postoperative nausea and vomiting, urinary retention, ileus, and respiratory depression, which can delay discharge. Prolonged opioid use postoperatively can also be a "gateway" to opioid abuse disorder. The widespread use of these drugs has resulted in a national epidemic of opioid addiction and overdose deaths.

A great number of analgesic medications and techniques can be used to relieve acute postoperative pain. Some agents can be used preoperatively or during surgery to preempt postoperative pain. This technique prevents central sensitization by blocking the neural transmission of all noxious perioperative stimuli arising from the time of incision through wound healing.

In addition, experts recommend that health-care providers employ multimodal analgesia: the use of more than one type of analgesic modality to achieve effective pain control. Multimodal analgesia includes

---

BOX 6-3. Preemptive Multimodal Analgesics

- Preoperative use of NSAIDs, anxiolytics, and anticonvulsants
- Intraoperative use of neuraxial analgesia
- Continuous local anesthetic wound infusion
- Transversus abdominis plane (TAP) block
- Extended-release epidural morphine (EREM)
- Intravenous acetaminophen
- Intravenous ketamine
- Postoperative use of intravenous ibuprofen, newer opioids (e.g., tapentadol), opioid formulations (morphine-oxycodone)
- Patient-controlled analgesia (PCA) approaches

---

pharmacological and nonpharmacological therapies that achieve effective pain control. Multimodal analgesic techniques have demonstrated better pain control and fewer adverse effects than traditional approaches with oral opioid analgesics. Current preemptive multimodal analgesics are listed in Box 6-3.

Chapter Summary

- In a simple reflex arc, an afferent neuron carries sensory impulses into the dorsal horn of the spinal cord and connects with an interneuron, which connects to an efferent motor neuron that exits via the ventral horn.

- Nociceptors are receptors that respond to noxious stimuli.

- Afferent neurons, which are nociceptors, carry the sensations of touch, temperature, vibration, proprioception, and pain into the dorsal horn of the spinal cord.

- Afferent nerve fibers called A-delta and C fibers are sensory nerves that enter the spinal cord via the dorsal horn.

- A-delta fibers, large in diameter and myelinated, conduct impulses rapidly and cause the first, short-lived acute experience of pain.

- C fibers, smaller in diameter and unmyelinated, conduct impulses slowly and cause longer-lasting, persistent, dull pain.

- Efferent motor nerves exit the spinal cord via the ventral horn of the spinal cord and carry impulses to the muscles.

- Neurotransmitters are excitatory or inhibitory chemical mediators that are released from one neuron to stimulate another. Examples include norepinephrine, acetylcholine, dopamine, and serotonin.

- A dermatome is a skin area innervated by the sensory fibers of a single nerve root; a myotome is a group of muscles primarily innervated by the motor fibers of a single nerve root.

- The gate control theory focuses on peripheral tissue damage and acute stimulation of the spinal cord neurons.

- The neuromatrix theory emphasizes the role of the brain and the significant impression of chronic pain in the brain's neural network.

- Pain is regarded as the fifth vital sign, and specific assessment tools are used to evaluate its severity.

- To assess pain and its accompanying symptoms, the initial history can be obtained by using the OLDCART mnemonic: onset; location; duration; character; alleviating, aggravating, and accompanying factors; relieving factors; and treatment.

- When performing physical assessment, examine the area of pain last.

- It is difficult to quantify pain, but treating acute pain completely is advised in order to avoid development of intractable or chronic pain.

- The WHO recommends a step-ladder approach for prescribing opioid, nonopioid, and adjuvant medications. It has been updated with modifications to include nonpharmacological interventions.

- Opioids have a high potential for abuse, tolerance, and physical dependence and are designated as controlled substances by the FDA.
- Methadone and buprenorphine can be used in opioid abuse disorder.
- Naloxone is a drug that helps counter the effects of opiate overdose because it has an extremely high affinity for opioid receptors in the central nervous system. It takes the place of the opioid on the receptor.
- Naloxone use in a patient dependent on opioids will cause withdrawal symptoms.
- Antidepressants, anticonvulsants, and local anesthetics are commonly used as adjuvant pain treatment.
- Endocannabinoids are naturally produced in the CNS to dampen sensitivity to pain. The use of plant-based cannabinoids (marijuana) for medicinal purposes is a controversial subject, with evidential studies that both support and deny the efficacy of the agents in various disorders.
- Nonpharmacological treatment such as physiotherapy, acupuncture, and TENS have shown effectiveness for some kinds of pain.
- Integrative medicine includes alternative and complementary therapies in conjunction with traditional methods of pain relief.
- Disorders that have specific patterns and characteristics of pain include cancer, spinal nerve radiculopathy, diabetic peripheral neuropathy, CRPS, postherpetic neuralgia, fibromyalgia, trigeminal neuralgia, and postoperative pain.

Bibliography

Available online at fadavis.com

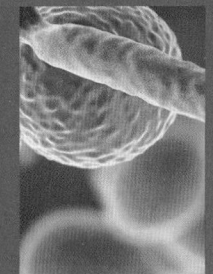

Fluid and Electrolyte Imbalances

Learning Objectives

Upon completion of this chapter, the student will be able to:

- Differentiate between the forces of osmotic pressure and hydrostatic pressure within the bloodstream.
- Describe Starling's Laws of Capillary Forces and factors influencing fluid movement between the intracellular and extracellular fluid compartments.
- Identify causes of abnormally low or elevated levels of significant electrolytes within the bloodstream.

- Recognize complications that can occur due to abnormally low or elevated levels of electrolytes within the bloodstream.
- Discuss how different intravenous fluid solutions can be used to create changes in fluid and electrolyte levels within the bloodstream.

Key Terms

Ascites
Atrial natriuretic peptide (ANP)
B type natriuretic peptide (brain natriuretic peptide) (BNP)
Dehydration
Diuresis
Edema
Effusion
Electrolyte
Extracellular fluid (ECF)
Hydrostatic pressure

Hypercalcemia
Hyperkalemia
Hypermagnesemia
Hypernatremia
Hyperphosphatemia
Hypocalcemia
Hypokalemia
Hypomagnesemia
Hyponatremia
Hypophosphatemia
Hypovolemia

Intake and output (I&O)
Interstitial fluid (ISF)
Intracellular fluid (ICF)
Oncotic pressure
Osmolality
Osmolarity
Osmotic pressure
Third-spacing
Tonicity

The human body is composed of approximately 60% water. It is the major constituent of the cells and bloodstream and acts as the body's solvent. **Electrolytes,** which are positively and negatively charged ions, are the body's solutes. Protein, specifically albumin, is the major solute in the bloodstream; body fluid, which is a solution largely composed of water, is the solvent. Electrolytes and protein, the solutes, have two main functions:

1. Deliver nutrients and electrolytes to cells
2. Carry away waste products from cellular metabolism

Basic Concepts of Fluid and Electrolyte Balance

Water is found in three different fluid compartments (see Fig. 7-1):

1. **Intracellular fluid (ICF)**
2. **Extracellular fluid (ECF)**
3. **Interstitial fluid (ISF)**

A constant state of fluid and electrolyte exchange occurs between the cell and its environment—mainly between the ICF and ECF. Two-thirds of the body's

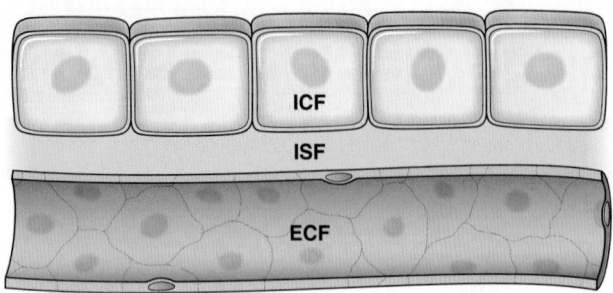

FIGURE 7-1. Water is located in the body in three basic fluid compartments. The ICF compartment is inside of the cells. The ECF compartment is within the bloodstream. The ISF compartment is between the intracellular and extracellular compartments.

water content is contained mainly within the ICF and one-third is within the ECF. Each cell is enveloped by a plasma membrane. This is a semipermeable membrane that allows passive movement of fluid and electrolytes back and forth but restricts larger particles. Table 7-1 describes the different transport mechanisms that maintain the concentration differences between ICF and ECF.

Fluid Balance

Intracellular Fluid Compartment
In the adult, 40% of total body weight is the water contained within the ICF compartment. Water can diffuse out of the ICF and cause cell shrinkage or cellular dehydration. Conversely, water can enter the ICF and cause cell swelling or cellular edema.

Extracellular Fluid Compartment
In the adult, 20% of total body weight is the water contained within the ECF compartment. Most of the ECF is found within the intravascular compartment or blood vessels. The ECF contains electrolytes, oxygen, glucose, and other nutrients to be delivered to cells, as well as cellular waste products designated for excretion.

Interstitial Fluid Compartment
ISF, which is a filtrate of the blood, is located between the cells and between the cells and capillaries. Like blood, it contains water and electrolytes, mainly sodium (Na^+). ISF lacks proteins because they are too large to diffuse out of the blood vessels into the interstitial spaces. However, during inflammation, capillary membranes become extrapermeable; the pores enlarge, allowing proteins such as white blood cells out to the tissues.

Hydrostatic Pressure

Hydrostatic pressure is the pushing force exerted by water in the bloodstream. The heart's pulsatile pumping action is the source of hydrostatic pressure, which exerts an outward force that pushes water through the capillary membrane pores into the ISF and ICF compartments (see Fig. 7-2).

TABLE 7-1. Transport Mechanisms		
Transport Mechanism	Description	Illustration
Diffusion	The process by which molecules passively spread from areas of high concentration to areas of low concentration. Water and electrolytes diffuse from high concentration to lower concentration until equilibrium is reached.	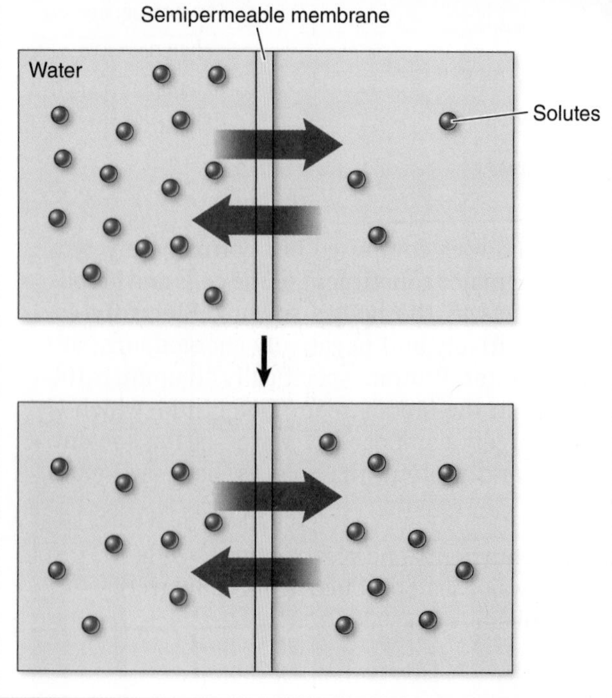 Semipermeable membrane / Water / Solutes

TABLE 7-1. Transport Mechanisms—cont'd

Transport Mechanism	Description	Illustration
Osmosis	The tendency of molecules of a solvent to pass through a semipermeable membrane from a less concentrated solution into a more concentrated one, equalizing the concentrations on each side of the membrane. Electrolytes and water move through the cell's semipermeable plasma membrane, but large proteins such as albumin cannot pass through the membrane. A semipermeable membrane selectively allows some molecules through its pores and obstructs others according to size.	ICF / ECF / ● Albumin / • Solutes
Facilitated transport	The passing of certain molecules through the plasma membrane with assistance from carrier proteins. Glucose undergoes facilitated transport into the cell by the carrier protein insulin.	ICF / ECF / ↻ Facilitated transport by insulin / ⬡ Glucose / ● Albumin / ●○ Various solutes
Active transport	Occurs when a substance requires energy to pass through a membrane against a concentration gradient. Sodium and potassium require active transport using the N^+/K^+ pump, which is within the plasma membrane to retain potassium as the major intracellular ion and sodium as the major extracellular ion. Sodium is a solute that draws water with it.	ATP pump keeps pumping Na^+ out of the cell… / …and K^+ into the cell. / ATP pump / ATP pump / ICF / ECF / ○ Sodium / ○ Potassium / ● Albumin

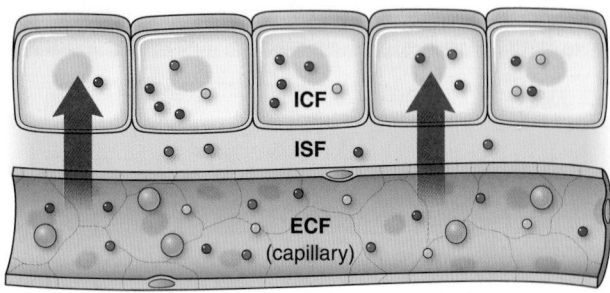

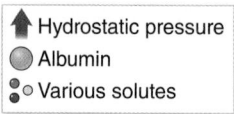
Hydrostatic pressure
Albumin
Various solutes

FIGURE 7-2. According to Starling's Law of Capillary Forces, hydrostatic pressure pushes water outward from the ECF to the ICF at the capillary–cell interface.

Osmotic Pressure

Osmotic pressure is the pressure exerted by the solutes in solution. In the bloodstream, osmotic pressure is exerted by electrolytes, mainly sodium ions and plasma proteins. Osmotic pressure is a force that pulls water into the bloodstream from the ICF and ISF and opposes hydrostatic pressure at all capillary membranes (see Fig. 7-3). Osmotic pressure is determined by the number of particles or their concentration within the solution. A solution with a greater number of particles has a higher osmotic pressure.

When a membrane such as a cell membrane separates two solutions with different osmotic pressures, fluid will move from the solution with lower osmotic pressure into the solution with the higher osmotic pressure, which is why a high osmotic pressure in the bloodstream favors fluid movement from the ICF and ISF into the bloodstream. Conversely, when the osmotic pressure is reduced, fluid moves out of the bloodstream and into interstitial and intracellular spaces (see Fig. 7-4).

Oncotic Pressure

Oncotic pressure, also called colloidal osmotic pressure, is a type of osmotic pressure exerted specifically by albumin in the bloodstream. Oncotic pressure and osmotic pressure exert the same type of pulling force from ICF to ECF. Albumin attracts water and helps keep it inside the blood vessel. Albumin is the main colloidal protein in the bloodstream and is essential for maintaining the oncotic pressure in the vascular system. Total albumin in the bloodstream is indicative of the body's protein nutritional status. The normal serum albumin level is 3.1 to 4.3 g/dL. Changes in this albumin level alter oncotic pressure. For example, in hypoalbuminemia (lack of sufficient albumin in the bloodstream), oncotic pressure is reduced. Hypoalbuminemia causes an imbalance in the oncotic pressure versus hydrostatic pressure forces. With reduced albumin, the oncotic pressure is low and the force exerted by hydrostatic pressure overwhelms the oncotic pressure. This causes water in the bloodstream to push outward from the capillary pores toward the ISF and ICF (see Fig. 7-5).

Osmolality

Osmolality is a measurement of the concentration of solutes per kg of solvent. It is based on 1 mole (or gram molecular weight equivalent) of a substance dissolved in 1 kilogram of water. In clinical practice, osmolality can be used to evaluate the body's hydration status based on the concentration of fluid and particles in solution. Normal plasma osmolality is 282

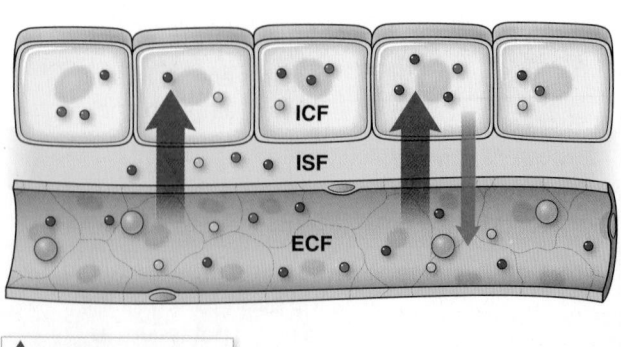

Hydrostatic pressure
Osmotic pressure
Albumin
Various solutes

FIGURE 7-3. According to Starling's Law of Capillary Forces, osmotic pressure pulls water from the ICF into the ECF at every cell–capillary interface. The osmotic pressure opposes the hydrostatic pressure; in healthy conditions, each force balances out the other.

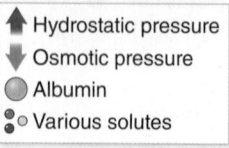
Hydrostatic pressure
Osmotic pressure
Albumin
Various solutes

FIGURE 7-4. According to Starling's Law of Capillary Forces, when osmotic pressure is lower than hydrostatic pressure, osmotic pressure is overwhelmed and hydrostatic pressure is an unopposed force, causing water to flow from the ECF to the ICF.

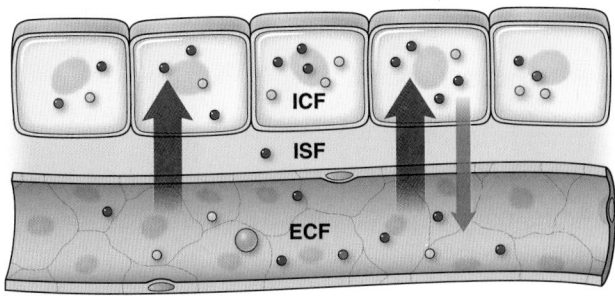

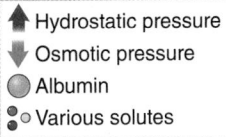
- ▲ Hydrostatic pressure
- ▼ Osmotic pressure
- ◯ Albumin
- ⦂∘ Various solutes

FIGURE 7-5. In hypoalbuminemia, there is a lack of sufficient albumin in the bloodstream. This causes a decrease in osmotic pressure. When osmotic pressure is lower than hydrostatic pressure, osmotic pressure is overwhelmed and hydrostatic pressure is an unopposed pushing force that pushes water from the ECF to the ICF. Cells will gain water and become edematous.

to 295 milliosmoles per kilogram of water. Low osmolality indicates a lesser amount of solutes in solution, whereas high osmolality indicates a greater amount of solutes. If the bloodstream is well hydrated, serum osmolality is 282 milliosmoles per kg of water or less. If the bloodstream is concentrated and has low water, the serum osmolality will be 295 milliosmoles per kg of water or greater. Serum osmolality can be calculated using the following mathematical formula:
milliosmoles of solute /kg of water $= 2 \times$ serum sodium + serum glucose /18 + BUN / 2.4.

Osmolarity

Osmolarity is the number of osmoles of solute per liter of solution; it is dependent on the number of particles suspended in a solution. In the body, the major solutes are albumin, sodium (Na^+), potassium (K^+), phosphate (Po_4^-), magnesium (Mg^{++}), calcium (Ca^{++}), bicarbonate (HCO_3^-), and glucose. The major protein within the bloodstream is albumin, which is the solute in the ECF that exerts the most osmotic pressure. Sodium, the main determinant of osmolarity, is a positive ion, also called a cation; it is found mostly in the ECF and assists in the maintenance of fluid balance and osmotic pressure. Potassium is the main intracellular cation; it assists in the maintenance of neuromuscular excitability and acid–base balance. Both sodium and potassium require the cell's Na^+/K^+ pump to maintain Na^+ as the extracellular ion and K^+ as the intracellular ion. Phosphate is an intracellular negative ion, also called an anion. Magnesium plays an important role in enzymatic systems within the body. Calcium plays an important role in neuromuscular irritability, blood clotting, and bone structure. Bicarbonate is responsible for acid–base balance.

> ### 🩺 CLINICAL CONCEPT
> The serum albumin level is a major protein in the bloodstream used to evaluate an individual's nutritional status.

Tonicity

Tonicity refers to the concentration of solutes in solution compared with the bloodstream. The term is also used to describe the various intravenous (IV) solutions used in the clinical setting (see Box 7-1). There are three types of IV solutions:

1. **Isotonic solution:** This has the same tonicity as blood; when infused as an IV solution, it does not cause fluid shifts or alter body cell size. It has a concentration of particles and fluid that is similar to blood and body fluids. A standard isotonic IV solution is 0.9% NaCl solution, also called normal saline. It is used frequently as a bloodstream volume expander. Often an isotonic solution is used to keep an open connection to the IV route for medication administration or a blood transfusion.

2. **Hypotonic solution:** This has fewer particles and more water than blood and body fluids. When a hypotonic solution is infused, water is added to the bloodstream and causes a fluid shift from ECF to ICF to deliver water to the body, as in dehydration treatment. A standard hypotonic solution is 0.45% NaCl and is also referred to as half normal saline.

3. **Hypertonic solution:** This contains more particles and less water than blood and body

---

BOX 7-1. Common Intravenous Solutions According to Tonicity

ISOTONIC	0.9% NaCl (normal saline solution [NSS]) Lactated Ringer's solution (LR)* Ringer's solution Dextrose 5% in water (D_5W)†
HYPOTONIC	0.45% NaCl (half normal saline) 0.33% NaCl 0.225% NaCl 2.5% dextrose in water
HYPERTONIC	3% NaCl IV Mannitol 10% Dextrose in water ($D_{10}W$) 20% Dextrose in water ($D_{20}W$) 50% Dextrose in water ($D_{50}W$)

*Also known as Hartmann solution.
†Provides free water after dextrose metabolized.

fluids. When a hypertonic solution is infused into the bloodstream, solutes are added to the bloodstream and cause fluids to shift from ICF to ECF, causing body cells to shrink. A commonly used hypertonic IV solution is mannitol. It can be used to diminish cell swelling, particularly in cerebral edema. Another hypertonic solution that is used less often is 3.0% NaCl.

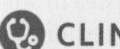 **CLINICAL CONCEPT**

To prevent hypoglycemia, 5% dextrose in water (D_5W) is often added to IV normal saline to deliver some glucose to the patient.

 CLINICAL CONCEPT

A solution often used as a temporary replacement for blood, called Ringer's lactate (also called lactated Ringer's solution), consists of similar physiological constituents as those found in blood.

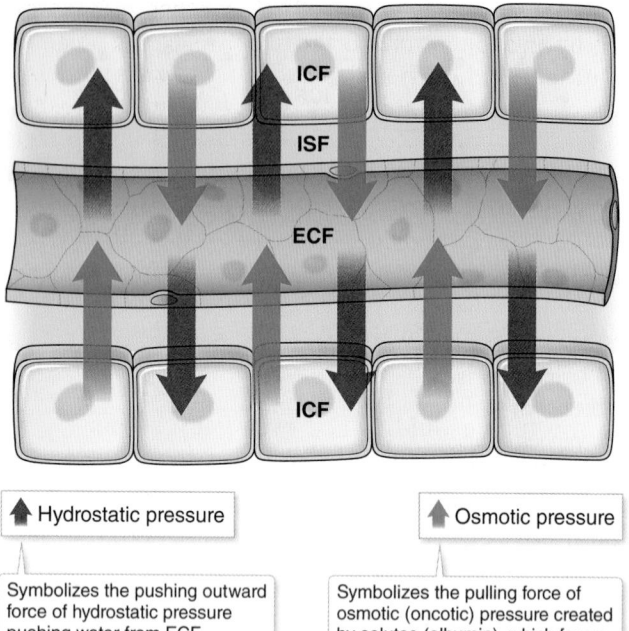

Hydrostatic pressure

Symbolizes the pushing outward force of hydrostatic pressure pushing water from ECF (capillary) into ICF.

Osmotic pressure

Symbolizes the pulling force of osmotic (oncotic) pressure created by solutes (albumin), which favors fluid movement from the ICF into the ECF (capillary).

FIGURE 7-6. According to Starling's Law of Capillary Forces, homeostasis exists when hydrostatic and osmotic pressures are equal at every capillary–cell interface.

Starling's Law of Capillary Forces

Starling's Law of Capillary Forces explains the movement of fluid that occurs at every capillary bed in the body. There are two major opposing forces at every capillary membrane:

1. Hydrostatic pressure
2. Osmotic pressure (includes oncotic pressure)

Within every capillary, electrolytes and proteins within the blood exert osmotic pressure. The fluid within the capillary exerts hydrostatic pressure. These pressure forces oppose each other and attempt to balance each other out at every capillary membrane, thereby creating a state of homeostasis (see Fig. 7-6).

 CLINICAL CONCEPT

Principles of Starling's Law can be applied in the clinical setting. For example, swelling can be reduced using an Epsom salt bath, which is a hypertonic magnesium salt solution. Placing a swollen finger in an Epsom salt bath will draw ICF from the finger into the Epsom salt solution, thereby reducing the finger's swelling.

Fluid Homeostasis

Various physiological mechanisms work together in order to maintain fluid homeostasis. In terms of fluid volume, both fluid intake and output must be regulated to prevent fluid volume overload, also known as edema, and fluid volume deficit, also known as dehydration. However, in addition to fluid volume status, the relative composition of body fluids, including electrolyte and acid or base concentrations, needs to be consistent. The kidney, renin–angiotensin–aldosterone system (RAAS), osmoreceptors, thirst sensation, antidiuretic hormone (ADH), and natriuretic peptides work together to maintain fluid homeostasis in the body.

Osmoreceptors, ADH, and Thirst. Changes in plasma osmolarity are responsible for both the sensation of thirst and the release of ADH, also called arginine vasopressin. High plasma osmolarity stimulates osmoreceptors in the hypothalamus. This stimulates the hypothalamic thirst center of the brain, as well as promoting the release of ADH from the posterior pituitary.

Thirst is a conscious desire to drink fluids. It is triggered by a response in the thirst center, which is located in the anterior hypothalamus. The osmoreceptors respond to changes in both blood osmolarity and blood fluid volume. When there is an increase in blood osmolarity, ICF shifts into ECF and the cells shrink, stimulating the thirst center. This center transmits signals to the cerebral cortex, promoting the sensation of thirst. Thirst causes a conscious desire to drink fluids, which brings water into the body's bloodstream to reduce osmolarity. Massive loss of blood and fluid volume, as is seen in severe trauma, will trigger the sense of thirst as well.

In a healthy person, osmoreceptors, ADH, and thirst responses work together. ADH is produced by the hypothalamus. Once the ADH is synthesized, it travels by an axonal transport mechanism to the posterior pituitary gland. When the bloodstream lacks sufficient water, plasma osmolarity is increased and the osmoreceptors shrink. This stimulates the ADH neurons to depolarize, releasing ADH from the posterior pituitary. In addition to changes in osmolarity, other factors such as pain, trauma, and medications stimulate the release of ADH.

After release into the bloodstream, ADH stimulates water reabsorption from the nephron tubule fluid at the collecting duct into the bloodstream. This raises the blood's water content and decreases the water in the tubule fluid, which eventually becomes concentrated urine. When there is enough water in the bloodstream, plasma osmolarity decreases, and ADH secretion is inhibited.

RAAS. Hypotension, hypovolemia, dehydration, and low cardiac output cause low circulation throughout the body. Reduced circulation causes low renal perfusion, which stimulates renin secretion by the kidney's juxtaglomerular apparatus. Renin initiates the RAAS, a compensatory mechanism used to replenish blood volume and raise blood pressure (see Fig. 7-7).

Renin is an enzyme released from the kidney in response to decreased renal perfusion. Renin converts angiotensinogen, a large protein produced by the liver, to angiotensin I. In the lungs, angiotensin-converting enzyme (ACE) changes angiotensin I into angiotensin II, a powerful vasoconstrictor. Angiotensin II binds to receptors in the adrenal cortex, stimulating the synthesis and secretion of aldosterone, a mineralocorticoid that increases sodium and water reabsorption into the bloodstream at the distal tubule of the nephrons. Aldosterone also stimulates the excretion of potassium into the nephron tubules, which eventually becomes urine. When blood volume decreases, aldosterone begins the reabsorption of sodium from the distal tubules into the bloodstream, bringing sodium back into the bloodstream. This causes more absorption of water and increased blood volume. When the blood volume returns to normal, aldosterone secretion is reduced.

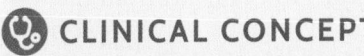

CLINICAL CONCEPT

Blocking ACE in the RAAS prevents angiotensin I from becoming angiotensin II; this prevents vasoconstriction and adrenal stimulation of aldosterone secretion.

Natriuretic Peptides. Natriuresis is the excretion of a large amount of both sodium and water by the kidneys in response to excess ECF volume. It is a process of natural diuresis initiated by the body.

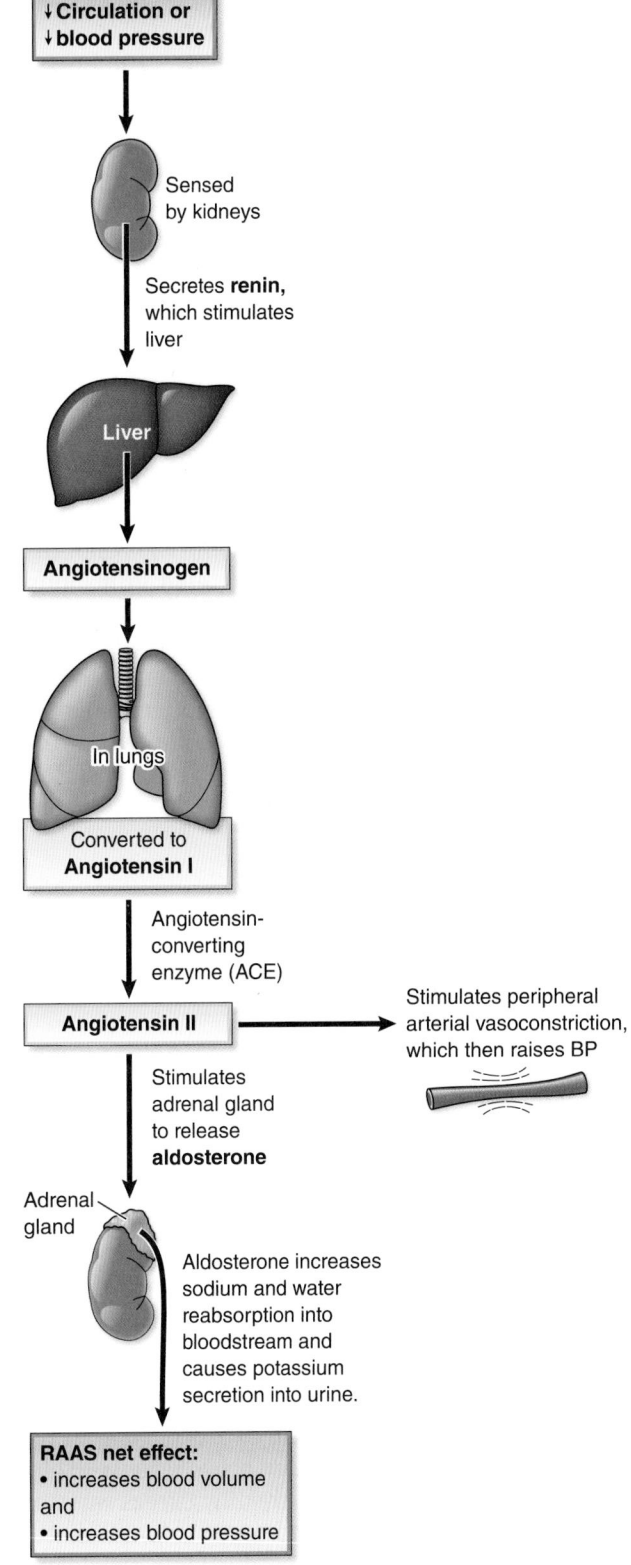

FIGURE 7-7. The RAAS. When there is a decrease in circulation or drop in blood pressure, the kidney senses decreased perfusion and releases renin. Renin stimulates the liver to release a protein called angiotensinogen. Angiotensinogen reaches the lungs and is transformed into angiotensin I. In the lungs, ACE transforms angiotensin I into angiotensin II. Angiotensin II is a potent arterial vasoconstrictor; it also stimulates the adrenal gland to release aldosterone. Aldosterone increases sodium and water reabsorption into the bloodstream at the nephron. It also causes potassium excretion from the bloodstream into the urine. The net effect of the RAAS is to raise blood volume and increase blood pressure.

> ### 🔬 CLINICAL CONCEPT
>
> **Diuresis** is the loss of water from the body. Furosemide (Lasix) and hydrochlorothiazide (HCTZ) are commonly prescribed diuretic agents.

Three major peptides promote natriuresis: **atrial natriuretic peptide (ANP), B-type natriuretic peptide) (BNP)** (also called brain natriuretic peptide), and C-type natriuretic peptide (CNP). ANP is produced by the heart's atria and is secreted in response to excess ECF volume that stretches the heart's atrial chambers. CNP is produced by endothelial cells of the arteries and ventricular cells of the heart.

BNP is produced in the heart's ventricles and, to a lesser extent, in the brain. It is excreted in response to fluid volume overload stretching the heart's ventricles—the more the ventricle is stretched by blood volume, the more BNP is secreted. Both ANP and BNP promote natriuresis at the glomerulus by increasing glomerular filtration rate. CNP has limited diuretic and natriuretic effects compared with ANP and BNP, but it has only been recently identified and is not completely understood.

Basic Pathophysiological Concepts of Fluid and Electrolyte Imbalance

Regulation of fluid balance is important for maintaining the body's normal homeostatic functioning. Alterations in fluid balance occur for a variety of reasons and can be related to illness or exposure to extreme heat. Because sodium is the major extracellular ion, it has a key role in fluid balance. Fluid volume deficit or excess fluid volume has ancillary effects on different systems of the body.

Edema

Edema occurs when there is an excess of fluid in the ISF and ICF compartments. It can occur because of elevated hydrostatic pressure created by excess water in the bloodstream or diminished osmotic force created by a low amount of solutes in the bloodstream. Edema can also occur because of inflammation, which causes increased capillary permeability; the capillary pores enlarge to allow fluid and cells out of the bloodstream to reach the site of injury. The fluid that moves into the ISF and ICF causes the edema.

When edema occurs because of high hydrostatic pressure in the bloodstream, the osmotic pressure force is overwhelmed and does not balance out the hydrostatic force. Consequently, according to Starling's Law of Capillary Forces, hydrostatic pressure pushes fluid out of the capillary membrane pores into the ISF and ICF. An example of this occurs in left-sided heart failure, where high hydrostatic pressure develops in the pulmonary bloodstream. The high hydrostatic pressure forces fluid out of the pulmonary blood vessels and into the alveolar spaces and the interstitial tissue. This is known as pulmonary edema. Edema can also occur in the peritoneal cavity as **ascites,** the pleural cavity as pleural effusion, and the lower extremities as ankle edema.

Edema can also occur because of a low amount of solute in the bloodstream. Low albumin in the blood, or hypoalbuminemia, causes an imbalance in capillary forces. Because albumin is the major source of oncotic pressure, hypoalbuminemia will cause low oncotic pressure in the bloodstream. According to Starling's Law of Capillary Forces, for homeostasis to occur, oncotic pressure must equal hydrostatic pressure. When oncotic pressure is low, hydrostatic pressure will be the overriding force and push fluid out of the capillary into the ISF and ICF compartments, thereby creating an edematous state.

An example of edema caused by hypoalbuminemia occurs in severe protein starvation. Without sufficient nutritional protein, blood albumin levels become extremely low and, consequently, oncotic pressure is diminished. An imbalance between oncotic pressure and hydrostatic pressure occurs at every capillary–cell interface. Hydrostatic pressure overwhelms oncotic pressure, and water is pushed out of the capillary into the ISF and ICF. Edema occurs throughout the body at every capillary–cell interface, and this is often most apparent in the peritoneal cavity as a swollen abdomen (termed *ascites*). In persons who are starving, the disorder of edema due to malnutrition is known as kwashiorkor.

Edema due to lack of albumin also occurs in patients with liver failure. Lack of liver function leads to decreased albumin synthesis, which in turn, causes hypoalbuminemia. Hypoalbuminemia causes decreased oncotic pressure, which leads to imbalanced capillary forces. The imbalanced hydrostatic pressure causes ascites. Generalized swelling occurring in the body is referred to as anasarca.

A specific kind of edema, called dependent edema, often forms in the lower extremities. Under healthy conditions, venous return to the heart from the lower extremities is assisted by venous valves and muscle contractions. A weakened venous valve system, lack of muscle contractions, and gravitational forces can allow venous blood to collect in the lower extremities. When an individual stands or sits in one position for an extended period, venous blood can pool in the lower extremities. Increased hydrostatic pressure in the veins allows fluid to flow out of the capillary into interstitial tissues. Fluid accumulates in the ankles and feet, which are the dependent parts of the body. To avoid dependent edema, brisk venous circulation back to the heart and vigorous muscle activity must be maintained in the lower extremities.

 CLINICAL CONCEPT

Thromboembolic stockings (TEDS) and pneumatic compression devices that surround the lower leg attempt to enhance venous return from the lower extremities up to the heart in patients on bedrest.

Sodium retention caused by illness or consumption of salty foods can also contribute to edema. Excess sodium in the ECF pulls fluid from the ICF into the ECF, causing cellular dehydration. Dehydration causes thirst, which, in turn, encourages the individual to drink water or other liquids. This ingestion and the movement of water from the ICF into the ECF cause an excess of water in the bloodstream, which increases hydrostatic pressure. As a result, hydrostatic pressure rises and overcomes osmotic pressure with resulting edema. This is also seen whenever there is increased activation of the RAAS. With increased cycling of the RAAS, enhanced sodium and water reabsorption into the bloodstream occurs, which raises blood volume and blood pressure.

 CLINICAL CONCEPT

Pitting edema occurs when pressure is applied to a small area and an indentation persists for some time after the release of the pressure. Depending on the severity, an individual can have +1, +2, or +3 pitting edema (see Fig. 7-8).

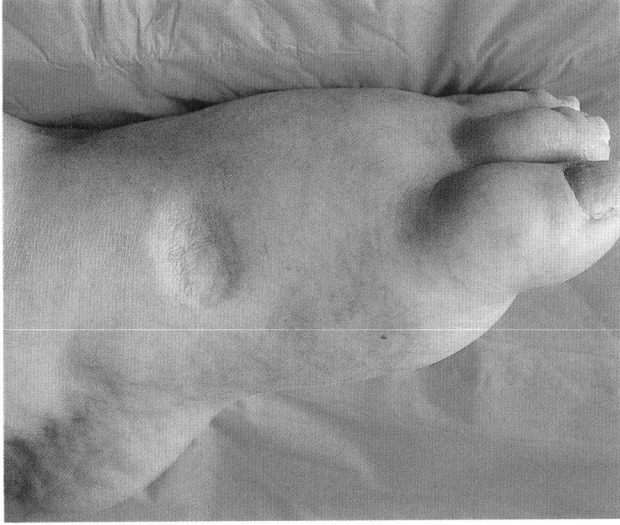

FIGURE 7-8. Pitting edema. Application of pressure over a bony area displaces the excess fluid, leaving an indentation or pit. *(From Williams, L., & Hopper, P. [2019]. Understanding medical-surgical nursing [6th ed.]. Philadelphia, PA: F. A. Davis Company, with permission.)*

Sequestered Fluids

During illness, fluids can become sequestered in body cavities that are normally free of fluids, such as the pericardial sac, peritoneal cavity, and pleural space. When this occurs, it is referred to as third-space accumulation of fluids; sometimes referred to as **third-spacing.** The fluid that accumulates in these cavities is commonly called an **effusion.** An effusion can be a transudate, which is a serous filtrate of blood, or an exudate, which contains material such as blood, lymph, proteins, pathogens, and inflammatory cells. Either type of effusion can surround organs and interfere with function. For example, a pleural effusion interferes with full lung expansion and ventilation, whereas a pericardial effusion can constrict the heart and prevent maximal filling of blood in the atria and ventricles.

 CLINICAL CONCEPT

A pericardial effusion can lead to cardiac tamponade, a disorder in which the heart's pumping action is restricted because of an accumulation of fluid surrounding it.

Fluid Volume Overload

Fluid volume overload occurs when the bloodstream has an excessive amount of water. One of the most common causes of fluid volume overload is heart failure. In heart failure, the RAAS is constantly cycling, which brings an excessive amount of water into the bloodstream. Blood volume increases, which increases the hydrostatic pressure. High hydrostatic pressure overwhelms osmotic pressure at every capillary bed, leading to edema in various places in the body. Ankle edema, peritoneal edema, and pulmonary edema all occur in heart failure.

Fluid volume overload can also be seen in certain cancers that secrete ADH, causing a disorder known as syndrome of inappropriate ADH (SIADH). Other causes of ADH-related fluid volume overload include cirrhosis of the liver, polycystic kidney disease, and some forms of hypertension. Disorders that cause constant secretion of ADH promote excess water reabsorption from the collecting duct of the nephrons into the bloodstream. Water reabsorption into the blood causes fluid volume overload. The concentration of sodium in the bloodstream is highly dependent on the volume of water in the bloodstream. High water volume in the blood decreases the concentration of sodium. This is called dilutional hyponatremia.

 CLINICAL CONCEPT

SIADH can occur in certain cancers, brain disorders, and after brain surgery.

Dehydration

Dehydration is a state of diminished water volume in the body. A deficit of intracellular fluid causes body cells to shrink. There is also a decreased amount of water in the extracellular fluid. Dehydration has many causes, including reduced fluid intake and excessive fluid loss caused by illness. Lack of sufficient ADH production or lack of renal stimulation by ADH can also lead to excessive fluid loss and dehydration, as can certain gastrointestinal disorders such as prolonged diarrhea. Burns, fever, and perspiration also commonly cause large fluid loss. Regardless of cause, dehydration causes **hypovolemia,** a diminished level of circulating blood volume that increases the osmolarity of the blood.

For example, in uncontrolled diabetes, glucose rises to high levels and acts as a solute in the blood. The high amount of solute in the blood raises osmotic pressure, which creates an imbalance in the capillary forces. If osmotic pressure rises to exceed hydrostatic pressure inside the capillary, then water from the ICF and ISF moves into the capillary and the cells lose water. This causes cells to shrink, a process known as cellular dehydration. The fluid shift into the circulation delivers more water to the kidneys, which is then excreted as excess urine (polyuria). Because of fluid shifts, the key symptoms of uncontrolled diabetes mellitus are thirst and polyuria.

Cellular dehydration can also occur because of hypernatremia (high sodium content of blood), which raises solute content and, in turn, raises osmotic pressure. High osmotic pressure causes water to shift from the ICF into the ECF. Cellular dehydration occurs with loss of ICF, causing the cells to shrink. The ECF gains fluid, which is excreted via the kidney; this leads to further dehydration. This situation continues until water is replenished.

> **ALERT!** There is a risk of renal dysfunction if the adult patient develops oliguria—urine output of less than 400 mL/day or less than 20 to 30 mL/hour. The kidney needs to yield a minimum of 400 mL of fluid daily to sufficiently excrete waste products.

The physiological response to dehydration is multifaceted. Osmoreceptors respond to the blood's high osmotic content and stimulate the thirst center in the hypothalamus. Thirst occurs, which stimulates the person to drink to replace fluid lost from the cells. The blood vessel baroreceptors sense a decreased blood pressure in dehydration. This, in turn, stimulates the sympathetic nervous system, which vasoconstricts arterial vessels and increases the heart rate to compensate. Additionally, osmoreceptors stimulate ADH secretion from the posterior pituitary gland. The ADH works at the nephron to increase water reabsorption into the bloodstream. Simultaneously, because the blood volume is low, circulation to the kidneys is decreased. Decreased kidney perfusion provokes renin secretion, which activates the RAAS, resulting in increased sodium and water in the bloodstream, raising blood volume. Additionally, angiotensin II acts as a potent vasoconstrictor, which raises blood pressure. These compensatory mechanisms restore fluid balance and maintain blood pressure in states of dehydration (see Fig. 7-9).

Assessment of Fluid Volume Status

Fluid losses and gains can be clinically assessed in many ways. A basic method to clinically assess an individual's fluid volume status is daily weight. When using daily weight to assess fluid volume status, it is important to take the measurement using the same scale, at the same time of day, every day. A weight change of 2 pounds from 1 day to the next is likely caused by fluid gained or lost.

A record of the patient's 24-hour **intake and output (I&O)** is another common way to monitor fluid status. The amount of fluid intake necessary for an adult with normal heart and renal function is 1500 mL/m^2 of body surface per day. On average, this is approximately 2 liters of fluid per day.

All fluids, including oral, IV, and tube feedings, are recorded as intake. All measurements should be recorded in milliliters (mL), so it is important to understand how to convert ounces to mL: *1 ounce of fluid is equal to 30 mL.* Water from ingested food can be estimated at approximately 500 to 1000 mL/day. Output includes urine; vomitus; wound or ostomy drainage; and insensible water losses through the lungs, sweat, and feces. Wound or ostomy drainage and vomitus must be estimated. Insensible water loss is usually 1000 mL/day, but it may be more if fever is present. Water requirements increase during specific conditions (see Box 7-2); for example, water requirements increase by 100 to 150 mL per day for each degree Celsius of body temperature elevation. I&O should be approximately equal over a 24-hour period. The daily I&O record can indicate fluid retention, which is a positive fluid balance, or fluid deficit, which is a negative fluid balance (see Fig. 7-10).

Another clinical assessment of fluid status involves the patient's vital signs. The patient who is dehydrated may have tachycardia and hypotension, particularly postural hypotension. To assess for postural hypotension, measure the blood pressure in the lying and standing positions.

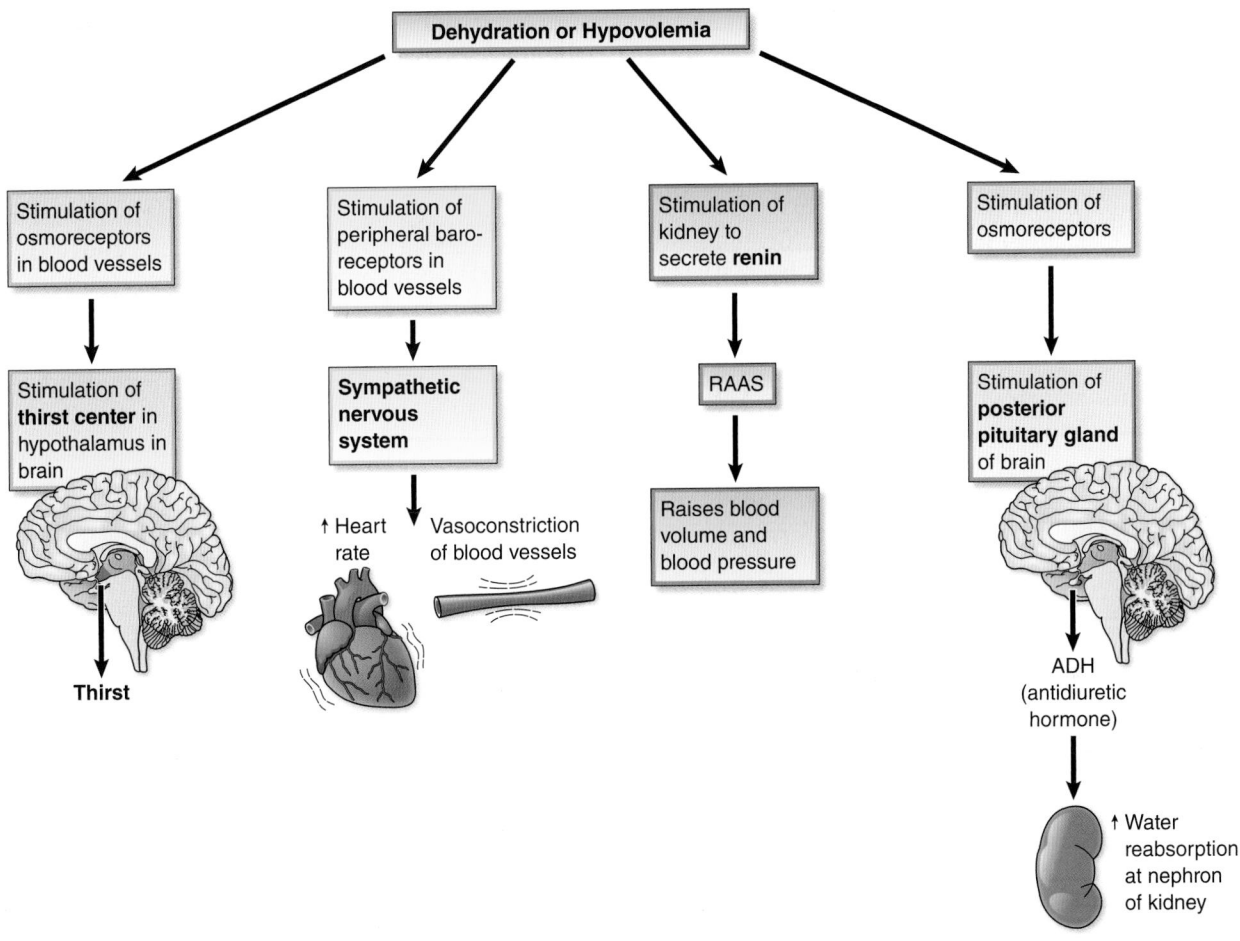

FIGURE 7-9. Physiological responses to dehydration. The body compensates for dehydration and hypovolemia (low blood volume) in various ways.

BOX 7-2. Conditions That Cause Dehydration and Increase Water Requirements

- Bleeding
- Breastfeeding
- Burns
- Fever
- Gastrointestinal (GI) fluid loss; vomiting, diarrhea
- Hypotension
- Nephrolithiasis
- Polyuria
- Surgical drains
- Sweating
- Tachypnea

🔬 **CLINICAL CONCEPT**

Orthostatic hypotension, which occurs in dehydration, is a systolic blood pressure decrease of at least 20 mm Hg or a diastolic blood pressure decrease of at least 10 mm Hg within 3 minutes when going from a lying to a standing position.

Finally, a patient with a fluid volume deficit will have a number of symptoms of dehydration, including thirst, dry mucous membranes, poor skin turgor, hypotension, low urine output, and dark-colored urine. Poor skin turgor is demonstrated through nonelasticity of the skin. When the skin is pinched, a small tent of the skin remains elevated for a few seconds.

A patient who has fluid volume excess will have edema, moist mucous membranes, and may have hypertension. With fluid excess, weight gain and possibly ascites, as well as pitting edema, can occur. In severe fluid volume excess, dyspnea may also be present because of pulmonary edema. Box 7-3 presents the different signs and symptoms of fluid volume deficit and excess.

Electrolyte Imbalances

For a cell to function properly, serum electrolytes must be within normal range. Sodium is the main extracellular electrolyte, whereas potassium is the main intracellular electrolyte. The cellular Na^+/K^+ pump is constantly at work to try to retain K^+ in the

INTAKE AND OUTPUT SHEET

Hospital # _____   Patient's name _____

Date _____   Room # _____

	INTAKE			OUTPUT			
				Urine		Gastric	
	By Mouth	Tube	Parenteral	Voided	Catheter	Emesis	Suction
Time 7–3	6 oz tea		IV 500 mL D5W in NaCl 0.9%	500 mL			
Time 3–11	6 oz tea		IV 500 mL D5W in NaCl 0.9%	500 mL			
Time 11–7	8 oz water			200 mL			
24-hour total	600 mL		1,000 mL				
24-hour grand total • Intake	1,600 mL			24-hour grand total • Output	1,200 mL		

FIGURE 7-10. Sample I&O record.
Remember: 1 ounce = 30 mL.

BOX 7-3. Signs and Symptoms of Fluid Volume Deficit and Excess

FLUID VOLUME DEFICIT
Dark urine with high specific gravity
Depressed fontanelles (infant)
Dry mucous membranes
Low urine output
Orthostatic hypotension
Poor skin turgor
Thirst
Weight loss

FLUID VOLUME EXCESS
Ascites
Crackles in lungs
Dyspnea caused by pulmonary fluid accumulation
Edema, either ankle or sacral
Weight gain (2 lb = 1 liter of fluid)

---

intracellular compartment and move Na^+ to the extracellular environment.

Many enzymatic, hormonal, and chemically mediated mechanisms are dependent on normal levels of serum electrolytes. These include the generation of adenosine triphosphate (ATP), transcription and translation of DNA and ribonucleic acid (RNA), neural transmission, and muscular contraction.

Alterations in sodium, potassium, and calcium ion levels have a major effect on neurotransmission and muscular contraction. Changes in nerve and muscle excitability are particularly important in cardiac muscle, where rhythm disruption and conduction disturbances can be life threatening.

Most cells maintain an electrochemical gradient because of the effect of intracellular and extracellular sodium and potassium. This is most apparent in cell-to-cell impulse propagation in neurotransmission. Without stimulation, cells maintain a resting membrane potential created by a set ratio of intracellular and extracellular sodium and potassium ions. Action potentials, the impulses generated along neuronal axons, are created by changes in sodium and potassium ions in ICF and ECF. During an action potential, sodium ion channels open in the plasma membrane, allowing the entry of sodium ions into the cell. This is followed by the opening of potassium ion channels that permit the exit of potassium ions from the cell. The inward flow of sodium ions increases the concentration of positively charged cations in the cell and causes depolarization, where the potential of the cell is higher than the cell's resting potential. The sodium channels close at the peak of the action potential, whereas potassium continues to leave the cell. The efflux of potassium ions decreases the membrane potential in the repolarization phase (see Fig. 7-11). With imbalances of sodium and potassium in the body, neural transmission in the body is widely disrupted. There is body-wide muscular weakness and changes in sensation such as paresthesias (numbness and tingling). The muscles of the gastrointestinal system dysfunction, causing nausea, constipation, and abdominal distention. Confusion and disorientation are common symptoms of central nervous system (CNS) dysfunction. Cardiac dysfunction is particularly apparent with potassium-level disruption. Electrocardiogram (ECG) changes, rhythm disturbances, and postural hypotension occur.

Cardiac muscle contractility is largely dependent on calcium ions. Like neurons and other muscles, a given cardiac muscle cell has a resting membrane potential. A notable difference between skeletal and cardiac muscle is how each depolarizes the muscle cells. When skeletal muscle is stimulated by motor nerves, an influx of Na^+ quickly depolarizes the skeletal muscle cell. In cardiac muscle cells, calcium influx through voltage-gated calcium channels on the plasma membrane causes muscle contraction. Changes in serum calcium levels can cause hypotension, cardiac dysrhythmias, heart failure, and diminished responsiveness to cardiac drugs.

Sodium Imbalances

Sodium is the main electrolyte in the ECF and is the primary determinant of the ECF's osmolarity and volume. It must constantly be pumped out of the cell into the bloodstream. Sodium has many important physiological roles. It controls the distribution of water, helps maintain normal fluid balance, and contributes to osmotic pressure. Sodium is also important to maintain the electrical gradient of neural membranes. However, because it is an extracellular ion, alterations in fluid balance can adversely affect its levels, which is why serum sodium levels need to be interpreted based on hydration status. Sodium is diluted by excess water in the bloodstream and concentrated when there is lack of sufficient water in the bloodstream.

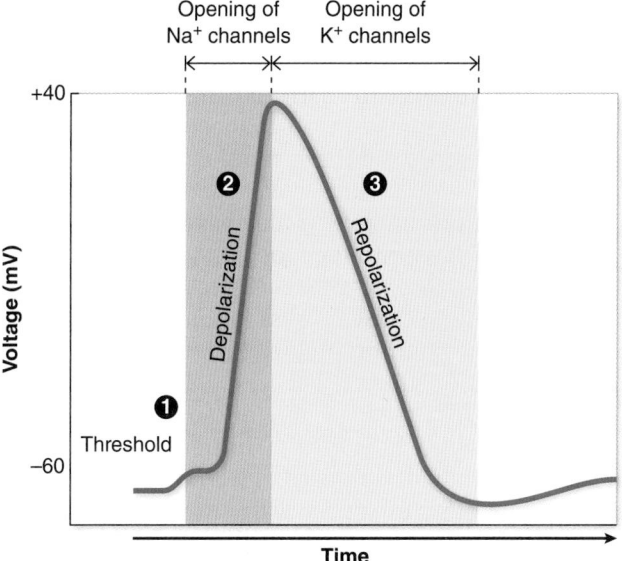

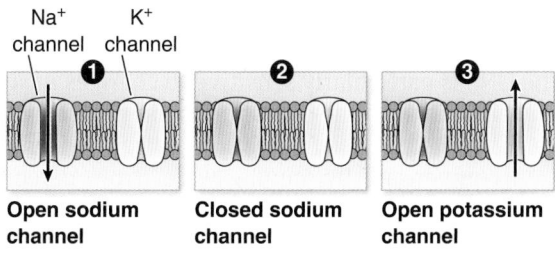

FIGURE 7-11. Nerve impulses are generated by action potentials within the neuron plasma membrane. Action potentials are generated by special types of ion channels embedded in a cell's plasma membrane. These channels are shut when the membrane potential is near the resting potential of the cell. (1) When the channels open, they allow an inward flow of sodium ions, which produces a rise in the membrane potential known as depolarization. This then causes more channels to open, and the process proceeds until all of the available sodium ion channels are open, resulting in a large upswing in the membrane potential. (2) The ion channels then close and sodium ions can no longer enter the neuron. (3) Potassium channels are then activated and there is an outward current of potassium ions, returning the electrochemical gradient to the resting state. This is called repolarization.

> ### 🩺 CLINICAL CONCEPT
>
> The average diet contains 1 to 3 grams of sodium per day. A low-sodium diet consists of less than 1500 mg of sodium per day. Low-sodium diets are recommended in hypertension and heart failure.

Hyponatremia

Hyponatremia is a sodium serum level of less than 135 mEq/L. The clinical picture of hyponatremia centers around water. When dehydration occurs because the body has lost sodium and fluid together, it is known as hypovolemic hyponatremia. This primarily happens due to losses from the kidney (renal) or GI tract (nonrenal).

The causes of renal hypovolemic hyponatremia include adrenal insufficiency, osmotic diuresis, diuretic use, and salt-losing nephritis. The causes of nonrenal hypovolemic hyponatremia include diarrhea, vomiting, excessive sweating, cystic fibrosis, gastric lavage, fistulas, burns, and wounds. In cases of dehydration caused by hypovolemic hyponatremia, the symptoms are thirst, dry mouth, orthostatic hypotension, tachycardia, azotemia (high blood urea nitrogen concentration), and oliguria. In the older adult, electrolyte imbalances, particularly hyponatremia, can occur due to side effects of medications, insensitivity of the thirst center, or inadequate hydration.

 CLINICAL CONCEPT

Neurological deficits, confusion, and behavioral changes are common effects of hyponatremia in the older adult. These CNS changes can lead to patient falls, which may be the first apparent sign of electrolyte imbalance.

Conversely, hyponatremia can occur in the presence of hypervolemia, or excess water. In this case, hyponatremia develops because sodium is diluted within an excess of water, which is why it is a dilutional hyponatremia. Symptoms include headache, lethargy, apathy, confusion, nausea, vomiting, diarrhea, muscle cramps, and muscle spasms.

Hyponatremia most commonly occurs when water excretion is impaired and sodium is diluted within a large volume of water in the bloodstream. This is clinically significant when hyponatremia is part of a drop in the serum total osmolality, which is measured by the calculation: $2(Na)\,mEq/L + serum\,glucose\,(mg/dL)/18 + BUN\,(mg/dL)/2.8$.

When there is an acute drop in the serum osmolality, neuronal cell swelling occurs because of the water shift from the extracellular space to the intracellular space. Swelling of the brain cells results in two consequences:

- It inhibits ADH secretion from neurons in the hypothalamus and hypothalamic thirst center, which leads to excess water elimination as dilute urine.
- There is an immediate cellular adaptation with loss of electrolytes, and over the next few days there is a more gradual loss of organic intracellular solutes.

Severe hyponatremia can cause seizures, coma, and irreversible neurological damage because of brain swelling.

Treatment of hyponatremia is based on its etiology. If the patient is dehydrated, slow replacement of sodium with adequate fluid intake is the easiest method. Slow treatment is necessary, as rapid correction of serum sodium can precipitate severe neurological complications. If that does not help, more aggressive measures will be needed, such as replacement with normal saline or hypertonic saline solution.

 CLINICAL CONCEPT

A patient who receives normal saline needs to be watched carefully for edema, particularly for pulmonary edema or other signs of fluid overload.

If the etiology of hyponatremia is SIADH, treatment requires restriction of water intake and investigating the source of ADH. If the etiology is fluid overload, diuretics will be used to remove excess water.

 CLINICAL CONCEPT

Severe hyponatremia (less than 125 mEq/L) has a high mortality rate. In instances when the serum sodium level is lower than 105 mEq/L, the mortality is over 50%. Postoperative and older patients have the highest incidence of hyponatremia.

Hypernatremia

Hypernatremia is a sodium level greater than 145 mEq/L. It can occur with an excess of sodium or decrease in body water (see Box 7-4). Most commonly, it is caused by water loss, although it can be caused by salt loading. With kidney dysfunction, other factors may be involved, such as the inability of the renal tubule to react to ADH, causing the kidneys to not reabsorb water. With an inadequate amount of water in the blood, sodium is more concentrated and presents as a high serum level. Also, if the kidneys' glomerular filtration rate is decreased, sodium and water reabsorption into the bloodstream is low, which stimulates the adrenal gland's secretion of aldosterone. Aldosterone causes reabsorption of sodium and water from the nephron tubule fluid into the circulation, raising the sodium level.

When hypernatremia of any etiology occurs, cells become dehydrated. The high osmotic load of the increased sodium acts to extract water from the cells. Dehydrated cells shrink from water extraction. In mild hypernatremia, individuals usually can drink water to lower the sodium level in the blood and the body regains equilibrium. However, severe hypernatremia often occurs in ill patients who cannot take oral fluids. The CNS is particularly sensitive to changes in sodium concentrations in the bloodstream. In severe hypernatremia, water is lost from brain cells. The brain cells then compensate by moving water from cerebrospinal fluid (CSF) into the brain cells. This also brings in solutes such as amino acids and other organic solutes from the CSF into the brain cells. These changes keep the brain cells from severely dehydrating. During the treatment of the hypernatremic patient, usually clinicians will use intravenous hypotonic solutions, which are high in water content. During treatment, if this water is infused too rapidly, it will move into the brain cells that are hypertonic compared with the hypotonic intravenous fluid. This can cause cerebral edema, leading to seizures, coma, and death. In treating severe hypernatremia, clinicians need to precisely calculate the free water deficit and replace water intravenously slowly over several hours to prevent cerebral edema from occurring.

BOX 7-4. Causes of Hyponatremia and Hypernatremia

CAUSES OF HYPONATREMIA
- Adrenal insufficiency
- Burns
- Cirrhosis
- Congestive heart failure
- Diaphoresis with more salt lost than water
- Diarrhea
- Diuretic therapy
- Excess hypotonic fluid administration (called *dilutional hyponatremia*)
- Hyperglycemia
- Hypoaldosteronism
- Laxatives
- Nasogastric suction
- Psychogenic polydipsia
- Renal disease
- SIADH, which causes excess reabsorption of water into the bloodstream at the nephron

CAUSES OF HYPERNATREMIA
- Certain medications such as osmotic diuretics, sodium bicarbonate, and sodium chloride
- Cushing's syndrome
- Diabetes insipidus (lack of antidiuretic hormone)
- Diarrhea
- Excess sodium administration
- Excessive adrenocortical secretion
- Hypercalcemia
- Impaired thirst
- Increased aldosterone
- Potassium depletion
- Profuse diaphoresis
- Tube feedings with lack of adequate water administration
- Uncontrolled diabetes mellitus
- Water deprivation

The clinical manifestations of hypernatremia can be divided into two distinct patterns, one with fluid overload and one without fluid overload. If hypernatremia causes water retention, then the picture is one of an edematous state: weight gain and hypertension. With severe edematous states, there may also be mental changes and pulmonary edema causing dyspnea. If the hypernatremia is that of sodium retention and water loss, the patient will appear to be dehydrated and demonstrate thirst, irritability, tachycardia, flushed skin, dry mucous membranes, and oliguria.

 CLINICAL CONCEPT

Hypernatremia risk is highest in breastfed infants and older adults.

Treatment of hypernatremia depends on the underlying cause. Replacement fluids can be given orally or parenterally if it is caused by fluid depletion. Oral glucose–electrolyte replacement solutions are available for infants and children. If excess water is present, diuretic therapy may be necessary.

The mortality rate from hypernatremia is high, especially among older patients. Mortality rates of 42% to 75% have been reported for acute changes and 10% to 60% for chronic hypernatremia.

Potassium Imbalances

Potassium is the main electrolyte of the ICF; adults require 40 to 60 mEq/L/day of K^+. Potassium is involved in a wide range of body functions, including conduction of nerve impulses in skeletal, cardiac, and smooth muscle; acid–base balance; synthesis of adenosine-5'-triphosphate (ATP); osmotic balance; and the kidney's ability to concentrate urine. The nephron regulates potassium because of the action of aldosterone, which absorbs sodium and water and excretes potassium at the distal tubule.

Muscle contains the bulk of the body's potassium, and alterations in potassium levels have neuromuscular effects. A decrease in serum potassium causes decreased neuromuscular excitability, resulting in muscle weakness. An increase in potassium causes increased neuromuscular excitability, resulting in muscle spasms. Changes in neuromuscular excitability are particularly important in the heart, where alterations in serum potassium can produce serious cardiac arrhythmias.

Fluid shifts between the ICF and ECF can cause temporary changes in plasma potassium levels. Additionally, potassium levels should be assessed in relation to acid–base balance. Potassium will move from the ICF to the ECF based on changes in the hydrogen ion (H^+) concentration in the bloodstream. When H^+ is high in the bloodstream, H^+ excretion takes precedence over K^+ excretion at the kidney. In acidosis, aldosterone stimulates excretion of H^+ ions from the bloodstream instead of K^+ ions. As a result, K^+ remains in the bloodstream, making it appear as though there is an excess of K^+ in the blood, but this is not true of hyperkalemia. When the acidosis is treated, K^+ will move into the ICF compartment, which will demonstrate that K^+ is actually low in the bloodstream. In diabetic ketoacidosis, when treatment is instituted using insulin, K^+ moves into the intracellular compartment. This movement of K^+ into the cells leaves an actual low K^+ level in the blood, thereby requiring administration of supplemental potassium.

Hypokalemia

Hypokalemia refers to a plasma concentration of potassium below 3.5 mEq/L. Diuretic therapy is the most common cause of hypokalemia; it is present in 20% to 50% of patients on non–potassium-sparing diuretics. African Americans and females are more susceptible. Risk is enhanced by concomitant illness such as heart failure or nephrotic syndrome. Both thiazide and loop diuretics increase the loss of K⁺ in the urine.

Inadequate intake is also a frequent cause of hypokalemia. Patients who are nothing-by-mouth status (NPO), people who abuse alcohol, patients who have undergone bariatric surgery, and those who suffer from eating disorders are at greatest risk. A daily potassium intake of at least 40 to 50 mEq is required for optimal cell function.

The body can also lose approximately 80% to 90% of potassium via the kidneys, with the remainder lost through sweat and feces. Renal losses are increased by stress, trauma, metabolic alkalosis, and increased levels of aldosterone. Skin and gastrointestinal losses of K⁺ can become excessive in burns, vomiting, nasogastric suctioning, and diarrhea. Severe diarrheal illness can cause a loss of potassium of 40 to 60 mEq/L.

The major signs and symptoms associated with hypokalemia include anorexia, nausea, vomiting, sluggish bowel, cardiac arrhythmias, postural hypotension, muscle fatigue, and weakness. Leg cramps are particularly common. Also, respiratory muscles can be weakened in severe hypokalemia. Deep tendon reflexes may be decreased or absent on physical examination. On ECG, there is a prolonged PR interval, flattened T wave, and prominent U wave (see Fig. 7-12).

Some specific clinical conditions can decrease potassium levels in the bloodstream. When large amounts of IV dextrose solution are administered to patients, the pancreas secretes excessive amounts of insulin; this can cause hypokalemia. The administration of adrenergic agents, such as epinephrine or albuterol, can also cause a drop in blood potassium levels. Commonly, diuretics also cause a loss of potassium from the bloodstream.

Digoxin (Lanoxin) toxicity often occurs when the patient is in the state of hypokalemia. Digoxin is a drug used when a patient is in heart failure. Heart failure often causes a loss of potassium because of the cycling of the RAAS when the heart is weakened.

When digoxin is administered to a patient, potassium and digoxin compete for binding sites in the heart. In hypokalemia, there are open binding sites for potassium in the heart, and digoxin binds to these sites. When a high number of binding sites become occupied by digoxin, the potential for toxicity increases.

CLINICAL CONCEPT

Diuretics and digoxin are often prescribed together in heart failure. Diuretics commonly cause urinary loss of potassium, leading to hypokalemia. Hypokalemia causes increased binding of digoxin in the heart, which increases susceptibility of toxicity, commonly demonstrated as arrhythmias. Potassium blood level and digoxin level need to be frequently monitored in heart failure.

Treatment of hypokalemia is accomplished by replacement of potassium with foods such as orange juice, bananas, dried fruits, meats, and oral or parenteral K⁺ preparations. Potassium can also be prescribed intravenously; commonly, 20 mEq of potassium chloride (KCl) per liter of IV solution is administered to NPO patients, not to exceed a total of 60 mEq/ day.

ALERT! Rapid administration of K⁺ can cause cardiac arrest. IV potassium must always be diluted and never given as an IV bolus. It is excoriating to the skin and blood vessels in large doses. In emergency cases, up to 40 mEq of potassium can be administered through a central venous line. A patient's ECG should be continuously monitored (telemetry) when given potassium.

Hyperkalemia

Hyperkalemia is a blood K⁺ level greater than 5.2 mEq/dL. Normal kidney function is important in the regulation of potassium. Renal failure is a major cause of hyperkalemia because the kidneys lose the ability to excrete K⁺. Any decrease in renal perfusion, such as decreased cardiac output, will diminish the kidney's ability to excrete K⁺, thus increasing the amount of potassium in the body. Hyperkalemia can also occur in major muscle trauma, such as a crushing injury, because potassium is released rapidly from muscle cells.

The clinical presentation of a patient with hyperkalemia will depend on the level of the potassium imbalance and if it is chronically or acutely elevated. Early symptoms of hyperkalemia include numbness or tingling of the extremities, muscle cramping, diarrhea, apathy, and mental confusion. The ECG will show

Hypokalemia

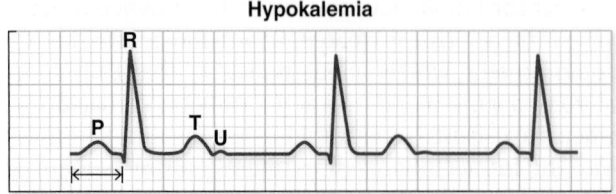

FIGURE 7-12. Electrocardiogram changes indicative of hypokalemia.

wide QRS complexes and tall, peaked T waves (see Fig. 7-13); as the potassium level rises, the ECG will show bradycardia, irregular pulse rate, and, ultimately, cardiac arrest.

Treatment of hyperkalemia is dependent on the cause. If hyperkalemia is severe (greater than 7.0 mEq/L), rapid treatment is needed to move K+ from ECF to ICF. Continuous ECG monitoring is necessary. An infusion of 50% dextrose, 10 units of regular insulin, and 75 mEq of sodium bicarbonate can be administered. If K+ levels continue to be elevated and the patient has normal renal function, a diuretic such as furosemide (Lasix) can be administered. Calcium chloride or calcium gluconate (Kalcinate) can also be administered. Albuterol and diuretics can be used to reduce high blood potassium. Another option for treatment is to give sodium polystyrene sulfonate (Kayexalate), which acts at the bowel to capture potassium and excrete it via feces. An oral suspension, called Patiromer (Veltassa), can enhance potassium excretion from the intestine into the feces. Alternatively, hemodialysis or renal replacement therapy can reduce K+ (see Box 7-5).

Calcium Imbalances

Calcium and phosphorus are the major mineral contents of bone. Small amounts of these electrolytes, which are regulated by vitamin D and parathyroid hormone (PTH), are found in the circulation. The major function of vitamin D is to facilitate the absorption of calcium from the gastrointestinal tract into the bloodstream; once in the bloodstream, PTH controls calcium levels. When the plasma calcium level is low, PTH is stimulated; when the plasma calcium level is high, PTH is inhibited.

PTH acts on bone to mobilize calcium and raise blood levels. Calcitonin, a hormone produced by the thyroid, acts at the bone and kidneys to remove calcium from the circulation.

Calcium is an important element in the body because of its role in the formation and function of bones and teeth, normal clotting, and regulation of neuromuscular irritability. It is stored in the bone, bound to plasma proteins, and bound with organic ions such as citrate. A small amount of calcium also remains free. This free, or ionized, calcium interacts in normal physiological functions. The ionized form participates in cellular activities such as enzymatic reactions; neuron excitability; muscle contraction; release of hormones, neurotransmitters, and other chemical messengers; blood vessel contractility; cardiac contractility and automaticity; and blood clotting. Calcium is found in both ECF and ICF.

Because calcium is highly protein bound, interpretation of calcium levels is based on serum albumin levels. About half of the calcium in the body is bound to

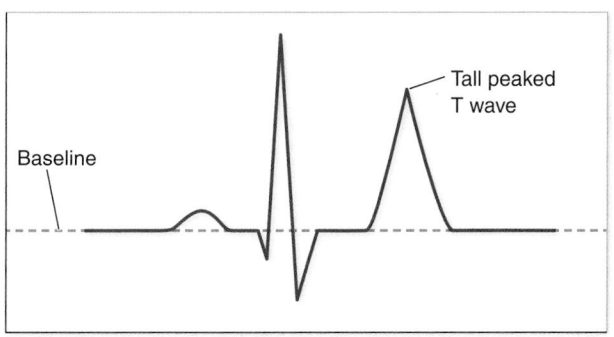

FIGURE 7-13. Electrocardiogram changes indicative of hyperkalemia.

BOX 7-5. Causes of Hypokalemia and Hyperkalemia

CAUSES OF HYPOKALEMIA
- Alkalosis
- Diuretic therapy
- Elevated glucocorticoids
- Excessive gastrointestinal, renal, or skin losses
- Hyperaldosteronism
- Inadequate intake
- Laxative abuse
- Nasogastric suction
- Redistribution of potassium (K+) between the intracellular and extracellular spaces

CAUSES OF HYPERKALEMIA
- Addison's disease
- Burns (can redistribute K+ into ECF from ICF)
- Digoxin toxicity
- Excessive administration of K+ sparing diuretics (spironolactone)
- Extreme exercise
- Hemolysis of red blood cells
- Hypoaldosteronism
- Medications: antibiotics such as sulfamethoxazole and trimethoprim (Bactrim), ACE inhibitors, chemotherapeutic agents, and immunosuppressive agents such as cyclosporine
- Metabolic acidosis
- Na+ depletion
- Renal failure
- Trauma (can redistribute K+ into ECF from ICF)

albumin. Hypoalbuminemia can cause the appearance of low calcium levels called pseudohypocalcemia. In pseudohypocalcemia, there is a normal level of body calcium with more in the ionized state than in the bound state because there is a diminished amount of albumin able to carry calcium. It is important to recognize that calcium and phosphate PO_4^- have an inverse relationship in the bloodstream. Both are bone-derived ions; when Ca^{++} rises in the bloodstream, PO_4^- diminishes in the bloodstream. When PO_4^- rises in the bloodstream, Ca^{++} diminishes in the bloodstream.

Hypocalcemia

Hypocalcemia occurs when the blood calcium level is less than 8.7 mg/dL in adults. It is most commonly caused by lack of sufficient Ca^{++} in the diet, vitamin D deficiency, renal disease, or hypoparathyroidism. Acute hypocalcemia is manifested by neuromuscular excitability, which is demonstrated in individuals as a subjective experience of paresthesias (numbness and tingling) around the mouth, hands, and feet. Chvostek's sign and Trousseau's sign are examples of neuromuscular irritability caused by chronically low calcium levels (see Fig. 7-14 and Fig. 7-15). Other signs may include muscle spasms of the face, hands, and feet; laryngeal spasm; seizures; and death. Cardiovascular effects of hypocalcemia include hypotension, arrhythmias (particularly heart block and ventricular fibrillation), and failure to respond to cardioactive drugs. Chronic hypocalcemia causes bone pain and fragility, dry skin and hair, cataracts, depression, and dementia. Because of the inverse relationship between calcium and phosphate in the blood, hypocalcemia will cause hyperphosphatemia.

Treatment of hypocalcemia requires calcium replacement. Oral calcium supplements with vitamin D are often used, as vitamin D is needed for calcium absorption from the intestine.

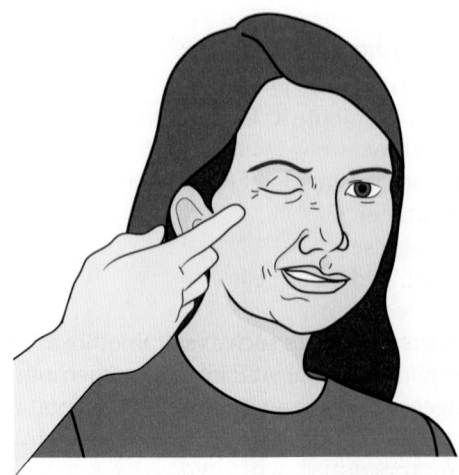

FIGURE 7-14. Chvostek's sign. Chvostek's sign is a clinical finding associated with hypocalcemia. A slight twitch of the facial muscles can be observed when tapping the facial nerve; a region in an individual's cheek, in front of the ear.

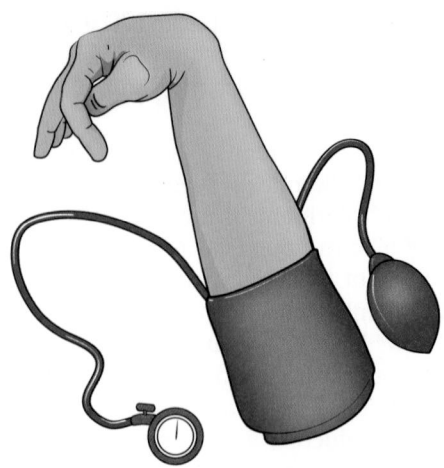

FIGURE 7-15. Trousseau's sign. A positive Trousseau's sign indicates hypocalcemia. It is a carpopedal spasm of the hand and wrist that occurs in response to having an inflated blood pressure cuff placed over the brachial artery for 2 to 3 minutes.

Hypercalcemia

Hypercalcemia is a calcium level greater than 10 mg/dL. Hypercalcemia occurs when the amount of calcium entering the ECF exceeds calcium excretion by the kidneys. The two most common causes are hyperparathyroidism and cancer. In hyperparathyroidism, PTH is overproduced, and the hormone pulls excessive amounts of calcium out of the bones and into the bloodstream. Cancer-related hypercalcemia is caused by malignant cells invading the bone, causing bone destruction. Cancer also releases a parathyroid-like hormone, causing an increase in serum calcium levels. Other causes of hypercalcemia are prolonged immobility that causes calcium to leach out of bone; excess calcium or vitamin D intake; toxic levels of drugs such as lithium, thiazide diuretics, and theophylline; aluminum-induced osteomalacia; and hypophosphatemia.

The signs and symptoms of hypercalcemia involve decreased neuromuscular excitability. Muscle flaccidity, proximal muscle weakness of the lower extremities, bone tenderness, and decreased neuromuscular activity of the bowel causing constipation are the main effects. High calcium concentrations in the urine increase susceptibility to renal calculi. The heart responds to hypercalcemia with increased contractility and ventricular arrhythmias. Other nonspecific effects include dulled consciousness, depression, anorexia, nausea, vomiting, and ulcers. Hyperreflexia and tongue fasciculations may also occur. Hypercalcemia also causes hypophosphatemia.

Treatment involves enhancement of urinary excretion of calcium and inhibition of bone breakdown. Increased fluids and loop diuretics enhance calcium excretion. Bisphosphonates, such as alendronate, and calcitonin are used to inhibit bone breakdown. Dialysis can be used in patients with kidney or heart failure (see Box 7-6).

BOX 7-6. Causes of Hypocalcemia and Hypercalcemia

CAUSES OF HYPOCALCEMIA
- Alcohol abuse
- Drugs: loop diuretics, anticonvulsants, calcitonin, gentamicin, phosphates
- Hyperphosphatemia
- Hypoalbuminemia
- Hypomagnesemia
- Hypoparathyroidism
- Inadequate dietary intake or inadequate vitamin D
- Malabsorption
- Pancreatitis
- Sepsis

CAUSES OF HYPERCALCEMIA
- Decreased elimination of calcium
- Drugs: diuretics, chemotherapy, androgens, estrogen, lithium, theophylline
- Excess vitamin D
- Hyperparathyroidism
- Increased bone resorption of calcium
- Increased intestinal absorption of calcium
- Malignancy such as bone, multiple myeloma, blood, breast, and lung cancer
- Prolonged immobility
- Renal insufficiency

Phosphorus Imbalances

Phosphorus is an essential component of bone, red blood cells, enzymatic processes, formation of ATP, acid–base balance, and cellular building blocks. Phosphorus is found in bone and circulates in the blood as phosphate (PO_4^-). Phosphates are incorporated into nucleic acids of DNA and RNA and the phospholipids of the cell membrane. The kidneys excrete phosphate, and the parathyroid glands regulate the phosphate level in the blood. Phosphate has a reciprocal relationship with calcium in the blood, meaning that when calcium is low in the bloodstream, phosphate is high and vice versa.

Hypophosphatemia

Hypophosphatemia occurs when the blood level of phosphate is lower than 2.5 mg/dL. There are three main causes of hypophosphatemia: decreased intestinal absorption of phosphorus, increased excretion of phosphorus by the kidneys, and an intracellular shift of phosphate. Low phosphate causes red blood cell, white blood cell, and platelet dysfunction, as well as neural dysfunction and disturbed musculoskeletal function. Lack of sufficient phosphate can cause tremors, paresthesias, hyporeflexia, anorexia, dysphagia, muscle weakness, joint stiffness, bone pain, and osteomalacia. Treatment of hypophosphatemia is replacement therapy.

Hyperphosphatemia

Hyperphosphatemia is a PO_4^- level of 4.5 mg/dL or greater in the blood. The most common cause is kidney failure, where the kidneys are unable to excrete excessive phosphorus. Hyperphosphatemia is usually accompanied by hypocalcemia, and many of its symptoms are related to low calcium levels. Treatment is directed at correcting the cause of the disorder. Calcium-based phosphate binders, such as sevelamer and lanthanum carbonate, inhibit gastrointestinal absorption of phosphate. Dialysis can also reduce hyperphosphatemia (see Box 7-7).

Magnesium Imbalances

Magnesium (Mg^{++}) is largely stored in bone and, like calcium, is protein bound within the bloodstream. About 60% of the body's magnesium is found in the bones. It is required for many cellular metabolic processes, such as functioning of nerve conduction, replication and transcription of DNA, translation of RNA, intracellular enzyme reactions, and all processes that require ATP. The cardiovascular system requires magnesium for vasodilation and normal functioning. Magnesium also affects sodium and potassium levels both inside and outside the cell membrane. In addition, magnesium can compete with and exert effects on calcium-mediated processes because of its effect on the parathyroid gland.

Magnesium is ingested from the diet in meats, seafood, green vegetables, and some sources of ground water. It is absorbed from the intestine, reabsorbed in the loop of Henle, and then excreted by the kidney. It is inhibited by high plasma calcium levels and high PTH levels. Magnesium also assists in the release of PTH. There is an interdependent relationship between Mg^{++} and K^+: when K^+ decreases, so does Mg^{++} and vice versa.

Hypomagnesemia

Hypomagnesemia is a magnesium blood level of less than 1.5 mEq/L. Hypomagnesemia occurs most commonly when Mg^{++} ions are released from bone in exchange for increased uptake of calcium. It usually occurs in conjunction with hypocalcemia and hypokalemia; however, recent studies show that magnesium deficiency is more common in the population than once thought. More than 50% of the population has inadequate levels of Mg^{++} (U.S. Department

---

BOX 7-7. Causes of Hypophosphatemia and Hyperphosphatemia

CAUSES OF HYPOPHOSPHATEMIA

- Recovery phase of diabetic ketoacidosis
- Acute alcoholism
- Severe burns
- Receiving total parenteral nutrition (TPN)
- Refeeding after prolonged undernutrition
- Severe respiratory alkalosis

Acute severe hypophosphatemia with serum phosphate < 1 mg/dL (<0.32 mmol/L) is most often caused by transcellular shifts of phosphate often superimposed on chronic phosphate depletion.

Chronic hypophosphatemia usually is the result of decreased renal phosphate reabsorption. Causes include the following:

- Increased parathyroid hormone levels, as in primary and secondary hyperparathyroidism
- Other hormonal disturbances, such as Cushing's syndrome and hypothyroidism
- Vitamin D deficiency
- Electrolyte disorders, such as hypomagnesemia and hypokalemia
- Theophylline intoxication
- Long-term diuretic use

Severe chronic hypophosphatemia usually results from a prolonged negative phosphate balance. Causes include:

- Chronic starvation or malabsorption, often in patients with alcoholism, especially when combined with vomiting or copious diarrhea
- Long-term ingestion of large amounts of phosphate-binding aluminum, usually in the form of antacids

CAUSES OF HYPERPHOSPHATEMIA
Increased intake of PO_4^-
This can result from the following:

- Excessive oral or rectal use of an oral phosphate-saline laxative (Phospho-soda[R])
- Excessive parenteral administration of phosphate
- Milk–alkali syndrome
- Vitamin D intoxication

Decreased excretion of PO_4^-
This can result from the following:

- Renal failure, acute or chronic
- Hypoparathyroidism
- Pseudohypoparathyroidism
- Severe hypomagnesemia
- Tumoral calcinosis
- Bisphosphonate therapy

Shift of phosphate from intracellular to extracellular space
This can result from the following:

- Rhabdomyolysis
- Tumor lysis
- Acute hemolysis
- Acute metabolic or respiratory acidosis

---

of Health and Human Services, 2015–2020). Also, more chronic conditions can cause hypomagnesemia than previously thought. Causes of hypomagnesemia include inadequate intake, chronic stress, alcoholism, chronic use of antacids, proton pump inhibitors, diuretics, prolonged diarrhea, laxative abuse, type 2 diabetes, sepsis, burns, and serious wounds requiring débridement. Also with advancing age, absorption of Mg++ decreases and renal loss increases (Rondanelli et al., 2021). Signs and symptoms of low Mg++ are similar to those of low Ca++ and K+ levels. These include neuromuscular manifestations such as tetany, Chvostek's sign, Trousseau's sign, tremors, muscle spasms, Babinski's sign, and cardiac arrhythmias. ECG changes similar to those of hypokalemia may be seen. More serious manifestations may be respiratory muscle paralysis, complete heart block, ventricular dysrhythmias, tachycardia, hypertension, osteoporosis with fracture, and coma. Treatment of hypomagnesemia is oral replacement therapy with a citrate, oxide, or carbonate compound.

Research is increasingly revealing that magnesium is a significant dietary nutrient and its deficiency can have widespread effects on the body. However, the U.S. Department of Agriculture dietary guidelines do not recommend supplementation of the diet with Mg++ because hypermagnesemia can have harmful effects.

Hypermagnesemia

Hypermagnesemia is a magnesium blood level of greater than 2.5 mEq/L. Magnesium is often used to treat cardiac disorders and pregnancy-related eclampsia, and levels must be carefully monitored. The most common cause of hypermagnesemia is renal dysfunction. High Mg++ inhibits acetylcholine release and can cause diminished neuromuscular function, demonstrated by hyporeflexia and muscle weakness. Magnesium also blocks calcium channels and can cause cardiovascular effects such as hypotension and arrhythmias. Severely high Mg++ levels (greater than 10 mEq/L) can cause cardiac arrest. Sedation, confusion, coma, and respiratory paralysis can occur. To counteract hypermagnesemia, IV calcium or dialysis can be used (see Box 7-8).

BOX 7-8. Causes of Hypermagnesemia and Hypomagnesemia

CAUSES OF HYPERMAGNESEMIA

- Renal failure
- Excessive intake
- Lithium therapy
- Hypothyroidism
- Addison disease
- Familial hypocalciuric hypercalcemia
- Milk-alkali syndrome
- Hyperparathyroidism
- Excessive Mg^{++} containing cathartics or laxatives
- Excessive M^{++} treatment for eclampsia
- Tumor lysis syndrome in chemotherapy
- Rhabdomyolysis

CAUSES OF HYPOMAGNESEMIA

Causes related to decreased magnesium intake include the following:

- Starvation
- Alcohol dependence and withdrawal
- Total parenteral nutrition

Causes related to the redistribution of magnesium from extracellular to intracellular space include the following:

- Hungry bone syndrome
- Treatment of diabetic ketoacidosis
- Refeeding syndrome
- Acute pancreatitis

Causes related to gastrointestinal magnesium loss include the following:

- Diarrhea
- Vomiting and nasogastric suction
- Gastrointestinal fistulas and ostomies
- Hypomagnesemia with secondary hypocalcemia (HSH)

Causes related to renal magnesium loss include the following:

- Renal tubular defects
- Gitelman's syndrome
- Classic Bartter's syndrome (type III Bartter's syndrome)
- Diuretics
- Antimicrobials: amphotericin B, aminoglycosides, pentamidine, capreomycin, viomycin, foscarnet
- Chemotherapeutic agents: cisplatin, cetuximab
- Immunosuppressants: tacrolimus, cyclosporine
- Proton pump inhibitors
- Primary hyperaldosteronism

Chapter Summary

- The human body is 60% water, and it is contained in three different compartments: intracellular, interstitial, and extracellular.
- The extracellular compartment is within the bloodstream, the intracellular compartment is within each cell, and the interstitial compartment is in the tissue between the cells and bloodstream.
- Hypovolemia, hypotension, or low perfusion of the kidney stimulates the RAAS.
- Signs of dehydration include thirst, dry mucous membranes, hypotension, poor skin turgor, dark-colored urine, and low urine volume.

- Hypovolemia or dehydration can cause oliguria (lack of adequate urine output), defined as less than 400 mL urine/day or less than 20 mL/urine per hour.
- Hypovolemia causes hypotension, which stimulates the baroreceptors to trigger the sympathetic nervous system to increase heart rate and arterial vasoconstriction.
- Blocking ACE inhibits the conversion of angiotensin I to angiotensin II in the RAAS.
- Angiotensin II is a potent vasoconstrictor and stimulates the adrenal gland to secrete aldosterone.

- ACE inhibitors and angiotensin receptor blockers are drugs that are commonly used to lower blood pressure and treat heart failure.
- Aldosterone increases sodium and water reabsorption into the bloodstream and excretes potassium into the urine.
- The RAAS is a compensatory mechanism of the body that will raise blood volume and stimulate arterial vasoconstriction, leading to an increase in blood pressure.
- The posterior pituitary can sense low blood volume and in response releases ADH, which causes water reabsorption into the bloodstream and raises water volume of blood.
- SIADH causes excess secretion of ADH and excess water reabsorption, which results in hypervolemia and dilutional hyponatremia.
- When the body has excessive water in the bloodstream, natriuretic peptides, ANP and BNP, are released by the heart tissue to increase water output into the urine.
- Diuresis means water loss from the body. The body contains natural diuretics, and many drugs act as diuretics. Major pharmacological diuretics include furosemide and hydrochlorothiazide.
- Starling's Law of Capillary Forces explains that there are two major forces at every capillary–cell interface in the body: hydrostatic and osmotic pressure. Hydrostatic pressure forces fluid out of the capillary pores into the tissues, and osmotic pressure pulls water from the tissues into the bloodstream.
- There are three types of IV solution: isotonic, hypotonic, and hypertonic. The most commonly used isotonic solution is 0.9% NaCl (normal saline).
- The loss of body water, whether acute or chronic, can cause a range of problems from mild lightheadedness to convulsions and coma. Conversely, the administration of excess water can be lethal to the patient.
- The electrolytes Na^+, K^+, Ca^{++}, Mg^{++}, and PO_4^- are the main ionic solutes in the blood.
- Sodium and water have a major influence on hydration status. Hydration status influences sodium concentration. Water follows sodium with fluid shifts.

- Hyponatremia can be due either to lack of sufficient sodium in the bloodstream or to excessive water in the bloodstream that dilutes the sodium content.
- Electrolyte imbalances, particularly hyponatremia, can cause behavioral changes such as disorientation and confusion in the older adult.
- Hypernatremia is associated with dehydration as a decrease in water level increases the sodium concentration.
- Potassium is one of the most important electrolytes to monitor in the body, particularly in patients with cardiac disease.
- Loop diuretics, often used in heart failure or edema, can cause hypokalemia.
- Hypokalemia can cause cardiac dysrhythmias and can cause digoxin toxicity.
- IV potassium must always be diluted because it is excoriating to skin and blood vessels. Commonly, 20 mEq of K^+ is added to a liter of IV fluid and administered over 8 hours.
- In emergency cases, up to 40 mEq of potassium can be administered through a central venous line.
- Hyperkalemia can cause cardiac arrest.
- Hypocalcemia can cause neuromuscular excitability, muscle cramping, and muscle spasms.
- Chvostek's and Trousseau's signs, both apparent muscle spasms, are indicative of hypocalcemia.
- Hypocalcemia and hypercalcemia can cause cardiac dysrhythmias (arrhythmias).
- Hypercalcemia causes sluggishness of muscles and can cause constipation due to slowed peristalsis and hardened stool. Hypercalcemia can also precipitate in the urine and cause kidney stones.
- Many types of cancers can secrete a parathyroid-like hormone that raises Ca^{++} levels in blood.
- Phosphate and calcium blood levels have an inverse relationship. When PO_4^- is high in bloodstream, calcium is low. When PO_4^- is low in bloodstream, calcium is high.
- Hypomagnesemia or hypermagnesemia can cause cardiac dysrhythmias (arrhythmias).

Making the Connections

Pathophysiology

Signs and Symptoms	Physical Assessment Findings	Diagnostic Testing	Treatment
Dehydration	Lack of body water in intracellular and extracellular fluid.			
Thirst. Dry mucous membranes. Weakness.	Low urine output. Dark urine. Poor skin turgor. Dry mucous membranes. Hypotension. In infants, depressed fontanelle.	High blood urea nitrogen (BUN). Oliguria. Hypernatremia caused by low water in blood.	Oral fluids. IV 0.45% NaCl.
Overhydration	Excess of body water in ICF and ECF.			
Edema. Weight gain.	Dyspnea caused by pulmonary fluid accumulation. Crackles in lungs. Edema, either ankle or sacral. Weight gain. Ascites.	Dilutional hyponatremia (excess water in the bloodstream causes a low sodium concentration in the bloodstream).	Diuretic.
Hyponatremia	Serum sodium lower than 135 mEq/L. Commonly caused by heart failure, diuretic therapy, cirrhosis, nephrosis, excess water intake, SIADH.			
Muscle cramps. Weakness. Headache. Depression. Anxiety. Lethargy. Confusion. Anorexia. Nausea. Vomiting.	Weakness. Depression. Anxiety. Lethargy. Confusion. Vomiting.	Serum sodium less than 135 mEq/L.	Depends on cause of low sodium. Slow replacement of sodium if true hyponatremia. Restriction of water intake if caused by dilutional hyponatremia.
Hypernatremia	Serum sodium greater than 145 mEq/L. Commonly caused by loss of water, fluid restriction, hypertonic IV fluids, diaphoresis with more water loss than sodium, tube feedings without adequate free water, Cushing's syndrome, diabetes insipidus.			
Decreased salivation. Thirst. Headache. Agitation. Seizures.	Decreased skin turgor if low water volume. Decreased reflexes. Tachycardia. Weak, thready pulse. Hypertension or hypotension depending on water volume.	Serum sodium greater than 145.	If caused by inadequate water: Replace with IV fluid 0.45% NaCl.
Hypokalemia	Serum potassium level less than 3.5 mEq/L. Commonly caused by dietary deficiency, diuretics, vomiting, diarrhea, nasogastric (NG) suction, hyperaldosteronism, salt wasting kidney disease, gastrointestinal (GI) surgery, alkalosis, laxative abuse.			
Anorexia, nausea, vomiting. Muscle weakness. Muscle cramps. Paresthesias. Confusion.	Postural hypotension. Increased sensitivity to digoxin toxicity. Muscle weakness.	Serum potassium level less than 3.5 mEq/L. ECG dysrhythmias. ECG: U wave.	Oral or parenteral K+.

Continued

Making the Connections—cont'd

Signs and Symptoms	Physical Assessment Findings	Diagnostic Testing	Treatment
Hyperkalemia | Serum potassium level greater than 5.2 mEq/L. Commonly caused by excessive intake, aldosterone deficiency, Na^+ depletion, acidosis, tissue trauma, burns, extreme exercise, renal failure, Addison's disease (lack of cortisol), hemolysis, potassium-sparing diuretics, ACE inhibitors.			
Nausea, vomiting. Intestinal cramping. Diarrhea. Paresthesias. Muscle weakness. Muscle cramping. Dizziness.	Muscle weakness. Dizziness.	Serum potassium level greater than 5.2 mEq/L. ECG changes, including peaked T wave. Risk of cardiac arrest with severe K^+ excess.	An infusion of 50% dextrose, 10 units of regular insulin, and 75 mEq of sodium bicarbonate. Furosemide (Lasix). Albuterol. Calcium chloride or calcium gluconate (Kalcinate). Sodium polystyrene sulfonate (Kayexalate). Patiromer.
Hypocalcemia | Serum calcium level less than 8.7 mg/dL. Commonly caused by hypoparathyroidism, malabsorption syndrome, hypomagnesemia, hyperphosphatemia, renal failure, insufficient vitamin D, hypoalbuminemia, diuretic therapy, diarrhea, acute pancreatitis, gastric surgery, massive blood transfusion.			
Body-wide muscle cramps (tetany). Laryngeal spasm. Paresthesias. Bone pain, deformities, fracture. Dry skin, hair. Confusion. Seizure.	Increased neuromuscular excitability (tetany). Hyperactive reflexes. Positive Chvostek's and Trousseau's sign. Hypotension. Seizure. Dementia possible.	Serum calcium level less than 8.7 mg/dL. Arrhythmias. Heart block. Ventricular fibrillation.	Administration of Ca^{++} and vitamin D.
Hypercalcemia | Serum calcium level greater than 10.0 mg/dL. Commonly caused by excessive calcium in diet, excessive vitamin D, immobility, bone breakdown, hyperparathyroidism, hypophosphatemia, diuretics, ACE inhibitors, lithium therapy, prolonged immobility, malignancy of bone or blood. Many types of cancer release a parathyroid-like substance that raises blood Ca^{++}.			
Anorexia. Nausea, vomiting. Constipation. Muscle weakness. Bone fracture possible.	Decreased neuromuscular excitability. Ataxia. Loss of muscle tone. Hypertension.	Serum calcium level greater than 10.0 mg/dL. Urine hematuria/calcium. Kidney stone possible. Bone breakdown may be apparent as source of high calcium in the bloodstream. Hypertension. Heart block.	Increased fluids and loop diuretics enhance calcium excretion. Bisphosphonates and calcitonin are used to inhibit bone breakdown. Dialysis may be necessary.
Hypophosphatemia | Serum phosphorus level less than 2.5 mg/dL. Can be caused by ingestion of excess antacids (aluminum and calcium), severe diarrhea, lack of vitamin D, hypercalcemia, alkalosis, hyperparathyroidism, diabetic ketoacidosis, alcoholism.			
Tremor. Lack of coordination. Paresthesias. Confusion. Seizures. Muscle weakness. Joint stiffness. Bone pain.	Tremor. Ataxia. Muscle weakness. Decreased reflexes.	Serum phosphorus level less than 2.5 mg/dL. Complete blood count; low hemoglobin, hematocrit, hemolytic anemia. Platelet dysfunction; bruising. White blood cell dysfunction; infections. Low bone density; osteomalacia.	Replacement of PO_4^-.

Making the Connections—cont'd

Signs and Symptoms	Physical Assessment Findings	Diagnostic Testing	Treatment
Hyperphosphatemia | Serum phosphorus level greater than 4.5 mg/dL. Can be caused by laxatives, enemas containing phosphate, massive trauma, heat stroke, rhabdomyolysis, tumor lysis syndrome, potassium deficiency, hypocalcemia, kidney failure, hypoparathyroidism.			
Paresthesias. Muscle cramps.	Tetany. Hypotension.	Serum phosphorus level greater than 4.5 mg/dL. Cardiac arrhythmias.	Calcium-based phosphate binders and dialysis reduce hyperphosphatemia.
Hypomagnesemia | Serum magnesium level less than 1.5 mg/dL. Can be caused by malnutrition/malabsorption, excessive loss of GI fluids, alcoholism/cirrhosis, diuretic therapy, hyperparathyroidism, hyperaldosteronism, diabetic ketoacidosis, thyroid malfunction, pancreatitis, NG suction, fistulas, renal diseases, proton pump inhibitors (PPIs), and certain antibiotic, immunosuppressive, and chemotherapeutic agents.			
Muscle cramps. Personality change. Uncontrollable movements.	Positive Chvostek's and Trousseau's sign. Nystagmus. Positive Babinski's sign. Hypertension.	Serum magnesium level less than 1.5 mg/dL. ECG: tachycardia, arrhythmias.	Replacement Mg^{++} therapy.
Hypermagnesemia | Serum magnesium level greater than 2.5 mg/dL. Can be caused by excessive use of Mg-containing antacids and laxatives, untreated diabetic ketoacidosis, excessive Mg infusion as in treatment of eclampsia of pregnancy, renal failure.			
Lethargy. Confusion. Weakness.	Decreased reflexes (hyporeflexia). Hypotension. Weak muscles.	Serum magnesium level greater than 2.5 mg/dL. ECG: Arrhythmias. Cardiac arrest possible.	IV calcium or dialysis.

Bibliography

Available online at fadavis.com

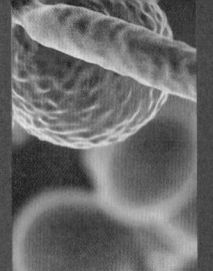

Acid–Base Imbalances

Learning Objectives

Upon completion of this chapter, the student will be able to:

- List the four primary types of acid–base disturbances.
- Name and describe the three primary buffer systems in the body.
- Explain how the lungs and kidneys compensate for acid–base disturbances.

- Describe how pH abnormalities may cause alterations in electrolyte levels.
- Interpret arterial blood gas values to identify acid–base disturbances.

Key Terms

Acid
Acidic
Acidosis
Acidemia
Alkaline
Alkalosis
Alkalemia
Anion gap (AG)
Arterial blood gas (ABG)
Base

Basic
Blood pH
Buffer
$CO_2 + H_2O \leftrightarrow H_2CO_3 \leftrightarrow H^+ + HCO_3^-$
Carbonic acid–bicarbonate system
Compensation
Metabolic acidosis
Metabolic alkalosis
Nonvolatile acid

Saturation of hemoglobin with oxygen
  (Sao_2)
Partial pressure of carbon dioxide (Pco_2)
Partial pressure of oxygen (Po_2)
pH
Pulse oximetry
Respiratory acidosis
Respiratory alkalosis
Volatile acid

Every second, a multitude of physiological and biochemical reactions occur within the body. As cells require sufficient oxygen and nutrients to function normally, they also require a suitable acid–base environment. The proteins within the body contain many acidic and basic groups; thus any alteration in pH disrupts protein structure and function. To prevent such changes in pH, the body employs **buffer** systems. The body utilizes three buffer systems: proteins, phosphates, and the carbonic acid–bicarbonate system. Although all of these systems are important, the majority of this chapter focuses on the carbonic acid–bicarbonate buffer system.

Basic Concepts of Acid–Base Balance

Knowing the chemistry of acids, bases, and buffers provides a means for understanding disturbances in the body.

Acids, Bases, and Buffers

An **acid** is any compound that donates hydrogen ions (H^+) in solution. When H^+ ions predominate in a solution, the solution is **acidic.** In the body, acids are present in two forms: volatile and nonvolatile. When CO_2, a volatile gas, combines with water, the **volatile acid,** carbonic acid (H_2CO_3), forms. Carbonic anhydrase, an enzyme present in large amounts in erythrocytes, helps to catalyze this reaction. H_2CO_3 can also dissociate into CO_2 and H_2O, with the CO_2 then being exhaled by the lungs. Other acids are not converted to CO_2 and thus are referred to as **nonvolatile** (or fixed) acids.

A **base** is a compound that accepts H^+ ions in solution. When basic ions predominate in a solution, the solution is **alkaline** or **basic.**

Metabolism and Acid–Base Levels

Various compounds in the body are acidic or basic. For example, cellular metabolism of fats and carbohydrates produces large quantities of CO_2. The CO_2 combines with H_2O in the bloodstream, forming the volatile acid, carbonic acid (H_2CO_3). Acidic products also form during hypoxic states when pyruvate converts to lactic acid during anaerobic metabolism. Metabolism of positively charged amino acids and hydrolysis of phosphates also produce acidic compounds. Most basic compounds form from the metabolism of negatively charged amino acids. By using buffers, the body counteracts potential pH changes brought on by these metabolic products.

pH Values

The H^+ ion is a very strong acid. In body fluids, however, the concentration of H^+ ions compared with other ions is extremely low. Because the hydrogen ion concentration is so small, it is expressed in terms of **pH.** The values for pH are calculated as the negative logarithm (p) of the H^+ ion concentration in mEq/L. For example, a pH value of 4 indicates that the H^+ concentration of a solution is 10^{-4} (0.00001 mEq/L). pH values and H^+ ion concentration are inversely related. A lower pH value indicates a higher concentration of H^+ ions and a more acidic solution, whereas a higher pH value represents a lower concentration of H^+ ions and a more alkaline solution (see Fig. 8-1).

Buffers

The normal range for **blood pH** is slightly basic at **7.35 to 7.45.** Deviations outside this normal range affect cellular function profoundly and are potentially life threatening. To prevent such large swings in blood pH, three buffer systems (protein, phosphate, and carbonic acid–bicarbonate) absorb excess H^+ ions or donate H^+ ions as needed.

Protein Buffering System
Because of their structure, almost all proteins can serve as functional buffers. Taken together, the proteins serve as the largest buffering system in the body. The amino and carboxyl groups found on amino acids enable proteins to absorb or donate H^+ ions as needed to maintain physiological pH. One of the primary proteins that carries out this function is hemoglobin.

Phosphate Buffering System
Phosphates play a key role in regulating pH in the intracellular environment. Phosphates (PO_4^-) can take on an acidic form, dihydrogen phosphate, or a basic form, hydrogen phosphate, to buffer pH changes.

Carbonic Acid–Bicarbonate System
The buffering system most commonly discussed is the **carbonic acid–bicarbonate system.** Carbon dioxide,

carbonic acid, hydrogen ions, and bicarbonate ions (HCO_3^-) all play a role in this buffering system. When CO_2 combines with water, H_2CO_3 (carbonic acid) is formed. The H_2CO_3 then dissociates, yielding H^+ (a strong acid) and HCO_3^- (a weak base). The chemical reaction of H_2CO_3 formation and dissociation is the following:

$$CO_2 + H_2O \leftrightarrow H_2CO_3 \leftrightarrow H^+ + HCO_3^-$$

The equation moves in both directions. When CO_2 levels are elevated, the equation *moves toward the right,* forming more H^+ and HCO_3^- ions. Likewise, when H^+ ion levels are elevated, the equation *moves toward the left,* as H^+ ions are converted to CO_2 and the CO_2 is exhaled. The carbonic acid–bicarbonate buffering system plays a significant role in the body, as two organs, the lungs and kidneys, use this buffering system to compensate for alterations in physiological pH. Because of this system, arterial blood gas (ABG) values include arterial carbon dioxide and bicarbonate levels, along with other factors (see Box 8-1).

Renal and Respiratory Compensations for Acid–Base Disturbances

As mentioned, the lungs and kidneys utilize the carbonic acid–bicarbonate buffering system to adjust any pH disturbances. Both organs relate to the environment in such a way that excretion or retention of acidic and basic compounds occurs in order to regulate blood pH. When the lungs and kidneys attempt to adjust pH disturbances, the process is called **compensation** (see Fig. 8-2). The lungs respond to acid–base disturbances within minutes, with the response reaching maximal levels by 24 hours. The response, though, cannot be maintained indefinitely. The kidneys require hours to a day to compensate; however, the response can be maintained for much longer.

Respiratory Compensation for Acid–Base Disturbances
Under normal conditions, the lungs correct pH imbalances by increasing or decreasing ventilation as needed. An increase in ventilation decreases CO_2. As CO_2 is exhaled, H^+ ion concentration falls (raising pH) by *moving the buffer equation toward the left:*

$$CO_2 + H_2O \Leftarrow H_2CO_3 \Leftarrow H^+ \text{ and } HCO_3^-$$

Decreased ventilation retains CO_2. The retention of CO_2 *moves the buffer equation toward the right,* resulting in an elevation of H^+ ion level and a decrease in pH (see Fig. 8-3).

$$CO_2 + H_2O \Rightarrow H_2CO_3 \Rightarrow H^+ \text{ and } HCO_3^-$$

Because of the link between ventilation, CO_2, and pH, carbon dioxide levels in the bloodstream are kept

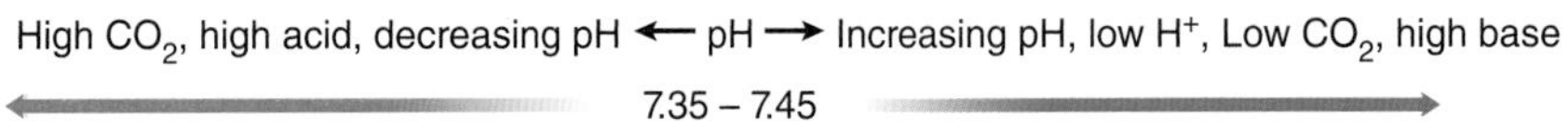

FIGURE 8-1. pH and relationship to H^+ and CO_2.

High CO_2, high acid, decreasing pH ← pH → Increasing pH, low H^+, Low CO_2, high base

7.35 – 7.45

BOX 8-1. The Carbonic Acid–Bicarbonate Chemical Reaction

This chemical reaction within the bloodstream can go back and forth according to the amount of acids or bases or CO_2 in the bloodstream.

$$CO_2 + H_2O \leftrightarrow H_2CO_3 \leftrightarrow H^+ \text{ and } HCO_3^-$$

Example 1: If there is excess CO_2 in the bloodstream, the equation moves toward the right, which shows that more acid (H +), which is a very strong acid, is created. The bloodstream becomes high in acid in a condition called acidemia (also called acidosis). [HCO_3^- *is a weak base and cannot neutralize* H^+]

$$CO_2 + H_2O \rightarrow H_2CO_3 \rightarrow H^+ \text{ and } HCO_3^-$$

Example 2: If there is an excess of H^+ in the bloodstream, the equation moves toward the left, which shows that more CO_2 is created and CO_2 is exhaled vigorously by the lungs. This reduction of H^+ then makes the blood alkalemic (also called alkalotic).

$$CO_2 + H_2O \leftarrow H_2CO_3^- \leftarrow H^+ \text{ and } HCO_3^-$$

in a narrow range. The normal range for **partial pressure of carbon dioxide (Pco_2) is 35 to 45 mm Hg.** Sometimes the Pco_2, specifically within the arterial blood, is written as $Paco_2$. Chemoreceptors in the brain closely monitor H^+ ion levels and send signals to the respiratory center in the medulla to adjust ventilation, and subsequently carbon dioxide levels, as needed. When the blood pH is too low (acidic), the ventilation rate increases, causing exhalation of CO_2, which in turn reduces acid in the blood and raises pH. The opposite occurs when blood pH is too high (alkaline). Ventilation is suppressed, increasing CO_2 levels in the bloodstream, which creates H^+ and lowers the pH (see Table 8-1).

🔬 CLINICAL CONCEPT

The two important premises to understand are:
1. Hyperventilation reduces CO_2, diminishing H^+ and raising pH.
2. Hypoventilation causes retention of CO_2, which increases H^+ ion levels and decreases pH.

Renal Compensation for Acid–Base Disturbances

The kidneys compensate for acid–base disturbances by regulating the excretion or reabsorption of two factors of the carbonic acid–bicarbonate system: H^+ and HCO_3^-. In conditions in which pH is too low, or acidic, the kidneys excrete more acid (H^+) and reabsorb more base (HCO_3^-). These actions lessen the amount of acid in the blood while adding more base (HCO_3^-), thereby raising blood pH and compensating for acidosis. Likewise, in conditions in which pH is too high, the kidneys reabsorb more H^+ and excrete more HCO_3^-, thereby lowering the pH, compensating for alkalosis. The kidneys' compensation is slow and may take days to reach maximal effectiveness. Therefore, medical interventions are commonly necessary to facilitate balancing the bloodstream's pH (see Table 8-2).

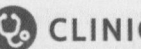

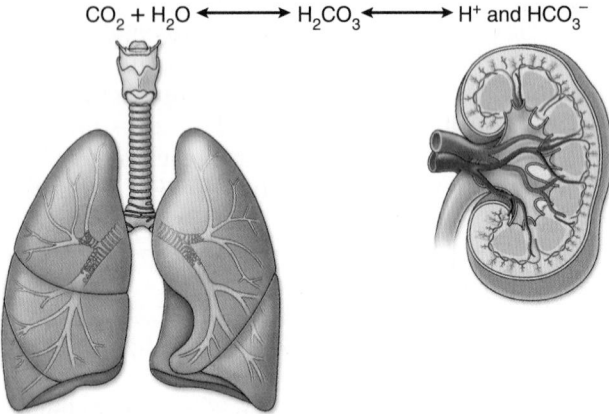

FIGURE 8-2. Acid–base balance via the lungs and kidneys.

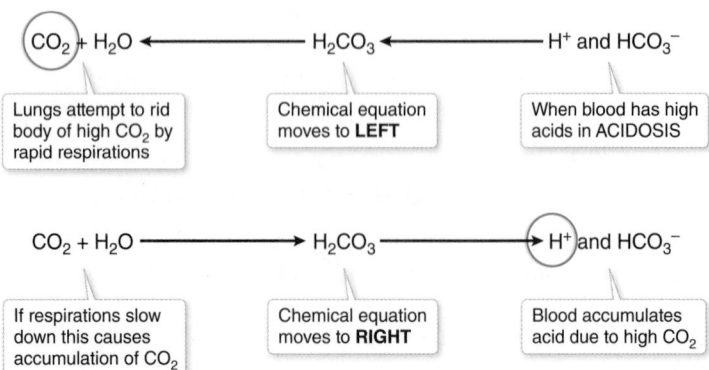

$$CO_2 + H_2O \longleftarrow H_2CO_3 \longleftarrow H^+ \text{ and } HCO_3^-$$

| Lungs attempt to rid body of high CO_2 by rapid respirations | Chemical equation moves to **LEFT** | When blood has high acids in ACIDOSIS |

$$CO_2 + H_2O \longrightarrow H_2CO_3 \longrightarrow H^+ \text{ and } HCO_3^-$$

| If respirations slow down this causes accumulation of CO_2 | Chemical equation moves to **RIGHT** | Blood accumulates acid due to high CO_2 |

FIGURE 8-3. Respiratory compensation for acid–base disturbances.

TABLE 8-1. Respiratory Compensation for Acid–Base Imbalances and Medical Intervention

The lungs attempt to correct metabolic acid–base disturbances when they occur but are often insufficient to complete compensation. This is when medical intervention is necessary.

Condition	Blood pH	Respiratory Compensation	Medical Intervention
Metabolic acidosis	<7.35	Respirations increase in depth and rate to blow off CO_2	Treatment to resolve the origin of the acid–base disturbance (e.g., insulin in DKA).
Excess H^+ or lack of base is in the bloodstream due to toxicity or illness			Sodium bicarbonate administration may be necessary.
Metabolic alkalosis	>7.45	Respirations slow down to increase CO_2 retention	Treatment to resolve the origin of the acid–base disturbance (e.g., in vomiting, administer antiemetic medication).
Excess base or lack of acids in blood due to toxicity or illness			Acetazolamide administration increases HCO_3^- excretion.

TABLE 8-2. Renal Compensation in Acid–Base Disturbances and Medical Intervention

The kidneys attempt to correct acid–base disturbances when they occur but are often too slow to reach complete compensation. This is when medical intervention is necessary.

Condition	Blood pH	Renal Compensation	Necessary Medical Intervention
Respiratory acidosis	<7.35	Kidneys attempt to excrete H^+ and conserve HCO_3^-	Patient may need assistance with ridding body of CO_2: • Requires intubation and mechanical ventilation • Can also administer sodium bicarbonate ($NaHCO_3$)
Excess CO_2 has accumulated, which is generating H^+			
Respiratory alkalosis	>7.45	Kidneys attempt to retain H^+ and excrete HCO_3^-	Patient may need assistance with retaining H^+ and conserving HCO_3^- • Patient can use a CO_2 rebreather mask to increase CO_2
Lungs blow off too much CO_2, creating less H^+ in blood			

🩺 CLINICAL CONCEPT

The lungs and kidneys are two organs that work to maintain acid–base balance. Therefore, if ventilation is suboptimal or if renal dysfunction occurs, acid–base imbalance can occur.

Arterial Blood Gases

In studying acid–base disturbances and compensation by the lungs and kidneys, **arterial blood gas (ABG)** levels are one of the most informative sets of values to consider. Analysis of ABGs helps determine the presence of acid–base imbalances within the bloodstream and whether the cause is respiratory or metabolic in nature. ABGs measure oxygenation, acidity, and alkalinity of the arterial blood. Blood pH, **partial pressure of oxygen (Po_2)**, Pco_2, and HCO_3^- are the values indicated by an ABG. The blood sample is commonly obtained from the radial or femoral artery. Alternatively, an indwelling arterial catheter is sometimes used for patients who require frequent ABG measurement. In addition to the values mentioned, **saturation of hemoglobin with oxygen (Sao_2)** may be reported. This measurement is obtained through a procedure called **pulse oximetry.** A pulse oximeter is a noninvasive sensor placed on the patient's finger. Normal ABG values are the following:

- **Blood pH:** 7.35 to 7.45
- **Pco_2:** 35 to 45 mm Hg
- **Po_2:** 90 to 100 mm Hg
- **HCO_3^-:** 22 to 26 mEq/L
- **Sao_2:** 95% to 100%

CLINICAL CONCEPT

When measuring ABGs, low Po_2 is classified as *hypoxia* or *hypoxemia*, elevated Pco_2 is termed *hypercapnia*, and diminished Pco_2 is termed *hypocapnia*.

Arterial Blood Gases and Acid–Base Disorders

The ability to interpret ABGs affords an understanding of the etiology behind acid–base disorders. The normal range for blood pH is 7.35 to 7.45. If blood pH is lower than 7.35, the bloodstream is acidic and the condition is termed **acidemia** (also called **acidosis).** If the blood pH is greater than 7.45, the bloodstream is basic and the condition is termed **alkalemia** (also called **alkalosis).** In addition to these classifications of acidosis and alkalosis, acid–base disturbances are categorized as respiratory or metabolic, based on the origin of the disturbance.

Respiratory Acid–Base Disturbances

Respiratory acidosis and alkalosis are marked by abnormalities in carbon dioxide levels, leading to the acid–base disturbance. For example, in **respiratory acidosis,** retention of CO_2 causes a reduction in pH. Often, respiratory acidosis arises with compromised gas exchange in the lungs, as may occur with chronic obstructive pulmonary disease (COPD), infection, foreign body obstruction, and asthma. In **respiratory alkalosis,** lower-than-normal CO_2 levels reduce H^+ ion levels and increase pH. Respiratory alkalosis occurs with hyperventilation.

Metabolic Acid–Base Disturbances

Metabolic acid–base disturbances involve an origin other than the pulmonary system and abnormal CO_2 levels. Metabolic acid–base disturbances may manifest for a variety of reasons, including toxicity, diabetes, renal failure, and excessive gastrointestinal (GI) losses. **Metabolic acidosis** may result from increased production of acids other than CO_2, as occurs in diabetic ketoacidosis (DKA), or from the excessive loss of a base, such as bicarbonate through, for example, prolonged diarrhea. **Metabolic alkalosis** develops from excess base, such as retention of sodium bicarbonate or from loss of H^+ ions, as may result from prolonged vomiting.

When interpreting ABGs, a clinician needs to determine whether the patient is enduring an acid–base imbalance and, if so, the source of the imbalance, whether respiratory or metabolic.

ABG values are not the whole story, however. They must be interpreted in relation to the patient's vital signs, history, and physical examination. When analyzing ABG results in conjunction with all other indicators, use questions in a step-by-step process (see Box 8-2). Remember to evaluate the whole clinical picture, including Po_2 and Sao_2.

Anion Gap

In addition to ABGs, another piece of information useful in determining the cause of an acid–base imbalance is the anion gap. The term **anion gap (AG)** represents the concentration of the *unmeasured* anions (negatively charged ions) in the bloodstream when comparing the *measured* cations (positively charged ions), $[Na^+]$ and $[K^+]$, and *measured* anions, $[Cl^-]$ and $[HCO_3^-]$, of the blood. The AG is calculated by summing the measured cations, $[Na^+]$ and $[K^+]$, and subtracting the measured anions, $[Cl^-]$ and $[HCO_3^-]$. To maintain electrochemical balance, the body's total number of cations should equal the total number of anions. Normally, though, a small number of unmeasured free anions exist in the bloodstream. These unmeasured anions comprise the normal AG between measured cations and anions (see Fig. 8-4). The major unmeasured anions include negatively charged plasma proteins (albumin), sulfates, and phosphates. The calculation of anion gap only applies to cases of metabolic acidosis.

Anion Gap Range

The normal range for the AG is 8 to 16 mEq/L, although laboratories may slightly differ in their reference range. The AG can be high, normal, or low. A normal AG has a small number of unmeasured anions in the bloodstream (see Fig. 8-4). A low AG is uncommon but can be caused by decreased unmeasured anions (usually low protein, especially hypoalbuminemia), increased unmeasured cations, or laboratory error. A high AG has a value between 16 and 20 mEq/L and may occur in specific instances of metabolic acidosis, such as DKA.

CLINICAL CONCEPT

The AG equation given by $[Na^+ + K^+] - [Cl^- + HCO_3^-]$ works on the assumption that a patient has a normal albumin level. Low serum albumin reduces the accuracy of the AG calculation.

Increased Anion Gap in Metabolic Acidosis

In certain instances of metabolic acidosis, the AG increases. The increase occurs when large amounts of unmeasured acids, such as ketones in DKA, are added to the blood. Ketones dissociate into H^+ ions and keto-anions. Bicarbonate, a measured anion, buffers the H^+ ions. As this buffering occurs, measured anions (bicarbonate) in the blood decrease, whereas unmeasured anions (keto-anions) increase. The AG, indicative of unmeasured anion, thus increases. The AG becomes important to clinicians in differentiating

BOX 8-2. Steps for Interpreting Basic Arterial Blood Gas Disturbances

When analyzing ABG laboratory results, remember that the patient's clinical condition must be taken into consideration. ABG laboratory results should not be analyzed alone apart from the patient condition. For example, ask if the patient is having difficulty breathing or is breathing rapidly. Look at the respiratory rate. Does the patient have a renal or gastrointestinal disorder? Is it possible that the patient has drug or chemical toxicity or DKA? Or lactic acidosis?

Step 1. Begin by asking if the blood pH is acidic, basic, or within the normal range.
- pH <7.35 indicates acidosis
- pH >7.45 indicates alkalosis
- pH 7.35–7.45
- Normal if Pco_2 and HCO_3^- are normal
- Normal but compensations are occurring if Pco_2 and HCO_3^- are abnormal

Step 2. Identify the Pco_2 level. Is it high, low, or normal?
- Normal = 35–45 mm Hg
- High >45 mm Hg
- Low <35 mm Hg

Step 3. Determine whether the acid–base disturbance is respiratory or metabolic.

Comparing the pH and Pco_2 levels enables you to determine whether the respiratory system is the origin of the acid–base imbalance or if the acid–base imbalance is metabolic in origin. Examine both the pH and the Pco_2 levels and use these rules:

- If **pH and Pco_2 are moving in opposite directions,** meaning if the Pco_2 is high and the pH is low, then the Pco_2 levels <u>are</u> contributing to the acid–base disturbance and thus it is **respiratory in nature.** If the Pco_2 is low and the pH is high, the Pco_2 levels <u>are</u> contributing to the acid–base disturbance and thus it is **respiratory in nature.**
- If **Pco_2 is normal or is moving in the same direction as pH, meaning if the Pco_2 is normal or high and the pH is high,** the condition is metabolic in nature (i.e., not due to respiratory involvement). If the Pco_2 is normal or low and pH is low, the condition is **metabolic in nature** and is not due to respiratory involvement.

Examples of Step 3:

Respiratory acidosis: pH <7.35 and Pco_2 >45 mm Hg
- pH is low = acidosis, Pco_2 is high
- pH and CO_2 are moving in opposite directions. The high CO_2 is contributing to the acidic pH; thus the acid–base imbalance is respiratory in origin.

Respiratory alkalosis: pH >7.45 and Pco_2 <35 mm Hg
- pH is high = alkalosis, Pco_2 is low
- pH and CO_2 are moving in opposite directions. The low CO_2 is contributing to the basic pH; thus the acid–base imbalance is respiratory in origin.

Metabolic acidosis: pH <7.35 and Pco_2 <35 mm Hg or normal
- pH is low = acidosis, Pco_2 is low
- pH and CO_2 are moving in the same direction. The pH is low (acidic) and CO_2 is low; thus CO_2 <u>is not</u> causing the acidic pH so the disturbance is metabolic in origin.

Metabolic alkalosis: pH >7.45 and Pco_2 >45 mm Hg
- pH is high = alkalosis, Pco_2 is high
- pH and CO_2 are moving in the same direction. The pH is high (basic) and CO_2 is high; thus CO_2 <u>is not</u> causing the alkaline pH, so the disturbance is metabolic in origin.

Step 4. Determine whether the condition is a compensated or uncompensated condition.

Uncompensated: pH will be abnormal
- Use the previous steps to determine whether the condition is respiratory or metabolic in nature.

Compensated: pH is normal or nearing normal
- Use the previous steps to determine whether Pco_2 is contributing to the original acid–base disturbance. If so, a compensated respiratory condition is present. If not, the disorder is metabolic in nature, and Pco_2 is compensating.

COMPENSATED RESPIRATORY ACIDOSIS

pH = initially low, elevating to normal, Pco_2 >45 mm Hg, HCO_3^- (>26 mEq/L)
- pH = initially low, Pco_2 = high
- pH and Pco_2 are initially in opposite direction, so it is respiratory in nature
- High bicarbonate compensating for high CO_2 and acidic pH

COMPENSATED RESPIRATORY ALKALOSIS

pH = initially high, lowering to normal, Pco_2 <35 mm Hg, HCO_3^- (<22 mEq/L)
- pH = initially high, Pco_2 = low
- pH and Pco_2 are initially in opposite direction, so it is respiratory in nature
- Low HCO_3^- compensating for low CO_2 and basic pH

COMPENSATED METABOLIC ACIDOSIS

pH = initially low, elevating to normal, Pco_2 <35 mm Hg, HCO_3^- (<22 mEq/L)
- pH = initially low, Pco_2 = low
- pH and Pco_2 are initially in same direction, so it is metabolic in nature
- Original acidity of blood not due to CO_2, low CO_2 is compensating for low base (i.e., acidic pH).

COMPENSATED METABOLIC ALKALOSIS

pH = initially high or lowering to normal, Pco_2 >45 mm Hg, HCO_3^- (>26mEq/L)
- pH = initially high, Pco_2 = high
- pH and Pco_2 are initially in same direction, so it is metabolic in nature
- Original alkalinity of blood not due to high CO_2, high CO_2 is compensating for alkalinity of the blood

Continued

BOX 8-2. Steps for Interpreting Basic Arterial Blood Gas Disturbances—cont'd

CASE STUDY 1

Patient A is enduring an asthma attack and is brought into the emergency department. The patient's vital signs are: Temp: 98.4°F, Pulse: 110 beats/min, Resp rate: 24 shallow breaths/min, BP: 136/86 mm Hg.

ABGs are:
- Blood pH: 7.30
- PCO_2: 58 mm Hg
- PO_2: 88 mm Hg
- HCO_3^-: 28 mEq/L
- SaO_2: 88%.

Step 1. Does the blood pH show an acidotic, alkalotic, or normal bloodstream?

In this problem, the blood is acidic at pH 7.30, which is less than 7.35; therefore the condition is acidosis.

Step 2. What is the PCO_2?

A PCO_2 of 58 mm Hg is elevated beyond the normal range of 35–45 mm Hg.

Step 3. Is the acid-base imbalance caused by a respiratory or metabolic source?

pH (low) and PCO_2 (high) are moving in opposite directions. The high PCO_2 is causing the low pH, indicating it is a respiratory disturbance and therefore respiratory acidosis.

The high PCO_2 indicates a ventilation problem, and the PO_2 and SaO_2 are also low, further confirming a lung problem.

Step 4. Is this a compensated or uncompensated problem?

The pH is abnormal; therefore the condition is uncompensated. The body is attempting to compensate by reabsorption of HCO_3^- at the kidney. HCO_3^- is slightly elevated at 28 mEq/L vs. the normal range of 22–26 mEq/L.

Result

Because of the low blood pH and high PCO_2, this is **uncompensated respiratory acidosis**. The kidney is attempting to compensate through the reabsorption of HCO_3^-.

CASE STUDY 2

Patient B is unconscious and brought into the emergency department because of suspected drug toxicity. Vital signs include: Temp: 97.8°F, Pulse: 90 beats/min, Resp rate: 12 breaths/min, BP: 100/70 mm Hg.

The patient's ABGs are:
- Blood pH: 7.29
- PCO_2: 32 mm Hg
- PO_2: 95 mm Hg
- HCO_3^-: 13 mEq/L
- SaO_2: 98%.

Using the previous step-by-step process:

Step 1. Does the blood pH show an acidotic, alkalotic, or normal bloodstream?

In this problem, the pH is less than 7.35; therefore the condition is acidosis.

Step 2. What is the PCO_2?

The PCO_2 is 32 mm Hg, which is low. This indicates the lungs are eliminating CO_2 excessively.

Step 3. Is the acid-base imbalance caused by a respiratory or metabolic source?

As pH (low) and PCO_2 (low) are moving in the same direction, PCO_2 is not contributing to the acid-base imbalance. The acid-base disturbance is metabolic in nature. Also, because the PO_2 and SaO_2 are normal, the lungs are functioning well.

Step 4. Is this a compensated or uncompensated problem?

The pH is abnormal, so the condition is uncompensated. The lungs in this case are trying to compensate for the low pH in the bloodstream by exhaling CO_2, but the compensation is inadequate.

Result

Because of the low blood pH and low PCO_2, the condition is uncompensated metabolic acidosis. The lungs attempt to compensate for the acidosis by increasing ventilation to decrease CO_2. In cases of metabolic acidosis, a further step would be to calculate the anion gap to help narrow the list of possible causes.

CASE STUDY 3

Patient C is having an anxiety attack and comes to the emergency department. Vital signs are as follows: Temp: 98.1°F, Pulse: 121 beats/min, Resp rate: 28 breaths/min, and BP: 138/88 mm Hg.

The patient's ABGs are:
- Blood pH: 7.58 mm Hg
- PCO_2: 28 mm Hg
- PO_2: 93 mm Hg
- HCO_3^-: 22 mEq/L
- SaO_2: 92%.

Step 1. Does the blood pH show an acidotic, alkalotic, or normal bloodstream?

The pH is greater than 7.45; therefore the condition is alkalosis.

Step 2. What is the PCO_2?

The PCO_2 is 28 mm Hg, which is low. The lungs are hyperventilating, exhaling CO_2.

Step 3. Is the acid-base imbalance caused by a respiratory or metabolic source?

As pH (high) and PCO_2 (low) are moving in opposite directions, a respiratory condition is occurring. The PO_2 and SaO_2 are on the low side, additionally indicating a pulmonary problem.

Step 4. Is this a compensated or uncompensated problem?

The pH is abnormal; therefore this is uncompensated. The hyperventilation is causing a reduction in CO_2, elevating pH. The kidneys are attempting to compensate by excreting HCO_3^-.

BOX 8-2. Steps for Interpreting Basic Arterial Blood Gas Disturbances–cont'd

Result

Because of the high blood pH, low Pco_2, and low HCO_3^-, this is uncompensated respiratory alkalosis.

CASE STUDY 4

Patient D has endured 3 days of nausea and vomiting caused by a virus. Vital signs are as follows: Temp: 101.1°F, Pulse: 98 beats/min, Resp rate: 12 breaths/min, BP: 90/60 mm Hg.

The patient's ABGs are:
- Blood pH: 7.61 mm Hg
- Pco_2: 49 mm Hg
- Po_2: 99 mm Hg
- HCO_3^-: 49 mEq/L
- Sao_2: 99%.

Step 1. Does the blood pH show an acidotic, alkalotic, or normal bloodstream?

A pH of 7.61 indicates alkalosis.

Step 2. What is the Pco_2?

The Pco_2 is high.

Step 3. Is the acid–base imbalance caused by a respiratory or metabolic source?

In this case, pH (high) and Pco_2 (high) are moving in the same direction, thus indicating a metabolic acid–base disturbance. The high CO_2 is not causing the alkaline pH. Also, the Po_2 and Sao_2 are normal, indicating normal lung function. Therefore the lungs are not causing the alkalosis.

Step 4. Is this a compensated or uncompensated problem?

The pH is abnormal, so this is uncompensated. The body is attempting to retain acids in the bloodstream by slow respirations (which increases CO_2) and neutralize the elevated bicarbonate levels.

Result

Because of a high blood pH and high Pco_2, this is an uncompensated metabolic alkalosis. The lungs are attempting to compensate by breathing slowly but cannot accomplish full compensation.

CASE STUDY 5

Patient E presents to the emergency department in a coma with no history. The ABGs are:
- Blood pH: 7.37
- Pco_2: 47 mm Hg
- Po_2: 85 mm Hg
- HCO_3^-: 28 mEq/L
- Sao_2: 87%.

Step 1. Does the blood pH show an acidotic, alkalotic, or normal bloodstream?

In this problem, the blood pH is between 7.35 and 7.45, which is within the normal range. However, both Pco_2 and HCO_3^- values are abnormal, indicating some type of compensation.

Step 2. What is the Pco_2?

The Pco_2 is 47 mm Hg. This is a high Pco_2, which means the lungs are hypoventilating and retaining CO_2.

Step 3. Is the acid–base imbalance caused by a respiratory or metabolic source?

pH is normal, but Pco_2 is high, as is HCO_3^-, so further analysis is required. Compensation for an acid–base disturbance is likely occurring. The low Po_2 and Sao_2, coupled with the high Pco_2, indicate a pulmonary problem is likely. The elevated bicarbonate levels are indicative of a compensation to address the higher-than-normal Pco_2 due to respiratory problems.

Step 4. Is this a compensated or uncompensated problem?

The blood pH is normal, whereas Pco_2 and HCO_3^- are abnormal, indicating a compensated condition. The kidneys are trying to reabsorb enough HCO_3^- to neutralize the H^+ caused by high Pco_2.

Result

Because of the normal pH, high Pco_2, and high HCO_3^-, this is compensated respiratory acidosis.

---

underlying causes of metabolic acidosis, as some causes of metabolic acidosis, such as GI loss of bicarbonate, do not present with an elevated AG.

 CLINICAL CONCEPT

Calculating the AG is clinically useful, as it helps differentiate types of metabolic acidosis disease states.

Metabolic acidosis with an elevated AG is found in the following conditions:

- Lactic acidosis
- Ketoacidosis
- Renal failure
- Overdose of aspirin (acetylsalicylic acid [ASA])
- Ingestion of methanol or ethylene glycol

Metabolic acidosis with a normal AG is found in the following conditions:

- GI loss of HCO_3^-
- Increased renal HCO_3^- loss
- Hypoaldosteronism
- Ingestion of ammonium chloride
- Hyperalimentation

Acid–Base Disturbances and Electrolytes

Changes in pH can influence the movement of ions between the intracellular fluid (ICF) and extracellular

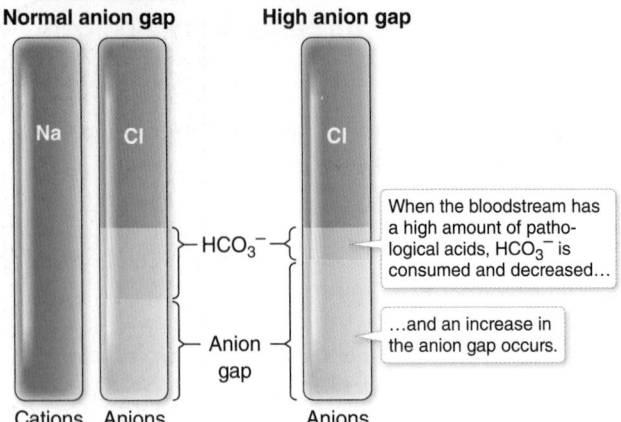

Normal anion gap High anion gap

When the bloodstream has a high amount of pathological acids, HCO_3^- is consumed and decreased...

...and an increase in the anion gap occurs.

Cations Anions Anions

FIGURE 8-4. The normal anion gap versus high anion gap within the bloodstream. The bloodstream normally has a certain level of unbound anions, called the normal anion gap. When the bloodstream has an increased amount of acids, as in DKA, the anion gap is increased.

fluid (ECF), and vice versa, and changes in electrolyte levels can influence the pH state. Ion movement is driven by the electrochemical gradient. Changes in this gradient, due to changes in one or more ions, can profoundly affect the movement of other ions. Two of the ions most affected by alterations in pH levels are K^+ and Ca^{++}. Many of the systemic signs and symptoms of acid–base disturbances are not simply due to pH changes, but rather the impact of H^+ ion concentration on electrolyte movement.

Relationship Between H^+ and K^+

Both K^+ and H^+ ions are positively charged, and both ions move freely between the ICF and ECF. As such, these ions are often exchanged for one another, and changes in H^+ concentration can affect the movement of K^+ ions and vice versa. In the case of acid–base disturbances, shifts in potassium are more pronounced in acidosis than alkalosis and are also greater in metabolic acidosis than respiratory acidosis.

Acidosis and Hyperkalemia In the intracellular and extracellular electrolyte environment, excess H^+ in the bloodstream causes ion movements. H^+ ions move into the cells, and K^+ ions move out of the cells into the bloodstream. The bloodstream thus becomes high in K^+, causing *hyperkalemia*. However, the total body level of K^+ is unchanged. The bloodstream appears as though it is hyperkalemic. As soon as the state of acidosis resolves, the K^+ levels reequilibrate between the intracellular and extracellular environment.

Also, in acidosis, the kidney, which usually excretes K^+, is inundated with H^+ and selectively excretes H^+ in lieu of K^+. This causes K^+ to accumulate in the bloodstream because the kidney is not excreting it. Therefore although the blood may seem to have high potassium levels, the body content of K^+ is not changed. However, high levels of K^+ retained in the blood (hyperkalemia) are a serious complication of acidosis because this has

effects on cardiac tissue. Hyperkalemia can cause dysrhythmias, or in severe cases, cardiac arrest. As soon as the acidosis condition is resolved, K^+ is once again excreted by the kidney and blood levels equilibrate back to normal.

CLINICAL CONCEPT
Intravenous (IV) fluid replacement with K^+ may be needed in some states of acidosis due to the shift of K^+ from the intracellular to the extracellular space and potential K^+ ion loss in the urine.

Alkalosis and Hypokalemia. As acidosis may lead to hyperkalemia, alkalosis is linked to hypokalemia, as K^+ ions shift into the cells from the plasma. This movement of potassium from the ECF to the ICF lowers serum potassium, resulting in *hypokalemia*. Also, in alkalosis, transport mechanisms in the kidneys result in additional K^+ loss in the urine.

The Effect of Potassium Levels on pH. Because of the interrelatedness of H^+ and K^+ ion movements, changes in K^+ ion levels can lead to acid–base disturbances. Hypokalemia may cause alkalosis, as H^+ shifts into cells to compensate for lower-than-normal K^+ levels, whereas hyperkalemia may cause acidosis as H^+ ions enter the bloodstream.

The Effect of pH on Calcium Levels. Calcium ion levels are also affected by pH disturbances. Calcium is transported in the blood in a free, ionized form or attached to the plasma protein albumin. The binding and transport of calcium by albumin is a reversible process influenced by H^+ ion concentration. In acidosis, H^+ ions compete with Ca^{++} ions for binding sites on albumin. Thus in acidosis, free, ionized forms of calcium increase, leading to hypercalcemia. In alkalosis, with fewer H^+ ions to compete for binding sites on albumin, free, ionized calcium levels decrease as more calcium binds to albumin. Alkalosis is thus associated with hypocalcemia.

pH, Electrolyte Levels, and Cellular Functioning. Electrolyte disturbances due to changes in pH can have a profound impact on several cellular processes, particularly in excitable cells such as neurons and muscle cells, including the cells of the heart. Potassium, in particular, affects the resting membrane potential of myocardial cells.

In acidosis, which may result in hyperkalemia, the increased K^+ ion levels cause the resting membrane potential of cells to become more positive, making them hyperexcitable. In hypokalemia associated with alkalosis, reduced K^+ ion levels cause the resting membrane potential to become less positive and the cells less excitable. Changes in the resting membrane potential affect the functioning of the heart, neurons, and muscles. The heart's functionality can be compromised to the point that severe arrhythmias, and even cardiac arrest, develop.

pH-induced changes in albumin binding affinity for calcium and the subsequent changes in free, ionized calcium also negatively affect cells. Hypercalcemia, which can develop in acidosis, increases the threshold for depolarization, making cells less excitable. In hypocalcemia due to alkalosis, lower-than-normal Ca^{++} levels increase the excitability of cells. The link between pH, K$^+$, and Ca$^+$ levels and cell excitability provides yet another example of the critical importance of maintaining these factors within a narrow range.

Pathophysiological Concepts Regarding Acid–Base Imbalances

There are four states of acid–base imbalance in the bloodstream:

1. Respiratory acidosis
2. Respiratory alkalosis
3. Metabolic acidosis
4. Metabolic alkalosis

Each has a different etiology, clinical presentation, compensatory mechanism, and treatment.

Respiratory Acidosis

Respiratory acidosis occurs when the body accumulates too much CO_2 and cannot exhale it sufficiently. The development of respiratory acidosis indicates inadequate exchange of carbon dioxide within the lungs, leading to an elevation in CO_2 known as *hypercapnia*. Hypercapnia pushes the carbonic acid–bicarbonate buffer equation to the right, producing more H$^+$ and HCO$_3^-$:

$$CO_2 + H^2O \Rightarrow H2CO_3^- \Rightarrow H^+ \text{ and } HCO_3^-$$

As CO_2 converts into H$^+$ ions, pH levels fall. The shift in pH due to elevated CO_2 can occur rapidly or over an extended period. The hallmark of respiratory acidosis is a pH below 7.35 and a PCO_2 above 45 mm Hg.

Epidemiology
The incidence of respiratory acidosis is different for its varied etiologies.

Etiology
Box 8-3 lists common causes of respiratory acidosis.

Pathophysiology
Respiratory acidosis develops when the lungs are unable to remove sufficient CO_2, causing it to accumulate

---

BOX 8-3. Causes of Respiratory Acidosis

PULMONARY
- Chronic obstructive lung disease, such as asthma, emphysema, and bronchiectasis
- Pulmonary edema
- Pneumonia
- Airway obstruction, such as laryngospasm, bronchospasm, and aspiration
- Underventilation by mechanical ventilation
- Hypoventilation secondary to obesity, postoperative pain, abdominal distention, or use of abdominal binders
- Excessive fatigue or weakness of rib cage muscles
- Cystic fibrosis

NONPULMONARY
- Overdosage of anesthetic, sedatives, and narcotics
- Neuromuscular disorders, such as Guillain-Barré, myasthenia gravis, and advanced multiple sclerosis
- Severe spinal deformities
- Central nervous system depression related to cerebral infarct, meningitis, or trauma
- Cardiopulmonary arrest

---

in the bloodstream. When CO_2 is high, the **$CO_2 + H_2O \rightarrow$ $H_2CO_3 \rightarrow$ H$^+$ and HCO$_3^-$** shifts to the right, creating increased acid (H$^+$). Higher H$^+$ ion levels reduce the pH. In respiratory acidosis, insufficient CO_2 elimination leads to CO_2 levels rising above 45 mm Hg.

Chemoreceptors in Chronic Respiratory Acidosis
In chronic respiratory acidosis, as may occur with COPD, the respiratory center in the medulla becomes insensitive to high CO_2 levels. Normally when CO_2 rises in the bloodstream, the chemoreceptors in the medulla stimulate increased ventilation to rid the body of CO_2. However, in long-term COPD, high CO_2 levels do not stimulate the medulla and respirations as expected. Patients with long-term COPD live with hypercapnia and precariously balanced blood pH values because of this adaptation.

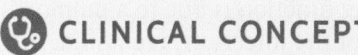 CLINICAL CONCEPT

Patients with long-term COPD retain CO_2, which increases susceptibility to respiratory acidosis.

Clinical Presentation
Patients in respiratory acidosis complain of anxiety, restlessness, headache, lethargy, fatigue, shortness of breath, rapid breathing, and cough. Advanced respiratory acidosis leads to confusion, somnolence, and

possible coma. The effects of excess CO_2 are commonly referred to as "carbon dioxide narcosis."

Physical Examination Findings

The thoracic examination of patients with respiratory acidosis usually reveals obstructive lung disease with compromised air exchange. The signs include diffuse wheezing, hyperinflation of the lungs, barrel-shaped chest in emphysema, decreased breath sounds, hyper-resonance on percussion, and prolonged expiration. Rhonchi may also be heard. Cyanosis and clubbing may indicate the presence of chronic hypoxia. Confusion, disorientation, somnolence, or stupor can be present with high levels of P_{CO_2}.

> **ALERT!** Respiratory acidosis can occur with severe asthma despite the patient having tachypnea. The breathing rate is increased, but the breaths are very shallow and do not eliminate CO_2. CO_2 accumulates, causing increased production of acids in the bloodstream.

Compensatory Mechanisms and Values

As discussed, the kidneys are the primary means of compensation when an acid–base imbalance is respiratory in nature. In respiratory acidosis, respiratory compensation is incapable of totally counteracting the pH disturbance. In acute respiratory acidosis, the kidneys attempt to compensate by reabsorbing HCO_3^- and excreting H^+. ABG values for *uncompensated respiratory acidosis* reveal a pH less than 7.35 and a CO_2 level greater than 45 mm Hg. If the kidneys can successfully compensate for the pH abnormality by reabsorbing additional bicarbonate (HCO_3^-), then pH value normalizes. ABG values for *compensated respiratory acidosis* reveal a pH that is normal, CO_2 level greater than 45 mm Hg.

Treatment

Treatment of respiratory acidosis centers on improving gas exchange. Oxygenation of blood may be maintained by administering oxygen. Bronchodilation is attempted via oral and parenteral adrenergic agents. If the compromised lung function is due to a pulmonary infection, treatment of the infection is required. If gas exchange does not improve, endotracheal intubation with mechanical ventilation is necessary.

Respiratory Alkalosis

Respiratory alkalosis occurs when CO_2 levels in the blood are low, often due to hyperventilation. Causes of hyperventilation include stress and anxiety, drug toxicity, and head injuries. The reduction in CO_2 resulting from hyperventilation lowers H^+ ion levels and elevates pH, shifting the carbonic acid–bicarbonate buffer equation toward the left:

$$CO_2 + H_2O \Leftarrow H_2CO_3^- \Leftarrow H^+ \text{ and } HCO_3^-$$

Etiology

Respiratory alkalosis is a common acid–base abnormality observed in critically ill patients. It is also common in patients with hyperventilation due to anxiety. Box 8-4 lists common causes of respiratory alkalosis.

Pathophysiology

Hyperventilation, with a subsequent reduction in CO_2 and H^+ ion levels, causes respiratory alkalosis. Many of the signs and symptoms present in persons with respiratory alkalosis relate to the ion disturbances that may develop with hypocapnia, such as hypocalcemia and hypokalemia.

Clinical Presentation

In respiratory alkalosis, tingling of extremities (paresthesia), muscle cramps, tetany, dizziness and/or syncope, confusion, anxiety, seizures, and coma may occur. Cardiac symptoms include palpitations, dysrhythmias, and hypotension. Many patients with hyperventilation due to anxiety feel as though they are enduring a cardiac problem.

Physical Assessment Findings

Many patients enduring hyperventilation appear anxious and are frequently tachycardic. With acute hyperventilation, obvious chest wall movements and use of intercostal muscles to breathe are visible. Hypocalcemia may elicit muscle spasms, as well as Chvostek's

---

BOX 8-4. Causes of Respiratory Alkalosis

PULMONARY
- Pneumonia
- Pulmonary edema
- Pulmonary embolus
- Asthma
- Lung disease with shortness of breath (asthma, pneumonia, acute respiratory distress syndrome [ARDS], fibrosis, pulmonary embolism)
- Hypoxia with hyperventilation
- Overventilation by mechanical ventilation

NONPULMONARY
- Anxiety
- Pain
- Liver disease
- Fever/infection/sepsis
- Central nervous system disorders (tumors, cerebrovascular accidents)
- Salicylate intoxication
- Alcohol intoxication

and Trousseau's signs. Underlying pulmonary disease may be present with signs such as crackles and rhonchi. If the patient is hypoxic, cyanosis may be apparent. The patient may have focal neurological signs or a depressed level of consciousness. Cardiac rhythm disturbances often occur.

Compensatory Mechanisms and Values

Because the lungs cannot adequately compensate for the acid–base disturbance, as indicated by the low CO_2, the kidneys carry out the majority of compensation by reabsorbing H+ into the bloodstream and excreting HCO_3^-. The compensation can take hours to days to accomplish, so medical intervention is needed. In *uncompensated respiratory alkalosis,* blood pH is above 7.45 with a CO_2 level lower than 35 mm Hg. If the kidneys compensate successfully through absorption of H+ and excretion of HCO_3^- ions, ABG values reveal a pH that is normalizing or decreasing toward normal and CO_2 less than 35 mm Hg.

Treatment

Treatment of respiratory alkalosis lies in identifying the underlying trigger that has produced hyperventilation. Pain management or sedation may be required to slow and control the respiratory rate. One common treatment for respiratory alkalosis involves patients breathing into a paper bag. This allows for rebreathing of exhaled CO_2 to bring CO_2 levels back up to a normal range. A CO_2 rebreather, available in the clinical setting, is a type of breathing apparatus that recycles the exhaled CO_2 and adds O_2 to compensate for the oxygen consumed by the user.

 CLINICAL CONCEPT

Hyperventilation is the most common cause of respiratory alkalosis. Simply rebreathing into a paper bag can replace lost CO_2.

Metabolic Acidosis

Metabolic acidosis is due to an excess of acid not related to CO_2. The primary findings are a pH below 7.35 but with normal or lower-than-normal CO_2 levels, indicating that CO_2 is not driving the reduction in pH. One of the primary causes of metabolic acidosis is a metabolic condition that leads to acidic end products, such as ketones or lactic acid. Alternatively, excessive bicarbonate loss due to kidney or GI tract disorders can reduce pH levels.

Metabolic acidosis is mainly divided into processes associated with a normal (8 to 16 mEq/L) or an elevated AG (greater than 16 mEq/L) (see the section on the AG). Addition of acids, such as ketones, increases the anion gap, whereas loss of a base, such as bicarbonate, does not alter it.

Epidemiology

Morbidity and mortality in metabolic acidosis are dependent on the underlying condition. If severe forms of metabolic acidosis go untreated, death may result.

Etiology

Box 8-5 contains a list of common causes of metabolic acidosis.

Pathophysiology

Metabolic acidosis is a condition characterized by an arterial pH lower than 7.35 in the absence of an elevated P_{CO_2}. Three primary mechanisms may lead to the condition of metabolic acidosis:

1. Increased level of acids in the bloodstream
2. Decreased excretion of acids
3. Loss of base from the bloodstream

Increased production of acids that occurs under certain metabolic conditions may lead to metabolic acidosis. DKA is one of the most common causes of metabolic acidosis. In DKA, an accumulation of keto-acids leads to widespread metabolic acidosis. In another example, when widespread ischemia is present, cells with the capacity to rely on anaerobic metabolism produce lactic acid. The accumulation of lactic acid leads to the development of lactic acidosis, which is a type of metabolic acidosis. Alternatively, toxic ingestion or medication overdoses with acidic substances can cause metabolic acidosis. An example is aspirin toxicity, which causes ASA accumulation in the bloodstream. Metabolic acidosis may also develop when there is a reduction in the ability of the kidneys to excrete H+ or to reabsorb HCO_3^-. For example, prolonged diarrhea, in which intestinal contents, including bicarbonate, are lost, can also result in metabolic acidosis.

As previously discussed, acid–base imbalances alter electrolyte levels. In metabolic acidosis, the kidneys

---

BOX 8-5. Causes of Metabolic Acidosis

INCREASED NONCARBONIC ACIDS
- DKA
- Lactic acidosis
- Alcoholic ketoacidosis
- Uremic acidosis
- Ingestion of toxic substances (antifreeze, aspirin)
- Intestinal, biliary, or pancreatic fistulas
- Hypocalcemia, hypokalemia, or hypomagnesemia

BICARBONATE LOSS
- Prolonged diarrhea
- Renal tubular acidosis
- Interstitial renal disease
- Ureterosigmoid loop
- Ingestion of acetazolamide or ammonium chloride

excrete H^+ in lieu of K^+. Thus K^+ accumulates in the bloodstream. Hyperkalemia develops and potentially disrupts the functioning of the heart. Arrhythmias, peaked T waves, QRS widening, and ventricular fibrillation may manifest. Tachycardia is the most common cardiovascular effect seen with mild metabolic acidosis, as hypotension from decreased contractility of the heart may develop. Serum calcium levels elevate in metabolic acidosis due to reduced binding of Ca^{++} to albumin. Hypercalcemia causes muscle weakness, confusion, and lethargy.

Clinical Presentation

The signs and symptoms of metabolic acidosis are widespread and are often due to abnormal serum potassium and calcium levels. The patient complains of respiratory distress as the lungs attempt to compensate for the acidosis. Neurological symptoms include headache, drowsiness, confusion, seizures, neuromuscular fatigue, twitching, and coma. GI symptoms such as nausea, vomiting, and anorexia are common. Cardiovascular symptoms present as hypotension, dysrhythmias, and decreased cardiac contractility.

Physical Assessment Findings

The patient is tachypneic and in respiratory distress. Cardiovascular signs may include weak pulses, tachycardia, hypotension, and arrhythmia. The patient may have GI pain and vomiting. Excessive vomiting can lead to dehydration. Signs of dehydration may include tachycardia, dry mucous membranes, and delayed capillary refill. Patients with DKA may present with fruity odor to their breath due to ketone production. Metabolic acidosis can also cause confusion, lethargy, and possibly coma or seizures.

Compensatory Mechanisms and Values

Unlike respiratory acidosis, in which the kidneys attempt to excrete excess acids, in metabolic acidosis, the lungs, along with the kidneys, attempt to compensate. In metabolic acidosis, the high H^+ ion levels stimulate chemoreceptors, which in turn stimulate the respiratory center to increase the respiratory rate. Elimination of CO_2 pulls H^+ ions out of the bloodstream, increasing the blood pH. This is evident in the carbonic-bicarbonate equation as it moves to the left:

$$CO_2 + H_2O \leftarrow H_2CO_3 \leftarrow H + \text{ and } HCO_3^-$$

Deep, rapid breathing due to metabolic acidosis is referred to as Kussmaul's breathing. Kussmaul's breathing is particularly common in DKA. The lungs ventilate rapidly to attempt to rid the body of CO_2 and, consequently, decrease H^+ levels. In addition, to compensate for metabolic acidosis, the kidneys, if healthy, reabsorb HCO_3^- and excrete H^+. Compensatory mechanisms require hours to days to remedy the condition, often necessitating medical intervention. The hallmark of *uncompensated metabolic acidosis* is pH less than 7.35 with normal to low CO_2 levels, indicating CO_2 is not the reason for the acidic pH. HCO_3^- values will also be lower than normal (<22 mEq/L).

A higher-than-normal AG is due to excess acids, as may occur in DKA or ingestion of acidic compounds. A normal AG indicates the reduced pH is due to loss of basic compounds, such as bicarbonate.

In *compensated metabolic acidosis,* pH is normal or rising toward normal. P_{CO_2} is lower than normal (<35 mm Hg) as CO_2 is exhaled to compensate for the acidic pH. The kidneys reabsorb more HCO_3^- and excrete H^+ ions to compensate.

Treatment

All types of metabolic acidosis require treating the underlying cause. For example, if the cause is DKA, insulin is needed. If the metabolic acidosis is caused by kidney failure, in which the kidneys cannot effectively remove H^+ ions from the blood, hemodialysis is required. Correcting the underlying disorders and restoring electrolyte and fluid balance are critical. IV sodium bicarbonate may be utilized in severe cases of metabolic acidosis when pH is lower than 7.20. Caution is needed, as excessive use of sodium bicarbonate may produce a rebound metabolic alkalosis.

Metabolic Alkalosis

Metabolic alkalosis is a blood pH greater than 7.45 with a normal or higher-than-normal CO_2 level. It is caused by excessive loss of acids unrelated to CO_2 or an increase in bicarbonate levels, such as with retention of sodium bicarbonate. Loss of acids can take many forms, including intracellular shift of H^+ ions from the plasma, as occurs with hypokalemia, or loss of H^+ through the GI tract, as occurs with severe vomiting. The use of certain diuretics can result in the loss of H^+ ions by the kidneys, resulting in alkalosis. Administration of excess sodium bicarbonate and volume depletion are the primary reasons for bicarbonate excess, which also results in metabolic acidosis.

Epidemiology

Metabolic alkalosis is an acid–base disturbance that commonly occurs in hospitalized patients. The more elevated the pH beyond the normal range, the higher the morality rate.

Etiology

Box 8-6 lists common causes of metabolic alkalosis.

Pathophysiology

The most common cause of metabolic alkalosis is depletion of H^+ ions. Loss of H^+ ions occurs primarily through the kidneys and GI tract. Gastric secretions contain large amounts of hydrochloric acid (HCl). Any process that depletes gastric fluid, such as severe vomiting or GI tract suctioning, can result in metabolic alkalosis. Development of metabolic alkalosis due to

BOX 8-6. Causes of Metabolic Alkalosis

- Bicarbonate ingestion
- Excess IV sodium bicarbonate
- Potassium-wasting diuretics
- Loss of gastric fluids from vomiting, gastric suctioning, diarrhea, or binge–purge syndrome
- Cushing's syndrome
- Primary hyperaldosteronism
- Secondary hyperaldosteronism

gastric loss of H^+ ions is a concern for individuals suffering from bulimia, who frequently induce vomiting. The kidneys may contribute to metabolic alkalosis if they are unable to retain adequate H^+ or excrete HCO_3^- at the necessary level.

As observed with the other acid–base disturbances, electrolyte imbalances may play a role in pH abnormalities and vice versa. Metabolic alkalosis may develop in response to hypokalemia. Hypokalemia may develop with the use of certain diuretics or in Cushing's syndrome, in which elevated amounts of aldosterone increase K^+ ion excretion by the kidneys. With the loss of potassium ions, H^+ ions shift into the intracellular space, depleting H^+ ion levels in the bloodstream. Metabolic alkalosis also commonly occurs in cardiac resuscitation. Administration of large amounts of sodium bicarbonate is needed to neutralize the lactic acidosis that forms in cardiac arrest. Excessive amounts of sodium bicarbonate in the bloodstream can exceed the capacity of the kidneys to excrete the bicarbonate. Finally, metabolic alkalosis can lead to hypokalemia and hypocalcemia. These electrolyte disturbances account for some of the signs and symptoms associated with metabolic alkalosis.

Clinical Presentation

The symptoms of metabolic alkalosis are widespread, affecting the neurological, cardiovascular, GI, and musculoskeletal systems, primarily through alteration in ion levels. Patients may present with confusion, dizziness, agitation, weakness, vomiting, diarrhea, and possibly seizures.

Physical Assessment Findings

The physical signs of metabolic alkalosis are nonspecific and multisystemic. Hypokalemia due to metabolic alkalosis can cause muscular weakness, myalgia, muscle spasms, and cardiac arrhythmias. Hypocalcemia may also develop and present as tetany, Chvostek's sign, and Trousseau's sign. Fluid volume status can also change. Evaluation of this status includes assessment of orthostatic changes in blood pressure and heart rate, mucous membranes, presence or absence of edema, skin turgor, weight change, and urine output. In patients with metabolic alkalosis who are suffering from bulimia, erosion of the teeth enamel and dental caries may be present.

Compensatory Mechanisms and Values

Similar to metabolic acidosis, both the lungs and kidneys attempt to compensate in states of metabolic alkalosis. Chemoreceptors detect the higher-than-normal pH of the blood and induce a reduction in ventilation. By slowing the breathing rate, the lungs retain CO_2, thereby raising H^+ content of the blood and lowering pH. The kidneys compensate by reabsorbing H^+ into the bloodstream and excreting HCO_3^-. This can take days to reach the point of adequate compensation; therefore, medical intervention is necessary. In *uncompensated metabolic alkalosis,* pH is greater than 7.45 with normal-to-high CO_2 levels, indicating CO_2 is not causing the elevation in pH. Elevated HCO_3^- values are present (>26 mEq/L). pH will be normal or reducing toward normal in *compensated metabolic alkalosis,* with an elevated P_{CO_2} (>45 mm Hg). CO_2 retention by slow ventilation of the lungs helps reduce pH levels.

Treatment

Treatment of metabolic alkalosis includes electrolyte and fluid replacement. Potassium-sparing diuretics may be administered if the cause of alkalosis is diuretic use. Acetazolamide, which reduces HCO_3^- reabsorption in the kidneys, may also be used to treat conditions of moderate to severe metabolic or respiratory alkalosis.

Mixed Disorders

Clinicians must also be aware that more than one type of acid–base disturbance can be present at any given time. These mixed acid–base disorders manifest when more than one underlying condition disrupts pH. Analysis of ABG values, AG, and patient presentation are critical in determining the course of the acid–base disturbance and the underlying causes of the coexisting disturbances.

Chapter Summary

- An acid is defined as any compound that donates hydrogen ions (H^+) in solution.
- A base is a compound that accepts H^+ ions in solution.
- When H^+ ions predominate in a solution, the solution is acidic. When basic ions predominate in a solution, the solution is alkaline.
- Buffers resist changes in pH by donating or accepting H^+ ions as needed.
- Three main buffer systems that exist in the body are protein, phosphate, and carbonic acid-bicarbonate system.
- The lungs and the kidneys regulate the body's acid-base balance through use of the carbonic acid-bicarbonate buffer system.
- Blood pH, partial pressure of oxygen (Po_2), partial pressure of carbon dioxide (Pco_2), and bicarbonate ion concentration (HCO_3^-) are the values indicated by an ABG.
- The normal pH of blood is 7.35 to 7.45. A pH level lower than 7.35 is acidemia (also called acidosis); a level greater than 7.45 is alkalemia (also called alkalosis).
- A chemical buffering system used by the body is the carbonic acid-bicarbonate system: $CO_2 + H_2O \leftrightarrow H_2CO_3 \leftrightarrow H^+$ and HCO_3^-. Both the lungs and kidneys utilize this system to compensate for acid-base disturbances.

- During hypoventilation, the lungs retain CO_2; during hyperventilation, the lungs blow off CO_2.
- The greater the amount of CO_2 in the body, the greater the formation of H^+ ions.
- Four possible acid-base disturbances occur in the body: respiratory acidosis, respiratory alkalosis, metabolic acidosis, and metabolic alkalosis.
- Hypoventilation, which causes Pco_2 greater than 45 mm Hg, results in respiratory acidosis; hyperventilation, which causes Pco_2 less than 35 mm Hg, results in respiratory alkalosis.
- An excess of acid or a loss of HCO_3^- in the blood causes metabolic acidosis. In uncompensated metabolic acidosis, HCO_3^- will be lower than 22 mEq/L and the pH will be lower than 7.35.
- Metabolic alkalosis is caused by excessive loss of acids, shift of H^+ ions into the intracellular space, or increase in bicarbonate in the bloodstream. In uncompensated forms, the blood pH will be greater than 7.45 and the bicarbonate concentration greater than 26 mEq/L.
- Acid-base imbalances affect serum electrolyte levels. Acidosis is generally associated with hyperkalemia, and alkalosis with hypokalemia. Due to altered albumin-binding affinity for Ca^{++} with pH changes, acidosis may cause hypercalcemia and alkalosis may cause hypocalcemia.

Making the Connections

Disorder and Pathophysiology

Signs and Symptoms	Physical Assessment Findings	Diagnostic Testing	Treatment
Respiratory Acidosis | Lungs are not ventilating; retaining too much CO_2, creating too much H^+. Commonly due to COPD, severe asthma, or any cause of reduced ventilation.			
Dyspnea. Respiratory distress. Patient may be lethargic, stuporous, or comatose.	Diminished respiratory rate. Cyanosis. Clubbing if chronic hypoxia.	Uncompensated: blood pH less than 7.35. Pco_2 greater than 45 mm Hg. Po_2: low. Urine: acidic.	Treat the lung disorder for better ventilation. Bronchodilation. Antibiotics if pneumonia. Intubation and mechanical ventilation if needed.
Respiratory Alkalosis | Lungs are hyperventilating; losing too much CO_2 creates too little H^+ in the blood. Commonly due to hyperventilation secondary to anxiety or shallow respirations in asthma.			
Hyperventilation. Anxiety. Palpitations. Paresthesia. Patient may have pain.	High respiratory rate. Tachycardia.	Uncompensated: blood pH greater than 7.45. Pco_2 less than 35 mm Hg. Urine: basic.	Slow the breathing rate; CO_2 rebreather. Patient may need sedative.

Making the Connections—cont'd

Signs and Symptoms	Physical Assessment Findings	Diagnostic Testing	Treatment
Metabolic Acidosis | Excessive acid in the bloodstream (e.g., ketoacids or lactic acid) or excessive loss of HCO_3^- (e.g., GI tract loss). Commonly due to DKA, lactic acidosis, drug toxicity, or GI loss of excessive HCO_3^- as in diarrheal illness.			
Symptoms according to etiology of disorder: respiratory distress, headache, drowsiness, confusion, seizures, fatigue. GI symptoms of nausea, vomiting, and anorexia are common.	Tachycardia. Hypotension, weak pulses. Dehydration signs may be present: dry mucous membranes, poor skin turgor, and delayed capillary refill. Patients with DKA may present with fruity odor to their breath. Metabolic acidosis can also cause confusion, lethargy, and possibly coma or seizures.	Uncompensated: blood pH less than 7.35. PCO_2 normal or slightly low. Serum K^+: high. Urine: acidic. Electrocardiogram (ECG) changes caused by hyperkalemia: arrhythmias, peaked T waves, QRS widening, and ventricular fibrillation possible.	Sodium bicarbonate IV. Treat etiological disorder (for example, if DKA, treat diabetes).
Metabolic Alkalosis | Excessive base in the bloodstream (such as toxic ingestion) or lack of sufficient acid in the bloodstream caused by high loss of H^+ (such as loss of HCl with excessive vomiting).			
Symptoms according to etiology of disorder; often related to decreased calcium ionization resulting from low H^+ level. Low Ca^{++} levels cause tetany, irritability, disorientation, and seizures. Prolonged vomiting may be the cause.	Chvostek's sign. Trousseau's sign. Hypotension or hypertension may be present. Patients with bulimia often have erosions of teeth enamel and dental caries.	Uncompensated: blood pH greater than 7.45. PCO_2 normal or slightly high. Urine: basic. Serum ionized Ca^{++} low. ECG may show dysrhythmias.	IV acetazolamide.

Bibliography

Available online at fadavis.com

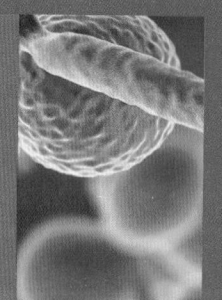

CHAPTER
9

Inflammation and Dysfunctional Wound Healing

Learning Objectives

Upon completion of this chapter, the student will be able to:

- Describe the phases of inflammation and the mediators and cells involved in the reaction.
- List the types of white blood cells involved in inflammation.
- Identify the laboratory tests that are involved in diagnosis of inflammation.

- Discuss the different systemic reactions that occur due to inflammation.
- Distinguish among primary, secondary, and tertiary wound healing.
- Identify major factors that affect the process of healing.
- Recognize complications of wound healing.

Key Terms

Abscess
Acute phase proteins
Angiogenesis
Chemokines
Chemotaxis
Contracture
C-reactive protein (CRP)
Cytokines
Effusion
Erythrocyte sedimentation rate (ESR)
Eschar
Fibroblast

Fibrinogen
Granuloma
Histamine
Inflammation
Interleukins (ILs)
Keloid
Leukemoid reaction
Leukocytosis
Lymph node
Lymphocytes
Nitrogen balance
Phagocytosis

Primary intention
Prostaglandins (PGs)
Purulent exudate
Pyrogens
Secondary intention
Stricture
Tertiary intention
Transudate
Tumor necrosis factor (TNF) alpha
White blood cell (WBC) differential
Wound dehiscence
Wound evisceration

Inflammation is a protective, coordinated response of the body to an injurious agent. It involves many cell types and inflammatory mediators that initiate, modulate, amplify, and terminate this response. Characteristic cellular products, tissue changes, and systemic responses are associated with inflammation. The intensity of the inflammatory reaction is usually proportional to the extent of the tissue injury. The major aims of inflammation are to wall off the area of injury, prevent spread of the injurious agent, and bring the body's defenses to the region under attack.

Inflammation and the Inflammatory Response

The inflammatory response is a multistage process that involves vascular and cellular changes but may also include systemic changes. White blood cells (WBCs) are brought to the damaged area, and they secrete mediators that control the process from initial injury to resolution or long-term inflammation. The inflammatory response is most efficient when it rids the body of injury, enhances healing processes, and resolves. In some disorders, such as rheumatoid arthritis (RA), tuberculosis (TB), and atherosclerosis, inflammation can persist and ultimately cause unremitting damaging effects on the body; these are considered chronic inflammatory conditions. See Box 9-1 for examples of inflammatory conditions.

Inflammatory conditions can cause discomfort, organ dysfunction, and diminished quality of life. Cell biologists continue to uncover micromolecular-level mediators of inflammation, which could be precise targets for drugs. Our current knowledge base regarding inflammation is incomplete, but research continues to enhance our understanding of this complex physiological response.

Types of Inflammation

There are two types of inflammation: acute and chronic. Acute inflammation occurs rapidly in reaction to cell injury, rids the body of the offending agent, enhances healing, and terminates after a short period, either hours or a few days. Chronic inflammation occurs when the inflammatory reaction persists, inhibits healing, and causes continual cellular damage and organ dysfunction.

Acute Inflammation

Acute inflammation can be triggered by various injurious stimuli, such as infections, microbial toxins, physical injury, surgery, cancer, chemical agents, tissue necrosis, foreign bodies, and immune reactions. Regardless of etiology, all acute inflammatory reactions cause the same characteristic vascular, cellular, and systemic changes. These reactions are orchestrated by responses to various inflammatory mediators. The acute inflammatory reaction involves two main phases:

1. Vascular phase: momentary vascular constriction followed by a long period of vascular permeability
2. Cellular phase: attraction and rush of WBCs to area of injury

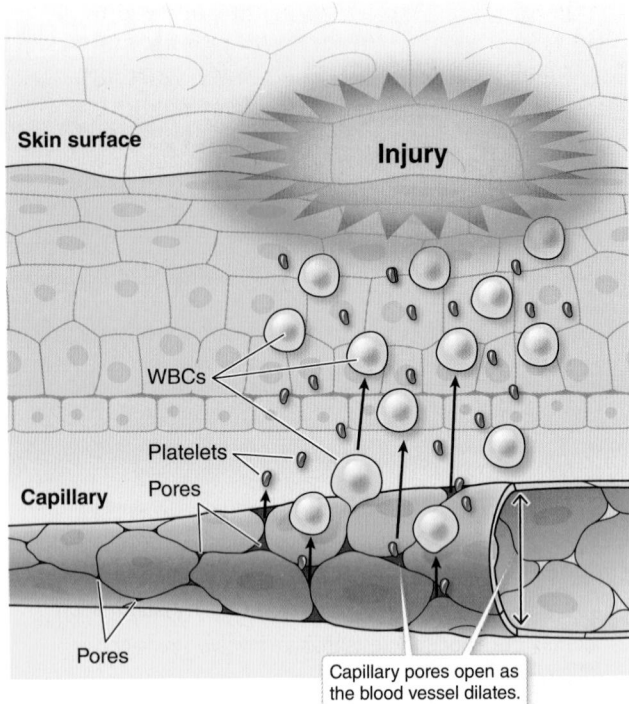

FIGURE 9-1. The vascular permeability phase of inflammation. Inflammation stimulates dilation of blood vessels and the opening of capillary pores. The capillary pores allow fluid and cells, such as WBCs and platelets, out to the area of injury.

Vascular Permeability. During the vascular phase, there is transient vasoconstriction followed by a prolonged period of vascular permeability. At a site of inflammation, inflammatory mediators such as histamine and bradykinin cause the blood vessels to dilate and become more permeable. Capillary pores open and allow fluids, WBCs, and platelets to travel to the site of injury or infection (Fig. 9-1). The increased fluid in the tissues dilutes the toxin and lowers the pH of the surrounding fluids so they are not conducive to microbial growth.

The inflamed area immediately starts to become congested, warm, red, and swollen from the vasodilation and fluid extravasation into the tissues from the capillaries. These effects can occur internally within an organ or externally on the surface of the body, depending on where the cell injury and inflammation are occurring.

BOX 9-1. Inflammatory Conditions

In most cases, the terminology that indicates inflammation of tissue or an organ uses the suffix *-itis*. For example, the term *acute pharyngitis* means inflammation of the pharynx; it is commonly known as sore throat.

Other inflammatory conditions include:
- **Appendicitis:** inflammation of the appendix
- **Hepatitis:** inflammation of the hepatocytes or liver
- **Colitis:** inflammation of the colon
- **Arthritis:** inflammation of Arthus tissue or joints

 CLINICAL CONCEPT

The classic external signs of inflammation are known as the five cardinal signs: rubor (redness), tumor (swelling), calor (heat), dolor (pain), and loss of function (functio laesa).

The fluid that leaves the capillaries is a protein-rich filtrate of blood that contains WBCs. As the WBCs perform defensive activities, the fluid increases within the tissue spaces and causes edema, or swelling. If the fluid is rich in protein from WBCs, microbial organisms, and cellular debris, it is called **purulent exudate,** or pus. An **abscess** is a localized, walled-off collection of purulent exudate within tissue. In contrast, fluid that contains little protein and is mainly a watery filtrate of blood is called **transudate.** Other types of exudates include serous (clear, watery fluid), sanguineous (blood), serosanguineous (bloody/watery fluid), or fibrinous (thick, fibrin-rich fluid).

Any accumulation of fluid in a body cavity is called an **effusion.** An effusion can occur due to inflammatory or noninflammatory processes.

CLINICAL CONCEPT

An example of purulent exudate is the whitish-green drainage emitted from an infected wound. An example of a transudate is the clear fluid contained within a noninfected blister. Both are types of fluid that result from inflammation.

Leukocytosis. During the cellular phase of inflammation, a chemical signal from microbial agents, endothelial cells, and WBCs attracts platelets and other WBCs to the site of injury. This is referred to as **chemotaxis.** During this phase, an increased number of leukocytes (WBCs) are released from the bone marrow into the bloodstream, a process known as **leukocytosis.** During inflammation, the WBC count in the blood commonly increases from a normal baseline of 4000 to 10,000 cells/mL to 15,000 to 20,000 cells/mL. The clinician can use the number of WBCs to determine the severity of the infectious process that the patient is experiencing.

Once the WBCs arrive at the site of inflammation, they line up along the endothelium in the area of inflammation in a process called margination. At the site of injury, the leukocytes adhere to the endothelial lining of the blood vessels, held by adhesion molecules called selectins and integrins (Fig. 9-2).

The term **leukemoid reaction** is used to describe an extreme, extraordinary elevation in the number of WBCs. Leukemoid reactions can raise the WBC count to 50,000 cells/microliter or more. These reactions can occur in conditions such as leukemia.

CLINICAL CONCEPT

Some genetic disorders such as severe combined immunodeficiency syndrome cause a deficiency in selectins and integrins, leading to immunodeficiency and increased risk of infection.

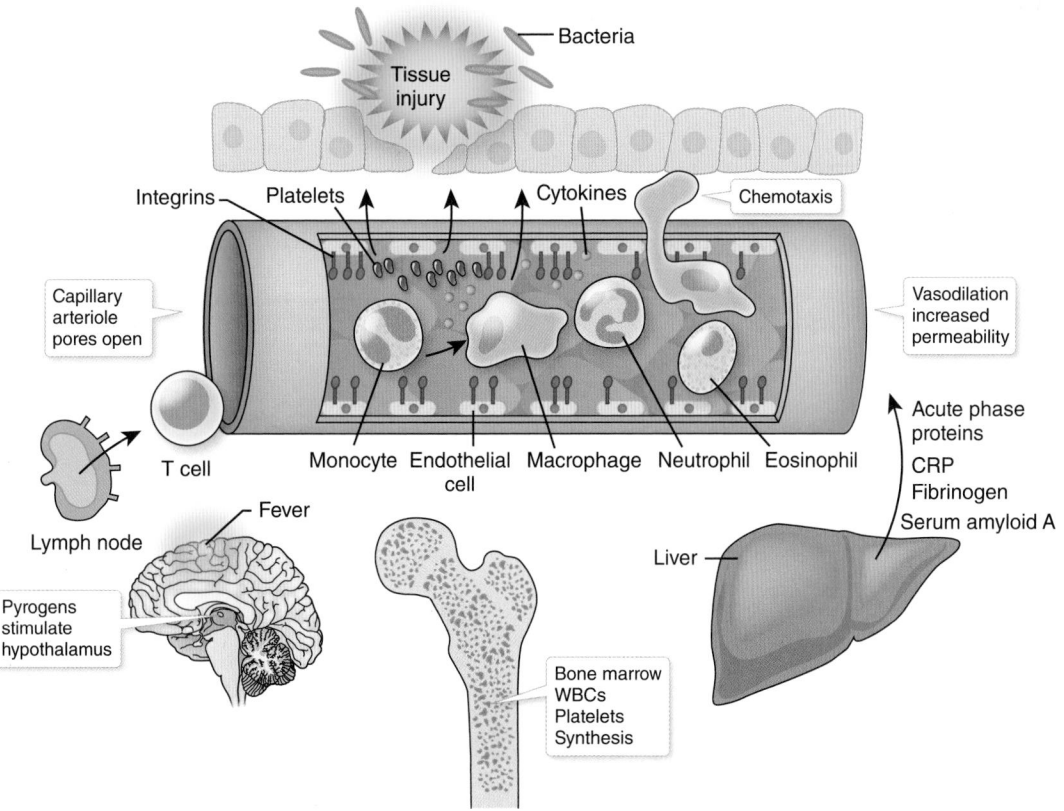

FIGURE 9-2. Acute inflammation.

After binding to the endothelial surfaces of the blood vessels, the WBCs then squeeze through pores in the capillaries to arrive at the tissues of injury. The type of WBC varies as time passes in the process of inflammation. During the first 6 to 24 hours, neutrophils predominate in the inflammatory infiltrate. Neutrophils undergo apoptosis and are gradually replaced by monocytes. Over the next 24 to 48 hours, monocytes change into macrophages. Macrophages then survive for long periods (weeks to months) and are the predominant type of WBC in persistent inflammatory reactions. There are some exceptions to this pattern. In certain infections—such as those caused by *Pseudomonas* bacteria—the cellular infiltrate is dominated by neutrophils for several days; in viral infections, lymphocytes dominate as the WBCs in the infiltrate. In allergic reactions, eosinophils are the dominant type of WBC in the infiltrate. Analysis of the type of WBC in the infiltrate can assist the clinician to determine the etiology of the inflammatory reaction.

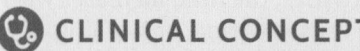 CLINICAL CONCEPT

Some infections—such as typhoid fever and infections caused by *Rickettsia*, protozoa, and viruses—cause a decreased number of WBCs, termed leukopenia.

WBCs and injured tissue release many different inflammatory mediators that act in various ways. Some mediators amplify the inflammatory process, recruiting more WBCs to the area of injury, and others attempt to stop the inflammatory process.

Mediators of Inflammation

The mediators of inflammation are substances that promote or inhibit inflammatory reactions. These include interleukins (ILs) and tumor necrosis factor alpha (TNF-alpha). Inflammatory mediators are summarized in Table 9-1. Many anti-inflammatory

Patho-Pharm Connection

Tissue Injury and Inflammation

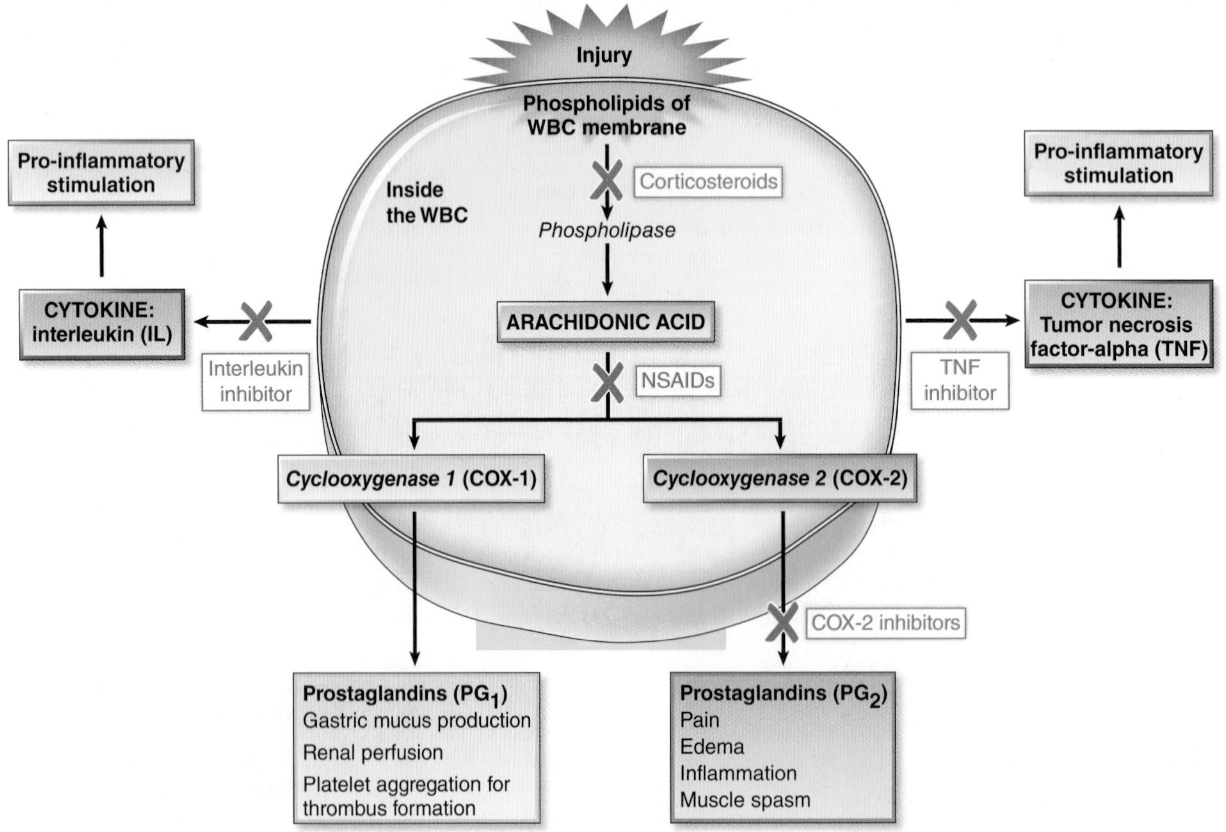

Injury

Phospholipids of WBC membrane

Inside the WBC

Corticosteroids

Phospholipase

Pro-inflammatory stimulation

CYTOKINE: interleukin (IL)

Interleukin inhibitor

ARACHIDONIC ACID

NSAIDs

Pro-inflammatory stimulation

CYTOKINE: Tumor necrosis factor-alpha (TNF)

TNF inhibitor

Cyclooxygenase 1 (COX-1)

Cyclooxygenase 2 (COX-2)

COX-2 inhibitors

Prostaglandins (PG$_1$)
Gastric mucus production
Renal perfusion
Platelet aggregation for thrombus formation

Prostaglandins (PG$_2$)
Pain
Edema
Inflammation
Muscle spasm

Tissue injury stimulates inflammation reaction in the white blood cell. Injury stimulates the action of the phospholipase enzyme that breaks down phospholipids, which are key components of the white blood cell membrane. This enzymatic action yields arachidonic acid. [See how phospholipase is blocked by corticosteroids. Note the side effects of not producing "good PGs1": decreased gastric mucus, kidney perfusion, and platelet aggregation.] NSAIDs stop

Patho-Pharm Connection–cont'd

arachidonic breakdown and inhibit both cyclooxygenase 1 and cyclooxygenase 2 pathways. This inhibition, in turn, inhibits production of both PG1 and PG2 prostaglandins. [Note that PG1 prostaglandins are "good PGs," which enhance body processes such as production of gastric mucus, renal perfusion, and platelet aggregation/clot formation.] Cyclooxygenase 2 (COX-2) inhibitors block

production of solely PG2 prostaglandins, which block the edema, inflammation, pain, and muscle spasms. TNF inhibitors and IL inhibitors block production of the cytokines, TNF alpha, and interleukins. These are released by white blood cells and promote the inflammation reaction. Blockade or inhibition of interleukins decreases inflammation.

pharmaceutical agents have been devised to counteract different types of inflammatory-promoting mediators (see Patho-Pharm Connection).

Cytokines, Chemokines, and Acute Phase Proteins.
Some of the inflammatory mediators released by WBCs are referred to as **cytokines;** the most common are **tumor necrosis factor (TNF) alpha** and **interleukins (ILs).** Cytokines modulate the inflammatory reaction by amplifying or deactivating the process. Simultaneously, they cause localized and systemic effects. **Chemokines** are proteins that attract leukocytes to the endothelium at the area of injury. Cytokines cause stimulation of the liver to release substances called **acute phase proteins.** Acute phase proteins include **C-reactive protein (CRP),** fibrinogen, serum amyloid A, and hepcidin. Acute phase proteins facilitate WBC phagocytosis of microbes and other foreign material and assist in the analysis of the inflammation process occurring in the body.

CRP is a key acute phase protein that is integral to marking foreign material for phagocytosis; activating

the complement system, which augments immunity; and stimulating other inflammatory cytokines. Elevation of CRP in the bloodstream indicates that active inflammation is occurring. Elevation of a specific type of CRP, identified by a laboratory test called high sensitivity CRP, is a marker for increased risk of myocardial infarction in patients with coronary artery disease.

Fibrinogen binds to red blood cells (RBCs) and fixes them into stacks that precipitate rapidly in the blood through processes called rouleaux and sedimentation. This is the basis for a laboratory test called **erythrocyte sedimentation rate (ESR)** that, if elevated, indicates active inflammation. Elevated CRP, fibrinogen, and ESR alert the clinician that an active process of inflammation is occurring currently. Prolonged secretion of serum amyloid A causes a condition called amyloidosis, which indicates chronic inflammation and alerts the clinician that the patient has endured a long-term inflammatory process. Elevated hepcidin levels in the bloodstream indicate diminished iron storage in the body—a process that leads to anemia in chronic inflammatory conditions.

TABLE 9-1. Major Proinflammatory Mediators

Inflammatory Mediator	Origin	Effects
Tumor necrosis factor-alpha	Macrophages	Fever, lack of appetite, raises metabolism to cause cachexia, hypotension
Interleukins	Macrophages	Fever, stimulates platelet production, fatigue, anemia, headache
Histamine	Mast cells, basophils, platelets	Vasodilation, increases vascular permeability, activates endothelium
Kinins	Liver, lungs, kidneys	Increases vascular permeability, smooth muscle contraction, pain, natriuresis, hypotension
Platelet-activating factor	Platelets, leukocytes, mast cells	Vasodilation, increases vascular permeability, platelet aggregation, angiogenesis (formation of new blood vessels), leukocyte adhesion to endothelium
Prostaglandins	Leukocytes	Pain, fever, vasodilation, muscle spasm
Leukotrienes	Leukocytes, mast cells	Bronchospasm, increased vascular permeability
Substance P	Neurons	Pain, hypotension, enhances vascular permeability

CLINICAL CONCEPT

Laboratory tests that demonstrate elevated CRP, ESR, and fibrinogen levels in the bloodstream are indicators that the patient is enduring an active inflammatory process.

CLINICAL CONCEPT

Neutrophils are also referred to as polymorphonuclear leukocytes (PMNs); in their immature form, they are called bands or stabs.

Types of White Blood Cells. There are five basic types of WBCs: neutrophils, lymphocytes, eosinophils, basophils, and monocytes (see Fig. 9-3).

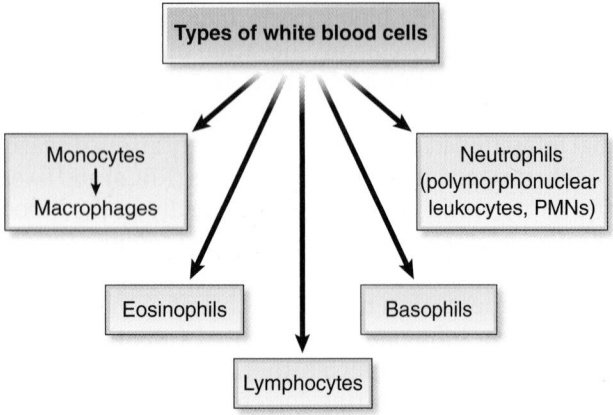

FIGURE 9-3. Types of WBCs.

Neutrophils, basophils, and eosinophils are referred to as granulocytes because obvious cytoplasmic granules can be seen when examined under the microscope. These cytoplasmic granules contain important enzymes and antimicrobial proteins that support the inflammatory process and fight infection. Neutrophils have a short life span ranging from approximately 10 hours to a few days. Mature neutrophils have distinctive multisegmented nuclei and are sometimes known as segmented neutrophils (segs). As mature neutrophils die off and the supply becomes exhausted, the bone marrow responds with a rapid release of immature neutrophils (bands).

Neutrophils begin the process of phagocytosis of the foreign matter immediately. **Phagocytosis** involves recognition and attachment of the leukocyte to the foreign matter, engulfment, and degradation or killing of the ingested matter (Fig. 9-4). During engulfment, extensions of the cytoplasm called pseudopods surround the foreign matter and pinch off, forming a phagosome. The phagosome then contains the foreign matter, and lysosomal and granular enzymes break it down.

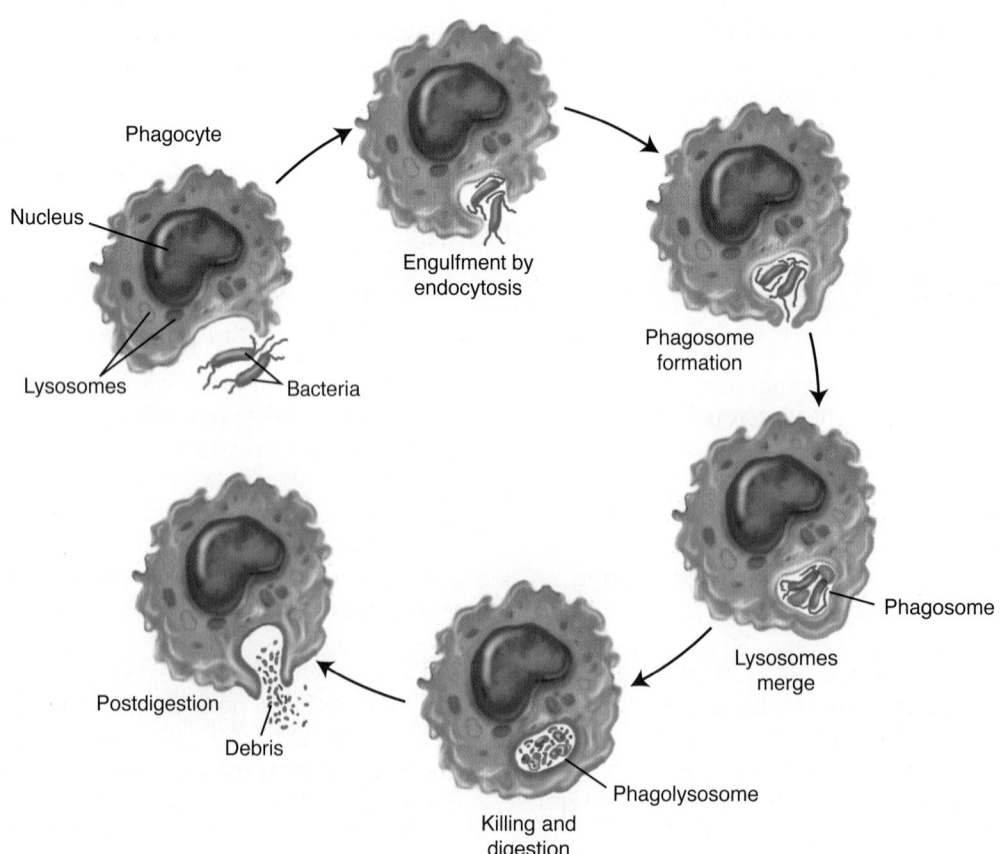

FIGURE 9-4. Phagocytosis.

While the neutrophils are involved in phagocytosis of microbial organisms and cellular debris, there is a respiratory burst from the mitochondria. This burst releases free radicals (also called superoxides or reactive oxygen species) that disrupt microbial membranes, leading to their destruction. Free radicals contain a superoxide anion (O_2), which is an oxygen molecule with a free electron that is drawn to elements in tissue. Using different terminology, free radicals oxidize microbial membranes and some of the surrounding host tissue cell membranes. However, host cells contain antioxidants that protect against extensive tissue damage. A genetic disorder called chronic granulomatous disease causes a deficiency of free radicals, which leads to immunodeficiency and increased risk of infections.

CLINICAL CONCEPT

Antioxidant vitamins A, C, E, and beta carotene can counteract collateral free radical oxidizing damage of healthy tissue in inflammatory processes.

A laboratory test called a **white blood cell (WBC) differential** is used in the diagnosis of infection and inflammation. This test is part of a complete blood count (CBC) with differential, which quantifies RBCs and WBCs. A WBC with differential measures the total number of WBCs and calculates the percentages of specific types of WBCs within the total. The result of the laboratory test shows the predominant type of WBC responding to the infectious agent and can be used to indicate the etiology of inflammation. For example, a patient with pneumonia who has an elevated total WBC count of 16,000 with 90% neutrophils most likely has bacterial pneumonia, whereas a patient with pneumonia and an elevated WBC with 90% lymphocytes most likely has viral pneumonia.

The WBC count with differential can also indicate an acute inflammatory reaction by quantifying the number of bands in the bloodstream. When a high number of bands are present, clinicians often use the phrase "shift to the left," indicating an increase in newly formed neutrophils. An elevated WBC count with a "shift to the left" indicates that an acute inflammatory process is occurring. As inflammation resolves, immature neutrophils become less numerous and the WBC count returns to normal.

Systemic Responses. Persons enduring acute inflammation experience symptoms throughout the whole body, such as fever, pain, lymphadenopathy (swollen lymph nodes), anorexia, sleepiness, lethargy, anemia, and weight loss. These are known as systemic responses. Inflammatory mediators such as prostaglandins (PGs), TNF-alpha, and ILs are responsible for many of these systemic effects. Studies also show that inflammatory mediators are elevated in older adults suffering from frailty. Progressive increases in frailty severity are correlated with inflammatory mediator concentrations, particularly IL and TNF.

Fever. Fever, an increase in body temperature, is a common manifestation of inflammation and infection. Microbial organisms, bacterial products, and cytokines all act as **pyrogens,** which are substances that cause fever. Pyrogens activate PGs to reset the hypothalamic temperature-regulating center in the brain to a higher level. A higher body temperature is theorized to increase the efficiency of WBCs in their defense of the body against foreign invaders (see Fig. 9-5).

CLINICAL CONCEPT

Fever, although advantageous to the immune system, can reach levels high enough to cause seizures and brain damage. Therefore, it is recommended to keep fever below 102°F through the use of antipyretic medications such as aspirin, ibuprofen, or acetaminophen. These medications inhibit PG formation and thus reduce fever.

ALERT! Never give children or adolescents aspirin or any salicylate-containing products to control a fever. Research has demonstrated a link between salicylate use and Reye's syndrome in children and adolescents who have viral infections. Reye's syndrome is a life-threatening disorder in which mitochondrial failure leads to liver failure and encephalopathy.

The sensation of chills often accompanies fever. When the set point of the hypothalamic temperature-control center is suddenly changed from normal (98.6°F) to a higher temperature, it takes some time before the body reaches the new higher set point. Initially, the blood temperature is less than the new higher set point and the person has a sensation of being cold. The blood vessels constrict and the body attempts to conserve and generate heat. To reach the new hypothalamic temperature set point, the muscles shiver to generate body heat. The sensation of cold and muscle shivering are experienced as chills, which continue until the body reaches the higher hypothalamic temperature set point. When the stimulus for the fever resolves, pyrogens stop stimulating PGs and the hypothalamic temperature returns to normal levels. The feverish body must adapt to the new, lower hypothalamic set point. In response, vasodilation and intense sweating (diaphoresis) occur to dissipate the

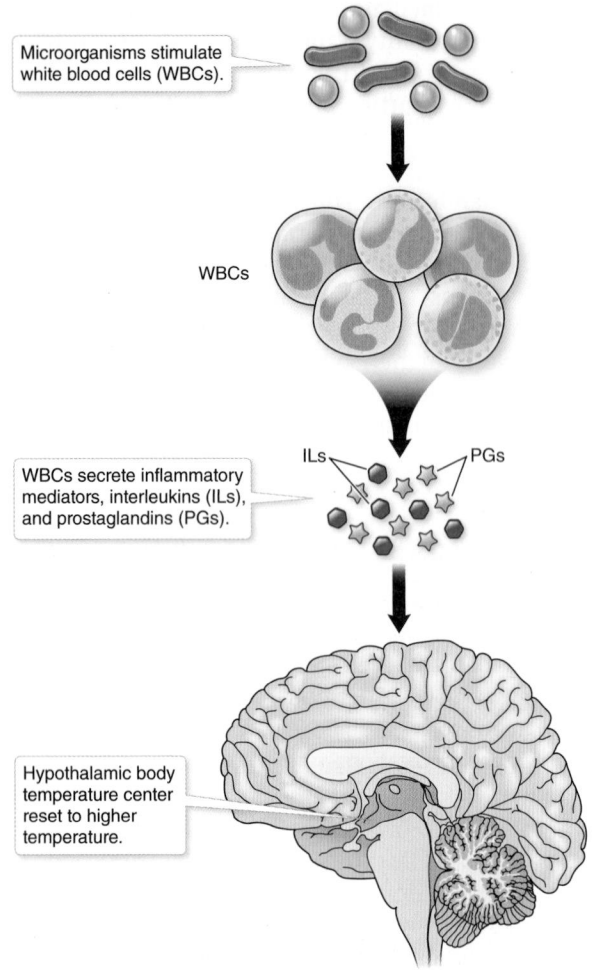

FIGURE 9-5. The fever response. Microorganisms enter the body and stimulate WBCs. Pyrogens are inflammatory mediators that are released by WBCs. Pyrogens reset the hypothalamic temperature center in the brain to create fever. Fever assists the WBCs in performing their activities in infection.

body heat. As body temperature declines, the patient appears flushed and diaphoretic because of widespread vasodilation.

Lymphadenopathy. Lymphadenopathy, or lymphadenitis, is a term used to describe the enlargement of lymph nodes because of inflammatory processes. **Lymph nodes** are small, bean-sized masses of tissue located in various regions of the body, including the neck, axillary regions, central thoracic region, inguinal areas, and gastrointestinal tract (Fig. 9-6). **Lymphocytes** mature within a lymph node, and during an inflammatory process, lymph nodes become enlarged. Because of the active proliferation of lymphocytes, lymph nodes enlarge, which stretches their capsule and causes tenderness. Lymphatic fluid or lymph circulates around body tissues and collects debris. The injurious agents that cause the inflammation can invade lymph and then spread to other lymph nodes.

Histamine Release. **Histamine,** an inflammatory mediator released from basophils, platelets, and

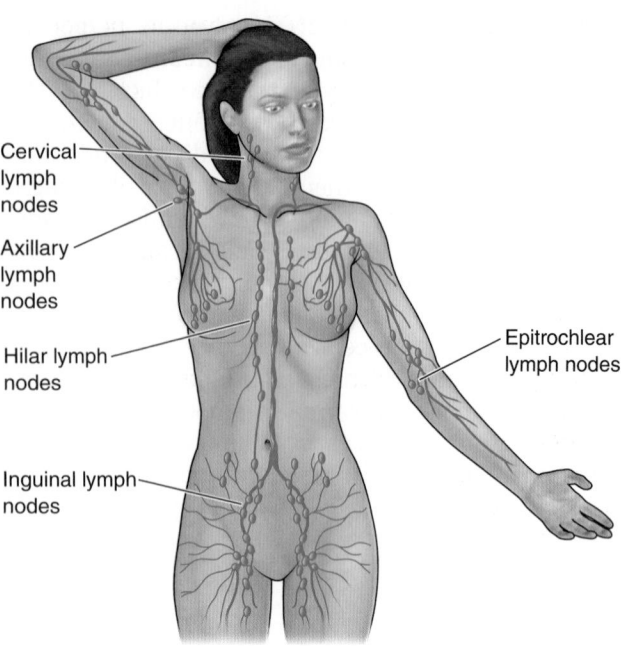

FIGURE 9-6. Regions of the lymph nodes in the body.

mast cells, has many systemic effects. It causes arteriolar vasodilation, large artery vasoconstriction, and increased permeability of venules.

Mast cells, located in tissues adjacent to blood vessels, are the richest source of histamine. Physical injury, immune reactions, cytokines, and other inflammatory mediators stimulate histamine release. Commonly, sneezing, rhinorrhea (runny nose), eye tearing, sinus inflammation, and pharyngeal irritation are consequences of histamine released in the upper respiratory tract.

Effects of Prostaglandins, Leukotrienes, and Their Enzymatic Pathways. **Prostaglandins (PGs)** are released from WBCs and other cell membranes through a series of reactions. During inflammation, an enzyme called phospholipase is stimulated and acts on phospholipids, constituents of the WBC cell membrane. Phospholipids are broken down into arachidonic acid, which undergoes further enzymatic action by cyclooxygenase and lipoxygenase. The cyclooxygenase pathways produce PGs, and the lipoxygenase pathway produces leukotrienes. Some PGs perpetuate negative effects of inflammation, and other PGs are needed for protective bodily functions. Leukotrienes provoke bronchiole inflammation in asthma.

Two different enzymes are involved in the formation of PGs from arachidonic acid: cyclooxygenase-1 (COX-1) and cyclooxygenase-2 (COX-2). Each pathway yields a different type of PG. The COX-1 pathway breaks down arachidonic acid enzymatically into helpful PGs, and the COX-2 pathway yields harmful PGs. The PGs formed from the COX-1 pathway stimulate gastric mucus production, enhance renal perfusion, and assist platelets to aggregate and form clots.

The PGs formed by the COX-2 pathway perpetuate inflammation; cause pain, fever, swelling, and muscle contractions; and potentiate the effects of other inflammatory mediators (see Fig. 9-7).

Systemic Effects of TNF-alpha and ILs. TNF-alpha, IL-1, and IL-6 are major cytokines produced by macrophages in the inflammation reaction and have been shown to induce fever, loss of appetite, and lethargy. TNF-alpha also promotes lipid and protein mobilization, which causes weight loss and cachexia, the wasting of lean body mass. TNF-alpha can enhance release of WBCs into the bloodstream and facilitate the release of pituitary corticotropin and adrenal corticosteroids in the body. In an infected bloodstream, a condition known as sepsis, TNF-alpha provokes hypotension, widespread vasodilation, increased heart rate, and decreased blood pH.

CLINICAL CONCEPT

In severe sepsis, large amounts of bacteria stimulate enormous quantities of cytokines, notably TNF and ILs, which cause shock, disseminated intravascular coagulation, and possible death.

Outcomes of Acute Inflammation. Acute inflammation will result in one of three outcomes:

1. Complete resolution
2. Healing by connective tissue
3. Chronic, persistent inflammation that does not recede

Ideally, acute inflammation is a short-lived reaction that eliminates an injurious agent, allows little tissue destruction, and terminates by facilitating the regeneration of normal tissue. Resolution involves normalization of vascular permeability, deactivation of chemical mediators, elimination of cellular debris and edema, and apoptosis of WBCs.

At times, severe tissue injury and a large acute inflammatory reaction preclude the regeneration of normal cells. This happens when inflammation involves tissues incapable of regenerating cells or when inflammatory exudates and cellular debris cannot be adequately cleared at the conclusion of the inflammatory reaction. At these times, resolution and healing occur through the proliferation of connective tissue. Cellular debris and exudates are reabsorbed, and fibrous scar tissue, rather than regenerated cells, replaces damaged cells. Finally, there are times when acute inflammation cannot be resolved because of persistence of the injurious agent or other interference with healing. In these cases, inflammation becomes a chronic, persistent condition with failure to resolve and extensive tissue damage.

Chronic Inflammation

An inflammatory reaction that persists for a prolonged time, from weeks to months, without resolution or healing is considered a chronic inflammatory disorder. Specific etiological agents are known to cause chronic inflammation, but a persistent, unremitting inflammatory reaction can also occur for unknown reasons.

Etiologies of Chronic Inflammation

Causes of chronic inflammation include:

- Persistent infection by microorganisms that are difficult to eradicate (e.g., *Mycobacterium tuberculosis* [TB]).
- Hypersensitivity disorders, which cause excessive activation of the immune system. Examples of these disorders include autoimmune diseases

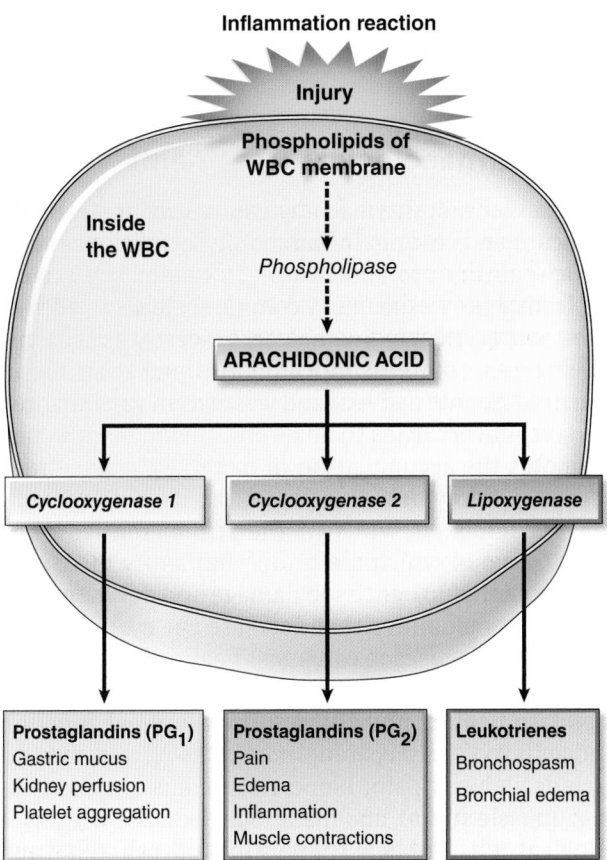

FIGURE 9-7. Prostaglandin and leukotriene synthesis pathways within the WBC. Injury stimulates inflammation, which attracts WBCs to the area of injury. Within the WBC, phospholipase acts upon phospholipids to yield arachidonic acid, which is then converted to PGs via the COX-1 or COX-2 pathway or to leukotrienes via the lipoxygenase pathway. The PGs created by the COX-1 pathway are needed to secrete gastric mucus and enhance renal perfusion and thrombus formation. The PGs created by the COX-2 pathway cause uncomfortable symptoms of inflammation, such as fever, edema, and pain. Leukotrienes cause bronchospasm and bronchiole edema.

such as RA, multiple sclerosis (MS), or systemic lupus erythematosus (SLE).
- Prolonged exposure to potentially toxic agents such as coal dust, which causes anthracosis (black lung).

Atherosclerosis is also a chronic inflammatory disease affecting the arterial wall that is caused by agents that damage the endothelial cells. Some agents that cause endothelial injury include hypertension, free radicals (superoxide molecules), and high blood glucose. Some cancers, such as basal cell carcinoma—a type of skin cancer caused by excessive sun damage, are promoted by chronic inflammatory reactions.

In contrast to acute inflammation, which is manifested by vascular permeability and neutrophil proliferation, chronic inflammation is characterized by the predominance of monocytes, lymphocytes, and macrophages. In acute inflammation, the products of activated macrophages eliminate injurious agents such as microbes and initiate the process of healing. In chronic inflammation, however, these same products, when constantly secreted by macrophages, cause tissue damage. The destructive macrophage products include free radicals, proteases, cytokines, angiogenesis growth factors, and fibroblast activators. Tissue is repeatedly damaged, healing is delayed, and connective tissue replaces injured cells. As tissue damage causes cell death, necrotic tissue stimulates an inflammatory reaction. As a result, tissues undergoing chronic inflammation can have regions demonstrating acute inflammation as well.

T and B lymphocytes commonly amplify and perpetuate chronic inflammation. These are the cells found in chronic autoimmune disorders. T lymphocytes are particularly involved in chronic inflammatory conditions, as they produce ILs and interferon, which recruit macrophages.

Chronic inflammation often causes a distinctive histological pattern of granulomatous changes. A **granuloma** is an area where macrophages have aggregated and are transformed into epithelial-like or epithelioid cells. The epithelioid cells are surrounded by lymphocytes, fibroblasts, and connective tissue. Frequently, the epithelioid cells fuse to form giant cells within the granuloma. TB is the prototypical granulomatous chronic inflammatory disease. On histological examination of the lungs, a TB granuloma is characterized by an aggregate of macrophages surrounding TB organisms. After acute infection, neutrophils and monocytes surround, but cannot kill, TB bacteria. The WBCs attracted to the area of infection can only wall off the bacteria. Eventually this region, infiltrated with macrophages, becomes a chronic inflammatory granuloma called a tubercle. The tubercle can be identified on histological examination and x-ray of the lungs (see Fig. 9-8).

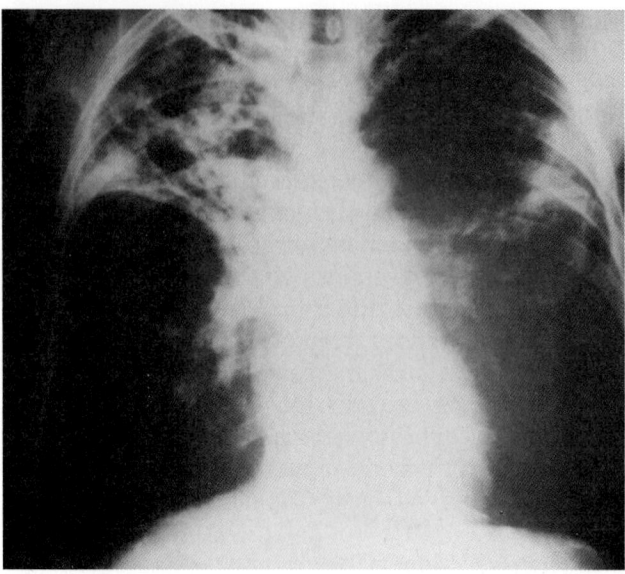

FIGURE 9-8. Chest x-ray showing TB. *(Courtesy of CDC.)*

Treatments to Counteract Inflammation

Nonpharmacological Treatments

The goals of nonpharmacological treatment strategies for acute and chronic inflammatory conditions are to reduce pain and promote healing. Inflammation resulting from acute tissue injury commonly leads to edema, pain, and erythema. Edema can exacerbate mechanical stresses, compressing capillaries and resulting in impaired oxygen delivery and waste removal. Impaired oxygen delivery leads to anaerobic metabolism, which promotes the accumulation of metabolic waste products (e.g., inorganic phosphate, lactic acid, and H^+). The accumulated WBCs in the region release cytokines, some of which are proinflammatory mediators that promote further tissue damage and delay healing. Therefore, modalities that decrease the cycling of the inflammatory cascade can assist healing.

Heat and cold therapy modalities are often used to facilitate healing and the return to normal function and activity. The physiological effects of cold therapy include reduced pain, blood flow, edema, inflammation, muscle spasm, and metabolic demand. The physiological effects of heat therapy include pain relief and increased blood flow, metabolism, and elasticity of connective tissues.

Cold therapy, also known as cryotherapy, is the application of any substance or physical medium to the body that removes heat, decreasing the temperature of the contact area and adjacent tissues. Ice packs, commercially available cold gel packs, ice massage, cold compression units, and cold whirlpool can be used. Cold therapy is usually recommended in the management of acute injury/trauma that causes acute inflammation, muscle spasm, pain and tenderness, and edema. Decreasing temperatures of skin, soft tissue, and muscle reduces blood flow to the cooled tissues, reduces edema, and slows delivery of inflammatory mediators to the region. Intermittent application of cold therapy is commonly recommended (10 minutes ice, 10 minutes room temperature, 10 minutes ice, every 2 hours) with rest for the first 48 hours postinjury (Malanga et al., 2015).

Heat therapy is the application of heat to the tissue. Superficial modes of heat therapy include hot water bottles, heat pads, electric heat pads, heat wraps, heated stones, soft heated packs filled with grain, poultices, hot towels, hot baths, sauna, paraffin, steam, ultrasound diathermy, and infrared heat lamps. Physiological effects of heat therapy include pain relief, increased blood flow, enhanced tissue metabolism, decreased muscle spasm, and increased elasticity of connective tissue. Heat therapy, along with mild physical activity, is often recommended for chronic inflammation. According to Hoekstra et al. (2020), studies show a reduction in basal concentrations of proinflammatory markers following chronic exercise training. Therefore, heat therapy along with regular exercise is often recommended to decrease chronic, low-grade inflammatory conditions.

Some medicinal herbs and alternative medical treatments possess anti-inflammatory activity. Steroids, glycosides, phenolics, flavonoids, alkaloids, polysaccharides, terpenoids, cannabinoids, and fatty acids are common phytoconstituents that have anti-inflammatory potential. Different mechanisms have been explored for the anti-inflammatory effects of these active ingredients (Yatoo et al., 2018). Complementary and alternative medical therapies such as chiropractic, osteopathic manipulation, acupuncture, Tai Chi, Qigong, and yoga have also been effective in the reduction of symptoms of various inflammatory disorders (Bower & Irwin, 2016; Zhang et al., 2014; Urits et al., 2021). Many studies of the beneficial effects of alternative therapies are based on empirical experience, with limited evidence-based research to support efficacy. However, an evidence-based research basis for these alternative therapies is in development.

Pharmacological Treatments

There are numerous kinds of pharmacological agents available that counteract inflammation. In order to understand the action of anti-inflammatory agents, the pathways and substances involved in the inflammation reaction need explanation (see Patho-Pharm Connection).

Phospholipids, which are major components of cell membranes, are damaged during the acute and chronic inflammation reaction. Tissue injury stimulates the enzyme phospholipase. Phospholipase breaks down the cell membranes of various tissues during inflammation. Corticosteroids, the most potent anti-inflammatory agents (e.g., dexamethasone, prednisone), act by inhibiting the phospholipase enzyme. The inhibition of this enzyme, in turn, diminishes the inflammation reaction at an initial step in the process. Although corticosteroids are highly effective at counteracting the initial steps in the inflammatory reaction, they have potential to cause a multitude of adverse side effects (see Table 9-2). Therefore, corticosteroids should only be used for short-term treatment of inflammatory conditions.

NSAIDs (e.g., ibuprofen, naproxen, aspirin) do not contain a steroid component, and act by blocking both cyclooxygenase pathways that produce the cytokines known as prostaglandins (PGs). The COX-1 pathway leads to production of prostaglandin 1 cytokines and the COX-2 pathway leads to production of prostaglandin 2 cytokines. Prostaglandin 1 (PG1) cytokines are integral to maintenance of some significant physiological processes. PG1s are needed to manufacture gastric mucus for protection of the stomach lining. PG1s also enhance renal perfusion, which maintains circulation within the kidney. PG1s also enhance platelet aggregation that contributes to clot formation. However, prostaglandin 2 (PG2) cytokines promote inflammation,

TABLE 9-2. Potential Adverse Effects of Prolonged Corticosteroid Use

Cardiovascular	Hypertension, fluid retention, weight gain
Gastrointestinal	Peptic ulcer
Musculoskeletal	Osteoporosis, growth retardation
Endocrine	Glucose intolerance; hyperglycemia, hyperlipidemia, Cushingoid facies, menstrual irregularities, adrenal atrophy
Skin	Bruising, striae, acne, impaired wound healing
Immunity	Immunosuppression with increased risk of infection
Neurological	Psychiatric disturbances, mood disturbances
Ophthalmological	Cataracts, increased intraocular pressure (glaucoma)

trigger pain, intensify edema, and cause muscle spasm. NSAIDs block both cyclooxygenase pathways, thereby blocking both the formation of PG1s and PG2s. NSAIDs, when blocking PG1s, can cause lack of gastric mucus production, diminished renal perfusion, and decreased platelet aggregation. Thus, overuse of NSAIDs can lead to the detrimental side effects of gastric irritation and ulceration: renal dysfunction, and decreased clotting.

COX-2 inhibitors (e.g., celecoxib) are drugs that solely block the COX-2 pathway. Therefore these agents mainly block PG2s, which perpetuates the adverse effects of inflammation: pain, edema, and muscle spasm.

WBCs release other cytokines such as TNF-alpha and ILs, which also perpetuate inflammation. Newer drugs that are laboratory-synthesized antibodies called monoclonal antibodies (mAbs) (also called biological agents) are recent additions to the pharmacological arsenal of anti-inflammatory agents. The monoclonal antibody pharmacological agents, known as tumor necrosis factor inhibitors and interleukin inhibitors, are used in various types of inflammatory disorders. Monoclonal antibody agents are commonly used in treatment of RA, psoriatic arthritis, and inflammatory bowel disease. Some commonly prescribed TNF inhibitors include adalimumab, infliximab, etanercept, golimumab, and certoliumab. Interleukin inhibitors include anakinra, secukinumab, upadacitinib, ixekizumab, and daclizumab. The research area focusing on anti-inflammatory pharmaceuticals, particularly biological agents, is a burgeoning field with increasing numbers of agents being released each year.

Tissue Repair and Wound Healing

Tissue healing and regeneration are the desirable outcomes of cell injury and inflammation. Optimal regenerative healing occurs when injured cells are replaced by cells of the same type, leaving no trace of residual injury. Certain tissue injuries, such as those involving loss of tissue because of gouging injuries, cannot heal by cellular replacement. In situations such as this, cells are replaced by connective tissue, which leaves a scar.

Normal Wound Healing

Wound healing can be divided into four phases:

1. Hemostasis
2. Inflammation
3. Proliferation, granulation tissue formation, angiogenesis, and epithelialization
4. Wound contraction and remodeling

Hemostasis occurs shortly after injury as exposed collagen surfaces attract platelets. Platelets aggregate and secrete inflammatory mediators such as serotonin, histamine, and platelet-derived growth factor. Vasoactive amines such as epinephrine cause short-term vasoconstriction, which limits blood loss.

Inflammation occurs next in the acute phase, after injury, and has been described previously. Vasodilation, increased vascular permeability, and chemotaxis occur during this phase.

In the subsequent proliferation phase, granulation tissue forms. The **fibroblast,** a connective tissue cell that synthesizes collagen and provides the extracellular matrix in wound healing, is the key cell involved in this process. As early as 24 to 48 hours after injury, fibroblasts form the granulation tissue that serves as the foundation of scar tissue. Vascular endothelial cells create new blood vessels in a process called **angiogenesis.** The granulation tissue then secretes growth factors and cytokines such as vascular endothelial growth factor (VEGF), platelet-derived growth factor (PDGF), fibroblast growth factor (FGF), tissue growth factor-beta (TGF-beta), and IL-1. Also, during this phase, epithelial cells migrate and proliferate to form a new surface and fill in the gap between the wound edges. Fibroblasts produce collagen for days, weeks, or months, depending on the wound size. Approximately 3 weeks after injury, the remodeling phase begins, where the scar tissue is structurally refined and reshaped by fibroblasts and myofibroblasts (see Fig. 9-9).

Primary, Secondary, and Tertiary Intention

Skin wounds heal by either of three processes: primary, secondary, or tertiary intention (see Fig. 9-10). The nature of the wound determines the process the body uses. Healing by **primary intention,** also called primary union, is the least complicated type of wound repair. The edges of the wound are clearly demarcated, cleanly lacerated, and easily brought together, and there is no missing tissue within the injured area. A surgical wound is the best example of this type of injury, which usually undergoes a simple, rapid healing process. Surgical wounds can be closed with sutures, staples, or adhesive. Sutures are the gold standard and can be made of absorbable or nonabsorbable material. Within 24 hours, WBCs congregate and a fibrin clot develops at the site. After 24 to 48 hours, simple epithelialization predominates as the major process that closes the wound. By day 5, granulation tissue progressively fills in the incision space and new blood vessel growth is maximal. During the second week, there is accumulation of collagen and proliferation of fibroblasts within the incisional scar. By the end of the first month, inflammation has subsided, and connective tissue covered by an intact epidermis makes up the wound site.

> ### 🔬 CLINICAL CONCEPT
>
> Primary intention is best exemplified by healing of a clean, surgical laceration. It requires predominately surface reepithelialization and reestablishment of tissue integrity of the approximated edges.

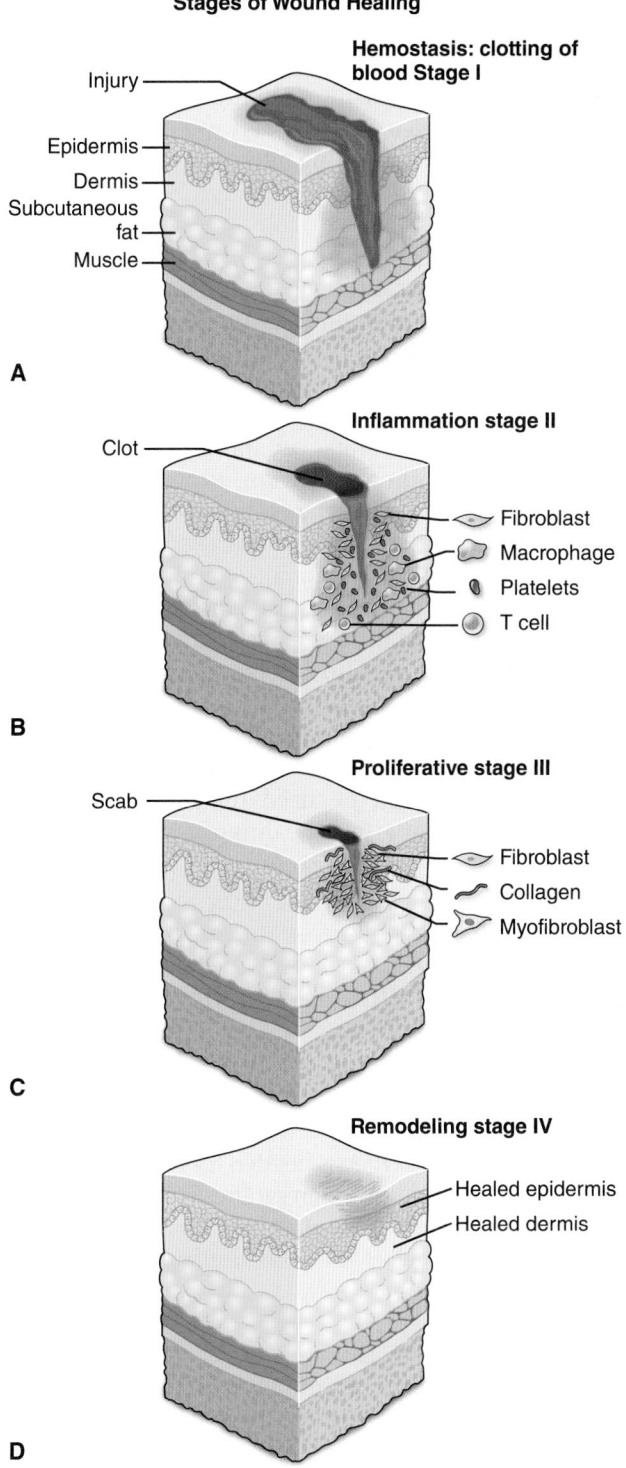

Stages of Wound Healing

Hemostasis: clotting of blood Stage I

Injury

Epidermis

Dermis

Subcutaneous fat

Muscle

A

Inflammation stage II

Clot

Fibroblast

Macrophage

Platelets

T cell

B

Proliferative stage III

Scab

Fibroblast

Collagen

Myofibroblast

C

Remodeling stage IV

Healed epidermis

Healed dermis

D

FIGURE 9-9. Stages of wound healing. (A) Hemostasis. (B) Inflammatory stage. (C) Proliferative stage. (D) Remodeling.

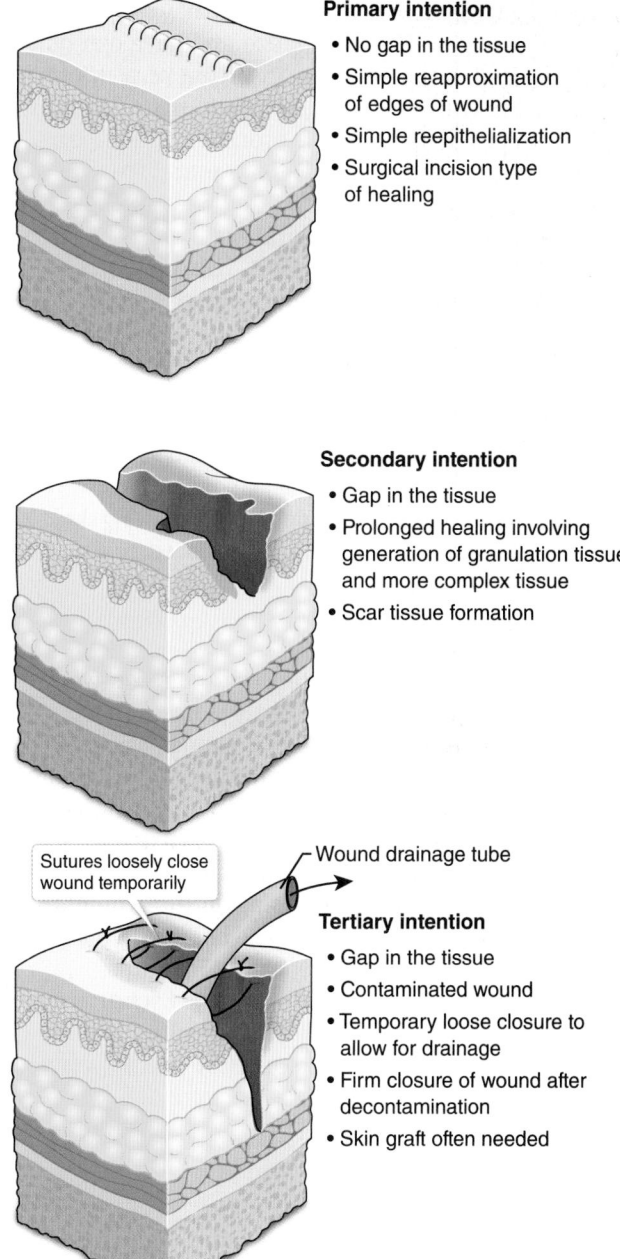

Primary intention

- No gap in the tissue
- Simple reapproximation of edges of wound
- Simple reepithelialization
- Surgical incision type of healing

Secondary intention

- Gap in the tissue
- Prolonged healing involving generation of granulation tissue and more complex tissue
- Scar tissue formation

Sutures loosely close wound temporarily

Wound drainage tube

Tertiary intention

- Gap in the tissue
- Contaminated wound
- Temporary loose closure to allow for drainage
- Firm closure of wound after decontamination
- Skin graft often needed

FIGURE 9-10. Primary, secondary, and tertiary intention healing.

When there is extensive loss of tissue within a wound, the repair process is more complex; in this case, **secondary intention,** also called secondary union, healing begins (see Fig. 9-10). Regeneration of the same cells to replace lost tissue is not possible. Abundant granulation and fibrous tissue are necessary to fill the defect and restore the original structure of tissue. The inflammation process within this type of wound is more intense and longer in duration. The formation of granulation tissue requires extensive time and support for the healing process.

The phase that differentiates primary from secondary intention is wound contraction. Wound contraction occurs because of myofibroblasts, which are connective tissue cells with smooth muscle characteristics. These specialized cells cause the contraction of the wound's edges to close the tissue gap. Substantial scar formation and thinning of the epidermis occurs. Wounds of this type are highly susceptible to infection, complications, and deformity.

In **tertiary intention,** also called tertiary union, the wound is missing a large amount of deep tissue and is contaminated. It is cleaned and left open for

4 to 5 days before closure. The wound may require temporary packing with sterile gauze and have extensive drainage that often requires insertion of a drainage tube. By the fifth day, WBC phagocytosis of contaminated tissues occurs and the processes of epithelialization, collagen deposition, and maturation take place. Foreign materials are walled off by macrophages and other types of leukocytes to form granulomas. There is prominent scarring with healing. This type of wound commonly requires a skin graft.

 CLINICAL CONCEPT

Pressure injuries and severe burns are examples of wounds that require secondary and tertiary intention healing. These wounds have large areas of missing skin, dermis, and deeper tissue, which are replaced by scar tissue (see Fig. 9-11).

Primary, secondary, and tertiary intention wounds do not regain full tensile strength of unwounded skin after healing is completed. Clinicians and patients need to be aware of the weakened integrity of the skin and underlying tissues. Careful support of the area to facilitate healing is necessary during the first few weeks after surgery. After sutures are removed, usually 1 to 2 weeks later, wounded skin is again in a vulnerable, weakened state. The healed wound builds to a maximal tensile strength of 70% to 80% after 3 months.

Some wounds develop eschar tissue. **Eschar** is dead tissue that sheds or falls off from healthy skin. It is common in burn wounds and pressure injuries. Eschar is typically tan, brown, or black and often has a crusty top layer.

CLINICAL CONCEPT

To perpetuate and stimulate healing, débridement of a wound is often necessary. Débridement is the removal of necrotic tissue to promote and enable reepithelialization and new growth of tissue.

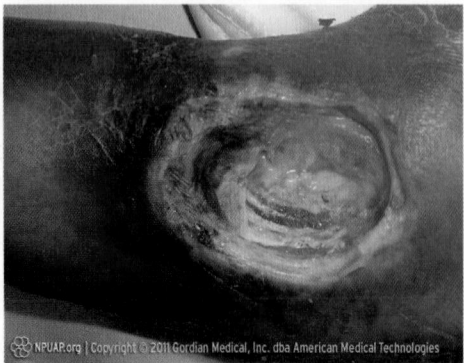

FIGURE 9-11. Stage IV pressure injury.

Factors That Affect Wound Healing

Wound healing is a complex phenomenon involving many body systems. Healing requires a sufficient supply of nutrients and oxygen, as well as efficient removal of tissue debris and invading microorganisms. Box 9-2 summarizes the positive and negative factors involved in wound healing; each is discussed in detail in the following text. All of these effects can delay wound healing, increase risk for infection, decrease wound tensile strength, and lead to wound rupture.

Nutrition

Successful wound healing depends on adequate protein, carbohydrates, fats, vitamins, and minerals obtained from optimal nutrition. Protein is particularly necessary for cellular regeneration and synthesis of connective tissue. For wounds to heal, a patient must be in a state of positive nitrogen balance. **Nitrogen balance** is defined as the difference between nitrogen intake and nitrogen excretion. Protein is the best source of nitrogen in the diet. When a patient's nitrogen intake exceeds nitrogen excretion, the resultant positive nitrogen balance suggests the availability of protein for wound repair.

Carbohydrates can be used for energy to spare protein sources for tissue healing. Fats are essential

---

BOX 9-2. Factors Involved in Wound Healing

- **Nutrition:** Lack of adequate nutrients, particularly protein, decreases cellular regeneration and metabolic function.
- **Oxygenation:** Oxygen is needed for neutrophil phagocytosis and collagen synthesis.
- **Circulation:** Lack of adequate circulation predisposes the individual to ischemia, infarction, and consequent infection of necrotic tissue, also known as gangrene.
- **Immune strength:** Diabetes, corticosteroid use, cancer, HIV, aging, and immunosuppressant agents diminish WBC activity, delay wound healing, and predispose to infection.
- **Contamination:** Foreign bodies present in a wound diminish healing ability and predispose to infection. Foreign bodies include sutures that remain in place too long, surgically inserted devices such as pacemakers, heart valves, and orthopedic or prosthetic implants.
- **Mechanical factors:** Includes increased localized pressure, torsion, and excessive fat tissue.
- **Age:** The regeneration process of infants and young children is superior to that of adults. Studies show that fetal wounds heal without fibrosis or scarring. Older adults have the slowest healing process.

components of cell membranes that are synthesized during the healing process.

Most vitamins are essential cofactors for the body's metabolic activities. They are particularly important in wound healing. The role of vitamins and other trace elements in successful wound healing is listed in Table 9-3.

Blood Flow and Oxygen Delivery

Arterial and venous circulation should be optimal in the region that requires healing, as healing tissue needs a rich supply of nutrients and oxygen delivered via arterial blood flow, as well as adequate waste removal provided by efficient venous flow. Bacteria, cellular debris, necrotic tissue, and local toxins need to be eliminated as tissue regenerates. Wounds that attempt to heal under ischemic conditions require lengthier periods and are susceptible to infection. Ischemia fosters the growth of anaerobic bacteria such as *Clostridium perfringens,* the microorganism that causes gangrene.

Obesity tends to impair wound healing because adipose tissue is less vascular and, in turn, deficient in oxygen.

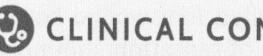

CLINICAL CONCEPT

Gangrene occurs when ischemic tissue undergoes bacterial infection leading to tissue necrosis.

Brisk arterial blood flow is needed to deliver maximal oxygen to the area. Oxygen facilitates collagen synthesis and WBC function. Without oxygen, WBCs cannot kill phagocytosed microorganisms, and collagen growth is deficient. Hyperbaric oxygen, which is 100% oxygen delivered at two times normal atmospheric pressure, facilitates collagen synthesis, angiogenesis, neutrophil phagocytic activity, and fibroblast proliferation.

Smoking has a deleterious effect on wound healing. Nicotine in cigarettes acts as a vasoconstrictor, which decreases circulation and subsequent oxygenation. The smoke also contains free radicals, which are oxidizing agents that damage cell membranes.

Immune Strength

Optimal wound healing requires a strong immune system that is capable of eliminating dead tissue, walling off foreign matter, and killing microorganisms. A brisk inflammatory response is needed in the initial stages of tissue injury, followed by efficient phagocytic WBC function and strong acquired immune reactions. The infant who is naïve immunologically and the older adult patient who is naturally immunosuppressed are vulnerable to suboptimal wound healing because of susceptibility to infection. However, in general, immunocompetent children have more efficient healing processes than adults. Studies show that fetal wounds heal without fibrosis or scarring. Compared with adult wounds, fetal wounds are richer in hyaluronic acid, a component thought to facilitate cellular regeneration and collagen synthesis. Older patients heal less efficiently because of aged skin, a thinned dermal layer, reduced collagen and fibroblast synthesis, and greater potential for secondary conditions that reduce blood flow to the area.

Conditions that cause immunosuppression, such as cancer, HIV, diabetes mellitus, and corticosteroid use, may delay healing. Diabetes mellitus decreases the phagocytic ability of neutrophils and macrophages, which hinders the inflammation response in wound healing. Diabetes mellitus also injures small arterial blood vessels, diminishing peripheral circulation. Decreased peripheral circulation diminishes the arteriolar blood flow to peripheral nerves, which, in turn, decreases sensation. Individuals with diabetes mellitus gradually develop increasing sensory deficit of the lower extremities, particularly of the feet. Lack of sensation and circulation in the feet predispose the

TABLE 9-3. Vitamins, Minerals, and Wound Healing	
Substance	**Function in Wound Healing**
Vitamins A and C	• Build proteins • Fortify epithelial mucous membranes • Increase collagen strength
Vitamin B_{12}	• Enable cell replication • Support growth of RBCs • Maintain nervous system • Enable synthesis of nucleic acids
Vitamin D	• Foster absorption of calcium from gastrointestinal tract
Vitamin K	• Enable synthesis of coagulation factors
Folate	• With vitamin B_{12}, enable synthesis of nucleic acids
Calcium, phosphorus	• Support bone growth
Iron	• Essential for synthesis of hemoglobin and RBCs • Required for mitochondrial functioning
Zinc, copper, manganese	• Needed for cellular metabolism

individual to wound formation. For example, a person with diabetes mellitus who wears an ill-fitting shoe can develop a blister that goes unrecognized because of lack of pain sensation in the feet. This simple blister can quickly become an infected foot wound because of the diabetic patient's lack of sensation, diminished circulation, and decreased WBC function.

Corticosteroids, potent anti-inflammatory agents, suppress the inflammation phase of wound healing. These drugs also inhibit collagen synthesis, which is integral to the proliferative and remodeling phases of wound healing. Therefore, patients on corticosteroids can become immunosuppressed and experience poor wound healing.

Infection is the single most important cause of delayed healing. A wound's susceptibility to infection is influenced by the patient's immune strength, the type of wound present, and conditions of injury. The presence of infection perpetuates the inflammation phase and delays the formation of granulation tissue and collagen synthesis. Foreign bodies present within the wound are major impediments to the healing process and increase risk of infection. Vigorous irrigation, cleansing, and removal of necrotic tissue and foreign matter are necessary to facilitate optimal wound healing.

Foreign Bodies

Any fragments or debris left inside the wound due to traumatic injury can impede healing. Examples include bullets, glass, steel, wood, or bone. Sutures can act as foreign bodies if they are not removed in a timely manner from the healing wound site. Surgically inserted devices such as pacemakers, heart valves, and orthopedic or prosthetic implants can become sources of infection and predispose the patient to sepsis.

Mechanical Factors

Increased localized pressure, torsion, or excessive fat tissue can cause wound dehiscence. Adipose tissue is difficult to close surgically. Surgical procedures on obese patients require more time and cause more tissue trauma. In addition, surgical wound closure is more difficult in obese patients because of the tension on the sutures.

The abdomen is a surgical site where sutured wounds need support. The patient should be taught how to splint the surgical site during coughing or movement.

Dysfunctional Wound Healing

Wounds can fail to heal properly if the factors needed to support healing are lacking. Individuals who are poorly nourished or immunocompromised are at risk for suboptimal wound outcomes. In addition, the healing wound must be protected if it is to close properly. Finally, the processes involved in functional wound healing may become overly aggressive and lead to complications (see Box 9-3).

BOX 9-3. Possible Complications of Wound Healing

- **Keloid:** hyperplasia of scar tissue
- **Contractures:** inflexible shrinkage of wound tissue that pulls the edges toward the center of the wound
- **Dehiscence:** opening of a wound's suture line
- **Evisceration:** opening of wound with extrusion of tissue and organs
- **Stricture:** an abnormal narrowing of a tubular body passage from the formation of scar tissue (e.g., esophageal stricture)
- **Fistula:** an abnormal connection between two epithelium-lined organs or vessels that normally do not connect (e.g., tracheoesophageal fistula)
- **Adhesions:** internal scar tissue between tissues or organs

---

Wound Rupture

Most wounds require structural support and immobility for the initial healing period. Undue tension on the wound can inhibit the approximation of edges and epithelialization of the surface. There is particularly high tension on the edges of abdominal wall wounds because of the mechanical stresses of coughing, vomiting, and the Valsalva maneuver. When previously closed wound edges open and rupture, the condition is called **wound dehiscence.** In rare cases, internal tissues and organs can extrude from the open wound, a condition called **wound evisceration.** Abdominal wounds are most susceptible to these conditions (see Fig. 9-12).

ALERT! Wound dehiscence and evisceration require immediate wound protection with sterile, saline-moistened dressings and prompt surgical evaluation.

Keloid Formation

Wound healing can be complicated by hyperplastic epithelialization and collagen formation. The excessive accumulation of epithelium and collagen can form a hypertrophic scar, also called a keloid. The etiology of keloid formation is unknown; however, it is more common in persons of African descent. Keloids can be reduced by cosmetic surgery.

Contractures

Wound contraction, the last step in second intention healing, can become exaggerated and result in a deformity called a **contracture,** an inflexible shrinkage of wound tissue that pulls the edges toward the center of the wound. Contractures often occur in burn wounds

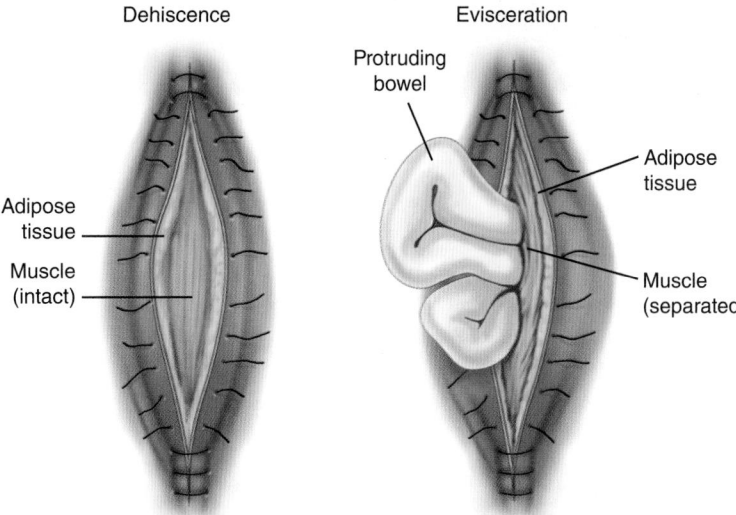

FIGURE 9-12. Wound dehiscence and evisceration.

and limit mobility when they occur across a joint surface. A related type of wound complication is a **stricture,** a complication of wound healing that causes narrowing or closure of an open area of the body. A duct, canal, or tube may develop a stricture caused by scar tissue. For example, if the esophagus is injured, a stricture would reduce the diameter and narrow or completely close off the tubular open area for passage of food.

Fistula

A fistula is an abnormal connection between two different areas of tissue or organs. A fistula can form with abnormal wound healing and cause complications. An example is a tracheoesophageal fistula, which is a connection between trachea and esophagus. Aspiration of contents from the esophagus can obstruct the trachea.

Adhesions

Adhesions are abnormal bands of internal scar tissue that can form after invasive surgical procedures. These bands of scar tissue can limit mobility if they form within a joint, as in adhesive capsulitis of the shoulder (frozen shoulder). Alternatively, adhesions can form around internal organs, where they can cause pain or obstruction, and require surgical excision.

Chapter Summary

- Inflammation is an essential process for protecting the body during injury or infection.
- In the initial phase, WBCs are attracted to the site of the injury in a process called chemotaxis.
- Blood vessel walls become more permeable so fluid and WBCs can move out of the bloodstream to the site of injury.
- Types of WBCs include neutrophils, eosinophils, basophils, lymphocytes, and monocytes, which turn into macrophages.
- The five cardinal signs of inflammation are rubor (redness), tumor (swelling), calor (heat), dolor (pain), and loss of function (functio laesa).

- CRP and ESR increase in acute inflammation.
- Inflammation can either undergo healing and resolution or persist as chronic inflammation.
- Wound healing consists of four phases: hemostasis, inflammation, proliferation, and remodeling.
- Healing involves one of three processes: primary, secondary, or tertiary intention.
- Nutrition status, oxygen supply, steroid use, diabetes, and immunosuppression affect the process of healing.
- There are many possible complications of wound healing, including keloid formation, contracture, stricture and fistula formation, wound dehiscence, and wound evisceration.

Bibliography

Available online at fadavis.com

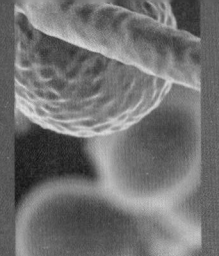

Infectious Diseases

Learning Objectives

Upon completion of this chapter, the student will be able to:

- Identify the most common types of microorganisms that cause infection.
- Recognize stages of infection, portals of entry, and modes of transmission of infection.
- Differentiate between the innate and adaptive immune responses to infection.

- Describe laboratory studies that assist in the diagnosis of infection.
- Recognize common bacterial, viral, fungal, parasitic, and prion-mediated infections.
- Discuss methods of prevention, eradication, and treatment of infection.

Key Terms

Antibody titer

Colonization

Community-acquired pneumonia (CAP)

Congenital

Dermatophytes

Endemic

Epidemic

Epidemiology

Exanthem

Gram-negative

Gram-positive

Group A beta hemolytic streptococcus (GABHS)

Health-care-acquired or hospital-acquired infection

Host

Immunocompetence

Immunosuppression

Incidence

Infection

Inoculum

Methicillin-resistant *Staphylococcus aureus* (MRSA)

Opportunistic infection

Pandemic

Pathogen

Portal of entry

Prevalence

Reservoir

Septicemia (Sepsis)

Vancomycin-resistant *Staphylococcus aureus* (VRSA)

Vector

Virulence

Infectious diseases are found among people of all ages, races, and geographic locations. They can be difficult to manage because of human susceptibilities, environmental factors, and their ability to evolve and develop resistance to antibiotics. Across the world, infectious disease is a significant cause of morbidity, disability, and death.

Many infectious diseases of viral origin, such as measles, mumps, and rubella, were once the bane of childhood, but the advent of mandatory immunizations has helped lessen their impact. Parasitic infections, such as malaria, are present in developing countries but are uncommon in industrialized regions. With the increase in international travel, however, diseases previously endemic to specific regions have the potential to spread across the globe.

Clinical settings contain different populations of bacteria, viruses, fungi, and parasites, many of which are resistant to drugs. All patients, particularly those who are immunosuppressed, are susceptible to microbial invasions developing into health-care–acquired (previously called nosocomial) infections. Therefore

all clinicians, regardless of setting, need to be aware of prevention, pathophysiology, diagnosis, and treatment of infectious disease.

Basic Concepts of Infection

Humans are constantly exposed to microorganisms. Pathogens, specific microorganisms that are capable of causing infectious disease, are categorized mainly as viruses, bacteria, fungi, and parasites. These pathogens are capable of invading, colonizing, and stimulating an inflammatory reaction in host tissues. **Host** is the term used to describe the human or animal invaded and colonized by a **pathogen**, whereas **infection** describes the invasion, colonization, and multiplication of pathogens within the host. **Colonization** indicates that a pathogen is living within the host, but does not mean infection exists. Infection is diagnosed when there is isolation of a pathogen or evidence of its presence and pathogen-related host symptoms.

Different pathogens have varying disease-producing potential, which is called **virulence**. Various virulence factors enhance the pathogen's ability to infect the host. Examples of virulence factors include pathogenic toxins that destroy host cells, adhesion factors that enhance attachment of the pathogen to the host cells, and evasive factors that shield or hide the pathogen from the host's immune system. The severity of infection depends on the pathogen's virulence and the strength of the host's defenses at the time of infection.

A reservoir and a vector may also be involved in infection transmission. A **reservoir** is a source of a pathogenic organism that may or may not be suffering from the disease caused by the pathogen. A child suffering from chickenpox would be considered a reservoir because they harbor the transmissible microorganism. Environmental objects, called fomites, can also act as reservoirs of microorganisms. An unsanitary bathroom surface is an example of a fomite.

A **vector** is a living being that can carry the pathogenic organism from the reservoir to the host. Commonly a vector is an insect, such as a mosquito, tick, or housefly. A vector is not considered infected with the organism but is needed to transmit the pathogen to the host (see Fig. 10-1).

The study of infectious disease requires an understanding of pathogens at the population, individual, cellular, and molecular levels. For example, HIV has infected so many people across the world that it has decreased the immune strength of the population as a whole. At the individual level, HIV causes immunosuppression and consequent susceptibility to opportunistic infections, which can be transmitted from individual to individual. At the cellular level, HIV attacks CD4 cells (also known as T helper cells) and macrophages, which are integral to the immune response. Loss of CD4 cells and macrophages causes dysfunction of other body systems. Finally, at the molecular level, there is a gene that confers resistance to HIV in certain individuals. Study of this gene may lead to the development of a vaccine that could prevent HIV infection.

Epidemiology is the study of disease distributions in human populations. Epidemiological data include **incidence**, which is the number of new cases of infection within a population, and **prevalence**, which is the number of active ongoing cases of infection at any given time. A disease is considered **endemic** if the incidence and prevalence are relatively stable; an **epidemic** is an abrupt increase in the incidence of disease within a geographic region. A **pandemic** is a term used for global spread of a specific disease.

Normal Microbial Flora Versus Pathogens

The human body contains numerous species of bacteria that are considered normal flora. Normal microbial flora are organisms that perform advantageous functions for

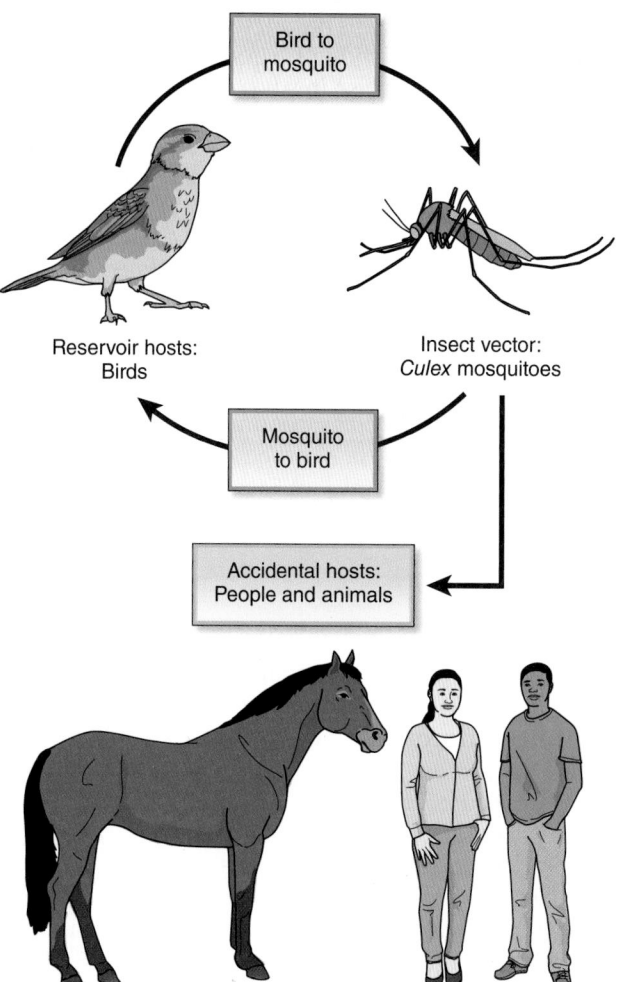

FIGURE 10-1. Example of the infection transmission cycle. *(From California West Nile Virus website, http://westnile.ca.gov/)*

the life of the host and reside in a specific niche in the human body. Staphylococci live on skin surfaces; lactobacilli, *Escherichia coli,* and bacteroides reside within the gastrointestinal (GI) tract; and streptococci are normal inhabitants of the vagina. Microorganisms that serve as normal flora secrete needed nutrients, perform necessary metabolic activities, and help defend the body against other microorganisms. Normal flora do not cause infection when they remain within the strict boundaries of their anatomical niche in the body. However, if normal flora bacteria invade noncolonized areas of the body, they can cause infection.

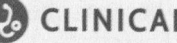 CLINICAL CONCEPT

Clinicians must be careful to not allow normal flora to invade sterile areas of the body when performing invasive procedures. For example, if an intravenous catheter is inserted without properly disinfecting the skin, staphylococci from the skin can be transferred into the bloodstream. Infection of the bloodstream is termed **septicemia (sepsis)**.

In general, all humans harbor the same normal flora. However, some individuals carry specific microbes that do not cause disease for them but can cause infection in others. These individuals, who can carry certain bacteria and transmit infection to susceptible individuals, are known as carriers.

🔬 CLINICAL CONCEPT

Mary Mallon was a cook for a number of families in New York in the early 1900s. Although healthy herself, Mary was a carrier of the bacteria that cause typhoid fever. Many members of the families she worked for became ill with typhoid, and several died. Each time, Mary moved onto another job, and the cycle repeated itself. Because of this, history remembers her as Typhoid Mary.

Individuals are exposed to many common microorganisms within the environment on a daily basis. The term **immunocompetence** refers to an individual's ability to protect herself or himself from infectious agents because of a strong immune system. **Immunosuppression** indicates that there is a defective immune system that is placing a person at risk for infections. From a young age, an immunocompetent person builds immune defenses and swiftly eliminates many microorganisms as threats of infection. However, if the individual becomes immunosuppressed, common microorganisms can overwhelm the weakened immune defenses and multiply within the body to cause an **opportunistic infection**, which is an infection caused by a microorganism that flourishes because of a host's deficient immune system.

Hospitalized patients are in a precarious situation with respect to pathogenic microorganisms. The hospital environment exposes bacteria to a wide variety of antibiotics. Bacteria can adapt to many antibiotics, resulting in a high number of bacteria within the hospital environment that are antibiotic-resistant. Hospitalized patients are vulnerable to infection because of illness, surgery, and other invasive procedures. A patient infection caused by microorganisms that originated within the clinical environment is called a **hospital-acquired** or **health-care–acquired infection** (previously termed nosocomial infection). These infections may be difficult to treat because they are often caused by antibiotic-resistant bacteria.

ALERT!

ALERT! Hospital personnel often inadvertently spread microbes from one patient to another because of lack of proper hand washing and poor sterile technique. Careful hand washing is critical to patients' health.

Types of Microorganisms

Many types of pathogenic microorganisms are capable of causing infectious disease. Each microorganism has unique characteristics, mechanisms of disease, and methods of elimination. The clinician needs a broad understanding of the agents of infectious disease, diagnostic methods, and the antibiotics that can be used to eliminate them.

Bacteria

Bacteria are ubiquitous, free-living microorganisms within the environment that can be either advantageous or harmful to humans. The human body is colonized with bacteria as normal flora on the skin and within the oropharynx, GI tract, and vaginal canal. Bacteria are categorized according to their shape, aerobic or anaerobic respiratory capability, and the laboratory staining of their cell wall structure.

The common shapes of bacterial microorganisms are round, called cocci, and rod-shaped, called bacilli. A small number of bacteria, called spirochetes, are spiral-shaped (Fig. 10-2). Chlamydiae, rickettsiae, and mycoplasma are unique types of bacteria that have distinctive features and cannot be categorized according to their shape.

Cocci bacteria can be found living unattached to each other in the environment in clusters. Alternatively, they can be found in chains, called streptococci, or in duos, called diplococci.

Gram staining is a laboratory procedure used to identify and highlight bacterial organisms within infected tissue. Bacteria stain differently depending on the composition of their cell wall. The cell wall of bacterial organisms is made up of different percentages of peptidoglycan, an amino acid and sugar complex. **Gram-positive** bacteria have a thick, peptidoglycan-rich cell wall that takes on a characteristic purple color when subjected to the staining procedure in the laboratory. **Gram-negative** bacteria have a thin cell wall that contains less peptidoglycan and takes on a pink-colored stain.

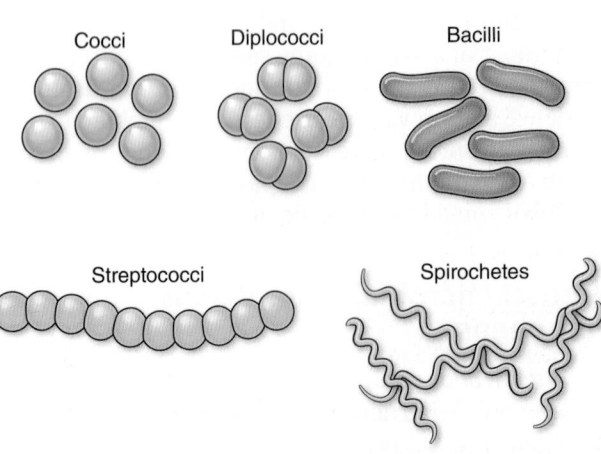

FIGURE 10-2. Categories of bacteria according to shape.

There are certain bacteria that cause common infectious diseases. Clinicians should be familiar with names and characteristic features associated with these bacteria (Table 10-1). Bacteria are usually referred to by the genus to which they belong, followed by the species, or name of the specific bacteria. For example, the bacterium that causes gonorrhea is called *Neisseria gonorrhoeae,* meaning it belongs to the genus *Neisseria* and the species *gonorrhoeae*. It is common to abbreviate the names of bacteria by using the capitalized initial of the genus, followed by the species name, such as *N. gonorrhoeae*. Both genus and species terms are italicized.

Viruses

Viruses are microorganisms that depend on a host cell's metabolic processes for their life cycle. They consist of a DNA or ribonucleic acid (RNA) genome surrounded by a protein coat (see Fig. 10-3). In general, a virus enters a human cell and reprograms the

TABLE 10-1. Common Disease-Causing Bacteria

Species Name	Common Disease Presentation
Staphylococcus aureus	Skin and wound infections, impetigo, pneumonia, septicemia
Streptococcus pyogenes or group A beta-hemolytic *Streptococcus* (GABHS)	Pharyngitis, impetigo, upper respiratory tract infection, rheumatic fever, scarlet fever, glomerulonephritis
Streptococcus pneumoniae (pneumococcus)	Community-acquired pneumonia
Escherichia coli	Urinary tract infection, wound infection, pneumonia, septicemia
Klebsiella pneumoniae	
Enterobacter aerogenes	
Pseudomonas aeruginosa	
Haemophilus influenzae	Meningitis, upper and lower respiratory tract infection
Legionella pneumophila	Legionnaire's disease
Bordetella pertussis	Whooping cough
Shigella	Gastroenterocolitis
Vibrio cholerae	
Campylobacter jejuni	
Enteropathogenic E. coli	
Salmonella	
Clostridium tetani	Tetanus
Clostridium botulinum	Botulism
Clostridium perfringens	Gas gangrene, necrotizing cellulitis
Clostridium difficile	Pseudomembranous colitis
Mycobacterium tuberculosis	Tuberculosis
Bacillus anthracis	Anthrax
Borrelia burgdorferi	Lyme disease
Treponema pallidum	Syphilis
Neisseria meningitidis (meningococcus)	Meningitis
Neisseria gonorrhoeae	Gonorrhea

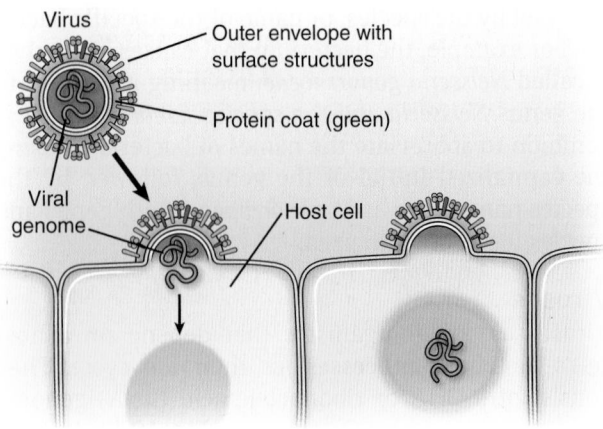

FIGURE 10-3. A typical virus has an outer envelope with specific surface structures designed to attach to a host cell surface. A protein coat lies beneath the envelope, and the viral genome in the form of DNA or RNA is in the center. The goal of the virus is to inject its DNA or RNA into a host cell. The viral DNA or RNA can then direct the activities of the host cell and manufacture more viral particles.

infected cell to synthesize viral particles. This viral replication continues for the virus's life cycle, a time frame that varies for different types of viruses. Most viruses, such as influenza and rhinovirus, cause transient, acute illnesses. However, certain viruses, such as hepatitis B, can persist and cause chronic infection, which damages tissues. Other viruses can cause acute illness; enter a dormant, nonreplicating stage; and then reactivate at a later time. The most common example of this type of viral infection involves herpes viruses.

CLINICAL CONCEPT

Varicella zoster causes an acute, transient illness commonly known as chickenpox that consists of a blister-like rash and an upper respiratory infection. After resolution of the illness, the virus is able to remain dormant within the dorsal ganglia of the spinal cord. Later in life, when immunity is weakened, this blister-like illness can reactivate and cause a condition called herpes zoster, also known as shingles. The adult endures painful, blister-like lesions along the distribution of the involved spinal nerve.

In addition to causing infections, some viruses can initiate cancer cell growth in host cells. An example of this type of virus is human papillomavirus, which can cause cervical cancer.

At present, antibiotic medications are able to kill various kinds of bacteria, but not viruses. Some antiviral drugs are available that can inhibit certain metabolic actions of viruses within host cells. A number of

viruses commonly cause human illness, and clinicians should be familiar with the names of these organisms (see Table 10-2).

Fungi

Fungi are moldlike organisms that can live on human tissue and cause infectious disease. They are diagnosed by the characteristic appearance of filamentous, or string-like, structures found on culture. Fungal

TABLE 10-2. Common Viruses That Cause Disease

Viral Pathogen	Common Disease Presentation
Adenovirus	Upper respiratory tract infection
Rhinovirus	Upper respiratory infection
Coronavirus	Upper respiratory infection
Influenza virus	Influenza
Respiratory syncytial virus (RSV)	Bronchiolitis, pneumonia
Mumps virus	Mumps, pancreatitis, orchitis
Norovirus	Gastroenteritis
Hepatitis A, B, C, D, and E virus	Acute or chronic hepatitis
Measles virus	Rubeola
Rubella virus	Rubella
Varicella zoster virus	Chickenpox, shingles
Herpes simplex virus 1	Cold sores
Herpes simplex virus 2	Genital herpes
Parvovirus	Erythema infectiosum
Coxsackie virus	Hand–foot–mouth disease, herpangina, severe acute respiratory syndrome (SARS)
Epstein-Barr virus	Infectious mononucleosis
Human papillomavirus	Condyloma accuminata; oral, throat, and anal cancer
HIV1 and HIV2	HIV infection and AIDS
Regional hemorrhagic fever virus	Ebola, Marburg disease
Arboviral encephalitis viruses	Eastern equine encephalitis, Western equine encephalitis, Venezuelan equine encephalitis, St. Louis encephalitis

infections, also called mycoses, are classified as superficial or deep infections. **Dermatophytes**, such as tinea (ringworm), are fungi that cause superficial infections involving the skin, hair, or nails. Invasive, systemic mycoses, such as *Candida albicans,* occur most often in an immunocompromised host and can cause fatal disseminated infection. The clinician should be familiar with a number of significant disease-causing fungi (see Table 10-3).

Parasites

Protozoa, helminths, and insects are parasites capable of causing infection in humans. Protozoa are single-celled organisms present within the environment that can infect the body through the skin and genitourinary and GI tracts. Contaminated water, food, or disease-carrying insects can transmit protozoa. Mosquitoes that carry the *Plasmodium* protozoan organism transmit malaria by injecting it into the human bloodstream. Other common clinical examples of protozoan infections are amebiasis and giardiasis, which are both acquired from contaminated water. Helminths are worms that can invade the body via the skin or GI tract; examples include pinworms, tapeworms, and roundworms.

Insects can be the direct cause of disease or be a vector of disease. An insect that acts as a vector harbors a pathogen and transmits the pathogen to humans via its sting or bite. The deer tick acts as a vector, harboring the *Borrelia burgdorferi* bacterium that causes Lyme disease in humans. A few of the many significant disease-producing parasites are listed in Table 10-4.

Prions

Prions are unique proteinaceous infectious agents capable of causing brain diseases in animals and humans. They are resistant to human proteases and have the ability to confer this resistance to other proteins in human cells. It is believed that prions enter neurons in the brain and convert existing proteins into prion-type protein. These abnormal proteins accumulate within large areas of brain tissue, causing distinctive histological changes within brain tissue and

TABLE 10-4. Common Parasites That Cause Disease

Protozoan Parasites	Common Disease Presentation
Entamoeba histolytica	Amebic dysentery, liver abscess
Giardia lamblia	Giardiasis diarrheal illness
Trichomonas vaginalis	Vaginitis
Cryptosporidium	Enterocolitis
Toxoplasma gondii	Toxoplasmosis
Plasmodium	Malaria
Helminth Parasites	**Common Disease Presentation**
Taenia saginata	Tapeworm infection
Trichinella spiralis	Trichinosis
Schistosoma	Schistosomiasis
Trichuris trichiura	Whipworm
Enterobius vermicularis	Pinworms

a condition called spongiform encephalopathy, literally meaning sponge-like damage to the brain. Prions cause animal diseases such as bovine spongiform encephalopathy (BSE; "mad cow disease") and scrapie, which is a disease in sheep. Among humans, prions cause Creutzfeldt-Jakob disease, an encephalopathy transmitted through infected beef.

All the spongiform encephalopathies are untreatable and fatal. Some forms of prion disease are inherited because of a defective gene that allows normal brain cell proteins to transform into abnormal prion-type proteins. Currently, prion-induced diseases are not fully understood.

Mechanisms of Infection

To gain entry and infect the host, pathogenic organisms must penetrate or overwhelm the host's defensive barriers. The human body has two primary levels of defenses:

1. Innate immunity
2. Adaptive immunity

The innate defensive barriers include the skin, mucous membranes, phagocytic cells, ciliated cells, and mediators of the inflammatory reaction. Innate immunity is a nonspecific mechanism that defends the body immediately against all types of pathogens. Sensitized T lymphocytes and B lymphocytes, which have memory for specific antigens, comprise the defenses known as adaptive immunity. Adaptive immunity is developed with exposure to antigens and targets precise pathogens.

TABLE 10-3. Common Fungi That Cause Disease

Fungus	Common Disease Presentation
Candida	Candidiasis
Trichophyton	Tinea
Histoplasma	Histoplasmosis
Pneumocystis jirovecii	Pneumonia
Aspergillus	Aspergillosis
Coccidioides	Coccidioidomycosis

Portals of Entry

Pathogens can infect the body by skin contact, inhalation, ingestion, sexual transmission, insect or animal bites, or injection. The **portal of entry** for microorganisms can be the skin, respiratory, GI, or urogenital tracts.

Skin. Skin is naturally resistant to infection because of its thick, dense composition and low pH (5.5). The health and integrity of skin is influenced by nutrition, hormones, physical activity, environmental exposures, and systemic disorders. External trauma, burns, insect bites, and other conditions, such as acute and chronic dermatoses, can cause breaks in skin integrity. Urticaria, eczema, acne, and psoriasis are examples of conditions that can cause breaches in intact skin.

The skin surface is inhabited by resident normal flora that include *Staphylococcus epidermidis, Staphylococcus aureus,* Corynebacterium, and *C. albicans.* The skin is most vulnerable to infection when there is a break in the integrity of the surface. Keeping the skin intact, dry, and clean can prevent most skin infections.

Persons with limited mobility should not put pressure on one area of the skin surface for a prolonged period. Pressure on areas of the skin that lie over bony prominences can cause an individual to develop pressure injuries (previously called pressure ulcers or decubitus ulcers), which are breaks in the skin that can evolve into wounds.

Dermatophytes, which cause fungal infections of the hair, nails, and skin, often occur without a breach in the integrity of the skin surface. Dermatophytes, like all fungi, thrive in moist, dark areas; spread from person to person; and are difficult to eliminate once established. A common dermatophyte is tinea or ringworm. There are many types of tinea infection, including *Tinea cruris,* which affects the groin region; *Tinea versicolor,* which affects the whole body; *Tinea capitis,* which affects the scalp; and *Tinea pedis,* commonly called "athlete's foot."

🔬 CLINICAL CONCEPT

Lack of position changes can lead to skin breakdown and pressure injuries, which are vulnerable to infection.

Respiratory Tract. Thousands of different microorganisms are inhaled into the respiratory tract every day. Many of these pathogens are transmitted by droplet infection. Droplets of fluid emitted from sneezes and coughs of infected individuals contain large inoculums (volume of infectious material) of pathogens; when emitted into the air, these droplets are inhaled by individuals who then can become infected and transmit the pathogens to others.

Several defense mechanisms protect the respiratory portal of entry. After inhalation, large microorganisms are trapped by the mucous membranes and mucous secretions and swept away by the ciliated respiratory tract cells. These mechanisms are referred to as mucociliary defenses. Sneezing and coughing are reflexive defensive actions that attempt to expel infectious agents in response to irritation of the respiratory tract. Alveolar macrophages are present to phagocytose small microorganisms that penetrate beyond the mucociliary defenses. The respiratory epithelial cells also secrete interferon, which is the body's natural antiviral cytokine. Immunoglobulin A (IgA) is found in large amounts in the B lymphocytes of the respiratory tract and defends the body against inhaled antigens. Numerous cervical lymph nodes located within the oropharyngeal region store white blood cells (WBCs) to defend against inhaled infectious agents.

Certain microorganisms are capable of evading the first line of defense of the respiratory tract. They accomplish this through a variety of mechanisms. The influenza virus, *Haemophilus influenzae, Bordetella pertussis, Pseudomonas aeruginosa,* and *Mycoplasma pneumoniae* are able to bypass the mucociliary defenses. *Streptococcus pneumoniae* and *S. aureus* often invade a host after a viral infection has impaired the mucociliary defenses. They then enter the alveoli and cause pneumonia consisting of widespread inflammation and infiltration of exudative fluid in the alveolar regions of the lungs. This infiltration is often referred to as a consolidation. *Mycobacterium tuberculosis* is unique because it can evade the phagocytic and killing effects of respiratory tract macrophages in the alveolar regions. Rhinoviruses, which cause the common cold, are able to thrive within the nasal passages and upper respiratory tract, despite the defense mechanisms. Inhaled fungi, such as *Pneumocystis jirovecii* (previously called *Pneumocystis carinii*) and *C. albicans,* can become infectious agents when persons are immunosuppressed.

Gastrointestinal Tract. Most GI pathogens are transmitted by food or drink contaminated with infectious agents. The fecal–oral route is often described as the method of transmission of GI pathogens, which indicates that ingested material was contaminated by fecal matter. Fecal matter contains a large **inoculum** of *E. coli* and *Enterococcus faecalis* and may harbor hepatitis A; many bacteria in the *Shigella* and *Salmonella* geni; *Vibrio cholerae;* or any number of other bacteria, viruses, or parasites. Fecal contamination of drinking water reservoirs may occur because of problems in sewage systems. This contamination may lead to significant levels of bacteria in drinking water. It is therefore necessary to perform frequent analysis of bacteria counts. Transmission of disease by the fecal–oral route may also be the result of food preparation by persons with poor hygiene or lack of sanitary food preparation methods.

The acidic conditions and mucous lining of the stomach and intestine protect the body from invasion by many pathogens. Pancreatic enzymes, bile, mucosal antimicrobial peptides, normal bacterial flora, and lymphoid tissue secretions of IgA antibodies also serve to defend the body against ingested pathogens. Infections via the GI tract usually occur when defenses are weakened. Some microorganisms are relatively resistant to the body's protective mechanisms and may cause infection in an otherwise healthy host. *Helicobacter pylori, Shigella,* and *Giardia* cysts, for example, can resist the acidic environment of the stomach. Viruses such as rotavirus, hepatitis A, and Norwalk virus (also called Norovirus) can resist bile and pancreatic enzymes. Staphylococcus can grow on foods and secrete an enterotoxin, a toxic secretion that targets the gastrointestinal mucosa. The staphylococcal enterotoxin causes a diarrheal illness commonly called food poisoning. *Salmonella typhi,* bacteria found on some foods, can be absorbed from the GI tract, enter the lymphatic system and bloodstream, and cause a systemic infection. *Entamoeba histolytica,* found in contaminated water, erodes the intestinal mucosa and causes a hemorrhagic, diarrheal illness called dysentery. Intestinal parasites can live in the intestine and absorb the host's nutrients.

Genitourinary Tract. Urogenital infections most commonly originate from entry of pathogens into the urethra. Urine outflow through the urethra serves as a protective mechanism that constantly flushes microorganisms out of the body. Certain organisms such as gonococcus and *E. coli* are capable of adhering to bladder mucosa epithelium and thus evade the protective mechanisms afforded by urine outflow.

Female anatomy predisposes to urinary tract infection (UTI) because of the close proximity of the rectal mucosa and urethra. The bowel is the natural habitat for *E. coli,* and urethral invasion into the bladder is common. UTIs can spread retrograde from the urethra and bladder and into the ureter and kidney. Pyelonephritis is an upper UTI that can occur in this manner.

Lactobacilli are colonized in the vaginal canal as normal flora. They break down glycogen stores and keep the vaginal pH low. The low pH is a defensive mechanism that wards off other microbial invaders. The vaginal pH can be altered if the normal flora are eradicated, which can occur as a side effect of antibiotic use. The vaginal canal then becomes susceptible to infection. Vaginal candidiasis is a common side effect of long-term antibiotic use.

Male semen and female vaginal fluids can also transmit microorganisms. Unsafe sexual practices allow for the spread of these microorganisms and the passage of sexually transmitted diseases, which are commonly viral and bacterial infections, between individuals.

Blood–Blood Transmission. Blood transfusion is the most common method of transmission of bloodborne infections, although blood donations are vigilantly screened to prevent transfusion of infected blood. Exposure to bloodborne pathogens can also occur through a needlestick or lacerating injury with a sharp instrument contaminated with infected blood. Intravenous (IV) drug users can contract infection from unsterile needles. Bloodborne pathogens can also enter the body via the eye, naso-oral mucous membranes, and skin. For this reason, universal precautions should be followed when handling patient body fluids and biohazardous material.

Following exposure to bloodborne pathogens, risk of infection depends on the type of exposure, amount of infected blood transferred to the recipient, and the number of pathogens contained in the infected blood. The most commonly transmitted bloodborne pathogens are hepatitis B, hepatitis C, and HIV.

CLINICAL CONCEPT
Health-care and emergency personnel are at highest risk for the occupational hazard of bloodborne infections caused by accidental needlesticks or sharp instrument contamination. This is why it is so important for clinicians to follow all universal precautions.

Maternal–Fetal Transmission. Some pathogens that cause infection in a pregnant woman can be transmitted to the developing fetus in two ways:

1. Pathogens that invade the maternal bloodstream and placenta can pass into the fetal circulation.
2. Maternal infection can be transferred during childbirth when infected vaginal secretions and membranes come in contact with the newborn.

When an infectious disease is passed from mother to newborn, it is called a **congenital** infection. Certain microorganisms are common causes of congenital infection, including cytomegalovirus (CMV), *Toxoplasma gondii, Treponema pallidum* (syphilis), rubella, herpes simplex virus, varicella zoster, parvovirus B19, group B streptococci, and HIV.

Stages of Infection

After a pathogen enters a host, there are five distinct stages of infection:

1. Incubation period
2. Prodromal stage
3. Acute stage
4. Convalescent stage
5. Resolution phase

Different pathogens have distinctive time periods for each stage (see Fig. 10-4).

The incubation period is the phase when the microorganism begins active replication without producing

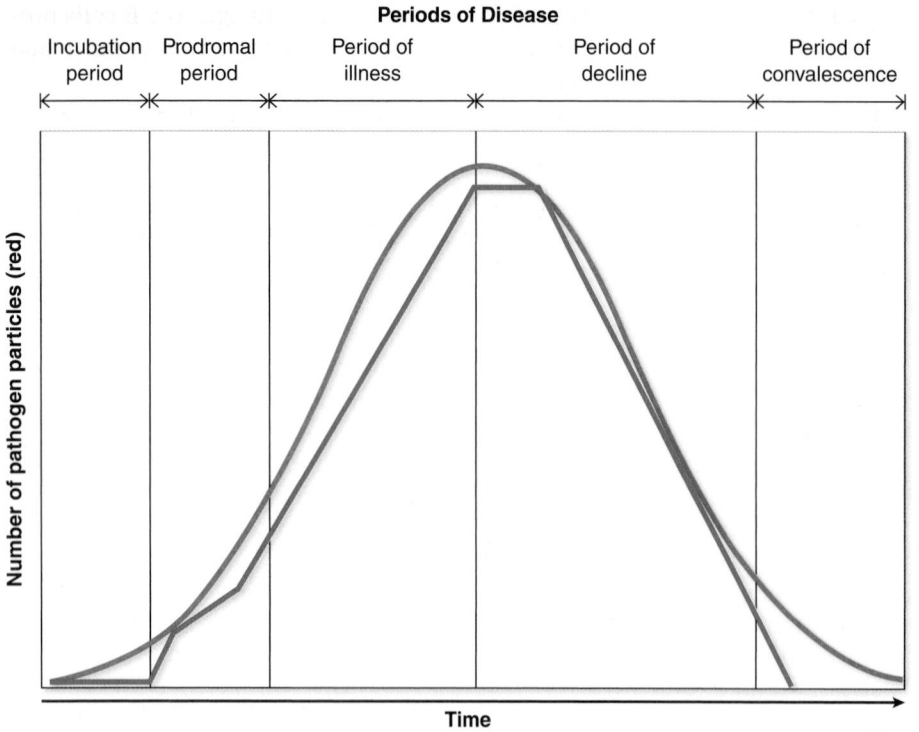

FIGURE 10-4. Stages of infection. (© Nov 1, 2016 OpenStax. Textbook content produced by OpenStax is licensed under a Creative Commons Attribution License 4.0 license.)

identifiable symptoms in the host. Its duration may be short, as in the case of rhinovirus, which causes the common cold and lasts about 24 hours, or prolonged, as in hepatitis B infection, which can last between 1 and 3 months. Some infections are highly contagious during this phase, and the host is usually unaware of the developing illness.

The prodromal stage occurs when the initial appearance of symptoms is apparent in the host. During this time, the host may have only a vague sense of illness with general malaise, myalgias, headache, or fatigue. It is also a time when the host is highly contagious to others.

The acute stage is the period during which the host experiences the full infectious disease with rapid proliferation of the pathogen. The host's defenses are in full force and the inflammation reaction is fully engaged. The host's symptoms are heightened and more specific than in the prodromal stage. The patient remains contagious during this stage.

The convalescent stage is characterized by the body's attempt to contain the infection and progressively eliminate the pathogen. Resolution of symptoms begins to occur and may stretch over days, weeks, or months, depending on the pathogen.

The resolution phase is the time when there is total elimination of the pathogen from the body without residual signs or symptoms.

Immune Responses to Infection

Infection stimulates the body's immune system to defend against an invading pathogen. The two major types of immunity are innate immunity and adaptive immunity. Innate immunity consists of nonspecific, cellular reactions that protect an individual who is exposed to a pathogen. Adaptive immunity consists of specific cellular responses that are stimulated when the body recognizes a pathogen it has encountered in the past. Adaptive immunity most effectively defends the body upon reexposure to a pathogen, whereas innate immunity defends the body in a general manner, regardless of history of exposure to the pathogen.

The innate system is the first level of defense against invasion by pathogens. It consists of anatomical barriers, antipathogenic chemicals, and cellular reactions. The anatomical barriers of the innate immune system include the intact epithelial surface of the skin, as well as the respiratory, GI, and genitourinary tracts. The skin and mucous membranes provide a mechanical and chemical barrier to pathogens. Skin and mucous membranes are protective coverings that secrete certain peptides and enzymes that have antibacterial, antifungal, and antiviral properties. The low pH of sweat also acts as a chemical antipathogenic barrier. In the nose and lungs, cilia act as anatomical barriers to sweep away debris and keep the airways clear. Tears, secreted by the lacrimal glands around the eyes, contain enzymes that help flush pathogens away. The acidic pH of gastric secretions acts as an antipathogenic barrier. In the lower GI and genitourinary tract, mucus traps any ingested pathogens and expels them in the stool or urine.

An acute inflammatory reaction is triggered when the innate immune system is stimulated. The components of the inflammatory reaction act as cellular barriers in the innate immune system. These include

WBCs, the complement system, coagulation system, and cytokines, which are active during the chemotaxis phase of an acute inflammatory reaction.

The complement system also responds to pathogens in the innate and adaptive immune systems. It is composed of enzymes, proteins, and chemical mediators that target and attack pathogens. The complement system acts to mediate antigen–antibody reactions in the adaptive immune responses and enhances the inflammatory reaction.

The adaptive immune system is the second line of defense against the invasion of pathogens. It is slower to respond than the innate system of defense. The adaptive immune system is antigen-specific, reacts to a pathogen that it recognizes, and has a memory for the pathogen. The main cells within this system are the lymphocytes, also called B and T cells. T cells are produced primarily in the thymus, and B cells arise primarily from the bone marrow. Different types of T cells take part in the adaptive immune response. These include cytotoxic and helper T cells. Cytotoxic T cells, also called CD8 cells, directly attack the pathogen, whereas helper T cells, also called CD4 cells, assist CD8 cells and stimulate the proliferation of B cells. B cells produce specialized glycoproteins known as immunoglobulins (Igs) that attack antigens. Igs may be undifferentiated and provide general defense against infection by binding to microbes. These non-specific Igs, also called immunoglobulin D (IgD), are found on the surface of B cells. Once the invading antigens have been bound by the IgD, the B cells produce specific Igs that recognize and bind to particular foreign antigens.

Immunoglobulin M (IgM) is the earliest specific Ig to appear in response to exposure to antigen in the bloodstream. It is responsible for initiating further immune reactions. Immunoglobulin G (IgG) develops later in the course of infection and predominates for many years after exposure, conferring some long-lasting immunity against the specific antigen. Secretory IgA is found on mucosal surfaces and in the bloodstream, and immunoglobulin E (IgE) is produced in response to allergies and parasitic infections. Table 10-5 summarizes these Ig functions.

Importantly, the function of the adaptive immune system is dependent on an intact innate immune system. Toll-like receptors (TLRs) are proteins on the surface of many cells of the innate immune system that detect specific pathogens and play a critical role in stimulating the adaptive immune response. When a TLR detects a pathogen, it relays a signal to the cell's nucleus. The signal switches on specific genes that code for release of substances that perpetuate the innate immune response and stimulate the adaptive immune response.

Diagnosis of Infection

Distinctive signs and symptoms are exhibited by the host during specific infectious processes. Most

TABLE 10-5. Immunoglobulins and Their Functions

Immunoglobulin	Location	Function	Most Active Phase of Infection
IgA	Breast milk, tears	Protect mucous membranes of genitourinary, gastrointestinal, and pulmonary systems	Activity not related to infection; has a protective and preventive role
IgD	Attached to surface of B cells	Binds antigens to B cells	Early stage, when antigen has first entered the body
IgE	Found on mast cells in pulmonary and gastrointestinal tracts	Active in allergic reactions; binds to mast cells and basophils to release histamine and leukotrienes	Not related to infection, found in persons with allergies
IgG	Throughout the bloodstream	Activates complement to release inflammatory and bactericidal mediators Confers long-term immunity, active against viruses, bacteria, antitoxins; moves across maternal–fetal barrier	Late disease, recovery, and long after
IgM	Throughout bloodstream	Initiates complement activity and further immune responses Controls ABO blood reactions	Early infection

infections present with nonspecific symptoms, such as fever, myalgias, lethargy, and anorexia. However, the specific symptoms experienced by the patient often reflect the specific system that is infected. For example, hepatitis presents with jaundice, a sign of liver dysfunction. *Salmonella* infection presents with intestinal symptoms such as nausea, vomiting, and diarrhea. Diagnosis of infection is based on the history, clinical symptoms, physical examination findings, and laboratory testing.

Laboratory Studies

Specimens of infectious material can be subjected to microscopic staining and culture procedures. Bacteria can be classified according to how their cell membrane absorbs a dye such as a Gram stain or acid-fast stain. A culture of the infected tissues or body fluids involves growing the microbes on a specific medium, such as agar, so they can be studied and identified. The extent of infection may be inferred from the number of microorganisms seen per microscopic high-power field or in a specific volume of substrate, such as 1 milliliter. A culture can also be used to yield information about the organism's antibiotic susceptibility. Culture media can be infused with different antibiotics, and growth or suppression of microbes can be observed.

At times, infection is difficult to diagnose and a biopsy of tissue may be needed for histological study. In histological study of tissue, the cells within a biopsy are examined under a microscope for signs of inflammation and infection. The tissue is scrutinized for evidence of the pathogenic organism or characteristic cell changes associated with the pathogen.

Infection can also be confirmed through serological testing that studies the blood serum for the existence of antibodies to the microorganism in the bloodstream. A sample of blood is withdrawn from the patient and tested for the presence of specific antibodies. For example, a person infected with syphilis would develop antibodies to *T. pallidum,* which can be confirmed in a serological study. The level of antibody within the bloodstream is called an **antibody titer**, and usually the titer corresponds to the level of exposure to the microbe. Serological testing can also assist in the staging of infection because levels of IgG and IgM can be measured. IgM is the first Ig to rise in response to infection; IgG rises later.

Direct antigen identification is another method that combines culture and microscopic procedures. The infectious agent is fused with artificially synthesized antibodies that are fluorescent. When the artificial antibody attaches to the antigen, the antigen–antibody complex fluoresces under the microscope, making them easier to identify and quantify.

Yet another technique for identifying an infectious agent is the polymerase chain reaction (PCR) technique, which detects a microorganism's genetic material (DNA or RNA). A specimen containing the infectious agent is mixed with a reagent that targets the pathogen's DNA or RNA. The method can accurately detect extremely low levels of pathogen within a specimen. For example, the HIV RNA assay is a type of PCR diagnostic technique that can determine the number of HIV particles present in the bloodstream.

Treatment and Eradication of Infection

Most infections are self-limiting and will resolve if allowed to progress through the stages of infection. However, when the infectious disease manifestations are prolonged or cause undue risk for the patient or those in contact with the patient, medical therapy is recommended. The treatment may involve antimicrobial agents, immunological boosting agents, or surgical removal of infected tissues.

Antimicrobial agents consist of a wide array of antibacterial, antiviral, antifungal, antiprotozoal, and anthelmintic medications. The most numerous among the antimicrobial agents are antibiotics or antibacterial medications. Bacteria are highly adaptable and commonly develop resistance to available antibiotics when exposed for a prolonged period. This resistance creates a continual need for development of new antibiotic agents.

Prevention of Infection Through Immunization

Prevention of infectious disease through administration of vaccines is the most efficient method of controlling contagious disease within a population. Some infectious diseases, such as smallpox, have been virtually eliminated through the use of vaccines. Although vaccines offer long-term immunity, few confer lifelong immunity and must be readministered at intervals (booster doses) to maintain protection. Recommended immunizations vary by age, health status, and exposure risk of the individual, but are based on protecting public health by decreasing the number of susceptible persons in a population.

Emerging Infectious Diseases

Emerging infectious diseases are diseases that have appeared recently in the population and those that are rapidly increasing in incidence or geographic range. Emergence may be caused by the spread of a new agent, by recognizing an infection that has been present in the population but has gone undetected, or by realizing that an established disease has an infectious origin. Emergence may also be used to describe the reappearance of a known infection after a decline in incidence.

Emergence Versus Reemergence

With the modern ability to travel anywhere in the world in 36 hours or less, unique infections can easily and unknowingly be transmitted to areas where they previously had not been found. Governments have regulations that bar individuals with certain infectious diseases from traveling, but it is nearly impossible to adequately screen every passenger. Furthermore, some diseases are contagious during the incubation and prodromal phases when there are no obvious signs of sickness. In addition, some microbes can survive on inanimate objects, such as doorknobs, keyboards, and telephones, and are transported in this manner. Many emerging diseases arise when infectious agents in animals are passed to humans; these transmitted diseases are called zoonoses. As the human population expands into new geographical regions, the possibility that humans will come into close contact with animal species that are potential hosts of an infectious agent increases. When that factor is combined with increases in human density and mobility, it is easy to see that this combination poses a serious threat to human health.

Another factor that is especially important in the reemergence of disease is the acquired resistance of pathogens to antimicrobial medications such as antibiotics. Over time, bacteria and viruses can change and develop resistance to antimicrobial medications, resulting in the forced disuse of treatments that were once effective in controlling disease. A wide variety of antibiotic-resistant bacteria that are currently challenging clinicians include **methicillin-resistant *Staphylococcus aureus* (MRSA), vancomycin-resistant *Staphylococcus aureus* (VRSA)**, vancomycin-resistant enterococcus (VRE), drug-resistant *Streptococcus pneumoniae* (DRSP), and drug-resistant *Clostridium difficile*. See Table 10-6 for current Centers for Disease Control (CDC) drug-resistant microbial threats.

Reappearance may also occur because of breakdowns in public health measures that had previously controlled a particular infection. For example, if a significant sector of the population refrains from rubella immunization, this can raise the incidence of rubella infection in the total population.

TABLE 10-6. Drug-Resistant Microbial Threats Listed by CDC

Hazard Level	Description	Examples
Urgent	These are high-consequence antibiotic-resistant threats because of significant risks identified across several criteria. These threats may not be currently widespread but have the potential to become so and require urgent public health attention to identify infection and to limit transmission.	*Clostridium difficile* Carbapenem-resistant Enterobacteriaceae (CRE) Drug-resistant *Neisseria gonorrhoeae* (cephalosporin resistance)
Serious	These are significant antibiotic-resistant threats. For varying reasons (e.g., low or declining domestic incidence or reasonable availability of therapeutic agents), they are not considered urgent, but these threats will worsen and may become urgent without ongoing public health monitoring and prevention activities.	Multidrug-resistant *Acinetobacter* Drug-resistant *Campylobacter* Fluconazole-resistant *Candida* (a fungus) Extended-spectrum b-lactamase–producing Enterobacteriaceae (ESBL) Vancomycin-resistant *Enterococcus* (VRE) Multidrug-resistant *Pseudomonas aeruginosa* Drug-resistant nontyphoidal *Salmonella* Drug-resistant *Salmonella typhi* Drug-resistant *Shigella* Methicillin-resistant *Staphylococcus aureus* (MRSA) Drug-resistant *Streptococcus pneumonia* Drug-resistant tuberculosis (MDR and XDR)
Concerning	These are bacteria for which the threat of antibiotic resistance is low and/or there are multiple therapeutic options for resistant infections. These bacterial pathogens cause severe illness. Threats in this category require monitoring and, in some cases, rapid incident or outbreak response.	Vancomycin-resistant *Staphylococcus aureus* (VRSA) Erythromycin-resistant *Streptococcus* group A Clindamycin-resistant *Streptococcus* group B

Adapted from https://www.cdc.gov/drugresistance/biggest_threats.html

Infectious Agents and Bioterrorism

The world has become highly vigilant of the threat of bioterrorism in recent years. Some infectious agents can be used as weapons and harm large segments of the population. Biological agents with the potential to be used as weapons can be classified based on ease of dissemination or transmission, potential for major public health impact, and requirements for public health preparedness. Agents of high concern include:

- *Bacillus anthracis* (anthrax)
- *Yersinia pestis* (plague)
- *Variola major* (smallpox)
- *Clostridium botulinum* toxin (botulism)
- *Francisella tularensis* (tularemia)
- Filoviruses (Ebola hemorrhagic fever, Marburg hemorrhagic fever)

Many governments are engaged in research on how to protect their populations from this particular form of warfare.

Selected Bacterial Infections

Staphylococcus and streptococcus are two kinds of bacteria that are normal flora of the human body as well as instigators of infectious disease. In recent years, these bacteria have become major challenges to clinicians because of antibiotic resistance. *Neisseria meningitidis,* also known as meningococcus, resides within the nasopharynx and can cause a serious bloodstream infection as well as meningitis. It is important to keep a high index of suspicion for meningococcal infection when examining schoolchildren, college students, and military recruits with flulike illness who live in close quarters such as dormitories.

Staphylococcal Infections

Staphylococci are hardy, gram-positive, round microorganisms that form clusters. They are capable of surviving for prolonged periods on inanimate surfaces in variable conditions. One of the most important and ubiquitous strains is *S. aureus,* which colonizes the skin, vagina, nares, and oropharynx as normal flora. *S. aureus* can change from normal flora to an infectious agent and has become the leading cause of health-care–associated infection and surgical wound infection. In the community, *S. aureus* is a major cause of skin and soft tissue infections, osteomyelitis, respiratory infections, and among IV drug abusers, endocarditis. *S. aureus* can also cause food contamination leading to staphylococcal food poisoning (SFP). The toxins secreted by the staphylococcus bacteria can cause severe GI illness. Toxins are heat-resistant and can contaminate meats, dairy products, and leafy green vegetables.

S. aureus has developed resistance to many antibiotics, and strains such as MRSA and VRSA are commonly encountered in clinical settings. Because of an ability to produce three types of toxins, *S. aureus* can cause life-threatening illness such as septicemia. *S. aureus* can also cause a wide range of infections affecting almost every body system.

S. epidermidis, also a constituent of normal flora, and *S. saprophyticus* are other staph organisms that normally colonize the skin and can cause infection. However, *S. aureus* is a most virulent strain because it secretes proteases, produces hemolytic toxins that degrade host cells, and has the genetic ability to develop antibiotic resistance.

Antibiotic-Resistant Staphylococcus Aureus

The introduction of the antibiotic penicillin in the 1940s dramatically reduced the morbidity and mortality associated with bacterial infections. Penicillin seemed to be a panacea until strains of penicillin-resistant organisms evolved. Some strains of *S. aureus* developed genetic changes that enabled the organism to secrete penicillinase, also called *beta lactamase,* an enzyme that destroys penicillin and allows the organism to resist the antibiotic. The emergence of penicillin-resistant *S. aureus* created a need to develop new antibiotics that could resist beta lactamase. Methicillin had been the most commonly used drug for that purpose. However, within 1 year after the introduction of methicillin, methicillin-resistant strains of *S. aureus* were found. Despite a steady, slow increase in the number of methicillin-resistant strains of *S. aureus,* methicillin and its derivatives, oxacillin, nafcillin, cloxacillin, and dicloxacillin, were effective against *S. aureus* for many years. A dramatic rise in methicillin-resistant strains of *S. aureus* occurred in the 1990s.

Approximately 40% to 50% of *S. aureus* strains found in hospitals are resistant to methicillin, as well as to many other antibiotics. As resistant strains increased, vancomycin became the sole antibiotic effective against MRSA. However, with time and exposure to vancomycin, some strains of *S. aureus* have become resistant to vancomycin and its derivatives. Identifying an antibiotic to kill VRSA became the challenge for pharmacologists.

MRSA infection is especially problematic in hospitals and other congregate settings. Strict isolation procedures and universal precautions by health-care providers are necessary to prevent transmission of the infection. Scrupulous hand washing practices among health-care personnel is a key prevention strategy. Health-care providers should be vigilant about disinfecting diagnostic equipment such as stethoscopes when using them for multiple patients in the hospital environment. Patients with antibiotic-resistant infections should have dedicated equipment that is not used for any other patients.

Community-acquired MRSA infections are a treatment challenge. The widespread use of broad-spectrum antibiotics in health care and the addition of antibiotics in livestock feed exposes bacteria to our arsenal of antibiotics. This exposure allows bacteria to develop genetic changes leading to resistance.

Presently, *S. aureus,* enterococcus, and *S. pneumoniae* are the bacterial organisms most resistant to available antibiotics. It is a constant challenge for researchers to develop newer and more effective antibiotics in this era of continuing bacterial resistance.

Streptococcal Infections

A number of streptococcal organisms cause human disease. **Group A beta hemolytic streptococcus (GABHS),** also called *Streptococcus pyogenes,* is a bacterium that causes many different infections. These bacteria have capsules that resist WBC phagocytosis and secrete substances that degrade tissue membranes. Streptococci can also release an exotoxin that can cause fever and rash.

Streptococci are gram-positive, spherical organisms in chains that produce zones of hemolysis when cultured on blood agar, referred to as beta hemolysis. GABHS secretes large numbers of extracellular products that enhance its toxicity in the spread of infection through tissues. These products include streptolysins S and O, streptokinase, DNAases, protease, and exotoxins. GABHS can infect almost every body system; before the advent of antibiotics, it commonly caused serious complications. Rheumatic fever, streptococcal pharyngitis (strep throat), scarlet fever, glomerulonephritis, skin infections, pneumonia, necrotizing fasciitis, and toxic shock syndrome are among the many possible diseases caused by GABHS (see Fig. 10-5).

GABHS infection is also associated with pediatric autoimmune neuropsychiatric disorder associated with Streptococcus (PANDAS). Children are diagnosed with PANDAS when obsessive-compulsive disorder or tics appear shortly after sustaining a streptococcal infection. Usually sudden in onset, children can become anxious, irritable, and develop vocal or motor tics. Sleep problems, hyperactivity, emotional lability, joint pain, and motor difficulties can also occur.

Other streptococcal bacteria can cause a number of significant diseases. *S. pneumoniae* is the major cause of community-acquired pneumonia and can cause meningitis. *S. faecalis,* also called *E. faecalis,* is a major cause of UTIs, health-care–acquired bacteremia, and endocarditis. *S. viridans* can also cause infective endocarditis.

 CLINICAL CONCEPT

In persons suffering from sore throat, a throat culture is the only method that can accurately diagnose or rule out GABHS pharyngitis. In some individuals, GABHS can cause rheumatic fever and rheumatic heart disease (RHD), a condition involving the development of a heart murmur. In RHD, an immune reaction occurs; antibodies developed against GABHS mistakenly attack heart valve tissue and cause valvular deformities.

Bacterial Pneumonias

Bacteria are hardy microorganisms that commonly invade the respiratory tract via the nasopharynx. Bacteria can invade lower respiratory tract tissues, stimulate inflammation, and create an exudative fluid that hinders oxygen exchange at the alveoli. Exudative fluid in and around the alveoli is referred to as a consolidation when seen on chest x-ray, but is most commonly known as pneumonia.

Streptococcus Pneumoniae
S. pneumoniae (Pneumococcus) is the most common cause of **community-acquired pneumonia (CAP)**. This is a gram-positive, diplococcal bacterium that colonizes the nasopharynx. After colonization, organisms may gain access to areas of the upper and lower respiratory tracts by direct extension. Under normal conditions in a healthy host, anatomical and ciliary clearance mechanisms prevent clinical infection. However, clearance may be inhibited by chronic factors such as smoking, allergies, and bronchitis, as well as acute factors such as viral infection and allergies, both of which can lead to infection. Influenza is a common precursor of streptococcal pneumonia. Alternatively, pneumococci may reach normally sterile areas, such as the blood, peritoneum, cerebrospinal fluid (CSF), or joint fluid, by hematogenous spread after mucosal invasion. The most vulnerable individuals are children younger than 2 years old and adults aged 60 years and older. Pneumococcal pneumonia affects approximately 100 per 100,000 adults each year and has a mortality rate of 20% annually.

Classically, pneumonia is preceded by a viral illness that is followed by an acute onset of high fever—often with rigors, productive cough, pleuritic chest pain, dyspnea, tachypnea, tachycardia, sweats, malaise, and fatigue. The patient may report blood-tinged sputum.

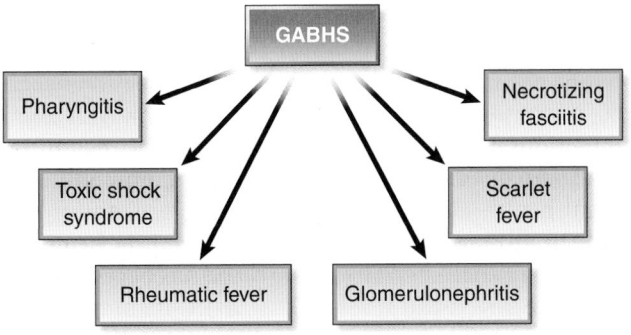

FIGURE 10-5. Diseases caused by GABHS.

Patients typically appear ill and may have an anxious appearance. On physical examination, crackles can be heard in the lung region affected by the pneumonia. About half of all patients exhibit dullness to percussion over the involved lung region. Diagnostic tests include chest x-ray and sputum culture. Chest x-ray shows consolidation in the region of pneumonia (see Fig. 10-6). A serotype-specific urinary antigen test can also be used to diagnose pneumonia due to *S. pneumoniae.*

Another laboratory test that measures procalcitonin levels in the blood is used in the diagnosis of bacterial infections. Antibiotic susceptibilities should be obtained routinely on all cultures with growth of *S. pneumoniae.* Antibiotic resistance to penicillin and erythromycin is commonly encountered with these bacteria.

Pneumococcal vaccine every 5 to 10 years has been recommended for older adults and has greatly reduced infections. Routine childhood pneumococcal conjugate vaccine, introduced in 2000, has decreased rates of invasive pneumococcal infections by greater than 90%.

Mycoplasma Pneumoniae

Mycoplasma pneumonia is an infection of the lungs from *M. pneumoniae,* a very small bacterium without a cell wall. It causes an atypical pneumonia that commonly affects people younger than 40 years. This type of pneumonia is often referred to as "walking pneumonia" because the affected individual does not appear very ill. Various studies suggest that it makes up 15% to 50% of all pneumonia cases in adults and even more in school-aged children. People at highest risk for mycoplasma pneumonia include those living or working in crowded areas such as schools and homeless shelters, although many people who contract mycoplasma pneumonia have no identifiable risk factor. It is spread by droplet infection. The symptoms are generally mild and appear over a period of 1 to 3 weeks. Common symptoms include fever, sore throat, chills, cough, myalgias, headache, and earache. In this type of pneumonia, headache and earache are unique symptoms. A complete physical examination and a chest x-ray are necessary. Sputum culture may be necessary. Treatment includes specific antibiotics that affect bacteria without a cell wall, such as tetracyclines, and supportive measures.

Legionnaire's Disease

Legionnaire's disease is an acute respiratory infection caused by gram-negative bacteria called *Legionella pneumophila.* The bacterium was named in 1976 when people who attended a Philadelphia convention of the American Legion suffered an outbreak of this disease. These bacteria are found most often in the warm, moist air conditioning systems of large buildings, though they have also been found in water delivery systems. The microbe is transmitted via aerosolized mist in the air. Person-to-person transmission has not been shown. Most infections occur in middle-aged or older people, although they also have been reported in children. Risk factors include alcoholism; cigarette smoking; diseases such as kidney failure or diabetes; diseases or medications that weaken the immune system, including cancer and steroids; long-term (chronic) lung disease such as chronic obstructive pulmonary disease (COPD); and use of a ventilator. Symptoms include dyspnea, chest pain, nonproductive cough, chills, hemoptysis, fever, nausea, vomiting, diarrhea, headache, arthralgias, and possible ataxia. These symptoms tend to get worse during the first 4 to 6 days and typically improve in another 4 to 5 days. Diagnostic tests include chest x-ray, sputum culture, and urine antigen test. Antibiotics are the major treatment measure.

Pseudomonas Infection

Pseudomonas is a gram-negative rod that is widespread in nature, inhabiting soil, water, plants, and animals, including humans. *P. aeruginosa* has become an important cause of infection, especially in patients with compromised host defense mechanisms. It is the most common pathogen isolated from patients who have been hospitalized longer than 1 week. It is a frequent cause of health-care–acquired infections such as pneumonia, UTIs, and bacteremia. Pseudomonal infections are complicated and can be life threatening.

P. aeruginosa is also the fourth most commonly isolated health-care–acquired pathogen, accounting for 10% of all hospital-acquired infections. It is found on the skin of some healthy persons and has been isolated from the throat and stool of 5% and 3% of nonhospitalized patients, respectively. The GI carriage rate among hospitalized patients increases to 20% within 72 hours

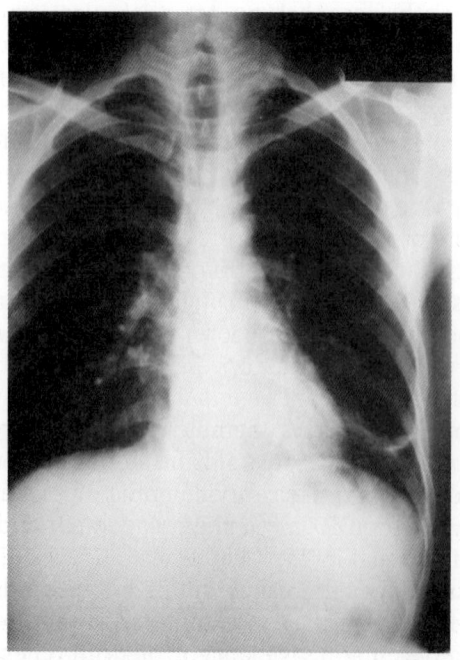

FIGURE 10-6. Chest x-ray showing lobar pneumonia. *(Courtesy of CDC/Dr. Thomas Hooten.)*

of admission. Predisposing conditions include placement of IV lines, severe burns, urinary tract catheterization, surgery, trauma, and premature birth (in infants).

In pseudomonas pneumonia, patients have crackles, rhonchi, fever, cyanosis, retractions, and hypoxia. Shock may develop in patients with bacteremic pneumonia. Pseudomonal bacteremia occurs in association with malignancy, chemotherapy, AIDS, burn wounds, and diabetes.

Diagnostic procedures depend on the site of *Pseudomonas* infection. In pneumonia, sputum culture, chest x-ray, and blood cultures are necessary. Double antibiotic therapy is needed for treatment.

Bacterial Meningitis Infection

Meningitis is a potentially fatal infectious disease caused by inflammation of the meningeal layers that surround and protect the brain and spinal cord. Meningitis is most commonly caused by viruses or strains of bacteria. *S. pneumoniae* (pneumococcus), *Neisseria meningitides* (meningococcus), and *H. influenzae* are bacterial causes of meningitis. Bacterial meningitis is a very serious illness, whereas viral meningitis, also called aseptic meningitis, is usually a milder disorder.

The key signs of meningitis are fever, nuchal rigidity (stiff neck), and headache. Certain kinds of meningitis can present with an accompanying rash. Kernig's and Brudzinski's signs are commonly exhibited by the patient during physical examination (see Fig. 10-7). The diagnosis of meningitis requires a lumbar puncture, a test that allows sampling and culturing of the CSF. High-dose antibiotic therapy is necessary for bacterial meningitis. Viral meningitis usually resolves by

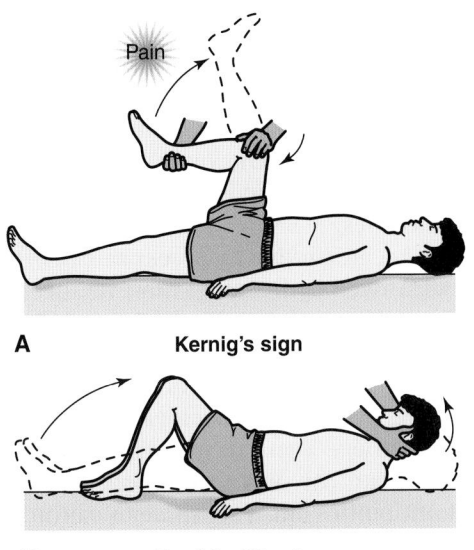

A **Kernig's sign**

B **Brudzinski's sign**

FIGURE 10-7. (A) In Kernig's sign, attempt to extend the leg at the knee. The patient feels pain in the neck and leg. (B) In Brudzinski's sign, the patient flexes knees and hips when you flex the neck.

itself and requires supportive treatment. Complications of meningitis include seizures, brain damage, ischemia of extremities, and visual or hearing losses. Bacterial meningitis can be prevented by immunization with *Haemophilus influenzae* b (Hib), meningococcal, and pneumococcal vaccines.

Neisseria Meningitidis

Meningitis is commonly caused by the bacterium *N. meningitidis*, which is also known as meningococcus, a gram-negative, diplococcus bacteria. The human nasopharynx is a known reservoir for *N. meningitidis*. Meningococci spread from person to person by droplet infection. The prevalence is approximately 1 to 2 cases per 100,000 population, but outbreaks of meningococcal disease have occurred in some specific populations. Outbreaks often involve persons living in close quarters, such as those who are incarcerated, college students living in dormitories, and military recruit populations. Although not common, school-age children have spread meningococcal infection to each other. Exposure of school-age children to meningococcus commonly requires prophylactic antibiotic treatment.

Meningococcal infection usually first occurs in the bloodstream as meningococcemia. This infection can range in severity from a transient bacteremia that is benign to an overwhelming infection that is rapidly fatal. Meningitis commonly occurs during the course of meningococcemia. At first, meningitis may seem like an upper respiratory illness with pharyngitis, fever, and chills. However, the disorder rapidly deteriorates into more severe symptoms such as high fever, malaise, weakness, myalgias, headache, nausea, vomiting, and arthralgias. Nuchal rigidity (stiff neck), photophobia, and headache are signs of meningitis. Nuchal rigidity can be confirmed on physical assessment by Kernig's and Brudzinski's signs. Lethargy, drowsiness, or coma, which is an ominous sign, can occur. Alternatively, apprehension, restlessness, and, frequently, delirium can occur. Encephalopathy refers to mental status changes that can occur, such as disorientation, confusion, and memory loss. A skin rash accompanies meningococcemia as a characteristic manifestation. The skin rash may advance from a few ill-defined petechial lesions to widespread purpura and ecchymotic areas within a few hours. Disseminated intravascular coagulation, vascular collapse, and ischemic necrosis of extremities can develop. Gangrene of extremities requires amputation.

Rapid diagnosis and treatment initiation are critical in meningitis because it is potentially fatal. Lumbar puncture is a necessary diagnostic procedure for analysis of the CSF in meningitis. Protein and WBCs will be elevated in the CSF because of the microbes. Glucose will be diminished in CSF because it is being utilized by the microbes. Bacteria can be cultured from the CSF. Magnetic resonance imaging (MRI) or computed tomography (CT) scan of the head can evaluate complications.

Treatment involves high doses of IV antibiotics, antiemetics, analgesics, corticosteroids, hydration, and antipyretics. The patient should be placed in isolation. Seizure precautions are necessary. Surgical amputation of gangrenous extremities may be required. Meningitis can leave a patient with complications of cognitive problems, as well as vision and hearing loss. Rifampin is advised for all those who have come in close contact with the person suffering from meningococcal infection. Meningococcal vaccine is recommended for adolescents and young adults, particularly those entering college who live in dormitories.

> **ALERT!** Nuchal rigidity, headache, photophobia, and high fever are key signs of meningitis.

 CLINICAL CONCEPT

Patients with meningitis may exhibit opisthotonus—spasm of the whole body that causes legs, head, and neck to hyperextend and the body to arch backward.

Haemophilus Influenzae

H. influenzae is a small, gram-negative, coccobacillus-shaped bacterium. The most virulent strain is type b (Hib), which has a characteristic outer capsule. It accounts for more than 95% of *H. influenzae* invasive diseases in children and half of invasive diseases in adults. It can be manifested as bacteremia, meningitis, cellulitis, epiglottitis, septic arthritis, or pneumonia. Hib conjugate vaccine has led to dramatic declines in incidence and prevalence of these diseases. The most vulnerable populations include children and older adults. Before Hib immunization programs, *H. influenzae* was a major cause of meningitis in children and adults. Because of successful immunization of children in the United States, *H. influenzae* accounts for only 5% to 10% of cases of adult meningitis. Transmission is by direct contact or by inhalation of respiratory tract droplets. The incubation period is not known. The presence of a concomitant viral infection can potentiate the infection. The colonizing bacteria invade the mucosa and enter the bloodstream.

Meningitis is the most serious manifestation of Hib infection. Symptoms of upper respiratory infection before *H. influenzae* meningitis are common. Headache, nuchal rigidity, photophobia, altered mental status, and fever are the most common presenting features. Infants demonstrate irritability, fever, lethargy, poor feeding, and vomiting. As with other types of bacterial meningitis, diagnosis requires lumbar puncture, and treatment involves high-dose antibiotics. Complications include brain damage, as well as vision and hearing losses.

Gastrointestinal Bacterial Infections

Salmonella, Shigella, E. coli, and Campylobacter are leading bacterial causes of gastroenteritis worldwide. They cause severe diarrheal illness and can be serious in infants and older adults. *E. coli* is also the most common cause of UTI typically affecting women.

Salmonella

Salmonella are rod-shaped, gram-negative, non–spore-forming, motile enterobacteria with flagella. *Salmonella* can be found in uncooked foods, contaminated water, contaminated kitchen utensils, and in some animals, such as reptiles. Animal fecal matter that contaminates eggs or vegetation can cause disease. It can also be caused by unsanitary food preparation by carriers of the organism. *Salmonella* can be transmitted between animals and humans, but most infections are caused by ingestion of contaminated food.

The two main types of organism are *Salmonella enterica,* which causes gastroenteritis, and *Salmonella typhi,* which causes typhoid fever. Both types secrete endotoxins that affect the GI tract. The organism enters through the digestive tract and must be ingested in large numbers to cause disease in healthy adults. After a short incubation period of a few hours to a day, the organism multiplies in the intestinal lumen, causing fever, vomiting, and intestinal inflammation with diarrhea that is often mucopurulent and bloody. In infants and older adults, severe dehydration can occur.

S. typhi is particularly spread by human carriers. There are an estimated 16 to 33 million cases of typhoid fever annually, resulting in 216,000 deaths in endemic areas of Africa, Asia, and South America. Typhoid fever is a potentially fatal disease that causes high fever, cough, abdominal pain, watery diarrhea, and cardiac problems that include bradycardia and endocarditis. Liver involvement and intestinal perforation are common. Neuropsychiatric symptoms such as delirium also can occur. A distinctive rash called rose spots may occur on the lower chest and abdomen. Diagnosis is made by blood or stool culture and serological antibodies.

Salmonella can survive for weeks outside the body. It is not destroyed by freezing; however, heat can kill the organism after at least 10 minutes at 167°F.

According to the CDC, approximately 5% of people who contract typhoid continue to carry the disease after they recover. These persons can transmit the infection to others. Two vaccines are available to prevent the disease. The organism is resistant to several different antibiotics but is sensitive to azithromycin.

Shigella

Shigella are gram-negative, non–spore-forming, non-motile, rod-shaped bacteria related to *E. coli* and *Salmonella. Shigella* infection, called shigellosis, is an intestinal disease that causes severe diarrhea that is often bloody, a condition referred to as dysentery. *Shigella* causes approximately 90 million cases of severe dysentery, with at least 100,000 of these resulting in death each year, mostly among children in the developing world.

There are several different types of *Shigella* bacteria. Some secrete toxins; these can cause hemolytic-uremic syndrome (HUS), a disorder of acute renal failure. The most common symptoms are diarrhea, fever, nausea, vomiting, stomach cramps, and flatulence. The stool may contain blood, mucus, or pus. In rare cases, young children may have seizures. Symptoms often begin 2 to 4 days after ingestion of contaminated food or water and last for weeks. A common cause of *Shigella* is direct contact of the bacteria in stool with diaper changes in a child care setting. *Shigella* can also be spread by anal sexual activity. Treatment consists of antibiotic therapy with agents such as ampicillin or fluoroquinolones.

Escherichia coli

E. coli are gram-negative, rod-shaped bacteria that inhabit the human intestine. There are multiple different strains. Although most strains of *E. coli* are harmless, the organisms can cause cholecystitis, bacteremia, cholangitis, UTI, traveler's diarrhea, neonatal meningitis, and pneumonia.

Several types are known to produce toxins that can cause severe gastroenteritis, diarrhea, and renal failure. A specific strain called *E. coli* O157:H7 causes severe gastroenteritis and can cause HUS. This specific bacterium is one of the enterohemorrhagic *Escherichia coli* (EHEC). The EHEC bacteria are acquired by the fecal–oral route, usually in food or contaminated water. The bacteria live in the intestines of healthy cattle, and contamination of the meat can occur in the slaughtering process. Eating infected meat that is rare or undercooked is the most common way of acquiring the infection. Infection can also occur after consuming fecal-contaminated vegetation or unpasteurized milk, juice, or cider. In addition, person-to-person transmission can occur. Infants and older adults are most susceptible to illness caused by *E. coli* O157:H7.

Infected persons can develop mild to severe diarrhea with abdominal cramps and blood in the stool. Usually little or no fever is present. In some people, particularly children younger than 5 years of age, the infection can cause HUS. The patient has high amounts of red blood cell (RBC) and platelet breakdown and renal failure. Diagnosis is made by stool culture or PCR. Transfusions of blood or blood clotting factors as well as kidney dialysis may be necessary. IV antibiotics and hospitalization are usually required, and most patients recover completely.

E. coli UTIs are caused by uropathogenic strains of *E. coli*. Uncomplicated lower UTIs, also called cystitis, occur primarily in females who are sexually active and are colonized by a uropathogenic strain of *E. coli*. The periurethral region is colonized from contamination with colonic bacteria, and the organism reaches the bladder during sexual intercourse. Males can develop UTI when urine stasis develops in the bladder, commonly caused by benign prostatic hyperplasia (BPH). The prostate obstructs urine outflow, and static urine serves as a perfect medium for bacterial growth. The most prominent symptoms are dysuria (burning on urination), frequency, and urgency. Fever is not an aspect of lower UTI. If fever is present, pyelonephritis should be ruled out.

An *E. coli* UTI can be treated with antibiotics and usually causes no complications. However, in older adults, UTI can become a serious bloodstream infection called urosepsis. Patients can develop acute illness with fever and severe hypotension. IV antibiotics are required for urosepsis.

Campylobacter Jejuni

Campylobacter jejuni is a gram-negative, helical-shaped bacterium found in animal feces, particularly those of birds. It is one of the most common causes of gastroenteritis in the world and usually produces diarrheal illness that is self-limited. Contaminated food, particularly poultry, is a common source, though cattle infection can lead to infected beef. Improper meat or poultry preparation is the usual cause of infection. The illness can spread person to person. Men who have sex with men (MSM) and immunosuppressed patients are at increased risk. The disorder causes abdominal pain, fever, and diarrhea, often containing blood. It can last 24 hours to a week. Specific culture media is required to diagnose the illness. Antibiotic treatment with erythromycin or ciprofloxacin is usually sufficient. Guillain-Barré syndrome is a rare complication that can develop 2 to 3 weeks after the gastroenteritis.

Cholera

Cholera is an infection of the small intestine caused by *Vibrio cholerae*, a toxin-producing, flagellated bacterium. Cholera affects an estimated 3 to 5 million people worldwide and causes 100,000 to 130,000 deaths a year. It is endemic in Africa and parts of Asia. The organism lives in nature, but can reach high levels in fecal-contaminated water. Transmission occurs primarily by drinking water or eating food that has been contaminated by the feces of an infected person. For reasons that are not understood, persons with O blood type are more susceptible than others. The main symptoms are profuse, watery diarrhea and vomiting. The diarrhea is extremely watery and has been referred to as "rice water" diarrhea. Some patients can lose 10 to 20 liters of fluid per day, so rehydration is continually needed. The severity of the diarrhea and vomiting can lead to rapid dehydration, electrolyte imbalance, and, in some cases, death.

A dipstick test is available for diagnosis of cholera, and a positive test should be confirmed with a stool culture. A number of safe vaccines are available. Water sanitation is the most effective means of prevention. Fluids, electrolytes, and doxycycline have been effective treatments.

Other Bacterial Infections

Bacteria such as diphtheria, tetanus, and pertussis are less common causes of infection, mainly because of decades of successful immunization policies. However, because of a recent movement against vaccination, these microorganisms and their infections are reemerging. *Clostridium botulinum* and *Clostridium tetani* are neurotoxic bacteria that rarely cause disease. A tetanus booster every 10 years virtually eradicates the threat of *C. tetani*. *C. difficile,* however, has become a dreaded source of health-care–acquired infection.

Diphtheria, Pertussis, and Tetanus

Diphtheria, pertussis, and tetanus are uncommon diseases in industrialized countries because of the success of routine immunization of children. Epidemics, however, can occur when immunization rates decline, as happened in Russia in the 1990s. A massive diphtheria epidemic occurred and caused more than 5,000 deaths.

Corynebacterium diphtheriae is a toxin-producing bacterium that infects mucous membranes in the respiratory tract. It causes a distinctive gray-colored pseudomembrane consisting of sloughed epithelium, necrotic debris, WBCs, and bacteria that line the respiratory tract. It presents with a sore throat, fever, and tonsillar exudate. Obstruction of the respiratory tract can occur, caused by the extensive pseudomembrane formation. Diphtheria antitoxin is administered to those who are infected. A combination of antibiotics, such as penicillin and erythromycin, is also administered. Other treatments may include IV fluids and oxygen; heart monitoring and intubation may be needed in severe cases. Individuals who come into contact with persons infected with *C. diphtheriae* should receive an immunization or booster shot against diphtheria. Protective immunity lasts only 10 years from the time of vaccination, so it is important for adults to get a booster of tetanus-diphtheria (Td) vaccine every 10 years.

Pertussis, also called whooping cough, is an infection of the respiratory tract caused by *Bordetella pertussis.* Bordetella is a toxin-producing bacterium that allows the binding of bacteria to respiratory ciliated cells. Other toxins produced by *B. pertussis* cause tissue necrosis and impairment of the immune responses mounted by the body. The infected individual has episodes of spasmodic, forceful coughing with an audible whoop. The cough may be so forceful that it causes vomiting, subconjunctival hemorrhages, bulging eyes, and neck vein distention. Infants need hospitalization and have the highest mortality rate. Early treatment with antibiotics, IV fluids, and oxygen is necessary. Cough elixirs and expectorants are contraindicated.

Diphtheria-tetanus-pertussis (DTaP) vaccine is administered in five doses to infants at 2 months, 4 months, 6 months, and 15 to 18 months and then children at age 6 years. A booster vaccine should be administered to children at age 10 to 12 years and every 10 years thereafter. In a pertussis outbreak, children younger than age 7 years should be kept away from those suspected of disease. Complications include pneumonia, convulsions, cerebral hemorrhage, and apnea.

Tetanus is a neurological disorder characterized by intense muscle spasms caused by *C. tetani,* a toxin-producing, spore-forming anaerobic bacterium. *C. tetani* is a common organism found in soil, and its spores can survive for many years under harsh conditions. Tetanus infection can occur after a penetrating injury such as a puncture wound or laceration. *C. tetani* toxin is released in the wound, binds to peripheral motor neurons, and is then transported to the spinal cord. The toxin blocks inhibitory neurotransmitters, causing hyperactivity of neurons. Infected persons may first notice increased muscle tone, particularly in the masseter muscles and jaw. For this reason, the term *lockjaw* has been used to describe the initial sign of tetanus infection. Generalized muscle spasms with the uncontrollable, rigid arching of the back may occur. Respiratory arrest, hypertension or hypotension, tachycardia or bradycardia, profuse sweating, and hyperpyrexia may result. Antibiotics are of little value in the treatment of tetanus; tetanus immunoglobulin (TIG), aggressive wound care, and tetanus toxoid booster are required.

> ### 🔎 CLINICAL CONCEPT
>
> Children should receive five doses of DTaP vaccine before age 7. These are usually given at 2, 4, 6, and 15 to 18 months of age and 4 to 6 years of age. At age 11 to 12 years preteens should receive DTaP. Adults should receive tetanus (Td) vaccination every 10 years (www.cdc.gov/tetanus).

Botulism

C. botulinum is a spore-producing, toxin-secreting bacterium found in soil. The toxin can be ingested or inhaled, or it can invade the body through breaches in the skin. In industrialized countries, most cases are foodborne and result from improper storage and packaging of canned foods. However, contaminated water, fish, cured ham, honey, and corn syrup also have been sources. Approximately 100 cases occur per year in the United States, with the majority in infants. The botulinum toxin affects neurons and causes a descending paralysis, initially affecting the cranial nerves. Weakness progresses rapidly from the head down into the neck, arms, trunk, and legs. Nausea, vomiting, and abdominal pain may occur, as may dizziness, blurred vision, dry mouth, and a change in mental status. Pupillary reflexes may be absent in some patients.

Botulism is a reportable disease, and clinicians should contact the CDC to obtain appropriate directions for treatment with antitoxin. Because botulinum toxin can be widely dispersed as an aerosol or food contaminant, it has the potential as a weapon in bioterrorism and biological warfare. Botulinum toxin can also be injected therapeutically to relieve muscle spasm, migraine headache, and cosmetically for reduction of facial wrinkles. The toxin used for cosmetic purposes is known as onabotulinumtoxinA (Botox).

Clostridium Difficile

C. difficile is a spore-forming, toxin-secreting anaerobic bacterium. Spores of *C. difficile* are ingested and germinate in the small and large intestine. The organisms emit toxins that disrupt the intestinal mucosa, erode the intestinal epithelial cells, and form pseudomembranes that contain necrotic tissue, WBCs, and mucus.

C. difficile is shed in feces. Any surface, device, or material (e.g., toilets, bathing tubs, and electronic rectal thermometers) that becomes contaminated with feces may serve as a reservoir for the *C. difficile* spores. *C. difficile* spores can be transferred to patients via the hands of health-care personnel and is a common hospital-acquired (nosocomial) infection. *C. difficile* can also be community acquired, as it can be airborne, and some individuals are asymptomatic carriers. Prolonged, frequent diarrhea; fever; and abdominal pain are the most common presenting symptoms. Stool culture to identify the presence of *C. difficile* is diagnostic of the condition. Because the most common predisposing factor is long-term antibiotic use that alters the normal flora in the gut, discontinuation of the antibiotic in use is necessary, and supportive treatments, such as rehydration, may be initiated. Treatment with metronidazole, vancomycin, or fidaxomicin is recommended. Transplanting stool from a healthy person to the colon of a patient with repeat *C. difficile* infections has been shown to successfully treat *C. difficile.* These "fecal transplants" appear to be the most effective method for helping patients with repeat infections.

Clostridial Gas Gangrene

Clostridium perfringens, previously known as *Clostridium welchii,* is the most common cause (80% to 90% of cases) of clostridial gas gangrene. Clostridial organisms can be found in soil and isolated from normal human colonic flora, skin, and the vagina. *C. perfringens* is a highly lethal organism that causes myonecrosis, a rapidly spreading necrotizing infection of skeletal muscle and surrounding tissue. The destruction of tissue is caused by toxins secreted by the organism. The toxin causes direct vascular injury, cellular necrosis, hemolysis, leukocyte degeneration, and polymorphonuclear cell damage. The process of myonecrosis can spread as

fast as 2 cm per hour. Spreading infection often results in systemic toxicity and shock that can be fatal within 12 hours. If properly treated, the overall mortality rate is 20% to 30%. If untreated, the process is 100% fatal.

Clostridial infection usually occurs in a wound after trauma or surgery. The symptom that should alert the clinician to clostridial infection is severe, sudden pain that is out of proportion to physical findings at the wound site (see Box 10-1). On physical examination, the involved body part commonly demonstrates the following characteristics:

- Edema
- Erythema with purplish-black discoloration
- Extreme tenderness
- Brownish skin discoloration (bronzing, brawny) with bullae
- Profuse, "dish-watery," serous drainage from ruptured bullae
- Discharge that may have a peculiar, "mousy," sweet odor
- Crepitant tissue that may extend well beyond any skin discoloration or edema

X-rays reveal fine gas bubbles within the soft tissues, dissecting into the intramuscular fascial planes and muscles. The wound discharge should be collected for culture and sensitivity. Penicillin is the preferred drug for clostridial infections. Patients allergic to penicillin may be treated with clindamycin or chloramphenicol. Surgical consultation is necessary and may result in amputation of the involved area.

Tick-Borne Bacterial Disease

Lyme disease and Rocky Mountain spotted fever (RMSF) are the most common tick-borne illnesses in the United States. Both diseases are caused by bacterial parasites that are harbored by forest animals, such as deer. A tick feeds off the animal and then carries the

---

BOX 10-1. Risk Factors for Clostridial Infection

Clostridia are bacterial organisms that can cause gangrene in ischemic tissue. The following risk factors make one susceptible to clostridial infection:

- Diabetes mellitus
- Peripheral vascular disease
- Alcoholism
- Drug abuse
- Advanced age
- Chronic debilitating disease(s)
- Immunocompromised state caused by:
  - Steroid use
  - Malnutrition
  - Malignancy
  - AIDS

bacterial parasite. Humans come in contact with the pin-sized ticks in forested regions and are commonly bitten without awareness. Lyme disease and RMSF tick bites cause debilitating symptoms. Despite its name, RMSF can occur throughout the United States. Lyme disease is mainly found in the northeastern United States.

Lyme Disease. Lyme disease is caused by a bacterial spirochete called *Borrelia burgdorferi,* a microorganism found in forest animals such as squirrels, rodents, and the white-tailed deer. A tick that feeds off one of these animals can harbor the microorganism. Neither the reservoir (deer) nor vector (tick) becomes ill because of the microorganism. However, the tick can bite a human, who can become infected with the microorganism and develop illness. Deer ticks can be tiny, no larger than the point of a pencil, and the infected individual frequently cannot remember being bitten (see Fig. 10-8). The tick must be embedded in the skin for 36 to 48 hours or more to transmit disease. After a lengthy incubation period ranging from 3 to 32 days, a rash known as *erythema migrans* begins as a painless, red macule that expands slowly to form a target-like lesion (see Fig. 10-9). Within a few days, the center of the lesion can become extremely erythematous, vesicular, and ulcerated. The legs, thighs, groin, scalp, and

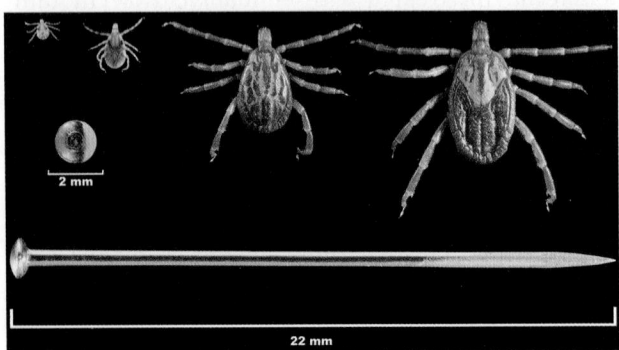

FIGURE 10-8. Relative sizes of ticks at different life stages. *(Courtesy of CDC/Dr. Christopher Paddock.)*

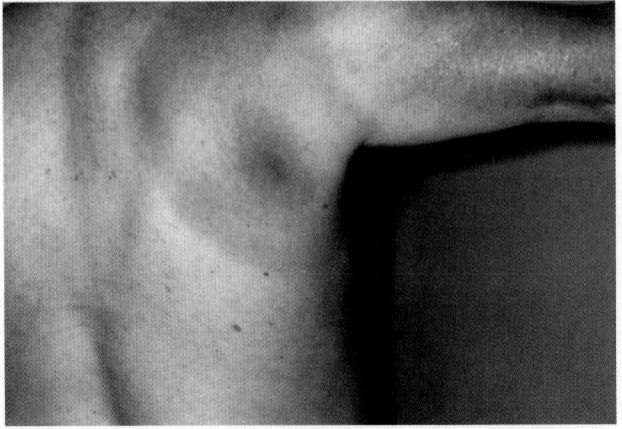

FIGURE 10-9. Erythema migrans. *(Courtesy of CDC.)*

axilla are common sites of the lesion. However, almost 20% of infected persons do not exhibit the characteristic skin lesion.

Skin involvement is usually followed by headache, mild stiffness of the neck, fever, chills, migratory musculoskeletal pain, arthralgias, and extreme fatigue. Early symptoms usually wane within several weeks. Cranial neuritis, or inflammation of the facial nerve, can develop in some patients, causing one side of the face to be paralyzed—a condition called Bell's palsy. The patient exhibits a one-sided facial droop when smiling and is unable to close the eye on the affected side. Months after the onset of *Borrelia* infection, approximately 60% of patients develop arthritis, usually of the large joints, particularly the knees.

Diagnosis of Lyme disease is difficult because positive cultures are only obtained early in the disease when most infected persons are unaware of the infection. Biopsy samples of the erythema migrans lesion or involved joint fluid may reveal evidence of the *B. burgdorferi* organism. However, Lyme disease is usually diagnosed by the characteristic history and clinical presentation of the patient, in addition to serological testing for the antibody to *B. burgdorferi.* The test for the antibody may be negative in the initial period of the disease, but after several weeks, most patients develop a positive antibody titer. Serological tests cannot distinguish between active and inactive infection. Patients can remain seropositive for many years after initial infection, even after antibiotic treatment.

Lyme disease is best treated early in the disease with oral doxycycline for 21 days.

CLINICAL CONCEPT

Typhus and typhoid fever are not the same disease. Typhus is caused by any one of a number of *Rickettsia* bacteria, whereas typhoid fever is caused by *Salmonella typhi.*

Rickettsia. Rickettsia comprise a specific type of bacteria known as obligate intracellular parasites because they must be within a living cell in order to reproduce. They can be transmitted only via vectors, usually fleas, ticks, or mites. As a class, rickettsia are responsible for a number of significant human diseases, including RMSF, typhus, and Q fever.

Rocky Mountain Spotted Fever. The bacterium *Rickettsia rickettsii* is a small, gram-negative bacillus that may be harbored in a dog tick or a wood tick. *R. rickettsii* enters the skin through a tick bite and spreads along the lymphatic system. Initially, the classic triad of symptoms is fever, rash, and history of a tick bite. However, as with Lyme disease, most individuals do not recall being bitten. After entry into the lymphatic system, *R. rickettsii* rapidly infects the endothelial cells and causes increased vascular permeability, with resulting edema. Vascular permeability also causes hypoalbuminemia, hypovolemia, hypotension, and reduced serum oncotic pressure. An inflammatory reaction follows, including activation of platelets and the fibrinolytic system. Various organ systems may be involved, including the pulmonary, cardiac, nervous, renal, hematopoietic, and hepatic systems.

Initial symptoms may include nonspecific systemic signs such as fever, nausea, vomiting, severe headache, muscle pain, and lack of appetite. Later signs and symptoms include rash, abdominal pain, joint pain, and diarrhea. The characteristic red, spotted (petechial) rash of RMSF is usually not seen until the sixth day or later after onset of symptoms. The rash involves the palms of the hands or soles of the feet, but 10% of patients may never develop it.

Serological or antibody testing is the most frequently used method for confirming cases of RMSF. The indirect immunofluorescence assay is a type of serology test that is generally considered the reference standard in RMSF.

Patients with RMSF are critically ill and require immediate intensive care and antibiotic treatment. Cardiac monitoring, hemodialysis, blood transfusion, and endotracheal intubation with ventilatory support may be required. Long-term health problems after acute infection may follow.

Selected Viral Infections

Viruses are ubiquitous and have the ability to mutate, which confounds treatment. They spread most often from human to human by droplet infection or via contact, and they require the cellular machinery of a living organism in order to reproduce. The common cold is a typical viral disorder.

Common Cold Viruses

Acute upper respiratory illnesses are the most common of human diseases. On average, adults suffer three to four upper respiratory illnesses per person per year. It is estimated that two-thirds to three-fourths of acute respiratory illnesses are caused by viruses. Rhinovirus, coronavirus, and adenovirus are the major causes of the common cold, and all present in a similar manner. These viruses spread through direct contact or droplet infection. Frequently, the virus is transmitted from hands that have been in contact with respiratory secretions. They can survive for 1 to 3 hours on environmental surfaces, such as keyboards.

The incubation period for rhinovirus is 1 to 2 days, and symptoms usually begin with rhinorrhea and sneezing. Illness generally lasts 4 to 9 days and resolves spontaneously. Rhinovirus infection can lead to otitis media and sinusitis or can stimulate asthma in those who are susceptible to these conditions. Diagnosis is usually made on clinical presentation alone. Treatment is supportive, consisting of antihistamines and decongestants. Thorough hand washing and environmental disinfection can help prevent spread of the infection to others.

Influenza Virus

The three major types of influenza virus—A, B, and C—are among the most common causes of upper and lower respiratory tract infection affecting all age groups. Influenza viruses have been responsible for many pandemics and epidemics across the world. Some epidemics have been notable, such as the "Spanish flu" of 1918 that took many lives.

Outbreaks of influenza occur annually and are particularly worrisome for the very young, older adults, and those with chronic disease. These viruses possess surface antigens known as hemagglutinin and neuraminidase, proteins that facilitate entry into respiratory cells and enhance release of viral particles. The most extensive and severe outbreaks are caused by influenza A viruses because of their ability to undergo mutation. From year to year, the hemagglutinin and neuraminidase antigens of influenza A change because of genetic mutations. Influenza B virus causes outbreaks that are associated with less severe disease because genetic mutation causing variation in their hemagglutinin and neuraminidase antigens is less common. The periodic genetic mutations that occur in influenza viruses require new vaccine development each year.

Transmission of influenza occurs through droplet infection and aerosols generated by coughs and sneezes of individuals. Fomites and hand-to-hand contact also can spread the virus. Initially the virus enters the upper respiratory tract and then invades the lower respiratory tract mucous gland cells, alveolar cells, and macrophages. The infection usually presents as abrupt onset of fever, chills, headache, myalgias, arthralgias, cough, and sore throat. Uncomplicated influenza generally resolves over a 1-week period, although cough may persist for 2 weeks or longer. In older adults, postinfluenza weakness and fatigue can persist for several weeks. Influenza in older adults also increases susceptibility to pneumonia.

Influenza virus can be isolated from throat culture, nasopharyngeal secretions, or sputum. Treatment consists of antipyretic medications, hydration, and rest. Amantadine, rimantadine, zanamivir, and oseltamivir are antiviral medications that can be used to shorten the disease's course. Influenza vaccine is recommended annually for all persons older than age 6 months, but it is particularly important for older adults and people with chronic illnesses. The influenza vaccine may not prevent an individual from developing active disease, but it is highly effective at preventing severe disease and complications. Health-care workers need to get annual immunization, because unimmunized persons can transmit the virus even if they do not become symptomatic themselves.

SARS-CoV-2 (COVID-19)

Severe acute respiratory syndrome coronavirus 2 (SARS-CoV-2) became known as COVID-19 during the worldwide pandemic of 2019. SARS-CoV-2 is an RNA virus with distinctive surface spikes that give the organism the appearance of a solar corona. It is mainly transmitted person to person via droplet infection from sneezes or coughs; however, it can survive on inanimate surfaces for up to 3 to 4 days. Maternal COVID-19 is currently believed to be associated with low risk for vertical transmission to the fetus.

Early in infection, the virus targets nasal and bronchial epithelial cells and pneumocytes. The infection may be asymptomatic or it may cause a wide spectrum of symptoms, including mild upper respiratory tract infection, pneumonia, acute respiratory distress syndrome (ARDS), and life-threatening sepsis. The incubation period is approximately 10 days, then a symptomatic period occurs. Viral shedding begins approximately 2 to 3 days before the onset of symptoms, and viral load in the upper respiratory tract appears to peak around the time of symptoms. Asymptomatic and presymptomatic carriers can transmit the virus.

The clinical presentation of COVID-19 begins within 14 days of exposure. Most patients exhibit a mild upper respiratory infection. Persons with comorbidities or immunosuppression are at highest risk for more severe disease. Common symptoms in patients include fever, rhinorrhea, dry cough, shortness of breath, weakness, fatigue, myalgias, and headache. Anosmia (lack of sense of smell) or ageusia (lack of sense of taste) are common symptoms. Gastrointestinal symptoms of nausea, vomiting, and diarrhea can also occur.

In later stages of infection when viral replication accelerates, SARS-CoV-2 infects pulmonary capillary endothelial cells, leading to an inflammatory reaction and triggering an influx of monocytes, T cells, and neutrophils. There is diffuse thickening of the alveolar walls with inflammatory exudates and consequent reduced alveolar–capillary diffusion of oxygen. It is believed that proteins secreted by the coronavirus may disable the immune response of some patients. This process results in a severe immunopathological cascade, with the release of many proinflammatory cytokines, referred to as a cytokine storm or cytokine release syndrome.

In severe COVID-19, fulminant activation of coagulation and consumption of coagulation factors can occur. Disseminated intravascular coagulation (DIC) and microthrombi formation can lead to venous and arterial thrombotic complications (e.g., venous thrombosis, pulmonary embolism, limb ischemia, ischemic stroke, myocardial infarction). In critically ill patients, there can be life-threatening multiple organ failure.

Common laboratory abnormalities among hospitalized patients include lymphopenia, elevated inflammatory markers (e.g., erythrocyte sedimentation rate, C-reactive protein, ferritin, tumor necrosis factor alpha, interleukin-1, interleukin-6), elevated liver enzymes alanine aminotransferase and aspartate aminotransferase, and abnormal coagulation parameters (e.g., prolonged prothrombin time, thrombocytopenia, elevated D-dimer, low fibrinogen). Common chest x-ray findings include bilateral lower-lobe infiltrates. CT scan reveals bilateral, peripheral, lower-lobe ground-glass opacities.

Diagnosis of COVID-19 is typically made using polymerase chain reaction (PCR) testing via nasal swab. IgM antibodies are detectable within 5 days of infection, with rising IgM levels during weeks 2 to 3 of illness. An IgG response is first seen approximately 14 days after symptom onset.

Patients should be placed in isolation and clinicians should use full personal protective equipment when performing care. Currently, supportive care measures such as oxygenation and fluid management are the standard of care.

Other treatments have been used based on preliminary research and continue to be investigated. Convalescent plasma, which contains antibodies from recovered patients, can suppress viremia if administered early. Remdesivir, an RNA-dependent polymerase inhibitor, has demonstrated some efficacy. Interferon beta-1b has been used in combination with protease inhibitors, lopinavir-ritonavir, showing some promising results. Some centers have proposed therapeutic anticoagulation using heparin or direct-acting oral anticoagulants for critically ill patients. In cytokine release syndrome, some protocols include recommendations for the use of tocilizumab, a monoclonal IL-6 antibody. Intravenous systemic corticosteroids, particularly high-dose dexamethasone, are recommended to counteract pulmonary and systemic inflammation. For patients requiring invasive mechanical ventilation, lung-protective ventilation with low tidal volumes is effective. Additionally, prone positioning, a higher positive end-expiratory pressure strategy, and short-term neuromuscular blockade are recommended.

Currently, there are vaccines and boosters available to prevent SARS-CoV-2 disease. The COVID-19 pandemic inspired researchers to develop a novel experimental mRNA-based vaccine which uses part of the spike protein's genetic code. Vaccination, vigilant hand hygiene, N95 respirator mask use, and social distancing have become the recommended public health measures to protect against the spread of disease.

Epstein-Barr Virus

Epstein-Barr virus (EBV) is the cause of infectious mononucleosis, a common infection of adolescents and young adults. By adulthood, more than 90% of individuals have been infected with EBV and have developed antibodies to the virus.

EBV is spread by oral secretions because the virus infects the epithelium of the oropharynx and salivary glands. The virus is frequently spread from asymptomatic adults to children by transfer of saliva. Among adolescents and young adults, the virus is most often spread by kissing, and so infectious mononucleosis has the nickname "the kissing disease." The virus initially binds to and infects the cells of the oropharynx. After the virus enters the oropharynx, it invades the bloodstream and has a predilection for B lymphocytes. The virus incites an immune response that causes proliferation of B lymphocytes within lymphoid tissue, resulting in lymphadenopathy. The cervical lymph nodes, which are most commonly involved, are tender and symmetrically enlarged. Pharyngitis, fatigue, headache, fever, chills, abdominal pain, nausea, and vomiting are usually presenting symptoms. Pharyngitis is often the most prominent sign with tonsillar enlargement and exudate. Some individuals develop periorbital edema and a papular rash on the trunk and arms. Administration of ampicillin during infection with EBV can provoke development of an erythematous maculopapular rash. Enlargement of the liver and spleen can also occur. Hepatomegaly can cause elevated liver enzymes and jaundice, whereas splenomegaly can predispose the patient to splenic rupture. Symptoms of infectious mononucleosis are self-limited and usually resolve within 4 weeks, although some individuals may require up to 6 months for full recovery.

WBC counts with examination of the cells show a lymphocytosis with atypical lymphocytes. These atypical cells are larger than normal lymphocytes and contain large vacuoles in their cytoplasm. The heterophile antibody test is a specialized diagnostic test that can detect antibodies in acute EBV infection. Repeated testing may be necessary because antibodies develop throughout the illness and are most easily detected during the third week of infection. Heterophile tests usually remain positive for 3 months, although antibodies can persist for up to a year. A rapid monospot test is often used clinically, but it is not as accurate as the heterophile test.

After recovery from infectious mononucleosis, the virus is shed from the oropharynx for as long as 18 months after acute infection and may continue to be shed intermittently for many years in healthy EBV-positive individuals. As long as the virus is shedding, it may be transmitted to another individual. Furthermore, EBV has a unique ability to remain dormant within the body after recovery from acute infection. EBV remains in a dormant form within lymphoid tissue for life, and reactivation is possible.

Treatment is supportive, which includes adequate hydration, nutrition, and rest. Splenomegaly increases the chance of splenic rupture and internal bleeding. Aspirin should be avoided to decrease the chance of bleeding. Other antipyretic medications such as acetaminophen are recommended for fever and sore throat. Corticosteroids may be necessary if there is severe tonsillar enlargement with impending airway obstruction. Antiviral medications have not shown to be effective for treating infectious mononucleosis.

Although rare, EBV is associated with nasopharyngeal cancer. It has also been implicated in chronic fatigue syndrome.

ALERT! The individual with EBV infection and splenomegaly should not participate in strenuous activities or contact sports for at least 3 weeks or until the spleen returns to normal size.

Cytomegalovirus

CMV is capable of causing a wide range of disorders in all age groups. It can cause an asymptomatic infection, birth defects in the fetus, mononucleosis-type syndrome in adults, and severe disseminated infection in immunosuppressed individuals. Initially, the virus infects the salivary epithelial cells and is shed in the saliva. CMV also commonly infects the genitourinary tract, shedding in the urine. In immunocompetent persons, CMV infection may be asymptomatic or present as a mild flu-like illness or a mononucleosis-like illness. The most common symptoms are extreme fatigue, fever, pharyngitis, lymphadenopathy, and, in some cases, splenomegaly.

In comparison to EBV mononucleosis, CMV mononucleosis has a lower incidence of cervical lymphadenopathy and negative heterophile test. CMV can cause pneumonia and hepatitis, which is usually self-limited and resolves without complication in immunocompetent individuals. However, CMV can cause more serious disseminated bloodstream infection of the immunosuppressed patient. Once in the bloodstream, the virus can be found in breast milk, saliva, feces, urine, cervical secretions, and semen. Transmission of the virus from person to person is facilitated by close living conditions and poor personal hygiene. It can be transmitted sexually, through blood transfusion, and by transplantation. In the immunocompromised individual, CMV can cause life-threatening pneumonitis, GI disease, retinitis, hepatitis, encephalitis, and myeloradiculitis.

CMV antibodies are found in the bloodstream 4 to 7 weeks after infection and may persist for as long as 20 weeks. CMV antigen can also be isolated from tissue culture or from the bloodstream.

CMV is the most common congenitally acquired infection in infants. During pregnancy, women without immunity are susceptible to disseminated infection, which affects the placenta and is transferred to the fetus. Cervical excretion of the virus is common during pregnancy and can be transferred to the infant during delivery. CMV may also be transmitted to the infant through breast milk. Most children infected in utero appear healthy but may demonstrate symptoms of disease later in development. Ten percent are born with cytomegalic inclusion disease. The symptoms of cytomegalic inclusion disease include jaundice, splenomegaly, thrombocytopenia, intrauterine growth retardation, microcephaly, and retinitis. Children born with cytomegalic inclusion disease commonly develop neurological or cognitive impairment.

CMV is within the herpes family of viruses; like all herpes viruses, it has the potential to remain dormant in the body after the acute infection subsides.

Cell-mediated immunity is the most important defense mechanism against CMV. Patients with AIDS and immunosuppressed transplant recipients are most vulnerable.

At present, there are no sufficiently effective antiviral medications to combat CMV infection.

Measles, Mumps, and Rubella

Measles, mumps, and rubella (MMR) were common childhood illnesses less than 50 years ago, but are now less common because of widespread vaccination. Rubella and measles (also called rubeola) are referred to as viral **exanthems**, a term indicating rash. The clinical significance of MMR now lies mainly in their public health implications. As immunization has become mandatory in many economically developed countries, public knowledge and concern about these serious diseases have decreased dramatically. In some instances, a false sense of security has occurred, and people have become lax in adhering to recommendations for immunization. Some parents are refusing vaccination of their children because of fear of dangerous side effects, which is increasing the incidence of MMR. Localized outbreaks of MMR are now common due to lack of vaccination. Health-care providers have an important role in educating the public about diseases that have become uncommon because of immunization programs. Additionally, people need accurate, easily understood information on the actual risks and benefits of vaccination. The CDC recommends 1 dose of MMR vaccine at 12 to 15 months of age; followed by a second dose at 4 to 6 years of age; and a booster at 18 years of age. Postexposure prophylaxis is also available.

Measles

The measles virus is an RNA virus of the genus *Morbillivirus* within the family Paramyxoviridae. Humans are hosts, and infection is transmitted via respiratory droplets, which can remain active and contagious, either airborne or on surfaces, for up to 2 hours. The measles virus, once acquired, establishes a localized infection at the respiratory epithelium, after which the virus infects regional lymph nodes and endothelial cells and then disseminates to distant organs. In immunocompetent individuals, measles virus infection induces an

effective immune response, which clears the virus and results in lifelong immunity. The MMR vaccination virtually eliminates the risk of disease.

The CDC reports the childhood mortality rate from measles infection in the United States to be 0.1% to 0.2%. Globally, however, measles remains one of the leading causes of death in young children. According to the CDC, an estimated 10 million cases and 197,000 deaths caused by measles occur in children worldwide each year.

Measles has an incubation period of 7 to 14 days and a prodromal stage of 4 to 7 days. High fever, cough, upper respiratory illness, conjunctivitis with periorbital edema, and photophobia are major symptoms. There are unique white areas in the oral buccal mucosa called Koplik's spots that appear in the prodromal stage. Koplik's spots are considered pathognomonic for measles. After the appearance of Koplik's spots, the characteristic tiny maculopapular, mildly pruritic rash appears on the body (see Fig. 10-10). The rash develops from head to toe and then fades after 5 to 7 days.

Diagnosis is usually made by clinical history and physical examination, PCR testing, and specific measles IgM and IgG immunoglobulins can be found in the blood. Rest, hydration, antipyretics, oatmeal baths for pruritus, and other supportive therapy are required for treatment. Vitamin A supplements are also recommended because they have been found to decrease mortality and complications by 50%. Complications, which are more likely to occur in persons younger than 5 years or older than 20 years, include bacterial pneumonia, eye damage, and blindness.

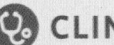

CLINICAL CONCEPT

Children should get two doses of MMR vaccine, starting with the first dose at 12 to 15 months of age, and the second dose at 4 to 6 years of age. Teens and adults should also be up to date on their MMR vaccination.

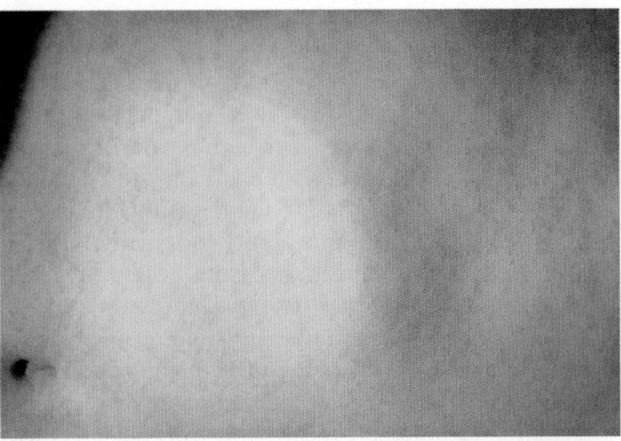

FIGURE 10-10. Measles rash. *(Courtesy of CDC/Dr. Heinz F. Eichenwald.)*

Rubella

Rubella, also known as German measles, is an RNA virus classified as a *Rubivirus* in the Togaviridae family. Before the rubella vaccine, epidemics of the disease were seen in young children, adolescents, and young adults in winter and early spring. Since development of the rubella vaccine, the number of cases has decreased significantly. One major focus of infection is now unvaccinated adults.

The disease is spread by droplet infection from cough or sneeze and infects the respiratory epithelium. It has an incubation period of 14 to 19 days, with onset of a rash usually on the 15th day. The disease can be spread from a few days before the rash appears to 5 to 7 days after its appearance. Patients are most contagious when the rash is erupting and are noncontagious after 7 days of rash.

The rash may be the first manifestation, followed by fever, sore throat, and rhinitis. The rash begins as discrete, red macules on the face that spread to the neck, trunk, and extremities. The macules may coalesce on the trunk. Appearance of the rash corresponds with the appearance of the rubella-specific antibody. The rash lasts 1 to 3 days, first leaving the face. Forchheimer's spots, which are pinpoint red macules and petechiae over the soft palate and the uvula, can be seen just before or with the rash.

The hallmark of rubella is generalized, tender lymphadenopathy that involves all nodes, but particularly the suboccipital, postauricular, and anterior and posterior cervical nodes. Although less common in children, polyarthralgia and even polyarthritis may occur in adults and rarely may persist longer than 2 weeks. Serological studies show a rise in IgM antibodies in the beginning of the disease and IgG later in the disease. IgG remains and confers long-term immunity. PCR testing can also detect the viral RNA.

The major complication of rubella is its teratogenic effects when pregnant women contract the disease, especially in the early weeks of gestation. The virus can be transmitted to the fetus through the placenta and can cause serious congenital defects, spontaneous abortions, and stillbirths. Congenital rubella syndrome (CRS) can cause microcephaly, blindness, hearing impairment, heart defects, diabetes, and bone disease in the fetus.

Treatment for rubella involves supportive therapy with antipyretics, hydration, and oatmeal baths, which can be used to soothe the pruritic rash. The MMR vaccine is usually administered to infants at 12 to 15 months, and again at 4 to 6 years old.

Mumps

Mumps is a paramyxovirus transmitted by droplet infection of a cough or sneeze. It has an incubation period of 14 to 25 days, after which time prodromal symptoms occur and last anywhere from 3 to 5 days. The most common presentation is parotitis, or swollen parotid salivary glands, which occur in 30% to 40% of patients. Other reported sites of infection are the testes, pancreas, eyes, ovaries, central nervous system (CNS), joints, and kidneys. A patient is considered infectious from about 3 days before the onset to up to 4 days after the start of active parotitis. Infections can be asymptomatic in up to 20% of persons.

The most common symptoms are parotitis, submaxillary/submandibular gland swelling, fever, and sore throat. The average length of illness is 5 days. Complications, including encephalitis and orchitis, are reported in 5% of patients. In the male, orchitis can result in sterility. Diagnosis is based on clinical examination, and mumps-specific IgG can be detected in the bloodstream. PCR testing for the virus can also be done. Testicular ultrasonography is needed to diagnose orchitis, whereas lumbar puncture is necessary for symptomatic meningitis or encephalitis. Treatment is supportive, including anti-inflammatory agents, IV hydration, and use of ice packs to decrease parotid or scrotal swelling. Vaccination with the MMR vaccine is usually administered to infants at 12 to 15 months, and again at 4 to 6 years old.

Varicella Zoster

The varicella zoster virus (VZV) causes the clinical syndrome varicella, more widely known as chickenpox. Varicella is largely a childhood disease, with more than 90% of cases occurring in children younger than 10 years old. As with MMR, varicella is becoming a less common disease because of immunization programs. The disease is benign in the healthy child, whereas increased morbidity is seen in adults and in patients who are immunocompromised. The adult who has not developed varicella as a child is susceptible to varicella pneumonia, which is a serious illness with prolonged recovery and potential complications.

Varicella is usually acquired by the inhalation of airborne respiratory droplets from an infected host. A history of exposure to an infected contact within the incubation period of 10 to 21 days is an important clue in the diagnosis. It is a highly contagious virus and is usually diagnosed on the basis of the characteristic rash and successive crops of lesions. The typical patient is infectious for 1 to 2 days before the development of rash and until the last vesicles have crusted over. The triad of rash, malaise, and low-grade fever are typical signs. The characteristic chickenpox vesicle, surrounded by an erythematous halo, is described as a "dewdrop on a rose petal" (see Fig. 10-11). Small, erythematous macules often first appear on the scalp, face, trunk, and proximal limbs, with rapid sequential progression over 12 to 14 hours to papules, clear vesicles, and pustules, with subsequent central umbilication and crust formation. Vesicles may appear on the palms and soles and on the mucous membranes, with painful, shallow, oropharyngeal, or urogenital ulcers. Intense pruritus commonly accompanies the vesicular stage of the rash. Diagnosis is most commonly based

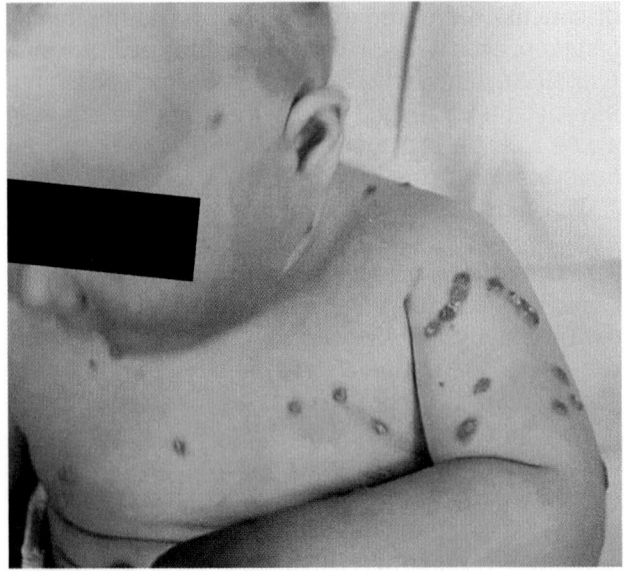

FIGURE 10-11. Varicella. *(Courtesy of CDC/Susan Lindsley.)*

on history and physical examination. PCR testing of skin lesions can detect the virus. Treatment consists mainly of supportive measures such as antipyretics, hydration, oatmeal baths, and antihistamines for the pruritic rash. Oral acyclovir is used for persons at increased risk of severe varicella infections, most notably people older than 12 years. To prevent the disease, VZV vaccine is recommended in childhood.

Herpes zoster infection, also known as shingles, is a reactivation of varicella zoster. After resolution of varicella, the varicella virus lies dormant in the dorsal root ganglia of the spinal nerves. In adulthood, during times of extreme stress or immunosuppression, the virus can become reactivated and cause herpes zoster infection. Upon reactivation, the virus migrates down the sensory nerve to the skin, causing a characteristic line of vesicular lesions, usually along a single dermatome. It may be followed by painful postherpetic neuralgia (PHN) for up to a year after the initial shingles infection.

The incidence of herpes zoster increases with age, with older adults being disproportionately affected. Immunization with two doses of herpes zoster vaccine at 2 to 6 months apart is advised for persons age 50 and older. Antiviral agents such as acyclovir can be prescribed to lessen the severity of the disorder.

Erythema Infectiosum

Erythema infectiosum (fifth disease) is a common childhood viral exanthem caused by human parvovirus B19. Acute infection involves an adaptive immune response, with the production of specific IgM antibodies and subsequent formation of immune complexes that deposit in skin and joints. The infection tends to occur in the late winter or early spring.

Erythema infectiosum typically has an incubation period of 4 to 14 days and is spread primarily via droplet infection during this period. The prodromal phase may include headache, low-grade fever, pharyngitis, and malaise. Classic skin rash follows within 3 to 7 days. The facial skin develops a classic slapped-cheek appearance that may appear like a sunburn and typically fades over 2 to 4 days (see Fig. 10-12). It is occasionally edematous.

Within 1 to 4 days of the rash appearing on the cheeks, the second-stage skin rash develops. It is an erythematous macular-to-morbilliform rash over the extremity extensor surfaces that can involve the palms and soles.

After several days, most of the second-stage skin rash fades into a lacy pattern, with particular emphasis on the proximal extremities. After starting to fade, the rash may recur over several weeks after physical stimuli such as exercise, sun exposure, friction, bathing in hot water, or stress.

Diagnosis is most commonly made by history and physical examination. It is a self-limited disorder. Treatment involves mainly supportive measures such as antipyretics, antihistamines, and hydration.

Monkeypox

Monkeypox is an emerging zoonotic disease caused by monkeypox virus (MPXV), a member of the *Orthopoxvirus* genus, which is similar to smallpox. At the time of this writing in 2022, monkeypox outbreaks have occurred globally. As of December 2022, this viral infection reached a peak of 29,700 cases in the United States and 80,000 cases globally, and then quickly declined. Deaths from monkeypox were rare.

The monkeypox virus is transmitted mainly by close intimate contact. The highest-risk population is MSM. Monkeypox can spread to anyone through close, skin-to-skin contact, particularly contact with rash lesions, body fluids, or respiratory secretions. Also, the virus can be spread via objects or surfaces in close contact with the person with monkeypox. It can be transmitted through oral, anal, or vaginal sexual activity. Prolonged face-to-face contact and kissing can also transmit the virus. A pregnant person can spread the virus to their fetus through the placenta.

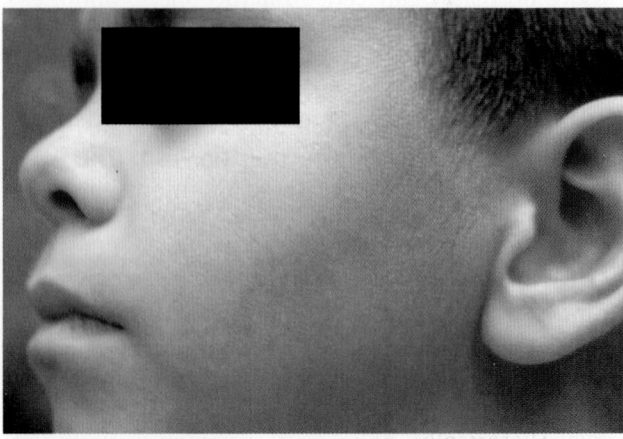

FIGURE 10-12. Erythema infectiosum. *(Courtesy of CDC.)*

The clinical presentation closely resembles smallpox; however, there is early lymph node enlargement at the onset of fever. A rash usually appears 1 to 3 days after onset of fever, with vesicular lesions appearing simultaneously. The distribution of the rash is mainly peripheral but can occur anywhere on the body. The infection lasts approximately 4 weeks as the lesions desquamate. Patients can suffer from a range of complications including secondary bacterial infections, respiratory distress, bronchopneumonia, gastrointestinal involvement, dehydration, sepsis, encephalitis, and corneal infection with ensuing loss of vision.

There is currently no specific treatment for monkeypox virus infection, and patients are managed with supportive care and symptomatic treatment. Smallpox vaccine is administered as prevention for those at high risk.

Herpes Simplex Virus

There are two herpes simplex viruses (HSV): HSV-1 and HSV-2. The two viruses cause disease in the same manner but are distinctly categorized because they usually infect different parts of the body. HSV-1 is the common cold sore virus, whereas HSV-2 is the cause of genital herpes infection.

Both HSV-1 and HSV-2 cause acute and latent infection. Acute infection is characterized by abrupt onset of vesicular lesions within the epidermis and mucous membranes. The fluid-filled vesicles contain active viral particles; transmission of the virus to others during this phase is common. After a few weeks, the acute phase ceases and is followed by a period of dormancy when there are no apparent lesions and the virus is inactive. During the latent period, the herpes viral DNA remains dormant within the nucleus of the affected individual's neurons and evades immune destruction. Reactivation of HSV frequently occurs during periods of stress, illness, or immunosuppression.

In active HSV-2, the lesions occur in the genital region and perineal area. During sexual activity or close skin contact, the virus can spread from these lesions to partners. At times, the affected individual may not have apparent symptoms of active lesions and can unknowingly spread the virus (see Chapter 28 for more on HSV-2).

The characteristic cytological changes induced by HSV can be demonstrated in a specialized culture called a Tzanck smear. Alternatively, HSV DNA can be extracted from lesions by PCR. Supportive measures are used for treatment. Acyclovir is an antiviral medication often used to lessen the severity of the outbreak of HSV infection.

Poliomyelitis

Poliomyelitis is a disease that is caused by the polio virus. Historically, polio caused epidemics resulting in high death rates and disability. Since the 1950s, the disease has been preventable through routine immunization. Jonas Salk developed the first polio vaccine in 1955; since then, the disease has been eradicated in areas where immunization is routine and widespread. There are two types of vaccines. The inactivated polio vaccine is an injectable vaccine that is given at 2 months and 4 months of age, then again between 6 and 18 months. It is followed by another dose at 4 to 6 years. Boosters are recommended for world travelers. Oral polio vaccine is given in other countries.

Polio enters the body through the fecal–oral route, usually from contaminated eating utensils, water sources, or through hand contamination from the stool of an infected person. The virus lives in the throat and intestinal tract of the infected person for approximately 1 to 6 weeks. Ninety percent of individuals will have no symptoms for the first 2 weeks after initial infection. Others will have short-term symptoms of headache, tiredness, fever, stiff neck and back, and generalized muscle pain. Unfortunately, the infected person is most contagious before the symptoms manifest.

Polio causes damage to the motor neurons of the CNS. There are three related syndromes for polio. Abortive poliomyelitis is a nonspecific disease with a fever for 2 to 3 days. There is no CNS involvement, and the patient may not even seek medical attention. The second syndrome is aseptic meningitis. Again, there is fever, but recovery is rapid and complete, without any complications. The third syndrome is paralytic poliomyelitis, which is the classic presentation. At one time the disease was called infantile paralysis. There is asymmetrical flaccid paralysis, deep tendon reflexes are decreased or absent, and sensation remains intact. Complications of poliomyelitis mostly affect the legs, although paralysis of the diaphragm muscle and swallowing mechanisms may be seen in cases called bulbar paralytic poliomyelitis.

There is no treatment for polio. Therapy is supportive and consists of mobility, support of the work of breathing, and prevention of complications such as aspiration.

Postpolio syndrome (PPS) can occur in older adults who are polio survivors. Affected persons experience increased weakness and atrophy in muscles that were previously affected. Slowly progressive new muscle weakness, joint disorders, and scoliosis can occur. Respiratory and esophageal muscles can be affected, causing breathing and swallowing difficulty. Swallowing muscle weakness can cause aspiration. Treatment of PPS using corticosteroids, IV immunoglobulin, and anticonvulsant medication is under investigation.

Hantavirus

Hantaviruses, which belong to the Bunyaviridae family of viruses, were first recognized in the 1950s during the Korean War. There are five different viruses within the Bunyaviridae family; each is made up of a single-stranded RNA virus. They are rodent-borne viruses transmitted via inhalation. Humans breathe in the aerosolized virus from infected rodents' urine, droppings, or saliva.

The incidence of hantavirus infection varies depending on geography. In China and Russia, 20,000 to 100,000 cases are reported annually. In the United States, approximately 400 cases are reported annually, mostly in the states of New Mexico, California, Washington, and Texas.

Hantavirus can cause two separate syndromes: hemorrhagic fever with renal syndrome (HFRS) and hantavirus cardiopulmonary syndrome (HCPS). They have different symptoms.

HFRS has five phases, which occur after the incubation period of 2 to 4 weeks:

1. **Febrile phase:** characterized by fever and flu-like symptoms lasting 3 to 7 days.
2. **Hypotensive phase:** characterized by decreasing platelets, tachycardia, and hypotension. This phase lasts for approximately 2 days.
3. **Oliguric phase:** features the onset of acute renal failure and proteinuria and lasts 3 to 7 days.
4. **Diuretic phase:** characterized by urine output of 3 to 6 liters/day and may last for a few days or several weeks.
5. **Convalescent phase:** characterized by recovery of renal and respiratory function. This phase may last for a couple of weeks.

HCPS is the more fatal form of the hantavirus. If contracted, the symptoms are similar to the HFRS, but the cardiovascular shock is potentially fatal.

Serological testing is the method for a definitive diagnosis. IgG and specific kinds of IgM antibodies will be present upon testing. Treatment is based on symptomatology. Support of the respiratory system with early mechanical ventilation and administration of antiviral medications may be helpful. The earlier the disease is recognized and treated, the better the outcome for the patient. Environmental rodent control is the principal strategy for preventing the virus.

West Nile Virus

West Nile virus (WNV) was first diagnosed in 1937 in Uganda, Africa, but did not appear in the United States until 1999. WNV is within the family of Flaviviridae, part of the Japanese encephalitis antigenic complex of viruses. The virus is spread when a mosquito bites an infected bird, ingests its blood, and then bites a person. Mosquitoes carry the highest amount of viral load in the early fall. The risk of disease decreases in cold weather.

People who are infected with WNV may have one of three different syndromes, ranging from an asymptomatic infection, to a mild febrile syndrome, to the virus entering the brain. In this last case, WNV may be deadly, causing encephalitis or meningitis. The highest-risk groups are older individuals, those with compromised immune systems, and pregnant women.

Diagnosis of WNV is by complete blood count, which will indicate an elevated leukocyte count; lumbar puncture with CSF testing, which will show a predominance of lymphocytes as well as elevated protein levels; head CT scan and head MRI, which usually return negative findings; electroencephalogram (EEG), which may show generalized slowing in the frontal or temporal regions; and serology, checking for antibodies against the virus. The IgM antibody assay is most often used for diagnosis. PCR testing of serum, CSF, or tissue can be useful early in infection. WNV should be suspected if the patient presents with an acute febrile episode and symptoms suggestive of meningitis or flaccid paralysis during mosquito season.

There are no vaccines or treatments for WNV, but antiviral medications may be used. Complications are rare, but in severe cases permanent brain damage, muscle weakness, and death can occur.

The principal method of control is to avoid mosquitoes by using insect repellent and eradicating the mosquito breeding sites.

Hemorrhagic Viruses

Ebola and Marburg viruses belong to the family of viruses known as the filoviruses. They are responsible for severe hemorrhagic fever. Both the Ebola and the Marburg viruses are classified as Category A bioterrorism agents because of their virulence, stability, and high infectivity as small-particle aerosols.

Ebola Virus

Ebola virus is extremely lethal and rapid in onset. It was first isolated in the Congo region of Africa and causes a hemorrhagic fever. It is hypothesized that the virus is a zoonosis, appearing first in animals, then spread to humans by contact. Primates and fruit bats can carry the disease. Transmission is by direct contact with the virus through blood and body fluids. Humans spread it to each other when in close contact or commonly in unsterile clinic conditions. The incubation period is from 2 to 21 days. The mechanism of entry into the body is unknown. The virus is activated and then begins to release its own genetic material, causing the host to produce proteins for viral replication. It then rapidly spreads to other cells and continues to spread until all the cells have the virus. Ebola hemorrhagic fever symptoms range from vomiting, diarrhea, and general body malaise to internal bleeding from organs and fever. Mortality rates are high, up to 90%, and death occurs within 7 to 14 days. The cause of death has been attributed to shock and organ dysfunction.

Diagnosis is through PCR and enzyme-linked immunosorbent array (ELISA) testing. Immediate isolation of the affected patient is necessary. Health-care providers should isolate the affected patient and use specialized protective hoods, masks, gloves, gowns, boot covers, and goggles when caring for patients. It is also important to prevent close contact with bodies of the deceased. An experimental vaccine called rVSV-ZEBOV was found to be highly protective against the virus in a trial conducted by the World Health Organization (WHO) in 2015. Food and Drug Administration (FDA) licensure for the vaccine is expected.

Marburg Virus

Marburg virus causes Marburg hemorrhagic fever. Similar to Ebola virus, it begins with infection of animals, such as nonhuman primates. The African fruit bat is a known reservoir of the virus. The disease occurs in sporadic outbreaks within Africa. It has also occurred in laboratory workers in Europe working with primate blood samples.

The disease is transmitted via contact with infected bodily fluids. The incubation period is 3 to 9 days. Early symptoms are fever, headache, and general malaise. After 5 days, a rash is noted on the trunk. Symptoms of late-stage Marburg hemorrhagic fever include jaundice, pancreatitis, weight loss, delirium, neuropsychiatric symptoms, and hemorrhage. Diagnosis is made using PCR testing. The mortality rate has been reported as high as 90%. There is no standard treatment. Health-care providers need to use full-body protection precautions, similar to the Ebola virus.

Zika Virus

Zika virus is transmitted via infected mosquitoes and most commonly causes severe fetal defects if a pregnant woman is bitten. Microcephaly and brain defects occur in the fetus of infected pregnant women. The Zika virus is prevalent in parts of South America, Puerto Rico, Virgin Islands, Mexico, and Africa. In 2018, sporadic cases were reported in the United States, with the highest number of cases in Florida and California.

Zika virus can also be spread via sexual transmission: oral, anal, or vaginal. Persons can be asymptomatic or sustain fever, rash, muscle and joint pain, conjunctivitis, and headache for a few days to a week. Guillain-Barré syndrome, a disorder of ascending neurological paralysis, has also been associated with Zika infection. Zika virus remains in the blood for approximately a week. It is unclear whether the virus can be transmitted via blood transfusion. Zika virus RNA has been detected in a number of body fluids, including blood, urine, saliva, and amniotic fluid. Laboratory testing of whole blood, serum, or plasma is recommended to detect virus, viral nucleic acid, or virus-specific immunoglobulin M and neutralizing antibodies. There are no specific treatments for the viral syndrome other than supportive measures. The CDC recommends standard precautions in all health-care settings to protect both health-care personnel and patients from infection with Zika virus, as well as from blood-borne pathogens. Zika infection is a nationally notifiable condition. Health-care providers should report suspected cases to their state or local health departments to facilitate diagnosis and mitigate the risk of local transmission.

Selected Fungal Infections

Fungi are plant-like organisms that live in air, soil, plants, water, and even the human body. Fungi reproduce through tiny spores in the air. Fungal infections often affect those with a weakened immune system and those who are on prolonged antibiotics. They can affect the skin and nails, or they can infect the lungs, GI tract, genitourinary tract, or vaginal tract. Some fungal infections are difficult to eradicate. Some common fungal infections include tinea (also called ringworm) infections, yeast infections, and skin and nail infections. Fungus that grows on skin, nails, and mucous membranes are also called dermatophytes.

Candida

Candida is a common fungus in our environment and part of the normal flora. *C. albicans*, normally found in the GI and vaginal tracts, is the most common type of *Candida* infection. *Candida* becomes pathogenic when an overgrowth of the fungus occurs, commonly causing superficial diseases. The host immune response is one of the most important determinants of the type of infection that will be caused by *Candida*. An immunocompromised host can develop widespread dissemination of *Candida* within the body, which can then progress to overwhelming sepsis. A bloodstream infection with *Candida* is known as systemic candidiasis.

Oropharyngeal candidiasis, or thrush, is commonly seen in infants, denture wearers, and those individuals who are immunosuppressed, either because of chemotherapy or because of a primary immunocompromising disease such as AIDS. The common symptoms of thrush are dry mouth, the presence of fluffy white lesions on the tongue and buccal surfaces, and loss of taste. In more severe cases, patients may have difficulty eating and swallowing. Scraping the lesions and conducting microscopic examination can confirm the diagnosis; however, the presence of the characteristic white plaque lesions is usually diagnostic. Treatment consists of oral agents, such as a swish and swallow of an antifungal agent or an antifungal lozenge.

A more severe type of oral candidiasis is esophageal candidiasis, which is found in patients who are immunocompromised and patients who have hematological malignancies. The major symptom is painful swallowing, known as odynophagia. Endoscopic examination of the esophagus is the definitive diagnosis, but most often the diagnosis is made by history and clinical signs and symptoms.

Vulvovaginal candidiasis is yeast infection of the female outer genitalia and vaginal canal. It is commonly seen in women with increased estrogen levels, such as those taking oral contraceptives, estrogen therapy, and those who are pregnant. Other risk factors for vulvovaginitis include medications such as antibiotics and steroids, and comorbid conditions of diabetes and HIV infection. Women who use intrauterine devices and diaphragms are also at higher risk for vulvovaginitis. Clinical manifestations include itching and discharge, dyspareunia, dysuria, and vaginal irritation. Physical examination shows a classic white, curd-like watery discharge. Vulvular erythema and swelling may also be present.

Balanitis is a *Candida* infection of the penis that is associated with severe burning and itching. The infection can also be found on the thighs, gluteal folds, buttocks, and scrotum.

Treatment for all the local *Candida* infections is antifungal medication, either orally or topically.

Aspergillus

Aspergillus is a fungus that grows on carbon sources, such as plants and starchy foods like bread and potatoes. The most common species of *Aspergillus* that may cause invasive disease are *A. fumigatus* and *A. flavus*. Aspergillosis is the term used for a group of fungal diseases caused by *Aspergillus*. It is an infection that occurs in immunocompromised, critically ill patients. Patients suffering from hematological malignancies are particularly vulnerable to invasive fungal infections of the *Aspergillus* type. Mainly a disease of the pulmonary system, it is characterized by a flu-like illness, fever, cough, chest pain, dyspnea, and infiltrates on chest x-ray. The major forms of the disease are allergic bronchopulmonary aspergillosis, acute invasive aspergillosis, and disseminated invasive aspergillosis. Exposure to *Aspergillus* can also cause a syndrome termed hypersensitivity pneumonitis, a pulmonary infection that is difficult to diagnose. Aspergillosis is treated with antifungals such as amphotericin B or itraconazole.

Cryptococcus

Cryptococcus is encapsulated yeast that causes meningitis or disseminated disease. There are 19 species in the genus *Cryptococcus*, but only *C. neoformans* is associated with disease in humans. Cryptococcosis is an invasive fungal infection seen in patients who are immunocompromised.

Disseminated cryptococcosis begins with infection of the lungs via inhalation. The infection moves from the lungs into the bloodstream, allowing dissemination to the brain and CNS. Cryptococcus is capable of secreting potent enzymes that allow for its penetration through the blood–brain barrier. The organism's thick polysaccharide capsule protects it from phagocytosis by macrophages. Cryptococcal infection of the brain is rare but has arisen in patients with AIDS. Diagnosis is by culture confirmation. Infection requires aggressive treatment with antifungal medications, surgical intervention, and supportive treatments.

Histoplasmosis

Histoplasmosis, also known as Darling's disease, is a fungal disease caused by *Histoplasma capsulatum*, a dimorphic fungus that is found in the soil of areas inhabited by bats and birds. It is the most prevalent endemic mycosis in the United States. Most cases of histoplasmosis are self-limiting, but some may develop into systemic infection, especially in patients who are immunocompromised. There are approximately 2,000 cases of acute infections per year in the United States.

Histoplasmosis enters the body through inhalation into the respiratory tract. It is then germinated into yeast. Neutrophils, macrophages, lymphocytes, and natural killer cells are attracted to the site of infection. These defense mechanisms are usually adequate to control the infections, except in immunosuppressed individuals, who usually have a more severe disease course. However, the macrophage infiltration leads to the translocation of the fungus via the lymphatics to other areas. At autopsy, patients with disseminated histoplasmosis have involvement of the liver, spleen, bone marrow, adrenal glands, and the GI tract. Lesions have also been noted in the CNS.

Risk factors for severe disease include patients who are immunocompromised by disease or via treatment with immunosuppressive medications, such as corticosteroids, methotrexate, and tumor necrosis factor-alpha inhibitor therapies.

Pneumocystis

Pneumocystis jirovecii, previously known as *Pneumocystis carinii*, is the organism responsible for *Pneumocystis* pneumonia (PCP), the most common opportunistic infection in patients with HIV. The organism has been recently renamed *Pneumocystis jirovecii* for the researcher, Otto Jirovec, who discovered the microbe as a cause of human infection. The organism, mistaken as a protozoan in the past, is now categorized as a fungus.

Pneumocystis infection occurs most often in patients who are immunocompromised by AIDS, chemotherapy, or immunosuppressive agents for solid organ transplant recipients. The fungal organism is a normal inhabitant of the respiratory tract and in healthy individuals does not cause disease. Severe immunosuppression allows proliferation, and macrophages cannot eradicate the organism. The fungal organism produces hardy spores. When the organism proliferates in the lungs, patients exhibit signs and symptoms of pneumonia that include fever, dyspnea, cough, crackles, hemoptysis, and pulmonary infiltrates on chest x-ray.

Diagnosis of PCP requires sputum analysis obtained by bronchoalveolar lavage, staining procedures that highlight *Pneumocystis* cysts found in sputum samples, and lactic dehydrogenase levels, which indicate degree of lung involvement. Treatment requires antibiotic medication.

Coccidioidomycosis

Coccidioides immitis is a fungal organism that resides in the soil of the western United States, Mexico, Central America, and South America. Coccidioidomycosis is a fungal infection that is also known as valley fever. The fungus is usually dormant but develops long filaments that break off into airborne spores in the rainy season. The spores disperse into the air with any disruption of the soil, such as during construction. Infection is caused by inhalation of the particles. It affects humans and animals; however, the disease is not transmitted from person to person. Immunosuppressed persons are more susceptible than others.

Initially the infection begins similar to the flu, with coughing, fever, muscle aches, and headache. A macular skin rash can occur. It is self-limited in most persons; however, some can develop pneumonia, meningitis, bone and joint infection, or bloodstream infection. Chest x-ray, CT scan, serology, and blood culture are often done to diagnose the disease. Tissue biopsy may be required. Treatment consists of antifungal medications such as fluconazole.

Selected Parasitic Infections

Parasitic infections are uncommon in the United States but frequently affect individuals in underdeveloped countries. Diagnosis is a challenge for the clinician; however, antiparasitic agents are widely available and effective. Some parasitic infections, such as malaria, are endemic to certain areas of the world. With worldwide travel, persons of these areas often bring parasitic diseases to distant regions.

Malaria

There are four protozoan organisms that can infect humans and cause malaria:

1. *Plasmodium falciparum*
2. *Plasmodium vivax*
3. *Plasmodium ovale*
4. *Plasmodium malariae*

All of these parasites are transmitted to humans via the *Anopheles* mosquito. Through widespread pesticide utilization in the 1950s, mosquito control has led to malaria eradication in North America, Russia, and Europe; however, it remains a problem in Africa, South and Central America, and parts of Asia.

Malaria most commonly occurs when the female *Anopheles* mosquito bites a human and injects the microscopic *Plasmodium* parasites into the bloodstream. However, malaria can be transmitted to individuals from blood products, contaminated needlesticks, or organ transplantation. From the bloodstream, the parasites invade the liver and multiply within the hepatocytes, which then burst and release the organisms into the blood. The organisms enter RBCs, where they multiply vigorously and degrade the blood cell constituents, particularly hemoglobin. In fulminant malaria parasitemia, RBCs become deformed, obstruct small blood vessels, die, and accumulate within the spleen. This destruction of RBCs causes accumulation of bilirubin from hemoglobin breakdown, resulting in jaundice. Hemoglobinuria can also cause renal damage. The sequelae of malaria may also include hemolytic anemia, hepatomegaly, splenomegaly, and eventual splenic rupture.

The release of *Plasmodium* organisms from dead RBCs induces an immune response within the host that includes a characteristic pattern of fever and chills occurring every 2 to 3 days. Headache, myalgia, nausea, vomiting, and orthostatic hypotension are common. In many individuals, a strong immune response can suppress the disease so that the individual has asymptomatic periods in life.

Diagnosis of malaria is based on demonstration of the parasite within RBCs on a peripheral blood smear. Repeat blood smears are necessary to obtain a sample with proof of the organism. In general, patients with more than 105 parasites per microliter are considered to have a poor prognosis. Serological testing that demonstrates the specific antibody against *Plasmodium* is also used to diagnose malaria.

Chloroquine is the major medication used to treat malaria; however, resistant strains are widespread. Other medication regimens such as sulfadoxine plus pyrimethamine or quinine plus tetracycline are used for resistant organisms. Mefloquine is a prophylactic medication that is recommended for those who travel to areas where malaria remains a transmissible disease. Travelers are advised to consult the CDC for up-to-date recommendations about malaria prophylaxis.

Toxoplasmosis

Toxoplasmosis is a disease caused by the parasite protozoan *Toxoplasma gondii*. It infects warm-blooded animals, including humans, but the primary host is the cat. Pregnant women and immunosuppressed individuals are at high risk for toxoplasmosis infection. In the pregnant woman, the infection may cause congenital disease in the fetus. The newborn can experience complications that range from vision impairment to significant learning disabilities or death. Most infants born with toxoplasmosis are asymptomatic at birth, though some have fever, maculopapular rash, hepatosplenomegaly, microcephaly, seizures, jaundice, thrombocytopenia, and rarely generalized lymphadenopathy. The symptoms of chorioretinitis, hydrocephalus, and intracranial calcifications have been considered the classic triad.

In the immunosuppressed adult, toxoplasmosis infection symptoms are similar to those of a mild flu-like illness. The parasite can cause encephalitis and progressive neurological diseases that can also extend to the heart, liver, and eyes. Transmission can occur through the ingestion of raw or partly cooked meat, specifically pork, lamb, and venison. Oocysts (eggs of the organism) may be found on hands of people who handle the meat or on contaminated cooking utensils. Contamination can also occur by ingestion of toxoplasmosis-contaminated cat feces. For this reason, pregnant women and immunosuppressed individuals are cautioned against handling cat litter boxes. The infection can also be contracted from contaminated drinking water and infected organ transplant or blood transfusion.

Amebiasis and Giardiasis

Amebiasis and giardiasis are both water-borne protozoan infections. Amebiasis is caused by the protozoan parasite *Entamoeba histolytica*. Giardiasis is caused by *Giardia lamblia*. Amebiasis and giardiasis are contracted by consuming contaminated food or water containing the cyst stage of the parasite. The cyst stage is a hardy form of the organism that is resistant to gastric acid. After ingestion, the cysts can develop into the motile organism referred to as the trophozoite form. Trophozoites adhere to and lyse the epithelial cells of the GI tract and cause necrosis. Organisms are commonly transmitted via contaminated water or the fecal–oral route. Anal–oral sexual activity can also transmit the organisms.

Individuals can carry the parasite for weeks to years, often without symptoms. The majority of cases of amebiasis and giardiasis are asymptomatic; however, significant morbidity and mortality are associated with the dysentery form of illness. The trophozoite form of the protozoan (motile organism) is responsible for the clinical syndrome referred to as dysentery. This syndrome includes nausea, vomiting, intense abdominal pain, tenderness, and copious diarrhea of watery stool, sometimes with blood. Microscopic identification of *E. histolytica* or *G. lamblia* in stool culture is the basis for diagnosis. Amebic dysentery is treated with metronidazole, amebicides, and supportive measures. Giardiasis is treated with metronidazole.

Leishmaniasis

Leishmaniasis is a disease caused by a protozoan of the genus *Leishmania* that infects mammalian reservoir hosts, particularly rodents. The prevalence among soldiers returning from the Persian Gulf is higher than in the general population because sandflies that bite the infected rodents act as vectors by then biting humans. The protozoan invades the bloodstream and can then invade body organs. Asymptomatic infection is common, though the protozoan can cause fever, splenomegaly, lymphadenopathy, hepatomegaly, cachexia, and gray discoloration of the skin. Diagnosis is made by demonstration of the organism from microscopic staining, histological tissue sampling, or culture. Serological testing for *Leishmania*-specific cell-mediated immunity is also used. Vector control with pesticides, protective garments, and insect repellents are the best methods to prevent infection. Different types of antibiotic agents have been moderately effective for treatment.

Helminth Infections

Parasitic helminths, commonly known as worms, cause infectious disease in animals and humans. The parasite's life cycle, which progresses from egg to larva to adult stages, influences the clinical course and manifestations of the infection. Some of these infections can be transmitted directly from infected to uninfected persons; in others, eggs must mature outside the human host before the larva enters the host. Alternatively, some parasitic worms mature from egg to adult and spend a part of their life cycle in the soil before becoming infective to humans.

In general, repeated or intense exposure to a multitude of helminths in the infective stage is required for infection to be established and disease to arise. Significant helminthic diseases include enterobiasis (pinworms), trichuriasis, ascariasis (roundworm), hookworm, strongyloides, trichinosis, filariasis, schistosomiasis, and tapeworm infection.

Many helminth infections are more prevalent in tropical areas with warm, moist climates. Trichuriasis, an infection with the helminth *Trichuris trichiura,* is one of the most prevalent worldwide; infection rates of up to 75% have been found in young schoolchildren in Puerto Rico. Ascariasis, hookworm infection, and strongyloidiasis are common infections in tropical countries with poor sanitation.

Enterobiasis is caused by pinworms and is a highly prevalent disease throughout the world, particularly in children. Unsanitary hygiene measures that spread the helminth via the fecal–oral route perpetuate the infection. Typically, children are infected by unknowingly touching pinworm eggs and putting their fingers in their mouths. The eggs are swallowed and hatch in the small intestine before maturing in the colon. Female worms then move to the child's anal area, especially at night, and deposit eggs. This usually causes intense itching. When the child scratches the perianal area, the eggs can get under the child's fingernails. These eggs can be transferred to other children, family members, and items in the house. A tape test can be done where a piece of cellophane tape is pressed against the skin around the anus and removed. This should be done in the morning before bathing or using the toilet, because bathing and wiping may remove eggs. The tape is then placed on a slide to review with a microscope to look for eggs. The anthelmintic medication mebendazole is used to eradicate the infection.

Helminths can also be transmitted in undercooked food. Trichinosis is a disease caused by the *Trichinella* worm that is harbored within carnivorous animals. Contraction of the infection occurs by ingestion of the helminth in uncooked or undercooked meat. When a person eats meat from an infected animal, *Trichinella* cysts break open in the intestines and grow into adult roundworms. The infection can move through the GI wall and into the bloodstream. These organisms tend to invade muscle tissues, including the heart and diaphragm. They can also affect the lungs and brain. Intense abdominal pain, diarrhea, fever, and muscle pain occur. A muscle biopsy is needed to confirm diagnosis. The anthelmintic medication mebendazole is used for treatment. Avoiding raw meat and cooking meat well enough (to greater than 160°F) will prevent infection.

Taenia saginata, commonly known as the tapeworm, causes infection of humans mainly by ingestion of *Taenia* eggs contained in undercooked beef or contaminated vegetation. After ingestion, the tapeworm attaches to the intestinal wall. The worm then depletes the patient of nutrients to support its own growth. Tapeworms can grow to as long as 8 meters within the digestive tract and can live for years. Clinical signs and symptoms include abdominal pain, nausea, anorexia, weight loss, and passage of eggs in the stool. Segments of the worm can be passed in stool as well. If pork tapeworm larvae move out of the intestine, they can cause local growths and damage tissues such as the brain, eye, or heart. This condition is called cysticercosis. Infection of the brain can cause seizures and other nervous system problems. Avoiding raw meat and cooking meat well enough (to greater than 160°F) will prevent tapeworm infection. Freezing meats to −4°F for 24 hours also kills tapeworm eggs. Anthelmintic medications praziquantel and niclosamide are used for treatment.

Prion Infectious Disease

Prions are infectious agents composed of abnormal proteins. Similar to viruses, prions require a host, where they use the host cell machinery to replicate itself. How a prion is formed is not completely understood. However, it is known that when a prion enters a healthy organism, it induces existing, properly formed proteins to convert into the disease-associated prion forms. Newly synthesized prions then go on to convert more proteins into prions. Prion agents cause several diseases, and the diseases share a common symptom: progressive neurological deterioration of the brain.

Creutzfeldt-Jakob Disease

Creutzfeldt-Jakob disease (CJD) is a rare but fatal degenerative neurological disease caused by a prion. CJD causes progressive death of the brain's nerve cells; brain tissue pathology demonstrates a spongiform appearance of the brain tissue. It affects people between the ages of 45 and 75 years. The duration of the disease varies, but it is fatal within months or even weeks. In more than 85% of the cases, the duration of CJD is less than 1 year after onset of symptoms.

The first symptom of CJD is rapidly progressive dementia, with memory loss, personality changes, and hallucinations. This is accompanied by speech impairment, myoclonus (involuntary jerky muscle movements), ataxia, and seizures. The tests for the diagnosis of CJD are electroencephalography (triphasic spikes seen), CSF analysis for 14-3-3 proteins, and brain MRI, which shows high signal intensity bilaterally in the caudate nucleus and putamen. The only definitive diagnostic test, however, is biopsy of the brain. There is no treatment or cure.

Variant Creutzfeldt-Jakob Disease

Variant Creutzfeldt-Jakob disease is a new form of CJD that has been noted mostly in the United Kingdom and France. It differs from CJD in that it affects younger people, with the average age of onset at 33 years. It is believed to be caused by the same infectious agent that causes bovine spongiform encephalopathy (BSE), also called "mad cow disease." The symptoms begin with psychiatric problems or problems with hearing, seeing, or smelling. The first symptoms are seen for weeks or months and then progress to poor muscle coordination, muscle spasms, and mental confusion. Death occurs an average of 13 months after the first symptoms are noted.

Bovine Spongiform Encephalopathy

BSE is a progressive neurological disorder of cattle. The infectious agent is unknown, but the most accepted theory is that the agent is a prion.

The vast majority of cases of BSE have been reported from the United Kingdom, but other cases have been reported throughout Europe—and both Canada and the United States have reported at least one case.

The disease is spread via meat-and-bone meal fed to cattle. The mechanism of disease is unknown; however, the natural diet of cows is not meat, and this type of feed may be causative. In response to a BSE outbreak, the United Kingdom placed many restrictions on the meat industry, from the slaughter of cattle to the restriction of feed and how the meat is cooked. In the United States, the U.S. Department of Agriculture has placed a prohibition on the importation of livestock from countries where BSE is known to exist.

Chapter Summary

- The body's normal flora are organisms that colonize the body but do not normally cause infection.
- The body has both innate and adaptive immune responses for defending against invading pathogens.
- An antibody titer is the level of antibodies against the pathogen in the bloodstream.
- When defense mechanisms fail, the body is susceptible to colonization and infection by bacteria, viruses, prions, fungi, or parasites.
- In infectious disease, the host is the infected being, the reservoir is the source of pathogens, and the vector is the organism that can transmit the pathogen.
- Microorganisms gain entry via a portal such as skin; the respiratory, GI, or genitourinary tracts; or are transmitted via blood or maternal–fetal pathways.
- Bacteria are categorized as cocci, streptococci, bacillus, and spirochetes.
- Bacteria are categorized as gram-negative or gram-positive according to how their membranes take up Gram stain. Specific antibiotics are effective against each.
- The five distinct phases of infection are incubation, prodrome, infection, convalescence, and resolution.
- Culture and sensitivity is the common method of diagnosis in bacterial disease.
- Viral exanthems are specific rash-inducing infections that occur in childhood and include measles, rubella, fifth disease, and varicella.
- An opportunistic infection occurs in an immunosuppressed patient.
- A hospital-acquired or health-care–acquired infection (previously called a nosocomial infection) is an infection contracted from the clinical setting.
- MRSA, VRSA, VRE, DRSP, and *Clostridium difficile* are known as antibiotic-resistant bacteria. Many other antibiotic-resistant microbial organisms are considered threats by the CDC. An updated list of resistant bacteria can be found on the CDC website at https://www.cdc.gov/drugresistance/biggest_threats.html.
- In the United States, a wide number of antibiotic medications are available to treat infectious diseases. There are also many immunizations in the arsenal against infections.
- Many infectious diseases have been virtually eradicated in the United States because of successful vaccination campaigns.
- Microorganisms are constantly mutating and developing resistance to the available antibiotics. In addition, some individuals choose to not get immunized. These factors increase the susceptibility of the population to infectious disease.
- Certain highly virulent pathogens are considered possible bioterrorist weapons.

Bibliography

Available online at fadavis.com

Immune System Disorders

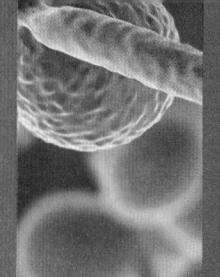

Learning Objectives

Upon completion of this chapter, the student will be able to:

- Differentiate between innate and adaptive immunity, which are the two levels of the immune system.
- Compare and contrast the mechanisms of antibody-mediated immunity versus cell-mediated immunity.
- Describe the different mechanisms of the four hypersensitivity reactions.
- Discuss the mechanisms of significant autoimmune diseases.

- Identify the three stages of HIV infection and the clinical presentation of each stage.
- Define the significant laboratory tests involved in the diagnosis of HIV infection and AIDS.
- Recognize significant opportunistic infections associated with AIDS.
- Discuss mechanisms of different drugs known as antiretroviral drug treatment and preventive HIV drugs.

Key Terms

Active acquired adaptive immunity
Adaptive immunity
AIDS
Allergy
Amnestic response
Anaphylaxis
Anergy panel
Angioedema
Antibody-mediated immunity
Antibody titer
Antigen
Antiretroviral therapy (ART)
Atopic disorder
Autoimmune disease

Autoimmunity
B lymphocyte
Booster
CCR5 receptor
CD4 cell
CD8 cell
Cell-mediated immunity
CXCR4 receptor
Dendritic cell
HIV
HIV RNA assay
Humoral immunity
Hypersensitivity
Immunization

Immunodeficiency
Immunoglobulins (Igs)
Innate immunity
Major histocompatibility complexes (MHCs)
Molecular mimicry
Opportunistic infection
Passive acquired adaptive immunity
Raynaud's phenomenon
T lymphocyte
Toxoid
Urticaria
Vaccine
Vaccination

The immune system is a complex defense mechanism that protects humans from a constant barrage of injurious agents in the environment, including microbes such as viruses, bacteria, fungi, and parasites. In addition, many foreign substances that are ingested, inhaled, and absorbed are potentially damaging agents. The immune system can decipher which substances are "self" versus "non-self." Non-self substances, which are identified as foreign **antigens**, are the targets of the immune system. A vital immune system, in conjunction with the inflammatory reaction of the body, rapidly identifies an antigen and subjects it to barriers and protective cellular forces that destroy the threat.

The immune system has two basic parts:

1. **Innate immunity**
2. **Adaptive immunity**

The innate immune mechanism comes to the body's defense first and immediately. It is composed of the body's natural anatomical barriers, normal flora, white blood cells (WBCs), and protective enzymes and chemicals. Natural anatomical barriers include skin and mucous membranes, whereas normal flora includes bacteria that live on the skin and within the gastrointestinal (GI) tract. The WBCs are macrophages that phagocytose foreign debris and antigens. Interferon, cytokines, and hydrochloric acid are some of the protective enzymes and chemicals that protect the body from bacteria and viruses.

The adaptive immune system comes to the body's defense after the innate system. A more specific form of protection, the adaptive immune line of defense is developed after exposure to antigens. However, after exposure, the adaptive immune mechanisms act rapidly, specifically, destructively, and with memory for every individual antigen it has encountered.

In a type of immune dysfunction called **immunodeficiency**, the immune system can weaken to the extent that it cannot destroy foreign invaders, and antigens can overwhelm the body. Alternatively, in a type of immune dysfunction called **autoimmunity**, the immune system can no longer distinguish between self and non-self. In autoimmune disorders, the immune system attacks non-self and self antigens indiscriminately. Lastly, in **hypersensitivity** disorders, which can take the form of a simple case of hives to life-threatening transplant rejection, the immune system can become overreactive against foreign invaders.

Basic Concepts of Immunity

Immunity is the way the body defends itself against injurious agents in the environment. To understand the mechanism of immunity, basic concepts of immunology need to be introduced first.

Innate Immunity

Innate immunity refers to natural mechanisms that ward off invaders as a first line of defense. The major component of innate immunity consists of anatomical barriers that block entry of environmental antigens, such as the nasal epithelium, which consists of mucus-producing cells and hairs that trap inhaled substances before they enter the respiratory tract. Innate immunity also consists of phagocytic cells that engulf and ingest microorganisms and other noxious substances. These cells, known as macrophages, provide constant surveillance in different organ systems; they are recruited to sites of infection and stimulate the inflammation reaction. Examples include alveolar macrophages in the lungs, Kupffer's cells in the liver, and microglial cells in the brain. Innate barriers also include natural killer (NK) cells, which are a specific kind of T lymphocyte that directly attacks antigens, and the complement system of the inflammation reaction, which is a legion of proteins that bind to antigens in the innate system and to antibodies in the adaptive system. Lastly, innate immunity includes natural enzymes, bactericidal and antiviral substances, and acidic secretions that make the skin and mucous membranes inhospitable to pathogens.

If a foreign invader attempts to enter the body, it must deal with the innate immune system first. For example, when an individual inhales infectious bacteria, mucus and ciliated epithelium trap the pathogen in the respiratory tract, allowing the cough reflex to expel the microbe.

Other innate mechanisms of defense include processes within the GI tract. Within the initial section of the GI tract, pathogens are weakened by enzymes and antibacterial substances in the saliva. Farther along in the GI tract, gastric mucus traps pathogens and destroys them with hydrochloric acid. Should the pathogen survive these innate defenses and make its way into the intestine and bowel, the body defends itself with normal flora—natural bacterial colonies that live in symbiosis with the body. Other innate barriers include tears, which flush pathogens out of the eyes; urine, which eliminates antigens from the genitourinary tract; and sweat, which acts as an antibacterial barrier on skin.

Once the innate line of defense is compromised, the inflammatory reaction begins within seconds and has the potential to last minutes or even days. If the innate defense mechanisms prove inadequate to deal with a foreign invader, the second line of defense, the adaptive immune system, is activated.

Monocyte–Macrophages

Macrophages arise from WBCs called monocytes. Monocytes leave the peripheral circulation and migrate to the tissues. Common locations where tissue macrophages are found include the lymph nodes, spleen, bone marrow, perivascular connective tissue, skin, lungs, liver, bone, central nervous system (CNS), synovial membranes, and serous cavities such as the peritoneal and pleural spaces. Macrophages mediate innate immune functions, such as destruction of bacteria and tumor cells. The macrophages ingest bacteria or viruses and then undergo apoptosis, or self-degeneration. Macrophages that are infected and apoptotic are phagocytosed by dendritic antigen-presenting cells (APCs). The destruction of pathogens by phagocytosis is largely mediated by cytokines.

Macrophage secretory products, which are more diverse than those of any other cells, have the ability to break down various types of antigens. Secretory products include hydrolytic enzymes, oxidative metabolites, tumor necrosis factor (TNF)–alpha, interleukins (ILs), and other cytokines.

Cytokines

Cytokines are inflammatory mediators produced by WBCs, mainly macrophages and lymphocytes. These inflammatory mediators promote leukocyte recruitment and acute inflammation reactions; regulate lymphocyte growth, activation, and differentiation; activate macrophages; and stimulate growth and production of new blood cells.

Natural Killer Cells

NK cells are lymphocytes that contain cytoplasmic granules; however, they are not considered typical granulocytes. They are part of the innate immune response and act as a first line of defense. NK cells can destroy tumor cells and virus-infected cells without previous exposure.

Adaptive Immunity

The adaptive immune system allows the body to recognize an antigen, target the specific antigen, limit its response to that antigen, and develop memory for the antigen for future reference. The adaptive immune system's ability to recognize and remember specific antigens is called specificity. The ability to respond again and again to specific antigens is caused by a memory response, which develops after a second exposure to an antigen.

The ability to distinguish self from non-self is another vital function of the adaptive immune system. Every human cell has surface antigens called **major histocompatibility complexes (MHCs)**, also called human leukocyte antigens (HLAs). The adaptive immune system allows the body to distinguish between antigens that belong to the host versus foreign antigens that are from an invader.

B Lymphocytes and T Lymphocytes

The two major categories of adaptive immunity are:

1. B lymphocyte immunity, also known as **humoral immunity**
2. T lymphocyte immunity, also known as **cell-mediated immunity**

In both categories of adaptive immunity, the lymphocyte is the primary cell. Lymphocytes originate in the bone marrow in immature form and cannot initiate immunity until they mature, which occurs as they pass through lymphoid tissues such as the thymus, spleen, and lymph nodes. **T lymphocytes**, also called T cells, mature within the thymus gland, a small gland located in the midchest. The thymus gland degenerates with age, contributing to decreased immunocompetence in old age. After maturation in the thymus, mature T cells are found in the bloodstream and T-cell zones of lymph nodes. **B lymphocytes**, also called B cells, mature within the bone marrow, spleen, and lymph nodes.

CD4 and CD8 Cells

During the maturation process in the thymus, T cells begin developing surface antigens that differentiate them from one another. These are called cluster of differentiation (CD) antigens. The most common T cells that take part in cell-mediated immunity are called CD4 cells, also called T helper cells, and CD8 cells,

also called cytotoxic T cells. CD4 cells and CD8 cells perform distinct but overlapping functions. The **CD4 cell** influences all other cells of the immune system, including other T cells, B lymphocytes, macrophages, and NK cells. The CD4 cells are involved in cell-mediated immunity and assist in antibody-mediated adaptive immunity. The **CD8 cell** directly attacks an antigen. HIV targets CD4 cells. By targeting CD4 cells, HIV defeats both cell-mediated and antibody-mediated immune responses, the human body's strongest two defense mechanisms.

Antigen-Presenting Cells

T cells cannot be activated by antigen alone; APCs process the antigen first and induce cell-mediated immunity (see Fig. 11-1). APCs capture and attach to antigen and process it before the antigen is attacked. APCs include dendritic cells and macrophages. **Dendritic cells**, which are named for their numerous fine

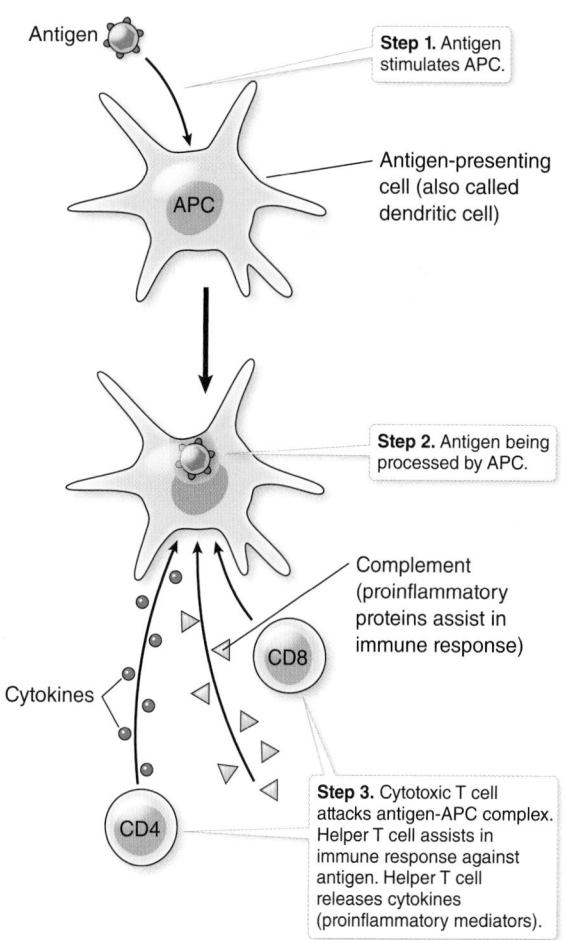

FIGURE 11-1. Cell-mediated immunity is an immune response that involves the activation of cytotoxic T lymphocytes, called CD8 cells. **Step 1.** An antigen provokes an antigen-presenting cell (APC). **Step 2.** The APC processes the antigen. **Step 3.** CD8 cells attack the antigen processed by the APC. Concurrently, a helper T cell assists the CD8 cell in the attack and yields cytokines that promote an inflammatory reaction. Proteins called complement also take part in the proinflammatory process.

dendritic cytoplasmic projections, attach to the broadest range of antigens. They are located within the epidermis and mucous membranes, where antigens enter the body. When dendritic cells come in contact with bacteria or viruses, they release cytokines that stimulate cells of the innate and adaptive immune systems to respond.

Plasma Cells

B lymphocytes, also called B cells, are naïve or immature until they encounter antigens. After exposure to an antigen, B cells are stimulated to further mature into plasma cells. As plasma cells, they have the ability to produce specific proteins called **immunoglobulins (Igs)**, also called antibodies, which attack the antigen. The process of B-cell maturation into plasma cells and Ig production comprises **antibody-mediated immunity**, also called humoral immunity (see Fig. 11-2). Antibody-mediated immunity confers long-term immunity, though full initiation of this immune response takes time.

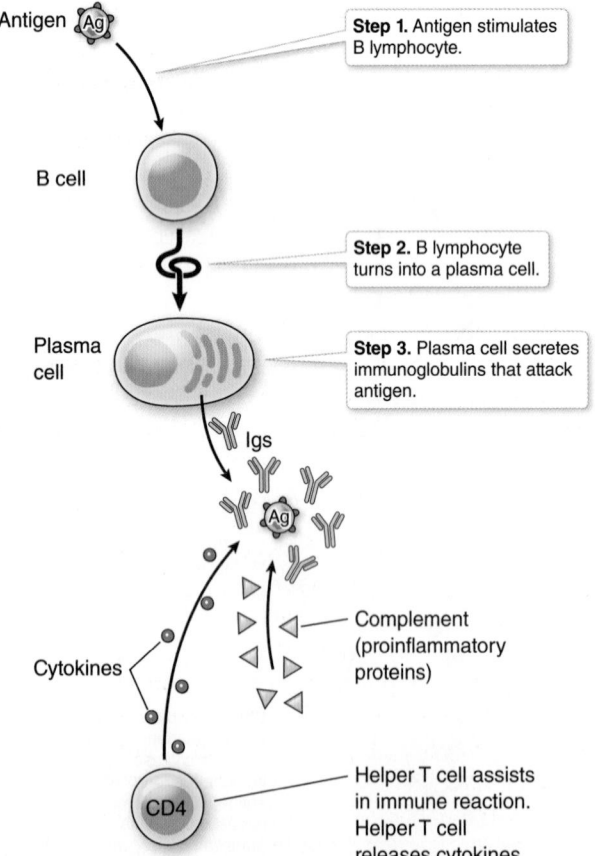

FIGURE 11-2. Antibody-mediated immunity is an immune response that involves the activation of B lymphocytes and Igs. **Step 1.** The antigen stimulates a B lymphocyte. **Step 2.** The B lymphocyte transforms into a plasma cell. **Step 3.** The plasma cell secretes Igs. Concurrently, a helper T cell assists in the attack and yields cytokines that promote an inflammatory reaction. Proteins called complement also take part in the proinflammatory process.

Upon first exposure to the antigen, the process of B-cell maturation into plasma cells that synthesize immunoglobulins takes days to initiate. Problems can occur when pathogens overwhelm the body before the antibody-mediated immune response is fully initiated. The components of the T-cell–mediated immune response become activated more quickly than the antibody-mediated immune response. During the lag time of B-cell maturation, CD4 cells attack antigens to blunt the pathogen effect on the body. In this manner, CD4 cells are integral to the antibody-mediated immune response.

Immunoglobulins

The terms *antibody* and *immunoglobulin* are interchangeable. An Ig is a product of a plasma cell that is derived from a B lymphocyte. An antigen stimulates a B lymphocyte to mature into a plasma cell, which, in turn, develops the ability to synthesize Igs. Antibody-mediated immunity involves five subtypes of Igs: IgM, IgG, IgA, IgE, and IgD (see Table 11-1). These Igs are categorized by structural and functional differences. As a group, Igs are responsible for neutralizing bacterial toxins, attacking viruses, promoting phagocytosis of bacteria, and activating and reactivating the immune response.

Igs circulate within the bloodstream and body fluids, including the lymph system, bone marrow, and other lymphoid organs. Once an antigen is recognized by a B cell, the B cells transform into plasma cells that secrete Igs. Igs are activated and attack the antigen directly. The initiation of the response begins with the binding of the immunoglobulin to antigen. Physically, once bound, the antigen is no longer able to bind to another cell and therefore cannot infect any other cell or reproduce its antigenic parts. Chemically, the antigen is targeted for phagocytosis, and proliferation of B cells begins with development of plasma cells ready to destroy the antigenic invader.

The body's antibody-mediated response to an antigen consists of two phases: primary and secondary. The primary phase occurs when the host cell is exposed to an antigenic invader and there is a lag time between recognition and proliferation of Igs to neutralize the invader. There can be a lag time of 5 to 7 days before an increase in IgM, the primary immunoglobulin responder, can be detected. The increase in IgM marks the primary response. Once the pathogen is eradicated, the existing Igs degrade and immunoglobulin levels return to normal.

A second exposure to the same antigen initiates a secondary immune response, known as an **amnestic response**, that stimulates a quick increase in levels of Igs. During this time, an increase in IgG occurs, comprising approximately 75% to 85% of total serum Igs. IgG is the predominant immunoglobulin made after the host's reexposure to antigen. IgA comprises 7% to 15% of total serum Igs, but it is mainly found within

TABLE 11-1. Classes of Immunoglobulin and Clinical Significance

Immunoglobulin	Clinical Significance
IgM	Also called macroglobulin due to large size. Earliest immunoglobulin to respond to infection.
IgG	Most abundant immunoglobulin in the bloodstream. Most important antipathogenic immunoglobulin in infections and commonly involved in autoimmune diseases.
IgA	Most abundant in mucosal secretions; sweat, saliva, tears, breast milk, nasal, bronchial, and digestive tract secretions.
IgE	Abundant in skin, mucous membranes, and respiratory tract. Responds to antigens that commonly cause allergic reactions (e.g., pollen, animal dander, dust).
IgD	Binds to basophils and mast cells in hypersensitivity reactions. Found in skin and digestive and respiratory tracts.

Adapted from Immunoglobulins: Test overview. https://www.uofmhealth.org/health-library/hw41342

secretions, such as tears, saliva, nasal and respiratory secretions, GI fluid, and breast milk. IgE is usually present in very low concentrations in the blood, but it rises to high levels in allergic reactions. IgD, which binds to basophils and mast cells in hypersensitivity reactions, comprises only 1% of Igs.

 CLINICAL CONCEPT

IgM immunoglobulins are large antibodies that increase in the bloodstream after the first exposure to an antigen. During a pregnancy in which the mother and fetus have incompatible blood types, IgM antibodies are developed by the mother against the fetus's blood cells. However, because of their large size, they cannot cross the placenta and the fetus is protected.

Active Acquired Versus Passive Acquired Immunity

Adaptive immunity can be categorized as actively acquired or passively acquired. **Active acquired adaptive immunity** is obtained through exposure to an antigen (which commonly causes an illness) or through a **vaccination** that provides **immunization**. For example, after a child contracts measles infection (rubeola), the child develops active acquired adaptive immunity: The child's body has to process the antigen and develop B cells and plasma cells that secrete Igs while enduring the disease. The child develops all the symptoms of disease but at the same time develops significant Igs for life. The Igs are specific for measles and are remembered by the B cells. Because the child's body actively developed immunity, future exposure to measles will be dealt with by the preformed Igs.

Alternatively, a child can develop active acquired adaptive immunity by receiving a measles vaccine. A **vaccine** is a specific formulation that contains a weakened, non–disease-producing pathogen. It cannot cause actual disease, but it can stimulate the adaptive immune system. The vaccine is "seen" by the adaptive immune system as an actual antigen, despite its non–disease-producing attributes. The body recognizes the vaccine as an antigen and develops an immune response and memory of the antigen without direct disease contraction. Also, any future exposure to the antigen will be dealt with by the preformed Igs.

In both forms of active acquired immunity, the body recognizes an antigen, develops immune cells specifically against the antigen, attacks and neutralizes the antigen, remembers the antigen, and develops long-lasting immunity. The body has to perform the activities needed to develop immunity in both forms of active acquired adaptive immunity.

The other type of adaptive immunity is called **passive acquired adaptive immunity**. To gain this form of immunity, an individual is given premade, fully formed antibodies against an antigen. The patient is a passive recipient of the antibodies, and their body does not have to perform the actions needed to develop immunity. This provides immediate immunity, but short term, not long lasting. An example involves hepatitis B immunoglobulin (called HBIg). If a member of a family develops hepatitis B infection, the other family members need immediate immunity, which can be conferred through administration of HBIg. The family members receive an injection of preformed IgG against hepatitis B for instant, short-term immunity. The family members are then protected during their exposure to the infected individual.

 CLINICAL CONCEPT

An example of passive acquired adaptive immunity occurs when an infant is breastfed and receives fully formed maternally produced antibodies in breast milk.

Active acquired adaptive immunity is longer lasting than passive acquired adaptive immunity. Passive immunity is short-lived immunity that exists for only a finite period; it is not permanent.

Vaccines

A vaccine can consist of either viral or bacterial components. Most viral vaccines consist of a live virus that has been inactivated. The inactivated viruses exhibit antigenic properties and stimulate an immune response but do not transfer disease to the host. Live virus vaccines have the potential, although rare, to mutate into a disease-causing strain. This has been seen with the oral poliovirus vaccine; therefore, vaccines derived from live viruses should not be administered to those with compromised immune systems.

Another type of vaccine, termed mRNA vaccine, was developed during the COVID-19 pandemic. These vaccines are synthesized from a section of messenger RNA of the viral pathogen. The mRNA that codes for a surface protein from the virus is administered to the patient. The patient's body then manufactures the protein. The protein is recognized as a "non-self" antigen and triggers the patient's immune system. The patient, in turn, develops antibodies to the viral protein and these antibodies are prepared to attack the virus.

It is important to recognize that some vaccine immunity can wear off after a certain period of time. This often requires administration of another dose of vaccine to stimulate the immune system's antigen memory; this is known as a **booster** vaccination.

Bacterial vaccines are derivatives of killed microorganisms or extracts of antigens or toxins. Some bacteria damage a host through injurious secreted exotoxins rather than cellular invasion. The vaccines produced against these toxin-producing bacteria are called **toxoids**. The toxoid type of vaccine is a modified form of the bacterial toxin that has no disease-producing effects. An example of a toxoid type of vaccine is the tetanus toxoid, which should be administered every 10 years.

In general, vaccines allow the body to recognize exposure and develop a response and memory of the antigen without direct disease contraction. Primary immune responses stimulated by vaccines are long lasting. However, some first responses are inadequate and boosters are required to obtain full immunity. Boosters restimulate the body to initiate immune responses and confer longer-lasting active immunity. To accomplish this long-term resistance, vaccines are often given to children in a series (see Chapter 10). Hepatitis B vaccine and human papillomavirus (HPV) vaccine are examples of vaccines that require a series of doses for full immunity. Certain immunizations, such as tetanus toxoid, require routine boosters.

Anergy Panel

An **anergy panel** is a test of immunocompetence; it consists of common antigens to which individuals are exposed, such as mumps, *Candida,* or *Trichophyton.* These antigens are injected intradermally, just under the skin. The clinician inspects the patient's reaction to these antigens after a set period. A positive skin reaction to one or more of these antigens indicates general immunocompetence. No reaction to the skin test indicates a lack of immune responsiveness and immunodeficiency.

Antibody Screening and Titer

Antibody screening tests, referred to as **antibody titers**, are laboratory tests used to confirm adequate immune protection against a particular antigen by measuring IgM and IgG. Because IgM is the immunoglobulin that responds first in infection, elevated IgM levels indicate a recent or current infection. IgG is a secondary responder, which means that levels rise after a second exposure to an antigen. IgG levels indicate previous exposure and immune competence to a particular antigen. The antibody screening test identifies the presence of the immunoglobulin, and the titer provides a measurement of the amount of immunoglobulin.

It is common to screen for rubella virus immunity through a blood test that measures IgG antibody. Women planning to become pregnant have a rubella titer drawn to check if they have immunity because maternal rubella infection can cause multiple birth defects in the fetus. A positive IgG rubella titer indicates the person has immunity against rubella virus through past infection or vaccine. A negative rubella titer indicates that there is no immunity to rubella. The pregnant woman may be advised to obtain a rubella vaccine based on the discretion of the health-care provider.

To prevent health-care providers from transmitting the rubella virus to pregnant patients, they are required to obtain a rubella titer to determine whether they have immunity. Those who do not have a positive rubella titer are required to obtain the rubella vaccine.

> ### 🔬 CLINICAL CONCEPT
>
> Health-care providers, particularly those engaged in maternal–child health care, should have a rubella titer to ensure their own immunity to rubella. Without immunity, the health-care provider can transmit rubella to patients. Rubella can cause serious disease in a fetus.

Allergy Testing

Allergy testing includes skin tests and serology blood tests. Skin tests measure the body's IgE reaction to an allergen by scratching or injecting a small amount of the allergen into the skin. Allergen preparations such as pollen, grass, or peanut extracts are used. The testing is considered positive for the allergen if the skin becomes red, swollen, and itchy.

Serology testing measures the presence of IgE, which is associated with allergic or hypersensitivity reactions. These serology tests are called the enzyme-linked immunosorbent assay (ELISA), radioallergosorbent test (RAST), and ImmunoCAP IgE test; they can evaluate the severity of allergy by measuring how much IgE reacts with allergen.

Hypersensitivity

The development of immunity can come with unintended consequences. Immune responses to environmental antigens lead to induction of protective defense mechanisms, but they can also cause reactions that are injurious to tissues. Injurious immune reactions can range from a mild allergic rash to life-threatening diseases. The various damaging immune reactions are called hypersensitivity reactions, and they involve either cell-mediated or antibody-mediated immune mechanisms. There are four types of hypersensitivity reactions:

1. Type I immediate hypersensitivity
2. Type II cytotoxic hypersensitivity
3. Type III immune complex disorders
4. Type IV delayed hypersensitivity

Type I Immediate Hypersensitivity

Type I immediate hypersensitivity is a rapidly developing immune reaction that occurs after IgE binds to mast cells and combines with antigen. This type of reaction, also called an **allergy** or **atopic disorder**, occurs in individuals previously exposed to an antigen.

Mast cells are key components in type I immediate hypersensitivity. These cells are widely distributed in the tissues—particularly the respiratory, nasal, and conjunctival epithelium. Mast cells have cytoplasmic granules that contain histamine, a potent vasodilator of arterioles and venules.

Immediate hypersensitivity reactions can present as local or systemic disorders. The nature of the local reaction depends on the portal of entry of an allergen. Common localized reactions include hives, a skin rash also called **urticaria**; nasal and conjunctival discharge; bronchial asthma; and allergic gastroenteritis. Common allergens include pollen, animal dander, dust, shellfish, peanuts, chocolate, and medications such as penicillin.

The mechanism of type I immediate hypersensitivity reactions involves CD4 cells, IgE antibodies, eosinophils, and mast cells (see Fig. 11-3). The first step

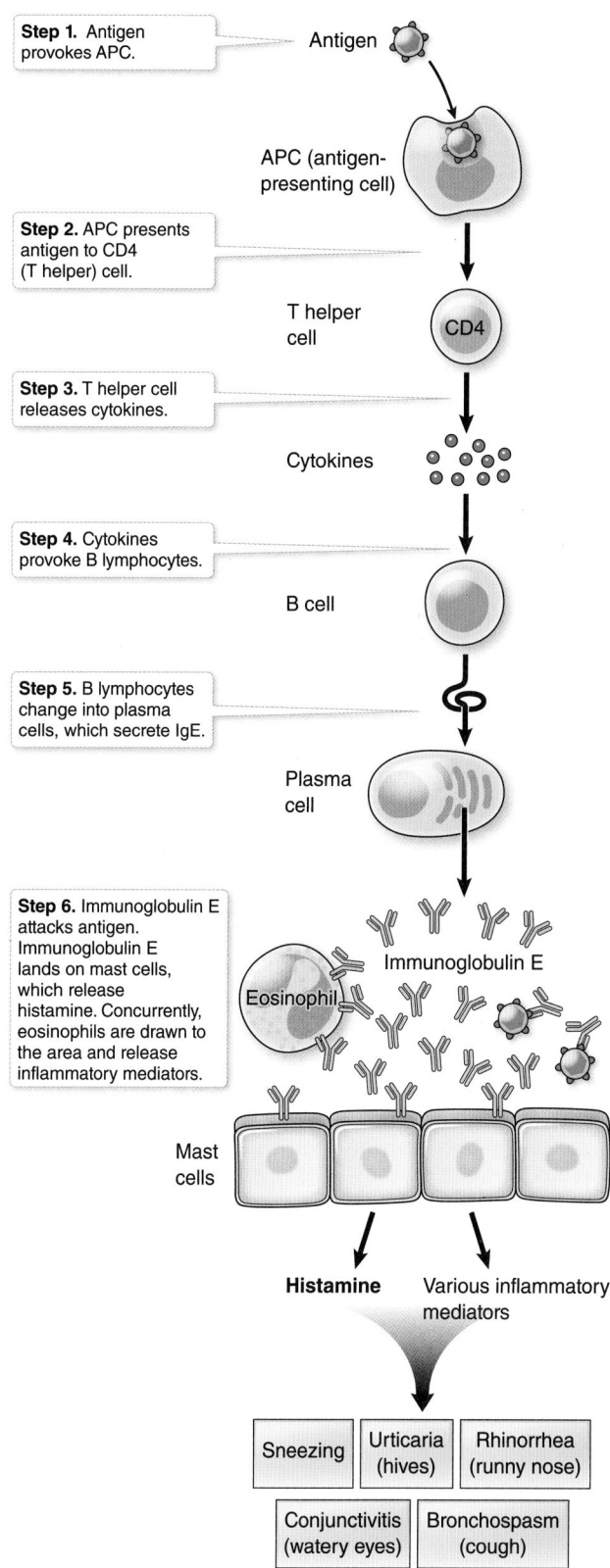

FIGURE 11-3. Immediate hypersensitivity reaction. **Step 1.** Antigen provokes an antigen-presenting cell. **Step 2.** Antigen is presented to CD4 cell. **Step 3.** CD4 cell releases cytokines. **Step 4.** Cytokines provoke a B lymphocyte. **Step 5.** B lymphocyte turns into a plasma cell that secretes immunoglobulin E. **Step 6.** Igs attack antigen. Igs land on mast cells and provoke release of histamine. Eosinophils are attracted to the area and release other inflammatory mediators. Within minutes, symptoms of allergy result, including sneezing, urticaria, rhinorrhea, conjunctivitis, pharyngitis, and cough.

in the synthesis of IgE is the presentation of the antigen to CD4 cells by dendritic APCs. The CD4 cells produce cytokines, which stimulate IgE-producing B lymphocytes and attract eosinophils to the area. Mast cells bind with the IgE antibodies and, in turn, the IgE antibodies bind to the allergen. This stimulates the release of histamine from mast cells. Other inflammatory mediators such as proteases, heparin, leukotrienes, prostaglandins, and platelet-activating factor (PAF) also are involved in the reaction. Within minutes, symptoms of allergy, including urticaria, allergic rhinitis, conjunctivitis, and bronchospasm, result.

Allergic Rhinitis

Exposure to allergens such as mold, animal dander, or pollen leads to the development of allergic rhinitis, a type I immediate hypersensitivity response. The incidence of allergic rhinitis is increasing, and it is now one of the most common medical disorders. Approximately 50% of people in the United States have a positive skin test to one of the 10 most common allergens that lead to the development of allergic rhinitis (see Box 11-1). Allergic rhinitis is also associated with the development of asthma, sinusitis, and respiratory infections.

Exposure to the allergen triggers the production of IgE and the release of inflammatory mediators. These mediators include histamine, prostaglandins, and leukotrienes. The result is vasodilation, smooth muscle constriction of the bronchioles, and mucus hypersecretion. The most common symptoms include watery eyes, sneezing, and rhinorrhea. The secretions are white or clear in an allergic response. Symptoms may progress to coughing and bronchospasm. Nasal polyps may develop in chronic cases of allergic rhinitis.

It is important to ask if there is a personal or family history of asthma or other allergic illnesses. Nasal secretions demonstrate the presence of eosinophils. Diagnostic testing can determine the presence of IgE antibodies to common allergens. Treatment involves the use of antihistamines, intranasal corticosteroids, and decongestants.

BOX 11-1. Most Common Allergens

- Milk (mostly in children)
- Eggs
- Peanuts
- Tree nuts, like walnuts, almonds, pine nuts, brazil nuts, and pecans
- Soy
- Wheat and other grains with gluten, including barley, rye, and oats
- Fish (mostly in adults)
- Shellfish (lobster, crab, shrimp) (mostly in adults)

Source: U.S. Department of Health and Human Services. Food and Drug Administration (FDA). Food allergies: What you need to know. https://www.fda.gov/food/buy-store-serve-safe-food/food-allergies-what-you-need-know

---

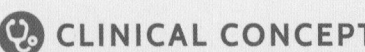

CLINICAL CONCEPT

During a physical examination, the nasal mucosa appears pale because of the swelling from an allergic response. The mucosa is erythematous if the symptoms are caused by an infection.

Systemic Anaphylaxis

Systemic **anaphylaxis** is a severe, life-threatening type I immediate hypersensitivity reaction. Extremely small doses of an allergen can trigger this overwhelming allergic reaction within minutes after exposure. Although patients at risk can generally be identified by a previous history of allergy, any individual can endure an anaphylactic reaction at any time in life.

Within minutes after exposure, itching, urticaria, and skin erythema appear, followed by bronchoconstriction. Laryngeal edema, tongue swelling, and **angioedema**, a swelling of the facial regions—particularly the lips, mouth, and periorbital regions—can occur. Because of widespread vasodilation, blood pressure drops and can induce vascular shock, at which point the disorder is anaphylactic shock. The patient may lose consciousness and require cardiac monitoring. This is a medical emergency and requires rapid response from emergency medical personnel. IV or intramuscular (IM) antihistamines, glucocorticoids, and epinephrine are required immediately. The patient needs cardiac monitoring and periodic blood pressure measurement until recovery. Patients should be aware of the allergen that triggered the reaction and wear a medical alert bracelet or necklace. Also, for prophylaxis, the patient should carry an EpiPen (predrawn syringe of epinephrine) at all times.

ALERT! Patients with allergic urticaria should be carefully observed for signs of anaphylaxis. Anaphylaxis is a medical emergency that requires vigilant monitoring of the patient's vital signs, respiratory status, and electrocardiogram. Immediate injection of epinephrine is required.

Type II Cytotoxic Hypersensitivity

Type II cytotoxic hypersensitivity is mediated by Igs directed toward antigens present on cell surfaces. The antigens may be intrinsic to the cell membrane, or they may take the form of an exogenous antigen, such as a drug metabolite, that is attached to a cell surface. In simpler terms, Igs target cells coated with antigen in type II cytotoxic hypersensitivity. Antibody-mediated cell destruction and phagocytosis occur in these reactions (see Fig. 11-4).

The classic type II hypersensitivity reaction is a transfusion reaction in which cells from an incompatible

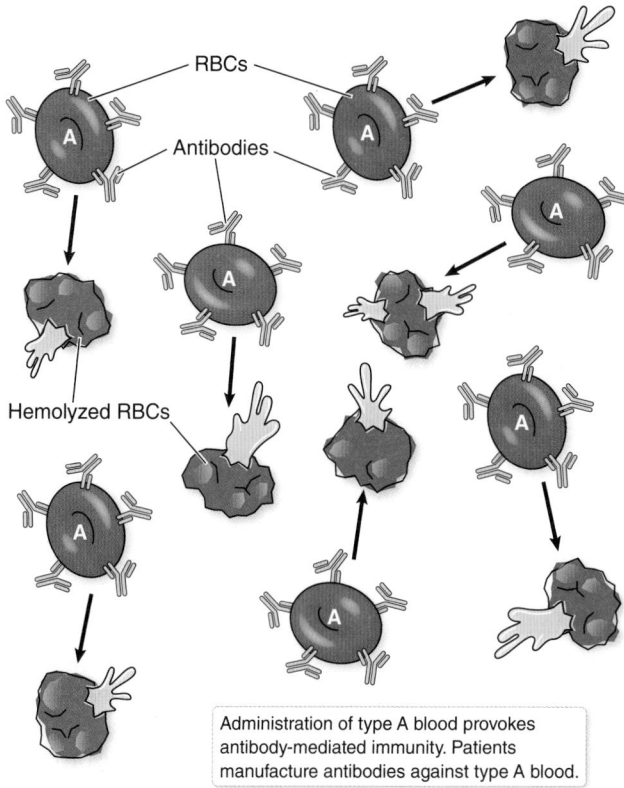

FIGURE 11-4. Type II cytotoxic hypersensitivity reaction. A patient has type B blood and is mistakenly administered a transfusion with type A blood. The donor RBCs stimulate antibody formation by the patient against the transfused blood. Patient anti-A antibodies attack the transfused type A red blood cells, causing hemolysis.

Administration of type A blood provokes antibody-mediated immunity. Patients manufacture antibodies against type A blood.

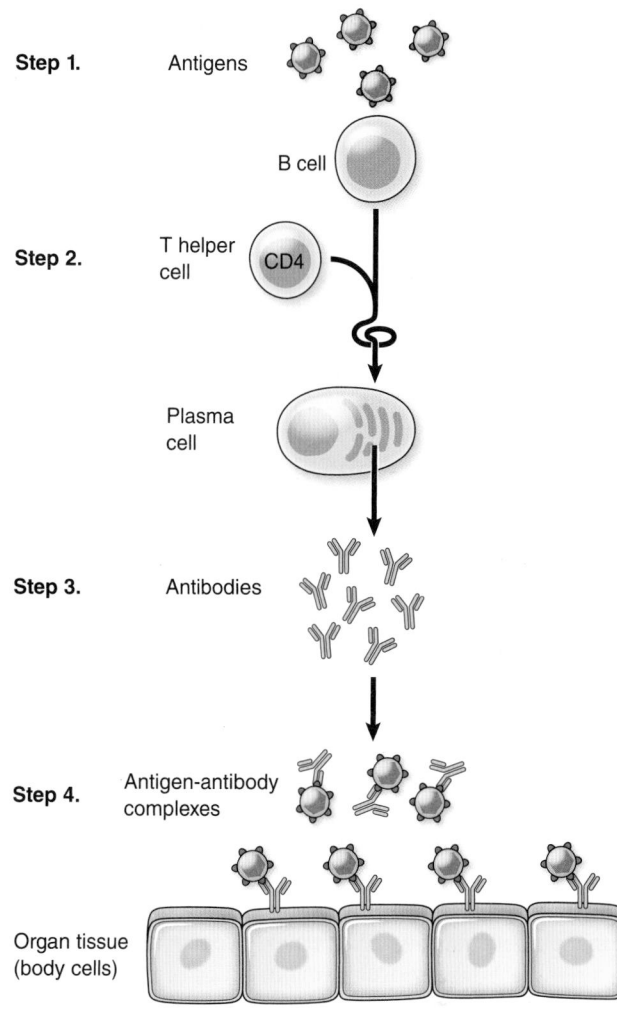

FIGURE 11-5. Type III hypersensitivity reactions involve the antigenic stimulation of Igs that combine with the antigen to form immune complexes. **Step 1.** Antigen provokes B cells. **Step 2.** The B cells transform into plasma cells with the assistance of CD4 cells. **Step 3.** Plasma cells secrete Igs. **Step 4.** Antigen combines with Igs within circulation, and these complexes are then deposited in tissues. The deposition of the antigen–Ig complexes within tissue membranes causes organ dysfunction.

donor react with host Igs. For example, if type A blood from a donor is administered to a type B recipient, the anti-A Igs of the recipient will attack and destroy the type A red blood cells, causing a massive hemolytic reaction. Another example includes certain drug reactions in which Igs are produced that react with a drug that has coated host cells. The Igs attack and destroy the drug-coated cells.

CLINICAL CONCEPT

Health-care providers need to be vigilant when administering blood products. The donor and recipient blood type must match to avoid a transfusion reaction or type II cytotoxic hypersensitivity reaction. At least two different clinicians should confirm that the patient's blood type and the blood to be infused are the same.

Type III Immune Complex Hypersensitivity

Type III hypersensitivity reactions occur when antigen combines with Ig within circulation and these complexes are then deposited in tissues (see Fig. 11-5). The deposition of the antigen–Ig complexes, also referred to

as immune complexes, within tissue membranes causes organ dysfunction. Immune-complex disorders can be systemwide, a situation in which immune complexes are deposited in many different organs. An example of this occurs in systemic lupus erythematosus (SLE), where complexes are deposited in the kidney, blood vessels, lung, and skin. Immune complex–mediated disorders can also be localized to specific tissues in the body, such as the joints in rheumatoid arthritis (RA). The antigen of an immune-complex disease may not be identifiable. There is an unidentifiable antigen that triggers the type III hypersensitivity reactions in SLE and RA.

Type IV Delayed Hypersensitivity

Type IV delayed hypersensitivity is initiated by T lymphocytes that have had previous exposure to an antigen. The T lymphocytes that are sensitized to the antigen do not attack the antigen until days after initial exposure. The inflammatory reaction that occurs in delayed hypersensitivity is referred to as contact dermatitis.

Because the inflammation reaction occurs days after exposure to the antigen, it is sometimes difficult to diagnose the source of the antigen. A classic example of this type of delayed hypersensitivity reaction occurs with exposure to poison ivy, a plant that usually grows wild in grassy fields and gardens in the United States. The person's exposure to poison ivy occurs days before the appearance of a vesicular, erythematous rash on the hands or other part of the body. At times, the patient may not be able to recall exposure to the antigen.

Another important example of type IV delayed hypersensitivity occurs in transplant rejection. Donor tissue has MHCs on its cells that differ from a recipient's MHCs. The donor tissue cells are antigenic to the recipient, and the recipient's T cells target the donor tissue. The T cells destroy the donor's foreign MHC-bearing transplant cells and cause rejection of the transplant. This usually takes a few days to become apparent.

CLINICAL CONCEPT

The Mantoux test is a tuberculosis (TB) screening test that demonstrates type IV delayed hypersensitivity. The patient receives a subcutaneous injection of tuberculin, which is a protein component of *Mycobacterium tuberculosis*, on the forearm and then waits 48 hours for a result. If there is a reaction of erythema and induration of 10 mm or larger, active TB disease is probable. If the reaction is 5 mm or smaller, there has probably been exposure to TB in the past. If there is no erythema, there has been no exposure to TB or infection. There is also a blood test called the interferon gamma release assay (IGRA). A positive blood test indicates that the person has been infected with the TB mycobacterium. Additional testing is necessary to determine whether the person has latent or active TB.

Pathophysiology of Selected Autoimmune Disorders

Autoimmune disease encompasses immune reactions against self antigens that result from the loss of self-tolerance. Under normal conditions, the immune system is vigilant in its surveillance and recognition of non-self antigens. The healthy immune system can precisely distinguish self from non-self, and its purpose is to preserve and protect the body from injurious non-self invaders. In autoimmune disease, T cells or Igs cannot make a distinction between nonantigenic cell surface markers and antigenic foreign cell surface markers. The body's own immune system becomes intolerant to its own cells, attacks its own tissues, and renders organs dysfunctional. The body develops Igs against its own tissues, known as autoantibodies.

Autoimmune disorders can be organ-specific or widespread and generalized. An example of organ-specific autoimmunity is type 1 diabetes. The body's own T cells and Igs attack beta cells of the pancreas and cause an inflammatory response that renders these insulin-producing cells nonfunctional. The patient incurs an unrecoverable insulin deficiency and contracts a permanent condition of diabetes. In multiple sclerosis, another autoimmune disease, the body's T cells attack myelin, the white matter of the CNS. Individuals suffer neuropathy of motor and sensory neurons that results in gait disturbance and loss of sensation.

An example of a generalized autoimmune disease is SLE. In SLE, Igs are developed against the body's DNA, cell membranes, and blood cells. Individuals with SLE endure a classic facial skin rash, kidney dysfunction, joint inflammation, or cardiac and lung dysfunction.

The underlying etiological mechanisms of autoimmune diseases remain unclear. However, some autoimmune disorders are associated with infectious disease. It is theorized that a mechanism called **molecular mimicry** is involved in some autoimmune disorders. Molecular mimicry occurs when an infectious agent is composed of antigens that have the same amino acid sequences as some self-antigens. Immune responses are mounted against the foreign microbial antigens, and the immune cells mistake the body's own tissues for foreign antigens. Although the immune cells attack antigen, they also attack the normal tissue with the similar composition.

An example of molecular mimicry occurs in rheumatic fever (see Fig. 11-6). In this disease, group A beta hemolytic streptococcus (GABHS) infects the throat, causing a disorder called streptococcal pharyngitis, commonly known as strep throat. The body reacts by developing Igs against the streptococcal proteins and destroys the strep organisms. In a small percentage of individuals, the body's antistreptococcal Igs not only attack the strep organisms, they also attack myocardial proteins, specifically cardiac valvular tissue. The antistrep Igs are subjected to molecular mimicry as the myocardial proteins are mistakenly attacked along with the strep organisms. There is a molecular similarity of the myocardial cell protein structure and strep organism cell structure. The result is that antistrep Igs attack the microbes but also attack heart tissue, which, in turn, results in myocarditis with irreversible valvular deformity, also known as rheumatic heart disease.

Systemic Lupus Erythematosus

SLE, commonly called lupus, is a multisystem autoimmune disease characterized by autoantibodies, particularly antinuclear antibodies (ANAs). SLE is a chronic

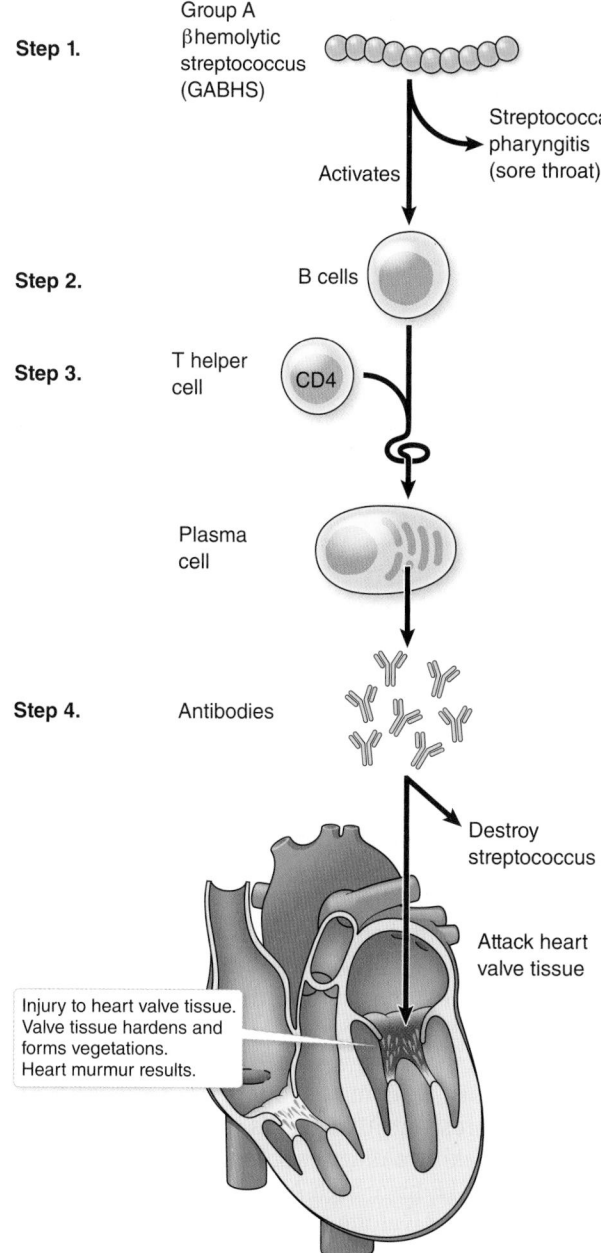

Step 1. Group A βhemolytic streptococcus (GABHS)

Streptococcal pharyngitis (sore throat)

Activates

Step 2. B cells

Step 3. T helper cell — CD4

Plasma cell

Step 4. Antibodies

Destroy streptococcus

Attack heart valve tissue

Injury to heart valve tissue. Valve tissue hardens and forms vegetations. Heart murmur results.

FIGURE 11-6. The process of rheumatic heart disease: Molecular mimicry. An example of molecular mimicry occurs in rheumatic fever. **Step 1.** In this disease, GABHS infects the throat. **Step 2. Streptococcus** activates B cells. **Step 3.** The B cells transform into plasma cells that secrete antibodies. CD4 cells assist in this reaction. **Step 4.** The antibodies destroy the Streptococcus organisms. In a small percentage of individuals, the body's antistreptococcal antibodies not only attack the strep organisms, they also attack myocardial proteins, specifically cardiac valvular tissue, resulting in heart murmur.

disease that can have an acute or insidious onset. It is characterized by remissions and exacerbations with fever; skin rash; joint inflammation; and damage to the kidney, lungs, and serosal membranes.

Epidemiology

The prevalence of SLE is 81 to 144 per 100,000 population in the United States. It is mainly a disease of women, as women are 5.5 to 6.5 times more likely to develop SLE than men. Women of child-bearing age account for 65% of all SLE cases. African American women are two to three times more likely to develop SLE than European Americans; those of Asian and Hispanic descent are also diagnosed more frequently than those of European ancestry.

Etiology/Risk Factors

The cause of SLE is unknown. Risk factors include genetic predisposition and environmental, hormonal, and immunological elements. In the majority of individuals, multiple genetic alterations are most likely responsible. Genome-wide association studies have identified approximately 90 gene loci with polymorphisms (variants) that predispose to SLE. However, genetic predisposition accounts for only 28% of susceptibility to SLE. Therefore, it is believed that environmental or epigenetic influences or undiscovered genes are involved in the etiology of SLE. Genetic factors that confer the highest susceptibility are deficiencies of complement proteins C1q, C4A and B, C2, or the presence of a mutated *TREX1* gene on the X chromosome. Also, approximately 50% of known predisposing genes enhance interferon function or production.

Some environmental and hormonal factors can trigger SLE. The hormone estrogen and genes on the X chromosome are thought to increase risk of SLE. Women, in general, have higher risk of SLE and women on estrogenic compounds have been found to have significant risk. Genes on the X chromosome are thought to be related to development of SLE as persons with XXY karyotype have increased risk. The presence of Epstein-Barr virus (EBV) antibodies also increases the risk of SLE. The risk is noted to be more intense in African Americans, as EBV increases risk five- to six-fold in this racial group. Drugs such as hydralazine, procainamide, quinidine, phenytoin, isoniazid, and penicillamine can also induce SLE-like reactions. Exposure to ultraviolet (UV) light exacerbates the disease. Tobacco smoking and exposure to silica dust also increase risk of SLE.

Pathophysiology

The pathological process of SLE involves formation of autoantibodies, particularly ANAs. Specific types of autoantibodies include anti–double-stranded DNA antibodies (antidsDNA), antihistone, antierythrocyte, antineuronal, and anti-Smith (anti-Sm) antibodies. Antiphospholipid antibodies are present in some patients with SLE, who then have an increased risk of arterial and venous thromboembolism. Anticomplement C1q antibodies increase risk of nephritis in SLE patients.

SLE can affect practically every organ system due to destruction of the microvasculature within the organs. Antibodies form immune complexes that are deposited in organs and tissues such as the skin, heart, joint synovial membranes, glomeruli of the kidney, and lungs. The deposition of immune complexes triggers an inflammation reaction that damages small blood vessels and various organ membranes. The kidneys are particularly susceptible to inflammation in SLE, termed lupus nephritis. The lungs also commonly succumb to inflammatory changes such as pneumonitis, pleuritis, and pulmonary hypertension. Cardiac involvement in individuals with SLE can cause pericarditis, endocarditis, and coronary artery disease. Hematological manifestations include anemia, lymphopenia, and thrombocytopenia. Gastrointestinal involvement can cause autoimmune peritonitis, intestinal perforation, and ischemia. Sicca syndrome (dry eye disease), conjunctivitis, retinal vasculitis, and optic neuritis can affect the eyes.

 CLINICAL CONCEPT

The kidneys are commonly affected in SLE, as deposition of immune complexes leads to glomerular damage, called lupus nephritis.

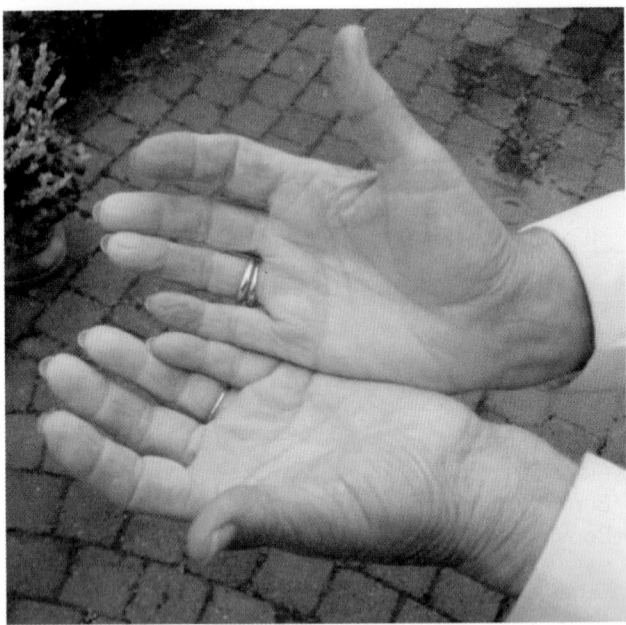

FIGURE 11-7. Raynaud's phenomenon. *(Wikipedia: Courtesy of Jamclaassen.)*

Clinical Presentation

The symptoms of SLE vary depending on the organs that are affected. General symptoms include fever, fatigue, myalgias, and arthralgias, but these symptoms are vague and often lead to misdiagnosis. A classic butterfly rash across the bridge of the nose and cheeks is pathognomonic for SLE. Joint inflammation and musculoskeletal symptoms occur in 90% of patients. Other signs include splenic enlargement, pleural effusion, vasculitis, pericarditis, anemia, and thrombocytopenia.

The kidneys are notably the organ most severely affected in SLE. Nephrotic syndrome with hypertension and hematuria are common manifestations. Nephrotic syndrome often causes edema; periorbital or peripheral edema is common. **Raynaud's phenomenon**, episodic vasospasm of the arteries supplying the fingers, is common; it is observed as a tricolor change in the fingers from cyanosis to pallor to rubor particularly upon exposure to the cold (see Fig. 11-7).

Accelerated ischemic coronary artery disease can also develop in patients with SLE. This may present as atypical chest pain and needs to be distinguished from pulmonary symptoms of SLE. Pleuritis and pleural effusion are also frequently endured by patients with SLE. Lung manifestations such as coughing and dyspnea occur and can be confused with symptoms of infection. Leukopenia, anemia, and thrombocytopenia can develop in SLE because of antibody targeting of blood cells. Leukopenia predisposes the patient to infection, and thrombocytopenia increases risk of bleeding. However, in patients with aPl antibodies, thrombus formation is more common.

Diagnosis

The diagnosis of SLE is based on a detailed patient history, physical examination, and laboratory tests. Clinicians should use the 2019 EULAR/ACR Classification Criteria for SLE. The algorithm gives a score based on the patient's history and clinical features. The patients must be + for ANA (antinuclear antibodies) and have a score of 10 for diagnosis. In some patients, the criteria can accrue over time (see Box 11-2).

No single laboratory test can diagnose SLE, but several laboratory tests may support the diagnosis. The immunofluorescent ANA test is most commonly performed in making a diagnosis. More than 95% of individuals with SLE have high ANA levels, though ANA is not specific to SLE alone. Other autoimmune diseases, cancers, inflammatory disorders, and chronic renal and liver disease can also cause elevated ANA.

The ANA test should be followed by antidsDNA and anti-Sm antibody levels, which are more specific to patients with SLE. There are three widely accepted tests to measure different autoantibodies: anticardiolipin, antibeta2-glycoprotein, and lupus anticoagulant. Other antibodies are also frequently present in SLE, including anti-Ro and antiphospholipid antibodies. Complement levels C3 and C4 are often diminished in SLE because they are consumed by immune complexes formed in the disease. Erythrocyte sedimentation rate (ESR) and C-reactive protein (CRP) are elevated in SLE due to inflammation. A complete blood count (CBC) with differential often reveals anemia, leukopenia, and thrombocytopenia, as antibodies can attack blood cells. Urinalysis may show proteinuria, hematuria, casts, or pyuria due to lupus nephritis. Serum creatinine level is needed to monitor renal involvement of SLE. Liver enzymes may be elevated in acute SLE or

BOX 11-2. Diagnostic Criteria for Systemic Lupus Erythematosus (SLE)

To diagnose a patient with systemic lupus erythematosus, the following criteria are recommended:

Serum antinuclear antibodies (ANAs) ≥1: 80 on HEp-2 cells or an equivalent positive test

and

SIGNS AND SYMPTOMS (EACH WEIGHTED DIFFERENTLY)	LABORATORY TESTS (EACH WEIGHTED DIFFERENTLY)
Fever	Leukopenia
Oral ulcers	Thrombocytopenia
Alopecia	Autoimmune hemolysis
Butterfly malar rash	Proteinuria
Body rash	Renal biopsy shows nephritis
Pleural or Pericardial effusion	Anticardiolipin antibodies or antibeta 2GP1 antibodies or lupus anticoagulant
Joint involvement; arthralgias	Low complement proteins 3 and 4
	Anti-DS DNA antibodies or anti-Smith antibodies

Adapted from: EULAR/ACR Criteria; Aringer, M., Costenbader, K., Daikh, D., Brinks, R., Mosca, M., et al. (2019). European League Against Rheumatism/American College of Rheumatology. https://www.rheumatology.org/Portals/0/Files/Classification-Criteria-Systemic-Lupus-Erythematosus.pdf

in response to medications. Creatinine phosphokinase levels may be elevated in cases of SLE-induced myositis (inflammation of muscle).

X-rays may show joint and soft tissue swelling and osteopenia. Chest x-ray is necessary to rule out pleuritic involvement and pneumonitis. Magnetic resonance imaging of the brain may show changes consistent with SLE of the CNS. Skin biopsy of the butterfly rash can also help diagnose SLE.

Treatment

The course of SLE is unpredictable, with remissions and exacerbations occurring over many years. The goals of therapy for patients with SLE are to ensure long-term survival, achieve the lowest possible disease activity, prevent organ damage, minimize drug toxicity, improve quality of life, and educate patients about their role in disease management. The Systemic Lupus Erythematosus Disease Activity Score-2K (SLE-DAI-2K) is widely used to monitor disease activity based on clinical features with scores.

Nonpharmacological therapy includes advising the patient to avoid prolonged exposure to sunlight and/or UV light, as these can exacerbate symptoms. Sunscreen protectants with a sun protection factor (SPF) factor of greater than 55 are recommended. Supplemental vitamin D may be necessary due to lack of sun exposure.

Exercise and dietary measures should be used to maintain bone and cardiovascular health: low-fat, high-fiber, low-salt diet and daily exercise. Smoking cessation is necessary, as this can aggravate the disease. Immunizations should be kept up to date before any immunosuppressive therapies. Live virus vaccines should be avoided in persons on immunosuppressive treatment such as corticosteroids. Sulfonamide and tetracycline medications should be avoided, as they can cause exacerbations. Pregnancy should be avoided in active disease, as there is high incidence of miscarriage. Women of childbearing age should be counseled that pregnancy is safest after remission of disease for at least 6 months.

Pharmacological treatment for SLE includes hydroxychloroquine or chloroquine (antimalarial drugs), NSAIDs, and short-term corticosteroids. To spare the use of corticosteroids, biological and/or targeted therapeutic agents can be added to the regimen. Biological agents are laboratory-synthesized monoclonal antibodies that target inflammatory mediators, auto-antibodies, and/or lymphocytes. Belimumab and anifrolumab are the biological agents currently showing efficacy for patients with persistent disease. Agents that target tyrosine kinases are under study. Tyrosine kinases are enzymes that enhance proliferation of inflammatory mediators, auto-antibodies, and T cells. Baricitinib, which inhibits Janus kinase, is demonstrating effectiveness. Immunosuppressive agents such as azathioprine, methotrexate, cyclophosphamide, or mycophenolate may be added to the regimen in those patients with therapy-resistant SLE and life-threatening lupus nephritis.

> ALERT! Those treated with immunosuppressant drugs for inflammatory disorders are at increased risk for developing infections.

Rheumatoid Arthritis

RA is a chronic autoimmune inflammatory disorder that affects the joints and may have systemic effects. It is the most common type of chronic inflammatory arthritis that can cause functional disability. RA causes symmetric polyarthritis and systemic manifestations of fatigue, peripheral neuropathy, vasculitis, pericarditis, and lung involvement. There are specific criteria for diagnosis of this disorder. Research over the past two decades has revolutionized the diagnosis and treatment of RA. Earlier, proactive intervention and expanded treatment options have resulted in improved outcomes in patients with RA.

Epidemiology

The prevalence of RA in the adult population is fairly constant at 0.5% to 1%. Prevalence increases with age, and the disorder is two to three times more common in females than in males. Incidence of RA increases between 25 and 55 years of age, then decreases after age 75.

Etiology

The cause of RA is unknown. Autoimmune mechanisms are notable in RA; however, what instigates the immune reaction is unclear. Genetic, environmental, hormonal, immunological, and infectious factors may play significant roles. Genetic factors account for 50% of the risk for developing RA. Several genes are being studied. Genetic variations that program for MHCs confer the greatest risk of RA. There is an allelic variation in the HLA-DRB1 gene, which encodes for the MHC molecule associated with disease. This genetic variation is associated with production of circulating anticitrullinated protein antibodies (ACPAs) that are involved in the dysregulated immune response of RA. Another genetic variation that increases risk of RA is *PTPN22,* which is involved in coding for B and T cell function and ACPAs. The *PAD14* gene, which is associated with a two-fold risk for RA, is also involved with production of ACPAs. Epigenetic changes such as post-translational histone modifications and DNA methylation are also likely involved in the chronic inflammatory dysregulation in RA.

In addition to genetic predisposing factors, environmental influences are involved in pathogenesis of RA. Cigarette smoking confers a 1.5 to 3.5 increased risk of RA, particularly in women. Certain pathogenic organisms including EBV and the oral bacterium that causes periodontal disease, *Porphyromonas gingivalis,* have been implicated in the development of disease.

Pathophysiology

In RA, the body's immune system attacks its own synovial tissues, stimulating an inflammatory process that results in destruction of cartilage, bone, tendons, and ligaments (see Fig. 11-8). A hypertrophied, inflamed, swollen synovial membrane is termed a pannus. A hallmark of RA is the development of bone erosions due to activation of osteoclasts and invasive synovial pannus formation in the involved joints.

The sequence of events in the RA inflammation cascade begins when an unknown, initial antigenic stimulus provokes an APC. APCs activate T cells (T lymphocytes), which play a key role in the destruction of joint components. Following activation, T cells secrete cytokines, which recruit other WBCs to the synovial regions, escalating the inflammatory process. Once set in motion, the inflammation becomes persistently fueled by reactivated T cells and cytokines that constantly attract other WBCs into the joint space.

Among the other WBCs recruited are B cells (B lymphocytes), which transform into plasma cells that secrete Igs. Plasma cells secrete the autoantibody commonly referred to as rheumatoid factor (RF), which can be found in large quantities in the synovial fluid. Plasma cells also produce ACPAs, which are also found in synovial fluid and serve as prognostic biomarkers.

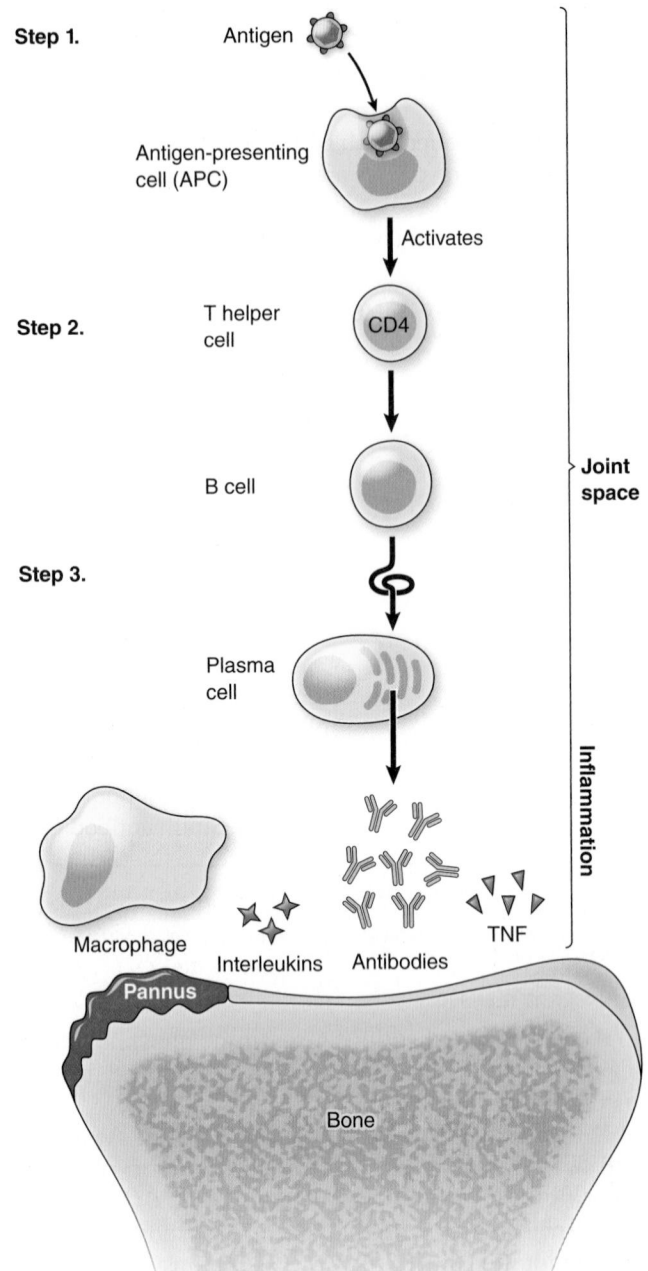

FIGURE 11-8. The inflammatory process in rheumatoid arthritis. **Step 1.** Within the joint space, an unknown antigenic stimulus provokes antigen-presenting cells (APCs). **Step 2.** The APCs process T cells and other WBCs, including B cells and macrophages, which are attracted to the joint space. **Step 3.** B cells transform into plasma cells, which secrete destructive antibodies, and macrophages secrete proinflammatory, damaging cytokines, including tumor necrosis factor (TNF), interleukins (ILs), and metalloproteases (MPs), which persistently fuel the inflammatory process.

Concurrently, WBCs such as macrophages and monocytes produce proinflammatory cytokines such as TNF-alpha, ILs, and matrix metalloproteases. Together with the cellular components involved in RA, these cytokines incite the inflammation, causing a chronic, persistent destructive, autoimmune process.

Continual inflammation of the synovial membrane causes hypertrophy; this region of the joint becomes known as the pannus in RA. Osteoclast activation at the site of the pannus causes bone erosions. TNF-alpha, in particular, suppresses osteoblast activity and counteracts bone formation.

The autoimmune process leads to deformity through the stretching of tendons and ligaments and destruction of joints through the erosion of cartilage and bone. If untreated or unresponsive to therapy, inflammation and joint destruction lead to loss of physical function. In more severe cases of RA, which affect approximately 40% of patients, there is involvement of the musculoskeletal system other than joints (e.g., bone and muscle) and of organs (e.g., skin, eye, lung, heart, kidney, blood vessels, salivary glands, central and peripheral nervous systems, and bone marrow).

Clinical Presentation

Classic symptoms of RA include symmetrical, tender, swollen joints, most commonly of the fingers, wrists, knees, hips, and feet. In addition, patients often experience fatigue, fever, and general malaise. Patients commonly report painful, stiff joints lasting approximately 30 minutes to an hour in the morning or after a period of prolonged rest. The chronic joint inflammation experienced by RA patients results in permanent damage of the surfaces of joints. Most patients show fluctuation of disease activity over periods lasting weeks to months. RA is characterized by phases of quiescent disease versus active disease. During active disease, there is a flare-up in symptoms of arthritis. Although the disease has a variable course, damage to bone and joints is cumulative and irreversible. As the disease progresses and more joints are involved, RA patients become increasingly limited in their mobility.

Characteristic deformities occur in the joints of the hands due to the swelling of joint spaces, erosion of bone, and stretching of ligaments and tendons. Involvement includes the metacarpal and proximal interphalangeal (PIP) joints, with sparing of the distal interphalangeal joints (DIP) in the fingers. The two classic rheumatoid deformities in the fingers are boutonnière deformity and swan neck deformity. With severe hand deformity, there is a distinctive ulnar deviation of the metacarpal bones (see Fig. 11-9). Also, a cystic nodule in the popliteal region called a baker's cyst is common.

In severe cases of RA, the patient can experience osteopenia or osteoporosis with vertebral compression fractures and increased risk of hip fracture.

Although musculoskeletal and joint conditions are most prominent in RA, there are many extra-articular manifestations of the disease. Accelerated atherosclerosis occurs in RA and is a major cause of death. Pulmonary disorders are also associated with RA; including interstitial lung disease, pneumoconiosis, pleural effusion, and pulmonary fibrotic nodules. Cervical myelopathy caused

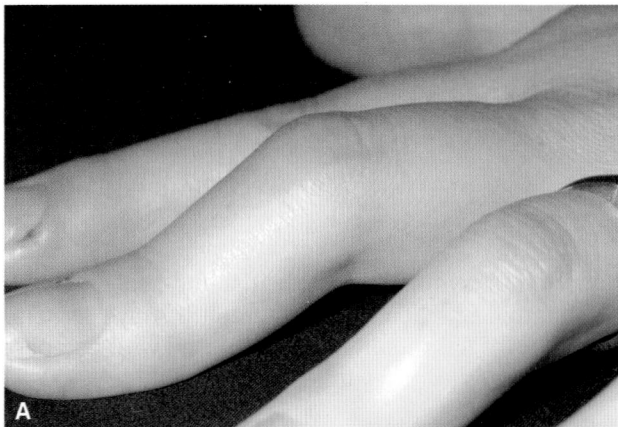

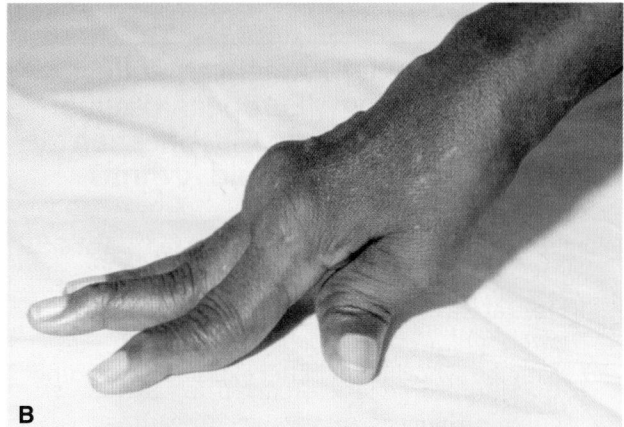

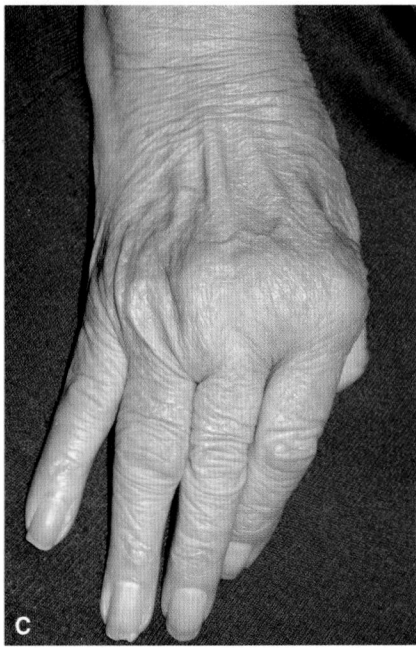

FIGURE 11-9. Classic rheumatoid deformities in the fingers. **(A)** Boutonnière deformity. *(From Dr. P. Marazzi/Science Source.)* **(B)** Swan neck deformity. *(From Sue Ford/Science Source.)* **(C)** Ulnar deviation of the fingers on the hand. *(From SPL/Science Source.)*

by vertebral subluxation and carpal tunnel syndrome can occur. Ocular manifestations include keratoconjunctivitis sicca, keratitis, and scleritis. Amyloidosis and Felty's syndrome, which includes splenomegaly, leukopenia, and thrombocytopenia, can occur.

Diagnosis

The diagnosis of RA is made according to a set of specific criteria developed by the American College of Rheumatology (ACR)/European League Against Rheumatism (EULAR) classification system (see Box 11-3) and is based on several clinical criteria and laboratory tests. Clinical criteria include the presence of morning stiffness in the joints; polyarthritis, which includes the hand joints; symmetrical arthritis; and subcutaneous rheumatoid nodules for a minimum of 6 weeks. The diagnosis of RA should not be confused with osteoarthritis, as there are key differences (see Table 11-2).

BOX 11-3. **The 2010 American College of Rheumatology/European League Against Rheumatism Classification Criteria for Rheumatoid Arthritis**

Target population (Who should be tested?): Patients who
1. Have at least 1 joint with definite clinical synovitis (swelling)
2. With the synovitis not better explained by another disease

Classification criteria for RA (score-based algorithm: add score of categories A–D; a score of 6/10 is needed for classification of a patient as having definite RA).

CLINICAL SIGN	SCORE
A. Joint Involvement	
1 large joint*	0
2–10 large joints	1
1–3 small joints %	2
4–10 small joints	3
>10 small joints	5
B. Serology	
Negative RF and negative ACPA	0
Low positive RF and low positive anti-CCP antibodies	2
High positive RF or high positive anti-CCP antibodies	3
C. Acute Phase Reactants	
Normal CRP and normal ESR	0
Abnormal CRP or abnormal ESR	1
D. Duration of Symptoms	
<6 weeks	0
>6 weeks	1

*"Large joints" refers to shoulders, elbows, hips, knees, and ankles.
%"Small joints" refers to the metacarpophalangeal joints, proximal interphalangeal joints, second through fifth metatarsophalangeal joints, thumb interphalangeal joints, and wrists.
ACPA: anticitrullinated peptide antibodies, anti-CCP: anticyclic citrullinated peptides, CRP: C-reactive protein, ESR: erythrocyte sedimentation rate, RF: rheumatoid factor.
Adapted from Aletaha, D., Neogi, T., Silman, A. J., et al. (2010). 2010 Rheumatoid Arthritis Classification Criteria: An American College of Rheumatology/European League Against Rheumatism Collaborative Initiative. *Arthritis & Rheumatism, 62*(9), 2569–2581.

Major diagnostic evidence includes elevated serum RF, ESR, and CRP. RF can be negative in up to 30% of patients. ACPAs, biomarkers that indicate erosion of the synovial membrane of joints, are present in up to 70% of patients. The presence of serum ACPAs in the presence of early inflammatory arthritis is highly diagnostic of RA. Other biomarkers may be used to assess disease activity as the patient undergoes treatment. Monitoring the various levels can be done by an RA multibiomarker disease activity (MBDA) laboratory test. X-rays of the hands, wrists, and feet are usually done to follow progression of the disease. Periodic monitoring of inflammatory biomarkers, CRP and ESR, is necessary to assess disease activity.

Treatment

Early diagnosis and treatment are key to reducing disability due to RA. Nonpharmacological treatment includes patient education regarding RA. Regular aerobic exercise is recommended. A diet and exercise regimen should be prescribed to promote cardiovascular and bone health. Weight loss is recommended for patients with obesity, as obesity increases stress on joints and can worsen disease. Physical therapy can provide passive and active range of motion to decrease pain and preserve joint movement. Application of heat and cold, splints, and ultrasound can decrease joint and tendon inflammation. Occupational therapy can instruct patients how to use assistive devices to accomplish tasks. Patients should be kept up to date on immunizations, particularly influenza, pneumococcal, and hepatitis B. Live virus vaccines should not be used in patients on immunosuppressive therapy.

The pharmacological treatment goal is remission or a state of at least low disease activity, which should be attained within 6 months. Methotrexate (MTX) is first-line therapy and should be prescribed at an optimal dose of 20 mg weekly and in combination with glucocorticoids. MTX suppresses overactive T-cell and B-cell activity that is causing joint pain and inflammation. It can be given orally or subcutaneously once weekly. Because MTX interferes with metabolism of folic acid, folic acid must be given. With this regimen, 40% to 50% of patients reach remission or at least low disease activity. If this treatment fails, sequential application of targeted therapies, such as biological disease-modifying antirheumatic drugs (DMARDs) or Janus kinase inhibitors in combination with MTX, have allowed up to 75% of these patients to reach the treatment target over time.

Biological DMARDs target cytokines and other inflammatory mediators. Major cytokines targeted are TNF-alpha and ILs. The biological DMARDs include TNF inhibitors: etanercept, infliximab, adalimumab, golimumab, and certolizumab pegol; the IL-1 receptor antagonist anakinra; and the IL-6 receptor antagonist tocilizumab. They also include other biological response modifiers such as the T-cell costimulation blocker abatacept and the anti-CD20 B-cell–depleting

TABLE 11-2. Rheumatoid Arthritis Versus Osteoarthritis

	Rheumatoid Arthritis	Osteoarthritis
Etiology	Autoimmune disease	Wear and tear or overuse of joints caused by excessive weight-bearing
		Traumatic injury can predispose to osteoarthritis
Age	20 to 40 years old	Older than age 50
Population affected	Women are predominately affected	Both women and men affected
Pain	Stiffness in morning but better with use of joint	Stiffness in morning and worse with use of joint Rest decreases pain
Movement	Movement of joint decreases pain	Movement of joint increases pain
Joints	Symmetrical involvement of joints; hands most commonly affected initially	Symmetrical or asymmetrical involvement of small and large joints
Diagnosis	Specific rheumatological association criteria and x-ray	x-ray
Time frame	Gradual with exacerbations and remissions	Gradual over years and steady decline of health of joints
Associated symptoms	Systemic disease; feeling of being ill, fever, elevated WBC count	Limited to the joint pain
Key characteristics	Swan neck and boutonnière deformity of fingers with ulnar deviation of metacarpal bones	Heberden's and Bouchard's nodes of fingers
	Rheumatoid nodule in lung; baker's cyst in popliteal space	

monoclonal antibody, rituximab. Tofacitinib is another DMARD that targets other inflammatory mediators called Janus kinases. Before administration of MTX or DMARDs, the patient should be tested for tuberculosis, hepatitis B, and hepatitis C.

Anti-inflammatory therapies, including systemic and intra-articular glucocorticoids and NSAIDs, are also used as adjuncts for temporary control of disease activity in patients in whom treatment is being started with DMARDs, in patients in whom the DMARD regimen requires modification, or in patients who are experiencing disease flares. Intra-articular injections of long-acting glucocorticoids are used to reduce synovitis in particular joints that are more inflamed than others.

Sarcoidosis

Sarcoidosis is a chronic, autoimmune multisystem disorder of unknown origin characterized by an accumulation of T lymphocytes, macrophages, and epithelioid granulomas in various organs. Any organ can be involved, although the most frequently affected is the lung. Other organs that can be involved include the skin, eye, liver, and lymph nodes. The disease can be episodic with relapses and remissions over many years.

Epidemiology

Sarcoidosis affects females more commonly than males with a prevalence of 10 to 20 per 100,000 in the United States. African American females are more commonly affected than European American females. For women, peak incidence of sarcoidosis occurs at ages 50 to 69; for men, peak incidence occurs at age 40 to 59. African American individuals tend to contract the disease at younger ages than European American persons.

Pathophysiology

Macrophages, CD8 and CD4 T cells, and inflammatory mediators accumulate in affected organs. It is believed that sarcoidosis is triggered by a foreign antigen that stimulates monocytes to transform into antigen-presenting cells (APCs), such as macrophages. The macrophages stimulate helper T cells, which activate inflammatory cytokines, including TNF-alpha and ILs.

The acute inflammatory process is followed by a chronic form of the disease in 20% of those affected. During the chronic inflammation phase, granulomas form; these are aggregates of macrophages, epithelial-like cells, and other inflammatory mediators surrounded by

T cells, B cells, mast cells, fibroblasts, and hyaline cartilage. Characteristic multinucleated giant cells are found within the granulomas. The presence of granulomatous inflammation is theorized to result from an exaggerated cell-mediated immune response to one or more unidentified antigen(s). No single etiological agent and no genetic locus has been clearly implicated in the pathogenesis of sarcoidosis. The granulomas and inflammatory changes cause structural distortions within organs and may cause organ dysfunction, particularly of lungs, liver, and lymph nodes.

Clinical Presentation

Sarcoidosis can range from an asymptomatic disorder to a disease with extensive organ dysfunction. It is unclear why some patients are mildly affected and others are severely affected. Symptoms include fever, fatigue, malaise, anorexia, and weight loss. The fatigue can be overwhelming for many patients. Some patients may develop arthritis in the ankles, wrists, knees, and elbows. Over 90% of those affected have lung disease presenting as cough, dyspnea, and chest discomfort. Wheezes, due to hyperreactive airways, are often auscultated over the lung fields. Respiratory tract abnormalities, which mainly consist of interstitial lung disease, cause most of the morbidity and mortality in sarcoidosis.

Patients often develop a characteristic skin rash called erythema nodosum (EN), which manifests as tender, erythematous nodules on the anterior surface of the legs. A nonspecific maculopapular rash can develop on the face around the eyes and nose, on the back, and on the extremities. This dermatological manifestation is termed lupus pernio.

Löfgren's syndrome (LS) is a clinically distinct syndrome in sarcoidosis. Patients experience acute onset of the disease with fever, bilateral hilar lymphadenopathy, arthritis, and EN.

Parotid gland and lymph node enlargement are commonly found in patients with sarcoidosis. Ocular manifestations include uveitis, retinitis, and pars planitis. Uveoparotid fever, also known as Heerfordt's syndrome, is a specific subtype of sarcoidosis characterized by a combination of facial palsy, or trigeminal nerve involvement, parotid gland enlargement, uveitis, and low-grade fever.

The most common hematological problems are anemia and lymphopenia. Lymphopenia is caused by sequestration of lymphocytes within the granulomas in the body. The spleen, liver, kidney, bone, muscle, and heart can also develop granulomatous lesions, which lead to organ dysfunction. Hypercalcemia and hypercalciuria occur due to excessive production of vitamin D by granulomas. These metabolic imbalances can lead to kidney stone formation. Sarcoidosis can affect the neurological system, manifesting as cranial nerve dysfunction, optic neuritis, or granulomatous inflammation of the meninges.

Diagnosis

The diagnosis of sarcoidosis is not standardized but is based on three major criteria: clinical presentation, finding nonnecrotizing granulomatous inflammation in one or more tissue samples, and the exclusion of alternative causes of granulomatous disease.

Bilateral hilar lymphadenopathy (swelling of lymph nodes in the mediastinum) is a hallmark of sarcoidosis and is seen in 90% of persons with the disease. This is demonstrated on chest x-ray or pulmonary computed tomography (CT) scan. The lungs also show "ground glass" opacities, nodular consolidations, and cystic scarring. Chest x-ray assists in the staging of disease, which consists of Stages 1 through 4 depending on the severity of pulmonary findings. Pulmonary function tests (PFTs), including spirometry, lung volumes, and diffusing capacity for carbon monoxide (DLCO), demonstrate a restrictive disease. The patient commonly is given a 6-minute walk test (6MWT) to assess for breathing impairment. PFTs can be used to assess the severity of respiratory impairment and to monitor the course of disease. No specific blood tests are diagnostic of sarcoidosis, though most affected individuals have elevated levels of angiotensin-converting enzyme (ACE). A biopsy of a sarcoid lesion in a lymph node or in cells recovered from bronchoalveolar lavage is essential to make a definitive diagnosis.

Treatment

In most patients with sarcoidosis, the disease resolves spontaneously and does not require systemic therapy. Patients with severe disease that is causing organ dysfunction need treatment. Treatment focuses on suppression of inflammation using short-term glucocorticoid therapy, chemotherapeutic agents, immunosuppressive drugs, and immunomodulators. For patients requiring long-term suppression of inflammation, early institution of antisarcoidosis agents is recommended, either alone as first-line treatment or in combination with tapered doses of a glucocorticoid. Commonly used agents include MTX, azathioprine, leflunomide, and mycophenolate. An alternative is the antimalarial agent hydroxychloroquine. If antisarcoidosis agents, administered alone or in combination with glucocorticoids, are toxic or ineffective or if the disease is severe and progressive, treatment with immunomodulators is considered. Infliximab and adalimumab are immunomodulators (monoclonal antibody agents) that inhibit TNF-alpha. TNF-alpha is a cytokine released by WBCs that causes persistence of the inflammatory reaction in sarcoidosis. Since immunomodulators cause immunosuppression, vaccination and other measures for preventing infection are necessary in patients treated with these agents. In addition to pharmacological treatment, the clinician should encourage lifestyle changes, such as physical training for patients with fatigue or deconditioning. Dietary modifications may also be beneficial, as suggested by studies indicating that antioxidants may relieve chronic cough and reduce reliance on glucocorticoids.

Sjögren's Syndrome

Sjögren's syndrome (SS) is a chronic autoimmune disease characterized by dry eyes, also called keratoconjunctivitis sicca, and dry mouth, also called xerostomia. These major symptoms occur because of immunologically mediated destruction of lacrimal and salivary glands. Other disease manifestations affecting multiple organ systems may occur. It can present as an isolated disorder or in combination with other autoimmune diseases, particularly RA and SLE.

Epidemiology

SS occurs most commonly in women between ages 50 and 60 years. Approximately 60% of individuals with SS also suffer from RA. There is a familial tendency to develop SS along with an increased risk of other autoimmune disorders in relatives of patients with SS. There is no specific gene linked to the disease; the strongest associations are with MHC genes, including those in the HLA-DR region.

Pathophysiology

SS is characterized by a lymphocytic infiltration of many of the body's exocrine glands. The infiltrate consists mainly of T cells, B cells, plasma cells, and inflammatory mediators. Excess proliferation of lymphocytes interferes with glandular function. The main targets are salivary and lacrimal glands; however, respiratory and GI involvement is also seen. The infiltrate mainly surrounds ducts and vessels within glandular tissue. Ductal epithelial cells show hyperplasia, which eventually protrude into the lumen of the ducts. The hyperplastic cells obstruct the lumen of the ducts, preventing secretions such as tears and saliva from releasing. Regions of lymphocytic infiltration in glands eventually undergo fibrosis and atrophy. The lack of secretions from affected glands can cause complications. Lack of tears causes drying of the cornea, and lack of saliva causes dryness and breakdown of the oral mucosa.

Clinical Presentation

Fatigue and fibromyalgia are common in SS. Other common symptoms include blurred vision, burning and itching of the eyes, and thickened secretions that can block tear ducts. Dry mouth makes swallowing difficult and renders the patient with a decreased ability to taste. Oral mucous membranes become cracked and fissured. Skin dryness, EN, cutaneous vasculitis with palpable purpura, and Raynaud's phenomenon can be evident. EN is tender, red nodules on the shins that are caused by a type 4 hypersensitivity reaction due to exposure to certain antigens. Specific antigens that stimulate EN are unknown. Manifestations of extraglandular involvement, such as synovitis (inflammation of joints), pulmonary fibrosis, and peripheral neuropathy, are seen in a third of patients. Approximately 50% of patients have arthralgias, with the hands, wrists, and knees most commonly affected. Parotid gland enlargement can sometimes be evident. Thyroid abnormalities, GI inflammation and celiac disease, nephritis, anemia, leukopenia, hypergamma globulinemia, and depression often occur.

Diagnosis

Autoantibodies are a key characteristic of SS. ANAs and antibodies referred to as anti-Ro/SSA and anti-La/SSB are diagnostic of the syndrome and are detected in up to 90% of those affected. Laboratory tests may demonstrate leukopenia, thrombocytopenia, anemia, hyperglobulinemia, and elevated ESR. Diagnosis requires a biopsy of the lip tissue to examine minor salivary glands. The patient also requires an ophthalmological examination. Tear production is measured using the Schirmer test and fluorescein staining of the cornea is commonly performed. The 2016 ACR/EULAR classification criteria for SS are based on clinical features that are weighted with a score.

The lymph nodes are commonly enlarged and infiltrated with dysplastic B cells. Because of lymphocytic proliferation, persons with SS have a 40-fold increased risk of developing lymphoid malignancies, such as non-Hodgkin's lymphoma.

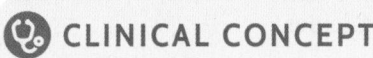

> ### 🔬 CLINICAL CONCEPT
>
> Antinuclear antibodies (ANAs) are commonly present in autoimmune disease.

Treatment

Treatment is aimed at symptomatic relief and limiting the damaging effects of xerostomia and keratoconjunctivitis sicca. Ophthalmic solutions to replace tears and medications that stimulate salivary gland function are used. Treatment of glandular lymphoproliferation and more severe extraglandular manifestations includes the use of glucocorticoids; antimalarials (hydroxychloroquine); nonbiological DMARDs such as MTX, leflunomide, azathioprine, sulfasalazine, mycophenolic acid, and cyclosporine; and other potent agents, including the alkylating agent cyclophosphamide and the anti-CD20 antibody rituximab, which targets B cells.

Scleroderma

Scleroderma, also known as systemic sclerosis (SSc), is a chronic, autoimmune disease of unknown origin characterized by abnormal accumulation of fibrous tissue in the skin and various organs. The skin is most noticeably affected, but the GI tract, kidneys, muscles, and lungs are frequently involved as well. Progressive skin fibrosis of the face, hands, and fingers occurs in early disease. Scleroderma is categorized as either localized (skin only) or systemic disease. SSc is the term more commonly used when the disease involves internal organs. The esophagus is commonly affected by gastroesophageal reflux and lungs can be affected by fibrosis.

Epidemiology

An estimated 40,000 to 165,000 persons in the United States are affected by scleroderma. Women between 30 and 50 years old are most commonly affected, and the disorder occurs more often in African American women than European American women.

Etiology

The cause of scleroderma is unclear; however, numerous gene mutations are associated with it. Genetic mutations that produce abnormal B cells, T-cell components, and cytokines have been implicated. Among the many genes under scrutiny are *BANK1,* a gene located at 4q24; *BLK,* located at 8p23; and *CD247,* located at 1q22. There is a strong consistent association with HLA subtype genes, *NOTCH4,* and *PSORSC1* on chromosome 6. Other genetic variants in SSc are involved in innate immunity and interferon signaling (*IRF5, IRF7, STAT4,* and *TLR2*). Exposure to toxic substances has also been associated with scleroderma. These include silica, organic solvents, hydrocarbons, epoxy resins, and pesticides.

Pathophysiology

The pathophysiological mechanism in SSc involves environmental factors that trigger epigenetic changes in a genetically susceptible individual. These changes cause alterations in the behavior of multiple types of cells. There are three major pathological mechanisms: widespread microangiopathy, inflammation and autoimmunity, and visceral and vascular fibrosis affecting multiple organs. The microangiopathy is an inflammatory reaction in the endothelial lining of blood vessels. The endothelial reaction leads to a cascade of changes that involve fibroblasts, T lymphocytes, macrophages, and mast cells. These activated cells infiltrate the vasculature, skin, and some organs in an autoimmune reaction. Inflammatory mediators that play an important part in the reaction include IL-4, transforming growth factors, platelet-derived growth factor, and connective tissue growth factor. Visceral and vascular fibrosis involves the extensive deposition of collagen in organs, resulting in fibrosis of the skin, subcutaneous tissues, and deep tissues. A diminished number of capillary branches are noted in the affected tissue as well. The disorder may present as a diffuse, widespread disease or a localized disease limited to the skin of the face, arms, hands, and fingers.

Extracutaneous scleroderma can involve the lungs, GI system (particularly the esophagus), kidneys,

musculoskeletal system, and heart. Pulmonary interstitial fibrosis and pulmonary hypertension are common. Compared with the general population, persons with scleroderma have an increased risk of lung cancer. Kidney damage is manifested by hypertension, proteinuria, and elevated serum creatinine. Possible cardiac complications include myocardial fibrosis, myocardial ischemia, dysrhythmias, and pericarditis. Musculoskeletal symptoms include arthralgia, myalgia, and swelling of the hands.

Clinical Presentation

Initial complaints are vague at times because of scleroderma's widespread involvement of the body. The disorder can present as an inflammatory musculoskeletal problem. The patient commonly complains of chronic fatigue, muscle aches, joint pain, and swelling with limited range of motion. The most noticeable sign is skin involvement, which renders skin shiny, smooth, and stretched in appearance, particularly on the face and hands. There is a facial mask-like appearance with loss of normal wrinkles and nasolabial folds. The skin on the hands can become so stiff as to cause contractures of the fingers.

As the disorder continues, dysphagia is common because of esophageal dysmotility. Abdominal pain, intestinal obstruction, and malabsorption with weight loss and anemia can occur, as can cardiac dysfunction and malignant hypertension.

Some persons develop CREST syndrome, which is a type of scleroderma. Its name is an acronym for the cardinal clinical features of the syndrome: calcinosis, Raynaud's phenomenon, esophageal dysmotility, sclerodactyly, and telangiectasia syndrome. Calcinosis is the deposition of calcium deposits in skin, subcutaneous tissues, and organs. Calcium deposits may be particularly visible in the fingertips. Raynaud's phenomenon is the vasospasm and vasoconstriction of the small blood vessels in the fingers that can cause ischemia. Esophageal dysmotility can cause gastroesophageal reflux disease (GERD). Sclerodactyly is the contracture of fingers caused by the tightening of the skin covering the hands. Telangiectasias are dilated, small venules that appear as spider veins in various places on the body.

Diagnosis

Diagnosis of scleroderma is based on patient symptoms and physical examination findings. The skin fibrosis with characteristic symmetric involvement of the hands and fingers along with history of Raynaud's phenomenon and GERD symptoms, helps establish the diagnosis. ANAs are commonly elevated. Antibodies called antitopoisomerase-1 and anticentromere antibodies are highly specific for SSc. Other diagnostic tests include pulmonary spirometry, chest x-ray, electrocardiogram, echocardiogram, and 24-hour Holter monitoring when scleroderma is widespread. CT of the lungs demonstrates a "ground glass" or "honeycomb" appearance because of development of pulmonary fibrosis. Esophageal manometry, which measures pressure and motility, shows esophageal involvement in 90% of patients.

Treatment

Currently there is no specific treatment for scleroderma. The management of the disease is individualized depending on patient symptoms and the specific organ involvement. For example, patients with GERD are treated with proton-pump inhibitors, patients with Raynaud's phenomenon are frequently treated with calcium channel blockers, and patients with hypertension due to renal involvement are treated with ACE inhibitors. Patients with severe skin involvement can be treated with immunosuppressive therapy such as MTX, mycophenolate, or rituximab. Cyclophosphamide can be used in patients with severe pulmonary involvement. Hydroxychloroquine and short-term corticosteroids can be used if there is inflammatory joint disease. Biological agents used to treat RA, including TNF inhibitors, rituximab, abatacept, and tocilizumab, can be used if other drugs are ineffective.

CLINICAL CONCEPT

Upon exposure to cold, many persons with an autoimmune disorder exhibit Raynaud's phenomenon, a vasospasm of small blood vessels in the fingers. A tricolor change of blue (cyanosis) to red (erythema) to white (pallor) is characteristic of this phenomenon (see Fig. 11-7).

Polyarteritis Nodosa

Polyarteritis nodosa (PAN) is a disease characterized by necrotizing inflammation of blood vessel walls. The vascular lesions resemble those found in type III hypersensitivity reactions, which are caused by immune complex deposition. The trigger or etiological agent is unknown, but any type of blood vessel can be involved: arteries, arterioles, veins, or venules. Tissue ischemia can occur distal to the inflamed blood vessel. Hepatitis B and C and leukemia can often cause secondary PAN.

PAN can involve any organ; however, it usually spares the lungs. Typically the disease affects renal and visceral blood supply. There is thickening of inflamed arterial walls that can cause narrowing of the blood vessel, reducing blood flow and predisposing to thrombosis of affected vessels. The resulting ischemia or infarction of tissue causes various clinical manifestations depending on the organ involved. Arteriogram findings include aneurysms in the small- and medium-sized arteries of organs, particularly the liver and kidney. Biopsy of tissue showing the typical vascular inflammatory changes commonly confirms the diagnosis. Typically a disease of young adults, it can be episodic and remitting with long symptom-free intervals. Clinical manifestations include fever, myalgias, arthralgias, skin lesions, hypertension, abdominal pain, peripheral neuritis, and malaise. Renal involvement is often severe and the cause of death. Treatment involves the use of corticosteroids and immunosuppressive agents. MTX, azathioprine, and mycophenolate are often used, with the goal of suppressing the disease into remission. Cyclophosphamide is often used in severe disease. If hepatitis is involved, antiviral medications are needed.

Pathophysiology of Selected Immunodeficiency Disorders

Immunodeficiencies can be divided into primary, or congenital, and secondary, or acquired, disorders. Most primary immunodeficiency diseases are genetic, and most manifest during infancy, between the ages of 6 months and 2 years. These patients may show deficiencies of innate or adaptive immunity. Many of the primary immunodeficiency disorders are X-linked, which is why they mostly manifest in males.

The major acquired immunodeficiency disorders develop after birth because of disorders with immunosuppressive effects. These include lymphoma, leukemia, and HIV infection.

Severe Combined Immunodeficiency Disease

Severe combined immunodeficiency disease (SCID) is a constellation of genetically distinct syndromes, all of which have defects of both antibody-mediated and cell-mediated immune responses. Of the 16 genetic SCID diseases, X-linked SCID and adenosine deaminase (ADA) deficiency are the most frequent types.

T-cell lymphopenia is the chief disorder in SCID, which leads to widespread immune deficiency. Because T cells are integral to the mechanisms in antibody-mediated, cell-mediated, and innate immunity, there is complete absence of immune defenses in the newborn with SCID. In the absence of immune defenses, the newborn is susceptible to life-threatening bacterial, fungal, and viral infections. SCID is a recessive genetic disorder and common in cultures where consanguineous marriage is practiced. The most common form is X-linked, which is why the disease presents most frequently in males. The incidence is 1 case per 50,000 to 75,000 births.

A newborn screening test for SCID—the T-cell receptor excision circle (TREC) assay utilizing dried blood spots—is used in the United States and internationally. If this test is abnormal, an infant can receive further diagnostic testing for SCID, before onset of infectious complications. This early screening test allows for immediate institution of protective measures and definitive, life-saving treatment.

Infants with SCID usually present with many different kinds of infection during early weeks of life. Patients are susceptible to a wide array of pathogens; community-acquired infections and opportunistic infections are common. T-cell counts are less than 300 cells/microliter (average normal range is 800 to 1200 cells/microliter). Oral candidiasis (thrush), diarrheal illness, pneumonia, and failure to thrive (FTT) are common initial manifestations. Infections with common viral pathogens, such as adenovirus, cytomegalovirus (CMV), EBV, rotavirus, norovirus, respiratory syncytial virus (RSV), varicella zoster virus (VZV), herpes simplex virus (HSV), measles, influenza, and parainfluenza 3, are frequently fatal. Pneumonia caused by *Pneumocystis jirovecii* is common. Without treatment, death from infection usually occurs within the first 2 years of life.

Live vaccines must not be administered because these can cause life-threatening illness in immunosuppressed individuals. Infants with suspected SCID should be kept in protective isolation until they receive definitive treatment. Diagnosis must be made before severe life-threatening infections occur so that the immunity can be restored with bone marrow transplant, which can lead to long-term survival. With bone marrow and other stem cell reconstitution techniques, many patients with SCID can develop normal immunocompetence. Gene therapy has also been shown to correct the T cell immunodeficiency caused by SCID. Lentivirus vectors carrying the corrected gene have been shown to normalize T lymphocyte counts, which in turn, reconstitute B cell and natural killer cells. Genome editing of the mutated gene is envisioned as another strategy to treat SCID in the future.

Selective IgA Deficiency

Selective IgA deficiency (sIgAD) is one of the most common primary immune deficiencies. Prevalence ranges from 1 in 100 to 1 in 1,000 persons per year in the United States. It is theorized that sIgAD is most likely caused by a genetic defect, because first-degree relatives of affected individuals are 50 times more likely to have the disease. It is also known that affected mothers are more likely than affected fathers to transmit the disorder to their offspring. Although many instances of sIgAD are caused by a genetic defect, the deficiency can be acquired as well.

Medications that can cause sIgAD include D-penicillamine, sulfasalazine, fenclofenac, gold, captopril, chloroquine, phenytoin, and valproic acid. In addition, some infections, including rubella, CMV, *Toxoplasma gondii,* and EBV, can increase susceptibility to sIgAD. Benzene exposure has also been associated with sIgAD.

The pathogenesis of sIgAD remains incompletely understood and multiple mechanisms are involved, including defective B cell maturation, decreased or impaired helper T cells and/or abnormal cytokine signaling.

IgA is the most numerous immunoglobulin in the body. It is found in saliva, milk, colostrum, tears, and mucosal secretions from the respiratory tract, genitourinary tract, and prostate. It is called secretory IgA because of its presence in mucosal surfaces, assisting in the process of phagocytosis by macrophages. In sIgAD, B cells that produce IgA are dysfunctional.

In most cases, individuals affected with sIgAD are asymptomatic but are at higher risk for atopic diseases and autoimmune diseases. Sinus and pulmonary infections are more common in adults with sIgAD than in the general population. Children experience recurrent otitis media, sinusitis, and/or pneumonia. Those older than 6 months who have recurrent upper and lower respiratory tract infections with encapsulated bacteria (e.g., *Haemophilus influenzae, Streptococcus pneumoniae*) should be evaluated for sIgAD. GI disorders such as celiac disease and inflammatory bowel disease are more common in persons with sIgAD. Intestinal *Giardia lamblia* infections are also more common. Lack of secretory IgA has been hypothesized to compromise the defense against infection with *Helicobacter pylori,* which is thought to be a cause of stomach cancer. Food allergies, respiratory allergies, and anaphylactic reactions to blood products are common in patients. Approximately 20% of those affected by sIgAD develop an autoimmune disease such as SLE, Graves' disease, myasthenia gravis, and RA. Some patients with chronic obstructive pulmonary disease (COPD) have been found to have sIgAD.

Persons with absent IgA can present with recurrent respiratory tract infections, including swelling, pain, or tenderness upon palpation over the maxillary and frontal sinuses; chronic otorrhea, scarred or perforated tympanic membranes, and decreased auditory acuity or even deafness; chronic nasal discharge; fever; nonproductive or productive cough; and dyspnea. GI findings may include abdominal distention, cramps after eating, diffuse pain, and increased peristalsis.

Diagnosis of sIgAD is made when serum IgA level is less than 7 mg/dL in patients older than 4 years old with normal levels of IgG and IgM and normal vaccine response. Secondary causes of hypogammaglobulinemia and T-cell defects need to be excluded. sIgAD is usually diagnosed through routine screening of family members of individuals with another primary immune deficiency. Normal levels of IgM and IgG and undetectable levels of serum IgA are diagnostic of the disorder. In children younger than 4 years, the diagnosis should be considered preliminary, and the child should be monitored over time to see if IgA levels normalize. IgA levels may normalize as late as adolescence. Pulmonary function tests (PFTs) may show an obstructive pattern in adults with sIgAD, and jejunal biopsy specimens of patients with chronic diarrhea and malabsorption may show blunting of the villi.

If patients are symptomatic with increased infections, monthly immunoglobulin injections can be administered IV, IM, or subcutaneously. Prophylactic antibiotics may also be warranted. Sinus surgery can frequently help relieve chronic obstruction and promote drainage. Tympanostomy tubes may also be helpful in reducing the risk of decreased hearing and secondary defective speech development in children with chronic otitis. Live virus vaccines should be avoided in persons with symptomatic sIgAD.

Chronic Mucocutaneous Candidiasis

Chronic mucocutaneous candidiasis (CMCC) is a disease in which patients develop persistent, noninvasive *Candida* infections of the skin, mucous membranes, and nails, as well as autoimmune disorders, most commonly involving the endocrine system. CMCC is referred to as an autoimmune regulator (AIRE) deficiency due to a genetic mutation at 21q 22.3, commonly called the AIRE gene, and the signal transducer and activator of transcription 1 gene (*STAT1*). CMCC is sometimes referred to as AIRE deficiency/autoimmune polyendocrinopathy–candidiasis–ectodermal dystrophy (APECED). In CMCC the T lymphocyte is unable to respond to challenges of *Candida albicans,* a common fungal organism found on the skin and in the GI tract and vaginal canal. *Candida* infections are one of the most common signs of the disease. CMCC is also associated with autoimmune disorders, which include adrenal insufficiency, thyroid disease, myasthenia gravis, thymoma, hypoparathyroidism, autoimmune hemolytic anemia, immune thrombocytopenia purpura, autoimmune neutropenia, and RA. Hypoparathyroidism, which causes hypocalcemia, is another common sign of the disease. The classic triad of conditions in CMCC is mucocutaneous candidiasis, hypoparathyroidism, and adrenal failure.

Eighty percent of CMCC cases present in children younger than 3 years of age. Children often present with persistent oral candidiasis (thrush) and *Candida* dermatitis and autoimmune endocrine disorders.

The only definitive laboratory test for the diagnosis of CMCC is the genetic analysis of relevant genes. Autoantibodies against interferon (IFN)-alpha, IFN-omega, and interleukins (IL-17 and IL 22) are also consistently high in the patient. Evaluation of the immune system may identify a selective inability to respond to *C. albicans,* especially in patients with AIRE deficiency. Standard laboratory tests are necessary to evaluate for endocrine disorders; hypoparathyroidism and adrenal insufficiency. Antifungal therapy is part of the treatment. Candidiasis usually clears with the medication fluconazole. The Janus kinase inhibitors ruxolitinib and baricitinib have also been effective in treating oral, esophageal, and vaginal candidiasis. Endocrine abnormalities should be treated with replacement therapy, when possible. In cases of hypoparathyroidism, calcium levels should be carefully monitored, and calcium supplementation should be given. Frequently, magnesium must be given to avoid seizures that can be caused by hypomagnesemia. Antibody deficiency, if severe, should be treated with immunoglobulin replacement. Short-term prednisone, tacrolimus, and mycophenolate mofetil can reverse multiple autoimmune manifestations and reduce levels of autoantibodies.

Hypogammaglobulinemia

Hypogammaglobulinemia is a condition of decreased number of Igs related to a defect in B-cell development and maturation. With this decreased production, the immune system cannot respond to and initiate the immune/inflammatory response. The disorder can be caused by genetic defects or can be acquired. Acquired hypogammaglobulinemia can be caused by immunomodulator treatments, renal loss of Igs, GI immunoglobulin loss, B-cell–related malignancies, and severe burns. Renal loss of Igs occurs in nephrotic syndrome, in which IgG loss is usually accompanied by albumin loss. GI loss occurs in protein-losing enteropathies and intestinal lymphangiectasia. Recent studies show that the immunomodulator agent that targets B cells, rituximab, can cause acquired hypogammaglobulinemia (Alhassan et al., 2020; Labrosse et al., 2021; Tieu et al., 2021).

Patients with hypogammaglobulinemia experience an increased incidence of infections starting at an early age. Symptoms typically begin at 6 months of age when maternal antibodies start to wane in the newborn. Severe candidiasis and *P. jiroveci* pneumonia are common before 2 years of age. Encapsulated bacteria such as *Streptococcus pneumoniae, S. pyogenes, H. influenzae,* and *Staphylococcus aureus* are pathogens that commonly cause respiratory infections. Diarrhea with malabsorption syndrome is reported in more than 50% of patients. Gastritis with achlorhydria and pernicious anemia may occur. *G. lamblia* and *Campylobacter* species are the pathogens involved in the GI manifestations in many of these patients.

The diagnosis of hypogammaglobulinemia is made after a child is 2 years of age. Before age 2, low immunoglobulin levels in the blood can be caused by a normal delay of B-cell maturation. Although no pathognomonic physical examination finding is typical, lymphadenopathy, splenomegaly, and hepatomegaly can all be present. Failure to thrive is a common diagnosis. Abnormal lung examination indicating bronchiectasis caused by frequent respiratory infections is common. A patient could also have a positive fecal occult blood test secondary to invasive bacterial infection.

Hallmarks of the disease are a lack of Igs and an impaired antibody response to vaccination. IgG levels persistently below the fifth percentile for age are usually present in this disorder. Decreased levels of IgA are also common in this group, and low IgM levels may be seen, but less frequently. Most infants have normal lymphocyte counts for age.

Treatment consists of bone marrow transplantation, immunoglobulin transfusions, and prophylactic antibiotics. Live vaccines should not be administered to the patient or family members.

Wiskott-Aldrich Syndrome

Wiskott-Aldrich syndrome (WAS) is an X-linked recessive disease caused by a mutation in the gene that encodes for Wiskott-Aldrich protein (WASp) found at Xp11.22. Because this disease is X-linked, it is found almost exclusively in boys. It is an uncommon disorder with an incidence of 1 in 100,000 live births. The gene mutation affects development of T cells, platelets, and Igs. In WAS, T cells and IgM are usually deficient, and thrombocytopenia is common.

Because of a lack of platelets, WAS usually presents with bleeding; in male infants, prolonged bleeding from circumcision is commonly one of the first symptoms. Purpura or unusual bruising and blood in the stool can occur early. Because of IgM deficiency, infections caused by encapsulated organisms can cause life-threatening complications, including pneumonia, meningitis, and sepsis. P. jiroveci and viral infections are also seen. Eczema develops in 81% of patients. Patients frequently become anergic (completely immuno-incompetent) and are vulnerable to overwhelming infections and sepsis. Autoimmune diseases have been reported in 26% to 70% of WAS patients. Patients are also found to have hemolytic anemia, neutropenia, vasculitis involving both small and large vessels, inflammatory bowel disease, and renal diseases. There is an increased risk of malignancies, such as lymphoma and leukemia, in adolescents and adults with WAS.

Diagnosis is made by testing for the presence of the WASp gene mutation. Absolute lymphocyte counts are usually normal during infancy, but T- and B-cell numbers decrease later in life in patients. Decreased lymphocyte proliferation in response to antigens occurs in approximately 50% of patients. Delayed-type hypersensitivity skin testing is abnormal in 90% of affected individuals. There are variations in the levels of Ig, including normal levels of serum IgG, decreased levels of IgM, and elevated levels of IgA and IgE. There are also low platelet counts.

Treatment consists of prophylactic antibiotics, such as trimethoprim sulfamethoxazole, to prevent P. jirovecii pneumonia in infants and children younger than 3 to 4 years with classic WAS. Prophylactic acyclovir is given to patients with recurrent HSV infections. Live vaccines should not be administered to the patient or family members. Platelet transfusions can treat major bleeding episodes. Intravenous immunoglobulin (IVIG) therapy is indicated in WAS patients with significant antibody deficiency. Immunosuppressive treatment may be required for autoimmune manifestations. Life expectancy of patients with WAS is reduced, with premature death resulting from infections, hemorrhage, autoimmune disease, and malignancies. Bleeding is the main cause of death. Malignancies in patients with WAS are often fatal. However, bone marrow transplant is a mainstay of treatment for patients with WAS and has resulted in a cure for many patients.

DiGeorge Syndrome

DiGeorge (22q11.2 deletion) syndrome (DGS) is an isolated T-cell deficiency that results from maldevelopment of the thymus gland. The disease is caused by a genetic deletion at 22q11.2. The infants born with this genetic mutation may present with a spectrum of conditions that can include congenital cardiac abnormalities, parathyroid gland maldevelopment with hypocalcemic tetany, and absence of the thymus gland. Facial abnormalities characteristic of the disease may include cleft palate, micrognathia (underdeveloped jaw), hypertelorism (eyes that are wide apart), and a shortened philtrum (top lip disfigurement). Individuals with 22q11.2 deletion syndrome may have several of the different conditions, whereas others may be only mildly affected. Incidence is approximately 1 per 4,000 to 5,000 live births.

Eighty percent of affected infants have congenital heart defects, such as tetralogy of Fallot and ventricular septal defects. Recurrent infections usually present in patients older than 3 to 6 months. The facial features of this syndrome are often subtle and may go unnoticed until later in childhood. The overall incidence of immune dysfunction is 77%, and recurrent infections are usually observed. Autoimmune diseases such as juvenile RA often occur with the disease. Hypocalcemia can cause seizures early in development. Developmental delay and learning difficulties are observed in 70% to 90% of patients.

To diagnose the syndrome, a karyotype can reveal the characteristic gene deletion at 22q11.2. Lymphocyte count and serum calcium will be abnormal. Cardiac catheterization can demonstrate the cardiac defects.

Multidisciplinary coordinated health care with use of multiple specialists is necessary to ensure that these patients receive optimal medical care. The patient often needs consultations from a cardiac surgeon, immunologist, endocrinologist, developmental psychologist, and craniofacial surgical specialist. The patient's immunoglobulin levels are normal; however, because of the deficiency of CD3 T cells, immune responses are impaired. Live vaccines are contraindicated in patients with DGS. Treatment requires immediate protection with strict isolation, cardiac surgery, craniofacial surgery, infusions of IVIG, and anti-infective prophylaxis, followed by thymic or bone marrow transplantation.

HIV Infection

HIV infection is a disease that has three stages: acute HIV infection, chronic HIV infection, and a third stage termed AIDS. If HIV infection progresses without treatment, it can advance to AIDS; however, highly effective antiretroviral medications are protecting many individuals from reaching this stage.

HIV first came to the public's attention because of an unusual outbreak of disease among homosexual males in Los Angeles in 1981. At that time, there was no name for the disease, but it was known to be associated with severe immune deficiency, *Pneumocystis carinii* pneumonia, and Kaposi's sarcoma, which were highly unusual diseases contracted by healthy homosexual males. The Centers for Disease Control (CDC) took intense interest in examining the outbreaks, and by 1983 a new organism, HIV, was isolated. By 1984, HIV was confirmed as the causative agent of AIDS. The infection quickly became an epidemic and pandemic before it was known that sexual contact and blood products transmit the disease. Before treatments were discovered, many individuals died, and HIV infection was thought to be fatal. Today, thanks to advances in diagnostic testing and treatment, many individuals with HIV never see the disease progress to AIDS, allowing them to live a normal life with chronic HIV infection.

Epidemiology

In 2019, 36,801 people received an HIV diagnosis in the United States. The annual number of new diagnoses decreased 9% from 2015 to 2019. Although there has been a decrease in the incidence of HIV since 2015, progress within different sectors of the U.S. population is unequal. Black people account for 42% of the diagnoses, yet they comprise only 12% of the U.S. population. In the United States, gay and bisexual men accounted for 83% (6,385) of all new HIV diagnoses in people aged 13 to 24 in 2019. Specifically, young Black/African American gay and bisexual men are most affected, as they represented 50% (3,209) of new HIV diagnoses among young gay and bisexual men. Persons who are IV drug users make up 7% of those affected by HIV infection.

Globally, in 2020, there were approximately 38 million people living with HIV and 680,000 AIDS-related deaths. Worldwide, deaths due to HIV have decreased due to higher rates of HIV testing and greater numbers of persons receiving life-saving treatment. In 2020, more than 75% of the 38 million people living with HIV were in treatment. More than half of all people living with HIV in treatment had suppressed viral loads (UNAIDS, 2022). The UNAIDS organization has established a global strategy toward ending AIDS; *Global AIDS Strategy 2021–2026: End Inequalities*. End AIDS is a program that aims to prioritize people who are not accessing life-saving HIV services. Its goal is to end AIDS as a public health threat by 2030.

Interestingly, there is a segment of the population that is completely resistant to HIV infection. Due to a gene mutation, these persons lack a key surface receptor on T cells and macrophages, called the CCR5 receptor. Without this receptor, HIV cannot attach or fuse with a T cell or macrophage. These persons are termed HIV resistors (see Box 11-4).

BOX 11-4. Human Immunodeficiency Virus Resistors

C-C chemokine receptor type 5 (CCR5) is a protein that is encoded by the *CCR5* gene. The *CCR5* gene codes for a receptor on CD4 cells that binds with HIV. Certain populations, however, have inherited a mutation resulting in the deletion of the *CCR5* gene; these individuals do not have a receptor for HIV on their CD4 cells. Homozygous carriers of this mutation are resistant to HIV-1 infection.

 CLINICAL CONCEPT

Because of the success of drug therapy, chronic HIV infection is becoming the most common form of HIV infection, allowing for long survival rates for affected individuals.

Etiology

HIV is a retrovirus within the genus *Lentivirus*. Lentiviruses have a long latency period and a slowly progressing disease course. There are two major strains of HIV. HIV-1 is the type that infects most individuals in the United States, and HIV-2 is the strain most common in West Africa.

HIV targets cells that express the CD4 receptor and the chemokine receptors CCR5 or CXCR4. These include T lymphocytes (called T helper cells or CD4 T cells), monocytes, and macrophages in the lymph nodes, spleen, bone marrow, lung and brain and dendritic cells in lymphoepithelial tissue in the vagina, rectum, and tonsils.

A retrovirus has RNA as its genetic material and comes equipped with its own enzyme, called reverse transcriptase, that can convert its RNA into DNA so that the virus can give genetic instructions to the host cell. The human host cells are mainly the CD4 T cell and macrophage. The host cell then uses the DNA for instructions to manufacture more viruses.

Pathophysiology

The hallmark of HIV is a progressive depletion of CD4 T cells, which are integral to both cell-mediated and antibody-mediated immune mechanisms. CD4 cells are necessary components for a fully functioning immune system, and their depletion leads to immunodeficiency. Attacking CD4 cells allows the virus to destroy both immune mechanisms of the body. Macrophages act as reservoirs of HIV, allowing for viral persistence that can be undetectable in laboratory tests. Macrophages are believed to serve as vehicles for dissemination. Mucous membranes throughout the body are rich in macrophages. HIV sequentially attaches to the CD4 surface receptor and CCR5 or CXCR4 (or fusin) chemokine coreceptors on host cells. The virus then uses reverse transcriptase to change its RNA into DNA. An enzyme called integrase then allows the viral DNA to be integrated into the host cell DNA. Integrase secreted by HIV incorporates the genetic directions for synthesis of viruses into the genome of the host cell. The host cell becomes a "factory" for manufacturing more viruses. Protease is an HIV enzyme that assists in the assembly of protein components to construct new viruses.

After HIV uses the CD4 cell for replication of itself, it eventually destroys the cell and moves on. Viruses move from one CD4 cell to another, using them as "factories," and then leave CD4 cells to die. The infected CD4 cell can no longer function within cell-mediated immune responses or assist antibody-mediated immune responses, which weakens the body's two categories of adaptive immunity. By destroying macrophages, HIV weakens the body's innate immunity as well (see Fig. 11-10).

As viremia, the number of viruses in the bloodstream, increases, more host cells are attacked and the number of CD4 cells in the blood decreases. The viral load increases as the CD4 cell count gradually drops, weakening the body's immune response. This usually occurs over a number of years. The CD4 cell count is used to monitor the course of the disease. If the CD4 + cell count drops below 200 cells/mm^3, severe immune dysfunction occurs and a diagnosis of AIDS is made. If left untreated, people at this stage of the disease usually succumb to opportunistic infections.

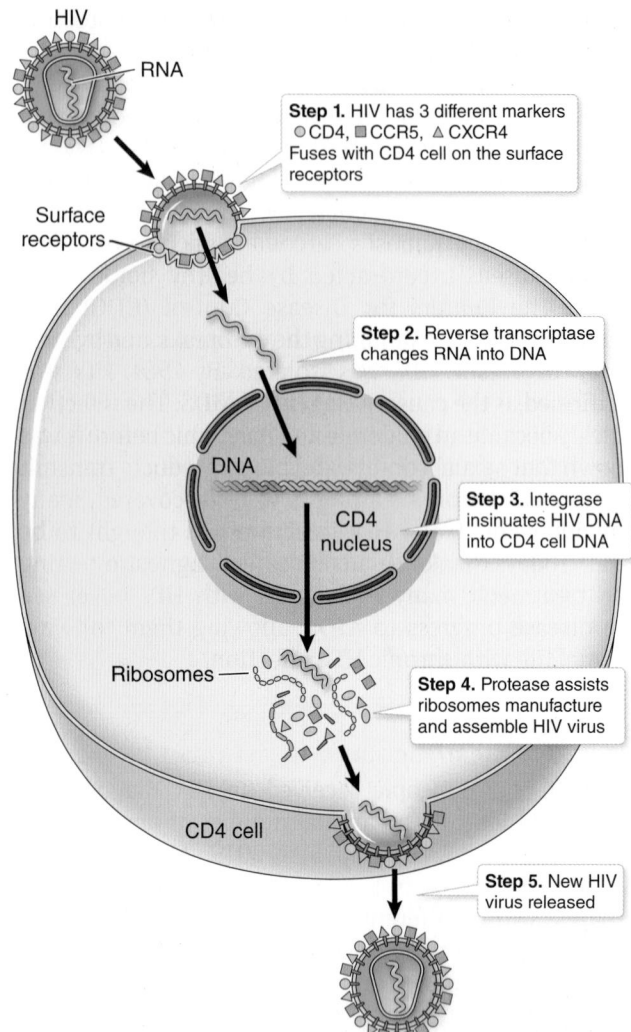

FIGURE 11-10. The life cycle of HIV. **Step 1.** The virus fuses with CD4, CCR5, and CXCR4 surface receptors located on the CD4 cell (T helper cell). **Step 2.** After fusion, HIV inserts its RNA into the cell. Through the use of a viral enzyme, reverse transcriptase, viral RNA is transformed into DNA. **Step 3.** The enzyme integrase facilitates the HIV DNA to insinuate into the CD4 cell DNA. **Step 4.** At the ribosomes, the CD4 cell uses the enzyme protease to synthesize and assemble new HIV virus particles. **Step 5.** Newly assembled HIV viruses are released.

CLINICAL CONCEPT

The enzyme reverse transcriptase enables HIV to transform its RNA into DNA. The enzyme integrase allows insertion of the viral DNA into the CD4 cell's DNA. Thus, major categories of anti-HIV drugs are reverse transcriptase inhibitors and integrase inhibitors.

Clinical Presentation

After contraction of the virus, acute HIV infection presents as a mononucleosis-like viral syndrome consisting of fever, headache, fatigue, pharyngitis, GI symptoms, lymphadenopathy, arthralgias, and myalgia. This early disorder, referred to as acute retroviral syndrome, occurs within 28 days of contracting the virus. The acute retroviral syndrome lasts a couple of weeks and then resolves. Many persons disregard the early symptoms as a mild viral syndrome and do not seek medical attention. After the acute retroviral syndrome resolves, the patient becomes asymptomatic. However, the virus can

remain dormant within CD4 cells and macrophages. This period of dormancy is one of the reasons HIV is difficult to treat.

During the initial phase of infection, there is no rise in antibodies or serological representation of disease. Time is needed for the immune system to recognize the invader and begin making antibodies against the virus. For most individuals, the development of antibodies to HIV requires from 2 weeks to 6 months. Early in the disease, HIV is a silent, asymptomatic infection, and the physical examination may be completely normal. The patient appears healthy, and antibody tests are usually negative. Although antibodies are not present early in the infection, viral particles can be detected in the bloodstream. During this time, individuals with the virus can transmit it to others without knowing that they have an infection. Up to 38% of new HIV infections are transmitted by persons who are unaware of their HIV status (Li et al., 2019).

After resolution of the acute retroviral syndrome, the infection enters a latent stage, referred to as chronic HIV infection. If the infection is untreated, increasing levels of viremia and decreasing numbers of CD4 cells occur, usually over a number of years. This period can last from 6 months to 10 years, depending on the individual.

As the virus replicates, the CD4 cell count begins to show a slow steady decline due to destruction by the virus. Normal range of CD4 cells is 800 to 1200 cells/mm³. Immunological impairment becomes significant when the CD4 cell count goes below 500 and an affected individual starts to become susceptible to **opportunistic infections**. An opportunistic infection is an illness caused by a pathogen that takes advantage of the lack of immune defenses within the host (see Box 11-5).

A CD4 cell count below 200/mm³ indicates an AIDS-defining disorder, thus the diagnosis of AIDS is made. Without intervention, the strength of the immune system continues to decline, the opportunistic infection or disorder overwhelms the body, and death is imminent (see Fig. 11-11).

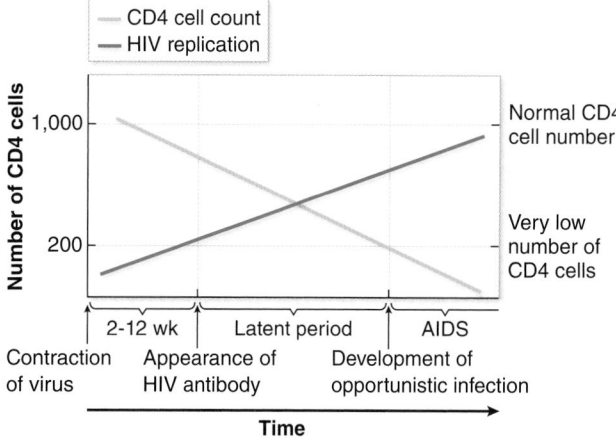

FIGURE 11-11. The clinical course of HIV infection. There is a 2-week to 6-month period from the time of contraction of the virus to the appearance of the HIV antibody. This is called the window, when the blood does not demonstrate any HIV antibody. After the virus is contracted, the virus replicates by infecting an increasing number of CD4 cells. As time goes on, the CD4 cell number decreases. The latent period is a span of time of increasing viremia when the patient is asymptomatic but the virus is gradually destroying CD4 cells. When there is a low number of CD4 cells, the patient is immunosuppressed and susceptible to opportunistic infection. When the patient has developed an opportunistic infection and has fewer than 200 CD4 cells, the HIV infection is then termed AIDS.

CLINICAL CONCEPT

Kaposi's sarcoma is an AIDS-defining disorder associated with HIV infection. It is a cancerous condition of the endothelium caused by a type of herpes virus, exhibited by red to purple papular lesions on the skin and mucous membranes.

BOX 11-5. Common Opportunistic Infections and Diseases Associated With HIV Infection

Candidiasis (thrush)
Cryptosporidiosis
Cryptococcal meningitis
Cytomegalovirus (CMV)
Hepatitis A, B, and C
Herpes simplex (cold sores and genital herpes)
Herpes zoster (shingles)
Human papillomavirus (HPV)
Kaposi's sarcoma (KS)
Molluscum contagiosum
Mycobacterium avium complex (MAC)
Pneumocystis jirovecii pneumonia
Progressive multifocal leukoencephalopathy (PML)
Toxoplasmosis
Tuberculosis (TB)

Risk of Transmission

High-risk behaviors such as unprotected sexual activity, anal intercourse, and IV drug abuse should alert the health-care provider of the patient's susceptibility to HIV infection. Currently, the most at-risk population is men who have sex with men (MSM), particularly African American and Hispanic males. The activity of anal intercourse is a particularly high-risk behavior. The receptive partner is at higher risk than the insertive partner. Other at-risk populations include IV drug users and heterosexuals who engage in unprotected sexual activity. Heterosexual females are at higher risk of HIV infection than heterosexual males. Persons with a history of sexually transmitted disease (STD) are also at high risk. Despite the fact that donor blood and donor organs are screened for HIV, persons who require frequent transfusions, such as hemophiliacs or those who have undergone transplantation, are also at risk for HIV infection. Offspring of HIV-positive mothers can contract infection during pregnancy or through breastfeeding. Although not a common occurrence, HIV transmission is also possible through unsanitary tattooing, piercing, dental, and manicure instruments. People with substance use disorders who share instruments such as spoons or straws are also at risk. Though the risk of HIV transmission through oral sex is low, several factors may increase that risk, including open sores in the mouth or vagina or on the penis, bleeding gums, oral contact with menstrual blood, and the presence of other STDs.

CLINICAL CONCEPT

CDC recommends that everyone between the ages of 13 and 64 get tested for HIV at least once as part of routine health care. For those at higher risk, CDC recommends getting tested at least once a year.

Screening Tests for HIV Infection

Mass screening tests are available for HIV infection. These rapid tests require a swab of cheek cells, saliva, or a small sample of blood and are based on detection of the p24 antigen/antibody combination or antibody alone. The p24 antigen is a protein within the capsid of HIV. Viral antigen (p24 protein) can be detected at approximately day 14 after contraction of the virus. High levels of p24 are present in the bloodstream of newly infected individuals; however, antibodies to p24 are produced during seroconversion, rendering p24 antigen undetectable after seroconversion in most cases. Testing for p24 antigen is not reliable for diagnosing HIV infection; it still requires a confirmatory laboratory HIV RNA assay blood test.

CLINICAL CONCEPT

Blood donations are screened for HIV using the p24 antigen test. The risk of contracting HIV infection from donor units of blood is between 1 in 1.4 million and 1 in 1.5 million units.

Diagnosis

Precise diagnostic laboratory testing for HIV infection includes CD4 count, HIV viral load (also called **HIV RNA assay** or HIV nucleic acid test), HIV antibody, and HIV drug-resistance testing.

In the clinical setting, if a health-care provider deems that an HIV test is necessary, written consent by the patient is not necessary. However, after a patient is notified that an HIV test is recommended by the health-care provider, the patient can choose to opt out of testing.

The HIV RNA blood test (also called viral load or HIV nucleic acid test) is the most accurate measure of the number of viruses in the bloodstream. The results of a viral load test are described as the number of copies of HIV RNA in a milliliter of blood. There is an "eclipse period" of approximately 3 to 4 days from the point of contraction of the virus to the ability to detect HIV RNA in the bloodstream. The virus is usually detectable by an HIV RNA blood assay within 4 to 11 days of contraction. A viral load of less than 10,000 is considered low risk for development of AIDS. A viral load greater than 100,000 is considered at risk for AIDS.

HIV antibody is not present in the bloodstream immediately after contraction of the virus. HIV antibody develops slowly after contraction of the virus. In most persons, HIV antibody is not present until 2 weeks to 6 months after contraction of the virus. In some persons, HIV antibody may not be detectable until later than 6 months after contraction of the virus. Therefore, the HIV antibody test cannot detect early HIV infection. There is a "window period" when the patient is antibody negative, also called serologically negative. Seroconversion occurs when antibody appears in the bloodstream, at which time, the person is considered seropositive. It is during this window period when there is no discernible antibody in the bloodstream and no symptoms of disease that infected individuals often unknowingly transmit the virus to others. After seroconversion, the presence of HIV antibody can be detected by enzyme-linked immunosorbent assay (ELISA).

Inversion of the CD4 to CD8 ratio occurs early in infection. This occurs because there is a decrease in the number of CD4 cells and the CD8 cells remain unaffected. Normally, in an infection the CD4 to CD8 ratio is 2:1. This ratio reverses with HIV infection: the CD4 to CD8 ratio becomes 1:2.

An HIV RNA blood test should be initiated before **antiretroviral therapy (ART)** and again after ART is initiated 2 to 8 weeks later. If the viral load remains detectable, it is recommended that a repeat test is done every 4 to 8 weeks until the viral load drops below 200 copies/mL. Viral load testing can be repeated every 3 to 6 months thereafter.

Viral load indicates the severity of the disease and susceptibility to AIDS. It is important to note that if the viral load falls to undetectable levels, the virus is still present in the body in tissue reservoirs and the patient can still transmit the virus to others—it is just not measurable by current blood tests. The HIV drug-resistance test is also done to check if the virus has a mutation that endows it with resistance to specific types of ART. This test can guide choice of treatment regimen. The HIV drug-resistance test can be done if the viral load is above 500 copies/mL. Clinicians also test for HLA B*5701, which detects a gene that predisposes to an allergic reaction to the specific ART medication abacavir. This test also guides the choice of treatment.

The HIV enters cells by attaching to the CD4 receptor, followed by binding to either the **CCR5** or **CXCR4 receptor**. A blood test can determine the specific coreceptor affinity (i.e., CCR5, CXCR4, or both) of the patient's virus.

Because HIV often occurs due to unprotected sexual activity, clinicians should also test for STDs, mainly syphilis, gonorrhea, and chlamydia. Hepatitis B and hepatitis C blood testing is also recommended. The individual with HIV is highly susceptible to TB, so testing in the form of a purified protein derivative (PPD) or a blood test called interferon gamma release assay is done.

When the CD4 cell count falls to 200 cells/mm³ or below, opportunistic infections can be contracted. The patient commonly experiences symptoms of persistent fever, night sweats, weight loss, and opportunistic infections. Kaposi's sarcoma, which causes tumors on the linings of blood vessels, can develop and leave purple-blue blotches on the skin. These tumors can also develop within organs. Common opportunistic infections associated with HIV include recurring *Candida* infection, *Pneumocystis jirovecii* pneumonia, toxoplasmosis, cryptococcus, and TB.

 CLINICAL CONCEPT

To be diagnosed with AIDS, a person with HIV must have an AIDS-defining condition or have a CD4 count less than 200 cells/mm³.

Treatment

Treatment of HIV and AIDS has posed a great deal of difficulty for the health-care community for a number of reasons. Because of the latency of the disease, an infected individual commonly does not seek treatment until symptomatic with an opportunistic disorder, at which time the immune system is already greatly compromised. HIV is highly mutatable, and development of a vaccine or an effective antibody has proved impossible to date. Although the body produces antibodies to the disease, they are not effective combatants in the fight against it. Also, HIV can remain dormant in the body within nonreplicating CD4 cells.

Only ART has been successful in the long-term treatment of HIV infection. During this therapy, different kinds of antiretroviral medications are used to attack the virus at various stages of its life cycle. Early initiation of ART is recommended. Recent studies have shown that very early initiation of ART can preserve immune function and reduce complications of HIV-1 infection. More than 85% of patients who consistently receive ART have sustained virological suppression indefinitely (CDC, 2020a).

Types of ART currently available include (see Table 11-3):

- Fusion inhibitors
- CCR5 antagonists (CCR5s) (also called entry inhibitors)
- Nonnucleoside reverse transcriptase inhibitors (NNRTIs)
- Nucleoside reverse transcriptase inhibitors (NRTIs)
- Integrase strand transfer inhibitors (INSTIs)
- Protease inhibitors (PIs)

Fusion inhibitors act by blocking HIV from attaching to the surface the CD4 cell. Chemokine coreceptor 5 (CCR5) antagonists are also entry inhibitors that

TABLE 11-3. Types of Antiretroviral Agents (current as of 2018)	
Fusion Inhibitors	Enfuvirtide (Fuzeon)
CCR5 antagonists	Maraviroc (Selzentry)
NRTIs	Emtricitabine (Emtriva)
	Lamivudine (Epivir)
	Zidovudine (Retrovir)
	Didanosine (Videx)
	Tenofovir (Viread)
	Stavudine (Zerit)
	Abacavir (Zigen)
NNRTIs	Rilpivirine (Edurant)
	Etravirine (Intelence)
	Delavirdine (Rescriptor)
	Efavirenz (Sustiva)
	Nevirapine (Viramune)
INSTIs	Raltegravir (Isentress)
	Dolutegravir (Tivicay)
	Elvitegravir (Vitekta)* requires a booster
Protease inhibitors	Tipranavir (Aptivus)
	Indinavir (Crixivan)
	Saquinavir (Invirase)
	Ritonavir (Norvir)
	Darunavir (Prezista)
	Atazanavir (Reyataz)
	Nelfinavir (Viracept)
	Fosamprenavir (Lexiva)
	Lopinavir + ritonavir (Kaletra)

Note. Several of the NRTI drugs may be combined into one tablet to make it easier to take the medications. These drugs are known as fixed-dose combinations. Adapted from U.S. Department of Health and Human Services (2018). HIV treatment. What to start: Choosing an HIV regimen. https://aidsinfo.nih. gov/understanding-hiv-aids/fact-sheets/21/53/what-to-start–choosing–an-hiv-regimen; U.S. Department of Health and Human Services. (2018). HIV treatment. FDA-approved HIV medicines. Retrieved from https://hivinfo. nih.gov/understanding-hiv/fact-sheets/fda-approved-hiv-medicines; U.S. Department of Health and Human Services. (2017). Guidelines for the use of antiretroviral agents in adults and adolescents living with HIV. Retrieved from https://clinicalinfo.hiv.gov/en/guidelines/hiv-clinical-guidelines-adult-and-adolescent-arv/whats-new-guidelines

block HIV from latching onto the CCR5 receptor and entering the host cell. Both NRTIs and NNRTIs act by blocking the HIV enzyme reverse transcriptase. Reverse transcriptase is a viral enzyme that allows HIV to transform its RNA into DNA. Thus, NRTIs and

NNRTIs prevent HIV from changing its RNA into DNA, and HIV therefore cannot give genetic directions to the CD4 cell. INSTIs block HIV from inserting its viral DNA into the host cell DNA. This in turn blocks HIV from replicating itself inside the CD4 cell. PIs block HIV from synthesizing the protein pieces that are needed to synthesize more HIV particles in the host cell.

When HIV was first discovered in the 1980s, the life expectancy of patients with the disease was 2 years at most. Today, with ART treatment approaches and the prevention of opportunistic infections, patients with HIV can live a long life from their date of diagnosis. HIV is no longer a life-threatening illness; it is a chronic disease with effective treatment.

Preventive Treatment

Currently, there are two forms of preventive treatment: pre-exposure prophylaxis (PrEP) and postexposure prophylaxis (PEP). PrEP is the use of antiretroviral medications in highly susceptible uninfected individuals. It requires taking a single combination pill daily consisting of emtricitabine and tenofovir (Truvada). PrEP is a strategy used with partners when one is HIV positive and the other is HIV negative. Persons who use PrEP must take the drug every day, use condoms, and follow up with their health-care provider every 3 months. When taken consistently, PrEP has been shown to reduce the risk of HIV infection in persons at high risk. PrEP reduces the risk of getting HIV from sex by about 99% and reduces the risk of getting HIV from injection drug use by at least 74% (CDC, 2023).

PEP is the use of antiretroviral drugs after a single high-risk event to prevent contraction of HIV. After exposure to HIV, PEP must be started within 72 hours to be effective. It includes a 28-day course of triple ART that includes tenofovir and emtricitabine (Truvada) with raltegravir or dolutegravir.

Complications of HIV

Opportunistic Infections Associated With HIV

Prophylaxis against specific opportunistic infections is indicated for patients with substantial immunosuppression. With effective ART, immune function can be restored and prophylaxis can be discontinued.

Prophylaxis against the opportunistic infections *P. jirovecii, T. gondii,* and *Mycobacterium avium* should begin depending on CD4 counts.

Malignancies Associated With HIV

HIV does not cause cancer directly; however, over time it weakens the immune system, which can lead to increased cancer risk in people living with HIV. AIDS-defining malignancies include Kaposi's sarcoma, non-Hodgkin's lymphoma, and invasive cervical cancer. Other types of cancer that are increasing in incidence in people living with HIV include anal cancer, Hodgkin's lymphoma, hepatocellular carcinoma, skin cancer, head and neck cancer, and lung cancer. Clinicians should perform routine malignancy screening and should be alert for symptoms in people living with HIV infection. A baseline anal Papanicolaou (Pap) test should be done in all patients with HIV. Women living with HIV should have a baseline cervical Pap test and, if normal, a second one 6 months later. If the second is normal, annual Pap smears are recommended.

Paradoxical Response to ART: Immune Reconstitution Inflammatory Syndrome

After initiation of ART, immune restoration is not always a smooth transition to health. Starting ART may be initially accompanied by an aberrant inflammatory response termed immune reconstitution inflammatory syndrome (IRIS), wherein patients experience deterioration in response to ART, despite efficient control of HIV viral replication and no apparent drug toxicity. The hallmark of the syndrome is paradoxical worsening of an existing infection or disease process or appearance of a new infection/disease process soon after initiation of therapy. The most common forms of IRIS are associated with mycobacterial infections, fungi, CMV, and herpes viruses.

AIDS

The most advanced stage of HIV infection is AIDS (the third stage). At this stage, the patient has 200 CD4 cells/mm^3 or less and/or an opportunistic infection or HIV-associated malignancy. The immune system is severely weakened, and the patient requires treatment for HIV as well as the associated infection or cancer. If treatments are unsuccessful, AIDS is commonly fatal.

Chapter Summary

- The immune system is a complex defense mechanism that protects humans from a constant barrage of injurious agents in the environment.
- The immune system deciphers which substances are "self" versus "non-self." Non-self substances, also called foreign antigens, are the targets of the immune system.
- The innate line of immunity is the nonspecific defenses that act against all antigens. Innate immunity includes defenses provided by skin, mucous membranes, enzymes, and macrophages.
- The adaptive immune line of defense is developed after exposure to antigens and has memory for antigens.

Specific T-cell and B-cell antibodies are synthesized against specific antigens.

- Adaptive immunity has two categories: cell-mediated (T lymphocyte) and antibody-mediated (B lymphocyte). After exposure, the adaptive immune mechanisms act rapidly, specifically, destructively, and with memory for every individual antigen it has encountered.

- After exposure to antigen, T lymphocytes attack antigens themselves.

- After exposure to antigens, B lymphocytes are transformed into plasma cells that release antigen-attacking Igs.

- There are two types of adaptive immunity: active and passive. Active adaptive immunity occurs when an individual contracts a disease and builds Igs against the antigen or when an individual receives a vaccine. Passive adaptive immunity occurs when an individual receives fully formed antibodies to use against antigen.

- Although the immune system is designed for protection, dysfunction of the immune system can wreak havoc within the body. Immunodeficiency, immune hypersensitivity, and autoimmunity can occur when the immune system dysfunctions.

- There are four types of hypersensitivity reactions. Type I is immediate hypersensitivity, which is an allergic or atopic reaction. Type II is a cytotoxic reaction, such as a transfusion reaction. Type III occurs by immune complex deposition, as in RA. Type IV is delayed hypersensitivity, such as the body's delayed reaction to the Mantoux TB test, which develops after 48 hours.

- Autoimmune disease occurs when the body cannot decipher between self and non-self and antibodies attack the body's own tissues.

- Disorders of the immune system can be categorized as autoimmune disorders or immunodeficiency disorders. Autoimmune disorders include SLE, RA, sarcoidosis, SS, scleroderma, and PAN. Immunodeficiency disorders include SCID, selective IgA deficiency, chronic mucocutaneous candidiasis, hypogammaglobulinemia, WAS, and DGS.

- There are three stages of HIV infection: acute HIV infection, chronic HIV infection, and AIDS.

- HIV mainly attacks CD4 cells (T helper cells) and macrophages.

- HIV is able to undermine both the cell-mediated and antibody-mediated protective defenses of the body by attacking the CD4 cell.

- HIV can be transmitted via semen, vaginal secretions, breast milk, blood, and transplanted tissues.

- The HIV antibody requires 2 weeks to 6 months for development. The window of HIV infection occurs from the time of contraction of the virus to antibody development.

- The patient is termed seronegative when there is no antibody and seropositive when antibody appears.

- The HIV RNA assay (HIV nucleic acid test) is the earliest and most sensitive test of HIV. It measures viral particles or viral load.

- To be diagnosed with AIDS, a person with HIV must have an AIDS-defining condition or have a CD4 count less than 200 cells/mm^3.

- Key opportunistic disorders that are associated with HIV infection include TB and other mycobacterial diseases, candidiasis, *P. jirovecii,* Kaposi's sarcoma, and toxoplasmosis.

- Although there is no cure at present, millions are living with and managing their chronic HIV infection due to the availability of ART.

- Different types of ART attack HIV in different stages of its life cycle. Combinations of drugs are used, which strike the virus at different stages.

- PrEP is a strategy to prevent HIV infection in uninfected but highly vulnerable persons such as partners of HIV-positive individuals. PrEP is showing efficacy in IV drug users and MSM.

- PEP is a strategy used to treat persons who had known exposure to HIV infection. It must be initiated within 72 hours of contraction of the virus.

 Making the Connections

Disorder and Pathophysiology

Signs and Symptoms	Physical Assessment Findings	Diagnostic Testing	Treatment
Allergic Rhinitis (Type 1 Immediate Hypersensitivity) | Exposure to allergen triggers B cells to produce plasma cells, which in turn secrete Igs. IgE, eosinophils, and mast cells interact to release inflammatory mediators such as histamine, leading to tissue edema.			
Sneezing. Conjunctivitis. Rhinorrhea.	Copious clear secretions from nose. Pale nasal mucous membranes. Erythema of conjunctiva.	Nasal secretions containing eosinophils. Skin testing to identify specific allergens.	Antihistamines. Intranasal anti-inflammatory corticosteroid.

Continued

Making the Connections–cont'd

Signs and Symptoms	Physical Assessment Findings	Diagnostic Testing	Treatment
Systemic Anaphylaxis (Severe Type I Immediate Hypersensitivity) | Anaphylaxis is an exaggerated allergic reaction that is a medical emergency. Exposure to allergen triggers B cells to produce plasma cells, which in turn secrete Igs. IgE, eosinophils, and mast cells interact to release a persistent high amount of inflammatory mediators such as histamine, leading to tissue edema.			
Pruritic urticaria (itchy hives). Coughing. Stridor. Asthma attack. Extreme anxiety. Fainting.	Urticaria. Edema of tongue. Bronchospasm. Laryngeal edema. Facial edema (angioedema). Hypotension.	Elevated IgE level. Eosinophils in nasal and bronchial secretions. Severe hypotension.	Medical emergency. IV or IM antihistamines, corticosteroids, and epinephrine required.
Rheumatoid Arthritis | Autoimmune disease mainly involving T cells and inflammatory mediators that attack joints and synovial membranes.			
Painful, tender joints, particularly of hands, wrists, and fingers. Extra-articular manifestations; possible pulmonary involvement, bone erosions, coronary artery disease. Systemic symptoms such as fever, malaise, fatigue, and anorexia may be present.	Joint swelling. Joint deformities, particularly of metacarpal joints and proximal interphalangeal joints of fingers. Swan's and boutonnière deformity. Ulnar deviation of hands.	Elevated ESR, CRP, leukocyte count. RF may be positive. Anticyclic citrullinated peptide (anti-CCP) antibodies. X-ray of regions of joint destruction and pannus formation.	Anti-inflammatory medications: NSAIDs, MTX, and biological DMARDs, which include TNF inhibitors: etanercept, infliximab, adalimumab, golimumab, and certolizumab pegol; the interleukin (IL)-1 receptor antagonist anakinra; and the IL-6 receptor antagonist tocilizumab. Others include abatacept, rituximab, and tofacitinib. Intra-articular glucocorticoids are used to reduce synovitis in particular joints that are more inflamed than others.
Systemic Lupus Erythematosus | Chronic autoimmune inflammatory disease with unclear antigen that triggers innate and adaptive immune reactions. Affects skin, heart, lungs, kidneys, and blood cells. Patients can experience remissions and exacerbations.			
Classic butterfly rash across the bridge of nose and cheeks. Fever. Joint pain and swelling. Fatigue. Weight loss.	Rash. Fever. Weight loss. Joint inflammation. Myositis. Splenic enlargement. Pneumonitis. Pleural effusion. Vasculitis. Pericarditis. Anemia. Thrombocytopenia. Cardiac valve deformities and renal dysfunction are common. Renal inflammation is common; lupus nephritis.	ANA antibodies and specific antibodies to double stranded-DNA, Smith antigen, antiribosomal, antihistone, antierythrocyte, antineuronal, anticardiolipin, and antiphospholipid antibodies. Lupus anticoagulant, anticomplement antibody. Complement levels in blood are decreased. Elevated ESR, CRP. Elevated CPK possible if myositis. Liver enzymes necessary. Serum creatinine may be elevated in lupus nephritis. Urinalysis may show hematuria and proteinuria. Biopsy of rash can diagnose SLE. Chest x-ray may show pleuritis or pneumonitis.	Hydroxychloroquine or chloroquine (antimalarial drugs), NSAIDS, and short-term corticosteroids. Biological agents: belimumab, anifrolumab, baricitinib. Other immunosuppressive agents that may be used include azathioprine, rituximab, methotrexate, cyclophosphamide, or mycophenolate.

Making the Connections–cont'd

Signs and Symptoms	Physical Assessment Findings	Diagnostic Testing	Treatment
Severe Combined Immunodeficiency Disease | Genetically distinct syndromes with defects of both humoral and cell-mediated immune responses.			
Chronic viral infection symptoms. Candidiasis. Severe diaper rash. Failure to thrive.	Chronic infections. Candidiasis. *Pneumocystis jirovecii* pneumonia. Severe diaper rash. Failure to thrive.	TREC assay. Low immunoglobulin level. Low T-cell level.	Bone marrow transplant. Gene therapy.
DiGeorge Syndrome (22q11.2 deletion syndrome) | Isolated T-cell deficiency that results from maldevelopment of the thymus gland. Caused by a genetic deletion mapped to 22q11.			
Chronic infections.	Infant has facial abnormalities characteristic of the disease: cleft palate, micrognathia, hypertelorism, and a shortened philtrum. Absence of thymus gland. Hypoparathyroid hypocalcemic muscle tetany. Congenital cardiac defects.	Lack of T lymphocytes. Hypocalcemia due to hypoparathyroidism.	Thymus gland or bone marrow transplant. Ig infusions. Antibiotics.
Sarcoidosis | Chronic multisystem autoimmune disorder of unknown origin characterized by an accumulation of T lymphocytes and macrophages and epithelioid granulomas in various organs.			
Fever. Fatigue. Malaise. Anorexia. Weight loss. Some patients may develop arthritis at the ankles, wrists, knees, and elbows. Many patients have cough, dyspnea, and chest discomfort if the respiratory system is affected.	Characteristic skin rash called erythema nodosum, which are tender, erythematous nodules on the anterior surface of the legs. Nonspecific maculopapular rash can develop on the face, around eyes and nose, on the back, and on the extremities. Parotid gland and lymph node enlargement.	Histological examination of lymph nodes and bronchoalveolar cells. Chest x-ray shows characteristic bilateral hilar lymphadenopathy.	Anti-inflammatory and immunosuppressive agents. Oral prednisone for 4 to 6 weeks and then the patient is reassessed. Immunosuppressive agents that may be used include methotrexate, azathioprine, leflunomide, or TNF-alpha inhibitors; infliximab, adalumimab.
Scleroderma | Autoimmune disease mainly involving collagen infiltration of skin and some organs, particularly esophagus.			
Appearance of shiny, stretched skin, particularly of face and hands. Esophageal dysmotility causes GERD. Myocardial ischemia, dysrhythmias, and pericarditis. Arthralgias and myalgias.	Appearance of shiny, stretched skin, particularly of face and hands. Finger contractures. Hypertension. GERD symptoms such as epigastric pain, burning, and regurgitation. Raynaud's phenomenon. Telangiectasias. Pulmonary symptoms such as cough. Chest pain due to myocardial ischemia or pericarditis. Calcinosis; fingertips and swelling of the hands.	Histological examination of skin. Antinuclear antibodies. Antitopoisomerase, anticentromere antibodies. Renal damage may be indicated by increased serum creatinine and proteinuria.	Individualized according to patient symptoms. GERD: proton pump inhibitors. Raynaud's phenomenon: calcium channel blockers. Hypertension: ACE inhibitors. Severe skin involvement: immunosuppressive therapy such as methotrexate, mycophenolate, or rituximab. Pulmonary involvement: cyclophosphamide. Arthritis: hydroxychloroquine and short-term corticosteroids. Biological agents, including TNF inhibitors, rituximab, abatacept, and tocilizumab, can be used if other drugs are ineffective.

Continued

Making the Connections—cont'd

Signs and Symptoms	Physical Assessment Findings	Diagnostic Testing	Treatment
HIV/AIDS | HIV is contracted via blood, sexual activity, transplacental route, or breastfeeding. HIV replicates mainly within the CD4 cells and kills them. As virus increases in the blood, CD4 cell count decreases, which diminishes both humoral and cell-mediated immunity, leaving the patient susceptible to opportunistic infections.			
Early symptoms may include a flu-like syndrome. Late symptoms may include weight loss and symptoms of opportunistic infections.	Signs may be absent if early in disease. Late in disease, signs are those of the opportunistic infections such as lymph-adenopathy, fever.	HIV RNA assay. HIV antibody: ELISA test CD4 cell count. CD4:CD8 ratio. HIV drug-resistance test. Test for HLA B*5701 gene that predisposes to an allergic reaction to the specific ART medication abacavir. A blood test to determine the specific coreceptor affinity (i.e., CCR5, CXCR4, or both) of the patient's virus. STD testing. Hepatitis testing. TB testing.	ART triple-drug regimen. Several categories of ART: fusion inhibitors, CCR5 antagonists, reverse transcriptase inhibitors, integrase inhibitors, and protease inhibitors. Pre-exposure prophylaxis. Postexposure prophylaxis. Prophylactic antibiotics.

Bibliography

Available online at fadavis.com

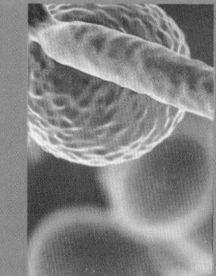

CHAPTER

12

White Blood Cell Disorders

Learning Objectives

After completion of this chapter, the student will be able to:

- Compare and contrast different types of white blood cells and their role in defending the body.
- Identify normal versus abnormal laboratory values of white blood cells on complete blood count.
- Describe the synthesis and maturation of white blood cells in the bone marrow and lymph nodes.

- Discuss the basic pathological mechanisms that occur in hematological neoplastic disease.
- Recognize the clinical manifestations of bone marrow dysfunction in hematological neoplastic disease.
- List various types of treatment modalities used for hematological neoplastic disease.

Key Terms

Agranulocytes
Allogeneic hematological stem cell transplant
Autologous hematological stem cell transplant
Bands
Basophil
BCR-ABL oncogene
Bence Jones proteins
Blast cells
B lymphocyte (B cell)
CAR-T cell therapy
Dendritic cell
Differentiation syndrome
Eosinophil

Granulocyte
Immunophenotyping
Immunotherapy
Leukapheresis
Leukemia
Leukemoid reaction
Leukocytosis
Leukopenia
Lymphoma
Macrophage
Monoclonal antibodies
Multiple myeloma (MM)
Myelodysplastic syndrome (MDS)
Neutropenia (leukopenia)

Neutrophilia
Ph chromosome
Plasma cells
Plasmacytoma
Pluripotent stem cells
Polymerase chain reaction (PCR)
Polymorphonuclear (PMN) WBC
Richter's transformation
Segs
Shift to the left
Targeting therapies
T lymphocyte (T cell)
Tumor lysis syndrome
Tyrosine kinase

White blood cells (WBCs), also called leukocytes, protect the body against infection. They function within the innate and adaptive divisions of the immune system. Those found in the innate division, known as **macrophages**, are the first line of defense against foreign invaders, or antigens. They engulf, ingest, and enzymatically break down foreign matter such as bacteria, pollen, viruses, and fungi that enter the body. Other WBCs of the innate system include neutrophils, eosinophils, basophils, and natural killer (NK) cells. In the adaptive

division, specialized WBCs called **B lymphocytes** and **T lymphocytes** attack specific antigens while maintaining a memory of these antigens for future defensive action.

All WBCs are manufactured in the bone marrow and released. Lymphocytes mature further within lymphoid tissue, such as the lymph nodes, tonsils, adenoids, thymus gland, and spleen.

Infections, immune diseases, and hematological neoplasms are the main disorders that affect WBCs. Hematological neoplasms, the major disorder of WBCs reviewed in this chapter, include leukemias, lymphomas, myelodysplastic syndrome, and multiple myeloma. These cancerous disorders target WBCs, but they also have effects on red blood cells (RBCs) and platelets. Hematology, the study of the blood cells, and oncology, the study of cancers, are closely related fields, and specialist clinicians are usually skilled in both types of disease.

Epidemiology

Leukemias, lymphomas, myelodysplastic syndrome (MDS), and **multiple myeloma (MM)** are the most common neoplastic disorders that affect WBCs. Lymphomas are solid tumors of proliferating lymphoid cells such as T cells and B cells. There are two main types: Hodgkin's and non-Hodgkin's lymphoma. Lymphomas affect approximately 3% of the U.S. population per year. Hodgkin's lymphoma affects persons primarily between ages 15 and 20 and 50 to 70 years. It is one of the most curable of the hematological cancers and affects 1 in 25,000 people annually.

Leukemias cause proliferation of cancerous WBCs, which in turn leads to hypercellular bone marrow that crowds out healthy blood cells. Proliferation of cancerous WBCs leads to immunosuppression and consequent infection. Worldwide, leukemia affects approximately 350,000 people per year, with 90% of those cases diagnosed in adults. It is, however, the third most common cancer in children.

Myelodysplastic syndrome (MDS) is the dysplastic development of one or more stem cell lineages within the bone marrow—either RBC, WBC, or platelet lineage. An uncommon disorder, it affects approximately 10,000 persons a year in the United States, the majority older than 70 years.

MM causes excessive proliferation of **plasma cells**, which are immunoglobulin-producing blood cells derived from B lymphocytes. It is a relatively uncommon cancer in the United States, mainly affecting males older than age 65. Approximately 32,000 persons per year are affected by MM.

Basic Concepts of White Blood Cell Function

WBCs are the major defenders of the body. The bone marrow produces them in response to inflammation or infection. Macrophages are WBCs of the innate immune system, which are always ready and waiting to defend. Lymphocytes, part of the adaptive immune system, act against specific antigens for which they have memory.

Categories of White Blood Cells

The normal range of total WBCs in the body is between 4,000 and 10,000 cells per microliter (mcL) (different laboratories vary slightly). They are divided into three major categories: monocytes (also known as macrophages), lymphocytes, and **granulocytes**. There are also three types of granulocytes: neutrophils, eosinophils, and basophils, with neutrophils comprising the majority of the granulocytes. Neutrophils are also referred to as **polymorphonuclear (PMN) WBCs**. WBCs without granules such as monocytes and lymphocytes are sometimes called **agranulocytes**. There are two types of lymphocytes: T cells and B cells. Each type of WBC has its own normal range (see Table 12-1).

Synthesis and Maturation of White Blood Cells

All blood cells arise from a small number of undeveloped, precursor cells in the bone marrow called **pluripotent stem cells** during the process of hematopoiesis. These precursor cells have the potential to become any type of blood cell. The bone marrow is stimulated to produce specific types of blood cells according to the body's needs. WBCs have a short life span and need constant replenishment by the bone marrow. To produce WBCs, the bone marrow begins with pluripotent stem cells called myeloid and lymphoid stem cells. Granulocyte and monocyte cells are derived from myeloid stem cells, and lymphocytes from lymphoid stem cells. Immature precursor cells for each WBC cell line are called **blast cells**. From the blast cell stage, each type of WBC begins to differentiate and mature along a committed cell line (see Fig. 12-1).

Lymphocytes mature to a certain extent in the bone marrow, but then leave and complete the maturation process in lymphoid tissue (see Fig. 12-2). B lymphocytes develop into plasma cells, which are antibody-producing cells, within lymph nodes.

TABLE 12-1. White Blood Cell Differential	
WBC Count	**4,000–10,000 cells/mcL (different laboratories may vary slightly)**
• Neutrophils (also called polymorphonuclear WBCS or PMNs)	• 40% to 80%
• Immature neutrophils (bands)	• 0% to 10%
• Lymphocytes	• 20% to 40%
• Monocytes	• 2% to 10%
• Eosinophils	• 1% to 7%
• Basophils	• 0% to 2%

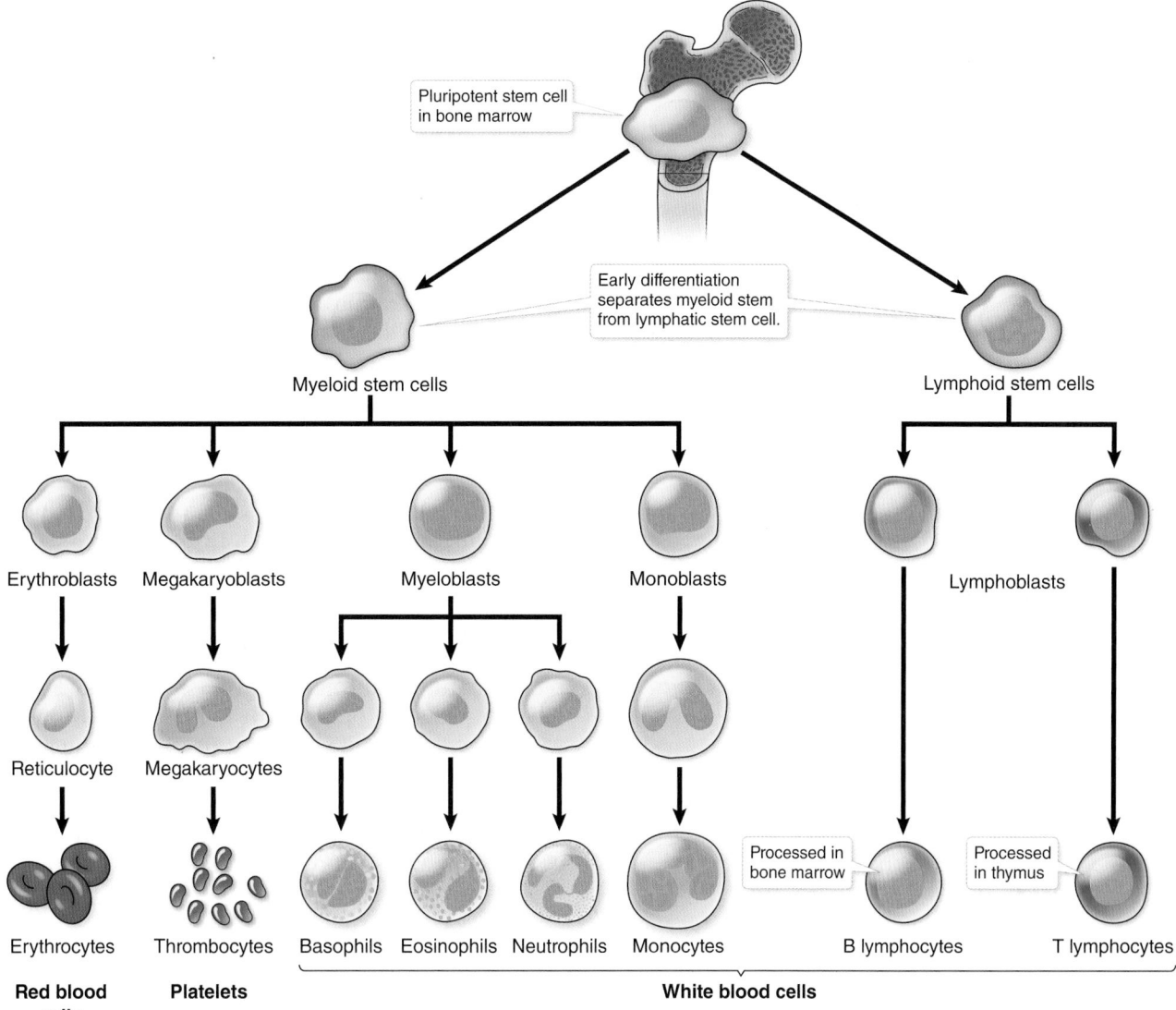

FIGURE 12-1. Hematopoiesis. All blood cells are derived from a pluripotent stem cell that has the ability to become any kind of blood cell. From the pluripotent stem cell, there is a differentiation into either a myeloid or a lymphoid line of stem cells. From the myeloid stem cell line, erythroblasts, myeloblasts, monoblasts, and megakaryoblasts can form and develop into mature cells. Erythroblasts develop into RBCs. Myeloblasts and monoblasts develop into different types of WBCs. Megakaryoblasts develop into platelets. From the lymphatic stem cell line, lymphoblasts can form and develop into mature lymphocytes.

T lymphocytes continue the maturation process mainly within the thymus gland, where they become T helper (CD4) and cytotoxic T cells (CD8) and then move into lymph nodes for proliferation.

Lymphoid tissue is located at various sites throughout the body. The spleen is an organ rich in lymphoid tissue, as are the tonsils in the pharynx. In addition, the gastrointestinal, respiratory, and genitourinary tracts are guarded by zones of lymphoid tissue and high numbers of macrophages.

Monocytes

Monocytes make up 2% to 10% of circulating WBCs. When they leave the circulation and enter tissue, they mature into macrophages, which are found in large quantities in the spleen and other organs. They have the ability to exit and reenter circulation while maintaining their primary function, which is phagocytosis. In this process, the macrophage engulfs, ingests, and enzymatically destroys antigenic substances and cellular debris. Macrophages are a major component of the innate immune system and are the primary immunological response to a foreign invader, termed an antigen. Another important function of monocytes is their ability to synthesize and secrete cytokines, substances that enhance inflammation and stimulate function of other WBCs. Monocytes can also become **dendritic cells**, which are specialized cells that present antigens to T cells. In this way, monocytes as dendritic cells link the innate immune system to the adaptive immune system.

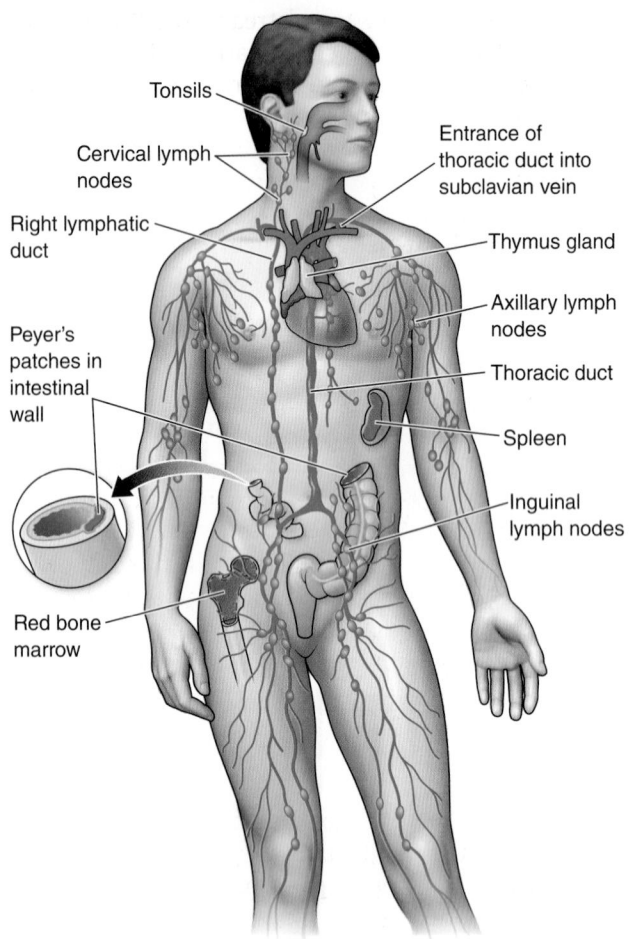

FIGURE 12-2. The lymphatic system.

and then catabolizing debris during phagocytosis. The three types of granulocytes—eosinophils, basophils, and neutrophils—are classified by the chemical makeup of their granules. Laboratory differentiation is possible because different granules stain differently when dye is applied.

Neutrophils. Neutrophils make up 40% to 80% of the WBCs in circulation. Like macrophages, they are the first responders to an infection, stressful event, or inflammatory reaction. Antigens, epinephrine, and corticosteroids stimulate generation and release of neutrophils in the bloodstream. At the first sign of cell injury, neutrophils leave the circulation and enter the tissues, where they lyse (break down) bacteria by releasing enzymes stored in their granules. When a neutrophil phagocytizes an invading organism or cellular debris, it releases a respiratory burst of free radicals called superoxides $[O_2^-]$ that contribute to injury of surrounding tissues (see Fig. 12-3).

Mature neutrophils, also called polymorphonuclear (PMN) leukocytes, have a life span of 1 to 2 days, and new recruits from the bone marrow are necessary during infection or inflammation. Under the microscope, mature neutrophils have a segmented, multilobed nucleus, as opposed to immature neutrophils, which have a bandlike nucleus. Because of the shape of their nucleus, mature neutrophils are referred to as **segs**, whereas immature neutrophils are called **bands**. The bone marrow releases immature neutrophils when the mature neutrophil supply in circulation is

🔬 CLINICAL CONCEPT

Macrophages function within the innate immune system and are the first responders in the defense against antigens. They also act as dendritic cells that present antigens to T cells.

Lymphocytes

Lymphocytes make up 20% to 40% of circulating WBCs. The two main types of lymphocytes are B cells and T cells. Lymphocytes are part of the adaptive branch of the immune system. After exposure to an antigen, lymphocytes recognize, target, and have memory for specific antigens. The stimulus of an antigen transforms a B cell into a plasma cell, which produces immunoglobulins (Igs) that attack antigens. In contrast, the stimulus of an antigen activates a T cell to directly attack the antigen. B and T cells endow the body with long-term immunity (see Chapter 11 for more information).

Granulocytes

Granulocytes are WBCs with chemical-containing granules in their cytoplasm. Their granules contain powerful digestive enzymes capable of killing microorganisms

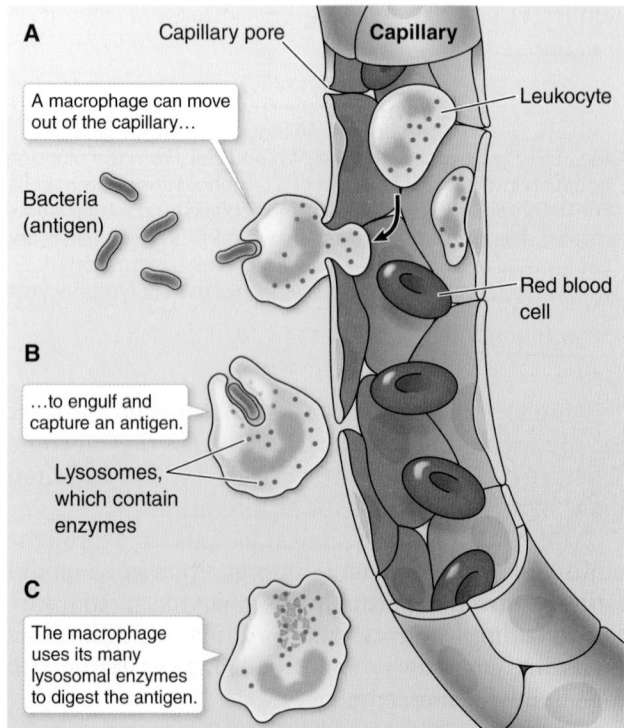

FIGURE 12-3. Phagocytosis of bacteria by a macrophage. A macrophage can move out of the capillary to engulf and capture an antigen. The macrophage uses its many lysosomal enzymes to digest the antigen.

exhausted. Bands in circulation indicate that the bone marrow is working very hard to manufacture enough WBCs for the infection or inflammatory disorder in the body. In severe acute infection or inflammation, the bone marrow cannot keep up with the body's need for mature neutrophils, so it releases bands. A laboratory test indicating a high number of bands in circulation is referred to as a **shift to the left**. This indicates there is a high ratio of immature neutrophils (young neutrophils coming from the bone marrow) to mature neutrophils in circulation, which occurs in acute inflammation.

 CLINICAL CONCEPT

Purulent exudate, commonly called pus, is a whitish-green–colored discharge from a site of injury that contains dead neutrophils, infectious material, and cellular debris.

Eosinophils. **Eosinophils** are WBCs that are generated by the bone marrow and released mainly during allergic reactions and parasitic infection. They include granules in the cytoplasm that contain chemical mediators and enzymes, such as histamine, eosinophil peroxidase, ribonuclease, deoxyribonuclease, lipase, and plasminogen. These mediators are released following activation of the eosinophil and are toxic to both parasites and host tissues. In healthy individuals, eosinophils make up about 1% to 7% of all WBCs, but their number rises during allergic reactions or parasitic infection.

Basophils. **Basophils** make up fewer than 2% of circulating WBCs but rise in response to infection or allergy. Their granules have chemical mediators, including histamine, prostaglandin, leukotrienes, and heparin. Basophils are generated and released by the bone marrow in response to many inflammatory reactions, particularly parasitic infection. The mediators histamine and heparin assist in the migration of neutrophils to an inflammatory site.

Basic Concepts of White Blood Cell Pathophysiology

WBCs can rise or become deficient in number, indicating a specific pathophysiological condition and corresponding side effects. Additionally, there are conditions of neoplastic proliferation of WBCs that can disrupt normal immune function.

Alterations in White Blood Cell Number

Pathological conditions, mainly infection, inflammation, and extreme stress, stimulate the rise in the

number of WBCs in the bloodstream (see Table 12-2). However, neoplasms or bone marrow disorders can also increase WBC count. A rise in WBC count above 11,000/mcL is called **leukocytosis**.

A **leukemoid reaction** is leukocytosis in excess of 50,000/mcL because of disorders other than leukemia. In a leukemoid reaction, there is an excess of normal, early neutrophil precursors: myelocytes, metamyelocytes, and promyelocytes. In contrast, acute leukemia shows a predominance of cancerous, immature WBCs called blasts. Leukemoid reactions occur for various reasons, including hemorrhage, specific infections, splenic dysfunction, and organ necrosis.

A decrease in WBC count below 4000/mcL is **leukopenia**, a general term that describes a decrease in all types of WBCs. Any agent that diminishes bone marrow function or any condition that causes destruction of WBCs causes leukopenia. Leukopenia increases risk of infection, decreases signs of infection, and diminishes healing ability. Neutrophils are the most common type of WBC affected in leukopenia.

Neutrophils
The type of WBC that most commonly rises in leukocytosis is the neutrophil. **Neutrophilia** is the term used for neutrophil predominance in the WBC count; it is defined as a neutrophil count above 7000/mcL in patients with a total WBC count of fewer than 11,000/mcL. Neutrophilia commonly occurs in response to bacterial infection. It is secondary to infection, inflammation, or malignancy, but it can also be caused by additional factors, such as smoking, stress, and drugs. In fact, cigarette smoking has been estimated to raise the WBC count in smokers by about 25%, and the total WBC count may remain elevated for up to 5 years after cessation. The rise in neutrophil levels is theorized to occur as the result of smoking-related inflammation. Drugs that cause neutrophilia include glucocorticoids, lithium, and epinephrine.

TABLE 12-2. Common Causes of Elevated Levels of White Blood Cells	
WBC	Common Cause of Elevation
Neutrophils	Bacterial infection
Lymphocytes	Viral infection
Eosinophils	Allergic reaction
Basophils	Parasitic infection or allergic reaction
Monocytes (macrophages)	Inflammation, chronic infection, malignancy, autoimmune disease

CLINICAL CONCEPT

WBC count is measured using a laboratory test called a complete blood count with differential (CBC with differential). It measures total RBCs, hemoglobin (Hgb), hematocrit (Hct), platelets, total WBCs, and the percentage of each type of WBC present. When the WBC count contains a large number of immature neutrophil bands, this is referred to as a "shift to the left."

Neutropenia, the lack of a sufficient number of neutrophils, is the most frequent kind of leukopenia. It is diagnosed in patients with fewer than 1500 neutrophils/mcL. A decrease in neutrophil number can occur rapidly and may occur because of deficient marrow function, WBC destruction, or a shift of neutrophils into various tissues.

There are many causes of neutropenia (see Box 12-1). With moderate-to-severe neutropenia (less than 1000/mcL), the body's immune defenses are significantly impaired, though monocytes are still active and will cause a rise in body temperature. Neutropenia with fever is evidence of infection. Filgrastim (Neupogen) is a stimulant of the bone marrow that can increase leukocyte synthesis, specifically neutrophils.

BOX 12-1. Common Causes of Neutropenia

Infections, more commonly viral infections, but also bacterial or parasitic infections

Medications, including those that may damage the bone marrow or neutrophils, including cancer chemotherapy, chloramphenicol, phenothiazines, allopurinol, carbamazepine, and phenylbutazone

Vitamin deficiencies, including megaloblastic anemia caused by vitamin B_{12} or folate deficiency

Diseases of the bone marrow, including leukemias, myelodysplastic syndrome, aplastic anemia, myelofibrosis, and any cause of bone marrow suppression

Radiation therapy

Hemodialysis machinery

Heart–lung machinery used in cardiac bypass

Congenital (inborn) disorders of bone marrow function or of neutrophil production, such as Kostmann's syndrome

Autoimmune destruction of neutrophils (either as a primary condition or associated with another disease such as Felty's syndrome) or from drugs stimulating the immune system to attack the cells

Hypersplenism, which refers to the increased sequestration and/or destruction of blood cells by the spleen

---

CLINICAL CONCEPT

Neutropenia increases susceptibility to infection and diminishes the external signs of inflammation. Persons with neutropenia require isolation and protective clinical precautions due to immunosuppression.

Monocytes

Monocytic leukocytosis is defined as a monocyte count above 800 mcL, or more than 8% of total WBC count. An elevated monocyte count in the presence of a normal total WBC count is called monocytosis. It is seen in a wide range of disorders, including acute infection or inflammation, chronic infection, malignancy, and autoimmune disease. Monocytopenia, an abnormally low number of monocytes, can be caused by high-dose steroids but is usually a result of a malignancy.

Eosinophils

Eosinophilia is an abnormally high number of eosinophils in the blood. Normally, there are no more than a few hundred eosinophils among all WBCs. In eosinophilia, there are more than 600 cells/mcL in the bloodstream. Eosinophilia is usually a result of an allergy or parasitic infection. Leukemia, as well as certain medications, toxins, and autoimmune disease, can cause eosinophilia.

Basophils

Basophilic leukocytosis is a rare condition most often associated with basophilic or mast cell types of acute or chronic leukemia. Other causes include hypersensitivity or inflammatory reactions, parasitic infection, hypothyroidism, ulcerative colitis, and varicella virus. Basopenia, an abnormally low number of basophils, is usually the result of a malignant disorder.

Lymphocytes

Lymphocytosis is an increase in lymphocytes within the bloodstream. B lymphocytes are produced in the bone marrow and mature in the spleen. T lymphocytes are produced by bone marrow and mature within the thymus gland. The thymus gland, however, degenerates over time, producing diminishing numbers of T cells with age. Because thymus-derived T cells decrease in number as a person ages, the definition of lymphocytosis also changes as a person ages:

- **Infant:** lymphocyte count greater than 9000/mcL
- **Children:** lymphocyte count greater than 7000/mcL
- **Adults:** lymphocyte count greater than 4000/mcL

Lymphocytosis is a sign of infection, particularly viral infection. In older individuals, lymphoproliferative disorders, including chronic lymphocytic leukemia (CLL) and lymphomas, often present with lymphadenopathy and lymphocytosis.

Lymphocytopenia, a decrease in lymphocytes, is a result of decreased production in the bone marrow because of an acquired or inherited immunodeficiency. Alternatively, it can occur because of lymphocyte destruction from radiation or chemotherapy. It, too, is diagnosed at different levels at different ages:

- **Children:** lymphocyte count lower than 3000/mcL
- **Adults:** lymphocyte level lower than 1500/mcL
- **Older adults:** lymphocyte count lower than 1400/mcL

In some cases, lymphocytopenia can be further classified according to the kind of lymphocytes that are reduced. In T lymphocytopenia, there are too few T lymphocytes but a normal number of other lymphocytes. This is usually caused by HIV infection, an inherited disorder, severe infection, radiation, or chemotherapy. In B lymphocytopenia, there are too few B lymphocytes but normal numbers of other lymphocytes. This is usually caused by medications that suppress the immune system. In NK lymphocytopenia, a rare disorder, there are too few NK cells but normal numbers of other lymphocytes.

Myelodysplastic Syndrome

Myelodysplastic syndrome (MDS) is a broad term used for disorders of the stem cells in the bone marrow. In this syndrome, all or part of bone marrow hematopoiesis is dysfunctional and ineffective, and differentiation of all or one category of precursor stem cells into committed cell lines is impaired. The patient sustains deficient numbers of all blood cells or one type of blood cell: WBCs, RBCs, or platelets.

The mean age at onset is older than 70 years with a slight male predominance. MDS is rare in children. Estimates of incidence are approximately 30,000 to 40,000 new cases per year in the United States, with incidence increasing as the age of the population increases.

MDS is caused by environmental exposures such as radiation and benzene; other risk factors have been reported inconsistently. Secondary MDS occurs as a toxic effect of prior radiation or cytotoxic cancer treatment. Signs and symptoms are nonspecific and generally related to a diminished number of blood cells. The clinical presentation is similar to that of hematological neoplasms. Lack of RBCs causes anemia, lack of WBCs causes infections, and lack of platelets causes increased susceptibility to bleeding and bruising.

Accurate diagnosis of MDS requires peripheral blood (PB) smear, bone marrow aspirate, and bone marrow biopsy. A full bone marrow karyotype, molecular genetic testing, flow cytometry, immunophenotyping, and clinical information such as any prior exposure to cytotoxic therapies are key to diagnosis. It is important to demonstrate persistent and clinically unexplained blood cell cytopenia and significant morphological dysplasia of the blood cells. MDS

may be triggered by the cytogenetic abnormality termed del 5q. This is a gene deletion at the q arm of the 5th chromosome.

MDS is classified into low- or high-risk disease. High-risk MDS can transition to acute myelogenous leukemia or complete bone marrow failure. In a substantial number of patients with low-risk MDS in which cytopenias are mild and asymptomatic, no treatment is required. In high-risk MDS, erythropoiesis-stimulating agents are used first to counteract anemia. Transfusion of the deficient type of blood cells and chemotherapy are commonly required. Lenalidomide (Revlimid, Celgene) is a chemotherapeutic agent that inhibits the cell cycle in malignant cells in high-risk MDS. Allogenic stem cell transplantation may also be indicated in high-risk MDS.

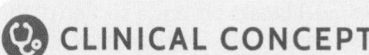

CLINICAL CONCEPT

High-risk MDS often leads to leukemia or bone marrow failure.

Hematological Neoplasms

Leukemia, lymphoma, MM, and MDS are the hematological neoplasms that affect the bone marrow, blood cells, lymph nodes, and other parts of the lymphatic system. They account for 9.8% of new cancer diagnoses in the United States.

Leukemias commonly develop in precursor stem cells of the bone marrow from a specific cell line. The abnormal cells appear similar to the immature forms of these cells, also called blasts. These blasts continue to proliferate and do not differentiate into mature cells.

Lymphomas are hematological neoplasms that specifically arise from abnormal proliferation of B or T lymphocytes. The tumors typically begin in the lymph nodes but can develop from any lymphoid tissue.

MM arises due to abnormal proliferation of plasma cells, which yield excessive immunoglobulins and immunoglobulin fragments. MDS is the abnormal development of one stem cell lineage within the bone marrow—RBCs, WBCs, or platelets.

Etiology

Hematological cancers can develop from any agent that damages the DNA of developing cells in the bone marrow. The damage turns on oncogenes or turns off tumor suppressor genes in the individual's genome, causing abnormal blood cell development. These malignancies are sometimes associated with a single gene abnormality, such as the **Ph chromosome** (formerly the Philadelphia chromosome), or changes to whole chromosomes, such as trisomy (three chromosomes instead of two) or monosomy (one chromosome instead of a pair).

The Ph chromosome is an abnormality that results from a translocation of a gene (see Fig. 12-4). The

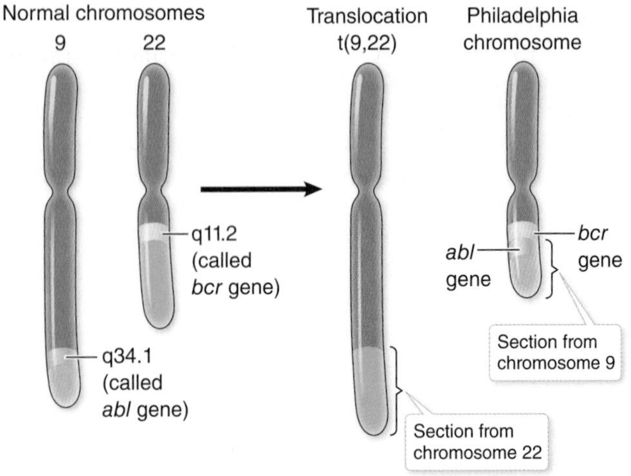

Normal chromosomes
9   22

Translocation
t(9,22)

Philadelphia
chromosome

q11.2
(called
bcr gene)

q34.1
(called
abl gene)

abl
gene

bcr
gene

Section from
chromosome 9

Section from
chromosome 22

FIGURE 12-4. Formation of the Ph chromosome. A section of the long arm of chromosome 9 breaks off, and a section of the long arm of chromosome 22 breaks off. The broken sections from each chromosome switch positions. The section from chromosome 9 binds to chromosome 22, whereas the broken section from chromosome 22 binds to chromosome 9. The translocation of these chromosomes is involved in the etiology of chronic myelogenous leukemia.

translocation is between chromosome 9 and chromosome 22; parts of chromosomes 9 and 22 actually change places with each other. The translocation causes a fusion of the parts of the two genes. A gene called the break point cluster (BCR) gene on chromosome 22 fuses with the Abelson leukemia virus (ABL) gene on chromosome 9. This translocation is commonly referred to as the **BCR-ABL** oncogene. The protein formed by the directions of these genes is the enzyme **tyrosine kinase**, which causes leukemia in hematopoietic cells. Many new drugs used to treat leukemias are tyrosine kinase inhibitors that prevent BCR-ABL from inciting leukemic changes.

Risk Factors

Exposure to any agent that can damage DNA is a risk for a hematological cancer. Exposure to intense radiation and contact with benzene are known predisposing factors for leukemia. Some viruses have been found to predispose to hematological cancers, such as Epstein–Barr virus (EBV), HIV, and human T-lymphotropic virus (HTLV). Chronic gastric infection with *Helicobacter pylori* is also associated with lymphoma.

Lymphomas have also been associated with congenital or acquired immunodeficiency disorders, including those resulting from immunosuppression treatment. See Box 12-2 for a list of common risk factors for hematological malignancies.

Pathophysiology

Leukemias are states of neoplastic proliferation involving WBCs. Lymphomas are neoplasms of lymphocytes and are commonly solid tumors found in lymphoid tissue. Each specific type of leukemia or lymphoma

has a specific pathophysiological process. Regardless of the type of neoplasm, leukemias and lymphomas cause similar pathophysiological conditions in the body. Nonfunctional, cancerous WBCs proliferate and overwhelm the bone marrow and other lymphoid tissue. The cancerous WBCs increase to excess numbers, and they crowd and suppress development of the other blood cells in the bone marrow—healthy WBCs, RBCs, and platelets.

Clinical Presentation

As with any illness, assessment begins with a complete history and physical examination. A complete list of all medications, including over-the-counter medications and supplements, should be obtained, as many medications and supplements can alter the production and number of WBCs. Past history of toxic or occupational exposures should be assessed to investigate possible risk factors associated with hematological disorders. For example, history of benzene exposure is related to leukemia. History of herbicide or insecticide exposure is associated with some types of lymphoma. Past medical and surgical disorders are important because some illnesses predispose to leukemias or lymphomas. For example, persons with EBV are at risk for development of Burkitt's lymphoma.

Family history and psychosocial history are important because many hematological disorders can be caused by genetic abnormalities or behavioral risk factors. For example, chronic lymphocytic leukemia (CLL) is often found among family members. Unsafe sexual practices can predispose individuals to HIV infection, which is a risk factor for lymphoma.

Signs and Symptoms. Key symptoms seen in patients with leukemia or lymphoma are those related to bone marrow suppression. Bone marrow becomes overwhelmed by the proliferation of neoplastic blood cells that crowd out healthy blood cells. The symptoms are related to low RBC count (anemia), WBC count (leukopenia), or platelets (thrombocytopenia) (see Box 12-3 for symptoms of hematological neoplasms).

Physical examination may reveal enlarged lymph nodes, splenomegaly, or both. An enlarged lymph node is the result of proliferative neoplastic WBCs and may be noticed by the patient or clinician on a physical examination. Splenomegaly may be present, the result of excessive infiltration of neoplastic WBCs or excessive hemolysis performed by an overactive spleen. In leukemia or lymphoma, splenomegaly is often the initial symptom.

BOX 12-3. Common Signs and Symptoms of Hematological Neoplasms

Common signs and symptoms of hematological neoplasms are caused by the excessive proliferation of neoplastic blood cells that overwhelm the bone marrow and crowd out and suppress development of healthy RBCs, WBCs, and platelets. Neoplastic cells also invade the lymph nodes, spleen, and liver.

- **Anemia:** caused by decreased red blood cells; chronic tiredness, shortness of breath, pallor, and sometimes chest pain
- **Neutropenia:** decreased normal WBCs, which causes increased susceptibility to infections
- **Thrombocytopenia:** decreased platelets, which increases susceptibility to bleeding and ecchymosis (bruising), nosebleeds (epistaxis), gingival bleeding, or subcutaneous hemorrhaging resulting in purpura or petechiae
- **Bone pain:** caused by excessive proliferation of neoplastic cells inside the bone marrow of many different bones, most commonly the sternum, femur, and tibia
- **Lymphadenopathy (enlarged lymph nodes):** excessive proliferation of abnormal lymphocytes within lymph nodes causes enlargement
- **Splenomegaly (enlargement of spleen):** excessive proliferation of abnormal lymphocytes within the spleen causes enlargement
- **Hepatomegaly (enlargement of the liver):** excessive proliferation of lymphocytes within the liver causes enlargement
- **Abdominal feeling of fullness:** caused by an enlarged spleen or liver putting pressure on the stomach
- **Unintentional weight loss:** caused by decreased appetite and hypermetabolism
- **Fever, chills:** caused by hypermetabolic state resulting from constant neoplastic cell production

Diagnosis

CBC with differential is usually the initial laboratory test with abnormal findings that begins the investigation into hematological malignancy. Bone marrow or lymph node biopsy and genome investigation of abnormal cells follow.

CBC With Differential. A CBC with differential is an important initial diagnostic test used to identify which specific type of WBC is causing the neoplastic disorder. The CBC identifies RBC number, Hgb, Hct, platelet number, and proportions of specific WBCs in the bloodstream. This is the basic diagnostic test that most often initiates further investigation into a hematological neoplasm.

Marrow Aspiration. Blood cells develop from their precursor cells in the bone marrow. It is through aspirating and examining this marrow that the etiology of the illness can be determined. Most aspiration procedures use a large-bore needle that extracts cells from the hip bone as the source of bone marrow. Normal results of bone marrow aspiration, also known as bone marrow biopsy, would demonstrate an adequate amount of precursor cells with other cells in various stages of maturation. Changes in the cell types or increased presence of immature cells are often seen in hematological disorders.

Cytogenetic Testing. Tissue samples, cell biopsies, and blood cells can undergo chromosomal analysis by cytogenetic testing. Cytogenetic testing analyzes the cell's chromosome number and chromosome structure. Chromosomal disorders such as aneuploidy, gene deletions, duplications, translocations, insertions, or inversions can be identified. Cytogenetic analysis is used in determining specific diagnosis, prognosis, and appropriate therapy.

Fluorescence in Situ Hybridization. Fluorescence in situ hybridization (FISH) is used to analyze cells for chromosome defects. It can be performed on tissue, peripheral blood, or bone marrow, where it detects and localizes the presence or absence of specific DNA sequences on chromosomes. This diagnostic test can be used to identify a specific chromosome, show translocations and deletions, or identify extrachromosomal fragments of chromatin.

Polymerase Chain Reaction. The **polymerase chain reaction (PCR)** can amplify small sections of DNA for molecular and genetic analysis. The DNA section amplified by PCR can be used in many different laboratory procedures.

Flow Cytometry. Flow cytometry is a diagnostic technique for examining cells and analyzing DNA by suspending tissue in fluid and passing it through an electronic detection apparatus that uses laser light. It is used frequently in leukemia diagnosis, as it aids in staging and prognosis.

Immunophenotyping. **Immunophenotyping** is the analysis of cancer cells to identify specific surface antigens. This results in an immunological subtype classification of the cancer for diagnostic, prognostic, and therapeutic purposes. The possession of certain cell surface antigens often correlates with effectiveness of specific immunotherapeutic agents.

Lymph node biopsy. Lymph node biopsy is the microscopic examination of lymphoid tissue for cellular changes. Lymph node tissue can be extracted by needle aspiration or open surgical removal. This is commonly done in lymphoma or to assess for metastasis in other types of malignancies.

Lumbar puncture. Lumbar puncture allows extraction of a sample of cerebrospinal fluid (CSF). The CSF can contain evidence of metastatic cancer cells in the brain. The brain can be a sanctuary site for metastatic cancer cells as it is protected by the blood-brain barrier, which can inhibit the penetration of chemotherapy agents.

Treatment for Different Types of Hematological Cancer

The treatment regimens for hematological neoplasms are based on the type of disorder. The basic types of treatment commonly utilized include chemotherapy, monoclonal antibodies, radiation, stem cell transplants, and surgery. Cancer **immunotherapy** (also called CAR-T therapy) is a new treatment modality that uses the patient's own T cells to attack cancer cells.

Chemotherapy. Most chemotherapeutic agents target rapidly dividing cells, including cancer cells. However, chemotherapy causes ancillary effects on rapidly dividing healthy cells such as skin, gastric mucosa, and bone marrow. Hair loss, disruption of the gastric lining, and bone marrow suppression occur in chemotherapy. **Neutropenia** (also called leukopenia) is a major complication of chemotherapy with its associated risk of life-threatening infection. This threat can be reduced by the administration of a neutrophil stimulant such as filgrastim (Neupogen) to increase the production of neutrophils.

Monoclonal Antibodies. **Monoclonal antibodies** are highly specific antibodies that can each target a single antigen; in this case, specific types of cancer cells. In the laboratory, a tumor antigen is identified and introduced to myeloma cells, which are cells that continually synthesize antibodies. The myeloma cells are genetically reprogrammed so that they do not cause disease but act to continually synthesize antibodies specifically against an antigen on the tumor cells. As a result, monoclonal antibodies are a supply of genetically engineered antibodies that can hone in on the cancer cells and destroy them. Some monoclonal antibody agents are attached to chemotherapeutic agents. In these cases, the engineered monoclonal antibodies bring the chemotherapeutic agent directly to the tumor for precise targeted treatment.

Radiation. Radiation therapy is the use of high-dose x-rays to destroy cancer cells, particularly those cells that are not totally removed by surgery. Radiation therapy is often used to treat non-Hodgkin's lymphoma (NHL), Hodgkin's lymphoma (HL), and all types of leukemia. Radiation therapy may be used alone or in combination with chemotherapy. For lymphoma or leukemia, radiation therapy may be administered from a machine outside the body that directs radiation to the cancer (external radiation). Alternatively, it may be given as internal radiation through seeds, wires, or catheters that are implanted in the body. The method of radiation depends on the type and stage of cancer being treated.

Bone Marrow Stem Cell Transplants. Bone marrow stem cell transplantation has long been used as a treatment for hematological malignancies. Initially in this procedure, the patient's diseased bone marrow is completely or partially ablated. Ablation destroys the patient's diseased bone marrow using intense chemotherapy, radiation, or both. During ablation, the patient is severely immunosuppressed and highly susceptible to infection. After ablation is achieved, healthy bone marrow stem cells that were harvested from a donor whose tissue type matches the recipient are infused into the patient. These are called **allogeneic hematological stem cell transplants**. The donor's healthy bone marrow is obtained through a large-bore needle inserted into the donor's pelvis, and cells are then administered to the recipient. When successful, the donor's healthy bone marrow cells replace the recipient's cancerous bone marrow. However, bone marrow transplant rejection occurs frequently. Siblings are most often found to have matching types of tissue for bone marrow transplant.

An alternative procedure that is commonly used is **autologous hematological stem cell transplant**. This kind of transplant involves initial extraction of healthy hematopoietic stem cells from the patient and storage of the harvested cells in a freezer. The patient is then treated with high-dose chemotherapy with or without radiation to destroy the patient's malignant cell population at the cost of partial or complete bone marrow ablation. In partial bone marrow ablation, the patient is not completely immunosuppressed. After complete or partial bone marrow ablation, the patient's own stored healthy stem cells are returned to his or her body, where they replace destroyed tissue and resume the patient's normal blood cell production. Autologous transplants have the advantage of lower risk of infection during the immunocompromised portion of the treatment because the recovery of immune function is rapid. Also, the incidence of patients experiencing rejection is very rare because the donor and recipient are the same individual.

 CLINICAL CONCEPT

An allogeneic hematological stem cell transplant uses donor cells from another individual's bone marrow implanted in the patient. An autologous hematological stem cell transplant reimplants the patient's own healthy bone marrow cells into the patient.

Umbilical cord stem cells are also being used as stem cell transplants for hematological cancers with varying rates of success. Cord blood has a higher concentration of hematological stem cells than is normally found in adult blood. However, the small quantity of blood obtained from an umbilical cord (typically about 50 mL) makes it more suitable for transplantation into small children than into adults.

CAR-T Cell Cancer Immunotherapy

A recent advance in cancer immunotherapy, called **CAR-T cell therapy**, is showing promising results in treating patients with leukemia or lymphoma. Cancer immunotherapy uses the natural ability of the body's own T cells to attack and kill tumor cells. Some of the patient's T cells are harvested and genetically engineered to target cancer cell antigens. After exposure of the patient's T cells to the cancer cells in the laboratory, the T cells develop special receptors that allow them to recognize and attach to a specific antigen on the tumor cells. These specialized T cells are called chimeric antigen-receptor modified T cells (CAR-T cells). In 2017, two CAR-T cell therapies were approved by the Food and Drug Administration (FDA), one for the treatment of children with acute lymphoblastic leukemia (ALL) and the other for adults with advanced lymphomas.

Complications of Cancer Treatment

Serious complications of cancer treatment are always a possibility, regardless of the method used. Standard chemotherapy can cause immunosuppression, which can increase susceptibility to infection. Rapidly dividing cells of the skin, gastrointestinal lining, and bone marrow are affected by standard chemotherapy. This causes hair loss, anorexia, nausea, and vomiting. The patient can become anemic, which requires blood transfusion. The patient can also become thrombocytopenic, which may require platelet infusion. Leukopenia often occurs; therefore growth factors called filgrastim (Neupogen), pegfilgrastim (Neulasta), or sargramostim (Leukine) may be administered to boost WBC count. Patients who receive allogeneic stem cell bone marrow transplant can experience graft rejection, where the body rejects the transplant.

Tumor Lysis Syndrome. Another possible side effect of cancer chemotherapy is a serious complication called **tumor lysis syndrome**. It results from rapid destruction of a large number of tumor cells all at once. The lysed cells release their intracellular contents into the surrounding tissues and circulation, causing hyperuricemia (from purine breakdown), hyperkalemia, and hyperphosphatemia with secondary hypocalcemia. The uric acid crystals can cause damage to the glomeruli and nephron tubules, causing acute kidney injury.

 CLINICAL CONCEPT

Tumor lysis syndrome is most often seen 48 to 72 hours after initiation of cancer treatment and can cause acute kidney injury. Excessive tumor cell breakdown products overwhelm the nephrons.

Differentiation Syndrome. An important side effect of specific chemotherapy with retinoic acid is called **differentiation syndrome**. This occurs when the leukemia cells release certain chemicals into the blood. It is most often seen during the first couple of weeks of treatment and in patients with a high white blood cell count. Symptoms can include fever, dyspnea due to fluid buildup in the lungs and around the heart, low blood pressure, kidney damage, and severe fluid buildup elsewhere in the body. Although differentiation syndrome can be serious, it can often be treated by stopping the drugs temporarily and administering a steroid such as dexamethasone.

Cytokine Release Syndrome. T-cell **targeting therapies** such as the monoclonal antibody treatment and CAR-T have revolutionized the approach to patients with acute leukemia. However, the products of the cells involved in the immune mechanisms of these treatments can cause cytokine release syndrome (CRS). CRS is cancer treatment–related toxicity. The clinical signs of CRS include fever, hemodynamic instability, and capillary leak, which correlate with T-cell activation and elevated cytokine levels. Tocilizumab, an anti–IL-6 receptor antagonist, provides control of severe CRS induced by CAR-T cells without being directly T-cell toxic. Corticosteroids are also used in CRS.

Pathophysiology of Selected White Blood Cell Disorders

Leukemia

Leukemia is a cancer of developing WBCs within the bone marrow. The cancerous WBCs are arrested at an early stage of development, proliferate uncontrollably, and do not function. As discussed previously, the two basic categories of cells within the bone marrow are myeloid and lymphoid cells. Leukemias that affect the myeloid lineage are called myelocytic leukemias. Leukemias that affect the lymphoid lineage are called lymphoblastic or lymphogenous leukemias. There are four classifications of leukemia: acute lymphoblastic leukemia (ALL), chronic lymphocytic leukemia (CLL), acute myelogenous leukemia (AML), and chronic myelogenous leukemia (CML).

> ### CLINICAL CONCEPT
>
> Myelocytic leukemias are also called myelogenous, myeloblastic, or nonlymphocytic leukemias, whereas lymphocytic leukemias are also called lymphoblastic or lymphogenous leukemias.

Acute Lymphoblastic Leukemia

ALL is an aggressive cancer that is more common in children than adults. It is the most frequent neoplastic disease in children with an early peak at the age of 3 to 4 years. ALL accounts for 75% of all pediatric leukemia cases, with most affected children younger than age 5. There is a bimodal epidemiological distribution with highest incidence in young children, lowest incidence in young adults, then increased incidence in older adults. The risk of ALL declines until age 20 then increases in adults older than age 50.

Etiology. It is believed that leukemias originate from a complex interaction between environmental and genetic factors, which in combination lead to cellular modifications. Many chromosomal and genetic alterations are associated with ALL. Aneuploidy, an abnormal number of chromosomes, is found in the ALL cancer cells in many patients. There are genetic translocations on some chromosomes, including the Ph chromosome. The Ph chromosome is a rearrangement of genes at chromosome numbers 9 and 22, referred to as the BCR-ABL translocation or t;(9:22) (see Fig 12-4). This form of ALL is referred to as Ph+ ALL. There is also a form of ALL referred to as Ph-like ALL because it has genetic alterations similar to Ph+ ALL.

Risk Factors There is no known cause of ALL, but previous chemotherapy or radiation therapy for other diseases increases the risk. In children, prenatal exposure to high doses of radiation is thought to be a common risk factor. Adult risk factors include being male, white, older than 70 years, and having radiation exposure. Other predisposing factors include exposure to pesticides and genetic disorders such as Down syndrome, Klinefelter's syndrome, neurofibromatosis, ataxia-telangiectasia, Fanconi's anemia, or Bloom's syndrome. Some viruses, such as EBV and the human

T cell lymphotropic virus 1 (HTLV-1), are also risk factors for ALL. There is evidence that advanced parental age is associated with increased childhood ALL risk, and this association is most marked among children aged 1 to 5 years.

Pathophysiology. In ALL, the stem cell precursors for T or B lymphocytes in the bone marrow do not function and do not mature beyond the lymphoblast stage (also referred to as the blast stage). As the lymphoblasts become more numerous, there is less room for healthy WBCs, RBCs, and platelets within the bone marrow. The lack of healthy WBCs leads to neutropenia, which increases risk of infection. A low RBC count leads to anemia, and a low platelet count leads to thrombocytopenia. Lymph nodes also contain large numbers of lymphoblast cells, which can enlarge the lymph nodes and crowd out healthy lymphocytes.

The central nervous system (CNS), kidneys, and testicles can be infiltrated with lymphoblast cells. The brain's meningeal layers can be involved in as much as 85% of patients, especially with T-cell ALL.

Clinical Presentation. It is important to gather a complete history and perform a comprehensive physical examination on the patient with signs of ALL. However, the patient's initial history may not prompt quick recognition of ALL because symptoms can be vague and mistakenly attributed to other disorders. Frequently, the patient presents with a nonspecific array of symptoms that is erroneously attributed to a viral syndrome. The medical, surgical, and family history are frequently unremarkable. The psychosocial history may include occupational exposure to toxins such as benzene or radiation, which increases risk. Past use of chemotherapy agents for cancer and lifestyle factors such as smoking can also increase risk of ALL.

Signs and Symptoms. Clinical signs and symptoms of ALL are related to the extent of replacement of the bone marrow with cancerous lymphoblast cells. Because cancerous lymphoblasts do not function and crowd out healthy WBCs in the bone marrow, patients may present with frequent infection, ranging from infected tonsils, canker sores, and diarrhea to life-threatening pneumonia or opportunistic infections.

Also because of cancerous lymphoblasts crowding out healthy RBCs in the bone marrow, the patient may present with anemia, which causes fatigue, weakness, dizziness, dyspnea, and pallor. Some patients experience other vague symptoms, such as fevers, chills, night sweats, and other flu-like symptoms. Additionally, cancerous lymphoblast cells proliferate within lymph nodes and the spleen and liver, increasing the size of these organs. An enlarged lymph node or spleen is often the initial sign of ALL. Some patients experience nausea or a feeling of fullness caused by an enlarged liver and spleen that places pressure on the stomach; this can result in unintentional weight loss.

Cancerous lymphoblast cell proliferation within the marrow stretches the interior of bones and leads to persistent bone pain, which is most pronounced at the sternum, tibia, and femur. Because of the crowding out of healthy platelets by cancerous lymphoblasts, patients will have unexplained bruising, gingival bleeding, epistaxis (nosebleeds), and extremely heavy bleeding with menstrual periods. If the cancerous lymphoblast cells invade the CNS, neurological symptoms such as headaches can occur.

Diagnosis. Diagnosing ALL based on history and physical assessment alone is difficult. The first diagnostic sign of ALL is an unusually high WBC count, which may be seen on a CBC with differential. A bone marrow biopsy demonstrates hypercellularity with predominantly lymphoblasts. Normally healthy bone marrow has only about 5% lymphocytes. A bone marrow lymphoblast count of over 20% of total WBC is sufficient for a diagnosis of ALL.

A lumbar puncture to examine the cerebrospinal fluid (CSF) for leukemic blast cells is necessary. Immunophenotype testing identifies specific antigens expressed on the surface of the leukemic cells. The type of cell surface antigens has therapeutic implications. Cytogenetic and molecular analyses are important to specify the subtype of ALL; this has prognostic and therapeutic implications.

Treatment. The aims of ALL treatment regimens are rapid restoration of bone marrow function, adequate prophylactic treatment of sanctuary sites (sites that may have concealed cancerous lymphoblast cells such as the CNS), and maintenance therapy to eliminate minimal or undetectable disease. The overall goal is to put the patient into remission, which is a period of undetectable or no disease. The faster the response to treatment, the better the prognosis for ALL. Bone marrow transplantation from a tissue-matched sibling or donor and chemotherapy are commonly used treatments in children and young adults. Older adults are mainly treated with chemotherapy agents. Chemotherapy for ALL is a multidrug regimen that consists of several phases: prephase therapy, induction therapy, consolidation cycles, and maintenance treatment. Various different chemotherapeutic drugs and targeted therapies are used. Prephase therapy decreases tumor cell volume, treats any existing infection, and reconstitutes platelet or erythrocyte deficiencies. The goal of induction therapy is to achieve complete remission. Consolidation cycles aim to eliminate sanctuary sites. Maintenance treatment is the final phase, which often includes targeted therapy. Targeted therapy with tyrosine kinase inhibitors (TKIs) (e.g., imatinib, dasatinib, nilotinib, ponatinib) is commonly part of the regimen. TKIs effectively inhibit the enzyme that allows for the excessive proliferation of ALL cells. Immunotherapeutic approaches using laboratory synthesized monoclonal antibodies may also be used. Monoclonal antibodies target specific ALL cell surface antigens (e.g., rituximab, inotuzumab, blinatumomab).

CAR-T cell therapy is a new immunotherapy approach to the treatment of ALL. A small number of the patient's own T cells are removed and genetically reprogrammed to attack the ALL cells. These reprogrammed T cells are then intravenously administered back to the patient, where they target and destroy the ALL cells.

The effectiveness of ALL treatment is related to the age of the patient, with cure rates of approximately 90% in children. Age-adapted treatment regimens that match the ALL subtype with targeted therapy are allowing high rates of complete, durable remission in adults as well.

Chronic Lymphocytic Leukemia

Chronic lymphocytic leukemia (CLL) is the most common type of leukemia in the United States and other Western countries. CLL is a B-cell lymphocyte malignancy, with more than 17,000 people diagnosed yearly in the United States. The disease is found in older adults, with a median age at diagnosis of 70 years. The male-to-female ratio is 2:1. One of the primary risk factors appears to be family history of CLL or any B-cell malignancy. As the population ages, the incidence of CLL is expected to rise.

Risk Factors. Male gender, advanced age, Caucasian race, and family history of hematological cancer are risk factors for CLL. There is an inherited genetic predisposition, with a six-fold to nine-fold increased risk for family members of patients with CLL. Exposure to certain herbicides and insecticides, including Agent Orange used during the Vietnam War, has also been linked to an increased risk of CLL. Reduced recreational sun exposure, medical history of atopic health conditions, and exposure to hepatitis C virus are also risk factors.

Etiology. Genetic changes are the fundamental cause of CLL. Exposure to any agent that can disrupt DNA is an etiological agent. The disease is initiated by the loss or addition of large amounts of chromosomal material (e.g., deletion 13q, deletion 11q, trisomy 12), followed by additional mutations that may render the leukemia more aggressive. Over 80% of patients with CLL have some type of chromosomal abnormality, with trisomy 12 being the most common. Other common abnormalities include genetic deletions at 13q4, 17p13, and 11q22-23. Studies also demonstrate alterations in genes that code for antiapoptotic proteins. Antiapoptotic proteins allow unrelenting proliferation of cancerous B cells. There are also genetic mutations in the *NOTCH1, SF3B1, MYD88, ATM,* and *TP53* genes. These genetic mutations allow cancerous B cells to resist many chemotherapy and targeted therapy agents.

Pathophysiology. Chronic lymphocytic leukemia is characterized by the proliferation of mature, functionally incompetent CD5-positive B cells within the blood, bone marrow, lymph nodes, and spleen. They are referred to as B-CLL lymphocytes. B-CLL lymphocytes contain genes that code for the BCL2 protein that allows constant proliferation of B-CLL precursor cells in the bone marrow. In the peripheral blood, these cells resemble mature B cells, but they synthesize and release low levels of immunoglobulin (Ig), mutated Igs, or no Ig at all. CLL is classified into two subgroups based on the presence of mutations within the variable regions of the immunoglobulin heavy chain gene (IGHV). Patients with CLL with mutated IGHV (IGHV-M CLL) have a more favorable prognosis than those with unmutated IGHV (IGHV-UM CLL).

CLL causes inadequate humoral immunity and accumulation of B-CLL cells results in crowding of the bone marrow and consequent decreased development of healthy RBCs, WBCs, and platelets. Therefore, the lack of RBCs causes anemia, lack of WBCs cause neutropenia, and lack of platelets causes thrombocytopenia. Anemia causes weakness and fatigue. Neutropenia causes increased risk of infections, and thrombocytopenia causes spontaneous bleeding and bruising. The proliferation of B-CLL cells also occurs in the lymph nodes and spleen, causing lymphadenopathy (enlarged lymph nodes) and splenomegaly (enlarged spleen).

Clinical Presentation. Early in the disorder, patients commonly have an unremarkable history that does not include any diagnostic clues for CLL. Twenty-five to fifty percent of patients will be asymptomatic at the time of presentation. Onset is often subtle, and CLL is often discovered incidentally after a blood cell count is performed for another reason.

Later in the disease, patients may present with complaints of enlarged, painless lymph nodes; fatigue; fever; and pain in the upper-left portion of the abdomen, which may be caused by an enlarged spleen. Night sweats, weight loss, and frequent infections are common. Patients may report a family history of hematological cancer. Occupational history is important, because CLL is associated with exposure to certain herbicides and insecticides, particularly Agent Orange, which was used by the military in the past.

Signs and Symptoms. Most people do not have symptoms early in CLL, but a routine blood test returns a high WBC count, and further investigation reveals the disorder. As the disease advances, the patient suffers lymphadenopathy, splenomegaly, hepatomegaly, and, eventually, anemia and infections. The patient typically suffers from symptoms similar to those of other hematological neoplasms.

Diagnosis. CLL is usually first detected by the presence of a lymphocytosis on a CBC with differential test. This abnormality is frequently an incidental finding during a routine medical visit. The hallmark of CLL is lymphocytosis with a total WBC count of greater than 20,000/mcL. The diagnosis of CLL requires the presence of specifically greater than 5,000 B-lymphocytes/μL in the peripheral blood for the duration of at least 3 months. The presence of lymphocytosis in an older adult should raise strong suspicion for CLL, and a confirmatory diagnostic test, in particular, flow cytometry, should be performed.

The humoral immune system in CLL is dysregulated with very few normal B lymphocytes (B cells) and lack of functioning immunoglobulins (hypogamma globulinemia). The bone marrow is hypercellular with normal blood cells crowded out by the abnormal B cells. Immunophenotyping is done to identify specific surface antigens on the B-CLL cell. B-CLL cells commonly coexpress the CD5 antigen, as well as CD19, CD20, CD22, CD23, and CD52 antigens. These CD antigens have prognostic and therapeutic implications. Lumbar puncture and computed tomography (CT) scan are done to check for spread of disease to organs. Genetic and chromosomal testing reveals deletions in parts of chromosomes 13, 11, or 17. Other, less common chromosome changes include an extra copy of chromosome 12 (trisomy 12) or a translocation (genes change places) between chromosomes 11 and 14 [written as t (11;14)].

Staging of CLL. There are two widely accepted clinical staging systems: the Rai and Binet systems. CLL is staged according to both these systems (see Box 12-4). The system designates severity of disease according to the extent of lymphocytosis and characteristics of the cancerous lymphocytes.

Treatment. Treatment of CLL varies with the clinical stage and the presence or absence of symptoms. Asymptomatic patients with early stage disease (e.g., Rai 0, Binet A) should be monitored without therapy unless they have evidence of rapid disease progression. When patients progress or present with progressive or symptomatic/active disease, treatment should be initiated. With the ability to identify cell mutations using flow cytometry, PCR, FISH, and immunophenotyping, treatment is commonly specific to the B-CLL cell mutation. Leukapheresis, a procedure that extracts and removes excess WBCs, may be needed initially if there is an extremely high number of B-CLL cells. This process can decrease the B-CLL numbers.

Chemotherapy can be curative or palliative. Early chemotherapy is considered for all patients with high-risk biological or genetic markers predicting a poor long-term prognosis. Combinations of different agents is a common treatment strategy. The major types of drugs most commonly used to treat CLL include: __

- **Purine analogs:** fludarabine (Fludara), pentostatin (Nipent), and cladribine (2-CdA, Leustatin). Fludarabine is often one of the first drugs used against CLL. (It is administered with cyclophosphamide and rituximab. This combination is called FCR.)

BOX 12-4. Rai and Binet Staging of Chronic Lymphocytic Leukemia

RAI STAGING SYSTEM

Rai stage 0: High lymphocyte count but no enlargement of the lymph nodes, spleen, or liver. The red blood cell and platelet counts are near normal.

Rai stage I: High lymphocyte count with enlarged lymph nodes. The spleen and liver are not enlarged. The red blood cell and platelet counts are near normal.

Rai stage II: High lymphocyte count with enlarged spleen and an enlarged liver may be involved. The lymph nodes may or may not be enlarged. The red blood cell and platelet counts are near normal.

Rai stage III: High lymphocyte count and the lymph nodes, spleen, or liver may or may not be enlarged. The red blood cell count is low, which indicates anemia. The platelet count is near normal.

Rai stage IV: High lymphocyte count and enlarged lymph nodes, spleen, or liver. The red blood cell counts may be low or near normal. The platelet count is low, which indicates thrombocytopenia.

The Rai stages also classify CLL as low-, intermediate-, or high-risk groups, which are factors in the determination of treatment options.
- Stage 0 is low risk.
- Stages I and II are intermediate risk.
- Stages III and IV are high risk.

BINET STAGING SYSTEM

Binet stage A: Fewer than three areas of lymphoid tissue are enlarged, with no anemia or thrombocytopenia.

Binet stage B: Three or more areas of lymphoid tissue are enlarged, with no anemia or thrombocytopenia.

Binet stage C: Anemia and/or thrombocytopenia are present. Any number of lymphoid tissue areas may be enlarged.

From American Cancer Society (2018). How is chronic lymphocytic leukemia staged? https://www.cancer.org/cancer/chronic-lymphocytic-leukemia/detection-diagnosis-staging/staging.html

- **Alkylating agents:** chlorambucil (Leukeran), bendamustine (Treanda), and cyclophosphamide (Cytoxan). They are often given along with a monoclonal antibody.
- **Corticosteroids** such as prednisone, methylprednisolone, and dexamethasone.
- **Monoclonal antibody agents** target the CD20 protein found on the surface of B lymphocytes. These drugs include:
  - Rituximab (Rituxan)
  - Obinutuzumab (Gazyva)
  - Ofatumumab (Arzerra)

Alemtuzumab (Campath) is a monoclonal antibody that targets the CD52 antigen, which is found on the surface of CLL cells and many T lymphocytes. It is used mainly if CLL is no longer responding to standard treatments.

Another monoclonal antibody that targets the CD22 protein found on B lymphocytes is moxetumomab pasudotox (Lumoxiti). This drug is known as an antibody–drug conjugate. The monoclonal antibody acts like a homing device that targets the cells, and a toxin is attached that kills the cancer cells.

TKIs are revolutionizing therapy of B-cell lymphoid malignancies. Tyrosine kinases are enzymes produced by the cancer cell that allow continuous, unrelenting B cell proliferation. In CLL, these include Bruton tyrosine kinase (BTK), spleen tyrosine kinase (Syk), ZAP70, Src family kinases, and PI3K. Blocking the action of these enzymes inhibits the growth of the B-CLL cells. The TKIs that are proving to be effective in treatment of CLL include idelalisib (Zydelig) and ibrutinib (Imbruvica).

BCL-2 inhibitors are agents that block BCL-2 proteins that are secreted by B-CLL cancer cells. These proteins, encoded by the BCL-2 gene in the B-CLL cells, allow cancer cells to evade apoptosis, which in turn leads to their unrelenting proliferation. Venetoclax (Venclexta), a BCL-2 inhibitor that blocks the function of the BCL-2 protein, is a new therapeutic option proving effective in stopping growth of B-CLL cells.

Allogeneic bone marrow stem cell transplantation is considered for relapsing patients or patients who are refractory to other inhibitor therapy.

Complications of CLL. One of the most serious complications of CLL is a change (transformation) of the leukemia to a high-grade or aggressive type of non-Hodgkin's lymphoma (NHL) called diffuse large B-cell lymphoma (DLBCL) or to Hodgkin's lymphoma (HL). This happens in 2% to 10% of CLL cases, and is known as **Richter's transformation**. Treatment is often the same as it would be for lymphoma and might include stem cell transplant because these cases are often hard to treat.

Less often, CLL may progress to prolymphocytic leukemia. As with Richter's syndrome, this, too, can be hard to treat. Some studies have suggested that certain drugs such as cladribine (2-CdA) and alemtuzumab may be helpful.

Acute Myelogenous Leukemia

Acute myelogenous leukemia (AML), also called acute myeloid leukemia, is caused by the proliferation of undifferentiated WBCs (excluding lymphocytes) in the myeloblast stage within the bone marrow. The bone marrow will have more than 20% myeloblasts (referred to as blast cells), which is abnormally high. With the proliferation of blasts, the production of healthy blood cells by the bone marrow is reduced. As with other hematological neoplasms, the consequences include anemia from lack of RBCs, bleeding disorders from lack of platelets, and infections from neutropenia. Mutations that turn on oncogenes or turn off tumor suppressor genes within the myeloblast cells cause overproliferation of cancer cells. For instance, oncogenes such as *FLT3, c-KIT,* and *RAS* are common in AML cells. Also, tumor suppressor genes such as *RUNX1* and *RARa* are turned off in AML.

The proliferation of the blasts continues, with infiltration beyond the bone marrow to the blood, tissues, spleen, and liver. AML can also invade the skin, with the myeloid blasts causing a diffuse rash or raised nodules. If the blasts invade the lungs, symptoms are similar to those of pneumonia.

Etiology and Risk Factors. Previous chemotherapy and radiation therapy for a variety of cancers, including breast cancer and HL, have been a cause of AML. The increased incidence of AML following the 1986 Chernobyl nuclear disaster in Russia was directly proportional to the radiation exposure. Other risk factors include male gender, smoking, childhood ALL or myelodysplastic syndrome (MDS), and benzene exposure. Also, some genetic diseases can increase susceptibility to AML: Down syndrome, trisomy 8, Fanconi's anemia, Bloom's syndrome, ataxia-telangiectasia, Diamond-Blackfan anemia, Schwachman-Diamond syndrome, Li-Fraumeni syndrome, neurofibromatosis type 1, and severe congenital neutropenia (also called Kostmann's syndrome). Other factors that have been studied for a possible link to AML include exposure to electromagnetic fields (such as living near power lines); workplace exposure to diesel, gasoline, and certain other chemicals and solvents; and exposure to herbicides or pesticides.

Signs and Symptoms. Due to neutropenia, the patient may experience symptoms of infection that include fever, chills, and night sweats. Extreme fatigue, weakness, and dizziness are common due to anemia.

Easy bruising, nosebleeds, and gingival bleeding can occur due to thrombocytopenia. Swollen lymph nodes and enlarged spleen or liver can occur. Because the enlarged liver and spleen put pressure on the stomach, appetite is poor, weight loss may occur, and the patient may have abdominal pain. The patient's immune system sometimes synthesizes antibodies against the patient's own body cells, which is called autoimmunity. Autoimmune hemolytic anemia can occur due to antibodies made against the patient's RBCs.

Diagnostic Testing. Diagnostic testing includes CBC with differential, bone marrow biopsy, FISH, and PCR to look for genetic and chromosomal abnormalities. Genetic translocation between chromosome 8 and 12, referred to as t(8;21), is common. Also a translocation between chromosomes 15 and 17, referred to as t(15;17), is seen. A chromosomal inversion at chromosome 16, referred to as inv(16), can be found. A deletion of part of chromosome 7—written as del (7)—is common. Also, aneuploidy, a duplication of chromosome 8, is found. Some common oncogenes found in AML include the *FLT3, IDH1,* and *IDH2* genes; *c-Kit;* and *RAS.* These oncogenes cause the AML cells to proliferate uncontrollably. Some AML cells are found to have a biomarker called the CD33 protein.

Treatment. As with other hematological neoplasms, standard chemotherapy, targeted chemotherapy, radiation, and bone marrow stem cell transplant are the main treatment modalities. Treatment for most patients with AML is divided into two standard chemotherapy phases:

- Remission induction
- Consolidation (also called postremission therapy)
- Some patients who have extremely high numbers of cancerous WBCs require **leukapheresis**, which reduces the number of WBCs. This may be needed before remission induction chemotherapy.
- In patients younger than age 60, the induction treatment begins with cytarabine (ara-C) and is followed by an anthracycline drug such as daunorubicin (daunomycin) or idarubicin. This is sometimes called a 7 + 3 regimen, because it consists of cytarabine continuously for 7 days, along with short infusions of an anthracycline on each of the first 3 days. Induction is considered successful if remission is achieved.
- In the consolidation phase, several cycles of chemotherapy with high-dose cytarabine (ara-C) (sometimes known as HiDAC) is administered. Then either an allogeneic (donor) or autologous stem cell transplant is administered.

In some patients with AML, targeted therapy with TKIs or monoclonal antibodies is added to the chemotherapy regimen. Targeted TKI therapy includes midostaurin (Rydapt), which blocks the FLT3 protein that is produced in AML cells with the *FLT3* gene. Targeted

TKI therapy also includes the *IDH* inhibitors ivosidenib (Tibsovo) and enasidenib (Idhifa), which block IDH proteins produced by AML cells containing the *IDH* gene. Gemtuzumab (Mylotarg) is a monoclonal antibody that is attached to a chemotherapeutic agent that targets cancer cells with the CD33 protein, a common biomarker on AML cells.

Venetoclax is an oral highly selective inhibitor of the antiapoptotic protein BCL-2. BCL-2 is thought to cause resistance to standard therapy in some patients with AML. Venetoclax (Venclexta) is often administered with decitabine (Dacogen) and azacitadine (Vidaza) in resistant cases.

Chronic Myelogenous Leukemia

Chronic myelogenous leukemia (CML), also called chronic myeloid leukemia, is a disorder characterized by an overproduction of mature myeloid cells in the bone marrow. The myeloid cells look mature but they do not function. Most affected persons are age 65 or over. CML accounts for about 15% to 20% of leukemia in adults, with slightly more males than females diagnosed.

Etiology and Risk Factors. Like other leukemias, exposure to ionizing radiation is a known risk. Ninety-five percent of adults with CML have the Ph chromosome, which is a BCR-ABL oncogene mutation in a single pluripotent hematopoietic stem cell. There is a translocation of genes on chromosomes 9 and 22 [referred to as (t:9:22)] (see Fig 12-4). This genetic change in myeloid cancer cells triggers production of tyrosine kinase. Tyrosine kinase is an enzyme that causes inhibition of cellular apoptosis. Tyrosine kinase allows for the unrelenting proliferation of cancer cells.

Clinical Phases of CML. The clinical course is divided into three phases:

1. Chronic phase. Patients have less than 10% immature neutrophils (referred to as blasts) in the bloodstream and bone marrow. Symptoms are usually mild at this time. Patients are often diagnosed in this phase and respond to treatment.
2. Accelerated phase. Patients have less than 30% immature neutrophils (blasts) in the bloodstream and bone marrow, very low platelet counts, and the Ph chromosome is apparent on genetic testing. Moderate symptoms such as fever, loss of appetite, and weight loss occur. Patients are less responsive to treatment.
3. Blast crisis phase. Large clusters of blast cells are present in bone marrow, and the bloodstream has a high percentage of blasts. Blast cells have spread to organs such as the spleen and liver. Patients have severe symptoms due to a decreased number of healthy WBCs, RBCs, and platelets in the bone marrow.

Signs and Symptoms. Signs and symptoms occur due to anemia, leukopenia, and thrombocytopenia. Extreme fatigue and weakness occur due to anemia. Leukopenia causes increased susceptibility to infection with fever, chills, and night sweats. Thrombocytopenia causes bleeding and bruising. Bone pain occurs due to widespread proliferation of myeloid cells within the bone marrow that stretches the interior of bones. Other symptoms include abdominal fullness from hepatomegaly and splenomegaly, which put pressure on the stomach. WBC count can rise to more than 100,000 cells. As the WBC count increases, patients may have respiratory distress because of accumulation of blasts in the lungs.

Factors that commonly indicate a poor prognosis include splenomegaly, older age, genetic mutations in addition to the Ph chromosome, basophilia, and eosinophilia (see Box 12-5).

Diagnostic Testing. Diagnostic tests for CML are similar to those used for other types of leukemia: CBC with differential, bone marrow biopsy, FISH, PCR, magnetic resonance imaging (MRI), and CT scan. The FISH and PCR tests find the Ph chromosome translocation.

Treatment. TKIs are standard treatment in CML. Due to the Ph chromosome, the CML cells secrete the enzyme tyrosine kinase. This enzyme allows for unrestrained proliferation of the CML cells. TKIs such as ponatinib (Inclusig) inhibit the enzyme and can induce

---

BOX 12-5. Prognostic Factors in Chronic Myelogenous Leukemia

Poor CML prognosis occurs with:
- Accelerated phase, also called the "blast" phase
- Enlarged spleen
- Regions of bone damage from growth of leukemia
- Increased number of basophils and eosinophils in blood
- Very high or very low platelet counts
- Age 60 years or older
- Multiple chromosome changes in the CML cells

These factors are used in the Sokal system, which calculates a score used to help predict prognosis. This system considers the person's age, the percentage of blasts in the blood, the size of the spleen, and the number of platelets. These factors are used to categorize patients into low-, intermediate-, or high-risk groups. Another system, called the Euro score, includes the other factors, as well as the percentage of blood basophils and eosinophils. Having more of these cells indicates a poorer outlook.

From American Cancer Society (2018). Phases of chronic myeloid leukemia. https://www.cancer.org/cancer/chronic-myeloid-leukemia/detection-diagnosis-staging/staging.html

a complete remission in over 90% of treated patients. There are different kinds of responses to the TKI agents (see Box 12-6). Surgery to remove the spleen may be necessary if splenomegaly is present. Allogeneic bone marrow transplantation is also indicated for some patients with CML.

Lymphomas

Lymphoma is the most common type of blood cancer in the United States. Lymphoma falls into one of two major categories:

1. Hodgkin's lymphoma (HL), previously called Hodgkin's disease
2. Non-Hodgkin's lymphoma (NHL)

NHL accounts for 83% of lymphoma cases, with HL accounting for the other 17%. In the United States, about 77,000 new cases of NHL and 8,500 new cases of HL occur per year. Lymphoma can occur at any age, including childhood. HL is most common in two age groups: adults 15 to 20 years of age and people 50 years of age and older. NHL is more likely to occur in older people.

NHL and HL may be associated with the same symptoms and often have similar appearance on physical examination. However, they are readily distinguishable via microscopic examination. HL develops from a specific abnormal B lymphocyte line, whereas NHL may derive from either abnormal B or T cells. Both are distinguished by unique genetic markers.

There are five subtypes of HL and about 30 subtypes of NHL. The different subtypes and the classification are based on microscopic appearance, as well as genetic and molecular markers. Many of the NHL subtypes look similar, but they are functionally different and respond to different therapies. HL subtypes are microscopically distinct, and typing is based upon the microscopic differences as well as extent of disease. The risk factors, signs, and symptoms are similar for all lymphomas (see Box 12-7 and Box 12-8).

Staging of Lymphoma

Lymphomas are evaluated and classified according to size, spread, microscopic appearance, and genetic and molecular markers and then assigned a stage. The Lugano Staging System is based on the Ann Arbor Staging System that was used in the past. Staging is used to classify lymphomas and assist in determining prognosis and treatment (see Box 12-9).

BOX 12-6. Responses of Chronic Myeloid Leukemia to Medications: Tyrosine Kinase Inhibitors

HEMATOLOGICAL RESPONSE
The hematological response is based on the number of CML cells found in the bloodstream.

Complete hematological response (also called CHR): all blood cell counts have returned to normal, there are no CML cells seen in the bloodstream, and the spleen is normal in size. There are no symptoms of CML.
Partial hematological response: all blood counts have improved, but there are still signs or symptoms of CML. The CML cells are less than half the number of cells that were found before treatment with the TKI. The spleen has noticeably shrunk but is still enlarged.

CYTOGENETIC RESPONSE
This test is done on a bone marrow biopsy to look for mutated chromosomes within the cells.

A complete cytogenetic response (CCyR): there are no cells with the Philadelphia chromosome found in the bone marrow.
A partial cytogenetic response (PCyR): 1% to 34% of the cells in the bone marrow still have the Philadelphia chromosome.
A major cytogenetic response (MCyR): less than 35% of the cells in the bone marrow have the Philadelphia chromosome.

A minor cytogenetic response: more than 35% of the cells in the bone marrow still have the Philadelphia chromosome.

MOLECULAR RESPONSE
The molecular response uses the PCR test, which evaluates the DNA found in the cells of the blood or bone marrow. It is based on the number of CML cells found in the bloodstream.

A complete molecular response (CMR): PCR test does not find the BCR-ABL gene in any of the cells within the bloodstream.
A major molecular response (MMR): PCR test finds the amount of BCR-ABL gene in the cells within the bloodstream is decreased to 1/1000th (or less) of what it was before treatment for CML.
An early molecular response (EMR): PCR test finds that there is 10% or less BCR-ABL gene within the cells in the bloodstream after 3 months and 6 months of treatment.

The terms *long-term deep molecular response* and *durable complete molecular response* indicate a long-lasting complete molecular response and is the goal of CML treatment.

From American Cancer Society (2018). How do you know if treatment for chronic myeloid leukemia is working? https://www.cancer.org/cancer/chronic-myeloid-leukemia/treating/is-treatment-working.html

BOX 12-7. Risk Factors for Lymphomas

Age older than 60 years
Male
Caucasian
Autoimmune disorders
Infections:
- HIV
- EBV
- *H. pylori*
- *Chlamydia psittaci*
- *Campylobacter jejuni*
- Human herpesvirus 8 (HHV-8)
- Human T-cell lymphotropic virus (HTLV-1)
- Hepatitis C

Radiation exposure
Immunosuppressive therapy
Occupational exposure to toxic chemicals, such as pesticides, herbicides, benzene, and other solvents
Family history of lymphoma

BOX 12-8. Signs and Symptoms of Lymphoma

The first sign of lymphoma is often a painless, enlarged lymph node in the neck, under an arm, or in the groin. The enlarged lymph node sometimes causes other symptoms by pressing against a vein or lymphatic vessel (swelling of an arm or leg), nerve (pain, numbness, or tingling), or the stomach (early feeling of fullness). Other signs and symptoms of lymphoma include:
- Splenomegaly
- Hepatomegaly
- Abdominal pain or discomfort, nausea, and vomiting caused by splenomegaly and hepatomegaly
- Fevers
- Chills
- Unexplained weight loss
- Headache, seizure, vision impairment, facial numbness, weakness of part of body, behavior changes caused by pressure on brain from lymphoma
- Superior vena cava syndrome: lymphoma can exert pressure on SVC, leading to swelling of upper chest, head, and arms
- Frequent infections
- Chest pain or pressure
- Shortness of breath due to pressure on trachea from lymphoma
- Easy bruising or bleeding
- Night sweats
- Lack of energy
- Rash and itching, most commonly in the lower extremity, but can occur anywhere, be local, or spread over the whole body

BOX 12-9. Lugano Staging System Based on Ann Arbor Staging for Lymphoma*

STAGE I (EARLY DISEASE)
- The lymphoma is limited to one lymph node (stage I) or a single extranodal site (stage IE).

STAGE II (LOCALLY ADVANCED DISEASE)
- The lymphoma is located within two or more groups of lymph nodes on the same side of (above or below) the diaphragm (called stage II).
- The lymphoma is in a group of lymph node(s) and in a region of a nearby organ on the same side as the diaphragm (called stage IIE).

STAGE III (ADVANCED DISEASE)
- The lymphoma is in lymph node regions that are located on both sides of (above and below) the diaphragm which may include the spleen (stage IIIS) or limited, contiguous, extralymphatic organ or tissue (IIIE) or both (IIIES).

STAGE IV (WIDESPREAD OR DISSEMINATED)
- The lymphoma is spread throughout multiple organs within the body such as lungs, liver, and bone marrow.

*All stages are further subdivided according to the absence (A) or presence (B) of systemic symptoms including fevers, night sweats, and/or weight loss (>10% of loss of body weight over 6 months before diagnosis).
From American Cancer Society. (2022). Non-Hodgkin lymphoma stages. https://www.cancer.org/cancer/nonhodgkin-lymphoma/detection-diagnosis-staging/staging.html

Non-Hodgkin's Lymphoma

NHLs can be caused by cancerous T cells, B cells, or NK cells and are classified according to cell type and aggressiveness. Most types of NHL are of B cell origin. They usually develop among middle-aged and older adults and are 50% more frequent in men than in women. The incidence of NHL rises steadily with age. The incidence of NHL has almost doubled over the past 20 to 40 years. Persons with immune dysregulation are most susceptible to NHL.

Etiology. Chromosomal translocations are the genetic hallmark of lymphomas. A common translocation in NHL is the translocation of genes at 14q32 and 18q21, termed t(8:14), present in 85% of follicular lymphomas. However, there are numerous other common gene translocations associated with development of NHL [e.g., t(14:18), t(11:14), t(2:5), and t(11:18)]. Why the translocations occur is unknown, although there is evidence that oncogenic pathogens may be involved. Some pathogens that have been associated with the development of NHL include HIV, EBV, *H. pylori*, human T cell leukemia virus-1 (HTLV-1), hepatitis C, and human herpesvirus-8.

The viral pathogens introduce their genes into affected lymphocytes, causing mutations in the genome of the affected cells. The mutations involve either stimulation of oncogenes or inhibition of tumor suppressor genes, either of which causes uncontrolled proliferation of the affected lymphocytes. HIV specifically causes lymphoma of the brain, which causes focal neurological signs and mental status changes. It is a late complication of HIV infection. Hepatitis C increases the risk of B-cell NHL by 30%. Chronic infection with *H. pylori* in the stomach is associated with gastric mucosa-associated lymphocytic tumor (MALT).

Risk Factors. The risk factors for NHL are similar to those for all lymphomas (see Box 12-7).

Pathophysiology. NHLs consist of over 20 different lymphomas, each of which has a distinct microscopic appearance. About 85% of NHLs form in lymph tissue from mutated B cells, 15% develop from T-cell mutations, and fewer than 1% arise from NK cells. Lymphomas are also grouped by certain properties, such as size, shape, and appearance of cells within a lymph node. The appearance within a lymph node is described as follicular (round clusters of abnormal cells) or diffuse (abnormal cells spread throughout the node). The most common type of NHL is diffuse large B-cell lymphoma (DLBCL).

Tumors are characterized by the level of differentiation, the size of the cell of origin, the origin cell's rate of proliferation, and the histological pattern of growth. For many of the B-cell NHL subtypes, the pattern of growth and cell size may be important determinants of tumor aggressiveness. Tumors that grow in a nodular or follicular pattern are generally less aggressive than lymphomas that proliferate in a diffuse pattern. Lymphomas of small lymphocytes generally have a milder course than those of large lymphocytes, which may have intermediate-grade or high-grade aggressiveness.

Clinical Presentation. The patient with NHL may present with a variety of different symptoms (see Box 12-8). The patient should be questioned about past medical history, particularly infection with EBV, HIV, hepatitis C, or gastric ulcer (caused by *H. pylori*). Immunosuppressive treatments can also predispose individuals to NHL. Persons who have immunosuppression for organ transplantation or due to HIV, and persons with autoimmune disease are most susceptible to NHL. Occupational exposures and family and psychosocial history are also important. Toxic exposure to herbicides, pesticides, benzene, and radiation are known risk factors. Unsafe sex practices or illicit IV drug use can predispose individuals to HIV, HBV, or HCV infection, which are risk factors.

Signs and Symptoms. In patients with NHL, the patient or clinician often notices an enlarged, painless lymph node, which initiates further investigation. Other signs and symptoms of NHL are listed in Box 12-8.

Diagnosis. Although a variety of laboratory and imaging studies are used in the evaluation and staging of suspected NHL, a lymph node biopsy is the mainstay of diagnosis. The diagnostic studies commonly performed for a patient with suspected NHL include CBC with differential, liver function tests, serum protein electrophoresis, serum beta-2 microglobulin level, lactate dehydrogenase levels, HIV, and hepatitis laboratory testing; bone marrow aspiration; and nuclear medicine studies. Lumbar puncture, pleural fluid sampling (thoracentesis), and peritoneal fluid sampling (paracentesis) may be necessary. FISH and PCR are also commonly done to check for chromosomal or genetic defects. Immunophenotyping of the cancer cells is also done as it allows the identification of specific NHL subtypes. Gene expression profiling is also part of the cellular analysis in NHL. This technology allows identification of patterns of gene expression in the cancer cells that can influence type of treatment. Imaging tests include CT scan, chest x-ray, MRI, ultrasound, positron emission tomography (PET) scan, and bone scan. F-fluorodeoxyglucose (FDG)-PET scanning is highly sensitive for detecting both nodal and extranodal sites involved in NHL.

Treatment. Treatment of NHL depends on how aggressive the disease is and the symptoms of the patient. Aggressive types of NHL require immediate treatment with combination therapy regimens. Forms of NHL that are less intense can be observed and treated only when they cause symptoms or organ dysfunction. Depending on the type and stage (extent) of the lymphoma and other factors, treatment options for people with NHL might include:

- **Chemotherapy:** One of the most common combinations is called CHOP. This includes the drugs **c**yclophosphamide, doxorubicin (also known as **h**ydroxydaunorubicin), vincristine (**O**ncovin), and **p**rednisone. Bendamustine is a chemotherapeutic alkylating agent that is also used in NHL.
- **Immunotherapy:** Chemotherapy is often combined with an immunotherapy drug, especially rituximab (Rituxan). The combination is known as R-CHOP (rituximab, cyclophosphamide, hydroxydaunorubicin, oncovin, prednisone). Monoclonal antibody treatment that targets the cancer cell surface antigen CD19 is used in chemotherapy-resistant disease. Tafasitamab in combination with lenalidomide is used.
- **Targeted therapy:** TKIs, proteasome inhibitors, histone deacetylase inhibitors, and PI3k inhibitors are often used. These different medications inhibit proteins and enzymes that are integral to the growth of the lymphoma. Ibrutinib is a TKI that has been used.
- **Chimeric antigen receptor T-cell (CAR-T) treatment**: CAR-T cell treatment is used particularly for chemotherapy-resistant B-cell lymphomas that express CD19, such as DLBCL.

- **Radiation therapy:** Usually given 5 days a week for a few weeks.
- **Stem cell transplant:** Autologous stem cell transplant (bone marrow cells from the patient) or allogeneic stem cell transplant (bone marrow cells from a donor) can be used.
- **Surgery:** This is rarely used but may be needed if lymphoma starts in the spleen, thyroid, or stomach.

The prognosis for NHL is based on specific factors (see Box 12-10).

Hodgkin's Lymphoma

Hodgkin's lymphoma (HL), a malignancy of B lymphocytes, is the most common lymphoma in adolescents and young adults. HL has a worldwide incidence of 62,000 cases per year. Overall, HL is somewhat more common in males than in females. Age-specific incidence rates of HL peak in young adults (aged 15 to 34 years) and older individuals (older than 55 years). HL is subdivided into classic Hodgkin lymphoma (cHL) and nodular lymphocyte predominant (NLPHL) based on cellular analysis. Over 90% of cases are of cHL, which behaves as an aggressive neoplasm, whereas NLPHL has a less aggressive course. Classic HL is further subdivided into four subtypes: nodular sclerosis (NSCHL), mixed cellularity (MCCHL), lymphocyte rich (LRCHL), and lymphocyte deficient (LDCHL). NSCHL is the most common subtype of cHL.

Etiology. The cause of HL is unknown, but EBV has been found in malignant B lymphocytes. Also, persons who are immunosuppressed have a higher risk of HL. Exposure to carcinogens, viruses, and genetic and immune mechanisms have been proposed as etiologies, but none have been proven.

Pathophysiology. Classic HL is commonly diagnosed by the presence of Reed-Sternberg (RS) cells in the lymphoid tissue (see Fig. 12-5). The RS cell is a large malignant B cell with two nuclei that give the cell the appearance of owl's eyes. About 50% of patients have EBV in their RS cells.

The malignancy is thought to start in one area, such as a lymph node, and then spread throughout the lymphatic system. The cervical lymph nodes, mediastinal nodes, and spleen are involved in most cases. There are various types of HL, each with different growth patterns and required treatments.

Clinical Presentation. The patient with HL usually has no dramatic symptoms. The patient or clinician may discover a painless, enlarged lymph node. Painless lymphadenopathy enlarging over months is the common mode of presentation. The three most common sites of disease presentation are mediastinal node involvement (chest), left neck cervical nodal enlargement, or right neck cervical nodal enlargement.

BOX 12-10. Prognostic Indicators for Non-Hodgkin's Lymphoma

The International Prognostic Index (IPI) is used to determine the prognosis for people with aggressive lymphomas that are fast-growing cancers. The index depends on the following five factors:
- The patient's age
- The stage of the lymphoma
- Whether the lymphoma is in organs outside the lymphatic system
- Performance status (PS)—how well a person can complete normal activities of daily living
- The blood level of lactate dehydrogenase (LDH), which increases congruent with the increasing amount of lymphoma in the body

Good Prognostic Factors	Poor Prognostic Factors
Age 60 or younger	Age older than 60
Stage I or II	Stage III or IV
Lymphoma limited to lymph nodes, or lymphoma in only one region of the body outside of the lymph nodes	Lymphoma is in more than one organ of the body outside of the lymph nodes
Performance status: able to function normally	Performance status: lack of independence with daily activities
Serum lactate dehydrogenase is normal	Serum lactate dehydrogenase is high

Each poor prognostic factor is counted as 1 point. For example, patients with no poor prognostic factors would have a score of 0, whereas those with all of the poor prognostic factors would have a score of 5. Higher score indicates poorer prognosis.

The number of prognostic factors determines a classification system of four risk groups for lymphoma:
- Low risk (none or one poor prognostic factor)
- Low-intermediate risk (two poor prognostic factors)
- High-intermediate risk (three poor prognostic factors)
- High risk (four or five poor prognostic factors)

From American Cancer Society (2022). Survival rates and factors that affect prognosis (outlook) for non-Hodgkin lymphoma. https://www.cancer.org/cancer/nonhodgkin-lymphoma/detection-diagnosis-staging/factors-prognosis.html

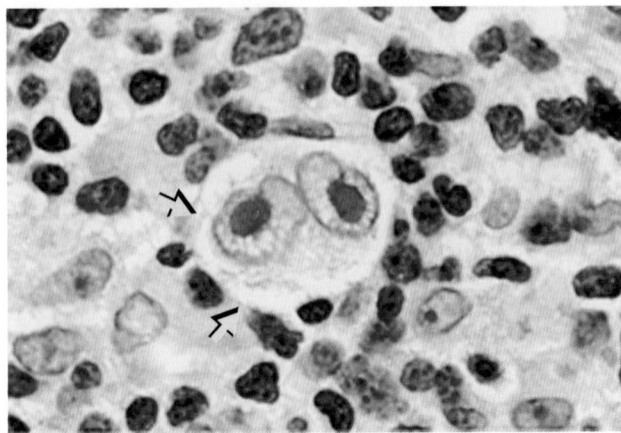

FIGURE 12-5. Reed-Sternberg cell. Reed-Sternberg cells are large abnormal lymphocytes with multiple nuclei, which are characteristic cells found in Hodgkin's lymphoma (HL).

Alternatively, the patient can experience symptoms of sore throat, fever, trouble swallowing, shortness of breath, abdominal pain, or other various symptoms associated with the enlargement of lymphoid tissue in the body. As with all cancer patients, a complete history and physical are necessary.

Signs and Symptoms. Patients with HL present with solid tumors of lymphoid tissue. Enlargement of lymphoid tissue at lymph nodes or extranodal sites such as the thymus gland, spleen, liver, or tonsils usually occurs. Symptoms depend on the affected site. Waldeyer's ring, a circular arrangement of lymphoid tissue in the pharynx, which includes the palatine, pharyngeal, and lingual tonsils, is a common site of involvement.

CLINICAL CONCEPT

A lymphoma in the thymus gland may produce chest pain or pressure from an enlarging tumor. A lymphoma can also place pressure on the trachea, possibly causing shortness of breath or coughing. If a lymphoma is placing pressure on the superior vena cava (SVC), it may cause SVC syndrome with edema of the head and arms. If a lymphoma involves lymphatic tissue below the diaphragm, there may be abdominal distention with splenomegaly.

Diagnosis. Diagnosis is made after biopsy of nodal and extranodal sites. Flow cytometry and DNA analysis identify chromosomal translocations and molecular rearrangements. Bone marrow biopsy to rule out leukemia is done in the presence of anemia, leukopenia, or thrombocytopenia. Fluorodeoxyglucose (FDG) positron emission tomography (PET)–computed tomography (CT) has very high sensitivity and specificity in HL and can be used to stage the disease. Immunophenotyping tests check for certain cell surface antigens,

such as CD15 and CD30, which are found on the surface of the RS cells. Clinical staging is done after history and physical examination; laboratory studies; and thoracic, pelvic, and abdominal CT scans. PET scans can also be used to evaluate response to treatment. For clinical staging of HL, see Box 12-11.

Treatment. Chemotherapy and radiation are the mainstays of cHL treatment. Treatment options will depend on multiple factors, including type and stage of the lymphoma.

- **Combination chemotherapy:** Combinations of different chemotherapy agents are used for HL because different drugs can attack the cancer in different ways. A combination of Adriamycin (doxorubicin), Bleomycin, Vinblastine, and Dacarbazine (ABVD) has become the standard chemotherapeutic regimen used to treat cHL in the United States Common chemotherapy regimens are summarized in Box 12-12.
- **Radiation therapy:** Different types of radiation therapy are used for HL. The most commonly used type is called involved site radiotherapy (ISRT), which limits the radiation to the specific region of the cancer cells.
- **Immunotherapy:** Monoclonal antibody therapy involves using genetically engineered antibodies to target specific surface antigens on cancer cells. The engineered antibody can carry a drug into cancer cells. Brentuximab vedotin (Adcetris) is an example of a monoclonal antibody that targets CD30 surface markers on HL cells. The monoclonal antibody is attached to a chemotherapeutic drug, which then enters the cells and kills them. Rituximab (Rituxan) is another monoclonal antibody that is used to treat nodular lymphocyte-predominant Hodgkin's lymphoma (NLPHL). This monoclonal antibody attaches to a substance called CD20 on some types of lymphoma cells. Other monoclonal antibodies being investigated are nivolumab (Opdivo) and pembrolizumab (Keytruda), which target specific checkpoint pathways in cellular development and lead to programmed degeneration.
- **High-dose chemotherapy and stem cell transplant:** After high-dose combination chemotherapy, bone marrow stem cell transplant can be used in treatment of HL. Either an autologous stem cell transplant involving the patient's own bone marrow or allogeneic stem cell transplant using donor bone marrow cells may be performed.

Prognosis for HL is based on specific factors (see Box 12-13).

Multiple Myeloma

Multiple myeloma (MM) is a hematological neoplasm that arises in B lymphocytes. In normal conditions, B lymphocytes transform into plasma cells, which then

BOX 12-11. Lugano Stage Classification of Hodgkin's Lymphoma

For limited stage (I or II) HL that affects an organ outside of the lymph system, the letter E is added to the stage (for example, stage IE or IIE).

STAGE I: Either of the following means that the HL is stage I:
- HL is found in only 1 lymph node area or lymphoid organ such as the thymus (I).
- The cancer is found only in 1 part of 1 organ outside the lymph system (IE).

STAGE II: Either of the following means that the HL is stage II:
- HL is found in 2 or more lymph node areas on the same side of (above or below) the diaphragm, which is the thin muscle beneath the lungs that separates the chest and abdomen (II).
- The cancer extends locally from one lymph node area into a nearby organ (IIE).

STAGE III: Either of the following means that the HL is stage III:
- HL is found in lymph node areas on both sides of (above and below) the diaphragm (III).
- HL is in lymph nodes above the diaphragm and in the spleen.

STAGE IV: HL has spread widely into at least one organ outside of the lymph system, such as the liver, bone marrow, or lungs.

Other modifiers may also be used to describe the Hodgkin lymphoma stage:

BULKY DISEASE
This term is used to describe tumors in the chest that are at least one-third as wide as the chest, or tumors in other areas that are at least 10 centimeters (about 4 inches) across. It's usually labeled by adding the letter X to the stage. It's especially important for stage II lymphomas, because bulky disease may require more intensive treatment.

A VS. B
Each stage may also be assigned a letter (A or B). B is added (stage IIIB, for example) if a person has any of these **B symptoms:**
- Loss of more than 10% of body weight over the previous 6 months (without dieting)
- Unexplained fever of at least 100.4°F (38°C)
- Drenching night sweats

If a person has any B symptoms, it usually means the lymphoma is more advanced, and more intensive treatment is often recommended. If no B symptoms are present, the letter A is added to the stage.

From American Cancer Society (2022). Hodgkin lymphoma staging. https://www.cancer.org/cancer/hodgkin-lymphoma/detection-diagnosis-staging/staging.html

BOX 12-12. Combination Chemotherapy for Hodgkin's Lymphoma

The combinations used to treat HL are often referred to by abbreviations.

ABVD is the most common regimen used in the United States
- Adriamycin (doxorubicin)
- Bleomycin
- Vinblastine
- Dacarbazine (DTIC)
- Chemotherapy is given in cycles that include a period of treatment followed by a rest period to give the body time to recover. In general, each cycle lasts for several weeks.

Adapted from American Cancer Society. (2022). Treating Hodgkin lymphoma. Retrieved from https://www.cancer.org/cancer/hodgkin-lymphoma/treating/chemotherapy.html

BOX 12-13. Prognostic Factors Used in Hodgkin's Lymphoma

The following factors are used to determine severity of illness and intensity of treatment. Possessing some of these factors indicates the disease is more serious.
- Male
- Older than age 45
- Stage of the disease (earlier stages have better prognosis)
- Bulky disease: tumor in chest is one-third as wide as the chest, or tumors in other areas are 10 cm or more in width (indicates more serious disease)
- Constitutional symptoms: fever, night sweats, weight loss
- Elevated WBC count greater than 15,000
- Low RBC hemoglobin level less than 10.5
- Low lymphocyte count greater than 600
- Low blood albumin level less than 4
- High erythrocyte sedimentation rate (ESR) greater than 30

From American Cancer Society. (2022). Survival rates for Hodgkin lymphoma by stage. https://www.cancer.org/cancer/hodgkin-lymphoma/detection-diagnosis-staging/survival-rates.html

secrete immunoglobulins (Igs). In MM, the B lymphocytes that become plasma cells proliferate uncontrollably within the bone marrow. As a consequence, an excessive number of Igs are secreted by the plethora of plasma cells. There are large numbers of abnormal Igs and Ig fragments.

MM is a B-cell malignancy that affects approximately 35,000 people in the United States yearly. It accounts for 1.1% of all malignancies and is the second most common hematological neoplasm in the United States. MM has a higher incidence in men than in women (2:1) and in African Americans than in European Americans (2:1). It is most prevalent in persons older than 65 years.

Etiology

The triggering factor in MM is unknown, although genetic and chromosomal changes are found in affected patients. Myeloma cells show abnormalities in their chromosomes. Some myeloma cells have extra chromosomes (called a duplication) or are missing all or part of a chromosome (called a deletion). Chromosomal deletions appear to make the myeloma more aggressive and resistant to treatment. In about half of all people with myeloma, part of one chromosome has switched with part of another chromosome in the myeloma cells, called translocation (t). The following findings are considered high-risk chromosomal changes: 1q +, t(4;14), t(14;16), t(14;20), and del(17p) (TP53 mutation). Additional chromosomal changes may include hyperdiploidy, defined as trisomy of chromosomes 3, 5, 7, 9, 11, 15, 19, and/or 21 or the translocation t(11;14). Translocations including t(4;14), t(6;14), t(11;14), t(14;16), and t(14;20) are associated with oncogenes, MMSET/FGFR3, CCND3, CCND1, MAF, and MAFB, respectively, which ultimately drive plasma cell hyperproliferation.

There is also excessive production of a cytokine called interleukin-6 (IL-6), which stimulates excessive numbers of plasma cells to proliferate.

Risk Factors

The cause of MM is unknown. In the United States, risk factors for MM include male sex, occupation as a firefighter, obesity, exposure to the chemicals dioxin/Agent Orange, and being a World Trade Center 9/11 first responder. Agent Orange was used extensively by the military in the past; therefore, older military veterans may have higher risk. Also, there were known and unknown chemical exposures for those involved in the New York City 9/11/2001 World Trade Center disaster. Studies show rescue and recovery workers at the World Trade Center site appear to be at higher risk of developing multiple myeloma (Landgren et al., 2018).

Pathophysiology

In almost all patients, MM begins as monoclonal gammopathy of undetermined significance (MGUS). MGUS progresses to MM in approximately 1% to 2% of persons over a course of 20 years. Smoldering multiple myeloma (SMM) is a more advanced plasma cell disorder, with approximately 10% of patients progressing to MM each year. Periodic clinical monitoring of those with MGUS or SMM is recommended.

Treatment may not be necessary. For some high-risk patients with SMM, active treatment versus observation is under study.

MM is characterized by neoplastic plasma cells (derived from abnormal B cells) that proliferate within the bone marrow. In the bloodstream, these aberrant plasma cells synthesize abnormal Ig proteins that precipitate out of the blood and become filtered by the kidneys into the urine. The overproliferation of plasma cells within the bone marrow leads to crowding out of healthy RBCs, WBCs, and platelets. This leads to anemia, leukopenia, and thrombocytopenia. The Igs in the blood can overwhelm the kidney filtration system and cause renal failure. The cytokines in the myeloma cells stimulate osteoclastic activity and inhibit osteoblastic activity, causing bone destruction and inhibition of bone formation. Hypercalcemia due to bone breakdown occurs. Vertebral bone deterioration and compression fracture can occur. A frequent neurological occurrence called radiculopathy is caused by compression of a spinal nerve by a paravertebral plasmacytoma (neoplastic plasma cell tumor) in the lumbosacral area.

The pathology of myeloma depends on the neoplastic plasma cell identified on bone marrow biopsy. Normally, each type of plasma cell produces only one type of Ig. Healthy Ig proteins are composed of two identical heavy chains and two identical light chains (see Fig. 12-6). However, in MM, plasma cells can produce excessive whole Igs or Ig fragments such as light chains. The abnormal Ig fragments are referred to as monoclonal proteins or M-proteins. Bence Jones myeloma, identified in 1848 by Dr. Henry Bence Jones, is a myeloma in which only the light chains of Ig structure are produced; these light chains are also called **Bence Jones proteins**.

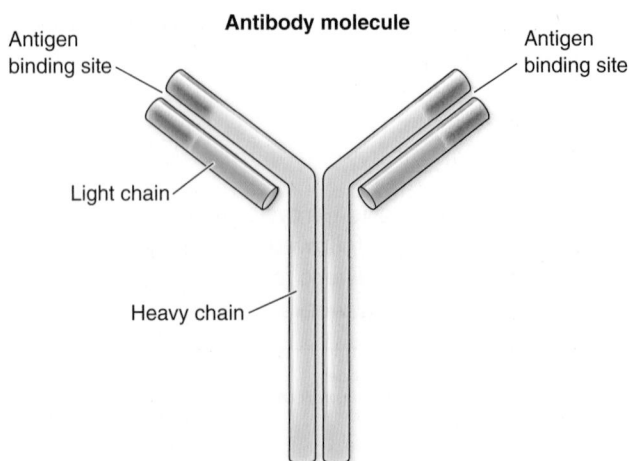

Antibody molecule

Antigen binding site

Antigen binding site

Light chain

Heavy chain

FIGURE 12-6. Antibody structure. Antibodies, also called immunoglobulins (Igs), are proteins synthesized by plasma cells. Plasma cells are formed from B cells. Each antibody consists of four polypeptides—two heavy chains and two light chains joined to form a Y-shaped molecule. The polypeptide tips of the Y vary among different antibodies and give the antibody its specificity for antigen.

The most common MM proliferative Igs are IgG and IgA. Proliferation of IgG accounts for about 60% to 70% of all myeloma, and IgA accounts for about 20%. IgD and IgE rarely proliferate in MM. IgM can be proliferative in MM, but high amounts of IgM are usually related to another disease called Waldenstrom's macroglobulinemia. With high amounts of circulating Igs, hyperviscosity of the blood can occur. Because Igs are of differing size, with IgM being very large, it causes the greatest increase in viscosity. IgG and IgE are smaller and cause less of a problem.

Clinical Presentation

Clinical symptoms are the result of the disease progression. Bone pain, especially in the back, is a common complaint at diagnosis. It is a result of bone destruction and the formation of **plasmacytomas**, which are tumors of plasma cells within the bone. Bone lesions are rounded, punched-out areas of bone found most commonly in the vertebra, skull, ribs, humerus, and femur. Bone scans may not reflect the lytic destruction seen on x-ray. Osteopenia is seen on bone density study.

Weakness, pallor, and fatigue associated with anemia occur. The anemia is a normocytic, normochromic anemia. There may be a decreased vitamin B_{12} level and Rouleaux formation of RBCs. Rouleaux formation is a phenomenon in which RBCs collect in clumps and appear as stacks of coins. It is found in patients with elevated serum protein levels.

Infection frequently occurs because of the deficiency in healthy WBCs and lack of antibody-mediated immunity. The myeloma cells outnumber and crowd out normal plasma cells, which causes low levels of normal Igs. The risk of infection is greatest at the time of diagnosis and will decrease as the disease responds to treatment. Most deaths from infection occur early during treatment, when the body has little natural immunity available.

Renal disease is present in one-half of patients at the time of diagnosis and contributes to a poor prognosis. The two major causes of renal insufficiency are hypercalcemia and myeloma cast nephropathy. Hypercalcemia occurs because of bone breakdown, and calcium can precipitate in the kidney, causing kidney stones. Myeloma cast nephropathy is characterized by the presence of large, waxy, laminated casts or deposits in the distal and collecting tubules of the kidneys.

They are formed from precipitated abnormal Ig light chain fragments that have collected in the nephron tubules. Proximal tubules are also damaged by the large protein load. Hypercalciuria as well as hyperuricemia also contribute to kidney damage.

Approximately 10% to 15% of patients with MM are diagnosed with concurrent immunoglobulin light chain amyloidosis during the course of their disease. Light chain amyloidosis is protein deposition in vital organs. These proteins cause organ dysfunction, particularly in the heart and kidney. These complications are termed amyloid cardiomyopathy and nephropathy.

Approximately 3.3% of patients endure extramedullary disease. Extramedullary disease can present as plasmacytomas outside of the bone marrow, central nervous system involvement, or plasma cell leukemia. Extramedullary disease is associated with a more aggressive disease course.

Diagnosis

MM is diagnosed as having 10% or more plasma cells in the bone marrow and organ or tissue damage resulting from the proliferation of the plasma cells. Plasmacytomas, or tumors made up of plasma cells, may be found on tissue biopsy.

The most critical criterion in the diagnosis of MM is the evidence of multiple myeloma–related organ damage. The acronym CRAB is a mnemonic for the end-organ damage caused by plasma cell hyperproliferation. CRAB stands for **c**alcium elevation, **r**enal dysfunction, **a**nemia, and **b**one disease. In addition to CRAB, infection is also a clinically significant symptom. Bone end-organ damage is detected in 70% of patients with MM at diagnosis (see Box 12-14).

Required diagnostic tests include CBC with differential, blood chemistry panel, serum protein electrophoresis to check Ig blood levels, urine electrophoresis to check for Bence Jones proteins, and beta-2-microglobulin level (a biomarker of MM). During treatment, monitoring the urine and blood levels of Ig fragments can gauge efficacy of therapy.

Flow cytometry should be done to identify abnormal circulating plasma cells to exclude plasma cell leukemia. Genetic analysis of the malignant plasma cells can be performed using fluorescent in situ

BOX 12-14. End Organ Damage in Multiple Myeloma–CRAB

C calcium elevation
R renal dysfunction
A anemia
B bone disease

Adapted From: International Myeloma Working Group. (2003). Criteria for the classification of monoclonal gammopathies, multiple myeloma and related disorders: a report of the International Myeloma Working Group. *Br J Haematol.* 2003 121(5), 749-757.

hybridization (FISH), in which fluorescent probes bind to chromosomal changes in the abnormal cells. This can identify genetic factors that assist in prognosis and treatment decisions.

A bone marrow aspirate and biopsy should be performed. The bone marrow is analyzed for morphology of plasma cells and quantification of the surface antigen CD138 +.

Imaging studies should include CT, MRI, and PET scans to exclude lytic lesions in bone, vertebral compression, or pathological fractures. An echocardiogram of the heart is necessary to check for amyloid protein infiltration of the heart muscle.

Staging of MM

MM is staged according to the Revised International Staging System (see Table 12-3). The disease is staged according to the amount of albumin, beta-2-microglobulin, and lactate dehydrogenase in the blood and genetic abnormalities found in

cancer cells. Specific chromosome changes can indicate poor outcome. For example, gene deletion found within chromosome 17 and translocation of genes between chromosomes 4 and 14 and 4 and 16 indicate high risk for a poor prognosis.

Treatment

Treatment of asymptomatic patients with MGUS is usually deferred and patients are monitored periodically for evidence of worsening disease. If disease converts to MM, treatment is initiated. In patients with SMM, early intervention may or may not be indicated. Some patients may be treated with lenalidomide (Revlimid), an immunomodulatory agent, and dexamethasone (a corticosteroid) to prevent progression of disease. Lenalidomide (Revlimid) is an immunodulator similar to the drug thalidomide. Lenalidomide inhibits the production of proinflammatory cytokines and enhances immunity by stimulating the body's own T cells and NK cells.

Patients with symptomatic MM require treatment to control proliferation of cancerous plasma cells and supportive care to ameliorate complications and adverse effects of therapy. Treatment includes an initial induction process followed by consolidation, maintenance regimen, and relapse management. Treatment is influenced by the patient's age and existing comorbidities. Once initiated, treatment commonly consists of chemotherapy, followed by autologous stem cell transplantation.

Chemotherapy includes immunomodulatory agents, proteasome inhibitors, and targeted monoclonal antibodies. Lenalidomide (Revlimid), bortezomib (Velcade), and dexamethasone are commonly used in combination before stem cell transplantation. Bortezomib (Velcade) is a proteasome inhibitor that blocks degradation of proteins that trigger cellular apoptosis in cancer cells. Thus, bortezomib (Velcade) enhances cancer cell apoptosis, which is cancer cell degeneration.

In patients who are not candidates for stem cell transplantation because of age or other comorbidities, initial combination therapy is administered for approximately 8 to 12 cycles, followed by maintenance therapy with lenalidomide (Revlimid). For high-risk patients, bortezomib-based maintenance is considered.

Almost all patients with MM eventually relapse. In relapsed patients, daratumumab (Darzalex)-based combination regimens have shown efficacy. Daratumumab (Darzalex) is a monoclonal antibody that targets the surface antigen CD38, which is overexpressed on MM cells. Other treatments used for relapse include panobinostat (Farydak) and bendamustine (Treanda, Bendeka)-based regimens. Panobinostat is a potent inhibitor of histone deacetylase, which is responsible for the regulation of gene transcription, cellular differentiation, cell-cycle progression, and apoptosis. In MM cells, the inhibition of histone deacetylase damages DNA and upregulates proteins that promote apoptosis

TABLE 12-3. The Revised International Staging System of Multiple Myeloma

Multiple myeloma is staged using the Revised International Staging System (RISS) based on four factors:
- The amount of albumin in the blood
- The amount of beta-2-microglobulin in the blood
- The amount of LDH in the blood
- The specific gene abnormalities (cytogenetics) of the cancer

Stage	Factors
Stage I	Serum beta-2 microglobulin is less than 3.5 (mg/L) **AND** Albumin level is 3.5 (g/dL) or greater **AND** Cytogenetics (chromosomal abnormalities) that are considered "not high risk" **AND** LDH levels are normal
Stage II	The associated factors do not match those in stage I or stage III
Stage III	Serum beta-2 microglobulin is 5.5 (mg/L) or greater **AND** Cytogenetics (chromosomal changes) that are considered "high-risk"* **AND/OR** LDH levels are high

*See Etiology section. Chromosomal translocations and deletions are considered high risk.
From American Cancer Society. (2022). Multiple myeloma stages. Retrieved from https://www.cancer.org/cancer/multiple-myeloma/detection-diagnosis-staging/staging.html

and cell-cycle arrest. Bendamustine (Treanda, Bendeka) is an alkylating, cytotoxic agent that attacks the rapidly dividing MM cells. Currently, chimeric antigen receptor T cell (CAR-T) therapy that targets B cell antigens is under investigation for MM.

Supportive treatment of the patient with MM is necessary due to susceptibility to infection, bone degeneration, renal dysfunction, anemia, pain, and adverse effects of chemotherapeutic agents. The patient requires calcium supplementation and vitamin D to strengthen bone. Bisphosphonates (e.g., pamidronate [Aredia] or Denosumab [Prolia]) are also administered to inhibit osteoclastic activity. Kyphoplasty or vertebroplasty surgical procedures are considered for patients with collapsed vertebrae. High fluid intake is necessary to preserve renal function. Plasmapheresis is a treatment that can clear some of the immunoglobulin fragments from the bloodstream that can reduce hyperviscosity of the blood. Prophylactic administration of gamma globulin may be needed to boost immunity to infections. Pneumococcal vaccine should be considered to decrease risk of pneumonia. Erythropoetin, vitamin B_{12}, and folic acid can be administered to boost red blood cell production. Bone pain requires analgesics or may respond to localized radiation. Preventive treatment of deep vein thrombosis with aspirin or anticoagulants is necessary for patients on lenalidomide.

Chapter Summary

- WBCs are an integral part of the body's defense against antigens.
- WBCs are born in the bone marrow and released in response to the body's needs. After bone marrow synthesis, lymphocytes, also called B cells and T cells, need to mature within lymphoid tissue that includes the lymph nodes, tonsils, adenoids, thymus gland, and spleen.
- All WBC synthesis is stimulated by infections, inflammatory reactions, extreme stress, and neoplasms.
- Bacterial infections particularly stimulate neutrophil synthesis, whereas allergic reactions and parasitic infections provoke eosinophil and basophil production.
- Lymphocytes classically respond to viral infection.
- Leukocytosis greater than 11,000/mcL is most commonly indicative of infection; however, neoplastic disease causes a rise in the number of WBCs, but neoplastic WBCs do not function and multiply uncontrollably.
- Myelodysplastic syndrome (MDS) is a hematological disease where a specific stem cell line of immature blood cells within the bone marrow does not develop properly. This can lead to defective maturation of WBCs, RBCs, or platelets.
- Neoplastic diseases of WBCs are termed leukemias and lymphomas.
- In leukemia, there is a neoplastic proliferation of WBCs that are stopped from maturation in early development within the bone marrow. These immature leukemic WBCs are referred to as blast cells.
- Lymphoma is a cancerous proliferation of lymphocytes within lymphoid tissue, often first presenting as an enlarged lymph node.
- Cancerous WBCs are nonfunctioning cells that crowd out healthy WBC, RBC, and platelet production in the bone marrow. Lack of healthy WBCs leads to infection,

lack of healthy RBCs leads to anemia, and lack of healthy platelets leads to thrombocytopenia.
- The classic signs of hematological neoplastic disease are infection, anemia, and thrombocytopenia. Infection often causes fever, anemia causes extreme fatigue, and thrombocytopenia leads to easy bruising and spontaneous bleeding.
- There are four classifications of leukemia: acute lymphoblastic leukemia (ALL), chronic lymphocytic leukemia (CLL), acute myelogenous leukemia (AML), and chronic myelogenous leukemia (CML).
- There are two major types of lymphoma: non-Hodgkin's lymphoma and Hodgkin's lymphoma.
- There are different types of leukemia and lymphoma, but all cause the same basic condition: immunosuppression because the cancerous WBCs do not function to defend the body and they crowd out all healthy WBCs.
- The etiology of most leukemias and lymphomas is unclear. Radiation and chemical exposures are common risk factors. Some viral pathogens such as HIV, EBV, herpesvirus 8, and HTLV-1 can increase susceptibility to some types of leukemia and lymphoma.
- Polymerase chain reaction (PCR), fluorescent in situ hybridization (FISH), and flow cytometry are procedures used to examine DNA and are commonly used in cancer diagnosis.
- Cytogenetic analysis identifies precise genetic changes of cancer cells. This procedure allows specific diagnosis, prognosis, and targeted treatments.
- Immunophenotyping identifies specific cell surface antigens on cancer cells. This procedure enables specific diagnosis, prognosis, and targeted treatments.
- Many leukemias are caused by genetic and chromosomal changes such as translocation, deletion, and

inversion of genes; and aneuploidy, the duplication of chromosomes.

- The **Ph (Philadelphia)** chromosome is a common genetic mutation found in CML and ALL due to translocation of genes on chromosome numbers 9 and 22; referred to as t(9:22).

- Multiple myeloma (MM) is a unique kind of neoplastic condition involving overproliferation of plasma cells, which leads to excessive production of Ig fragments that accumulate in the bloodstream.

- Cancerous MM cells overwhelm the bone marrow and lead to clinical manifestations known by the acronym CRAB. CRAB stands for calcium elevation, renal failure, anemia, and bone disease. MM commonly spreads to the vertebrae and can present as lumbosacral pain.

- Similar treatments are used to combat leukemias and lymphomas: standard chemotherapy, immunotherapy, different types of targeted therapies, radiation, and bone marrow transplantation (also called stem cell transplantation).

- Standard chemotherapeutic agents work by destroying rapidly dividing cells, which includes the cancer cells as well as normal skin, gastrointestinal cells, and bone marrow. Due to these widespread effects, standard chemotherapeutic agents cause many noxious adverse effects and collateral damage to healthy cells.

- Standard chemotherapeutic agents cause bone marrow suppression, which in turn leads to lack of healthy WBCs (leukopenia), RBCs (anemia), and platelets (thrombocytopenia). Other side effects of standard chemotherapy include anorexia, nausea, vomiting, hair loss, and sore mucous membranes of the mouth.

- Standard chemotherapy treatment for leukemias and lymphomas is increasingly being replaced by immunotherapy and targeted therapy regimens that have fewer adverse effects.

- Tyrosine kinase inhibitors (TKIs) are a form of targeted hematological cancer treatment that only affects the TK enzyme that allows for constant proliferation of cancer cells.

- Immunotherapy consists of laboratory-synthesized monoclonal antibodies that target specific surface antigens only present on cancer cells.

- CAR-T immunotherapy is a process that extracts the patient's own T cells and reprograms the T cells to specifically attack an antigen on the cancer cells. These reprogrammed T cells are then readministered to the patient to kill the hematological cancer cells.

- Tumor lysis syndrome can occur when a large number of cancer cells are killed all at once by chemotherapy. The cells release their breakdown products—uric acid, calcium, and phosphorus—which can overwhelm the kidneys and cause acute kidney injury.

- Filgrastim (Neupogen) is a stimulant of the bone marrow that can increase leukocyte synthesis, specifically neutrophils, when a patient has leukopenia due to chemotherapy.

Making the Connections

Pathophysiology

Signs and Symptoms	Physical Assessment Findings	Diagnostic Testing	Treatment
Myelodysplastic Syndrome | Disorder of one or more stem cell lines in the bone marrow; RBCs, WBCs, or platelets; can lead to complete bone marrow suppression.			
Deficient number of healthy WBCs causes infection and lack of signs of inflammation. Deficient healthy RBCs cause fatigue, weakness, pallor. Deficient healthy platelets cause bruising and bleeding, such as nosebleeds.	Infection, fever, or lack of signs of inflammation. Bruises or nosebleeds caused by thrombocytopenia. Pallor, tachycardia, fatigue, weakness caused by anemia.	CBC with differential, bone marrow flow cytometry, PCR, FISH, karyotype, molecular genetic testing, immunophenotyping. The finding of an unexplained blood cell cytopenia and significant morphological dysplasia of the blood cells. Cytogenetic abnormality del 5q.	Erythropoiesis-stimulating agents are used to counteract anemia. Transfusion of the deficient type of blood cells. Chemotherapy. Allogenic stem cell transplantation may be indicated.

Making the Connections–cont'd

Signs and Symptoms	Physical Assessment Findings	Diagnostic Testing	Treatment

Acute Lymphoblastic Leukemia | Stem cell precursors of B cells or T cells do not function and do not mature beyond lymphoblast stage (referred to as blasts).

Frequent infection, fatigue, dyspnea, fever, chills, night sweats, other flu-like symptoms. Bone pain caused by overproliferation of lymphoblasts in bone marrow. Bleeding and bruising due to thrombocytopenia. Anemia causes weakness, dizziness, shortness of breath, abdominal feeling of "fullness" if spleen is enlarged, unintentional weight loss.	Infection and fever caused by inadequate healthy WBCs. Blast cell proliferation in spleen and liver causes hepatomegaly and splenomegaly. Deficient platelets cause signs of bruising and nosebleeds. Anemia causes pallor, tachycardia, weakness. Lymph node or spleen enlargement. Unintentional weight loss.	CBC with differential and bone marrow aspiration show immature lymphoblast count greater than 20%. Lymph node biopsy. Flow cytometry, FISH, PCR, cytogenetic testing show the Ph chromosome; translocation of genes at chromosome 9 and 22 termed Ph + ALL. Also Ph-like ALL. Aneuploidy is often found in ALL cells. Immunophenotyping identifies cell surface antigens. LP, CT, MRI, chest x-ray, and bone scan.	Combination of standard chemotherapy to induce remission and maintenance. TKI targeted therapy. Monoclonal antibody targeted therapy. CAR-T immunotherapy. Allogenic stem cell transplantation.

Chronic Lymphocytic Leukemia | Proliferation of mature, functionally incompetent CD5-positive B-cells within the blood, bone marrow, lymph nodes, and spleen. CLL B cells do not synthesize normal immunoglobulins.

Frequent infection caused by deficient healthy WBCs, fatigue, dyspnea caused by anemia, fever, chills, night sweats, and other flu-like symptoms caused by deficient WBCs. Spontaneous bruising caused by lack of platelets. Bone pain caused by overproliferation of lymphoblasts in bone marrow. Enlarged spleen that can cause feeling of stomach fullness.	Infections. Pallor. Bruises. Nosebleeds. Lymphadenopathy, splenomegaly, and hepatomegaly. Autoimmune hemolytic anemia can occur.	CBC with differential; lymphocytosis greater than 20,000 cells/mcL. Presence of specifically greater than 5,000 B-lymphocytes/µL in the peripheral blood for the duration of at least 3 months. Flow cytometry, FISH, and PCR tests show deletions in parts of chromosomes 13, 11, or 17. Other less common chromosome changes trisomy 12 or a translocation between chromosomes 11. Immunophenotyping shows B-CLL cells coexpress the CD5 antigen, CD19, CD20, CD22, CD23, and CD52 antigens.	Standard chemotherapy. Corticosteroids. Targeted therapy with TKIs and P13K inhibitors. Venetoclax targets BCL-2 protein in CLL cells. Monoclonal antibodies target CD surface antigens. Allogenic stem cell transplantation.

Continued

Making the Connections—cont'd

Signs and Symptoms	Physical Assessment Findings	Diagnostic Testing	Treatment
Acute Myelogenous Leukemia | Proliferation of myeloid blast cells in bone marrow. Overproliferation of myeloblasts in organs such as lymph nodes, spleen, and liver.			
Frequent infection caused by deficient healthy WBCs. Fatigue and dyspnea caused by anemia. Spontaneous bruising caused by lack of platelets. Bone pain caused by overproliferation of lymphoblasts in bone marrow. Lymphadenopathy, infiltration of skin, lungs, and other organs with lymphoblast cells.	Infections. Pallor. Bruises. Nosebleeds. Lymphadenopathy, splenomegaly, and hepatomegaly.	CBC with differential; bone marrow aspiration with lymphocytosis greater than 20%. Bone marrow biopsy, FISH, and PCR show genetic translocation t(8;21) and t(15;17), and inversion at chromosome 16. Also a deletion at chromosome del (7). Aneuploidy at chromosome 8. Common oncogenes include *FLT3, IDH1,* and *IDH2* genes; *c-Kit*; and *RAS*. Immunophenotyping shows CD33 surface antigen.	Standard chemotherapy. Radiation. Targeted therapy; TKIs. Monoclonal antibodies target CD surface antigen. Allogenic stem cell transplantation.
Chronic Myelogenous Leukemia | Overproliferation of mature myeloid cells in bone marrow that do not function. Overproliferation of myeloid cells invade organs such as lymph nodes, spleen, and liver; leading to lymphadenopathy, splenomegaly, and hepatomegaly.			
Frequent infection caused by deficient healthy WBCs. Fatigue and dyspnea caused by anemia. Spontaneous bruising caused by lack of platelets. Bone pain caused by overproliferation of myeloid cells in bone marrow. Abdominal fullness caused by liver and spleen pressure on stomach, causing decreased appetite.	Infections. Pallor. Bruises. Nosebleeds. Lymphadenopathy, splenomegaly, and hepatomegaly.	CBC with differential, bone marrow aspiration shows excessive WBCs. PCR, FISH, flow cytometry show 95% of adults with CML have the Ph chromosome, which is a BCR-ABL oncogene mutation caused by translocation of genes between chromosome 9 and 22 [t(9;22)].	Targeted therapy with TKI. Allogenic stem cell transplantation. Splenectomy if splenic dysfunction occurs.
Non-Hodgkin's Lymphoma (NHL) | Proliferation of abnormal B cells, T cells, or NK cells. Most common type is diffuse large B-cell lymphoma (DLCL)			
Fever, chills, night sweats, weight loss, fatigue. Lymphatic blockage causing lymphedema or nerve impingement, which causes numbness and tingling caused by enlarged lymph node.	Painless enlarged lymph node, splenomegaly, hepatomegaly. Lymphedema. Nerve impingement can cause weakness and sensory loss in an extremity.	Lymph node biopsy; main diagnostic procedure. CBC with differential, liver function tests, serum protein electrophoresis, serum beta-2 microglobulin level, lactate dehydrogenase levels, HIV, and hepatitis laboratory testing. Bone marrow aspiration; abdominal CT scan, LP, pleural fluid sampling (thoracocentesis), and peritoneal fluid sampling (paracentesis). FISH, PCR, flow cytometry, immunophenotyping, gene expression profiling chest x-ray, MRI, ultrasound, bone scan, and FDG-PET scanning.	Standard chemotherapy combination regimens + monoclonal antibody, rituximab. **Targeted therapy:** TKIs, proteasome inhibitors, histone deacetylase inhibitors, and PI3k inhibitors. CAR-T cell treatment. Allogenic stem cell transplantation. Radiation. Surgery may be necessary.

Making the Connections—cont'd

Signs and Symptoms	Physical Assessment Findings	Diagnostic Testing	Treatment

Hodgkin's Lymphoma | Enlarged, malignant B cells called RS cells that may contain EBV.

Signs and Symptoms	Physical Assessment Findings	Diagnostic Testing	Treatment
Enlarged lymph node. Sore throat, fever, trouble swallowing, shortness of breath, abdominal pain.	Pharyngeal edema and erythema. Painless, enlarged lymph node, signs of infection, splenomegaly, enlarged thymus. Enlarged mediastinal lymph node can cause SVC syndrome.	CBC with differential, biopsy of lymph node; PCR, FISH, immunophenotyping, flow cytometry, bone marrow aspirate and biopsy, CT of abdomen, thorax, or pelvis; PET scan.	Combination standard chemotherapy. Radiation. Allogenic stem cell transplantation. Immunotherapy (specific monoclonal antibody agents).

Multiple Myeloma | Neoplastic excessive numbers of plasma cells proliferate in bone marrow that synthesize excessive abnormal Igs and Ig fragments. Excessive cytokine production causes deterioration of bone.

Signs and Symptoms	Physical Assessment Findings	Diagnostic Testing	Treatment
Infections due to immunosuppression. Fatigue, weakness, dizziness due to anemia. Thrombocytopenia leads to bleeding and bruising. Bone pain/decreased bone density particularly of vertebrae. Nerve pain, numbness, and tingling can occur if spinal nerve impingement occurs due to vertebral compression. Back and abdominal pain due to kidney stones.	Fever due to infection. Bruising and bleeding due to thrombocytopenia. Pallor, weakness due to anemia. Tenderness over involved bone; commonly vertebrae in lumbosacral area. Vertebral bone fracture common. Nerve impingement can cause weakness and sensory loss in an extremity. Costovertebral angle tenderness due to kidney stones.	CRAB criteria; calcium elevation, renal dysfunction, anemia, bone degeneration. CBC shows excessive WBCs. Lactate dehydrogenase and beta-2-microglobulin level (a biomarker of MM). PCR, FISH, flow cytometry. Cytogenetic testing demonstrates different genetic abnormalities including del 17 (gene deletion within chromosome 17) and t(4:14) and t(4:16) translocation of genes between chromosomes 4 and 14 and 4 and 16. Serum and urine electrophoresis. Bone marrow aspirate and biopsy shows excessive WBCs. Immunophenotyping for CD + 138. Elevated serum creatinine. Urine shows fragmented Igs called M-proteins or Bence Jones proteins. Hypercalciuria, myeloma casts, and proteinuria. CT, MRI, PET scans, echocardiogram.	Chemotherapy includes lenalidomide, bendamustine. Targeted therapy with proteasome inhibitor. Inhibitor of histone deacetylase; Panobinostat. Immunotherapy (monoclonal antibody) aimed at CD 38. Allogenic stem cell transplantation. Supportive treatments include bisphosphonates, denosumab, plasmapheresis, erythropoietin-stimulating agents, vaccines.

Bibliography

Available online at fadavis.com

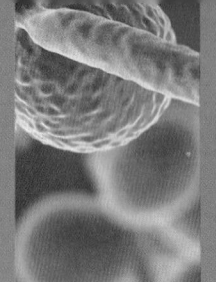

Red Blood Cell Disorders

Learning Objectives

Upon completion of this chapter, the student will be able to:

- Differentiate between normal red blood cell count, anemia, and polycythemia.
- Recognize the various etiologies of common types of anemia.
- Describe the mechanisms of common types of anemia.

- List the signs and symptoms of various causes of anemia.
- Identify the laboratory tests used in the diagnosis of anemia.
- Discuss the treatment of common types of anemia.

Key Terms

Agglutinogens
Alloimmune hemolysis
Anemia
Aplastic anemia
Cold agglutinin syndrome
Erythroblastosis fetalis
Erythrocytosis
Erythropoiesis
Erythropoietin (EPO)
Hematochezia

Hematopoiesis
Hemoglobinopathy
Hemolysis
Hemolytic disease of the newborn (HDN)
Hyperbilirubinemia
Intrinsic factor (IF)
Melena
Oxyhemoglobin dissociation curve
Pernicious anemia
Pica

Polycythemia
Reticulocyte
Reticulocytosis
Serum ferritin
Sickle cell anemia (SCA)
Subacute combined degeneration
Total iron binding capacity (TIBC)
Transferrin
Vaso-occlusive crisis
Warm agglutinin syndrome

The main function of the red blood cell (RBC), also called an erythrocyte or corpuscle, is to deliver oxygen to the body's tissues. It is solely designed to carry oxygen on its large hemoglobin (Hgb) molecule. The major pathophysiological condition involving RBCs is **anemia**, a condition in which there is insufficient delivery of oxygen to the tissues caused by an inadequate number of mature, healthy RBCs in the blood. Insufficient oxygen delivery to the tissues produces signs and symptoms related to cellular hypoxia and lack of cell energy.

Anemia has various causes, including blood loss, nutritional deficiencies, defective Hgb, bone marrow failure, and chronic disease. It is a common disorder that affects more than 3 million people in the United States across all age, ethnic, and racial groups. Although anemia occurs in both men and women, women of childbearing age are at higher risk than men. Older adults, especially those with chronic medical problems, are also at increased risk.

Another less common disorder of RBCs is **polycythemia**, a disorder characterized by overproliferation of all blood cells in the bone marrow.

Epidemiology

Anemia is the most common problem associated with RBCs. In the United States, approximately 6.6% of men and 12.4% of women have anemia. The prevalence of the disorder increases with age and is prevalent in 44.4% of men 85 years and older. In underdeveloped countries, prevalence of anemia is estimated to be two to five times greater than in the United States. Growing children in undeveloped countries commonly suffer from anemia.

Certain races and ethnic groups have an increased prevalence of genetic factors associated with particular anemias. For example, **sickle cell anemia (SCA)** is common in Africa, the Middle East, and the Mediterranean region. In areas of poor socioeconomic conditions, a deficient diet leads to an increased prevalence of anemia. For instance, iron-deficiency anemia is much more prevalent in countries where there is little meat in the diet. Anemia of chronic disease (ACD) is commonplace in populations with a high incidence of chronic infectious diseases, such as malaria, tuberculosis, and AIDS. Although most prominent in older individuals, anemia also occurs during infancy and adolescence. Growth spurts in adolescence predispose to anemia. Infants weaned from breast milk to cow's milk also are at risk.

Basic Concepts of Red Blood Cell Physiology

Hematopoiesis is the process by which all blood cells are formed in the bone marrow. The bone marrow is in a constant state of synthesis of RBCs, white blood cells (WBCs), and platelets. RBCs, the only cells that carry oxygen, have a life span of 120 days. Therefore, the body is constantly renewing the RBC supply.

Synthesis of Erythrocytes

Erythropoiesis is the specific series of steps in the bone marrow that leads to the synthesis of mature RBCs. All RBCs begin as pluripotent stem cells in the bone marrow that are stimulated to become erythroid precursor cells. Each precursor goes through a series of changes until it becomes a mature erythrocyte released by the bone marrow (see Fig. 13-1). The nucleus of the RBC is expelled in one of the last stages of erythropoiesis, which is why the RBC has no genetic material in its mature state.

The last stage of erythropoiesis involves formation of the **reticulocyte**, an immature RBC. Reticulocytes usually remain in the bone marrow until fully matured as RBCs. Normally, the reticulocyte count in the bloodstream is approximately 1%, reflecting the daily replacement of approximately 1% of the RBC population. However, when the bone marrow cannot synthesize enough RBCs to keep up with their loss, as in excessive blood loss or **hemolysis**, more reticulocytes are released into the circulation. The markedly higher percentage of reticulocytes in the bloodstream is called **reticulocytosis**. High numbers of reticulocytes in the bloodstream commonly indicate bleeding or brisk RBC destruction. Conversely, abnormally low numbers of reticulocytes occur in conditions of bone marrow suppression or other causes of poor RBC production.

Hypoxia is the major stimulus for erythropoiesis. The kidney senses hypoxia in the bloodstream and releases the hormone **erythropoietin (EPO)**, which stimulates the bone marrow. When stimulated by erythropoietin, the bone marrow synthesizes RBCs from stem cell erythroid precursors. The resulting increase in the number of RBCs reverses the hypoxia (see Fig. 13-2).

Substances needed for adequate synthesis of healthy RBCs include protein, iron, vitamin B_{12}, and folic acid (see Box 13.1). Iron is the main nutritional element needed for Hgb synthesis. Hgb is composed of a heme and globin compound. Heme is composed of iron (Fe^{++}) and a protein called porphyrin. Porphyrin is metabolized into a protein called biliverdin, a green-colored compound that colors bile, feces, and

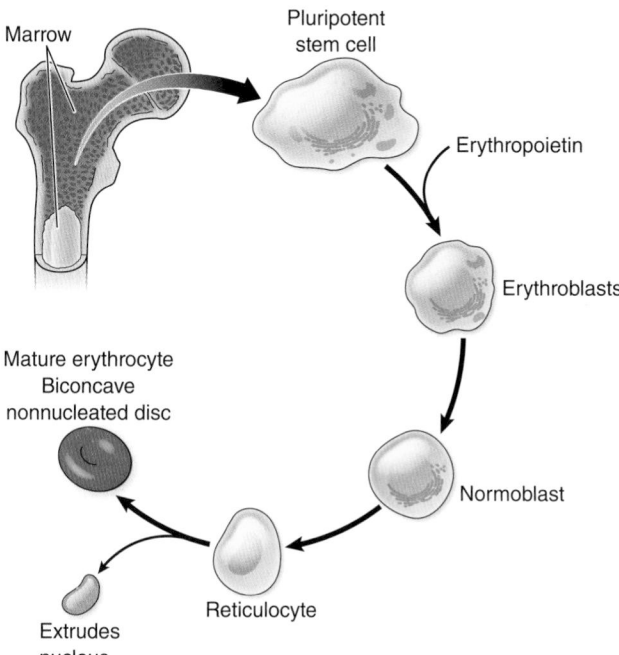

FIGURE 13-1. Erythropoiesis is the process of maturation of a pluripotent stem cell into mature erythrocytes in the bone marrow. Under the influence of EPO, the pluripotent stem cell in the bone marrow develops into a nucleated erythroblast and then into a normoblast. The normoblast extrudes its nucleus to become a reticulocyte and then fully matures into a nonnucleated erythrocyte.

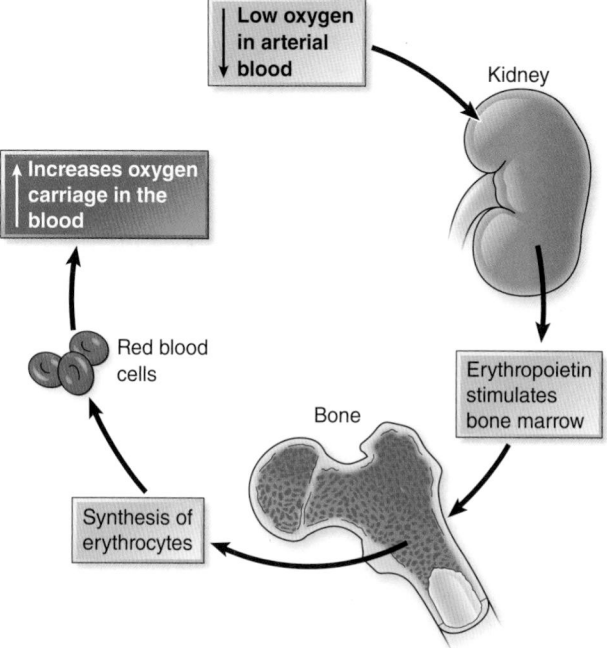

FIGURE 13-2. Synthesis of erythrocytes. The kidney releases the hormone erythropoietin (EPO) in response to hypoxia sensed in the bloodstream. EPO activates the bone marrow to synthesize erythrocytes. The extra erythrocytes raise the blood's oxygen-carrying ability; this is sensed by the kidney, which in turn shuts down EPO synthesis.

BOX 13-1. Constituents Needed for Healthy RBC Production

Protein
Iron
Vitamin B_{12}
Folic acid
Healthy bone marrow
Healthy kidney; erythropoietin

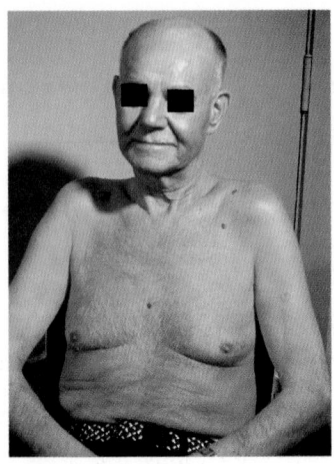

FIGURE 13-4. Person with jaundice.

ecchymoses. Biliverdin is further broken down into bilirubin, a yellow-colored compound that is a constituent of bile. In conditions where there is a high amount of breakdown of RBCs, bilirubin accumulates in the bloodstream, a condition called **hyperbilirubinemia** (see Fig. 13-3). Bilirubin adheres to elastin, a component of connective tissue contained in the skin and sclera of the eye. The skin and sclera take on an obvious yellow stain, resulting in a condition called jaundice (also called icterus) (see Fig. 13-4). Jaundice is often a sign of a high amount of RBC breakdown but can also occur in liver disorders.

🩺 CLINICAL CONCEPT

The number of reticulocytes is a good indicator of bone marrow activity, because it represents recent production of RBCs. A high reticulocyte count indicates that the bone marrow is working hard to keep up with RBC loss.

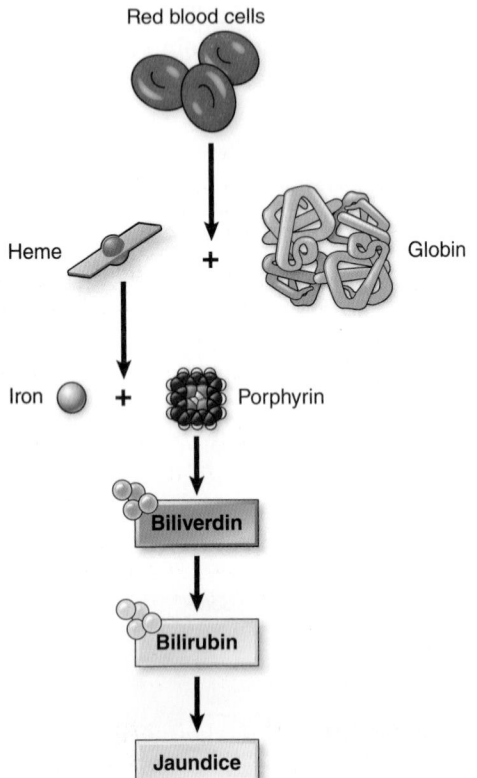

FIGURE 13-3. Hgb breakdown from erythrocytes. Hemoglobin breaks down into heme + globin. Heme further breaks down into iron (Fe^{++}) and porphyrin. Porphyrin breaks down into biliverdin, which is transformed into a yellow substance called bilirubin. High bilirubin levels in the bloodstream cause jaundice, which is a yellowish color obvious in the skin and sclera of the eyes. Therefore, a large amount of RBC breakdown (hemolysis) causes jaundice.

The Erythrocyte

The unique design of the erythrocyte produces efficient transport of oxygen. The lack of a nucleus allows more room for Hgb, which fills the erythrocyte and produces its red color. Erythrocytes are biconcave discs, providing a large surface area for diffusion (see Fig. 13-5). Erythrocytes are very flexible and easily change shape in order to pass through small capillaries. They have a limited life expectancy, generally lasting about 120 days. The spleen removes aged, lysed, and dead RBCs from circulation. In the spleen, RBCs are broken down into their component parts, which are recycled to make new red blood cells.

Approximately 95% of oxygen travels in the circulation attached to Hgb, whereas only 5% is directly dissolved in the plasma. Hgb also carries carbon dioxide away from tissues, but most carbon dioxide travels in the form of soluble bicarbonate (HCO_3^-) in the plasma.

🩺 CLINICAL CONCEPT

The spleen, a highly vascular organ, is the "graveyard of RBCs" and an organ of immunity. It sequesters abnormally shaped and hemolyzed RBCs and destroys them. Splenomegaly occurs when there is a large amount of RBC breakdown occurring in the body.

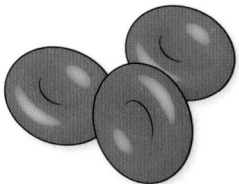

FIGURE 13-5. The RBC is a biconcave disk with no nucleus and is red in color.

Hemoglobin

The RBC carries oxygen because of the affinity of Hgb for oxygen. In adults, the Hgb molecule is composed of four polypeptide chains referred to as alpha 1, alpha 2, beta 1, and beta 2. Each chain has an atom of iron that can carry one oxygen atom, allowing for each Hgb molecule to carry four oxygen atoms (see Fig. 13-6). Oxygen attaches to Hgb in the pulmonary capillaries, and from there it is delivered to tissues. Hgb carries oxygen to cells and carries some carbon dioxide away from cells and back to pulmonary circulation. The synthesis of Hgb is greatly dependent on the availability of iron. A lack of iron results in small amounts of Hgb in each RBC and a resulting low amount of oxygen carriage in the blood.

Normal Hgb is called Hgb A. In the fetus until early infancy there is a specific kind of Hgb called Hgb F. Hgb F has four alpha chains and a very high affinity for oxygen. It can facilitate transfer of oxygen across the placenta. Hgb F is replaced by Hgb A by 6 months of age.

The formation of the four polypeptide chains that make up Hgb is directed by genes within the DNA of the early RBC. In disorders called hemoglobinopathies, Hgb structure is abnormal because of a genetic mutation. For example, in SCA, there is a mutation in one of the genes that directs the synthesis of the beta polypeptide chains. Within one of the beta chains there is

an abnormal substitution of the amino acid valine for glutamic acid. Because of this mutation, persons with SCA have a different Hgb called Hgb S.

Iron Metabolism

Iron is needed in the diet to synthesize Hgb in RBCs and myoglobin, a component of muscle cells. Cellular enzymes, used in various metabolic processes, also require iron for optimal function. Iron is absorbed primarily in the duodenum and upper jejunum. Some iron is sequestered within the intestinal cells, and some is released into the bloodstream. The epithelial intestinal cells are constantly sloughed and excreted, and with loss of the cells, there is loss of iron. When absorbed into the bloodstream from the gastrointestinal (GI) system, iron is transported by a protein called **transferrin**. Iron that is bound to transferrin and other sites in the body is represented within the measurement called **total iron binding capacity (TIBC)**.

Transferrin carries iron to the bone marrow for erythropoiesis. Membrane receptors on erythroid precursors in the bone marrow avidly bind transferrin. About 10% to 20% of absorbed iron goes into a storage pool in cells of the reticuloendothelial system, which is made up of the macrophages throughout the body. The storage of iron occurs in ferritin complexes that are present in all cells, but most commonly found in the bone marrow, liver, and spleen. The liver's stores of ferritin are the primary physiological source of reserve iron in the body.

The composition of the diet influences iron absorption. Citrate and vitamin C can form complexes with iron that increase absorption, whereas tannates in tea can decrease its absorption. The iron in heme found in meat is the most readily absorbed kind of iron. Iron homeostasis is closely regulated via intestinal absorption. Increased absorption is signaled by decreasing iron stores, hypoxia, inflammation, and erythropoietic activity (see Fig. 13-7).

Only a small fraction of the body's iron is gained or lost each day. Most of the iron in the body is recycled when old RBCs are taken out of circulation and destroyed. The RBC iron is scavenged by macrophages within the reticuloendothelial system and spleen and returned to the storage pool for reuse.

Oxyhemoglobin Dissociation

The sole purpose of the RBC is to transport oxygen from the pulmonary capillaries to the cells and carbon dioxide away from the cells back to the lungs. At high levels of arterial oxygen pressure (PO_2), Hgb has a strong affinity for oxygen and it is fully saturated. However, as PO_2 diminishes, Hgb sites for oxygen go unfilled, and Hgb becomes less attracted to oxygen. Hgb starts to drop all its oxygen as PO_2 falls below 60 mm Hg.

The **oxyhemoglobin dissociation curve** is an important tool for understanding how blood carries

Hemoglobin

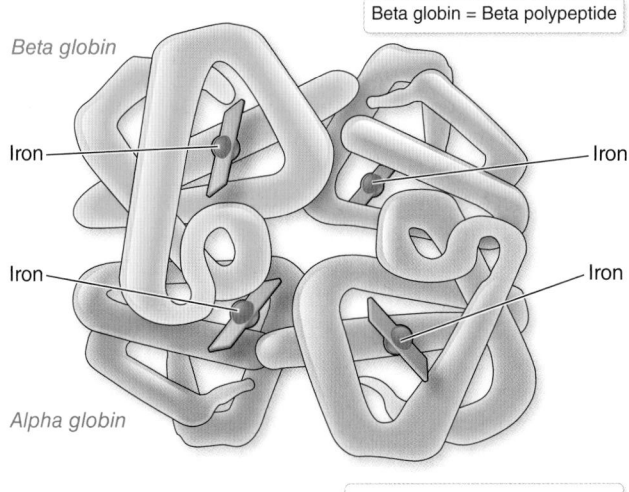

Beta globin = Beta polypeptide

Beta globin

Iron — — Iron

Iron — — Iron

Alpha globin

Alpha globin = Alpha polypeptide

FIGURE 13-6. Structure of Hgb. The Hgb molecule consists of two beta polypeptide chains and two alpha polypeptide chains. There are four iron atoms that bind to oxygen.

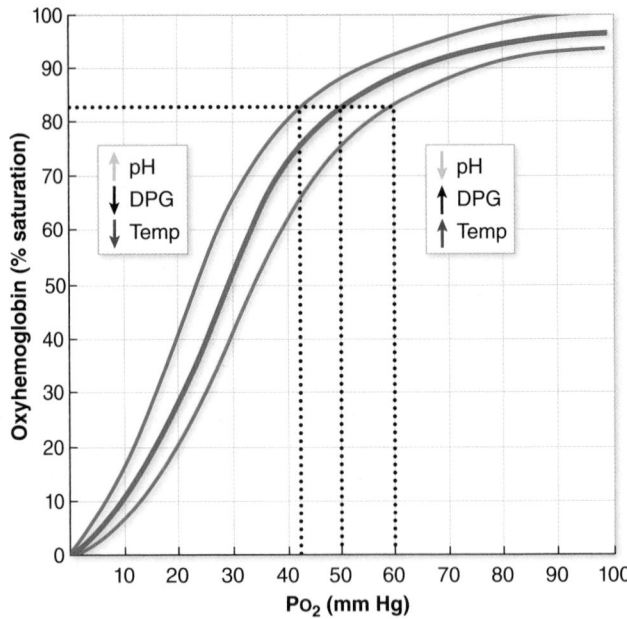

FIGURE 13-7. Normal iron absorption and metabolism. Iron is absorbed from the diet in the duodenum and jejunum. Only 10% of iron in the diet is absorbed, and it is in the intestinal epithelium until absorption into the bloodstream. Some of the intestinal epithelium is sloughed daily, and so some iron is lost in the feces daily. After absorption into the bloodstream, iron is carried by a protein called transferrin, which carries iron in the bloodstream to the bone marrow. In the bone marrow, iron is used for the synthesis of red blood cells. Iron is also delivered to the liver for storage as ferritin. Some iron is also used in cellular processes. As RBCs die, they are transported to the spleen for breakdown; the iron is absorbed back into the bloodstream and recycled in the body.

and releases oxygen (see Fig. 13-8). The oxyhemoglobin dissociation curve represents the relationship between Po_2 and the affinity of Hgb to oxygen. When Po_2 is 100 mm Hg, Hgb is totally saturated with oxygen atoms. This is the ideal and highest level of oxygen–hemoglobin affinity. However, at a Po_2 of approximately 60 mm Hg, Hgb affinity for oxygen dramatically falls and oxygen is given up to the tissues.

FIGURE 13-8. Oxygen–hemoglobin dissociation curve. The normal binding of Hgb to oxygen (O_2) is depicted in blue. Normally, when the partial pressure of oxygen (Po_2) in blood is 100 mm Hg, there is great affinity of Hgb for oxygen and great saturation. At approximately Po_2 60 mm Hg there is a dramatic drop in affinity of Hgb for oxygen (blue). In fever, high carbon dioxide, acidosis, and high DPG, there is less affinity of Hgb for O_2 and less saturation (red). In alkalosis, hypothermia, and low DPG, there is greater affinity of Hgb for O_2 and greater saturation (green).

Some conditions decrease or increase affinity of Hgb for oxygen. An increase of carbon dioxide in the blood, fever, increased 2,3 diphosphoglycerate (2,3 DPG), and a decrease in pH (acidosis) result in a reduction of the affinity of Hgb for oxygen. These conditions shift the sigmoid-shaped oxy–Hgb dissociation curve to the right, showing less affinity of Hgb for oxygen. Because Hgb has less affinity, it gives up oxygen to the tissues easily. Conversely, an increase of pH in the blood (alkalosis), decreased 2,3 DPG, and hypothermia increase Hgb affinity for oxygen. These conditions shift the oxy–Hgb dissociation curve to the left, showing greater affinity of Hgb for oxygen. Oxygen is held by Hgb more tightly than normal and less is given up to the tissues.

The effect of pH on Hgb's ability to bind oxygen is called the Bohr effect. When pH is low (acidosis), Hgb binds oxygen less strongly, and when pH is high (alkalosis), Hgb binds more tightly to oxygen. Because of the Bohr effect, Hgb gives up oxygen to tissue easily during low pH. Alternatively, the Haldane effect occurs when oxygen is high in concentration in the bloodstream and it saturates Hgb sites. Hgb binds oxygen tightly, and O_2 displaces carbon dioxide from Hgb. In deoxygenated blood, Hgb has free sites for binding to carbon dioxide.

2,3 DPG is an organic phosphate bound to Hgb in RBCs. It is a by-product of the breakdown of glycogen to glucose. It reduces the affinity of Hgb for oxygen, shifting the oxygen dissociation curve to the right and thereby assisting the unloading of oxygen to tissues.

CLINICAL CONCEPT

Oxygen delivery to tissues is affected by both oxy–Hgb saturation and the amount of Hgb in the blood. If the oxygen saturation is 100% and Hgb level is normal, oxygen delivery to the tissues is ideal. However, if oxygen saturation of blood is 100% and Hgb is low (as in anemia), oxygen delivery will be inadequate and cellular hypoxia will result.

ALERT! Hgb has greater affinity for carbon monoxide (CO) compared with oxygen. If there are high levels of CO in the environment, oxygen will be displaced off Hgb sites and hemoglobin will be saturated with CO. This deoxygenated state is often fatal.

Blood Types

All body cells, including RBCs, contain surface antigens. Specific types of antigens on the surface of RBCs are called **agglutinogens**. There are two different types of agglutinogens: type A and type B. The ABO blood type classification system categorizes blood into four types according to these agglutinogens: types A, B, AB, and O.

Another antigen on the surface of RBCs is Rh factor, also called D antigen. If the RBC surface has the Rh factor, it is categorized as positive (Rh+); if it does not have the Rh factor, it is called negative (Rh–). All blood types are either Rh+ or Rh–. Individuals inherit their blood type from their parents. The A and B antigens are encoded by different alleles, one from the mother and the other from the father. A gene called the O allele codes for a nonfunctional protein that does not produce surface molecules. The person with O blood has no antigens on their RBCs. The possible combinations of alleles that can yield the blood type of offspring can be configured with a Punnett square (see Fig. 13-9).

Individuals develop antibodies to blood antigens that are not the same as their own. For example, a person with type A blood has antibodies against type B blood called anti-B antibodies. A person with type O blood has no antigens on the surface of their RBCs; however, they have both anti-A and anti-B antibodies (see Table 13-1).

The ABO system is the blood-group system used to categorize human blood, mainly for the purpose of blood transfusion. If a person receives blood from a donor that is a different type than their own, antibodies attack the infused RBCs and cause a transfusion reaction that involves hemolysis. For example, if a person with type A blood receives a type B blood

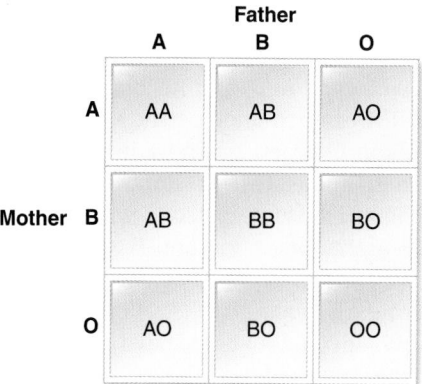

FIGURE 13-9. Punnett square for inheritance of blood types.

transfusion, the anti-B antibodies of the recipient will attack the type B RBCs of the donor blood. The person with type O negative blood can donate blood to persons with any type of blood because they have no surface antigens on their RBCs. Individuals with type AB positive blood can accept any kind of foreign blood because they do not have antibodies.

CLINICAL CONCEPT

A person with type O negative blood is known as a universal donor, whereas a person with AB positive blood is known as a universal recipient.

Basic Concepts of Red Blood Cell Pathophysiology

Anemia is the most common disorder that affects RBCs. Oxygen delivery to the tissues is inadequate either because of deficient Hgb, abnormal Hgb, or a low number of RBCs. Polycythemia, the opposite kind of disorder, is a condition of too many RBCs in circulation.

Anemia

Anemia is the major pathophysiological condition affecting RBCs. It can be defined as a decreased RBC mass that becomes clinically apparent when levels of Hgb and hematocrit (Hct) are less than normal. A complete blood count (CBC) measures all RBCs and RBC characteristics. Different types of anemia produce different CBC results.

CLINICAL CONCEPT

The World Health Organization defines anemia as an Hgb level lower than 13 g/dL in men and lower than 12 g/dL in women.

TABLE 13-1. Blood Types and Antibodies

Persons with type A, B, and AB blood have antigens on their RBC surface and specific antibodies in their plasma. Type O blood has no antigens on the RBC surface and stimulates no antibody formation in the recipient. However, persons with type O blood have anti-A antibodies and anti-B antibodies in their plasma. Therefore, type O persons cannot receive type A or type B blood.

Persons with type AB blood have both A and B antigens on the surface of the RBCs and have no antibodies in their plasma.

Blood cells are also categorized according to an Rh factor; some blood cells are Rh-positive, which means they have a D antigen on their surface. Rh-negative blood cells have no D antigen on their surface. Persons with Rh-positive blood have no antibodies in their plasma. Rh-positive blood cells can stimulate an antibody reaction in the recipient of this blood.

A transfusion will work if a person who is going to receive blood has a blood group that doesn't have any antibodies against the donor blood's antigens. If a person who is going to receive blood has antibodies against the donor blood's antigens, the red blood cells in the donated blood will agglutinate.

Example 1: Type O negative blood can be given to all persons because there are no antigens on the blood cells, so the recipient will not build antibodies against any antigen. However, only type O negative blood can be given to type O negative recipients because O negative persons have anti-A and anti-B antibodies and Rh antibodies.

Example 2: Type A blood individuals cannot give blood to type B recipients because the recipient has anti-A antibodies. Type B blood individuals cannot give blood to type A recipients because the recipient has anti-B antibodies.

Blood Type	Antibody
A	Anti-B antibody
B	Anti-A antibody
AB (both surface antigens)	No antibodies
O (no surface antigens)	Anti-A antibody, anti-B antibody
Rh-negative (no surface D antigen)	Anti-Rh antibody
Rh-positive (D antigen)	No Rh antibodies

Complete Blood Count

The CBC is one of the basic diagnostic procedures used when investigating any disorder in the body. The CBC includes Hgb, Hct, a number of RBCs, mean corpuscular volume (MCV), mean corpuscular hemoglobin (MCH),

and MCH concentration (MCHC) (see Table 13-2). It can be ordered as a CBC with differential when the measure of WBCs is also needed.

Hemoglobin

Hgb is a direct measure of the amount of Hgb in a given volume of blood. Normal values differ for men and women. The normal range for men is 13 to 18 gm/dL, whereas the normal range for women is 12 to 16 gm/dL. Females and African American males usually have levels 1 to 2 g lower than European American males. Women have lower Hgb and Hct than men because of monthly menstrual blood loss. Men have higher Hgb also because testosterone enhances erythropoiesis. Persons who live at high altitudes normally have higher Hgb and Hct because their environment naturally has lower oxygen concentration. The low oxygen in their bloodstream constantly stimulates renal erythropoietin (EPO), which in turn, stimulates the bone marrow to synthesize RBCs. A high number of RBCs is called secondary polycythemia or erythrocytosis.

Hematocrit

Hct is the percentage of blood that consists of RBCs. The normal range for men is 45% to 52%, whereas the normal range for women is 37% to 48%.

Total Red Blood Cell Count

Total RBC count is a measure of the number of RBCs in a given volume of blood. This value is usually between 4.5 and 5.5×10^6 cells per cubic millimeter for males and 4.0 to 4.9×10^6 cells per cubic millimeter for females.

Mean Corpuscular Volume

MCV is the volume of one RBC or corpuscle. This value reflects red blood cell size as seen under the microscope. It is used to classify the anemia as either microcytic, megaloblastic (also called macrocytic), or normocytic. The normal value of MCV is 80 to 100 femtoliters.

 CLINICAL CONCEPT

Microcytic cells are smaller than normal, megaloblastic cells are larger than normal, and normocytic cells are normal size.

Mean Corpuscular Hemoglobin and Mean Corpuscular Hemoglobin Concentration

MCH is the average amount of Hgb in an average RBC. Normal MCH is 27 to 32 picograms. MCHC is the average concentration of Hgb in a given volume of RBCs. The normal range is 32% to 36%.

TABLE 13-2. CBC Normal Values*

Parameter	Definition	Normal Levels
Total red blood cells × 106	Number of RBCs per liter	Males: 4.5 to 5.5
		Females: 4.0 to 4.9
Hemoglobin (Hgb)	Amount of Hgb in blood g/dL	Males: 13 to 18
		Females: 12 to 16
Hematocrit (Hct)	Packed RBC volume; fraction of the whole blood that consists of RBC	45% to 52% males, 37% to 48% females
Mean corpuscular volume (MCV)	Size of the RBC	80 to 100
Mean corpuscular hemoglobin (MCH)	Mass of the RBC	27 to 32
Mean corpuscular hemoglobin concentration (MCHC)	Concentration of Hgb (color)	32% to 36%
RBC distribution width	Measures the variation in RBC size and shape	11 to 15
Platelets	Cells that assist clotting	90,000 to 450,000
Reticulocytes	Immature RBCs	1%

*Different laboratories have minor differences in normal values.

 CLINICAL CONCEPT

MCH and MCHC can be used to indicate the color of the RBCs. A low value for either indicates that cells are pale or hypochromic.

In anemia, when MCV is normal and MCHC is normal, size and color of the RBCs are normal. This is characterized as a normocytic normochromic (NCNC) anemia. The most common cause of NCNC anemia is blood loss, as the lack of RBC mass and low Hgb and Hct occur because there is a deficient number of RBCs.

When MCV and MCHC are both decreased, the size and color of the RBCs are abnormal. A low MCV indicates small size of RBCs, and a low MCHC indicates a pale color of RBCs. This is categorized as microcytic hypochromic anemia. This most commonly occurs with iron deficiency.

When MCV is high, the RBCs are abnormally large; this is also referred to as megaloblastic or macrocytic anemia. This most commonly occurs in vitamin B_{12} and folic acid deficiency.

Red Blood Cell Distribution

RBC distribution width (RDW) measures the variation in RBC size and width.

Platelets

Platelets are the blood cells that cause clotting of the blood. If the total amount of platelets is too low, bleeding or bruising can occur; if it is too high, clotting can occur. The normal value is 90,000 to 450,000 platelets per microliter of blood.

Reticulocyte Count

Reticulocyte count measures the number of new RBCs in the blood and helps determine whether the bone marrow is producing new red blood cells at an appropriate rate. Increased reticulocyte numbers associated with anemia suggest accelerated destruction or loss of RBCs. Normal reticulocyte count is approximately 1% of total RBCs.

Basic Pathophysiological Concepts Related to Anemia

There are various possible etiologies for anemia. The physiological response to anemia varies according to the etiology and rate of onset. With anemia caused by acute blood loss, a sudden reduction in oxygen-carrying capacity occurs, along with a rapid decrease in intravascular volume, with resultant hypoxia and hypovolemia. Hypovolemia will trigger baroreceptors and the activity of the sympathetic nervous system. The heart will beat faster in an attempt to accomplish greater blood oxygenation. Also, the renin–angiotensin–aldosterone system (RAAS) is provoked to remedy the hypovolemia and hypotension. The RAAS raises blood pressure, and volume of the bloodstream increases. The hypoxia in the bloodstream stimulates the kidney to release erythropoietin, which stimulates the bone marrow to synthesize more RBCs. Acute blood loss incites emergency responses by the body.

In chronic blood loss, the body loses RBCs slowly over a long period. The blood volume lost may not be perceptible by the patient, and the small blood volume lost is not the main problem, as the body can replace it. However, the body is unable to synthesize healthy RBCs, which requires iron, vitamin B_{12}, and folic acid. The stores of these nutrients slowly become exhausted because of loss of the blood's nutrients. In other words, the RBCs are slowly, constantly lost, along with the iron, vitamin B_{12}, and folic acid that they contain. Normally, after the RBC's death, the components are recycled in the spleen. In chronic blood loss, however, there is no recycling; the RBCs produced by the bone marrow become deficient in these nutrients. The RBCs become particularly iron deficient because iron stores become exhausted more quickly than stores of vitamin B_{12} and folic acid. Iron-poor RBCs cannot carry oxygen required by the tissue. Tissue hypoxia results, which can cause ischemia of the heart muscle and weakening of peripheral musculature. Cerebral hypoxia occurs, and organs become dysfunctional because of the lack of tissue oxygenation. A similar process of dysfunctional erythropoiesis occurs when anemia is caused by vitamin B_{12} or folic acid deficiency.

With hemolytic anemias, the RBCs are destroyed prematurely and dead RBCs accumulate in the spleen, causing splenomegaly. The circulation contains fewer RBCs and less oxygen delivery occurs, resulting in diminished tissue oxygenation.

Diagnosis of Anemia

A thorough history and physical examination are needed to diagnose anemia. Commonly, anemia causes subtle symptoms, and the patient may be unaware of the disorder. In addition, physical findings can be understated. Incidental findings on a laboratory test are often the way individuals discover that they have anemia.

History

Asymptomatic anemia is common, as it usually occurs gradually over a long period without an obvious initiating event. Patients may complain of fatigue and being generally run down. The patient's medication list should be reviewed because some drugs can cause hemolytic anemia, folic acid deficiency, or bone marrow suppression. It is important to ask about diet and nutritional intake, especially in older patients, where lack of adequate diet and impaired absorption play a role in the development of anemia.

The GI tract is a common site for slow blood loss, and it is important to ask about the appearance of the stool, especially the color, and any history of stomach or intestinal disorders, such as gastric ulcers or inflammatory bowel disease, which can produce bleeding. Black tarry stools, also called **melena**, contain blood from GI bleeding. **Hematochezia** is the passage of red blood via the anus or within the stool.

In women of childbearing age, it is important to ask about menstrual periods and any history of uterine problems. Menorrhagia, or excess menstrual blood loss, often goes unreported and is a common cause of iron-deficiency anemia. The date of the last menstrual period is important because ectopic pregnancy or spontaneous abortion can cause acute blood loss.

Past medical history is important, as certain diseases such as kidney problems or chronic disorders can cause anemia. Some infections, such as infectious mononucleosis, mycoplasma, and malaria, predispose to anemia. Family history is important, as certain anemias such as sickle cell anemia, hereditary spherocytosis, and thalassemia are inherited disorders. Social habits should be investigated, as lifestyle factors such as alcohol misuse can lead to anemia.

Signs and Symptoms

The appearance and severity of symptoms depend on whether the anemia developed rapidly or slowly. Symptoms of anemia are frequently overlooked by the patient and attributed to tiredness. For a list of the common symptoms associated with all anemias, see Box 13-2.

Physical Examination

The vital signs in anemia may reveal tachypnea and tachycardia. The patient's complexion may be pale, as also may be the conjunctiva of the eye, nailbeds, creases in the palm of the hand, and the buccal mucosa. Persons with hemolytic anemia may exhibit jaundice. Jaundice is best observed in the sclera of the eyes in dark-skinned persons. Splenomegaly is a sign that the spleen is hyperactive, which would occur in hemolytic anemia.

BOX 13-2. Common Signs and Symptoms of Anemia

Different types of anemia have distinctive symptoms. However, the signs and symptoms common to all types of anemia include:
- Pallor of skin, conjunctiva, nailbeds, and buccal mucosa
- Excessive fatigue
- Weakness
- Shortness of breath, especially with activity
- Exercise intolerance
- Palpitations (tachycardia)
- Chest pain
- Dizziness or feeling faint
- Headache
- Nutritional anemias can cause glossitis, cheilitis, koilonychia, or pica

Some types of chronic anemia cause hair loss, koilonychia, cheilitis, and glossitis. Koilonychia is an abnormal spoon shape of the nails. Cheilitis is presence of fissured sores on the corners of the mouth. Glossitis is a smooth, swollen red tongue.

Diagnostic Tests

The diagnostic tests used in the investigation of all anemias are the CBC, discussed earlier in the chapter, and the peripheral blood smear, which allows microscopic visualization of blood cells, including their size, shape, color, coating, and any abnormal fragments or cellular material. If anemia is difficult to diagnose, a bone marrow aspiration or biopsy is performed. The bone marrow is usually taken from the hip bone and examined for abnormalities such as signs of neoplastic disease.

A cardiovascular examination is needed with anemia. Echocardiogram and electrocardiogram (ECG) are needed to assess cardiovascular health. Additional diagnostic tests are indicated based on the type of anemia. For more specific diagnostic studies, see each type of anemia.

Treatment

There are many different treatments because there are a wide range of causes of anemia. In anemia caused by blood loss, transfusion may be the only treatment. For treatment of specific anemias, see their respective sections.

Pathophysiology of Selected Red Blood Cell Disorders

Different types of anemia can be categorized according to etiology. Anemia caused by decreased RBC mass includes acute and chronic blood loss and RBC loss caused by hemolysis. Anemia can also be caused by lack of sufficient RBC synthesis. Iron, vitamin B_{12}, and folic acid deficiencies cause insufficient synthesis of RBCs. Hemoglobinopathies cause anemia because of abnormal Hgb structure, which causes deficient oxygen carriage. Hemolysis can be caused by hemoglobinopathy, medication side effects, transfusion reaction, and autoimmune reactions against RBCs.

Anemias Caused by a Decrease in RBC Mass

A decrease in RBC mass can occur mainly through acute blood loss, chronic blood loss, or hemolysis. The adult has a total blood volume of approximately 5 liters and can usually lose 500 mL of blood without serious or lasting effects. However, if the loss reaches 1,000 mL or more, serious adverse effects such as hypovolemic shock

and cerebral hypoperfusion can occur. Blood loss can be acute or chronic, and hemolysis can be mild or severe.

Anemia of Acute Blood Loss

Anemia of acute blood loss is a precipitous drop in the RBC population caused by hemorrhage. Trauma is the most common cause of acute hemorrhage. Acute anemia can also result from significant acute internal blood loss into the thoracic and abdominal cavities caused by rupture of an artery or an organ. Older adults and children are at highest risk of death from acute external blood loss because of less resilience. There are many different traumatic causes of anemia caused by blood loss; incidence depends on the etiology.

Risk Factors

Recent trauma is the major risk factor for acute blood loss, and the blood loss can be either overt or occult. Abdominal trauma predisposes to rupture of the spleen, a highly vascular organ. Head trauma can predispose to epidural or subdural hematoma, which is blood loss between the layers of meninges in the cranium. History of aortic aneurysm can predispose to rupture of the aorta. Anticoagulants increase the risk of blood loss because of the prolonged clotting time of the blood. History of hematological neoplasms increases the risk of bleeding because of lack of platelets. A family history of hereditary blood disorders that cause bleeding such as von Willebrand's disease or hemophilia increases risk. Alcohol use disorder can cause formation of esophageal varices, which are fragile and cause acute blood loss. In females, acute blood loss can occur during pregnancy, particularly early when the patient may not be aware of the pregnancy. Ectopic pregnancy and spontaneous abortion, also called miscarriage, are common causes of acute blood loss.

Etiology

Acute blood loss is a rapid loss of blood as in hemorrhage caused by trauma, childbirth, or rupture of a major blood vessel or organ. Severe GI bleeding can occur in disorders such as esophageal varices or penetrating peptic ulcer.

Pathophysiology

In acute blood loss, large numbers of blood cells and plasma volume are lost. It is a rapid development of an NCNC anemia because cells are normal in size and color but deficient in number. The lack of a sufficient number of RBCs to carry oxygen causes tissue hypoxia. The severity of the signs and symptoms of NCNC anemia depends on the amount of blood loss. When Hgb falls below 12 g/L, erythropoiesis is activated and the bone marrow starts to synthesize RBCs. With acute hemorrhage, the loss of RBCs can be too fast for the bone marrow to replace them with mature RBCs, so reticulocytes are released into the bloodstream. Reticulocytosis and other compensatory mechanisms are activated. Because of the fluid lost from the bloodstream, there is compensatory stimulation of the sympathetic nervous system, systemic arterial vasoconstriction, fluid shift from tissues into the capillaries, stimulation of the RAAS, and antidiuretic hormone (ADH) release. These mechanisms attempt to diminish the effect of the lost blood volume, and they all act to increase fluid volume in the bloodstream. The increase in fluid volume within the bloodstream can result in hemodilution. Hemodilution of the circulating blood is exhibited by a decrease in Hct.

Clinical Presentation

A thorough history and physical examination are needed in acute blood loss. If trauma is the etiology, the patient often is not able to give the history. Clinicians must use physical assessment skills to assess bleeding source and volume lost. If the patient is able to give a history, there are specific questions to ask in regard to possible causes of acute blood loss.

History

If there is obvious trauma, the patient should be asked about the incidents that led to the trauma. This can give the clinician specific guidance for the physical examination. With acute blood loss, time is of the essence, and finding the source of bleeding is a priority. The manner in which the trauma occurred can give clues as to the presence of internal bleeding.

If the patient is not in an acute state of traumatic blood loss, more detailed questions can be asked. The patient should be asked about current medications. Often the medication list can give the clinician clues as to what is causing the acute blood loss. It is important to ask about use of aspirin, NSAIDs, or corticosteroids. When used long term, these drugs are common causes of GI ulceration and bleeding. Past medical history can give information about risk factors for bleeding. For example, does the patient have a history of hematological malignancy or clotting disorder? Is the patient on anticoagulant medications? Social habits are also important, as these can cause increased risk of bleeding. For example, alcohol use disorder can lead to bleeding from esophageal varices.

> ALERT! Chronic use of aspirin, NSAIDs, or corticosteroids can cause GI ulceration with bleeding.

Signs and Symptoms

Signs and symptoms seen with acute blood loss depend on the volume lost:

- Loss of less than 15% of total blood volume causes orthostatic hypotension and anxiety.
- Loss of 15% to 30% of total blood volume results in the activation of compensatory mechanisms designed to increase blood volume and oxygen delivery to vital organs. Baroreceptors in the arteries sense a drop in blood pressure (BP) and stimulate the sympathetic nervous system to increase heart rate and vasoconstrict arteries. The kidney senses the low volume of blood and releases renin, which kicks off the RAAS. Water is conserved by ADH, which decreases urine output to fewer than 30 mL/hr. Restlessness and changes in level of consciousness occur as perfusion of the brain is decreased.
- Loss of 30% to 40% of total volume results in worsening of the previous signs, with tachycardia above 120 beats per minute; weak, rapid pulse associated with the loss of Hgb and plasma volume; cool, pale skin; hypotension; and urine output of 5 to 15 mL/hr.
- Loss greater than 40% of total volume causes profound shock (severe hypotension) with confusion and decreased level of consciousness, heart rate above 140 beats per minute, scant or no urine output, and profound hypotension. Shock can reach an irreversible stage when compensatory mechanisms become exhausted.

Vital signs in acute blood loss include hypotension, tachycardia, and tachypnea. Pallor; cool, clammy skin; and loss of consciousness develop as bleeding worsens. If bleeding is apparent, then a complete examination of the region of trauma is needed. If bleeding is occult, a complete physical examination is necessary to rule out internal bleeding. The left upper quadrant of the abdomen should be palpated to assess the spleen, as splenic rupture is often the source of bleeding caused by abdominal trauma. In head trauma, the clinician should rule out epidural and subdural hematoma, as these are sources of occult bleeding. Patients with severe GI bleeding will vomit blood or excrete blood in the stool. Patients with blood loss require a thorough chest, abdomen, and pelvic examination. Digital rectal examination with fecal occult blood test (FOBT) can detect signs of GI bleeding.

> ALERT! When rapid bleeding is overt or suspected, danger signs include hypotension, heart rate above 110 bpm, complaints of thirst, and urine output of less than 30 mL/hr.

CLINICAL CONCEPT

Patients bleeding because of esophageal varices often exhibit a large loss of blood via vomiting, which is referred to as hematemesis. Blood mixed with stomach acid and mucus in vomitus is referred to as "coffee ground" emesis. Patients losing large amounts of blood via the rectum exhibit hematochezia, which is bright red blood in the stool.

Diagnosis

Hemorrhage that is overt or occult will cause a rapid NCNC anemia with reticulocytosis (high reticulocyte count) on a CBC. Platelet count should be reviewed on the CBC to assess clotting ability. Blood pressure may be in the hypotensive range of less than 100 mm Hg systolic. In cases where acute blood loss is occult, reticulocytosis is an important diagnostic sign indicating the bone marrow is rapidly generating RBCs to replace those lost. Blood chemistry studies, serum creatinine, and arterial blood gases (ABGs) are important because acute blood loss can cause abnormalities in these values. The patient should have an FOBT to investigate the possibility of bleeding from the GI tract. A pregnancy test should be performed on women of childbearing age. The patient should have laboratory testing for blood type and crossmatching in case of the need for transfusion. A computed tomography (CT) scan of the abdomen and pelvis can assist with recognition of occult internal bleeding. If the patient has head trauma or is unconscious, a CT scan of the head is important.

Treatment

Immediate treatment includes establishing hemostasis, restoring blood volume, and treating shock. An IV normal saline solution should be infused until a matching blood product can be infused. Transfusion is currently the only reliable way to restore blood volume and oxygen-carrying capacity. If blood is not immediately available, plasma is the most suitable substitute. If the amount of blood lost is not large, erythropoiesis will restore normal volume and Hgb over time. After the patient is stabilized, endoscopy and colonoscopy should be done to investigate GI bleeding.

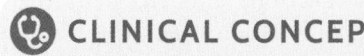 **CLINICAL CONCEPT**

Reticulocytosis indicates that the bone marrow is synthesizing a large number of RBCs, usually because of rapid blood loss. Mature RBCS are being lost faster than the bone marrow can supply them.

Anemia of Chronic Blood Loss

Anemia of chronic blood loss occurs when the patient endures a slow, gradual blood loss via the GI tract or excessive monthly menstrual loss. Alternatively, there may be hemolysis of blood cells, which slowly diminishes blood cell mass. Chronic blood loss is usually subtle and asymptomatic.

The incidence of anemia caused by chronic blood loss depends on the underlying cause. Approximately 100,000 patients are admitted to U.S. hospitals annually for upper GI bleeding, of which peptic ulcer is a common cause. Lower GI bleeding accounts for approximately 20% to 33% of episodes of GI bleeding,

with an annual incidence of about 20 to 27 cases per 100,000 population in Western countries. Colon cancer is a common cause of lower GI bleeding.

Excessive monthly menstrual blood loss, known as menorrhagia, is another common cause of chronic blood loss. Menorrhagia affects nearly 2 million women each year in the United States. Heavy menstrual bleeding has been reported in approximately 10% to 15% of all women at some point during their life. Among these women, as many as 20% will go on to develop anemia.

Risk Factors

Risk factors for chronic blood loss include GI disorders such as gastric ulceration, inflammatory bowel disease, and colon cancer. The chronic use of aspirin or NSAIDs can predispose individuals to gastric ulceration and slow bleeding. In females, chronic blood loss commonly occurs because of menorrhagia; large losses of menstrual blood monthly can lead to anemia.

Pathophysiology

The major problem that arises with chronic blood loss is iron-deficiency anemia. The RBCs are the largest iron depot in the body. When RBCs are lost, iron is lost and not recycled in the body. Slow loss of RBCs gradually depletes the body's iron stores.

Clinical Presentation

In chronic blood loss, patients may not complain of symptoms, which then requires investigation into possible unrecognized problems. It is important to obtain a list of medications. The patient may not be aware of overuse of aspirin and NSAIDs that can lead to gastric ulceration. The patient may report use of over-the-counter antacids, proton pump inhibitors such as lansoprazole (Prilosec), or acid suppressants such as ranitidine (Zantac). Frequent use of these medications can indicate the patient is attempting to treat gastric ulceration.

History

The patient should be asked about dark stools (melena), as these can indicate GI blood loss. Past medical and surgical history is important, especially regarding GI problems. Women may report episodes of excessive menstrual bleeding. The patient should also be questioned about the last menstrual period to investigate the possibility of pregnancy. Social habits such as smoking, caffeine, and alcohol use are important because these are risk factors for development of gastric ulcer. Chronic alcohol misuse can lead to bleeding from esophageal varices.

Signs and Symptoms

Signs and symptoms of anemia such as pallor, weakness, exercise intolerance, and fatigue may not develop in an obvious manner. The patient is usually not aware of the slow decrease in Hgb and Hct. Also, physical signs and symptoms are not as dramatic as in acute blood loss. GI symptoms may be present, such as those of esophagitis and gastric ulceration. Gastric ulcer symptoms include epigastric burning and a gnawing pain that occurs between meals. The patient may have melena. Women may not have apparent signs of excessive menstrual blood loss and should be questioned about this. Soaking through one menstrual pad or one tampon per hour is usually indicative of menorrhagia. Alternatively, a menstrual period that lasts longer than 1 week can be indicative of menorrhagia.

 CLINICAL CONCEPT

In chronic, slow blood loss, the physical examination is often unremarkable. Alternatively, the patient may show general signs of anemia such as pallor, tachycardia, and tachypnea.

Diagnosis

In chronic blood loss, the CBC commonly demonstrates MCHC anemia. The slow bleeding gradually depletes Hgb, Hct, and iron stores. Iron deficiency anemia is commonly caused by slow, chronic GI blood loss. Therefore, blood tests should include serum Fe^{++}, **serum ferritin**, TIBC, and serum transferrin. Blood chemistry, serum creatinine, and liver function tests should be done. An endoscopy can view disorders in the upper GI tract such as bleeding ulcer. A colonoscopy can examine any disorders of the lower GI tract such as inflammatory bowel disease, polyps, or colon cancer. An FOBT is important to investigate GI bleeding that is exhibited in the stool. In women of childbearing age, a pregnancy test is necessary. Women may require an abdominal or pelvic image study as well.

Treatment

For chronic blood loss, treatment consists of remedying the source of bleeding. The patient may need gastric ulcer medications or inflammatory bowel treatment. If the patient has a severe GI ulceration, polyp, or colon cancer, a gastroenterologist and surgeon should be consulted. A colonoscopy is commonly indicated if GI blood loss is suspected. For women with probable excessive menstrual blood loss, a gynecologist should be consulted. Commonly, the patient needs iron replacement treatment; usually, oral ferrous sulfate or intramuscular iron administration is sufficient to rebuild the Hgb and Hct. In rare cases, the person with chronic blood loss requires blood transfusion. When Hgb falls below 7 g/dL, transfusion is commonly considered.

Hemolytic Anemia

Hemolysis, another cause of decreased RBC mass, can occur because of various disorders, including hemoglobinopathies, medication side effects, autoimmune disorders, hereditary spherocytosis, blood transfusion reactions, and **hemolytic disease of the newborn (HDN)**. They represent 5% of all anemias.

Hemolytic anemias can be categorized as acute or chronic and intravascular or extravascular. Intravascular hemolytic anemia occurs within the circulating blood. Extravascular hemolytic anemia occurs because of splenic destruction of the RBCs, RBC lysis in the reticuloendothelial system, or mechanical destruction as in prosthetic valve damage of RBCs.

 CLINICAL CONCEPT

Drugs that are known to trigger hemolytic anemia include cephalosporins, quinidine, penicillins, levodopa, methyldopa, and NSAIDs.

Hemolytic anemia occurs when erythrocyte destruction outpaces RBC synthesis by the bone marrow. When RBC destruction occurs in autoimmune disorders, the body's immune system acts as though the RBCs are antigens and produces antibodies against them. This most often occurs in systemic autoimmune problems such as systemic lupus erythematosus or vasculitis. If the antibody causing the destruction of the RBCs is of the IgG class, the hemolysis will occur at any temperature, which is called **warm agglutinin syndrome**. If the antibody against the RBCs is of the IgM class, this is called **cold agglutinin syndrome**, in which hemolysis occurs at low temperatures. There are also drugs that are known to produce hemolytic anemia, which disappears when the drug is withdrawn.

Alloimmune hemolysis occurs when antibodies are formed against antigens on the RBC surface. This occurs in transfusion reactions and HDN. In HDN, the mother forms antibodies that attack the RBCs of the fetus. This is most commonly associated with Rh incompatibility, but may also occur in ABO incompatibility. The same mechanism occurs in the hemolysis that occurs with the transfusion of incompatible blood.

Signs and Symptoms

Signs and symptoms include the general signs of anemia: fatigue, pallor, shortness of breath, and tachycardia. Additional signs and symptoms related to the hemolysis include chills, jaundice (caused by increased bilirubin levels produced by the breakdown of the RBCs), dark urine (caused by increased urobilinogen), and an enlarged spleen, which occurs as a result of the spleen's efforts to remove the increased numbers of damaged and broken RBCs from the circulation.

Diagnosis

Diagnosis involves assessing the CBC and bone marrow response through evaluation of the reticulocyte count. Reticulocyte count is elevated when the bone marrow cannot keep up with RBC destruction. It is also important to measure the products of erythrocyte destruction such as methemoglobin and bilirubin. The peripheral smear in hemolytic anemia will show anisocytosis, poikilocytosis, and spherocytosis. These are terms that indicate misshapen and damaged RBCs, which is the appearance of lysed RBCs. Once the presence of hemolysis has been established, a variety of tests are performed to determine the exact cause. These include Hgb electrophoresis, bone marrow examination, and tests for the presence of autoantibodies.

Treatment

Treatment depends on the type and cause of the hemolytic anemia and may include folic acid and iron replacement, corticosteroids, and, in some emergent situations, transfusions. In cases of autoimmunity, treatments may include immunosuppressive drugs and splenectomy.

Specific Types of Hemolytic Anemias

Hemoglobinopathies, hereditary spherocytosis, HDN, lead poisoning, and transfusion reactions are all causes of hemolytic anemia. Certain hemoglobinopathies are prevalent among people of different cultures. HDN commonly occurs due to ABO incompatibility of the mother and infant, but usually causes very mild hemolysis. Lead destabilizes RBC structure, leading to hemolytic anemia; interferes with Hgb synthesis; and shortens the life span of RBCs.

Hemoglobinopathy

A **hemoglobinopathy** is an inherited disorder of the structure of the Hgb molecule that can lead to destruction of the RBC. The abnormal Hgb cannot carry oxygen efficiently, and the blood undergoes frequent hemolysis. SCA and thalassemia are common hemoglobinopathies.

Sickle Cell Anemia

SCA is one of the most common inherited hemoglobinopathies. It is a disease found mainly in those of African, Middle Eastern, and Mediterranean ancestry. In the United States, the SCA gene is present in approximately 8% of African Americans. More than 2 million people in the United States, nearly all of them of African ancestry, carry the sickle cell gene. SCA occurs in 1 in every 500 African Americans. Individuals with one sickle cell gene carry the trait but do not endure full sickle cell disease. Individuals with two sickle cell genes, one from the mother and one from the father, experience the full severity of the disease.

For centuries, it has been known that individuals with SCA are resistant to malaria. In the past, malaria was a major cause of death in the regions where SCA is prominent—Africa and the Middle East. Even today, malaria infects more than 300 million persons every year. Malaria organisms live within RBCs but cannot thrive in RBCs carrying the Hgb defect of SCA.

Over the years, SCA carriers living in malaria-ridden locales have had a survival benefit compared with noncarriers, allowing them to live longer and have more children. This benefit is what evolutionary biologists call heterozygote advantage, and it explains why the sickle cell trait has persisted in areas where malaria is common.

SCA is caused by an abnormal kind of Hgb called Hgb S that distorts the RBC's shape upon exposure to hypoxia or severe stress. These RBCs are less able to deliver oxygen to tissues and are fragile when they change into a characteristic sickle shape. Some sickled RBCs are destroyed by the immune system, causing hemolysis. These sickled RBCs can also occlude capillaries and cause ischemia in various organs throughout the body.

Individuals can be heterozygous for the SCA genetic mutation, where they only carry the trait. Carriers have different amounts of Hgb S in their circulation, which causes a spectrum of clinical disease presentations. Some carriers do not have enough Hgb S to suffer any symptoms; however, some carriers do have enough Hgb S to exhibit symptoms of disease. Some persons who only carry the trait can manifest all the complications of SCA when exposed to high stress, hypoxia, dehydration, or infection. More than 30,000 patients have homozygous Hgb S disease, which indicates that both alleles have the genetic mutation; these patients have the most severe form of the disease. Males and females are affected equally.

Although hematological changes indicative of the disorder are evident as early as the age of 10 weeks, clinical signs of SCA usually do not appear until the first year of life. This is because fetal Hgb levels decline at approximately 6 months of age and then Hgb S starts to control oxygen transport. SCA persists for the entire life span, which is shortened for those with the full spectrum of clinical disease. Rates of complications increase after age 10. Renal disease is one of the major complications of SCA. The average survival time after the diagnosis of renal disease is about 4 years, and the median age of death is 27 years, despite dialysis treatment.

Etiology. SCA occurs because of a genetic mutation that directs abnormal synthesis of the Hgb molecule. Normally, the Hgb molecule is composed of four polypeptide chains: a pair of alpha chains and a pair of beta chains. The SCA gene mutation causes one of the beta polypeptide chains to be abnormal, as one of the amino acids in the chain, valine, is substituted for glutamic acid. This changes the Hgb molecule into Hgb S, the major type of Hgb in SCA. This mutation causes structural fragility of the SCA RBCs, whereupon exposure to hypoxia or stress causes the RBC to contort into a sickle shape.

SCA is transmitted by a recessive trait. Some individuals are homozygous (two traits for Hgb S) and endure severe disease, and some are heterozygous (one trait for Hgb S and one trait for normal Hgb A) and only carry the trait. Chances for offspring to be born with SCA can be configured on a Punnett square (see Fig. 13-10).

Persons with SCA have both Hgb S and normal Hgb A in their bloodstream. There is a spectrum of the degree of severity of disease depending on the amount of Hgb S in the circulation. Those who are homozygous for the disorder have the majority of their RBCs in the form of Hgb S. Persons with sickle cell trait can possess up to 40% Hgb S in their circulation. These individuals tend to suffer mild anemia but upon exposure to extreme stress can develop symptoms of severe SCA.

Pathophysiology. The genetic mutation in SCA causes synthesis of Hgb that is more fragile and inefficient at carrying oxygen. Under conditions of hypoxia, severe stress, infection, or dehydration, the SCA Hgb tends to polymerize and become distorted in shape, which in turn causes the RBC to change into a crescent or sickle-shaped cell (see Fig. 13-11). The RBCs can reoxygenate and resume normal condition, but with frequent episodes of sickling, they remain distorted. These abnormal RBCs have a severely shortened life span of only 10 to 20 days. Because they are broken down by the spleen at a rate much faster than the bone marrow can replace them, the result is severe hemolytic anemia.

The misshapen RBCs also cannot pass easily through capillaries. They become trapped, blocking blood flow and creating obstructions to distal tissues and organs. The occlusion in these vessels causes ischemia and consequent tissue hypoxia, which leads to organ damage and possible infarction. The episodes of ischemia, called **vaso-occlusive crises**, can occur in various organs of the body. Common sites obstructed by sickled RBCs are the chest, abdomen, long bones, and joints. Multiple sites are often involved simultaneously.

> ### 🔍 CLINICAL CONCEPT
> Vaso-occlusive episodes are extremely painful for the patient. Ischemia and infarction cause chronic damage of the liver, spleen, heart, kidneys, and retina.

The spleen can become ischemic and dysfunction can begin early in childhood because of the high number of lysed RBCs that must be processed. This diminishes the spleen's immune function, which increases the risk of infection in the patient with SCA. Children are particularly vulnerable to severe bacterial infections and sepsis.

Clinical Presentation. The common signs of anemia are present, particularly fatigue and exercise intolerance. The frequent hemolysis of RBCs causes a high amount of heme breakdown in circulation with concomitant hyperbilirubinemia. High bilirubin in the bloodstream causes jaundice and bile concentration in the gallbladder, often leading to gallstones.

Episodes of vaso-occlusion cause severe pain, fever, tachycardia, and anxiety. Vaso-occlusive crises can be triggered by different stressors, including exposure to cold, hypoxia, infection, dehydration, acidosis, emotional stress, high exertion, and pregnancy. The pain's location will vary with the area of the circulation affected. Multiple sites of pain occurring simultaneously are common. Repeated crises can require three to four hospitalizations a year.

Chest pain can occur with tachypnea, fever, cough, and low arterial saturation. The chest pain can mimic myocardial infarction, pulmonary embolism, or pneumonia. Commonly experienced by sufferers of SCA, this is called acute chest syndrome and leads to pulmonary infarction and possible respiratory failure.

Children are particularly susceptible to severe infections, growth retardation, osteomyelitis, and stroke. Children commonly suffer repeated strokes due to cerebral infarction, with resulting neurological sequelae such as paralysis.

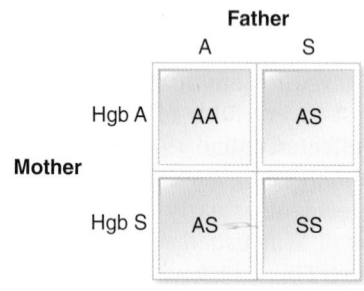

Father

	A	S
Hgb A	AA	AS
Hgb S	AS	SS

Mother

FIGURE 13-10. Punnett square for offspring of parents who are carriers of the SCA trait. Hgb AA represents normal Hgb. Hgb AS represents SCA trait. Hgb SS is SCA disease. When the Punnett square is configured for two parents with sickle cell trait, the following are the risks for having an affected offspring: 25% chance of having a child with full SCA disease, 50% chance of having a child with the SCA trait, and 25% chance of having a child with normal Hgb.

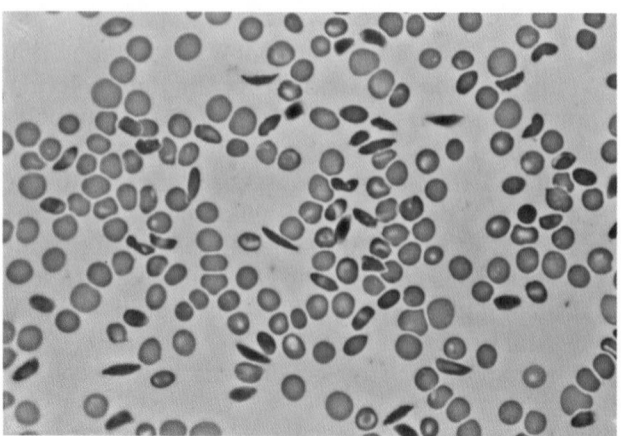

FIGURE 13-11. Peripheral smear with sickled cells. *(From Biology Pics/Science Source.)*

Hand–foot syndrome is a complication that occurs because of painful ischemia and infarctions in the hands and fingers. The formation of ischemic ulcerations of the lower extremities is common. A painful disorder of male patients called priapism can occur because of blockage of veins in the penis. Renal necrosis can also occur with all the signs and symptoms of renal failure. Retinal ischemia and hemorrhages can lead to retinal detachment with its symptoms of partial blindness.

Diagnosis. A blood sample is screened for the presence of Hgb S as part of the routine screening of newborns, but it can also be done on patients of any age. Early identification of these infants, along with improved treatments, has more than doubled the life expectancy of these patients. Hgb electrophoresis can differentiate which patients with Hgb S are homozygous and which are heterozygous. A CBC can assess for anemia, and a peripheral blood smear can show the typical sickle-shaped cells. Reticulocytosis indicates a high amount of hemolysis is occurring. Genetic counseling of parents who are carriers or sufferers of SCA is necessary to discuss the chance of passing the gene to offspring.

Treatment. The combination of oxygen, hydration, pain medications, and prophylactic antibiotics is used to treat vaso-occlusive crises and complications. A high amount of fluid is administered by IV in an effort to flush out occlusive areas of cells. Pain medications, such as opiates, are commonly needed, but these are problematic, as they can lead to dependence.

Hydroxyurea, an antitumor drug, has proven effective in decreasing vaso-occlusive episodes. It increases the level of fetal Hgb in erythrocytes; this treatment does not cure the disease but does help decrease the disorder's severity and the occurrence of occlusive episodes.

Much of the treatment for SCA is directed at preventing and managing the disease's complications. Prophylactic antibiotics are used to prevent infection. All required immunizations are administered. Patients take folic acid supplements to prevent aplastic crisis in the bone marrow. Patients are also educated to avoid the triggers that cause crises. Splenic sequestration crisis is a disorder of ischemia and occlusion of vessels in the spleen. This usually requires splenectomy, which in turn, increases the risk of infection.

Bone marrow transplant allows replacement of defective bone marrow with healthy marrow. However, finding a matching bone marrow donor is challenging. Blood transfusions can increase the number of normal RBCs and help reduce the anemia. It is important to recognize that because blood transfusions contain iron, chronic use of transfusions can lead to iron overload, which is toxic to the body and requires the use of iron-chelating agents.

Other experimental treatments include gene therapy to replace the defective gene with a corrected copy to promote the production of normal Hgb by the bone marrow (termed CRISPR-Cas9 technology). Researchers are also exploring ways to suppress the defective gene and to reactivate the gene responsible for producing fetal Hgb. Nitric acid, which helps keep blood vessels open and reduces the adhesiveness of RBCs, is low in persons with SCA, and replacement may help decrease the formation of the sickle cells.

 CLINICAL CONCEPT

Splenectomy causes immunodeficiency and increased risk of infection with encapsulated bacteria such as *Streptococcus pneumoniae*, *Haemophilus influenzae* type B, *Klebsiella*, and *Salmonella*.

Thalassemia

Thalassemia resembles SCA, in that it is a genetic disorder that causes defects in Hgb synthesis. The similarity of the two diseases extends to the cultural background of affected individuals. Thalassemia mainly affects persons of Mediterranean, African, and Southeast Asian descent. It affects 200 million persons worldwide and is one of the most common genetic disorders in the world. Approximately 15% of African Americans are carriers of the trait. The minor form of disease occurs in 3% of African Americans, whereas the major form of disease occurs in fewer than 1%.

Etiology. Thalassemia is caused by a genetic defect. Thalassemia minor occurs if one defective gene is inherited from one parent. Persons with this form of the disorder are carriers of the disease and usually have no or mild symptoms. Risk factors for thalassemia include being of Asian, Chinese, Mediterranean, or African ancestry and having a family history of the disorder.

Thalassemia affects the alpha and beta polypeptide chains of the Hgb molecule. The genes that code for Hgb formation are missing or variant; consequently, some proteins needed for Hgb synthesis are abnormal or absent. The two main types of the disease are alpha and beta thalassemia. In alpha thalassemia, an alpha chain is missing, and in beta thalassemia, a beta chain is absent. Sometimes the disease is called alpha thalassemia or beta thalassemia, depending on the specific Hgb component affected.

Thalassemia has an autosomal-recessive inheritance pattern similar to that seen in sickle cell disease. A child who inherits defective genes from both parents is homozygous for the abnormal Hgb and exhibits moderate-to-severe disease. Homozygotes have a form of the disease called thalassemia major. Those who are heterozygous for the defective Hgb are carriers; they can have a mild form of the disease called thalassemia minor. Beta thalassemia major, also called Cooley's anemia, is the most severe form of the disease.

Pathophysiology. In both thalassemia major and minor, one of the polypeptide chains of the Hgb structure is deficient, leading to reduced Hgb synthesis and decreased RBC production. However, within the RBC, the unaffected polypeptide chains continue to be synthesized and accumulate. The accumulation of polypeptide chains interferes with normal maturation of the RBC. The affected RBCs become defective and destroyed in the bone marrow or spleen, which leads to large amounts of hemolysis. The accumulations of normal polypeptide chains within the RBCs develop into pathological fragments called Heinz bodies, which are pathognomonic for thalassemia.

The bone marrow also attempts to compensate for the loss of RBCs with an exaggerated rate of erythropoiesis in the bone marrow. Osteopenia of bone marrow occurs because of the large amount of space taken by maturing erythrocytes.

Clinical Presentation. The signs and symptoms of thalassemia include the expected signs of anemia: fatigue, weakness, pallor, and exercise intolerance. Those who are homozygous for the trait usually have no overt symptoms and endure a mild anemia. In the more severe forms of disease, the signs and symptoms appear in early childhood and require frequent transfusions.

Because of the high amount of erythropoiesis needed to replace lysed RBCs, the bone marrow expands inside all the bones, causing pain. The bones become weak, enlarged, and distorted, particularly the cranial bones. Children often develop a characteristic chipmunk-cheeked appearance because of hyperplasia of the marrow in the cheekbones. The skull develops tiny bone deformities that resemble "hair on end" in an x-ray (see Fig. 13-12).

The spleen and liver become filled with dead RBCs and enlarged because of the high amount of RBC destruction. The hepatomegaly and splenomegaly cause a protuberant abdomen. The large amount of hemolysis and required transfusions cause iron overload, also called hemochromatosis. The myocardium, liver, kidney, and pancreas can be affected by iron overload. Also, the great amount of hemolysis in the bloodstream causes hyperbilirubinemia with resulting jaundice and dark urine. Concentrated bile in the gallbladder can form gallstones with right upper quadrant abdominal pain and tenderness.

Diagnosis. Diagnostic studies include a CBC, which reveals a microcytic hypochromic anemia. Hgb electrophoresis provides additional information about the types of Hgb present in the RBCs. The abnormal Hgb found in beta thalassemia is termed Hgb A2. It is important to distinguish alpha thalassemias from iron-deficiency anemia to avoid inappropriate treatment with iron, so tests of iron levels in the blood and iron stores are needed.

There are numerous types of molecular diagnostic tests that can determine the exact nucleotide sequence of one or more globin genes as well as the presence of copy number variations (e.g., deletions, duplications) and complex chromosomal rearrangements. These genetic tests are done on leukocytes within the bloodstream.

Genetic testing is especially important in precise diagnosis, carrier detection, prenatal testing, and genetic counseling. Prenatal genetic tests can be done using amniotic fluid cells or chorionic villus samples.

Radiographically, the skeletal response to marrow proliferation consists of thinning of cortical bone and resorption of cancellous bone, which results in a generalized loss of bone density.

Treatment. Treatment depends on the severity of the disease. Those who have the trait but are asymptomatic require no treatment. However, genetic counseling is necessary so individuals understand the chance of passing the trait on to offspring. The mainstays of treatment for those with the more severe forms of the disease are transfusions and prevention of infection. All immunizations should be administered as required. If splenomegaly occurs, splenectomy becomes necessary, increasing the risk of infection. As with SCA, the regular transfusions lead to iron buildup in the body and necessitate iron chelation treatments to avoid the toxic effects of the iron. Folic acid supplementation helps the body build normal red cells. As with SCA, enhancement of fetal Hgb levels lessens the disease's severity. Gene therapy in which the abnormal gene or genes are replaced with normal genes is being studied as a way to cure the disease. Bone marrow or stem cell transplants have cured thalassemias in some children but are still considered experimental. Gene therapy using lentiviruses that carry an appropriate gene is under investigation. Gene editing to disrupt the BCL11A gene is under investigation as a means of

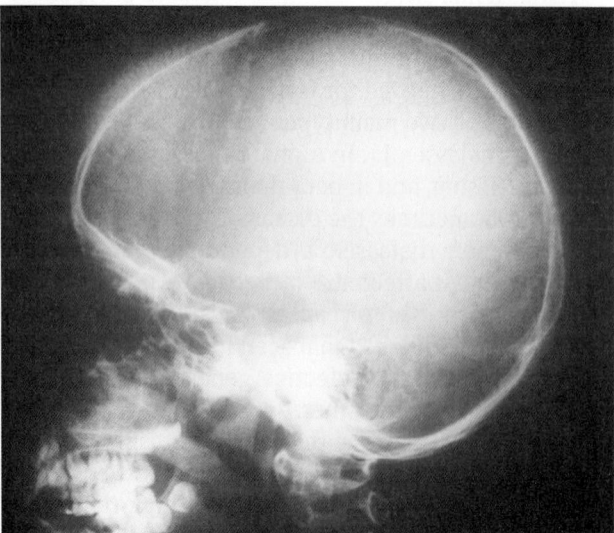

FIGURE 13-12. Hair-on-end appearance of skull bone formation in thalassemia. *(From Biophoto Associates/Science Source.)*

increasing fetal hemoglobin (Hb F) to treat beta thalassemia. Luspatercept is a subcutaneous agent that improves RBC maturation by an incompletely understood mechanism. It was approved for the treatment of adults with transfusion-dependent beta thalassemia in November 2019.

Hereditary Spherocytosis

Hereditary spherocytosis is a familial hemolytic disorder caused by a lack of membrane proteins in RBCs. The lack of membrane integrity causes fragility and gives RBCs a characteristic spherical shape. It is most common among people of Northern European descent. In the United States, the disorder's incidence is approximately 1 case in 5,000 people.

Hereditary spherocytosis is an autosomal-dominant disorder. Only heterozygous individuals have been identified in the population, suggesting that the homozygous state is incompatible with life. The major problem in this disorder involves the spleen and fragile RBCs. Spherocytic RBCs are sequestered and destroyed, after which they accumulate in the spleen. The disease's expression varies in individuals. Some of those affected have no symptoms, whereas others can have anemia, splenomegaly, jaundice, and bilirubin gallstones.

The major complications are aplastic anemia crisis, megaloblastic anemia, hemolytic anemia, cholecystitis and cholelithiasis, and severe neonatal hemolysis. Aplastic anemia crisis occurs when Hgb levels fall rapidly and severely because ongoing destruction of spherocytes is not balanced with new RBC production. Blood transfusions and splenectomy are required treatment. Megaloblastic anemia crisis can also occur where there is inadequate folic acid for erythropoiesis. Patients with hereditary spherocytosis are instructed to take supplementary folic acid (1 mg/dL) for life in order to prevent a megaloblastic crisis. Severe neonatal hemolysis requires transfusion and phototherapy to rid the body of bilirubin.

Blood Transfusion Reactions

Hemolytic transfusion reactions are the result of antibodies in the recipient's blood directed against antigens on the donor's erythrocytes. This results in rapid intravascular hemolysis of the donor RBCs. ABO incompatibility caused by clerical error is the most frequent cause. In hemolytic transfusion reactions, symptoms usually occur after a small amount of blood has been transfused and almost always before the unit is transfused completely (see Box 13-3). Hemolytic transfusion reactions occur in 1 per 40,000 transfused units of packed RBCs.

Nonhemolytic febrile reactions and minor allergic reactions are the most common transfusion reactions, each occurring in 3% to 4% of all transfusions. Nonhemolytic febrile reactions and extravascular hemolysis are observed more commonly in patients who have developed antibodies from prior transfusions.

BOX 13-3. Signs and Symptoms of Hemolytic Transfusion Reaction

Hemolytic transfusion reactions occur when the wrong blood type is administered to a patient. The wrong type of donor blood will stimulate the recipient's development of antibodies against the donor blood cells. The following are symptoms of this hemolytic reaction:

- Fever
- Chills
- Flushing
- Nausea
- Burning at IV line
- Chest tightness
- Restlessness
- Apprehension
- Joint pain
- Back pain
- Tachycardia
- Tachypnea

In severe cases of hemolytic transfusion reaction, hypotension, oozing from the IV site, diffuse bleeding, hemoglobinuria, oliguria, shock, and renal failure can occur.

Proteins in the donor plasma can also cause minor allergic reactions.

Nonhemolytic febrile reactions are thought to stem from the formation of cytokines during the storage of the blood. This anaphylactoid nonhemolytic reaction is observed more frequently with components containing large amounts of plasma, such as whole blood, pooled platelets, and fresh frozen plasma. Minor allergic reactions are associated with urticaria.

Nonhemolytic febrile reactions do not occur as rapidly as acute hemolytic reactions. They occur between 1 and 6 hours after transfusions and are associated with the nonspecific symptoms of fever, chills, and malaise. Some patients may complain of dyspnea. These nonspecific symptoms also occur with a hemolytic transfusion reaction. These reactions seldom proceed to hypotension or respiratory distress.

Anaphylactic reactions occur in 1 per 20,000 transfused units. Risk of transfusion-related hepatitis B is approximately 1 per 350,000 units transfused. Risk for hepatitis C is 1 per 2 million units transfused. Risk of transfusion-related HIV infection is 1 per 2 million units transfused.

Anaphylactic reactions most often are observed in those patients with a hereditary immunoglobulin A (IgA) deficiency. Some of these patients have developed complement-binding anti-IgA antibodies that cause anaphylaxis when exposed to donor IgA. In anaphylactic reactions, symptoms usually occur with fewer than 10 mL of blood transfused and only rarely occur more insidiously. Anaphylactic reactions to blood transfusion are associated with rapid development of dyspnea, flushing, urticaria, abdominal pain, bronchospasm, hypotension, facial swelling, and edema of the tongue.

In hemolytic transfusion reactions, pharmacological treatment is aimed at increasing renal blood flow and preserving urinary output. The transfusion should be stopped immediately when a reaction is suspected. A normal saline IV drip should be substituted for the blood. Acetaminophen is given for fever. Diuretics such as furosemide, antihistamines such as diphenhydramine, and steroids such as Solu-Medrol can be used. In anaphylaxis, the goals of therapy are to maintain airway and hemodynamic stability and reverse the underlying process. Commonly required medications include epinephrine, corticosteroids, antihistamines, and vasopressors such as dobutamine.

 CLINICAL CONCEPT

It is mandatory for two clinicians to double-check the patient blood type and donor blood type before administration of a transfusion. All patients receiving blood products should be placed on continuous cardiac monitoring and pulse oximetry.

Hemolytic Disease of the Newborn

HDN involves an antigen–antibody reaction between a mother's antibodies and the newborn infant's RBCs at the time of birth. The mechanism of HDN involves maternal synthesis of antibodies against the surface A, B, or Rh antigens, also called D antigens, on fetal or neonatal RBCs. Antibodies that react against ABO blood antigens are of the IgM class, which are large in size and cannot pass through the placenta during pregnancy. Therefore, a mother whose blood type is different from the fetus can carry the pregnancy without problems. It is common during delivery, when maternal and infant blood may mix, that ABO incompatibility can occur between mother and infant. Some of the infant's RBCs can enter the maternal circulation and stimulate an antibody reaction in the mother. The mother's antibodies, in turn, can enter the infant's circulation and attack infant RBCs. In these cases, the infant may experience a mild hemolysis because of ABO incompatibility. The infant endures a mild hyperbilirubinemia caused by RBC breakdown and exhibits mild jaundice, but it is usually short-lived. Exposure to sunlight or phototherapy is used to break down the bilirubin in the infant. A severe hemolytic reaction called **erythroblastosis fetalis** can occur if a fetus is Rh-positive and the mother is Rh-negative (see Box 13-4).

Anemia Due to Lead Poisoning

Anemia can develop with lead poisoning, which is often due to environmental sources of organic lead. Lead paint, lead pottery or toys, batteries, and aging lead plumbing fixtures are sources of lead. They can allow lead to accumulate in the water supply, which can cause lead toxicity. Lead impairs hemoglobin synthesis; destabilizes RBC structure, which triggers hemolysis; and shortens RBC life span. Lead is most toxic to the neurological system, particularly in children. Children can develop central nervous system (CNS) symptoms such as irritability, behavioral changes, hyperactivity or hypoactivity, delays in developmental milestones, and learning disabilities. Lead also interferes with iron metabolism and can cause iron-deficiency anemia. A simple blood test can assess for lead blood levels. Chelation therapy is used if blood lead levels are greater than 45 mcg/dL. Calcium disodium ethylenediaminetetraacetic acid (EDTA) is one of the chelation agents used that is administered by injection. EDTA binds with lead and then is excreted in the urine. Succimer and D-penicillamine are oral chelation agents. Patients who have undergone chelation therapy need follow-up assessment, as bone stores of lead can be released into blood. Prevention of lead exposure is the best method to eliminate lead poisoning. The Centers for Disease Control (CDC) recommends screening of all children in high-risk environments. Children who have been exposed to lead should have long-term follow-up. Any sources of lead in households, schools, workplaces, or other environments should be removed through lead abatement procedures.

Red Blood Cell Maturation Defects

Nutrients necessary for synthesizing RBCs include protein, iron, vitamin B_{12}, and folic acid. Iron is an essential element of Hgb synthesis and multiple metabolic processes, and vitamin B_{12} and folic acid are necessary components of DNA synthesis. Any deficiency of these components can lead to decreased erythropoiesis in the bone marrow, which in turn leads to anemia. The bone marrow is constantly generating new blood cells: RBCs, WBCs, and platelets. Disturbance of bone marrow function can lead to anemia, leukopenia, and thrombocytopenia. Complete disruption of bone marrow function inhibits manufacture of all blood cells, a condition called **aplastic anemia**. Aplastic anemia is a life-threatening disorder that can be caused by cancer, sepsis, or radiation exposure.

Iron-Deficiency Anemia

Iron deficiency is the most common cause of anemia worldwide. Its prevalence is approximately 50% in underdeveloped countries and 10% in developed countries. In countries where little meat is in the diet, iron-deficiency anemia is six to eight times more prevalent than in North America and Europe. The highest prevalence of iron deficiency occurs in women of childbearing age and older adults. Approximately 15% of women between ages 20 and 45 years are iron deficient. Prevalence of anemia in older adults ranges from 8% to 44%, with the highest prevalence in men aged 85 years and older.

BOX 13-4. Erythroblastosis Fetalis

Erythroblastosis fetalis can occur if a fetus is Rh-positive and the mother is Rh-negative. It is a severe hemolytic reaction in the Rh-positive fetus caused by anti-Rh antibodies from the mother. This usually occurs in cases where the mother has had prior exposure to the Rh antigen and has formed Rh antibodies.

The mother was most likely sensitized to Rh-positive blood during a previous pregnancy at delivery, when mixing of maternal and infant blood occur. Other ways in which the mother could have been exposed to the Rh-positive antigen include fetal–maternal hemorrhage caused by trauma, abortion, childbirth, ruptures in the placenta during pregnancy, or medical procedures carried out during pregnancy that breach the uterine wall. Once the Rh antibodies are formed in the mother, they cross the placenta into the fetal circulation and attack the fetal RBCs, causing a high amount of hemolysis. The fetus suffers hemolytic anemia, which can be severe. Severe hemolytic anemia of the fetus can cause heart failure with hepatomegaly, splenomegaly, hyperbilirubinemia, and possible death. The infant can be stillborn. However, if the fetus can survive the hemolysis, hyperbilirubinemia occurs because of the large amount of RBC lysis. The neonate exhibits high bilirubin at birth, which can lead to kernicterus. At delivery, RhoGAM, a medication that coats Rh-positive RBCs, is administered to mothers to prevent the mother from developing Rh antibodies. This prevents erythroblastosis fetalis from occurring in future pregnancies.

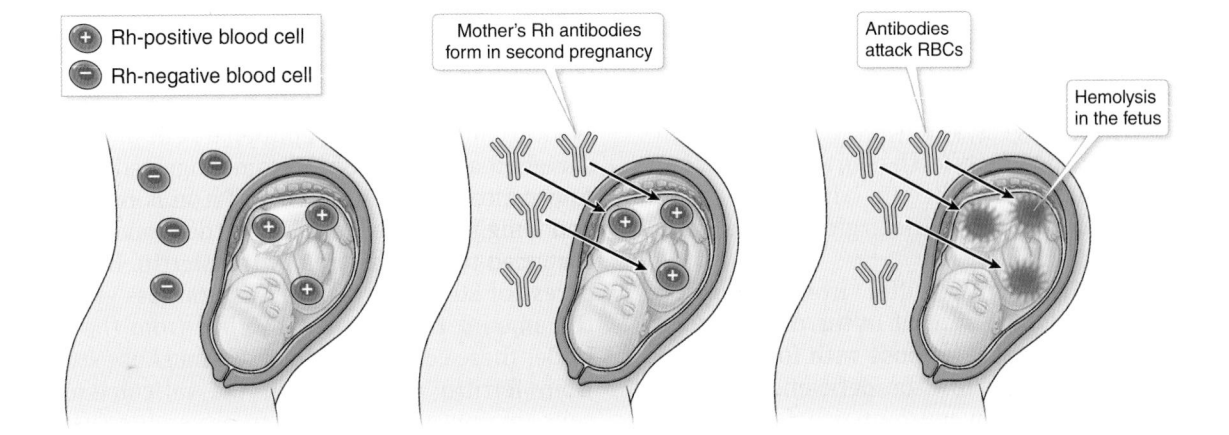

Slow, chronic loss of blood can cause iron deficiency. Slow GI bleeding from peptic ulcer or colon cancer and excessive monthly menstrual blood loss are common imperceptible causes of iron deficiency. A recent study showed that 60% of individuals with colon cancer have iron deficiency.

The following groups of people have an increased risk of iron-deficiency anemia:

- Women of childbearing age: Because women lose blood during menstruation, women in general are at greater risk of iron-deficiency anemia. Heavy menstrual bleeding, a total blood loss of greater than 80 mL per menstrual cycle, is a common cause of iron deficiency. Prolonged monthly menstrual blood loss of duration greater than 7 days can also cause iron deficiency. Pregnancy, delivery, and breastfeeding also utilize a high amount of maternal iron stores.
- Infants and children: Infants who are weaned from formula to cow's milk may need extra iron because of the low iron in cow's milk. Children and adolescents need extra iron during growth spurts, as extra iron is metabolized at these times.

- Vegetarians: Individuals who don't eat meat may have a greater risk of iron-deficiency anemia if they don't supplement their diet with iron-rich foods.
- Persons who lack the ability to obtain recommended daily nutrient-rich food; commonly in populations with food insecurity secondary to lack of resources.
- Older adults: Poor diet and lack of stomach acid can cause iron deficiency. Atrophic gastritis or frequent use of proton pump inhibitors can lead to low acidity and poor gastric iron absorption.
- Persons with celiac disease or inflammatory bowel disease may have decreased ability to absorb iron.
- Individuals with GI bleeding: Persons with peptic ulcer, esophageal varices, or cancer of the GI tract can lose blood in the stool. Persons who frequently use aspirin or NSAIDs are also at risk for gastric bleeding, which leads to iron deficiency.
- Persons with malabsorption due to bariatric surgery.

Etiology. The most common causes of iron deficiency are inadequate intake, excessive menstrual blood loss, and GI blood loss. Meats contain the most absorbable kind of iron compared with plants, so vegetarians have to be vigilant about eating iron sources such as green leafy vegetables, beans, mushrooms, and soy.

The adult male absorbs and loses about 1 mg of iron from an average diet containing 10 to 20 mg daily. During childbearing years, an adult female loses an average of 2 mg of iron daily and must absorb a similar quantity of iron in order to maintain equilibrium. With each pregnancy, a woman loses about 500 mg of iron. In menstruating women, menstrual blood loss is highly variable, ranging from 4 to 100 mg of iron lost per period.

Healthy newborn infants have a total body iron of 250 mg, which is obtained transplacentally from maternal sources. Breastfeeding mothers need considerably more iron in the diet because the growing infant draws from the maternal storage. For the infant, breast milk and formula have adequate iron, but when the child is weaned, iron deficiency often occurs because cow's milk is iron deficient.

Iron deficiency is also the most common type of anemia seen in teenagers, as it is related to increased demand for RBCs during growth spurts, which occur during these years. Adolescents also suffer iron deficiency because of poor diet; girls particularly are at risk.

Older adults frequently suffer from poor iron nutrition caused by lack of meat in the diet. Persons who live in "food deserts" or those with food insecurity are also at high risk for iron deficiency because of the inability to obtain nutrient-rich foods. Also, older adults commonly have achlorhydria, or a lack of hydrochloric acid (HCl), of the stomach, a natural physiological change of aging that decreases iron absorption in the stomach. Persons who frequently use antacids such as histamine-2 antagonists or proton pump inhibitors are also at risk for iron deficiency caused by lack of gastric HCl. For men, loss of blood from the GI tract is the most common cause for iron-deficiency anemia. GI problems that can cause bleeding include gastritis, ulcerations, esophageal varices, and carcinomas. Frequent use of aspirin or NSAIDs can increase risk of gastric bleeding. In both men and postmenopausal women, colon cancer frequently presents with iron-deficiency anemia caused by undetected chronic blood loss from the GI tract. Causes of iron deficiency due to GI malabsorption include bariatric surgery, celiac disease, and inflammatory bowel disease. Persons taking erythropoietin to stimulate red blood cell production can rapidly develop iron deficiency. The high synthesis of RBCs requires more iron than can be supplied by diet alone. Persons with chronic inflammatory disorders can also be iron deficient. High hepcidin levels in inflammation can inhibit iron absorption. In certain geographic areas, intestinal parasites, particularly hookworm, cause iron deficiency because of blood loss from the GI tract.

CLINICAL CONCEPT

The majority of patients with a new diagnosis of colorectal cancer are iron deficient at presentation. Adult males or postmenopausal females with iron deficiency require colonoscopy to screen for colon cancer.

ALERT! The appearance of iron deficiency in an adult male means that the clinician should suspect GI blood loss until ruled out.

Pathophysiology. Iron is needed in the diet to synthesize Hgb. The heme portion of Hgb contains iron that carries oxygen atoms. Lack of sufficient iron leads to poor oxygen transport by iron-deficient Hgb molecules. Iron is absorbed from the GI tract, and some is stored in the intestinal cells before crossing into the bloodstream. Intestinal epithelial cells are constantly sloughed and excreted, so some ingested iron is lost. Approximately 0.5 to 1.5 mg of iron is ingested daily and 1 mg is lost in the feces. In the bloodstream, iron is carried to storage sites by transferrin. Blood loss in excess of 20 mL per day causes iron loss greater than the amount that can be absorbed from the GI tract. Under these conditions, the body must use stored iron from ferritin complexes in the reticuloendothelial cells (mainly macrophages from various sites), bone marrow, liver, and spleen. When iron stores become depleted, serum ferritin complexes and transferrin become depleted. Once the circulating transferrin becomes depleted of iron, Hgb synthesis is impaired and iron-deficient erythropoiesis starts to occur. As Hgb synthesis decreases, RBC numbers diminish. The RBCs that are synthesized are abnormally small (microcytic) and pale (hypochromic). When iron deficiency is severe, the process of erythropoiesis in the bone marrow is affected and fewer RBCs are produced.

Clinical Presentation. A thorough history and physical examination are important in a patient suspected of iron-deficiency anemia. Questions of particular importance to ask include age; current medications, including over-the-counter drugs; current history of GI symptoms; current menstrual history in women; history of past health disorders; and social habits. Current medications can give some information about the patient's current health disorders. For example, frequent use of NSAIDs can cause gastric ulceration with slow, gradual GI blood loss. It is important to know the frequency of alcohol misuse and if the patient smokes. These activities predispose to GI bleeding as well. Menstruating women should be asked about the duration and volume of menstrual blood loss. Use of more than one tampon per hour indicates excessive menstrual blood loss. Women with menstrual blood loss for more than 7 days may also be at risk for iron deficiency. All patients should be asked about dark stool, which can indicate melena (blood in stool).

Signs and Symptoms. The signs and symptoms of iron-deficiency anemia are those of anemia in general: fatigue, weakness, and exercise intolerance. If iron deficiency is caused by GI blood loss, the patient may have melena. Women of childbearing age may have menorrhagia.

Iron deficiency also has some specific signs, including hair loss; cheilitis; glossitis; nail changes called koilonychias, which are spoon-shaped nails; and pica. **Pica,** a unique sign of iron deficiency, is a craving for nonfood substances such as ice, clay, starch, chalk, dirt, or other material. At times, an individual craves specific food items to excess, such as carbohydrates. Cold intolerance and feeling of tingling or numbness in the fingers occur in many who are iron deficient.

Physical Examination. The physical examination is commonly unremarkable except for pallor of the conjunctiva, nailbeds, and palms. In severe cases of anemia, splenomegaly may be found on the abdominal examination.

Diagnosis. Iron-deficiency anemia is primarily a laboratory diagnosis. Useful tests include a CBC, peripheral smear, serum iron, TIBC, and serum ferritin (see Box 13-5). Serum iron and ferritin are decreased, but TIBC is high because there are many free iron-binding sites in the body. A peripheral blood smear will often show signs of iron deficiency before the CBC exhibits abnormalities. Because GI blood loss is often the reason for iron-deficiency anemia, an FOBT should be done along with other diagnostic tests. A colonoscopy or endoscopy is indicated if the FOBT is positive.

When iron and folic acid (also called folate) deficiency occur together, a peripheral smear reveals a population of macrocytes among the microcytic hypochromic RBCs. This combination of microcytes and macrocytes can erroneously normalize the MCV.

Chronic lead poisoning may produce a CBC with mild microcytosis. The incidence of lead poisoning is greater in individuals who are iron deficient than in healthy subjects because increased absorption of lead occurs in individuals who are iron deficient.

Treatment. In most patients, the iron deficiency should be treated with oral iron therapy (ferrous sulfate), and the underlying etiology should be corrected to avoid recurrence of anemia. Vitamin C enhances absorption of iron. Oral iron can cause gastritis and constipation. Parenteral iron therapy, either intramuscular or IV, is an option, but anaphylaxis is a risk factor. The patient can be advised to use iron cookware, as iron can naturally seep into foods prepared in this way.

Vitamin B₁₂ Deficiency

Vitamin B_{12}, also called cyanocobalamin or cobalamin, is a cofactor for two important processes: synthesis of DNA in RBCs and normal synthesis of the myelin cells that surround neurons. Lack of vitamin B_{12} results in an inability of the body to make enough mature RBCs and allows breakdown of the myelin sheaths surrounding some of the body's sensory and motor nerves.

The exact prevalence of vitamin B_{12} deficiency is unknown, but it is known that **pernicious anemia,** which results from vitamin B_{12} deficiency, is a common cause of anemia throughout the world, especially in persons of European or African descent. Pernicious anemia is an autoimmune disease that causes destruction of intrinsic factor that allows GI absorption of vitamin B_{12}. Dietary deficiency of vitamin B_{12} is also a common cause, particularly in vegetarians and in populations with food insecurity due to lack of resources. Globally, according to various studies, low vitamin B_{12} is prevalent in 25% to 70% of persons in underdeveloped countries. It is a severe problem in India, Mexico, Central and South America, and selected areas in Africa.

According to the U.S. Framingham Offspring Study, up to 39% of adults in the United States are vitamin B_{12} deficient, particularly older adults. Prevalence is greater than 20% in the older adult population, commonly caused by intestinal malabsorption. Malabsorption caused by gastric bypass surgery is also an increasingly common cause of vitamin B_{12} deficiency as the gastric bypass procedure is becoming more frequently performed for treatment of obesity. Alcohol use disorder and a specific oral antidiabetic agent called metformin can deplete vitamin B_{12} stores as well.

BOX 13-5. Diagnosis of Iron-Deficiency Anemia

The following laboratory test results are indicative of iron-deficiency anemia:

CBC RESULTS
- Hgb: low
- Hct: low
- MCV: low (microcytic)
- MCH: low
- MCHC: low (hypochromic)

ADDITIONAL LABORATORY TESTS
- Serum Fe⁺⁺: low
- Serum ferritin: low
- Total iron binding capacity: high
- Peripheral blood smear: shows small, pale blood cells
- FOBT should be done

Etiology. The most absorbable sources of vitamin B_{12} are in animal products such as meat and dairy foods. Therefore, vitamin B_{12} deficiency is common in persons who lack meat in the diet. Those who follow a strict vegetarian diet are at risk, as are those with poor diets related to aging, chronic alcohol use disorder, and economic factors.

Vitamin B_{12} stores in the liver can last for years. An average diet contains between 5 and 30 micrograms per day, with the daily requirement being 1 to 3 micrograms per day. Body stores of vitamin B_{12} are approximately 2 to 3 mg, sufficient for 3 to 4 years if supply is cut off.

In older patients, vitamin B_{12} deficiency is caused primarily by food–cobalamin malabsorption or pernicious anemia. Food–cobalamin malabsorption syndrome is characterized by the inability to release vitamin B_{12} from food or from intestinal transport proteins. This syndrome is defined by vitamin B_{12} deficiency in the presence of sufficient food and B_{12} intake.

Pernicious anemia, another disorder common in older adults, occurs as a result of a lack of **intrinsic factor (IF)**, an essential carrier protein of vitamin B_{12} in the stomach. Without IF, vitamin B_{12} is not absorbed into the bloodstream (see Fig. 13-13). Achlorhydria can also be responsible for vitamin B_{12} deficiency. Frequent use of proton pump inhibitors such as omeprazole (Prilosec), which can cause achlorhydria, also have been found to be a cause of vitamin B_{12} deficiency. Persons who do not obtain enough of the recommended daily allowance of nutrient-rich food, as in areas termed "food deserts" or those who are food insecure, can also develop vitamin B_{12} deficiency. Vegans are particularly susceptible to vitamin B_{12} deficiency if they do not consume plant sources such as legumes. Persons who have undergone bariatric surgery may also become vitamin B_{12} deficient if not given supplements. Persons with *Helicobacter pylori* gastric infection, achlorhydria, or excessive use of antacids or proton pump inhibitors can have vitamin B_{12} deficiency. Celiac disease or inflammatory bowel disease are also risk factors for vitamin B_{12} deficiency.

Pathophysiology. Food–cobalamin malabsorption is caused primarily by gastric atrophy. Over 40% of patients older than 80 years have gastric atrophy and achlorhydria. Normally, the absorption of vitamin B_{12} from the stomach into the bloodstream requires adequate gastric HCl and IF. Gastric mucosal atrophy, common in older adults, causes a decrease in the number of cells that secrete HCl and IF.

In pernicious anemia, for unclear reasons, the body develops antibodies to IF. The antibodies destroy the IF, and consequently vitamin B_{12} cannot be absorbed into the bloodstream. This autoimmune destruction of IF is most commonly seen in older adults. Oral sources of vitamin B_{12} are not absorbed with complete IF deficiency.

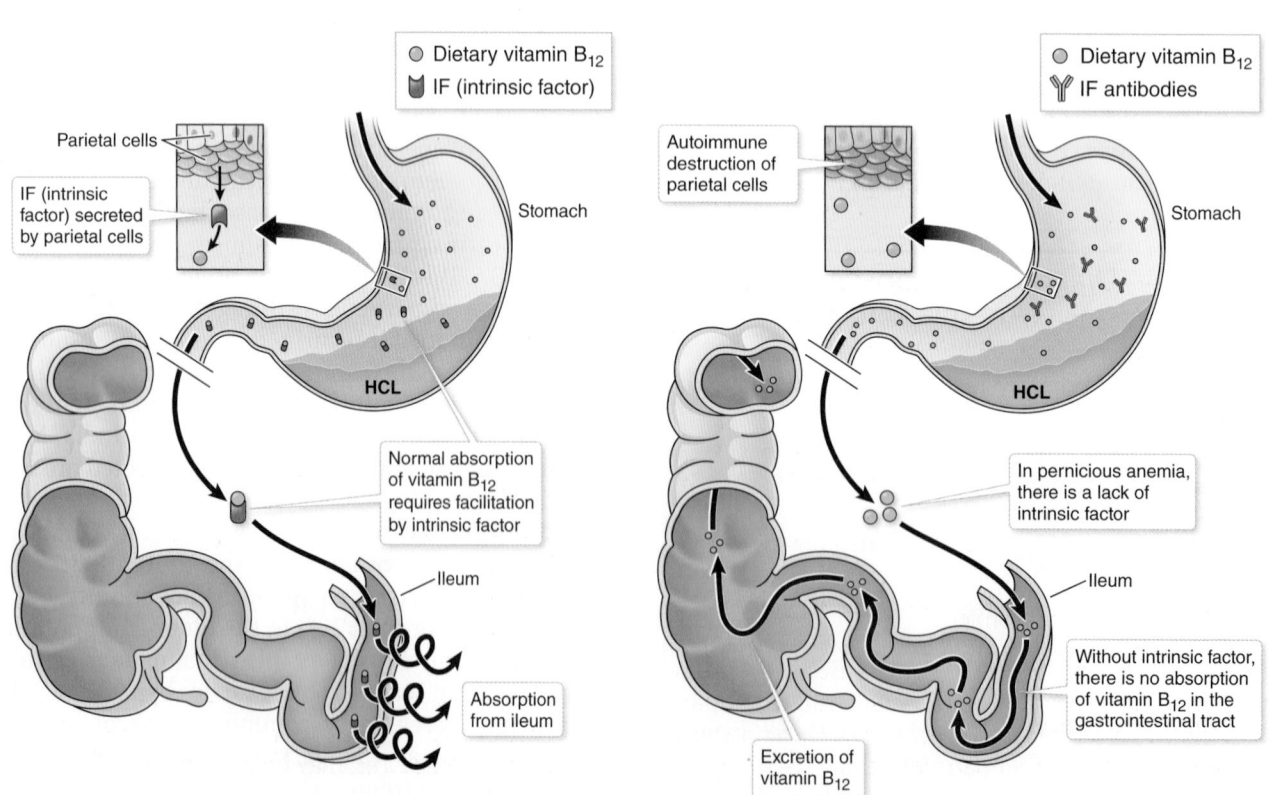

FIGURE 13-13. In pernicious anemia, there is autoimmune destruction of IF in the stomach. IF is necessary for absorption of vitamin B_{12} in the gastrointestinal tract; without IF, vitamin B_{12} is not absorbed.

Other factors that contribute to malabsorption of vitamin B_{12} in older adults include chronic carriage of *H. pylori*. The proliferation of the bacteria in the stomach, a common cause of gastric ulceration, can interfere with vitamin B_{12} absorption into the bloodstream.

Vitamin B_{12} Deficiency: Effects on the Body. Both vitamin B_{12} and folic acid are necessary for DNA synthesis. The rapidly dividing blood cell precursors of the bone marrow are constantly synthesizing DNA, so deficiency of either vitamin B_{12} or folic acid negatively affects hematopoiesis. Vitamin B_{12} is a vital factor in folic acid metabolism.

Vitamin B_{12} deficiency also has an effect on the neurological system, but the mechanism is not well understood. CNS demyelination occurs, but how vitamin B_{12} deficiency exactly leads to demyelination remains unclear. Myelin defects and abnormal neural conduction occur mainly in the dorsal horns and corticospinal tract of the spinal cord. The disorder is referred to as **subacute combined degeneration**, which is manifested as numbness and weakness in the extremities and gait disturbance. In addition, synthesis of serotonin, norepinephrine, and dopamine is affected by lack of vitamin B_{12}. This suggests that vitamin B_{12} deficiency affects neurotransmitter synthesis and may be relevant to mental status changes, such as depression and memory loss.

CLINICAL CONCEPT

Vitamin B_{12} deficiency can have widespread neurological effects; sensory, motor, and cognitive problems.

Clinical Presentation. The history and physical examination may or may not cause the clinician to suspect vitamin B_{12} deficiency. This is often not readily apparent to the patient through symptoms or to the clinician via physical assessment findings. Those patients at highest risk include vegetarians and older adults.

Signs and Symptoms. Signs and symptoms of vitamin B_{12}–deficiency anemia include those of other anemias: fatigue, exercise intolerance, dyspnea, weakness, and tachycardia. The patient may also have glossitis. Symptoms usually develop slowly over time, with nervous system changes such as numbness and tingling in the hands and feet, unsteady gait, balance problems, and mental changes possibly being noticed first. Mental changes such as depression and memory impairment that mimic dementia can occur. Optic atrophy and consequent visual impairment can also occur.

Physical Examination. The physical examination of the patient with vitamin B_{12} deficiency may be unremarkable. The examination should involve assessment for signs of anemia such as pallor and tachycardia. The conjunctiva and palms of the hand should be inspected for signs of pallor. The tongue should be inspected for glossitis. Patients can develop cheilosis, which is the presence of fissures in the corners of the mouth. The cranial nerves should be examined. Sensation of the extremities should be assessed. Gait and balance should be observed. Romberg's sign, imbalance with eyes closed in a standing position, may be positive. There may be a loss of deep tendon reflexes and a positive Babinski's sign. If the patient exhibits mental changes, a depression and dementia assessment tool may be useful.

Diagnosis. Diagnosis begins with establishing that anemia is present, based on the CBC. Additional tests should be done to assess vitamin B_{12} levels, as well as folic acid, homocysteine (tHcy), and methylmalonic acid (MMA) levels (see Box 13-6). The concentration of total tHcy is elevated in both folic acid and cobalamin deficiencies. To differentiate between folic acid and vitamin B_{12} deficiency, an MMA level is necessary. Vitamin B_{12} is specifically needed to break down MMA. Elevated MMA specifically indicates vitamin B_{12} deficiency. The CBC will show decreased Hgb, decreased Hct, and increased MCV, which indicate megaloblastic anemia. There is also a deficiency of reticulocytes, as the bone marrow is weakly producing RBCs. Peripheral blood smear demonstrates enlarged oval RBCs, referred to as macrocytosis, and some misshapen RBCs, conditions referred to as anisocytosis and poikilocytosis. Leukopenia may be present. Neutrophils have nuclei that are characteristically hypersegmented

BOX 13-6. Diagnosis of Pernicious Anemia

Pernicious anemia is a specific type of vitamin B_{12} deficiency. The following laboratory test results are indicative of pernicious anemia:

CBC RESULTS
- Hgb: low
- Hct: low
- MCV: high
- MCH: normal
- MCHC: normal
- Reticulocytes: low

ADDITIONAL LABORATORY TESTS
- Vitamin B_{12} assay: low
- IF antibodies: positive
- Parietal cell antibodies: positive
- Gastrin: high
- *H. pylori* antibodies: may be positive
- tHcy: high
- MMA: high
- Folic acid: low

and multilobed. A low serum B_{12} assay indicates a low amount of vitamin B_{12} in the bloodstream; however, in vitamin B_{12} deficiency, there may be a normal vitamin B_{12} level in the bloodstream. Other blood tests include bilirubin levels and presence of IF antibodies and parietal cell antibodies, though these antibodies are not always exhibited in a blood test. Bilirubin may be elevated because of death of immature RBCs in the bone marrow.

Treatment. The main goal of treatment is correction of the anemia, which is accomplished by first remedying the underlying cause, such as poor nutrition. If the cause is not readily remedied, the patient needs administration of vitamin B_{12} intramuscularly. Insufficient dietary intake is corrected by recommending a diet rich in sources of vitamin B_{12} and through the use of oral supplements. Replenishment of body stores can be accomplished with six 1,000-mcg intramuscular injections of hydroxocobalamin given at 3- to 7-day intervals. For maintenance therapy, 1,000 mcg of vitamin B_{12} intramuscularly every 3 months is sufficient. If an intramuscular regimen is not possible, the patient can take large oral doses of vitamin B_{12}. For pernicious anemia, the dosage is 1,000 to 2,000 mcg daily. For food–cobalamin malabsorption syndrome, 250 mcg daily is recommended.

Before administering vitamin B_{12} replacement, it is important to assess folic acid levels to assess the need for folic acid supplementation. Synthesis of folic acid is mediated by vitamin B_{12}; therefore, the lack of vitamin B_{12} will cause diminished folic acid.

Folic Acid Deficiency

A deficiency of folic acid results in a megaloblastic anemia similar to that seen with vitamin B_{12} deficiency. Folic acid is a form of B vitamin found in a variety of foods, including whole grains, beans, and green leafy vegetables such as spinach. In the United States and developed countries, foods are fortified with folic acid, so in these countries folic acid deficiency is uncommon; however, underdeveloped countries that do not have fortified food have higher rates of folic acid deficiency. In the United States, patients at risk for folic acid deficiency include:

- Pregnant and lactating women
- Patients with alcohol use disorder
- Chronic use of NSAIDs
- Patients taking certain drugs, such as phenytoin, sulfonamides, oral contraceptives, anticonvulsants, or methotrexate
- Older adults, because of malnutrition and comorbid medical conditions
- Individuals with celiac disease or inflammatory bowel disease
- Patients with chronic inflammatory disorders such as rheumatoid arthritis, tuberculosis, psoriasis, bacterial endocarditis, and systemic infections.

Etiology. A healthy individual has about 500 to 20,000 mcg of folic acid in body stores and needs 50 to 100 mcg of folic acid per day in order to replenish the daily degradation and loss through urine and bile. Although folic acid deficiency from malnutrition can occur, malabsorption of folic acid from the GI tract is a much more common cause. Folic acid deficiency occurs in gluten-induced intestinal disorders, intestinal resection surgery, Crohn's disease, and celiac disease. It is also seen in patients taking certain drugs, such as methotrexate, triamterene, trimethoprim, anticonvulsants, certain antibiotics, and oral contraceptives. Chronic use of NSAIDs can also deplete folic acid stores.

Increased demand for folic acid, which plays a vital role in neural development in the fetus, occurs with pregnancy, as well as during lactation. During pregnancy, up to 400 mcg of folic acid is needed daily; prenatal vitamins are a good source. Newborn infants have a demand for folic acid that is 10 times that of an adult.

Because folic acid is loosely bound to plasma proteins, dialysis can remove it, causing deficiency in patients with renal failure. Chronic intake of alcohol other than beer causes folic acid depletion, though the mechanism is unknown. Alcohol use disorder also causes significant depletion of thiamine, or vitamin B_1. Thiamine deficiency can cause a dementia-like syndrome.

Hematological disorders such as chronic hemolytic anemia, particularly SCA, can also cause folic acid deficiency.

Pathophysiology. In order to understand folic acid deficiency, it is necessary to comprehend the synthesis of activated folic acid, as well as the effects of folic acid deficiency on DNA synthesis.

Folic Acid and DNA Synthesis. The common feature of all megaloblastic anemias is a defect in DNA synthesis that affects rapidly dividing cells in the bone marrow. Folic acid is needed in reactions that lead to DNA synthesis. Within the plasma, folic acid is present, mostly in the 5-methyltetrahydrofolate (5-methyl THFA) form, and is loosely associated with plasma proteins in circulation. The 5-methyl THFA enters the cell via a diverse range of folic acid transporters with differing affinities and mechanisms. Once inside the cell, 5-methyl THFA must be demethylated to THFA, the active form participating in folic acid–dependent enzymatic reactions. Vitamin B_{12} is required in this conversion, and in its absence, folic acid is trapped as 5-methyl THFA. This is referred to as folic acid trapping. Without vitamin B_{12}, folic acid cannot become active to participate in DNA synthesis.

Folic Acid and Prevention of Fetal Neural Tube Defects. Spina bifida is a disorder of the spinal cord that can develop in the fetus during the first month of gestation. In spina bifida, some vertebrae overlying the spinal cord are underdeveloped and do not fuse around the spinal cord. There are varying degrees of spina bifida. The most severe form is myelomeningocele, in which the spinal cord and meningeal membranes protrude through an opening in the spine. Other neural tube defects include anencephaly (absence of portions of the brain) and encephalocele, conditions in which a portion of the cerebral neural tube protrudes through the skull. Anencephaly is not compatible with life.

If not severe, spina bifida can be surgically repaired after birth, but this usually does not restore complete normal function to the affected part of the spinal cord. Intrauterine surgery for spina bifida is also performed. The mechanism by which folic acid prevents spinal cord deformities is unclear, but the incidence of spina bifida can be decreased by up to 70% when daily folic acid supplements are taken before conception.

Folic Acid and Prevention of Cardiovascular Disease. Homocysteine (tHCy) is an amino acid that requires folic acid for its breakdown. Without sufficient folic acid, tHCy levels accumulate and can cause injury to the endothelial lining of arteries. Some studies have linked elevated blood levels of tHCy to increased risk of premature coronary artery disease, stroke, and venous blood clots. These studies have led to speculations that high tHCy levels could contribute to arteriosclerosis, which is why some clinicians are prescribing folic acid to prevent cardiac disease and arteriosclerosis.

Clinical Presentation. A thorough history and physical examination is necessary if folic acid deficiency is suspected. However, the deficiency does not cause overt symptomatology, nor does it cause obvious physical assessment findings. In patients with alcohol use disorder and those who are malnourished, folic acid deficiency is probable.

Signs and Symptoms. Folic acid anemia usually progresses over several months, and the patient typically does not exhibit symptoms until the Hct reaches very low levels, below 20%. At that point, symptoms such as weakness, fatigue, difficulty concentrating, irritability, headache, palpitations, and shortness of breath can occur. Heart failure can develop in light of high-output cardiac compensation for the decreased tissue oxygenation. Angina pectoris may occur in predisposed individuals because of increased cardiac work demand. Tachycardia, postural hypotension, and lactic acidosis are other common findings.

Physical Examination. The physical examination of the patient with folic acid deficiency may be unremarkable. Signs of anemia such as pallor, tachycardia, and cheilitis may or may not be present.

Diagnosis. Blood and bone marrow findings exhibit megaloblastic anemia that is indistinguishable from vitamin B_{12} deficiency. It is important to distinguish folic acid from vitamin B_{12} deficiency (see Box 13-7). Because vitamin B_{12} is necessary for activation of folic

---

BOX 13-7. Diagnosis of Folic Acid Deficiency

- Hgb: low
- Hct: low
- MCV: high
- MCH: normal
- MCHC: normal
- Folic acid level: low
- tHCy: high
- MMA level: normal

---

acid, simply supplementing the diet with folic acid alone can bypass the need for vitamin B_{12}. Administering folic acid can mask the vitamin B_{12} deficiency. However, vitamin B_{12} is necessary for neurological health and it needs to be replaced as well.

A vitamin B_{12} assay and folic acid level should be done together. However, blood folic acid levels have false-positive and false-negative results. The best test for folic acid deficiency as the cause of megaloblastic anemia is a comparison of serum tHCy level and a level of its metabolite, MMA. A normal MMA level with an elevated tHCy level indicates that folic acid is not assisting in the metabolism of homocysteine, which is diagnostic for folic acid deficiency.

Treatment. Treatment commonly consists of oral replacement of folic acid at the dose of 1 mg/day. This will restore tissue levels. Oral doses of 5 to 15 mg of folic acid can be absorbed in those with malabsorption. Long-term therapy is needed when the underlying cause cannot be corrected. It is important to measure vitamin B_{12} levels to investigate if treatment with B_{12} is also needed. In pregnant women, folic acid supplementation should begin as soon as pregnancy is discovered. Infants also should have vitamins containing folic acid.

ALERT! Before treating a patient with folic acid in megaloblastic anemia, it is important to exclude vitamin B_{12} deficiency. Treating the patient with only folic acid would correct the anemia but not prevent the neurological damage associated with vitamin B_{12} deficiency.

Lack of Bone Marrow Production of Red Blood Cells

The lack of bone marrow synthesis of RBCs is another possible cause of anemia. Although uncommon, when this type of anemia occurs, it often involves WBCs and platelets as well. Therefore, infection and lack of clotting are accompanying symptoms. Anemias due to lack of bone marrow production include those caused by a lack of EPO, aplastic anemia, and anemia of chronic disease.

Lack of Erythropoietin

Lack of EPO causes anemia, as there is a lack of stimulation of the bone marrow to synthesize RBCs. The anemia will be NCNC, because although the RBCs that are synthesized are normal, there is a scarcity of them. There is also a lack of reticulocytes in the peripheral blood and bone marrow because the progenitor cells and immature forms of RBCs are deficient.

The most common cause of EPO deficiency is renal failure. In renal failure, the degree of anemia depends on the severity of the renal dysfunction. However, hypometabolic states such as hypothyroidism and hypopituitarism, as well as protein deficiency, also decrease production of EPO.

Therapy is directed at the underlying cause. In cases like chronic renal disease where normal function cannot be reestablished, recombinant EPO can be administered to stimulate production of a normal level of RBCs. Transfusion is usually not required.

CLINICAL CONCEPT

In renal failure, EPO is currently used to stimulate RBC production and correct the anemia.

Aplastic Anemia

Aplastic anemia occurs when the bone marrow fails, resulting in hypocellular bone marrow and pancytopenia, which is a deficiency of all blood cells. There is a deficiency of all hematopoietic stem cells. Approximately 80% of the time, the problem is acquired because of infections such as hepatitis, HIV, or Epstein–Barr virus; exposure to toxic levels of radiation or chemicals such as benzene; certain drugs; or immune disease. The disease can also be inherited due to genetic mutations. Aplastic anemia can coexist with or evolve into myelodysplastic syndrome or acute myeloid leukemia. Aplastic anemia is rare, occurring in 2 persons per million in the United States. It can occur at any age, but incidence increases in people older than 60 years. The major causes of death among this population are infection caused by lack of WBCs and bleeding caused by lack of platelets.

Etiology. In bone marrow failure, early forms of hematopoietic cells are greatly diminished; the stem cell pool is reduced to less than 1%. The bone marrow often contains fat instead of blood cells.

In drug-induced or chemical damage of the bone marrow, direct tissue injury occurs because of toxic metabolites. High doses of radiation also cause direct cell injury. However, in cases caused by other agents, the disorder may be immune mediated. Activated cytotoxic T cells are present in patients with aplastic anemia, and these diminish with immunosuppressive therapy. However, the sustained autoimmune response is not well understood. There are chromosomal abnormalities associated with aplastic anemia at 6p, 7, and/or 13. Gene mutations are commonly found, including the *PIGA, BCOR, BCORL1, DMNT3A,* and *ASLX1*. Epigenetic changes can also cause the disease with mutation in the TP53 gene. In addition, acquired mutations in the *TERT* gene, which is involved in the telomere repair pathway, appear to be a genetic risk factor.

Clinical Presentation. Signs and symptoms can develop abruptly or gradually. Symptoms caused by thrombocytopenia are petechiae, bleeding gums, easy bruising, nosebleeds, and heavy menstrual bleeding. The lack of RBCs will produce the typical symptoms of anemia, including fatigue, pallor, tachycardia, and tachypnea. Lack of WBCs increases the risk for infections. Short stature, microcephaly, skeletal abnormalities, and developmental delays may be apparent in children. There may be abnormalities in the heart, kidneys, and lungs, and pancreatic insufficiency.

Diagnosis. Diagnosis begins with a CBC, which will reveal pancytopenia. Some small amounts of enlarged RBCs may be found, making for a mild megaloblastic anemia. The reticulocyte, WBC, and platelet counts will be low. Bone marrow examination reveals severe hypocellularity with lack of hematopoietic cells and a predominance of fat cells. It is important to establish the cause of aplastic anemia as an inherited or an acquired disease as this determines treatment options. Therefore, additional tests are needed to identify the cause such as genetic testing, flow cytometry, karyotype, HLA typing, % of fetal HgbF in the bloodstream, hepatitis panel, HIV, CMV, EBV, and parvovirus serologies, lactic dehydrogenase, antinuclear antibody, and haptoglobin levels, vitamin B_{12}, folic acid, copper, and pancreatic enzymes. Aplastic anemia can be mild, moderate, or severe. The severe form is life-threatening with extremely low blood cell counts and requires immediate hospitalization.

Treatment. Blood transfusions are required until the diagnosis is confirmed and specific treatment is started. However, the goal of treatment is to achieve independence from transfusions. The use of transfusions should be limited where possible to decrease the occurrence of sensitization, which would increase the risk of rejection in candidates for bone marrow transplantation. Infections are the major cause of mortality, so preventive use of broad-spectrum antibiotic therapy is recommended, particularly for those patients with indwelling catheters. Early use of antifungal agents should be considered for those with persistent fever.

Bone marrow transplantation from a human leukocyte antigen (HLA)–matched sibling donor is the preferred treatment. The risk of rejection, also called graft versus host disease (GVHD), increases with the patient's age. Immunosuppressive drugs may be recommended including antithymocyte globulin, cyclosporine, and eltrombopag (a bone-stimulating agent). Prophylactic antibiotics and platelet, RBC, and WBC transfusions are necessary. Bone marrow stimulants such as filgrastim (Neupogen) and epoetin-alfa (Epogen) can be used to stimulate the marrow to produce more cells and provide symptom relief.

In cases of aplastic anemia caused by radiation or chemotherapy, the marrow usually recovers once the treatment is stopped. Bone marrow–stimulating drugs (filgrastim and epoetin-alfa) are used to relieve symptoms until the marrow recovers.

Anemia of Chronic Disease

ACD develops as a result of chronic disorders such as infection, inflammation, cancer, heart failure, diabetes, and stroke. It is a side effect of a long-term disorder that weakens the body. The long-term disorders often associated with anemia include rheumatoid arthritis or other autoimmune disease; tuberculosis or other chronic infection; and inflammatory bowel disease, chronic heart failure, and kidney failure. It is particularly common among older adult patients, as they often have one or more chronic diseases and take multiple medications that may contribute to their anemia. The mechanisms of ACD include a decrease in RBC survival time, blunted erythropoietic response in the bone marrow, and impaired iron metabolism in the cell, resulting in inefficient recycling of iron from old RBCs. Therefore, there is a lack of available iron for erythropoiesis. The clinician will need to distinguish this anemia from iron-deficiency anemia, though this can be difficult, as ACD and iron-deficiency anemia frequently coexist in older individuals. The serum ferritin and transferrin levels are recommended to evaluate iron levels.

Signs and symptoms are usually those of the underlying disease accompanied by signs and symptoms of anemia, principally fatigue, pallor, and tachycardia. The anemia is usually NCNC but may become microcytic over time.

Treatment should focus on the underlying disease. Transfusions are not recommended, but the use of recombinant EPO has been effective. Because of the blunted response to EPO, higher-than-usual doses are needed to be effective.

Polycythemia

Polycythemia can be described as the opposite of anemia. Instead of a deficit of RBCs, there is an overabundance of RBCs. In primary polycythemia, there is hyperproliferation of all blood cells. Secondary polycythemia is more common and is a hyperproliferation of only the RBCs. Secondary polycythemia occurs in response to chronic blood hypoxia.

Primary Polycythemia

Primary polycythemia, also called polycythemia vera, occurs when there is an excess of all blood cell types—RBCs, WBCs, and platelets—in the bone marrow. The excess RBCs make the blood viscous and it flows slowly, especially through small vessels. The slow blood flow and thrombocytosis result in the formation of clots, which can incite a number of serious problems, including heart attack and stroke. The etiology of primary polycythemia is unknown, but chromosomal abnormalities are associated with 30% of cases. These include gene deletions at 20q and 13q, trisomy 9, and a mutation at the JAK2 gene locus on 9p. A mutation in JAK2, a tyrosine kinase enzyme that allows for hyperproliferation of blood cells, is found in 90% to 95% of patients with primary polycythemia. In addition to the erythrocytosis, leukocytosis and thrombocytosis occur. Primary polycythemia is rare, more often seen in adults older than 60 years and rarely in persons younger than 20 years. It occurs more often in men than in women. Primary polycythemia is usually diagnosed by an incidental finding on a CBC. Hgb can be as high as 20 g/dL and Hct greater than 60%. Symptoms are usually related to hyperviscosity of the blood. Systolic hypertension and deep venous thrombosis may be presenting signs. Patients experience neurological symptoms related to cerebral blood flow, such as vertigo, tinnitus, headache, visual disturbances, and transient ischemic attacks. Ischemia of organs, easy bruising, nosebleeds, or GI bleeding may occur because of vascular stasis. A complication called erythromelalgia causes ischemia and infarction in the lower extremities. The patient experiences pain, numbness, erythema, and digital necrosis. Body-wide pruritus is a chronic problem, and antihistamines do not provide relief. Splenomegaly can occur because of the constant breakdown of blood cells. Because the patient has an excess of blood cells, a large amount of cellular breakdown occurs daily. The large amount of cellular DNA further breaks down into purines, which become uric acids. The patient often develops hyperuricemia and gout.

The diagnostic tests for primary polycythemia include EPO level, abdominal ultrasound to assess size of the spleen, and assessment for JAK2 mutations. A normal level of EPO is an indication that the polycythemia is occurring without any stimulus from EPO. For treatment, patients require periodic phlebotomy (drawing of blood). Thrombosis due to thrombocytosis is the most significant complication. Therefore, aspirin or anticoagulants are given to prevent clots. Allopurinol is a medication that keeps uric acid low to prevent development of gout. Splenectomy may be required. Myelosuppressive agents may be ordered to reduce the overproduction of cells by the bone marrow. Hydroxyurea is a commonly used myelosuppressive agent. Anagrelide, a phosphodiesterase inhibitor, can reduce platelet count and is less toxic than hydroxyurea. Pegylated interferon-alpha has been shown to induce hematological remission in 20% of patients with primary polycythemia. Ruxolitinib, a JAK2 inhibitor, is a new agent that is increasingly prescribed. It alleviates constitutional symptoms such as pruritus, reduces spleen size, and decreases need for phlebotomy. Most persons with primary polycythemia can live long lives without functional impairment with the described treatments.

Secondary Polycythemia

Secondary polycythemia, also called **erythrocytosis**, is a more common disorder than primary polycythemia. It is caused by prolonged hypoxia as a compensatory effort by the body to improve oxygen delivery. Hypoxia constantly stimulates EPO, which in turn provokes the bone marrow to produce RBCs. Persons with chronic hypoxia, such as those who suffer from chronic obstructive pulmonary disease (COPD), spend long periods at high altitudes, or have severe heart or lung disease are most likely to have secondary polycythemia.

The signs and symptoms develop slowly, and the patient can be asymptomatic for years. The various symptoms include headache; dizziness; weakness; shortness of breath, especially when lying down (called orthopnea); feelings of fullness on the left side of the abdomen caused by splenic enlargement; vision changes; redness and itching of the skin; and unexplained bleeding. The person may also experience angina and abdominal pain.

Secondary polycythemia is often an incidental finding on a CBC. Hgb levels usually do not become greater than 17 or 18 g/dL. It should be suspected when the person has an abnormally high Hgb or Hct level and a high EPO level. Secondary polycythemia may be reversed depending on whether the underlying cause of hypoxia can be eliminated.

Chapter Summary

- RBCs are synthesized in the bone marrow in response to EPO secretion by the kidneys.
- RBCs are nonnucleated cells that carry oxygen on an Hgb molecule. Iron is necessary to form Hgb.
- Reticulocytes are immature RBCs that are produced in high numbers by active bone marrow.
- Bilirubin is a breakdown product of RBCs. Jaundice occurs when there is a high amount of bilirubin in the bloodstream.
- The spleen is the graveyard of RBCs. Splenomegaly and splenic dysfunction can occur if a constant number of RBCs need to be processed by the spleen.
- Anemias are disorders in which there is a lack of mature, healthy RBCs, leading to impaired oxygen delivery to cells and tissues.
- Causes of anemia include blood loss, accelerated destruction of erythrocytes, and failure of erythrocyte production.
- Common symptoms of anemia include fatigue, dyspnea, exercise intolerance, pallor, and tachycardia.
- Diagnosis of anemia begins with a CBC, which establishes the presence of the disorder. The indices MCV, MCH, and MCHC provide information about possible causes.
- The MCV index indicates the size of the RBC. Normal MCV indicates normal-sized RBCs. Low MCV indicates small RBCS called microcytic cells. High MCV indicates megaloblastic or macrocytic cells. The MCHC indicates the color of the RBCs. Normal MCHC indicates normal color of cells. Low MCHC indicates pale cells.
- Anemias can be categorized according to how they appear on a peripheral blood smear. The various descriptive categories include normocytic normochromic (NCNC), microcytic hypochromic (MCHC), or megaloblastic (also called macrocytic).
- A large amount of blood loss causes NCNC anemia.
- Iron deficiency is the most common cause of anemia. It is MCHC anemia commonly caused by menorrhagia and GI bleeding in adults.
- Iron deficiency is caused by a slow loss of RBCs from the body. With this slow loss, the body gradually loses Hgb, which is the main source of iron in the body and therefore causes iron deficiency.
- Iron deficiency in a male or postmenopausal female should increase the clinician's suspicion of GI bleeding due to ulcer or colon cancer.
- Serum ferritin, transferrin, TIBC, and FOBT are tests needed in iron deficiency.
- Iron deficiency in adult males and postmenopausal females requires colonoscopy to assess for colon cancer.
- Vitamin B_{12} deficiency causes megaloblastic anemia and neurological dysfunction of the spinal cord. Older adults can develop gait dysfunction, sensory loss in the feet, and dementia-like symptoms.
- Pernicious anemia is a vitamin B_{12} deficiency caused by autoimmune destruction of IF in the stomach. Vitamin B_{12} requires IF for absorption. Therefore, pernicious anemia is best treated with parenteral vitamin B_{12}.
- Folic acid deficiency also causes megaloblastic anemia. This deficiency allows accumulation of homocysteine, an amino acid that causes endothelial damage leading to arteriosclerosis.

- Folic acid deficiency in pregnant women can cause spinal cord and CNS abnormalities in the fetus.
- SCA and thalassemia are the most common disorders of Hgb structure (termed hemoglobinopathy).
- Vaso-occlusive crises can occur when individuals with SCA endure hypoxia, stress, or infection. Children often suffer numerous vaso-occlusive crises as they grow.
- Vaso-occlusive crises are severely painful episodes that often occur in the long bones or organs. Opiate medications are commonly needed for episodes, which can lead to dependence.
- Vaso-occlusive crises can lead to ischemia of an organ. Ischemia of the brain can cause stroke.
- Transfusion, a mainstay of treatment in anemia, is commonly used when Hgb is 7 g/dL.

- Type O blood is the universal donor; type AB is the universal recipient.
- HDN commonly occurs at birth due to ABO incompatibility of the mother and infant when a small quantity of blood from the mother can enter fetal circulation. The maternal antibodies destroy some infant RBCs. This causes a mild anemia with jaundice in the infant.
- Secondary polycythemia is stimulated by chronic hypoxia of the bloodstream.
- Polycythemia vera is a cancerous condition of the blood cells that causes excessive accumulation of RBCs, WBCs, and platelets in the bloodstream.
- Bone marrow transplantation requires a donor with matching tissue type of the recipient.

 ## Making the Connections

Pathophysiology

Signs and Symptoms	Physical Assessment Findings	Diagnosis	Treatment
Anemia | Lack of adequate numbers of mature, healthy RBCs results in insufficient oxygen delivery to tissues. The cells are unable to meet the demand for oxygen, causing an oxygen deficit. Because oxygen demand is higher with activity, the deficit is worse with increased activity or stress.			
Unusual fatigue. Decreased ability to carry out activities of daily living. Shortness of breath that worsens with activity. Dizziness. Cold intolerance. Headache possible. Chest pain possible.	Pallor. Tachypnea. Tachycardia. Cold extremities.	Decreased Hgb and Hct levels. Decreased RBC count. Increased reticulocyte count if there is a normal bone marrow response to rapid blood loss. MCV and MCHC parameters can assist diagnosis of cause of anemia.	Depends on the cause of the anemia: Standard treatment is blood transfusion. Avoidance of stress and increased activity. Oxygen.
Anemia Caused by Hemorrhage, Rapid Blood Loss | Trauma or severe GI bleeding causes the body to lose large amounts of blood. Sympathetic nervous system response causes increased heart rate and peripheral vasoconstriction. Activation of the renin–angiotensin system results in retention of water by the kidney, which increases blood volume and blood pressure.			
Depends on volume of blood loss. • Less than 15% loss: anxiety and orthostatic hypotension. • 15% to 30% loss: restlessness, changes in level of consciousness (LOC). • 30% to 40% loss: further decrease in LOC. Faint, dizziness, apprehension. Feels cold. • Greater than 40% loss: profound shock. Patient may report hematemesis if blood loss is from esophageal varices. Melena and hematochezia if blood loss from lower GI tract.	Postural blood pressure drops. Changes in LOC. Narrowed pulse pressure. Urine output lower than 30 mL/hr. Tachycardia greater than 120. Weak pulse, hypotension, cool, pale. Heart rate greater than 140. Scant or no urine output. Profound hypotension.	Low Hgb and Hct. Low RBC count. Normochromic, normocytic anemia. High reticulocyte count. FOBT may be positive if GI bleed.	Identify the bleeding site and restore hemostasis. Transfusion to restore RBCs and blood volume. Avoid inotropic drugs in the setting of low blood volume. Oxygen. Elevate feet.

Continued

Making the Connections—cont'd

Signs and Symptoms	Physical Assessment Findings	Diagnosis	Treatment
Anemia Caused by Chronic Blood Loss | Gradual, slow blood loss from GI tract or caused by heavy menses. Colon cancer is a common cause of chronic blood loss via the GI tract. Slow loss of blood depletes the body of iron.			
Fatigue, weakness, or no symptoms. Some shortness of breath with activity. Dark stool possible (melena). If excessive menstrual blood loss, the patient uses an excessive number of pads or tampons per day.	Mild tachycardia. Pallor. Melena: FOBT positive stools if GI bleed. Unusually heavy menses if caused by menorrhagia.	Low Hgb and Hct. Microcytic hypochromic anemia. Low RBC count. Low serum iron and ferritin levels caused by loss of iron stores and inability to recycle iron.	Identify the site of the blood loss and establish hemostasis. If blood loss has been severe, transfusions are required. Iron replacement therapy is needed for hemopoiesis.
Hemolytic Anemia | Accelerated RBC destruction exceeds erythrocyte production. Causes: mechanical turbulence caused by prosthetic cardiac valves; autoimmune response leading to destruction of RBCs by antibodies. Can be an adverse effect of medication. The spleen enlarges because it is working hard to remove damaged RBCs.			
Fatigue, pallor, shortness of breath. Chills, jaundice possible.	Tachycardia as compensatory response to anemia. Pallor. Jaundice caused by excess breakdown on RBCs, which releases bilirubin into blood. Dark urine caused by bilirubin in urine. Enlarged spleen caused by high activity.	Decrease in Hgb and Hct. Increased reticulocyte count. Increased bilirubin, methemoglobin, and urobilinogen levels, which are breakdown products of RBCs. Tests for autoantibodies: IgM class is called cold agglutinins; IgG class is called warm agglutinins.	If medication suspected as etiology, stop medication. Folic acid and iron replacement. Corticosteroids. Autoimmune diagnosis may require immunosuppressive drugs and splenectomy.
Pernicious Anemia | A specific type of vitamin B_{12} anemia caused by a lack of IF. Lack of IF results in impaired absorption of vitamin B_{12} from stomach. Autoimmune destruction of IF by antibodies is the cause of IF deficiency. Nerve and blood cells need vitamin B_{12} to function properly, so neurological functions are impaired. RBCs cannot be properly synthesized, and neurons in the dorsal columns of the spinal cord show loss of myelination.			
Usual symptoms of anemia: pallor, shortness of breath with activity, fatigue. Vitamin B_{12} deficiency. Neurological symptoms, including numbness and tingling of hands and feet, gait disturbances, and lack of coordination. Depression and dementia also may be caused by vitamin B_{12} deficit.	Unsteady gait. Sensory loss in feet. Positive Babinski's reflex. Loss of deep tendon reflexes. Personality changes; dementialike symptoms and depression. Neurological changes are often seen before the anemia is diagnosed. Red, smooth tongue; glossitis. Sore mouth; cheilitis.	Enlarged oval-shaped RBCs. Hgb and Hct may be low or normal. Megaloblastic, macrocytic anemia. Low serum levels of vitamin B_{12} and folic acid. High levels of total homocysteine (tHCy) in blood. Elevated MMA levels.	Treatment with vitamin B_{12}. Replacement of parenteral vitamin B_{12}; intramuscular injection every 3 months. Nasal spray available. Diet rich in meat, eggs, milk, and dairy products.

Making the Connections—cont'd

Folic Acid Deficiency Anemia | Lack of sufficient folic acid in diet results in a megaloblastic anemia very similar to vitamin B_{12} deficiency.

Signs and Symptoms	Physical Assessment Findings	Diagnosis	Treatment
Usual signs and symptoms of anemia: pallor, fatigue, shortness of breath with activity, possible dizziness.	Patient is usually asymptomatic except for anemia signs; pallor, cold extremities may be present. Fetal adverse effects; lack of full spinal cord development; open neural tube defect. Infant often born with spina bifida, which causes paraplegia. Can also cause encephalocele or anencephaly. Folic acid deficiency is a risk factor for arteriosclerosis.	Folic acid levels lower than 4 mcg/mL. Low Hgb and Hct levels. MCV high. Megaloblastic anemia. Elevated tHCy levels.	Oral replacement of 1 mg folate/day. Diet rich in breads, pasta, asparagus, green leafy vegetables such as spinach, and beans.

Iron-Deficiency Anemia | Most common cause of anemia in general. Iron is essential for the formation of heme, the part of Hgb responsible for attaching oxygen for transport. Normal erythropoiesis cannot occur.

Signs and Symptoms	Physical Assessment Findings	Diagnosis	Treatment
Usual signs and symptoms of anemia: pallor, fatigue, shortness of breath, dizziness. Pica. Patients may have melena (dark, tarry stools) from slowly losing blood from GI tract. Women may have menorrhagia with each menstrual cycle.	Pallor. Tachycardia. Red, swollen tongue; glossitis. Sores of mouth; cheilitis. Enlarged spleen.	Microcytic. Hypochromic anemia. Decreased Hgb and Hct. Low serum iron and serum ferritin levels. Increased total iron binding capacity. Absence of iron in the bone marrow. Fecal occult blood test should be done to check for GI blood loss.	Oral supplements such as ferrous sulfate. If iron malabsorption is present, parenteral forms of iron are recommended. Vitamin C helps the body absorb oral iron.

Aplastic Anemia | Deficiency of all cells produced by the bone marrow, including RBCs, WBCs, and platelets. Radiation, severe infection, or cancer chemotherapy can cause this deficiency of bone marrow. Aplastic anemia can also be inherited via gene mutation.

Signs and Symptoms	Physical Assessment Findings	Diagnosis	Treatment
Severe signs and symptoms of anemia: high output heart failure can occur. Increased susceptibility to infections caused by WBC deficiency. Increased bleeding risk caused by platelet deficiency.	Severe pallor. Easy bruising, petechiae, and easy bleeding that is hard to stop, such as nosebleeds. Severe infections. Short stature. Microcephaly may be present. Skeletal abnormalities. Slow developmental milestones. Some organ anomalies may be present.	CBC reveals pancytopenia; no synthesis of any type of blood cell. Panel of laboratory testing to rule out genetic mutations, autoimmunity, hemolytic anemia. Low reticulocyte count indicates failure of marrow response. Bone marrow examination reveals hypocellularity with lack of hematopoietic cells and predominance of fat cells.	Transfusions. Leuko-poor blood transfusions preferred because fewer WBCs will allow for less chance of hypersensitivity. Bone marrow stimulants such as filgrastim and epoetin. Bone marrow transplant. Prophylactic broad-spectrum antibiotic. Immunosuppressive therapy.

Continued

Making the Connections–cont'd

Signs and Symptoms	Physical Assessment Findings	Diagnosis	Treatment
Anemia of Chronic Disease | Results from a chronic disorder that leads to decreased RBC survival time, blunted erythropoietic response in the bone marrow, impaired cellular iron metabolism, and inefficient recycling of iron from old RBCs. The chronic disease, which is often an autoimmune disorder, chronic infection, or chronic cause of inflammation, causes a weakening of the bone marrow.			
Signs and symptoms of the underlying disease along with the symptoms of anemia.	Pallor. Fatigue. Tachycardia. Shortness of breath with activity. Signs of the chronic disease, which is the etiology.	NCNC anemia. Iron stores are normal, unlike those in a patient with iron-deficiency anemia. Serum transferrin levels and transferrin receptor levels are normal.	Treatment focuses on the underlying disease. Recombinant EPO has been successful.
Sickle Cell Anemia | Most common hemoglobinopathy; a genetic disorder that causes production of flawed Hgb structure: Hgb S is produced instead of normal Hgb. Flawed Hgb provokes a hemolytic reaction by the body and poor oxygen carriage by the abnormal RBCs. Autosomal-recessive inheritance pattern. RBCs polymerize or clump under certain conditions such as hypoxia or dehydration. Distorted RBCs block blood flow in the microcirculation, leading to ischemia and damage to tissues and organs. These RBCs also have a shortened life span, leading to a secondary anemia.			
Usual signs and symptoms of anemia, particularly fatigue and reduced activity tolerance. During vaso-occlusive episodes, severe pain. Long bones often affected. Pain can be in any area of body. Stroke and myocardial infarction can occur early in childhood.	Weakness caused by anemia. Shortness of breath with activity. Stunted growth. Jaundice caused by accelerated breakdown of abnormal cells. Increased infections caused by splenic dysfunction. Enlargement of the spleen.	CBC to assess for anemia: low Hgb and Hct. Commonly a normocytic normochromic or microcytic hypochromic. Peripheral blood smear shows crescent-shaped RBCs. Screen blood sample for presence of Hgb S, the altered sickle cell Hgb. Part of routine screening of newborns. RBC breakdown causes hyperbilirubinemia. Infections with encapsulated bacterial organisms is common because of splenic dysfunction.	IV fluids to flush out clogged RBCs. Prevention and management of pain; opiates commonly needed. Prophylactic antibiotics to reduce infections. Educate patients to avoid triggers that cause crises. Bone marrow transplant if suitable donor available. Transfusions to increase numbers of normal cells. Hydroxyurea given during crisis. Gene therapy and CRISPR-Cas9 technology under investigation.
Thalassemia | A common hemoglobinopathy. Abnormal Hgb structure; two types of disease: alpha or beta. Genetic disorder with autosomal-recessive inheritance. Hemolysis of abnormal RBCs occurs and large amounts of erythropoiesis in the bone marrow leads to deformities and weakening of bones. Spleen enlarges because of hyperactivity.			
Usual signs of anemia; can be severe depending on Hgb and Hct deficiency. Can have heart failure if severe anemia. Weakness. Pallor. Shortness of breath with activity. Tachycardia. Palpitations. Hemolysis causes high bilirubin levels, which leads to jaundice.	Stunted growth. Enlarged spleen and liver. Jaundice. Dark urine. Characteristic bone abnormalities: chipmunk cheeks and hair on end skull deformities.	CBC; low Hgb and Hct, microcytic hyperchromic anemia. Electrophoresis to determine type of Hgb present. Splenomegaly. X-ray shows osteopenia, characteristic bone deformity.	Genetic counseling. Transfusions. Bone marrow transplant. Prophylactic antibiotics to reduce infections.

Making the Connections–cont'd

Signs and Symptoms	Physical Assessment Findings	Diagnosis	Treatment
Polycythemia | An excess of RBCs causes blood to be more viscous and increases peripheral vascular resistance. Blood flow slows, especially in smaller vessels, leading to increased clotting. **Primary polycythemia** results from a gene mutation that occurs after conception. High numbers of RBCs, WBCs, and platelets cause high viscosity of blood. **Secondary polycythemia** is a compensatory response to chronic hypoxia associated with smoking, living at high altitudes, and chronic diseases of the lungs and heart.			
Headache. Dizziness. Weakness. Shortness of breath, especially when lying down. Feeling of fullness on the left side of the abdomen. May have angina and abdominal pain.	Enlarged spleen and liver. Redness and itching of the skin. Unexplained bleeding or clotting. Flushed face caused by excessive numbers of RBCs.	CBC reveals abnormally high Hgb and Hct, with high WBC and platelet counts. Increased vitamin B_{12} and uric acid levels. Serum EPO is very low in primary polycythemia vera but high in secondary polycythemia.	Periodic phlebotomy. Myelosuppressive agents such as hydroxyurea. Low-dose aspirin to reduce clotting. In secondary polycythemia, control or elimination of cause.

Bibliography

Available online at fadavis.com

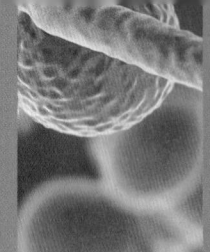

Platelet, Hemostasis, and Coagulation Disorders

Learning Objectives

Upon completion of this chapter, the student will be able to:

- Explain the process of hemostasis, including platelet aggregation and activation, and the coagulation cascade.
- Distinguish between causes of activation of the intrinsic and extrinsic pathways in the coagulation cascade.
- Describe pathological disorders caused by excessive clotting.

- Describe disorders of defective hemostasis or coagulation that cause excessive bleeding.
- List the various pharmacological agents that can be used to counteract platelet aggregation or inhibit the coagulation cascade.
- Identify the laboratory test procedures needed to monitor coagulation during some forms of anticoagulation treatment.

Key Terms

Activated partial thromboplastin time (aPTT)

Antiphospholipid syndrome

Antithrombin (AT) deficiency

Coagulation factors

Disseminated intravascular coagulation (DIC)

Extrinsic pathway

Factor V Leiden mutation

Fibrinolysis

Glycoprotein (GP) IIb/IIIa receptor

Hemostasis

Heparin

Immune thrombocytopenic purpura (ITP)

International normalized ratio (INR)

Intrinsic pathway

Low molecular weight heparin (LMWH)

Megakaryocytes

Plasmin

Prothrombin time (PT)

Prothrombin G20210A mutation (PGM)

Protein C deficiency

Protein S deficiency

Reverse cholesterol transport

Thrombocytopenia

Thrombocytosis

Thrombopoietin

Thrombosis

Thrombotic thrombocytopenic purpura (TTP)

Thrombus

Tissue plasminogen activator

Hemostasis is the physiological process that stops bleeding at the site of an injury. Blood vessels in the area of injury are torn open and leak blood; therefore, there is a need to stop blood loss. At the area of injury in the blood vessel, the endothelium stimulates the two main processes of hemostasis to initiate formation of a blood clot. This consists of platelet aggregation, or primary hemostasis, and fibrin formation, or secondary hemostasis.

During primary hemostasis, platelets aggregate to form a platelet plug and adhere to the site of injury. Secondary hemostasis refers to the deposition of fibrin, which is generated by the coagulation cascade. Fibrin forms a mesh that is incorporated into and around the platelet plug to strengthen and stabilize the blood clot. These two processes happen simultaneously and interweave to create a durable blood clot, or **thrombus**, that will stop bleeding at a site of injury.

Although blood clotting is a necessary body function, pathological thrombus formation can be detrimental

to the health of an individual. For example, a thrombus can form in the lower extremity and travel up into the inferior vena cava, then to the right atrium leading to the pulmonary artery, which creates a pulmonary embolism. Conversely, hemostasis can be dysfunctional due to inadequate platelet activity or coagulation cascade impairment, which can cause excessive bleeding.

Platelets and coagulation factors are the major elements involved in blood clotting, and an abnormality in either can cause either excessive bleeding or excessive clotting. The normal range of platelets is 150,000 to 400,000/uL. **Thrombocytopenia** is the term for a low number of platelets, fewer than 100,000/uL, which can cause bleeding. **Thrombocytosis** is the term for an excessive number of platelets, more than 750,000/uL, which can cause excessive clotting. A wide number of medications can trigger an antibody reaction to platelets, causing lysis of platelets and thrombocytopenia. A viral or bacterial infection can also stimulate antibody destruction of platelets for unknown reasons. In disorders such as polycythemia, a hyperactive disorder of the bone marrow, too many platelets can lead to development of thrombi (clots); as a result, occlusion of blood vessels can occur, and this can give rise to stroke, myocardial infarction, deep venous thrombosis, pulmonary emboli, and peripheral arterial disease.

Epidemiology

Platelet or coagulation disorders are uncommon in clinical practice. Thrombocytopenia can often be a side effect of a medication or can accompany hematological cancers such as leukemia, which inhibits development of all blood cells in the bone marrow. **Immune thrombocytopenic purpura (ITP)**, a disorder in which the immune system specifically targets platelets, can be triggered by a wide variety of medications and has an incidence of 66 cases per million persons per year. Because coagulation factors are synthesized by the liver, cirrhosis caused by alcohol use disorder is probably the most common cause of deficient coagulation. Up to 20% of heavy drinkers develop cirrhosis and consequent risk of bleeding.

Disseminated intravascular coagulation (DIC) is the most commonly acquired disorder of coagulation. Often triggered by sepsis, it occurs in 1% of all hospitalized patients. The most common genetic disease of coagulation, hemophilia A, affects 1 out of 5,000 male newborns per year. Hemophilia B, also called Christmas disease, is less common and affects 1 out of 30,000 male babies per year.

Basic Concepts of Bleeding and Clotting Physiology

The process of clotting involves the process of hemostasis, the function of platelets, and the activated coagulation cascade. An understanding of all these concepts is necessary to comprehend pathological conditions of clotting and bleeding.

Hemostasis

Hemostasis is a protective mechanism whereby the formation of a thrombus prevents excessive blood loss from the body. It has three major steps:

1. Vasoconstriction
2. Development of a platelet plug
3. Blood coagulation

Platelets, also called thrombocytes, are the cells in the body that make up clots and assist in hemostasis. Hemostasis is divided into two stages: primary hemostasis and secondary hemostasis. In primary hemostasis, platelets form a fundamental platelet plug. In secondary hemostasis, coagulation factors undergo a process known as the coagulation cascade, which leads

to fibrin formation, and eventually, a finished fibrin clot or thrombus. A thrombus is a collection of aggregated platelets reinforced by fibrin. Platelets and coagulation factors are activated to form a thrombus when the body is injured, a blood vessel wall is damaged, or blood flow is sluggish or stagnant. The coagulation system's formation of fibrin is counterbalanced by a system of fibrinolytic (clot-dissolving) mechanisms that ensure that the hemostatic effect is regulated and does not extend inappropriately.

In pathological states, hemostatic events can escape normal control mechanisms because of either inherited or acquired defects, resulting in **thrombosis**, the generation of an occlusive thrombus (clot) that obstructs blood flow in an artery or vein. Coronary, cerebrovascular, and venous thromboses are some of the consequences.

Platelets

Platelets begin as immature cells called **megakaryocytes** in the bone marrow. Megakaryocytes have no nucleus, DNA, or ribosomes, and they cannot synthesize proteins. However, they mature into platelets that have powerful granules, which contain procoagulant substances.

Platelet formation is stimulated by the hormone **thrombopoietin**, which is synthesized by the liver. A reduction in platelet numbers in the bone marrow stimulates this hormone. The normal platelet has a life span of 7 to 10 days. Almost one-third of all platelets reside in the spleen, but when enlarged and hyperactive, the spleen can sequester up to 80% of platelets.

Under normal conditions, the endothelial lining of blood vessels is a smooth, antithrombotic surface. However, when injured, inflammatory mediators and prothrombotic substances released by the endothelium draw platelets to the area. Exposed collagen and von Willebrand factor (vWF) released by the endothelium activate platelets, which in turn stimulate coagulation factors and draw additional platelets to the site. Platelet adhesion results in the activation of the **glycoprotein (GP) IIb/IIIa receptor**, which binds to fibrinogen from the coagulation cascade and enhances further platelet aggregation. Activated platelets release adhesive proteins, growth factors, and thromboxane A2 that promote platelet aggregation, draw more platelets to the site, and facilitate blood clot formation. This leads to formation of an occlusive platelet thrombus that is stabilized by fibrin.

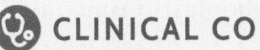

CLINICAL CONCEPT

Some antiplatelet agents work as GPIIb/IIIa receptor blockers to diminish platelet and fibrinogen linkage and inhibit clot formation. Abciximab (ReoPro) is an example of a GPIIb/IIIa inhibitor.

The Coagulation Factors

Secondary hemostasis requires a stepwise activation of proteins in the blood called **coagulation factors** that take part in a complex cascade. The cascade ultimately forms fibrin strands, which strengthen the platelet plug formed in primary hemostasis. The coagulation cascade has two pathways: the **intrinsic pathway**, also known as the contact activation pathway, and the **extrinsic pathway**, also known as the tissue factor (TF) pathway. The pathways are triggered by different events but ultimately end in the same final pathway that synthesizes fibrin. The two pathways both terminate in the same steps: the activation of factor X, which converts prothrombin to thrombin and, in turn, converts fibrinogen to fibrin. The coagulation cascade is best understood by reviewing the various step-by-step reactions portrayed in Figure 14-1.

Extrinsic Pathway

The extrinsic pathway is stimulated by trauma to a blood vessel occurring from an external injury such as a laceration. Factor VII is activated and comes into contact with TF located on injured membrane components such as fibroblasts and leukocytes. The two components form an activated complex called TF-factor VII. TF-factor VII activates factor IX and factor X. The activation of factor X by TF-factor VII is almost immediately impeded by an extrinsic pathway inhibitor. Factor X and its cofactor, factor V, form a complex that activates prothrombin to thrombin. Both the extrinsic and intrinsic pathways arrive at this significant step, which leads to the ultimate conversion of fibrinogen into fibrin (see Fig. 14-1). The clotting time of the extrinsic pathway can be measured by the **prothrombin time (PT)** diagnostic test or **International Normalized Ratio (INR)**.

Intrinsic Pathway

The intrinsic pathway is stimulated by tissue damage incurred by injury to the endothelial lining of a blood vessel, as in inflammation or atherosclerosis. The pathway can also be triggered by stasis of blood, as occurs in atrial fibrillation. The pathway begins with activation of factor XII; from there, activation of a number of factors occurs until factor X is reached (see Fig. 14-1). Factor X activates the conversion of prothrombin to thrombin, which leads to the ultimate conversion of fibrinogen into fibrin. The blood clotting time of the intrinsic pathway can be measured by the **activated partial thromboplastin time (aPTT)** diagnostic test.

Final Pathway in the Coagulation Cascade

Both intrinsic and extrinsic pathways go through an array of complex step-by-step reactions to arrive at a common final pathway: conversion of prothrombin

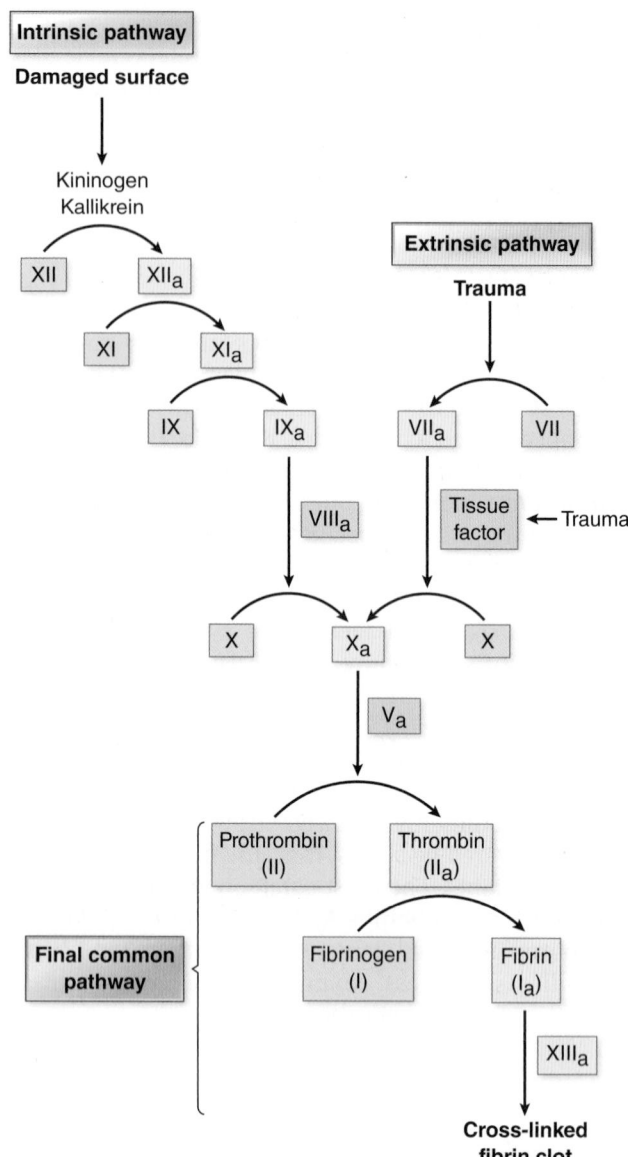

FIGURE 14-1. The coagulation cascade is a sequence of coagulation factors, synthesized by the liver, that form a clot. Two different pathways can activate the coagulation cascade: the intrinsic and extrinsic pathways, both of which end in a final common pathway that stimulates prothrombin to form thrombin and fibrinogen to form fibrin. The intrinsic pathway is stimulated by any damage to the endothelial surface of a blood vessel, as in arteriosclerosis, or any turbulence in blood flow, as in atrial fibrillation. The extrinsic pathway is stimulated by external trauma to a blood vessel, as happens in a laceration.

into thrombin. Thrombin has many functions, mainly the conversion of fibrinogen to fibrin, the major building block of a clot. Calcium and vitamin K are required for the proper functioning of the coagulation cascade. These can be obtained from the diet through consumption of sources of calcium (e.g., dairy foods) and vitamin K (e.g., green leafy vegetables). Some vitamin K is produced by intestinal bacteria. Vitamin K is fat soluble, meaning it is stored in fatty tissue. Any disorder that decreases absorption of fat will decrease absorption of vitamin K.

Clot Dissolution

Three substances act to decrease clot formation and dissolve clots:

1. Plasmin
2. Plasminogen
3. Tissue plasminogen activator (tPA)

These substances are involved in limiting the size of the clot and act to eventually dissolve it. Blood clots are dissolved by a process termed **fibrinolysis**. The main enzyme responsible for fibrinolysis is **plasmin**, which breaks down clots. Plasmin is derived from a large protein called plasminogen. **Tissue plasminogen activator (tPA)** enzymatically changes plasminogen into plasmin. Plasmin then breaks down the clot. After the clot is dissolved, blood flow can be reestablished (see Fig. 14-2). A drug called recombinant tissue plasminogen activator (rtPA) (alteplase [Activase]) is often used therapeutically to perform this same reaction to break down a clot.

 CLINICAL CONCEPT

Arterial thrombi are referred to as white thrombi because they are rich in platelets but scarce in red blood cells (RBCs). Venous thrombi are referred to as red thrombi because they have a large number of RBCs and small number of platelets.

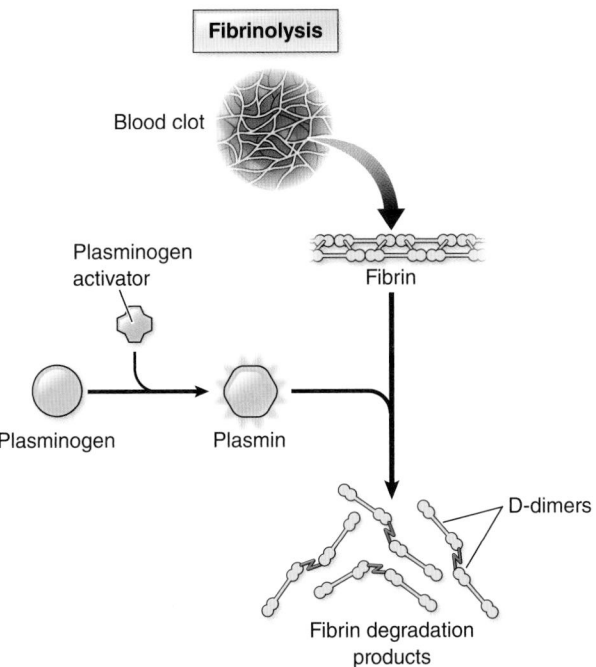

Fibrinolysis

Blood clot

Plasminogen activator

Fibrin

Plasminogen

Plasmin

D-dimers

Fibrin degradation products

FIGURE 14-2. Fibrinolysis. After a clot is formed, the body can dissolve it using plasmin. Plasminogen activator is a natural enzyme that catalyzes the transformation of a large protein called plasminogen into plasmin. Plasmin then catalyzes the breakdown of fibrin inside the clot into fibrin degradation products, also called D-dimers.

Basic Concepts of Bleeding and Clotting Pathophysiology

Pathophysiological problems of clotting can develop because of inadequate or excessive platelet numbers, platelet dysfunction, inadequate coagulation factors, or defective coagulation cascade activity. Inadequate platelet numbers, missing coagulation factors, and decreased coagulation activity can lead to bleeding problems, whereas excessive platelet numbers and enhanced coagulation activity can lead to hypercoagulability and complications of excessive thrombus formation (see Box 14-1).

Clotting Disorders

A susceptibility to clot formation occurs with thrombocytosis, enhanced platelet activity, or increased activation of coagulation factors. Enhanced platelet activity can occur with disturbances in blood flow and endothelial damage. Increased activation of coagulation factors occurs with stasis of blood flow, increase in procoagulation factors, or decrease in anticoagulation factors.

Increased Platelet Number and Activity

Thrombocytosis, which describes an increased number of platelets in excess of 750,000/uL, is a disorder that can occur after splenectomy, because the spleen sequesters and lyses dead platelets; without the spleen, the body is unable to eliminate platelets. Platelet excess also occurs in myeloproliferative disorders such as polycythemia or leukemia, where the bone marrow is hyperactive.

BOX 14-1. Conditions Associated With Hypercoagulability

Specific conditions that increase platelet activity or enhance coagulation factor production increase the blood's susceptibility to clotting.

INCREASED PLATELET ACTIVITY
- Atherosclerosis
- Diabetes mellitus
- Elevated blood lipid and cholesterol levels
- Increased number of platelets
- Smoking
- Splenectomy

ENHANCED COAGULATION FACTOR FORMATION
- Atrial fibrillation
- Cancer
- Heart failure
- Immobility
- Postsurgical state
- Pregnancy and postpartum period
- Use of oral contraceptives

There are two types of thrombocytosis: primary and secondary. Primary thrombocytosis, also known as essential thrombocytosis (ET), occurs in the bone marrow. The cause is unknown, but the increased number of platelets enhances the risk of clot formation. Secondary thrombocytosis, also called reactive thrombocytosis, is an elevated platelet count caused by another primary condition, such as iron-deficiency anemia, cancer, inflammation, infection, surgery, or myeloproliferative disorders. In secondary thrombocytosis, the exact mechanism for development of thrombocytosis is unclear, but the excessive number of platelets does not cause excessive clotting. In fact, in myeloproliferative disorders such as polycythemia vera, elevated platelet count leads to bleeding. Platelet counts can rise into the millions, causing a paradoxical risk of bleeding. Although there are excessive numbers of platelets, many are dysfunctional.

Aside from an excessive number of platelets, increased platelet activity can lead to enhanced platelet aggregation and increased susceptibility to blood clot formation. Increased platelet activation most commonly occurs with disturbances in blood flow and endothelial damage. Atherosclerotic plaques disrupt smooth blood flow through arteries, and plaque rupture exposes an irregular surface that attracts platelets and promotes clot formation. Causes of vessel injury that draw platelets to the site and predispose to platelet aggregation and thrombus formation include smoking, elevated lipids and cholesterol, hypertension, diabetes, and immune reactions.

Increased Coagulation Activity

Increased activation of the coagulation system is caused by stasis of blood flow, increase in procoagulation factors, or decrease in anticoagulation factors. Sluggish or stagnant blood flow is a common cause of venous thrombus formation, which often occurs in the lower extremities of immobile, sedentary, or postoperative patients. A deep vein thrombosis (DVT) in the femoral vein can travel into the inferior vena cava and flow into the right atrium and ventricle and then into the pulmonary artery, causing a pulmonary embolism (see Fig. 14-3). Heart failure, which causes weakened pumping of blood, can also lead to venous stasis in the lower extremities, which predisposes to thrombus formation. Atrial fibrillation, which causes a quivering, noncontracting atrium, leads to stagnation of arterial blood in the left atrium. Stagnant blood tends to form arterial thrombi that then travel to the left ventricle, then to the aorta, and into any systemic artery. Commonly, an arterial thrombus from the left atrium travels up to the carotid arteries and into the brain, causing ischemic stroke (see Fig. 14-4).

High estrogen levels increase hepatic synthesis of coagulation factors and decreased antithrombotic factors, which is why oral contraceptives, the high estrogen levels of pregnancy, and the postpartum period are risk factors for the formation of a venous thrombus.

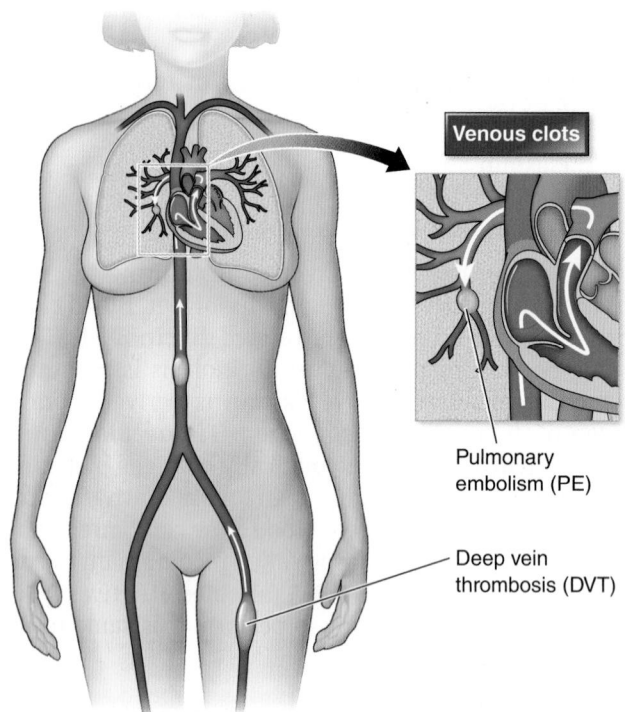

FIGURE 14-3. A femoral DVT can break away from the leg vein, ascend into the interior vena cava, and then enter the heart's right atrium. From the right atrium, the thrombus enters the right ventricle, and then flows into the pulmonary artery and into the lung's arterial system. It lodges in a pulmonary arterial vessel and blocks the circulation from becoming oxygenated.

> ### CLINICAL CONCEPT
>
> The incidence of stroke, thromboemboli, and myocardial infarction is greater in women who use oral contraceptives, particularly those women aged 35 years and older and persons who smoke.

A hypercoagulability state is also common in cancer because tumor cells secrete prothrombotic substances. A reduction in the body's natural anticoagulants, antithrombin (AT) and protein C, predisposes to arterial and venous thromboses. Deficiencies of AT or protein C occur as genetic disorders. Elevated homocysteine levels, which occur along with vitamin B and folic acid deficiencies, have also been associated with increased venous and arterial thrombi.

Antiphospholipid syndrome is a condition associated with the formation of multiple clots. The cause of this disorder is unknown, but there is a high prevalence in persons with autoimmune disease. Antiphospholipid antibodies are found in the bloodstream, but it is unclear how the antibodies lead to the formation of clots. In this syndrome, thrombosis can be precipitated by trauma, surgical procedures, use of drugs such as oral contraceptives, or abrupt withdrawal of anticoagulant drugs. Increased predisposition to clot formation increases the incidence of stroke, myocardial

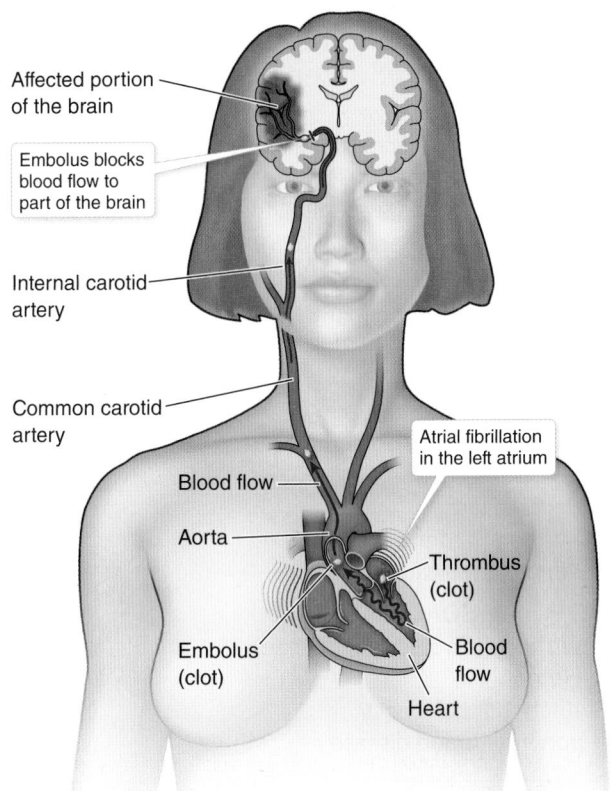

FIGURE 14-4. How atrial fibrillation leads to cerebral embolism that causes ischemic stroke. The fibrillating left atrium is not contracting, and stasis of blood in the atrium leads to clot formation. The clot travels from the left atrium to the left ventricle and into the aorta before moving up the brachiocephalic artery to the common carotid artery; at this point, it is referred to as an embolism. The common carotid artery divides into the internal and external carotid artery. The clot travels up the internal carotid artery and then lodges in a section of the middle cerebral artery, causing ischemic stroke.

infarction, ischemia, and gangrene of the lower extremities. Glomerular and renal arterial clots often lead to renal failure. Women with antiphospholipid syndrome often have a history of recurrent pregnancy loss because of clotting of the placenta. In catastrophic antiphospholipid syndrome, multiple thrombotic events with resulting vascular occlusions occur simultaneously in the body over a period of days. Multiple organ infarctions can also occur, and are often fatal.

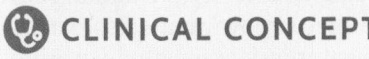

CLINICAL CONCEPT

Women with antiphospholipid syndrome tend to have repeated miscarriages.

Thrombophilic Disorders

A thrombophilic disorder is a hereditary or acquired condition that increases the risk of thrombosis. The most common hereditary thrombophilias that predispose to venous thrombosis are antithrombin (AT) deficiency, protein C deficiency, protein S deficiency,

prothrombin G20210A mutation (PGM), and factor V Leiden mutation.

Antithrombin Deficiency

Antithrombin (AT) deficiency is a genetic disorder that causes lack of antithrombin. Antithrombin is a natural anticoagulant that inhibits thrombin, which is required for the development of blood clots. Antithrombin also is the primary inhibitor of two other clotting factors, factor Xa and factor IXa, that are required for the generation of thrombin. Therefore, a deficiency of antithrombin creates risk for development of thrombotic disorders.

There is large variability among patients with AT deficiency with regard to genetic penetrance and clinical severity of the disease. Those who are heterozygous for AT deficiency do not have high risk of thrombotic disease. However, persons with homozygous AT deficiency are at increased risk of arterial thrombosis, venous thromboembolism, and pregnancy complications. Antithrombin deficiency may also be acquired by causes other than genetic. Conditions that can cause AT deficiency include leukemia treatment with L-asparaginase, heparin treatment, DIC, severe trauma, or severe burns.

Anticoagulant treatment is highly specific in patients with AT deficiency. Heparin resistance is common; therefore, another type of anticoagulant treatment is necessary. The vitamin K antagonist warfarin can counteract formation of clots. The direct oral anticoagulant apixaban (Eliquis) has also been effective.

Protein C and Protein S Deficiency

Protein C and protein S deficiency are genetic hypercoagulability disorders. Deficiency of these proteins causes an inability to deactivate coagulation factors V and VIII in the coagulation cascade. Therefore, persons with these deficiencies are at risk for the formation of venous thromboembolism. Protein C deficiency is caused by an alteration (mutation) in the *PROC* gene. Persons with two *PROC* genes who are considered homozygous are at higher risk than those who are heterozygous. Protein C deficiency can also be acquired from causes other than genetic. These people acquire the disease at some point in their lives due to various conditions that include vitamin K deficiency, warfarin therapy, severe liver disease, DIC, severe bacterial infections in the young, and some chemotherapy drugs. Protein S deficiency can be genetic due to a mutation in the *PROS1* gene or acquired due to hepatic disease, nephrotic syndrome, or vitamin K deficiency.

Persons with protein C or S deficiency can develop venous thrombotic events (VTE) including parenchymal thrombi, deep vein thrombosis (DVT), pulmonary emboli (PE), and DIC.

Treatment for persons with thrombotic disorders due to protein C or S deficiency includes anticoagulation therapies such as heparin (low molecular weight heparin or unfractionated), vitamin K antagonist (VKA), or direct oral anticoagulant (DOAC).

CLINICAL CONCEPT

Some women may have fetal loss as their only manifestation of protein C or S deficiency.

Prothrombin G20210A Mutation

Prothrombin G20210A mutation (PGM), also called factor II mutation, is a genetic disorder that causes excessive formation of prothrombin. Prothrombin protein enhances the formation of fibrin, which is a fundamental constituent of clots. Having the prothrombin G20210A mutation increases the likelihood of developing venous thromboemboli and pulmonary emboli. Women who have the prothrombin mutation have increased risk of developing a DVT or stroke if they use estrogen-containing oral contraceptives. Women also have risk for developing clots during pregnancy and the postpartum period. Persons with prothrombin G20210A mutation should take all measures to prevent development of venous thromboembolism. These persons should not use estrogenic agents, not smoke, and avoid conditions that predispose to venous stasis. Anticoagulant treatment is prescribed for those affected by active clots.

Factor V Leiden Mutation

Factor V Leiden (FVL) mutation is a genetic disorder that causes a lack of cleavage of factor V and factor Va in the coagulation cascade. Genetic penetrance varies among those affected, and severity of the condition is influenced by penetrance. FVL mutation leads to an increased risk of formation of thrombi, particularly venous thromboembolism and pulmonary emboli. FVL mutation is considered the most common inherited thrombophilia. Persons with the heterozygous combination of genes have a 7-fold increased risk of development of venous thrombi. Persons with the homozygous combination of genes have 20-fold increased risk of development of venous thrombi. However, many persons with FVL mutation do not ever endure thrombotic events. Generally, DOACs are used for patients with typical venous thromboembolism presentation.

Bleeding Disorders

Bleeding disorders and impairment of blood clotting occur because of decreased platelet number, defects associated with platelets, coagulation factors, and vascular integrity (see Box 14-2). The normal number of platelets (150,000 to 450,000/uL) must be severely depleted to levels between 10,000 and 20,000/uL before hemorrhagic problems or spontaneous bleeding arise.

> **BOX 14-2. Conditions Associated With Increased Susceptibility to Bleeding**
>
> Conditions that decrease platelet number, diminish platelet activity, or cause defective coagulation can increase the blood's susceptibility to bleeding.
>
> **DECREASED PLATELET NUMBER OR ACTIVITY**
> - Aplastic anemia
> - Cancer in the bone marrow
> - Extracorporeal circulation
> - Folate deficiency
> - Hypersplenism
> - Infections in the bone marrow (very rare)
> - Myelodysplasia
> - Renal failure
> - Vitamin B_{12} deficiency
> - Various medications
>
> **DEFECTIVE COAGULATION**
> - Cirrhosis (chronic liver disease)
> - Hemophilia
> - Vitamin K deficiency
> - von Willebrand disease

Decreased Platelet Number and Activity

Thrombocytopenia can result from decreased platelet synthesis in the bone marrow, increased sequestering of platelets in the spleen, or decreased platelet life span. Dilutional thrombocytopenia can occur from multiple transfusions because blood stored for more than 24 hours has few or no platelets.

Decreased platelet production can result from suppression of bone marrow, as occurs in aplastic anemia, or from replacement of bone marrow by cancer cells, as in leukemia. Reduced synthesis of platelets can also occur with HIV infection, exposure to radiation, or use of antineoplastic drugs.

There may be normal production of platelets with excessive pooling of platelets in the spleen. A majority of platelets can be sequestered when the spleen is enlarged. Decreased platelet survival is an important cause of thrombocytopenia. In many cases, premature destruction of platelets is caused by antiplatelet antibodies. Antibody-mediated platelet destruction occurs in ITP. Decreased platelet survival may also occur as the result of mechanical injury associated with prosthetic heart valves or cardiopulmonary bypass surgery.

Impaired Platelet Activity

Acquired platelet dysfunction is common and usually caused by antiplatelet therapy agents or as a side effect of other drugs. The most common cause of impaired platelet function is the use of aspirin and other NSAIDs. Aspirin (acetylsalicylic acid) produces irreversible acetylation of platelet cyclooxygenase, the enzyme required for synthesis of the procoagulant, thromboxane A2, in inflammation. The antiplatelet effects of aspirin last for the life of the platelet, usually 7 to 10 days. The antiplatelet effects of other NSAIDs are reversible and last only for the duration of the drug action.

Acquired platelet dysfunction commonly occurs in renal failure. The high level of nitrogenous waste products in the bloodstream causes decreased adhesion and lysis of platelets. Impaired platelet function may also result from inherited disorders of adhesion or acquired defects caused by drugs, disease, or extracorporeal circulation, as occurs in hemodialysis.

> **CLINICAL CONCEPT**
>
> Aspirin prolongs bleeding time for up to 7 days and so it should be avoided for a week before surgery.

Defective Coagulation

Impairment of blood coagulation can result from deficiencies of one or more of the known clotting factors. Deficiencies can arise because of defective synthesis, inherited defects, or increased consumption of the clotting factors. The most commonly known inherited disorders of coagulation are hemophilia A, hemophilia B, and von Willebrand disease (vWD). The most common acquired deficiency of coagulation factors occurs in liver disease, such as alcohol-related cirrhosis. In defective coagulation, prolonged bleeding is provoked by injury or trauma. Large bruises, hematomas, or prolonged bleeding into the gastrointestinal or urinary tract or joints are common. Head trauma can cause bleeding between the layers of the meninges, called a subdural hematoma.

Impaired Synthesis of Coagulation Factors. The coagulation factors are synthesized in the liver; therefore, blood clotting depends on a healthy liver. In liver disease, such as cirrhosis, coagulation factors are not manufactured, and bleeding often results. Some coagulation factors require vitamin K for normal function, which is why vitamin K deficiency can cause the liver to produce dysfunctional clotting factors. Vitamin K is a fat-soluble vitamin produced by intestinal bacteria. When the intestinal flora is disrupted, as with broad-spectrum antibiotic treatment, vitamin K is not produced and coagulation can be impaired. Impaired fat absorption caused by liver or gallbladder disease also leads to vitamin K deficiency and possible clotting dysfunction.

> 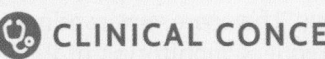 **CLINICAL CONCEPT**
>
> Vitamin K is administered to newborns because they have undeveloped intestinal flora to synthesize the vitamin.

Assessment of Bleeding and Clotting Disorders

The patient with a suspected bleeding or clotting disorder should have a complete history and physical examination. Specific questions regarding occurrences of nosebleeds, spontaneous bruising, or prolonged bleeding with trauma should be asked. The patient's body should be examined for any clues to bleeding susceptibility, such as bruises. Clotting disorders are more difficult to assess because the effects of hypercoagulability are coronary, cerebrovascular, venous, and peripheral arterial thromboses or organ infarction.

History

Patient history can reveal risk factors of bleeding and clotting disorders. Patient medications should be reviewed because many drugs can cause thrombocytopenia (see Box 14-3). Vitamin K deficiency can diminish clotting ability. Oral contraceptives and estrogen can increase clotting risk.

> ### BOX 14-3. Drugs Associated With Thrombocytopenia
>
> A wide variety of drugs can destroy platelets and decrease platelet number, including:
> - Antidepressants
> - Antiepileptic drugs
> - Antihistamines
> - Anti-inflammatory drugs
> - Antimicrobials
> - Antineoplastic drugs
> - Benzodiazepines
> - Cardiac medications and diuretics
> - Gold salts
> - Heparin
> - Histamine-2 antagonists
> - Illicit drugs, including cocaine and heroin
> - Iodinated contrast agents
> - Quinine/quinidine group
> - Retinoids
> - Sulfonylurea drugs
> - Miscellaneous drugs, including:
>   - Actinomycin-D
>   - Aminoglutethimide
>   - Danazol
>   - Desferrioxamine
>   - Levamisole
>   - Lidocaine
>   - Morphine
>   - Papaverine
>   - Tamoxifen
>   - Ticlopidine

Past medical history is important because cancer and other disorders can lead to clotting problems. Malignant tumors often secrete prothrombotic substances, leading to thrombi. DVTs are common in patients with cancer. Venous stasis, peripheral arterial disease, atherosclerosis, and atrial fibrillation all increase susceptibility to clot formation. On the other hand, hematological cancers of the bone marrow, such as leukemia, can inhibit the synthesis of platelets in the bone marrow and lead to bleeding. A recent viral or bacterial infection can be a catalyst for thrombocytopenia. Spleen, kidney, and autoimmune disease commonly cause platelet destruction. Liver disease can cause coagulation factor deficiency. Cushing's disease, Marfan's syndrome, Ehlers-Danlos disorder, and connective tissue diseases can all cause a tendency for bleeding that initially appears with bruising.

Women should be questioned about menorrhagia, excessive loss of blood at menses, as it is an initial symptom of vWD. Pregnancy and the postpartum period are associated with hypercoagulability, and DVT formation is common. Repeat miscarriages can indicate antiphospholipid syndrome, a disorder that causes multiple clots. Social habits such as smoking and alcohol misuse can contribute to coagulation disorders. Smoking increases coagulability, whereas alcohol misuse can lead to cirrhosis of the liver, resulting in decreased coagulation factors. Family history is important in assessment because many bleeding disorders have an inheritance pattern, including the X-linked recessive hemophilias.

Signs and Symptoms

During the physical examination, the clinician should look for signs of bleeding. Ecchymoses or large bruises may be the first symptom of platelet deficiency. Less remarkable bleeding such as petechiae or purpura may also be apparent (see Fig. 14-5). Spontaneous bleeding such as nosebleeds (epistaxis), bleeding from the gums, and abnormal vaginal bleeding can occur when the platelet count decreases to fewer than 20,000/uL. Other signs of bleeding to look for include excessive bleeding with trauma and occult bleeding from the gastrointestinal tract. In addition to signs of bleeding, the spleen may be enlarged because of increased activity.

🩺 CLINICAL CONCEPT

Petechiae, pinpoint red-purple areas of bleeding that resemble a rash, can be the first sign of thrombocytopenia.

Clotting disorders are more difficult to diagnose based on physical examination. Coronary and cerebrovascular thromboses, stroke, myocardial infarction, DVT, pulmonary embolism, and arterial thrombi of the extremities are the most common disorders associated

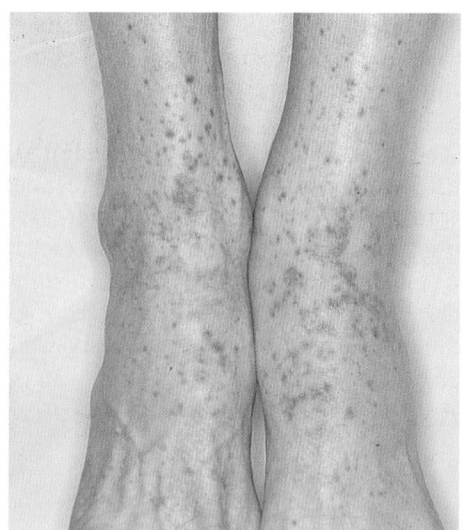

FIGURE 14-5. Petechiae.

with increased formation of clots. All of these disorders have a wide variety of symptoms and physical assessment findings.

Diagnosis

Complete blood count (CBC) with platelet count, peripheral blood smear, prothrombin time (PT), and activated partial thromboplastin time (aPTT) are all key components in the evaluation of the patient with a bleeding or clotting disorder. PT reflects the activity of coagulation factors I, II, V, VII, and X, which measures the integrity of the extrinsic pathway of coagulation. It also measures the clotting time from the activation of factor VII through the formation of the fibrin clot. The aPTT measures the function of factor XII through the fibrin clot in the intrinsic pathway.

Both PT and aPTT are measured in seconds—the time it takes for the blood to clot. For PT, the approximate normal range is 10 to 14 seconds. For the aPTT, the approximate normal range is 30 to 40 seconds. The greater the patient's PT or aPTT compared with normal values, the longer it takes for the patient's blood to clot. Anticoagulants prolong the time needed for blood to clot and thereby hinder clot formation. To acquire an anticoagulant therapeutic effect on the blood, the clinician aims for the PT and aPTT to be prolonged. For example, a clinician can administer an anticoagulant with the aim of prolonging clotting time to two times normal. Because normal PT is 10 to 14 seconds, the clinician would want to see the PT at 20 to 28 seconds to ensure the therapeutic effect of the anticoagulant. It is important to recognize that a prolonged clotting time can lead to the undesired complication of bleeding. Therefore, when administering anticoagulants, frequent monitoring of PT and aPTT is required.

A test used in place of PT is the INR, which is a method of standardizing the measurement of clotting.

The INR is calculated from the PT, while avoiding the wide difference in normal ranges for PT. If a blood sample has an INR of 1, this indicates the blood has a normal clotting time. The greater the INR, the longer it takes for the blood to clot. For example, an INR of 3 indicates that the blood is taking three times the normal time to clot. A common target range for INR in anticoagulant use (e.g., warfarin) is 2 to 3. In some cases, if more intense anticoagulation is required, the target range may be as high as 3 to 4. PT, aPTT, and INR laboratory tests are most commonly monitored when a patient is on anticoagulation medications. Other specific laboratory tests that assist in the diagnosis of clotting and bleeding disorders are listed in Table 14-1.

Treatment

Various types of anticoagulants are commonly used in clinical practice. Some agents inhibit platelet aggregation, whereas others block the activity of vitamin K. A few different agents work by impeding the steps of the coagulation cascade. Thrombolytic agents are used in emergency situations to travel directly to a clot and dissolve it.

TABLE 14-1. Common Laboratory Tests for Platelets, Coagulation Activity, and Bleeding Disorders

Laboratory Test	What Does It Measure?	Meaning of Abnormal Results
CBC	Counts and evaluates size and shape of platelets. RBCs and WBCs. Proportions of the different types of WBCs in circulation. Measures hemoglobin (Hgb), hematocrit (Hct), and size and color of RBCs.	Decreased Hgb/Hct indicates anemia. Increased WBCs indicates inflammation or infection. Decreased platelet number indicates increased bleeding tendency.
D-dimer	Measures fibrin degradation products.	If elevated, indicates recent clotting activity may be caused by acute or chronic condition, such as a thromboembolism, DIC, or pulmonary embolism.
Fibrin degradation products	Reflects clotting activity.	If increased, indicates recent blood clot formation and breakdown.
Fibrinogen	Reflects clotting ability and activity.	If low, may indicate decreased production or increased use of fibrinogen; may be elevated with infection and inflammation.
aPTT	Measures time to clot; evaluates the intrinsic pathway of coagulation cascade.	Prolonged aPTT suggests need for further tests. May indicate: • Coagulation factor deficiency • Inhibition of factor VIII • Nonspecific inhibitor, such as lupus anticoagulant • Patient on heparin
Platelet aggregation	Evaluates platelet's ability to adhere and form clumps.	If abnormal, there is an increased risk of excessive bleeding; may indicate presence of one of several disorders such as von Willebrand disease.
PT	Measures time to clot; evaluates the extrinsic pathway of coagulation cascade.	Most common use is monitoring warfarin anticoagulant therapy. Prolonged PT may suggest need for further tests. May be elevated in inherited or acquired coagulation disorders.
INR	Time for patient's blood to clot compared with normal time for blood to clot.	Any result >1 indicates prolonged time of clotting of blood.

Antiplatelet, Anticoagulation, and Thrombolytic Therapy

Antithrombotic drugs that decrease the body's ability to form clots include antiplatelet, anticoagulant, and thrombolytic agents. Thrombolytic agents are also called fibrinolytic agents or "clot-busters." Arterial and venous clots are major causes of morbidity and mortality. Arterial clots lead to obstruction of arterial blood supply, thereby causing ischemia and infarction of major organs. Stroke, myocardial infarction, and limb ischemia are the result of clots that form in arterial vessels. DVT, a clot that forms in the deep veins of the lower extremities, can lead to pulmonary embolism, which is often fatal. Platelets, coagulation factors, and the endothelium of blood vessels interact to generate clots. Arterial clots are rich in platelets, whereas venous clots are predominately composed of fibrin and trapped RBCs. Thrombolytic agents are used to directly dissolve arterial or venous clots, such as obstructive coronary artery clots that cause myocardial infarction, cerebral clots that cause ischemic stroke, and venous clots that form pulmonary emboli.

 CLINICAL CONCEPT

Antiplatelet agents are the main agents used to prevent arterial clots, whereas anticoagulants are more effective to prevent venous clots and clots formed due to left atrial fibrillation. Thrombolytic agents are used to dissolve arterial or venous clots.

Antiplatelet Drugs

Platelets adhere to the exposed collagen surface of the injured endothelial lining of arterial vessels. They synthesize and release adenosine diphosphate (ADP) and thromboxane A2, which activate other circulating platelets and recruit them to the site of injury. Disruption of the endothelial lining also exposes tissue factor (TF), which initiates the coagulation cascade. Activated platelets bind to the coagulation factors for assembly of a thrombus that attracts more platelets, enhancing clot formation. When platelets are activated, the GPIIb/IIIa receptor on the platelet surface binds to fibrinogen and acts as a bridge between adjacent platelets, increasing the size of the clot. Aspirin is the most commonly used antiplatelet medication; it is recommended in small doses of 70 to 150 mg daily to prevent myocardial infarction. Other antiplatelet drugs, which target different steps in the process of platelet aggregation, are listed in Box 14-4.

ALERT! NSAIDs compete with aspirin for the cyclooxygenase sites on platelets.

BOX 14-4. Antiplatelet Drugs

P2Y12 RECEPTOR INHIBITORS
- Clopidogrel (Plavix)
- Ticagrelor (Brilinta)
- Ticlopidine (Ticlid)
- Prasugrel (Effient)
- Cangrelor (Kengreal)

THROMBIN RECEPTOR INHIBITOR
- Vorapaxar (Zontivity)

PLATELET AGGREGATOR INHIBITOR
- Dipyridamole (Persantine)

GPIIb/IIIa RECEPTOR ANTAGONISTS
- Abciximab (ReoPro)
- Eptifibatide (Integrilin)
- Tirofiban (Aggrastat)

In cases where there are an excessive number of platelets, such as essential thrombocythemia (ET), medications such as hydroxyurea are used to suppress platelet production by the bone marrow. In cases of severe life-threatening thrombocytosis, a procedure called platelet pheresis is performed to immediately lower the platelet count to safer levels. In this procedure, blood is removed from the patient, the platelets are removed, and the blood is returned to the patient.

ALERT! Patients experiencing acute coronary syndrome should be told to chew 162 to 325 mg of uncoated aspirin, which can reduce platelet aggregation.

Anticoagulant Drugs

There are parenteral and oral forms of anticoagulants. Parenteral agents include unfractionated heparin, **low molecular weight heparin (LMWH)**, and fondaparinux (Arixtra). The oral anticoagulants include warfarin (Coumadin), dabigatran (Pradaxa), rivaroxaban (Xarelto), apixaban (Eliquis), edoxaban (Savaysa), and betrixaban (Bevyxxa). The choice of anticoagulant depends on the disorder that is being treated. For prophylaxis of clot formation in the clinical setting, unfractionated heparin (UFH), LMWH, or fondaparinux may be used initially. For long-term anticoagulation the oral vitamin K antagonist, warfarin, or DOACs are used.

Heparin. **Heparin** acts as an anticoagulant by activating AT, the body's natural clot-dissolving substance. It acts to prevent clot formation or limit the extension of a clot, but it does not dissolve clots. It can be administered intravenously or subcutaneously.

Heparin binds to plasma proteins in circulation, which causes reduced anticoagulant activity. Because levels of plasma proteins vary from person to person, heparin has an unpredictable anticoagulant response. The blood level of heparin must be titrated individually for each patient, and careful coagulation monitoring is essential. Subtherapeutic levels predispose the patient to additional clot formation, whereas excessive levels subject the patient to bleeding episodes. The aPTT laboratory test monitors heparin activity. Antifactor X levels can also be used to monitor heparin therapy.

UFH is administered intravenously, takes time to rise to a therapeutic level, and requires frequent monitoring of its level in the bloodstream. A therapeutic heparin dose is based on a control aPTT (approximately 30 to 40 seconds), and the aim is to keep heparin at a level that maintains aPTT at two to three times the control value.

There are some drawbacks to using UFH. It has an unpredictable anticoagulant response, it requires monitoring, and it takes time to reach therapeutic levels in the blood. Also, side effects include thrombocytopenia, osteoporosis, elevated liver enzymes, and bleeding. However, a positive feature is that protamine sulfate can be used to neutralize heparin if bleeding occurs.

Low Molecular Weight Heparin. LMWH has a shorter half-life and fewer side effects than UFH. It consists of small fragments of heparin and exerts its anticoagulant effect by activating AT. It binds to plasma proteins, but not as strongly as UFH; this allows LMWH to have a more predictable anticoagulant response. It can be administered, usually subcutaneously, once or twice a day without coagulation monitoring. Fixed dosages are recommended for venous versus arterial clots. The LMWH agent commonly used is enoxaparin (Lovenox), and it can be counteracted by protamine sulfate. Other LMWH agents are listed in Box 14-5.

 CLINICAL CONCEPT

If bleeding occurs in a patient on UFH, the antidote, protamine sulfate, is necessary. To counteract bleeding in a patient on LMWH, simply stopping the drug is usually all that is necessary.

BOX 14-5. Low Molecular Weight Heparins (LMWHs)

- Dalteparin
- Tinzaparin
- Certoparin
- Reviparin
- Bemiparin
- Nadroparin

Fondaparinux. Fondaparinux (Arixtra) causes factor Xa inhibition, which inhibits prothrombin from forming thrombin. It is a subcutaneous agent given once daily and is used most commonly for thromboprophylaxis in general surgical and high-risk orthopedic patients. It produces a predictable anticoagulant effect after administration in fixed doses because it does not bind to plasma protein. It has few side effects and is counteracted by an inactive antithrombin agent.

Vitamin K Antagonists. Warfarin (Coumadin) interferes with the synthesis of the vitamin K–dependent clotting factors prothrombin and factors VII, IX, and X. Warfarin is almost completely absorbed by the gastrointestinal tract, and levels peak in the blood about 90 minutes after drug administration.

 CLINICAL CONCEPT

Warfarin (Coumadin) requires frequent monitoring of PT or INR. Genetic factors that involve liver metabolism may make some individuals require smaller doses of warfarin. Fluctuations in dietary vitamin K intake can also affect warfarin level.

A wide variety of drugs and various disease states can modify the anticoagulant effect of warfarin, so close monitoring of warfarin levels is necessary. PT has been the laboratory test used to monitor warfarin levels in the past, but the INR is preferable. When using the PT test, the normal value is approximately 10 to 14 seconds, and for adequate anticoagulation, the aim is to keep the PT between 1.5 and 2 times the normal value. For example, if a patient's normal PT is 12 seconds and warfarin is administered to inhibit clotting, a PT value of 18 to 24 seconds would be considered in the therapeutic range. When using the INR laboratory test, the aim is to keep the therapeutic level between two and three times the normal value of 1 for adequate coagulation. An INR of 2 or 3 would indicate prolonged clotting time, which is the therapeutic goal.

Warfarin is usually started at a dose of 5 to 10 mg; when at the therapeutic level, monitoring is advised every 2 to 3 weeks. The major side effect is bleeding, which can be reversed by administering vitamin K. It is contraindicated in pregnancy. A rare complication is skin necrosis of the body's fatty areas.

Direct-Acting Oral Anticoagulants

DOACs are agents that specifically target one of the coagulation factors within the coagulation cascade. Dabigatran (Pradaxa) is a direct thrombin (also called factor IIa) inhibitor that is given orally. It can be used to prevent stroke in patients with atrial fibrillation that is not caused by a heart valve disorder. Venous thrombi are also inhibited by dabigatran, and

Patho-Pharm Connection

Clotting and Platelet Disorders

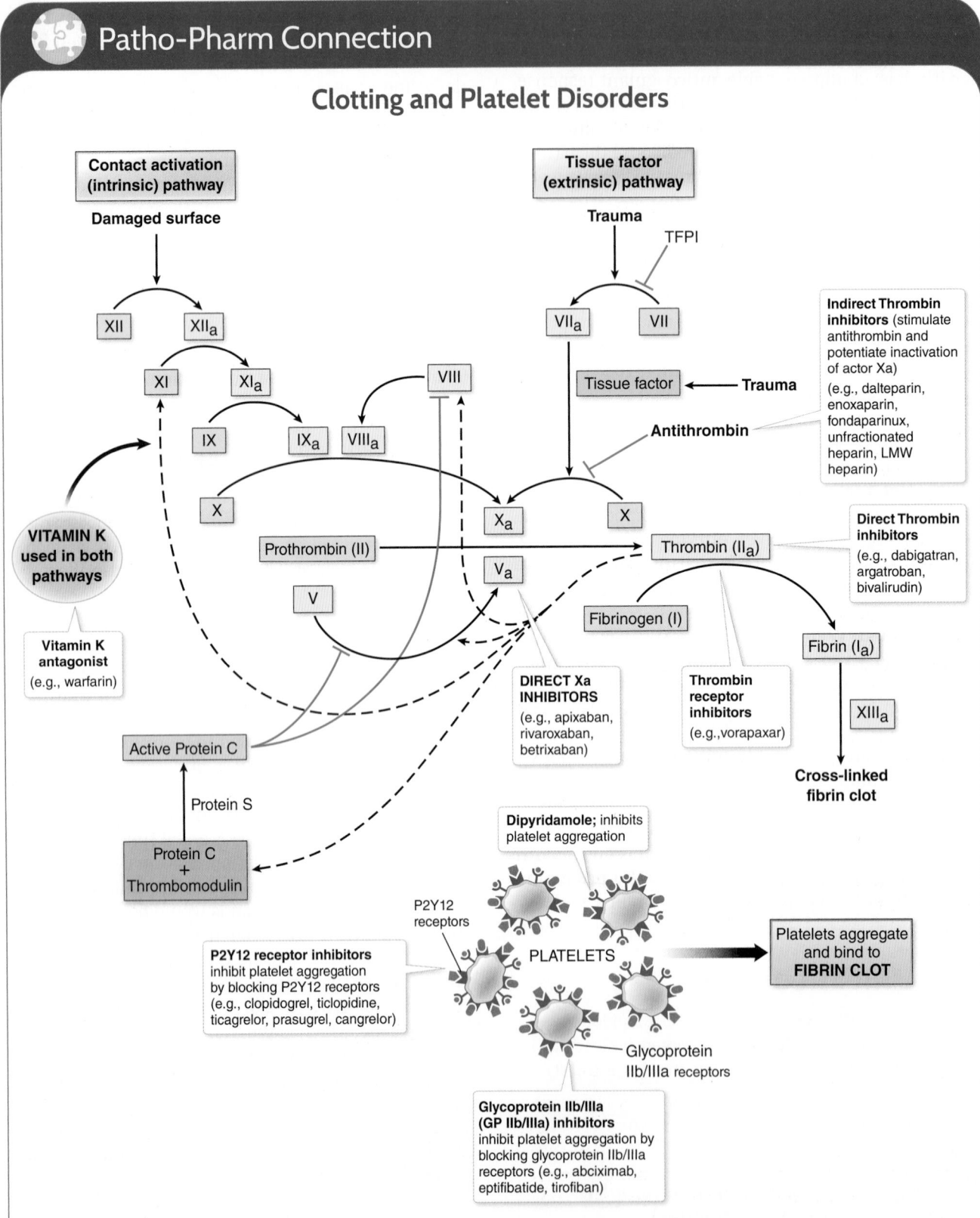

This is a diagram of how and where anticoagulant and antiplatelet medications act within the process of coagulation and platelet aggregation. The coagulation factors are synthesized by the liver and require vitamin K for their production. Warfarin is a vitamin K antagonist and thus affects the production of all coagulation factors. Direct factor Xa inhibitors include apixaban, rivaroxaban, edoxaban, and betrixaban. Indirect thrombin inhibitors are agents that stimulate antithrombin and potentiate inactivation of factor Xa. These include dalteparin, enoxaparin, fondaparinux, unfractionated heparin, and low molecular weight (LMW) heparin. Thrombin is one of the end

Patho-Pharm Connection–cont'd

products of the coagulation cascade and is inhibited directly by dabigatran, argatroban, and bivalirudin. A thrombin receptor inhibitor is vorapaxar.

Platelets aggregate and then bind to reinforce the fibrin plug formed by the coagulation cascade. Platelets have specific types of receptors, including P2Y12 and GPIIb/IIA, that enhance their aggregation. Inhibitors of these receptors can diminish ability of platelets to combine and aggregate to form a clot. P2Y12 receptor inhibitors include clopidogrel, ticlopidine, ticagrelor, prasugrel, and cangrelor. Glycoprotein IIb/IIIa (GP IIb/IIIa) receptor inhibitors include abciximab, tirofiban, and eptifibatide. Dipyridamole inhibits the enzymes adenosine deaminase and phosphodiesterase, which in turn block biochemical pathways that degrade cyclic adenosine monophospate (cAMP). The potentiation of cAMP levels in platelets inhibits platelet function and stimulates vascular vasodilation.

perioperative administration is common. Its effects last 24 hours and it does not require monitoring of INR, PT, or PTT. Idarucizumab (Praxbind) is a reversal agent for dabigatran.

Rivaroxaban (Xarelto) is an oral factor Xa inhibitor that is well absorbed from the gastrointestinal tract and peaks approximately 4 hours after a dose. It is recommended for nonvalvular atrial fibrillation and can prevent arterial and venous clots. The effects of rivaroxaban can last up to 24 hours, and once-daily dosing is recommended. It does not require monitoring of INR, PT, or PTT.

Other DOACs that inhibit factor Xa include apixaban (Eliquis), edoxaban (Savaysa), and betrixaban (Bevyxxa). Andexanet alfa (Andexxa) is a reversal agent for the DOACs rivaroxaban and apixaban. Other antidotes for DOACs are under investigation.

 CLINICAL CONCEPT

Individuals on anticoagulants who sustain trauma or head injury should be thoroughly assessed for signs of intracranial or internal bleeding. Subdural hematoma is commonly caused by head trauma.

Thrombolytic Agents

Thrombolytic agents, also called "clot-busters," can be used to dissolve thrombi. They can be administered systemically or delivered via catheters directly into the thrombus. Systemic delivery is used in acute myocardial infarction, acute ischemic stroke, and pulmonary emboli. The goal is to dissolve the clot and reestablish blood flow.

Thrombolytic agents include tissue plasminogen activator (tPA), alteplase, and recombinant tissue-type plasminogen activators reteplase and tenecteplase. Streptokinase, urokinase, prourokinase, and anistreplase are other less commonly used thrombolytic agents. All of these agents convert plasminogen to plasmin, and plasmin then degrades the fibrin matrix of a thrombus. With ischemic stroke, ideally, the goal is to treat the patient in less than 3 to 4 hours from the time of the acute event. Thrombolytic therapy is indicated in patients with evidence of ST segment elevation myocardial infarction (STEMI) or new left bundle branch block presenting within 12 hours of the onset of symptoms if there are no contraindications to fibrinolysis.

Pathophysiology of Selected Coagulation Disorders

Important disorders that cause bleeding due to thrombocytopenia include drug-induced thrombocytopenia, heparin-induced thrombocytopenia (HIT), ITP, **thrombotic thrombocytopenic purpura (TTP)**, essential thrombocytopenia, and hemolytic uremic syndrome. Hemophilia and vWD also cause bleeding, but in these disorders the bleeding is caused by coagulation factor problems. DIC is severe malfunction of the coagulation system, which causes unpredictable episodes of both bleeding and clotting.

Drug-Induced Thrombocytopenia

Drug-induced thrombocytopenia has been associated with more than 1,500 medications. Heparin, antimalarial drugs, and sulfonamides are some of the most common causes of the disorder. Because many drugs are associated with thrombocytopenia, all drugs should be suspect in a patient without another apparent cause of thrombocytopenia. Herbal and over-the-counter medications are included as possible causes.

 CLINICAL CONCEPT

Often drug-induced thrombocytopenia is misdiagnosed as autoimmune disease because the drugs induce antigen–antibody reactions.

Typically, a patient will have taken the offending drug for about 1 week or intermittently over a longer period before presenting with petechial hemorrhages and purpura that are indicative of thrombocytopenia. Occasionally, symptoms develop within 1 or 2 days after the first exposure to a drug. Platelet counts can decrease to levels of 20,000/uL or lower. Systemic symptoms such as lightheadedness, chills, fever, nausea, and vomiting often precede bleeding symptoms. Severely affected patients have epistaxis or bleeding from the gums, gastrointestinal tract, or urinary tract. If the causative medication is stopped, symptoms usually resolve within 2 days, and the platelet count returns to normal in less than a week.

Heparin-Induced Thrombocytopenia

HIT is different from thrombocytopenia induced by other drugs because it is not associated with bleeding, but it is paradoxically associated with increased risk of thrombosis. The disorder results from the development of an antibody to heparin. Some individuals who develop the antibody do develop low platelet count, but the majority develops clots. HIT can occur with standard heparin or LMWH and develops approximately 5 to 10 days after exposure. Thrombi can develop in the arterial or venous vessels. Direct thrombin inhibitors are used in the treatment of HIT.

Immune Thrombocytopenic Purpura

ITP is one of the most common autoimmune disorders. It is caused by autoantibodies that develop against platelets. The antigenic target in most patients appears to be the platelet GPIIb/IIIa complex. The complex is attacked by IgG antibodies, and these platelet–antibody complexes are phagocytosed by macrophages and destroyed by the spleen.

Acute ITP is more common in children and usually follows a viral infection. It is characterized by a sudden onset of petechiae and purpura and is a self-limited disorder for which treatment is usually not needed. In contrast, a chronic form of the disorder is usually seen in adults, with a peak incidence between ages 20 and 50 years; it is usually seen twice as often in women as it is in men. It may be associated with other immune disorders such as AIDS or systemic lupus erythematosus.

ITP is a diagnosis of exclusion; all other possible diagnoses should be investigated, particularly drug-induced thrombocytopenia. The condition presents with signs of bleeding, such as petechiae, purpura, bleeding from the gums, epistaxis, and abnormal menstrual bleeding. Because the spleen is the site of platelet destruction, splenic enlargement may occur. Hemorrhage represents the most serious complication; intracranial hemorrhage is the most lethal. Diagnosis usually is based on severe thrombocytopenia (fewer than 20,000/uL) and exclusion of other causes. Treatment includes use of corticosteroid drugs, IV immunoglobulin (IVIg), platelet transfusion, and the use of immunosuppressive drugs. Splenectomy may be necessary.

Thrombotic Thrombocytopenic Purpura

TTP is a combination of thrombocytopenia, hemolytic anemia, thrombotic vascular occlusions, fever, and neurological abnormalities. It is caused by a deficiency of a metalloprotease enzyme that acts on vWF. Specifically, the metalloprotease called ADAMTS13 (A Disintegrin-like And Metalloprotease with ThromboSpondin type 1 motif 13) is destroyed by autoantibodies—antibodies that the body generates against its own cells. The lack of this metalloprotease leads to unmodified vWF, which causes platelet adhesion and aggregation. This platelet aggregation leads to widespread clot formation. The exact etiology of TTP is unclear. For unknown reasons, it is common in persons with HIV infection, as well as in pregnant women.

TTP consists of five specific signs and symptoms:

- Microangiopathic hemolytic anemia
- Thrombocytopenic purpura
- Neurological abnormalities
- Fever
- Renal disease

The onset is abrupt, and the outcome can be fatal. Widespread vascular occlusions consist of clots in arterioles and capillaries of many organs, including the heart, brain, and kidneys. Ischemia of heart, brain, and kidneys can occur. Erythrocytes become fragmented as they circulate through the partly occluded vessels and cause hemolytic anemia. The damaged erythrocytes, called schistocytes, are apparent on peripheral blood analysis. Bilirubin levels in the blood rise due to the decomposition of hemoglobin, causing jaundice and dark urine (hemoglobinuria). The clinical manifestations include purpura, petechiae, and neurological symptoms ranging from headache to seizures and altered consciousness.

Although the etiology of TTP is unknown, the initiating event seems to be widespread endothelial damage and activation of intravascular thrombosis. Toxins produced by certain strains of *Escherichia coli* (*E. coli* O157:H7) are a trigger for endothelial damage and an associated condition called hemolytic-uremic syndrome (HUS) that is characterized by acute renal failure, hemolytic anemia, and thrombocytopenia. However, TTP is distinguished from HUS by the specific antibody to the ADAMTS13 metalloprotease and large number of large unmodified vWF proteins in the blood.

Treatment for TTP includes plasmapheresis (plasma exchange), a procedure that involves removing the blood's plasma portion and replacing it with fresh frozen plasma; this treatment is continued until remission occurs. With plasmapheresis, there is a complete recovery in 80% to 90% of cases. Another treatment modality is the use of Octaplas, a sterile solution of treated human plasma from multiple blood donors. If these treatments do not work, a cryoprecipitate-poor plasma with the vWF removed is used. Corticosteroids are used in conjunction with the treatment. Rituximab, a monoclonal antibody type of medication, has also been effective. However, this is an off-label use of rituximab, meaning it is not specifically approved by the Food and Drug Administration (FDA) for TTP.

Potential complications of TTP include disorders caused by clot formation, including myocardial infarction, ischemic stroke, and transient ischemic attack (TIA). Pregnant women often sustain miscarriage or fetal loss. If untreated, TTP has a high mortality rate; however, plasmapheresis and other treatments lower the mortality rate to 10% to 20%.

Hemophilia

There are two major forms of hemophilia based on the deficiency of a specific coagulation factor. Hemophilia A is caused by a deficiency of factor VIII, whereas hemophilia B is caused by a lack of factor IX. Both are X-linked, recessive disorders that primarily affect males. Women can carry the trait for either disease but do not suffer the bleeding problems. Hemophilia A is the more common form, comprising 80% of hemophilia cases. Both diseases have similar pathophysiological mechanisms and symptoms because of a deficient or dysfunctional coagulation factor.

Hemophilia A is mainly a hereditary disorder, but there is no familial history of it in approximately 30% of newly diagnosed cases. Approximately 90% of persons with hemophilia A produce insufficient quantities of factor VIII, with the remaining 10% producing a defective form of factor VIII. There is a wide spectrum of the severity of disease, with up to 50% affected by mild hemophilia.

In mild or moderate forms of the disease, bleeding usually does not occur unless trauma provokes it. The mild disorder may not be detected in childhood. In severe hemophilia, bleeding can be spontaneous. The hallmark of hemophilia is spontaneous acute hemarthrosis, which is bleeding into a joint space. Characteristically, bleeding occurs in soft tissue; the gastrointestinal tract; and the hip, knee, elbow, and ankle joints. Bleeding into muscle tissue can compress arteries and veins and cause compartment syndrome. Joint bleeding usually begins when a child starts to walk. After a joint is affected, it is commonly subjected to repeated bleeding, causing inflammation of the synovium with acute pain and swelling. Common symptoms of hemophilia in different body systems due to bleeding, which can be occult, are listed in Box 14-6.

Without proper treatment, chronic bleeding and inflammation can cause joint fibrosis and contractures, resulting in major disability. Bleeding into the oropharyngeal spaces, central nervous system, or retroperitoneum can be fatal and requires immediate treatment.

When hemophilia is a known familial disorder, carrier detection and prenatal diagnosis should be performed. Diagnosis of the disease involves a CBC, coagulation studies, a factor VIII assay for hemophilia A, and a factor IX assay for hemophilia B. The hemoglobin/hematocrit usually show normal or low values. Platelet counts are normal. On coagulation studies, the PT, which assesses the extrinsic coagulation pathway, is normal, whereas the aPTT, which assesses the intrinsic coagulation pathway, is prolonged.

Factor VIII replacement therapy is initiated in hemophilia A when bleeding occurs. Factor IX is the replacement treatment for persons with hemophilia B. Recombinant factor VIII and recombinant factor IX are synthetic forms of the coagulation factors, and these are the preferred treatments to reduce the risk of transmitting HIV or other viruses from donor pools of coagulation factors. Although donor pools of coagulation factors are screened, there is a slight risk of contamination with HIV or hepatitis infection. For this reason, individuals with hemophilia should receive the hepatitis B vaccine.

Desmopressin acetate (DDAVP), which is a synthetic analog of vasopressin, may be used to prevent bleeding in persons with mild hemophilia A. This synthetic vasopressin stimulates the release of vWF, a carrier of factor VIII, from the endothelium, thus increasing factor VIII levels twofold to threefold for several hours. Antifibrinolytic agents such as aminocaproic acid or tranexamic acid can be used to stop bleeding episodes. Monoclonal antibody–type medications, such as rituximab or emicizumab, have also been used in patients who have evidence of factor VIII or IX inhibitory antibodies in the bloodstream.

The cloning of the factor VIII and factor IX genes has led to the hope that hemophilia A and B may be cured by gene therapy.

BOX 14-6. Common Symptoms of Hemophilia by Body System

General: weakness, tachycardia, tachypnea, spontaneous or easy bruising
Nose/throat: epistaxis, hemoptysis, bleeding gums, excessive bleeding with dental procedures
Musculoskeletal: joint pain and stiffness (due to hemarthrosis), compartment syndrome
Central nervous system: headache, stiff neck, spinal cord syndromes (bleeding into spinal cord), intracranial hemorrhage (subdural or epidural hematoma)
Gastrointestinal: abdominal pain, hematemesis (blood in vomitus), melena (blood in stool)
Genitourinary: back pain, hematuria, postcircumcision bleeding in infant

Essential Thrombocytosis

ET (also called primary thrombocythemia) is a rare, chronic disorder of the bone marrow. It is a disorder of megakaryocyte proliferation that increases the number of circulating platelets. The excess of platelets increases susceptibility to clot formation. However, many of the excessive platelets do not function; consequently, there can be an increased susceptibility to bleeding. The disorder causes a platelet count greater than 600,000/uL, splenomegaly, and a tendency for coagulation or bleeding episodes.

Epidemiology

There is an incidence of approximately 6,000 cases of ET each year in the United States. ET is more frequent in older patients, with a median age at diagnosis of 60 years. Both sexes are affected equally. Death commonly occurs from clotting episodes that lead to myocardial infarction or stroke. For unclear reasons, some patients with ET develop the complication of acute myelogenous leukemia (AML).

Etiology/Pathophysiology

There is no known etiology of ET. The presence of a gene mutation called JAK2 on chromosome 9p is present in 50% of patients with ET. Other mutations occur in the calreticulin (CALR) gene or myeloproliferative leukemia virus oncogene (MPL). There is an excessive number of platelets; some show less ability to aggregate, leading to susceptibility to bleeding. Other platelets show hyperaggregation tendencies, which leads to clot formation.

Clinical Presentation

Approximately 25% to 33% of patients with ET are asymptomatic at diagnosis. Most symptomatic patients present with clots in small or large blood vessels. However, some patients may present with bleeding because of dysfunctional platelets. Neurological symptoms include headache and paresthesias of the fingers and toes. Some patients suffer ischemia of the fingers and toes that causes burning and erythema, a condition called erythromelalgia. Patients often report symptoms associated with TIAs caused by clots that lodge in a cerebral artery. Symptoms of TIAs include unsteadiness, vertigo, dizziness, syncope, seizures, and dysarthria.

Clots in the large veins and arteries are common and may result in occlusion of the leg, coronary, and renal arteries. Clots can also develop in the splenic, hepatic, leg, and pelvic veins. Pulmonary hypertension can result because of clotting in the pulmonary vasculature. In contrast, the gastrointestinal tract, gums, urinary tract, joints, and brain are susceptible to bleeding. Patients also report fever, diaphoresis, and pruritus. ET is also known to cause complications during pregnancy, such as an increase in spontaneous abortions, ischemia of the placenta, intrauterine growth retardation, and fetal death.

Diagnosis

A CBC count is necessary for the diagnosis of ET and shows an unexplained, excessive number of platelets. There may also be an excessive number of white blood cells (WBCs) and RBCs. On bone marrow biopsy, megakaryocytic hyperplasia is common. The PT and aPTT studies are usually within reference ranges. The bleeding time may or may not be prolonged. Blood chemistry studies reveal elevated uric acid (UA) levels in 25% of patients at diagnosis. Computed tomography (CT) scan or ultrasound of the spleen may reveal splenomegaly.

Treatment

Medications used in ET are those that inhibit megakaryocyte maturation into platelets. Some medications include hydroxyurea, anagrelide, interferon alfa, busulfan, and ruxolitinib. Hydroxyurea is an antimetabolite type of antineoplastic agent that inhibits cellular proliferation of platelets. Anagrelide is a phosphodiesterase-3 inhibitor that decreases megakaryocyte production, thereby decreasing platelet numbers. Interferon alfa is a biological response modifier that also reduces platelet count and is safest to use in pregnant women. Busulfan suppresses bone marrow activity, thereby reducing platelet production. Ruxolitinib is a kinase inhibitor that blocks mediators that stimulate bone marrow hyperactivity. Low-dose aspirin may be useful in treating patients with symptoms of microvascular clotting. In emergencies, plateletpheresis, a procedure that removes excess platelets from the bloodstream, may be useful if there is severe thrombocytosis.

von Willebrand Disease

vWD is a genetic disorder transmitted as an autosomal trait that causes a deficiency or defect of vWF. vWF is a protein that connects platelets to the endothelial lining of blood vessels and binds to factor VIII of the coagulation cascade. vWF deficiency causes decreased platelet adhesion and reduced levels of active factor VIII, which result in defective clot formation.

Epidemiology

vWD has an incidence of approximately 125 persons per million. Males and females are equally affected; however, females have a more evident course of disease because vWD causes severe menstrual bleeding. vWD presents as a spectrum from mild to severe forms of the disorder.

Etiology/Pathophysiology

The etiology of vWD is a genetic mutation on the short arm of chromosome 12. The gene is expressed in megakaryocytes and endothelial cells. vWF functions to enhance platelet aggregation and platelet adhesion to endothelium and stops the degradation of factor VIII. Consequently, without vWF there is defective hemostasis and lack of factor VIII, which increases the patient's susceptibility to bleeding and hemorrhage.

Clinical Presentation

Symptoms of vWD include easy bruising; excessive menstrual blood loss; and bleeding from the nose, mouth, and gastrointestinal tract. Many persons are unaware of the disorder until a surgical or dental procedure results in abnormally prolonged bleeding.

Diagnosis

In order to diagnose vWD, laboratory tests need to demonstrate a deficiency of vWF. This may be difficult to obtain, as many conditions can stimulate production of vWF. Stress, estrogen, growth hormone, and vasopressin can stimulate vWF production and increase amounts in the blood. The patient's amount of vWF can fluctuate, so obtaining an accurate result can be difficult. Laboratory tests include PT, aPTT, factor VIII activity, and concentration of vWF antigen in the bloodstream (vWF:Ag). The aPTT is usually prolonged because of low levels of factor VIII. Another laboratory test called the ristocetin cofactor (RCoF) assay can be used to estimate vWF activity in the blood. Sometimes RCoF assay is difficult to interpret, and another laboratory test called gain-of-function GPIbα mutants can be a more accurate assessment of vWF activity.

Treatment

Most cases of vWD are mild and do not require treatment. In severe cases, factor VIII products that contain vWF are infused to replace the deficient clotting factors. The disorder is also treated with desmopressin (DDAVP), a synthetic form of vasopressin, which stimulates the endothelial cells to release vWF and plasminogen activator. Antifibrinolytic agents, such as aminocaproic acid or tranexamic acid, can be used to limit bleeding. Patients should avoid aspirin and activities that place them at risk for injury. In women, menorrhagia (excessive menstrual bleeding) can be counteracted using estrogen/levonorgestrel, which inhibits luteinizing and follicular stimulating hormones.

Hemolytic-Uremic Syndrome

HUS is a disorder that causes progressive renal failure, hemolytic anemia, and thrombocytopenia. It is the most common cause of acute renal failure in children and is increasingly occurring in adults. The two forms of the disorder are Shiga toxin–producing HUS (Stx-HUS) and non–Shiga toxin–producing HUS (non–Stx-HUS). Stx-HUS is often referred to as typical HUS, whereas non–Stx-HUS is atypical.

Epidemiology

Stx-HUS is the more common form of the disease, with an incidence of 0.5 to 2.1 cases per 100,000 persons per year. However, in children younger than 5 years, the incidence is 6.1 cases per 100,000 persons per year. Non–Stx-HUS accounts for 5% to 10% of all cases of HUS, and the incidence in children is about one-tenth that of Stx-HUS. Non–Stx-HUS has a worse prognosis than Stx-HUS.

Etiology

In North America and Western Europe, 70% of cases of Stx-HUS are caused by E. coli serotype O157:H7. Although most strains of E. coli are harmless and live in the intestines of healthy humans and animals, E. coli O157:H7 produces a powerful toxin (called Shiga toxin or Stx) and is considered an enterohemorrhagic strain. E. coli O157:H7 is found in the environment and in animal intestines, particularly cattle. Most illness is caused by ingestion of contaminated produce, water, or undercooked meat. Other sources include unpasteurized milk and juice and contact with infected live animals. Waterborne transmission can occur by swimming in contaminated lakes or pools or by drinking inadequately treated water. Flies have been shown to carry E. coli O157:H7 as well. The organism is easily transmitted from person to person via the fecal–oral route and has caused epidemics in child day-care centers.

Shiga toxin–producing E. coli is often referred to as STEC. In Asia and Africa, HUS is often caused by Stx-producing Shigella dysenteriae serotype 1. Streptococcus pneumoniae infection accounts for 40% of all cases of non–Stx-HUS in the United States. Other causes of non–Stx-HUS include other strains of bacteria, viruses, fungi, drugs, malignancies, vaccinations, transplantation, pregnancy, and other underlying medical conditions such as antiphospholipid syndrome and systemic lupus erythematosus (see Box 14-7). Non–Stx-HUS can also be a familial disease due to a factor H1 gene mutation, or nonfamilial due to a sporadic mutation in the factor H1 gene. The factor H1 gene is involved in the production of complement proteins, which are integral to the immune response.

Pathophysiology

Once ingested, the E. coli O157: H7 bacterium closely adheres to the mucosal lining of the human intestine. It irritates the intestinal mucosa and causes a bloody diarrheal illness. When in the bloodstream, the E. coli O157:H7 toxin directly damages endothelial cells and binds to WBCs. The toxin causes the lysis of RBCs and the formation of arteriolar and capillary microthrombi. The route by which the toxin is transported from the intestine to the kidney is unclear.

Clinical Presentation

The patient usually reports gastroenteritis, fever, and bloody diarrhea for 2 to 7 days. The disorder causes abdominal pain, dehydration, fatigue, and a very low urine output. Acute renal failure is diagnosed soon after infection. The physical findings commonly include hypertension, edema, lethargy, and pallor.

The source of the gastroenteritis is not always clear. Patients should be questioned about recent foods eaten and sources of the food. The patient needs to recall ingestion of any raw foods, untreated water, or recent association with sick individuals.

BOX 14-7. Etiologies of Hemolytic-Uremic Syndrome

Causes of Stx-HUS include bacterial infections, viral infections, and vaccinations.

BACTERIAL INFECTIONS
- *Campylobacter jejuni*
- *Escherichia coli* O157:H7
- *Legionella pneumophila*
- *Mycoplasma* species
- *Neisseria meningitidis*
- *Shigella dysenteriae*
- *Streptococcus pneumoniae*
- *Salmonella typhi*
- *Yersinia pseudotuberculosis*

VIRAL INFECTIONS
- Coxsackievirus
- Echovirus
- Epstein–Barr virus
- Herpes simplex virus
- HIV
- Influenza virus

VACCINATIONS
- Influenza triple-antigen vaccine
- Polio vaccine
- Typhoid–paratyphoid A and B (TAB) vaccine

Causes of non-Stx-HUS syndrome include conditions, disorders, and medications. No cause is identified in about 50% of all cases of sporadic non–Stx-HUS.

CONDITIONS AND DISORDERS
- Allogenic hematopoietic cell transplantation
- Cancers, chiefly mucin-producing adenocarcinomas
- Collagen–vascular disorders, such as systemic lupus erythematosus and antiphospholipid antibody syndrome
- Malignant hypertension
- Pregnancy and postpartum period
- Primary glomerulopathies
- Transplantation

MEDICATIONS
- Anticancer agents, including mitomycin, cisplatin, bleomycin, and gemcitabine
- Antiplatelet agents, including ticlopidine and clopidogrel
- Chemotherapeutic agents, including mitomycin-C, cisplatin, bleomycin, gemcitabine, carmustine, oxaliplatin, pentostatin, bevacizumab, and sunitinib
- Immunotherapeutic agents, including cyclosporine and tacrolimus
- Oral contraceptives
- Quinine

Diagnostic Tests

In the diagnosis of HUS, a urinalysis will reveal mild proteinuria and hematuria. Blood urea nitrogen and serum creatinine may be high, which indicate renal insufficiency. On the peripheral blood smear, fragmented RBCs are seen, as well as thrombocytopenia. Bilirubin levels may be elevated because of a large amount of hemoglobin breakdown. Stool culture should be done to check for *E. coli* O157:H7 and *Shigella* bacteria. The ADAMTS13 test should be done to rule out TTP, which can often present similarly to HUS. Genetic studies for the factor H1 gene are also important in non–Stx-HUS, as this form of HUS requires different treatment than Stx-HUS.

Study of kidney tissue will reveal the characteristic findings of HUS: obstructive microthrombi of the capillaries and arterioles in the kidney. These are small clots that cause ischemia and infarctions of renal tissue. In HUS, microthrombi are limited mainly to the kidney, whereas in TTP, microthrombi occur throughout the body.

Treatment

Supportive therapy, the major form of treatment, includes maintenance of fluid and electrolyte balance, blood pressure control, and dietary protein restriction. If diarrhea is severe, parenteral nutrition may be necessary. Between 20% and 40% of patients develop seizures, so prophylactic treatment with phenytoin (Dilantin) may be necessary.

Antibiotics are used if the patient is septic, in which case azithromycin may be effective. If end-stage renal disease (ESRD) develops, hemodialysis and renal transplantation are recommended.

Treatment of non–Stx-HUS requires plasma exchange (plasmapheresis) early in the course of the disease, where the patient's plasma component of blood is removed and replaced with donor plasma. Plasma exchange treatment should be started within the first 24 hours of the patient's illness and then continued once or twice a day for at least 2 days after complete recovery. Aspirin to inhibit platelet aggregation is used in combination with plasma exchange. Eculizumab is the only drug approved for treatment of non–Stx-HUS. It is a monoclonal antibody–type medication that inhibits activation of complement in the immune response. By inhibiting the activity of complement, the immune response is suppressed, which in turn reduces the hemolysis that occurs in the disease.

In *S. pneumoniae* non–Stx-HUS, plasma treatment is contraindicated. Renal transplantation is not an option for non–Stx-HUS because there is a 50% recurrence rate in the transplanted kidney and 90% chance of transplant failure. This failure of transplantation is particularly common in patients with the factor H1 gene mutation.

Disseminated Intravascular Coagulation

DIC is a disorder of both clot formation and bleeding episodes in critically ill patients. It is sometimes referred to as a consumptive coagulopathy. There is active stimulation of the coagulation cascade with formation of fibrin clots. Simultaneously, there is depletion of coagulation factors with unrestrained fibrinolysis causing bleeding. In addition, fibrinolysis is suppressed. The resultant clinical condition is characterized by episodes of both coagulation and hemorrhage. The patient unpredictably begins to form clots, which can lead to ischemia of organs and multiple organ dysfunction syndrome (MODS). The patient also undergoes random periods of spontaneous bleeding.

Epidemiology

DIC is a critical illness that is always secondary to another formidable disorder. DIC occurs in 30% to 50% of patients with sepsis. It can occur in all races and affects males and females equally. The presence of DIC can double the risk of death in sepsis. In cases of major trauma, the occurrence doubles the mortality rate.

Etiology

DIC occurs in critically ill patients and is a complication of a wide number of conditions (see Box 14-8). It is most commonly observed in patients with sepsis and septic shock. Sepsis, caused by both gram-positive and gram-negative organisms, is commonly associated with DIC; however, other organisms—including viruses, fungi, and parasites—may cause it as well. In infections caused by gram-negative bacteria, endotoxins released from the bacteria activate both the intrinsic and extrinsic pathways of coagulation. In addition, endotoxins inhibit the anticoagulant activity of protein C. In obstetrical conditions, particularly those involving shock, hypoxia, acidosis, and fetal death can provoke DIC. Other clinical conditions that can trigger DIC include massive trauma, burns, transfusion, anaphylaxis, shock, meningococcemia, and malignant disease. In particular, neurotrauma and systemic inflammatory response syndrome (SIRS) can provoke DIC.

Pathophysiology

The main mechanisms of DIC are uncontrolled synthesis of thrombin, suppression of anticoagulant mechanisms, and abnormal fibrinolysis. Together, these abnormalities lead to excessive fibrin deposition in small and midsized blood vessels. The fibrin deposition in blood vessels obstructs the blood supply to organs, particularly the lungs, kidneys, and brain, with consequent organ failure. Persistent activation of coagulation results in the depletion of clotting factors

---

BOX 14-8. Conditions Associated With DIC

Many types of conditions can trigger DIC. These include obstetric disorders, cancers, infections, shock, transfusion reactions, trauma, or surgery.

CANCER
- Leukemia
- Metastatic cancer

HEMATOLOGICAL CONDITIONS
- Blood transfusion reactions

INFECTIONS
- Acute bacterial infections such as meningococcal meningitis
- Acute viral infections
- Rickettsial infection such as Rocky Mountain spotted fever
- Parasitic infection such as malaria

OBSTETRIC CONDITIONS
- Abruptio placentae
- Dead fetus syndrome
- Preeclampsia or eclampsia
- Amniotic fluid embolism

SHOCK
- Septic shock
- Severe hypovolemic shock

TRAUMA OR SURGERY
- Burns
- Massive trauma
- Surgery involving extracorporeal circulation
- Snakebite
- Heatstroke

---

and platelets, which, in turn, leads to bleeding. Further aggravation of bleeding occurs because of increased fibrinolysis. The coagulation system is severely dysfunctional, swinging from extreme clotting activity to severe anticoagulant activity.

Activation of the TF/factor VIIa pathway (extrinsic pathway of coagulation) has been implicated as the central mediator of intravascular coagulation in sepsis. Injured endothelium and polymorphonuclear leukocytes produce TF. Once DIC begins, antithrombin levels, which would normally inhibit clot formation, become markedly reduced. Low antithrombin levels are associated with high mortality in DIC. Also the protein C and protein S pathways, which are major natural anticoagulant systems, are disabled. TF pathway inhibitor, another anticoagulant system, is also disabled. The fibrinolytic pathway, which reduces the body's ability to dissolve clots, is shut down as well.

Blood vessel endothelium also plays a role in DIC. Endothelial cells normally secrete vWF, which enhances adhesion between platelets and vessel walls. In DIC this adhesion propensity is increased, causing clot formation. Also, in DIC, inflammation and coagulation pathways invigorate each other. Many of the coagulation factors stimulate the endothelial cell release of inflammatory cytokines.

In general, if the underlying condition is self-limited or can be appropriately treated, DIC will resolve and the coagulation status will return to normal. For example, a patient with acute DIC associated with abruptio placentae (impaired placental connection to the uterus) needs quick delivery of the fetus and placenta, and the DIC will resolve with the treatment. However, a patient with acute DIC that is stimulated by metastatic gastric carcinoma likely has a fatal condition that will not be altered, regardless of treatment.

Clinical Presentation

Although coagulation and formation of microemboli may characterize DIC in the initial phase, its most harmful effects are more directly related to the bleeding problems that occur. The bleeding may be present as petechiae, purpura, oozing from puncture sites, severe hemorrhage, or uncontrolled postpartum bleeding. Bleeding can occur internally within serous cavities. Gastrointestinal bleeding, bleeding from gums, spontaneous bruising, hemoptysis, hematuria, and jaundice often occur. Specific thrombotic complications commonly seen in DIC are distal extremity cyanosis, hemorrhagic skin infarctions, limb ischemia, and gangrene. Patients can experience loss of limbs and/or organ infarctions. Cardiovascular shock is a common complication causing severe hypotension and tachycardia. Microthrombi may obstruct blood vessels and cause ischemia and infarction of the kidneys, heart, lungs, and brain. As a result, renal, circulatory, or respiratory failure can occur. Effects on the central nervous system include transient neurological deficits, lethargy, stupor, or coma.

Diagnosis

Platelet counts are moderately to severely reduced in DIC. Hemolytic anemia can develop as RBCs become damaged when passing through vessels obstructed by thrombi. The peripheral blood smear can demonstrate evidence of abnormally shaped RBCs caused by hemolysis. Fibrinolysis is also an important feature of DIC, and fibrin breakdown is demonstrated by elevations in the D-dimer laboratory test, the most sensitive test for DIC. Clotting times (both aPTT and PT/INR) are elevated. Fibrinogen, antithrombin levels, and individual coagulation factors are diminished in DIC. The International Society on Thrombosis and Hemostasis (ISTH) DIC scoring system is an assessment tool based on platelet count, fibrinogen levels, fibrin split products, and PT that can help in diagnosis.

Treatment

To treat DIC, it is necessary to control the primary disease, replace clotting factors, and prevent further activation of clotting mechanisms. Transfusions of fresh frozen plasma, platelets, or fibrinogen-containing cryoprecipitate may correct the clotting factor deficiency. Heparin may be given to decrease blood coagulation, thereby interrupting the clotting process. The use of antifibrinolytic agents may reduce bleeding episodes, and protein C concentrates can be effective. Activated protein C and protein C products have shown promising results in sepsis-related DIC with resolution of the coagulopathy and correction of hemostasis.

Chapter Summary

- Platelet formation is stimulated by the hormone thrombopoietin, which is synthesized by the liver.
- The normal platelet count is 150,000 to 450,000/uL, and a platelet's life span is 7 to 10 days.
- Almost one-third of all platelets reside in the spleen; when enlarged and hyperactive, the spleen can sequester up to 80% of platelets.
- Numerous GP receptors (GPIIb/IIIa) on the surface of a platelet assist in clot formation. Some antiplatelet agents work as GPIIb/IIIa receptor blockers to diminish platelet aggregation.
- The activated platelet surface provides the major physiological site for coagulation factor activation.
- Coagulation factors are produced in the liver and require vitamin K.

- Clots formed because of stasis of blood or endothelial injury are created via the intrinsic pathway.
- Clots formed because of external trauma to a blood vessel are created via the extrinsic pathway.
- Acquired deficiencies of coagulation are the most frequently encountered disorders in the clinical area. Causes include liver disease, vitamin K deficiency, and DIC.
- The most common hereditary bleeding disorder is hemophilia. In these disorders, blood coagulation is hindered. Bleeding can be occult, as in gastrointestinal blood loss, or apparent, as in traumatic hemorrhage.
- Many different drugs can cause thrombocytopenia.
- In platelet dysfunction or deficiency, lesions such as petechiae may be seen on physical examination.

Spontaneous bleeding can occur as bruises, nose-bleeds, bleeding from the gums, or vaginal bleeding.

- Hypercoagulability of the blood causes susceptibility to clotting. Clots can occlude blood vessels and cause tissue ischemia, infarction, or gangrene. Stroke, myocardial infarction, peripheral arterial disease, DVT, and pulmonary embolism are all caused by blood clots.

- Thrombophilic disorders are conditions that predispose a person to arterial and/or venous clot formation. Thrombophilic disorders can be inherited due to genetic mutations or acquired.

- The INR is a standard measurement of clotting. If a blood sample has an INR of 1, this indicates normal clotting. The greater the INR, the longer it takes for the blood to clot.

- For adequate anticoagulation, an INR should be maintained between 2 and 3.

- The greater the patient's PT or aPTT compared with normal values, the longer it takes for the patient's blood to clot, which can increase risk for bleeding.

- Aspirin is commonly used to decrease platelet aggregation.

- Protamine sulfate is a heparin antagonist.

- Vitamin K antagonizes warfarin.

- Patients on warfarin should avoid eating excessive amounts of green leafy vegetables.

- DIC, where the coagulation system dysfunctions and causes both clotting and bleeding, can occur in critically ill patients, particularly those who have sepsis.

Making the Connections

Pathophysiology

Signs and Symptoms	Physical Assessment Findings	Diagnostic Tests	Treatment
Immune Thrombocytopenic Purpura (ITP) | Antibody destruction of platelets triggered by an antigen because of an unknown cause. The antigenic target appears to be the platelet GPIIb/IIIa complex. The complex is attacked by IgG antibodies.			
Purpura. Petechiae. Mucosal bleeding. Ecchymoses. GI bleeding. Heavy menstrual blood loss.	Mucocutaneous bleeding, ecchymoses, gastrointestinal or excessive menstrual bleeding. Retinal hemorrhages possible.	Decreased platelet count. Peripheral smear may show enlarged platelets. Iron deficiency may be present. Serum protein electrophoresis and immunoglobulin levels to detect possible hypogamma globulinemia, and a direct antiglobulin test (also called Coomb's test).	Corticosteroid, IV immunoglobulin, immunosuppressive agents, platelet transfusion.
Thrombotic Thrombocytopenic Purpura (TTP) | Deficiency of or antibodies to metalloproteases that cleave vWF. The persistence of vWF causes platelet adhesion and aggregation.			
Five specific signs and symptoms: • Microangiopathic hemolytic anemia • Thrombocytopenic purpura • Neurological abnormalities • Fever • Renal disease	Petechiae and purpura of lower extremities. Fever.	Decreased platelet count caused by platelet adhesion. Hemolysis. Microvascular thrombosis. Increased bilirubin caused by breakdown of RBCs. Increased reticulocyte count caused by increased bone marrow activity to replace lysed RBCs. Negative direct antiglobulin test. Peripheral smear has schistocytes, which are odd-shaped RBCs caused by hemolysis.	Plasma exchange, immunomodulatory medications, splenectomy, glucocorticoids. Octaplas.

Continued

Making the Connections—cont'd

Signs and Symptoms	Physical Assessment Findings	Diagnostic Tests	Treatment
Drug-Induced Thrombocytopenia | Antibody attack on platelets in the presence of certain drugs.			
Petechiae. Purpura.	Petechiae. Purpura.	Decreased platelet count and antibodies to drug metabolites.	Stop medications.
Hemolytic-Uremic Syndrome (HUS) | Renal failure, hemolytic anemia, thrombocytopenia commonly preceded by *E. coli* O157:H7 infection.			
Fever, abdominal pain, pale skin, fatigue and irritability, bruising or bleeding of nose and mouth, reduced urination, edema.	History of diarrheal illness caused by *E. coli* O157:H7; may have blood in urine because of large amount of hemolysis; bloody diarrhea.	Decreased platelet count, normal aPTT, and normal PT; low RBC caused by hemolysis; high bilirubin caused by RBC breakdown. Stool culture for *E. coli* O157:H7. Increased serum creatinine caused by renal insufficiency and renal failure.	Supportive treatment with dialysis, plasma exchange may be used.
Essential Thrombocytosis | High platelet number because of an unknown cause.			
Secondary Thrombocytosis | Almost always caused by iron deficiency; inflammation, cancer, or infection; or underlying myelodysplastic disorder. The patient may have had a splenectomy.			
May have no symptoms. When symptoms do appear, they can be caused by abnormal blood clotting and cause stroke, heart attack, or deep venous thrombosis.	May have no physical assessment abnormalities. Possible signs include stroke, heart attack, or deep venous thrombosis.	Increased platelet count. May have low iron, low serum ferritin, or high total iron-binding capacity indicating iron-deficiency anemia. Erythrocyte sedimentation rate and C-reactive protein may be elevated because of inflammation. Bone marrow shows excessive platelets. Splenectomy may be evident through imaging studies.	Aspirin or antiplatelet drugs. Plateletpheresis.
von Willebrand Disease | A major adhesion molecule that ties platelets to exposed endothelial tissue. Hereditary and involves diminished vWF protein, decreased function of vWF, and decreased factor VIII levels.			
Excessive bleeding caused by trauma, surgical procedures, or at menses.	Excessive bruising or bleeding with minor trauma, spontaneous nosebleeds, bleeding from gums, or menorrhagia.	CBC, decreased platelet count, aPTT, and PT show prolonged bleeding time. Diminished vWF.	Desmopressin acetate, which releases vWF and factor VIII from endothelial stores. vWF replacement. Antifibrinolytic agents.
Disseminated Intravascular Coagulation (DIC) | Secondary to another disease. Overactivation of the clotting mechanism. Commonly caused by sepsis.			
Petechiae. Purpura. Hematomas. Shortness of breath. Severe pain in back, chest, and muscles. Vomiting.	Clotting and bleeding occur at the same time. Severe hypotension.	Increased PT, increased aPTT, CBC. Increased fibrin-split products. Decreased fibrinogen. D-dimer level increased.	Fresh frozen plasma transfusion for bleeding (has most amount of coagulation factors), heparin, fibrinolytic drugs for excessive clotting, and treatment underlying disease.

Making the Connections—cont'd

Signs and Symptoms	Physical Assessment Findings	Diagnostic Tests	Treatment
Hemophilia A | Genetic disorder; lack of factor VIII causes decreased clotting ability.			
Bruises. Nosebleeds. Gum bleeds. Hemarthrosis. Common symptoms in different body systems due to bleeding, which can be occult: • General: weakness, tachycardia, tachypnea, spontaneous or easy bruising. • Nose/throat: epistaxis, hemoptysis, bleeding gums, excessive bleeding with dental procedures. • Musculoskeletal: joint pain and stiffness (due to hemarthrosis), compartment syndrome. • Central nervous system: headache, stiff neck, spinal cord syndromes (bleeding into spinal cord), intracranial hemorrhage (subdural or epidural hematoma). • Gastrointestinal: abdominal pain, hematemesis (blood in vomitus), melena (blood in stool). • Genitourinary: back pain, hematuria, postcircumcision bleeding in infant.	Excessive bruising or bleeding with minor trauma, spontaneous nosebleeds, bleeding from gums, or menorrhagia.	Normal PT. Increased PTT. Normal platelet count. Decreased factor VIII levels.	Factor VIII transfusion until bleeding stops; genetic counseling.
Hemophilia B | Genetic disorder; lack of factor IX causes decreased clotting ability.			
Bruises. Nosebleeds. Gum bleeds. Hemarthroses.	Excessive bruising or bleeding with minor trauma, spontaneous nosebleeds, bleeding from gums, or menorrhagia.	Normal PT. Increased PTT. Normal platelet count. Decreased factor IX levels.	Factor IX transfusion until bleeding stops; genetic counseling.

Bibliography

Available online at fadavis.com

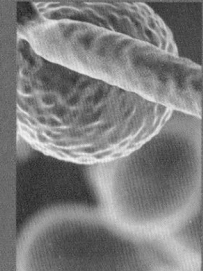

Arterial Disorders

Learning Objectives

After completion of this chapter, the student will be able to:

- Describe the pathological process of each arterial disorder.
- Identify agents that cause endothelial injury and contribute to the formation of atherosclerosis.
- List the risk factors that lead to each arterial disorder.

- Explain the assessment of the patient with arterial disorders.
- Recognize the various complications that can result from arterial disorders.
- Discuss effective modalities to prevent and treat each arterial disorder.

Key Terms

Abdominal aortic aneurysm (AAA)

Aneurysm

Ankle–brachial index (ABI)

Artery

Arteriosclerosis

Atherosclerosis

Baroreceptor

Cardiac output (CO)

Cholesterol

Diastole

Dyslipidemia

Endothelium

Familial hypercholesterolemia

Free radical

Glycosylation (glycation)

High-density lipoprotein (HDL)

Hyperlipidemia

Hypertension (HTN)

Intermittent claudication

Low-density lipoprotein (LDL)

Natriuresis

Peripheral arterial disease (PAD)

Pulse pressure

Renin

Renin-angiotensin-aldosterone system (RAAS)

Reverse cholesterol transport

Stroke volume (SV)

Systole

Triglyceride

The arterial system is composed of large- and medium-sized arteries and arterioles. **Arteries** are muscular-walled blood vessels with large amounts of elastic fibers; this built-in elasticity allows for pulsatile flow. The heart's pumping action is reflected in the arteries—a large volume of blood is pumped through the arteries with the heart's contraction; when the heart relaxes, the arteries rest.

Arteries direct blood out of the heart to the tissues of the rest of the body, thereby supplying the tissues with oxygenated blood and nutrients. A key concept to understand is that the greater the pressure of blood within the arteries and arterioles, the higher the resistance the heart must pump against. The main artery that arises from the heart is the aorta, the body's largest and most muscular arterial vessel.

Basic Physiological Concepts of Arterial Structure and Function

Cardiovascular health depends mainly on the heart and the arteries. The arteries are muscular blood vessels that maintain blood pressure (BP) throughout the body. Their composition is significant because their inner lining, called **endothelium**, can undergo key changes that predispose individuals to **arteriosclerosis** and **atherosclerosis** leading to cardiovascular disease (CVD). The muscular walls of the arteries respond to autonomic impulses that signal blood flow needs; sensors in the arterial walls largely regulate blood flow and BP, and pulsations in the arteries are reflective of the heart's contractile function. Heart function is most commonly assessed through the pulses of the radial, carotid, and brachial arteries. Blood constituents, such as lipids, glucose, nicotine, and others, can affect the artery's reactivity and undermine the health of the endothelium, resulting in arteriosclerosis and atherosclerosis. Understanding the artery's structure and function is fundamental to full comprehension of the workings of the cardiovascular system.

🩺 CLINICAL CONCEPT

Arteriosclerosis is the hardening and narrowing of the arteries. With atherosclerosis, plaque builds up on the artery walls and restricts blood flow.

The Composition of the Arterial Wall

Artery walls are composed of three layers (see Fig. 15-1):

1. **Tunica intima**: The innermost layer of the artery wall. It is composed of a thin layer of endothelial cells that lie adjacent to each other and have contact with the blood. The endothelium is a smooth, contiguous surface of cells that blankets all the inner linings of the arteries. It is a metabolically active tissue that releases substances, reacts to chemical mediators, and responds to blood contents. The endothelium is the primary site of damage of arteriosclerosis and atherosclerosis.
2. **Tunica media**: The middle layer of the artery wall. It is composed of smooth muscle that can constrict and dilate to change the artery's diameter. The smooth muscle is innervated by autonomic nerves, which are the sympathetic (also called adrenergic) and parasympathetic (also called cholinergic) nerve fibers. There are alpha-adrenergic and beta-adrenergic nerves. Alpha-adrenergic nerve fibers are excitatory and cause vasoconstriction, whereas beta-adrenergic fibers are inhibitory and cause vasodilation. The vascular smooth muscle relies on extracellular calcium for depolarization. Calcium enters membrane channels to evoke contraction and vasoconstriction.
3. **Tunica externa**: The outermost covering of the artery wall; it is also called the tunica adventitia. It is largely composed of connective tissue that provides support for the artery.

🩺 CLINICAL CONCEPT

Calcium channel blocker (CCB) medications block vasoconstriction of arteries and are used in the management of elevated BP, also known as hypertension.

The Endothelium as Active Tissue

The endothelium is composed of a blanket of endothelial cells, which are specialized squamous epithelial cells. These cells line the interior surface of arteries, from the heart to the smallest arterioles and capillaries. The endothelium forms an interface between the blood and the artery walls. The endothelium of the interior surfaces of the heart chambers is called the endocardium.

Endothelial cells have distinct metabolic functions, including fluid filtration, maintenance of blood vessel tone, hemostasis, angiogenesis (the formation of new blood vessel growth), neutrophil chemotaxis, and hormone secretion (Fig. 15-2). The endothelium

The artery is a muscular tube composed of three distinct layers.

Tunica adventitia	Tunica media	Tunica intima
Connective tissue	Smooth muscle	Interior lining of artery: Basement membrane Endothelial cells

FIGURE 15-1. The three layers of arteries: tunica intima (endothelium), tunica media (smooth muscle), and tunica adventitia (outer connective tissue).

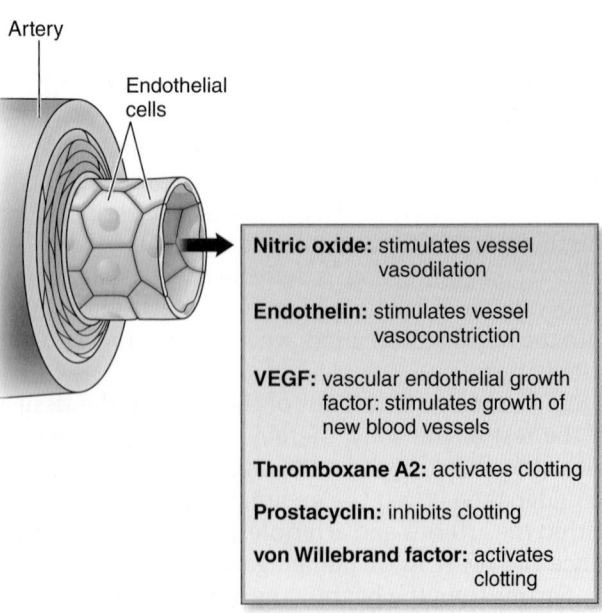

Artery

Endothelial cells

Nitric oxide: stimulates vessel vasodilation

Endothelin: stimulates vessel vasoconstriction

VEGF: vascular endothelial growth factor: stimulates growth of new blood vessels

Thromboxane A2: activates clotting

Prostacyclin: inhibits clotting

von Willebrand factor: activates clotting

FIGURE 15-2. The endothelium is a metabolically active tissue. It can secrete chemical mediators that activate vasodilation, vasoconstriction, clotting, and new growth of blood vessels. It can also secrete factors that inhibit clotting.

acts as a semipermeable barrier between the vessel lumen and surrounding tissue, controlling the passage of biochemical substances and the transit of white blood cells (WBCs) into and out of the bloodstream. Endothelial cells also produce nitric oxide (NO), which stimulates dilation of blood vessels, and endothelin, which provokes constriction of vessels.

To stimulate angiogenesis, endothelial cells produce vascular endothelial growth factor (VEGF). Collateral branches of arterioles form in response to VEGF. Studies show exercise stimulates VEGF, which in turn enhances angiogenesis. Angiogenesis is cardioprotective because it enhances vascularity, which increases collateral blood vessels and lowers blood pressure over time (Gorski & DeBock, 2019).

When blood volume is excessive, endothelial cells produce C-type natriuretic peptide to cause diuresis, which is excretion of excess water.

Substances that oppose each other are produced by the endothelium. Prostacyclin, which breaks down clots, and thromboxane A2 (TXA2), which enhances clot formation, are also secreted by the endothelial cells.

Some organs contain highly differentiated endothelial cells that perform filtering functions. Examples of such unique endothelial structures include the renal glomerulus and the blood–brain barrier.

Endothelial injury causes endothelial dysfunction, which is the key early event in the development of arteriosclerosis and atherosclerosis. Endothelial injury incites the inflammation reaction, which brings WBCs to the site of damage. The WBCs engulf and phagocytose lipids in the region and form lipid-laden macrophages called foam cells. This inhibits the release of NO, which decreases blood vessel vasodilation capability. Recent studies show that autoimmunity is involved in the process of atherogenesis. The WBCs induced by the inflammation cascade include T lymphocytes that react against oxidized low-density lipoprotein (oxLDL) as if it was antigenic. Also, B lymphocytes produce antibodies that react against oxLDL as though it were an antigen (Kobiyama & Ley, 2018; Wolf & Ley, 2019).

Simultaneously, excessive quantities of von Willebrand factor are released, which promote platelet aggregation and adhesion to the endothelial surface. These reactions together provide the elements for vascular dysfunction and atherosclerotic plaque construction.

CLINICAL CONCEPT

Dysfunctional endothelium is seen in patients with coronary artery disease (CAD), diabetes mellitus, hypertension, and hypercholesterolemia, as well as in people who smoke.

Blood Flow Regulation

In the cardiovascular system, the arteries are the most influential structures in control of blood flow. The arteries are vessels of high volume, high pressure, and high or low resistance, depending on their state of vasoconstriction or vasodilation. The elements of volume, pressure, and resistance regulate the blood flow through the arteries. Optimal circulatory function requires volume that fills the blood vessel and pressure to move the blood into all areas of body tissues. In the arterial system, areas of large artery diameter gradually feed into areas of smaller artery diameter. Blood flow is inversely related to the diameter of the blood vessel. When blood flows from an area of larger vessel diameter to an area of smaller vessel diameter, flow is reduced and pressure is increased in the vessel. Resistance is the amount of obstruction to blood flow caused by vessel diameter, vessel length, and blood viscosity, which is the thickness of the fluid caused by the particles in solution. In the bloodstream, viscosity is fairly constant. The relation of pressure, resistance, and blood flow is expressed in the equation:

$$\text{Blood flow} = \text{Pressure of blood}/\text{Resistance of blood}$$

In the circulatory system, blood flow is analogous to **cardiac output (CO)**, which is the amount of blood that flows from the heart's left ventricle per minute. The pressure of blood is the arterial BP, which measures the force against the walls of arteries as the heart pumps blood through the body. The resistance is the total peripheral vascular resistance (PVR) caused by the blood vessels within the circulatory system. The mathematical calculation of blood flow is:

$$CO = BP / PVR$$

This can also be expressed as:

$$CO \times PVR = BP$$

The relationship between the variables of blood flow, blood pressure, and resistance can be observed in these mathematical relationships. The body is able to adjust the factors independently to maintain homeostasis. For example, if BP decreases, the body can both increase CO and PVR to elevate the BP.

Blood flow normally is laminar, meaning that the flow is smooth and parallel to the horizontal lines of the vessels. This allows a smooth, low-friction flow of blood and is a hallmark of a healthy endothelium. In areas where the endothelium is rough, injured, or inflamed, blood flow tends to become turbulent. Turbulent blood flow causes areas of blood to move perpendicular to vessel walls and predisposes the formation of small areas of stagnant blood (see Fig. 15-3). The nonstreamlined and stagnant movement of blood causes blood constituents, such as red blood cells, WBCs, platelets, and coagulation factors, to come in contact with the arterial endothelial lining. The stasis

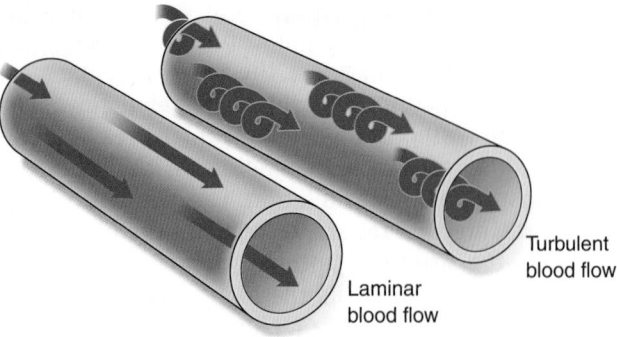

FIGURE 15-3. Laminar versus turbulent blood flow in a blood vessel.

of blood and stimulation of endothelium predisposes to thrombus (clot) formation. Areas of turbulence often occur in damaged and arteriosclerotic sections of artery walls, leading to thrombus formation.

> ### 🔬 CLINICAL CONCEPT
>
> Turbulent blood flow often produces whooshing sounds called bruits that can be heard through the stethoscope.

Arterial Wall Tension

In a blood vessel, wall tension is the force in the vessel wall that opposes the distending pressure inside the vessel. The internal pressure expands the vessel until it is inhibited by the tension in the vessel wall. The smaller the vessel's radius, the greater the pressure needed to overcome wall tension. Laplace's law expresses the effect of the radius on wall tension:

$$\text{Intraluminal pressure} = \text{Tension} / \text{radius}$$

or

$$\text{Tension} = \text{Pressure} \times \text{radius}$$

or

$$P = T / r$$

or

$$T = P \times r$$

Wall tension is also inversely related to wall thickness: the thicker the vessel wall, the lower the tension, and vice versa. This can be expressed as the following mathematical equation:

$$\text{Tension} = \text{Pressure} \times \text{radius} / \text{wall thickness}$$

or

$$T = P \times r / \text{wall thickness}$$

In **hypertension (HTN)**, arterial vessel walls hypertrophy and become thicker, thereby reducing the tension and minimizing the wall stress. Laplace's law can be applied to the pressure required to maintain the patency of small blood vessels. When the thickness of the vessel wall remains constant, it takes more pressure to overcome wall tension and keep the vessel open as its radius decreases in size. There is a critical pressure where the vessels collapse and blood can no longer flow through them.

Distention and Compliance

Compliance is the distention capacity of a blood vessel; distention capacity allows for increased blood flow with each mm Hg rise in blood pressure. The high distention capacity of the aorta and large arteries allows them to accommodate the high output of the heart.

Blood Pressure Regulation

Arterial BP reflects the cardiac cycles of systole and diastole. **Systole** is the period of cardiac contraction, and **diastole** is the period of cardiac relaxation. In the arteries, BP rises when the left ventricle contracts in systole and ejects blood from the chamber. This is followed by the decline of blood pressure when the left ventricle ends its contraction in diastole. In healthy adults, the systolic pressure is ideally lower than 120 mm Hg and the diastolic pressure is ideally lower than 80 mm Hg. Numerous research investigations, such as the Framingham Heart Study, have demonstrated that when systolic and diastolic pressure are maintained at these values, there is a diminished risk of cardiovascular disease (CVD) (see Box 15-1). The difference between

> ### BOX 15-1. The Framingham Heart Study
>
> In 1948, the Framingham Heart Study, under the direction of the National Institutes of Health, began a novel research project. At the time, little was known about the causes of heart disease and stroke, but the death rates for CVD had been increasing steadily since the beginning of the century and had become an American epidemic. The objective of the study was to identify the common factors that contribute to CVD by following a group of 5,209 men and women between the ages of 30 and 62 from the town of Framingham, Massachusetts. These participants were the first to undergo extensive physical examinations and interviews about factors related to CVD development. Since 1948, the subjects have continued to return to the study every 2 years for a detailed medical history, physical examination, and laboratory tests. In 1971, the study enrolled a second generation–5,124 of the original participants' adult children and their spouses–to participate in similar examinations. A wealth of information has been revealed about CVD risk factors from this study. In 2002, the study entered a new phase, the enrollment of a third generation of participants, the grandchildren of the original participants. The study continues today.

the systolic and diastolic arterial BP is called the **pulse pressure**, which ideally is approximately 40 mm Hg.

In a healthy adult, approximately 70% of the blood in the left ventricle is ejected during systole; this volume ejected per contraction is called the **stroke volume (SV)**. Within the left ventricle, there is approximately 100 mL of blood and 70% of this volume is ejected; therefore, SV is approximately 70 mL.

The average heart rate (HR) is 70 beats per minute. Mathematically, one can multiply SV by HR to obtain the volume of blood per minute ejected from the left ventricle. The volume of blood ejected by the left ventricle per minute is the cardiac output (CO). Therefore, SV multiplied by HR is equal to CO (SV × HR = CO). In the healthy adult, 70 mL of SV × 70 heart beats/minute = 4900 mL blood/minute (approximately 5 liters).

 CLINICAL CONCEPT

Normal CO at rest is approximately 5 liters blood/minute.

The systolic and diastolic components of BP are determined by CO and peripheral vascular resistance (PVR). This is mathematically expressed as BP = CO × PVR. The PVR is mainly influenced by the diameter of the arterial blood vessel. The diameter is regulated by the autonomic nervous system innervation of the smooth muscle wall of the artery and arteriole. Arteries and arterioles are frequently referred to as resistance vessels because they constrict or relax to control the outflow of blood into the capillaries. Mathematical relationships of BP, CO, and PVR can be expressed as:

$$CO \times PVR = BP$$

or

$$CO / BP = PVR$$

or

$$CO = BP / PVR$$

CO is determined by BP and PVR. The body has to adjust PVR and BP inversely to maintain CO. For example, to maintain CO when BP decreases, the body has to raise peripheral vascular resistance by arterial vasoconstriction.

 CLINICAL CONCEPT

Cardiac output (CO) varies reciprocally with changes in peripheral vascular resistance (PVR) when BP is unchanged.

Given the mathematical relationship discussed earlier (CO = BP / PVR), the interrelation of blood flow,

BP, and resistance is clear. Several systemic mechanisms are in place to regulate BP and, subsequently, blood flow. BP-regulating mechanisms include baroreceptors, the renin–angiotensin–aldosterone system (RAAS), the posterior pituitary–antidiuretic hormone (ADH) mechanism, and natriuresis (see Fig. 15-4).

Baroreceptors: Neural Mechanisms of Blood Pressure Regulation

Short-term regulation of BP is aimed at correcting temporary imbalances that occur when the body changes position or endures exercise. The cardiovascular regulation center in the brain is in the lower pons and medulla, where modulation of the autonomic nervous system occurs. The center transmits sympathetic and parasympathetic signals to the heart and blood

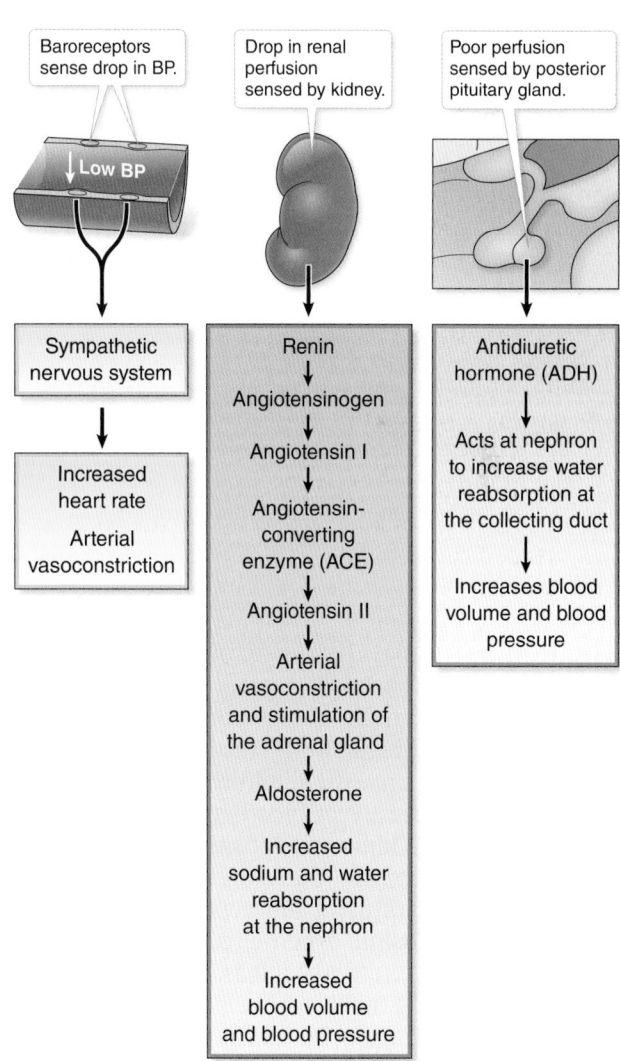

FIGURE 15-4. Body mechanisms that maintain blood pressure. 1. Baroreceptors located in the arterial wall sense decreases in BP and stimulate the SNS. The SNS stimulates the heart to increase rate and activates arterial vasoconstriction. 2. The RAAS is activated when the kidneys sense low blood pressure. The effect of the RAAS is increased blood volume and vasoconstriction. 3. The posterior pituitary gland senses low perfusion and secretes ADH, which acts at the nephron to increase water reabsorption; this raises blood volume and blood pressure.

vessels. The parasympathetic impulses are transmitted via the vagus nerve to the heart and some blood vessels. The sympathetic impulses travel to the heart and blood vessels via the spinal cord and peripheral nerves. The vagus nerve slows down HR, and the sympathetic stimulation increases HR and contractility. The sympathetic stimulation also causes vasoconstriction of the arteries.

Within the walls of arteries, particularly the carotid artery and aortic arch, are BP sensors known as **baroreceptors**. When baroreceptors detect a drop in BP, they respond rapidly by stimulating the sympathetic nervous system (SNS). The SNS stimulates an increase in HR and contractility and stimulates contraction of vascular smooth muscle in the arteries. The increase in HR, contractility, and vasoconstriction causes BP to quickly increase in response to the drop in BP. This baroreceptor reflex is commonly exhibited when an individual goes from a lying position to a sitting or standing position; this change in position causes a brief drop in BP that is sensed by the baroreceptors, which in turn stimulate the SNS to enact a reflexive increase in HR and vasoconstriction. The sensitivity of baroreceptors is key to the maintenance of BP. As individuals age, baroreceptor sensitivity decreases.

 CLINICAL CONCEPT

Orthostatic hypotension is a drop in BP that occurs when changing position from lying to standing. The drop in BP causes decreased cerebral perfusion, which leads to dizziness. This is often experienced by older adults and individuals on antihypertensive medications.

The Renin–Angiotensin–Aldosterone System

The **renin-angiotensin–aldosterone system (RAAS)** is a key part of BP regulation. This multistep reaction raises BP in response to diminished circulation in the body. When the BP or blood volume in the body is diminished, the kidney is sensitive to the drop in BP. **Renin** is an enzyme that is released by the juxtaglomerular apparatus of the nephrons in response to decreased perfusion. When circulation to the kidney is diminished, renin is released into the bloodstream, stimulating the liver to release a large protein called angiotensinogen. In the lungs, angiotensinogen is transformed into angiotensin I; angiotensin-converting enzyme (ACE) changes angiotensin I into angiotensin II. Angiotensin II is a potent arterial vasoconstrictor and stimulates the adrenal gland to release the hormone aldosterone. The arterial vasoconstriction raises BP. Aldosterone works at the nephron to increase sodium and water reabsorption into the bloodstream and secrete potassium into the nephron tubules. Retention of sodium and water increases the

volume of the bloodstream and BP, which may lead to an increase in BP.

The Posterior Pituitary–Antidiuretic Hormone Mechanism

Another important hormone secreted in response to diminished BP is ADH, also called vasopressin. The posterior pituitary secretes ADH when it senses a drop in blood volume or BP or an increase in blood osmolarity. ADH acts at the nephron to increase water reabsorption into the bloodstream, thereby raising blood volume and BP. ADH only reabsorbs water into the bloodstream, not sodium.

Natriuresis

Natriuresis is natural diuresis promoted by the heart. In response to excess water in the bloodstream, the ventricles of the heart stretch. This triggers release of atrial natriuretic peptide (ANP) and B type natriuretic peptide (BNP). The natriuretic peptides act at the nephrons to release excess water into the urine. Natriuresis decreases the water content in the blood, and sodium follows water out into the urine. The reduction of blood volume can contribute to a lowering of BP. When BP and blood volume return to normal, water and sodium excretion cease.

The Effect of Blood Composition on Arteries

The endothelial lining of the arteries consists of metabolically active cells that are influenced by the constituents of the bloodstream. Common constituents of the blood include lipids, glucose, and free radicals. High levels of any of these components have a negative effect on the endothelium.

Lipids

Lipids are fats that circulate in the bloodstream and make up the cell membranes in the body. Lipids are mainly composed of **cholesterol**, a fatty steroidal substance that is ingested from the diet and synthesized by the liver. Cholesterol is an essential structural component of cell membranes, and it assists in the maintenance of proper membrane permeability. In addition to its importance within cells, cholesterol is an important component in the body's hormonal systems for the manufacture of bile acids, steroid hormones, and vitamin D. Cholesterol is ingested via animal products, such as meat, milk, butter, and cheese; it is insoluble in blood but is carried by proteins to form soluble lipoproteins. There are different types of lipoproteins: some contain cholesterol and others contain triglycerides. **Triglycerides** are large lipid molecules acquired through diet and stored as fat tissue. Lipoproteins are classified by size and lipid content into **low-density lipoproteins (LDLs)** and **high-density lipoproteins (HDLs)**. HDL is excreted from the body, which is why it is considered "good" cholesterol, whereas LDL is deposited on artery walls, which is why it is considered "bad" cholesterol. The deposition occurs at areas of endothelial injury where inflammation is occurring. WBCs phagocytose the LDL and form lipid-laden macrophages called foam cells; the foam cell is the preliminary change in the endothelium that leads to larger collections of fat, inflammatory mediators, and platelets called atherosclerotic plaque (see the "Hyperlipidemia" section).

Glucose

Chronically high circulating levels of glucose in the bloodstream cause harm to the endothelial lining of arteries. Glucose reacts with the cell membranes of endothelial cells in a process called **glycosylation** (also called **glycation**). The glucose reacts with vessel wall proteins and forms advanced glycosylation end products (AGEs), which injure the smooth endothelial surface. This type of endothelial injury is a precursor to endothelial inflammation and formation of atherosclerotic plaque. In addition, the stimulation by AGEs causes endothelium to secrete endothelin, a hormone that causes potent vasoconstriction. Continuous high glucose levels, like those that occur in uncontrolled diabetes, predispose to arteriosclerosis, atherosclerosis, and vasoconstricted arteries. These changes occur throughout the body, which is the reason diabetes is a risk factor for acute cardiovascular events, such as stroke and myocardial infarction (MI).

Free Radicals

Free radicals are chemical compounds with an unpaired electron. They have a strong affinity for cell membranes and cause damage to the artery endothelial lining. These molecules have an oxidative effect and set up areas of inflammation in the artery. The areas of inflammation become the preliminary change that sets up formation of atherosclerotic plaque.

Nicotine

Nicotine, a common ingredient in cigarettes, is a potent vasoconstrictor of arteries, particularly the coronary arteries. Nicotine is known to immediately increase BP, and significant remnants of nicotine remain in the body for 6 to 8 hours after smoking a cigarette. It also activates the SNS, acting via splanchnic nerves to the adrenal medulla, and stimulates the release of epinephrine, which increases HR and causes central nervous system stimulation.

Homocysteine

Homocysteine is an amino acid that is integrally involved in the metabolism of folic acid and B vitamins. Deficiencies of folic acid and B vitamins cause decreased breakdown of homocysteine. Elevated levels of homocysteine in the bloodstream lead to damage of the endothelial lining of the arteries. High homocysteine levels are linked to thrombosis formation and CVD.

Pathophysiology of Arterial Disorders

CVD begins in the body's arteries. Arteriosclerosis and atherosclerosis are the fundamental changes in the body that initiate widespread CVD. Many agents can injure the endothelial lining of arteries, and this damage is the inciting event for arteriosclerosis, which may lead to atherosclerosis. Many conditions, such as HTN, hyperlipidemia, and diabetes mellitus, may predispose patients to arteriosclerotic and atherosclerotic damage.

Hyperlipidemia

Hyperlipidemia refers to elevated levels of lipids, mainly cholesterol and triglycerides, in the bloodstream. In more precise terms, hypercholesterolemia refers to elevated cholesterol levels, whereas hypertriglyceridemia refers to elevated triglyceride levels. Hyperlipidemia is one of the major conditions that lead to atherosclerosis, a contributing factor to all forms of CVD. The specific type of cholesterol that contributes to atherosclerosis is LDL. Elevated levels of LDL cholesterol are often accompanied by decreased levels of HDL cholesterol. High levels of LDL cholesterol and low levels of HDL cholesterol predispose to CVD. The term **dyslipidemia** describes a disorder combining hypertriglyceridemia, elevated LDL cholesterol levels, and decreased HDL levels.

Familial hypercholesterolemia (FH) is a specific type of hyperlipidemia that causes elevated levels of blood cholesterol. FH is a genetic condition that results in premature atherosclerotic cardiovascular disease due to lifelong exposure to elevated low-density lipoprotein cholesterol (LDL-C) levels. There are two forms of FH: homozygous FH is rare, and heterozygous FH is more common in the population. Specific gene variants have been correlated with homozygous and heterozygous FH and additional gene variants under investigation. Heterozygous FH is the most common genetic cause of cardiovascular disease, with an estimated prevalence of ~1 in 220 persons and more common in certain ethnic groups. If not identified and appropriately treated from an early age, studies show that untreated male subjects are at a 50% risk for a fatal or nonfatal coronary event by 50 years of age and untreated female subjects are at a 30% risk by 60 years of age. FH is believed to be an underrecognized condition with millions of affected persons in the United States who are undiagnosed.

Etiology

Cholesterol is a necessary lipid component of body structures. It is a major component of all cell membranes, is needed to maintain cell stability, and is a basic constituent of steroid hormones and bile acids, two components involved in many physiological functions. All cells are capable of synthesizing cholesterol, but the liver is most effective at its production, metabolism, and excretion. Cholesterol is largely acquired by the body via diet and liver production.

FH is most commonly a polygenic condition associated with genetic variants in one or more of specifically identified genes. These specific genes include the low-density receptor *(LDLR)* gene and the genes encoding apolipoprotein B *(APOB),* apolipoprotein E *(APOE),* and proprotein convertase subtilisin/kexin 9 *(PCSK9).* The *LDLR* gene codes for the number of LDL receptors in the liver. The *APOB* and *APOE* genes code for how the body handles cholesterol metabolism. The *PCSK9* gene codes for how the PCSK9 enzyme degrades LDL receptors. Other genes have been implicated and continue to be investigated in FH.

Liver Synthesis of Cholesterol. The liver is the principal organ for maintaining cholesterol homeostasis in the body. The hepatic mechanisms in cholesterol homeostasis include:

- Biosynthesis of cholesterol via the enzyme HMG-CoA reductase
- Uptake of cholesterol through LDL receptors; hepatic LDL receptors bind plasma LDL particles, thus lowering blood cholesterol levels
- Lipoprotein release into the bloodstream
- Storage of cholesterol
- Degradation and conversion of cholesterol into bile acids.

It is important to note that the enzyme HMG-CoA reductase stimulates cholesterol synthesis in the liver. This enzyme is inhibited by the most commonly prescribed lipid-lowering medications called statins. Statins are highly effective at lowering blood LDL cholesterol levels.

LDL receptors in the liver play a major role in determining LDL levels in the bloodstream. A low number of hepatic LDL receptors is associated with high LDL levels in the bloodstream, while a high number of hepatic LDL receptors is associated with low LDL levels in the bloodstream. The number of LDL receptors in the liver is regulated by the cholesterol content of the liver cell and is influenced by the genetics of the individual.

When cellular cholesterol levels are decreased, LDL receptors are highly expressed by the liver. Conversely, when cellular cholesterol levels are high, the expression of hepatic LDL receptors is low. In individuals with genetic variants that cause a low number of hepatic LDL receptors, blood LDL cholesterol levels are high.

It is important to note that the PCSK9 enzyme regulates the rate of degradation of LDL receptors. Studies show that inhibiting this PCSK9 enzyme lowers LDL cholesterol levels in the bloodstream. This enzyme is inhibited by the new monoclonal antibody–type lipid-lowering medication evolocumab.

After the liver synthesizes cholesterol, it is released into the bloodstream as apolipoproteins including chylomicrons (contain triglycerides), VLDL, IDL, LDL, HDL, and Lp (a). Chylomicrons, VLDL, IDL, LDL, and Lp (a) are all proatherogenic while HDL is antiatherogenic. LDL transports cholesterol to the tissues, where it is deposited within artery walls. HDL transports cholesterol back to the liver or into the intestine for excretion via feces.

Reverse cholesterol transport occurs when HDL takes cholesterol from the bloodstream and returns it to the liver for excretion. HDLs maintain low levels of tissue and plasma cholesterol, so high levels of HDL keep overall cholesterol levels in check. HDL also enhances excretion of cholesterol. However, with low levels of HDL, the body cannot initiate sufficient reverse cholesterol transport. Low HDL allows cholesterol-rich atherosclerotic plaques to accumulate on arterial walls. High levels of HDL have a protective effect against atherosclerosis.

CLINICAL CONCEPT

HDL cholesterol is cardioprotective because it carries cholesterol away from artery walls to be excreted.

Dietary Sources of Lipids. Dietary sources of lipids include saturated and unsaturated fats, as well as transfatty acids. A saturated fat is a fatty acid with a single carbon chain and every available bonding site filled or bonded with hydrogen ions. Saturated fats are usually solid forms of animal fat. The most visible example is the fat contained in meats. Other sources of saturated fats are animal products, such as eggs, butter, cheese, and dairy products. A diet high in saturated fat raises blood cholesterol levels.

An unsaturated fatty acid is chemically a carbon chain with one or more unsaturated double bonds. Compared with saturated bonds, unsaturated double bonds are easily broken down. Commonly, unsaturated fats are liquid forms of fat. If there is only one unsaturated double bond, it is called a monounsaturated fatty acid; if there is more than one double bond, it is a polyunsaturated fat. Dietary sources of monounsaturated fats include olive oil, peanut oil, and canola oil. Vegetable oils, such as sesame, corn, and safflower oils; fish; and margarine represent polyunsaturated fats. Monounsaturated and polyunsaturated fat in the diet are advised for keeping blood cholesterol levels low.

Transfatty acids are manufactured and used to extend the life of polyunsaturated fats in processed foods. This is done by taking the polyunsaturated double-bonded carbon chain and forcing the double bond to break so that hydrogen ions can be introduced at these sites, thereby "transforming" the polyunsaturated fats into transfats via the hydrogenation process. Transfats have been linked to increased levels of LDL and the formation of plaque in the arterial vessels, as well as decreased levels of HDL.

Risk Factors

Several conditions can increase lipid levels in the bloodstream. The genetic disorder FH causes elevated levels of cholesterol in the bloodstream. One in 220 persons is affected by heterozygous FH. In FH, the LDLR gene mutation on the short arm of chromosome 19 at 19p13.2 causes a deficiency of LDL receptors in the body. Without LDL receptors, the liver cannot efficiently metabolize LDL cholesterol, so high levels of LDL cholesterol accumulate in the bloodstream. Extremely high cholesterol levels and premature CVD occur in affected persons. Most cases of FH are due to more than one genetic variant. The condition is the result of a number of different gene mutations and is influenced by diet. The genetic mutations commonly associated with FH hyperlipidemia are found at chromosomes 1q21-23, 11p14.1-q12.1, 19p13.2, 19p.13.32, and 16q22-24.1.

 CLINICAL CONCEPT

Persons with FH develop severely elevated blood cholesterol levels, atherosclerosis, and MI (heart attack) at an early age.

Diabetes mellitus, both type 1 and type 2, are associated with elevated lipid levels. In diabetes mellitus, there is decreased hepatic removal of LDL from the circulation, as well as increased levels of free fatty acids (FFA). The increased FFAs are the result of enhanced lipolysis, an action that enables fat stores to be used as the cells' alternative energy source. Elevated levels of blood glucose, associated with poorly managed diabetes mellitus, cause glycosylation of endothelial cells, which has a damaging effect on the arterial lining. The high blood glucose levels associated with diabetes mellitus accelerate the widespread development of arterial plaque buildup, leading to atherosclerosis.

Obesity is a condition that causes excess cutaneous body fat, visceral fat accumulation, and elevated blood lipid levels. Hypercholesterolemia and hypertriglyceridemia are common in obese individuals, increasing the risk for atherosclerosis.

Hypothyroidism is associated with decreased LDL receptors in the liver. Fewer liver receptors for LDL cause less LDL metabolism and excretion. This, in turn, leads to elevated LDL levels, which enhances development of atherosclerosis. Increased synthesis of lipids also occurs with the kidney disorder called nephrotic syndrome. Therefore, it is important to identify and treat disorders that lead to elevated lipid levels.

Other factors, such as physical activity, diet, and medications, may affect lipid levels. Low physical activity or sedentary lifestyle predisposes to hyperlipidemia. LDL cholesterol increases and HDL levels decrease with lack of physical activity. A diet that is high in cholesterol, saturated fats, and transfats will increase LDL levels. In addition, certain medications increase lipid levels in the bloodstream. These drugs include progestins, anabolic steroids, corticosteroids, diuretics, and beta-adrenergic blockers.

Pathophysiology

The finding of LDL cholesterol and triglyceride-rich lipoproteins in atherosclerotic plaque has provided substantial evidence for their direct role in atherosclerosis, which begins with injury of the endothelium. Endothelial inflammation occurs and macrophages rush to the area along with platelets. The prelude to atherosclerosis occurs as macrophages engulf and ingest LDLs. As LDLs accumulate within the WBCs, the WBCs develop a foamy appearance and are referred to as foam cells. Foam cells deposited along the vessel wall accumulate and form fatty streaks; this is a preliminary stage in the development of atherosclerotic plaque.

 CLINICAL CONCEPT

Hyperlipidemia is the fundamental condition that causes atherosclerosis.

Clinical Presentation

Clinicians seeking diagnostic signs of hyperlipidemia should interview the patient about the existence of other cardiovascular problems, such as HTN, angina, or MI. Thorough descriptions of diet and activity level are also key elements in the patient history. Commonly, individuals with hyperlipidemia report a diet high in fat. In addition, patients often describe a sedentary lifestyle and lack of exercise in the daily routine.

A family history of CVD is also frequently reported. Parents, siblings, or other relatives commonly have HTN, high cholesterol, MI, angina, or stroke. A family history of premature MI, which occurs in persons younger than age 45 years, is particularly indicative of FH. The patient should also be questioned about current medications and the existence of predisposing disorders, such as hypothyroidism, diabetes, or kidney disease.

Signs and Symptoms. Patients do not usually report any symptoms associated with hyperlipidemia because it is largely a silent disorder. Persons may report symptoms related to angina or MI.

Physical Examination. Physical examination findings often include xanthoma and xanthelasma—yellowish cholesterol deposits under the skin and around the eyes (see Fig. 15-5). Arcus senilis may be noted in the ophthalmological examination. This is a yellow-white ring around the cornea of the eye that

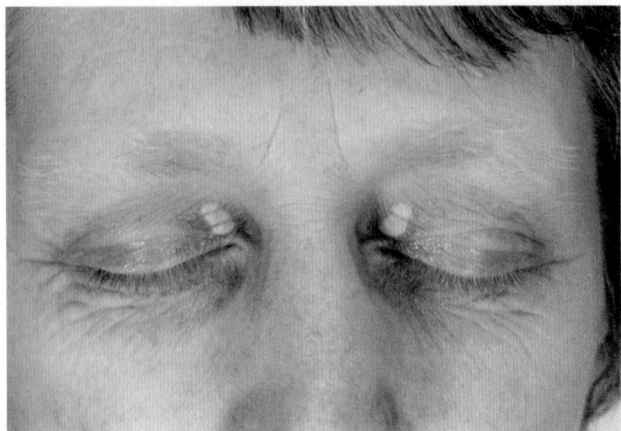

FIGURE 15-5. Xanthoma/xanthelasma. *(From Biophoto Associates/ Science Source.)*

consists of cholesterol deposits. The patient may also exhibit signs and symptoms of metabolic syndrome, which is a constellation of disorders that include central obesity, glucose intolerance, hyperinsulinemia, HTN, and hyperlipidemia.

Diagnosis

In addition to a history and physical examination, blood samples for lipoproteins, cholesterol, and triglycerides should be obtained. To reduce atherosclerotic CVD risk in adults, the 2018 American College of Cardiology (ACC) and American Heart Association (AHA) established specific categories for evaluating blood lipid levels. These guidelines are largely based on the 10-year atherosclerotic cardiovascular disease (ASCVD) risk of the patient, which should be calculated using the ACC Risk Estimator App found at http://tools.acc.org/ASCVD-Risk-Estimator-Plus/#!/calculate/estimate/. This peer-reviewed online calculator uses the Pooled Cohort Equations to estimate the 10-year primary risk of ASCVD among patients without preexisting CVD who are between 40 and 79 years of age (see Table 15-1). According to the AHA/ACC some persons are considered high risk for ASCVD; these include persons with a 10-year ASCVD risk score ≥7.5%. Also those with a history of multiple major ASCVD events or one major ASCVD event and multiple high-risk conditions are at high risk. High-risk conditions include established CVD, such as stable or unstable coronary artery disease (CAD), ischemic stroke, transient ischemic attack (TIA), or peripheral arterial disease (PAD). Also anyone with the following conditions:

- Acute coronary syndrome within the past year
- FH
- Diabetes mellitus
- Chronic kidney disease stages 3, 4, or 5
- Recurrent atherosclerotic CVD event or need for revascularization while on statin therapy
- Polyvascular disease

TABLE 15-1. AHA/ACA Cholesterol Management Guidelines

The 2018 American Heart Association (AHA)/American College of Cardiology (ACC) Cholesterol Management Guidelines are largely based on the 10-year ASCVD risk of the patient using the ACC Risk Estimator App found at http://tools.acc.org/ASCVD-Risk-Estimator-Plus/#!/calculate/estimate/.

Total Cholesterol	Category
<150 mg/dL	Ideal for persons with high ASCVD risk*
<200 mg/dL	Optimal
200 to 239 mg/dL	Borderline high
≥240 mg/dL	High

LDL Cholesterol	Category
<70 mg/dL	Ideal for persons with high ASCVD risk*
<100 mg/dL	Optimal for persons with average ASCVD risk
100 to 129 mg/dL	Above optimal
130 to 159 mg/dL	Borderline high
160 to 189 mg/dL	High
≥190 mg/dL	Very high

HDL Cholesterol	Category
>60 mg/dL	Ideal; considered cardioprotective
<50 mg/dL	Women low
<40 mg/dL	Men low

Triglycerides	Category
<150 mg/dL	Ideal
150 to 199 mg/dL	Borderline high
200 to 499 mg/dL	High
>500 mg/dL	Very high

*Persons with 10-year risk score >7.5%; also see major risk factors listed in text. Adapted from Grundy, S. M., Stone, N. J., Bailey, A. L., Beam, C., Birtcher, K. K., et al. (2018). AHA/ACC/AACVPR/AAPA/ABC/ACPM/ADA/AGS/APhA/ASPC/NLA/PCNA guideline on the management of blood cholesterol: A report of the American College of Cardiology/American Heart Association Task Force on Clinical Practice Guidelines. *J Amer Coll Cardiol.* pii: S0735-1097(18)39034-X. doi: 10.1016/j.jacc.2018.11.003

Some other measurements may be considered in estimating ASCVD risk. These measures may be used in the evaluation of patients without known CVD who are at intermediate risk for CVD and for whom a more definite estimate of CVD risk would change management:

- High-sensitivity C-reactive protein (hs-CRP)
- Carotid artery intima-media thickness
- Coronary artery calcification by computed tomography (CT)

• Homocysteine blood level
• Lipoprotein(a)

Laboratory testing must also be used to rule out possible causes of elevated lipid levels, such as hypothyroidism, diabetes mellitus, obstructive liver disease, and kidney disease. Therefore, blood glucose, thyroid-stimulating hormone, blood urea nitrogen (BUN), serum creatinine, and liver enzymes should be checked. Because cholesterol levels are affected by food, a complete lipoprotein analysis must be drawn following a 9- to 12-hour fast.

Genetic Testing for Familial Hypercholesterolemia. Historically, the diagnosis of FH has been based on clinical criteria that include elevated LDL-C levels, clinical history of premature CVD, family history of hypercholesterolemia and/or CVD, and physical examination findings (e.g., tendon xanthomas and corneal arcus). However, the 2018 AHA/ACC Expert Consensus Panel recommends that FH genetic testing become the standard of care for those patients with probable or definite FH as well as for their at-risk relatives. Testing should include the genes encoding the low-density lipoprotein receptor (*LDLR*) located at 19p13.2, apolipoprotein B (*APOB*) located at 2p24.1, apoprotein E (*APOE*) located at 19q13.32, and proprotein convertase subtilisin/kexin 9 (*PCSK9*) located at 1p32.3.

Treatment

Lifestyle changes are a fundamental part of hyperlipidemia treatment. A low-fat diet that is particularly low in cholesterol is necessary. The patient should aim to keep dietary cholesterol lower than 300 mg per day. Fats should be limited to fewer than 30% of total dietary calories. Saturated fat must be strictly limited. Monounsaturated fats, such as olive oil and polyunsaturated fats such as vegetable oil, are preferable. Physical activity should be included in the daily routine; usually 30 minutes of vigorous walking is sufficient. Exercise has been shown to raise HDL ("good" cholesterol) levels in the bloodstream, which enhances excretion of cholesterol. Also, the individual should refrain from smoking and limit alcohol use. A glass of red wine daily has been shown to reduce CVD risk in some individuals. Fish oils, also known as omega-3 fatty acids, have been shown to reduce triglycerides. Fish oil can be taken as a supplement or obtained through fish, such as mackerel, tuna, salmon, bluefish, anchovy, sardines, herring, and trout. High fiber is also a recommended component of the diet to reduce hyperlipidemia.

There are different classes of lipid-lowering medications (see Patho-Pharm Connection). Medications called statins or HMG-CoA reductase inhibitors, such as atorvastatin (Lipitor), rosuvastatin (Crestor), and simvastatin (Zocor), are recommended as first-line agents if diet and exercise do not lower bloodstream lipids to desired levels. These agents block the liver enzyme that assists in the manufacture of cholesterol. Statins diminish cholesterol synthesis and can reverse atherosclerotic plaque formation. Preexistent atherosclerotic plaque has been shown to diminish with statin treatment.

Bile acid sequestrants such as cholestyramine (Questran) are second-line agents for the treatment of elevated LDL cholesterol. These block bile acid absorption in the gastrointestinal (GI) tract. The main component of bile acids is cholesterol; therefore, these agents prevent cholesterol absorption from the intestine into the bloodstream. Fibrates such as gemfibrozil (Lopid) and fenofibrate (Tricor) are used as first-line treatment for elevated triglyceride concentrations and may be prescribed in combination with the other drug classes. These medications decrease triglyceride secretion by the liver. Ezetimibe (Zetia), another type of medication, decreases intestinal absorption of fat and is used because of its effectiveness, safety, and lack of side effects. Ezetimibe is often added to a statin medication regimen in patients with hypercholesterolemia.

In patients with severe atherosclerotic disease or FH who have not been successful at reducing LDL sufficiently with standard lipid-lowering agents, the monoclonal antibody type medications evolocumab or alirocumab can be used. These medications have been shown to reduce serum LDL cholesterol values by 50% to 75%. These injectable medications block the enzyme PCSK9, which breaks down LDL receptors. LDL receptors are found on the liver and are needed to metabolize and process LDL molecules. By inhibiting the PCSK9 enzyme, LDL receptors are not broken down and remain available to connect to LDL molecules so they can be processed by the liver. By enhancing the LDL receptor–LDL molecule connection, these medications promote metabolism of LDL and decrease blood levels of LDL.

Hypertension

HTN is the elevation of BP to values that are correlated with cardiovascular damage. It is called the "silent killer" because it has no symptoms and can lead to fatal CVD. The AHA and ACC have established that HTN exists when two or more diastolic BP measurements on at least two or more clinical visits are 80 mm Hg or greater, or when the systolic BP readings on two or more clinical visits are consistently 130 mm Hg or greater. According to the AHA and ACC, there are five different categories of BP according to numerical values: normal BP, elevated BP, stage 1 HTN, stage 2 HTN, and hypertensive crisis (see Table 15-2).

Controversy currently exists between the recommended BP goals of the AHA; ACA; and Joint National Committee on Prevention, Detection, Evaluation, and Treatment of Hypertension. There is ongoing investigation into the optimal BP management for older

Patho-Pharm Connection

Hyperlipidemia

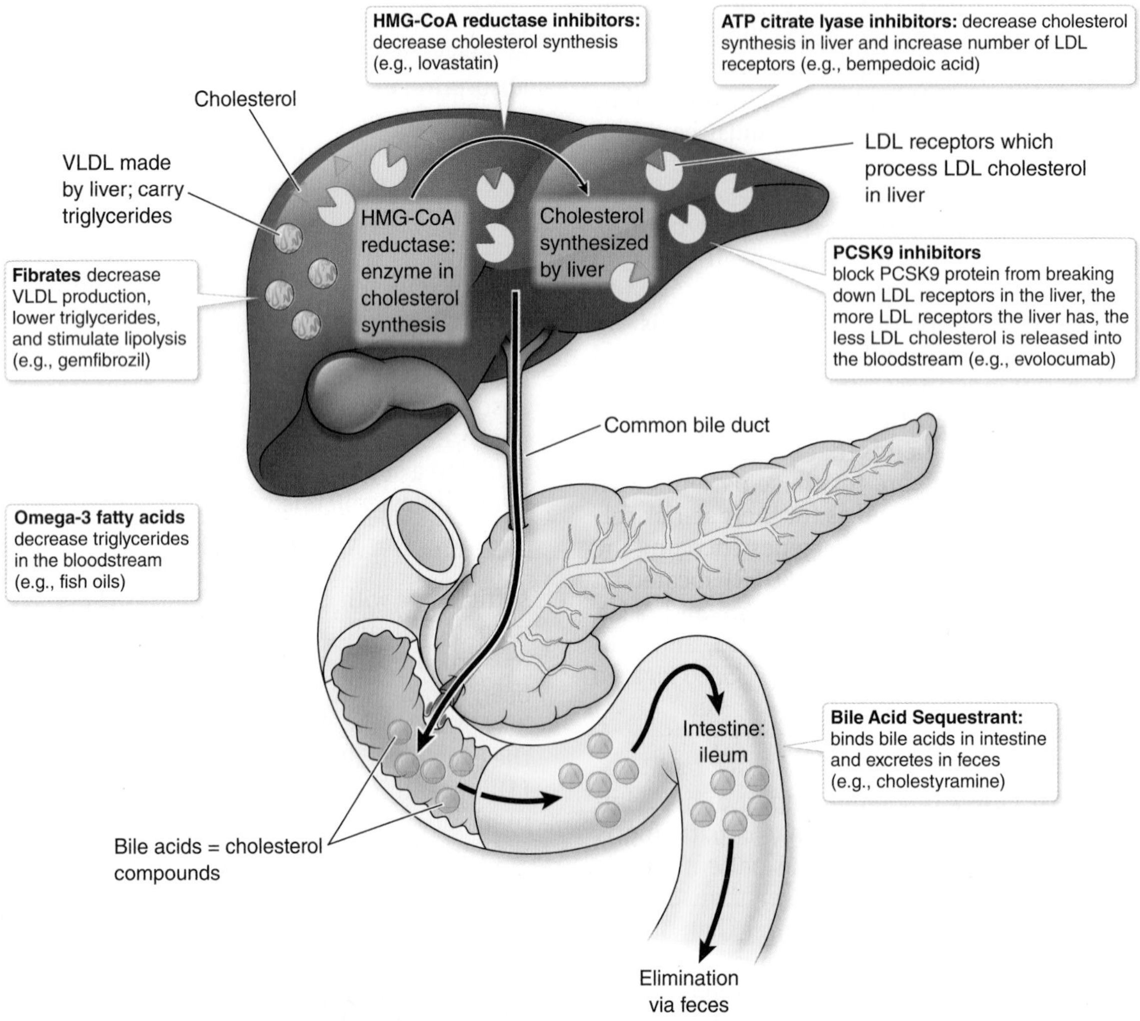

HMG-CoA reductase inhibitors: decrease cholesterol synthesis (e.g., lovastatin)

ATP citrate lyase inhibitors: decrease cholesterol synthesis in liver and increase number of LDL receptors (e.g., bempedoic acid)

Cholesterol

VLDL made by liver; carry triglycerides

Fibrates decrease VLDL production, lower triglycerides, and stimulate lipolysis (e.g., gemfibrozil)

HMG-CoA reductase: enzyme in cholesterol synthesis

Cholesterol synthesized by liver

LDL receptors which process LDL cholesterol in liver

PCSK9 inhibitors block PCSK9 protein from breaking down LDL receptors in the liver, the more LDL receptors the liver has, the less LDL cholesterol is released into the bloodstream (e.g., evolocumab)

Common bile duct

Omega-3 fatty acids decrease triglycerides in the bloodstream (e.g., fish oils)

Intestine: ileum

Bile Acid Sequestrant: binds bile acids in intestine and excretes in feces (e.g., cholestyramine)

Bile acids = cholesterol compounds

Elimination via feces

The most commonly prescribed lipid-lowering agents are the HMG-CoA reductase inhibitors called statins. These agents block the enzyme that catalyzes the production of cholesterol by the liver, thereby decreasing cholesterol in the bloodstream. Examples include lovastatin, atorvastatin, simvastatin, and rosuvastatin.

Bile acids are substances created by the liver that contain cholesterol. Bile acid sequestrants attach to bile acids and enhance their gastrointestinal excretion into feces. An example is cholestyramine.

Fibrates are substances that inhibit triglyceride production by the liver, enhance excretion of LDL cholesterol, raise HDL cholesterol levels, and stimulate lipolysis. Examples include clofibrate, gemfibrozil, and fenofibrate.

PCSK9 inhibitors are monoclonal antibodies that block the PCSK9 protein that breaks down LDL receptors in the liver. Inhibiting this process enhances LDL receptors in the liver that attach to the LDL cholesterol and lower blood cholesterol levels. Examples include evolocumab and alirocumab.

Drug Class	Action	Examples
HMG-CoA reductase inhibitors	Inhibit the enzyme that stimulates synthesis of cholesterol in liver	"Statins": Simvastatin, Lovastatin, Atorvastatin, Rosuvastatin
Cholesterol absorption inhibitor	Blocks intestinal absorption of cholesterol	Ezetimbe
Fibrate	Enhances triglyceride excretion and raise HDL	Gemfibrozil, Fenofibrate, Clofibrate
Bile acid sequestrant	Bind to bile acids (bile acids contain cholesterol) in intestine and promote excretion (inhibiting reabsorption in ileum for bile acid recycling)	Cholestyramine, Colestipol, Colesevelam

Patho-Pharm Connection–cont'd

Drug Class	Action	Examples
PCSK9 inhibitor	Monoclonal antibody type of medication which blocks enzyme that degrades LDL receptors in liver; lowers LDL in bloodstream	Evolocumab
ATP citrate lyase inhibitor	Blocks cholesterol synthesis in liver and increases number of LDL receptors in liver	Bempedoic acid
Omega 3 fatty acids (fish oils)	Lower triglycerides in blood	Eicosapentaenoic acid (EPA), Docosahexaenoic acid (DHA)

Original table; adapted from: Rader, D. (2022). Chap 407 Disorders of lipoprotein metabolism. In Loscalzo, J., Fauci, A., Kasper, D., Hauser, S., Longo, D., & Jameson, J. L. (2022). *Harrison's principles of internal medicine,* Vol II. New York: McGraw Hill.

TABLE 15-2. Blood Pressure Classification

BP Classification	Systolic BP (mm Hg)	Diastolic BP (mm Hg)
Normal	Less than 120	And less than 80
Elevated	120 to 129	And less than 80
Stage 1 HTN	130 to 139	Or 80 to 89
Stage 2 HTN	140 or greater	Or 90 or greater
Hypertensive crisis*	>180	And/or >120

Immediate hospitalization required if there are signs of organ damage.
Whelton, et al. (2018). ACC/AHA/AAPA/ABC/ACPM/AGS/APhA/ASH/ASPC/NMA/PCNA guideline for the prevention, detection, evaluation, and management of high blood pressure in adults: A report of the American College of Cardiology/American Heart Association Task Force on Clinical Practice Guidelines. *Hypertension, 71*(6), 1269–1324.

adults. The JNC-8 made the following recommendations for the management of HTN in certain groups of adults:

- Adults age 60 and older with high BP: optimal BP is less than 150/90
- Adults age 30 to 59 with high BP: optimal BP is less than 140/90
- Adults with diabetes or chronic kidney disease: optimal BP is less than 140/90

It is noteworthy that for older adults, JNC-8 BP recommendations are less than 150/90 mm Hg. This recommendation is likely based on the physiological need for higher BPs among older adults to attain cerebral perfusion and circulation to organs. In other words, higher BP is necessary in older adults for blood to reach the brain and other organs. As adults age, blood vessels become less elastic and stiffer, which physiologically raises BP. Organ circulation requires higher pressure in old age. Therefore, the baseline recommendation of BP for older adults is higher than for younger adults.

These recommendations of the JNC-8 differ from the BP goals recommended by the AHA and ACC (see Table 15-2). The AHA/ACC recommendations do not take age of adults into account and do not advise any different BP values for older adults. To fully understand the difference, compare the AHA/ACC guidelines with the JNC-8 guidelines. There is some controversy regarding the AHA/ACC recommendations for BP in older adults. Some experts recommend a return to BP <140/90 mm Hg for older subjects with uncomplicated HTN, particularly for frail older adults.

The JNC-8 expert panel also recommended how to achieve optimal BP measurements. It recommended that persons with high BP adopt healthy lifestyle changes. These include weight loss; limitation of daily salt intake to 1,500 mg; a diet rich in fruits, vegetables, and whole grains; and at least 30 minutes of physical activity daily. The JNC-8 also recommends specific drug therapy for African Americans and all persons with diabetes. For European Americans, an ACE inhibitor, angiotensin-receptor blocker (ARB), calcium channel blocker (CCB), and thiazide-type diuretic are the best medications for control of HTN. For African Americans, a CCB or thiazide-type diuretic is the best initial medication for HTN. Among individuals with declining kidney function or diabetes, a low dose of an ACE inhibitor or ARB is the preferred treatment for HTN. ACE inhibitors and ARB medications protect the kidneys from further damage.

The strong association between HTN and CAD has been well established by epidemiological studies. HTN is a major independent risk factor for CAD, stroke, and renal failure. The diagnosis and consequent treatment of HTN over the past 50 years has resulted in major reductions in cardiovascular morbidity and mortality. There are two main categories of HTN: primary HTN, also called essential HTN, and secondary HTN. Primary HTN is the most common type, but its etiology is unknown. Secondary HTN affects a much smaller percentage of the population and is the result of some pathology in another system or organ.

Epidemiology

HTN is one of the most common worldwide diseases. Because of the associated morbidity and mortality and the cost to society, it is an important public health challenge. According to the Centers for Disease Control and Prevention, approximately 78 million people in the United States are affected by HTN; this is one in three adults. Substantial improvements have been made with regard to increasing awareness and treatment of the disorder, but only 54% of adults have their high BP under control. Also, many younger people have unrecognized HTN.

Etiology

Primary HTN accounts for 90% to 95% of adult cases; a small percentage of patients have a secondary cause. Primary HTN has no known cause. Secondary HTN is a side effect of another systemic disorder, such as Cushing's disease, pheochromocytoma, kidney disease, or hyperaldosteronism (see Box 15-2). Treating the systemic disorder will lower BP in secondary HTN.

Risk Factors

There are many risk factors for HTN, including:

- Male sex
- Age
- African American ethnicity
- Family history
- Obesity (body mass index [BMI] >30)
- Diabetes mellitus (fasting blood glucose ≥126 mg/dL on multiple office visits or A1c ≥6.5%)
- Sedentary behavior
- Tobacco use
- Excess sodium in diet (<1500 mg sodium = low-salt diet)
- Insufficient potassium in diet (approx. 4700 mg K + needed/day)
- Insufficient vitamin D in diet (approx. 400 to 800 units vitamin D needed/day)
- Excess alcohol (>1 alcohol drink/day women or >2 alcohol drinks/day men)
- Stress

Pathophysiology

HTN has two major negative effects on the cardiovascular system. It exerts high damaging forces against all the endothelial linings of the arteries. It also causes high resistance against the heart's left ventricle. BP in the aorta is elevated when there is HTN in the systemic arteries. High aortic pressure places an excessive workload on the heart's left ventricle, raising the intramyocardial wall tension in the ventricular muscle. Over time, this results in left ventricular hypertrophy (LVH) as the muscle works harder to eject blood into the aorta (see Fig. 15-6). The enlarged left ventricle develops into a prominent muscle that requires increased circulation and oxygen. However, the coronary blood flow available is inadequate for the enlarged ventricular muscle. The enlarged left ventricle, which hypertrophied because of HTN, becomes susceptible to ischemia, infarction, and heart failure.

HTN predisposes all the systemic arteries to injury. It creates a high shearing force against all arterial vessel walls, which causes weakening and injury of the endothelium. Arteries particularly damaged by HTN include those of the retina, kidneys, brain, and

---

BOX 15-2. Causes of Secondary Hypertension

Secondary HTN occurs when a disorder causes elevated BP as a side effect.

RENAL CAUSES
- Chronic kidney disease
- Liddle syndrome
- Polycystic kidney disease
- Renin-producing tumor
- Urinary tract obstruction

CARDIOVASCULAR CAUSES
- Coarctation of aorta
- Collagen-vascular disease
- Vasculitis

ENDOCRINE CAUSES
- Acromegaly
- Congenital adrenal hyperplasia
- Cushing's syndrome
- Hyperaldosteronism, primary
- Pheochromocytoma
- Hyperparathyroidism
- Hyperthyroidism and hypothyroidism

NEUROGENIC CAUSES
- Brain tumor
- Bulbar poliomyelitis
- Intracranial HTN

DRUGS AND TOXINS
- Adrenergic medications
- Alcohol
- Cocaine
- Cyclosporine, tacrolimus
- Decongestants containing ephedrine
- Erythropoietin
- Herbal remedies containing licorice or ephedrine
- NSAIDs
- Oral contraceptives

OTHER CAUSES
- Hypercalcemia
- Obstructive sleep apnea
- Pregnancy-induced HTN

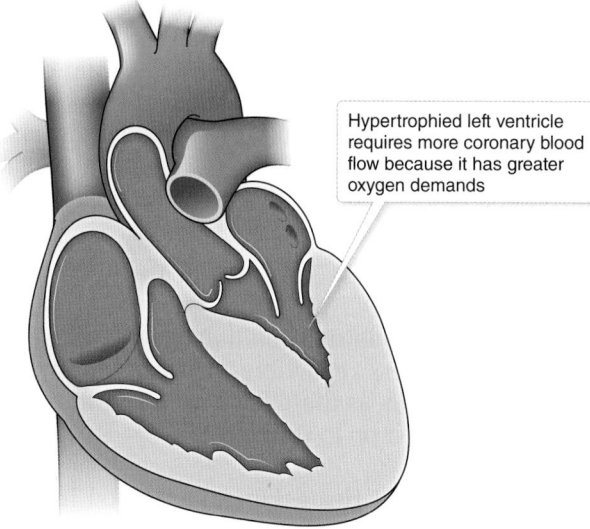

Hypertrophied left ventricle requires more coronary blood flow because it has greater oxygen demands

FIGURE 15-6. Long-term HTN leads to left ventricular hypertrophy. The left ventricle hypertrophies because of the excessive resistance in the aorta in HTN. The enlarged muscle of the left ventricle then requires extra coronary artery blood flow because of the increased energy needs of the large muscle. However, an extra supply of coronary artery blood flow is unavailable and so the left ventricle is susceptible to ischemia and infarction.

lower extremities. Damaged retinal arteries can lead to blindness, injured renal arteries can lead to renal failure, and damaged cerebral arteries can lead to hemorrhagic stroke.

The RAAS plays a role in the regulation of BP and its elevation. In certain circumstances, hypersensitivity to angiotensin II, with its resulting arterial vasoconstriction and increased blood volume, is believed to contribute to primary HTN. Research has also shown that stress can cause persistently elevated levels of angiotensin II. Chronic stress stimulates renin and sets off the RAAS, which increases total blood volume and causes widespread arterial vasoconstriction. The result of chronic stimulation of the RAAS is HTN.

CLINICAL CONCEPT

In population studies, African American individuals have higher BP measurements on average compared with European Americans. Many African American individuals have been identified as having high sensitivity to sodium. The AHA recommends a daily dietary sodium intake of 1500 mg. However, the average daily American diet consists of more than double this amount (3400 mg), mainly because of the sodium contained in many processed foods. In the body, excess sodium increases water content of the blood, which results in high blood volume and elevated BP. In persons with high sensitivity to sodium, any excess sodium in the diet intensely increases blood volume and BP.

Other studies have examined renin activity in the body. Some individuals are known to be high renin secretors. High renin activity results in the same outcomes as discussed with angiotensin II sensitivity, such as chronic cycling of the RAAS. This cycling causes widespread arterial vasoconstriction, increases circulating blood volume, and elevates BP.

Clinical Manifestations

HTN is a silent, gradual process that most commonly has no symptoms until it causes organ dysfunction. In reviewing the patient's history, it is important to determine whether any disorders are present that can predispose to HTN, such as Cushing's disease, pheochromocytoma, diabetes, kidney disease, or hyperaldosteronism. The patient's list of medications should be checked for possible medication-induced HTN. Such medications include steroids, sympathetic stimulants, NSAIDs, or monoamine oxidase (MAO) inhibitor antidepressants.

The clinician should ask the patient about symptoms correlated with target organ damage of HTN. The target organs of HTN are the heart, brain, extremities, retina, and kidney. Symptoms such as chest pain, dyspnea on exertion, palpitations, headache, vision disturbances, dizziness, weakness in an extremity, leg pain, or edema can be indications of target organ damage. Additionally, if the patient indicates that these symptoms are present, it is necessary to determine the quality, character, duration, and associated symptoms. The patient should also be asked about diet, physical activity, and smoking. Foods that are high in saturated fat and salt, such as fast foods and processed foods, raise BP. Sedentary activity and excessive alcohol use are also associated with HTN.

Signs and Symptoms. Primary HTN commonly has no signs or symptoms. The disease may be quite advanced before it is detected or diagnosed and may have already caused target organ damage. Rarely, persons with HTN complain of headache, nosebleeds, blurred vision, or palpitations.

Physical Examination. A complete physical examination of the patient should be completed with focus on the cardiovascular system. Accurate measurement of both the systolic and diastolic BP is needed to identify those at risk and to monitor the success of therapy. The individual should be comfortably seated for at least 5 minutes. There should be no caffeine, exercise, or smoking within 30 minutes of taking the measurement. The arm should be supported and the cuff large enough for the bladder to cover 80% of the upper arm. The accurate calibration of the sphygmomanometer is critical. At least two measurements should be taken and the average recorded. To diagnose HTN, there should be at least two separate measurements of high BP on two different days.

The United States Preventive Services Task Force recommends confirming a diagnosis of HTN with ambulatory BP monitoring. Ambulatory 24-hour BP monitoring is an effective means of measuring BP during daily activities and sleep. An accurate assessment of BP can be made taking the average of daily BP readings. This is a more accurate assessment, because up to 30% of individuals suffer from "white coat HTN," which is an elevated BP in the clinical setting compared with the home setting. This is commonly due to anxiety and can lead to a misdiagnosis of HTN. Conversely, 20% of individuals have lower BP while in the clinical setting compared with home. This effect can cause unrecognized HTN. Ambulatory 24-hour BP can also indicate if antihypertensive medications are effective throughout the day and night.

Fundoscopic examination is a procedure that uses an ophthalmoscope to assess the retina and optic nerve. There are characteristic changes in the retinal vessels caused by HTN. This is the only place the clinician can gather direct information about the health of the body's arteries using physical examination techniques.

The chest should be examined for indications of HTN. The clinician should palpate the chest for the point of maximal impulse (PMI). In long-term untreated HTN, the left ventricle hypertrophies. This causes the PMI to be palpable farther left in the chest, at the fifth intercostal space toward the axillary line. There also may be a visible left ventricular lift of the chest. When listening to the heart, the clinician may hear an S4 sound, which occurs before S1 because of a less compliant left ventricle in LVH.

The health of the peripheral arteries is essential when assessing a patient for HTN. The clinician should use the stethoscope to listen for bruits over the aorta, carotid, and renal arteries. Bruits are indicative of turbulent blood flow caused by an aneurysm or arterial stenosis (narrowing).

Examination of the peripheral arteries of the lower extremities is also important in patients with HTN. Inspect and palpate the lower extremities for signs of peripheral arterial obstruction. The clinician should focus on the color, temperature, sensation, and pulses in the lower legs and feet. Pallor, coolness, decreased sensation, and weak pulses are indications of peripheral arterial obstruction.

Diagnosis

Diagnostic evaluation of HTN should rule out any potential causes of an elevated BP and determine whether there is any target organ damage. Testing includes a 12-lead electrocardiogram (ECG), urinalysis, complete blood count (CBC), blood glucose, serum potassium, serum creatinine, and serum calcium. An ECG can provide information about hypertensive cardiac effects, such as LVH. The urinalysis, BUN, and serum creatinine levels can identify early indications of hypertensive injury to the kidneys. The presence of protein in the urine, a condition known as proteinuria, in conjunction with elevated BUN and serum creatinine level, is indicative of renal damage.

Diagnostic testing should rule out such disorders as hyperthyroidism, kidney disease, diabetes, pheochromocytoma, and Cushing's disease, which cause secondary HTN.

Treatment

Treatment focuses initially on lifestyle modifications, such as diet, stress reduction, physical activity, and smoking cessation, as these have been shown to have a significant effect on lowering BP.

Diet. The National Heart, Lung, and Blood Institute advocates the DASH diet, which stands for Dietary Approaches to Stop Hypertension. The DASH diet includes low sodium (1,500 mg) and low-fat foods—mainly fruits, vegetables, whole grains, poultry, fish, and low-fat dairy products. The benefits of reducing saturated and transfats in the diet and reducing sodium have repeatedly been proven to be effective. Also beneficial is a diet rich in folic acid, as folic acid has been shown to reduce homocysteine, which at high levels causes endothelial injury.

Stress Reduction and Physical Activity. Stress has been proven to play a significant role in the development of HTN. Complementary medicine or healing modalities have long established the powerful connection between the mind and body. Biofeedback, relaxation techniques, and yoga are all methods of stress reduction. A sedentary lifestyle has been shown to predispose individuals to HTN. Thirty minutes of vigorous physical activity at least 5 days per week is also advocated as a way to lower CVD risk and deal with stress. Endorphins are released with physical activity, and these help to reduce stress. Exercise also stimulates angiogenesis, which is the building of collateral blood vessels. Over time, angiogenesis effects will lower blood pressure within the arterial system.

Smoking Cessation. Smoking cessation is recommended for cardiovascular health. Nicotine is an arterial vasoconstrictor that raises BP and increases resistance to blood flow. The left ventricle must contract with greater force, thereby causing it to hypertrophy when there is arterial vasoconstriction. The left ventricle can become exhausted by the high resistance it must pump against in the aorta; eventually, heart failure occurs. In addition, free radicals contained in cigarette smoke are known to damage the endothelial linings of the arteries. The endothelial damage initiates the development of arteriosclerosis and atherosclerosis. By stopping smoking, the nicotine stimulus for vasoconstriction and the free radical damage can be eliminated. Also, the arterial resistance against the left ventricle can be relieved.

Pharmacological Treatment. It is important to note that lifestyle modifications and pharmacological agents are both needed in the management plan when diet and exercise alone are not enough to lower BP. Pharmacological agents, such as diuretics, renin inhibitors, ACE inhibitors, ARBs, CCBs, or beta-adrenergic blockers, may need to be added to the regimen. There are many different classes of antihypertensive drugs (see Table 15.3). Diuretics decrease the water content of the bloodstream. Renin inhibitors block renin, which initiates the RAAS. ACE inhibitors block ACE that changes angiotensin I into angiotensin II in the RAAS. ARBs diminish angiotensin II activity. CCBs block the molecular stimulus of calcium that causes vasoconstriction. Beta blockers diminish the effects of the SNS on the heart and arteries, thereby decreasing HR and blocking vasoconstriction. See Patho-Pharm Connection below.

Complications

HTN is responsible for damage to target organs, which include the heart, retina, kidney, brain, and peripheral arteries. When it is not well controlled, it contributes to the development of hypertensive heart disease, heart

TABLE 15-3 Drugs Used to Treat Hypertension

Drug Class	Action	Examples
Diuretics	Enhance loss of water from bloodstream at the nephrons into the urine	Furosemide Butmetanide Hydrochorothiazide
Beta adrenergic blockers • Cardioselective; beta 1 blocker • Nonselective: beta 1 and beta 1 blocker • Combined: beta and alpha blocker	Inhibit sympathetic stimulation of heart and blood vessels	Atenolol (beta 1 blocker) Metoprolol (beta 1 and beta 2 blocker) Labetolol (beta and alpha adrenergic blocker) Carvedilol (beta and alpha adrenergic blocker)
ACE inhibitors	Block the angiotensin converting enzyme from turning angiotensin I into angiotensin II in the RAAS	Lisinopril Ramipril
Angiotensin II receptor blockers	Block angiotensin II actions (inhibits vasoconstriction and adrenal gland stimulation)	Losartan Valsartan Candesartan
Aldosterone antagonist	Blocks action of aldosterone; blocks sodium and water reabsorption into bloodstream at nephron; inhibits excretion of potassium out of blood	Spironolactone
Renin inhibitor	Blocks release of renin from kidney	Aliskiren
Calcium channel antagonists	Inhibits peripheral arterial vasconstriction	Amlodipine Nifedipine Verapamil Diltiazem
Alpha adrenergic antagonist	Inhibits peripheral arterial vasoconstriction; relaxes prostate and bladder muscles around urethra (male)	Terazosin Doxazosin Prazosin
Central sympathetic blocker	Blocks central control in brain of sympathetic stimulation	Clonidine Methyldopa
Vasodilator	Vasodilates peripheral arteries	Hydralazine Minoxidil

Original table; adapted from: Kotchen, T. (2022). Chap 277 Hypertension. In Loscalzo, J., Fauci, A., Kasper, D., Hauser, S., Longo, D., & Jameson, J. L. (2022). *Harrison's principles of internal medicine*, Vol II. NY: McGraw Hill.

Patho-Pharm Connection

Hypertension

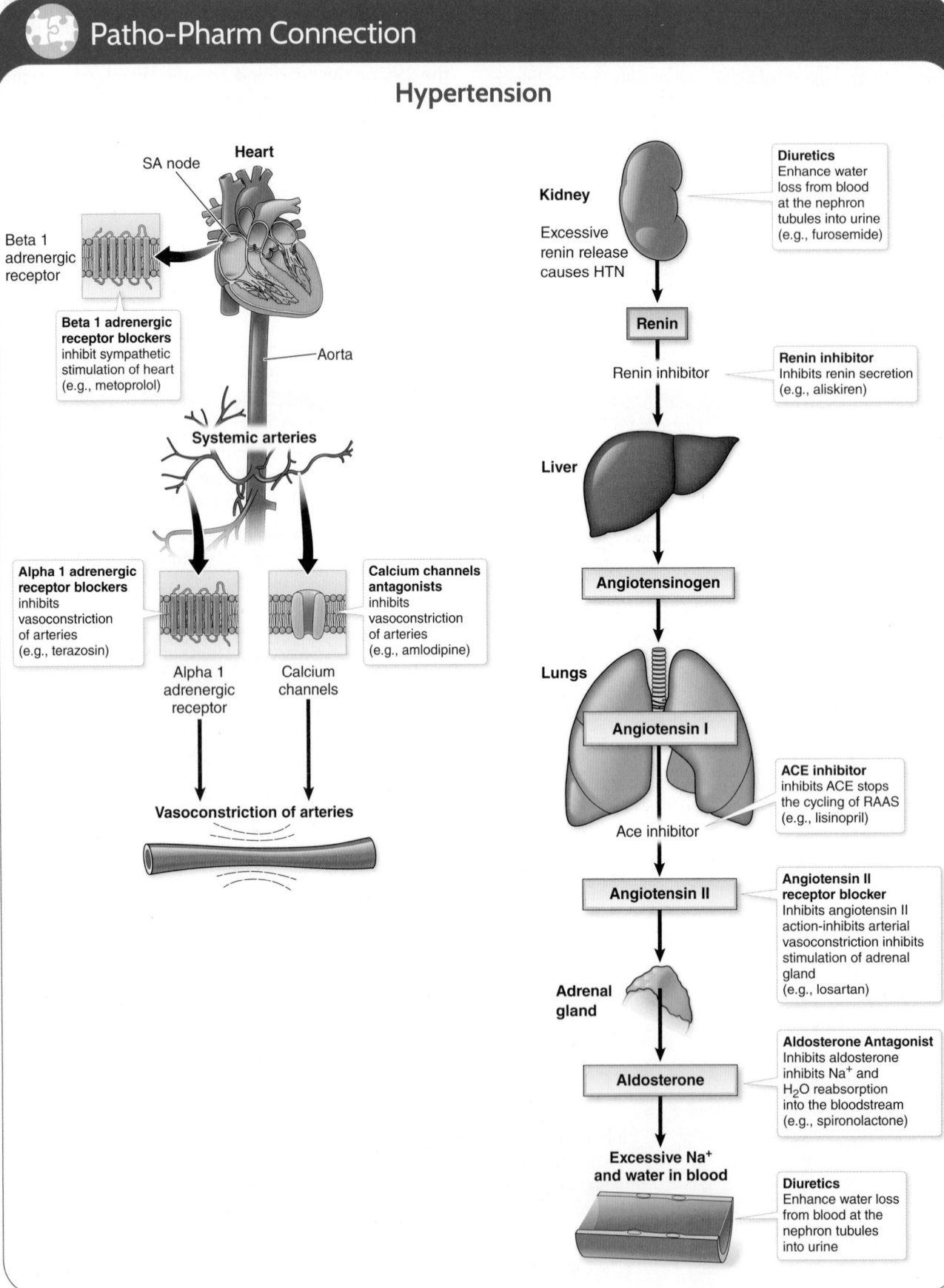

Heart

SA node

Beta 1 adrenergic receptor

Beta 1 adrenergic receptor blockers inhibit sympathetic stimulation of heart (e.g., metoprolol)

Aorta

Systemic arteries

Alpha 1 adrenergic receptor blockers inhibits vasoconstriction of arteries (e.g., terazosin)

Alpha 1 adrenergic receptor

Calcium channels antagonists inhibits vasoconstriction of arteries (e.g., amlodipine)

Calcium channels

Vasoconstriction of arteries

Kidney

Excessive renin release causes HTN

Diuretics Enhance water loss from blood at the nephron tubules into urine (e.g., furosemide)

Renin

Renin inhibitor

Renin inhibitor Inhibits renin secretion (e.g., aliskiren)

Liver

Angiotensinogen

Lungs

Angiotensin I

ACE inhibitor inhibits ACE stops the cycling of RAAS (e.g., lisinopril)

Ace inhibitor

Angiotensin II

Angiotensin II receptor blocker Inhibits angiotensin II action-inhibits arterial vasoconstriction inhibits stimulation of adrenal gland (e.g., losartan)

Adrenal gland

Aldosterone

Aldosterone Antagonist Inhibits aldosterone inhibits Na^+ and H_2O reabsorption into the bloodstream (e.g., spironolactone)

Excessive Na^+ and water in blood

Diuretics Enhance water loss from blood at the nephron tubules into urine

failure, and renal failure. Additionally, it is the major contributing factor to fatal intracerebral hemorrhage.

Hypertensive heart disease is a compensatory response to increased afterload, or the force against which the heart must pump in order to eject blood. LVH develops when the left ventricle must pump blood against excess arterial resistance for a prolonged period. The enlarged left ventricle muscle wall has an increased need for circulation and oxygen. However, the coronary artery blood supply is inadequate for the enlarged muscle; as a result, this region becomes susceptible to ischemia and infarction. Long-term HTN often leads to left ventricular myocardial ischemia and infarction. Also, as the left ventricle hypertrophies, the enlarged muscle protrudes into the left ventricular chamber, reducing the chamber's capacity. As a result, a reduced volume of blood fills the left ventricle, which reduces the volume of blood ejected with each contraction. At the same time, when the left ventricular wall hypertrophies, the interventricular septum also enlarges and diminishes the right ventricle's filling capacity. Both left and right ventricle SV decrease; as a result, there is an overall reduction in cardiac output. If this does not resolve with treatment, the heart fails to supply adequate circulation to the body. HTN is the most common predisposing factor for heart failure.

All arteries are subjected to the effect of hypertensive damage. HTN weakens the walls of arteries, increasing susceptibility to development of bulges in arterial walls called **aneurysms**. Aneurysms cause turbulent blood flow and are susceptible to rupture. The most common areas for aneurysm development are the aorta and cerebral arteries (see Fig. 15-7).

HTN has multiple effects on the brain. It places excess pressure on cerebral arteries and arterioles. The major concern is cerebral hemorrhage from hypertensive damage to small vessels within the brain. Acute elevations in BP can cause the rupture of cerebral blood vessels or hemorrhagic stroke. Although hemorrhagic stroke accounts for about 10% of all strokes, the mortality is very high. Also, because HTN accelerates the formation of atherosclerosis, there is an increased risk of plaque formation in the cerebral arteries, which leads to thrombotic or embolic obstruction within the brain. This can be manifested by a TIA or ischemic stroke.

Altered blood flow from HTN contributes to the development of hypertensive encephalopathy, which is described as a cerebral edema from arteriolar spasm. A patient who presents with this condition may display confusion, changing level of consciousness, and seizures.

HTN also contributes to retinal changes called hypertensive retinopathy (see Fig. 15-8). In response to HTN, the retinal vessels become thickened with a narrowing of the vessel lumen. Higher pressures make the vessels kinked and tortuous. This gives an appearance of arteriovenous nicking at points where arteries and veins cross. Increased pressure leads to microhemorrhages within the retina. Cholesterol deposits in arterioles give the vessels an appearance like copper–silver wiring. Small vessel infarcts in the retina give an appearance of cotton wool spots.

Renal disease is a common occurrence because of HTN. HTN is associated with an accelerated atherosclerosis; therefore, the afferent and efferent arterioles of the nephrons become obstructed by plaque. Also, the fragile capillaries of the glomeruli are damaged by the high BP. These detrimental changes of HTN decrease the glomerular filtration rate, which causes waste products to accumulate in the blood. Consequently, serum creatinine rises and BUN increases. Glomerular

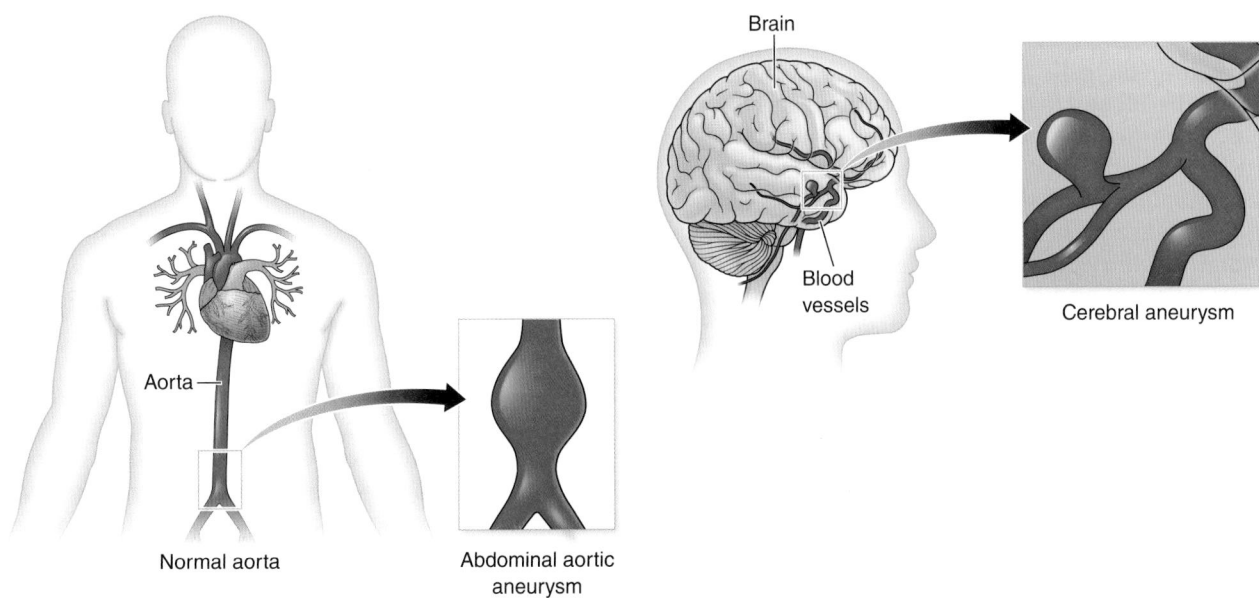

FIGURE 15-7. An aneurysm is a weakening in the wall of an artery. It is susceptible to rupture. 1. Abdominal aortic aneurysm. 2. Cerebral aneurysm.

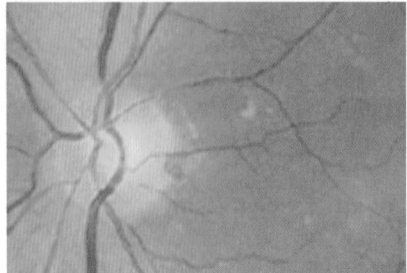

FIGURE 15-8. Hypertensive retinopathy.

injury increases glomerular permeability and loss of proteins into the urine, called proteinuria or microalbuminuria. As hypertensive disease continues, renal failure and end-stage renal disease can result.

Atherosclerosis

One basic physiological change that causes CVD is atherosclerosis, which is the gradual process by which atherosclerotic plaque builds up on the body's arterial walls. Atherosclerosis is a chronic, progressive disease with a long asymptomatic phase. It is a pathological series of changes that take place in the tunica intima, media, and adventitia of the artery, but primarily in the tunica intima, the innermost layer of the arterial wall. Spanning the whole arterial system, the endothelium sustains insults from many different agents and releases factors involved in atherogenesis (buildup of arterial plaque).

Epidemiology

Clinical manifestations of atherosclerosis, including CAD, cerebrovascular disease, and PAD, will occur in two out of three men and one in two women after age 40 years. Almost 60% of deaths are caused by CVD; this same death rate applies to atherosclerosis.

Etiology

The endothelial cells are exposed to all the constituents of the bloodstream, some of which can be injurious. Endothelial injury is the fundamental change that serves as the precursor of atherosclerosis. Agents that commonly harm the endothelium include oxidizing free radicals, the shearing force of high BP, high circulating glucose levels, and elevated levels of LDL. Their injurious influence is widespread, encompassing the extensive endothelial lining throughout the body. Endothelial injury, as with any injury in the body, stimulates the inflammatory reaction, a chain of events that involves WBCs, platelets, clotting factors, cytokines, and various other inflammatory mediators.

Risk Factors

The risk factors associated with atherosclerosis are categorized as modifiable or nonmodifiable (see Table 15-4). It is important to distinguish between the two because treatment can be implemented to counteract modifiable factors.

TABLE 15-4. Risk Factors of Cardiovascular Disease

Nonmodifiable	Modifiable
Age	**Diet**
Males older than 45 years Females older than 55 years (postmenopause)	Excess saturated fat and cholesterol Excess salt Lack of sufficient potassium Lack of folic acid
Gender	**Physical Activity**
Males greater than females Postmenopausal females have same risk as males	Lack of exercise
Race/Ethnicity	**Obesity**
African Americans greater than European Americans	Body mass index greater than 30 Triglycerides greater than 150 mg/dL Central adiposity
Family History	**Lifestyle Factors**
Familial hypercholesterolemia Genetic disposition to diabetes mellitus, HTN, MI, or stroke	Tobacco use Excessive alcohol use High stress
	Other Disorders That Accelerate CVD
	HTN BP greater than 140/90 mm Hg Diabetes mellitus

Gender. Gender is an important issue in the development of atherosclerosis. Atherosclerosis and CVD develop in men by age 45 years and in women by age 55 years. Men have a greater risk and incur MI earlier in life than do women. The reason for the difference in risk is that premenopausal women's estrogen activity is considered cardioprotective. Premenopausal estrogen levels in the female raise HDL. However, after menopause, women are more likely to die of MI than are men. In fact, CVD kills more women annually than breast cancer. A possible explanation for this is that women often present with symptoms of MI different from those seen in men. Additionally, the treatment of women with CVD is often less aggressive than that received by men.

Age. The physiological changes associated with age contribute to the development of arteriosclerosis and atherosclerosis. As people age, the blood vessels become less elastic and walls become fibrotic. In addition, arteries are more likely to develop atherosclerotic plaque formation with age.

Diabetes Mellitus. Diabetes mellitus accelerates the development of atherosclerosis. Patients with type 1 or type 2 diabetes mellitus often have significantly elevated triglycerides and LDL cholesterol levels, along with a lower level of HDL cholesterol. Therefore, patients with diabetes mellitus are at greater risk for developing atherosclerosis and cardiac pathology. Diabetes mellitus causes microvascular and macrovascular changes that compromise circulation to the myocardium, as well as other organs. Also, as blood glucose levels rise in poorly controlled diabetes mellitus, endothelial cells decrease their production of the vasodilatornitric oxide (NO). The endothelium also increases production of thromboxane A2 (TXA2), a clot enhancer. In addition, thrombolysis is diminished because of decreased plasminogen activator function. These conditions enhance clot formation, which could obstruct blood flow through arterial vessels. Finally, glucose interacts with the endothelium of the arterial wall through a process called glycosylation. Glycosylation stimulates endothelial cell secretion of endothelin, a potent vasoconstrictor. Therefore, diabetes promotes atherosclerosis, clot formation, and constriction of arteries. When the conditions of atherosclerosis, clot enhancement, and vasoconstriction occur in the coronary arteries or arteries of the extremities, there is an increased risk of heart attack and peripheral arterial occlusive disease.

Family History. Multiple genes are known to increase susceptibility to atherosclerosis and hyperlipidemia. However, the risk is not solely caused by genetics. Cultural and family influences on diet and lifestyle contribute to this risk factor as well.

Tobacco Use. Tobacco use has been identified as a risk factor for atherosclerosis. Cigarette smoke contains oxidizing free radicals that cause endothelial injury. Also, smoking decreases levels of HDL, which allows cholesterol to deposit on arterial walls and facilitate the formation of atherosclerotic plaque. Nicotine also contributes to occlusion of arteries and increased coagulability, both of which increase the risk for plaque formation.

Hypertension. HTN is an elevated arterial BP that causes direct and indirect cardiovascular damage. Increased pressure from within the arterial vessel causes endothelial injury, which initiates atherosclerosis. Also, within the damaged area of the endothelium there is decreased release of NO, the chemical of vasodilation, and increased release of endothelin, a potent vasoconstrictor. The net result is arterial vasoconstriction and initiation of atherosclerosis in the area subjected to high BP.

Once atherosclerotic plaque is fully developed, elevated pressure within the blood vessel increases the stress on the area of plaque and commonly causes plaque rupture. A piece of plaque travels to a more distal, narrower branch of the artery and creates an obstruction at this site. Ischemia of tissue is the end result. When this occurs in a coronary artery, it causes myocardial ischemia.

Obesity. Obesity is a global epidemic in both children and adults. It is associated with numerous disorders, such as atherosclerosis, diabetes, HTN, osteoarthritis, certain cancers, and sleep apnea. Obesity is an independent risk factor for CVD and is associated with an increased risk of morbidity and mortality. Excess adipose tissue places extra demands on the heart, as the heart must pump high amounts of blood to supply the excess body tissue. Excess adipose tissue is also known to be insulin resistant, which increases the risk of diabetes. In addition, obesity increases coagulation factors, thereby increasing the risk for thrombosis. Persons with obesity commonly have metabolic syndrome, which is a syndrome consisting of HTN, glucose intolerance, and hyperlipidemia.

The BMI calculation has been devised to evaluate an individual's body weight in relation to cardiovascular risk. A BMI greater than 30 is considered a cardiovascular health risk (see Chapter 5 for more information on BMI).

Lifestyle. A high-fat diet, high stress levels, and a sedentary lifestyle contribute to the development of atherosclerosis. A diet high in saturated fat, cholesterol, and transfatty acids brings more fat into the body for the manufacture of LDL cholesterol. LDL becomes the major component in atherosclerotic plaque, which eventually narrows and vasoconstricts the arteries.

Excessive stress elevates levels of hormones that initiate the fight-or-flight response. With acute stress, the endocrine system and SNS are stimulated, raising HR and vasoconstricting blood vessels. These conditions increase BP and pulse, which is detrimental if prolonged. Long-term stress also causes overactivation of the RAAS, which results in high BP. High BP damages the endothelium, and endothelial injury is the initial step in atherosclerosis.

Sedentary lifestyle and lack of exercise also increase the risk of atherosclerosis. Obesity and lower levels of HDL cholesterol are associated with sedentary behavior. Lower levels of HDL also decrease cholesterol excretion. Accumulation of cholesterol in the bloodstream enhances development of atherosclerotic plaque.

Pathophysiology

After endothelial injury, the development of atherosclerotic plaque begins in a sequential pattern (see

Fig. 15-9). Endothelial inflammation draws WBCs and platelets to the site of injury. One of the first changes in the endothelium involves WBCs that engulf and ingest LDL cholesterol. These lipid-rich WBCs form the foundation for atherosclerotic plaque.

Formation of Foam Cells. Injured endothelial cells produce molecules that have adhesive properties

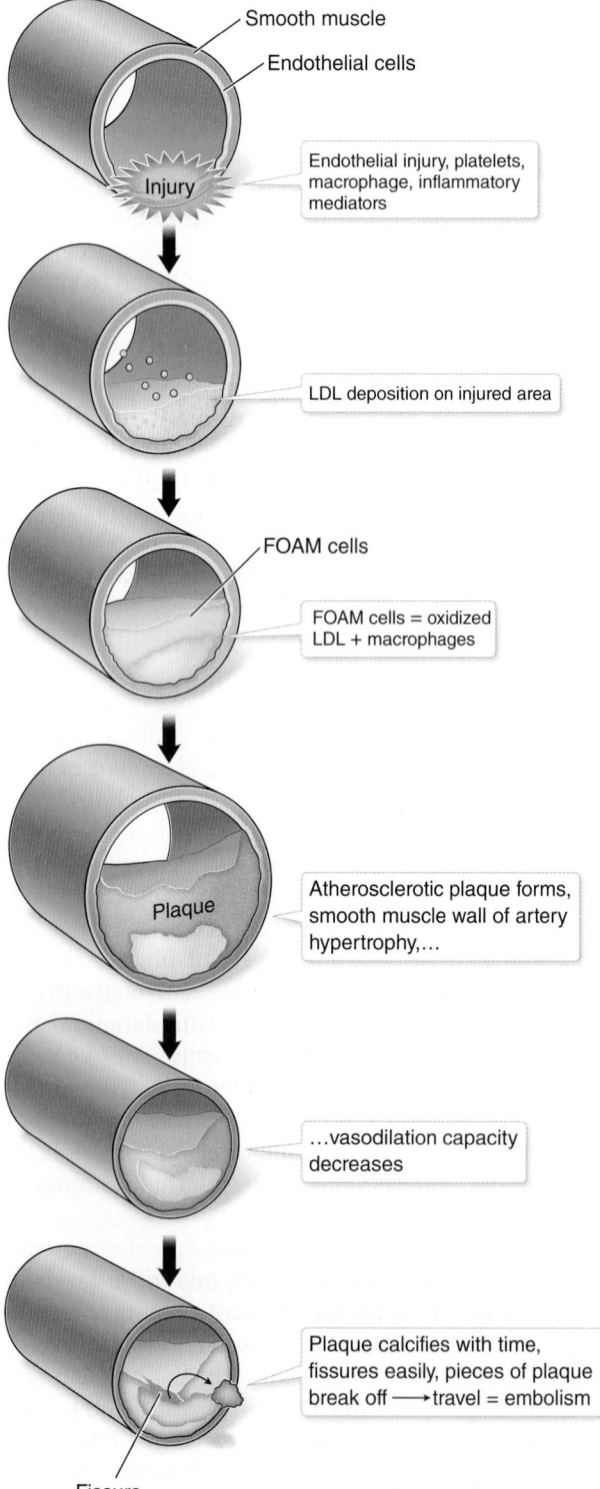

Smooth muscle

Endothelial cells

Injury

Endothelial injury, platelets, macrophage, inflammatory mediators

LDL deposition on injured area

FOAM cells

FOAM cells = oxidized LDL + macrophages

Plaque

Atherosclerotic plaque forms, smooth muscle wall of artery hypertrophy,...

...vasodilation capacity decreases

Plaque calcifies with time, fissures easily, pieces of plaque break off ⟶ travel = embolism

Fissure

FIGURE 15-9. The development of atherosclerotic plaque.

called vascular cell adhesion molecule 1 and chemoattractant protein-1. These adhesive molecules attract and bind circulating WBCs to the endothelium of arterial vessels. The adhered WBCs on the intima are then incorporated into the layer beneath the endothelium, the tunica media, where smooth muscle is located. The WBCs differentiate into macrophages that engulf and ingest LDL. At this point in atherogenesis, cholesterol is visible within the cytoplasm of macrophages. These LDL-laden macrophages become known as foam cells. Foam cells can accumulate LDL and create atherosclerotic plaque. However, foam cells can also transmit the cholesterol back to the bloodstream, where the circulating HDL could bind with it and transport it to the liver for excretion, a process called reverse cholesterol transport. If the level of LDL remains significantly elevated in the bloodstream, the stimulus for atherosclerosis remains, and the foam cells do not participate in reverse cholesterol transport.

Foam cells store cholesterol until they undergo apoptosis and release the stored lipid into the tunica media layer of the arterial wall. Macrophages release inflammatory cytokines that cause attraction of fibroblasts and increase the number of endothelial cell LDL receptors. This amplifies the binding of LDL to macrophages and creates more foam cells, which in turn leads to increased lipid deposits and fibrotic changes within the arterial wall.

Fibroblast activity is enhanced by inflammatory mediators: metalloproteinases, cytokines, growth factors, and plasmin. The arterial wall becomes less elastic because fibroblasts invade the vascular smooth muscle layer. Continual formation of foam cells and fibrosis within the vessel wall increases its thickness and promotes growth of foam cells that become fatty streaks. The fibrosis also diminishes the artery's vasodilation ability.

Formation of Fatty Streaks and Atherosclerotic Plaque. Lipid-rich, fibrotic changes of foam cells begin to form fatty streaks that are obvious on microscopic examination of the artery. As the lipid-rich fatty streak enlarges, it becomes an atherosclerotic plaque that protrudes into the vessel lumen, reducing the artery's diameter. Early in this process there may be no patient symptoms. However, with time, the plaque enlarges and becomes calcified and covered with a fibrous platelet cap. When this occurs, it is referred to as an atheroma. The vessel's elastic quality stretches to its limit to accommodate the expanding plaque, and the vessel becomes stiff or hardened. Some obstruction of the arterial lumen occurs, vasodilatory capacity of the artery is diminished, and the patient may begin to have symptoms, particularly during exertion. Exertion brings on symptoms because extra blood supply is needed and vasodilation is required during exercise; the stiff, atherosclerotic wall is less able to accommodate these needs. Over time, plaque calcifies, making it more fragile and susceptible to rupturing into pieces.

Plaque Rupture. An inflammatory sequence of events leads to plaque rupture. This is a complex process involving many mediators. Activated vascular endothelial cells and inflammatory WBCs secrete mediators that promote atheroma formation. Additionally, smooth muscle cells and platelets are a source of inflammatory mediators and clotting factors. The release of these mediators inhibits normal substances, such as NO, that should ordinarily prevent clot formation and vessel spasm. The plaque is constantly being remodeled, increasing the risk that plaque rupture will occur. The plaques that are most likely to rupture are those with large areas of extracellular lipids, foam cells, inflammatory cells, calcification, and those with a thin fibrous platelet cap. Although the actual trigger for plaque rupture is not clearly defined, once it occurs, there is bleeding into the atheroma. This is followed by the release of substances that draw platelets to the site and promote platelet aggregation. This is when a piece of plaque or clot generated by the plaque can break loose and travel to an arterial site, where it can obstruct blood flow. The vessel's subsequent occlusion leads to the signs and symptoms of ischemia and infarction.

 CLINICAL CONCEPT

CRP, a protein released with inflammation, is associated with increased risk of plaque rupture in atherosclerosis. This is measured as the hs-CRP blood level.

Clinical Manifestations

Atherosclerosis is a gradual process that has no symptoms until it causes organ dysfunction. In reviewing the patient's history, it is important to determine whether any complaints are present because of atherosclerosis. The clinician should ask the patient about episodes of chest pain, shortness of breath, palpitations, leg pain, or dependent edema. These questions are aimed at detecting atherosclerosis of the coronary arteries and peripheral arteries of the extremities. Additionally, if the patient indicates that these symptoms are present, it is necessary to determine the quality, character, duration, and associated symptoms. The patient should be asked about smoking, diet, and daily exercise.

Physical Examination

During physical examination, the clinician should look for clues of atherosclerosis and CVD. Examining a patient at rest can provide information about CVD status. As the clinician examines the patient, the following questions should be asked:

- Is the individual obese?
- Is the individual short of breath at rest?
- Are there changes in skin color indicating pallor or cyanosis?
- Are pulses weak in the lower extremities?
- Is the BP elevated?
- Is the pulse rapid?
- Does the patient have an S_4?
- Are bruits heard over the carotid arteries or aorta?
- Does the patient have apparent xanthoma or xanthelasma or arcus senilis?
- Is the PMI farther left of the midclavicular line toward the axilla?
- Do you hear a heart murmur?

If the answer to any of these questions is yes, then the patient likely has altered cardiovascular function. If on exertion the individual experiences chest pain or excessive dyspnea, cardiovascular function is probably compromised. A patient with chest pain may be pale and diaphoretic. Dependent edema could be indicative of heart failure. Cyanosis is indicative of decreased oxygen delivery to the tissues, another indication of heart failure.

There are few outward physical symptoms associated with atherosclerosis. However, physical examination should include assessment of BP. Additionally, a retina examination with an ophthalmoscope may reveal arteriosclerotic retinal artery changes indicative of arteriosclerosis and atherosclerosis. In the body, turbulent blood flow through narrow areas of arteriosclerotic arteries causes a unique sound called a bruit. Bruits may be heard with a stethoscope over the carotid arteries, abdominal aorta, and renal arteries. Arterial areas narrowed by arteriosclerosis and atherosclerosis are called areas of stenosis.

 CLINICAL CONCEPT

Arterial bruits and regions of arterial stenosis are signs of severe atherosclerosis.

Diagnosis

Various laboratory tests and procedures are used to diagnose CVD. The constituents of the blood, endothelial function, and inflammatory mediators can be measured to provide information about CVD risk. Cardiac catheterization is a widely used technique to diagnose coronary arteriosclerosis. CT calcium scan and ultrasound are also used in the investigation of CVD.

Lipid Profile. Atherosclerosis begins with elevated lipids circulating in the bloodstream. Therefore, diagnostic tests for atherosclerosis include those for hyperlipidemia: total cholesterol, LDL, HDL, and triglycerides. If hyperlipidemia is present, additional tests are needed for diabetes mellitus, hypothyroidism, and liver disease. BMI should be calculated because obesity is commonly present with hyperlipidemia and atherosclerosis.

Endothelial Function. The endothelium plays a key role in the development of atherosclerosis; endothelial injury and resultant dysfunction are often the catalysts for atherogenesis. Endothelium-dependent vasodilation can be assessed in the coronary and peripheral circulations, both invasively and noninvasively. Endothelial function of the coronary arteries can be assessed using intracoronary Doppler techniques to measure coronary blood flow in response to stimulation with acetylcholine. This can be accomplished during cardiac catheterization. In patients with healthy endothelial function, infusion of acetylcholine incites vasodilation. In patients with atherosclerosis, endothelial dysfunction becomes apparent by vasoconstriction or blunted responses to acetylcholine.

An ultrasound of the arm's brachial artery is also a noninvasive measure of endothelial cell function. A BP cuff is placed around the upper arm, which is then inflated and occludes blood flow to the forearm for 5 minutes. When the pressure is released, reactive hyperemia of the forearm should occur because of brisk vasodilation. If the forearm has delayed return of circulation, this is indicative of suboptimal arterial elasticity and endothelial injury. This technique has the advantage of being noninvasive and can readily identify populations with reduced endothelial function.

C-Reactive Protein. CRP is an acute-phase protein produced by the liver in response to inflammation in the body. It is produced in response to atherosclerosis, which is basically an inflammatory process. Studies have associated elevated CRP with high rates of cardiac events. According to the AHA, hs-CRP is a blood test that can help predict a cardiovascular event or stroke and help direct evaluation and therapy. People with elevated hs-CRP values have the highest risk of CVD; those with lower values have less of a risk.

🔬 CLINICAL CONCEPT

Individuals who have hs-CRP results in the high end of the normal range have 1.5 to 4 times the risk of having an MI as those with hs-CRP values at the low end of the normal range.

Homocysteine Level. Homocysteine is an amino acid that can be measured in the blood. The body uses folic acid to metabolize and break down homocysteine into usable amino acid components. Lack of sufficient folic acid causes accumulation of homocysteine in the bloodstream, called hyperhomocysteinemia. Hyperhomocysteinemia, in turn, causes endothelial injury. Lack of sources of folic acid in the diet can predispose individuals to this risk of endothelial injury leading to atherosclerosis.

Calcium Computed Tomography Scan. Calcification is part of the progression of atherosclerotic plaque lesions. Calcium is obvious on x-ray, and its deposition in vessels can be detected via a CT scan. These CT images may be just one sign of atherosclerosis, and clinicians need to review these scans along with patient symptoms and risk factors. Cardiac artery calcium CT scans are increasingly utilized to screen patients for potential cardiac episodes. Studies are being conducted to examine the relationship between the calcium scan value and its predictive worth in identifying patients who need to undergo cardiac catheterization or other invasive interventions.

Cardiac Angiography. Angiography is a radiopaque dye study using the cardiac catheterization procedure with x-rays to view blocked vessels (see Fig. 15-10). Sometimes referred to as cardiac catheterization, this test is the gold standard for diagnosing CAD, but it has risks because it is invasive and requires the introduction of a catheter, as well as a contrast medium, into the body.

Angiography can show the outline of a blood vessel, as well as how much an atherosclerotic lesion extends into the vessel's lumen. The health-care provider is given an outline but nothing more in terms of the constituents of the lesion; sometimes, the lesion may be missed. Results from cardiac angiography help determine whether treatment with coronary artery bypass graft (CABG) surgery or percutaneous coronary intervention (PCI), such as angioplasty, may be effective.

Intravascular Ultrasonography. Intravascular ultrasonography allows for detailed assessment of the coronary arteries. Intracoronary ultrasound, via small catheters, provides a cross-sectional image of the coronary arteries, thereby providing visualization and quantization of plaque. This technology can be used to determine whether a patient is a candidate for PCI. The calcium within the atherosclerotic plaque is echogenic, which allows it to be imaged on ultrasound.

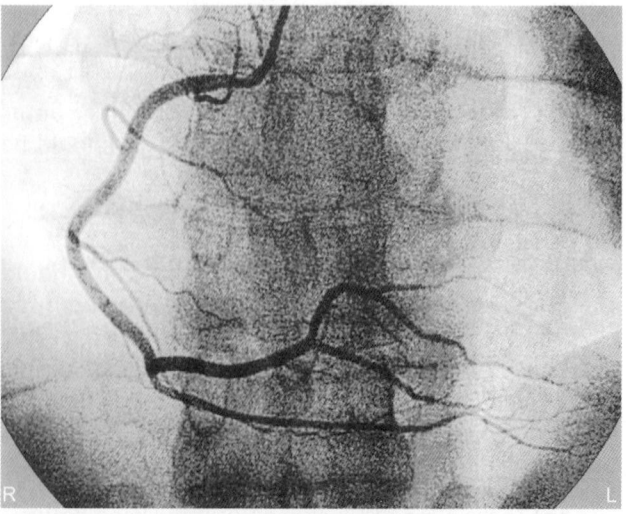

FIGURE 15-10. Coronary angiography. *(From BSIP/Science Source.)*

Treatment

The medical treatment for atherosclerosis is the same as that for hyperlipidemia. Surgical treatments are available for atherosclerosis of the coronary arteries and obstructed arteries of the extremities. CABG surgery and PCI are commonly implemented to reperfuse ischemic areas of the heart caused by obstructed coronary arteries. Angioplasty with stent placement is a common type of PCI. CABG surgery utilizes vessel grafts that are placed to circumvent areas of obstruction caused by coronary arteriosclerosis.

Peripheral Arterial Disease

Peripheral arterial disease (PAD) is a disorder that involves arteriosclerosis and atherosclerosis in the peripheral regions of the body outside the coronary arteries. It most often refers to arterial dysfunction and reduced blood flow within the lower extremities. PAD can be acute, but more often it is more gradual in nature. In an acute arterial obstruction, sudden disruption in blood flow leads to ischemia, which, if untreated, could result in infarction and necrosis of tissue. More often, PAD is a chronic disorder that can be silent for years. The most common site for an occlusion is the femoral artery located above the knee, though obstruction can occur in the iliac, popliteal, or tibial arterial vessels.

Epidemiology

PAD affects up to 20% of individuals aged 65 years and older. Before age 65, PAD is more common in men; after age 65, both sexes are affected equally. With advanced age, the incidence of PAD continues to rise, such that at age 85 years and older, 50% to 65% of the population is affected by the disorder. PAD is probably more prevalent than studies show because as PAD is developing, it is a silent disease.

In general, the incidence of PAD is higher among African Americans than among European Americans. Among persons who have a history of smoking and diabetes, the prevalence of PAD is as high as 50%.

Approximately 40% to 60% of persons with PAD also have CAD and cerebral artery disease, and patients who have PAD are three to four times more likely to suffer a stroke than the general population.

Etiology

Atherosclerosis is the most common cause of PAD. Similar to CAD, atherosclerotic plaque can accumulate in the peripheral arteries of the extremities. Diabetes mellitus accelerates development of PAD due to the uncontrolled glucose levels in the bloodstream causing endothelial injury. Blood vessel injury is particularly apparent in the lower extremities in diabetes.

Risk Factors

The risk factors for PAD are the same as those for general arteriosclerosis and atherosclerosis, including age older than 45 years for men and older than 55 years for women, HTN, high-fat diet, sedentary lifestyle, obesity, family history, and hyperlipidemia. Diabetes mellitus and smoking independently increase the risk of PAD by three to four times. Chronic kidney disease, cancer, hypercoagulable states, and obesity are other risks associated with increased incidence of PAD.

 CLINICAL CONCEPT

Individuals with uncontrolled diabetes commonly suffer peripheral neuropathy—loss of sensation in the lower extremities due to decreased circulation. A wound in an ischemic lower extremity cannot heal properly, and this increases the risk of infection, gangrene, and limb amputation.

Pathophysiology

PAD causes a reduction in arterial blood flow to the body's peripheral arteries. Arteries such as the carotid artery in the neck and femoral arteries in the legs are commonly affected. PAD typically develops gradually over time in persons with arteriosclerosis and atherosclerosis. PAD of the lower extremities causes characteristic symptoms. Reduced arterial blood flow leads to tissue ischemia, which presents as **intermittent claudication**, a cramping leg pain that occurs with exertion and is usually relieved by rest. Persons with PAD can often predict how much exercise of the leg will trigger pain.

The location of pain experienced with PAD varies depending on the vessels affected. In aortoiliac disease, the pain is often in the low back or across the buttocks, whereas in femoral or popliteal arterial disease, the pain or discomfort is usually in the calf.

Intermittent claudication is a classic symptom of PAD that occurs because of ischemia of muscle tissue. In arterial obstruction, lack of circulation causes an imbalance between tissue demand for oxygen and blood supply. During exertion, muscle tissue requires increased oxygenated blood, and an obstructed artery cannot meet this increased need. Therefore, muscle tissue undergoes anaerobic metabolism, which yields 2 adenosine triphosphate (ATP) and lactic acid. The 2 ATP are an inadequate amount of energy, and the lactic acid is noxious to muscle tissue and causes pain. If the demand for oxygen is reduced, the pain will subside. The patient can stop exercising to rest the muscle in order to reduce its oxygen demand and relieve the pain. Intermittent claudication is similar to angina, an episodic pain that occurs because of ischemia. However, the pain in PAD is caused by episodes of ischemia in the leg rather than in the chest.

The pathophysiology of intermittent claudication is not limited to an imbalance between oxygen supply and demand. Metabolic changes in skeletal muscle that occur with ischemic episodes contribute to the pain. Injury to endothelial cells, nerve cells, and muscle tissue may occur as a result of ischemia, followed by reperfusion of the tissue. During reperfusion, free radicals are produced, causing oxidative stress. Oxidative stress, in turn, results in injury to the vascular bed and alterations in muscle metabolism, which contribute to claudication.

Clinical Presentation

When assessing the patient who is suspected of having PAD, clinicians should focus on the signs of arteriosclerosis and atherosclerosis. Patients with signs of these conditions in the coronary arteries or cerebral arteries are likely to have arteriosclerosis and atherosclerosis of the extremities as well. Patient history of HTN, hyperlipidemia, diabetes mellitus, CAD, or MI are significant predisposing factors to PAD. The patient should be questioned about specific symptoms related to ischemia of the limbs, such as pain, numbness and tingling, and coolness of the extremities. It is important to ask if the patient has leg pain or numbness upon exertion. The pain or numbness associated with PAD in the lower extremities is intermittent, associated with exertion, and relieved by rest. The more severe the PAD, the less exertion is needed to cause claudication pain. Patients with pain at rest usually have critical limb ischemia, which can lead to necessary surgical amputation.

Clinical manifestations seen with PAD include diminished or absent pulses, palpable coolness, paresthesias, pallor, and pain of the lower extremity on exertion. The symptoms commonly worsen with elevation of the limb. Sensory assessments from distal to proximal should be carried out, including light touch, pain and temperature sensation, tactile discrimination, vibratory sensation, proprioception, and deep tendon reflexes. Loss of sensation in the feet is common in PAD; however, the patient may not be aware of this deficit. Patients who have PAD due to uncontrolled diabetes commonly suffer peripheral neuropathy—loss of sensation or tingling and burning sensation in the feet.

In PAD, one limb's pulses may be weakened or absent compared with the other limb's pulses, so peripheral pulses of the lower extremities should be compared. Lower extremity peripheral pulses include the femoral, popliteal, dorsalis pedis, and posterior tibial pulses.

🩺 CLINICAL CONCEPT

Symptoms of PAD are not usually present until approximately 70% of the arterial lumen is occluded, so it is important to remember that PAD may be present without apparent symptoms.

Diagnosis

In addition to peripheral pulse assessment, the **ankle–brachial index (ABI)** should be assessed to determine the severity of PAD. The ABI is a comparison of upper and lower extremity systolic BP whereby the ankle pressure is divided by the brachial pressure. When done properly, this noninvasive, inexpensive, simple test has become the diagnostic test of choice for detecting PAD. ABI measures are assessed when the patient has been supine for at least 5 minutes. To assess ABI, a Doppler sphygmomanometer device with pulse volume recording measures the systolic BP in the brachial artery of each arm and in the ankles. The ABI is calculated by first assessing the systolic BP in both upper extremities by auscultating the brachial artery with a Doppler. Next, the ankle systolic pressure is measured using a Doppler over either the posterior tibial artery or the dorsalis pedis artery, with the cuff firmly wrapped around the ankle above the malleolus. The ABI is calculated by dividing each ankle systolic pressure by the corresponding systolic brachial pressure. This will provide an ABI for both extremities.

Generally, the ABI in a healthy person is approximately 1 or slightly greater than 1, because the ankle pressure should be slightly higher than the brachial systolic pressure. For example, if the ankle systolic pressure is 140 mm Hg and the brachial systolic pressure is 120 mm Hg, then the ankle-to-brachial ratio is 140/120, which is greater than 1; this would be normal. However, if the ankle systolic pressure is 60 mm Hg and brachial systolic pressure is 120 mm Hg, the ratio of 60/120 is 0.5; this indicates moderate PAD (see Table 15-5 for the significance of ABI readings). An ABI lower than 1 indicates PAD.

Serum laboratory tests for PAD should include CBC, hemoglobin, hematocrit, platelet count, lipid profile, and nonspecific tests of inflammation, such as erythrocyte sedimentation rate (ESR) and CRP. Other useful diagnostic tests include impedance arterial plethysmography, pulse oximetry, ultrasonography, magnetic resonance angiography (MRA), conventional angiography, CT, and duplex ultrasonography. Plethysmography is a noninvasive diagnostic test used to measure changes in the size of blood vessels by determining blood volume. Impedance plethysmography diagnoses peripheral-arterial disease of the extremities through application of a series of BP cuffs that measure the amplitude of each pulse wave. An angiogram is an examination where dye is injected into the circulation and radiographic images are taken to determine the integrity of blood vessels. The arteriogram is invasive and carries some risk to the patient with compromised circulation. Consequently, better angiographic studies utilize CT or magnetic resonance imaging (MRI) to provide cross-sectional three-dimensional views of the vessel with or without use of contrast.

TABLE 15-5. Ankle–Brachial Index

The ABI is the ratio of the BP in the lower legs to the BP in the arms. Normally, BP is slightly higher in the legs compared with the arms. The ABI is calculated by dividing the systolic BP at the ankle by the systolic BP in the arm. An ABI that is greater than or equal to 1 is normal. An ABI that is lower than 1 indicates PAD. A Doppler ultrasound blood flow detector and a sphygmomanometer are usually needed to calculate ABI.

Category	ABI Calculation
Normal	1 or greater
Minimal PAD	0.8 to 0.95
Moderate PAD	0.4 to 0.8
Severe PAD	0.4 or lower

Right arm systolic pressure

Left arm systolic pressure

Right ankle systolic pressure

Left ankle systolic pressure

ALERT! In patients with suspected or confirmed PAD of the lower extremity, a pulse that is not palpable may indicate a critical lack of blood flow known as critical limb ischemia. This increases the patient's risk for lower extremity amputation.

 CLINICAL CONCEPT

Peripheral circulation can be assessed by checking capillary refill. Normal capillary refill time is less than 2 seconds.

Treatment

As in many disease processes, the initial focus of patient care in PAD should be on prevention and health promotion. Prudent lifestyle choices can prevent many of the vascular changes that occur over time. It is important to understand that a patient who has PAD likely has CAD and needs all CVD preventive measures. Regular exercise, weight control, abstention from smoking, maintenance of normal blood sugar levels in the presence of diabetes, and healthy cholesterol and lipoprotein levels reduce the risk of injury to the arteries that precedes disease. Exercise stimulates the growth of collateral vessels, which improves blood flow. Walking regimens of 30 minutes per day at least three times per week have been shown to provide significant benefits.

Pharmacological treatment generally includes medications to reduce blood cholesterol, control BP, inhibit platelet aggregation, and dilate peripheral vessels. The phosphodiesterase type-3 inhibitor cilostazol (Pletal) counteracts platelet aggregation and vasodilates peripheral arterial vessels. It has been shown to significantly increase walking distances and improve ABI in patients with PAD. Antiplatelet therapy with aspirin alone or clopidogrel alone is recommended to reduce the risk of MI, stroke, and vascular death in patients with symptomatic PAD. Thrombolytic agents (known as "clot busters") are also used in PAD. The best results occur when catheter-directed thrombolytic therapy takes place within 2 weeks of the onset of severe symptoms. Another drug, pentoxifylline (Trental), a blood viscosity reducing agent, has shown mixed results in the treatment of claudication.

Peripheral arterial revascularization procedures, which include endovascular and open surgical interventions, are used to improve circulation in the lower extremities. Endovascular procedures, interventions that insert a catheter into the artery of obstructed lower extremities, are effective treatments for patients with significant PAD. Types of endovascular procedures include standard percutaneous transluminal angioplasty (PTA; also called balloon angioplasty), drug-coated balloon angioplasty, atherectomy, stent insertion, and drug-eluting stent insertion. The addition of a drug to an angioplasty or stent has been shown to prevent restenosis of the obstructed artery. Drug-coated balloon angioplasty using the cytotoxic drug paclitaxel has been shown to be superior to standard PTA. Drug-eluting stents using paclitaxel have also proven to be superior to bare stents. Other drugs are under investigation for drug-eluting stents and drug-coated balloon angioplasty.

Instead of endovascular interventions, open surgical vascular bypass grafting can be performed. When open surgery is performed, a femoral-popliteal artery bypass is commonly inserted. The bypass graft can be constructed from a superficial leg vein or prosthetic graft material. Studies show that use of a superficial leg vein from the patient is the preferred type of graft (see Fig 15-11).

Aneurysm

An aneurysm is a weakening in an artery wall that causes a localized area of bulging or dilation. The weakened segment of the artery creates an outpouching that is susceptible to rupture. The disrupted wall can cause turbulent blood flow within the artery. The cerebral arteries and the aorta are the typical sites of aneurysms. Of the two sites, an **abdominal aortic aneurysm (AAA)** is the most common type (see Figure 15-7).

Epidemiology

An AAA is found in 5% to 7% of persons older than age 60 years. As the population ages, the incidence is expected to increase. Rupture of AAA causes 15,000 deaths each year. Compared with females, males have a three to eightfold higher risk of AAA formation.

AAAs are twice as prevalent in European Americans compared with African Americans. Males of European ancestry who are older than age 80 years with risk factors for heart disease have the highest incidence of AAA. Aortic aneurysm is often an incidental finding on examination when the patient presents to health care for another reason.

Cerebral aneurysms occur in about 1% to 5% of the U.S. population. Clinical manifestations increase with age, reaching a peak in people aged 55 to 60 years. Most patients with cerebral aneurysm are asymptomatic until the aneurysm ruptures, resulting in a subarachnoid hemorrhage (SAH). About 65% of individuals with an SAH from a cerebral aneurysm die suddenly before reaching health care; 25% die within a day of suffering an SAH. Cerebral aneurysms are more common in African Americans than European Americans. Approximately 2% of strokes are caused by ruptured cerebral aneurysms.

Etiology

Aneurysms are usually the result of damage to the artery lining from arteriosclerosis, but may also be caused by degenerative vascular disease, infection, collagen vascular disease, or trauma. There is a probable genetic predisposition to the development of intracerebral aneurysms; the existence in some families runs as high as 10%, approximately 10 times higher than that found in the general population. Two gene mutations, fibrillin-1, located on chromosome 15, and myofibril associated protein-5, located on chromosome 12, cause the faulty structural integrity of the aortic wall in familial aortic aneurysm. Risk for cerebral aneurysm has been observed in carriers of the *ADAMTS2* variant gene, which codes for defective structural components in the endothelium of cerebral arteries.

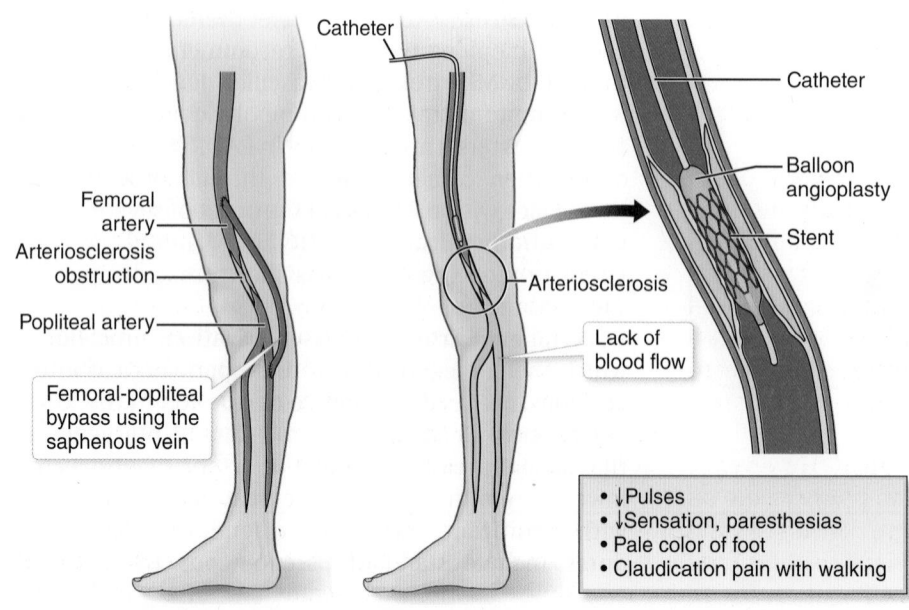

Femoral artery
Arteriosclerosis obstruction
Popliteal artery
Femoral-popliteal bypass using the saphenous vein

Catheter
Arteriosclerosis
Lack of blood flow

Catheter
Balloon angioplasty
Stent

• ↓Pulses
• ↓Sensation, paresthesias
• Pale color of foot
• Claudication pain with walking

FIGURE 15-11. Revascularization procedures in peripheral arterial disease.

Risk Factors

Atherosclerosis, smoking, and HTN are major risk factors for the formation and rupture of aneurysms. Genetic factors are likely involved, as there is a high incidence of aneurysm within families. Atherosclerotic plaque invades the wall of the artery and undermines its strength; in addition, blood flow rushing by this area of atherosclerosis contributes to the reduced strength of the wall. HTN is a constant force against arterial walls that also weakens the integrity of blood vessels. Connective tissue disorders, such as Marfan's syndrome or Ehlers–Danlos syndrome, increase the risk of aortic aneurysm.

Pathophysiology

In an aneurysm, a region of arterial wall bulges and contains an uneven interior surface. The wall becomes weaker as blood flows against it, and blood can collect within it. The dreaded sequela of an aneurysm is rupture, leading to internal hemorrhage. However, during the formation of an aneurysm, blood can enter the bulging pouch in the wall and become stagnant or turbulent. The stagnant blood inside the aneurysm can give rise to platelet aggregation, resulting in thrombus development. If thrombi embolize to other organs, they can lodge in small arterial vessels and cause ischemia, necrosis, or gangrene of those organs.

Aneurysms are classified by their size, shape, and location. Size and location may influence treatment and prognosis. Aneurysms may also be classified as either true aneurysms or false aneurysms. A true aneurysm involves all three layers of the vessel wall, whereas a false aneurysm is a hematoma where the clot is actually outside the arterial wall. Aneurysm shapes include fusiform and saccular. A fusiform aneurysm occurs when all the layers of the blood vessel's wall dilate equally, whereas a saccular aneurysm occurs when there is a weakness on only one side of the vessel with a pouchlike bulge.

Cerebral aneurysms, sometimes called berry aneurysms, are commonly small, berrylike outpouchings off the circle of Willis within the subarachnoid space (see Figure 15-7).

Clinical Presentation

Clinical presentation of an aneurysm depends on its size, location, and integrity. Aortic aneurysms tend to develop gradually, with 75% undetected until they rupture. Rupture may be the first sign of an AAA. Before rupture, symptoms that should raise suspicion of an AAA include abdominal, flank, or back pain. If the aneurysm is large, it can put pressure on adjacent organs. Nausea, vomiting, bowel, or ureteral compression symptoms can occur.

Cerebral aneurysms are usually silent. However, if the cerebral aneurysm is large, it can put pressure on adjacent tissues, such as cranial nerves. Headache and cranial nerve dysfunction can be signs of a cerebral aneurysm. Rupture of a cerebral aneurysm causes an SAH, and the classic symptom is a very severe headache. Most SAHs are fatal.

> **ALERT!** Individuals experiencing an SAH often refer to it as a sudden "thunderclap" headache or the worst headache of their lives.

No sound should be heard during assessment if blood flow in an artery is smooth. However, the turbulent blood flow through a large aneurysm may be heard with a stethoscope as a bruit.

In a thin patient, an AAA may be detected by inspection and palpation of the abdomen. A pulsatile mass may be evident in someone with a scaphoid abdomen. With rupture, circulation to the lower extremities will be diminished, resulting in cool, pale extremities with diminished or absent pulses. The patient will feel acute pain and go into shock. Manifestations of shock include cold, clammy skin; decreased BP; increased HR; and changes in the patient's level of consciousness.

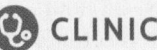
CLINICAL CONCEPT

Auscultation of a bruit over the abdominal aorta suggests the presence of an aneurysm.

> **ALERT!** If a pulsatile mass is evident in the abdomen during inspection or light palpation, deep palpation should not be performed until the possibility of AAA is ruled out.

Diagnosis

Most often, aneurysms are found incidentally because they are usually silent until they rupture. Ultrasonography is the diagnostic test of choice for detection and follow-up of suspected AAAs. Ultrasound can indicate the size, location, and progression of the AAA. Advantages are its lack of invasiveness, lack of a need for contrast, and its sensitivity between 95% and 100%. In comparison, x-rays can only show a large calcified aortic silhouette and do not indicate the size of the AAA. Contrast CT scan provides detailed information on the size and location of an aneurysm but requires use of a contrast medium. MRA, which can indicate the size and location of AAAs, does not require contrast, but it is less accurate than a CT or ultrasound. MRI can also indicate the size and location of AAAs.

Treatment

Preventive medical treatment for an aneurysm includes smoking cessation and reductions in BP and blood volume. After initial identification of an AAA, periodic follow-up is needed to assess progression and susceptibility to rupture. Because of the significant risks associated with surgery, AAAs are not usually operated on until the aortic diameter exceeds 4.5 cm.

Surgical treatment usually involves endovascular repair with graft or stent placement. Endovascular repair is performed by removing the aneurysm and replacing that section of the aorta with a synthetic graft or stent. For cerebral aneurysms, microsurgical and endovascular procedures aim to impede the blood flow from the cerebral circulation into the aneurysm. This is accomplished by inserting a clip, coil, or band around the neck of the aneurysm.

Aortic Dissection

Aortic dissection is a potentially lethal disorder of the aorta that involves a tear in the arterial lining between the tunica media and intima. Blood flows within the tear and commonly forms a hematoma within the wall.

Epidemiology

Aortic dissection is two to three times more common than rupture of the abdominal aorta. When left untreated, about 33% of patients die within the first 24 hours, and 50% die within 48 hours. The 2-week mortality rate approaches 75% in patients with undiagnosed ascending aortic dissection. African Americans are affected more than European Americans. Males are affected more than females. Affected persons are commonly in the 50- to 65-year-old age range. Approximately 2,000 cases are reported in the United States annually.

Etiology

Aortic dissection is influenced by genetic predisposition, HTN, and arteriosclerosis. Aortic dissection is more common in patients with connective tissue disorders, congenital aortic stenosis, or a bicuspid aortic valve. Individuals with Marfan's syndrome are particularly at risk for the disorder. More than 70% of patients with aortic dissection have HTN. It is also common in those with a family history of aortic dissection. Individuals with *MYLK* and *ACTA2* mutations, which confer smooth muscle defects in the wall of the aorta, have been shown to have aortic dissections.

Pathophysiology

The wall of the aorta is composed of collagen, elastin, and smooth muscle. With aging, collagen breakdown and arteriosclerotic changes weaken the wall of the aorta. Because the aorta is under constant pulsatile stress, it is prone to injury and disease. If an aneurysm is present, the aorta is particularly susceptible to rupture because of high wall tension.

In aortic dissection, the aortic wall undergoes a splitting of the layers between the inner lining and the middle muscular wall. Blood starts to flow between the layers, which traumatizes the region and causes more of a gap between the wall layers. Eventually, a hematoma develops in the region that protrudes into the lumen. The dissection of the aortic wall forms a false lumen in the aorta, which ends in a blind pouch that collects blood and can reduce blood flow to the major arteries arising from the aorta. Several classification systems have been developed for thoracic aortic dissection. The Stanford system classified aortic dissections as type A or B. The Stanford type A aortic dissection involves the ascending aorta, which is a proximal dissection. The Stanford type B aortic dissection is limited to the arch or descending aorta, which is a distal dissection. Aortic dissection occurs most commonly in the first few centimeters of the aortic arch, with 90% occurring within 10 cm of the aortic valve (see Fig. 15-12).

Clinical Presentation

With aortic dissection, onset of symptoms is usually sudden. The patient may complain of severe pain in the chest or back associated with a ripping or tearing sound. Pallor, tachycardia, and diaphoresis may be present. BP elevation or difference from one side to the other may be evident. The pain of aortic dissection is similar to that of MI.

HTN may result from the patient's anxious state or underlying essential HTN. However, with severe aortic dissection, HTN is usually present. There may be a difference in BP in the right and left arm; a difference of greater than 20 mm Hg should increase the suspicion of aortic dissection.

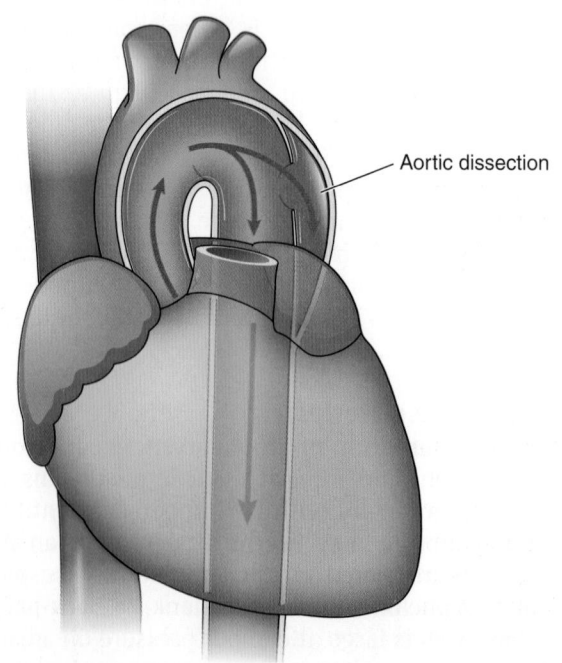

Aortic dissection

FIGURE 15-12. Aortic dissection occurs when there is a tear in the inner wall of the aorta, which causes blood to flow between the layers of the wall of the aorta, forcing the layers apart. The separation of the layers of the aorta creates another lumen, where blood flows and widens the tear in the layers. Aortic dissection increases risk of aortic rupture and is a medical emergency.

Signs of aortic regurgitation caused by dysfunction of the aortic valve, including bounding pulses, wide pulse pressure, and diastolic murmur, may be present. Acute, severe aortic regurgitation may result in heart failure. Signs of heart failure include dyspnea, orthopnea, bibasilar crackles, or elevated jugular venous pressure.

Other cardiovascular manifestations include findings suggestive of cardiac tamponade, a condition caused by pressure around the heart, limiting its pumping action. Signs of cardiac tamponade include muffled heart sounds, hypotension, jugular venous distention, wide pulse pressure, and pulse deficit or asymmetry of pulses.

Neurological deficits occur in up to 20% of cases. The most common neurological deficits are syncope (fainting, loss of consciousness) and decreased level of consciousness. Syncope may be the result of increased stimulation of the vagus nerve, hypovolemia, or dysrhythmia. Other causes of syncope or altered mental status include stroke from compromised blood flow to the brain or spinal cord.

Diagnosis

Patients require an ECG and chest x-ray. CT and MRI of the chest are also usually performed to reveal aortic dissection. Some studies have shown use of transesophageal echocardiogram (TEE) is best because it can best visualize the aortic arch. Intravascular ultrasound and angiography are also sometimes used to guide surgical repair.

Treatment

Medical therapy in an intensive care unit with hemodynamic monitoring should be initiated as soon as aortic dissection is considered. Blood pressure reduction to decrease shear stress on the aortic wall is necessary. Beta adrenergic blockers, sodium nitroprusside, or calcium channel antagonists should be used. Aortic dissection is treated by surgery to repair the tear in the aorta with a graft. Aortic stenting is also done when the dissection is in the thoracic aorta.

Vasculitis

Vasculitis, the inflammation of arterial vessels, most often occurs as a result of an autoimmune disorder. Many of the vasculitis disorders are considered to be immune complex–mediated diseases where antigens and antibodies are formed. An excess number of antigens is deposited in the vessel walls, leading to inflammation. With some disorders, the antigen has not been clearly identified. Vasculitis disorders are categorized according to their involvement of either large, medium, or small arterial vessels.

Large-vessel vasculitis includes temporal arteritis (TA) and Takayasu's arteritis. TA generally affects the branches of the aorta that supply the head. Takayasu's arteritis typically involves the aorta and its main branches. Vasculitis affecting medium-sized blood vessels include polyarteritis nodosa (PAN) and Kawasaki's disease. PAN is an inflammatory condition of arteries and arterioles that can occur in any organ of the body. Kawasaki's disease is a disease that mainly affects children and causes problems in the heart. The most common types of vasculitis of small-sized arterioles include Raynaud's disease and thromboangiitis obliterans (TAO). Other types of vasculitis are summarized in Table 15-6.

Temporal Arteritis

TA, also called giant cell arteritis, is a common type of vasculitis primarily affecting patients older than 50 years. The disorder mainly involves inflammation

TABLE 15-6. Types of Vasculitis	
Type of Vasculitis	**Description**
Wegener's granulomatosis	Vasculitis of small arterioles and venules. It can affect many organs of the body, but it usually involves the kidneys, the lungs, and the upper respiratory tract. Certain antibodies, such as antineutrophil cytoplasmic antibodies, are associated with Wegener's disease and may be detected in the blood in these patients.
Henoch-Schönlein purpura	A small-vessel vasculitis that also affects many different organs. This vasculitis is seen in infants, children, and adults, but it is more common in children between ages 4 and 7 years.
Hypersensitivity vasculitis	A small-vessel vasculitis that may be related to an allergic insult to blood vessels. The main areas of involvement are cutaneous, as they damage the small vessels of the skin; therefore, they may also be called predominantly cutaneous vasculitis or cutaneous leukocytoclastic vasculitis.
Essential cryo-globulinemia vasculitis	A small-vessel vasculitis related to cryoglobulins, which are small protein complexes that can precipitate in cold temperatures. They may cause vascular inflammation by depositing in the vessel walls.

of the superficial temporal arteries; however, the aorta, carotid, subclavian, vertebral, and iliac arteries are often affected as well.

Epidemiology. TA typically occurs in older adult patients of European descent. Women are affected two to three times more frequently than men. The average age of onset is 72 years, rarely affecting individuals younger than age 50 years. Incidence increases with age and can range from 1 in 10,000 to 5 in 10,000 annually in the United States. The most serious complication of TA is blindness. Studies show bilateral visual loss occurs in up to 33% of patients.

Etiology. The exact etiology of TA is unknown. The inflammation cascade is involved, although the event that triggers the cascade remains uncertain. On biopsy, there is a preponderance of T cells that attack the arterial wall, suggesting that it may be an autoimmune disease. Many infectious pathogens have been suggested as triggers, such as herpes simplex virus, parvovirus B19, Epstein–Barr virus, and *Chlamydia* species, but the involvement of microbial pathogens is still unclear.

Risk Factors. The etiology of TA involves both genetic and environmental influences. There is some evidence that persons with human leukocyte surface antigens HLA-DR4 and HLA-DRB104 are more susceptible than others.

Pathophysiology. TA is a chronic, systemic vasculitis, primarily affecting the walls of medium and large arteries. Inflammation is apparent across all layers of the artery wall with infiltration by lymphocytes, macrophages, and multinucleated giant cells. The arterial walls become thickened and arterial lumens become narrowed, causing distal ischemia of tissues.

The temporal artery is affected, often resulting in headache in the region of the artery. Other commonly affected vessels include the ophthalmic artery and the central retinal artery, which causes visual impairment.

The inflammatory changes seen in TA are also seen in polymyalgia rheumatica (PMR). PMR and TA may have the same underlying disease process. The symptoms of PMR include pain and stiffness in the shoulder and pelvic musculature, as well as systemic signs of fever, malaise, and weight loss. Approximately half of patients initially presenting with TA also develop PMR.

Clinical Presentation. Headache is the most common symptom reported and occurs in over two-thirds of patients with TA. The headache tends to be sudden in onset and localized to the temporal region. The headache pain of TA is unique and unlike past headaches, according to the patient. Therefore, TA should be considered a diagnosis in any new type of headache in patients older than 50 years.

TA tends to affect the branches of the carotid artery, and symptoms vary depending on the region of the ischemic artery. Superficial temporal artery involvement can cause severe scalp tenderness. Patients may also present with apparent areas of scalp ischemia and necrosis. Pain in the jaw often occurs in patients with involvement of the maxillary artery. There is often a prominent, beaded, pulseless, tender temporal artery.

Sudden loss of vision may also be an initial symptom. Initial visual symptoms are usually episodic, occurring as unilateral visual loss or diplopia. If left untreated, permanent blindness can result.

Systemic symptoms caused by widespread inflammation are common. Fever, malaise, memory impairment, anorexia, weight loss, fatigue, and depression are often reported. The pain and stiffness of PMR is an initial symptom in about half of all cases of temporal arteritis. Peripheral musculoskeletal manifestations are reported in both TA and PMR, including arthritis, swelling of the distal extremities with pitting edema, tenosynovitis, and carpal tunnel syndrome.

Diagnosis. Elevated ESR and CRP are signs of inflammation in temporal arteritis. However, up to 20% of patients with TA do not present with these inflammatory indices. CBC may show leukocytosis, anemia, or thrombocytosis. Elevated liver enzymes, particularly alkaline phosphatase, are present in about one-half of patients with TA. Color duplex ultrasound of the temporal arteries show a "halo" sign around the temporal artery. A definitive diagnosis is based on a temporal artery biopsy.

Treatment. Steroid treatment is the most common therapy used in TA. Low-dose aspirin is recommended as well. The patient may require oral steroids for 1 to 2 years. TA commonly relapses when corticosteroids are tapered; corticosteroid use cannot be prolonged due to side effects that include glucose intolerance, osteoporosis, gastric ulceration, and immune deficiency. The interleukin-6 (IL-6) receptor alpha inhibitor tocilizumab has been effective in reducing the rates of relapse during the tapering of corticosteroid medication. However, more studies of this medication are needed.

Takayasu's Arteritis

Takayasu's arteritis is a rare, systemic, large-vessel vasculitis of unknown cause that most commonly affects women younger than 50 years. It is defined as granulomatous inflammation of the aorta and its major branches. Arteries throughout the body can be involved, with multiorgan effects.

Epidemiology. Takayasu's arteritis affects approximately 2.6 persons per million per year worldwide. It is observed more frequently in patients of Asian or Indian descent. Approximately 80% of patients with Takayasu's arteritis are women approximately 30 years old.

Etiology. The etiology of Takayasu's arteritis is unclear; however, it is an autoimmune, inflammatory disorder. Microorganisms proposed as etiological agents that may trigger the disease include spirochetes, *Mycobacterium* tuberculosis, and streptococcal organisms. Genetic factors may play a role in the pathogenesis. Individuals with the human leukocyte surface antigen HLA-Bw52 are particularly affected.

Pathophysiology. Takayasu's arteritis is an inflammatory disease of large and medium arteries that particularly affects the aorta and its branches. The inflammatory process affects the wall of the aorta, causing narrowing, obstruction, or aneurysms. Vascular complications include HTN, most often caused by renal artery stenosis, aortic insufficiency, pulmonary HTN, and aortic aneurysm.

Clinical Presentation. There are three stages of disease. During the first stage, the patient suffers a flu-like illness that includes fever, general malaise, and fatigue. This stage occurs before the inflammatory changes of the arteries.

The second stage involves inflammatory changes of the arteries that cause stenosis, aneurysms, and ischemia of tissue. The patient has various complaints, including pain in the extremities and joints, dyspnea, palpitations, headaches, rash, hemoptysis, and weight loss. The patient can also suffer various symptoms of arterial insufficiency and ischemia, including arm numbness, claudication in the legs, visual impairment, stroke, TIA, seizures, and paralysis of the extremities.

The third stage of Takayasu's arteritis is referred to as the burned-out stage, when fibrosis develops in the arteries and symptoms subside. However, this stage does not occur in all patients and does not indicate full recovery. Patients in remission can suffer a relapse of severe illness.

Diagnosis. Laboratory tests indicative of inflammation, such as ESR and CRP, are elevated. Leukocyte count may be normal or slightly elevated. Normochromic, normocytic anemia may be present. Antiendothelial antibodies may be present in the blood. Angiography is the standard test for diagnosis and evaluation of the disease. CT scan, ultrasound, and MRA are also used in the diagnosis.

Treatment. Treatment for Takayasu's arteritis involves controlling the inflammatory process and controlling HTN. Corticosteroids are the mainstay of therapy for active disease. Use of cytotoxic agents methotrexate, azathioprine, and cyclophosphamide may allow tapering of chronic corticosteroid treatment. Relapse is common when corticosteroid doses are tapered. Antitumor necrosis factor (anti-TNF) agents such as etanercept and infliximab are sometimes effective. The IL-6 receptor alpha inhibitor tocilizumab has been found to be effective when corticosteroids are being tapered. However, more studies of this medication are needed.

Bypass graft surgery, aneurysm clipping, and percutaneous balloon angioplasty are used. Angioplasty and stenting are effective in treating recurrent stenosis; however, stroke can be a side effect.

HTN is treated with antihypertensive agents, and low-dose aspirin may have a therapeutic effect in large-vessel vasculitis. Antiplatelet agents, heparin, and warfarin can be used to prevent ischemic stroke.

CLINICAL CONCEPT

Pregnancy can exacerbate HTN and cardiovascular complications in Takayasu's arteritis, leading to high rates of morbidity and mortality.

Polyarteritis Nodosa

PAN is a rare, systemic, necrotizing inflammation of the small and medium arteries that can occur anywhere in the body. The vascular inflammation leads to aneurysms, thrombosis, ischemia, and infarction in the body's organs.

Epidemiology. PAN has an incidence of about 3 to 4.5 cases per 100,000 persons annually. It occurs in men more often than women and predominately affects individuals aged 45 to 65 years of age.

Etiology. The etiology of PAN is unknown. However, viral infections, including HIV infection, hepatitis C virus infection, and particularly hepatitis B virus (HBV) infection, have been associated with PAN. HBV was once the cause of up to 30% of PAN cases. However, with the advent of hepatitis B vaccine, the incidence of HBV-PAN has significantly decreased to fewer than 8% of all PAN cases. Other infectious organisms that are associated with PAN include tuberculosis, varicella-zoster virus, parvovirus B19, cytomegalovirus, human T-cell leukemia virus, streptococcal species, *Klebsiella* species, *Pseudomonas* species, *Yersinia* species, *Toxoplasma gondii, Rickettsia,* trichinosis, and sarcosporidiosis. It is unclear how these microorganisms may cause PAN. Malignancies, rheumatoid arthritis, and Sjögren's syndrome have also been associated with PAN.

Pathophysiology. PAN is an inflammatory disorder found in arteries, mainly at bifurcation points where arteries branch off from each other. Inflammation starts in the interior lining of the artery but eventually involves the entire arterial wall. The inflammation destroys the entire wall of the artery and leads to necrosis. The weakened arteries develop aneurysms that rupture and hemorrhage. Thrombi often develop at the sites of the inflammation. With progression of the disease, the arterial wall thickens and can protrude into the lumen to cause obstruction of the artery. Arterial obstruction can lead to tissue ischemia or infarction in organs.

Clinical Presentation. PAN is a spectrum of disease ranging from single-organ involvement to widespread multiorgan failure. The patient first presents with vague, flu-like symptoms of fever, malaise, fatigue, anorexia, myalgia, and arthralgias. With progression of the disorder, patients often complain of symptoms related to TIAs, particularly monocular blindness. Arteritis of the cerebral arteries can lead to cerebral hemorrhages, encephalopathy, and seizures.

Peripheral nerve inflammation develops in as many as 60% of patients. The neuropathy can involve motor or sensory nerves and is often asymmetrical, affecting one limb more than the other. Skin involvement that causes rash, cutaneous ischemia and infarction, gangrene, and Raynaud's phenomenon are common in PAN. GI involvement can present as abdominal pain, nausea, and vomiting, with or without obvious GI bleeding. Bowel ischemia and infarctions can occur.

Many patients with PAN suffer renal involvement. Renal ischemia causes flank pain and HTN. Renal failure develops in a small percentage of patients and may require dialysis. PAN can also affect the coronary arteries, leading to myocardial ischemia and infarction. Ophthalmic artery involvement presents as blurred vision. Infarction of genitourinary organs, such as the testicle and ovary, can occur.

Diagnosis. Angiography, CT, and MRI scans are used to examine the body for characteristic lesions. Aneurysms are often seen in the liver, kidney, and mesenteric arteries. When possible, a biopsy of involved tissue is collected to aid in the diagnosis. Biopsy reveals a necrotizing inflammation of the artery walls. Electromyography (EMG) studies may reveal neurological and muscle involvement. Nerve biopsy characteristically reveals axonal degeneration and fiber loss.

Treatment. Currently, corticosteroids are the standard treatment. The immunosuppressants cyclophosphamide, methotrexate, azathioprine, or mycophenolate mofetil can be added to the regimen when steroids do not yield results or when PAN includes major organ involvement. For patients with PAN associated with HBV, antiviral medications, steroids, and plasmapheresis are used. Rituximab, an anti–TNF-alfa medication, and tocilizumab, an anti-IL medication, are possible alternative treatments in cases of refractory or difficult-to-treat PAN.

Kawasaki's Disease

Kawasaki's disease, or Kawasaki's syndrome, is a type of vasculitis that affects children. The disorder has also been called mucocutaneous lymph node syndrome and infantile periarteritis nodosa.

Epidemiology. Epidemics of Kawasaki's disease primarily occur in the late winter and spring. In the United States, approximately 3,000 children are hospitalized annually for Kawasaki's disease. The disorder occurs most commonly in Asian children, especially those of Japanese descent, and is slightly more common in males than in females. Approximately 90% to 95% of cases occur in children younger than 10 years. In the United States, the incidence peaks in children aged 18 to 24 months.

Etiology. The etiology of Kawasaki's disease is unknown, but most evidence points to an infectious causative agent. Possible infectious causes include parvovirus B19, meningococcus, *Mycoplasma pneumoniae, Klebsiella pneumoniae* bacteremia, adenovirus, cytomegalovirus, parainfluenza type 3 virus, rotavirus infection, measles, Epstein–Barr virus, mite-associated bacteria, and tick-borne diseases. Some studies theorize that Kawasaki's disease is caused by a ribonucleic acid virus that enters through the respiratory route and causes disease in genetically predisposed individuals.

Studies also show that autoimmunity and genetic predisposition may be involved in the etiology. A genetic predisposition is based on the fact that siblings of affected children are 10 to 20 times more likely than the general population to develop Kawasaki's disease. Twenty-three genetic mutations are significantly correlated with Kawasaki's disease susceptibility. Ten genetic mutations are significantly associated with the incidence of coronary artery lesions in Kawasaki's disease.

Pathophysiology. Kawasaki's disease is a vascular inflammatory disease that occurs most prominently in the coronary arteries but also occurs in veins, capillaries, small arterioles, and larger arteries. Early in the disease, the arterial endothelium and muscle wall become edematous. WBCs rush to the area, followed by CD8 lymphocytes and immunoglobulin A–producing plasma cells. The WBCs secrete various cytokines, including TNF; VEGF; IL-1, IL-4, and IL-6; and metalloproteinases that target the endothelium of arteries and cause vascular damage.

In severely affected vessels, necrosis occurs in smooth muscle cells in the walls. The artery walls weaken and layers can separate and split, leading to aneurysms. With time, the active inflammatory cells are replaced by fibroblasts and monocytes. Fibrous tissue begins to form within the vessel wall, and the inner lining thickens. The arterial vessel eventually becomes narrowed and obstructed by a thrombus. Commonly, death occurs from an MI secondary to thrombosis of a coronary aneurysm or from rupture of a large coronary aneurysm.

Clinical Presentation. Most children with Kawasaki's disease present with fever. Affected children are usually treated with antibiotics, but fever persists. Fever can be accompanied by vomiting, decreased oral intake, cough, diarrhea, rhinorrhea, abdominal pain, and joint pain. There are four stages: acute, subacute, convalescent, and chronic (see Box 15-3).

BOX 15-3. The Four Stages of Kawasaki's Disease

STAGE 1: ACUTE FEBRILE STAGE

The acute stage begins with an abrupt onset of fever and lasts approximately 7 to 14 days. The fever is typically high-spiking and remittent, with peak temperatures ranging from 102°F to 104°F (39°C to 40°C) or higher. This fever may not be responsive to antibiotics or antipyretics and can persist for up to 3 to 4 weeks if untreated. However, with appropriate therapy, high-dose aspirin, and IV immunoglobulin, the fever typically remits within 48 hours.

In addition to fever, signs and symptoms may include bilateral conjunctivitis (90%), anterior uveitis (70%), perianal erythema (70%), erythema and edema on the hands and feet, strawberry tongue, and lip fissures. Hepatic, renal, and gastrointestinal dysfunction can occur. Myocarditis, pericarditis, and lymphadenopathy (75%) occur. Commonly there is a single, enlarged, cervical lymph node measuring approximately 1.5 cm.

STAGE 2: SUBACUTE STAGE

The subacute stage begins when the fevers have abated, and it continues until week 4 to 6. The hallmarks of this stage are desquamation of the digits, thrombocytosis (the platelet count may exceed 1 million/mcL), and the development of coronary aneurysms. The risk for sudden death is highest at this stage.

Other characteristics of the subacute stage are persistent irritability, anorexia, and conjunctival injection.

Persistence of fever beyond 2 to 3 weeks may be an indication of recrudescent Kawasaki's disease. If fever persists, the outcome is less favorable because of a greater risk of cardiac complications.

STAGE 3: CONVALESCENT PHASE

The convalescent phase is marked by complete resolution of clinical signs of the illness, usually within 3 months of presentation. During this stage, most of the clinical findings resolve; however, deep transverse grooves across the nails (Beau's lines) may become apparent 1 to 2 months after the onset of fever.

During the convalescent stage, cardiac abnormalities may still be apparent. Smaller coronary artery aneurysms tend to resolve on their own (60% of cases), but larger aneurysms may expand, and MI may occur. In patients whose echocardiograms were previously normal, however, detection of new aneurysms is unusual after week 8 of the illness.

STAGE 4: CHRONIC PHASE

This stage is of clinical importance only in patients who have developed cardiac complications. Its duration is of lifetime significance because an aneurysm formed in childhood may rupture in adulthood. In some cases of aneurysms rupturing in adult life, careful reviews of past medical histories have revealed febrile childhood illnesses of unknown etiology.

Diagnosis. No specific laboratory test is used to diagnose Kawasaki's disease; however, ESR, CRP, and alpha 1–antitrypsin levels are elevated at first. They usually return to normal 6 to 10 weeks after the onset of the illness. On CBC, mild-to-moderate, normocytic, normochromic anemia is observed in the acute stage. The WBC is moderate to high, with 50% of patients having a WBC count greater than 15,000/mcL. The CBC shows a left shift, which indicates immature WBCs are rising within the bloodstream in an acute infection.

During the subacute stage, platelet count increases in the second and third week. Platelet counts average 700,000/mcL, but levels as high as 2 million have been observed.

In the convalescent stage, the levels of platelets and other inflammatory mediators begin to return to normal values. Laboratory values may require 6 to 8 weeks to normalize.

Levels of antineutrophil cytoplasmic antibodies, antiendothelial cell antibodies, antinuclear antibody, and rheumatoid factor are all within the reference range. Culture results are negative, as are tests for adenovirus. Urinalysis may show mild-to-moderate numbers of WBCs and proteinuria. Two urine biomarkers—proteins called meprin and filamin—may be present.

Echocardiography is the main diagnostic study used to evaluate for coronary artery aneurysms. ECGs should be obtained at the time of Kawasaki's disease diagnosis, at 2 weeks, and at 6 to 8 weeks after the onset of the illness. These may need to be performed more frequently in high-risk patients. MRI, MRA, and CT scanning are other noninvasive tests that can be used to evaluate coronary artery abnormalities.

On ECG, tachycardia, prolonged PR interval, ST-T wave changes, and decreased R waves may indicate myocarditis. Q waves or ST-T wave changes may indicate MI. Cardiac enzyme and troponin levels are elevated if MI is present.

Some patients may require cardiac catheterization and angiography. Coronary CT angiography and MRA may also be used to evaluate the coronary arteries.

Liver enzyme tests may show elevated serum transaminase values in 40% of affected patients. Elevated alanine aminotransferase levels can indicate serious disease. Bilirubin values are elevated in 10% of affected patients.

A chest x-ray should be done to evaluate for cardiomegaly or pneumonitis or to confirm existence of heart failure.

If the patient has joint involvement, an arthrocentesis may be indicated to analyze synovial fluid. Synovial fluid analysis in patients usually shows numerous WBCs, ranging from 125,000 to 300,000/mcL, with normal glucose levels and negative culture results.

Lumbar puncture may be indicated in patients with signs of meningitis; 50% of children with Kawasaki's disease show evidence of aseptic meningitis on lumbar puncture.

Some children present with many of the clinical signs of Kawasaki's disease but do not have all the required diagnostic criteria. These children are diagnosed with "incomplete" Kawasaki's disease.

Treatment. The aim of treatment for Kawasaki's disease is to prevent CAD and to relieve symptoms. Intravenous immunoglobulin (IVIg) and aspirin are the major treatments and have been shown to decrease autoantibodies, decrease platelet aggregation, and diminish the proliferation of inflammatory mediators. If IVIg is not successful, corticosteroids and the anti-TNF agent infliximab (Remicade) are used. Cyclophosphamide and methotrexate have also been used with some success in IVIg-resistant disease. Antiplatelets and anticoagulants may be needed to prevent thromboses.

Raynaud's Disease

Raynaud's disease causes vasospasm of the arterioles of the hands and sometimes the feet. It is a primary disorder, whereas Raynaud's phenomenon is secondary to other diseases. Raynaud's phenomenon can also occur from exposure to cold or vibration.

Epidemiology. Raynaud's disease occurs in 11% of women and 8% of men and does not usually cause serious complications. However, in rare cases, it can cause ischemia of an affected body part. Raynaud's disease usually occurs in the second or third decade of life. Raynaud's phenomenon is commonly a sign of autoimmune disease, including scleroderma (progressive systemic sclerosis), systemic lupus erythematosus, and hyperviscosity syndromes.

Etiology. The disease affects primarily young women and is often precipitated by cold temperature or stress. There may also be a genetic predisposition to the disorder.

Pathophysiology. The pathophysiology is unclear in Raynaud's disease, but it is theorized to be an exaggerated reflex sympathetic stimulus that causes vasoconstriction. There is endothelial dysfunction, deficiency of the vasodilatory mediator NO, and high levels of endothelin-1, a potent vasoconstrictor. High levels of circulating angiotensin are also present, which have vasoconstrictive effects. Research indicates that patients with Raynaud's disease or phenomenon repeatedly undergo cutaneous vasoconstriction in response to many stressful stimuli.

An important neuropeptide, calcitonin gene–related peptide, is a potent vasodilator secreted by nerves that supply blood vessels. In patients with Raynaud's disease, there is a diminished number of calcitonin gene–related peptide–releasing neurons in skin biopsy samples. Neuropeptide Y, a potent vasoconstrictor, is increased in Raynaud's phenomenon secondary to scleroderma.

In Raynaud's disease, there is increased platelet activation and aggregation. In addition, an increased production of platelet thromboxane A2, a potent vasoconstrictor, has been found in patients. There is also an impaired fibrolytic system that contributes to vascular obstruction.

Clinical Presentation. Signs of disease occur bilaterally and include pain, blanching of the skin, and numbness and coolness of the fingers and toes. Lack of oxygen to the tissue can cause cyanosis. When vasospasm subsides, blood flow returns to the extremity, causing rubor, paresthesia, and throbbing pain.

 CLINICAL CONCEPT

In both Raynaud's disease and Raynaud's phenomenon, there is a classic tricolor change of white (pallor), blue (cyanosis), and red (rubor) in the fingers.

Diagnosis/Treatment. Diagnosis involves a wide variety of laboratory tests to rule out autoimmune disease. Treatment is aimed at prevention of vasospasm by avoiding precipitating factors. Smoking cigarettes and exposure to cold should be avoided. Stress-reduction practices, such as yoga or meditation, are recommended. CCBs have been shown to be most effective; high doses may be necessary.

Thromboangiitis Obliterans

TAO, also known as Buerger's disease, is an inflammatory disorder of unknown etiology where the small and medium arteries and veins of the hands and feet are affected by inflammation, vasospasm, and thrombus formation. Thrombus formation most likely occurs as a result of reduced blood flow through the spasmodic, inflamed vessels. There may also be an autoimmune component to this disorder.

Epidemiology. TAO is mostly found in young adult males between ages 20 and 45 years who smoke. Its prevalence has been estimated at 12.6 to 20 cases per 100,000 population. Incidence has been decreasing because of the overall trend of smoking cessation in the United States; 43% of patients with the disease who continue to smoke develop ischemia, necrosis, and gangrene of the fingers, which then require amputation. Amputation risk in long-term management of

TAO is 25% 5 years after diagnosis, 38% after 10 years, and 46% after 20 years.

Etiology. The etiology of TAO is unknown; however, cigarette smoking is known to initiate the disease. Studies show that individuals with the genetic mutation MyD88 (myeloid differentiation factor-88) have a defect in innate immunity and high susceptibility to endothelial injury.

Pathophysiology. The disease mechanism underlying TAO is unknown. It is theorized that smoking is a trigger of an immunological reaction that leads to vasospasms and inflammatory thrombi of the fingers. The pathological processes in TAO include endothelial cell injury, inflammation, autoimmunity, and thrombosis. There is migratory thrombophlebitis and hypercoagulability, which can cause limb ischemia. Patients demonstrate hypersensitivity to tobacco, elevated antiendothelial cell antibody titers, antineutrophil antibody titers, and impaired peripheral vasodilation.

Clinical Presentation. Symptoms include a deep red skin color caused by increased capillary blood flow. Dusky or cyanotic skin color also occurs as deoxygenated blood collects in the tissues. Thin, shiny skin is a result of chronic nutrient deficiency to the tissues. There is palpable coolness of the extremities and pain. Raynaud's phenomenon is often seen with the disorder. Patients may also complain of claudication of the hands, feet, forearm, and calves. Other signs include severe ischemia of fingertips, trophic nail changes, painful ulcerations, and susceptibility to gangrene.

Diagnosis. No specific laboratory tests confirm or exclude the diagnosis of TAO. The primary goal of the laboratory tests is to exclude other disease processes. Tests for antinuclear antibody, rheumatoid factor, anticentromere antibody, and antiphospholipid antibodies are done.

Angiogram is the best diagnostic test in TAO because it demonstrates the occlusive lesions of the small and medium vessels. Angiogram can show that arteriosclerosis is not the primary disease causing the vascular occlusion. There are characteristic branches of blood vessels around areas of occlusion in TAO known as "corkscrew" collaterals.

Treatment. Treatment for TAO includes smoking cessation, vasodilators to reduce vasospasm, and exercises to promote blood flow. Iloprost, a prostacyclin analogue, is widely used to reduce pain due to ischemia. Antiplatelet agents and anticoagulants are also used to counteract the hypercoagulability. CCBs and pentoxifylline can reduce vasospasms. Bosentan, an endothelial blocking agent, may be effective, but more studies are necessary. Sympathectomy can relieve pain. Revascularization procedures, such as surgical bypass grafts, have also been used to enhance circulation in limb ischemia. Necrosis and gangrene of the fingers or toes require amputation.

Arterial Ulcers

Arterial ulcers are ischemic skin wounds that develop gradually because of lack of blood flow to the extremity. Obstructive arteriosclerosis causes lack of oxygen and blood delivered to the lower extremity. The extremity is pale, and pulses may be absent or diminished. Toenails are thickened and yellowed, and capillary refill is delayed. The leg is often painful, and elevation worsens pain. Dangling the leg brings circulation into the leg and improves pain and circulation. Arterial ulcers are usually located distally at the tips of the toes, the heel, or the lateral malleolus. Diagnosis is usually made by clinical examination in a patient with known PAD. Patients often have diabetes and require strict glucose control. Treatments for arterial ulcers vary, depending on the severity of the arterial disease. Antibiotics may be needed to prevent infection. Endovascular therapy or bypass surgery to restore circulation to the affected leg may be required. It is important to protect the skin from further injury and breakdown. The patient should avoid pressure and weight-bearing on the affected leg. Surgical débridement, which is the removal of necrotic tissue from wounds, is commonly done to accelerate healing. Frequently, special shoes or orthotic devices are required.

Chapter Summary

- The artery wall is composed of three distinct layers: tunica intima, tunica media, and tunica externa.
- The tunica intima is composed of endothelial cells that are metabolically active and exposed to blood constituents that are potentially damaging.

- High BP, high lipids, high glucose levels, free radicals, and high homocysteine levels in the blood can cause endothelial injury, which is the inciting event that starts the process of atherogenesis.
- LDL is the type of cholesterol that is deposited on artery walls. Optimally, levels should be less than 100 mg/dL.

- HDL is the type of cholesterol that is excreted. Optimally, levels should be greater than or equal to 60 mg/dL. HDL of greater than or equal to 60 mg/dL is cardioprotective.
- Hyperlipidemia, which consists of high total cholesterol, high LDL, and elevated triglycerides, predisposes individuals to atherosclerosis.
- The therapeutic value of exercise includes raising HDL ("good cholesterol") and stimulating angiogenesis (building of collateral blood vessels), which over time lowers BP.
- 2017 AHA/ACC Blood Pressure Categories include:
  - Normal: Less than 120/80 mm Hg
  - Elevated: Systolic between 120 and 129 **and** diastolic less than 80
  - Stage 1 HTN: Systolic between 130 and 139 **or** diastolic between 80 and 89
  - Stage 2 HTN: Systolic at least 140 **or** diastolic at least 90 mm Hg
  - Hypertensive crisis: Systolic over 180 and/or diastolic over 120, with patients needing prompt changes in medication if there are no other indications of problems, or immediate hospitalization if there are signs of organ damage
- According to the JNC-8 BP guidelines, the BP goal for individuals older than age 60 years is <150/90.
- The target organs of HTN include the retina, kidney, heart, brain, and peripheral arteries of the extremities.
- HTN causes arterial damage throughout the body, LVH, hemorrhagic stroke, retinopathy, and glomerular injury.
- Many individuals with HTN require two or more types of medications to control their BP, and individuals tend to prefer it if multiple medications are combined into a single pill.
- Artery walls can become weakened and form aneurysms. Turbulent blood flow within an aneurysm can be heard as a bruit through the stethoscope.
- An AAA, the most common type of aneurysm, is usually asymptomatic until the time of rupture.
- Aortic dissection is a disorder where the layers of the wall of the aorta tear and split apart. Blood then collects in between the walls of the aorta.
- PAD, arterial disease in a lower extremity, is common in hyperlipidemia, HTN, and diabetes.
- The symptoms of PAD in a lower extremity include pulselessness, intermittent claudication (pain), pallor, paresthesias, paresis (weakness), and palpable coolness.
- An ABI of less than 1 indicates PAD.
- Vasculitis is inflammation of the arterial vessels that is often caused by autoimmune disease.
- Raynaud's phenomenon is a tricolor change in the fingertips from white (pallor), to blue (cyanosis), and then to red (erythema) when exposed to cold or stress.
- TAO is a vasculitis that is exacerbated by cigarette smoking.

Making the Connections

Disorder and Pathophysiology

Hyperlipidemia | Elevated total cholesterol in the bloodstream caused by excess ingestion of fatty foods or liver synthesis of cholesterol. Specifically, elevated LDL and elevated triglycerides in the bloodstream are harmful to cardiovascular health. LDL is deposited on arterial walls, leading to the formation of atherosclerotic plaque. Low HDL in the bloodstream is also harmful because HDL normally carries cholesterol away to be excreted. All these conditions predispose individuals to atherosclerosis and cardiovascular disease.

Signs and Symptoms	Physical Assessment Findings	Diagnostic Testing	Treatment
None.	Xanthoma. Xanthelasma. Retinal blood vessel changes in some affected persons—copper-silver wiring, cotton wool spots. Arcus senilis.	Total cholesterol greater than 200 mg/dL. LDL greater than 100 mg/dL. HDL less than 40 mg/dL. Triglycerides greater than 150 mg/dL.	Diet low in fat to reduce cholesterol ingested. Exercise daily to raise HDL. Antilipidemia agents, such as statin medications, that reduce liver synthesis of cholesterol.

Making the Connections—cont'd

Signs and Symptoms	Physical Assessment Findings	Diagnostic Testing	Treatment
Hypertension	Elevated BP, which causes endothelial injury and increases susceptibility to atherosclerosis. HTN directly targets the small arteries of the retina, glomerulus, and brain, as well as peripheral arteries throughout the body. High pressure in cerebral arteries can cause stroke. It targets the heart by causing high aortic resistance against the left ventricle, which causes LVH. LVH is a risk factor for MI.			
None.	Headache in some affected persons. BP greater than 130/80 mm Hg.* According to JNC-8, HTN in adults older than age 60 years is ≥150/90. S_4 heart sound. Retinal blood vessel changes in some affected persons—arteriovenous nicking, flame hemorrhages caused by retinal artery rupture.	Increased renin levels in some affected persons, which in turn will cause constant cycling of the RAAS. ECG shows LVH in some affected persons.	Low-salt, low-fat diet. Daily exercise will lower BP over the long term. Antihypertensive agents, such as beta blockers, decrease HR and inhibit vasoconstriction. Diuretics decrease the water content of blood. Calcium antagonists inhibit vasoconstriction. ACE inhibitors, renin inhibitors, or ARBs are used.
Atherosclerosis	Widespread arterial wall plaque composed of lipid, platelets, fibroblasts, and WBCs, which protrudes into arterial lumen. The arteriosclerotic plaque hardens over time and calcifies. It then can rupture into pieces that travel as emboli and can lodge in smaller-diameter arteries to cause ischemia in tissue.			
None.	Retinal blood vessel changes in some affected persons—copper-silver wiring, cotton wool spots. Carotid, aortic, or renal artery bruits are found in some affected persons.	Elevated hs-CRP. Total cholesterol greater than 200 mg/dL. LDL greater than 130 mg/dL in most affected persons. HDL less than 40 mg/dL in most affected persons. Elevated blood homocysteine level.	Diet low in fat, low in salt to diminish formation of cholesterol and decrease BP. Antilipidemic medications. Folic acid to lower homocysteine. Anticoagulant, such as aspirin. Keep BP low. Exercise daily.
Peripheral Arterial Disease	Arteriosclerosis within the lower extremities that obstructs blood flow to the legs.			
Pain: Intermittent claudication, especially with muscle activity. Pallor of leg. Paresthesia. Palpable coolness of leg.	Pallor. Palpable coolness. Pulselessness. Paresis or paralysis. Pain with activity and on elevation.	Elevated hs-CRP. Total cholesterol greater than 200 mg/dL. LDL greater than 130 mg/dL in most affected persons. HDL less than 40 mg/dL in most affected persons. Elevated blood homocysteine level. ABI less than 1.	Diet low in fat, low in salt to diminish formation of cholesterol and decrease BP. Antilipidemic medications. Folic acid to lower homocysteine. Anticoagulant, such as aspirin. Keep BP low. Exercise daily to build collateral branches of leg arteries. Vasodilator medications. Revascularization treatments; endovascular angioplasty or surgical bypass graft.

Continued

Making the Connections—cont'd

Signs and Symptoms	Physical Assessment Findings	Diagnostic Testing	Treatment
Aneurysm | Weakening of an arterial wall with a localized area of dilation. Blood flow is turbulent in these areas, thrombosis is more common in these areas, and rupture of the aneurysm can be fatal.			
Cerebral aneurysm most commonly has no symptoms. Headache, seizure, or abrupt loss of consciousness occurs with rupture. If aneurysm places pressure on cranial nerve, then there will be cranial nerve dysfunction. AAA: nausea; vomiting; bowel or bladder disturbances; back, flank, or abdominal pain. May have sudden severe pain and symptoms of shock with rupture.	Cerebral aneurysm: Presentation may include headache or cranial nerve dysfunction. May have seizure activity or abrupt loss of consciousness with rupture. In AAA, pulsatile mass may be palpated or visible.	Bruit may be heard over an aortic aneurysm. Chest x-ray can often show thoracic aortic aneurysm. CT scan can show aortic aneurysm. MRA can show cerebral arterial aneurysm.	Keep BP low. Use surgical intervention to clip off cerebral aneurysm or place stent or graft within aorta to repair aneurysm.
Aortic Dissection | A disorder that causes splitting of layers of the wall of the aorta. The wall develops a gap that fills with blood.			
Sudden chest pain that radiates to the back. Possible loss of consciousness.	Sudden hypotension, loss of consciousness. Pallor. Tachycardia. Difference of 20 mm Hg BP over brachial arteries of two arms.	Chest x-ray. TEE. Angiography. MRI.	Regulate BP. Pain medication. Immediate surgery to repair aortic wall.
Raynaud's Disease | Vasospastic disorder of the arterioles and arteries of the hands and feet. Often vasospasms occur because of autoimmune disease; antigen–antibody complexes are deposited in tissues.			
Pain, numbness, and coolness of the extremity, beginning distally.	Tricolor changes, blanching, and cyanosis followed by rubor with return of blood flow when vasospasm abates.	Diagnostic studies should investigate if an autoimmune disorder is present: CBC with differential, liver function tests, renal function tests, serum glucose (fasting), ESR, CRP, antinuclear antibody, rheumatoid factor, anti-centromere antibody, and antiphospholipid antibodies. Angiogram: best diagnostic imaging test.	Smoking cigarettes and exposure to cold should be avoided. CCBs and other vasodilators are used. Sympathectomy may be carried out if noninvasive medical measures are unsuccessful.

Making the Connections–cont'd

Signs and Symptoms	Physical Assessment Findings	Diagnostic Testing	Treatment

Vasculitis | Inflammation and vasospastic condition of small and medium arteries, which can be caused by bacteria, virus, or autoimmune disease. The walls of the arteries become degraded, necrotic, and develop thrombi and aneurysms. Examples of vasculitis include PAN, Kawasaki's disease, and TAO.

Signs and Symptoms	Physical Assessment Findings	Diagnostic Testing	Treatment
Depending on the location of vasculitis, symptoms usually include systemic manifestations, such as fever, and symptoms localized to the artery involved.	Signs and symptoms depend on the specific arteries involved. Coronary artery vasculitis can cause MI. Vasculitis of a cerebral artery can cause stroke and seizures. Vasculitis of the renal artery can cause renal failure. Vasculitis of the fingers and toes can cause ischemia and gangrene.	Angiography. MRI. CT scan. EMG. Biopsy of vessel.	PAN: Immunosuppressive agents; rituximab, an anti-TNF alfa medication; and tocilizumab, an anti-interleukin medication. Kawasaki's disease: IVIg and aspirin; corticosteroids; anti-TNF agent, infliximab; cyclophosphamide, and methotrexate. Antiplatelets and anticoagulants. TAO: Iloprost, antiplatelet agents and anticoagulants, CCBs, pentoxifylline, bosentan, sympathectomy. Revascularization.

Bibliography

Available online at fadavis.com

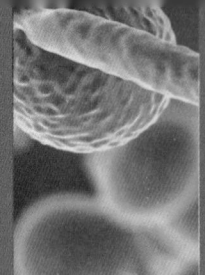

Ischemic Heart Disease and Conduction Disorders

Learning Objectives

Upon completion of this chapter, the student will be able to:

- Describe the coronary arteries and how the processes of arteriosclerosis and atherosclerosis lead to ischemic heart disease.
- Identify the risk factors of ischemic heart disease.
- Differentiate between the specific disorders that can cause acute coronary syndrome.
- Distinguish between the signs and symptoms of acute coronary syndrome versus chronic stable coronary artery disease.

- Discuss the pathogenic mechanism of myocardial infarction and potential complications.
- Understand the laboratory tests and procedures used to diagnose myocardial infarction.
- List pharmacological agents used to treat acute angina pectoris, myocardial infarction, and chronic stable angina pectoris.
- Describe the inflammatory processes that can affect the heart and potential complications.

Key Terms

Action potential

Acute coronary syndrome (ACS)

Anginal equivalents

Angina pectoris

Beck triad

Cardiac tamponade

Cardiac troponin I (cTnI)

Chronic stable angina

Coronary artery bypass graft (CABG)

Coronary artery disease (CAD)

Coronary computed tomographic angiography (CCTA)

Depolarization

Dressler's syndrome

Dysrhythmias

Electrocardiogram (ECG)

Endocardium

Epicardium

High sensitivity cardiac troponin (hs-cTn) assay

Infective endocarditis (IE)

Ischemia with no obstructive coronary artery (INOCA)

Microvascular angina

Myocardial infarction (MI)

Myocardium

Non-ST segment elevation myocardial infarction (NSTEMI)

Percutaneous coronary intervention (PCI)

Percutaneous transluminal coronary angioplasty (PCTA)

Pericardial effusion

Premature ventricular contraction (PVC)

Pulsus paradoxus

Septic emboli

ST segment elevation myocardial infarction (STEMI)

Unstable angina

The heart is a muscular pump approximately the size of a fist. It sits left of the midline in the chest, within the mediastinum of the thoracic cavity, a space between the lungs and beneath the sternum. The broadest part of the heart, called the base, is at the upper right, where the great vessels, including the aortic arch and pulmonary arteries, enter and leave the heart. The pointed end of the heart, called the apex, is at the lower left.

Off the aortic arch are the coronary arteries, which perfuse the myocardium and supply the heart muscle with blood. Arteriosclerosis and atherosclerosis commonly affect these arteries and can obstruct vital blood to the heart muscle. Obstruction of a coronary artery can lead to **acute coronary syndrome (ACS)**, which is a disorder caused by myocardial ischemia. If myocardial ischemia is prolonged, **myocardial infarction (MI)** occurs, which can cause death.

Researchers have been investigating coronary arteriosclerosis, atherosclerosis, myocardial ischemia, and MI for more than 50 years. In that time, many technological advances have been made in the diagnosis and medical and surgical treatment of cardiovascular disease. In fact, many persons survive their first or second MI. However, despite the advances in medical technology, arteriosclerosis/atherosclerosis remains the number-one killer of much of the world's population. Heart disease is the cause of death in 25% of the U.S. population, and **coronary artery disease (CAD)** is the most common form of heart disease.

Structure and Function of the Heart

It is essential to understand the structure and function of the cardiovascular system in order to comprehend the consequences of heart disease.

Heart anatomy is sometimes difficult to understand because the aorta and pulmonary artery sit upon the base in a twisted fashion. To understand the heart's anatomy, it is useful to look at an image of the heart with the great vessels untangled (see Fig. 16-1).

The Heart Wall

The heart is composed of three layers of tissue: the epicardium, myocardium, and endocardium (Fig. 16-2). The **epicardium** is the outer layer that covers the heart and great vessels and then folds over to form the double-walled pericardium, which has two layers,

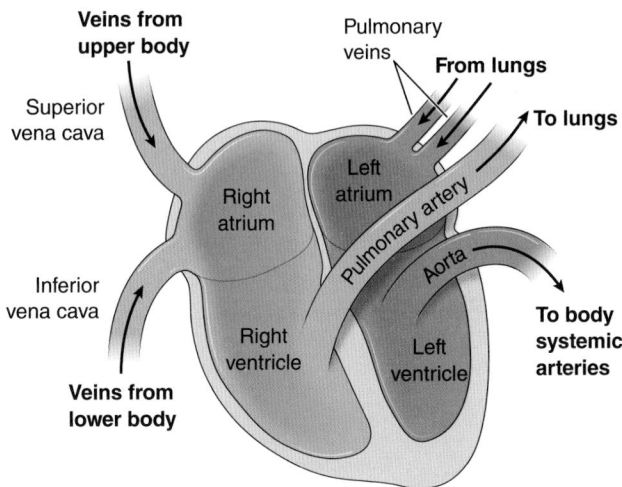

FIGURE 16-1. The SVC and IVC bring venous blood up from the body into the right atrium. The right atrium moves blood into the right ventricle, which pumps blood into the pulmonary artery, which then delivers it to the lungs for oxygenation. After oxygenation, the blood returns via the pulmonary veins into the left atrium, where it then moves into the left ventricle before being pumped into the aorta to the rest of the body. The arteries gradually become arterioles, which supply the capillary beds of all tissues; the veins then bring blood out of the tissues back up to the heart.

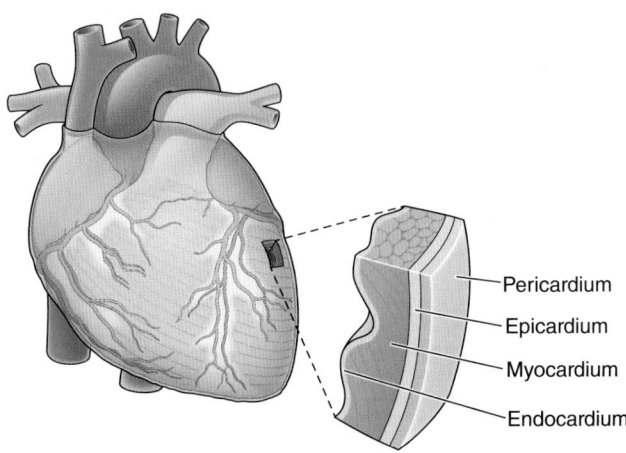

FIGURE 16-2. Dissection of the heart wall: pericardium, epicardium, myocardium, and endocardium.

the visceral and parietal layers. Between the visceral layer and parietal layer of pericardial membrane is the pericardial cavity. This space contains approximately 30 to 50 mL of serous fluid, which acts as a lubricant to minimize friction as the heart contracts and relaxes. When the chest is opened, the heart lies beneath the sternum, covered by the pericardium. The coronary arteries are interwoven within the heart's muscular layer and are vaguely apparent as they are covered by the translucent pericardial membrane.

The **myocardium** is the heart's muscular layer that contracts; it is controlled by the autonomic nervous system. This thick wall of cardiac muscle is different from smooth or skeletal muscle. Cardiac muscle cells are densely packed together and separated by gap junctions that are low-resistance pathways from one cardiac cell to another. When electrically stimulated, the myocardium behaves as a single unit rather than a group of isolated cells. An impulse travels rapidly so that the heart muscle contracts as one unit. Compared with other kinds of muscle, cardiac muscle can store very little calcium. It relies heavily on an influx of extracellular calcium ions for contraction.

The **endocardium** is a very thin, three-layered membrane that lines the interior heart and covers the valves. The innermost layer consists of endothelial cells supported by a thin layer of fibrous tissue, similar to the inner lining of an artery. The middle layer consists of dense fibrous tissue with elastin. The outer layer is denser connective tissue that contains blood vessels and nerves continuous with the myocardium. The four heart valves, which include the mitral, aortic, tricuspid, and pulmonic valves, are part of the endothelium.

Coronary Circulation

When the chest is opened and one can look straight down onto the heart, the coronary arteries are obvious as they pierce through the myocardium. There are two major coronary arteries: the right and the left main coronary artery. These arteries arise from the aortic arch just as the aorta arises from the left ventricle of the heart (see Fig. 16-3). The left main coronary artery branches off into the left anterior descending (LAD) artery, which travels down the heart's vertical axis along the left ventricle, and the circumflex artery, which travels toward the back of the heart. As the major arteries pass through the myocardium, they give rise to smaller branches that supply different areas of the muscle. The LAD artery supplies the left ventricle and is the artery most commonly involved in MI.

The right coronary artery arises from the aortic arch and travels down over the right atrium. It then moves down along the right ventricle and branches off into the posterior descending artery, which travels around to the back and supplies the posterior portion of the heart.

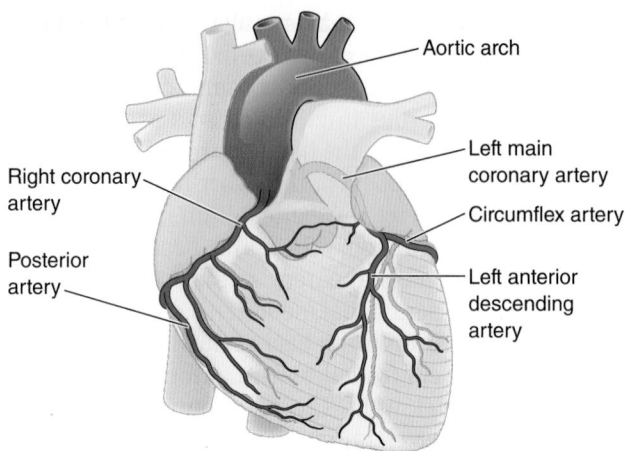

FIGURE 16-3. How the coronary arteries originate from the aorta.

Coronary artery anatomy is similar in most individuals. Athletic persons tend to have more branches off the left and right coronary artery, as exercise stimulates the construction of collateral vessels. These extra branches benefit the heart because the collaterals provide more avenues of circulation to the heart muscle. In arteriosclerosis and atherosclerosis, where there is possible obstruction of coronary blood vessels, the additional paths of circulation are of benefit (see Fig. 16-4).

The Chambers of the Heart

The heart contains four chambers:

1. Right atrium
2. Left atrium
3. Right ventricle
4. Left ventricle

Atria are thin-layered chambers that contract and relax. These chambers sit on top of the stronger-walled ventricles that also contract and relax. The right atrium

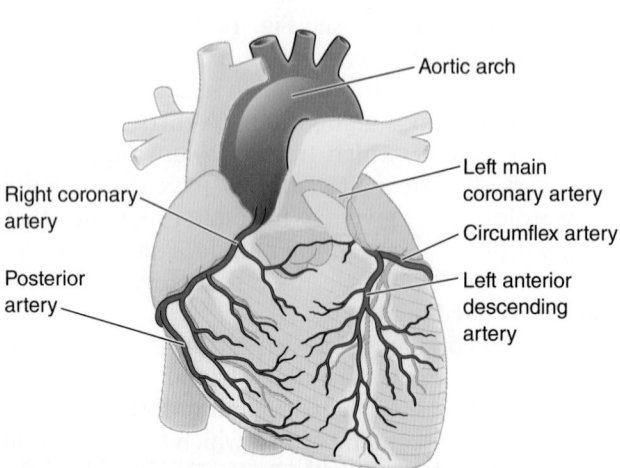

FIGURE 16-4. The physically fit heart has many collateral branches off the major coronary arteries.

collects blood from the superior vena cava (SVC) and inferior vena cava (IVC), the major veins of the body. The right atrium empties its blood into the right ventricle, which ejects its contents into the pulmonary artery. The left atrium empties its blood into the left ventricle, which ejects its contents into the aorta. The pulmonary artery is the entrance into the pulmonary circulatory system, and the aorta is the entrance into the systemic circulatory system (see Fig. 16-5).

Pulmonary and Systemic Circulation

The circulatory system can be divided into two parts: the pulmonary circulation and systemic circulation. The pulmonary system moves blood from the pulmonary artery into the lungs and allows oxygenation and gas exchange at the capillary bed. It then moves blood into the pulmonary vein, which empties into the left atrium. This is the only area in the body where an artery carries deoxygenated blood and a vein carries oxygenated blood (see Fig. 16-6).

The systemic circulation begins at the aorta, where blood from the left ventricle is moved into the tissues for oxygenation. The cells absorb the oxygen, and deoxygenated blood is carried back to the heart via the veins. The veins from the lower section of the

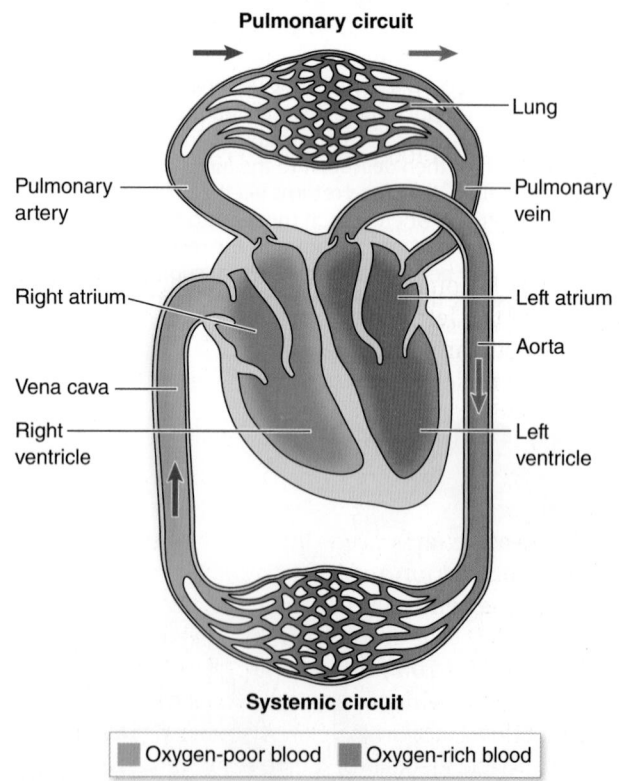

Oxygen-poor blood ■ Oxygen-rich blood

FIGURE 16-5. The heart showing the right ventricle pushing blood into the pulmonary arterial circulation and into the lungs. The pulmonary venous circulation brings blood back to the left atrium. The pulmonary artery carries blood to the lungs for oxygenation. The pulmonary veins carry oxygenated blood back to the heart from the lungs.

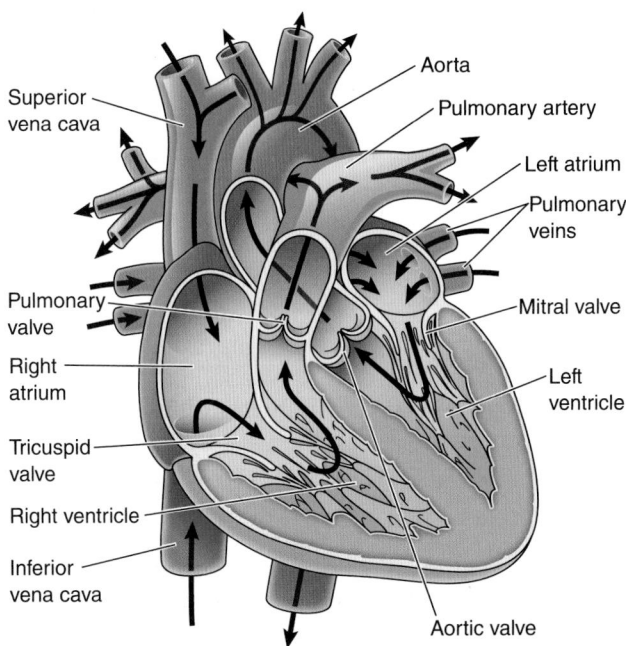

FIGURE 16-6. The heart with pulmonary and arterial circulation.

body drain into the IVC, and the veins from the upper section of the body drain into the SVC. Both the SVC and IVC empty into the right atrium.

The pulmonary circulatory system functions as a low-pressure system. The low pressure allows the blood to move through the lungs slowly, which is important for gas exchange. The systemic circulation is a high-pressure system. Its pulsations reflect the contractions of the left ventricle; it must work against gravity to move blood into the body's tissues.

Systolic and Diastolic Function

The heart is composed of two pumps: the right ventricle and the left ventricle. The right ventricle must push blood through the pulmonary circulation, and the left ventricle pushes blood through the aorta to all the body's peripheral tissues. Blood moves from the high-pressure left side of the heart through the tissues to the low-pressure right side of the heart and lungs.

The heart pumps according to a regular, rhythmic cycle of contraction and relaxation. Systole is the time in which the ventricles contract. During systole in the healthy adult, the left ventricle ejects a majority of its blood (50%–70%) into the aorta; this is called the stroke volume, which is also known as the left ventricular ejection fraction (LVEF). Also during systole, the right ventricle ejects blood into the pulmonary artery.

Diastole is the time when the ventricles relax. During diastole, the ventricles accept blood from atrial contraction. In the left ventricle, this is referred to as the LV end diastolic volume.

Contraction and relaxation occur because of the heart's neuromuscular system. The autonomic nervous

system innervates the heart muscle. Within each cardiac muscle cell, neural control is governed by the movement of ions at the cell membranes. The conduction system of the heart is constructed in a precise manner. The nerve tracts direct impulses in a specific direction from the atria down into the ventricles.

The Conduction System

Heart muscle is capable of generating and conducting its own nerve impulses. A specialized pathway of conductive tissue maintains an orderly impulse sequence for the heart's contraction and relaxation. The specialized conductive tissue includes the sinoatrial (SA) node, located in the right atrium; the atrioventricular (AV) node, located centrally in the heart in between the atria and ventricles; and the bundle of His (also called the atrioventricular bundle), which travels down the septum between the ventricles and Purkinje fibers (also called the subendocardial branches) in the walls of both ventricles (see Fig. 16-7). The conduction system can be divided into two systems: one that stimulates the atria and one that stimulates the ventricles. The impulse begins in the SA node within the right atrium, called the heart's pacemaker. It travels to the AV node, which provides one-way conduction of the impulse down into the ventricles through the bundle of His.

The transmission is slightly delayed at the AV node so that the atria can contract and eject their blood into the ventricles before the ventricular contraction. From the AV node, the impulse travels into the bundle of His and then into the Purkinje fibers. The Purkinje fibers divide into right and left bundles that fire rapidly to allow for simultaneous excitation of the right and left ventricles.

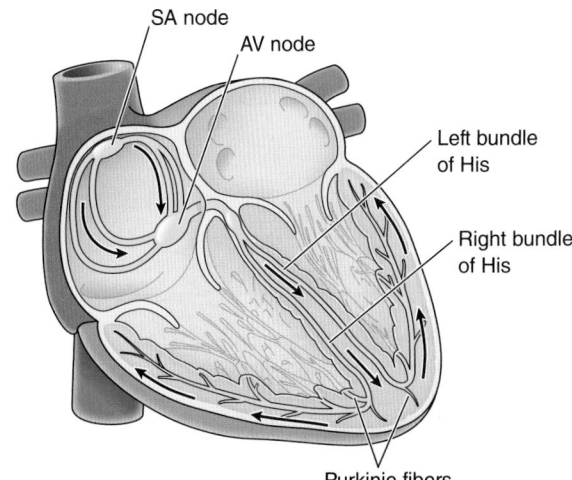

FIGURE 16-7. Conduction system through the heart. Impulses begin in the SA node of the right atrium and continue down into the AV node. The impulses then run down the right and left bundle of His to the Purkinje fibers.

Action Potential

A nerve impulse that occurs in cardiac tissue is called an **action potential**. Action potentials are electrical currents caused by the movement of positive and negative ions in and out of the cardiac cell membrane. When stimulated, the cardiac muscle generates a five-phase action potential. Initially, the action potential rises in voltage in the stage called **depolarization**, also referred to as phase 0. It reaches a maximal point and then slightly decreases in voltage, also called phase 1. After phase 1, there is a long plateau called phase 2. Phase 3 features rapid repolarization, until, in phase 4, it returns to baseline at the resting membrane potential (see Fig. 16-8).

The membrane of cardiac muscle has three types of ion channels that allow the voltage changes during the phases of the action potential. These are fast sodium channels, slow calcium–sodium channels, and potassium channels. At rest, the cardiac membrane is at –90 mV. In phase 0 the opening of fast sodium channels causes the initial upstroke of the action potential called depolarization. The entry of sodium ions into the cell causes a shift of electrical potential from –90 mV to +20 mV. Phase 1 occurs at the peak of the action potential; there is then an abrupt decrease in sodium permeability of the cardiac cell membrane. Phase 2 is the plateau of the action potential caused by the slow opening of sodium–calcium channels. Calcium ions enter the muscle cell and are integral to the contractile action of the cardiac muscle fibers. Phase 3 is the rapid repolarization that causes a decrease of the action potential down toward resting potential. During phase 3, the influx of calcium ceases and there is a sharp rise in potassium permeability of the cardiac cell membrane. Potassium ions move out of the cell, and the resting cell membrane potential is reestablished. In phase 4, the sodium–potassium pump is activated, moving sodium out of the cell and bringing potassium into the cell.

Absolute Refractory Period

The heart pump contracts and relaxes because of the ion channel movements of the action potential. There is a period in the action potential during which no stimuli can generate another action potential. This period is known as the absolute refractory period, and it includes phases 0, 1, 2, and part of phase 3. During this time, the cells cannot depolarize again under any circumstances. In other words, a second contraction cannot be stimulated until the first contraction's action potential phases are completed. The absolute refractory period maintains alternating periods of the heart's contraction and relaxation. This protects the heart from fatal rhythm disturbances called **dysrhythmias**. When a second impulse interferes with the phases of a first action potential in progress, dysrhythmias occur. Dysrhythmias are discussed later in the chapter.

Electrocardiogram

An **electrocardiogram (ECG)** is a recording of the electrical activity of the heart that can be measured from certain points on the body. Electrodes can be placed on the skin, and electrical current will project a pattern on a graph depicting the phases of resting potential, depolarization, plateau, and repolarization of the heart. Points designated as P, Q, R, S, and T represent different points within the phases of action potentials generated by cardiac muscle. The P wave represents the SA node and atrial depolarization, the QRS complex represents ventricular depolarization, and the T wave represents ventricular repolarization (see Fig. 16-9).

The horizontal axis of an ECG measures time in seconds, whereas the vertical axis measures amplitude of the impulse in millivolts (mV) (see Fig. 16-10). The ECG records the potential difference in charge between two electrodes as the depolarization and repolarization waves move through the heart. The shape of the tracing is determined by the direction in which the impulse spreads through the heart in relation to the electrode placement. A depolarization wave that moves toward the electrode registers positive or upward deflection. Conversely, a depolarization wave that moves away from the electrode registers negative or downward deflection.

Conventionally, 12 leads are recorded for a diagnostic ECG, each providing a view of the heart's electrical forces from a different position on the body (see Fig. 16-11).

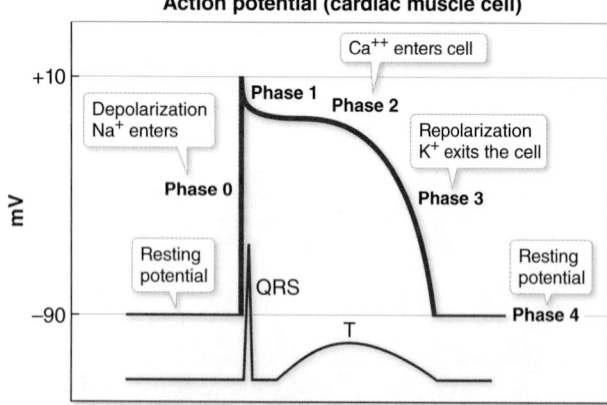

FIGURE 16-8. The cardiac action potential has five phases: During phase 0, membrane permeability to sodium ions increases, producing depolarization. During phase 1, there is partial repolarization because of a decrease in sodium permeability. Phase 2 is the plateau phase of the cardiac action potential. Membrane permeability to calcium increases during this phase, maintaining depolarization and prolonging the action potential. Membrane permeability to calcium decreases somewhat toward the end of phase 2. In phase 3, repolarization occurs, caused by the exit of potassium ions. At phase 4, there is a resting membrane potential.

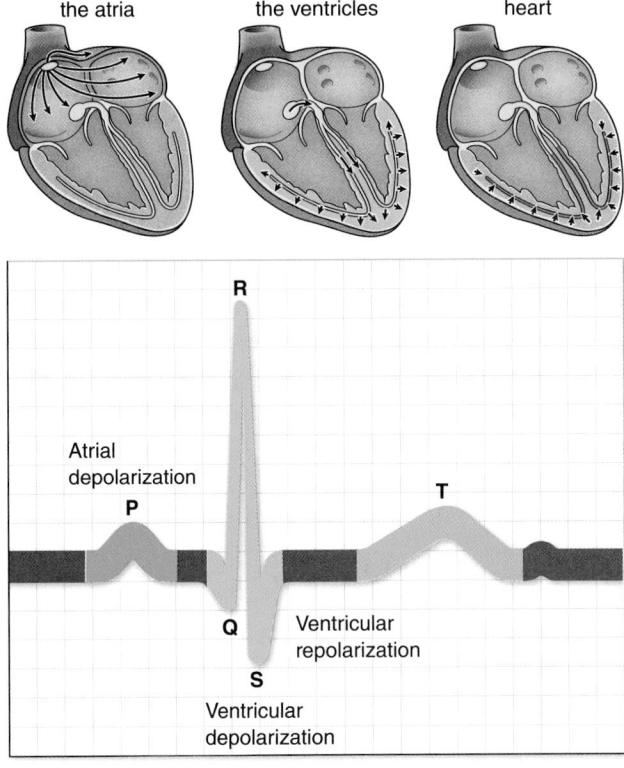

FIGURE 16-9. A basic ECG with corresponding parts of the heart activated during points on the ECG. The P wave represents atrial depolarization. The QRS complex represents ventricular depolarization. The T wave represents the phase of repolarization, or resting of the ventricles.

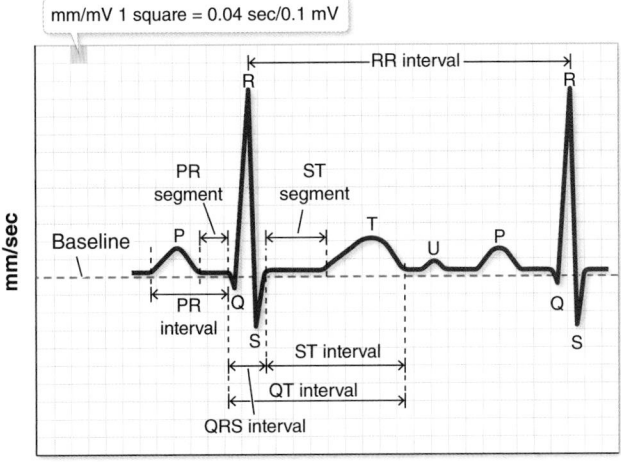

FIGURE 16-10. A detailed description of an ECG waveform. P wave = activation (depolarization) of atria. PR interval = time interval between onset of atrial depolarization and onset of ventricular depolarization. QRS complex = depolarization of ventricles, consisting of the Q, R, and S waves. QT interval = time interval between onset of ventricular depolarization and end of ventricular repolarization. R-R interval = time interval between two QRS complexes. T wave = ventricular repolarization. ST segment plus T wave (ST-T) = ventricular repolarization. U wave = time probably after depolarization (relaxation) of ventricles. The ST segment should be on the baseline in normal ECG, but above or below baseline in MI or myocardial ischemia.

Selected Pathophysiological Disorders of the Heart

The most common cardiac disorders cause ischemia of the heart muscle. Ischemic heart disease is caused by deprivation of circulation to the myocardium. Acute coronary syndrome (ACS) is a term used for ischemic disorders of the heart that occur suddenly and require immediate treatment. ACS is caused by either unstable angina or myocardial infarction. Angina (also called angina pectoris) is a term used to describe attacks of chest pain due to myocardial ischemia. There are two main types of angina: unstable angina and chronic stable angina. Other less common types of angina include Prinzmetal's and microvascular angina. Other disorders of the heart include infection and inflammatory conditions and dysrhythmias and conduction disorders.

Angina Pectoris

The term **angina pectoris** is derived from the Latin words *angere,* which means "to choke," and *pectus,* which translates as "chest." These two words aptly describe the sensations that many patients describe when explaining cardiac chest pain. **Angina pectoris** is the squeezing pain in the chest that occurs when there is lack of blood flow to the myocardium (termed myocardial ischemia). **Unstable angina (UA)** is cardiac chest pain that is occurring for the first time or is unlike prior episodes and is not relieved by rest. Unstable angina can lead to myocardial infarction (death of myocardial tissue). The severity of UA and potential for myocardial infarction are the reasons unstable angina is one of the disorders called an acute coronary syndrome. Angina is commonly described as stable or unstable; however, there are other less common variants such as Prinzmetal's angina and microvascular angina. **Chronic stable angina** is chronic chest pain that the patient has experienced in the past and feels similar to past episodes. The patient with chronic stable angina has had past experiences with the disorder and has been diagnosed and treated. The patient has a prescribed medication for episodes of chronic stable angina and self-medicates for treatment.

Unstable Angina

In the United States, the incidence of UA is increasing, and each year, nearly 1 million hospitalized patients have a primary diagnosis of UA. The mean age of persons presenting with UA is 62 years. On average, women with UA are 5 years older than men on presentation, with approximately half of women older than 65 years, as opposed to only about one-third of men. Black individuals tend to present at a slightly younger age than people of other races. UA is considered an acute coronary syndrome that requires immediate treatment.

12 leads

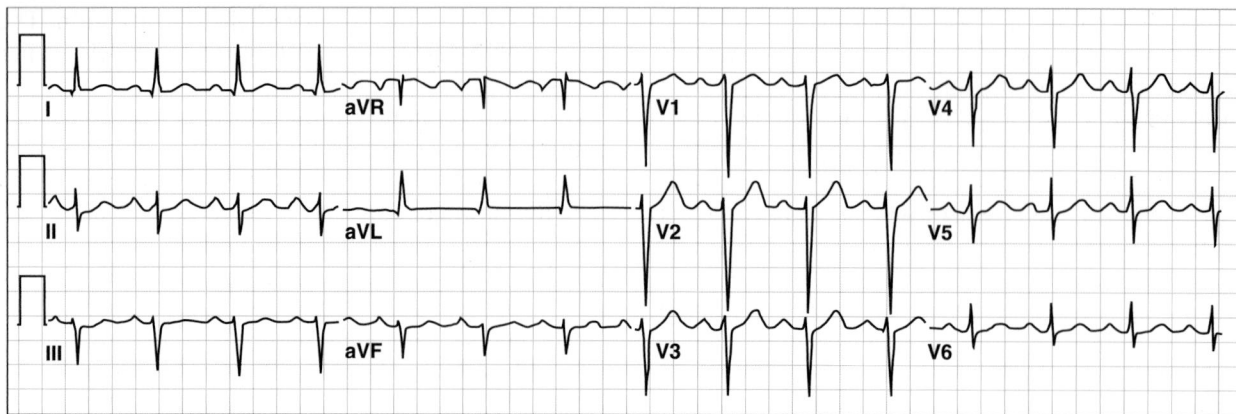

Rhythm strips lead II

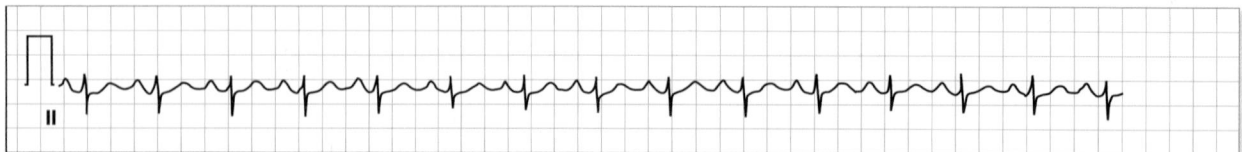

FIGURE 16-11. A 12-lead ECG will show a short segment of the recording of each of 12 leads placed on the patient's body. The ECG is arranged in a grid of four columns by three rows, the first column being the limb leads (I, II, and III), the second column the augmented limb leads (aVR, aVL, and aVF), and the last two columns being the chest leads (V1 to V6). Each column will usually record the same moment in time for the three leads; the recording will then switch to the next column, which will record the heartbeats after that point. Each of these segments is short, perhaps one to three heartbeats only, depending on the heart rate, and it can be difficult to analyze any heart rhythm that shows changes between heartbeats. To help with the analysis, it is common to print one or two rhythm strips as well. This will usually be lead II, which shows the electrical signal from the atria, and the P wave, which shows the rhythm for the whole time the ECG was recorded, usually 5 to 6 seconds.

Etiology and Risk Factors. The most common etiology of UA is myocardial ischemia as a result of coronary artery arteriosclerosis. Arteriosclerosis in the coronary arteries is a result of hyperlipidemia and endothelial injury. Arteriosclerotic plaque accumulation is the most common cause for obstruction of coronary artery blood flow. The large branches of the right or left coronary arteries are most commonly involved. The left anterior descending artery is the most common of the coronary arteries that become obstructed. However, there is evidence that UA can also be caused by obstruction of the microvascular branches of the coronary arteries, termed microvascular angina. UA can also be caused by coronary artery spasm, termed Prinzmetal's angina or variant angina. The risk factors for UA are the same as those for arteriosclerosis (see Chapter 15). These include cigarette smoking, diabetes mellitus (DM), hypercholesterolemia, and systemic hypertension. Other risk factors include LV hypertrophy; obesity; and elevated serum levels of homocysteine, triglycerides, and low-density lipoprotein (LDL), and low levels of high-density lipoprotein (HDL).

Metabolic syndrome is a constellation of symptoms that increase an individual's risk of CAD. These include apple-shaped obesity (waist circumference greater than 40 inches for men or greater than 35 inches for women), glucose intolerance (greater than 100 mg/mL fasting blood glucose), hyperinsulinemia, decreased HDL cholesterol levels (less than 40 mg/dL for men or 50 mg/dL for women), hypertriglyceridemia (greater than 150 mg/dL), and hypertension (greater than or equal to 130/85 mm Hg).

Pathophysiology. UA is most often experienced in relation to exertion when the heart muscle needs more coronary artery circulation to supply the cells with more oxygen. The ability of coronary arteries to increase blood flow in response to increased demand is termed coronary flow reserve. In healthy individuals, maximal coronary blood flow in response to exertional demand occurs with full dilation of the coronary arteries. It is roughly 4 to 6 times resting coronary artery blood flow. However, with exercise, arteriosclerotic plaque–filled coronary arteries cannot supply sufficient oxygenated blood to the cardiac muscle. Lack of circulation causes ischemia, which in turn leads to muscle cell hypoxia. This leads to anaerobic metabolism, which yields two adenosine triphosphate (ATP) and lactic acid. Studies show that the adenosine (from the breakdown of ATP) and lactic acid diffuse into the extracellular space and cause anginal pain.

There are several different pathophysiological processes by which cardiac muscle cells can suffer ischemia and lack of sufficient oxygen leading to UA. A coronary artery can be blocked by a thrombus (blood clot) that obstructs blood flow to the heart muscle. This is called a **coronary thrombosis** and is a common cause of myocardial ischemia. A coronary thrombosis is a consequence of endothelial injury and platelet aggregation. If the coronary artery diameter is blocked by 50% to 70%, an inadequate amount of blood flows past the blockage, resulting in ischemia. Another more common cause of myocardial ischemia is accumulation of hardened atherosclerotic plaque in a coronary artery (see Fig. 16-12). As atherosclerotic plaque ages, it calcifies and becomes fragile. A piece of calcified plaque often breaks off, embolizes (travels) downstream, and lodges in a small-diameter arteriole. After lodging in the arteriole, the piece of plaque obstructs blood flow to the distal myocardial tissue.

A third and less common way that myocardial ischemia can occur is by coronary artery vasospasm, which can lead to Prinzmetal's angina (also called vasospastic or variant angina; discussed in further detail below). The vascular spasm obstructs blood flow through the coronary artery, creating ischemia in the surrounding myocardial tissue. Prinzmetal's angina commonly occurs at rest and coronary artery spasm can be provoked with injection of acetylcholine, ergonovine, or methylergonovine.

A fourth type of myocardial ischemia or angina occurs without any apparent coronary artery obstruction on coronary angiography. According to many investigators, approximately 50% of patients with angina undergoing elective coronary angiography have no obstructive coronary artery disease (Aldiwani et al., 2020; Ong et al., 2018). **Ischemia with no obstructive coronary artery (INOCA)** is believed to be due to coronary microvascular dysfunction, termed **microvascular angina**. Persons with microvascular angina are at higher risk of developing major adverse cardiac events including MI, stroke, and heart failure with preserved ejection fraction. There are newly designated criteria for diagnosing microvascular angina (see Box 16-1).

A fifth possible cause of myocardial ischemia or angina, albeit uncommon, is anemia. In anemia, the cardiac and pulmonary systems are functioning normally; however, there is an inadequate number of red blood cells. Therefore, the lack of RBCs causes a deficiency of oxygen delivery to the myocardium. When the myocardium requires more oxygen, such as with exertion, there is insufficient oxygen supply, which causes angina.

Clinical Presentation. Patients with UA report retrosternal chest discomfort and use terms such as pressure, choking, squeezing, or heaviness on the chest to describe the sensation. Classic cardiac chest pain is a crushing sensation felt on the left side of the chest, radiating into the left shoulder down the left arm. Alternatively, cardiac pain can radiate to the jaw, back, neck, right arm, or epigastric region (see Fig. 16-13). A significant characteristic of angina is that it is precipitated by exertion or stress, and the pain lasts approximately 1 to 5 minutes. It can be relieved by rest and the use of medications called nitrates, if prescribed. Significantly, the intensity of pain does not change with respirations, cough, or change in position. Additional factors that can bring on angina include exposure to cold, eating a large meal, and emotional stress.

Symptoms referred to as **anginal equivalents** may occur instead of classic angina symptoms. Anginal equivalents often occur in women and include symptoms such as episodic dyspnea; dizziness; lightheadedness; feeling faint; pain of the jaw, epigastric region (heartburn), or back in response to exertion or stress.

Physical Examination. Some physical examination findings can be noted when observing patients with

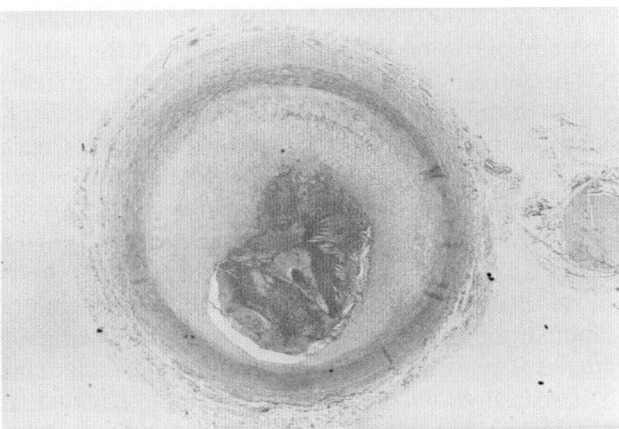

FIGURE 16-12. Coronary atherosclerosis. *(From Biophoto Associates/ Science Source.)*

> ## BOX 16-1. Criteria for Diagnosis of Microvascular Angina
>
> (1) Presence of symptoms suggestive of myocardial ischemia
> (2) Objective documentation of myocardial ischemia, as assessed by currently available techniques
> (3) Absence of obstructive CAD (coronary artery obstruction defined as <50% coronary diameter reduction and/or fractional flow reserve [FFR] >0.80)
> (4) Confirmation of a reduced coronary blood flow reserve and/or inducible microvascular spasm
>
> Adapted from Ong, P., Camici, P. G., Beltrame, J. F., Crea, F., Shimokawa, H., Sechtem, U., Kaski, J. C., Bairey Merz, C. N., & Coronary Vasomotion Disorders International Study Group (COVADIS). International standardization of diagnostic criteria for microvascular angina. *Int J Cardiol.* 2018 Jan 1;250:16–20. doi: 10.1016/j.ijcard.2017.08.068. Epub 2017 Sep 8. PMID: 29031990

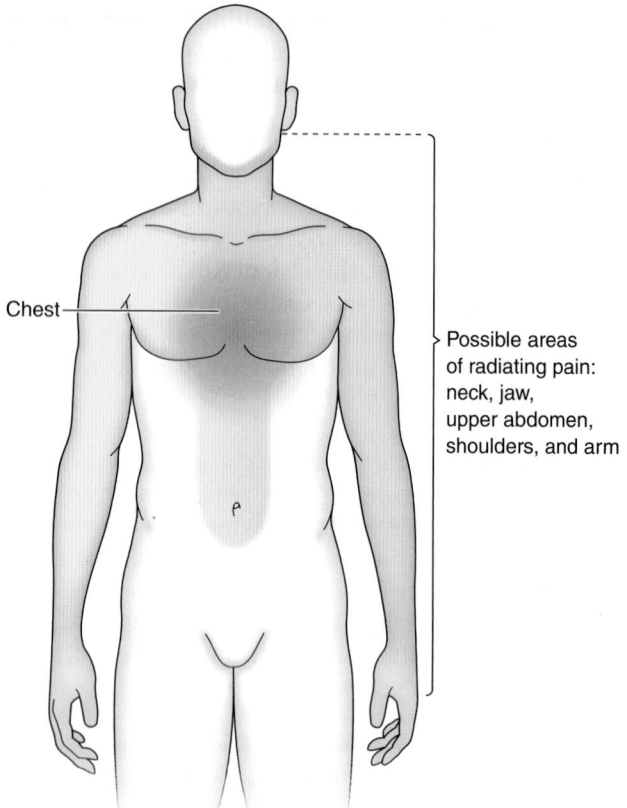

Chest

Possible areas of radiating pain: neck, jaw, upper abdomen, shoulders, and arm

FIGURE 16-13. Pain distribution of angina pectoris and myocardial infarction. The classic pain associated with ischemic heart disease is retrosternal, crushing chest pain that radiates down the left arm. Some patients describe a pressure-like pain, as if something is sitting on the chest. Pain can also radiate into the epigastric region, jaw, right arm, or back. Dyspnea, diaphoresis, pallor, and weakness are commonly associated with the pain.

angina. Commonly, individuals will clench a fist over the sternum when experiencing the pain of angina. This is known as a positive Levine's sign and is consistent with angina pectoris and MI. The individual may become pale, dyspneic, and diaphoretic. The pulses may be weak, and there may be signs of hyperlipidemia such as xanthomas or xanthelasmas. Heart rate may be normal, bradycardic, or tachycardic, and there may be extra beats or irregular rhythm.

Diagnosis. Diagnostic tests for angina are similar to those for arteriosclerosis (see Chapter 15). Blood pressure (BP) measurement, total blood cholesterol, low-density lipoprotein (LDL), HDL, and triglycerides are measured. Additional tests include ECG, serum electrolytes, high sensitivity C-reactive protein (hs-CRP), homocysteine, cardiac enzymes, lipoprotein (a), fibrinogen, high sensitivity cardiac troponin (hs-cTn), chest x-ray, calcium computed tomography (CT) scan, cardiac angiogram, cardiac catheterization, and intravascular ultrasonography.

In angina pectoris, the ECG can show ST depressions or ST elevations. Prinzmetal's angina can show reversible ST segment elevations, and acute MI is more commonly associated with ST elevations. It is important to recognize that cTn, not an ECG, is the confirmatory test of MI.

> ### 🩺 CLINICAL CONCEPT
>
> The ECG can appear similar in angina pectoris and MI, so hs-cTn is the laboratory test that is used to confirm diagnosis of MI.

A coronary artery calcium CT scan can show calcification in the coronary arteries that is indicative of atherosclerotic plaque. It provides a calcium score that indicates the extent of obstructive coronary arteriosclerosis.

Intravascular coronary angiography can show the internal atherosclerotic plaque within coronary arteries, and intravascular coronary angiography with ultrasound can measure the plaque thickness within the arteries. These have been gold standards in the diagnosis of CAD. However, these tests run the risk of rupturing atherosclerotic plaque. Noninvasive **coronary computed tomographic angiography (CCTA)** technology can demonstrate anatomy of the coronary arteries without invasive procedures and without the risk of rupturing atherosclerotic plaque.

Another diagnostic test specifically for angina is a graded exercise stress test used in conjunction with ECG, echocardiography, and radionuclide myocardial perfusion imaging. An echocardiogram, ECG, and imaging tests demonstrate coronary artery and LV function while the patient exercises to maximal level on a treadmill or stationary bicycle. Radionuclide myocardial perfusion imaging enables evaluation of cardiac perfusion and function at rest and during dynamic exercise or pharmacological stress for the diagnosis and management of patients with known or suspected coronary heart disease. Radioisotope is injected into the bloodstream and highlights the coronary artery blood flow to the heart stressed by exercise. This test is useful in patients suspected of having angina pectoris and can show the extent of coronary artery obstruction and perfusion defects in the heart. If the patient has had an MI, this scan will demonstrate the affected region of the heart. If a patient cannot exercise vigorously for the stress test, pharmacological agents, such as dobutamine or adenosine, can be administered to temporarily increase stress on the heart.

A resting ECG can be normal in a patient with angina pectoris. However, an ambulatory ECG can demonstrate changes that are missed with a resting ECG. Ambulatory ECG monitoring records the patient's ECG as they experience daily activities over 24 hours. It is measured with a portable, wearable device that can demonstrate key ECG changes indicative of CAD. Interestingly, ambulatory ECG monitoring has shown that silent ischemia is a common phenomenon among patients with established CAD. In one study, as many as 75% of episodes of ischemia (defined as transient ST depression of 1 mm or above persisting for at least 1 minute) occurring in patients with stable angina were clinically silent. Silent ischemia occurs most frequently in the early morning hours and may result in transient myocardial contractile dysfunction. The exact mechanisms for silent ischemia are not known.

After diagnostic tests are completed, angina pectoris can be categorized according to the stage of disease severity (see Box 16-2).

Treatment. The goals of UA treatment are to relieve symptoms, slow the progression of ischemic disease, and reduce future occurrences. Ultimately, the goal is to prevent an MI and premature death. Patients mainly need education and assistance to reduce modifiable risk factors such as smoking, stress, diet, and weight. Contributing pathology such as hypertension, DM, and hyperlipidemia must be addressed with patients to develop approaches that will reduce these risk factors. Patients who have not succeeded in reducing risk factors with lifestyle modification may require antihypertensive, antilipidemic, or antidiabetic medications.

Oxygen should be administered to the patient suffering from angina pectoris if oxygen saturation (SaO_2) is lower than 95%. Major medications used to treat angina pectoris include nitrates and aspirin. Nitrates are potent vasodilators that widen the coronary arteries to deliver optimal circulation to the myocardial muscle. They also reduce preload and afterload on the heart by stimulating venodilation and arterial dilation. Nitrates are available as a sublingual tablet, nasal spray, paste, patch, or IV preparation. Short-acting nitroglycerin (NTG) sublingual tablets have classically been used to immediately stimulate coronary vasodilation during episodes of acute angina. Long-acting nitrates, such as isosorbide, may be recommended in lieu of short-acting NTG preparations or in combination.

ALERT! For NTG sublingual 0.3 to 0.6 mg tablets, dosing is one tab SL, then repeat two additional doses 5 minutes apart during an acute attack, not to exceed three tablets within 15 minutes. If the patient with angina takes three NTG tablets within a 15-minute period without relief of chest pain, assume the patient is having an MI.

ALERT! NTG and other nitrate preparations can cause severe hypotension. NTG should not be administered with sildenafil (Viagra) because of the risk of severe hypotension.

Beta-adrenergic blockers, calcium antagonists, and angiotensin-converting enzyme (ACE) inhibitors have also been recommended for some patients with angina pectoris, regardless of the presence of hypertension or heart failure. Beta blockers counteract the sympathetic nervous system effect on the heart, reducing the myocardial oxygen needs. Calcium antagonists cause arterial dilation, which decreases resistance against the heart. ACE inhibitors reduce BP and lower resistance against the heart. Ranolazine is a cardioselective, anti-ischemic agent also used for patients with angina pectoris. It acts by disrupting sodium–calcium homeostasis within the cardiac muscle cell, which in turn inhibits myocardial ischemia.

Dual antiplatelet therapy, which includes aspirin (75 to 100 mg) and a P2Y12 receptor inhibitor (e.g., clopidogrel, prasugrel, or ticagrelor), is another treatment recommended for patients with CAD. However, the patient's risk for bleeding must be evaluated before administration of these medications.

Research studies have shown that microvascular angina (also referred to as INOCA) should be treated differently than other forms of angina. Antilipidemia statin agents in combination with ACE inhibitor or angiotensin receptor blockers (ARBs) at maximal doses appear to improve angina, stress testing, myocardial perfusion, coronary endothelial function, and microvascular function. Thromboxane A2 (TXA2)

BOX 16-2. Grading of Angina Pectoris

The Canadian Cardiovascular Society grading scale is used for classification of angina severity, as follows:

Class I: Ordinary physical activity does not cause angina, such as walking and climbing stairs. Angina with strenuous or rapid or prolonged exertion at work or recreation.

Class II: Slight limitation of ordinary activity. Walking or climbing stairs rapidly; walking uphill; walking or stair climbing after meals; or in cold or in wind, or under emotional stress, or only during the few hours after awakening. Walking more than two blocks on the level and climbing more than one flight of ordinary stairs at a normal pace and in normal conditions.

Class III: Marked limitation of ordinary physical activity. Walking one or two blocks on the level and climbing one flight of stairs in normal conditions and at normal pace.

Class IV: Inability to carry on any physical activity without discomfort; anginal syndrome may be present at rest.

Adapted from Campeau, L. (1976). Letter: Grading of angina pectoris. *Circulation,* *54*(3), 522–523. www.ccs.ca

inhibitors (low-dose aspirin and P2Y12 platelet inhibitors) are also likely useful in preventing adverse outcomes of INOCA patients (Bairey Merz et al., 2017; Bairey Merz et al., 2020).

Surgery and endovascular procedures are options, as **percutaneous coronary intervention (PCI)** or **coronary artery bypass graft (CABG)** are often used to treat angina pectoris and MI. These procedures aim to ensure perfusion in the areas of the myocardium denied circulation because of CAD. **Percutaneous transluminal coronary angioplasty (PCTA)** is a primary PCI that utilizes a catheter with a balloon at the tip (see Fig. 16-14). The catheter is inserted through a peripheral artery, such as the femoral artery in the leg or radial artery of the wrist. The catheter is inserted and threaded up the aorta into the obstructed coronary artery. At the point of obstruction, the balloon is inflated, pushing the plaque content against the walls of the artery, a procedure referred to as angioplasty. Alternatively, the plaque can be reduced using a specialized blade or laser tip on the catheter in a procedure referred to as an atherectomy. Often, a catheter is inserted with a stent at the end. A stent is a metal, meshlike, tubular structure that is inserted at the area of obstruction. The stent structurally reinforces the wall of the coronary artery, maintains an open vessel, and prevents reblockage with plaque. Drug-eluting stents that release sirolimus or paclitaxel can be used. These are timed-released drugs that limit proliferation of cells so narrowing doesn't recur and the vessel can remain open.

CABG surgery creates new routes around narrowed and blocked arteries, allowing sufficient blood flow to deliver oxygen and nutrients to the heart muscle (see Fig. 16-15). Traditionally, an incision is made down the middle of the chest through the sternum (sternotomy) for access to the heart. Alternatively, minimally invasive direct CABG procedures are performed via very small incisions in the chest.

The most commonly used vessel to act as a bypass is the saphenous vein, which is surgically excised from the leg. Bypass grafting involves sewing the graft vessels to the coronary arteries beyond the narrowing or blockage. The other end of this vein is attached to the aorta or left internal thoracic artery. Depending on the extent of obstructions in the coronary arteries, triple, quadruple, or quintuple bypasses can be performed. These types of revascularization procedures have increased survival for many individuals with CAD.

Traditionally, CABG is performed using a cardiopulmonary heart pump. The heart is stopped, and the heart pump keeps the blood oxygenated until surgery is completed. Alternatively, another procedure allows CABG without using a cardiopulmonary heart pump (referred to as "off pump"), with the heart still beating. This significantly minimizes the side effects and complications that may be seen after CABG.

Complications. Acute MI is a complication of angina pectoris, and it usually occurs in the same area of ST segment change as noted by the ECG. The greater the

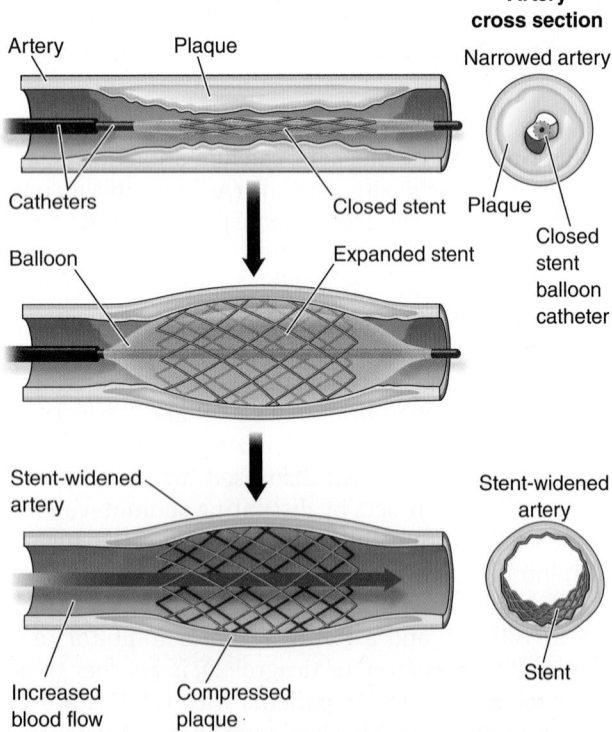

FIGURE 16-14. Percutaneous coronary transluminal angioplasty (PCTA) is the technique of mechanically widening narrowed or obstructed arteries that result from atherosclerosis. An empty and collapsed balloon on a guide wire, known as a balloon catheter, is passed into the narrowed coronary arteries and then inflated. The balloon compresses the plaque against the internal wall of the artery. The result is an opened blood vessel for improved flow; the balloon is then deflated and withdrawn. A stent may or may not be inserted at the time of the ballooning to ensure the vessel remains open.

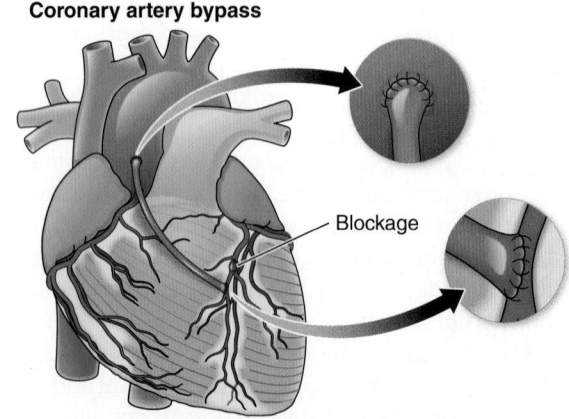

FIGURE 16-15. CABG is a surgical treatment for ischemic heart disease. During CABG, a healthy artery or vein from the body is connected, or grafted, to a blocked coronary artery. The grafted artery or vein goes around the blocked portion of the coronary artery. This creates a new path for oxygen-rich blood to flow to the heart muscle. Surgeons can bypass multiple coronary arteries during one surgery.

presence of atherosclerosis and coronary vessel stenosis in the patient's heart, the greater the incidence of MI for patients who have angina.

Prinzmetal's Angina (Vasospastic Angina)

Prinzmetal's angina, also known as variant or vasospastic angina, was originally described by Myron Prinzmetal in 1959. It is significantly different from classic angina because patients with Prinzmetal's angina have chest pain at rest. This type of angina is caused by coronary artery vasospasm. It can also be associated with MI, life-threatening ventricular arrhythmias, and sudden death.

Epidemiology. Prinzmetal's angina affects approximately 4 out of 100,000 people per year in the United States. Approximately 2% of patients with angina have coronary artery spasm; exact numbers are unknown, as many patients do not report episodes of coronary vasospasm. For unknown reasons, the prevalence of coronary spasm is higher in Japan and Korea than in Western countries.

Etiology. The etiology of coronary artery spasm is unclear, but there are several theories concerning this condition. Within the myocardium, there may be reduced amounts of the vasodilatory substance nitric oxide (NO). Elevated LDL cholesterol causes decreased production and inactivation of NO. Lack of NO is associated with coronary artery muscle thickening and enhanced sensitivity to vasoconstrictors. Also, the region of coronary artery spasm in Prinzmetal's angina typically occurs at or adjacent to atherosclerotic plaque. Because of this, endothelial dysfunction is hypothesized to be the cause of the spasm. Imbalances within the sympathetic and parasympathetic tone can also predispose to exaggerated vasoconstriction under normal circumstances and during exposure to acetylcholine and methacholine. As an alternative theory, abnormal magnesium metabolism, which results in the hypercontraction of smooth muscle cells in coronary artery walls, may be the cause of variant angina. Lastly, it is also proposed that hyperinsulinemia and insulin resistance are related to the etiology of variant angina, although the exact mechanisms of these associations have not been defined.

Risk Factors Typical cardiovascular risk factors have not directly been associated with the presence of vasospastic angina, except for cigarette smoking and inflammatory states, as evidenced by high levels of hs-CRP levels. It has been found that drugs such as ephedrine and sumatriptan can cause chest pain due to coronary spasm. Recreational drugs like cocaine, amphetamines, alcohol, and marijuana are also possible precipitating factors. Environmental factors such as external exposure to cold water can cause spasms in the coronaries. Valsalva maneuver, hyperventilation, and coronary manipulation through cardiac catheterization also can produce hyperreactivity of the coronaries.

Pathophysiology For reasons that are unclear, there is a localized area of vasospastic muscle wall in one or more coronary arteries. Coronary artery vasospasm obstructs blood flow to the myocardium, and the area undergoes temporary ischemia. Ischemia initiates anaerobic metabolism, which yields 2 ATP and lactic acid, an irritant to cardiac muscle cells. Vasospasm can occur at rest, last a few minutes, and cause the same squeezing chest pain as typical angina. Vasospasm can be mild with hardly any constriction apparent in the vessel wall or severe with tight spasm causing complete arterial obstruction. The vasospasm eventually subsides and the patient's symptoms are relieved.

Clinical Presentation. Patients with Prinzmetal's angina commonly do not have many cardiovascular risk factors. A history of episodes of squeezing chest pain may be all that the patient reports. However, the patient should be asked about cardiovascular risk factors such as hypertension, hyperlipidemia, fat and salt in the diet, sedentary lifestyle, and family history. The patient should be specifically asked about cigarette smoking because this is common in those with Prinzmetal's angina.

Another commonality in a small percentage of patients is the concurrent conditions of migraine headaches and Raynaud's phenomenon. As in Prinzmetal's angina, these two conditions are caused by an abnormality in the vasomotor tone of vessels.

The pain pattern for Prinzmetal's angina is unlike classic angina. Unlike the exercise intolerance observed with patients with typical angina, patients with Prinzmetal's angina have normal exercise tolerance. Most episodes of chest pain occur when the patient is at rest and in the early morning hours.

Diagnosis. Patients with Prinzmetal's angina are usually admitted to the hospital for observation, evaluation, and initiation of therapy. Diagnosis includes cardiac monitoring for 24 to 48 hours, coronary angiography, and serial cardiac enzyme assays. During angiography, coronary artery spasm is often provoked by chemical means, using acetylcholine, ergonovine, or methylergonovine as a vasoconstrictor. The coronary vasoconstriction of Prinzmetal's angina can be visualized by the angiographic demonstration of spontaneous or induced coronary vessel spasm that causes chest pain in patients at rest. The ECG may include ST-segment elevation or depression. Patients with Prinzmetal's angina may or may not have atherosclerosis of a major coronary artery.

If the patient is experiencing a prolonged period of chest pain, an ECG may show bradycardia, tachycardia, elevated ST segment, depressed ST segment, or dysrhythmias. The transient ECG changes and complaint of chest pain at rest provide the rationale for diagnosis of variant angina. An ambulatory ECG Holter monitor can demonstrate the cardiac irregularities of the patient during a 24- to 48-hour period.

Treatment. Initially, IV or sublingual NTG may be given, as well as a calcium blocker antagonist. A calcium channel antagonist is a first-line treatment due to a vasodilation effect in the coronary vasculature. A high dose of a long-acting calcium antagonist like diltiazem, amlodipine, nifedipine, or verapamil is recommended. Calcium antagonists are effective in alleviating symptoms in 90% of patients. Long-acting nitrates can be added to the treatment regimen if calcium antagonists alone are not completely effective. The use of fluvastatin has also been shown to be effective in preventing coronary spasm and may exert benefits via endothelial NO or direct effects on the vascular smooth muscle. Nicorandil, a nitrate and K-channel activator, can also suppress vasospastic attacks.

Complications. Acute MI is a complication of Prinzmetal's angina and is usually in the same area of ST-segment change as noted by the ECG during the prior anginal attack. The greater the involvement of the patient's heart with atherosclerosis and coronary vasospasm, the greater the incidence of MI. Patients can also have rhythm disturbances caused by the vasospasms and resulting ischemia of contractile tissue.

Chronic Stable Angina

Chronic coronary artery disease, also called chronic stable angina, is characterized by recurring episodes of chest pain caused by transient myocardial ischemia. It is estimated that 10 million adults in the United States have chronic stable angina. The prevalence of angina increases with age, ranging from 4% to 7% in adults aged 40 to 79 years to greater than 10% in those older than 80 years.

Etiology and Risk Factors. Persons with chronic stable angina usually have quiescent arteriosclerotic plaque. There is a fixed atherosclerotic coronary obstruction that is well established and longstanding. It is coronary obstruction that has progressed over years to the advanced stage of arterial lumen narrowing.

Patients with stable angina either cannot withstand surgical intervention for their CAD or have had surgical interventions that have not been successful to relieve their chest pain. They have chronic episodes of angina for which they self-medicate most commonly with nitroglycerin (NTG)-type medications. The risk factors for chronic stable angina are the same as those for arteriosclerosis (see Chapter 15).

Clinical Presentation. The chest pain of stable angina usually occurs during exertion or other conditions that increase the heart's work demands. It is similar to the chest pain of UA but has a predictable pattern that has been experienced by the patient. The patient can relieve the chest pain with medications. The patient is usually on a daily medication that aims to prevent angina episodes. Worsening of angina pain, sudden-onset angina at rest, and angina lasting more than 15 minutes are symptoms of UA. This requires immediate emergency intervention.

Diagnosis Diagnostic studies for chronic stable angina are similar to those for UA.

Treatment. Chronic stable angina treatment commonly consists of nitroglycerin preparations. Sublingual glyceryl trinitrate tablets or NTG spray remain the treatment of choice for rapid relief of acute symptoms and anticipated angina. Sublingual glyceryl trinitrate tablets are absorbed in the sublingual mucosa and take effect within a couple of minutes. Glyceryl trinitrate spray is equally effective, and due to its longer shelf-life, it is more convenient for those with infrequent symptoms of angina. Long-acting nitrates such as oral isosorbide mononitrate or transdermal patches are effective in relieving angina that occurs often and can improve exercise tolerance. Common adverse effects of nitrates include headache, hypotension, and lightheadedness. Nitrates should not be prescribed for patients taking phosphodiesterase-5 inhibitors such as sildenafil due to the risk of profound hypotension. Other contraindications include severe aortic stenosis and hypertrophic cardiomyopathy.

Nicorandil is a potassium channel activator that improves coronary flow as a result of both arterial and venous dilation. Ranolazine is another medication that can be used for chronic stable angina; it selectively inhibits the late sodium current in cardiomyocytes and has anti-ischemic and metabolic properties. Ranolazine improves myocardial relaxation and enhances myocardial perfusion. Ivabradine is a selective channel blocker that acts by reducing the firing rate of pacemaker cells in the SA node; the reduced heart rate increases the time for coronary blood flow by a prolongation of diastole. Ranolazine and ivabradine are useful in patients with chronic angina, whether at rest or during exercise. In addition, they can be used in monotherapy or in association with other conventional anti-ischemic drugs. Other medications include beta blockers and calcium channel antagonists for patients who are intolerant of nitrates.

Acute Myocardial Infarction

Acute MI is an acute coronary syndrome (ACS) that occurs when the heart tissue endures prolonged ischemia without recovery (see Fig. 16-16). Myocardial cells suffer irreversible damage because of hypoxia and die in a process referred to as infarction or ischemic necrosis. MIs are classified according to findings on an ECG such as **ST segment elevation myocardial infarction (STEMI)** or **non-ST segment elevation myocardial infarction (NSTEMI)**.

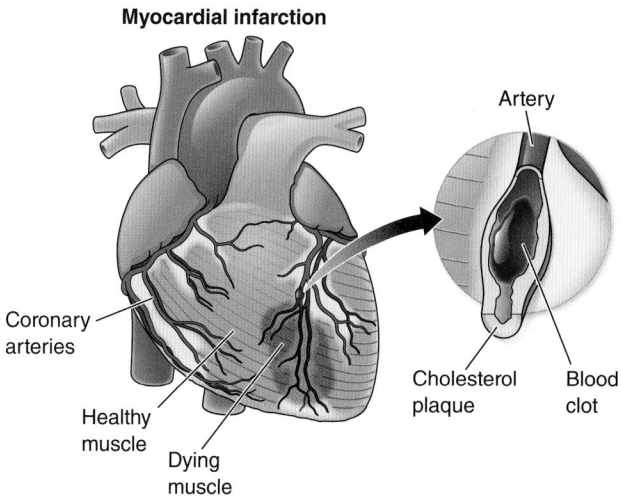

Myocardial infarction

Artery

Coronary arteries

Cholesterol plaque

Blood clot

Healthy muscle

Dying muscle

FIGURE 16-16. Prolonged ischemia leads to MI.

Frequently, acute MI occurs because a coronary artery is completely obstructed by atherosclerotic plaque or clot, and blood flow carrying oxygen to the myocardium is blocked. More commonly, a ruptured piece of atherosclerotic plaque breaks off and travels distally within a coronary artery to an area where it obstructs blood flow. Another common scenario of acute MI occurs when an atherosclerotic plaque ruptures and the exposed plaque area attracts platelets and forms a thrombus over the region. The thrombus then breaks off and travels within the bloodstream distally to a narrow area of a coronary artery and causes obstruction. Regardless of how it occurs, MI is a dead area of the cardiac muscle that is not perfused with coronary artery blood flow.

Acute MI can also result if the coronary artery supply remains constant but the myocardial metabolic demands increase, as in the case of severe hypertension, LV hypertrophy, or severe aortic valve stenosis. In all these cases, the left ventricle must pump against a great deal of resistance, which increases its need for extra coronary artery blood flow that is not available. The ventricle muscle endures ischemia; if ischemia is prolonged, infarction develops.

MI occurs because of a disparity between the oxygen needs of the myocardium and the oxygen available to it. The influences on the heart that increase myocardial oxygen demand include the following:

- Increased heart rate
- Increased muscle mass
- Increased systemic BP

MI can occur in different ways and can be classified according to how the injury occurred.

Epidemiology. Acute MI is the leading cause of death in the United States and in other industrialized nations throughout the world. Each year, approximately 1.5 million Americans suffer an MI, and 500,000 to 700,000 die of the event. It is the cause of death in

an estimated one-third of all deaths in those older than 35 years. The death rate related to acute MI is approximately three times higher in men than in women. It is also higher in Black patients compared with White patients. Approximately 50% of individuals who suffer an MI are younger than 65 years. Persons older than age 65 years often suffer silent, asymptomatic MI. Despite the public health service campaigns to educate the public about the signs and symptoms of MI and the importance of calling for medical assistance when experiencing the earliest symptoms, 250,000 individuals die of MI each year before arriving at a hospital. Hesitation and delayed requests for emergency care are major causes of death resulting from MI. Once patients are at the hospital and treated, survival rates for patients in the United States with acute MI are 90% to 95%.

Etiology. The most common etiology of MI is coronary artery atherosclerosis. MI usually develops due to coronary artery obstruction, which causes ischemia (see the section on angina pectoris). However, MI can have different causative factors, including evidence of biomarkers and cardiovascular procedures. There are five classifications of MI depending on the cause of the heart damage and conditions surrounding it:

- Type 1: MI occurring spontaneously due to atherosclerotic plaque rupture and thrombotic obstruction of a coronary artery.
- Type 2: MI due to oxygen supply/demand imbalance from causes other than atherothrombotic coronary disease.
- Type 3: MI resulting in death before cTn can be measured.
- Type 4: MI due to percutaneous coronary intervention/stent insertion (within 48 hours of the procedure).
- Type 5: MI due to CABG (within 48 hours of the procedure).

Pathophysiology. MI occurs because of prolonged ischemia of the cardiac tissue. Damage to myocardial cells occurs when needed oxygen is either not arriving at the cells or is inadequate in amount. The extent of damage caused by an MI is influenced by three factors:

1. Location or level of occlusion in the coronary artery
2. Length of time that the coronary artery has been occluded
3. Heart's availability of collateral circulation

These three factors play a significant role in determining whether the heart muscle will be able to survive an acute MI episode. The longer the period of coronary artery occlusion and the greater the area of myocardial ischemia, the more extensive the death of heart muscle. If, however, oxygen-enriched blood flow can be restored to the at-risk tissue, the heart muscle can be saved from necrosis, and the extent of damage to the myocardium can be reduced.

Prolonged ischemia of longer than 30 minutes usually causes irreversible cellular damage and necrosis, leading to decreased contractile force and alteration of conduction in the myocardium. The necrotic cells are inactive electrically and their cell membranes rupture, releasing their cellular contents into the interstitial spaces. These cellular contents can be measured and serve as diagnostic markers of myocardial injury. For example, creatinine phosphokinase MB (CPK-MB), also referred to as creatine kinase muscle/brain, is a cardiac isoenzyme released from dead myocardial cells.

Ischemic myocardial cells undergo changes associated with insufficient oxygen supply and anaerobic metabolism. Failure of the sodium–potassium pump occurs because of lack of energy. Potassium concentration increases in the extracellular space, and sodium remains inside the cell. There is also an increase in lactic acid from anaerobic metabolism, which leads to an increase in the hydrogen ion concentration surrounding the cell. Both of these changes contribute to changes in the myocardial cellular membrane potential and are seen on an ECG as ST segment changes.

MI tissue changes are evident within 12 to 24 hours. The myocardium becomes pale, progressing to a mottled appearance over the next 3 to 5 days. As phagocytic cells remove necrotic debris, the myocardial wall becomes soft and relatively thin. There is interstitial edema and evidence of microscopic hemorrhage. After 5 days, the fibroblasts begin collagen deposition and scar formation. Scar formation begins at the periphery of the infarcted tissue and gradually moves inward. The scar is well established at about 2 weeks. However, it can take as long as 2 months for completion of scar formation.

The area of infarct is surrounded by an area of injury and an ischemic zone. Some of the cells in the injured area will recover. The ischemic zone has relatively viable, salvageable tissue (see Fig. 16-17). The area of infarct and ischemic zone boundaries can change postinfarction depending on the success of

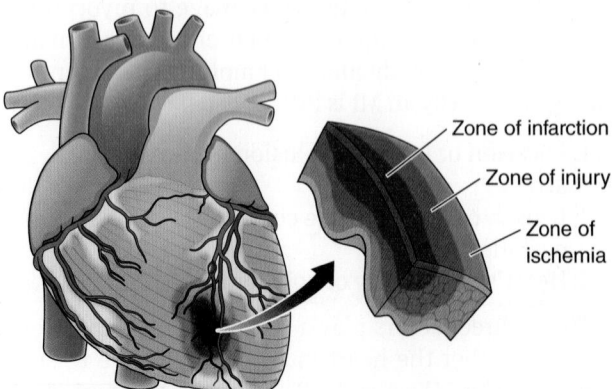

FIGURE 16-17. In acute MI, the infarcted region of the heart is surrounded by a zone of injury and a zone of ischemia. Zones surrounding the infarction are salvageable tissue that can be treated with reperfusion procedures.

measures to restore blood supply such as angioplasty and thrombolytic therapy.

The ultimate size of the infarct is dependent on the ischemic zone. Reversal of ischemia will decrease the amount of necrosis. The ischemic zone can be reduced by decreasing myocardial oxygen consumption and by increasing oxygen delivery to the tissues.

The location of the infarcted myocardium is important in terms of recovery and potential complications. For instance, inferior wall infarctions usually occur from right coronary artery occlusions and can be associated with variable degrees of heart block. The AV node usually receives its blood supply from the same vessel that nourishes the inferior wall. Thus, alterations in AV nodal conduction would be seen in an inferior-wall acute MI.

Reperfusion Injury. Early treatment of acute MI involves measures to restore myocardial blood flow. However, rapid restoration of blood flow to the myocardium also contributes to injury because ischemic myocardial tissue is less able to respond to normalized levels of oxygen and nutrients, a situation known as myocardial stunning. Reperfusion injury is most likely caused by oxidized free radicals generated by white blood cells (WBCs) and the cellular response to restored blood flow. Blood flow through damaged microvessels gives the tissue a hemorrhagic appearance. Clinically, reperfusion injury is characterized by arrhythmias and reduced contractile function.

Clinical Presentation. The patient suffering an MI commonly has risk factors in their history congruent with atherosclerosis and angina pectoris. Elevated blood cholesterol levels, in particular LDL, are associated with atherosclerosis and the occurrence of an MI. They also contribute to the development of angina pectoris, which can lead to MI. DM, both type 1 and type 2, causes an acceleration of atherosclerosis and hyperlipidemia. Patients with DM are at high risk for developing cardiac pathology and MI. They also have microvascular and macrovascular changes that compromise circulation of cardiac tissue. Hypertension is also consistently associated with a higher risk of MI. This risk can be reduced if patients maintain a regimen of medication and lifestyle modifications to lower BP.

Smoking or tobacco use has been identified as a cardiac risk factor for many years. The free radicals contained in the smoke cause endothelial injury, which kicks off the chain of events that lead to atherosclerosis. Nicotine in cigarettes causes arterial vasoconstriction. The combination of atherosclerosis and vasoconstriction of coronary arteries leads to myocardial ischemia; if ischemia is prolonged, the result is MI.

Another important risk factor is family history. Having a family history of coronary disease increases the patient's risk for MI. However, family history is not solely caused by genetic influences; lifestyle choices are influenced by family also. Diet, food preferences, food preparation, and exercise regimen are all part of family influence.

Signs and Symptoms. MI can present with very specific signs and symptoms, or no symptoms at all. Although each patient may experience unique symptoms, some are characteristic (see Box 16-3). When there are no signs or symptoms, it is referred to as a silent MI (see Box 16-4).

Physical Examination. During MI, if chest pain is ongoing, the patient may appear anxious, diaphoretic, and pale. They often demonstrate Levine's sign and respiratory distress. Peripheral pulses may be diminished and hypertension may be present. When hypotension is present, it usually indicates severe ventricular dysfunction caused by MI or acute valve dysfunction. After MI, the patient can present with signs of heart failure, which include jugular venous distention, pulmonary crackles, and a third heart sound (S_3). A new heart murmur may be present because of papillary muscle dysfunction, a common post-MI complication that causes valve dysfunction.

BOX 16-3. Signs and Symptoms of Myocardial Infarction

- Diaphoresis
- Dyspnea
- Extreme anxiety
- Levine's sign (fist to chest)
- Pallor
- Retrosternal crushing chest pain that radiates to shoulder, arm, jaw, or back
- Weak pulses

BOX 16-4. Silent Myocardial Infarction

Silent MI has been shown to occur far more frequently than anginal episodes in patients with CAD. Both an increase in myocardial oxygen demand and abnormalities of coronary vasomotor tone appear to play a significant role in the genesis of silent ischemia. Recent data show that in excess of 40% of patients with stable angina have frequent episodes of silent ischemia. Silent MI and asymptomatic MI affect older individuals and those with diabetes more than any other population of patients with cardiovascular disease risk. Most silent ischemic episodes occur during minimal or no physical exertion. Exercise testing appears to be the most suitable laboratory diagnostic test to document silent MI in asymptomatic individuals. An ECG will reveal a deep Q wave when performed on a person with a prior MI.

Diagnosis. Tests performed to diagnose an MI include an ECG, which assists in identifying an MI in progress or documenting an MI that has already occurred. The finding of ST elevation (see Fig. 16-18) or ST depression on the ECG is indicative of ACS, but ECG alone cannot confirm MI. Blood tests are needed for a definitive diagnosis.

When heart cells die, their membranes are disrupted and intracellular contents slowly spill into the bloodstream. To confirm if the patient is suffering from acute MI, blood is examined for specific cardiac enzymes and cardiac proteins, particularly CPK-MB fraction, a cardiac enzyme, and **cardiac troponin I (cTnI)**, a cardiac protein. CPK-MB levels begin to rise within 4 hours after an MI, peak between 18 and 24 hours, and subside over 3 to 4 days. The cardiac proteins are cardiac troponin I and troponin T. The **high**

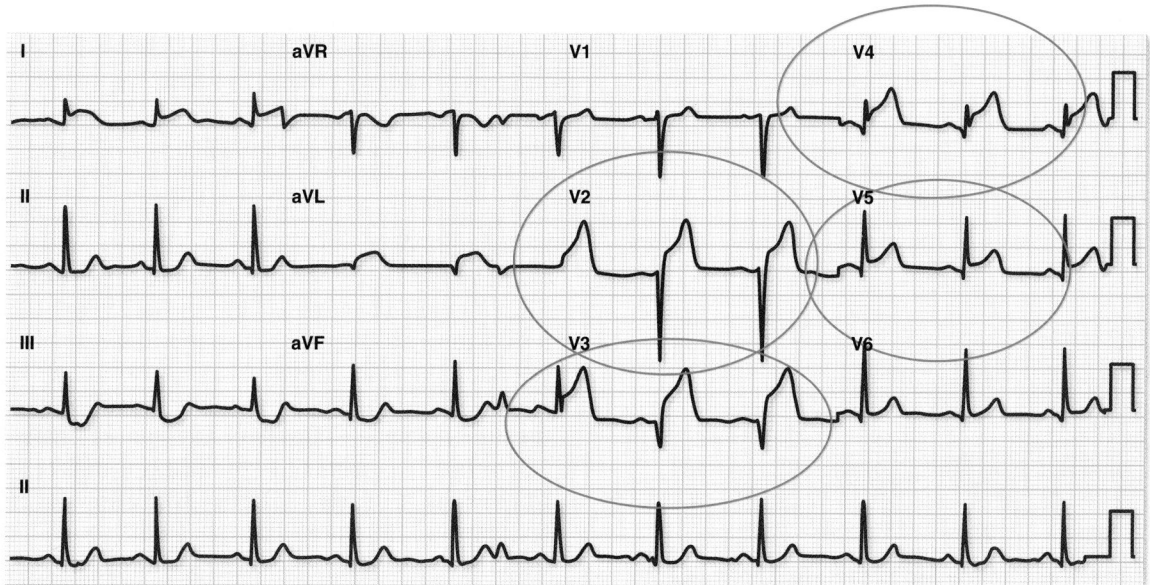

FIGURE 16-18. ECG showing ST-segment elevation MI.

sensitivity cardiac troponin (hs-cTn) assay is highly specific for cardiac muscle necrosis. The hs-cTn assay can be drawn on patient arrival to the clinical setting with a 1-hour turnaround time that is fairly accurate, and then a 3-hour level that is 100% final (Garg et al., 2017).

 CLINICAL CONCEPT

The hs-cTnI is considered the preferred biomarker for diagnosing MI.

High sensitivity cTnI is a cardiac-specific protein that is not normally found in serum and is released only when myocardial cell death has occurred. For early detection of myocardial necrosis, sensitivity of troponin is superior to that of the cardiac isoenzymes.

When MI is suspected, clinicians usually order serial cardiac CPK-MB and hs-cTnI to follow the progression of MI. The rise and fall of these biomarkers provide an indication of the extent of myocardial cell death (see Fig. 16-19).

CLINICAL CONCEPT

After confirming the presence of cardiac biomarkers indicative of MI, an MI can be categorized as STEMI or NSTEMI according to the ECG. An MI that is classified as STEMI indicates that the infarction is completely through the heart wall, whereas NSTEMI indicates that the MI is subendocardial and not completely through the heart wall.

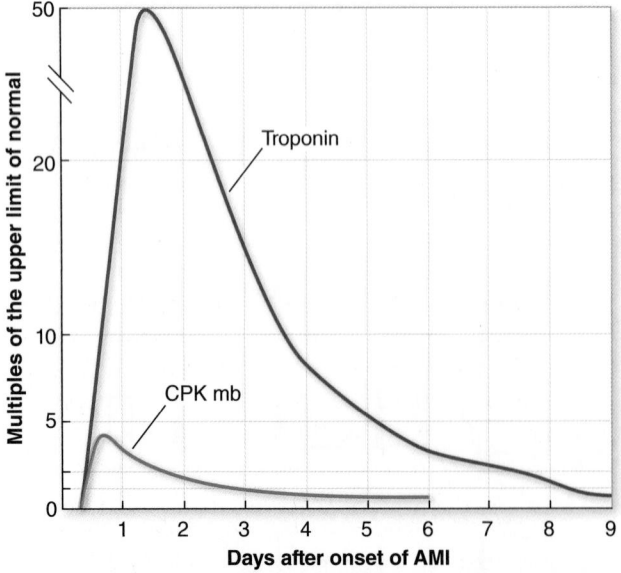

FIGURE 16-19. A graph of cardiac biomarkers that indicate MI. The most sensitive indicator of MI is cTn. The cardiac enzyme CPK-MB is also elevated.

An echocardiogram may also be done to identify what portion of the heart is affected by the MI. When the heart muscle has been injured by the restriction of its oxygenated blood supply, the immediate response of the heart cells is to cease muscle contraction in the region of infarction. Contractile dysfunction occurs at the area of vessel occlusion in the cardiac muscle, and the echocardiogram can identify abnormal wall motion within the infarcted portion of the heart. However, the information from an echocardiogram is limited because it cannot differentiate an acute MI from an old one. Therefore, an echocardiogram alone cannot diagnose acute MI.

Radionuclide myocardial perfusion imaging has excellent sensitivity to detect early acute MI. Perfusion imaging can be used to determine the extent and measurement of infarction. A radionuclide dye is injected into the bloodstream, and it highlights areas of the heart that lack perfusion.

Treatment. The main focus of treatment for an acute MI is to reestablish the flow of blood to the heart muscle to minimize damage. It is essential that patients seek medical assistance as soon as possible for reperfusion to be achieved.

An antiplatelet agent such as aspirin can be taken as soon as the patient experiences chest pain. A non–enteric-coated chewed aspirin is advised, as chewing the aspirin hastens absorption. Oxygen should be administered if the O_2 saturation is less than 95%. Nitrates are usually given as a 0.4-mg dose in a sublingual tablet, followed by close observation of the effect on chest pain and the hemodynamic response. If the initial dose is well tolerated, additional nitrates can be administered; three NTG sublingual tabs can be given over 10 minutes. The most common side effects of nitrates are hypotension and headache. Male patients must be asked if they are taking medications for erectile dysfunction (phosphodiesterase inhibitors such as sildenafil), because adding nitrates would result in severe hypotension or shock.

When chest pain persists or recurs, IV nitrates are indicated, usually started at a dose of 5 to 10 mcg/min and gradually increased until relief of chest pain is achieved.

Morphine sulfate is usually administered to relieve pain, improve gas exchange, and relieve anxiety.

Percutaneous Coronary Intervention (PCI). Early PCI or pharmacological reperfusion via a thrombolytic agent should be performed as soon as possible for patients with clinical presentation of STEMI and who have persistent ST-segment elevation or new or presumed new left bundle branch block, ideally within 12 hours of symptom onset. In addition, it is reasonable to consider an early reperfusion strategy for patients presenting after more than 12 hours, provided there is clinical and/or ECG evidence of ongoing ischemia, with primary PCI being the preferred method in this population. For patients presenting to a PCI-capable hospital, emergent coronary angiography and primary PCI should be accomplished within 90 minutes. PCI is defined as an emergent percutaneous coronary intervention in the setting of STEMI without previous thrombolytic treatment. It is the preferred reperfusion strategy in patients with STEMI, provided it can be performed expeditiously within clinical practice guidelines. PCI achieves superior reperfusion outcomes and is associated with a lower rate of complications, death, and long-term complications of STEMI compared with thrombolytic therapy.

PCI entails performing emergent coronary angiography after establishing arterial access, which can be achieved via the radial or femoral artery. After identifying the anatomy of the coronary circulation and determining the culprit vessel, coronary stents are placed to establish reperfusion. Drug-eluting stents or bare-metal stents are used. CABG surgery may also be an option in a patient who is stabilized; however, PCI with stent placement is preferred.

Thrombolytic Agents. Depending on the time between the onset of pain and the presentation in the emergency department, a thrombolytic agent (tissue plasminogen activator [tPA]) may be given. In some areas, paramedics can administer tPA within the first 90 minutes of the onset of MI. However, most patients need to wait until arrival at the emergency department before tPA can be administered. Thrombolytic therapy in patients with STEMI is highly effective in dissolving a clot and best administered early (within 12 hours after symptoms of MI began). Because of the risk for uncontrolled bleeding, there are strict contraindications regarding administration of thrombolytic agents (see Box 16-5).

Anticoagulant Medications. Anticoagulant agents are an important component in acute MI treatment along with other kinds of reperfusion treatments. For the patient undergoing PCI, unfractionated heparin, bivalirudin, and low molecular weight heparin (e.g., enoxaparin) are recommended.

Antiplatelet Medications. Dual antiplatelet therapy includes aspirin and P2Y12 receptor inhibitors (e.g., clopidogrel, ticagrelor, prasugrel). The patient receives these agents before or at the time of reperfusion and as a maintenance therapy thereafter, depending on the method of reperfusion. Other antiplatelet agents that may be used in STEMI management are the IV glycoprotein IIb/IIIa receptor antagonists, including abciximab, eptifibatide, and tirofiban.

Beta-Adrenergic Blocker Agents. Beta blockers reduce the sympathetic nervous system effects on the heart. They lower heart rate, BP, and myocardial contractility, decreasing the oxygen needs of the myocardium. They can also decrease reinfarction of the myocardium and inhibit ventricular arrhythmias. Preferred agents are metoprolol, carvedilol, and bisoprolol. It is recommended that they be given orally within the first 24 hours.

Calcium Channel Antagonists. The calcium channel antagonists verapamil or diltiazem may be administered for recurrent myocardial ischemia if there are contraindications to using beta blockers.

Complications. Complications can occur after a patient sustains an MI. Potential complications include dysrhythmia, papillary muscle rupture, thromboembolism, ventricular rupture, pericarditis, heart failure, and cardiogenic shock.

Post–Myocardial Infarction Dysrhythmias. The incidence of arrhythmias after MI is greatest early after the onset of MI symptoms. Within the first 24 hours of STEMI, ventricular tachycardia (VT) and ventricular fibrillation (VF) can occur without any preceding rhythm disturbance. The mechanisms responsible for infarction-related arrhythmias include autonomic nervous system imbalance, electrolyte disturbances, and ischemia of conductile cardiac tissue. Almost all post-MI arrhythmias are the result of a phenomenon known as reentry.

As described earlier, an electrical impulse is conducted through the healthy heart in an orderly, sequential manner, beginning at the SA node to AV node, through the bundle of His, and finally through the Purkinje fibers. The normal ECG demonstrates a P wave, representing atrial contraction; a QRS complex, representing ventricular contraction; and a T wave, which represents the heart's repolarization or refractory period.

Normally, the electrical impulse dies out after the sequence is completed and the refractory period takes place. However, ischemic and infarcted cardiac tissues do not conduct impulses; therefore, impulses are slowed or blocked at these areas. The slowing or blocking of impulses causes some impulses to change direction and travel antegrade or retrograde (see Fig. 16-20). This causes some depolarized areas to receive an extra impulse without refractory time, creating disrupted conduction and causing some of the cardiac conductile tissue to fire inappropriately. The heart develops excitable areas that begin to act as

---

BOX 16-5. Contraindications to the Use of tPA

The use of tissue plasminogen activator is contraindicated in the following situations in which the risk of bleeding is greater than the potential benefit:
- Active internal bleeding
- Recent history of stroke
- Recent (within 3 months) intracranial or intraspinal surgery or serious head trauma
- Presence of intracranial conditions that may increase the risk of bleeding, such as some neoplasms, arteriovenous malformations, or aneurysms
- Bleeding diathesis
- Current severe uncontrolled hypertension

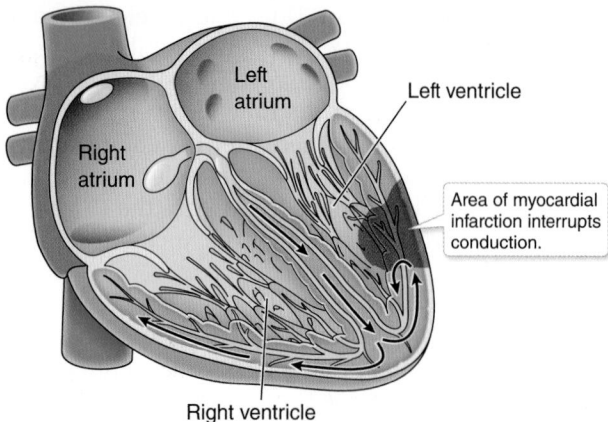

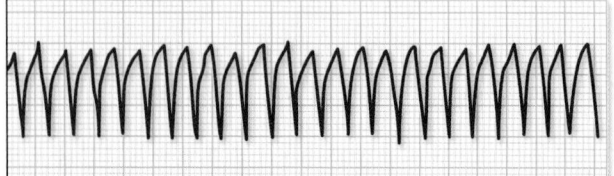

Ventricular tachycardia

FIGURE 16-20. Conduction disturbances are common complications of acute myocardial infarction. They are induced by ischemia and necrosis of the conduction system.

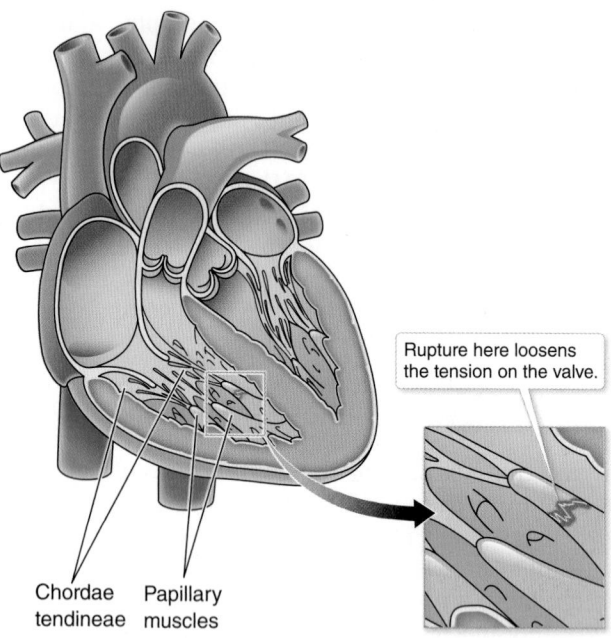

FIGURE 16-21. Papillary muscle rupture. A papillary muscle is attached to membranous strings called chordae tendineae, which are attached to the mitral and tricuspid valve leaflets. With MI, papillary muscle rupture can occur and the fixation of the valve leaflets comes loose. Blood then flows upward through the floppy valve with contraction of the ventricle, and this causes a regurgitant heart murmur.

ectopic pacemakers outside the normally functioning nodes (see the "Dysrhythmias and Conduction Disorders" section below).

Papillary Muscle Rupture. An MI in the left ventricle often involves injury to a papillary muscle. These small muscular projections are tethered to the heart valve leaflets via stringlike structures called chordae tendineae (see Fig. 16-21). In the left ventricle, papillary muscle rupture causes the mitral valve to be unable to close. With each contraction of the left ventricle, blood flows upward through the loose mitral valve into the left atrium. This causes a mitral valve regurgitation murmur, also called mitral insufficiency. As a consequence, mitral regurgitation often causes backup of blood and hydrostatic pressure into the left atrium, pulmonary veins, and pulmonary capillaries, causing pulmonary edema. Patient signs and symptoms include dyspnea, cough, pulmonary crackles, and heart murmur heard at the fifth intercostal space left midclavicular line. Treatment includes surgical valve repair and diuretic agents.

Thromboembolism. After MI, the atrial and ventricular muscles do not contract fully. The areas of infarction consist of dead tissue, which is noncontractile. In this noncontractile chamber, stagnant blood collects and is susceptible to clotting. A clot then can travel out of the heart into the pulmonary or aortic artery and become a thromboembolism, which can potentially obstruct blood flow through pulmonary or systemic arteries. Anticoagulant and thrombolytic therapies may be needed to break up the clot.

Ventricular Aneurysm and Rupture. After MI, a portion of the heart wall is infarcted and damaged so that it is noncontractile, necrotic, and scarred. The tensile strength of necrotic tissue is much less compared with normal myocardium. The weakened area is constantly exposed to the shearing force of blood and the pressure of adjacent contractile tissue. These conditions can contribute to the formation of a weakened bulging of the wall (see Fig. 16-22). When this occurs in the ventricle, the weakened area is a ventricular aneurysm with potential for rupture. Ventricular rupture causes a sudden drop in blood pressure and inadequate peripheral tissue perfusion. The patient loses consciousness and shows signs of shock. Surgical intervention to repair the rupture is needed immediately.

Pericarditis. Pericarditis is the inflammation of the pericardial membrane that surrounds the heart. It usually appears on the second or third day after MI. The patient experiences sharp, stabbing pain that is aggravated with deep inspiration and positional changes. The classic sound heard through the stethoscope is called a pericardial friction rub, which may or may not be present. Pericarditis can occur as a component of **Dressler's syndrome**, a hypersensitivity reaction to the tissue necrosis of MI. Dressler's syndrome includes pericarditis, pleuritis, and pneumonitis and is treated with anti-inflammatory agents.

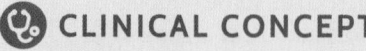

CLINICAL CONCEPT

The murmur of pericarditis, called pericardial friction rub, is a scratchy, rough sound.

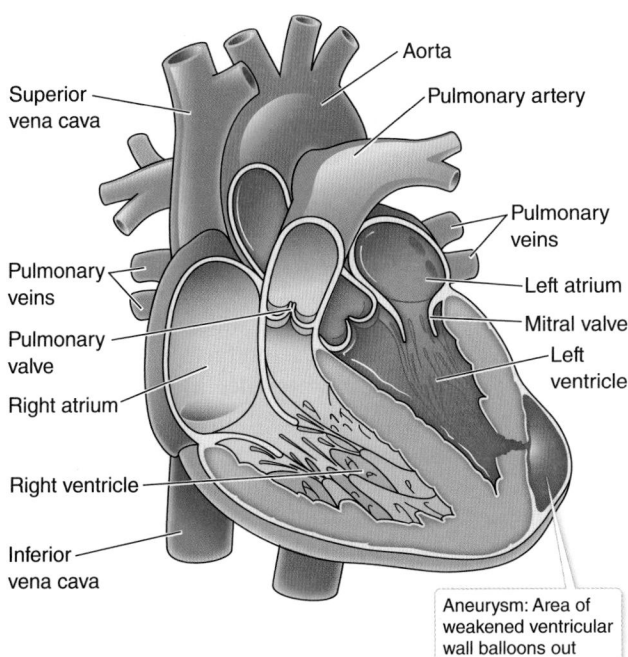

FIGURE 16-22. A ventricular aneurysm is a weakening in the ventricular wall that often occurs after myocardial infarction. This floppy area of dilated wall has turbulent blood flow within it. Thrombi often develop within the aneurysm.

Heart Failure. Heart failure, weakening of the ventricles of the heart, is a common complication of MI. The heart's pumping action becomes impaired, blood volume accumulates in the chambers, and hydrostatic pressure builds backward in the cardiovascular system. Hydrostatic pressure builds within the left ventricle, left atrium, pulmonary veins, and pulmonary capillaries. Pulmonary edema, a severe symptom of heart failure, develops. Symptoms include dyspnea, cough, pulmonary crackles, and peripheral edema.

Cardiogenic Shock. If the heart is severely damaged from an extensive MI, heart failure can worsen into cardiogenic shock, in which the ventricles are unable to pump sufficient blood to the rest of the body, causing blood pressure to drop abruptly (see Chapter 17). Acute myocardial infarction (MI) accounts for 81% of patients in cardiogenic shock. Due to severe impairment of the myocardium, there is left ventricular pump failure, diminished cardiac output, and multiple organ hypoperfusion, resulting in cellular hypoxia. Clinically, this presents as hypotension, which is refractory to volume resuscitation. Cardiogenic shock is a common cause of mortality.

Cardiac Inflammation and Infection

A few cardiac disorders are caused by inflammation and infection. Infective endocarditis (IE) is the most common type of cardiac infection. Heart valve disease occurs as a result of IE. Myocarditis is often caused by viruses that attack the cardiac muscle tissue. Pericarditis, which affects the outer layer around the heart, commonly occurs after MI.

Infective Endocarditis

Infective endocarditis (IE) is a noncontagious infection of the cardiac endothelium that most commonly affects the heart valves. It is caused mainly by bacteria, although fungi can also be the infection's etiological agent. Normally, the cardiac endothelium is a smooth membrane that helps regulate vascular tone, inflammation, thrombosis, and vascular remodeling. Damaged valves and turbulent blood flow within the heart create areas of impact that wear away at the smooth endothelial surface. These rough areas of the heart's membranous surface are prone to infection and provoke aggregation of platelets to form a thrombus. Intracardiac devices such as prosthetic valves and intravascular devices such as central venous catheters are significant risk factors for IE. IE is difficult to diagnose, and bacterial antibiotic resistance has become a significant obstacle in the treatment of this disease.

Epidemiology. The incidence of IE in the general population is estimated to be approximately 13 cases per 100,000, but incidence is greater among patients with underlying valvular heart disease and those who inject illicit IV drugs. More than 50% of IE cases occur in persons older than age 50 years. More than one-third of cases of IE are caused by hospital-acquired infections. The incidence of IE is rising because of longer survival of patients with degenerative heart diseases, increased use of intravascular devices, increased implantation of prosthetic heart valves, and aging of the population.

Etiology. The most common cause of IE is intravascular lines that introduce *Staphylococcus aureus* to the bloodstream. *S. aureus* has become the primary pathogen of endocarditis. As it evolves, IE continues to pose significant clinical challenges. The mortality rate within 1 year of acquiring infection is almost 30%. Prosthetic valves, pacemakers, and cardioverter defibrillators are commonly involved in IE. Prosthetic valve endocarditis is most commonly caused by *S. aureus.* Methicillin-resistant *S. aureus* (MRSA) infections are often present.

Endocarditis can be categorized as:

- Native valve endocarditis (NVE), acute and subacute
- Prosthetic valve endocarditis (PVE), early and late
- IV drug abuse (IVDA) endocarditis
- Pacemaker IE
- Health-care-acquired IE

The different types of IE have varying causes and involve different pathogens.

Native Valve Endocarditis (NVE). Rheumatic valvular disease, a complication of group A beta hemolytic Streptococcus (GABHS) infection, is responsible for 30% of cases of NVE. After GABHS, antibodies that developed against Streptococcus mistakenly attack heart valve tissue. The mitral valve is most commonly affected. Congenital heart disease is responsible for 15% of NVE, with patent ductus arteriosus and ventricular septal defect as leading causes. Mitral valve prolapse with murmur causes 20% of NVE. Degenerative heart diseases, such as calcific aortic stenosis, Marfan's syndrome, and syphilis, are also major causes. Approximately 70% of infections in NVE are caused by Streptococcus species, including *Streptococcus viridans, Streptococcus bovis,* and enterococci. *Staphylococcus* species cause 25% of cases and generally demonstrate a more aggressive acute course.

Prosthetic Valve Endocarditis (PVE). PVE associated with aortic valve prostheses is caused by a variety of pathogens, including *S. aureus* and *S. epidermidis.* These health-care-acquired organisms are often methicillin-resistant bacteria such as MRSA. Other causes include *Corynebacterium,* nonenterococcal streptococci, fungi (e.g., *Candida albicans, Candida stellatoidea, Aspergillus* species), Legionella, and the HACEK (i.e., *Haemophilus aphrophilus, Actinobacillus actinomycetemcomitans, Cardiobacterium hominis, Eikenella corrodens, Kingella kingae*) organisms.

IVDA Infective Endocarditis. Endocarditis in IV drug users is commonly caused by *S. aureus* and involves the tricuspid valve. Two-thirds of patients have no previous history of heart disease or murmur. Pulmonary manifestations may be most prominent in patients with tricuspid infection due to septic emboli of the lungs. MRSA accounts for an increasing proportion of *S. aureus* infections and has been associated with previous hospitalizations, long-term addiction, and nonprescribed antibiotic use. Groups A, C, and G streptococci and enterococci are also recovered from patients with IVDA IE. Fungal organisms (e.g., Candida), gram-negative organisms including *Pseudomonas aeruginosa,* and the HACEK microorganisms are also common etiologies.

Health-Care–Associated Infective Endocarditis. Health-care–associated IE commonly involves intravascular devices such as central or peripheral IV catheters, pacemakers and defibrillators, hemodialysis shunts and catheters, and chemotherapeutic and hyperalimentation IV lines. These patients tend to have infection with gram-positive cocci, enterococci, and nonenterococcal streptococci. Fungal endocarditis (e.g., Candida) is also associated with the health-care environment, particularly in those exposed to broad-spectrum antibiotics.

> ## CLINICAL CONCEPT
> Pacemaker-associated endocarditis can develop in patients with implantation of these devices caused by infection or because of erosion of pacemaker components.

Pathophysiology. Pneumonia, pyelonephritis, gingivitis, dental procedures, or other invasive procedures can be sources of microorganisms. Common ports of entry for *S. aureus* are the skin in IV drug use and intravascular lines. When microbes infect the bloodstream, bacteremia develops and allows microorganisms to travel into the heart, where they adhere to damaged endothelial tissue or attach to thrombi within the heart. Once adherent, the microorganisms multiply and attract WBCs and platelets, which release cytokines and coagulation factors. Stimulation of the coagulation cascade results in fibrin deposition and, eventually, development of a vegetation (see Fig. 16-23). A vegetation is a tiny mass that contains microorganisms, a meshwork of fibrin, and cellular components that are similar to thrombi. Microorganisms continually proliferate, are shed into the bloodstream, and stimulate development of additional vegetations. Cytokines attracted to the area provoke a persistent cycle of inflammation, which damages intracardiac structures, particularly heart valves. Vegetations are most commonly found on valve leaflets, and fragments of vegetations can embolize into the circulation. Carried by the bloodstream, these fragments, called **septic emboli**, can initiate infection or ischemia in remote tissues.

In approximately 10% of all cases of endocarditis, an infectious agent cannot be found. This can occur because of prior antibiotic treatment, difficulty isolating the microbial agent, or deeply lodged microbes within vegetations that are not released into the bloodstream.

Clinical Presentation. IE can occur as an acute or subacute infection. Subacute IE develops gradually, and initial symptoms may be subtle. Individuals with subacute infection may be unaware of the severity of the illness and delay obtaining medical attention. Acute IE develops suddenly, and the patient becomes

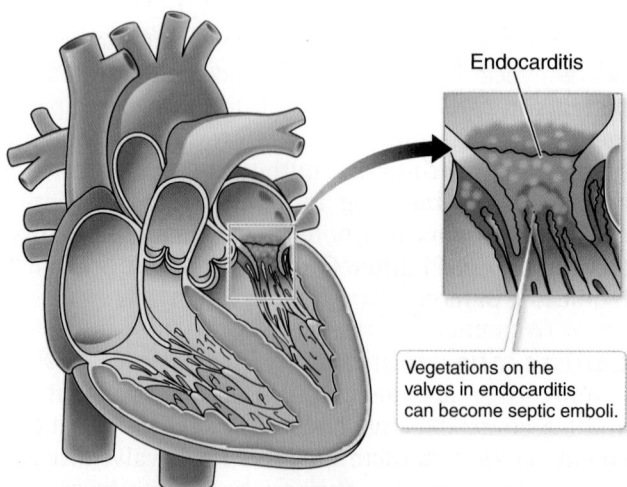

FIGURE 16-23. In infectious endocarditis, lesions called vegetations form on the heart valves. Vegetations on the valvular leaflets can become septic emboli.

critically ill and in need of medical attention. Individuals usually present with nonspecific symptoms, including fever, chills, anorexia, weight loss, myalgias, and arthralgias. Fever may be low or absent in older adults or severely debilitated persons. The development of a new heart murmur heard on auscultation with the stethoscope or worsening of a preexistent murmur are important diagnostic signs. With severe valvular dysfunction, signs of heart failure such as edema may be present.

Septic emboli can cause ischemia or infarction of the extremities, spleen, kidney, bowel, lungs, or brain. Signs consistent with ischemia of organs may be the initial clinical manifestations of IE. For example, septic emboli can lodge in a cerebral artery or arteriole and cause an ischemic stroke. Neurological symptoms from embolic stroke occur in up to 40% of patients with IE. Patients may also present with meningitis, seizures, encephalopathy, or abscesses of the brain. The kidney can also be damaged by septic emboli or immune-mediated glomerulonephritis. Septic emboli can lodge in the lungs, particularly in IV drug abusers. In IV drug abusers, the veins are the portal of entry; *S. aureus,* the flora of the skin, most commonly causes bacteremia. Septic emboli from *S. aureus* travel from the peripheral vein into the IVC and into the right side of the heart. As a result, tricuspid valve infection with evidence of tricuspid murmurs is most common in IV drug users. From the tricuspid valve, septic emboli travel easily into the right ventricle, then the pulmonary artery. The patient demonstrates cough, pleuritic chest pain, and a distinctive pneumonia on x-ray consisting of nodular infiltrates.

Classic clinical manifestations of IE caused by septic emboli include petechiae, splinter hemorrhages, Janeway lesions, Osler's nodes, and Roth spots. Splinter hemorrhages appear as red, linear streaks in the nailbeds. Janeway lesions are erythematous, nontender lesions on the palms and soles. Osler's nodes are subcutaneous nodules in the pulp of the fingertips that persist for hours or days. Roth spots are oval retinal hemorrhages with pale centers. These signs are pathognomonic for IE, and they are seen in persons who suffer prolonged illness without treatment.

Diagnosis. A definitive diagnosis of IE is based on a set of specific clinical signs, as well as laboratory and echocardiographic findings, called the Duke criteria (see Box 16-6). To diagnose IE, a patient must exhibit two major criteria, one major and three minor criteria, or five minor criteria. Assessment of a patient for the Duke criteria requires a thorough physical examination, multiple blood cultures, laboratory tests, and echocardiography. Multiple blood cultures are necessary because in IE there are fewer than 100 microorganisms per mL of blood, and it is difficult to obtain a sample of blood containing the etiological agent. At least three blood cultures drawn 12 hours apart is the preferred method.

BOX 16-6. Duke Major and Minor Diagnostic Criteria for Infective Endocarditis

MAJOR CRITERIA
- Blood cultures are positive for IE
- Evidence of endocardial involvement from diagnostic studies (particularly valuable is transesophageal echocardiography)

MINOR CRITERIA
- A predisposing factor is present (e.g., IV drug use, intravascular line)
- Fever
- Vascular phenomena (e.g., septic emboli, pulmonary infarct, mycotic aneurysm, intracranial hemorrhage, conjunctival hemorrhage, painless skin lesions, such as Janeway lesions)
- Immunological phenomena (e.g., Osler's nodes, glomerulonephritis, Roth spots, positive rheumatoid factor)
- Microbiological evidence (e.g., positive blood culture or serological evidence of infection)

DEFINITIVE DIAGNOSIS OF IE: Two major criteria met or one major and three minor criteria met or five minor criteria.

POSSIBLE DIAGNOSIS OF IE: One major and one minor criteria met or three minor criteria met

Adapted with permission from EBMcalc.com. Retrieved from https://www.merckmanuals.com/medical-calculators/EndocarditisMod.htm

---

Laboratory tests are necessary, including complete blood count, electrolytes, creatinine, blood urea nitrogen, glucose, erythrocyte sedimentation rate (ESR), coagulation panel, and urinalysis. Anemia is common in subacute endocarditis. Leukocytosis is observed in acute endocarditis. ESR, although not specific, is elevated in more than 90% of cases. Glomerulonephritis, which causes proteinuria and microscopic hematuria, is present in approximately 50% of cases. Decreased complement and the presence of rheumatoid factor are evident in subacute endocarditis.

A transthoracic ECG can demonstrate new-onset valvular dysfunction, vegetations, abscess, or prosthetic-valve dysfunction. New onset of regurgitant valvular dysfunction is particularly indicative of IE. Transesophageal echocardiography is significantly more accurate than transthoracic echocardiogram and is the preferred diagnostic procedure.

Additional cardiac imaging tools for diagnosis of IE include cardiac magnetic resonance imaging (MRI), cardiac CT, cardiac CT angiography (CTA), and fluorodeoxyglucose positron emission tomography with CT or CTA.

Treatment. Treatment of IE consists mainly of IV antibiotics for 6 weeks or longer. However, recent studies suggest that high doses of oral and depot antibiotics may be viable alternatives to conventional intravenous therapy (El-Dalati et al., 2020). The antibiotic should be precisely bactericidal for the cultured microorganism. Microbes within vegetations on infected valves are difficult to penetrate, necessitating high serum levels of antibiotics. Blood cultures should be repeated daily until sterile. Persistent fever despite antibiotic therapy often indicates paravalvular or extracardiac abscesses. Laboratory indicators of inflammation, such as elevated ESR, resolve slowly and do not reflect response to treatment. Vegetations may not change in size with treatment. Surgical intervention may be necessary in patients who do not respond to antibiotic therapy, those with heart failure, or those with persistent septic emboli. As many as 40% of patients with prosthetic-valve IE require surgical intervention.

After recovery from IE, the patient needs to be vigilant about prevention of recurrence. Prophylactic antibiotics are necessary in recovered patients anytime there is a risk for bacteremia, as in surgical procedures, certain invasive dental treatments, bronchoscopy, endoscopy, cystoscopy, or localized infections.

Complications. Regurgitant heart valve defects, intracardiac abscesses, and heart failure are the major cardiac complications of IE. Heart murmurs occur in 85% of affected individuals. Heart failure is usually the result of abnormal blood flow dynamics caused by valvular dysfunction, but it can also result from inflammation of the myocardium. Abscesses can form within the heart and erode through the endocardium or pericardium, causing pericarditis. Infection of the endocardium can also interrupt the cardiac conduction system and provoke dysrhythmias.

Extracardiac complications are most often caused by the septic valvular vegetations, which tend to break apart and embolize. Septic arterial emboli, which occur in 50% of patients, can lodge in remote tissues and form abscesses, particularly in the lungs, spleen, brain, and meninges. Septic emboli can also weaken the walls of arterial vessels and create mycotic aneurysms. Mycotic cerebral aneurysms form in 2% to 15% of patients, causing headaches, focal neurological signs, and cerebral artery rupture, leading to intracerebral hemorrhage. Septic emboli can also obstruct the circulation of extracardiac tissues and cause ischemia or infarction. This often occurs in the extremities, brain, lung, bowel, kidneys, and spleen. Ischemic stroke occurs in up to 40% of patients. The emboli can also lodge in the kidney and cause renal infarction and stimulate immune-mediated glomerulonephritis. When formed on the structures of the right side of the heart, septic emboli can cause pulmonary embolism.

Myocarditis

Myocarditis, also called inflammatory cardiomyopathy, is an inflammatory disease of the myocardium that can range from a mild disorder to a lethal condition. The myocardium undergoes inflammation with degeneration and necrosis of cardiac myocytes. It does not involve myocardial ischemia; however, conduction disruption is common.

Epidemiology. The incidence of myocarditis is estimated at 1 to 10 cases per 100,000 persons. As many as 1% to 5% of patients with acute viral infections may have involvement of the myocardium. The incidence of myocarditis is similar between males and females, although young males are particularly susceptible. Other susceptible populations include immunocompromised individuals, pregnant women, and infants.

Etiology. Viruses are common causes of myocarditis in the United States and Europe. Many different viruses, bacteria, fungi, and parasites, as well as drugs and toxins, can cause myocarditis. Influenza, adenovirus, parvovirus B19, enteroviruses, herpesvirus, diphtheria, viral exanthems such as rubella, Lyme disease, hepatitis, rheumatic carditis, *Trypanosoma cruzi* (which causes Chagas disease), and HIV/AIDS are common etiological agents. Other causes include radiation, hypersensitivity reactions, or exposure to toxic substances such as cocaine. Risk factors for myocarditis include viral infections; systemic infections caused by bacteria, fungi, or parasites; autoimmune disease; and a multitude of toxins, drugs, and chemotherapeutic agents. Myocarditis is the major cause of cardiac transplant rejection.

Pathophysiology. Myocarditis is inflammation of the muscle layer of the heart's wall. It can occur by direct invasion of a pathogen or a toxin that is liberated by a pathogen. It can also occur as an immunological mechanism initiated by an infectious agent. Cardiac myocytes undergo destruction with a large infiltration of T cells and WBCs that liberate tissue-damaging cytokines. Often the etiological organism is not found. It is believed that an organism often begins the process of cellular destruction; however, continued inflammation is then caused by an autoimmune mechanism.

Clinical Presentation. Patients with myocarditis can demonstrate varying clinical presentations, from no symptoms to severe chest pain, chills, fever, and dyspnea. Patients may report a flu-like syndrome of fever, myalgia, arthralgia, pharyngitis, tonsillitis, and upper respiratory infection. Symptoms of palpitations or syncope can occur. Sudden cardiac death can develop because of ventricular arrhythmias or AV block. Adults can develop heart failure years after an episode of myocarditis.

On physical examination, cardiac auscultation may reveal an S_3 gallop rhythm, which is an extra beat heard after S_2. A pericardial friction rub is also possible. Depending on the etiology, there may be various other signs, such as lymphadenopathy, rash, or those of the Jones criteria seen in rheumatic fever.

Diagnosis. Laboratory studies involved in the diagnosis include a complete blood count (CBC) that demonstrates leukocytosis, elevated ESR, and CRP, which indicates inflammation. The cTn and cardiac enzymes are elevated, indicating cardiac muscle damage. The blood is analyzed for various viral antibody titers such as enterovirus, adenovirus, HIV, influenza, hepatitis C, herpes virus, Coxsackievirus, Epstein–Barr virus, and cytomegalovirus. The presence of a viral genome within a biopsy of myocardium confirms a viral etiology. An ECG can reveal heart dysfunction and degree of heart failure, if present. A diagnostic test called antimyosin scintigraphy can identify myocardial inflammation. Gadolinium-enhanced MRI is used for assessment of the extent of inflammation and cellular edema. Cardiac magnetic resonance scanning and delayed-enhanced MRI are also used in diagnosis.

Treatment. Treatment focuses on symptom management and decreasing myocardial workload. Activity is restricted during a recovery period of 6 months or more. Treatment measures for heart failure such as diuretics, nitrates, ACE inhibitors, and inotropic agents are often necessary. Anti-infective agents are necessary for the underlying etiology. Pacemaker insertion may be needed. In severe cases of heart failure, cardiac transplantation is considered.

Pericarditis

Pericarditis is inflammation of the pericardium and epicardium, the folds of serous membrane that surround the heart's exterior. The pericardium is a tough, outer membrane that secures the heart in position and is attached to the sternum and thoracic structures. The inner layer is the epicardium, which is directly attached to the heart's surface. In between these layers is the pericardial space, which contains 30 to 50 mL of serous fluid that acts as a lubricant.

When the pericardium undergoes inflammation, additional fluid accumulates in the pericardial space. The fluid is called a **pericardial effusion**, and it surrounds the heart. If the fluid accumulates to high levels of 200 mL or greater, it can compress the heart, causing a condition called **cardiac tamponade** (see Fig. 16-24). In cardiac tamponade, the heart chambers are restricted by the surrounding pericardial fluid so they cannot stretch and fill with blood (see Box 16-7).

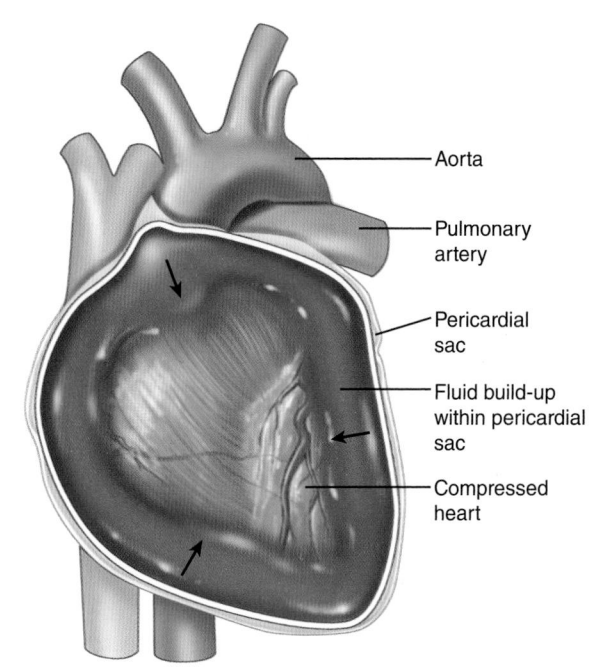

Aorta

Pulmonary artery

Pericardial sac

Fluid build-up within pericardial sac

Compressed heart

FIGURE 16-24. Cardiac tamponade.

BOX 16-7. Pericardial Effusion

Pericardial effusion is the presence of fluid in the pericardial cavity. Normally, the pericardial cavity contains approximately 40 mL of clear filtrate of blood. A small amount of pericardial fluid around the heart may not cause any symptoms. However, a large amount of fluid, such as 200 mL or more, causes compression against the heart, inhibiting filling of the chambers. Like pericarditis, pericardial effusions can be caused by disorders such as infection, autoimmune reactions, or systemic inflammatory conditions. To diagnose pericardial effusion, an echocardiogram is done. The echocardiogram will show the excess fluid surrounding the heart and can demonstrate the decrease in LV ejection volume. Treatment is aimed at removal of the pericardial fluid in a procedure called pericardiocentesis. Pericardial fluid analysis can assist in the determination of etiology. Treatment depends on the etiology of the effusion.

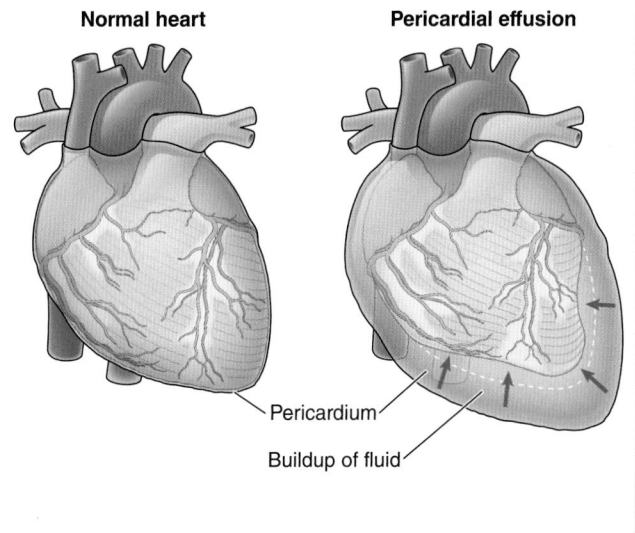

Normal heart   **Pericardial effusion**

Pericardium

Buildup of fluid

Epidemiology. Studies indicate that a diagnosis of acute pericarditis occurs in approximately 1 per 1,000 hospital admissions; however, this is thought to be a low estimate because many persons do not have symptoms with pericarditis. Acute pericarditis and MI present in a similar manner: chest pain and ST elevation on ECG. However, pericarditis occurs in only 1% of patients with acute chest pain and ST elevation. In general, males are affected more frequently than females by pericarditis. Pericarditis occurs in 6% to 20% of patients with advanced renal failure. Pericardial effusion occurs in 21% of patients with cancer and in up to 43% of patients with AIDS. After MI, Dressler's syndrome, a disorder that includes pericarditis, occurs in 5% to 6% of patients. Pericardial effusions, some of which go undetected, are estimated to occur in 28% of MI patients.

Etiology. Tuberculosis, viruses, radiation treatment of the chest, cardiac surgery, and connective tissue disease are the most common causes of pericarditis. Viruses such as Coxsackievirus, influenza, Epstein–Barr virus, varicella, hepatitis, mumps, and HIV cause pericarditis. Rheumatic fever; autoimmune inflammatory diseases such as systemic lupus erythematosus, rheumatoid arthritis, or Sjögren's syndrome; renal failure; and metabolic disorders can also cause pericarditis. Pericarditis commonly occurs after MI, a condition called Dressler's syndrome. Malignancies of the lung, breast, and skin, as well as leukemia and lymphoma, are associated with pericarditis.

Pathophysiology. In inflammation of the pericardium, the capillaries that supply the pericardial membrane become highly permeable. The capillary pores allow plasma proteins and fibrinogen to leave the bloodstream and enter the pericardial cavity. This creates a fibrin-rich, exudative edema that envelops the heart; as it heals, it forms scar tissue. Commonly, adhesions form between the layers of the pericardium, which can restrict optimal filling of the ventricles.

Dressler's syndrome is a specific type of pericarditis that develops in some person's post-MI. This autoimmune reaction may occur 2 to 3 weeks after an MI. Cardiac proteins released during an MI stimulate immunoglobulins that combine with the proteins to form immune complexes. The immune complexes are deposited in the pericardium, causing inflammation and fluid collection in the pericardial sac.

Clinical Presentation. The signs of acute pericarditis include chest pain, fever, dyspnea, pericardial friction rub, and specific ECG findings. The chest pain of pericarditis is described as sharp and sudden, and it worsens with deep breathing, swallowing, and coughing. The pain can radiate into the neck, jaw, abdomen, or back. A pericardial friction rub, which is a scratching sound, can be heard through the stethoscope. Symptoms of cardiac tamponade, called the **Beck triad**, can be present; they include hypotension, jugular vein distention, and muffled heart sounds. A finding called pulsus paradoxus occurs in 70% to 80% of patients with cardiac tamponade. **Pulsus paradoxus** is exhibited by a decrease in systolic blood pressure of 10 mm Hg or more with inspiration. In pulsus paradoxus, the thorax, which is full of air in inspiration, places pressure on the heart and diminishes the volume ejected from the left ventricle into the aorta.

Diagnosis. The ECG in pericarditis shows ST-segment elevations in multiple leads, which can appear as ECG changes of MI. Increased blood urea nitrogen and increased serum creatinine occur in pericarditis of renal failure. Otherwise, laboratory values can be normal, but if there is a concurrent MI or a great degree of cardiac stress, there may be elevated levels of cardiac markers such as cTn and CPK-MB. Echocardiogram, CT scan, and cardiac MRI are frequently done. Some patients require right-sided cardiac catheterization for hemodynamic studies of pressures within the heart chambers.

Treatment. Treatment depends on the etiology of pericarditis. If infection is present, antibiotics are administered. Pericardiectomy and surgical drainage of the pericardial space are necessary. Anti-inflammatory agents and heart failure medications such as diuretics are often necessary.

Dysrhythmias and Conduction Disorders

Dysrhythmias, also called arrhythmias, are disorders of cardiac rhythm. There are two categories of cardiac dysrhythmias: supraventricular and ventricular. The supraventricular dysrhythmias include those generated at the SA node, atria, and AV node. The ventricular dysrhythmias include those generated in the ventricular conduction system: bundle of His, Purkinje fibers, and ventricular muscle.

> **ALERT!** Ventricular dysrhythmias are potentially fatal.

The heart can beat excessively fast in tachyarrhythmias or excessively slow in bradyarrhythmias. Heart block occurs when impulses of the conduction system are blocked, most commonly at the AV node. In complete heart block, the atria and ventricles beat independently of each other.

An ectopic pacemaker is an excitable area outside the normal conduction pathway. A **premature ventricular contraction (PVC)** occurs when an ectopic pacemaker initiates a contraction. Several PVCs in a row lead to ventricular tachycardia, where the ventricle is beating independently without waiting for the completion of each action potential. This can lead to **ventricular fibrillation**, where the heart is beating so rapidly that the ventricle is actually quivering and not ejecting any blood.

Atrioventricular Block

AV block is associated with anterior- and inferior-wall MI. In anterior-wall infarction, heart block is related to ischemic malfunction of the conduction system, commonly caused by extensive myocardial damage. AV block occurs when the SA atrial impulse fails to be conducted to the ventricles, usually causing bradycardia. The ECG shows a prolonged PR interval with a slowed heart rate of fewer than 60 beats per minute. Temporary electrical pacing provides an effective means of raising heart rate in patients with bradycardia caused by AV block.

Atrial Fibrillation

Atrial fibrillation (AF) is the most commonly encountered arrhythmia in the clinical setting, with the highest prevalence within the older adult population. AF is present in almost 30% of those aged 80 to 89 years and complicates MI in 5% to 10% of cases. It is defined as the absence of coordinated, rhythmic atrial contractions. Multiple irregular fibrillatory P waves are seen on the ECG representing multiple, rapid reentrant impulses moving around in the atrial chamber. The multiple irregular P waves may or may not stimulate a concomitant irregular, rapid ventricular response.

When ventricular rate increases to tachycardic levels, AF can cause decompensation of the ventricle in the form of myocardial ischemia or heart failure. AF can also increase the risk of embolic stroke. The noncontracting, quivering atria in AF allow for stasis of blood and subsequent clot formation. A clot can form in the left atrium, travel into the left ventricle, then move into the aorta and up the subclavian artery to the internal carotid and middle cerebral artery of the brain. The rate of ischemic stroke in the presence of AF is two to seven times the rate of stroke in patients without AF.

Anticoagulant treatment is used to prevent clot formation and stroke. Warfarin, dabigatran, factor Xa inhibitors (e.g., rivaroxaban, apixaban, edoxaban), and aspirin are options for stroke prevention. Ablation therapy using a cardiac catheter is used to destroy abnormal regions in the left atrial wall responsible for stimulation of the abnormal rhythm of fibrillation. Surgical approaches that obliterate the left atrial appendage can be used to reduce stroke risk. The left atrial appendage is a small, pouchlike sac in the left atrium where stasis of blood can occur with clot formation. Surgical closure of this pouch can decrease clot formation in atrial fibrillation. Two implantable devices used to occlude the appendage, the Watchman and the Amplatzer Cardiac Plug, appear to be as effective as warfarin in preventing stroke.

> **ALERT!** AF can cause thrombus formation and embolism to the brain. It is a frequent cause of ischemic stroke.

Premature Ventricular Contractions

Sporadic PVCs are the most common arrhythmia occurring with MI. During PVCs, the ventricle beats independently without waiting for the sequential conduction initiated by the SA or AV nodes. PVCs do not have a P wave or T wave and are characterized by a wide, bizarre QRS. Their form on the ECG indicates that they do not follow an atrial contraction and do not allow for a refractory period. PVCs may occur singularly or in patterns of bigeminy, trigeminy, quadrigeminy, or other sequential patterns. In bigeminy, a PVC occurs every other beat. In trigeminy, a PVC occurs after every two normal beats. Sporadic, infrequent PVCs do not require treatment. However, two sequential PVCs are termed couplets and require vigilance because three PVCs in a row constitute ventricular tachycardia, a dangerous cardiac rhythm.

PVCs that are frequent, in that there are more than 10 per hour, or complex, such as those occurring in couplets, are associated with increased mortality. Cardiac mortality occurs in association with significantly impaired ventricular function. Patients may experience palpitations with PVCs. If frequent, PVCs can diminish cardiac output and cause fatigue, dizziness, and more severe arrhythmia.

Either medical treatment or catheter ablation are considered first-line therapies in most patients with PVCs associated with symptoms or heart failure. If medical treatment is selected, either beta blockers or nondihydropyridine calcium channel blockers are recommended for patients with normal ventricular systolic function.

Ventricular Tachycardia

Sustained VT is defined as VT that persists for longer than 30 seconds or associated with hemodynamic compromise. The ECG demonstrates a series of widened QRS waves without preceding P waves or any T waves that follow. With VT, the rate of the QRS waves, which represent rapid, ineffective ventricular contractions, is greater than 100 beats per minute. Also, the ventricular contractions do not allow for effective pumping of blood, severely diminishing cardiac output. Patients are aware of a sudden onset of rapid heart rate and may experience dyspnea, palpitations, and lightheadedness.

VT is often treated with antiarrhythmic drugs, but when VT causes significant hemodynamic compromise, cardioversion is necessary. Beta blockers are recommended and are highly beneficial in patients with reduced left ventricular function. Antiarrhythmic drugs can be used with amiodarone providing the most benefit. VT ablation targets clinical arrhythmias to prevent recurrence. Percutaneous ablation is a safe and effective catheter-based therapy to ablate myocardium from either the endocardial or the epicardial surface. Implantable cardioverter defibrillators (ICDs) reduce the mortality risk associated with recurrent VT and can terminate VT episodes.

Ventricular Fibrillation

VF is often precipitated by a single, early PVC falling on the T wave of a previous impulse. The T wave indicates repolarization or the refractory period for the ventricle. The lack of a refractory period is dangerous; often, the rhythm degenerates into a rapid, repetitive sequence of VT that deteriorates into VF. The word *fibrillation* means quivering; in VF; the ventricle is quivering and not contracting effectively to pump blood out of the chamber. The ECG shows bizarre waves with no discernible P, QRS, or T waves.

Onset of VF is rapidly followed by loss of consciousness and, if untreated, death. Most patients whose VF is treated successfully within the first 48 hours of the onset of acute MI have a good long-term prognosis with a low rate of recurrence or cardiac death. Cardiac pulmonary resuscitation and defibrillation are the treatments for VF. Patients can have cardioverters/defibrillators surgically implanted, which promptly recognize and terminate life-threatening ventricular arrhythmias.

Chapter Summary

- Three layers compose the wall of the heart: endocardium, myocardium, and epicardium.
- The two coronary arteries, the right and left main coronary arteries, are branches off the arch of the aorta.
- The LAD, which supplies the left ventricle with coronary blood flow, is most commonly affected by arteriosclerosis.
- Risk factors of CAD and MI include male gender, age greater than 45 years for males, age greater than 55 years for females, hyperlipidemia, hypertension, smoking, uncontrolled diabetes, high homocysteine level, obesity (particularly central obesity), sedentary lifestyle, and family history of cardiovascular disease.
- Cardiac chest pain is a crushing type of pain that usually radiates down the left arm and is accompanied by dyspnea, diaphoresis, and pallor. Alternatively, it can radiate into the epigastric region, back, right arm, or up to the jaw.
- Women often suffer anginal equivalents, signs of myocardial ischemia that differ from the classic chest pain. Anginal equivalents include dyspnea, diaphoresis, feeling faint, dizziness, extreme fatigue, and heartburn (epigastric pain).
- Prinzmetal's or vasospastic angina is caused by vasospasm of a coronary artery.
- ACS can take either of two forms: UA or myocardial infarction.
- There are two main types of myocardial infarction: STEMI and NSTEMI. However, angina can cause the same ST-segment changes on an ECG.

- Elevated cTnI is the confirmatory test indicating MI. The isoenzyme CPK-MB is also elevated. The high sensitivity cardiac troponin (hs-cTn) assay is the preferred test for diagnosis of MI.
- STEMI commonly indicates a transmural MI.
- The leading cause of IE is *S. aureus* bacteremia. Infection of intracardiac devices such as pacemakers, intravascular lines, intracardiac defibrillators, invasive procedures, prosthetic heart valves, and IV drug use are the most common causes of IE.
- Clinical manifestations of IE are heart murmur, petechiae, splinter hemorrhages, Janeway lesions, Osler's nodes, and Roth spots.
- Myocarditis is most often caused by a viral infection. Myocarditis is the major reason for cardiac transplant rejection.
- Pericarditis can be accompanied by a pericardial effusion that can cause cardiac tamponade.
- Cardiac tamponade is the compression of the heart by surrounding pericardial fluid that inhibits the heart chambers from completely filling with blood.
- Common complications of MI include dysrhythmias, heart failure, pericarditis, ventricular aneurysm, ventricular thrombosis, thromboembolism, and papillary muscle rupture.
- The most common rhythm disturbance post-MI is the PVC; three or more PVCs is called VT.
- VT predisposes to VF, which is considered cardiac arrest and requires defibrillation.

Making the Connections

Disorder and Pathophysiology	Signs and Symptoms	Physical Assessment Findings	Diagnostic Testing	Treatment

Unstable Angina Pectoris | UA pectoris, chest pain caused by myocardial ischemia, is part of ACS. There is inadequate coronary artery blood flow to the heart muscle. Ischemia develops, which causes myocardial cell hypoxia, triggering anaerobic metabolism. Anaerobic metabolism yields 2 ATP and lactic acid. Lactic acid is noxious to muscle cells, and 2 ATP is inadequate energy for the needs of the myocardial tissue. Other types of angina include:

- Stable angina: episodes of myocardial ischemia that are predictable and have the same pain pattern. Patient self-medicates with NTG.
- Prinzmetal's angina: caused by vasospasm of the coronary artery.
- Microvascular angina: a disorder of the microvasculature that causes angina pectoris.

| | An episode of retrosternal crushing, squeezing chest pain with radiation to the left arm, jaw, epigastric area, or back with a duration of 1 to 15 minutes. Chest pain most commonly occurs with exertion and is accompanied by dyspnea, diaphoresis, and pallor. | Vital signs show increased respiratory rate, slowed heart rate, and low BP. Patient often brings fist to chest (Levine's sign), indicating the crushing feeling on the chest. Pallor, dyspnea, and diaphoresis are apparent. Pulses are weak. | ECG shows ST depression or ST elevation or T-wave inversions. Cardiac catheterization with coronary angiogram will show areas of coronary artery occlusion caused by arteriosclerosis. Cardiac CT scan. Total cholesterol, HDL, LDL, hs-CRP, homocysteine, fibrinogen, lipoprotein (a). Calcium CT scan. Graded exercise stress test. ECG. Cardiac enzymes are used to rule out MI. The hs-cTn is used to rule out MI. | Low-fat diet. Daily exercise. Oxygen. Nitrates (NTG sublingual or nasal spray). One aspirin/day. Anticoagulants. Dual antiplatelet therapy. Ca++ antagonists. Beta-adrenergic blockers. Ranolazine. Possible PCI procedures include PCTA with stent placement in the affected coronary artery and CABG. |

Myocardial Infarction | Acute MI is an ACS that occurs when myocardial ischemia is prolonged and death of tissue (infarction) occurs. Can be a STEMI if it is a transmural MI or an NSTEMI if it is a subendocardial MI.

| | Steady retrosternal crushing, squeezing chest pain with radiation to the left arm, jaw, back, or epigastric region. Accompanied by pallor, dyspnea, and diaphoresis. Commonly occurs with exertion. Patient may lose consciousness. | Vital signs show increased respiratory rate, slowed heart rate, and low blood pressure. Levine's sign. Decreased level of consciousness (LOC) possible. Pallor. Diaphoresis. Respiratory distress. Diminished peripheral pulses. | Elevated hs-cTn assay. Elevated CPK-MB fraction. ECG shows ST elevation or ST depression, as well as inverted T waves. Cardiac catheterization with angiography shows coronary artery obstruction. Radionuclide angiogram. Cardiac CT scan. Calcium CT scan. Echocardiogram. | IV nitrates. Morphine. Aspirin. Oxygen. Heparin or another anticoagulant. Antiplatelet therapy. Beta blockers if stable. Ca++ antagonists. Thrombolytic agent to dissolve the clot for some eligible persons. PCI, which includes PTCA with stent placement or CABG. Cardiac rehabilitation. |

Continued

Making the Connections—cont'd

Disorder and Pathophysiology	Signs and Symptoms	Physical Assessment Findings	Diagnostic Testing	Treatment
Infective Endocarditis | A noncontagious infection of the cardiac endothelium that most commonly affects the heart valves. It is mainly caused by the bacteria *S. aureus*. Damaged valves are prone to infection and provoke aggregation of platelets to form a thrombus. Intracardiac devices such as prosthetic valves, pacemakers, cardiac defibrillators, or intravascular lines can incite the same conditions. IV drug use is also a common cause of IE.				
	Nonspecific symptoms, including fever, chills, anorexia, weight loss, myalgias, and arthralgias. Fever may be blunted or absent in older adults or severely debilitated persons.	Fever may be present. New heart murmur or changed preexistent heart murmur. Septic emboli form and can be manifested as infarction in organs such as the brain, which causes signs of stroke, such as neurological deficits. Clinical signs caused by septic emboli include petechiae, splinter hemorrhages, Janeway lesions, Osler's nodes, and Roth spots.	At least three blood cultures are performed at three different times of the day. See Duke Major and Minor criteria. Transthoracic echocardiogram or transesophageal echocardiogram is used to visualize heart valves. Laboratory tests are necessary, including CBC, electrolytes, serum creatinine, blood urea nitrogen, blood glucose, ESR, CRP, coagulation panel, and urinalysis. Leukocytosis is observed in acute endocarditis. ESR, although not specific, is elevated in more than 90% of cases. Glomerulonephritis, which elevates serum creatinine and causes proteinuria and microscopic hematuria, is present in approximately 50% of cases.	Treatment consists mainly of parenteral antibiotics for 6 weeks or a more prolonged course. Research studies show high doses of oral and depot forms of antibiotic are effective. Surgical removal of prosthetic valve, pacemaker, cardiac defibrillator, or intravascular line necessary. Patient needs antibiotics prophylactically any time there is an invasive procedure that can cause bacteremia.
Myocarditis | Myocarditis is inflammation of the muscle layer of the heart's wall. It can occur by direct invasion of a pathogen or a toxin that is liberated by a pathogen. It can also occur as an immunological mechanism initiated by an infectious agent or chest radiation. Myocarditis is also the major cause of cardiac transplant rejection.				
	Chest pain, chills, fever, and dyspnea. Patients may report a flu-like syndrome of fever, myalgia, arthralgia, pharyngitis, tonsillitis, and upper respiratory infection. Symptoms of palpitations or syncope can occur. Sudden cardiac death can develop because of ventricular arrhythmias or AV block. Adults can develop heart failure signs and symptoms, including ankle edema, ascites, and dyspnea with exertion. Patients may be asymptomatic.	On physical examination, cardiac auscultation may reveal an S_3 gallop rhythm indicative of heart failure. A pericardial friction rub and other signs such as lymphadenopathy and rash can be present, depending on etiology.	CBC, which demonstrates leukocytosis; elevated ESR and CRP, which indicate inflammation; and hs-cTn and cardiac enzymes, which are elevated with myocardial injury. Various viral antibody titers are drawn. Presence of a viral genome within a biopsy of endomyocardium is confirmatory. Echocardiogram can reveal heart function and degree of heart failure, if present. Antimyosin scintigraphy can identify myocardial inflammation. Cardiac MRI. Gadolinium MRI.	Decrease myocardial workload, including activity restrictions. Treatment measures for heart failure such as diuretics, nitrates, ACE inhibitors, and inotropic agents are often necessary. Antiarrhythmic agents. Pacemaker insertion may be needed. In severe cases of heart failure, cardiac transplantation is considered.

Making the Connections—cont'd

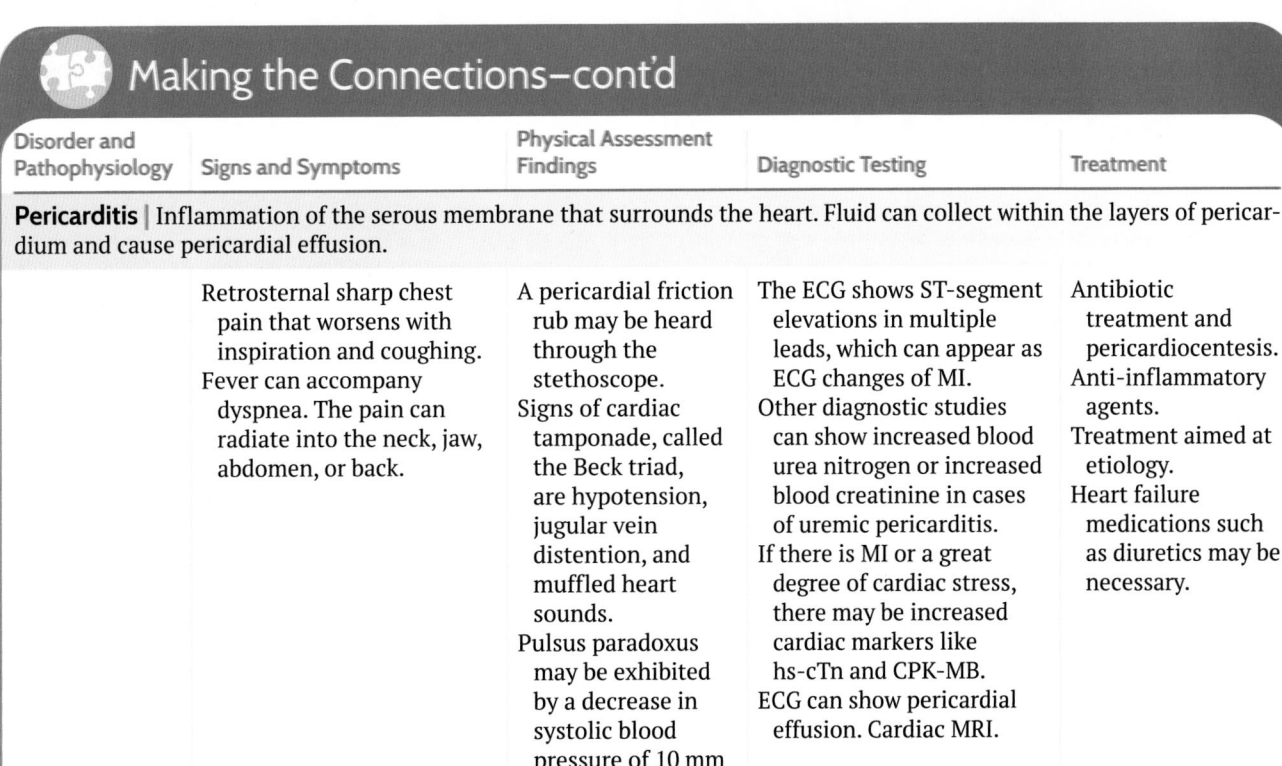

Disorder and Pathophysiology	Signs and Symptoms	Physical Assessment Findings	Diagnostic Testing	Treatment
Pericarditis | Inflammation of the serous membrane that surrounds the heart. Fluid can collect within the layers of pericardium and cause pericardial effusion.				
	Retrosternal sharp chest pain that worsens with inspiration and coughing. Fever can accompany dyspnea. The pain can radiate into the neck, jaw, abdomen, or back.	A pericardial friction rub may be heard through the stethoscope. Signs of cardiac tamponade, called the Beck triad, are hypotension, jugular vein distention, and muffled heart sounds. Pulsus paradoxus may be exhibited by a decrease in systolic blood pressure of 10 mm Hg or more with inspiration.	The ECG shows ST-segment elevations in multiple leads, which can appear as ECG changes of MI. Other diagnostic studies can show increased blood urea nitrogen or increased blood creatinine in cases of uremic pericarditis. If there is MI or a great degree of cardiac stress, there may be increased cardiac markers like hs-cTn and CPK-MB. ECG can show pericardial effusion. Cardiac MRI.	Antibiotic treatment and pericardiocentesis. Anti-inflammatory agents. Treatment aimed at etiology. Heart failure medications such as diuretics may be necessary.

Bibliography

Available online at fadavis.com

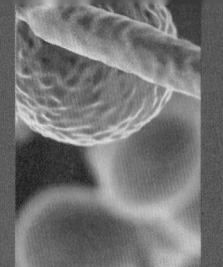

Heart Failure

Learning Objectives

Upon completion of this chapter, the student will be able to:

- Describe the physiological concepts of heart function that include preload, afterload, contractility, and left ventricular ejection fraction and how they are related.
- Recognize the risk factors and various etiologies of heart failure.
- Describe the mechanisms of left ventricular failure and right ventricular failure.

- Identify the signs, symptoms, and clinical manifestations of left ventricular failure and right ventricular failure.
- Recognize laboratory tests, procedures, and hemodynamic measures that are used to diagnose and monitor heart failure.
- Discuss pharmacological and nonpharmacological measures used to treat heart failure.

Key Terms

Afterload

Angiotensin-converting enzyme (ACE)

Ascites

Cardiac contractility

Cardiac resynchronization therapy (CRT)

Cardiomyopathy

Central venous pressure (CVP)

Chronotropic function

Heart failure (HF)

Heart failure with reduced ejection fraction (HFrEF)

Heart failure with preserved ejection fraction (HFpEF)

Hydrostatic pressure

Intra-aortic balloon pump

Inotropic function

Jugular venous distention (JVD)

Left ventricular assist device (LVAD)

Left ventricular ejection fraction (LVEF)

Orthopnea

Paroxysmal nocturnal dyspnea (PND)

Preload

Pulmonary capillary wedge pressure (PCWP)

Pulmonary edema

Pulmonary hypertension

Starling's capillary forces

Heart failure (HF) is defined as a syndrome characterized by elevated cardiac filling pressure and/or inadequate peripheral oxygen delivery, at rest or during stress, caused by cardiac dysfunction (Givertz & Mehra, 2022). The American Heart Association (AHA) and American College of Cardiology (ACC) define heart failure in terms of the heart's **left ventricular ejection fraction (LVEF)**, which is the percentage of blood propelled out of the left ventricle with each contraction. A normal ejection fraction in a healthy adult is 50% to 70% (American Heart Association, 2022). Most investigators divide heart failure into two categories: **heart failure with reduced ejection fraction (HFrEF)** and **heart failure with preserved ejection fraction (HFpEF)**. HFrEF is heart failure with a decreased ejection fraction of less than or equal to 40%. HFpEF is heart failure with a normal or near-normal ejection fraction of greater than or equal to 50%. Some investigators, particularly the European Society of Cardiology, identify a third category of heart failure: HF with mildly reduced or borderline ejection fraction (HFmrEF), where ejection fraction is 41% to 49% (Ponikowski et al., 2016).

Most epidemiological studies assert that approximately one-half of HF patients have HFrEF while the other half have HFpEF. The designation of HF according

to ejection fraction often has implications for types of effective treatment. There are also different etiologies associated with different types of HF. According to Li et al. (2021), HFrEF is most commonly associated with coronary artery disease, ischemic heart disease, and acute myocardial infarction, whereas HFpEF is associated with long-standing hypertension, atrial dysrhythmias, anemia, and chronic obstructive pulmonary disease (COPD). Also, HFpEF patients are more likely to be older, men are more likely to have HFrEF, and women are predisposed to HFpEF.

🩺 CLINICAL CONCEPT

Heart failure with reduced ejection fraction (HFrEF) is defined as heart failure with ejection fraction of less than or equal to 40%.

Heart failure with preserved ejection fraction (HFpEF) is defined as heart failure with ejection fraction of less than or equal to 50%.

Heart failure with mildly reduced ejection fraction (HFmrEF) is defined as heart failure with ejection fraction of 41% to 49%.

Regardless of ejection fraction, HF most commonly results from cardiac dysfunction; the ventricular muscle is unable to pump sufficient blood to meet the circulatory and oxygen needs of the tissues. A number of compensatory mechanisms become activated during heart failure that contribute to disease progression. There are hemodynamic abnormalities that cause both systolic and diastolic dysfunction. HF is most commonly a progressive disease that typically evolves from a sentinel event followed by months to years of structural and functional cardiovascular remodeling. Heart failure should not be confused with cardiac arrest, which is the cessation of all heart activity. A failing heart continues to pump but inadequately supplies the body with sufficient circulation. Commonly, this creates pressure changes within the heart's chambers that further weaken the heart muscle.

Heart failure is a disease of epidemic proportions within the United States, with more than 600,000 patients diagnosed with it each year. It affects 6.2 million Americans and causes 300,000 deaths annually. It also is the most common cause of hospitalization. Regardless of age, the lifetime risk of developing heart failure is approximately 20% for all patients older than 40 years, and its incidence in persons age 65 years and older is 10 per 1,000—numbers that are only expected to increase as the aged segment of the population grows. As the treatment for other cardiovascular diseases has improved, more persons are surviving into old age with chronic cardiovascular conditions. Mortality rates from ischemic heart disease, myocardial infarction (MI), and dysrhythmias have been significantly reduced over the past few decades, and the prevalence of cardiovascular morbidity has increased among survivors. Ironically, this has increased the prevalence of heart failure within the population. Persons with cardiovascular disease are surviving acute cardiac events and living longer with chronic cardiac disorders. In community-based studies, African Americans have the highest risk of developing HF, followed by Hispanic-, European-, and Asian Americans. HF hospitalizations are highest among African American men, followed by African American women, European American men, and European American women. In primary care, the overall 5-year survival following a diagnosis of HF is approximately 50%. In the United States, 1 in 8 deaths is from heart failure; most are from the consequences of progressive HF or sudden cardiac death.

Hypertension (HTN) is the greatest risk factor for the development of heart failure, as more than 75% of patients with heart failure are treated for HTN before developing it. About 22% of men and 46% of women will develop heart failure within 6 months following an acute MI. Other causes of heart failure include coronary artery disease and metabolic syndrome; a history of diabetes mellitus also increases the risk of developing the disorder. Women are often diagnosed with heart failure at an older age than men because natural estrogen is cardioprotective. After menopause,

the risk of cardiovascular disease for men and women is equal. Within the U.S. population, there is a greater prevalence of heart failure among African Americans compared with European Americans. Many researchers are investigating the causes for this disparity (see Box 17-1).

Basic Physiological Concepts of Heart Function

The heart's failure as a pump creates widespread consequences throughout the body and activates specific compensatory mechanisms. It is essential to understand the following key concepts related to the heart's physiology before understanding the pathophysiology of heart failure.

Cardiac Output

Cardiac output is the amount of blood that the heart pumps out of the left ventricle each minute. In general, cardiac output is diminished in heart failure, because the left ventricle is weakened and cannot adequately pump blood out of the chamber. It is based on heart rate (HR), the rate at which the heart beats, and stroke volume (SV), the volume of blood pumped out

---

BOX 17-1. Prevalence of Heart Failure Among African Americans

Mortality from heart failure is 2.5 times greater among African Americans compared with European Americans younger than 65 years of age. African Americans develop heart failure at an earlier age, and the hospitalization rates are substantially higher than those among European Americans. Between the ages of 45 and 64, African American males have a 70% higher risk for heart failure than European American males, and African American females between the ages of 45 and 54 have a 50% greater risk for developing heart failure than European American females of the same age range.

The reason for the increased morbidity and mortality in African American heart failure patients is unclear. Past research demonstrates that HTN is the specific cause for heart failure among a majority of African Americans, and conventional forms of antihypertensive medication are ineffective for this population. Current research focuses on specific pharmacological treatments that target the distinctive pathological mechanisms of heart failure and HTN in African Americans. The field of pharmacogenomics is in its infancy but can increase the efficacy of drugs by matching specific medications to specific patients.

of the ventricle with each contraction. In mathematical terms, cardiac output = HR × SV (see Box 17-2).

Because cardiac output varies by body size, a hemodynamic measurement termed cardiac index can be calculated to give a more accurate assessment of each individual's cardiac output. Cardiac output divided by an individual's body surface area yields the cardiac index.

HR is controlled by the sympathetic (adrenergic) and parasympathetic (cholinergic) nervous systems. Adrenergic stimulation raises HR, and cholinergic stimulation slows HR. Stroke volume is influenced by preload, afterload, and cardiac contractility.

Preload

Preload can be defined as the volume of blood in the heart at the end of diastole. Essentially, preload factors are those that affect cardiac output but occur before contraction. Most commonly, in clinical settings, preload refers to the volume of blood that enters the right atrium from the venous system (see Fig. 17-1).

As blood flows into the right atrium, it empties into the right ventricle during diastole. The preload volume of blood that originates from the venous system and ultimately empties into the right ventricle can also be called the ventricular end diastolic volume. Preload causes stretch and increased pressure within the ventricular chamber, which increases SV. With increased venous return, preload increases, and SV is enhanced. If venous return is diminished, preload decreases, and SV is reduced. However, excessive venous return can overload a weakened ventricle, resulting in decreased cardiac output and leading to heart failure. This relationship is described in the Frank–Starling law (see Box 17-3).

Afterload

Afterload can be described as the amount of resistance that the ventricle must overcome in order to

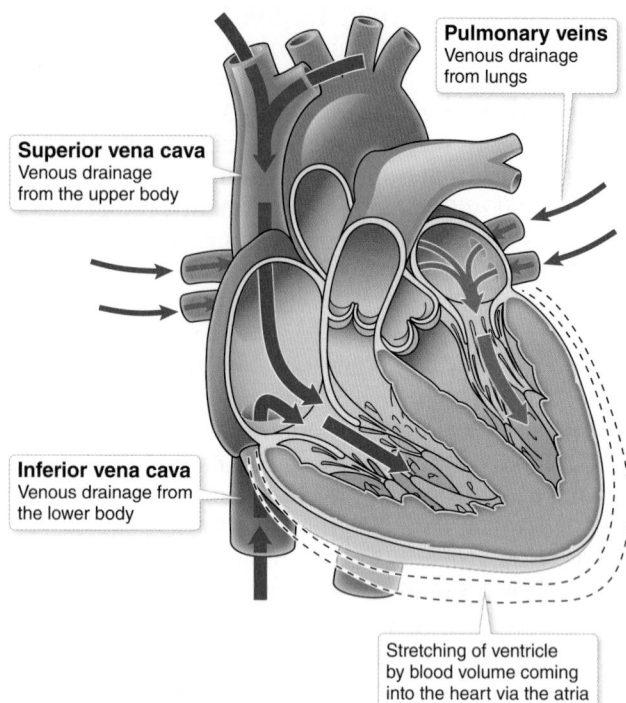

FIGURE 17-1. Cardiac preload. Preload is a volume of blood that stretches the right or left ventricle of the heart. It can be referred to as the ventricular end-diastolic volume that is achieved by the passive filling of the ventricle from the atria. In the clinical setting, the volume of blood entering the right atrium is most often referred to as preload.

pump blood out of the heart. The greater the pulmonary vascular resistance, the greater the afterload against the right ventricle. Pulmonary HTN, which is high pressure within the pulmonary arteries, creates high afterload for the right ventricle.

The greater the systemic arterial vascular resistance, the greater the afterload against the left ventricle. Most commonly, afterload describes the workload of the left ventricle, or resistance exerted by the pressure within the aorta against the left ventricle (see Fig. 17-2). Pressure within the aorta reflects systemic arterial blood pressure; therefore, systemic HTN creates high afterload for the left ventricle.

Cardiac Contractility

Cardiac contractility refers to the myocardium's ability to stretch and contract in response to the filling of the heart with blood. As blood fills the ventricle during diastole, tension in the heart muscle wall steadily increases, and stretching of the chamber occurs. Actin and myosin filaments of the myocardial muscle wall interact to create a force of contraction. The muscle filaments can change the force of contraction with varying amounts of stretch caused by blood volume or preload. SV is the amount of blood within the ventricle that is ejected with each contraction. Therefore, as preload increases, SV increases and the actin–myosin filaments in the heart wall stretch to accommodate the increased volume. These

---

BOX 17-2. Normal Cardiac Output

Cardiac output = SV × HR
SV = milliliters of blood ejected per ventricular contraction
HR = number of ventricular contractions per minute

In a healthy heart, SV equals approximately 70 mL of blood ejected per ventricular contraction. The average HR is 70 beats per minute or 70 contractions/minute. Therefore, cardiac output equals 70 mL/contraction × 70 contractions/minute or a blood volume of 4,900 mL/minute (approximately 5,000 mL or 5 liters/minute).

BOX 17-3. The Frank–Starling Law

The relationship between cardiac contractility, preload, afterload, SV, and cardiac output of the heart is called the Frank–Starling law. This mechanism describes how the ventricle can adjust its pumping force to accommodate various levels of preload and afterload. An increase in left ventricular end-diastolic volume (preload) will increase the blood volume in the ventricle, which in turn produces an increase in cardiac output. The force of contraction of the healthy heart is directly related to the blood volume that fills the ventricle in diastole (preload). The maximum force of contraction of the ventricle occurs when an increase in preload stretches muscle fibers to 2 ½ times their resting length.

Evaluating the heart's effectiveness as a pump is based on the relationship between preload and its SV. SV varies directly with preload and inversely with afterload. In the healthy heart, an increased volume of blood filling the ventricle stretches ventricular myocardial fibers and consequently increases cardiac contractility and SV. Cardiac output is enhanced by preload (see Fig. 17-1) and can be reduced by afterload (see Fig. 17-2).

The strength of the heart's cardiac contractility has a major effect on SV. As the heart pump fails, cardiac contractile strength diminishes, and the ventricle ejects a progressively decreased amount of SV from preload (see Fig. 17-3). Decreased SV, in turn, diminishes cardiac output. Cardiac contractile strength can be weakened by such conditions as direct injury of the myocardium, excessive afterload, or extremely low preload.

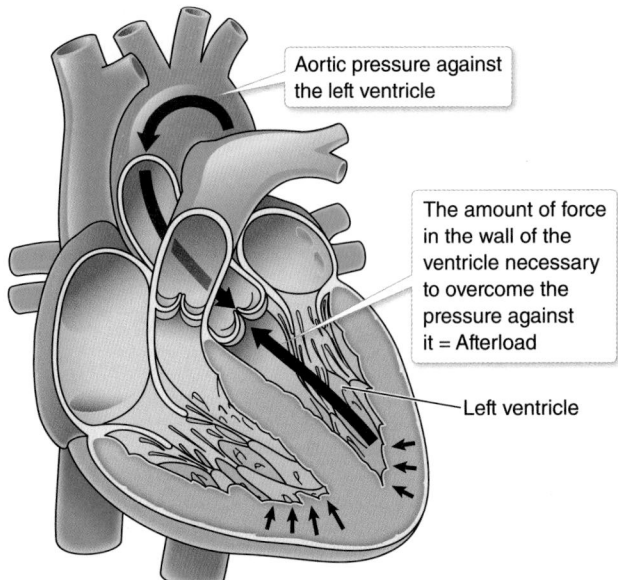

FIGURE 17-2. Cardiac afterload. Afterload is the force that the ventricle must overcome in order to eject its contents. It is the tension or stress developed in the wall of the ventricle during ejection. In the clinical setting, afterload is most commonly measured as the aortic pressure against the left ventricle. Aortic pressure reflects the systemic arterial pressure. Therefore, if there is high systemic arterial pressure (also referred to as HTN), this is considered high afterload.

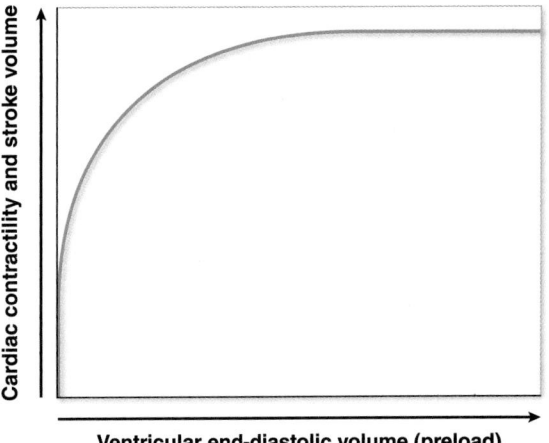

FIGURE 17-3. How changes in preload affect the contractility and SV of the healthy heart. As ventricular end-diastolic volume (preload) increases, myocardial contractility and SV increase until a maximal level is reached. In the healthy heart, cardiac contractility and SV increase until the stretch of myocardial muscle fibers is 2 ½ times their resting length.

conditions enhance contractility in a healthy heart (see Fig. 17-3).

Contractility can also be influenced by afterload. As afterload increases, the heart's workload increases, which can negatively affect contractility. If the afterload becomes excessive, the ventricle's ability to eject blood is lessened; consequently, SV is diminished. Also, the heart muscle is burdened with resistance and contractility decreases (see Fig. 17-4).

In the failing heart, an increase in preload causes high blood volume to fill the ventricle; however, the weakened ventricular muscle may not have the strength to pump the excessive volume out. SV decreases when the weakened ventricle cannot optimally eject its blood. Also, the ventricular muscle's fibers can become overly taxed by the burden of the excessive filling of blood in the chamber, and contractile force diminishes. Therefore, in a failing heart, with increased preload filling the weakened ventricle, contractility and SV can decrease (see Fig. 17-5).

Contractility is also influenced by the autonomic nervous system, acid–base balance, and electrolytes. Strong sympathetic nervous system (SNS) activity

provides enhanced contractility because of stimulation of beta-1 adrenergic receptors in the heart. Activation of the parasympathetic nervous system stimulates the vagal or cholinergic receptors in the heart, which decreases the force of contraction. Also, impaired calcium activity within cardiac ventricular muscle can negatively affect contractility.

Inotropic Versus Chronotropic Function of the Heart. The **inotropic function** of the heart refers to

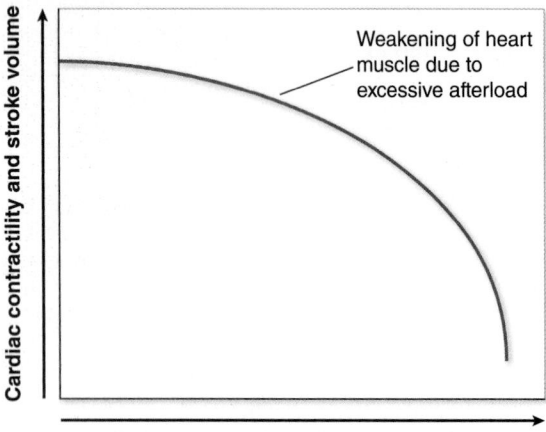

FIGURE 17-4. How changes in the afterload affect contractility and the heart's SV. As peripheral arterial resistance (afterload) increases, cardiac contractility and SV decrease. At a level of maximal afterload, the heart begins to weaken. In clinical settings, afterload is most commonly defined as the systemic arterial blood pressure or aortic pressure force exerted against the left ventricle.

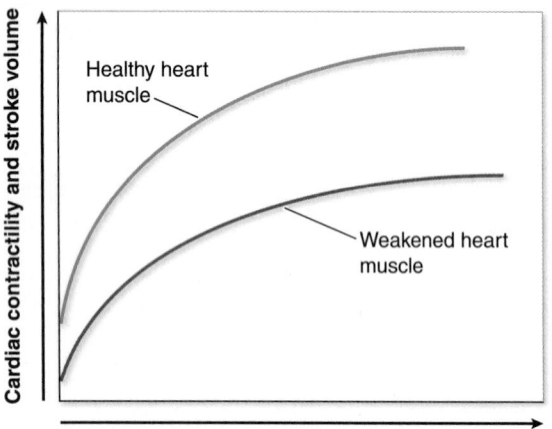

FIGURE 17-5. How increasing preload influences contractility and SV in the failing heart. As ventricular end-diastolic volume (preload) increases, a weakened heart muscle develops decreased cardiac contractility and SV.

the force of contraction of the cardiac muscle. The heart's contractility can be influenced by the amount of calcium available for interaction between the actin and myosin filaments of the cardiac muscle fibers. Sympathetic stimulation can increase force of contraction, which is referred to as a positive inotropic effect.

Chronotropic function refers to heart rate (HR). When digitalis is administered, it decreases HR by slowing conduction of impulses through the atrioventricular (AV) node; therefore, it has a negative chronotropic effect. Beta-adrenergic blocking agents antagonize the SNS effect on the heart by slowing impulses at the sinoatrial (SA) node, also a negative chronotropic effect. Conversely, epinephrine, an adrenergic or sympathetic stimulant, has positive

inotropic and positive chronotropic effects on the heart. Under the influence of epinephrine, the heart has a greater force of contraction and increased heart rate.

 CLINICAL CONCEPT

The cardiac glycoside drug digitalis is a positive inotropic agent and a negative chronotropic agent because it increases the force of ventricular contraction of the heart and decreases the HR. Before administering digitalis, the clinician needs to take an apical pulse; if the patient's pulse is less than 60 bpm, the clinician must hold the medication. It is also very important to monitor serum potassium when administering digitalis.

High Capillary Hydrostatic Pressure and Edema. There are two major opposing pressure forces at every capillary bed in the body: hydrostatic pressure and oncotic (osmotic) pressure. Together, these opposing pressure forces are known as **Starling's capillary forces**. At every capillary–cell interface, there are three fluid compartments: intracellular, extracellular, and interstitial. Intracellular fluid is found inside the cells, interstitial fluid surrounds the cells, and extracellular fluid is located inside the capillary.

Capillary membranes are semipermeable, which means they allow diffusion of fluid out of the blood through the capillary pores into the interstitial and intracellular spaces. Fluid within the blood exerts **hydrostatic pressure**, a force that attempts to push fluid out of the capillary pores into the interstitial and intracellular spaces. Particles within the blood, such as albumin, sodium, and glucose, exert oncotic or osmotic pressure.

Oncotic (osmotic) pressure is a force that attempts to pull fluid from the interstitial and intracellular spaces into the capillary. Oncotic pressure forces and hydrostatic pressure forces oppose each other at every capillary membrane. Under normal conditions, these forces balance each other, creating an equilibrium that exists at the capillary beds.

When hydrostatic pressure increases within the capillary, the forces become unbalanced. A high hydrostatic pressure force can overcome the opposing balancing effect of the oncotic pressure. High capillary hydrostatic pressure causes fluid to diffuse out of the capillary pores into the interstitial and intracellular spaces. This collection of fluid, which traverses into the interstitial and intracellular spaces, is called edema (see Fig. 17-6).

Hemodynamic Monitoring. A hemodynamic monitor measures pressures within the chambers and vessels of the right and left sides of the heart. Hemodynamic monitoring is accomplished by right-heart cardiac

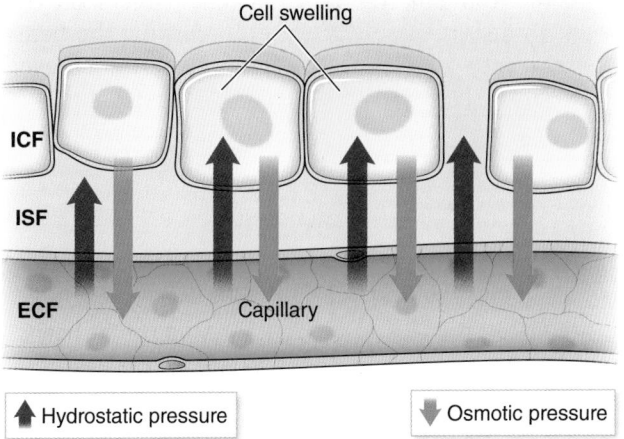

FIGURE 17-6. Edema fluid in interstitial fluid space and intracellular fluid space caused by high hydrostatic pressure. Edema occurs because of high hydrostatic pressure in capillary blood into interstitial spaces and intracellular spaces. Fluid accumulation in and around the cells is edema, which causes swelling.

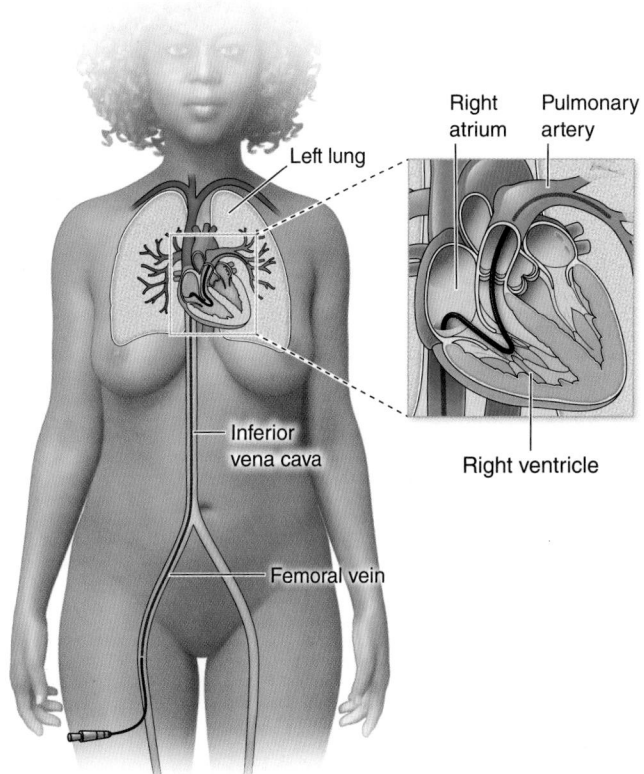

FIGURE 17-7. Right-heart cardiac catheterization to obtain pulmonary capillary pressure. Cardiac catheterization can be done via the venous system or the arterial system, depending on the goal of the procedure. In this diagram, right-sided cardiac catheterization is shown. The goal of right-sided cardiac catheterization is to obtain the pulmonary capillary wedge pressure (also called PCWP). The catheter is inserted via a peripheral vein, commonly the femoral vein. It is then threaded into the inferior vena cava, right atrium, right ventricle, and into the pulmonary artery. Finally, it is wedged in a pulmonary capillary. The PCWP is used to assess the severity of left ventricular failure.

catheterization or placement of a Swan–Ganz catheter. These are distinct invasive procedures that employ a specialized cardiac catheter device to diagnose heart disease and monitor treatment in heart failure.

A cardiac catheter is capable of measuring pressure and flow within the heart chambers. It is connected to a transducer that converts the pressure waves into a digital readout that can be seen on a monitor screen. The catheter is inserted into a large vein for right-heart hemodynamic assessment and the femoral artery for left-heart hemodynamic assessment.

To directly measure right-heart pressures, a Swan–Ganz catheter is threaded into the subclavian vein and advanced into the inferior vena cava (IVC) and right atrium. Pressure measurement within the IVC is referred to as **central venous pressure (CVP)**. The catheter can measure CVP, which is the same as right atrial pressure at this location. The catheter can be further advanced into the right ventricle and pulmonary artery and then wedged into a pulmonary capillary (see Fig. 17-7). Pressures within the right ventricle, pulmonary artery, and pulmonary capillary bed can be measured by the catheter at points along its path. When the catheter remains in place, it can provide a continuous measure of pulmonary capillary pressure. Upon inflation of the balloon on the tip of the Swan–Ganz catheter, the pressure reading is referred to as **pulmonary capillary wedge pressure (PCWP)**.

To directly measure left-heart pressures, a catheter is inserted into the femoral or radial artery and advanced against the flow of blood into the aorta; it is then further advanced into the left ventricle (see Fig. 17-8). Measurements can be taken of aortic pressure and systolic and diastolic pressures of the left ventricle from the catheter tip. LVEF, the volume of blood pumped with each ventricular contraction, can be approximated from the systolic and diastolic pressure measurements. In healthy individuals,

approximately 60% to 70% of blood volume in the left ventricle is pumped out with each contraction. An LVEF lower than 40% is indicative of heart failure.

The cardiac catheter inserted into a peripheral artery and into the aorta can be threaded into the coronary arteries. Radiopaque dye can be injected to illuminate the lumens of the coronary arteries and visualize blood flow. Obstruction to blood flow, thrombi, arteriosclerotic plaque, aneurysm, or other malformations of the arteries can be visualized through this procedure (see Fig. 17-9).

The healthy heart exhibits ranges of normal hemodynamic measurements. In the failing heart, these measurements become abnormal and can be used to differentiate right-sided versus left-sided heart dysfunction. Abnormal hemodynamic measurements obtained from cardiac catheterization can be used to diagnose right-sided versus left-sided ventricular failure. Cardiac catheterization is also used to diagnose coronary artery disease.

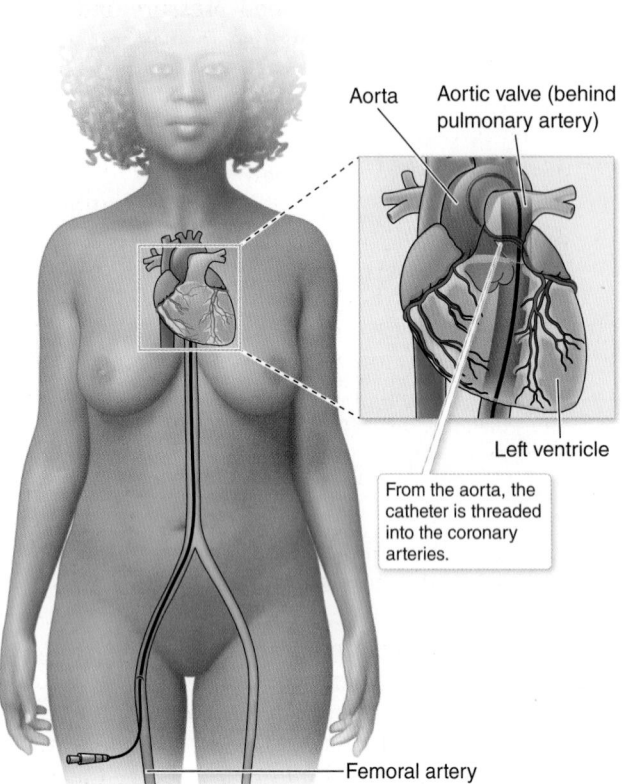

Aorta

Aortic valve (behind pulmonary artery)

Left ventricle

From the aorta, the catheter is threaded into the coronary arteries.

Femoral artery

FIGURE 17-8. Left-heart cardiac catheterization to visualize coronary arteries. Cardiac catheterization can be done via the venous system or the arterial system, depending on the goal of the procedure. In this diagram, left-sided cardiac catheterization is shown. The goal is visualization of the coronary arteries. The catheter is inserted via a peripheral artery, commonly the femoral artery. It is then threaded into the aorta and into the coronary arteries. An opaque dye is infused into the coronary arteries in order to highlight them in a specialized x-ray called a coronary angiogram. The interior structure of the coronary arteries can then be examined.

Cardiovascular Regulatory Mechanisms

Major sensors within the cardiovascular system respond to decreased blood pressure and blood volume. The major mechanisms include the renin–angiotensin–aldosterone system (RAAS), which the kidney triggers. The autonomic nervous system senses low circulation via baroreceptors that are embedded within the arteries. The posterior pituitary releases antidiuretic hormone (ADH) in response to decreased blood volume or blood pressure. In addition, there are substances in the body that regulate circulation to the tissues and cardiovascular changes: endothelin, nitric oxide (NO), natriuretic peptides, and tumor necrosis factor (TNF).

Renin–Angiotensin–Aldosterone System. The RAAS is a major mechanism in the regulation of arterial blood pressure. It is a compensatory mechanism that raises blood pressure and increases blood volume in response to decreased renal perfusion (see Fig. 17-10).

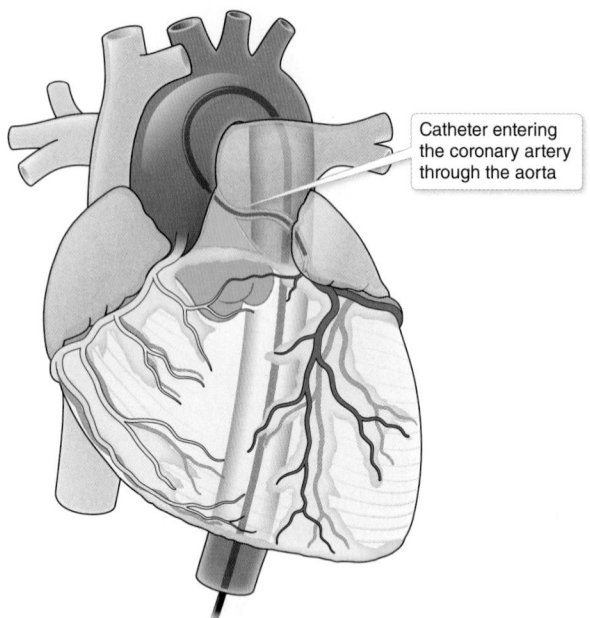

Catheter entering the coronary artery through the aorta

FIGURE 17-9. In left-sided cardiac catheterization, a catheter is inserted into a peripheral artery and then into the aorta. From the aorta, the catheter is threaded into the coronary arteries. At that point, an opaque dye is infused to outline the interior of the coronary arteries. A specialized x-ray called a coronary angiogram is then completed.

Renin is an enzyme that is released from the juxtaglomerular apparatus of the kidney in response to decreased renal perfusion. When blood pressure drops, renal perfusion diminishes, which, in turn, provokes renin release. After release, renin circulates and reacts with angiotensinogen, a protein synthesized by the liver. Angiotensinogen is then cleaved into a smaller protein, angiotensin I. Angiotensin I circulates, and in the lungs, **angiotensin-converting enzyme (ACE)** transforms angiotensin I into angiotensin II.

Angiotensin II is a potent arterial vasoconstrictor that raises blood pressure within the systemic arterial system. It is also a trigger for myocardial changes referred to as ventricular remodeling. Frequent stimulation of angiotensin II will activate genetic changes in the cardiac myocyte that lead to hypertrophy, apoptosis, and myocardial fibrosis. As some cardiac myocytes hypertrophy, the ventricular muscle enlarges. Other cardiac myocytes degenerate, causing ventricular muscle weakness. As the myocardium degenerates, it becomes infiltrated with collagenous fibrous tissue, which is noncontractile and nonconductive.

In addition, angiotensin II stimulates the adrenal gland to release aldosterone. Aldosterone is a hormone that acts at the nephron to increase sodium and water reabsorption from the distal tubule into the bloodstream. It also increases the secretion of potassium into the nephron tubule, resulting in potassium excretion. The sodium and water retention caused by aldosterone increases total blood volume and raises blood pressure.

Although the RAAS is a vital compensatory mechanism and major regulator of blood pressure, it has

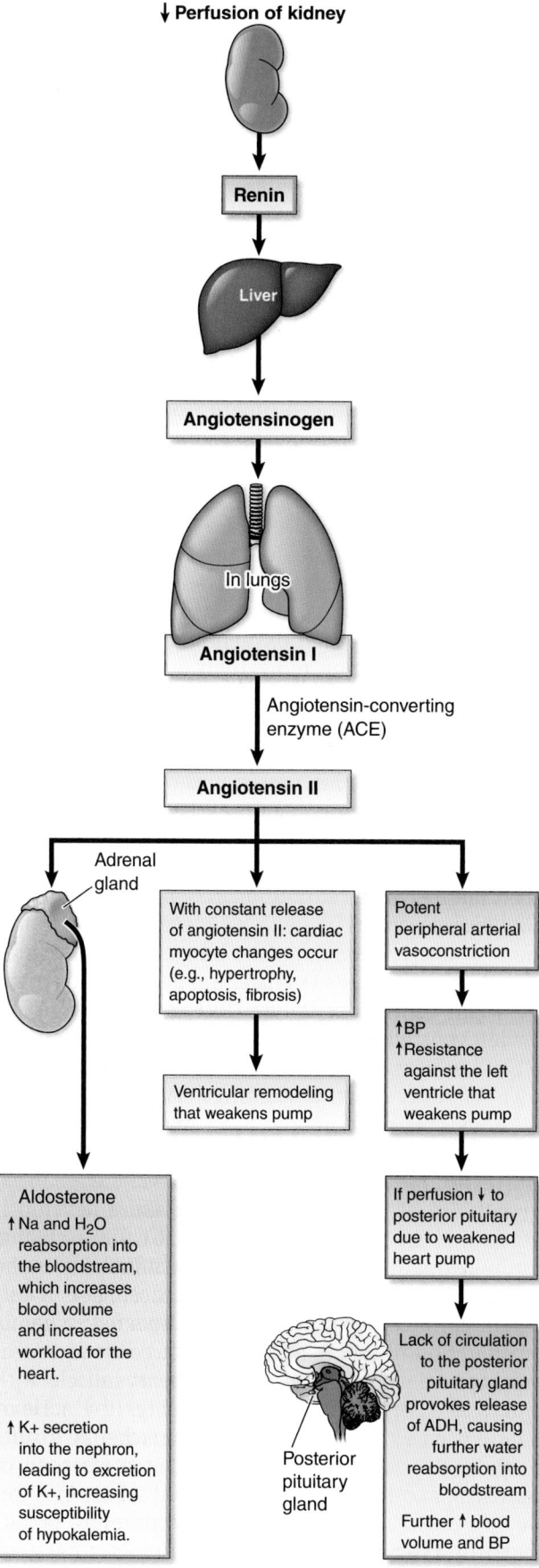

detrimental effects in heart failure. The net effects of the RAAS are elevated blood pressure and blood volume, which increase workload for the left ventricle. In left ventricular failure (LVF), this extra blood volume and high blood pressure further weaken the heart pump. Because this can be a vicious cycle, it can be said that heart failure begets heart failure. This mechanism is explained in more detail within the neurohormonal-forward failure effects of LVF.

Natriuretic Peptides. Within the circulatory system, increased water and sodium retention raises blood volume. High blood volume entering the heart stretches the heart's atrial chambers, which activates the release of natriuretic peptides from the atrial myocytes. Atrial natriuretic peptide (ANP) is a protein molecule that induces a process of natriuresis, which is increased excretion of sodium and water by the nephron. Release of ANP stimulates the glomerulus to increase filtration of the blood, inhibits reabsorption of sodium at the proximal tubule, blocks release of renin and aldosterone, and opposes the vasoconstrictive effects of angiotensin II. All these actions enhance the excretion of water from the body and decrease blood volume.

Similarly, when increased blood volume causes increased ventricular volume and stretch, the ventricular myocytes release B type natriuretic peptide (BNP). Elevated levels of BNP, or its precursor, N-terminal proBNP, indicate heart failure. BNP exerts the same effects as ANP, inducing the process of natural diuresis. In heart failure, both these natriuretic peptides are released because of the increased blood volume and edema.

Neprilysin. Neprilysin is an enzyme that breaks down atrial natriuretic peptide (ANP) and B-type natriuretic peptide (BNP). The natriuretic peptides are released by the heart muscle when intracardiac volume pressures are excessive. These are natural diuretic-type substances that enhance fluid loss at the kidney. Therapeutically, inhibiting neprilysin allows ANP and BNP to be continually active and allows for natriuresis. Therefore, pharmaceutical agents that inhibit neprilysin are effective at counteracting the excess fluid accumulation in heart failure.

Endothelin. Endothelin is a peptide that is secreted by the heart's endothelium and vasculature in heart failure. It is often elevated in heart failure following an acute MI. It stimulates vasoconstriction of the arterial blood vessels, which increases resistance against the left ventricle. Increased resistance causes high workload for the left ventricle. If resistance becomes excessive, the workload strains the heart. Endothelin also provokes fibrotic changes within the myocardium, which is part of the heart's ventricular remodeling, which occurs in heart failure.

Tumor Necrosis Factor-Alpha. In heart failure, elevated levels of TNF-alpha are present in the bloodstream and cardiac muscle. TNF-alpha is an inflammatory cytokine that stimulates hypertrophy, fibrotic changes, and cell death, or apoptosis of the myocardium. It also negatively affects the heart's inotropic function. This leads to dilation of the ventricle with decreasing cardiac output. Myocardial apoptosis, degeneration of heart muscle, puts further strain on the functional myocytes. The net effect is diminished strength of ventricular contraction, worsening heart failure, and detrimental remodeling of the heart.

Nitric Oxide. Nitric oxide is a potent vasodilator produced by vascular endothelial cells. Through its vasodilator action, it is a local regulator of blood flow to the tissues.

Antidiuretic Hormone. Another physiological response to decreased tissue perfusion is the release of ADH from the posterior pituitary gland. This hormone promotes water reabsorption into the bloodstream at the nephron in the kidneys and has vasoconstrictor effects.

Autonomic Nervous System Regulation. Cardiovascular homeostasis is promoted by the activity of the autonomic nervous system. The heart is richly innervated by both the sympathetic and parasympathetic neurons. The parasympathetic nervous system stimulates cholinergic receptors to slow the HR and decrease the force of contraction. Conversely, sympathetic stimulation of beta-1-adrenergic receptors results in an increase in HR and a strengthening of the force of contraction, which results in increased SV and cardiac output. However, sympathetic stimulation also leads to activation of alpha-adrenergic receptors within arterial vessel walls, which results in vasoconstriction.

Basic Pathophysiological Concepts of Heart Failure

Four major pathological changes can lead to the development of heart failure:

1. Increased fluid volume or volume overload
2. Impaired ventricular filling
3. Degeneration of ventricular muscle
4. Decreased ventricular contractile function

Any one of these can lead to a reduction in cardiac output and compensatory mechanisms associated with heart failure. Heart failure is initiated by a precipitating event, and the four pathological changes occur over time.

ⓠ CLINICAL CONCEPT

It is important to identify the most likely cause of heart failure, because it will guide treatment.

Epidemiology

Heart failure is the fastest-growing clinical cardiac disease entity in the United States, affecting approximately 2% of the population. It is the most frequent cause of hospitalization in individuals older than age 65 years. The AHA estimates that there are approximately 6.2 million people with heart failure in the United States and 26 million people with the disorder worldwide. The prevalence of heart failure and left ventricular dysfunction increases steeply with age. As the older segment of the population increases, heart failure prevalence is expected to increase to 8 million persons—an increase of 46% by 2030. The prevalence of heart failure in African Americans is reported to be 25% higher than in European Americans.

Etiology

There are many causes of heart failure; however, the most common cause is ischemic heart disease. Repeated episodes of coronary insufficiency deny the heart muscle of needed oxygen and nutrients. Many persons are surviving more than one MI, and many different areas of infarcted ventricular muscle cause a diminished contractile force. Chronic HTN is another major cause of heart failure because the left ventricle must overcome the high resistance of aortic pressure. Eventually, the ventricular muscle becomes exhausted. Chronic obstructive pulmonary disease (COPD) can cause right ventricular changes that lead to a type of heart failure called cor pulmonale. Obstructive pulmonary disease causes hypoxia, which constricts the pulmonary arterial vessels in the lungs. This pulmonary HTN eventually causes exhaustion of the right ventricle. Right ventricular failure (RVF) eventually affects the left ventricle, and heart failure develops. There are other, less common causes of heart failure, but they all have the same effect: weakening of the left ventricle—the body's main pump.

Ischemic Heart Disease

About 75% of patients with heart failure develop it because of ischemic heart disease, also called ischemic cardiomyopathy. Coronary artery insufficiency is the primary cause of ischemic heart disease. Lack of sufficient coronary circulation causes repeated ischemia or infarction of the myocardium. The consequence of repeated MI is a scarred, fibrotic heart muscle with diminished contractile strength (see Fig. 17-11). Heart failure occurs as a result of repeated ischemic insults to the myocardium, which weakens the strength of ventricular contractions.

Chronic Hypertension

Chronic HTN is the leading cause of LVF. Long-term high systemic arterial blood pressure causes high aortic pressure, which creates a high workload, or increased resistance for the left ventricle. In response

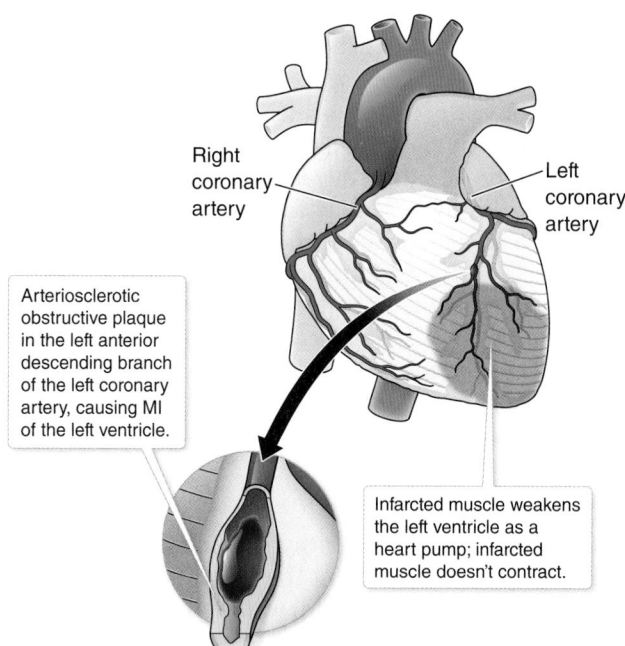

Right coronary artery

Left coronary artery

Arteriosclerotic obstructive plaque in the left anterior descending branch of the left coronary artery, causing MI of the left ventricle.

Infarcted muscle weakens the left ventricle as a heart pump; infarcted muscle doesn't contract.

FIGURE 17-11. Repeated episodes of ischemic heart disease (ischemic cardiomyopathy) lead to a weakened heart muscle or heart failure. Ischemic cardiomyopathy, or repeated episodes of ischemic heart disease, is a leading cause of heart failure. Repeated ischemic insults to the myocardial muscle weaken the heart muscle and create a suboptimal heart pump. One of the most common areas of arteriosclerosis is in the left coronary artery, a major arterial supply of the left ventricle (LV). The LV is the most common site of ischemia and MI. Infarcted heart muscle doesn't contract or conduct impulses. Repeated myocardial infarcts are extremely harmful to the strength of the ventricular muscle, which predisposes the individual to heart failure.

to the resistance caused by the high arterial pressure, the left ventricle hypertrophies. As the ventricular muscle increases in size, it requires increased circulation from the existing coronary artery supply. Eventually, the coronary artery supply cannot sufficiently perfuse the enlarged left ventricle. This condition predisposes the hypertrophied left ventricle to ischemic injury because of inadequate coronary arterial perfusion. A hypertrophied left ventricle is more apt to sustain ischemia and MI, which results in weakening of the muscle. Therefore, the hypertrophied left ventricle is detrimental to the heart's health.

In addition, the enlarged cardiac muscle wall encroaches on the left ventricular chamber. As the muscle wall enlarges, it leaves less filling space within the chamber, which results in a condition termed restrictive cardiomyopathy. Over time, the hypertrophied left ventricle impedes optimal ventricular filling and becomes increasingly predisposed to ischemia. These conditions lead to severely impaired left ventricular contractile function (see Box 17-4).

Chronic Pulmonary Disease

Chronic pulmonary disease is the leading cause of RVF. When pulmonary disease is the etiology of RVF,

BOX 17-4. How Chronic HTN Leads to Left Ventricular Failure

- High systemic arterial blood pressure is reflected in the aorta as high aortic pressure.
- High aortic pressure creates increased resistance against the left ventricle, which causes left ventricular hypertrophy.
- The hypertrophied left ventricle requires increased coronary circulation, and demand eventually exceeds coronary artery supply.
- The hypertrophied left ventricle becomes predisposed to ischemia and systolic dysfunction.
- The hypertrophied left ventricle impedes optimal ventricular filling, causing restrictive cardiomyopathy and a diastolic dysfunction type of heart failure.

the condition is referred to as cor pulmonale. In cor pulmonale, the initiating event of heart failure is a lung disease that causes chronic hypoxia. The heart starts out in good health until a lung disease exerts detrimental effects on the right ventricle.

To understand cor pulmonale, the basic premise to comprehend is that chronic hypoxia stimulates vasoconstriction of the pulmonary arterial circulation. In turn, vasoconstriction of the pulmonary arterial circulation creates high pulmonary artery pressure, or **pulmonary hypertension**. In pulmonary HTN, the right ventricle, which must pump its contents into the pulmonary artery, is confronted with increased resistance. This increased workload on the right ventricle eventually causes right ventricular hypertrophy. As the right ventricle muscle wall enlarges, it requires increased coronary circulation. Demand for coronary blood flow eventually exceeds supply, and the right ventricle sustains ischemia. Ischemic insults to the right ventricle consequently weaken the muscle, leading to RVF (see Fig. 17-12).

CLINICAL CONCEPT

Long-standing pulmonary disease that causes chronic hypoxia can lead to cor pulmonale; COPD is one of the most common lung conditions that lead to cor pulmonale.

Cardiomyopathies

The term **cardiomyopathy** is most commonly used to describe a disease that targets the heart muscle itself. Cardiomyopathy generally infers that the myocardium has been directly injured by an agent or damaged as a side effect of another disease process. Infections that cause myocarditis, autoimmune disorders such as

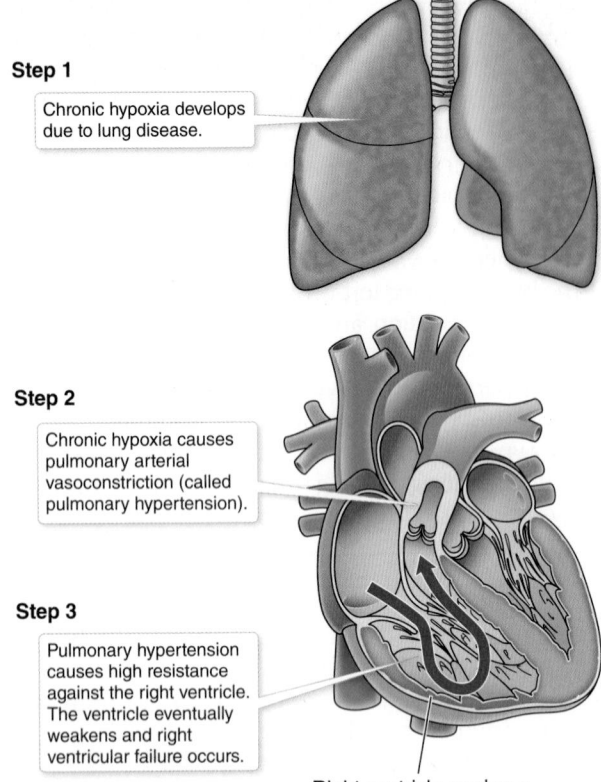

Step 1

Chronic hypoxia develops due to lung disease.

Step 2

Chronic hypoxia causes pulmonary arterial vasoconstriction (called pulmonary hypertension).

Step 3

Pulmonary hypertension causes high resistance against the right ventricle. The ventricle eventually weakens and right ventricular failure occurs.

Right ventricle weakens

FIGURE 17-12. Cor pulmonale. Cor pulmonale is right-sided heart failure that develops because of lung disease. The heart starts out healthy, but because of chronic lung disease, the right side of the heart weakens. The events occur as follows: Step 1: The lung is diseased and causes chronic hypoxia. Step 2: Chronic hypoxia causes pulmonary arterial vasoconstriction. Step 3: The pulmonary vasoconstriction causes high resistance against the right ventricle and eventually weakens the right ventricle.

sarcoidosis, neuromuscular diseases such as muscular dystrophy, and alcohol toxicity are examples of conditions that can directly injure the myocardium.

Ischemic cardiomyopathy is a term used to describe the diffuse myocardial fibrosis and scarring of the heart muscle caused by coronary artery insufficiency and MI. Dilated cardiomyopathy is another term used to describe enlargement and hypertrophy of the left or right ventricles in response to chronic injury. The distended ventricle loses contractile ability and exhibits poor systolic function. The enlarged ventricle becomes prone to dysrhythmias, stasis of blood, and consequent formation of emboli.

Cardiomyopathies are also described as restrictive or hypertrophic. In restrictive cardiomyopathy, the ventricle is impeded from filling to full capacity (see Box 17-5). Fibrotic changes of the myocardium, pericardial effusion, and pericarditis are disorders that restrict the ventricle's ability to fully expand. In hypertrophic cardiomyopathy, the left ventricular muscle is enlarged, usually on the side of the interventricular septum. The asymmetric hypertrophy of the left ventricle causes muscle wall stiffness and can obstruct the ejection of blood into the aorta during systole. Primary

---

BOX 17-5. Restrictive Cardiomyopathy

A minority of cases of heart failure result from diastolic dysfunction, an inability of the ventricle to relax, expand, and fill sufficiently during diastole. Restrictive cardiomyopathy occurs when the ventricle is unable to attain an adequate volume of blood because of a constrictive structural problem. This ventricular filling deficiency can occur in left ventricular hypertrophy, myocardial fibrosis, or pericarditis. Each of these conditions creates a smaller space within the ventricular chamber that cannot fill sufficiently with blood volume.

---

hypertrophic cardiomyopathy is commonly caused by a genetic predisposition for the muscular enlargement of the interventricular septal wall of the left ventricle.

Chronic HTN is referred to as a secondary cause of hypertrophic cardiomyopathy. HTN usually causes more diffuse enlargement of the left ventricle, not limited to the interventricular septal wall region, than is seen in primary hypertrophic cardiomyopathy.

Dysrhythmias

Dysrhythmias, also known as irregular heart rhythms, are common precipitating causes of heart failure. Tachydysrhythmias, rapid irregular rhythms of the ventricle, reduce the time available for ventricular filling, which can precipitate heart failure. Bradydysrhythmias, which are slow irregular rhythms of the ventricle, can slow the HR excessively, minimize cardiac output, and precipitate heart failure. Atrial dysrhythmias can diminish the atrial "kick" volume emptied into the ventricle, which in turn decreases SV. Decreased SV lessens the blood pumped out of the ventricle to meet the needs of the tissues.

Heart Valve Abnormalities and Cardiac Infections

Various heart valve disorders such as mitral regurgitation, which is insufficient closure of the mitral valve, and aortic stenosis, which is the narrowing of the aortic valve, cause pressure changes within the heart chambers, which can lead to heart failure.

Mitral Regurgitation. Mitral regurgitation, also known as mitral insufficiency, occurs when the mitral valve does not close completely during systole. As the left ventricle contracts, blood from the ventricle refluxes back into the left atrium. This increased blood volume in the left atrium increases backward pressure within the pulmonary veins. Pulmonary capillary hydrostatic pressure increases as a result, and fluid diffuses out of the capillaries into the pulmonary interstitium.

Mitral regurgitation commonly occurs after transmural MI of the left ventricle. The infarction commonly injures the papillary muscles, which are muscular projections that extend from the internal left ventricular wall. These small muscular projections are attached to the chorda tendineae, which are membranous, string-like cords that hold the heart valve leaflets in place. Chordae tendineae and papillary muscles assist in valve function. When rupture of a papillary muscle occurs because of MI of the left ventricle, the mitral valve becomes incompetent (see Fig. 17-13). The mitral valve leaflets become loose and do not come together to close off blood flow from the left atrium to the left ventricle. This dysfunction of the valve causes a classic holosystolic murmur heard loudest at the heart's apex. As the left ventricle contracts during systole, blood refluxes upward into the left atrium through the incompletely closed mitral valve. Consequently, backward pressure builds into the left atrium, pulmonary veins, and pulmonary interstitium leading to pulmonary edema.

Aortic Stenosis. Aortic stenosis is often caused by calcification of the aortic valve with aging, a process called aortic sclerosis. This produces a narrowing of the aortic valve that impedes the ejection of blood flow from the left ventricle into the aorta during systole (see Fig. 17-14). Aortic stenosis causes increased resistance against the left ventricle, which eventually causes left ventricular hypertrophy (LVH). As discussed previously, LVH is a precursor of events that lead to LVF.

Other Abnormalities. Aortic stenosis and mitral regurgitation are common heart valve disorders that lead to heart failure, but other disruptions of heart valve function can also lead to pressure changes within the heart chambers and eventual RVF or LVF.

Endocarditis and myocarditis, infections of the heart muscle, can cause detrimental biochemical and structural changes within the myocardium. These changes can lead to rapid deterioration of the contractile strength of the ventricular muscle. Rheumatic fever, a streptococcal infection, can lead to rheumatic heart disease, a cause of valve deformities.

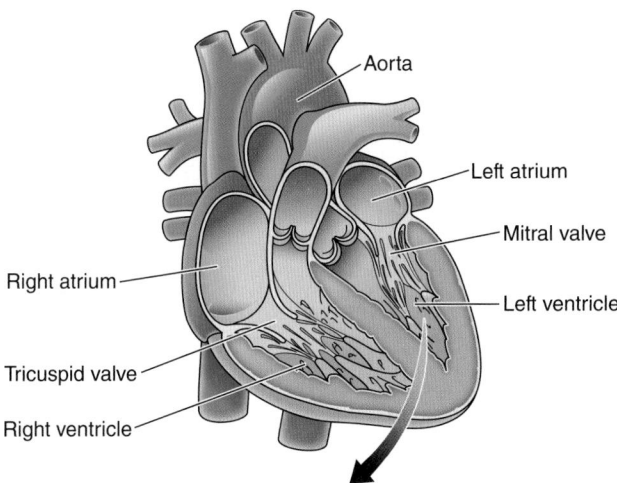

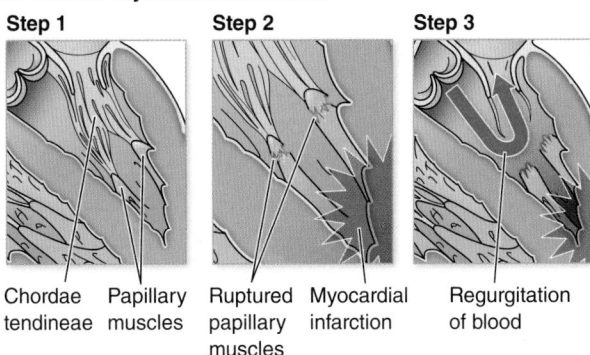

Left ventricle myocardial infarction:

Step 1	Step 2	Step 3

Chordae tendineae   Papillary muscles   Ruptured papillary muscles   Myocardial infarction   Regurgitation of blood

FIGURE 17-13. Papillary muscle rupture after MI with resulting mitral regurgitation. The event occurs as follows: Step 1: Papillary muscles are attached to the mitral valve leaflets by stringlike cords called chordae tendineae. Step 2: MI ruptures papillary muscles of the left ventricle. Step 3: The mitral valve leaflets become unattached to the ruptured papillary muscles, causing dysfunction of the mitral valve and regurgitation of blood up through the mitral valve into the left atrium.

> ### 🩺 CLINICAL CONCEPT
>
> A major cause of heart valve disease in the past, rheumatic fever has decreased in prevalence because of the widespread availability of antibiotics.

Pulmonary Embolism

A pulmonary embolism can cause acute RVF. An embolus lodged in the pulmonary artery suddenly raises pressure within the pulmonary artery. This acute rise in pulmonary artery pressure places an overwhelming amount of resistance against the right ventricle. This can rapidly and severely weaken the right ventricular muscle, causing acute RVF.

Risk Factors

There are a number of risk factors for heart failure, including the following:

- **Age:** Heart failure risk increases with advancing age. Heart failure is the most common reason for hospitalization in people age 65 years and older.
- **Ethnicity:** Heart failure occurs more often in African Americans than in European Americans. African Americans more often develop heart failure before age 50 years and die of the condition compared with European Americans.
- **Family history and genetics:** People with a family history of cardiomyopathies are at increased risk of developing heart failure. Cardiomyopathies are diseases of the heart that cause hypertrophy, dilation, or rigidity of myocardium. Currently, there are investigations into the genetic basis of these diseases.

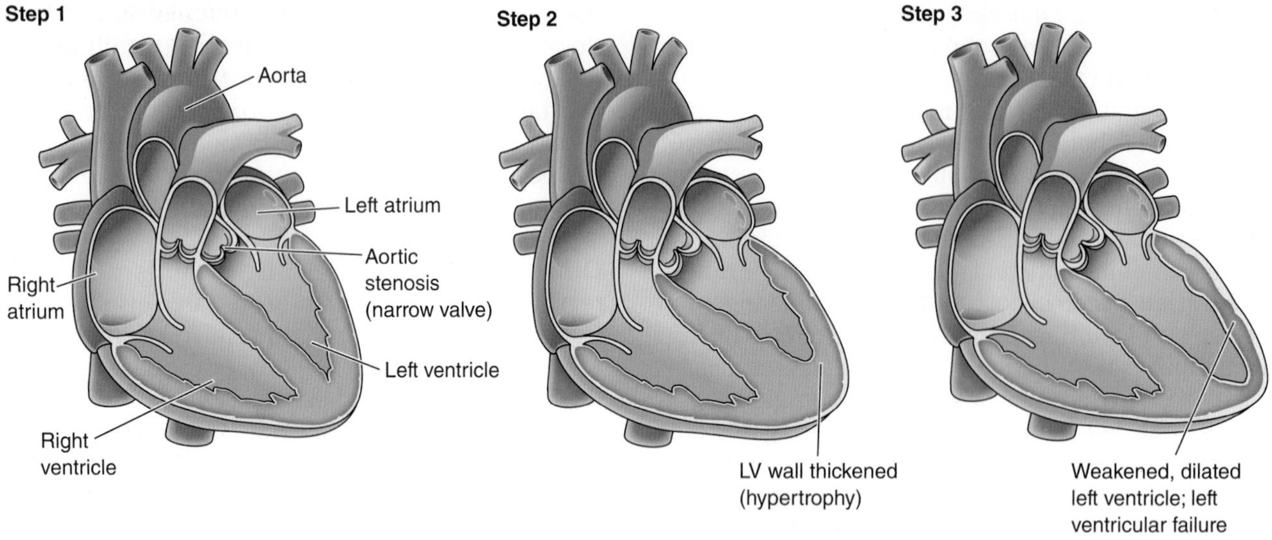

Step 1

Step 2

Step 3

FIGURE 17-14. Development of LVH and LVF caused by aortic stenosis. Aortic stenosis is the narrowing of the aortic valve. A narrowed aortic valve creates excessive resistance against the left ventricle. It is difficult for the left ventricle to pump its blood forward into the aorta. Step 1 shows aortic stenosis. Step 2 shows how the left ventricle hypertrophies because of the increased resistance. Step 3 shows how eventually the left ventricle fails when exhausted from excessive workload because of the narrowed aortic valve.

- **Diabetes:** Diabetes increases risk of arteriosclerosis throughout the body, including the coronary arteries. Coronary arteriosclerosis leads to coronary insufficiency, myocardial ischemia, and MI. These syndromes of ischemic heart disease weaken the heart muscle.
- **Obesity:** Obesity is associated with both HTN and type 2 diabetes, conditions that place the heart at risk for arteriosclerosis. HTN also causes development of LVH, with associated coronary insufficiency. These conditions together cause decreased strength of the heart muscle.
- **Lifestyle factors:** Smoking and sedentary lifestyle increase the risk for developing heart failure. Smoking and lack of physical activity increase the risk of arteriosclerosis. Smoking also causes vasoconstriction of arterial blood vessels. These problems lead to high workload and decreased coronary blood supply of the heart muscle.
- **Medications:** Long-term use of anabolic steroids, which are male hormones used to build muscle mass, increases the risk for heart failure. The drug itraconazole (Sporanox), used to treat skin, nail, or other fungal infections, has occasionally been linked to heart failure. The cancer drug imatinib (Gleevec) has been associated with heart failure cases, and other chemotherapy drugs, such as doxorubicin, can increase the risk for later developing heart failure years after cancer treatment. Cancer radiation therapy to the chest can also damage the heart muscle.
- **Sleep apnea:** Sleep apnea can cause hypoxia and increases the risk of rhythm disturbances.

Chronic hypoxia can lead to pulmonary artery vasoconstriction, which leads to pulmonary HTN. Pulmonary HTN increases the risk of RVF. Rhythm disturbances can weaken the heart muscle contractility.
- **Congenital heart defects:** Structural heart defects that occur in gestation and become apparent during the newborn period are called congenital heart defects. These defects may involve valvular abnormalities, imperfections in the heart wall, or anatomical problems with the aorta or pulmonary artery. These conditions cause changes in pressures within the heart chambers that can lead to excess workload for the heart and weakening of the heart muscle.
- **Viruses:** Although uncommon, certain viral infections can cause myocarditis, which weakens the heart muscle.
- **Alcohol abuse:** Excess long-term alcohol misuse can cause alcohol-related cardiomyopathy and lead to heart failure. Patients who consume more than two drinks per day have a 1.5- to 2-fold increase in HTN compared with persons who do not drink alcohol, and this effect is most prominent when the daily intake of alcohol exceeds five drinks. Long-term HTN causes increased resistance against the left ventricle, eventually causing heart failure. Alcohol itself also has a toxic effect on the heart muscle, causing a dilated, weak myocardium.
- **Kidney conditions:** Kidney conditions can cause excess blood volume, edema, HTN, and accumulation of nitrogenous waste. Excess blood volume and HTN can cause excess workload for the heart.

Excess nitrogen in the bloodstream is toxic to the heart muscle. These conditions will weaken the heart muscle.

Pathophysiology

Heart failure can be described in several ways: acute or chronic, systolic or diastolic dysfunction, HFrEF or HFpEF, high-output or low-output failure, right-sided or left-sided heart failure, and forward or backward failure. These contrasting descriptions are academic distinctions that explain the disorder's various mechanisms. However, these distinctions are often pertinent only early in the disease. Late in the course of heart failure, the distinctions become blurred.

The heart is a singular muscular organ that depends on the efficiency, rhythmicity, and strength of all its chambers. The biochemical and pressure changes that affect the myocardium in heart failure eventually affect both ventricles. A defect or weakness of one side of the heart will gradually lead to effects on the other side, causing a mixed clinical presentation of signs and symptoms late in the disease. Patients encountered in the clinical setting are often in the late stages of heart failure, when theoretical distinctions become less applicable. Clinically, most patients in heart failure present with a combination of right-sided and left-sided ventricular failure, systolic and diastolic dysfunction, and backward and forward failure effects. However, in order to better understand the complexities of this disorder, it is best to describe these mechanisms in terms of the previous distinctions.

Acute Versus Chronic Heart Failure

Acute heart failure describes the rapid, sudden development of heart failure that is often caused by substantial ventricular muscle injury as in massive MI.

Sudden, severe shock is often referred to as cardiogenic shock; it occurs when there is a significant loss of the ventricle's ability to pump blood adequately to maintain optimal blood pressure within the body. It often occurs because of extensive acute MI.

Chronic heart failure is a more common disorder, where the heart gradually suffers weakening over a long period.

Heart Failure With Reduced Ejection Fraction

In HFrEF, the weakened left ventricle has difficulty ejecting blood out of the chamber. The left ventricle is a poor forward pump, which in turn causes inadequate ventricular emptying (see Fig. 17-15). Stroke volume and cardiac output, both functions of forward heart-pumping action, are diminished. The LVEF, the amount of blood pumped out of the left ventricle, is less than 40% of the total left ventricular blood volume. Another similar type is HFmrEF. The amount of blood pumped out of the left ventricle with each contraction is 41% to 49%.

In both HFrEF and HFmrEF, blood accumulates in the weakened left ventricle, elevating pressure within the chamber. This causes a backup of hydrostatic pressure into the left atrium above it. The backward hydrostatic pressure in the left atrium causes further backup of pressure into the pulmonary veins, and ultimately the pulmonary capillaries. This excess hydrostatic pressure in the pulmonary capillaries causes **pulmonary edema**.

Also, with left ventricular pump weakening, there is activation of neurohormonal compensatory mechanisms that worsen heart failure. This neurohormonal mechanism involves the kidney and SNS. The kidney senses low perfusion, which stimulates the RAAS; this raises blood volume and peripheral arterial

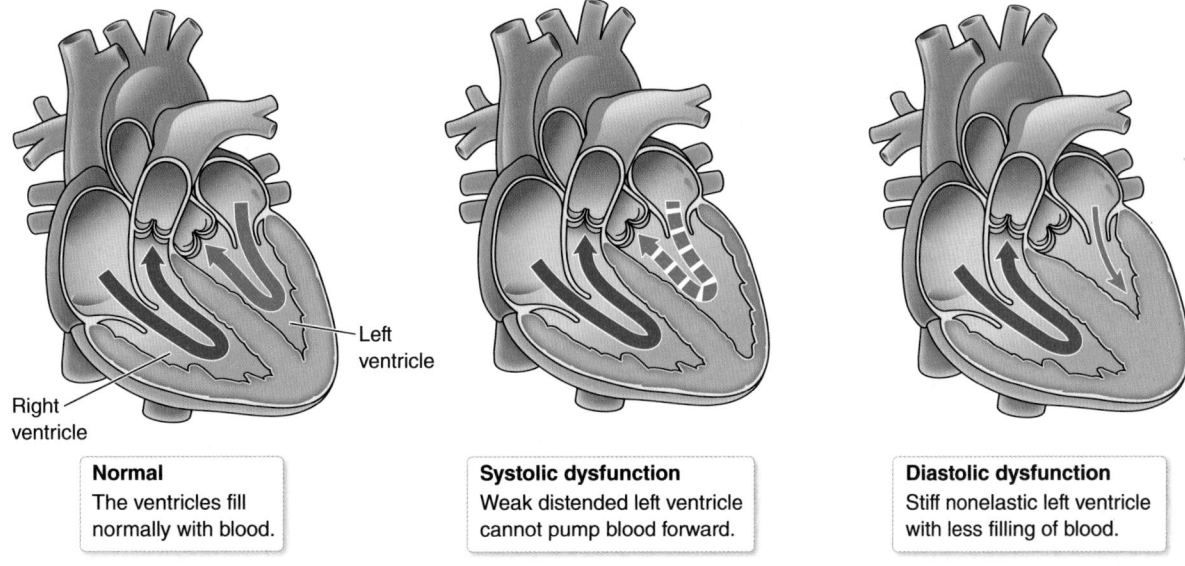

FIGURE 17-15. Normal heart function versus HFrEF versus HFpEF.

vasoconstriction (see Fig. 17-10). Extra blood volume places further strain on the weakened left ventricle. Peripheral arterial vasoconstriction places resistance against the left ventricle. In addition, the baroreceptors sense a drop in blood pressure as the heart pump fails, triggering the SNS to increase HR and further vasoconstrict peripheral arteries. The stimulus to increase HR strains the heart, and the additional peripheral vasoconstriction places more resistance against the left ventricle. These neurohormonal compensatory mechanisms further worsen the heart's ability to pump.

Heart Failure With Preserved Ejection Fraction

In HFpEF, the ventricle has difficulty relaxing, is less elastic, and cannot expand fully. The stiff ventricle cannot fill with blood adequately and therefore pumps out insufficient blood volume for the needs of the body's tissues. The percentage of the volume of blood ejected from the maximally filled total volume of the left ventricle is normal. In other words, the fraction of blood pumped out of the LV is greater than 50% of the total LV volume—this is called preserved ejection fraction (see Fig. 17-15).

High-Output Versus Low-Output Failure

High-output failure and low-output failure are less common mechanisms of heart failure. In high-output failure, the heart cannot pump sufficient amounts of blood to meet the high circulatory needs of the tissues. The heart is driven to high rates and contractile force to facilitate the delivery of blood to tissues demanding a greater amount of circulation. Under the strain of this effort, the heart can weaken and the ventricle can fail. High-output heart failure can be caused by systemic conditions that require increased arterial circulation caused by high metabolic demands, but this is a relatively uncommon occurrence. However, it is associated with thyrotoxicosis, AV shunting, severe anemia, Paget's disease of the bone, and thiamine deficiency.

In contrast, low-output failure occurs when the heart is unable to fill with adequate amounts of blood to pump out to the tissues. This is not a common cause of heart failure, but it can occur in conditions of impaired venous return to the heart. With less-than-adequate venous return, there is a lack of sufficient blood to recirculate through the heart and into the pulmonary and systemic arterial circulation. Consequently, in low-output failure, insufficient blood volume is pumped into the circulation, causing a lack of delivery of adequate oxygen to the tissues. For example, low-output failure can occur in traumatic injuries that block venous return from the legs up to the heart.

Left Ventricular Failure Versus Right Ventricular Failure

The simplest way to understand heart failure is by studying the process in terms of LVF and RVF. Failure of each side of the heart has distinctive consequences and can be simplified by visualizing each side of the weakened heart as having backward-failure and forward-failure effects (see Fig. 17-16 and Fig. 17-17). Essentially, backward effects are the result of a backup of hydrostatic pressure. Forward effects occur from decreased perfusion of the brain, kidney, and other vital organs. The heart is one organ; what happens to the right side will have consequences on the left side. Although heart failure usually involves both right and left ventricles, LVF and RVF will be explained individually for academic purposes in the following discussion.

Left Ventricular Failure. LVF can be explained in terms of systolic and diastolic dysfunction. Left ventricular diastolic dysfunction occurs from reduced relaxation or increased stiffness of the ventricular muscle. The increased afterload of HTN is commonly the cause for the development of these changes in the left ventricle. HTN causes increased resistance against the left ventricle, and the left ventricular muscle hypertrophies to compensate for the increased workload. LVF creates a noncompliant, enlarged, stiff-walled ventricular chamber. The thickened, muscular ventricular wall encroaches into the left ventricular chamber and diminishes the size of the left ventricle's interior. This leads to decreased left ventricular filling, as well as reduced SV and cardiac output. Because the ventricular filling or diastolic phase of heart function is most affected, this condition is often termed diastolic dysfunction.

Alternatively, left ventricular systolic dysfunction occurs when there is reduced forward pumping strength of the ventricular muscle. The left ventricle is weak and cannot eject its blood volume into the aorta, thereby decreasing SV and cardiac output. Systolic dysfunction of the left ventricle has two major consequences: backward effects and forward effects of failure. The backward effect of a failing left ventricle creates a buildup of hydrostatic pressure in the left atrium, pulmonary veins, and pulmonary capillaries. The forward failure effects cause decreased perfusion of the brain, kidneys, and other organs.

The backward effects consist of a buildup of hydrostatic pressure backward up into the left atrium and pulmonary vasculature, which causes fluid extravasation into the pulmonary interstitial and intracellular spaces leading to pulmonary edema. The opening and closing of alveoli against this fluid is heard as crackles through a stethoscope and is exhibited as cough, dyspnea, orthopnea, and **paroxysmal nocturnal dyspnea (PND)** by the patient.

The forward effects of the weak left ventricle cause inadequate ejection of blood into the aorta and diminished perfusion throughout the whole arterial circulatory system. The decreased perfusion of vital tissues activates a neurohormonal response that includes stimulation of the RAAS, ADH, and SNS (see Fig. 17-17).

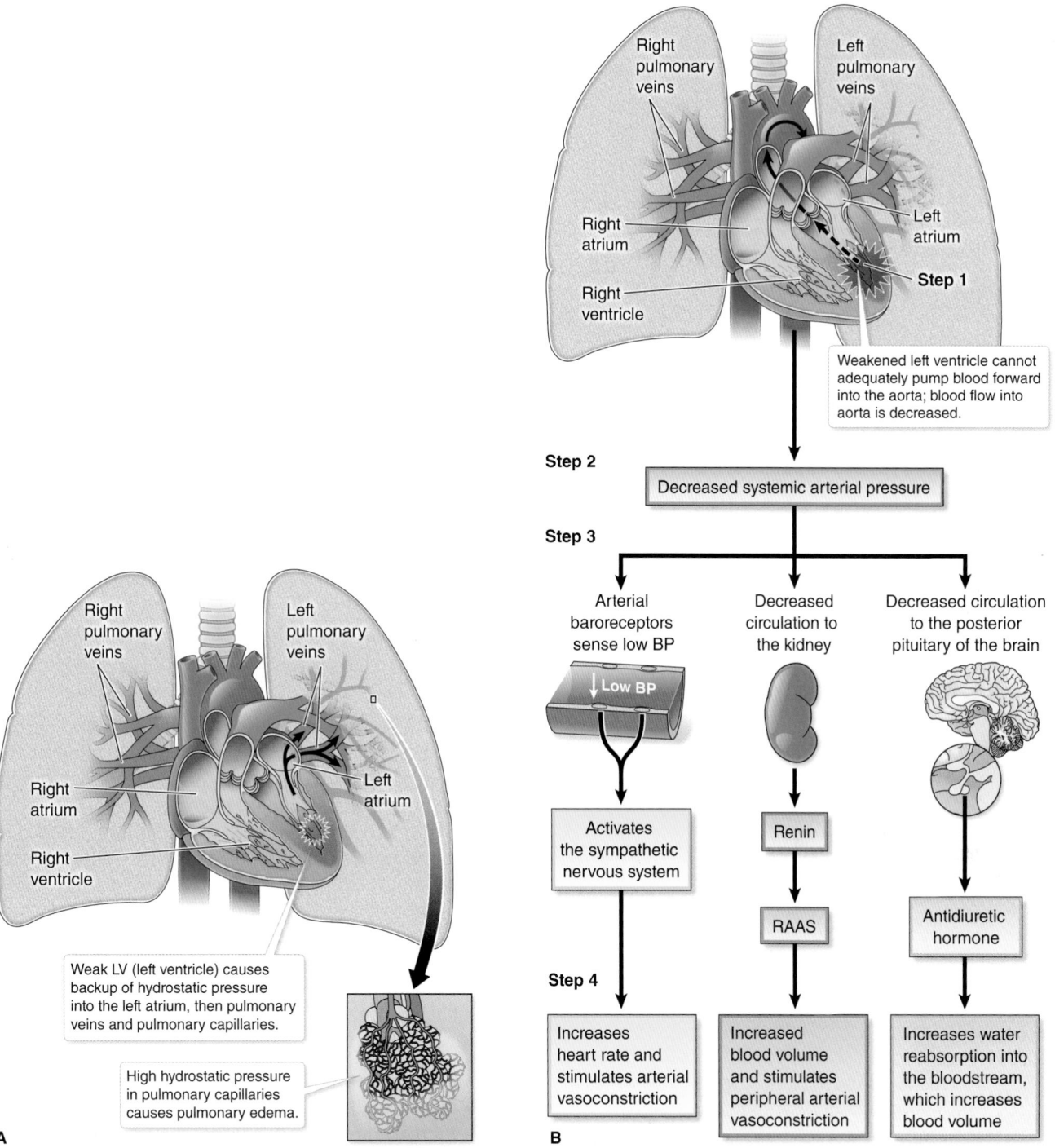

FIGURE 17-16. LVF. LVF can be studied by looking at the backward effects versus the forward effects of LVF. (A) Backward effects of left ventricular failure. A weakened left ventricle cannot pump all its blood forward into the aorta and consequently causes buildup of hydrostatic pressure in the left ventricle that is transmitted to the left atrium. The elevated hydrostatic pressure is further transmitted backward into the pulmonary veins and then pulmonary capillaries. High hydrostatic pressure within the pulmonary capillaries causes pulmonary edema. (B) Forward effects of left ventricular failure. Step 1: The failing left ventricle cannot adequately pump blood forward into the aorta. Step 2: Aortic pressure falls and systemic arterial pressure drops. Step 3a: Baroreceptors in the arteries sense a drop in BP and stimulate the SNS, which increases HR and stimulates peripheral arterial vasoconstriction. The increased HR further weakens the left ventricle. The increased arterial vasoconstriction increases resistance against the ventricle. Step 3b: As decreased blood flows into the systemic circulation and the kidney, the kidney secretes renin. Step 4: This stimulates the RAAS, which increases blood volume and blood pressure. This further increases the left ventricle's workload and weakens the ventricle more. Step 3c: Decreased circulation to the posterior pituitary gland of the brain causes secretion of ADH. ADH causes reabsorption of water into the bloodstream.

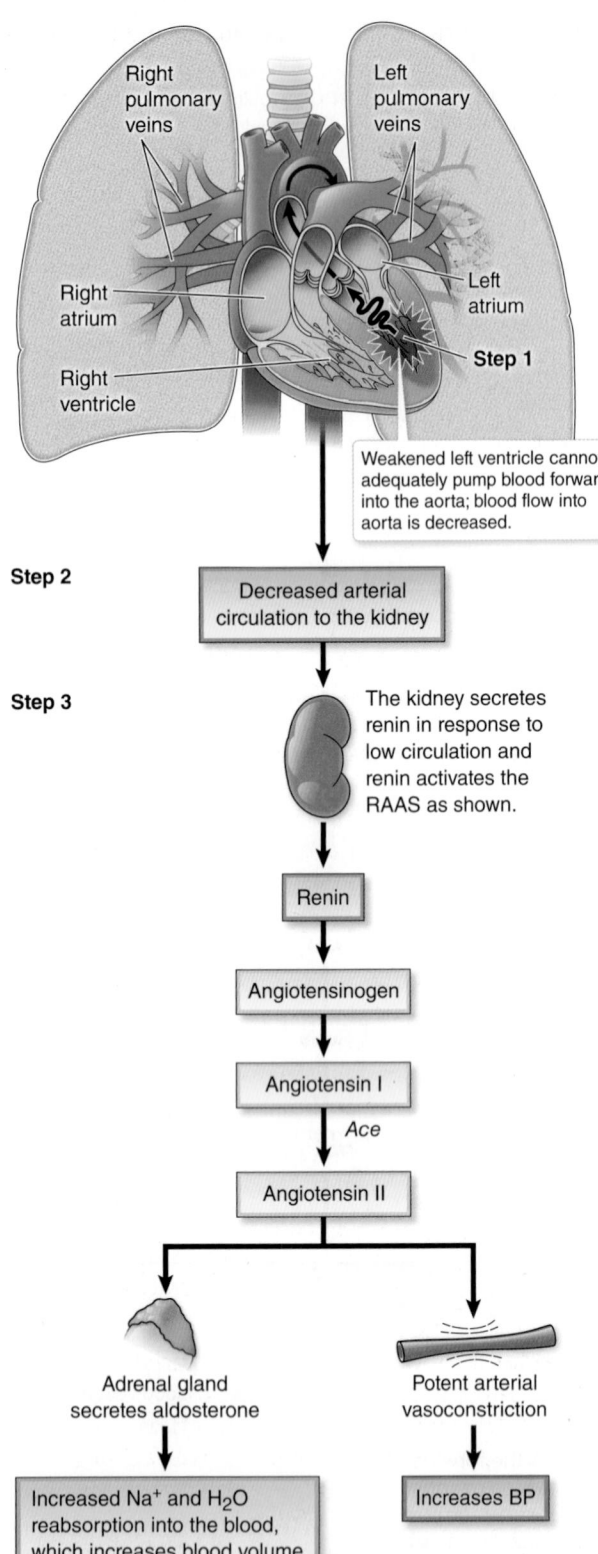

FIGURE 17-17. Forward failure effects of LVF stimulate the kidney to secrete renin and activate RAAS. Step 1: The failing left ventricle cannot adequately pump blood forward into the aorta. Step 2: Aortic pressure falls and systemic arterial pressure drops. Decreased blood flow to the kidney causes renin secretion. Step 3: This stimulates the RAAS, which increases blood volume and blood pressure. This further increases the workload of the left ventricle and weakens it more.

When the kidney senses decreased perfusion, it releases renin from the nephron juxtaglomerular apparatus and initiates cycling of the RAAS. Simultaneously, with decreased forward pumping of blood, the aorta and peripheral arteries experience diminished blood flow, which initiates other compensatory mechanisms.

The baroreceptors within the artery walls sense a drop in blood pressure, and this activates the SNS. The SNS stimulates adrenergic receptors in the heart and blood vessels to create further effects. Adrenergic stimulation of the heart increases HR, and adrenergic stimulation of the vasculature causes vasoconstriction (see Figs. 17-16 and 17-17).

Also, in response to diminished perfusion, the posterior pituitary gland releases ADH, which acts at the nephrons to increase water reabsorption into the bloodstream and, in turn, leads to increased blood volume (see Fig. 17-16).

> **ALERT!** Diminished perfusion of the kidney is particularly significant in LVF; it stimulates the secretion of renin from the juxtaglomerular apparatus of the nephron, which initiates cycling of the RAAS.

Pathophysiological Processes of LVF. The pathophysiological processes of LVF include cycling of the RAAS, adrenergic stimulation, progressive ventricular remodeling, and pulmonary edema.

Cycling of the RAAS. The RAAS plays a major role in the neurohormonal effects of heart failure. After release, renin circulates and reacts with angiotensinogen, a protein synthesized by the liver. Angiotensinogen is cleaved into a smaller protein: angiotensin I. Angiotensin I circulates, and ACE converts it into angiotensin II in the lungs. Angiotensin II has significant widespread systemic effects that worsen heart failure, including:

- Peripheral arterial vasoconstriction
- Increased blood pressure
- Increased resistance against the left ventricle
- Cardiac myocyte hypertrophy
- Detrimental ventricular remodeling
- Stimulation of adrenal aldosterone

Also, as mentioned previously, angiotensin II promotes the development of ventricular hypertrophy.

Angiotensin II is a potent arterial vasoconstrictor and exerts this effect on the systemic arterial system. This widespread vasoconstriction raises peripheral arterial resistance, which increases afterload for the weakened heart. The failing left ventricle, which is already weakened, is further challenged by the increased peripheral resistance against it. In addition,

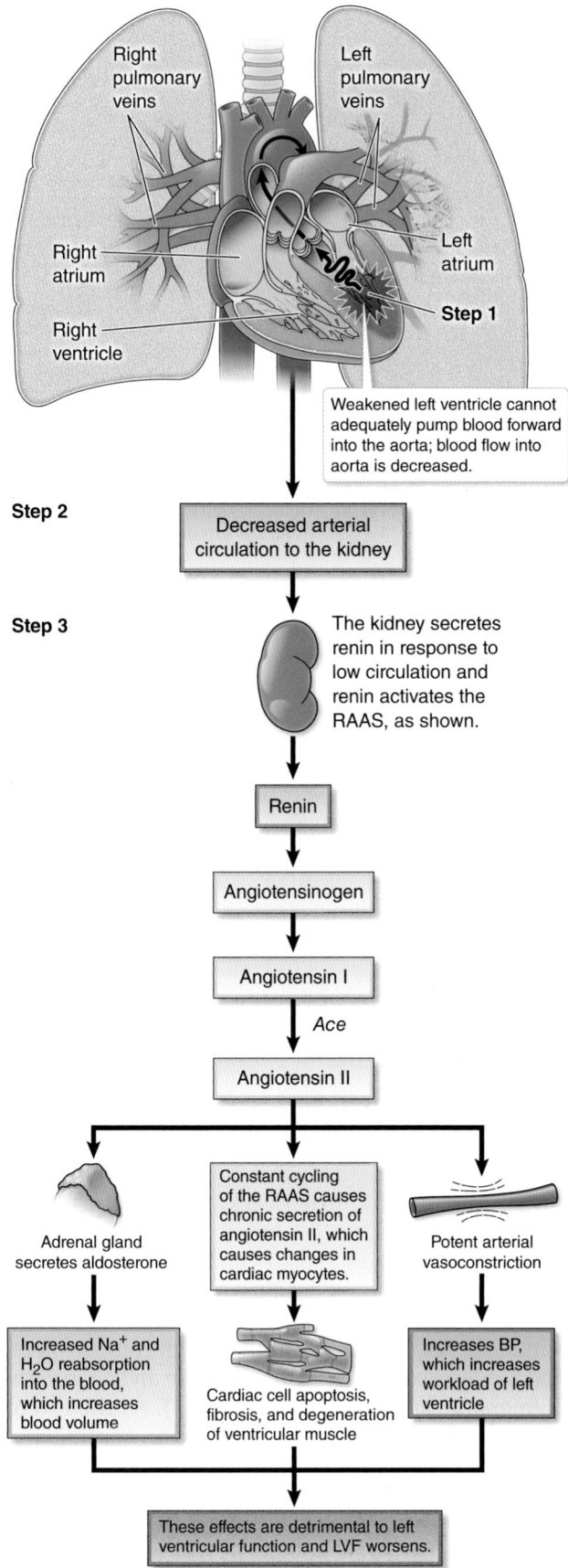

Step 1

Weakened left ventricle cannot adequately pump blood forward into the aorta; blood flow into aorta is decreased.

Step 2

Decreased arterial circulation to the kidney

Step 3

The kidney secretes renin in response to low circulation and renin activates the RAAS, as shown.

Renin

Angiotensinogen

Angiotensin I

Ace

Angiotensin II

Adrenal gland secretes aldosterone

Constant cycling of the RAAS causes chronic secretion of angiotensin II, which causes changes in cardiac myocytes.

Potent arterial vasoconstriction

Increased Na$^+$ and H$_2$O reabsorption into the blood, which increases blood volume

Cardiac cell apoptosis, fibrosis, and degeneration of ventricular muscle

Increases BP, which increases workload of left ventricle

These effects are detrimental to left ventricular function and LVF worsens.

FIGURE 17-18. There are many detrimental effects of activation of the RAAS in left ventricular failure.

angiotensin II stimulates the adrenal gland to release aldosterone (see Fig. 17-18).

Aldosterone causes sodium and water retention and potassium excretion from the bloodstream. The sodium and water retention increases total blood volume and raises blood pressure. Therefore, the stimulation of aldosterone by angiotensin II further challenges the weakened left ventricle.

ALERT! Hypokalemia, which increases the risk of cardiac dysrhythmias, can occur in heart failure caused by the constant stimulation of aldosterone.

The net effects of angiotensin II and aldosterone include an increased blood pressure and blood volume, as well as increased resistance against the left ventricle. These conditions require the failing ventricle to pump out a greater volume of blood against high resistance within the arterial circulation. As a result, the effects of angiotensin II and aldosterone further strain the weakened left ventricle, resulting in diminished forward pumping of blood into the aorta, which further diminishes arterial circulation and organ perfusion (see Fig. 17-18).

An increasingly weakened left ventricle further diminishes renal perfusion, which stimulates renin and provokes persistent cycling of the RAAS. As the RAAS cycles, the weakened heart continually deteriorates. Excess blood volume created by the constant cycling of the RAAS increases workload for the left ventricle, worsening heart failure. Without treatment, left ventricular heart failure leads to worsening LVF.

Adrenergic Stimulation. SNS activation occurs early in heart failure. Initially in LVF, there is a drop in arterial blood pressure caused by the inadequate forward pumping of blood into the aorta. The decline in blood pressure stimulates baroreceptors within arterial walls, which sense pressure changes. Baroreceptors, in turn, activate the SNS. Vasoconstriction of peripheral arteries occurs as a result of activation of the adrenergic (sympathetic) nervous system. This acts as a compensatory mechanism to raise blood pressure, but it also increases resistance within the arterial circulation. The increased resistance acts as increased afterload against the left ventricle, which further challenges the heart. Simultaneously, adrenergic stimulation increases HR by activating the SA node. The already failing heart is then stimulated to increase its rate, which further strains the ventricle (see Fig. 17-19).

Progressive Ventricular Remodeling. A weakened heart muscle activates the secretion of certain molecules that cause detrimental cellular changes within the myocardium. Molecular substances such as

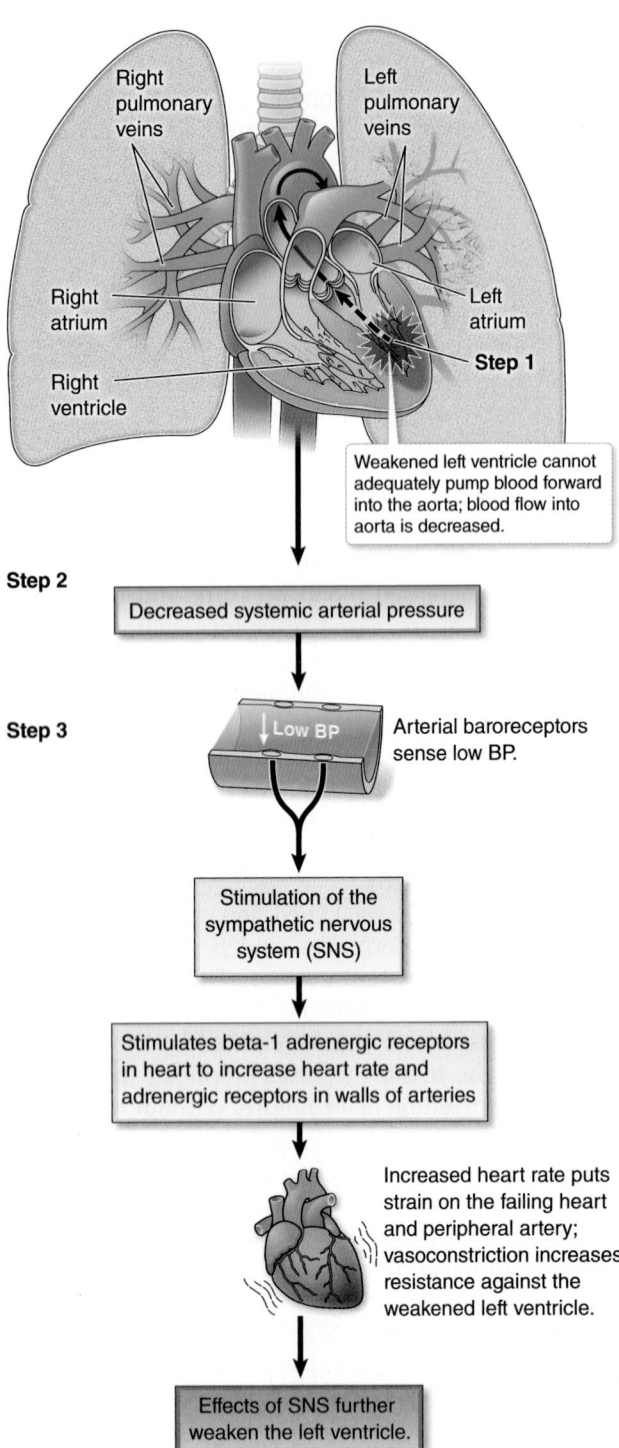

FIGURE 17-19. The effects of the SNS (adrenergic) stimulation in left ventricular failure. Step 1: The failing left ventricle cannot adequately pump blood forward into the aorta. Step 2: Aortic pressure falls and systemic arterial pressure drops. Step 3: Baroreceptors in the arteries sense a drop in BP. Step 4: Baroreceptors stimulate the SNS. Step 5: SNS stimulation increases HR and stimulates peripheral arterial vasoconstriction. The increased HR strains the weakened left ventricle. The increased arterial vasoconstriction increases resistance against the ventricle, weakening it further.

angiotensin II, aldosterone, endothelin, TNF-alpha, catecholamines, insulin-like growth factor, and growth hormone provoke genetic changes, apoptosis, and hypertrophy of cardiac myocytes, as well as collagen deposits and myocardial fibrosis (see Fig. 17-20).

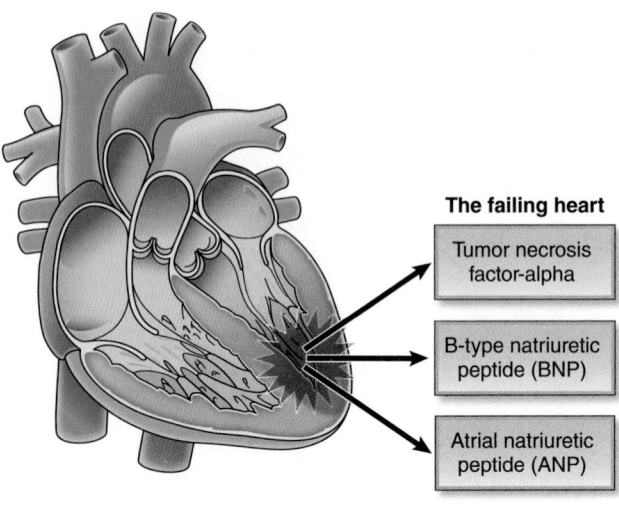

FIGURE 17-20. Molecular substances activated during heart failure. During heart failure, molecular substances are secreted. TNF-alpha, insulin-like growth factor, growth hormone, and endothelin cause detrimental ventricular remodeling. The ventricular cells undergo apoptosis, fibrosis, and degeneration. BNP secreted by the ventricles causes water loss from the body (called natriuresis). ANP secreted by the atria enhances water loss from the body (called natriuresis).

During the course of heart failure, these molecules cause changes in the heart that lead to enlargement and dilation of the left ventricle.

As these cellular changes occur, the ventricular myocardium progressively weakens. Additionally, there is impaired calcium utilization in the ventricular myocytes, leading to reduced contractile force. This triggers a vicious cycle with progressive weakening of the heart muscle, which continues to incite detrimental cellular changes. This cycle within the myocardium contributes to a continuous process of unfavorable progressive ventricular remodeling that worsens heart failure.

Pulmonary Edema. In LVF, as the forward ventricular pump is weakened, backward pressure builds within the left atrium, resulting in high hydrostatic pressure in the pulmonary veins. This high hydrostatic pressure is transmitted further backward into the pulmonary capillary bed. At the pulmonary capillaries, high hydrostatic pressure causes fluid extravasation into the interstitial spaces, leading to pulmonary edema. Edematous fluid builds within the pulmonary interstitial spaces and intracellular fluid compartments and hinders oxygen diffusion from the alveoli into the pulmonary capillaries (see Fig. 17-21). As the alveoli attempt to open and close against the accumulated fluid, crackles can be heard through a stethoscope. The patient experiences dyspnea and cough as fluid accumulates between the alveoli and capillary membranes.

Changes caused by pulmonary vascular congestion appear as vessel engorgement in the perihilar region on chest x-ray. High hydrostatic pressure within the pulmonary veins can also cause pleural effusion, which is edema accumulation in the pleural cavity. Pleural effusion can be identified on chest x-ray as a fluid level within the pleural cavity.

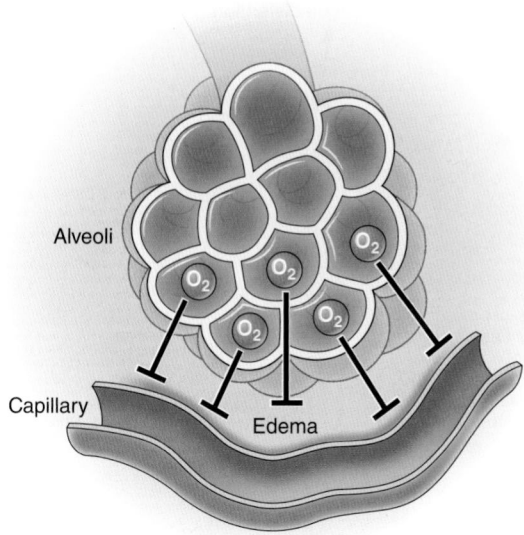

FIGURE 17-21. Pulmonary edema. Pulmonary edema is a fluid accumulation in the pulmonary interstitial spaces that hinders oxygen diffusion from alveoli to capillary. The blood cannot become sufficiently oxygenated and hypoxemia develops. The patient suffers severe dyspnea; cough; and pink, frothy sputum. Pulmonary edema can occur in left ventricular failure.

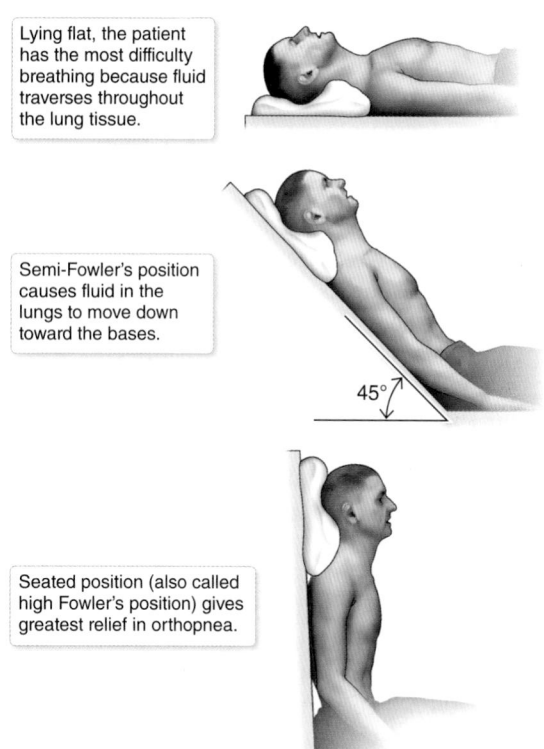

Lying flat, the patient has the most difficulty breathing because fluid traverses throughout the lung tissue.

Semi-Fowler's position causes fluid in the lungs to move down toward the bases.

45°

Seated position (also called high Fowler's position) gives greatest relief in orthopnea.

FIGURE 17-22. Orthopnea. Orthopnea is the feeling of shortness of breath when in a flat, supine position. Orthopnea most often occurs in LVF when fluid builds in the lungs. In the flat, supine position, the patient's pulmonary fluid traverses throughout the lung tissue. The person has the most difficulty breathing in this position. As the head of the bed is raised, orthopnea can be relieved because the fluid in the lungs is pulled downward to the bases of the lungs. Semi-Fowler's position (head at a 45-degree angle) can ease breathing, and the seated position can bring more relief because fluid is in the bases of the lungs. With fluid only in the bases of lungs, the patient can breathe easier.

Clinical Presentation. Patients with LVF may present with the following conditions.

Orthopnea. As fluid accumulates in the pulmonary interstitial spaces, the patient may experience **orthopnea,** which is a sensation of dyspnea when lying flat. When a patient is in the supine position, the fluid accumulation in the lungs becomes distributed throughout the lung fields. The supine position disperses the fluid within the lungs, which worsens the oxygen diffusion from the alveoli into the pulmonary capillaries. The standing position allows gravitational forces to pull fluid in the pulmonary interstitial spaces downward. While in this position, any fluid in the lungs is pulled toward the bases of the lungs. When a patient is supine or on bedrest, elevating the patient's head will redistribute pulmonary fluid downward toward the lung bases and ease breathing ability (see Fig. 17-22). For this reason, excess fluid caused by heart failure may be noticeable as pulmonary edema at night when the patient is supine. This can manifest as paroxysmal nocturnal dyspnea (PND). However, during the day when the patient is standing and fluid gravitates to the lung bases, there may be no respiratory difficulty.

Paroxysmal Nocturnal Dyspnea. PND is a unique symptom experienced by the patient who is experiencing the backward effects of LVF due to fluid accumulation in the lungs. PND is sudden shortness of breath that occurs in the middle of the night, disrupting a patient's sleep.

When the patient is in the supine position while asleep, any fluid in the pulmonary interstitium widely disperses over the lung fields. The fluid within the interstitial spaces hinders oxygen transfer from the alveoli into the capillaries, and the patient experiences hypoxia. When the patient is in the standing position, this same fluid accumulation in the lungs is less noticeable because gravitational forces pull it downward into the lung bases.

🩺 CLINICAL CONCEPT

Clinically, orthopnea can be described in terms of how many pillows the patient needs to breathe comfortably. For example, "two-pillow orthopnea" may be described in the clinical assessment of a patient. This term indicates that to breathe comfortably, the patient requires a head elevation at a level of two pillows.

🩺 CLINICAL CONCEPT

Patients often describe PND as nightmares or night terrors or feelings of strangulation that awaken them from sleep. Commonly, a patient is not able to accurately describe PND as shortness of breath because it occurs during sleep.

Cerebral Symptoms. With diminished strength of the left ventricle to pump blood into the arterial circulation, perfusion of the brain decreases. The patient may manifest decreased cerebral perfusion as confusion, headache, memory loss, insomnia, anxiety, or disorientation.

Constitutional Symptoms. Because of the diminished strength of the left ventricle, the organs receive less blood flow. Decreased gastrointestinal (GI) perfusion may cause anorexia, nausea, and abdominal discomfort. Reduced skeletal muscle perfusion can cause weakness and exercise intolerance. Poor urinary output and suboptimal filtration of blood can occur because of diminished renal perfusion. Diminished peripheral circulation results in decreased pulses bilaterally, as well as cold, pale extremities.

Right Ventricular Failure. In right-sided failure, the backward failure effects are most significant. In backward failure, the right ventricle is weak and has difficulty pumping all of its blood forward into the pulmonary artery. The ventricle's inability to pump its contents forward causes a backup of blood, raising hydrostatic pressure within the right heart chambers. Unejected blood accumulates in the right ventricle, increasing pressure within the ventricle, which in turn causes increased backward pressure in the right atrium. From the right atrium, backward hydrostatic pressure builds in the superior vena cava (SVC) and inferior vena cava (IVC) and consequently builds within the systemic venous system. Increased pressure within the venous system, also called central venous pressure, raises pressure in all the veins, which is transmitted as increased hydrostatic pressure in all peripheral capillary beds, causing edema. Continued backup of fluid contributes to organomegaly, or enlargement of the liver and spleen, and ascites, or fluid accumulation in the peritoneal cavity (see Fig. 17-23).

With weakening of the right ventricle, forward contractile force into the pulmonary artery is diminished. This decreases pulmonary arterial blood flow, which results in suboptimal alveolar–oxygen diffusion into the capillaries and, in turn, causes hypoxemia. The patient also may experience hypoxia and cyanosis. Compared with the backward failure effects of venous congestion and peripheral edema in RVF, forward failure effects are less dramatic.

Clinical Presentation. Patients with RVF may present with the following conditions.

Jugular Venous Distention. As the right ventricle weakens, pressure builds within the right atrium, SVC, and IVC. Demonstrable congestion within the SVC is exhibited in the jugular veins of the neck. **Jugular venous distention (JVD)**, or bilateral bulging blue neck veins, becomes the clinical sign of backward pressure within the SVC.

Elevated jugular venous pressure (JVP) is a classic sign of the backward effects of RVF (see Box 17-6).

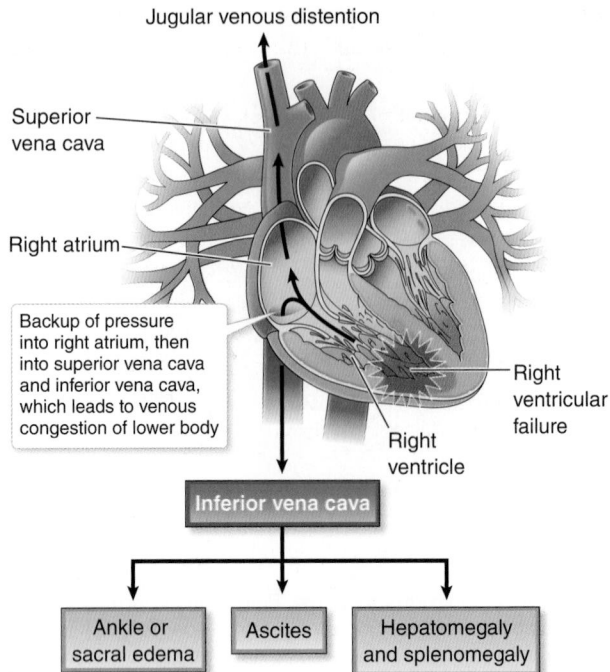

FIGURE 17-23. Right ventricular failure. The backward effects of RVF cause high hydrostatic failure in the right ventricle, which backs up into the right atrium and superior and inferior vena cava. From the vena cava, hydrostatic pressure builds throughout the body, causing widespread venous congestion. Venous congestion in the SVC is exhibited as JVD. Venous congestion in the gastrointestinal system is exhibited as peritoneal edema, which is called ascites. Venous congestion in the liver and spleen are exhibited as hepatomegaly and splenomegaly. Accumulation of hydrostatic pressure in the veins of the legs is exhibited as ankle edema. If the patient is in the supine position, sacral edema can occur.

BOX 17-6. Backward Effects of Right Ventricular Failure

- Jugular vein distention: result of high SVC pressure
- Elevated jugular venous pressure
- Elevated central venous pressure: high SVC and IVC pressure
- Ascites: backup of hydrostatic pressure in peritoneum
- Hepatomegaly: venous congestion/swelling of liver
- Splenomegaly: venous congestion/swelling of spleen
- Ankle or sacral edema

Pressure in the jugular veins reflects right atrial pressure and CVP, which are important clinical indicators of right ventricular function. As the right ventricle fails, right atrial pressure increases, which in turn increases CVP and JVP. Hence, RVF raises JVP.

Under normal conditions, jugular veins are collapsed and not visible in the seated or standing patient. Neck veins may be slightly distended under normal conditions when the patient is supine. However, in RVF, jugular veins are distended even when the patient is upright (see Box 17-7).

Venous Congestion of the Gastrointestinal Tract. As the right ventricle fails, hydrostatic pressure builds backward into the right atrium and throughout the venous system. As venous pressure rises, venous congestion in the GI tract occurs. Venous drainage diminishes within the GI tract. Anorexia, nausea, early satiety, postprandial fullness, indigestion, and impaired intestinal absorption are conditions associated with poor GI venous drainage. The liver and spleen endure venous congestion, which leads to engorgement within both organs.

Aside from organ dysfunction, venous engorgement leads to hepatomegaly and splenomegaly. Jaundice, coagulation problems, impaired drug metabolism, and elevated liver enzymes can develop because of the severe venous congestion of the liver. The liver's portal vein develops high pressure, which is referred to as high portal venous pressure. To confirm hepatic congestion caused by RVF, the clinician can elicit positive hepatojugular reflux.

> ### 🫀 CLINICAL CONCEPT
>
> In order to elicit hepatojugular reflux, the patient is supine, and the clinician presses on the liver. Pressure on the liver increases portal venous pressure and in turn raises JVP, producing visible JVD.

Increased hydrostatic pressure within all the GI veins is transmitted to the capillary beds, which creates edema within the peritoneal cavity, called **ascites**. In ascites, the patient develops a fluid-filled, distended abdomen. The abdominal distention of ascites can restrict full thoracic excursion during inspiration, impairing respiratory function.

Peripheral Edema. Venous congestion within the lower body causes high hydrostatic pressure within all the capillary beds of the extremities and leads to edema. Edematous fluid accumulation is influenced by gravitational forces. If the patient is supine or on bedrest, edema tends to accumulate around the sacral region. If the patient is in the supine position for prolonged periods, sacral edema increases the skin's fragility and can lead to skin breakdown. Erythema of the skin and edema in the sacral area is the first sign of pressure in this area. Sacral edema predisposes the patient to the formation of sacral decubitus ulcers. Because of the gravitational forces, dependent ankle edema develops in the standing or ambulatory patient. The feet and lower legs may also develop edema in RVF.

> **ALERT!** If RVF is severe, peripheral edema can be massive and gradually affect most of the tissues in the body, a condition called anasarca.

Biventricular Heart Failure. The heart is a single muscular organ that requires efficient functioning of all its chambers in a rhythmic, coordinated, and resilient manner. Dysfunction of any one chamber causes compensatory changes within the other chambers. If dysfunction of one heart chamber persists, compensatory mechanisms become exhausted and begin to diminish, and decompensation of the whole organ

---

BOX 17-7. Measuring Jugular Venous Pressure

To accurately assess JVP in a patient experiencing heart failure, the supine patient should have the head of the bed raised to a 45- to 60-degree angle. The clinician should place a centimeter ruler on the sternal angle of the patient's chest—the bony ridge of the sternum adjacent to the second rib. The sternal angle is approximately 5 cm above the right atrium. Using a straight edge, the clinician should measure the distance in centimeters from the sternal angle to the horizontal level of the highest visible pulsations of the distended neck veins. This measurement plus 5 cm provides an approximate measure of JVP. The following is an example of how JVP is clinically noted in patient assessment:

Neck:
+ JVD: jugular veins 9 cm from right atrium at
45 degrees alternatively
+ JVD: jugular veins 4 cm above sternal angle at
45 degrees

This assessment indicates that the clinician observed a level of jugular vein distention at 9 cm above the right atrium or 4 cm above the sternal angle, which is considered elevated JVP.

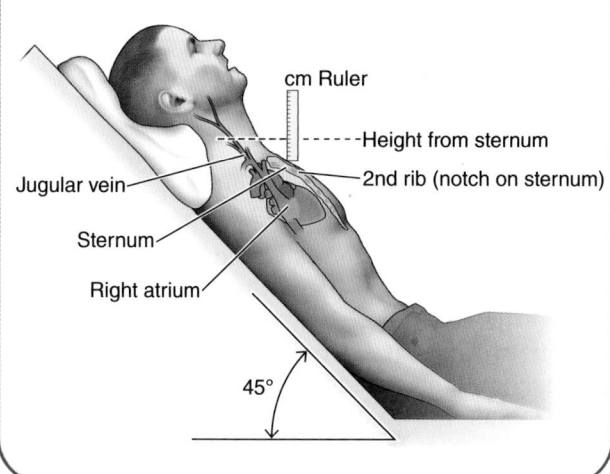

cm Ruler
Height from sternum
2nd rib (notch on sternum)
Jugular vein
Sternum
Right atrium
45°

occurs. Failure of one side of the heart ultimately results in damage to the other side of the heart.

In the clinical setting, a patient most often presents in biventricular failure, which is combined left- and right-sided heart failure. Depending on the extent of the disease, the patient commonly presents with a combination of the signs and symptoms of left and right ventricular failure. LVF produces pulmonary symptoms such as cough, dyspnea, and orthopnea, whereas RVF produces such systemic edema signs as JVD, ascites, hepatomegaly, and ankle edema. A patient in biventricular heart failure will exhibit a constellation of these signs and symptoms (see Box 17-8).

Clinical Presentation of Heart Failure

The diagnosis of heart failure is established by observable clinical manifestations, patient history, and laboratory findings. Patients commonly present to the clinician when combined RVF and LVF exist.

History

In mild to moderate heart failure, the patient may appear in no distress and clinical manifestations may be minimal at rest. However, the patient may report dyspnea upon exertion, dyspnea when lying flat for more than a few minutes, or a nocturnal cough. These are early signs of pulmonary interstitial fluid accumulation caused by failure of the left ventricle. Confusion, difficulty concentrating, and headache can occur with decreased cerebral perfusion. Cold, pale legs and feet may be noticeable to the patient, caused by diminished circulation in the extremities.

The patient may notice swelling in the ankles or fingers, which is indicative of increased venous pressure. Patients may report tight rings or shoes because of fluid retention. Abdominal swelling and GI symptoms, such as anorexia or a feeling of fullness, may be patient complaints associated with RVF. The patient may have increased frequency of urination and nocturia caused by excess fluid accumulation. Weight gain of 2 lb or more per day is often indicative of fluid retention.

Signs and Symptoms

Pulmonary crackles may not be audible in early LVF. With more moderate heart failure, as pulmonary capillary pressure rises, bilateral pulmonary crackles (indicative of pulmonary edema) can be heard farther and farther up from the bases of the lungs. Pulmonary edema can present with pink frothy sputum and coarse crackles.

In early stages of RVF, the jugular veins may not be visibly distended at rest. However, elevated venous pressure may become observable by positive hepatojugular reflux when the abdomen is deeply palpated over the liver. Ascites, hepatomegaly, and splenomegaly may not be present or will be minimally apparent in mild heart failure.

The diagnosis of mild to moderate heart failure is most often inferred by the patient history of risk factors, dyspnea on exertion, orthopnea, and PND episodes. PND is often described in terms of night terrors, nightmares, or a choking feeling that awakens one from sleep. Clinical manifestations may not be overtly apparent in the resting patient early in heart failure, so the patient history must be carefully evaluated.

In moderate to severe heart failure, the pulses are usually diminished, and cyanosis of the lips and nailbeds may be observed. Distended jugular neck veins are best observed with the patient in Fowler's position at a 45-degree angle.

Cardiomegaly, or left ventricular enlargement, may be demonstrated by a shifted point of maximal impulse or apical pulse. When the left ventricle is enlarged, the apical pulse, normally located at the left fifth intercostal space on the midclavicular line, can be palpated farther into the left axillary region.

Upon auscultation of the heart, a third and fourth heart sound may be heard through the stethoscope. The third heart sound (S_3) is a low-pitched sound heard after S_2, during rapid filling of the ventricle in the early part of diastole. In children and young adults, an S_3 may be normal. In adults older than age 40 years, the presence of an S_3 is abnormal and indicative of heart failure. High ventricular end diastolic volume and increased pressure within the chambers consequent to heart failure are responsible for a third heart sound.

A fourth heart sound (S_4) is heard when the atrium contracts against a noncompliant, stiff ventricle.

BOX 17-8. Signs and Symptoms of Biventricular Heart Failure

LEFT VENTRICULAR FAILURE
- Dyspnea
- Cough
- Orthopnea
- PND
- Weak peripheral pulses
- Decreased cerebral perfusion; confusion, disorientation

RIGHT VENTRICULAR FAILURE
- JVD
- Ascites
- Gastrointestinal disturbances caused by venous congestion
- Hepatojugular reflux
- Hepatomegaly
- Splenomegaly
- Peripheral edema; ankle or sacral edema; fingers, feet

Normally, when the atrium contracts, there is no sound. An S_4 is a low-pitched sound heard at the end of diastole, before S1. An S_4 commonly occurs in chronic HTN, caused by the structural changes that occur in the left ventricle as a result of high blood pressure. In HTN, high aortic pressure creates high resistance and hypertrophy of the left ventricle. The hypertrophic left ventricle is less elastic and distensible. Atrial contraction against this stiff left ventricle causes an audible S_4 during diastole.

Upon palpation of the pulse, resting tachycardia is often present in moderate or severe heart failure. Moist, inspiratory crackles may be heard over the lung bases bilaterally. Pulmonary edema is exhibited by coarse, bilateral crackles widely dispersed over the lung fields. A bilateral pleural effusion may develop as a result of high pulmonary venous pressure, causing diffusion of fluid into the pleural cavity.

Ascites occurs as a consequence of hepatic venous congestion, which causes diffusion of fluid into the peritoneal cavity. Fluid within the peritoneal cavity can be demonstrated by the finding of "shifting dullness" on physical examination. Turning patients on their side allows the clinician to percuss dullness over the dependent portion of the abdomen where peritoneal fluid has shifted. Tympany can be percussed at the superior aspect of the patient's abdomen, where there is no peritoneal fluid. A palpable, enlarged liver and spleen may be evident on examination of the abdomen. Pressure on the liver will transmit elevated venous pressure into the jugular veins as hepatojugular reflux.

Symmetric, dependent edema is often apparent in the ankles in the ambulatory patient and may be most observable in the evening. In bedridden patients, dependent edema accumulates over the sacral region. Patients sense edema when fingers or feet swell to cause rings or shoes to fit tightly. Edema can be exhibited as facial puffiness or periorbital swelling. Weight gain can occur when several liters of edematous fluid accumulate in interstitial spaces of the body.

Daily weight measurement is recommended in the clinical assessment of patients in heart failure. Weight fluctuation of 2 lb or more from day to day is often caused by fluid retention or edema. The skin over the extremities may be cool and pale because of decreased perfusion. The pulses of the extremities, particularly the dorsalis pedis pulses, are symmetrically diminished.

Diagnosis

To establish a diagnosis of heart failure, at least one of the major criteria and two of the minor criteria should be present from the Framingham Criteria for Diagnosis of Congestive Heart Failure (see Table 17-1).

Laboratory and Diagnostic Studies. There are a number of laboratory and diagnostic studies when it comes to diagnosing heart failure.

Brain Natriuretic Peptide (B-type Natriuretic Peptide). In heart failure, as the ventricle stretches in response to increased blood volume, the myocardium secretes BNP, a natural diuretic substance. This peptide, which is secreted by the heart, enhances the body's ability to allow water loss from the kidneys, which, in turn, decreases blood volume. BNP is elevated in the bloodstream in heart failure as well as other conditions, particularly pulmonary disease.

TABLE 17-1. Framingham Criteria for Diagnosis of Congestive Heart Failure

Major Criteria	Minor Criteria	Major or Minor Criteria
Paroxysmal nocturnal dyspnea	Bilateral extremity edema	Weight loss of 4.5 kg or more over 5 days of treatment for heart failure
Jugular vein distention	Nighttime cough	
Pulmonary crackles	Dyspnea on exertion	
Cardiomegaly	Hepatomegaly	
Auscultation of S_3 heart sound	Pleural effusion	
Increased CVP (greater than 16 cm H_2O)	Reduced pulmonary vital capacity by one-third from normal	
Positive hepatojugular reflux	Tachycardia (120 beats/min or greater)	

To establish a diagnosis of heart failure, at least one of the major criteria and two of the minor criteria should be present from the Framingham Criteria for Diagnosis of Heart Failure.

Adapted from Ho, K. K., Pinsky, J. L., Kannel, W. B., & Levy, D. (1993). The epidemiology of heart failure: The Framingham Study. *Journal of the American College of Cardiology, 22* (4 suppl A), 6A–13A.

ALERT! Levels of BNP greater than 500 are considered indicative of heart failure.

Serum Electrolytes. In heart failure, blood volume increases because of excess water within the bloodstream. This excess water commonly dilutes the serum sodium, causing dilutional hyponatremia. In addition, with the constant cycling of the RAAS in heart failure, aldosterone causes potassium excretion from the kidneys, which can lead to hypokalemia. The repeated simulation of the RAAS increases the risk of hypokalemia. Imbalances in serum electrolytes, particularly potassium, can have adverse effects on myocardial function. Hypokalemia predisposes the heart to dysrhythmias. In heart failure, serum electrolytes require periodic monitoring and correction if abnormal.

Chest X-Ray. A chest x-ray delineates the cardiac shadow and pulmonary fields. In heart failure, cardiomegaly, or enlargement of the heart, is commonly seen. Often the left ventricle is enlarged to a greater extent than the right ventricle. Cardiomegaly is often caused by LVH or dilation of the ventricles. The pulmonary fields may show vasculature congestion as increased opacity in the vessels.

Kerley A lines and Kerley B lines are specific pulmonary x-ray findings indicating the vasculature congestion of heart failure. These findings, interpreted by the radiologist, appear as opaque linear shadows representing the engorged blood vessels of the lungs. The chest x-ray of pulmonary edema shows dense opaque vessel shadows in the perihilar regions of the lung fields, called either "bat wing density" or "butterfly pattern" (see Fig. 17-24).

Electrocardiogram. The electrocardiogram (ECG) may demonstrate various abnormalities in heart failure. LVH or enlargement is exhibited by the waveforms derived from the chest leads. Other changes of the ST segment, T wave, or QRS complex may be apparent. There are no specific ECG signs of heart failure.

Echocardiogram. An echocardiogram is a type of non-invasive sonogram that can demonstrate the activity and structures of the heart. It is commonly used to evaluate the size and function of the ventricles, valve structure, and valve function. LVEF can be estimated using this diagnostic modality. Another type of echocardiogram is an ultrasonic cardiac output monitor (USCOM). It is a noninvasive transcutaneous continuous wave Doppler method for assessing hemodynamics. USCOM scans can measure stroke volume, cardiac output, and systemic vascular resistance.

Multiple-Gated Acquisition Scan. A multiple-gated acquisition scan, also known as radionuclide ventriculography, is a nuclear medicine procedure that involves injecting a small amount of radioactive dye into a peripheral vein. The radiopaque dye illuminates the

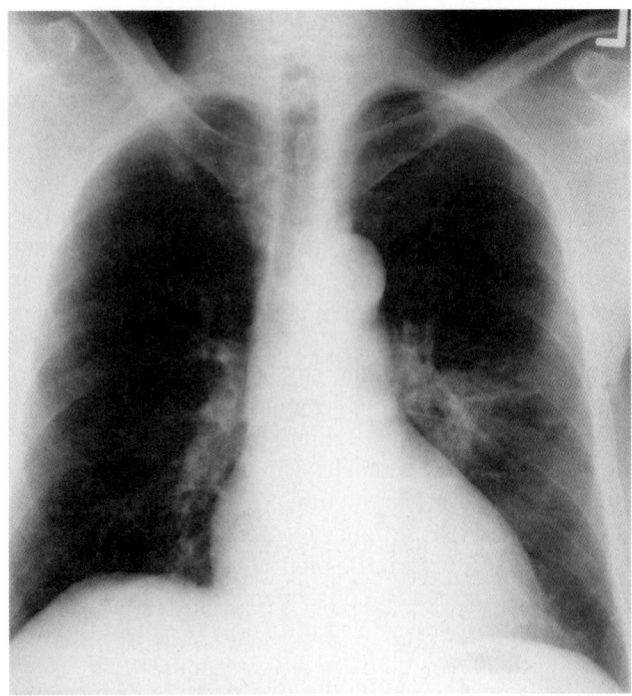

FIGURE 17-24. Chest x-ray showing heart failure. The heart is enlarged (cardiomegaly), and blood vessels are prominent in the hilar lung fields, which represents pulmonary venous congestion. Kerley lines are horizontal lines in the base of the lungs close to the chest wall. They are the result of interstitial edema in the lungs. *(From Southern Illinois University/Science Source.)*

heart on x-ray as it contracts. Similar to an echocardiogram, this procedure demonstrates the volume of blood pumped out of the ventricle with each contraction. The LVEF can be determined using this nuclear diagnostic procedure.

Cardiac Catheterization and Angiography. A specialized cardiac catheter can be used to perform hemodynamic monitoring within the heart or to study the coronary arteries. A cardiac catheter can be inserted via the femoral vein, femoral artery, or subclavian vein, depending on its intended purpose. If the goal is to measure hemodynamic pressures and volumes within the right side of the heart, a catheter can be inserted into the femoral vein, threaded into the IVC, and then moved into the right atrium and right ventricle. If the goal is to measure pressures and volumes within the left side of the heart, a catheter can be inserted into the femoral artery and then into the aorta and left ventricle.

A cardiac catheter can also be used to study the health of the coronary circulation. Commonly, a cardiac catheter is first inserted into the femoral artery in the leg and threaded into the aorta against the flow of blood and then into the openings of the coronary arteries.

The cardiac catheter can enter either the right or left coronary artery via the aorta. Radiopaque dye is injected via the catheter, which illuminates the coronary artery under study. The dye allows visibility of the artery structure on an x-ray called an angiogram or arteriogram. Angiography can be used to illuminate any artery in the body that is accessible via catheter.

Basic Hemodynamic Measurements of LVF Versus RVF.

In the failing heart, pressure changes within the heart chambers and great vessels cause abnormal hemodynamic measurements. Specific hemodynamic pressure changes occur that characterize right versus left heart failure. These values can be used to differentiate RVF from LVF or monitor the efficacy of heart failure treatment. These values are monitored in an intensive care setting (see Table 17-2).

Classification Systems of Heart Failure.

Two major classification systems describe the stages of heart failure according to the patient's symptoms: The New York Heart Association (NYHA) Classification and the ACA/AHA Classification. Each classification system aims to help clinicians evaluate the severity of heart failure in their patients (see Table 17-3 and Table 17-4).

Treatment

Different types of interventions are available for heart failure. Lifestyle modifications, such as changing to a low-fat diet, smoking cessation, and increasing physical activity, are basic health promotion strategies. Pharmacological agents, such as beta blockers and ACE inhibitors, are the cornerstone of treatment. Finally, there are intracardiac interventions, such as pacemakers, that can greatly improve the life of a patient with heart failure.

Lifestyle Modifications.

The patient with heart failure should limit fluid, salt, cholesterol, and alcohol consumption. A low-salt diet consisting of no more than 1.5 grams of sodium per day is commonly recommended. If the patient is ambulatory, a daily walking regimen is also recommended. If obese, the patient should begin a weight loss program that includes daily weight measurement.

Following a daily medication schedule, having periodic physical examinations, and performing laboratory

TABLE 17-2. Basic Hemodynamic Measurement Changes in Heart Failure

Hemodynamic Measure	Normal Value Range	Description	Hemodynamic Changes Occurring in Heart Failure
Central venous pressure (CVP)	1 to 5 mm Hg	Volume of blood returning to the right atrium from the venous circulation (e.g., can be referred to as preload)	In right ventricular failure, backward buildup of hydrostatic pressure increases right atrial pressure and CVP
Pulmonary artery pressure	17 to 32/4 to 13 mm Hg	Pressure within the pulmonary artery, which acts as resistance against the right ventricle	
Cardiac output	4 to 8 liters/min	Total volume of blood pumped out by the heart per minute	Decreases as ventricles fail
Systemic arterial blood pressure	90 to 140/60 to 80 mm Hg	Blood pressure within the arteries	Blood pressure decreases with left ventricular failure
Pulmonary capillary wedge pressure (PCWP)	12 to 15 mm Hg	Pressure within the pulmonary capillary bed	In LVF, backward failure effects cause backup of hydrostatic pressure in the pulmonary capillaries, which increases PCWP
Left ventricular ejection fraction (LVEF)	50% to 70% of blood in ventricle Lower than 40% indicative of LVF	The volume of blood ejected with each contraction of the left ventricle (can be referred to as stroke volume)	In LVF, LVEF is decreased

TABLE 17-3. The NYHA Classification of Heart Failure

Class	Patient Symptoms
Class I–Mild heart failure	No limitation of physical activity. Ordinary physical activity does not cause undue fatigue, palpitations, or dyspnea.
Class II–Mild heart failure	Slight limitation of physical activity. Comfortable at rest, but ordinary physical activity results in fatigue, palpitations, or dyspnea.
Class III–Moderate heart failure	Marked limitation of physical activity. Comfortable at rest, but more than ordinary physical activity causes fatigue, palpitations, or dyspnea.
Class IV–Severe heart failure	Unable to carry out any physical activity without discomfort. Symptoms of cardiac insufficiency at rest. If any physical activity is undertaken, discomfort is increased.

Source: American Heart Association. NYHA classification system. Retrieved from https://www.heart.org/en/health-topics/heart-failure/what-is-heart-failure/classes-of-heart-failure; adapted from Dolgin, M., Association NYH, Fox, A. C., Gorlin, R., Levin, R. I., New York Heart Association. Criteria Committee (1994). *Nomenclature and criteria for diagnosis of diseases of the heart and great vessels* (9th ed.). Boston, MA: Lippincott Williams and Wilkins; March 1, 1994. Original source: Criteria Committee, New York Heart Association, Inc. (1964). *Diseases of the heart and blood vessels; Nomenclature and criteria for diagnosis* (6th ed.). Boston, Little, Brown and Co., p. 114. ©1994 American Heart Association, Inc.

TABLE 17-4. ACC/AHA Classification of Heart Failure

Stage	Description	Examples
Stage A	Patients susceptible to heart failure because of the presence of conditions placing them at high risk. Patients have no identifiable structural or functional abnormalities of the myocardium, pericardium, or cardiac valves and have not shown heart failure signs or symptoms.	Systemic HTN, coronary artery disease, diabetes mellitus, history of cardiotoxic drugs, alcohol use disorder, rheumatic fever, or family history of cardiomyopathy.
Stage B	Patients who have developed structural heart disease strongly associated with heart failure development but who have not shown heart failure signs or symptoms.	LVH or fibrosis, left ventricular dilation or hypocontractility, asymptomatic valvular heart disease, or previous MI.
Stage C	Patients who have current or prior symptoms of heart failure associated with underlying structural heart disease.	Dyspnea or fatigue caused by systolic dysfunction or asymptomatic patients undergoing treatment for prior symptoms of heart failure.
Stage D	Patients with advanced structural heart disease and marked symptoms of heart failure at rest despite maximal medical therapy and who require specialized interventions.	Patients who are frequently hospitalized for heart failure and cannot be safely discharged from the hospital, patients in the hospital awaiting heart transplant, patients at home receiving continuous IV support for symptom relief or being supported with a mechanical circulatory assist device, or patients in a hospice setting for the management of heart failure.

tests are essential, as is smoking cessation if the patient smokes. A yearly flu vaccination and periodic pneumococcal vaccine are needed.

Pharmacological Therapies. Pharmacological therapies to treat patients with heart failure include diuretics, ACE inhibitors, angiotensin II receptor blockers (ARBs), aldosterone antagonists, beta-1-adrenergic blockers, inotropics, synthetic natriuretic peptides, ivabradine, neprilysin/ARB inhibitors, nitrates, and arterial vasodilators.

Diuretics. Diuretics enhance water loss from the body by decreasing blood volume and sodium retention, also called diuresis. This occurs through the induction of changes at the nephrons of the kidney, which decrease reabsorption of sodium and water into the bloodstream. The main effect of diuretics in heart failure is a reduction in pulmonary interstitial fluid and peripheral edema. Loop diuretics, such as furosemide, torsemide, and bumetanide, are commonly used and can have a dramatic initial effect when administered by IV. Patients are often maintained on low doses of oral diuretics, such as thiazides, to manage heart failure.

CLINICAL CONCEPT

Electrolyte imbalances, particularly hypokalemia, are a common side effect of diuretic therapy. Hypokalemia can worsen heart function and increase the risk of cardiac dysrhythmias. If hypokalemia becomes a problem, patients can be given potassium supplements or placed on potassium-sparing diuretics.

Aldosterone Antagonists. Spironolactone is an aldosterone antagonist that inhibits sodium and water reabsorption at the nephron. It is also referred to as a potassium-sparing diuretic, as it inhibits excretion of potassium at the nephron. Potassium is conserved within the bloodstream, and thus a highly important potential side effect of a potassium-sparing diuretic is hyperkalemia, which increases the risk of cardiac arrest.

ALERT! With all diuretics, the clinician needs to periodically monitor the patient's serum electrolytes, particularly serum potassium.

ACE Inhibitors. Many experts consider ACE inhibitors, such as ramipril, captopril, and lisinopril, the cornerstone of heart failure treatment. These drugs inhibit ACE, which in turn blocks the conversion of angiotensin I to angiotensin II in the RAAS. Blocking the formation of angiotensin II is key in heart failure because angiotensin II causes detrimental effects in heart failure, such as peripheral vasoconstriction, adrenal secretion of aldosterone, and hypertrophy of the myocardium. Thus, ACE inhibitors decrease peripheral arterial vasoconstriction, which, in turn, lowers resistance against the left ventricle. ACE inhibitors also block adrenal gland secretion of aldosterone, which, in turn, diminishes sodium and water retention in the bloodstream and lowers blood volume. In addition, ACE inhibitors block left ventricular hypertrophy. ACE inhibitors lower blood volume, decrease blood pressure, and stop the cycling of the RAAS to ease the heart's work.

ARBs perform similar actions as ACE inhibitors. ARBs restrict angiotensin II from binding to receptors on end organs. This blocks stimulation of arterial vasoconstriction and stops adrenal release of aldosterone. Similar to ACE inhibitors, ARBs also limit cycling of the RAAS. ARBs are frequently used in patients who cannot tolerate ACE inhibitors.

ALERT! Adverse effects of ACE inhibitors include hyperkalemia, angioedema, and cough.

Beta-1-Adrenergic Blockers. Beta-1-adrenergic blockers, such as metoprolol, bisoprolol, atenolol, and carvedilol, inhibit the effects of the SNS on the heart and vasculature. In heart failure, baroreceptors sense low arterial pressure caused by the heart's low contractile force and, in turn, stimulate the SNS. The SNS increases HR and stimulates peripheral vasoconstriction, both of which are detrimental to the failing heart. Stimulation of a weakened heart to pump faster further strains the heart.

Peripheral vasoconstriction increases resistance against the left ventricle (afterload). Beta-1-adrenergic blockers inhibit these processes and therefore reduce strain on the weakened heart.

ALERT! Beta-1-adrenergic blockers are contraindicated in patients with bradycardia, AV block, and hypotension; they should be used with caution in patients with asthma and diabetes.

CLINICAL CONCEPT

When beta blockers are not effective in reducing sympathetically driven increased heart rate, an alternative drug, ivabradine, is recommended. Ivabradine, a cardiotonic drug, decreases heart rate by directly inhibiting the SA node. Ivabradine is indicated in patients with an ejection fraction of 35% or less, persistent heart failure symptoms, sinus rhythm, and an HR of 70 bpm or more.

Inotropic Agents. Inotropic agents increase the contractile force of the heart muscle. Increasing the force of contraction of the heart muscle is called a positive inotropic effect. Additionally, inotropic agents often have chronotropic effects on the heart. Chronotropic effects influence HR. The most commonly used inotropic drugs are digitalis (digoxin), dobutamine, dopamine, and milrinone.

Digitalis exerts positive inotropic and negative chronotropic effects on the heart; it is a cardiac glycoside that increases the force of contraction of the ventricular muscle, thereby increasing the strength of the heart as a pump. Concurrently, digitalis slows conduction through the AV node, thereby slowing HR.

Heart Failure

JVD

SVC

Pulmonary veins

Backed-up pressure

Ivabradine
Blocks SA node stimulation

Diuretics
Decrease fluid accumulation
(e.g., furosemide)

Lungs

Pulmonary edema

Pulmonary edema

LA

RA

LV

RV

Inotropic agents
Enhance contractility of ventricles
(e.g., digoxin)

IVC

Neprilysin inhibitor/ARB
Block enzyme that destroys
ANP and BNP
Also blocks angiotensin II receptor
(e.g., sacubitril/valsartan)

ANP

BNP

Diuretics
Decrease fluid
accumulation
(e.g., furosemide)

Venous congestion:
Ascites
Hepatomegaly
Splenomegaly
Ankle edema

**Arterial system
decreased circulation**

**Stimulates
baroreceptors**

Kidney

Beta-1 adrenergic blocker
Blocks sympathetic stimulation
(e.g., metoprolol)

Renin

**SNS increases
heart rate**

Liver

Angiotensinogen

Angiotensin I

ACE inhibitor
Inhibits angiotensin converting
enzyme, which decreases cycling
of RAAS
(e.g., lisinopril)

Ace

Angiotensin II

Angiotensin II receptor blocker
Decreases angiotensin II action,
blocks peripheral vasoconstriction,
blocks stimulation of adrenal
(e.g., losartan)

Aldosterone antagonist
Blocks sodium and water
reabsorption into the bloodstream,
blocks excretion of K^+
(e.g., spironolactone)

Peripheral
vasoconstriction

Adrenal gland

Aldosterone:
↑ Sodium, H_2O reabsortion
into blood, excretes K^+

Patho-Pharm Connection—cont'd

Heart failure causes many systemic complications. Pharmacological agents are used to counteract these adverse effects. The heart is weakened in heart failure, and to increase the contractility of the ventricular muscle, inotropic agents such as digoxin can be used. Dobutamine and dopamine are also inotropic agents.

When the heart pump fails, peripheral arterial circulation decreases and the peripheral baroreceptors in the arteries sense this drop in blood pressure. The baroreceptors stimulate the sympathetic nervous system, causing vasoconstriction of arteries and increased heart rate. Beta-adrenergic blockers are often used to counteract this sympathetic stimulation. Another agent that counteracts the increased heart rate is ivabradine. Ivabradine can be used to slow the heart rate.

Also, when the peripheral circulation decreases, the kidney senses this drop in blood pressure. This stimulates renin secretion by the kidney, which triggers the renin-angiotensin-aldosterone system (RAAS). Pharmacological agents are used to counteract the constant cycling of the RAAS. ACE inhibitors (ACEi) are commonly used and angiotensin II receptor blockers (ARBs) may be used. Aldosterone antagonists can also be used to counteract constant aldosterone secretion by the adrenal gland. Excess fluid volume builds up in the body as the heart fails, causing hypervolemia, systemic edema, and pulmonary edema. Loop diuretics are commonly used to counteract the hypervolemia and edema.

When the heart fails, the heart muscle releases B type natriuretic peptide (BNP) and atrial natriuretic peptide (ANP) as natural diuretics. Neprilysin is an enzyme that breaks down the natriuretic peptides. Neprilysin inhibitors are agents that allow ANP and BNP to remain in the circulation longer. A medication called sacubitril/valsartan that combines a neprilysin inhibitor and an ARB is used.

Digitalis is most effective in persons with atrial fibrillation and heart failure.

Digitalis should be considered for those who remain symptomatic despite therapy with all other disease-modifying agents. Although it works as a positive inotrope, it can stimulate dysrhythmias. Clinicians need to monitor digitalis levels carefully, as high levels increase morbidity and mortality, particularly in women, older individuals, and those with compromised renal function.

> **ALERT!** Before administering digitalis, the clinician should measure the apical pulse for 1 full minute. Digitalis can slow the HR excessively and is contraindicated in patients with bradycardia.

> **ALERT!** The clinician should carefully monitor the patient's serum potassium level because digitalis in conjunction with hypokalemia causes cardiac dysfunction and serious dysrhythmias.

Dopamine is a catecholamine that stimulates the heart's beta-1 receptors. It increases both the inotropic and chronotropic responses of the heart, which increases contractility and HR. In addition, dopamine stimulates alpha-adrenergic receptors of arteries, causing vasodilation. Dopamine preserves perfusion of the peripheral organs, particularly the kidneys, as it increases the contractile force and rate of the heart. Dopamine is a preferred inotropic agent in patients with renal dysfunction.

Dobutamine, a synthetic catecholamine that is also a positive inotropic and chronotropic agent that acts on the heart's beta-1 receptors, increases contractility of the heart and HR.

Milrinone, a phosphodiesterase inhibitor, also increases contractility of the heart muscle, although through a different mechanism. This drug increases calcium availability to the cardiac myocytes, which increases the muscle's overall force of contraction.

> **ALERT!** All inotropic drugs may have negative side effects and require careful monitoring of the heart because they can induce dysrhythmias and tachycardia and activate the RAAS.

Synthetic Natriuretics. BNP is a natural substance secreted by the endothelium in heart failure to induce diuresis of the body. It is also available as nesiritide, a form of medication that acts at the renal vasculature to induce diuresis. Nesiritide, which is able to act rapidly, can decrease both pulmonary congestion and edema in heart failure when administered by IV.

> **ALERT!** Certain ancillary drugs, such as ACE inhibitors, antihypertensives, nitroglycerin, and some diuretics, should not be used in conjunction with nesiritide. Severe hypotension can result from the additive effects of potent diuresis and vasodilation when these drugs are used together.

Neprilysin Inhibitors. Neprilysin is an enzyme that breaks down BNP and ANP, which are the body's natriuretics; it also breaks down angiotensin II. Neprilysin inhibitors block the breakdown of BNP and ANP, allowing these substances to perform prolonged natriuresis in the patient with heart failure. However, neprilysin inhibitors also prevent the breakdown of angiotensin II. This effect is not advantageous in heart failure, as it allows angiotensin II to trigger arterial vasoconstriction and stimulate aldosterone. To avoid this action, a combination of ARBs and neprilysin inhibitors is effective in reducing symptoms in patients with systolic dysfunction. In studies, the combination of sacubitril (a neprilysin inhibitor) and valsartan (an ARB medication) has shown reduced severity of heart failure symptoms, hospital admissions, and death due to heart failure. According to the results of the PARADIGM-HF study, sacubitril/valsartan should be used as a substitute for ACE inhibitors or ARBs in patients with systolic dysfunction who experience persistent symptoms.

Nitrates. Nitrates are arterial and venous vasodilators that enhance coronary circulation, reduce systemic arterial blood pressure, and lower venous return. All of these actions decrease the heart's workload. Commonly used nitrates for heart failure are nitroglycerin, isosorbide dinitrate, and nitroprusside. Through stimulation of NO, nitrates promote widespread arterial vasodilation. These drugs significantly lower arterial blood pressure and thus decrease resistance against the heart. Through venous dilation, they also lower venous pressure, which decreases the volume of blood entering the heart. In addition, nitrates directly stimulate dilation of the coronary arteries, which enhances delivery of oxygenated blood to the heart muscle. Nitrates have been found to be more effective than other drugs for heart failure in African Americans.

> **ALERT!** Nitrates can exert a detrimental hypotensive effect if combined with sildenafil-type medications for erectile dysfunction.

Arterial Vasodilators. Dilation of the arterial circulation decreases aortic pressure and the resistance against the left ventricle. Arterial vasodilators significantly reduce workload for the weakened heart in heart failure and lower blood pressure. These medications facilitate the weakened heart's ability to pump more efficiently against reduced afterload. Isosorbide dinitrate/hydralazine is a combination of a nitrate and direct vasodilator that is an option for patients who are intolerant of ACE inhibitors and ARBs due to renal disease. The African American Heart Failure Trial showed that isosorbide dinitrate/hydralazine therapy provided significant mortality benefit in African Americans patients with systolic dysfunction. Retrospective

scrutiny found that African American patients have a genetic polymorphism that influences which drugs are effective in heart failure. If isosorbide dinitrate/hydralazine is recommended, however, it requires doses three times a day, which may be a drawback for some patients.

Devices and Cardiac Transplantation

Cardiac Resynchronization Therapy. In heart failure, the right and left ventricles may differ in the timing of their contraction. This asynchronous ventricular wall motion can contribute to a weakened force of contraction of the heart. **Cardiac resynchronization therapy (CRT)**, also known as biventricular pacing, is a technique that places a specialized pacemaker in a region that activates both the left ventricular wall and septum of the heart. CRT can optimize the pumping function of the heart by coordinating impulse conduction through both ventricles, thereby synchronizing their contraction.

An implantable cardiac defibrillator (ICD) can also be used in conjunction with CRT to counteract life-threatening rhythm disturbances. ICDs can prevent ventricular fibrillation and also serve as a pacemaker in episodes of bradycardia. Any patient with reduced ejection fraction and symptomatic heart failure or ischemic cardiomyopathy whose life expectancy is more than 1 year may be eligible for possible device therapy.

Intra-aortic Balloon Pump. In patients with severe heart failure, an **intra-aortic balloon pump** may be used in conjunction with interventional cardiac procedures, such as percutaneous transluminal angioplasty (PCTA). PCTA uses a catheter to clear the lumens of obstructed coronary arteries. An intra-aortic balloon pump may be needed during PCTA in patients with inadequate ventricular function for such a procedure.

An intra-aortic balloon pump may also be used in patients with end-stage heart failure awaiting transplant. A balloon pump attached to a cardiac catheter is inserted via a peripheral site into the thoracic aorta. The balloon is inflated during diastole, thus increasing aortic pressure during diastole and increasing coronary blood flow. The balloon is deflated before and during early left ventricular ejection, thus reducing aortic pressure and afterload.

Left Ventricular Assist Device. A **left ventricular assist device (LVAD)**, which has a pump that enhances the left ventricle's ejection of blood, can be used as temporary treatment until cardiac transplantation can occur, or can be used as treatment for end-stage heart failure. All LVADs consist of an inflow cannula that takes blood from the apex of the heart in the left ventricle, allows the blood to enter the LVAD pump, and then, using the pump, pushes blood through an outflow cannula in the aorta, right above the aortic valve, and out through the body (see Fig. 17-25).

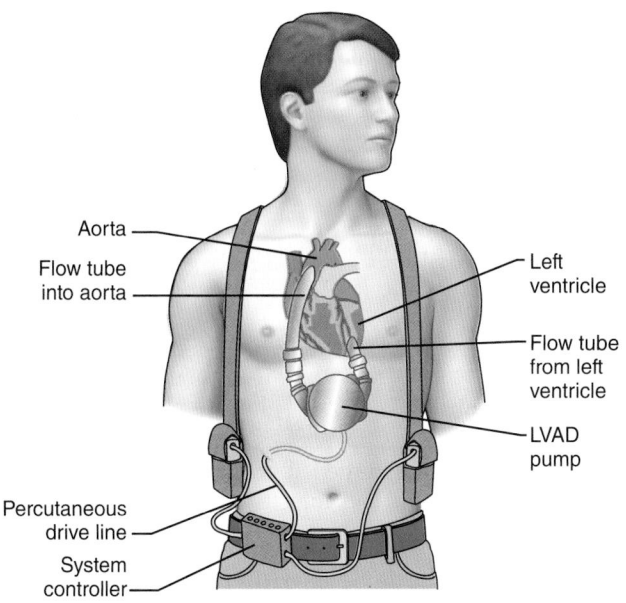

FIGURE 17-25. The left ventricular assist device (LVAD).

Labels: Aorta; Flow tube into aorta; Left ventricle; Flow tube from left ventricle; LVAD pump; Percutaneous drive line; System controller

The 2-year survival rate in patients given LVAD until transplantation occurs is 78%. In patients who opt to have the LVAD as end-stage treatment without transplant, the 2-year survival rate is 62%.

Cardiac Transplantation. It is estimated that 5% of patients with heart failure have end-stage (stage D) heart failure, carrying 1- and 5-year mortality rates of 28% and 80%, respectively. These patients may be candidates for cardiac transplantation. Eligibility for this surgical procedure is based on the age of the patient and the absence of comorbidities, such as peripheral or cerebrovascular disease, obesity, diabetes, or cancer. The United Network of Organ Sharing is a private organization under contract with the federal government that matches donors with heart transplant recipients. Allocation of donor hearts is decided by the network according to a set of conditions and priorities. A match of blood and tissue type, compatibility of gross body size between donor and recipient, and therapeutic immunosuppression of the recipient are some of the prerequisite conditions for heart transplant.

The International Society for Heart and Heart-Lung Transplantation monitors the survival of heart transplant patients. Over 90% of patients in the registry return to normal and unrestricted function following transplantation. About 67% of patients survive longer than 3 years. The average post-transplant survival time has been 9.3 years.

Chapter Summary

- The lifetime risk of developing heart failure is approximately 20% for all patients older than 40 years.
- Many individuals are surviving episodes of acute ischemic heart disease; eventually, the damage endured by these insults is demonstrated as chronic heart failure.
- Chronic heart failure is often the result of long-standing HTN, multiple MIs, or long-term diabetes mellitus.
- Heart failure can be categorized as LVF or RVF; it can also be categorized as systolic dysfunction versus diastolic dysfunction.
- Systolic dysfunction is also referred to as HFrEF; diastolic dysfunction is also referred to as HFpEF.
- LVF mainly causes pulmonary symptomatology: dyspnea on exertion, cough, orthopnea, PND, cyanosis, and crackles on auscultation.
- LVF can cause pulmonary edema, which can be exhibited by pink, frothy sputum, and loud, coarse crackles.
- In LVF, the RAAS is constantly stimulated, which increases blood volume, blood pressure, and left ventricular resistance; these compensatory mechanisms place more strain on the weak heart.
- Sympathetic stimulation occurs in LVF, which causes increased HR and further strain on the weak heart.

- When there is a question as to whether dyspnea is caused by a pulmonary origin or cardiovascular origin, the BNP diagnostic test is used.
- In RVF, symptoms are mainly caused by venous congestion in the body.
- The classic signs of RVF are JVD, ascites, hepatomegaly, splenomegaly, and ankle or sacral edema.
- An S_3 gallop rhythm is common in heart failure.
- A Swan–Ganz catheter is used to monitor the patient's cardiovascular hemodynamic measurements in cases of severe heart failure.
- Preload is the volume of blood that is returning to the heart—the right atrial volume.
- Afterload is the amount of resistance against the ventricle—commonly the aortic pressure.
- In LVF, LVEF is decreased and PCWP is increased.
- An LVEF of lower than 40% constitutes heart failure.
- Management of heart failure requires lifestyle modifications and pharmacological interventions. If heart failure is severe, interventional cardiovascular procedures are available.
- Some common agents used in heart failure include ACE inhibitors, beta blockers, diuretics, nitrates, vasodilators,

ivabradine, neprilysin inhibitors, digitalis, and the aldosterone antagonist spironolactone.

- An intra-aortic balloon pump may be used in patients with end-stage heart failure awaiting transplant.

- ICDs can prevent fatal cardiac dysrhythmias.

- The LVAD is a device that can sustain a person in end-stage heart failure until cardiac transplantation or can be used as a terminal treatment modality.

Making the Connections

Pathophysiology

Signs and Symptoms	Physical Assessment Findings	Diagnostic Testing	Treatment
LVF (backward effects)	Weak left ventricle causes a backup of hydrostatic pressure in the left atrium, pulmonary veins, and pulmonary capillaries. Hydrostatic pressure increases in lungs. Fluid builds in pulmonary interstitium, often to the point of pulmonary edema.		
Cough (cough with pink, frothy sputum equals pulmonary edema). Dyspnea. Orthopnea. PND.	Pulmonary bibasilar crackles (widespread pulmonary coarse, loud crackles equals pulmonary edema). Cyanosis. S_3 or S_4 audible through stethoscope.	Pulmonary congestion on chest x-ray (Kerley A and B lines) caused by pulmonary interstitial fluid. Cardiomegaly on chest x-ray caused by enlarged, dilated ventricles. Elevated BNP caused by elevated water volume in bloodstream. Elevated PCWP caused by backup of hydrostatic pressure.	Fowler's position to ease breathing. Oxygen for hypoxia caused by pulmonary edema. Low-sodium diet (<1,500 mg/day) to decrease water retention. Fluid restriction. Daily weight measurement to monitor water weight gain. Diuretics. Aldosterone antagonists. Beta-1-adrenregic blockers. Ivabradine. ACE inhibitors. Angiotensin II receptor blockers. Neprilysin inhibitor/ARD combination drug. Nitrates. Isosorbide dinitrate/ hydralazine. Digitalis or another inotropic drug.
LVF (forward effects)	Weak left ventricle forward pumping of blood into the aorta, peripheral, and cerebral arteries. Kidneys sense low circulation caused by weak forward pump of heart. Kidneys release renin. RAAS is triggered. Blood volume increases, blood pressure increases. Peripheral vasoconstriction occurs. The SNS is triggered by baroreceptors in the arterial walls caused by decreased blood pressure. SNS causes increased HR and vasoconstriction of peripheral arteries. These compensatory mechanisms worsen LVF.		
Cool, pale extremities. Confusion, disorientation. Edema. Nocturia.	Decreased peripheral pulses. Cool, pale extremities. Confusion, disorientation. S_3 or S_4 audible through stethoscope.	Decreased LVEF. HR may be high. Pulses weak.	Fowler's position. Oxygen. Diuretics. Low-sodium diet (<1,500 mg/day). Fluid restriction. Daily weight. ACE inhibitors or ARBs. Nitrates. Inotropic agents. Beta-adrenergic blockers.

Making the Connections–cont'd

Signs and Symptoms	Physical Assessment Findings	Diagnostic Testing	Treatment
RVF (backward effects) | Weak right ventricle causes backup of hydrostatic pressure into the right atrium, superior vena cava, and jugular veins, then into inferior vena cava, causing venous congestion in gastrointestinal, peritoneal, hepatic, and splenic veins.			
Jugular neck vein distention. Swelling (rings, shoes may feel tight). Anorexia, indigestion. Abdominal swelling.	JVD. Weight gain. Ascites. Hepatojugular reflux. Hepatomegaly. Splenomegaly. Ankle or sacral edema. Ascites; shifting dullness on abdominal examination. S_3 or S_4.	Elevated jugular venous pressure. Elevated central venous pressure. Dilutional hyponatremia. Hypokalemia.	Daily weight measurement. Low-sodium diet. Fluid restriction. Inotropic agents. Diuretics. Nitrates. ACE inhibitors and ARBs.

Bibliography

Available online at fadavis.com

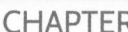
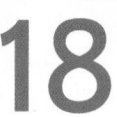
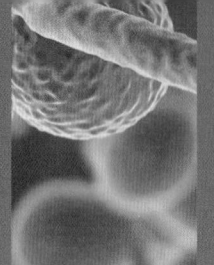

Valvular Heart Disease

Learning Objectives

Upon completion of this chapter, the student will be able to:

- Describe the normal blood flow through the heart and how valves open and close in relation to heart sounds.

- Recognize common types of valvular heart disorders and the etiologies of each disorder.

- Identify common signs, symptoms, and clinical manifestations of heart valve disorders.

- Recognize assessment techniques and common laboratory tests used to diagnose valvular disorders.

- Discuss various pharmacological and surgical modalities used to treat heart valve disorders.

- Explain preventive measures needed after valvular repair or prosthetic valve implantation.

Key Terms

Aortic sclerosis

Aortic stenosis

Aortic insufficiency (regurgitation)

Balloon valvotomy

Bioprosthetic valve

Bruit

Chordae tendineae

Doppler echocardiography

Echocardiography

Heart murmur

Hypertrophic cardiomyopathy (HCM)

Mechanical prosthetic valve

Mitral annular calcification (MAC)

Mitral insufficiency (mitral regurgitation)

Mitral stenosis

Mitral valve prolapse (MVP)

Papillary muscles

Percutaneous balloon valvuloplasty

Regurgitant

Rheumatic fever (RF)

Rheumatic heart disease (RHD)

S_3 gallop

Stenosis

Surgical valvular replacement

Thrill

Transcatheter valvular replacement (transcatheter valvular implantation)

Transesophageal echocardiography (TEE)

Transthoracic echocardiography (TTE)

Valve stress echocardiography

Valvotomy

The heart valves, made of specialized cardiac tissue, direct the flow of blood through the heart's chambers. They consist of thin leaflets of endothelium-covered, fibrous tissue that open and close in synchrony with the heart's contractions.

The heart valves can sustain injury that deforms their structure; this, in turn, can disrupt blood flow through the heart, alter chamber pressures, increase workload, incite thrombus formation or infection, and diminish the heart's pumping ability. Most valve disorders create turbulent blood flow that can be detected by auscultation as a heart murmur. **Echocardiography** is the gold standard for diagnosis of valve dysfunction.

Valvular heart disease can result from a number of disorders, including congenital defects, myocardial infarction (MI), trauma, infection, and inflammatory conditions. Valvular dysfunction can vary in degree from mild and asymptomatic to severe and rapidly fatal. Clinical consequences depend on the severity of valve impairment, rate of development of the dysfunction, and the heart's ability to compensate for

the impairment. Heart failure is a common result of untreated valvular disease.

Regardless of etiology, valvular disorders can be surgically repaired or replaced with mechanical or tissue-derived prosthetic valves. Because valvular disorders can cause turbulent or stagnant blood flow within the heart, prevention of clot formation is a key treatment modality. Also, because deformed or prosthetic valves can act as a site for infection, patients require prophylactic antibiotics before any invasive procedure.

Epidemiology

Acquired diseases of the aortic and mitral valves are the most common cause of morbidity and mortality among valvular heart diseases. The prevalence of valvular heart disease increases significantly with age. Valvular heart disease is estimated to affect up to 13% of adults older than age 75. Aortic stenosis (AS) is increasing in incidence due to the aging of the population. Calcification of the aortic valve, associated with atherosclerosis, is commonly the cause of aortic stenosis. This condition is termed aortic sclerosis.

Mitral insufficiency (also called mitral regurgitation) is the most common form of valvular heart disease in the United States. Mitral insufficiency is a common complication of acute myocardial infarction; it is also associated with atherosclerosis.

In the past, one of the major causes of heart valve disorders was **rheumatic fever (RF)**. It would begin as an acute streptococcal throat infection and eventually lead to **rheumatic heart disease (RHD)**, an inflammatory condition of the heart and heart valves. The heart's involvement was often silent in the acute phase of the disease, although heart valve deformities became obvious later in life. Commonly, there is a lengthy asymptomatic period of 30 to 40 years from onset of RF to the development of cardiac valve problems. With the widespread use of antibiotics, prevalence of RHD in the United States has declined, and the incidence is 1 in 100,000 persons. However, the prevalence of RHD remains high in underdeveloped nations. In India, for example, the prevalence is approximately 100 to 150 cases per 100,000, and in Africa the prevalence is 35 cases per 100,000.

Most valvular disorders in the United States and in developed nations are caused by congenital heart disease, myocardial infarction (MI), arteriosclerosis, and aging. Valvular abnormalities caused by congenital heart disease can remain silent and asymptomatic until adulthood. One of the most common congenital valvular diseases is a bicuspid aortic valve. Mitral insufficiency is common because it is often caused by MI. Infarction of the left ventricle often involves papillary muscle rupture, which causes a dysfunctional mitral valve. Up to 20% of individuals who suffer MI also endure the complication of mitral insufficiency. **Mitral valve prolapse (MVP)**, a type of mitral insufficiency, is diagnosed in 4% of the population but has been found to be asymptomatic in as many as 20% of the population. Myxomatous degenerative changes of the mitral valve leaflets often cause MVP; however, the etiology is unknown. Most persons with MVP are asymptomatic for their entire lives.

The incidence of infective endocarditis has also increased in the U.S. population and led to cases of valvular disease. This is due to widespread prevalence of vascular grafts and intracardiac devices, the emergence of more virulent multidrug-resistant microorganisms, the growing epidemic of diabetes mellitus, and the opioid crisis.

CLINICAL CONCEPT

Because of the expanding population of older adults, mitral and aortic valvular disorders are among the most common type of cardiac disorders encountered in the clinical area.

Basic Concepts of Cardiac Valve Function

The four chambers of the heart are separated from one another by atrioventricular valves. The tricuspid valve, located between the right atrium and right ventricle, is constructed of three valve leaflets. The mitral valve, between the left atrium and left ventricle, has two leaflets. The pulmonary artery and aorta each have a semilunar valve at their entry; the term *semilunar* describes their half-moon shape (see Fig. 18-1).

Anatomy and Function of Cardiac Valves

To understand valvular heart disease, a thorough knowledge of the anatomy and function of the heart's four valves is necessary. The mitral and tricuspid valves, located between the atria and ventricles, are attached to the myocardium via support structures called chordae tendineae and papillary muscles. **Chordae tendineae** are stringlike membranes that are tethered to the leaflets of the valve and anchored to tiny muscular projections of the myocardium, called **papillary muscles**. Damage to the chordae tendineae or papillary muscles can cause valvular instability.

During diastole, the ventricles fill with blood from the atria and pressure builds within the ventricular chamber. The increased pressure and enlargement of the ventricle causes tension in the ventricular wall and papillary muscles. As the tension builds in the ventricular wall, the chordae tendineae become taut and pull downward on the atrioventricular valve leaflets, keeping the valves closed. During systole, the mitral and tricuspid valves must remain closed despite the high pressure exerted by the contracting left and

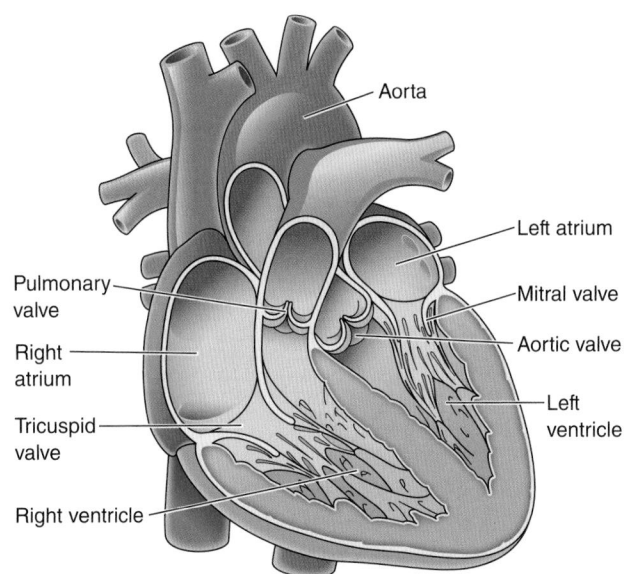

FIGURE 18-1. Heart anatomy showing the mitral, tricuspid, aortic, and pulmonic valves. In the diagram, the mitral and tricuspid valves are open; the aortic and pulmonic valves are closed.

right ventricles as they push blood into the aorta and pulmonary artery (see Fig. 18-2).

The open aortic valve allows blood to flow from the left ventricle into the aorta during systole, whereas the open pulmonic valve allows blood flow from the right ventricle into the pulmonary artery during systole. During diastole, the mitral and tricuspid valves open to allow blood to flow from the atria into the ventricles; the aortic and pulmonic valves must be closed for optimal ventricular chamber filling (see Fig. 18-3).

First and Second Heart Sounds

The first heart sound (S_1) and the second heart sound (S_2) are vibrations transmitted through the chest wall that are caused by the closure of the heart valves. They are sometimes referred to as sounding audibly as "lub-dub." Closure of the mitral and tricuspid valves transmit S_1, whereas closure of the aortic and pulmonic valves transmit S_2.

During systole, as the ventricles contract, the mitral and tricuspid valves close, creating S_1. During systole, the aortic and pulmonic valves are open, allowing blood to flow into the respective vessels through their openings. When normal valves are open, the blood flow through them usually does not transmit a sound. Only valve closure should cause the heart sounds. During diastole, as the ventricles fill with blood from the atria, the aortic and pulmonic valves close, creating S_2.

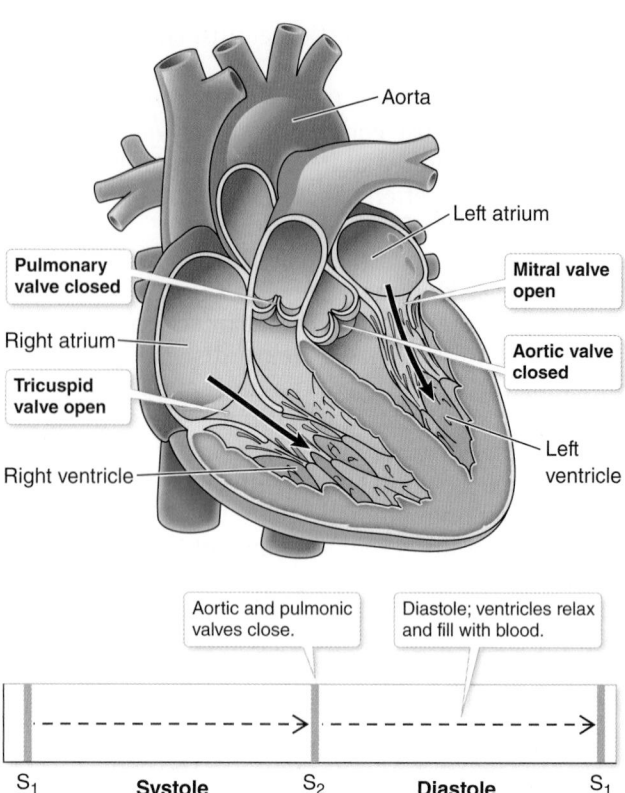

FIGURE 18-3. Normal valvular actions during diastole when the ventricles relax and fill with blood. When the ventricles relax, the aortic and pulmonic valves close; this causes the second heart sound (S_2). Blood can flow from atria to ventricles through open mitral and tricuspid valves.

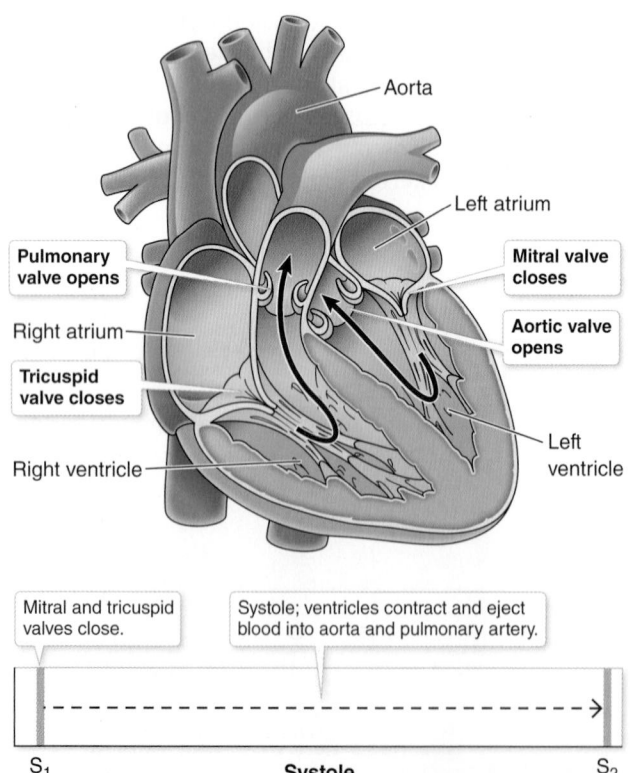

FIGURE 18-2. Normal valvular actions during systole when the ventricles contract. When the ventricles contract, the mitral and tricuspid valves close; this causes the first heart sound (S_1). Blood is then ejected from the ventricles into the open aortic and pulmonic valves.

Frequently, a split of the S_2 sound can be heard, created by the initial closure of the aortic valve and later closure of the pulmonic valve. This is a normal phenomenon often heard with deep inspiration and is referred to as an audible A_2 and P_2—a split S_2. A_2 refers to the aortic closure, and P_2 refers to the pulmonic valve closure. The split of S_2 occurs because, with deep inspiration, there is thoracic cage expansion that allows widening of the pulmonary arterial vessels. The widened arterial diameters enhance the capacity of the pulmonary artery, and an increased amount of blood can be accepted by the expanded vessel. The increased capacitance of the pulmonary artery allows more blood to enter from the right ventricle, and this prolongs the right ventricle's ejection time. Consequently, there is a slight delay in the pulmonic artery valve closure, causing the split of S_2, with the aorta closing first and the pulmonary valve closing later.

Third Heart Sound

At times during diastole, as blood flows rapidly from the atria into the ventricles, the vibrations of the blood flow against the ventricular wall can be heard as a third heart sound (S_3) (see Fig. 18-4). This can be a normal sound in children and young adults, but in older adults it can indicate decreased ventricular muscle elasticity; in this age group, S_3 is often called an **S_3 gallop** and may be present in heart failure.

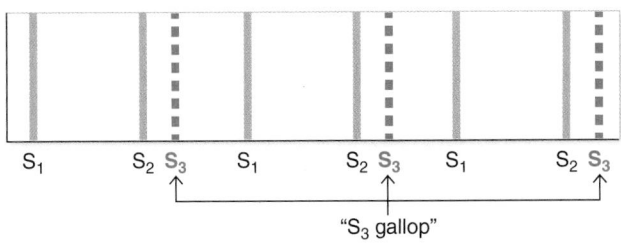

FIGURE 18-4. S_3 is a sound heard during diastole because of filling of the ventricle with a high amount of blood flow. This is commonly caused by heart failure. S_3 is heard after S_2 (closure of the aortic and pulmonic valves) and before S_1 (closure of the mitral and tricuspid valves). It is often referred to as an "S_3 gallop."

Fourth Heart Sound

Finally, although not usually heard in healthy individuals, atrial contraction may be auscultated as a fourth heart sound (S_4). At the end of diastole, the atria contract to eject an extra volume of blood into the ventricle; this is known as the atrial kick. This late diastolic phase immediately precedes systole and therefore occurs slightly before S_1.

An S_4 commonly occurs when the left atrium contracts against a noncompliant, stiff left ventricle. It is a low-pitched sound, best heard with the bell piece of the stethoscope. S_4 is associated with hypertension, because long-term hypertension causes left ventricular hypertrophy that creates a noncompliant, stiff left ventricle (see Fig. 18-5).

> ### ⊗ CLINICAL CONCEPT
>
> An S_3 sound is commonly heard in heart failure. An S_4 sound may be heard in left ventricular hypertrophy (LVH) due to hypertension.

Cardiac Valve Auscultation

There are anatomical sites on the chest where auscultation of the sounds created by a specific valve can be heard best. The mitral valve is best heard at the apex of the heart at the fifth intercostal space, midclavicular line. The tricuspid valve is heard best at the left sternal border, fourth intercostal space. The pulmonic valve is best heard at the base of the heart, at the second intercostal space, left sternal border; and the aortic valve, at the second intercostal space, right sternal border (see Fig. 18-6).

Basic Pathophysiological Concepts of Heart Valve Dysfunction

Heart murmurs are sounds transmitted through the chest wall heard with a stethoscope caused by turbulent blood flow through the heart or great vessels. Most commonly, they are caused by heart valve deformity, valve dysfunction, or defects in the heart wall.

Types of Heart Murmurs

There are two types of heart murmurs: pathological and physiological murmurs. Physiological heart murmurs, sometimes called innocent or functional heart murmurs, may be heard in states of high blood flow within the heart. Anxiety, stress, fever, anemia, overactive thyroid, and pregnancy will cause physiological murmurs. These heart murmurs are usually faint, intermittent, occur in a small area of the chest, and usually do not cause symptoms.

Pathological heart murmurs are sounds caused by abnormalities of the heart that include valvular deformities, valvular dysfunction, and heart wall defects. Cardiac valve problems commonly cause deleterious hemodynamic consequences such as heart failure. They also cause symptoms such as shortness of breath, dizziness, chest pains, or palpitations. Pathological heart murmurs usually require medical intervention to prevent complications, whereas physiological murmurs do not.

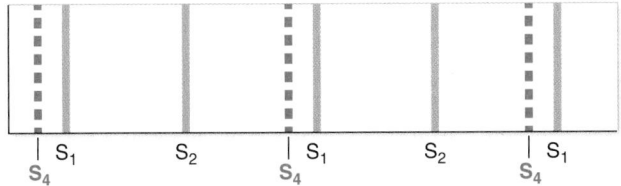

FIGURE 18-5. S_4 is an echo heard because of atrial contraction against a noncompliant, stiff left ventricle. This often occurs in left ventricular hypertrophy (LVH) created by long-term hypertension. S_4 is heard just before S_1.

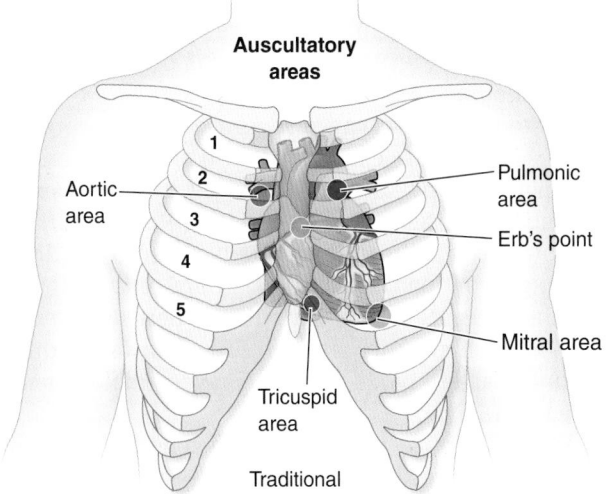

FIGURE 18-6. Cardiac auscultation sites where heart valves are heard best. Aortic valve: second intercostal space, right sternal border. Pulmonic valve: second intercostal space, left sternal border. Erb's point: third intercostal space, left sternal border. Tricuspid valve: fourth or fifth intercostal space, left sternal border. Mitral valve: fifth intercostal space, left midclavicular line.

Types of Valvular Dysfunction

Two major types of valvular dysfunction cause pathological heart murmurs. A valve may be narrowed, in which case it does not allow blood to flow freely across it. This abnormality is called **stenosis**, which is caused by a narrow valve orifice or a valve that does not open completely. The other type of valvular deformity is a **regurgitant**, or incompetent, valve. In this valvular abnormality, the valve does not close properly, which allows leakage of blood across it, a condition referred to as a valvular insufficiency.

 CLINICAL CONCEPT

Heart valves can cause heart murmurs due to stenosis (narrowing) or regurgitation (incomplete closure).

Hemodynamic Changes Caused by Valvular Dysfunction

Blood flow across a stenotic valve meets high resistance, which causes turbulent blood flow, less efficient movement of blood from one chamber to the other, and excess volume left behind. Blood is forced through a small space, which creates a heart murmur audible with the stethoscope. For example, in mitral stenosis, blood from the left atrium meets resistance when flowing through the narrowed mitral valve into the left ventricle. Blood flow through the stenotic valve is turbulent, and a diminished, limited volume moves from the left atrium into the left ventricle. As a result, the left ventricle has an inadequate volume of blood to eject forward and an excess volume of blood left behind. The volume left behind backs up and accumulates in the left atrium. The left atrium eventually is stretched and enlarged because of the greater amount of blood it has to accommodate.

A stenotic valve can also cause excess workload for the heart muscle, as in the case of aortic stenosis. When the aortic valve is narrowed, the left ventricle must push against high resistance created by the narrow aortic orifice to eject its blood into the aorta. The high workload causes hypertrophy of the left ventricular muscle. Left ventricular hypertrophy eventually leads to other problems, such as inadequate coronary artery blood flow and myocardial ischemia (see Fig. 18-7).

When there is valvular insufficiency, a different kind of turbulent blood flow occurs. A valve that does not make a firm seal will allow leakage of blood from one chamber to another. This occurs in regurgitant valves. For example, in mitral insufficiency, after the mitral valve closes and the left ventricle contracts during systole, the mitral valve leaflets do not close tightly. As the pressure builds within the left ventricle

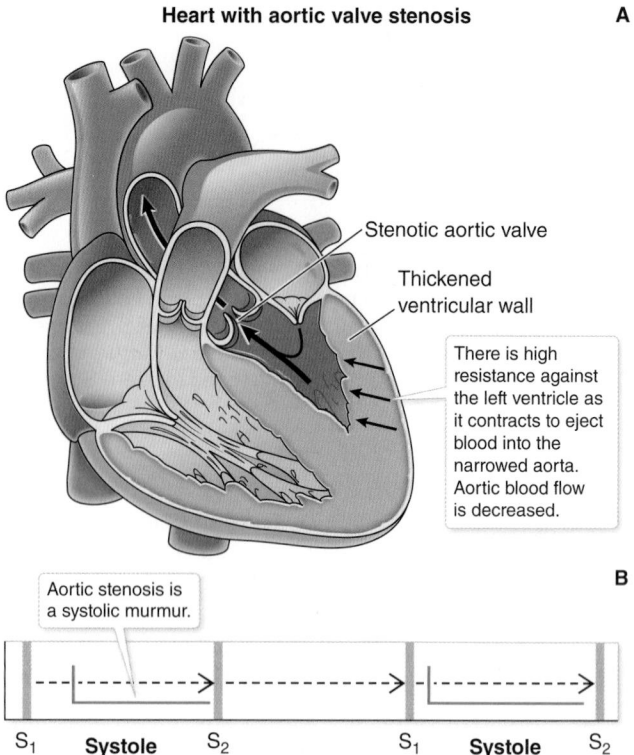

Heart with aortic valve stenosis **A**

Stenotic aortic valve

Thickened ventricular wall

There is high resistance against the left ventricle as it contracts to eject blood into the narrowed aorta. Aortic blood flow is decreased.

B

Aortic stenosis is a systolic murmur.

S_1 **Systole** S_2 S_1 **Systole** S_2

FIGURE 18-7. Aortic stenosis. (A) Aortic stenosis is narrowing of the aortic valve. Because of the narrowed valve, there is increased resistance against the left ventricle. The result is left ventricular hypertrophy and decreased aortic blood flow. (B) When blood flows into the narrowed aorta, there is a turbulent sound (heart murmur) heard through the stethoscope that occurs after S_1 systole. The murmur can be early, mid-, late, or holosystolic.

during systolic contraction, the mitral leaflets are pushed apart and blood regurgitates upward into the left atrium. This causes pressure changes within the left atrium and ventricle. Because some blood flows up into the left atrium, the left ventricle has less blood volume to eject into the aorta. Also, because of the loose valve leaflets, the left atrium collects and must accommodate extra accumulated blood volume. The extra blood volume causes dilation and stretching of the left atrium, which leads to stasis of blood and thrombus formation. Also, decreased blood flow ejected into the aorta causes less filling of the coronary arteries, which eventually causes ischemia of the myocardium (see Fig. 18-8).

Common Pathological Consequences of Valve Dysfunction

Heart valve deformities can lead to pressure changes within heart chambers, changes in blood fluidity, and disruption of cardiac function. Dysrhythmias, myocardial ischemia, stroke, and heart failure are consequences of valvular deformity. When valvular deformity causes distention and enlargement of a heart chamber, such as the right atrium, the conduction system is stretched and disrupted, causing dysrhythmia. Blood flow in the stretched atrium becomes nonlaminar, turbulent, and

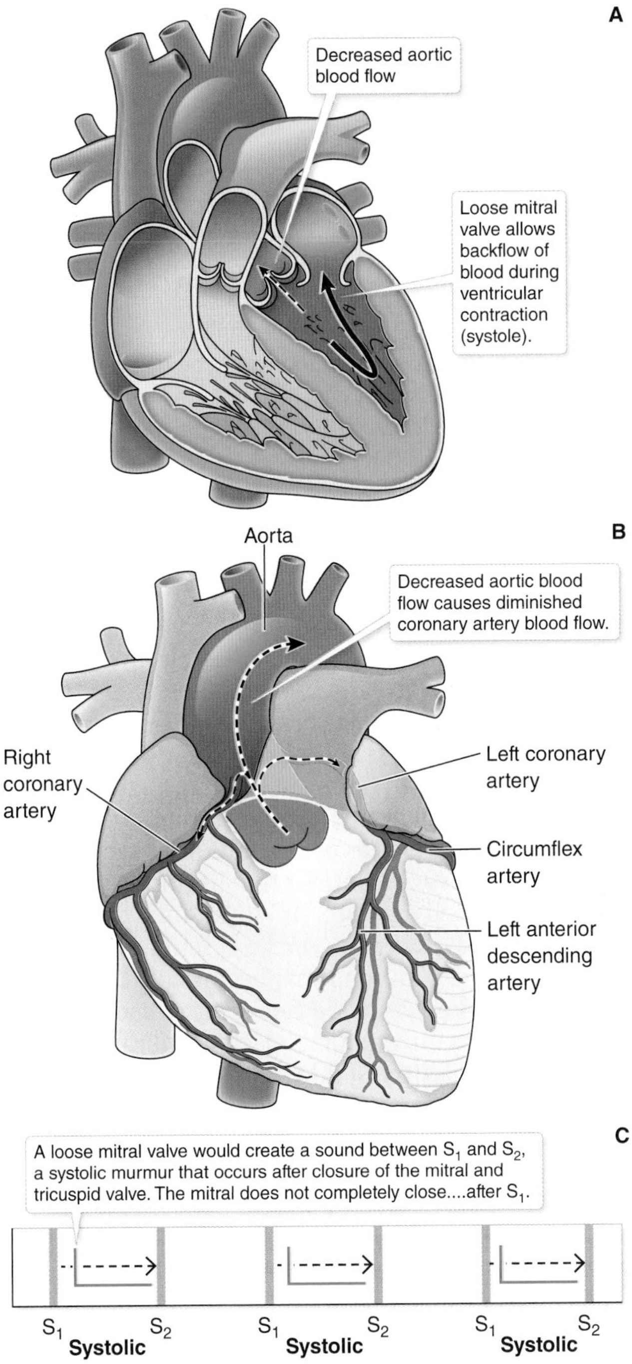

FIGURE 18-8. (A) Mitral insufficiency. In mitral insufficiency, the mitral valve leaflets are loose and allow blood to back up into the left atrium when the left ventricle contracts during systole. During systole, the blood flow into the aorta is decreased because some of the blood is flowing up into the left atrium. (B) Because the aorta has diminished blood flow, the coronary arteries, which come off the aorta, suffer from lack of blood flow. (C) The murmur of mitral insufficiency occurs after S$_1$ during systole as the left ventricle contracts, some blood regurgitates up through the loose mitral valve.

static—all conditions that predispose to thrombus formation. Thrombi travel in the bloodstream, where they become emboli. Once a thromboembolism is formed, it can lodge within a small-diameter vessel and cause obstruction and tissue ischemia anywhere in the body. A thromboembolism can lodge in the pulmonary arterial

vasculature or cerebral arteries, both of which are potentially fatal conditions.

Valvular stenosis can lead to MI and heart failure because it often causes hypertrophy of the myocardium, which leads to ischemia and eventual infarction. An example of this disorder occurs in pulmonic stenosis, where the right ventricle has to push its blood volume through the resistance of the narrow pulmonic valve. With time, right ventricular hypertrophy occurs, which eventually suffers inadequate coronary artery supply. This leads to ischemia, infarction, and right ventricular failure. Furthermore, there is a backup of blood from the failing right ventricle into the right atrium and venous vessels; the venous congestion causes all the classic signs of right ventricular failure.

Assessment of Cardiac Valve Dysfunction

Valvular dysfunction often occurs in patients who are unaware of a heart problem. A clinician often detects a heart murmur as an incidental finding on a physical examination. Alternatively, patients may present to a health-care provider because of symptoms of dizziness, chest pain, syncope, or heart failure. It may be these symptoms that lead to the diagnosis.

History

Rheumatic fever (RF) is a major risk factor for heart valve disorders. Acute RF can be a sequela of a previous group A beta hemolytic streptococcal infection of the upper respiratory tract called "strep throat." A small minority of those with untreated strep throat develop RF, which can progress to rheumatic heart disease (RHD). Although RF is a childhood disease, RHD does not become evident until adulthood. It usually becomes apparent as a heart murmur diagnosed as an incidental finding during a physical examination. Older adults who had undiagnosed or untreated RF as children may be suffering valvular dysfunction caused by RHD. However, widespread antibiotic use has decreased the incidence of valvular dysfunction caused by RF.

MI, particularly of the inferior wall, is a common cause of valvular dysfunction. In an inferior wall MI, the papillary muscles and chordae tendineae are commonly ruptured, which detaches the valve leaflets from their fixed position on the myocardial wall. The mitral valve leaflets become loose and do not close tightly, which allows backflow of blood into the left atrium.

Myxomatous degeneration of the mitral valve leaflets is another common cause of an incompetent mitral valve. Mitral insufficiency and mitral valve prolapse (MVP) occur in this manner. There is a genetic component to this disorder, and most individuals affected are unaware of the murmur until adulthood. There is a female predominance of MVP.

Arteriosclerotic calcification of heart valves caused by aging is also common. A disorder called **aortic sclerosis**, caused by a narrowed, calcified aortic valve, often presents as a new heart murmur in an older adult.

Signs and Symptoms

Patients with valvular disorders commonly become symptomatic upon physical exertion. Dyspnea, excessive fatigue, exercise intolerance, and syncope (fainting) are common symptoms. Severe valvular disorders can cause palpitations and symptoms of heart failure, such as cough, edema, ascites, orthopnea, or paroxysmal nocturnal dyspnea.

Physical Assessment

Heart murmurs should be carefully assessed and fully described to assist in identifying the cause. The clinician should begin with careful inspection of the anterior chest to look for the apical impulse. Palpation of the anterior chest can confirm the characteristics of the apical impulse and detect cardiac thrills, which are vibrations transmitted through the chest wall from turbulent blood flow. Percussion is usually not performed on the chest wall to detect murmurs. Auscultation, however, is the most valuable clinical assessment technique. The clinician can auscultate from the base of the heart to the apex or vice versa.

Both the diaphragm and the bell of the stethoscope are useful when assessing heart murmurs. The diaphragm best detects high-pitched sounds, whereas the bell is more sensitive to low-pitched sounds. The clinician should listen to the heart with the patient in the supine or seated position and inch the stethoscope carefully across the chest, listening for S_1, S_2, and any extra sound at every location. Throughout the examination, the clinician should decipher systole and diastole according to S_1 and S_2.

Auscultation at the anatomical sites of the valves on the chest is most important. However, heart murmurs can cause echoes and may radiate toward different areas, and these anatomical sites may not reflect the actual valvular origin of the murmur. In addition, the anatomical valve sites on the chest wall are inaccurate in individuals with an enlarged heart, heart anomalies, or dextrocardia.

Clinical Description of a Heart Murmur

To fully assess a heart murmur, the clinician needs to describe the following characteristics:

- **Grade (based on volume):** A heart murmur is subjectively graded according to its volume by the examiner. A murmur can be grade 1, where it is faintly audible with the stethoscope, to grade 6, where it is so loud it can be heard with the stethoscope off the surface of the chest (see Box 18-1).

BOX 18-1. Heart Murmur Grading

Heart murmurs are graded on a 6-point scale as follows:
- *Grade 1:* Very faint, heard only after listener has "tuned in"; may not be heard in all positions.
- *Grade 2:* Quiet, but heard immediately after placing the stethoscope on the chest.
- *Grade 3:* Moderately loud.
- *Grade 4:* Loud with a palpable thrill.
- *Grade 5:* Very loud, with thrill. May be heard when stethoscope is partly off the chest wall.
- *Grade 6:* Very loud, with thrill. May be heard with stethoscope off the chest wall.

- **Timing:** To describe the timing, the clinician must ascertain where the murmur occurs in relation to S_1 and S_2 to determine whether the murmur occurs in systole or diastole. Systolic murmurs can be early, late, or holosystolic. A murmur that begins after S_1 fades and stops before a clear S_2 is heard may be early systolic or midsystolic in timing. A murmur that begins simultaneously with S_1 and ends on S_2 without a gap is described as pansystolic or holosystolic (see Fig. 18-9). A murmur that begins shortly before S_2 and ends at S_2 is late systolic in timing.

  Similarly, murmurs can be described in terms of diastole. A murmur that begins at S_2 and fades before S_1 is heard can be described as early diastolic in timing. A middiastolic murmur starts a short time after S_2 is heard and fades before S_1. A late diastolic murmur starts after S_2 is clearly heard and continues up to S_1.

- **Location of maximal intensity:** The clinician should listen to all areas of the chest with the stethoscope to determine the location of maximal intensity of the heart murmur.

- **Radiation:** The clinician should listen around the area of maximal intensity to determine whether the murmur radiates to other regions, such as into the carotid arteries or into the axillary region.

- **Pitch:** The murmur's pitch should be described as high, medium, or low. A low-pitched sound is best heard with the bell piece of the stethoscope, whereas other sounds are heard well with the diaphragm.

- **Quality:** The quality of a murmur can be characterized as harsh, rough, blowing, rumbling, or musical.

- **Shape:** The shape of a murmur can be characterized as crescendo, which becomes louder in intensity over time; decrescendo, which becomes softer over time; or a steady plateau, which is unchanging in intensity (see Fig. 18-10).

A murmur may be accompanied by a **thrill**, which is a humming vibration over an area of the heart

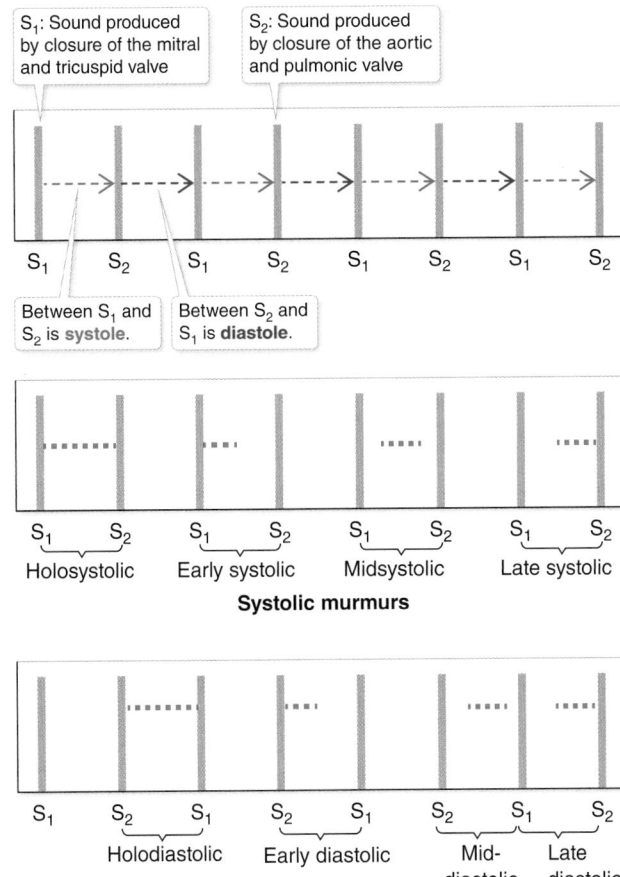

FIGURE 18-9. The timing of a heart murmur. A heart murmur can be heard during systole or diastole. The first heart sound (S_1) occurs when the mitral and tricuspid valves close. After S_1, systolic murmurs occur. The second heart sound (S_2) occurs when the aortic and pulmonic valves close. After S_2, diastolic murmurs occur. Heart murmurs can be described as early, mid-, late, or holosystolic. Alternatively, heart murmurs can be described as early, mid-, late, or holodiastolic.

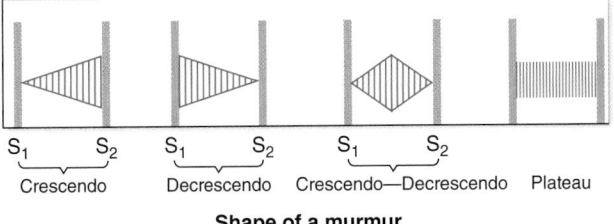

FIGURE 18-10. Describing a heart murmur.

that is palpable through the chest wall. At times a bruit may accompany a heart murmur. A **bruit** is a whooshing sound of turbulent blood flow heard through the stethoscope over an artery; a bruit may indicate an obstruction, aneurysm, or arterial malformation.

A fully described heart murmur may be documented as follows: "Grade 2/6, high pitched, harsh, decrescendo murmur heard best in the fifth intercostal space, left sternal border with radiation to the axilla."

Diagnosis

Echocardiography is the gold standard for the diagnosis of valvular heart disease. There are three types of echocardiographic techniques used for cardiac diagnostic study:

1. Transthoracic echocardiography (TTE)
2. Transesophageal echocardiography (TEE)
3. Doppler echocardiography

Transthoracic echocardiography (TTE) is a noninvasive technique that uses sound waves that reflect off cardiac structures to produce images of the heart. In TTE, an echocardiogram transducer is placed directly on the chest wall and moved to various locations on the chest surface to transmit images of the heart's interior structures.

Alternatively, in **transesophageal echocardiography (TEE)**, an ultrasound transducer is placed on an endoscope and inserted into the esophagus to obtain a closer image of the heart. In the sedated patient, TEE can provide visualization of heart structures because of the close proximity of the esophagus to the heart. TEE is more sensitive than TTE and is the preferred method to visualize heart valves and small intracardiac lesions.

Doppler echocardiography uses sound waves to measure the velocity of blood flow across valves and within cardiac chambers. It can visualize abnormal blood flow patterns in color. Echocardiograms are usually performed with the patient in the resting state. Further information can be obtained by visualizing cardiac structures during exercise or pharmacological-induced stress.

Echocardiograms are instantaneous images that enable clinicians to immediately determine cardiac structure abnormalities (see Fig. 18-11). They can be used to determine the etiology and morphology of valve disorders, estimate severity, and quantify left ventricular ejection fraction (LVEF). Echocardiograms can also detect regional wall abnormalities of the heart, which often indicate myocardial ischemia.

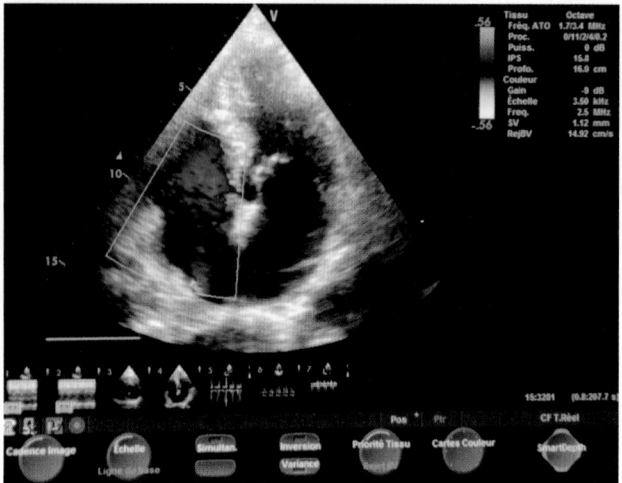

FIGURE 18-11. Example of an echocardiogram. *(From AJPhoto/ Science Source.)*

Patients with valvular disease often require echocardiograms annually, even in the absence of symptoms.

There are both two-dimensional (2D) and three-dimensional (3D) types of echocardiographic imaging studies available. Conventional 2D echocardiography may not provide enough detail and may be inadequate to study the anatomy and pathophysiological mechanisms of certain valvular disorders. Real-time 3D Doppler echocardiography provides superior visualization of AV and semilunar valves. Recent studies show that 3D echocardiograms can be used to reliably print AV and semilunar valve structures for design of valve models. The 3D models are highly accurate compared with the source echocardiographic images. This is a novel technique that adds valuable information on cardiac anatomy over current methods of imaging (Mowers et al., 2021).

When TTE and TEE echocardiography images are inadequate for evaluation of the valvular disorder, additional imaging modalities can play a complementary role in diagnosis. These include cardiac computed tomography (cardiac CT), cardiac magnetic resonance (CMR), and valve stress echocardiography (VSE). Cardiac CT can show 3D images of the heart from different angles. It is a primary tool for planning transcatheter valvular interventions because it allows precise measurements for device sizing and vascular access assessment.

CMR adds important advantages, particularly in the assessment of valvular disorders. It provides a view of the entire heart from different angles, is free of ionizing radiation, and does not require contrast administration. CMR has emerged as a useful second-line investigational tool providing quantitative assessments of valve disorders, heart chamber size, and systolic function. The ability of CMR to accurately assess the right ventricle, pulmonary, and tricuspid valves is a particular advantage in the assessment of right-sided valve lesions.

Valve stress echocardiography (VSE) can be performed as exercise or dobutamine stress echocardiography depending on the patient's clinical status and the severity and type of valve disease. Exercise stress echocardiography combines exercise testing with 2D and Doppler echocardiography during exercise. It provides objective assessment of exercise-induced changes in an individual's cardiac parameters. Dobutamine stress echocardiography is used on patients who cannot tolerate exercise. These tests assist in surgical risk assessment and determination of prognosis.

Cardiac catheterization and arteriography (angiography) are also used in patients with valvular disorders. A cardiac catheter can be threaded from a peripheral vein or artery into the right or left side of the heart to visualize the chambers and coronary arteries. Preoperatively, coronary angiography is advisable to determine left ventricular function and the health of the coronary arteries. Some patients may have coronary artery obstructions that can be surgically treated at the same time as valve repair or replacement.

Coronary computed tomography angiography (CCTA) is increasingly used as it is less invasive than the traditional cardiac catheterization procedure. The patient does not need any insertion of a catheter in this type of technology; only injection of contrast dye. High-resolution, 3D pictures of the moving heart and great vessels are produced during a coronary CCTA.

Treatment

There are a number of medical and surgical treatments for heart valve disorders. Individuals can be treated symptomatically with various pharmacological agents and lifestyle modifications. Medical therapies can remedy the symptoms of mild valvular disorders, but most patients require surgical treatment to repair or replace a dysfunctional heart valve.

Medication

Heart valve disorders often cause changes of the pressures within the heart chambers and major blood vessels such as the aorta. The pressure changes can cause a change in shape or conductivity within heart chambers. Thrombosis and dysrhythmias are often the result of these heart valve effects. Long-term changes in pressures can cause complications such as heart failure, ischemic heart disease, and stroke. To prevent these complications and to normalize the pressures and conduction within the heart, many different medications can be used.

Nitrates and vasodilators can reduce venous return, peripheral resistance, and ischemic chest pain. Beta-adrenergic blockers can prevent tachydysrhythmias and lower peripheral arterial resistance. Diuretics and salt restriction can treat volume overload associated with valve disorders. Exercise restrictions can limit strain on the heart. Anticoagulant therapy is commonly prescribed because deformed heart valves, stasis of blood, and turbulent blood flow can lead to thrombus formation. Atrial fibrillation, a common side effect of valvular dysfunction, particularly predisposes to thrombus formation. In left atrial fibrillation, a clot can easily form due to stasis of blood in the quivering, noncontracting atrium. The clot then travels from the left atrium into the left ventricle, which is then pumped into the aorta and arterial circulation. Often the clot lodges in a branch of a cerebral artery. This can cause ischemic stroke.

Anticoagulant therapy can prevent thromboembolism. Additionally, deformed or artificial valves can act as a site for bacterial growth if a patient develops bacteremia. Treatment regimens may require antibiotic prophylaxis whenever the patient undergoes dental treatment or other invasive procedures.

Surgery

Surgical treatment of valvular disorders can be lifesaving. However, surgical risk, morbidity, and mortality depend on the extent of the valvular disease, myocardial function, and general medical condition of the patient. When left ventricular function is impaired, surgical risk increases. Increased risk is also associated with advanced age, comorbidities such as diabetes or renal disease, and pulmonary hypertension.

Generally, there are two kinds of surgical procedures used in valvular disorders: surgical (open heart) interventions or transcatheter interventions. **Surgical valvular replacement** requires sternotomy (chest incision) or a minimal chest incision and open heart surgery. Some patients may have comorbidities or other risk factors that prohibit surgical interventions. In these cases, transcatheter interventions are done. However, **transcatheter valvular replacement (transcatheter valvular implantation)** is increasingly preferred to treat valvular disorders. Transcatheter interventions use a specialized catheter that contains the new collapsed valve. In this procedure, surgeons insert a catheter into the femoral artery in the groin or another approach such as transapical (through the apex of the left ventricle of the heart), subclavian artery, ascending aorta, or carotid artery, and then guide the catheter into the heart. The catheter contains a balloon and prosthetic valve. Valvotomy and valvuloplasty are the common surgical procedures done via a catheter. A balloon valvuloplasty valvotomy is commonly the first step to create an orifice of sufficient size for the valvular prosthesis. The balloon is expanded to press the valve into place, or in some cases, valves are self-expanding. The new valve is inserted without removal of the old, damaged valve.

A **percutaneous balloon valvuloplasty** is a procedure used when a patient has stenosis of a valve. A catheter is directed into the heart and threaded into the affected valvular region. Inflation of a balloon on the tip of the catheter pushes open a stenotic area.

Valvotomy is a surgical repair procedure that involves reshaping a heart valve by a commissurotomy, quadrangular resection, decalcification, annuloplasty, and leaflet patching. In a commissurotomy, narrowed valve leaflets are opened to allow for unrestricted blood flow through a valve. In a quadrangular resection, a floppy valve is stabilized to allow complete closure of the valve and limit regurgitation of blood flow. An annuloplasty reinforces a dilated valve ring, enhancing the heart valve's structural integrity.

Commonly, valvotomy is not a practical remedy, and a valve replacement is performed. A **bioprosthetic valve** or an artificial mechanical valve are options for valve replacement. A bioprosthetic valve is commonly made from porcine (pig), bovine (cow), or human cadaver tissue. Mechanical valves can last a lifetime for the patient; however, they act as a site for thrombus formation and predispose the patient to thromboembolism. Therefore, anticoagulation therapy is necessary for life with mechanical valves. Bioprosthetic valves are not associated with thrombus formation and therefore do not require anticoagulation therapy. However, bioprosthetic valves do not have the durability of mechanical valves. Studies show that 30% of patients need to replace their bioprosthetic heart valve after 10 years, and 50% need a replacement after 15 years.

Bioprosthetic Versus Mechanical Valve Replacement. The choice between a bioprosthetic valve or mechanical prosthetic valve requires consideration of multiple factors including age of the patient, comorbidities, etiology of the valve disorder, life expectancy, likelihood of future pregnancy for women, bleeding risk of the patient, and presence of other patient indications for anticoagulation. The advantage of bioprosthetic valves is that they do not require accompanying anticoagulant therapy. However, bioprosthetic valves often need reoperation and replacement after 10 years. **Mechanical prosthetic valves** have longer durability but require accompanying anticoagulant therapy.

Thus, for women who are expected to have a future pregnancy, the benefit of avoiding the risks of anticoagulation for a mechanical valve is weighed against the risk of reoperation if a bioprosthetic valve is placed. For patients who require valve replacement and are not expected to have future pregnancies (men and selected women), a mechanical prosthesis is commonly chosen because the patients are usually relatively young (younger than 65 to 70 years old), and some require chronic anticoagulation for atrial fibrillation.

> **ALERT!** Deformed or artificial valves can act as a site for bacterial growth.

🔬 CLINICAL CONCEPT

In many patients with valvular disorders, antibiotics should be administered prophylactically before any invasive treatment such as dental work or insertion of an IV catheter.

Pathophysiology of Selected Heart Valve Disorders

The most common valvular disorders are mitral and aortic stenosis, which account for two-thirds of all valvular disease. Calcific aortic sclerosis, which occurs because of atherosclerosis and aging, causes stenotic deformity of the aortic valve and is the most common valve disorder of all.

Mitral Valve Disorders

The mitral valve disorders include mitral stenosis, mitral insufficiency, and mitral valve prolapse (MVP). These are some of the most common heart murmurs heard in clinical practice.

Mitral Stenosis

Mitral stenosis is one of the most common heart valve disorders. It is a common sequela to RF or a consequence of calcification of the mitral valve, referred to as **mitral annular calcification (MAC)**. MAC is often a consequence of aging associated with long-standing atherosclerosis. Because it is associated with aging, it is commonly referred to as degenerative mitral valve stenosis.

Epidemiology. Patients with mitral stenosis due to RHD commonly become symptomatic between age 30 and 40 years old and are predominately female. The prevalence of RHD in developed nations is steadily declining, with an estimated incidence of 1 in 100,000. However, in underdeveloped countries, incidence of RF remains high.

Alternatively, the prevalence of MAC increases significantly with older age. Studies show that among individuals aged 60 to 70 years, 70 to 80 years, and 80 years and older, MAC accounted for 10%, 30%, and 60% of mitral stenosis cases, respectively.

Etiology. The most common risk factor for mitral stenosis is RF. In many individuals, RF leads to RHD if untreated. Most cases of mitral stenosis caused by RHD occur 10 to 30 years after RF. The patient may not recall having childhood RF.

MAC is caused by the development of fibrotic changes within the annulus of the mitral valve. It most commonly causes no symptoms and is discovered on chest x-ray or other imaging studies as an ancillary finding. Atherosclerosis, altered mineral metabolism, or increased mechanical stress can cause MAC.

Pathophysiology. In mitral stenosis, the mitral valve is thickened, fibrotic, and narrowed. With age, the valve can become calcified. The stiff valve impedes blood flow from the left atrium into the left ventricle. The murmur of mitral stenosis is heard when blood attempts to squeeze through the narrow mitral valve

during left ventricular filling or diastole. As the rigid mitral valve opens, often an opening snap (OS) can be heard, followed by a diastolic murmur (see Fig. 18-12).

The best location to hear the murmur of mitral stenosis is at the apex of the heart during diastole, after S_2 and before S_1. Placing the patient in the left lateral decubitus position can accentuate the murmur.

In the adult, the normal mitral valve orifice has a cross-sectional area of approximately 4.0 cm^2 to 6 cm^2. When the orifice is reduced to 2 cm^2, the pressure gradient across the valve begins to increase. Many patients develop symptoms when the mitral valve area is reduced to 1.5 cm^2, and nearly all patients become symptomatic when valve area is reduced to 1.0 cm^2 or less.

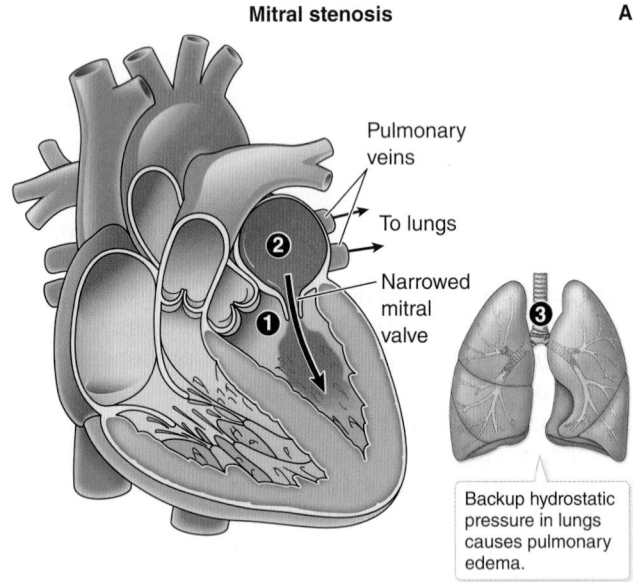

Mitral stenosis   **A**

1. Narrow mitral valve hinders blood flow into the left ventricle.

2. Blood backs up in the left atrium, causing left atrial enlargement.

3. Hydrostatic pressure builds backward into the pulmonary veins. Congested pulmonary veins cause pulmonary edema.

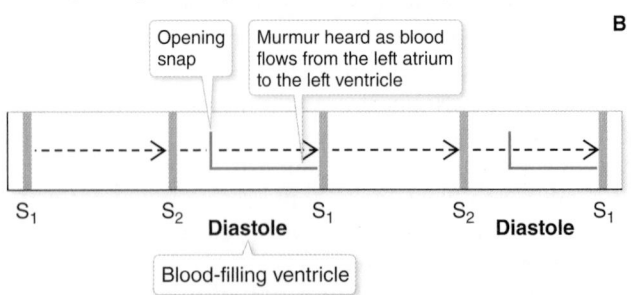

FIGURE 18-12. Mitral stenosis. (A) In mitral stenosis, the mitral valve is narrowed, and blood flow from the left atrium to the left ventricle is hindered. As a result, blood backs up into the left atrium and stretches the chamber, creating an enlarged left atrium. Hydrostatic pressure builds backward from the left atrium into the pulmonary veins, causing increased venous congestion of the lungs and pulmonary edema. (B) The murmur of mitral stenosis occurs after S_2 during diastole as the blood flows from the left atrium to fill the left ventricle. Commonly, an opening snap is heard when the stiff mitral valve opens.

In severe mitral stenosis, there is a lack of blood flow from the left atrium into the left ventricle, which diminishes cardiac output. When the mitral valve opening is severely narrowed, the left atrium becomes overloaded with blood and high hydrostatic pressure builds in the pulmonary veins. This creates high pulmonary capillary pressure, congestion of the pulmonary vessels, and pulmonary edema.

In long-standing mitral stenosis, the left atrium becomes volume overloaded, overstretched, and dilated. A distended atrial wall can stretch cardiac conduction fibers, causing episodes of atrial fibrillation. Atrial fibrillation causes stasis of blood in the left atrium and predisposes to thrombus formation. A thrombus that forms in the left atrium can travel into the left ventricle, aorta, and systemic circulation. An embolic thrombus commonly travels from the left atrium, into the left ventricle, and into the aorta. From the aorta, it can travel into the brachiocephalic artery, which leads to the common carotid and internal carotid artery. From the internal carotid artery it can then travel into a branch of the middle cerebral artery and cause an ischemic stroke.

Clinical Presentation. Dyspnea on exertion and cough are usually the initial symptoms associated with the pulmonary vascular congestion of mitral stenosis. Pulmonary edema can occur if hydrostatic pressure rises to high levels within the pulmonary capillaries. In the supine position, the patient experiences orthopnea. When the patient lies flat during sleep, hypoxia, which presents as paroxysmal nocturnal dyspnea (PND), may be experienced. A patient may describe PND as awakening in the middle of the night because of a night terror. With auscultation of the heart, an opening snap (OS) and diastolic murmur may be heard. An OS of the mitral valve is heard at the apex when the leaflets are still mobile. The OS is due to the halting leaflet motion of the inflexible mitral valve in early diastole. It is best heard at the apex and lower left sternal border. The murmur is a low-pitched diastolic rumble that is heard best with the patient lying on the left side and by using the bell of the stethoscope or the low-frequency range of an electronic stethoscope.

In long-standing mitral stenosis, there is increased hydrostatic pressure in the left atrium, which, over time, can cause enlargement of the left atrium. In the enlarged left atrium, atrial fibrillation can occur, which causes an irregular pulse, possible tachycardia, and thrombus formation in the left atrium. The patient may complain of palpitations. Atrial fibrillation, which is a quivering, noncontracting atrium, is a common predisposing condition to ischemic stroke. In the noncontracting left atrium, stasis of blood can lead to thrombus formation. The thrombus can travel from the left atrium into the left ventricle and into the arterial circulation, commonly into the cerebral circulation. The thrombus can cause obstruction of a branch of a cerebral artery and cause ischemic stroke. Symptoms of stroke, which include hemiparesis (weakness over half the body), facial droop, or slurring of speech, can occur.

Diagnosis. The best diagnostic studies for mitral stenosis include real-time 3D Doppler echocardiogram and cardiac computed tomography (CCT). Both transthoracic and transesophageal echocardiograms can assist in diagnosis; however, TEE may provide superior imaging. CCT provides superior ability to detect calcification in MAC and valuable information about the MV annulus, extent of calcification, and its relation to the adjacent structures. Cardiac magnetic resonance (CMR) imaging is also recommended, particularly for evaluation of rheumatic mitral stenosis. An electrocardiogram (ECG) and chest x-ray are necessary. Stress echocardiography is recommended particularly in asymptomatic patients or women with mitral valve disorders who are planning pregnancy. Pregnancy leads to an increase in cardiac output, heart rate, transmitral flow, and total blood volume, each of which can worsen mitral valve disease.

An ECG is recommended as it may reveal atrial fibrillation, which is demonstrated by rapidly repetitive P waves. Chest x-ray may reveal pulmonary congestion. Computed tomography (CT) scan and magnetic resonance imaging (MRI) scan of the brain should be done if atrial fibrillation is suspected. Based on analysis of valve anatomy, valve hemodynamics, secondary hemodynamic effects, and patient symptoms, mitral stenosis severity is graded as stage A, B, C, or D, according to valve diameter and diastolic blood flow (see Table 18-1).

Treatment. The formation of an atrial thrombus is a major complication of mitral stenosis and is the presenting event in some patients. Studies have shown that before anticoagulant therapy and surgical treatment in patients with mitral stenosis, as many as 30% of patients experienced an embolic event during the course of the disease. Therefore, anticoagulation is essential in mitral stenosis to prevent clot formation.

Diuretic therapy, usually with a loop diuretic, and dietary salt restriction are appropriate when there are manifestations of pulmonary vascular congestion such as exertional dyspnea. Beta blockers or calcium blockers are recommended to control atrial fibrillation.

TABLE 18-1. Stages of Mitral Stenosis	
STAGE	**MITRAL VALVE DIAMETER MEASUREMENT**
Stage A	Thickened mitral valve/no symptoms
Stage B	Mitral valve >1.5 cm^2
Stage C	Mitral valve ≤1.5 cm^2
Stage D	Mitra valve <1.0 cm^2

Adapted from Nishimura, R. A., & Carabello, B. (2016). Operationalizing the 2014 ACC/AHA guidelines for valvular heart disease: A guide for clinicians. *J Am Collf Cardiol, 67*(19), 2289–2294.

Percutaneous mitral **balloon valvotomy** is recommended for symptomatic patients with severe mitral stenosis (stage D) and in patients with favorable valve morphology, absence of left atrial thrombus, and absence of moderate to severe mitral regurgitation.

Surgical or transcatheter management of MAC is most commonly offered only for severe symptomatic mitral stenosis. Surgical management has been associated with high morbidity and mortality since most patients are older with multiple comorbidities. Technically, MV surgery for MAC is difficult due to high calcium build-up that can extend beyond the annulus and involve adjacent atrial or ventricular walls. Transcatheter mitral valve replacement (TMVR) has been proposed for the management of high surgical risk patients with MAC. Studies regarding this technique are in process.

For rheumatic mitral valve disease, open heart surgical techniques are recommended. Rheumatic mitral valve disease often includes shortening and fusion of chordae tendinae, and mitral regurgitation, as well as mitral stenosis. Visualization of the whole mitral valve is necessary. Mitral valve surgery, including repair, balloon valvotomy, commissurotomy, or valve replacement, is recommended in patients with severe mitral stenosis (stage D).

In mitral stenosis surgery, mechanical prosthetic valves are often recommended due to longer durability, and anticoagulation is needed anyway due to potential atrial fibrillation. Therefore, the patient with mitral stenosis with mechanical valve requires anticoagulant therapy and preventive antibiotics after dental treatment or invasive procedures.

Mitral Insufficiency

Mitral insufficiency (mitral regurgitation) valve disorders are most commonly due to myxomatous mitral valve disease and ischemic myocardial disease, mainly myocardial infarction. There are two types of mitral insufficiency; primary and secondary. Primary mitral insufficiency is due to abnormalities with the mitral valve itself such as myxomatous degeneration. Secondary mitral insufficiency (also called functional mitral insufficiency) is due to ischemia of the left ventricle, which causes papillary muscle dysfunction.

Secondary mitral insufficiency is most commonly caused by acute myocardial infarction. Papillary muscle in the left ventricle ruptures, which causes incomplete closure of the mitral valve during systole. Studies show that 50% to 60% of patients develop mitral insufficiency after MI. Mitral insufficiency after MI causes an increased risk of death and heart failure. The patient with mitral insufficiency due to MI is often clinically asymptomatic. Therefore, after MI, the heart should always be assessed using echocardiography. Echocardiograms show noncontractile areas of the ventricle, regurgitation of blood through the mitral valve, and estimates of LVEF.

Primary mitral insufficiency is one of the most common valve problems caused by myxomatous degeneration. Some rare cases are caused by genetic disorders such as Marfan's and Ehlers–Danlos syndromes, which cause connective tissue abnormalities. Myxomatous degeneration can also occur in persons without connective tissue disease; the etiology is unclear. Other causes of mitral insufficiency include rheumatic heart disease (RHD); mitral annular calcification (MAC); infective endocarditis (IE); and certain drugs, including ergotamine, bromocriptine, cabergoline, and fenfluramine. Mitral valve prolapse (MVP), often asymptomatic, is a condition that commonly causes intermittent episodes of mild mitral insufficiency. Previously thought to be benign, MVP can be a part of Barlow's disease. Barlow's disease is a clinical syndrome characterized by MVP and potentially fatal ventricular arrhythmias.

Epidemiology. The incidence of acute and chronic mitral insufficiency is approximately 5 in 10,000 people in the United States. In the past, RHD was the most common cause of mitral insufficiency. Antibiotic treatment has made RHD less common, and myxomatous disorders involving the mitral valve and MI are the leading causes of mitral insufficiency today. MVP has been estimated to affect as many as 20% of middle-aged and older adults, mostly women. Many have asymptomatic, undiagnosed MVP.

Etiology. The most common causes of mitral insufficiency include ischemic heart disease with MI, myxomatous mitral valve disease, MVP, RHD, IE, and MAC. In underdeveloped regions of the world, RHD is the major cause of mitral insufficiency. Risk factors for mitral insufficiency include female sex, lower body mass index, advanced age, renal dysfunction, prior MI, prior mitral stenosis, and prior MVP.

Pathophysiology. In mitral insufficiency, the mitral valve fails to close completely, allowing blood to back up into the left atrium as the left ventricle contracts. The two most common causes of mitral valve insufficiency are MI and myxomatous degeneration of the mitral valve.

In myocardial infarction (MI), when the left ventricular wall undergoes myocardial cell death, the papillary muscles, which are projections off the ventricular wall, commonly rupture. The papillary muscles are attached to the mitral valve leaflets via chordae tendinae strands. In MI, the ruptured papillary muscles lose their connection to a mitral valve leaflet or leaflets, which then leads to incomplete closure of the mitral valve, or mitral insufficiency.

In myxomatous degeneration of the mitral valve, there is anatomical abnormality of the mitral valve leaflets. In the majority of cases, the etiology is unclear; however, it includes mitral annular disjunction (MAD), a specific anatomical abnormality in which there is a distinct separation between the mitral annulus and the left atrial wall. Myxomatous degeneration commonly causes a spectrum of disease. It can cause infrequent MVP without symptoms to Barlow's syndrome, which is MVP with ventricular arrhythmias. Myxomatous degeneration of the mitral valve is also part of genetic disorders; for example, Ehlers–Danlos's and Marfan's syndromes, which are uncommon conditions.

With any kind of mitral insufficiency, each systolic contraction causes regurgitant blood flow back into the left atrium. Consequently, left atrial overload and distention are common. The left atrium stretches as it attempts to accommodate an increasingly larger volume of regurgitated blood into the chamber. This stretching of the chamber leads to conduction dysfunction in the form of atrial fibrillation. In atrial fibrillation, the left atrium quivers and does not contract. This noncontractile atrium allows blood to stagnate. Stagnation of blood leads to thrombus formation. A thrombus often travels from the left atrium into the left ventricle, then into the aorta. From the aorta, up into the carotid arteries, a thrombus can lodge in a cerebral artery. This thrombus can obstruct blood flow in the brain, leading to ischemic stroke.

The progressive accumulation of blood in the left atrium also causes backup of hydrostatic pressure into the pulmonary veins and pulmonary capillaries. This leads to pulmonary edema and consequent difficulty with breathing and air exchange.

In addition, more blood volume in the left atrium allows more blood to enter the left ventricle, which often causes dilation of the left ventricle. With time, the increasing enlargement and stretch of the left-sided heart chambers cause tension on the mitral valve leaflets, which worsens the incompetence of the mitral valve. Also, dilation of the left ventricle leads to decreased ventricular contractility, diminished pump strength, and heart failure.

Decreased blood volume pumped forward can lead to diminished aortic blood flow. Because the coronary arteries arise off the aorta, decreased aortic blood flow can cause lack of sufficient blood flow into the coronary arteries. This can cause coronary artery insufficiency and the associated symptoms of cardiac chest pain, particularly with exertion.

In sum, mitral valve insufficiency can lead to significant morbidity with the following sequelae:

- Coronary artery insufficiency
- Left atrial enlargement and atrial fibrillation, which can lead to ischemic stroke
- Diminished cardiac output and heart failure
- Left atrial volume accumulation and high pulmonary capillary pressure leading to pulmonary edema

Clinical Presentation. Patients with mitral insufficiency may be asymptomatic until the mitral valve allows so much blood to back up into the left atrium that there is not enough forward output into the aorta from the left ventricle. Because the coronary arteries branch off from the aorta, there is then diminished blood flow through the coronary arteries. The lack of sufficient coronary artery blood flow causes the patient to experience chest pain, pallor, diaphoresis, and dyspnea of myocardial ischemia. Along with coronary insufficiency, the aorta has diminished blood flow to pump forward from the left ventricle, thereby causing decreased cardiac output. Symptoms of diminished cardiac output include weakness, fatigue, and exercise intolerance. As the disease worsens, patients may present with symptomatic heart failure and pulmonary edema.

In mitral insufficiency, blood also backs up into the left atrium, which causes an overstretched, dilated left atrium. Within the dilated left atrium, the arrhythmia atrial fibrillation can develop. Atrial fibrillation creates a noncontracting left atrium and stagnation of blood. The stagnation of the blood often leads to thrombus formation. The thrombus can travel from the left atrium to the left ventricle and into the arterial circulation. Commonly, a thrombus due to atrial fibrillation travels from the left atrium into the left ventricle, then into the aorta and up into the carotid artery. From the carotid artery the thrombus travels into the cerebral arteries, causing obstruction and ischemic stroke.

On physical examination, the S_1 sound made by the closure of the mitral and tricuspid valve closure may be diminished. This is due to the lack of mitral valve leaflets coming together during closure. Also because of the incomplete closure of the mitral valve, there is leakage of blood back into the left atrium, which causes a holosystolic murmur. Classically, this holosystolic murmur is heard best at the apex. In MVP, there is typically a midsystolic click, which is due to the opening snap of the valve during midsystole. The murmur of MVP typically starts after a click during mid- to late systole.

Diagnosis. TTE and TEE are diagnostic tests that are used for mitral insufficiency. Cardiac magnetic resonance imaging has proved to be the best diagnostic test. These tests can accurately estimate the diminished left ventricular ejection fraction (LVEF) and decreased cardiac output present in mitral insufficiency. Chest x-ray may demonstrate cardiomegaly if there is left atrial dilation. ECG should be performed to rule out MI and atrial fibrillation.

Stress testing combined with Doppler echocardiography or cardiac catheterization is done in selected patients with chronic mitral insufficiency to evaluate exercise-induced changes in hemodynamics. Stress testing may be used to identify left ventricular ischemia.

Mitral insufficiency is categorized into stages A, B, C, and D, according to severity. Severity is based on the volume of blood that is regurgitated into the left atrium and left ventricle, LVEF, and pulmonary artery pressure. As the mitral valve disease worsens, the volume of regurgitated blood into the left atrium increases. This increases the size of the left atrium and increases the volume of blood accumulating backward into the pulmonary system, increasing pulmonary artery pressure. Also, the increased amount of blood in the left atrium causes increased volume entering the left ventricle, which in turn enlarges and dilates the ventricle. The enlarged, dilated left ventricle weakens with time. Heart failure often follows with decreased LVEF. Currently, severe mitral regurgitation is defined as an effective regurgitant orifice area of at least 0.4 cm² or a regurgitant blood volume of at least 60 mL.

The Mitral Regurgitation International Database (MIDA) score is a tool that can be used at diagnosis to help in risk stratification for patients with severe mitral regurgitation due to myxomatous disease (see Table 18-2). It delineates the clinical symptoms, echocardiographic parameters, and risk factors that are associated with adverse outcomes in patients with mitral valve disease. The score is meant to be used to determine whether a patient should be placed on medical therapy or undergo surgical intervention.

Staging of mitral insufficiency is based on symptoms, valve anatomy, hemodynamic changes based on left atrial and left ventricular size, and pulmonary artery pressure (see Table 18-3).

Treatment. Surgical treatment is preferred to medical therapy in mitral insufficiency. It is recognized that mitral valve repair is superior to mitral valve replacement in many patients with mitral insufficiency. Transcatheter mitral valve repair through the MitraClip procedure has become widely adopted in routine clinical practice. Designated as transcatheter edge-to-edge repair (TEER) with MitraClip, the surgeon accesses the mitral valve via a catheter, and then inserts a clip onto the mitral valve leaflet that tightens closure of the mitral valve.

However, mitral valve repair is not suitable for all patients, and some need mitral valve replacement. Between 60% and 70% of patients who undergo mitral valve replacement surgery receive a bioprosthetic valve. All bioprosthetic valves degenerate, affecting short- and long-term patient outcomes. Up to one-third of patients may require repeat mitral valve surgery after a median of 8 years. In patients with bioprosthetic MV failure or severe valve dysfunction, valve-in-valve (ViV) and valve-in-ring (ViR) transcatheter mitral valve procedures are done. In the ViV procedure, a new valve is inserted over the old dysfunctional valve. In ViR, the annulus of the mitral valve is repaired using prosthetic material.

Symptomatic patients with severe mitral insufficiency and LVEF less than 60% who are awaiting valve surgery or who are not candidates for valve surgery are treated with standard medical therapy for heart failure. Medications include angiotensin-converting enzyme (ACE) inhibitors, angiotensin II receptor blockers (ARBs), and angiotensin receptor–neprilysin inhibitors. Beta blockers, aldosterone antagonists, and diuretics are also indicated. Vasodilator treatment in select patients is recommended. If atrial fibrillation is present, direct cardioversion and antiarrhythmic medications are recommended.

Mitral Annular Calcification

Calcium deposits can develop in the rim, also called the annulus, of the mitral valve. Usually, this occurs with age and causes no dysfunction. At times, however, the irregular, hard calcifications can cause narrowing and rigidity of the mitral valve, causing incomplete emptying of the left atrium. Alternatively, the calcium deposits can cause the rigid valve leaflets to remain partially open and allow regurgitation of blood into the left atrium during left ventricular contraction. The calcium deposits can also become areas that harbor bacteria and predispose individuals to IE. Often, MAC can be visualized on a chest x-ray as an opacity surrounding the mitral valve. Echocardiography, CT, and MRI scans of the heart are used in the diagnosis. Asymptomatic MAC does not require specific medical therapy. However, blood can back up into the left atrium and pulmonary vasculature, causing pulmonary edema. Alternatively, the left atrium can become stretched out and susceptible to atrial fibrillation and thromboembolism formation. The possible consequence of pulmonary edema requires diuretics, and the prevention of thromboembolism requires anticoagulants. Surgery is usually not performed unless the mitral valve is severely affected.

Mitral Valve Prolapse

Often referred to as Barlow's syndrome, floppy valve syndrome, or systolic-click syndrome, MVP is a common cause of mitral insufficiency in the United States. It is a disorder that most commonly affects females ages 14 through 30 years. It is a frequent finding in persons

TABLE 18-2. Mitral Regurgitation International Database Score

SCORE FOR RISK STRATIFICATION WITH MYXOMATOUS MITRAL VALVE DISEASE

Factors	Points
Age >65	3
Clinical symptoms	3
Right ventricular systolic pressure >50 mm Hg	2
Atrial fibrillation	1
Left atrial diameter >55 mm	1
Left ventricular end systolic diameter greater than or equal to 40 mm	1
Left ventricular ejection fraction less than or equal to 60%	1

From Grigioni, F., Clavel, M. A., Vanoverschelde, J. L., et al.; MIDA Investigators (2018). The MIDA Mortality Risk Score: Development and external validation of a prognostic model for early and late death in degenerative mitral regurgitation. *Eur Heart J, 39*(15), 1281–1291. doi: 10.1093/eurheartj/ehx465

TABLE 18-3. Mitral Insufficiency Stages

Mitral Insufficiency Stage	Symptoms	Mitral Valve	Left Atrium Size	Left Ventricle Size	Pulmonary Artery Pressure
Stage A	No symptoms	Mild valvular prolapse	Normal	Normal	Normal
Stage B	No symptoms	Moderate mitral regurgitation with substantial valve abnormalities	Mild enlargement	No enlargement	Normal
Stage C	No symptoms	Severe mitral regurgitation with severe valve abnormalities	Atrial enlargement	Ventricular enlargement	High
Stage D	Symptoms of heart failure	Severe mitral regurgitation with severe valve abnormalities	Atrial enlargement	Ventricular enlargement	High

Adapted from: Gaasch, W. H. (2018). Management of chronic primary mitral regurgitation. www.uptodate.com

with genetic connective tissue disorders such as Marfan's syndrome, osteogenesis imperfecta, and Ehlers–Danlos syndrome. It can arise from RF, ischemic heart disease, or cardiomyopathies, but in most cases the cause is unknown. It often goes undetected because the disorder is commonly asymptomatic. It is known to exist in 4% of the population, but it is estimated that up to 20% have asymptomatic MVP.

In MVP, one or both mitral valve leaflets are loose and floppy because of myxomatous degeneration of the valve tissue—an excess of mucopolysaccharide. The mitral valve leaflets are thickened, and the attached chordae tendineae are thin and easily ruptured.

During left ventricular contraction, the loose mitral valve leaflets prolapse upward into the left atrium. The prolapse allows regurgitation of blood into the left atrium during systole. This causes a systolic murmur as blood flows out of an unsealed mitral valve. In some individuals, a midsystolic click may be heard, signaling the opening of the loose mitral valve leaflets. The tension in the wall of the contracting left ventricle pushes the incompetent mitral valve open into the left atrium. This turbulent, backward blood flow can create a midsystolic, holosystolic, or late systolic murmur, which is why the characteristic murmur heard in MVP is a midsystolic click followed by a systolic murmur (see Fig. 18-13).

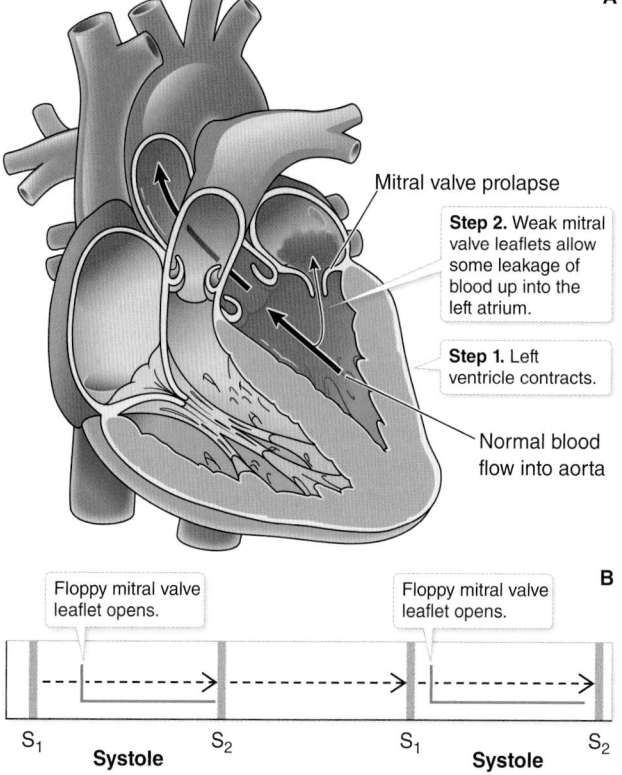

FIGURE 18-13. Mitral valve prolapse. (A) In mitral valve prolapse, there is a weak mitral valve. When the left ventricle contracts during systole, the mitral valve leaflets billow up and leak some blood backward into the left atrium. (B) The murmur of MVP occurs during systole.

CLINICAL CONCEPT

In many patients, there is benign MVP with sporadic episodes of prolapse of a leaflet of the mitral valve, referred to as MVP syndrome. The patient may describe episodes of palpitations, atypical chest pain, dyspnea, fatigue, dizziness, numbness and tingling, and anxiety.

Severe MVP is uncommon but can cause symptoms similar to angina. When MVP allows blood to flow backward into the left atrium, the blood volume within the left ventricle diminishes. This in turn decreases the blood volume into the aorta. With less aortic blood flow, there is diminished coronary artery blood flow. The affected individual can experience coronary insufficiency, which causes myocardial ischemia leading to chest pain, dyspnea, and fatigue.

Echocardiography is the major diagnostic procedure used in MVP. TTE or TEE can be used as with other valvular disorders, with noninvasive TTE usually used first. ECGs are indicated to assess for dysrhythmia. A 24-hour ambulatory ECG (Holter monitor) may be necessary. Cardiac MRI can be used if echocardiogram results are not optimal.

The majority of persons affected by MVP have a benign course and no hemodynamically significant effects. Education and reassurance about the nature of the disorder are often adequate to reduce patient concerns. Many patients benefit from a change in lifestyle, including aerobic exercise training; the avoidance of stimulants (caffeine, nicotine), alcohol, and undue fatigue; and a reduction in stress. Studies have shown that aerobic exercise decreases anxiety scores; increases general well-being; and decreases frequency of chest pain, fatigue, and dizziness. Magnesium supplementation may benefit a subset of patients with symptoms of MVP and magnesium deficiency.

A small percentage of patients with severe MVP can develop one of the following complications: IE, mitral insufficiency, dysrhythmias, or leaflet thrombi that embolize into the arterial circulation. MVP with accompanying dysrhythmias is often referred to as Barlow's syndrome. Dysrhythmias include premature atrial beats, paroxysmal supraventricular tachycardia, ventricular premature beats, and complex ventricular ectopy.

For patients who are symptomatic, beta blockers are often given to decrease heart rate. Also, anticoagulants may be recommended for those with atrial fibrillation. Oral contraceptives should not be used, as these can increase the risk of thrombus formation. If mitral prolapse is severe, surgery is similar to mitral regurgitation—either surgical repair through the percutaneous route or valve replacement.

Endocarditis prophylaxis is no longer recommended by the current American College of Cardiology/American Heart Association (ACC/AHA) guidelines for patients with MVP. Although MVP is associated with an increased risk of endocarditis, antibiotic prophylaxis is not effective in preventing episodes of endocarditis.

Aortic Valve Disorders

The aortic valve disorders include aortic stenosis and aortic insufficiency. Aortic stenosis is the most common valve disorder in older adults.

Aortic Stenosis

The most common cause of **aortic stenosis** is aortic sclerosis, which is the calcification of the aortic valve orifice that occurs in older adults. Also, a congenitally malformed bicuspid aortic valve is often responsible for many cases of aortic stenosis.

Epidemiology. Aortic sclerosis is the most common cause of aortic stenosis in the United States. The prevalence of aortic stenosis varies from 0.2% at ages 50 to 59 years, to 1.3% at ages 60 to 69 years, 3.9% at ages 70 to 79 years, and 9.8% at ages 80 to 89 years. A bicuspid aortic valve can cause a heart murmur in childhood. It is estimated that 2% of the population has this congenital valve structure. Males are more often affected than females.

Etiology. Aortic sclerosis, congenital bicuspid aortic valve, and childhood rheumatic fever leading to RHD are the most common causes of aortic stenosis. The valve in aortic sclerosis becomes inflamed, calcified, and rigid, demonstrating changes seen in atherosclerosis. Hypercholesterolemia accelerates sclerosis of the aortic valve, and individuals with aortic sclerosis usually suffer from coronary atherosclerosis as well. Endothelial dysfunction, lipid infiltration, calcification, and ossification are components of the disease process in aortic sclerosis. Aortic sclerosis is often referred to as calcific aortic valve disease or degenerative aortic stenosis.

In middle-aged adults, aortic stenosis is most commonly caused by a congenital bicuspid aortic valve, which, with its two leaflets, creates a significantly narrower opening than the normal three-leaflet aortic valve. A single gene defect to explain the majority of congenital bicuspid aortic valve cases has not been identified. This structural defect can cause a murmur in childhood but usually does not cause any hemodynamic problems or symptoms. It can be a silent condition that causes symptoms later in life. Symptoms often occur with aging when calcification and atherosclerotic plaque accumulate on the narrow bicuspid aortic valve, which further constricts the orifice.

Pathophysiology. Regardless of the etiology, in aortic stenosis the aortic valve is narrow and left ventricular outflow of blood is obstructed. The ejection of blood, which occurs during left ventricular contraction in systole, is hindered by the resistance of the distorted aortic valve.

In the majority of cases, as a compensatory mechanism to aortic stenosis, the left ventricle hypertrophies, and the patient can remain asymptomatic for many years. Eventually, the left ventricle muscle mass exceeds its coronary artery blood supply and myocardial ischemia can result. Therefore, left ventricular ischemia or angina pectoris is a common sequela of aortic stenosis.

Clinical Presentation. In most patients, aortic stenosis begins with a prolonged asymptomatic period. Persons may not become symptomatic until older age. Symptoms most commonly occur when the stenosis is severe (valve area is <1 cm^2). The classic clinical manifestations of aortic stenosis include dyspnea on exertion or exercise intolerance, exertional dizziness, and exertional angina. In severe aortic stenosis, there are symptoms of heart failure, syncope, and angina.

Exertional dyspnea occurs because in aortic stenosis the left ventricle is unable to empty all its blood into the narrowed aorta. The blood volume backs up into the left ventricle and atrium, resulting in overload of the left heart chambers. The hydrostatic pressure in the left atrium increases backward pressure in the pulmonary veins and pulmonary capillaries. High hydrostatic pressure in the pulmonary capillaries causes pulmonary edema. Consequently, the patient is short of breath, especially when there is stress on the heart. Exertional angina or chest pain occurs because there is a diminished volume of blood entering the narrowed aortic valve and the aortic blood volume is less than optimal. Less blood volume in the aorta causes less blood flow into the coronary arteries, and the result is coronary insufficiency and ischemia of heart muscle.

Exertional dizziness can occur because of the lack of sufficient blood volume entering the aorta and its branches. The blood volume in the brachiocephalic, common carotid, internal carotid, and cerebral arteries is diminished. Lack of sufficient cerebral artery blood flow can cause syncope.

Aortic stenosis is a systolic murmur, occurring after S_1 and before or into S_2. The murmur characteristically is an ejection murmur heard after S_1, which is crescendo, low pitched, and rough ending before S_2. It is heard best at the second right intercostal space with the patient in the seated position and leaning forward, as it commonly radiates up into the carotid arteries. An early systolic opening snap may be heard as the stiff aortic valve opens during systole.

On physical examination, a systolic thrill may be felt at the right intercostal space or at the sternal notch, especially during full expiration with the patient leaning forward. The S_2 may be loud as the aortic and pulmonic valves close simultaneously, or it may be a split S_2 in severe aortic stenosis, when the aortic valve closes after the pulmonic valve. The carotid arterial pulse rises slowly with a delayed peak. The left ventricular impulse may be displaced laterally due to left ventricular hypertrophy.

Diagnosis. Transthoracic or transesophgeal echocardiogram is done. Doppler echocardiography is the primary test for diagnosis and evaluation of aortic stenosis. Stress echocardiography may be used in those who are symptomatic. Exercise testing is contraindicated in patients with severe AS and symptoms related to the disease. At times, Doppler echocardiography images are inadequate to assess aortic sclerosis. For these cases, computed tomography–aortic valve calcium (CT-AVC) scan without contrast is widely used. Cardiac magnetic resonance (CMR) is recommended as it can add information about the structure and function of the left ventricle. It is important to evaluate left ventricular function as myocyte death and myocardial fibrosis are indicators of heart failure. Levels of high sensitivity troponin I (hsTnI) allow detection of low-level myocyte cell death and injury. ECG and hsTnI add to the assessment of the patient for appropriate treatment.

A B type natriuretic peptide (BNP) or N-terminal proBNP blood level is recommended because high or steadily rising BNP can be predictive of heart failure. Aortic stenosis is categorized according to severity as stage A, B, C, or D (see Table 18-4). Aortic transvalvular pressure measurement, symptoms, and LVEF are used to stage aortic stenosis.

Treatment. Medical treatment is recommended in patients without symptoms. The patient should not engage in strenuous physical activity, and hydration is important to maintain cardiac output. Medications may be necessary to treat hypertension or coronary artery disease. Patients with aortic sclerosis commonly have hyperlipidemia; therefore, statins are also commonly prescribed.

Surgical aortic valve replacement (SAVR) (open heart surgery) or transcatheter aortic valve implantation (TAVI) are two techniques used in patients with severe disease. A prosthetic aortic valve implantation is advised when valve area has diminished to less than 1 cm². Surgery or transcatheter intervention is also advised for those with left ventricular systolic dysfunction, bicuspid aortic valve, aneurysm, or those with coronary artery disease. Transcatheter aortic valve implantation has gained recognition as a preferable technique in many patients. It is recommended for

TABLE 18-4. Stages of Aortic Stenosis

Stages of Aortic Stenosis	Symptoms	Transvalvular Aortic Velocity Measurement	Left Ventricular Ejection Fraction
Stage A	No symptoms	<2 m/s	Normal
Stage B	Heart murmur present	2 to 3.9 m/s	Normal
Stage C	Heart murmur present	≥4 m/s	Normal to <50%
Stage D*	+ symptoms	≥4 m/s	<50%

*Stage D is divided into D1, D2, and D3 according to different parameters.
Adapted from Otto, C. M. (2018). Clinical manifestations and diagnosis of aortic stenosis in adults. www.uptodate.com

patients with prohibitive surgical risk and is reasonable in high-, intermediate-, and low-risk patients. It is most commonly preceded by balloon valvuloplasty to open up the aortic valve orifice. Compared with SAVR, TAVI results in fewer periprocedural deaths, and confers lower risk of stroke, major bleeding, and arrhythmias. TAVI is most commonly undertaken via the femoral artery, although trans-LV apical, subclavian, carotid, and ascending aortic routes have been used. Pharmacological treatments are under investigation for aortic sclerosis. Recent studies show that bisphosphonates are effective in aortic sclerosis, as they can decrease calcification of the aortic valve. Novel anti-inflammatory agents are under investigation as proinflammatory cytokines and fibrosis are major processes in aortic sclerosis. ACE inhibitors and ARBs are under investigation to reduce the left ventricular remodeling and fibrosis that accompany the aortic stenosis.

Hypertrophic Cardiomyopathy

Hypertrophic cardiomyopathy (HCM) is a disorder that inhibits ejection of blood from the left ventricle. In HCM, the interventricular septum of the left ventricle is disproportionately enlarged because of a structural derangement of muscle fibers. It is also referred to as hypertrophic obstructive cardiomyopathy (HOCM), asymmetric septal hypertrophy (ASH), and idiopathic subaortic stenosis (IHSS). It is a leading cause of sudden death in the young.

Etiology. HCM is a genetic disorder, affecting 1 in 500 adults in the United States. A sarcomere mutation is present in greater than 50% of those affected. More than nine different genes with numerous mutations have been implicated; however, 80% have a mutation in either MYH7 or MYBPC3. There is variable genetic penetrance and a consequent spectrum of disease severity. It is slightly more common in males than females and is the leading cause of sudden death in young athletes.

Pathophysiology. In HCM, the left ventricle is asymmetrically hypertrophied, which is different from the concentric hypertrophic changes that occur because of hypertension. There is misalignment and disarray of myofibrils and myocytes. Fibrotic changes and microvascular disease changes are present in the myocardium. The interventricular septum is the region of greatest hypertrophic change. The left ventricle is stiff and noncompliant, creating high diastolic filling pressure.

Obstruction to left ventricular outflow into the aorta is the major hallmark of the disease. Left ventricular outflow obstruction occurs because during systole, the anterior mitral valve leaflet opens against the enlarged interventricular septum. Both the septum and the mitral leaflet obstruct the outflow of blood from the left ventricle into the aorta (see Fig. 18-14). This obstruction causes a cascade of complications including smaller left ventricular chamber size and increased left ventricular systolic pressure. This leads

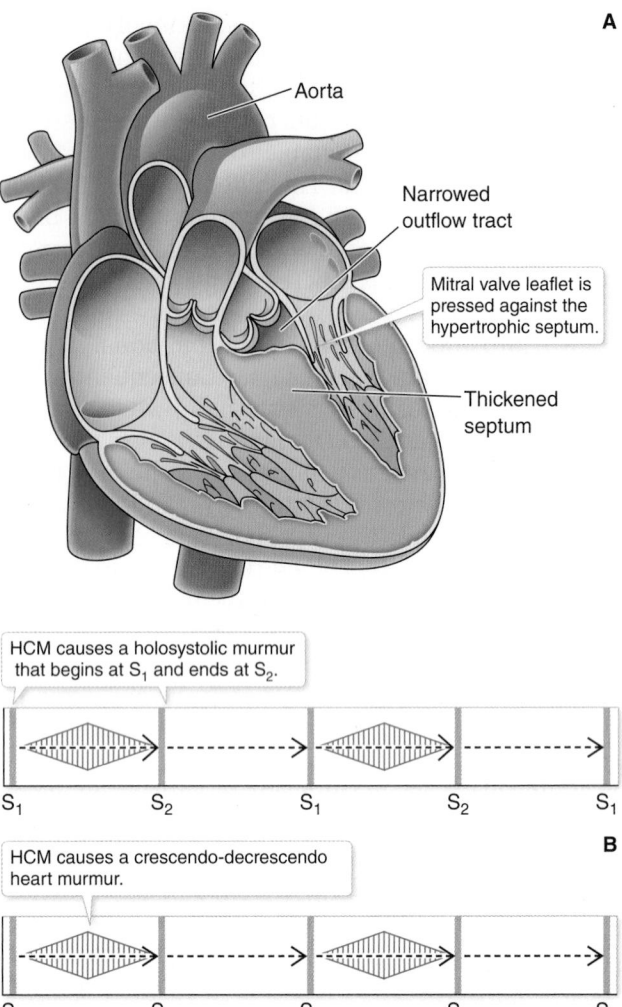

FIGURE 18-14. Hypertrophic cardiomyopathy. (A) In HCM, the interventricular septum is enlarged. When left ventricular contraction occurs, the enlarged septum obstructs blood flow into the aorta. As the left ventricle contracts, one of the leaflets of the mitral valve also obstructs blood flow into the aorta. With obstructed blood flow, the aorta receives decreased blood flow. (B) The heart murmur of HCM is a crescendo-decrescendo holosystolic murmur. It occurs after S_1 during left ventricular contraction as the blood from the ventricle squeezes through the obstruction into the aorta.

to high myocardial wall stress and myocardial oxygen demand, which can cause microvascular ischemia. There is decreased ventricular relaxation, impaired left ventricular filling, and decreased cardiac output.

Obstruction to left ventricular outflow of blood into the aorta is present at rest but worsened by exercise. Conditions such as dehydration and arterial vasodilation can lead to transient hypotensive episodes and syncope.

Patients with HCM have increased susceptibility to both atrial and ventricular dysrhythmias due to focal areas of fibrosis that are similar to scar tissue. It is hypothesized that microinfarctions of the hypertrophied myocardium cause formation of scar tissue. These scar tissue areas can cause conduction interruption and arrhythmias. Common dysrhythmias include atrial fibrillation, isolated premature ventricular contractions (PVCs), nonsustained ventricular tachycardia (NSVT) to sustained ventricular tachycardia, and ventricular fibrillation. Dysrhythmias can be asymptomatic or can be sufficiently severe to cause hemodynamic collapse, embolic stroke, and sudden cardiac death. Studies show that 88% of persons with HCM sustain isolated PVCs and 31% endure NSVT. Atrial fibrillation is four- to six-fold higher than in people of similar age in the general population. Atrial fibrillation, which is a quivering, noncontracting left atrium, is particularly problematic because it diminishes the "atrial kick" of blood into the left ventricle. Lack of atrial kick decreases left ventricular filling and reduces cardiac output. Therefore, one of the primary concerns of clinicians in the evaluation of patients with HCM is presence of dysrhythmias and their clinical consequences. Patients can also experience systolic and diastolic dysfunction, mitral regurgitation, and myocardial ischemia. Atrial fibrillation predisposes to thrombus formation in the left atrium. A thrombus in the left atrium can travel into the left ventricle, then into the aorta and arterial circulation. This increases susceptibility for a thrombus to travel into the cerebral circulation and cause ischemic stroke.

Clinical Presentation. Many patients with HCM are asymptomatic, and there is no associated hypertension or aortic valve deformity. However, this disorder can cause sudden death in children, adolescents, and young adults, often during or after physical exertion. Ventricular dysrhythmias, which are associated with HCM, are commonly the cause of death. Trained athletes with HCM may have no symptoms before sudden cardiac arrest during strenuous exercise. In symptomatic patients, the most common complaints are palpitations, dyspnea, chest pain, fatigue, dizziness, and syncope. Patients with dysrhythmias may have an irregular pulse.

Severe HCM causes a harsh, diamond-shaped systolic murmur, which begins after S_1 and is heard best at the lower left sternal border and apex. Ejection of blood flow is usually impeded in late systole, and the murmur occurs after a clear S_1 is heard. HCM may be accompanied by mitral insufficiency, which causes a holosystolic murmur.

Diagnosis. Echocardiography, color Doppler flow studies, CT, and MRI of the heart are performed to diagnose HCM. The hallmarks of the obstruction of HCM consist of systolic anterior motion of the anterior mitral valve leaflet, septal wall thickness of greater than 15 mm, and asymmetrical septal hypertrophy. Echocardiography also reveals diastolic dysfunction with decreased elasticity of the left ventricle. Systolic function is normal, and the LVEF may be high at the time of diagnosis. However, the left ventricular diameter is usually smaller than normal. A cardiac catheterization is useful to show the extent of outflow obstruction, hemodynamics within the atria and

ventricles, the characteristics of the left ventricle, and coronary artery anatomy. ECG and Holter monitoring for 48 hours are needed to study the electrical activity of the heart.

Treatment. Strenuous exercise is contraindicated in HCM. Medications usually include beta blockers and calcium channel blockers to decrease blood pressure and work of the heart. Beta blockers, nondihydropyridine calcium channel blockers (e.g., verapamil), or the two drugs in combination may be used to control the ventricular rate. Digitalis should be avoided, as well as nitrates, unless there is coronary artery disease. Sympathetic stimulants are avoided because of their effect of increasing heart rate. Anticoagulant treatment for atrial fibrillation is necessary. Cardioversion and/or catheter ablation may be needed for atrial fibrillation.

Surgical removal of excess septal muscle (septal or left ventricular myomectomy) via a thoracotomy can be performed. Septal myomectomy is highly effective with a greater than 90% relief of obstruction and improvement in symptoms. Transcatheter septal myocardial ablation, also referred to as alcohol septal ablation (ASA) or nonsurgical septal reduction therapy, can be performed as part of a cardiac catheterization procedure. Alcohol is injected into the area of septal hypertrophy to create a localized infarction, and septal remodeling occurs over time with widening of the left ventricular outflow tract. Replacement of the mitral valve may be necessary. Pacemaker insertion or an implantable cardioverter-defibrillator may be recommended because some patients are susceptible to ventricular arrhythmias. Septal myomectomy involves the discomfort and longer recovery time associated with open heart surgery, as opposed to the less invasive catheter-based therapy in ASA. In patients who are at higher risk for open heart surgery because of other comorbidities, ASA poses less overall risk. However, septal myomectomy can address other concomitant cardiovascular problems at the time of the procedure, such as mitral valve problems, coronary artery disease, and atrial arrhythmias.

Aortic Insufficiency

Aortic insufficiency (aortic regurgitation) is the incomplete closure of the aortic valve, which allows backward leakage of blood from the aorta into the left ventricle during diastole. Aortic insufficiency can be an acute or chronic disorder. Studies estimate the prevalence of aortic insufficiency as 5% in the population. It is more common in men than women. The incidence and severity of aortic insufficiency increases with age, peaking at 40 to 60 years.

Etiology. In the United States, acute aortic insufficiency is due to endocarditis and dissection of the aorta. Chronic aortic insufficiency is commonly due to aortic root dilation, congenital bicuspid aortic valve, and calcific valve disease. In undeveloped countries,

RF is the major cause of aortic insufficiency. Other causes include Marfan's syndrome, ankylosing spondylitis, long-term hypertension, syphilitic aortitis, and temporal and Takayasu's arteritis.

Pathophysiology. In aortic insufficiency, the aortic valve leaflets cannot remain closed due to deformity. As a result, after the left ventricle pumps its blood volume into the aorta, there is backflow of blood into the left ventricle from the incompetent aortic valve. When aortic insufficiency is severe, the regurgitant backflow of blood can cause volume overload in the left ventricle. As left ventricular end-diastolic volume increases, the left ventricle becomes dilated and loses contractile ability. As a result, stroke volume and LVEF can diminish, and the patient will start to show signs of left ventricular failure.

In advanced stages, there is an overloaded left ventricle with backward buildup of hydrostatic pressure into the left atrium, pulmonary veins, and pulmonary capillaries. Pulmonary edema can occur in severe cases. Volume overload within the pulmonary vasculature occurs, which, in turn, raises pressure within the pulmonary artery, leading to increased resistance against the right ventricle. The right ventricle then fails because of intense resistance.

Both left and right ventricular failure can occur in aortic insufficiency. In severe aortic insufficiency, the left ventricle can be stretched and dilated, causing the heart to become extremely large and overdistended. This enlarged myocardial muscle can eventually exceed coronary artery supply, causing myocardial ischemia. The patient then suffers angina pectoris and possibly MI.

Clinical Presentation. The murmur of aortic insufficiency is best heard in the third intercostal space along the left sternal border with the patient in the seated position, leaning forward. It is typically a high-pitched, blowing, decrescendo diastolic murmur. It is heard after the aortic valve closes at S_2.

During systole, S_1 is heard because of closure of the atrioventricular valves and the open aortic valve. During diastole, the ventricles are filling with blood and the aortic valve closes to produce an audible S_2. The regurgitant backflow from the aortic valve into the left ventricle is heard in diastole, after or coinciding with S_2. The backflow of blood can either continue until S_1 or cease before S_1 (see Fig. 18-15).

Another kind of sound, termed an Austin Flint murmur, can be heard in severe aortic insufficiency. This is a soft, low-pitched, rumbling, middiastolic bruit produced by regurgitant blood flow from the aorta, which disrupts the anterior mitral valve leaflet. This occurs when there is a large amount of regurgitant blood flowing into the left ventricle when the aortic valve should be closed, but is incompletely sealed, during diastole.

In advanced stages of aortic insufficiency, there is both left and right ventricular failure with symptoms

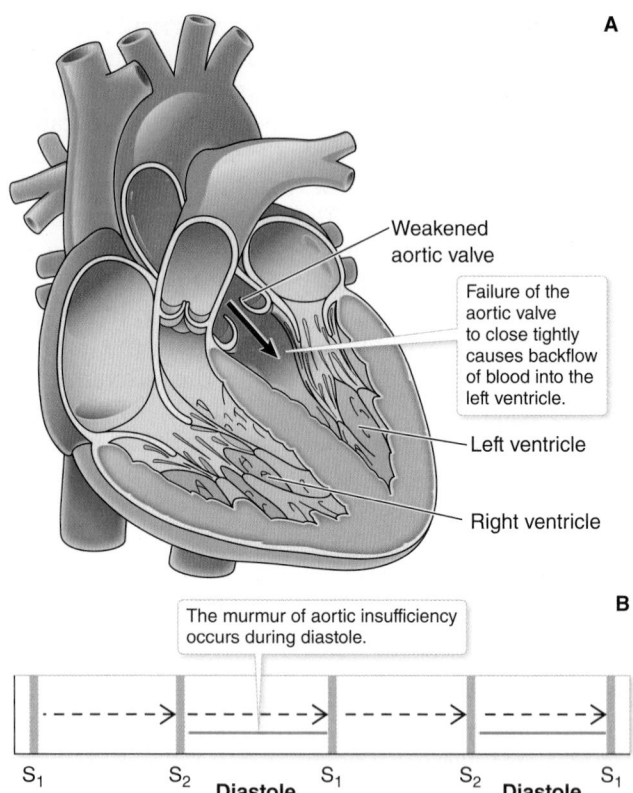

A

Weakened aortic valve

Failure of the aortic valve to close tightly causes backflow of blood into the left ventricle.

Left ventricle

Right ventricle

B

The murmur of aortic insufficiency occurs during diastole.

S_1 S_2 **Diastole** S_1 S_2 **Diastole** S_1

FIGURE 18-15. Aortic insufficiency. (A) In aortic insufficiency, the aortic valve is weak and does not close completely. In diastole, the aortic valve should be tightly closed. However, in diastole, as the left ventricle is filling with blood, the aorta leaks blood back into the ventricle. (B) The heart murmur of aortic insufficiency occurs after S_2 when the aortic valve should be closed. After S_2, there is a sound of the leakage of blood back into the left ventricle from the aorta.

such as orthopnea, paroxysmal dyspnea, diaphoresis, hepatomegaly, ascites, and peripheral edema.

In aortic insufficiency, the left ventricular impulse can often be visible through the chest wall and is usually displaced laterally and inferiorly. A diastolic thrill is often palpable along the left sternal border, and a systolic thrill may be palpable in the jugular notch of the sternum up toward the carotid arteries.

Diagnosis. Echocardiography is the major diagnostic test. Transthoracic echocardiogram is usually performed first, followed by transesophageal echocardiography. TEE can demonstrate more detail regarding valvular deformity. Color Doppler flow studies can visualize the retrograde jet of blood flow. A color jet area or jet width greater than 65% of left ventricular outflow tract (LVOT) diameter or area is indicative of severe aortic insufficiency. The regurgitant volume is greater than 60 mL/beat in severe aortic insufficiency. Both cardiac computed tomography (CCT) and cardiac magnetic resonance (CMR) imaging can provide important data regarding valve morphology and left ventricular function, dimensions, and volumes, as well as quantification of regurgitant volume and fraction. ECG commonly shows left ventricular hypertrophy. Chest x-ray shows the heart apex displaced downward and to the left in the frontal view. In lateral view, the left ventricle is displaced posteriorly toward the spine. When needed, right and left cardiac catheterization with contrast angiography can provide information about the magnitude of regurgitation and left ventricular function. Laboratory studies that pertain to the etiology of the valvular disorder, such as blood cultures in infectious endocarditis, should also be done. Exercise testing is useful to determine whether asymptomatic patients are symptomatic with stress of activity, and when patients have equivocal symptoms and borderline LV function and dimension.

Treatment. Aortic valve replacement is the main treatment for severe aortic insufficiency within 24 hours of diagnosis. For symptomatic patients with severe aortic insufficiency, medical treatment includes ACE inhibitor or ARB therapy because these medications decrease angiotensin's effect on the left ventricle. Angiotensin is found to cause structural remodeling of the left ventricle, leading to hypertrophy. Diuretics can decrease blood volume and stress on the left ventricle. Nitrates and hydralazine are vasodilators that can decrease the intensity of aortic regurgitation and improve left ventricular function. Nifedipine, a calcium antagonist, can decrease left ventricle wall stress and improve LVEF. Long-term medical management of aortic insufficiency is inadequate, as lifesaving treatment requires surgery. Aortic valve replacement is usually recommended; however, aortic valve repair may be possible in some cases. It may be possible to reduce regurgitation by narrowing the valve annulus or excising a portion of the aortic root without replacing the valve.

In most cases, surgical implantation of a mechanical or bioprosthetic aortic valve is performed. Transcatheter aortic valve implantation is not recommended for patients with severe aortic insufficiency. Mechanical valves are more durable but require long-term anticoagulation because of increased risk of thrombosis. Bioprosthetic valves are less durable and can deteriorate over time but avoid the need for long-term anticoagulation.

Pulmonic Valve Disorders

The pulmonic valve is not a common site of pathology, but it is associated with disorders such as pulmonary stenosis and pulmonary insufficiency. Pulmonic valve disorders can be caused by pulmonary hypertension, congenital heart disease, or carcinoid syndrome. The pulmonary valve is rarely affected by rheumatic heart disease.

Pulmonic Stenosis

Pulmonic stenosis is a narrowing of the pulmonic valve, the entrance to the pulmonary artery from the right ventricle.

Epidemiology and Etiology. It can occur in congenital heart disease known as tetralogy of Fallot, which occurs in 3 out of 10,000 live births. Pulmonic stenosis is also part of Noonan syndrome, which is a rare genetic disorder caused by a mutation in the PTPN1 gene at chromosome 12. Other causes include carcinoid syndrome, which is caused by a neuroendocrine tumor that releases excessive serotonin. Carcinoid tumors are most commonly located in the intestine or lung and occur in 3 out of 100,000 persons. Congenital rubella syndrome (CRS) can also cause pulmonic stenosis. CRS is uncommon, however, given the widespread use of measles, mumps, rubella vaccine. Pulmonic stenosis can also be benign without symptoms and without progression of disease.

Pathophysiology. In severe pulmonic stenosis, blood must squeeze through the restrictive opening into the pulmonary artery during systole. Right ventricular ejection is prolonged, and there is usually a delay in the closure of the pulmonic valve, causing a late P_2 component of S_2. The murmur is usually a harsh, systolic, crescendo-decrescendo sound heard best at the second intercostal space, left sternal border; this is commonly preceded by a systolic ejection sound. Pulmonic stenosis can cause high workload for the right ventricle leading to right ventricular failure. With right ventricular failure, the right atrium and ventricle enlarge and the patient experiences symptoms such as jugular venous distention, ascites, hepatomegaly, splenomegaly, and peripheral edema.

Diagnosis. Diagnosis involves use of echocardiography, ECG, cardiac catheterization, and pulmonary angiogram. Transthoracic echocardiography usually allows definitive diagnosis, showing the jet blood flow through the narrowed pulmonic valve and low pulmonary artery pressure. Transesophageal echocardiography may be better able to show details of the right ventricular outflow. ECG shows right axis deviation due to right ventricular hypertrophy and right atrial enlargement. Cardiac catheterization can demonstrate the pressures that are below and above the pulmonic valve.

Treatment. Medical treatment to diminish the effects of right ventricular failure includes diuretics and ACE inhibitors. Percutaneous balloon valvotomy to widen the pulmonic valve via a catheter is the most commonly recommended treatment. Surgical pulmonic valve replacement (SPVR), which is open heart surgery, has been the mainstay for patients with a dysplastic valve due to congenital heart disease. Transcatheter pulmonic valve implantation (TPVI) procedures are evolving and have been effective in managing patients with right ventricular outflow obstruction.

Pulmonic Insufficiency

Epidemiology and Etiology. The most common disease affecting the pulmonic valve is pulmonary insufficiency (also called pulmonary regurgitation). Mild pulmonary insufficiency is commonly encountered in adolescents and is considered benign. There are usually no symptoms and the patient may have a slight heart murmur.

Pulmonary insufficiency is also a disease of adults due to pulmonary hypertension, which is high blood pressure within the pulmonary arterial vasculature. Primary pulmonary hypertension is uncommon, affecting 15 to 50 persons per million within the United States. However, secondary pulmonary hypertension is more common. Lung diseases that cause chronic hypoxia often cause secondary pulmonary hypertension. Chronic hypoxia stimulates pulmonary arteriolar vasoconstriction, which in turn causes high pressure in the pulmonary artery. Chronic obstructive pulmonary disease (COPD) is an example of a disease that causes pulmonary hypertension. Other causes of pulmonary insufficiency are congenital heart disease, endocarditis, RHD, and carcinoid syndrome. Anorexogenic medications such as fenfluramine/phentermine can also cause pulmonary hypertension. Pulmonary insufficiency can also occur years after persons undergo percutaneous balloon valvotomy for pulmonary stenosis. For example, many patients develop pulmonary insufficiency after childhood surgery for tetralogy of Fallot up to 20 years later.

Because of the most common etiologies, prevalence of pulmonary insufficiency is thought to have two demographic peaks, first in young patients with repaired congenital pulmonary stenosis or benign pulmonary regurgitation, and second in older adult patients with pulmonary arterial hypertension.

Pathophysiology. In pulmonary insufficiency, the pulmonic valve is incompetent and does not close completely. Incomplete closure of the pulmonic valve causes regurgitation of pulmonary artery blood back into the right ventricle during diastole. The right ventricle becomes overloaded, and this causes backward pressure into the right atrium and vena cava, then into the venous system. Signs of right-sided heart failure are common. These include jugular venous distention, ascites, hepatomegaly, splenomegaly, and ankle or sacral edema. The right ventricle and right atrium enlarge and may sustain dysrhythmias. The overload in the right ventricle can lead to tricuspid valve incompetence. The murmur of pulmonary insufficiency produced by regurgitant blood flow is referred to as a Graham Steell murmur; it is a high-pitched, decrescendo, blowing diastolic murmur heard best at the second intercostal space, left sternal border, coinciding with or following S_2.

Diagnosis. Diagnosis involves use of color transthoracic Doppler echocardiography, CMR, ECG, and cardiac CT scan. Transthoracic Doppler echocardiography can demonstrate pulmonic valve structure and function. CMR can show the right side of the heart in greater detail and precise assessment of right ventricular volumes and function. ECG will show findings of right axis deviation in accordance with right atrial and ventricular enlargement. Cardiac stress testing and cardiac catheterization may be needed.

Treatment. Valve replacement and medical treatment for right-sided heart failure are recommended. Pharmacological vasodilator medications and diuretics can be used as medical treatment for pulmonary hypertension. Pulmonary artery vasodilators include phosphodiesterase-5 inhibitors such as sildenafil, endothelin receptor blockers such as bosentan, or prostacyclins such as epoprostenol. Transcatheter pulmonic valve implantation is recommended to replace the pulmonic valve. Bioprosthetic valves are preferred to mechanical valves in pulmonic insufficiency, but either can be used. Aspirin or anticoagulant treatment may be necessary with right atrial enlargement and dysrhythmias, regardless of the type of valve implanted.

Tricuspid Valve Disorders

Tricuspid valve disorders include tricuspid stenosis and insufficiency. These are the least common valve disorders. Because the tricuspid valve is located between the right atrium and right ventricle, it comes in contact with venous blood. Persons who use intravenous drugs can cause injection of bacteria into the venous circulation, and this can affect the tricuspid valve. Infectious endocarditis (IE) due to intravenous drug use or intravenous catheters is a common cause of tricuspid valve disease. Rheumatic heart disease is also a cause of tricuspid valve disorders; it commonly coexists with mitral valve disease.

Tricuspid Stenosis
Epidemiology and Etiology. Tricuspid stenosis can be due to rheumatic heart disease (RHD), infective endocarditis (IE), carcinoid syndrome, systemic lupus erythematosus (SLE), antiphospholipid antibody (APLA) syndrome, atrial myxomas, blunt trauma, metastasis of renal or ovarian tumors, congenital abnormalities, Fabry's disease, Whipple's disease, intravenous leiomyomatosis, ventriculoatrial shunts, and valvulopathy associated with drugs like fenfluramine/phentermine and methysergide.

Tricuspid stenosis is uncommon, causing 2.4% of all valvular disease. It is more common in women than men.

Tricuspid stenosis is mainly a sequela of RHD or IE. It is most commonly seen in IV drug abusers with IE. Staphylococcal organisms inhabit the skin, and needle puncture allows the organisms to invade the venous bloodstream, which empties into the right side of the heart. The infection is then within the bloodstream (sepsis) and affects the tricuspid valve. Staphylococcal emboli can develop and enter the lungs via the right ventricle and pulmonary artery.

Pathophysiology. Normal area of the tricuspid valve is 4.0 cm^2 and area less than 1.0 cm^2 is deemed severe tricuspid stenosis. In tricuspid stenosis, narrowing of the tricuspid valve hinders the free flow of blood from the right atrium into the right ventricle during diastole. During diastole, the tricuspid valve should be open and allow filling of the right ventricle. With obstructed outflow into the right ventricle, hydrostatic pressure builds in the right atrium and backward into the venous system.

High hydrostatic pressure builds in the superior and inferior vena cava, evidenced by peritoneal, hepatic, and splenic congestion and peripheral edema. High pressure in the superior vena cava is demonstrated by jugular vein distention, which appears as bulging, blue, enlarged veins in the neck. Peripheral edema is demonstrated by ascites, hepatomegaly, splenomegaly, and ankle or sacral edema.

Clinical Manifestations. The lungs are clear in patients with isolated tricuspid stenosis because the disease mainly affects the right side of the heart. However, in many patients there is combined mitral stenosis and tricuspid stenosis, which can cause pulmonary edema and crackles. The murmur of mitral stenosis can obscure the murmur of tricuspid stenosis.

On auscultation of the chest in isolated tricuspid stenosis, a low-frequency presystolic middiastolic murmur is heard at the lower-left sternal border in the fourth intercostal space. The murmur is heard as the blood squeezes through the narrowed tricuspid valve during filling of the right ventricle (diastole) after S_2. An opening snap of the narrowed tricuspid valve may be heard early in diastole after S_2 over the left-lower sternal border. The murmur is accentuated with inspiration because with chest expansion, there is distention and decreased resistance within the pulmonary arteries, which diminishes resistance against the right ventricle.

Diagnosis. ECG, echocardiography, and blood cultures are used in diagnosis. ECG commonly shows evidence of right atrial enlargement: prominent, peaked P waves. On transthoracic echocardiogram, the tricuspid valve is usually thickened and assumes a dome shape during diastole. The tricuspid valve area is diminished. The right atrium and inferior vena cava are enlarged. Cardiac catheterization is not routinely necessary. Blood cultures are necessary because infective endocarditis is a common cause of tricuspid valve disease.

Treatment. Persons with tricuspid stenosis exhibit marked venous congestion. Medical treatment includes salt restriction and diuretics. Surgery is commonly carried out to treat tricuspid stenosis because mitral valve disease is commonly present concurrently. Also tricuspid stenosis is almost always associated with some tricuspid regurgitation. Surgical valve repair or valve replacement is usually indicated. Transcatheter valve replacement is an option. Bioprosthetic valves are commonly used to replace tricuspid valves. Mechanical valves in the tricuspid position are more prone to thromboembolic complications than in other positions. Anticoagulants, mainly warfarin, are necessary with mechanical valves. Antibiotic medications are necessary if endocarditis is the origin of the valvular disease.

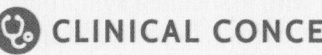

CLINICAL CONCEPT

Tricuspid valve abnormalities are commonly caused by infectious endocarditis due to illicit IV drug use.

Tricuspid Insufficiency

Epidemiology. Tricuspid insufficiency (also called tricuspid regurgitation) is increasing due to the aging of the population. Up to 5.6% of women and 1.5% of men have clinically significant tricuspid insufficiency by their eighth decade. Previously thought to be a benign disease, tricuspid insufficiency is often not diagnosed and not treated. It is a prevalent but underrecognized disease in the population, particularly in patients with left ventricular failure and atrial fibrillation. It is often undiagnosed but has a high mortality rate in untreated and treated individuals. A recent study reported a 42% mortality rate in untreated persons during a median follow-up of 2.9 years (Prihadi et al., 2018).

Etiology. Tricuspid insufficiency commonly occurs because of dilation of the tricuspid valve annulus, which hinders complete closure of the valve leaflets. It can be caused by several disorders, including right ventricular infarction, RF, IE, congenital heart disease, cardiomyopathy, pulmonary hypertension, and cor pulmonale.

Ebstein's anomaly is a congenital disorder that causes displacement of the tricuspid valve leaflets downward into the right ventricle. The tricuspid valve is placed low in the right ventricle, creating a small right ventricular chamber and large right atrium. Ebstein's anomaly commonly causes tricuspid insufficiency, atrial dysrhythmias, and right ventricular dysfunction.

Pathophysiology. Tricuspid insufficiency occurs because a loose tricuspid valve allows blood flow to back up from the right ventricle into the right atrium during systole.

The blood flow that backs up from the right ventricle into the right atrium causes distention and dilation of the right atrium. With stretching of the right atrial wall, the sinoatrial node and conductive tissue are disrupted and atrial fibrillation can develop. With time, volume overload of the right atrium and right ventricle causes right ventricular failure and associated symptoms. In right ventricular failure, venous congestion causes jugular venous distention, ascites, hepatomegaly, splenomegaly, and ankle or sacral edema.

Clinical Manifestations. Tricuspid insufficiency often coexists with left-sided heart valve lesions, left ventricular dysfunction, or pulmonary hypertension. Therefore, symptoms related to left-sided heart disease may dominate the clinical picture. Fatigue and exertional dyspnea due to decreased cardiac output are early symptoms of tricuspid insufficiency. As the disease worsens, the patient may experience worsening right-sided heart failure with associated symptoms of jugular venous distention, ascites, hepatic and splenic congestion, and ankle edema. The neck veins are particularly prominent. A prominent right ventricular pulsation in the left parasternal border may be seen.

The S_1 sound is created by the closure of the tricuspid and mitral valves. However, with incomplete closure of loose tricuspid valve leaflets in tricuspid insufficiency, a holosystolic murmur is heard that may make S_1 inaudible. The murmur is heard best along the left-lower sternal border, and a right ventricular thrill may be palpable along the sternal border on the chest wall. As with tricuspid stenosis, the murmur of tricuspid insufficiency is accentuated with inspiration because expansion of the thoracic cage allows increased venous return. The murmur of triscuspid insufficiency is often confused with mitral insufficiency.

Diagnosis. ECG, echocardiography, cardiac catheterization, and blood cultures are used in diagnosis. Blood cultures are necessary because IE is common. ECG may show evidence of past MI of the right ventricle, right atrial enlargement, right ventricular hypertrophy, or right bundle branch block. Atrial fibrillation is frequently noted. Transthoracic echocardiogram usually shows right atrial dilation; right ventricular overload; and prolapsing, displaced tricuspid valve leaflets. Real-time, 3D, color flow Doppler imaging is best used for visualizing the right side of the heart. CMR provides a more detailed image of the disease process.

A large number of patients with tricuspid insufficiency are illicit IV drug users. Vein puncture with unsterile needles frequently leads to infective endocarditis and blood infection (sepsis), particularly with staphylococcal microorganisms. Staphylococcal pulmonary emboli can be visualized on chest x-ray.

Antibiotic therapy is needed for infective endocarditis or sepsis. Diuretics are used to decrease volume overload in right ventricular failure. If pulmonary hypertension has caused the disorder, the goal is to reduce pressure in the pulmonary arterial circulation. Phosphodiesterase-5 (PDE5) inhibitors, such as sildenafil or tadalafil, decrease pulmonary arterial pressure. Milrinone, a selective phosphodiesterase-3 (PDE3) inhibitor, can improve contractility of the right ventricle and facilitate pulmonary vasodilation. There is a debate currently in the literature about the benefits of medical management versus surgical intervention. Surgical intervention for tricuspid valve repair is generally recommended. However, transcatheter tricuspid valve implantation is a procedure that is currently evolving and under study.

Chapter Summary

- Heart valves are structures composed of fibrous tissue covered by endothelial cardiac tissue.
- Heart valves direct the blood through the heart and great vessels.
- Heart valves can be damaged or deformed because of genetic disorders, infectious agents, RHD, MI, the aging process, and atherosclerosis.
- RHD rheumatic heart disease, a past common cause of valvular heart disease, was due to streptococcal disease. With the advent of antibiotics, streptococcal disease has diminished as a cause of RHD in developed countries.
- In underdeveloped and developing countries, RHD is still prevalent as a cause of valvular heart disease.
- Dysfunctional valvular consequences of RHD are commonly present many years later.
- A heart murmur is auscultated due to turbulent blood flow created by valvular heart disease.
- A heart murmur is the classic auscultatory finding indicative of valvular heart disease; it is described according to its occurrence in the cardiac cycle, volume, pitch, and location of auscultation on the chest wall.
- Currently, the most common valvular heart disorders affect the mitral and aortic valves.
- Aortic sclerosis is calcification of the aortic valve; it causes aortic stenosis and is common in older adults with atherosclerosis.
- Mitral insufficiency is a valvular disorder secondary to myocardial infarction that is common in adults suffering ischemic heart disease.
- Mitral annular calcification is also a common disorder causing mitral stenosis in older adults.
- Mitral valve prolapse is a common benign valvular disorder in adults, particularly females.
- There are classic landmarks on the chest wall where the sounds of specific heart valves can be heard best. The classic landmarks include aortic valve, R 2nd ICS RSB; pulmonic valve, L 2nd ICS LSB; Erb's point, 3rd ICS LSB; tricuspid valve, 4th ICS LCB; and mitral, 5th ICS MCL.

- Echocardiography is the method of choice to precisely diagnose valvular disease. TTE or TEE procedures can be done. Real-time 3D color Doppler flow echocardiographic studies are often used. Cardiac CT scan and cardiac magnetic resonance (CMR) are valuable tools that can avoid cardiac catheterization in some cases of valvular disease assessment.

- Damaged valves can cause a variety of complications, including blood flow turbulence and stasis, heart chamber pressure changes, arrhythmias, thrombi formation, heart failure, and sepsis.

- Stenotic valves are narrowed and restrict blood flow, whereas insufficient valves do not close completely, allowing regurgitant blood flow.

- HCM is the most common cause of sudden death of young athletes. It is often undiagnosed until the extreme stress and strain of athletic competition occurs.

- The excess tissue of the septum in HCM can be surgically reduced or ablated using injectable alcohol.

- IE in illicit IV drug users commonly causes tricuspid valvular dysfunction. Staphylococcus infective endocarditis can occur due to transfer of microorganisms from the skin into the venous system. Infective endocarditis can also cause pulmonary staphylococci emboli.

- Before any invasive procedure such as dental treatment or catheter placement, most patients with a valvular disorder should have antibiotics administered to prevent possible endocarditis and septicemia.

- Deformed natural valves and mechanical valves require anticoagulation, as these valves can develop thrombi.

- Bioprosthetic valves are made of porcine, bovine, or cadaver tissue and do not usually require anticoagulation.

- Bioprosthetic valves commonly require reoperation and replacement after 10 years.

- Surgical valve replacement, repair, or percutaneous balloon valvotomy are common procedures used for patients with valve disorders. Surgical valvular replacement requires open heart surgery. Transcatheter valve replacement is often performed and is less complicated than open heart surgery.

 Making the Connections

Disorder and Pathophysiology

Signs and Symptoms	Physical Assessment Findings	Diagnostic Testing	Treatment
Mitral Stenosis | Narrowed mitral valve opening; blood flow hindered from left atrium into left ventricle during diastole. Left atrial pressure builds and backs up into pulmonary veins to pulmonary capillaries, causing pulmonary edema.			
Dyspnea, cough, fatigue, orthopnea, PND.	Opening snap, diastolic murmur fifth intercostal space, left sternal border, after S_2 before S_1. If severe, bibasilar pulmonary crackles.	Transthoracic echocardiogram (TTE) or transeophageal echocardiogram (TEE) showing narrowed mitral valve; may show left atrial enlargement from backflow of blood. Real-time 3D Doppler color echocardiography provides best details if applicable. Stress echocardiography is often used in asymptomatic patients with valvular disease. ECG may show atrial fibrillation caused by enlarged left atrium. Cardiac CT (CCT) and cardiac magnetic resonance (CMR) imaging can provide best details and often avoid cardiac catheterization.	Oxygen. Anticoagulation to prevent clot formation in enlarged, stretched left atrium. Heart failure medications such as diuretics, ACE inhibitors, digitalis, or beta blockers. Surgical valve replacement, percutaneous balloon valvotomy, or transcatheter valvular implantation.

Continued

Making the Connections–cont'd

Signs and Symptoms	Physical Assessment Findings	Diagnostic Testing	Treatment

Mitral Insufficiency | Incompetent mitral valve leaflets that cannot close; during systolic contraction of left ventricle, blood regurgitates up into the left atrium. Left ventricular ejection is decreased, and backup of blood into the left atrium, pulmonary veins, and pulmonary capillaries occurs, which causes pulmonary edema. Aortic blood volume is diminished, as is blood volume entering coronary arteries. Myocardial ischemia results. Mitral insufficiency is the most common heart valve disorder that occurs with MI; papillary muscle rupture causes loosened valve leaflets.

Signs and Symptoms	Physical Assessment Findings	Diagnostic Testing	Treatment
Dyspnea, cough, fatigue, orthopnea, PND. Chest pain (angina).	Holosystolic murmur, fifth intercostal space, left sternal border, radiating into the axilla. S_3 may be heard. If severe, bibasilar pulmonary crackles heard. Pallor, diaphoresis, respiratory distress, fatigue, and exercise intolerance. Left atrial enlargement can lead to atrial fibrillation; irregular pulse.	TTE or TEE echocardiogram showing regurgitant mitral valve leaflets; may show left atrial and ventricular enlargement. LVEF and cardiac output (CO) can be reduced with subsequent heart failure. Real-time 3D Doppler color echocardiography provides details if applicable. Stress echocardiography is often used in asymptomatic patients with valvular disease. ECG may show atrial fibrillation. Cardiac CT (CCT) and cardiac magnetic resonance (CMR) imaging can provide best details and often avoid cardiac catheterization.	Oxygen. Anticoagulation to prevent clot formation in the left atrium. Heart failure medications such as diuretics, ACE inhibitors, digitalis, and beta blockers. Coronary artery disease medications such as oxygen, morphine, and nitrates if myocardial ischemia. Surgical valve replacement; open heart, percutaneous route, or transcatheter valve replacement. Mitral clip: noninvasive catheter insertion if surgery not an option.

Mitral Valve Prolapse | A disorder caused by a myxomatous degeneration of one or both mitral valve leaflets that makes them floppy. One or both mitral valve leaflets occasionally prolapse into the left atrium during systolic contraction of the left ventricle, allowing for some regurgitation of blood flow up into the left atrium.

Signs and Symptoms	Physical Assessment Findings	Diagnostic Testing	Treatment
Asymptomatic in many affected persons; some persons experience fatigue, dizziness, palpitations, and anxiety. If severe, ischemic chest pain, dyspnea, and fatigue occur.	Midsystolic or late systolic murmur heard after a midsystolic click at left lower sternal border.	TTE or TEE. Echocardiogram showing regurgitant mitral valve leaflet; may show left atrial and ventricular enlargement. Real-time 3D Doppler color echocardiography provides details if applicable. Stress echocardiography is often used in asymptomatic patients with valvular disease if there are indications. Cardiac CT (CCT) and cardiac magnetic resonance (CMR) imaging can provide best details and often avoid cardiac catheterization.	Commonly, no treatment is necessary. Patient education and reassurance that it is benign. Patient should refrain from caffeine, nicotine, and alcohol and any stimulants. Magnesium supplements may be necessary. If dysrhythmia is present, valve replacement can be done.

Making the Connections–cont'd

Signs and Symptoms	Physical Assessment Findings	Diagnostic Testing	Treatment

Aortic Stenosis | Narrowed aortic valve opening; blood flow hindered from fully ejecting into aorta from left ventricle; coronary arteries suffer lack of sufficient blood flow. Aortic blood flow is low and may diminish blood flow to cerebral arteries. Left ventricle can also fail because of high resistance of aortic opening. Aortic sclerosis, which is calcification of the valve due to aging, commonly causes aortic stenosis.

Signs and Symptoms	Physical Assessment Findings	Diagnostic Testing	Treatment
Chest pain (angina pectoris), fatigue, exertional dyspnea, exertional syncope (fainting caused by lack of cerebral blood flow).	Systolic ejection murmur, second intercostal space, right sternal border, opening snap, crescendo, low-pitched murmur after S_1 before S_2, split S_2 (P_2 A_2).	TTE or TEE. Echocardiogram showing narrowed aortic valve, left ventricular enlargement, left ventricular hypertrophy caused by excess resistance of aorta against left ventricle. Real-time 3D Doppler color echocardiography provides details. High-sensitivity cardiac troponin blood test. BNP level for heart failure and measurement of LVEF necessary. Cardiac catheterization to measure hemodynamic pressures in heart chambers. Cardiac CT (CCT) and cardiac magnetic resonance (CMR) imaging can provide best details and often avoid cardiac catheterization.	Treatment according to symptoms of angina or heart failure. Anticoagulation to prevent clot formation on valve deformity or left ventricular failure. Surgical valve replacement, percutaneous valvotomy, or transcatheter replacement.

Hypertrophic Cardiomyopathy | Interventricular septum is disproportionately enlarged, the left ventricle is eccentrically hypertrophied, and the anterior mitral leaflet opens against the enlarged septum, creating an obstructed outflow of blood from the left ventricle into the aorta.

Signs and Symptoms	Physical Assessment Findings	Diagnostic Testing	Treatment
Commonly asymptomatic. Atrial fibrillation, premature ventricular contractions, ventricular tachycardia, and ventricular fibrillation can occur. Few patients experience chest pain, dyspnea, and fatigue as warning signs.	Harsh, diamond-shaped systolic murmur; begins after S_1 at the lower left sternal border and apex. Ejection of blood flow is usually unimpeded until late in systole; therefore, the murmur occurs after a clear S_1. If atrial fibrillation is present, irregular pulse, palpitations, dyspnea on exertion, dizziness, and syncope can occur.	TTE and TEE. Echocardiogram shows an enlarged interventricular septum, left ventricular hypertrophy. Real-time 3D Doppler color echocardiography provides details. A 48-hour Holter ECG needed to check for ventricular dysrhythmias. Cardiac CT (CCT) and cardiac magnetic resonance (CMR) imaging can provide best details.	Surgical reduction of the interventricular septum (cardiac myomectomy). Nonsurgical injectable alcohol ablation of the septum is possible. Implantable cardioverter-defibrillator. Medications for angina or for heart failure, depending on patient condition; beta blockers, calcium antagonists can decrease heart rate and heart wall stress. Strenuous exercise should be avoided.

Continued

Making the Connections–cont'd

Signs and Symptoms	Physical Assessment Findings	Diagnostic Testing	Treatment
Aortic Insufficiency | Incompetent aortic valve allows leakage of blood back into left ventricle and possibly left atrium, insufficient blood flow forward into aorta.			
Chest pain (angina pectoris), fatigue, exertional dyspnea, exertional syncope (fainting), cough, dyspnea, PND, and orthopnea. Both right ventricular failure and left ventricular failure can occur in severe aortic insufficiency.	Diastolic murmur, third intercostal space, left sternal border, high-pitched, blowing, decrescendo. If severe, bibasilar pulmonary crackles.	TTE and TEE. Echocardiogram shows regurgitant aortic valve, left ventricular dilation from excess regurgitant blood volume. Real-time 3D Doppler color echocardiography provides details. ECG necessary. Cardiac CT (CCT) and cardiac magnetic resonance (CMR) imaging can provide best details. Cardiac catheterization may be required.	ACE inhibitor or ARB. Nitrates and hydralazine are vasodilators that can decrease the intensity of aortic regurgitation and improve left ventricular function. Nifedipine, a calcium antagonist, can decrease left ventricle wall stress and improve LVEF. Surgical valve replacement or repair or transcatheter valve replacement.
Pulmonic Stenosis | Narrowed pulmonic valve does not allow sufficient blood flow into the pulmonary artery; backup of blood into right ventricle, right ventricle hypertrophies against increased pulmonary artery resistance.			
Fatigue, dyspnea, signs of right ventricular failure; jugular venous distention, ascites, hepatomegaly, splenomegaly, or ankle or sacral edema.	Harsh, systolic, crescendo-decrescendo murmur at the second intercostal space, left sternal border, commonly preceded by a systolic ejection sound, split S_2 with delayed P_2.	TTE or TEE. Echocardiogram showing narrowed pulmonic valve, right ventricular hypertrophy, right ventricular and right atrial dilation from built-up blood, central veins congested. Real-time 3D Doppler color echocardiography provides details. ECG may show atrial fibrillation. Cardiac CT and cardiac magnetic resonance (CMR) imaging can provide best details. Cardiac catheterization may be necessary.	Anticoagulation to prevent clot formation. Heart failure medications. Surgical valve replacement or balloon valvotomy. Transcatheter valvular replacement procedures are currently under investigation.
Pulmonic Insufficiency | Incompetent pulmonic valve allows regurgitant blood flow from pulmonary artery into right ventricle; dilation of the right ventricle and right atrium possible with backup of hydrostatic pressure into the venous system.			
Fatigue, dyspnea, signs of right ventricular failure; jugular venous distention, ascites, hepatomegaly, splenomegaly, or ankle or sacral edema.	Graham Steell murmur; a high-pitched, decrescendo, blowing murmur heard best at the second intercostal space, left sternal border, coinciding with or following S_2.	TTE or TEE. Echocardiogram shows incompetent pulmonic valve, right ventricular and right atrial dilation from built-up blood, central vein congestion. Real-time 3D Doppler color echocardiography provides details. ECG may show atrial fibrillation. Cardiac CT and cardiac magnetic resonance (CMR) imaging can provide best details. Cardiac catheterization may be necessary.	Pharmacological vasodilator medications and diuretics can be used as treatment for pulmonary hypertension. Pulmonary artery vasodilators include phosphodiesterase-5 inhibitors, such as sildenafil, endothelin receptor blockers, such as bosentan, or prostacyclins, such as epoprostenol. Transcatheter pulmonic valve implantation is recommended to replace the pulmonic valve. Bioprosthetic valves are preferred. Anticoagulation to prevent clot formation. Heart failure medications if right ventricular failure present.

Making the Connections–cont'd

Signs and Symptoms	Physical Assessment Findings	Diagnostic Testing	Treatment
Tricuspid Stenosis | Narrowed tricuspid valve hinders free flow of blood into the right ventricle during diastole; blood damming in the right atrium causes high hydrostatic pressure to build backward into the venous system.			
Signs of increased venous pressure, jugular venous distention, ascites, hepatomegaly, splenomegaly, or ankle or sacral edema.	Opening snap after S_2, diastolic murmur over left lower sternal border, inspiration accentuates murmur.	TTE or TEE. Echocardiogram shows narrowed tricuspid valve, right atrial dilation from obstructed blood flow, central veins congested. Real-time 3D Doppler color echocardiography provides details. ECG may show atrial fibrillation. Blood cultures. Cardiac CT and cardiac magnetic resonance (CMR) imaging can provide best details. Cardiac catheterization may be necessary.	Anticoagulation to prevent clot formation. Heart failure medications: diuretics, ACE inhibitors. Surgical valve replacement or repair. Antibiotics if infectious endocarditis.
Tricuspid Insufficiency | Incompetent tricuspid valve does not close during right ventricular contraction, regurgitation of blood flow into the right atrium with each right ventricular contraction; increases backward pressure into the venous system.			
Signs of increased venous pressure, jugular venous distention, ascites, hepatomegaly, splenomegaly, or ankle or sacral edema.	Blowing, holosystolic murmur at lower left sternal border that may obscure S_1, prominent right ventricular pulsation, accentuated murmur with inspiration.	TTE or TEE. Echocardiogram showing incompetent tricuspid valve, right atrial dilation from regurgitant blood flow, central veins congested. Real-time 3D Doppler color echocardiography provides details. ECG may show right atrial fibrillation. Cardiac CT and cardiac magnetic resonance (CMR) imaging can provide best details. Cardiac catheterization may be necessary. Blood cultures.	Diuretics in right ventricular failure. If pulmonary hypertension has caused the disorder, PDE5 inhibitors, such as sildenafil or tadalafil, decrease pulmonary arterial pressure. Milrinone, a selective PDE3 inhibitor, can improve contractility of the right ventricle and facilitate pulmonary vasodilation. Surgical valve replacement. Antibiotics if infective endocarditis.

Bibliography

Available online at fadavis.com

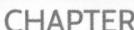
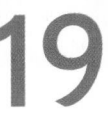
Venous System Disorders

Learning Objectives

Upon completion of this chapter, the student will be able to:

- Differentiate between the acute versus chronic disorders that affect the venous circulation.
- Identify signs and symptoms of venous insufficiency and deep venous thrombus.
- List the risk factors known as Virchow's triad that predispose an individual to deep venous thromboembolism.

- Explain the laboratory tests and procedures used to diagnose venous disorders.
- Describe how a deep venous thrombus evolves into a pulmonary embolism.
- Discuss the treatment modalities used in deep venous thrombus and pulmonary embolism.

Key Terms

D-dimer test

Deep venous thromboembolism (DVT)

Gradient compression stockings

Greenfield filter

Homan's sign

International normalized ratio (INR)

Pneumatic compression device

Pulmonary embolism (PE)

Sclerotherapy

Stasis dermatitis

Varicose veins

Venous ulcer

Ventilation-perfusion scan

Virchow's triad

Wells criteria

Chronic venous disorders of the lower limbs rank among the most common conditions affecting individuals. There is a wide spectrum of disease that varies from asymptomatic, minor varicose veins to disabling deep venous thromboembolism. In contrast to many other chronic conditions, patients often accept venous disease as a slowly progressive condition related to aging and do not seek health care for these disorders. Although venous disease is most common in adults older than age 50 years, immobility at any age increases susceptibility to **deep venous thromboembolism (DVT)**—a potentially fatal disease.

Epidemiology

There are mainly three different types of venous disease: venous insufficiency, DVT, and varicose veins. Venous disease is a common disorder that is more prevalent in females, increases in severity with age, and is a major cause of illness. Between 6% and 30% of all medical expenditures for cardiovascular disease are for venous disease. Chronic venous disease of the legs commonly occurs in the general population and is underreported. Studies estimate that the prevalence of varicose veins, the most common venous disorder, is as high as 56% in males and 60% in females. Venous ulcers are less common, affecting approximately 0.3%

of the adult population. Deep venous thrombosis is one of the most underdiagnosed diseases, but studies estimate it affects 80 persons per 100,000 annually.

Basic Concepts of Venous Structure and Function

Veins are thin-walled, flexible blood vessels that return blood to the heart. Their walls are composed of three layers: tunica intima, which is an endothelial cell lining; tunica media, a thin layer of smooth muscle; and tunica adventitia, an exterior layer of connective tissue (see Fig. 19-1).

There are two systems of veins: (1) superficial, small-diameter veins and (2) deep, large-diameter veins. Perforating veins connect the two systems. Blood from the skin and subcutaneous tissue collects in the superficial veins, which empty into the perforating veins. From the perforating veins, blood travels into the deep veins, which empty into the body's major venous vessels, the inferior and superior vena cava, which empty into the right atrium.

The venous system and right side of the heart are low-pressure regions. Veins do not pump blood as do arteries; instead, they direct blood toward the heart. In the extremities, veins rely on the supportive action of skeletal muscles that help pump the blood toward

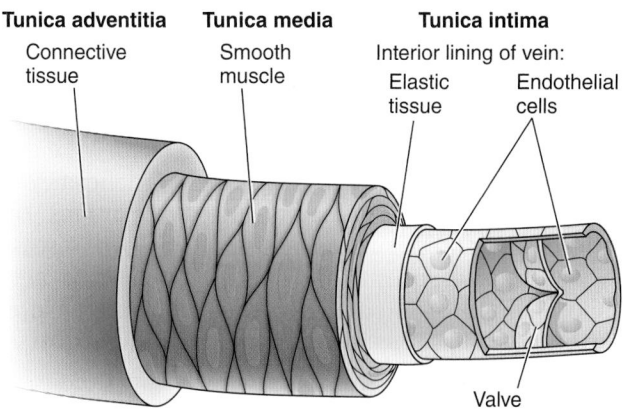

FIGURE 19-1. Anatomy of a vein. A vein is a collapsible, thin-walled vessel. Different from arteries, veins contain a thin wall of smooth muscle and valvular structures.

the heart. When an individual is walking, the gastrocnemius muscle in the calf provides pumping action for venous blood to return to the heart. Also, within the lumen of the veins are valves that prevent retrograde flow of venous blood (see Fig. 19-2).

Veins carry deoxygenated blood back to the right side of the heart and into the pulmonary artery, moving to the lungs for oxygenation. The exception to this rule occurs in the pulmonary veins and pulmonary artery. Pulmonary veins carry oxygenated blood from the lungs to the left atrium. The pulmonary artery carries the deoxygenated blood into the lungs from the right ventricle. The deoxygenated blood within the veins is a dark red color, which appears blue because of the light dispersion on the skin.

Veins are large-capacity vessels that carry almost two-thirds of the body's blood volume. Their walls can expand to hold a large volume of blood, which renders the system susceptible to stasis of blood. The number of valves and anatomy and structural strength of veins differ among people. The hardiness of the veins is an inheritable quality, which explains familial predisposition to the development of venous insufficiency.

Basic Pathophysiological Concepts of Venous Dysfunction

The return of venous blood to the heart constantly opposes the downward pull of gravity. The unidirectional blood flow up to the heart is dependent on valvular competence and skeletal muscle contraction against the vessel walls. Prolonged standing or any obstruction to upward blood flow from the lower extremities places excess pressure on the valves of the veins. Obesity and pregnancy are the two main conditions that cause weakness of the valve leaflets with resultant retrograde flow of venous blood. Retrograde blood flow leads to stasis of venous blood and susceptibility to thrombus formation, the conditions known as venous insufficiency.

Venous insufficiency occurs in the superficial or deep venous system. Superficial venous incompetence is the most common form of venous disease. In superficial venous insufficiency, the deep veins are normal, but venous blood flows backward through distended superficial veins in which the valves have failed. The superficial veins that become distended and distorted under the high pressure are termed **varicose veins**.

Venous insufficiency in the deep veins can also occur as in the superficial veins because of valvular dysfunction. In deep venous insufficiency, after prolonged standing, the veins are completely filled, and all the venous valves are open. Venous congestion and high hydrostatic capillary pressure develop in the lower extremities, which causes edema in the interstitial tissues. Within the tissue there is poor clearance of waste products, cellular debris, carbon dioxide, and lactic acid. Wounds in this area are difficult to heal.

Unlike superficial vein insufficiency, deep venous insufficiency can lead to deep venous thrombosis, a potentially fatal condition. Thrombus formation can occur in a deep vein in the leg and then travel within the bloodstream, at which point it is called DVT.

Pathophysiology of Selected Venous Disorders

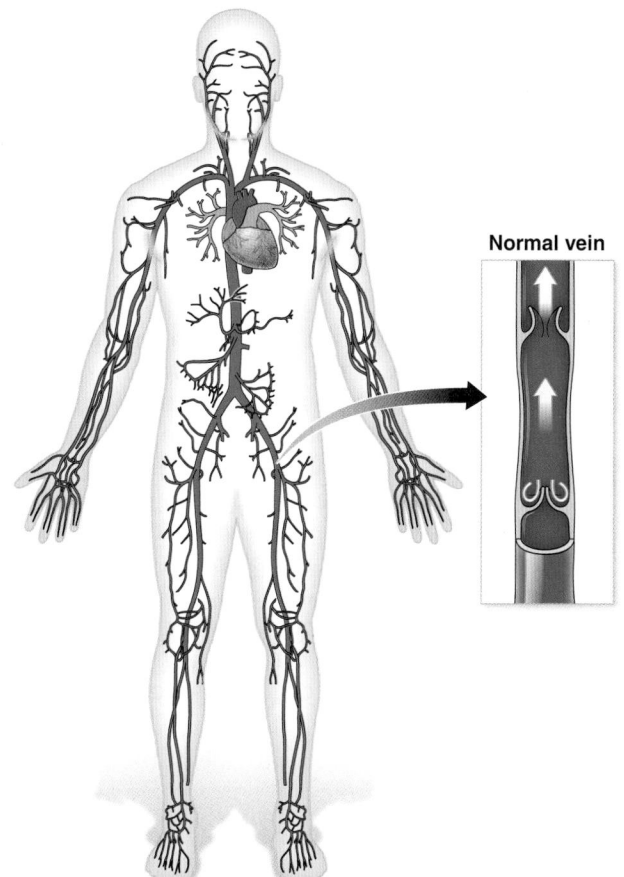

FIGURE 19-2. Valves of a deep vein. Valves keep the flow of venous blood up toward the heart.

The major venous disorders include chronic venous insufficiency, DVT, varicose veins, and venous ulcers.

Deep Venous Thromboembolism

Venous thromboembolism (VTE) is a term that is used to encompass both DVT and pulmonary embolism (PE). DVT occurs when a thrombus develops in a deep leg vein accompanied by inflammation. The thrombus can travel as an embolism within the venous system and then enter the lungs where it becomes a PE, a potentially fatal consequence.

Epidemiology

The exact incidence of DVT is unknown because many episodes go undiagnosed; however, data indicate that DVT occurs in 80 patients per 100,000 annually. It is estimated that approximately 1 person in 20 will develop DVT over the course of their lifetime. Hospital admissions for DVT have more than doubled over the past decade, mainly due to the greater sensitivity of new technology that can detect small, insignificant emboli, and approximately 900,000 new cases of DVT occur annually in the United States. According to the CDC (2022), 60,000 to 100,000 persons in the United States die of venous thromboembolism annually.

Etiology

The predisposing factors to DVT are venous stasis, vascular damage, and hypercoagulability, a trio of risk factors that together are known as **Virchow's triad** (see Fig. 19-3). Venous stasis occurs because of poor venous return associated with sedentary behavior, immobility, or valve dysfunction in the leg veins. Venous blood tends to pool in the lower extremities, and stagnant blood forms clots. Conditions that cause vascular damage such as surgery or trauma can also lead to DVT. Vein injury often leads to endothelial injury, inflammation, platelet aggregation, and stimulus of the coagulation cascade, which in turn causes formation of a clot. Any condition that causes hypercoagulability of blood can also lead to DVT. Cancers, which commonly secrete coagulation factors, and high estrogen states—which increase blood coagulability—increase risk of DVT as well. Other conditions that can contribute to formation of DVT are obesity and smoking, as both increase the risk of clot formation. Orthopedic surgery in particular causes a high risk of DVT because of vein injury during surgery and venous stasis, commonly associated with postoperative conditions. Some genetic conditions can increase predisposition to DVT and PE such as factor V Leiden, antithrombin, and protein S or protein C deficiency. In addition, some inflammatory-linked conditions can trigger DVT and PE such as inflammatory bowel disease, type 2 diabetes, obesity and metabolic syndrome, antiphospholipid syndrome, hyperlipidemia, rheumatoid arthritis, acute coronary syndrome, and acute stroke.

CLINICAL CONCEPT

DVT occurs in 30% to 80% of postoperative orthopedic surgery patients. Many of these DVTs are asymptomatic, and it is unknown what percentage become PEs. For this reason, prophylactic anticoagulant treatment is used after orthopedic surgery.

Pathophysiology

DVT occurs when a thrombus develops in a deep vein in the lower extremity. The thrombus forms at an area of inflammation in the vein. The sequela to DVT is **pulmonary embolism (PE)**. A venous thrombus can travel from the leg vein into the inferior vena cava (IVC) and then continue upward into the right side of the heart and into the pulmonary arterial circulation. When the thrombus enters the pulmonary circulation, it becomes a PE, which can cause pulmonary infarction and can be fatal (see Fig. 19-4). Venous thrombi often form silently and increase in size without producing manifestations. Deep venous thrombi can develop in the hips, knee, calf, or pelvic veins. Any condition that increases coagulation of the venous blood can cause DVT.

Clinical Presentation

The most common symptom of DVT is a cramp or "charley horse" in the lower calf that persists and intensifies. A large DVT can cause thigh swelling, tenderness, ropiness, and erythema along the course of a vein. The patient who develops DVT will commonly have a condition that causes venous stasis, venous injury, or hypercoagulability. A patient may have venous stasis caused by immobility or sedentary behavior. The patient may have a history of venous injury, such as trauma or recent surgery. The patient should be questioned about recent history of cancer, recent surgery, use of estrogen, and smoking, as these conditions increase the risk of DVT.

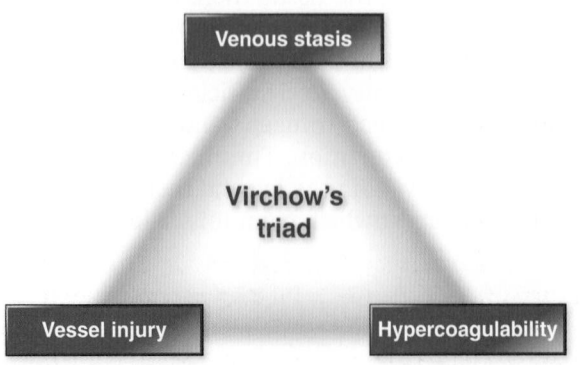

FIGURE 19-3. Virchow's triad. Virchow's triad describes the three risk factors that contribute to formation of a venous clot: hypercoagulability, venous stasis, and vascular damage.

CLINICAL CONCEPT

Patients who undergo orthopedic surgery are at high risk for DVT and PE.

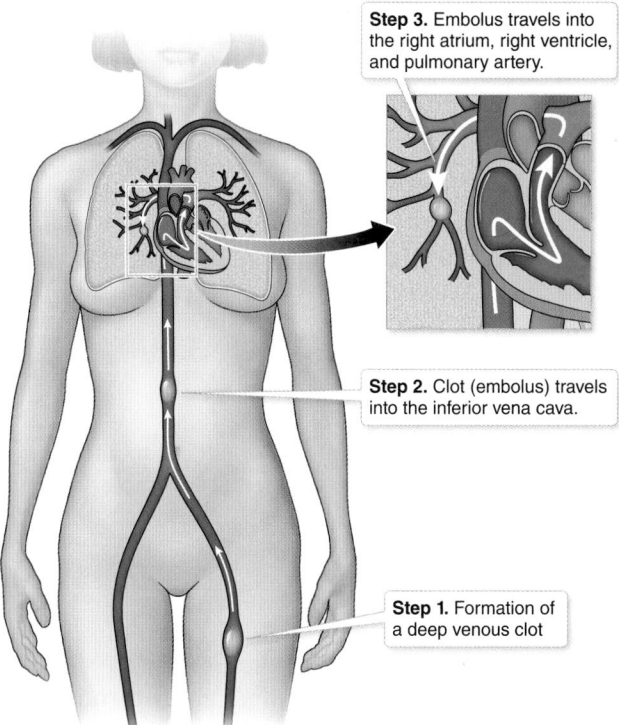

Step 3. Embolus travels into the right atrium, right ventricle, and pulmonary artery.

Step 2. Clot (embolus) travels into the inferior vena cava.

Step 1. Formation of a deep venous clot

FIGURE 19-4. Formation of a PE from a DVT. A clot (called a DVT) forms in the deep vein of a lower extremity and travels into the IVC. From the IVC, the clot travels into the right atrium of the heart, then right ventricle, and finally lodges in a pulmonary artery or arteriole. At the pulmonary arteriole, the PE can obstruct the diffusion of oxygen into the bloodstream.

> ### 🩺 CLINICAL CONCEPT
>
> The incidence of DVT in the lower extremity is 10 times the rate of DVT occurrence in the upper extremity. However, as peripherally inserted central catheter (PICC) use has increased, so has the rate of upper-extremity DVT.

The physical examination findings associated with DVT include unilateral leg pain, redness, ropiness, tenderness, and/or warmth over a vein; edema; and some may exhibit a positive **Homan's sign**, which is calf pain with dorsiflexion of the foot. Although Homan's sign can occur in DVT, 50% of persons can have the sign without DVT. PE presents with dyspnea, chest pain, tachycardia, hemoptysis, hypotension, and syncope, but both DVT and PE often can be silent without overt clinical symptoms.

> ### 🩺 CLINICAL CONCEPT
>
> Silent PE is very common in hospitalized patients. Preventive treatment of DVT and PE with anticoagulants is based on the patient's risk factors.

Diagnosis

DVT and PE cannot be diagnosed based on clinical symptoms because their symptoms often are not present, are subtle, or resemble other clinical disorders. DVT is frequently suspected but only diagnosed in 20% of cases. It is not ideal to perform imaging studies in every patient suspected of having DVT.

DVT is most commonly diagnosed through clinical criteria in conjunction with the **D-dimer test**, which is a blood test that detects the presence of fibrin clot degradation products in the blood. A positive D-dimer test is greater than 500 ng/mL. The sensitivity of the D-dimer test is greater than 80% for DVT and greater than 95% for PE. A normal D-dimer test is useful to rule out PE; however, D-dimer is not specific. D-dimer levels may be elevated in any medical condition where clots form, so the level is only used to rule out DVT, not to confirm diagnosis of DVT. D-dimer levels remain elevated in DVT and PE for about 7 days.

The **Wells criteria** are used to evaluate clinical signs of DVT, such as leg swelling and tenderness along a vein. The criteria summarize the risk of DVT with a score between 0 and 3 (see Table 19-1). A negative D-dimer assay in combination with a Wells criteria score of fewer than 2 rules out the possibility of DVT.

All patients with a positive D-dimer assay and a Wells criteria score of greater than or equal to 2 require venous duplex ultrasonography, which combines ultrasound images with Doppler blood flow studies. Venous duplex ultrasonography is the principal diagnostic test for suspected DVT. The absence of normal phasic Doppler signals arising from changes to venous flow in an extremity provides indirect evidence of venous occlusion.

Computed tomography (CT) of the chest with intravenous contrast is the principal imaging test for the diagnosis of PE. Lung scanning (**ventilation-perfusion scan**) is a second-line diagnostic test for PE, used mostly for patients who cannot tolerate intravenous contrast. When ultrasound is equivocal, magnetic resonance venography (MRV) with gadolinium contrast is an excellent imaging modality for diagnosis of DVT.

> ### 🩺 CLINICAL CONCEPT
>
> Venous duplex ultrasonography is the principal diagnostic test for DVT, and CT of the chest with intravenous contrast is the principal imaging test for diagnosing PE.

Treatment

Preventive strategies should be employed in all patients at increased risk for DVT. While a patient is immobile, sequential venous compression devices may be used to promote venous return. These devices are usually used with antiembolism stockings. They alternate inflation and deflation of chambers to provide sequential pressure over the lower extremity and promote venous

TABLE 19-1. Wells Criteria

Pretest – One point is given for each positive finding in the pretest, and 2 points are subtracted if an alternative diagnosis is likely as DVT is identified.

Finding	Point Value
Active cancer (treatment within last 6 months or palliative)	1
Calf swelling greater than 3 cm compared with other calf measured 10 cm below tibial tuberosity	1
Collateral superficial veins (nonvaricose)	1
Pitting edema (confined to symptomatic leg)	1
Previously documented DVT	1
Swelling of entire leg	1
Localized pain along distribution of deep venous system	1
Paralysis, paresis, or recent cast immobilization of lower extremities	1
Recently bedridden longer than 3 days, or major surgery requiring regional or general anesthetic in past 4 weeks	1
Alternative diagnosis at least as likely	2
DVT RISK CLASSIFICATION	
High probability	3 points
Moderate probability	2 points
Low probability	0 points

aPTT measures the intrinsic coagulation system. The actual blood clotting time is given in seconds, and the normal blood clotting time is given for comparison. The goal is to prolong clotting time in DVT, so a clotting time that is 1.5 to 2.5 times normal is achieved. For example, if normal clotting time is 30 seconds, a therapeutic level of anticoagulant would prolong clotting time to 45 to 75 seconds. While the patient is on anticoagulants, the PT and aPTT have to be measured often.

CLINICAL CONCEPT

When using warfarin, an effective INR is 2 to 3 for prophylaxis of DVT in most patients. Low molecular weight heparin, factor Xa inhibitors, and direct thrombin inhibitors do not require PT/aPTT or INR monitoring.

A simpler blood test called an **international normalized ratio (INR)** can also be used to monitor anticoagulant therapy. The INR indicates clotting time, which has to be kept in a specific range to avoid excessive anticoagulation. An INR result between 2 and 3 is commonly required for adequate anticoagulation.

Primary therapy for an existing DVT or PE consists of clot dissolution and pharmaco-mechanical therapy using catheter-directed thrombolytic agents. Catheter-directed treatment pulverizes the clot mechanically and pharmacologically dissolves the clot using tissue plasminogen activator (tPA). Ultrasound is used to facilitate catheter-directed surgery. Only patients with no risk of bleeding are eligible for this treatment.

A **Greenfield filter**, also known as an IVC filter, is often inserted to block clots from traveling up from the lower extremity to the pulmonary circulation (see Fig. 19-5). The IVC filter is used in persons with absolute contraindication to anticoagulant medication or those who have recurrent VTE despite anticoagulant treatment. These filters are inserted with the use of abdominal ultrasonography. The filter should be removed when the patient no longer requires it. Surgical removal of a thrombus, also called thrombectomy, may be used if other treatments prove ineffective or if risk of hemorrhage with anticoagulant is too great. Pulmonary embolectomy or pulmonary thromboendarterectomy are surgical procedures to remove PE.

Chronic Venous Insufficiency

Chronic venous insufficiency occurs as a result of damage to valves in the deep veins of the legs. Valves may become incompetent as a result of impaired venous return caused by trauma, central obesity, pregnancy,

return. When the patient is out of bed in a chair, their feet should be elevated to promote venous return. The patient should be taught not to stand for prolonged periods, to avoid constricting garments, to elevate legs periodically during the day, and to ambulate or do leg exercises that will promote blood flow and reduce venous stasis.

Patients are also treated prophylactically with drugs that interfere with clotting. Factor Xa inhibitors, direct thrombin inhibitors, low molecular weight heparin, unfractionated heparin, and warfarin are the medications used for DVT. To monitor the therapeutic effects of heparin and warfarin, prothrombin time (PT) and activated partial thromboplastin time (aPTT) laboratory tests have been used. Each of these tests measures the time it takes for the blood to clot; PT measures the extrinsic coagulation system, and

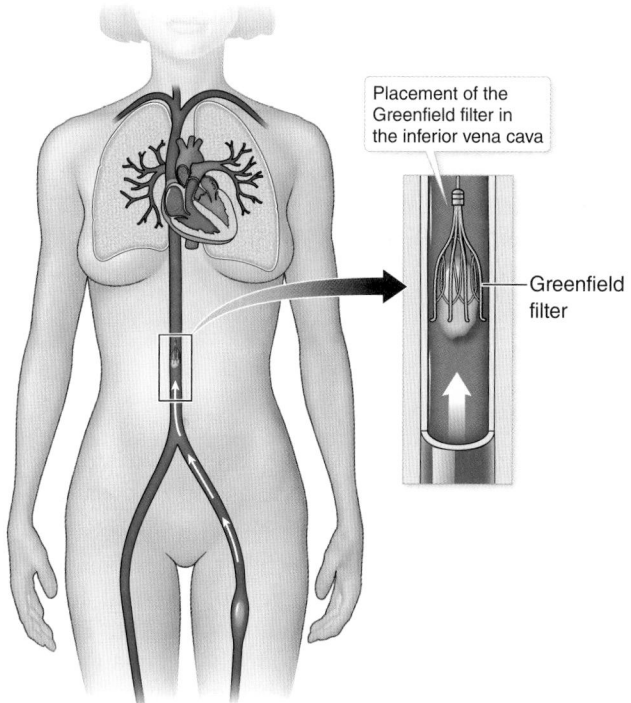

FIGURE 19-5. Greenfield filter. A Greenfield filter is an apparatus placed in the IVC that can trap a clot as it moves upward with venous flow. It can prevent a DVT from becoming a PE.

or prolonged standing. Genetic disorders can increase predisposition to venous insufficiency. Also, the left iliac vein can become occluded by extrinsic pressure from the overlapping right iliac artery in May-Thurner syndrome. Chronic venous insufficiency affects 7.5% of males and 5% of females in the United States. Valve damage leads to impaired venous return and abnormally high venous pressure in the venous system, which in turn leads to pooling and stasis of blood in the lower extremities. Venous congestion will affect capillary filtration by inhibiting movement of fluid and waste products out of the interstitial spaces. This usually causes edema in the lower extremities. Approximately 20% of patients with chronic venous insufficiency develop venous ulcers, which are shallow wounds near the medial and lateral malleoli of the ankle.

Clinical Presentation

Clinical presentation of venous insufficiency includes thin, shiny skin; dusky discoloration; edema; poor healing; and reduced or absent hair distribution. The patient often endures dull ache or heaviness in the legs with swelling typically after prolonged standing. These symptoms may be relieved by elevation of the leg. Other signs and symptoms include cramping, pruritus, telangiectasias, corona phlebectatica, and skin irritation that can lead to venous ulceration. Telangiectasias (commonly known as "spider veins") are dilated or broken blood vessels located near the surface of the skin or mucous membranes. Corona phlebectatica is a fan-shaped pattern of dilated veins near the ankle or foot. A circumferential dusky discoloration called **stasis dermatitis** is

often noted around the ankle, instep, and lower leg (see Fig. 19-6). The discoloration is caused by the buildup of hemosiderin in the tissues. Hemosiderin is the iron-containing pigment found in hemoglobin that is liberated from disintegration of red blood cells. Chronic venous congestion will lead to edema, waste product accumulation, and impaired healing. Edema occurs because stasis of blood increases hydrostatic pressure, resulting in fluid movement out of the vascular compartment into the interstitial spaces. A condition called lipodermatosclerosis can occur in severe venous insufficiency. Lipodermatosclerosis is the combination of inflammation, hemosiderin accumulation, and induration in the lower part of the leg just above the ankle.

Diagnosis

Key diagnostic tests for peripheral venous disorders include venous Doppler ultrasonography, photoplethysmography (PPG), and venography. Ultrasonography and PPG determine venous blood flow. PPG involves a noninvasive device that emits light that is applied to the skin. The device analyzes the light absorption in the region to determine the volume of blood in circulation. Venography, which requires injection of a radiopaque dye, can also be used to identify occlusions and patterns of collateral blood flow.

The severity of chronic venous disorders is classified according to the CEAP (clinical, etiological, anatomic, pathophysiologic) system. It broadly categorizes the patient's disease according to characteristics that allow more precise communication about the clinical status of the disease.

Treatment

Graduated compression is the main treatment of venous insufficiency. **Gradient compression stockings**

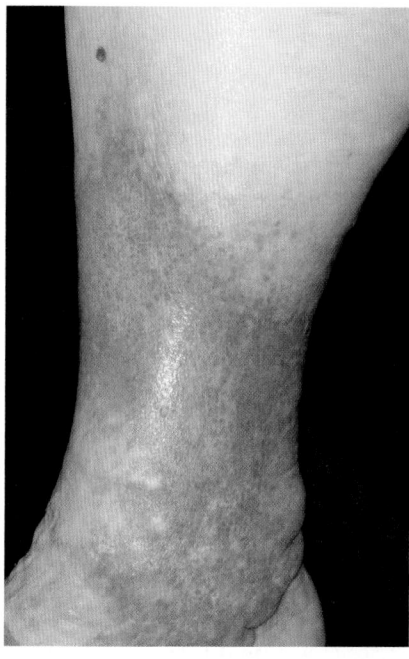

FIGURE 19-6. Stasis dermatitis. *(From Dr. P. Marazzi/Science Source.)*

are supportive hosiery that provide higher compression at the ankle than proximally up the leg. **Pneumatic compression devices** are also available that use inflatable compression sleeves on the legs to enhance venous blood flow. Graduated compression in combination with anticoagulant or antiplatelet medications is a common medical treatment. Catheter-delivered thrombolytic agents may also be used.

Surgical therapy can be used to improve venous circulation by removing the major reflux pathways through venoablation methods. **Sclerotherapy**, radio frequency ablation (RFA), and endovenous laser therapy are some venoablation procedures that aim to destroy the refluxing superficial veins by either injection of a sclerosing substance, passing a laser over the vein, or using thermal injury. Surgical therapy may also involve ligation and stripping of the great and small saphenous veins. Endovascular interventions, surgical bypass, and reconstruction of the valves of the deep veins can be performed in patients with severe venous insufficiency. Catheter-based stent placement may be considered to treat patients with chronic occlusion of the iliac vein. Valvuloplasty or valve transfer procedures may be performed in patients with severe venous ulcerations that do not heal. Valvuloplasty involves tightening of the valve leaflets surgically. Valve transfer involves taking another vein with competent valves and inserting into the segment of vein with incompetent valves.

Varicose Veins

A varicose vein, also called a varicosity, is an abnormally dilated superficial vein (see Fig. 19-7). Superficial leg veins are most commonly affected because they hold a large amount of blood. In the absence of disease, the action of muscles on the deep veins helps to promote venous return. The superficial veins have less supporting tissue than do deep veins; thus, varicosities are more likely in superficial veins.

Epidemiology

Studies show that the incidence of superficial varicose veins is twice as high in females compared with males. The hormone progesterone enhances relaxation of the

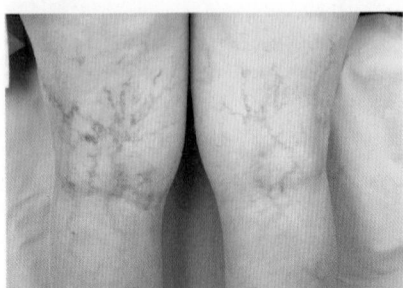

FIGURE 19-7. Varicose veins.

walls of veins in the lower extremities, which increases susceptibility to varicose veins in females.

 CLINICAL CONCEPT

The prevalence of varicose veins increases with age. In one study, 40-year-old individuals had a prevalence of 22%, 50-year-olds a prevalence of 35%, and 60-year-olds a prevalence of 41%.

Etiology

The cause of varicose veins is high pressure within the superficial veins that weaken venous valves. High pressure is known to occur in prolonged standing, sitting, pregnancy, and obesity. The Framingham Heart Study found that females with varicose veins generally are obese, have lower levels of physical activity, and have higher systolic blood pressure. Females who reported spending 8 or more hours in an average day in sedentary activities (sitting or standing) also had a significantly higher incidence of varicose veins than those who spent 4 or fewer hours a day in such activities. Pregnancy is a particular risk factor for varicose veins, as venous return is obstructed by the enlarged uterus.

For males, varicose veins were associated with lower levels of physical activity and higher smoking rates. These results suggest that increased physical activity, smoking cessation, and weight control may help prevent varicose veins among adults at high risk.

Pathophysiology

Varicose veins occur because of valvular incompetence in the legs. Valve incompetence occurs as a result of pressure on the valves over time. Gravitational pull and prolonged standing promote blood stagnation and pooling in the lower extremities. Valves are damaged from chronic pressure and become less competent at preventing backflow from one section of the vein into another. Venous valves are particularly stressed during pregnancy due to the venous pressure created by the gravid uterus. Also, the hormone progesterone in females causes blood vessel walls to relax. When these walls relax, the tiny valves within the vessels also relax and the pressure exerted by blood further weakens the vessels.

Diagnosis

Clinical examination of the legs in the standing position reveals the regions of varicose veins. The duplex ultrasound, which highlights the major superficial vein in the leg, the great saphenous vein, has become the most useful tool for diagnosing varicose veins.

Treatment

Treatment for varicose veins aims to remove the superficial veins either through surgery, endovenous ablation, or sclerotherapy ablation. Sclerotherapy is the most commonly used treatment. Under ultrasound guidance, a sclerosing substance is injected into the collapsed varicose veins, destroys the vessel's endothelial layer, and causes fibrosis of the remainder of the vessel. The body eventually reabsorbs all dead vascular tissue layers. Elastic supportive stockings, which compress the superficial veins, are also recommended.

Venous Ulcers

Venous ulcers, also called venous stasis ulcers, occur in lower extremities affected by venous insufficiency. They are wounds caused by trauma or pressure on the lower limbs. Skin breakdown, tissue damage, and necrosis occur because of lack of venous circulation.

Venous ulcers are the most common type of chronic lower extremity ulcers, affecting 1% to 3% of the U.S. population. In the United States, 10% to 35% of adults have chronic venous insufficiency, and 4% of adults 65 years or older have venous ulcers. Risk factors for venous ulcers include age 55 years or older, family history of chronic venous insufficiency, obesity, history of PE or superficial/deep venous thrombosis, lower extremity skeletal or joint disease, multiple pregnancies, parental history of ankle ulcers, physical inactivity, and venous reflux in deep veins.

Pathophysiology

Sluggish circulation, poor tissue oxygenation, deprivation of cellular nutrition, and impaired waste product removal are the pathophysiological changes found in venous stasis ulcers. Venous hypertension is defined as increased venous pressure resulting from venous reflux or obstruction. This process is thought to be the primary underlying mechanism for venous ulcer formation. Valve dysfunction, outflow obstruction, arteriovenous malformation, and calf muscle pump failure contribute to the pathogenesis of venous hypertension. Once skin breakdown occurs, tissue that is attempting to heal has high metabolic demands that cannot be met because of venous insufficiency.

Clinical Presentation

A venous ulcer is dark red in color, has an uneven margin, is usually painful, and is accompanied by a large amount of edema and drainage (see Fig. 19-8). Most ulcers are located medially over the ankle just above the medial malleolus of the lower leg. Pulses are usually present, and capillary refill time is normal. Other findings in the leg with venous ulceration include telangiectasias (spider veins), corona phlebectatica (fan-shaped dilated veins around the ankle and foot), atrophie blanche (atrophic, white

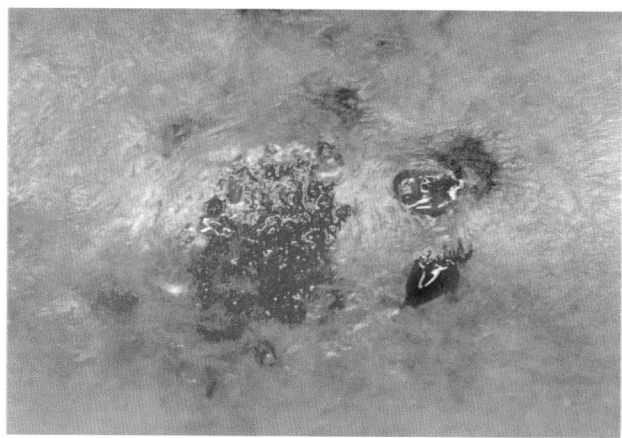

FIGURE 19-8. Venous ulcer. *(From Roberto A. Penne-Casanova/Science Source.)*

scarring of skin), and lipodermatosclerosis (indurated, hemosiderin-stained skin).

Diagnosis

Noninvasive imaging with venous duplex ultrasonography, arterial pulse examination, and measurement of ankle-brachial index is recommended for all patients with suspected venous ulcers. Ultrasonography should be used to assess for deep and superficial venous reflux and obstruction.

Treatment

Lifestyle modifications will reduce the pressure on the valves and may reduce edema. These modifications include avoidance of prolonged standing, institution of a regular exercise program, avoidance of constrictive clothing, and wearing elasticized compression gradient stockings. Measures are aimed at promoting venous return and decreasing venous pooling. Susceptibility to infection is high with venous ulcers because poor circulation impairs the immune and inflammatory response. Specialized wound care measures are usually necessary, such as antibiotic-impregnated semipermeable or occlusive dressings. Topical medications that contain epidermal, fibroblastic, and platelet-derived growth factors are used to assist chronic wounds with establishing healthy granulation tissue. Intermittent pneumatic compression has been shown to increase healing compared with no compression. Pentoxifylline, a vasoactive agent that improves blood flow by decreasing blood viscosity, is effective in some patients. An oral antibiotic is necessary if infection is suspected. Removal of necrotic tissue by débridement can facilitate healing. Early venous ablation and surgical intervention to correct superficial venous reflux can improve healing and decrease recurrence rates. Skin grafting may be required with large ulcerations.

Chapter Summary

- Veins bring blood back to the heart. The major vessels are the inferior and superior vena cava, which empty into the right atrium.
- Veins are unique in that they have valves that prevent retrograde blood flow.
- Venous insufficiency can occur in the superficial veins or deep veins.
- Venous insufficiency occurs because of incompetent venous valves, which allow for retrograde blood flow and stagnation.
- Superficial venous insufficiency causes varicose veins, a mainly cosmetic problem with no serious consequences.
- The major superficial vein in the leg is the great saphenous vein.
- Prolonged standing, sitting, sedentary behavior, obesity, and pregnancy increase susceptibility to varicose veins.
- Deep venous insufficiency causes edema, heaviness of the leg, and dusky color of the lower leg; these result from incomplete clearance of waste products, as well as accumulation of hemosiderin, carbon dioxide, and lactic acid.

- The most serious consequence of deep venous insufficiency is DVT, which is a thrombus of a leg vein that travels via the leg veins into the IVC, then into the right side of the heart into the pulmonary artery.
- Virchow's triad of venous stasis, vascular damage, and hypercoagulability are risk factors for DVT.
- The signs of DVT include tenderness, redness, ropiness, warmth, and swelling over a vein in the leg.
- DVT usually becomes a thromboembolism and can evolve into a PE.
- PE is often a cause of death in those who have an undiagnosed venous thrombus.
- Postoperative orthopedic patients, cancer patients, and sedentary hospitalized patients have high incidence of silent DVT and PE.
- Preventive treatment for DVT and PE with anticoagulant agents is commonly implemented based on the patient's risk factors.
- Venous ulcers occur because of trauma in areas of venous insufficiency.
- A common area for venous ulcer is the ankle area above the medial malleolus.

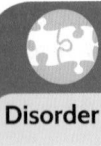 Making the Connections

Disorder and Pathophysiology

Signs and Symptoms	Physical Assessment Findings	Diagnostic Testing	Treatment
Chronic Venous Insufficiency | Veins are unable to keep blood moving in unidirectional flow up to the heart. Incompetent veins allow venous stasis and risk for thrombus formation.			
Heaviness of the legs. Sensation of fullness of the legs. Fatigue.	Edema and dusky, tan discoloration (hyperpigmentation) circumferentially with apparent distended veins.	Venous doppler ultrasonography demonstrates reduced blood flow in veins. CEAP classification of severity of venous insufficiency.	Graduated compression over the lower legs via support hosiery or pneumatic compression device. Endovascular interventions include thermal and nonthermal ablation, ligation and stripping of veins, endovenous stent placement, surgical bypass, and valve reconstruction. Educate patient on risk reduction and wearing of support hose. Teach patient not to stand for prolonged periods, to avoid constricting garments, to elevate legs periodically during the day, and to ambulate or perform leg exercises that will promote blood flow and reduce venous stasis.

Making the Connections–cont'd

Signs and Symptoms	Physical Assessment Findings	Diagnostic Testing	Treatment
Varicose Veins | Dilated, distended superficial veins that are incompetent and have retrograde blood flow.			
Heaviness and sensation of fullness in legs. Aching, muscle cramps, itching, and increased fatigue in lower leg muscles.	Visible tortuous, dilated blue or purple veins.	Duplex ultrasound highlights the anatomy of the major superficial vein in the leg, the great saphenous vein.	Sclerotherapy is commonly used to destroy the endothelial layer of the distended vein. The vein then fibroses and is reabsorbed by the body. Educate patient on risk reduction and wearing of support hose. Teach patient not to stand for prolonged periods, to avoid constricting garments, to elevate legs periodically during the day, and to ambulate or do leg exercises that will promote blood flow and reduce venous stasis.
Venous Thromboembolism (VTE) | VTE is combination of DVT and PE. Inflammation and thrombus formation in the vein is deep venous thrombosis (DVT). Thrombus becomes an embolism that can travel up into the IVC and into the right side of the heart and pulmonary artery to cause a pulmonary embolism (PE).			
Many times, there are no symptoms. Severe DVT can cause tenderness, warmth, redness, swelling, and ropiness over a vein in the leg.	Unilateral leg edema, tenderness, ropiness, warmth, and erythema over a vein. PE can present as sudden difficulty breathing, tachycardia, and chest pain.	D-dimer test (amount of fibrin breakdown products in blood) and Wells criteria can be used to assess probability of PE. Venous duplex ultrasonography is the principal diagnostic test for DVT, and CT of the chest with intravenous contrast is the principal imaging test for diagnosing PE. Follow clotting/bleeding time with either PT/aPTT or INR.	Unfractionated heparin, low molecular weight hepain, fondiparinux followed by warfarin (DVT therapy used in the past). Unfractionated heparin followed by oral direct-acting anticoagulant such as direct thrombin inhibitor (dabigatran) or Factor Xa inhibitor (edoxaban). Alternatively, monotherapy with direct oral anticoagulant medication such as rivaroxaban or apixaban. Monitor anticoagulant effects and levels. Monitor for signs of pulmonary embolus. Have antidote for anticoagulant available. If anticoagulation ineffective, IVC filter may be used and retrieved after use. Alternative for existing clot dissolution is "clot buster"—thrombolytic agent tissue plasminogen activator. Catheter-directed thrombolysis guided by ultrasound is recommended. Pulmonary embolectomy or pulmonary endarterectomy may be considered. Advise bedrest initially. Educate patient on risk reduction and wearing of support hose.

Continued

Making the Connections—cont'd

Signs and Symptoms	Physical Assessment Findings	Diagnostic Testing	Treatment
			Teach patient not to stand for prolonged periods, to avoid constricting garments, to elevate legs periodically during the day, and to ambulate or do leg exercises that will promote blood flow and reduce venous stasis.

Venous Ulcer | Venous ulcers are wounds caused by trauma or pressure on the lower limbs. Skin breakdown, tissue damage, and necrosis occur because of lack of venous circulation.

Signs and Symptoms	Physical Assessment Findings	Diagnostic Testing	Treatment
Dark red color, edema, and irregular margins of skin breakdown, often located around the medial ankle region.	Dark red color, edema, and irregular margins of skin breakdown, often located around the medial ankle region. Surrounding area has telangiectasias, dusky appearance, corona phlebectatica (fan-shaped dilated veins around the ankle and foot), atrophie blanche (atrophic, white scarring of skin), and lipodermatosclerosis.	Apparent findings on physical examination. Venous duplex ultrasound. Ankle-brachial index. Assess arterial pulses.	Measures are aimed at promoting venous return and decreasing infection. Surgical débridement assists healing. Antibiotic-impregnated semipermeable or occlusive dressings are used. Pentoxifylline can be used to enhance circulation. Topical medications that contain epidermal, fibroblastic, and platelet-derived growth factors are used to assist chronic wounds with establishing healthy granulation tissue. Intermittent pneumatic compression has been shown to increase healing compared with no compression.

Bibliography

Available online at fadavis.com

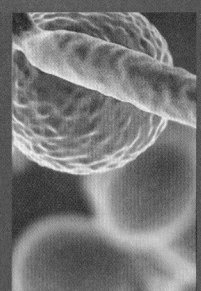

Respiratory Inflammation and Infection

Learning Objectives

After completion of this chapter, the student will be able to:

- Describe the physiological concepts of respiration and gas exchange.
- Describe mechanisms of inflammatory and infectious disorders in the respiratory tract.
- Recognize the signs and symptoms of inflammatory and infectious disorders of the respiratory tract.

- Describe assessment techniques and diagnostic testing used in inflammatory and infectious disorders of the respiratory tract.
- Identify common infectious disorders of the respiratory tract encountered in the clinical setting.
- Discuss treatment modalities of inflammatory and infectious disorders in the respiratory tract.

Key Terms

Acidosis

Adventitious breath sounds

Alkalosis

Arterial blood gases (ABGs)

Atelectasis

Bradypnea

Bronchitis

Bronchophony

Community-acquired pneumonia (CAP)

Diaphragm

Egophony

Epiglottitis

Expectoration

Expiration

Group A beta hemolytic streptococcus (GABHS) (*Streptococcus pyogenes*)

Hemoptysis

Hypercapnia

Hypoxemia

Hypoxia

Inspiration

Interferon gamma release assay (IGRA)

Mantoux tuberculin skin test

Mucociliary apparatus

Mycobacterium tuberculosis

Oxyhemoglobin

Oxyhemoglobin dissociation curve

Pressure of carbon dioxide in arterial blood ($PaCO_2$ or PCO_2)

Perfusion

Pneumonia

Pressure of oxygen in arterial blood (PaO_2 or PO_2)

PPD test

Pulmonary aspiration

Pulmonary embolus (PE)

Pulse oximeter

Retractions

Percentage of saturation of oxygen in the blood (SaO_2)

Streptococcus pneumoniae (pneumococcus)

Tachypnea

Tactile fremitus

Tuberculosis (TB)

Ventilation

Ventilation-perfusion (V-Q) ratio

Whispered pectoriloquy

Respiratory infections are common within the general population and range from the common cold to the life-threatening condition of **tuberculosis (TB)**. Noninfectious inflammatory conditions of the lung are less common but include autoimmune diseases, such as sarcoidosis, and pneumoconioses, such as asbestosis or anthracosis. Respiratory infections are highly contagious and often transmitted by casual contact. The most common route of transmission is droplet infection, which occurs through inhalation. Infected persons commonly transmit the disease to others by sneezing, coughing, or hand contact.

The lungs are also at risk for exposure to inhalants such as smoke, allergens, and pollutants. Pneumonia and influenza virus have long been a cause of death for many persons, especially older adults. However, immunizations such as pneumococcal and influenza vaccinations have reduced the frequency and severity of these respiratory infections. TB, a potentially fatal disease, remains a common respiratory infection worldwide. It has remained a scourge of the global population for centuries; over the years, the bacterium has developed resistance to many antibiotics.

Epidemiology

The most frequently occurring respiratory infection is the common cold. It can be caused by a variety of viruses found in the environment, such as rhinovirus, adenovirus, parainfluenza virus, respiratory syncytial virus, and coronavirus.

 CLINICAL CONCEPT

Rhinoviruses, one of the major causes of the common cold, are found worldwide and account for about 40% of colds.

In the primary care setting, upper respiratory infection (URI) is one of the most frequent reasons that patients seek care, with cough being one of the main symptoms. Cough is pathognomonic of acute bronchitis and pneumonia. Almost 5% of the general population in the United States develops acute bronchitis annually, with the highest incidence during the fall and winter months. Pneumonia, a more serious infection, affects 5 out of 1,000 adults each year in the United States, with up to a 28% mortality rate. It is one of the most common diagnoses in older adults and immunosuppressed individuals.

TB is a unique respiratory infection caused by a resilient bacterial organism that can remain dormant in the body as latent TB. A potentially fatal disease, TB affects 2 billion persons worldwide. This infectious disease remains in the individual for a lifetime. Those who are immunosuppressed, such as individuals with HIV, are highly susceptible to TB. The emergence of HIV infection in the 1980s led to a rise in TB as a global disease. TB remains a challenging infection to treat because of its ability to mutate and develop resistance to antibiotics.

Basic Physiological Concepts of Respiratory Function

The upper respiratory tract conducts air to the lower airways; protects the lungs from foreign matter; and warms, filters, and humidifies air as it enters the lungs. The lower respiratory tract participates in gas exchange by oxygenating blood and excreting carbon dioxide at the alveoli.

Lung Anatomy

The lungs sit in the center of the thoracic cage and receive air from the upper respiratory tract structures,

which include the nose, oropharynx, larynx, trachea, and two main bronchi and bronchioles. There are two lobes of lung tissue on the left (the upper and lower lobes) and three lobes of lung tissue on the right (the upper, middle, and lower lobes).

The trachea divides into two main bronchi, which are shaped differently. The left bronchus is curved as it enters the lung tissue, whereas the right bronchus is vertical and wider, providing a straight path downward into the right lung (see Fig. 20-1). The shape of the right bronchus increases susceptibility of aspiration into the right middle and right lower lobes of the lung. **Pulmonary aspiration** occurs when material from the oropharynx enters the lower respiratory tract. Aspiration occurs most frequently in patients who have trouble clearing their lungs, such as those with a diminished gag or cough reflex, and patients with a decreased level of consciousness. The consequences of pulmonary aspiration range from no injury at all to death within minutes from asphyxiation. Aspiration of small quantities of material is common, and healthy persons can cough forcefully to remove the material from the trachea. However, people with significant underlying disease are at greater risk for developing aspiration pneumonia.

CLINICAL CONCEPT

The right middle lobe, a common area for aspiration pneumonia, is auscultated under the patient's right arm in the axillary region.

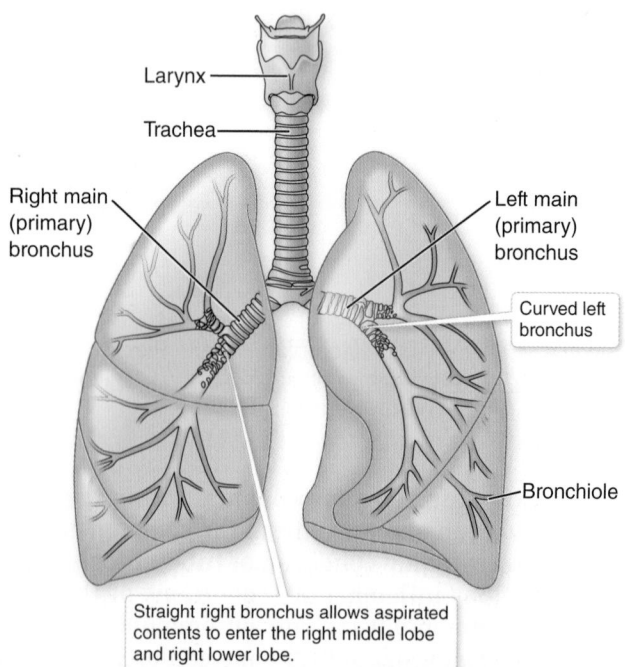

FIGURE 20-1. Shape of the bronchi. The left bronchus is curved, and the right bronchus is more vertical. Because of the anatomy, aspiration often occurs into the right lung because of the straight route downward from the right bronchus.

The two main bronchi branch into smaller bronchioles, which divide into respiratory bronchioles, terminal bronchioles, alveolar ducts, and alveoli. At the alveoli, transfer of oxygen occurs into the capillaries, and carbon dioxide transfers into the alveoli for exhalation.

Mucociliary Apparatus

During respiration, air enters the nasal passages and trachea and travels down to the lungs. The bronchioles contain a specialized cellular mechanism called the **mucociliary apparatus**. This consists of ciliated, pseudostratified columnar epithelial cells and goblet cells that secrete mucus. The wavelike motion of the cilia enables the movement of mucus downward from the nasal passages to the throat. Inhaled particles such as dust, pollen, and pathogens are trapped by the mucus and removed from the air passages. Upward motion of the cilia moves the mucus from the bronchioles up to the throat, where it is swallowed.

Because the mouth, nose, and throat are exposed to the outside environment, they are colonized with bacteria that are normal flora, organisms that do not cause illness in a healthy person. The lower respiratory tract and alveoli do not have normal flora. They are kept free of microorganisms by the mucociliary apparatus that sweeps away and traps organisms in the upper respiratory tract. If the ciliated respiratory epithelium becomes damaged, however, there is an increased risk of lower respiratory infection.

 CLINICAL CONCEPT

Smoking paralyzes the mucociliary apparatus, and inhaled particles stimulate smokers to forcibly cough to mobilize mucus. Failure to remove excess particles from the respiratory system increases the risk of infection.

Gas Exchange

Gas exchange of oxygen and carbon dioxide occurs within the respiratory bronchioles, alveolar ducts, and alveoli. Alveoli are thin-walled, balloon-like structures surrounded by pulmonary capillaries (see Fig. 20-2). This unique structure enables transfer of both oxygen and carbon dioxide. Air enters the alveolus, and oxygen moves across the alveolar membrane to the blood. At the same time, carbon dioxide moves from the blood into the alveolus to be excreted by exhalation.

Oxygen combines loosely with the heme portion of hemoglobin to form **oxyhemoglobin**. The most important function of hemoglobin is to combine with oxygen in the lungs and then release oxygen to the peripheral tissues. It then collects carbon dioxide

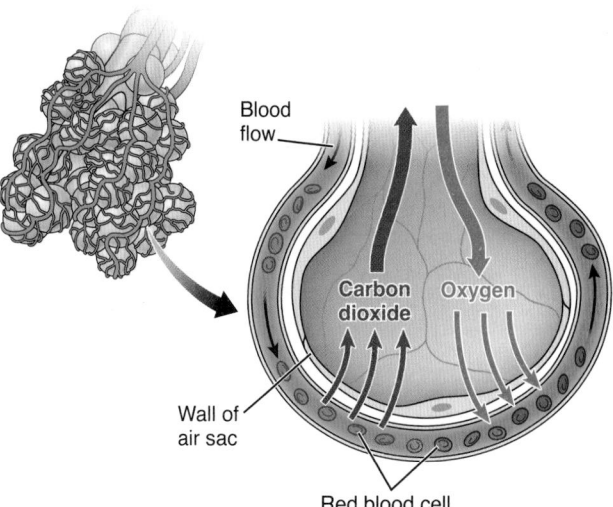

FIGURE 20-2. Oxygen and carbon dioxide gas exchange at alveoli.

from the tissues and carries it back to the lungs to be excreted. Each hemoglobin molecule can carry four oxygen molecules.

Hemoglobin holds onto oxygen and unloads its oxygen atoms to the tissue at certain PO_2 levels. Hemoglobin is fully saturated with oxygen atoms when the **pressure of oxygen in arterial blood (PaO_2 or PO_2)** is optimal at 100 mm Hg. However, hemoglobin affinity for oxygen dramatically decreases when PO_2 diminishes to approximately 60 mm Hg. When PO_2 decreases to 60 mm Hg, hemoglobin begins to unload *all* of its oxygen atoms.

The volume of oxygen dissolved in the plasma varies directly with the partial pressure of oxygen in the arteries. The relationship between the arterial pressure of oxygen and the **percentage of saturation of oxygen in the blood (SaO_2)** is shown in the **oxyhemoglobin dissociation curve**. The oxyhemoglobin dissociation curve illustrates the relationship of oxygen and hemoglobin. The curve shows that hemoglobin "lets go" of its oxygen and allows it out into the tissues when the PO_2 diminishes to the hypoxic level of 60 mm Hg. However, the affinity of hemoglobin for oxygen changes with various conditions (see Fig. 20-3). For example, in conditions of hyperthermia (fever), acidosis, and high PCO_2, the oxyhemoglobin curve shifts to the right; meaning hemoglobin lets go of oxygen earlier than a PO_2 of 60 mm Hg and higher PO_2 concentrations and allows it out into the tissues. In conditions of hypothermia, low CO_2, and alkalosis, hemoglobin has higher affinity for oxygen and lets go of its oxygen into the tissues at PO_2 lower than 60 mm Hg.

It is important to recognize that desaturation of hemoglobin leads to tissue hypoxia. To ensure optimal tissue oxygenation, it is important to keep hemoglobin fully saturated with oxygen above PO_2 of 90 mm Hg.

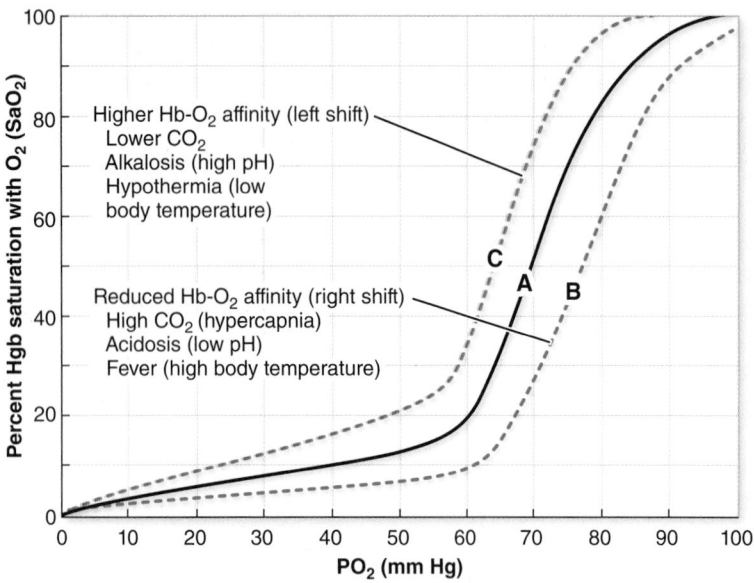

FIGURE 20-3. The oxyhemoglobin dissociation curve. The oxygen–hemoglobin dissociation curve demonstrates the proportion of hemoglobin that is saturated with oxygen on the vertical axis against the oxygen pressure in the bloodstream (PO_2) on the horizontal axis. Specifically, the oxyhemoglobin dissociation curve shows hemoglobin affinity for oxygen at different PO_2. (A) Under normal conditions, Hgb is fully saturated at the ideal PO_2 of 100 mm Hg; at approximately 60 mm Hg PO_2 in the blood, hemoglobin affinity dramatically diminishes. Hemoglobin unloads all of its oxygen. (B) Under conditions of hyperthermia (fever), low pH (acidosis), and high pressure of carbon dioxide in the blood (PCO_2), there is less saturation of hemoglobin. Hgb affinity for oxygen is less than normal. (C) Under conditions of hypothermia, low CO_2, and high pH (alkalosis), hemoglobin holds tighter to oxygen, until arterial oxygen is approximately 40 mm Hg, then unloads oxygen to the tissues. Hgb affinity for oxygen is greater than normal in those conditions.

 CLINICAL CONCEPT

The percentage of hemoglobin saturated by oxygen can be measured using a **pulse oximeter**, a monitor usually placed on the finger. This measures the peripheral oxygen concentration in the bloodstream.

Erythropoietin, which is responsible for the stimulation of red blood cell (RBC) production, is secreted by the kidneys in response to low oxygen levels in the bloodstream. Any condition that causes hypoxia, such as cardiac disease, lung disease, or changes in atmospheric pressure, will stimulate secretion of erythropoietin. Erythropoietin then stimulates the bone marrow to produce more RBCs that can carry more oxygen to the tissues.

 CLINICAL CONCEPT

At high altitude, the decreased air pressure causes decreased levels of PO_2, which stimulates erythropoietin. This, in turn, increases production of RBCs, which is why individuals who live in mountainous areas have higher-than-normal levels of hemoglobin and hematocrit.

Diaphragm and Respiratory Muscles

The **diaphragm** is a muscle that separates the abdomen from the thoracic cavity. It is composed of both skeletal and smooth muscle and is controlled both voluntarily and involuntarily. During inhalation, the diaphragm moves downward or contracts at the same time the rib cage is being pulled up, resulting in lung expansion. The incoming air movement as the lungs expand is **inspiration**. When the diaphragm ascends, the rib cage moves down and the diaphragm compresses the lungs, promoting exhalation. The accompanying air movement with lung deflation is referred to as **expiration**.

The phrenic nerve, which originates as the fourth cervical spinal nerve (C4), innervates the diaphragm. It originates in the neck and traverses downward between the lung and heart to reach the diaphragm. A spinal cord injury occurring at or above C4 causes motor and sensory conduction to the diaphragm to be interrupted and respirations to cease. The patient will require respiratory support to maintain life.

The other important respiratory muscles are the external and internal intercostal muscles and sternocleidomastoids. These muscles are used when an individual is short of breath. When an individual uses the intercostal muscles to breathe, the contractions are called **retractions**.

ALERT! It is critical to carefully assess all patients with spinal cord injuries for signs of respiratory distress. In spinal cord injuries affecting C4 or above, the patient needs rescue breathing or mechanical support.

Ventilation and Perfusion

Ventilation is the process of inspiration and expiration of air through the pulmonary airways. Physical factors affect the flow of air and oxygen content of the atmospheric air. At high altitudes, there is low atmospheric pressure and diminished oxygen content. The decreased O_2 levels trigger an increase in the rate and depth of respiration.

Perfusion is the movement of blood through the pulmonary circulation, eventually providing oxygen to every part of the body. Circulation to the lungs begins with the pulmonary artery, which arises from the right ventricle. The pulmonary artery divides into two trunks, which deliver blood to each lung. Oxygen and carbon dioxide are dissolved in the blood and transported throughout the body at the same time.

The **ventilation-perfusion (V-Q) ratio** is defined as the ratio of the amount of air reaching the alveoli to the amount of blood reaching the alveoli; it is measured with a ventilation-perfusion (V-Q) scan. The ideal V-Q ratio occurs when ventilation and perfusion are equal or when ventilation and perfusion match. When ventilation and perfusion are unequal, there is ventilation-perfusion imbalance. An area with no ventilation is termed a shunt. An area with no perfusion is termed dead space. The lungs have a built-in compensatory mechanism that attempts to match blood flow and ventilation: where there is little ventilation, pulmonary arterial vessels constrict. Pulmonary artery vasoconstriction leads to redistribution of blood flow to better-ventilated areas of the lung.

> 🩺 **CLINICAL CONCEPT**
>
> It is important that all functioning alveoli have adequate perfusion. Ventilation-perfusion imbalance occurs when air cannot flow into an alveolus or blood flow around an alveolus is altered. One of the most common etiologies for this is a blood clot in the lung, also called a **pulmonary embolus (PE)**. The clot prevents blood flow to the alveolus, and gas exchange cannot take place.

Control and Stimulus of Breathing

Various receptors control the process, rate, and depth of respirations during inspiration and expiration. Central chemoreceptors, located in the medulla, sense changes in carbon dioxide and blood pH and cause alterations in the rate and depth of respirations. An increase in CO_2 (**hypercapnia**) or a decrease in pH (**acidosis**) stimulates the central chemoreceptors, resulting in an increased rate of respirations. The end result is the return of the pH to normal.

Chemoreceptors in the medulla also sense the hydrogen (H^+) concentration of the cerebrospinal fluid (CSF). An increase or decrease of pH in the arterial blood is reflected in a chemical change in the CSF. When CO_2 is retained, carbonic acid (H_2CO_3) levels in the blood increase. This increases the **pressure of carbon dioxide in the blood (PaCO_2 or PCO_2)** level and lowers blood pH. In response to these changes, the respiratory center at the medulla stimulates respirations.

Peripheral chemoreceptors, found in the aortic arch and bifurcation of the carotid artery (called carotid bodies), respond primarily to a decrease in arterial oxygen. A decreased level of oxygen in the blood is sensed by the peripheral chemoreceptors, which stimulate respirations; this is referred to as a hypoxic drive. A hypoxic drive takes over when CO_2 accumulation is not stimulating the medulla to control respiration, as in diseases such as chronic obstructive pulmonary disease (COPD).

The normal stimulus to breathe is hypercapnia, an increase of carbon dioxide in the blood. The high CO_2 levels stimulate the central respiratory center in the medulla. However, when central chemoreceptors are exposed to high levels of CO_2 for extended periods, they become less responsive. The blunted response to CO_2 allows the peripheral chemoreceptors of low O_2 to take over as the stimulus of respirations. The hypoxic drive becomes the main trigger for breathing. This response correlates with a PaO_2 level of about 60 mm Hg, the point at which oxygen fully dissociates from hemoglobin.

> 🩺 **CLINICAL CONCEPT**
>
> In patients with long-term severe COPD, breathing is stimulated by low O_2 levels in the bloodstream instead of high CO_2 levels, as in healthy individuals.

Baroreceptors, sensors of blood pressure, are also located in the aortic arch and carotid artery. Baroreceptors send signals to the sympathetic nervous system, depending on blood pressure levels. When systolic blood pressure drops to 80 mm Hg or lower, the baroreceptors stimulate the sympathetic nervous system to increase heart and respiratory rate.

Proprioceptors, located in the muscles of movable joints, respond to body movement. When stimulated by exercise, respiratory rate and depth increase. The purpose of these receptors is to maintain adequate oxygen levels during periods of exertion.

The Hering–Breuer reflexes are stretch reflexes located in the bronchi and bronchioles. When the lungs inflate, neuronal impulses are sent up the vagus nerve to the medulla. The result is an inhibition of rate, rhythm, and duration of inspiration, which prevents the overdistention of the lungs.

Basic Pathophysiological Concepts of Respiratory Function

There are several signs of lung pathophysiology. Dyspnea, or shortness of breath, is the most common sign of a pulmonary problem. At times, it is difficult to decipher if dyspnea has a cardiac or pulmonary etiology. Cough, another common sign of pulmonary disease, usually develops because of an irritating stimulus in the bronchioles. However, heart failure can also be the cause of cough. Pulmonary symptoms must be considered in the context of the whole patient—the compilation of the history, signs, symptoms, and laboratory studies together will lead to an accurate pulmonary or cardiac diagnosis.

Dyspnea

Dyspnea is the sensation of being short of breath; it is a common symptom of pulmonary or cardiovascular disease. If dyspnea is sudden, it can be caused by PE, acute coronary syndrome, pneumothorax, or aspiration. Orthopnea, the sensation of dyspnea when lying flat, is a common indication of heart failure. Nocturnal dyspnea is particularly associated with heart failure but can be caused by asthma. Acute episodes of dyspnea are most often caused by bronchospasm of asthma, whereas chronic, persistent dyspnea is commonly caused by COPD.

Cough

A cough is an involuntary response to mechanical or chemical stimulation of the bronchial tree. It can occur as a result of a blockage in the airway caused by a foreign body, excess mucus, or aspirated fluids or foods. When this happens, coughing serves as a mechanism to eliminate the stimulant.

Coughing can be described as nonproductive or productive of mucus or sputum. The process of coughing up sputum is referred to as **expectoration**. Normal sputum is clear and thin in nature. In the presence of a bacterial infection, the production of sputum may become profuse and thick. The color may change to yellow or green. Pink-tinged, also called "rusty," sputum is often indicative of minor bleeding, as can occur when capillaries in the lungs rupture because of forceful coughing. Hemoptysis is the coughing up of a larger amount of blood, when the sputum clearly contains red blood. A cough with hemoptysis often is associated with TB or lung cancer. Grey-tinged sputum occurs from exposure to tobacco smoke.

Frequent, chronic coughing is a symptom that prompts individuals to see a health-care provider. It can be a sign of infection, inflammation, gastroesophageal reflux, bronchospasm, heart failure, or neoplastic disease. In healthy individuals, cough frequently occurs as a result of a respiratory tract infection. Asthma can also present as a chronic cough. In older adult patients, chronic cough is frequently caused by heart failure or COPD.

CLINICAL CONCEPT

Chronic cough is common in smokers. Exposure to secondhand smoke can trigger chronic coughing in children.

Hemoptysis

Hemoptysis is the production of blood-containing sputum. This is usually associated with serious illness such as infection, tumor, or TB. When assessing a patient complaining of hemoptysis, it is important to differentiate between blood in sputum versus blood from the gastrointestinal tract in vomitus. Blood from the gastrointestinal tract is referred to as hematemesis. Hematemesis usually consists of dark, coffee-colored blood, whereas hemoptysis contains bright red blood.

Atelectasis

Atelectasis is the collapse of a small number of alveoli resulting in reduced gas exchange. It can occur because of a compressive force on the alveoli, which may occur because of pressure from a mass. Alternatively, atelectasis can be caused by an obstruction of the bronchioles that inhibits the full inflation of alveoli. Atelectasis most commonly occurs postoperatively because of sedation. Under sedation, a patient's respiratory rate decreases and shallow breathing occurs. Some alveoli lack full inflation with shallow breathing, and atelectasis can occur. To treat atelectasis, the patient needs to cough and deep-breathe to open all the alveoli (see Fig. 20-4). Atelectasis predisposes individuals to pneumonia.

CLINICAL CONCEPT

Patients who undergo long surgical procedures often develop atelectasis. It is important to advise postoperative patients to cough, deep-breathe, and use an incentive spirometer to reverse atelectasis.

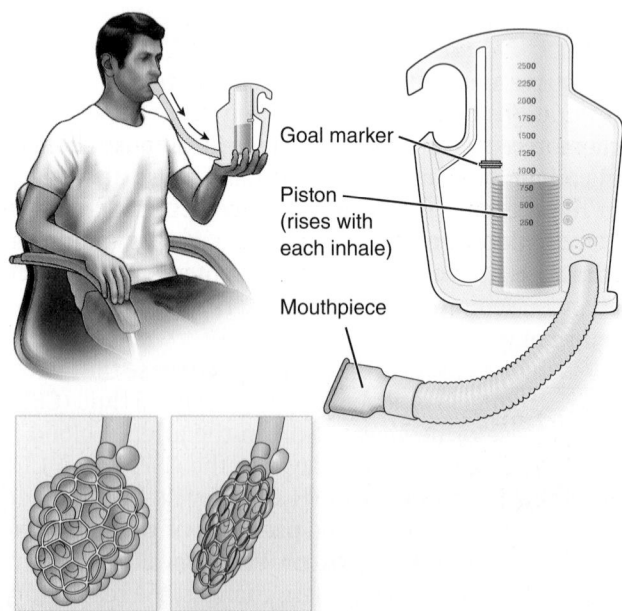

FIGURE 20-4. Atelectasis and incentive spirometer. Atelectasis is the collapse of a number of alveoli. Using an incentive spirometer, a patient is encouraged to breathe out into the device with effort. The piston rises and the patient tries to reach goal marker. This opens the alveoli.

Hypoxia

Hypoxia occurs when oxygen levels in the blood are insufficient to meet the needs of tissue. It can be caused by any number of conditions that alter gas exchange across the alveolar membrane. Pulmonary edema, for example, creates a fluid barrier to oxygen transfer across the alveolar–capillary interface. The term **hypoxemia** indicates a lack of sufficient oxygen in the arterial blood, whereas the term *anoxia* indicates a zero amount of oxygen in the blood.

Chemical poisoning, such as that seen in carbon monoxide poisoning, can cause hypoxia. In this case, carbon monoxide binds to hemoglobin as carboxyhemoglobin, which has a much higher affinity for hemoglobin than oxygen and prevents oxygen from binding to the hemoglobin molecule. High levels of carbon monoxide in the bloodstream can be fatal.

 CLINICAL CONCEPT

Hypoxia stimulates pulmonary arterial vasoconstriction. Patients with chronic hypoxia can develop chronic pulmonary vasoconstriction, which can result in pulmonary hypertension.

Impending Respiratory Failure

Respiratory failure occurs when the pulmonary system fails to oxygenate the blood or fails to sufficiently eliminate carbon dioxide. It is classified as either hypoxemic or hypercapnic respiratory failure.

Hypoxemic respiratory failure occurs when the pressure of oxygen in arterial blood (PaO_2 or PO_2) is lower than 60 mm Hg with normal arterial carbon dioxide ($PaCO_2$). Many acute diseases of the lung can cause respiratory failure, including pulmonary edema, PE, pneumonia, or pneumothorax.

Hypercapnic respiratory failure occurs when carbon dioxide in arterial blood ($PaCO_2$) is greater than 50 mm Hg. Common causes of hypercapnia include COPD and asthma. Hypoxemia commonly accompanies hypercapnic respiratory failure in persons who are breathing room air.

It is challenging to predict when a patient will cease independent breathing and incur respiratory failure. Serial **arterial blood gases (ABGs)** should be evaluated in all patients with respiratory problems. Usually, there is a gradual increase in arterial carbon dioxide and a decrease in arterial oxygen when a patient is developing respiratory failure (see Table 20-1). The patient typically appears distressed, may be using accessory respiratory muscles, and has difficulty maintaining a normal respiratory rate despite oxygen administration. Patients at risk of respiratory failure need intubation equipment ready at the bedside. The patient's whole clinical picture should be considered when deciding to intubate. After the patient's ventilatory status is corrected, the underlying pathophysiological process that led to respiratory failure needs investigation.

Assessment

A complete history and physical examination is necessary to diagnose a pulmonary disorder. Frequently, pulmonary and cardiac disorders present with the same symptoms.

History

A patient who presents with a pulmonary problem can have anything from a common cold to chronic heart failure. By asking specific questions in a thorough history, the clinician can try to categorize the symptoms as respiratory or cardiac in nature. The patient should be asked about risk factors such as smoking or occupational exposure to inhaled toxins. It is important to ask the patient to completely describe the symptom and associated features. When and how did the symptom occur? Suddenly or gradually? Has the symptom been present for a day, week, or month? The patient needs to be asked about symptoms of coronary artery disease to rule out dyspnea caused by cardiovascular

TABLE 20-1. Serial ABGs Demonstrating Trend Toward Respiratory Failure				
This chart shows how a patient's ABGs decompensated over the course of an hour and a half, from 9 a.m. to 10:30 a.m. At 11:00 a.m., the patient stopped breathing and went into respiratory failure, needing intubation.				
	9:00 A.M.	10:00 A.M.	10:30 A.M.	11:00 A.M.
BLOOD PH	7.36	7.35	7.32	7.30
PO$_2$	90 mm Hg	80 mm Hg	66 mm Hg	60 mm Hg
PCO$_2$	45 mm Hg	45 mm Hg	56 mm Hg	60 mm Hg
HCO$_3^-$	21 mg/dL	21 mg/dL	17 mg/dL	12 mg/dL
Interpretation of ABGs	Normal	Hypoxia	Hypoxia and hypercapnia	Respiratory failure

disease. For example, does the patient suffer dizziness or chest pain when they have dyspnea? Usually, dyspnea caused by cardiovascular disease worsens with exertion and is accompanied by diaphoresis and chest pain. The patient with dyspnea caused by heart failure commonly has edema. Ask the patient if lying flat causes difficulty breathing, called orthopnea, a classic symptom of heart failure. Nocturnal dyspnea is often a symptom of heart failure or asthma. If there is chest pain, the patient should fully describe it. Cardiac chest pain is crushing and a feeling of pressure. Pleuritic chest pain, caused by pleural membrane irritation, is sharp and worsens with deep breathing.

In respiratory infection, dyspnea and cough are often accompanied by fever and malaise. Sneezing, rhinorrhea, and a productive cough are classic features of URI. A patient who has audible wheezing is usually exhibiting bronchospasm that may be caused by asthma. Ask the patient about current medications. Does the patient have any allergies? Rhinitis and sinusitis can be caused by allergy as well as infection. Acute bronchitis commonly occurs after a URI. Pneumonia is commonly a secondary infection after a viral infection such as influenza.

Signs and Symptoms

The patient's symptoms can be thoroughly described in terms of the mnemonic "OLDCART"—onset, location, duration, character, aggravating or relieving factors, and treatment. It is important to assess if dyspnea occurs with exertion or in the presence of edema. Exertional dyspnea commonly occurs with a cardiac condition. The presence of ankle edema also often indicates a cardiac disorder.

The signs of pulmonary edema of cardiac origin can present similarly to pneumonia. Both of these disorders cause crackles indicative of fluid in the lung tissue. However, if fever is present, the fluid is usually caused by an exudate in pneumonia.

A chronic cough can be associated with asthma, heart failure, TB, lung cancer, or COPD. However, the patient usually demonstrates other symptoms that will narrow down the diagnosis. The chronic cough that is triggered by allergy is often asthma. A chronic cough that is accompanied by weight loss and hemoptysis is commonly caused by TB or lung cancer. A chronic cough in a smoker with cyanosis and a barrel-shaped chest is often indicative of COPD.

The patient with cough, pallor, weak pulse, and ankle edema probably has heart failure. An astute assessment of the whole patient from head to toe is necessary to distinguish a pulmonary, cardiac, or infectious origin of a cough or dyspnea.

Physical Examination

After taking the patient's vital signs, the clinician should conduct a thorough physical examination. Assessing the pulmonary system requires use of all the physical assessment techniques: inspection, palpation, percussion, and auscultation.

Inspection

The patient should be seated with relaxed posture and arms resting comfortably at the side or in the lap. Observe the patient's breathing pattern and excursion of the chest wall with inhalation and exhalation. The patient's skin should be warm and without cyanosis or pallor. Extremities should be inspected for normal brachial and radial pulses, and capillary refill in the fingernails should be less than 3 seconds. Clubbing of the fingertips can be a sign of chronic oxygen deprivation (see Fig. 21-2).

Assess the rate, rhythm, and depth of respirations by observing the rise and fall of the chest during breathing. The presence of retractions, visible indentation of the intercostal and supraclavicular spaces, is a sign of increased work of breathing and respiratory distress; it indicates that accessory muscles are necessary for inspiration. Nasal flaring is also a sign of respiratory distress. Normal respiratory rate is 12 to 20 breaths per minute. **Bradypnea**, or hypoventilation, is a respiratory rate less than 12 breaths per minute, whereas **tachypnea**, or hyperventilation, is a respiratory rate greater than 20 breaths per minute.

Palpation

Palpation involves examination of the chest wall with the fingers in order to identify areas of tenderness, changes in skin temperature, moisture, superficial lumps or masses, and skin lesions. Check symmetrical chest expansion by placing the hands on the posterior lateral chest wall with thumbs at the level of T9 or T10. Ask the patient to take a deep breath; the thumbs should move apart symmetrically.

Tactile fremitus is palpable vibration generated by the larynx and transmitted through the patient's bronchi to the chest wall. The examiner should place both hands on the patient's posterior chest and have the patient repeat the phrase "ninety-nine." The examiner then moves down the posterior chest wall in a systematic manner as the patient repeats "ninety-nine" (see Fig. 20-5). Vibration felt on the examiner's hands from both sides of the chest should be equal. An increased amount of vibration felt by one of the hands on the chest wall can indicate the presence of pneumonia in the region. A decreased amount of vibration can indicate pleural effusion.

Percussion

Percussion involves a specific technique of tapping tissues to elicit sounds. The examiner places a hand on the posterior chest wall between the patient's ribs. The examiner then takes their free hand and uses one or two fingers to strike the middle finger of the hand against the chest wall. The examiner does this down the back of the patient. The changes in the specific

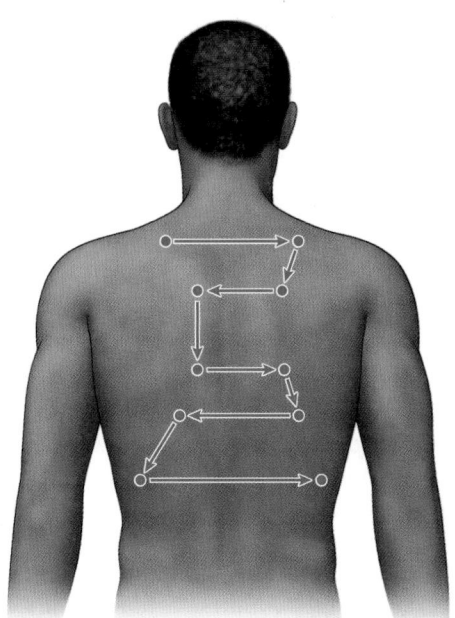

FIGURE 20-5. Palpation and auscultation of the chest in the systematic method.

tones are based on the density of the tissue. Tissues that contain air, such as the lungs, are described as resonant. Dull sounds indicate a solid mass or fluid consolidation. Hyperresonance indicates that the lungs are hyperinflated, which occurs in emphysema.

Auscultation

The flow of air through the bronchi, bronchioles, and into the alveoli can be assessed through auscultation of the lungs with a stethoscope. The presence of fluids or solid substances in the lung tissue can also be localized using auscultation.

Normal Breath Sounds. The characteristics of normal breath sounds vary according to the anatomical location within the lungs. Over the trachea, breath sounds are very loud, tubular, and high-pitched. They are called bronchial breath sounds; expiratory sounds last longer than inspiratory sounds. Over the bronchi, bronchovesicular sounds are heard, which are equal in inspiration and expiration and have an intermediate intensity and pitch. They can be heard over the main bronchi located in the first and second interspaces anteriorly and between the scapulae posteriorly. Vesicular breath sounds are longer in inspiration than expiration, low pitched, and heard over the peripheral lung fields.

Abnormal Breath Sounds. **Adventitious breath sounds** are extra lung sounds superimposed over normal breath sounds present in various kinds of pulmonary dysfunction. Crackles, sometimes called rales, are noncontinuous sounds that occur when deflated alveoli open and close against fluid. They are commonly present in heart failure or pneumonia. Wheezes are high-pitched, whistling sounds related to the constricted

diameter of the airways and may be inspiratory or expiratory in nature. Rhonchi are low-pitched, snore-like sounds present over inflamed bronchial airways. A friction rub is a grating, scratchy sound heard during inspiration and expiration with inflammation of the pleural surfaces.

Vocal resonance is the transmission of the sounds of speech through the lungs as heard when using the stethoscope. Listening for vocal resonance is a physical assessment technique that can be used in the diagnosis of pneumonia. To listen for vocal resonance in physical examination, the patient is asked to repeat a phrase such as "ninety-nine" as the clinician listens with a stethoscope over different regions of the lungs. In normal lungs, the sound of the patient's voice is muffled. In **bronchophony**, the patient's words become clearer and louder over areas of pneumonia. In **egophony**, the patient is asked to repeat "e" as the clinician listens over different regions of the lungs. Over areas of pneumonia, the "e" will sound like "a." In **whispered pectoriloquy**, over normal lungs, whispered words are usually muffled. However, when the clinician listens to areas of pneumonia, whispered sounds become clear and distinctive.

🔬 CLINICAL CONCEPT

When bronchial breath sounds are heard over the peripheral lung field, this commonly indicates pneumonia.

Diagnostic Testing

Diagnostic testing is an important component of respiratory assessment. Many tests are used to diagnose specific diseases, but discussion of all of them is beyond the scope of this text. The following are the most significant diagnostic tests used in respiratory disease. ABGs provide information about gas exchange. Chest x-rays can visualize the structure of the chest and lungs. If an infection is suspected, culture and sensitivity testing is performed on sputum or a swab of the throat. Computed tomography (CT) scanning and magnetic resonance imaging (MRI) demonstrate detailed cross-sectional views of the lungs and can be useful when chest x-ray is inadequate. A V-Q scan demonstrates the balance of ventilation and circulation within the lungs. It is commonly used to investigate PE if the CT scan is inadequate.

Arterial Blood Gases. ABGs are serum blood values obtained through an arterial puncture. They enable identification of alterations in acid–base balance caused by respiratory diseases. ABG results include blood pH, partial pressure of O_2, CO_2, bicarbonate ion, and the saturation of hemoglobin (Hgb) (see Table 20-2). A pH of more than 7.45 indicates **alkalosis**, and a pH of lower than 7.35 indicates acidosis (see Chapter 8).

The level of arterial oxygen (PaO_2) indicates the degree of oxygenation of the blood. Arterial oxygen

TABLE 20-2. Normal Values of Arterial Blood Gases

Value	Normal
pH	7.35 to 7.45
PCO_2	35 to 45 mm Hg
HCO_3^-	22 to 26 mEq/L
PO_2	90 to 100 mm Hg
% Hgb saturation with O_2	95% to 100%

may also be referred to as PO_2. The saturation of Hgb with oxygen (SaO_2) in the arterial blood also indicates the arterial oxygenation. The arterial carbon dioxide level ($PaCO_2$) is an indicator of alveolar ventilation. Arterial carbon dioxide may also be referred to as PCO_2. The PaO_2 and $PaCO_2$ values are useful in determining the ability of the lungs to provide oxygen and remove carbon dioxide. The pH of the blood is balanced by the lungs and the kidneys. The lungs regulate CO_2, and the kidneys regulate conservation and excretion of acid (H^+) and HCO_3^- (bicarbonate ion). The following equation demonstrates the chemical reaction occurring in the bloodstream in terms of CO_2, H^+ (acid) and HCO_3^- (base) (as discussed in Chapter 8):

$$CO_2 + H_2O \leftrightarrow H_2CO_3 \leftrightarrow H^+ + HCO_3^-$$

Culture and Sensitivity Testing. Culture and sensitivity testing of sputum samples can assist in the diagnosis of respiratory infection. Sputum that has been obtained by expectoration may be contaminated with normal flora from the mouth. Microscopic examination for the presence of epithelial cells from the oral mucosa can help determine whether it is contaminated. Sputum cultures obtained by suctioning the respiratory tract or through bronchoscopy are less likely to be contaminated by normal flora. Acid-fast smears and cultures of the sputum are used for TB. Nucleic acid amplification tests (NAAT) on sputum, also used to identify the presence of TB, can provide more rapid results than acid-fast smear and culture. NAAT can be used to diagnose other types of pathogens that cause respiratory infection or malignancy.

Pulse Oximetry. Pulse oximetry can continuously monitor the oxygen saturation of hemoglobin (SaO_2). A small probe is attached to an extremity, usually the fingertip, although the forehead, earlobe, or toe may also be used. Infrared light passes over the extremity, reflects the blood pulsing through the tissue, and senses changes in oxygen saturation. Normal SaO_2 is 95% to 100%. A saturation level lower than 95% indicates that tissues are not receiving enough oxygen.

Imaging Studies. Imaging studies used to diagnose lung disease include chest x-rays, CT, and MRI. Chest x-ray can demonstrate numerous abnormalities, including inadequate lung expansion, areas of consolidation, changes associated with COPD, tumor, pneumothorax, or the presence of fluid in or around the lungs. It is also often used to evaluate the response to treatment. A CT scan shows a more specific cross-sectional view of the respiratory system and can identify many different pathological conditions, such as lung abscesses, tumors, TB, and pleural effusion. A chest MRI can be used to provide more detail than a CT scan. Inhaled hyperpolarized gas MRI can use inhaled gases to evaluate ventilation and gas exchange in the lungs.

Bronchoscopy. Bronchoscopy allows for direct visualization of the larynx, trachea, and bronchi, which can then allow for biopsy and removal of foreign objects. Secretions may also be removed using suctioning during the test. Endobronchial ultrasound can be used with bronchoscopy to assist in the diagnosis of inflammatory, infectious, or cancerous respiratory conditions.

Thoracocentesis. Thoracocentesis is the removal of pleural fluid using a large-bore needle inserted through the chest wall into the pleural space. The procedure can be used to obtain specimens for culture and sensitivity or biopsy. Medication may also be inserted during the procedure.

Pulmonary Function Tests. Pulmonary function tests (also called spirometry) can be used in the diagnosis of inflammatory respiratory diseases. These tests evaluate lung volumes, such as inspiratory and expiratory flow and residual lung volume, and can differentiate between obstructive and restrictive diseases.

Treatment

Treatment of inflammatory and infectious pulmonary disease includes a variety of drugs and procedures. The following includes general treatment measures. Bronchodilators reduce bronchospasm, and antibiotics treat bacterial respiratory infections. PE can be treated with thrombolytic and anticoagulant medications. Decongestant medications cause vasoconstriction that helps to reduce the inflammation and edema in the nasal passage and relieve nasal congestion. Antihistamine medications block the inflammatory effects of histamine in the airways. Antitussive medications can be used to control coughs. A warm saltwater gargle and mild analgesics can be used to treat pharyngitis (sore throat). Antiviral drugs, such as amantadine, are available to lessen the effects of viral infection in the respiratory tract.

ALERT! Coughing is important for ridding the airways of secretions, so clinicians do not want to inhibit coughing or oversedate the patient to a point that weakens the cough.

Pulmonary hygiene measures are used to clear the respiratory tract of mucus and purulent drainage. Methods used for pulmonary hygiene include suctioning of the airways, chest physiotherapy, incentive spirometry, and nasotracheal suction. Percussion over the chest loosens secretions and allows the cilia of the airways to remove material. Positioning is another method for promoting drainage of secretions. Intermittent positive pressure breathing physiotherapy is often used in nonintubated patients. Nebulizers can deliver humidified air with medication. Supplemental oxygen and mechanical ventilation are used when hypoxia or respiratory failure occur.

Pathophysiology of Selected Upper Respiratory Tract Disorders

Respiratory tract infections affect airway clearance and breathing patterns by changing the amount and character of secretions produced in the airways. Risk factors for respiratory infection include stress and exposure to people infected with various microorganisms such as bacteria, viruses, and fungi. Any disease or condition that causes an immunocompromised state allows microorganisms to invade the body and proliferate rapidly, possibly resulting in infection.

More than 200 strains of viruses cause upper respiratory tract infections. A common method of spreading viruses is the release of airborne droplet nuclei when the infected individual coughs, laughs, or sneezes. Pathogens are also commonly spread by hand-to-hand contact.

Acute Rhinitis

Acute rhinitis is a disorder that results in inflammation and irritation of the mucous membranes of the nasal passages. Caused by rhinoviruses as well as other viruses, it is transmitted mainly through airborne droplets. The incubation period is approximately 2 to 4 days. Rhinovirus is shed in large amounts and is present a few days before cold symptoms are experienced by the patient. Viral shedding peaks on days 2 through 7 of the illness. A local inflammatory response to the virus in the respiratory tract leads to nasal discharge, nasal congestion, sneezing, and throat irritation. A slight fever may be present. Nasal mucociliary transport is markedly reduced during the illness and may be impaired for weeks. Diagnosis is mainly through physical examination and history. The nasal mucosa and nasal turbinates are red. The discharge from the nose can be clear, yellow, or green in color. Pharyngeal erythema and earache may also be present.

Complete blood count (CBC) may show a high number of lymphocytes with viral infection and a high number of neutrophils with bacterial infection. Both secretory immunoglobulin A and serum antibodies are involved in resolving the illness and protecting from reinfection.

Antihistamines, analgesics, and antipyretic medication such as acetaminophen are usually sufficient treatment. A corticosteroid nasal spray is often prescribed for allergic rhinitis.

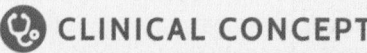

CLINICAL CONCEPT

Acute rhinitis can also be caused by allergies. In this case, it resembles the illness of the common cold; however, the interior nasal mucosa and turbinates are usually gray colored. Discharge from the nose is clear. The patient often has a crease at the tip of the nose from the constant maneuver of wiping upward from the nares, sometimes referred to as the "allergic salute." The patient's CBC usually shows a high number of eosinophils.

Acute Pharyngitis

Acute pharyngitis, an inflammation of the pharynx, is usually caused by a virus. If acute bacterial pharyngitis occurs, the cause can be **group A beta-hemolytic streptococcus (GABHS)**, also called *Streptococcus pyogenes*. The infection can spread from the pharynx to cause sinusitis and otitis media. In more severe cases, GABHS can cause bacteremia, pneumonia, meningitis, necrotizing fasciitis, rheumatic fever, rheumatic heart disease, scarlet fever, toxic shock syndrome, and glomerulonephritis.

In pharyngitis, assessment reveals red, swollen pharyngeal membranes and tonsils. The lymphoid follicles of the tonsils are swollen and often covered with white exudate; cervical lymph nodes may be enlarged and tender. The patient may have a fever, malaise, and a sore throat but typically has no cough.

Diagnosis is made by visual inspection and identification of the causative organism. A rapid screening test for streptococcal antigens and bacterial throat cultures are used to identify the organism causing the infection. To rule out Epstein–Barr virus (EBV), a heterophile antibody test is necessary. Penicillin, erythromycin, or cephalosporins may be used to treat a bacterial infection. Saltwater gargle, as well as antipyretic and analgesic medications, are used to treat the fever and sore throat.

Acute Sinusitis

Sinusitis is an infection of the facial sinuses and membranes of the nose. The sinuses are mucus-lined cavities filled with air that drain into the nose. Sinusitis may be acute, subacute, or chronic. Acute sinusitis often accompanies a URI or an allergic reaction and may be caused by a virus, bacteria, or both. Acute sinusitis caused by a virus usually lasts from 5 to 7 days. Bacterial sinusitis may last up to 4 weeks. Chronic sinusitis is an inflammation of the sinuses that persists for more than 12 weeks.

In sinusitis, the sinus cavity becomes obstructed because of accumulated fluid and edema caused by the inflammatory process. The fluid present in this area is an excellent medium for bacterial growth and infection. Symptoms include headache, facial pain or pressure over the sinus area, nasal obstruction, fatigue, purulent nasal discharge, fever, ear pain, dental pain, cough, decreased sense of smell, and sore throat. A sinus headache is usually made worse by the increased pressure that occurs when bending forward, coughing, or sneezing. Facial edema, nasal crusting, and purulent drainage in the nasal cavity may also be present.

Antimicrobial agents such as amoxicillin clavulanate (Augmentin), ampicillin (Ampicin), or third generation cephalosporins may be used to treat the infection. Decongestant and antihistamine medications, saline sprays, and heated mist may help relieve symptoms. Mucolytic agents may decrease secretions.

> **CLINICAL CONCEPT**
>
> A throat culture can confirm pharyngitis due to GABHS. A heterophile antibody test can confirm pharyngitis due to EBV.

Acute Tonsillitis

Acute tonsillitis is an acute infection of the tonsils and pharynx that is sometimes called pharyngotonsillitis. The most common causes of acute tonsillitis are GABHS or viruses such as EBV, adenovirus, herpes simplex virus, or cytomegalovirus. EBV is responsible for 19% of exudative tonsillitis in children; bacteria cause between 15% and 30% of the pharyngotonsillitis cases, and other cases are caused by other viruses. Sore throat, fever, and difficulty swallowing are the most common signs and symptoms. Cervical lymphadenopathy is a characteristic sign of EBV tonsillitis. EBV also can cause infectious mononucleosis.

The physical examination demonstrates erythema and swelling of the tonsillar tissue and pharynx. Severe swelling of the tonsils with abscess, called quinsy, can cause swallowing difficulty. Throat culture is the best diagnostic test. To rule out EBV, a heterophile antibody test is necessary. Some children are carriers of GABHS and do not develop pharyngotonsillitis but can transmit GABHS tonsillitis to others. These children can have a positive throat culture but do not have antibodies against GABHS. If there are recurrent infections or if severe tissue hypertrophy occurs, a tonsillectomy may be performed. If the infection is caused by GABHS, antibiotics are necessary.

Epiglottitis

Epiglottitis is the infection and inflammation of the epiglottis—the flap of tissue that sits atop the trachea

to keep food from going into the trachea during swallowing. When inflamed, the epiglottis can obstruct the trachea. It may be caused by a respiratory infection, exposure to chemical substances in the environment, trauma, and various organisms, including bacteria, viruses, and fungi. Common organisms that cause epiglottitis include *Streptococcus pneumoniae, Haemophilus influenzae,* parainfluenza, varicella zoster virus, herpes simplex virus type 1, and *Staphylococcus aureus.*

The disorder begins as inflammation and swelling between the base of the tongue and the epiglottis. The swelling pushes the epiglottis backward; as the process continues, complete blockage of the airway occurs, leading to suffocation and death.

X-rays and a laryngoscopic examination will show that the pharynx is inflamed, red, and stiff and that the epiglottis is swollen. Blood tests will show signs of infection or inflammation, ABGs will confirm lack of gas exchange, and cultures may grow bacteria and indicate the causative organism. Neck x-ray shows a characteristic swelling of the pharyngeal tissues called "steeple" sign.

Immediate hospitalization is usually necessary, as there is a danger of sudden and unpredictable closing of the airway. Initial treatment includes making the person as comfortable as possible, humidified oxygen, and IV fluids. Antibiotics are given to control inflammation and stop the infection after the causative organism has been identified.

> **ALERT!** Epiglottitis is a medical emergency. A laryngoscope and tracheostomy equipment should be available at the patient's bedside at all times, because intubation may be needed.

Laryngitis and Tracheitis

Laryngitis is inflammation of the larynx, whereas tracheitis is inflammation of the trachea. The infection that causes both is usually viral in nature, although bacteria such as *Haemophilus influenzae* can also cause the infection. Signs of acute laryngitis are hoarseness or complete loss of the voice. If the infection involves the larynx, trachea, and bronchi, then laryngotracheobronchitis, commonly called croup, occurs. Croup is mainly a children's disease.

In laryngitis, an irritating, high-pitched cough may be present. Tracheal involvement can produce a raspy cough or stridor, a high-pitched inhalation sound. Pleuritic chest pain may indicate pleural or other musculoskeletal involvement. The underlying cause of the cough is the irritation of the mucous membranes. Eventually, sputum will be produced in response to the chronic irritation. Sputum is usually thin and may be yellow or green when bacteria are causing the infection. Thin mucoid sputum may indicate a viral or bacterial infection. Foul-smelling sputum may indicate a lung abscess. As airways narrow, the patient begins to wheeze, mainly upon expiration.

There is no specific medical intervention for viral laryngitis other than resting the voice and managing the symptoms. If the infection has spread and proves to be bacterial, antibiotics may be administered. Bronchodilator medications are useful if the airway has narrowed and wheezing is present. Tracheitis can involve the epiglottis; if so, it can become a medical emergency.

Pathophysiology of Selected Lower Respiratory Tract Disorders

The lungs are constantly exposed to environmental pathogens and all types of pollutants, which increases susceptibility to infection. Aspiration of contents from the oropharynx can also increase the risk of respiratory infection. Infections of the lower respiratory tract hinder the exchange of oxygen and carbon dioxide, creating a vulnerability to hypoxia and hypercapnia.

Acute Bronchitis

Acute **bronchitis** is an inflammation of the bronchi and bronchioles caused by either bacterial or viral infection. Bronchitis can also be triggered by inhalation of toxic gases or chemicals.

Epidemiology
It is estimated that 44 out of 1000 adults suffer from acute bronchitis in the United States annually. This is likely a low estimate because not all individuals with acute bronchitis seek health care. Most episodes occur in fall or winter.

Etiology
Respiratory viruses are the most common causes of acute bronchitis. The most common viruses include influenza A and B, parainfluenza, respiratory syncytial virus, and coronavirus. Bacteria that cause acute bronchitis include *Mycoplasma* species, *Chlamydia pneumoniae, Streptococcus pneumoniae, Moraxella catarrhalis,* and *Haemophilus influenzae. Bordetella pertussis,* which causes whooping cough, is another microorganism that can cause bronchitis. *B. pertussis* has had a recent resurgence in incidence in the United States after many years of successful eradication because of pertussis vaccine.

Cigarette smoking and exposure to pollutants or chemical irritants increase susceptibility to bronchitis. URIs such as the common cold, sinusitis, and pharyngitis also increase susceptibility to acute bronchitis. Influenza is commonly complicated by acute bronchitis.

Pathophysiology
In acute bronchitis, the bronchial tree undergoes an inflammatory response to a pathogen or irritant. The cells of the bronchial tissue are irritated, and the mucous membrane becomes edematous, diminishing the bronchial mucociliary function. The air passages become obstructed by excessive mucus. Dysfunctional mucociliary movement and excess mucous secretion cause patients to frequently cough to clear the airway of secretions. Pleuritic chest pain with inhalation and exhalation, fever, and general malaise are also common.

Clinical Presentation
In the history, the patient may report that the illness began as a common cold. It is important to ask the patient when the symptoms began to exclude chronic bronchitis as the diagnosis. The clinician should ask about recent exposure of the patient to others who are ill, recent exposure to pollutants or occupational chemicals, and past medical history. It is important to know if the patient has a history of asthma because acute bronchitis sometimes presents with wheezing. The patient usually complains of sore throat, nasal discharge, muscle aches, and persistent cough. The initial days of infection can appear as the common cold and fever, and headache may occur. Cough becomes prominent as the disease progresses and can last from 10 to 20 days during the course of acute bronchitis. Sputum production is reported in most patients. Sputum may be clear, yellow, green, or even blood tinged. Purulent sputum is reported in 50% of persons with acute bronchitis. Sputum color is not indicative of bacterial versus viral infection.

On physical examination, the patient may exhibit pharyngeal erythema, localized lymphadenopathy, and rhinorrhea. Rhonchi and wheezes can be heard across all lung fields. In severe cases, diffuse wheezes, high-pitched continuous sounds, and the use of accessory muscles can be observed. Coughing can clear some of the rhonchi and wheezes. Inspiratory stridor indicates that there may be mucous obstruction within the trachea.

Diagnosis
Diagnosis is mainly based on symptomatology, although a culture of respiratory secretions may be done. A CBC may be useful to distinguish bacterial infections from nonbacterial infections. A chest x-ray is usually done to rule out pneumonia.

 CLINICAL CONCEPT

Chronic bronchitis is diagnosed when a patient reports a history of bronchitis for 3 months out of the year for at least 2 years.

Treatment
Broad-spectrum antibiotics are used to treat bacterial infections. Expectorant medications will assist the individual to cough up the exudate and mucus. Mucolytic agents can dissolve mucus. At times, a bronchodilator

is necessary if bronchospasm is present with cough. Cough suppressants may be needed at night to allow the individual to sleep.

Pneumonia

Pneumonia is inflammation of the lung tissue in which alveolar airspaces fill with purulent, inflammatory cells and fibrin. Infection by bacteria or viruses is the most common cause, although inhalation of chemicals, aspiration of contents from the oropharynx or stomach, or infection by other infectious agents such as rickettsiae and fungi may occur.

Epidemiology

Pneumonia causes more deaths in the United States than any other infection. There are various types of pneumonia, depending on the setting in which it occurs: community acquired, health-care acquired, and ventilator associated. Etiological pathogens vary widely, depending on the setting of the disease. In the United States, **community-acquired pneumonia (CAP)** accounts for over 4.5 million outpatient and emergency department visits annually. CAP is the second most common cause of hospitalization and the most common infectious cause of death. Approximately 650 adults are hospitalized with CAP every year per 100,000 population in the United States, corresponding to 1.5 million CAP hospitalizations each year. Nearly 9% of patients hospitalized with CAP will be rehospitalized due to a new episode of CAP during the same year.

Pneumonia is more prevalent during the winter months and in colder climates. The incidence of pneumonia is greater in males than in females. Advanced age increases the incidence of, and the mortality from, pneumonia. Comorbidity and a diminished immune response and defence against aspiration increase the risk of bacterial pneumonia. For adults in the United States, pneumonia is the most common cause of hospital admission other than women giving birth.

Pneumonia is often the cause of death in chronically ill patients. For individuals aged 65 years and older, pneumonia is the eighth leading cause of death. Health-care–associated pneumonia (also called hospital-associated pneumonia) (HAP) is a lung infection that is contracted after 48 hours of hospital admission. Among intubated and mechanically ventilated patients, the development of HAP is specifically called ventilator-associated pneumonia (VAP).

Etiological and Risk Factors

Bacteria are the most common etiological agents involved in pneumonia. Certain types of pneumonia are more common in specific settings and conditions. CAP is most often caused by *Streptococcus pneumoniae* (also called pneumococcus), *H. influenzae*, *Mycoplasma*, *Klebsiella*, *Staphylococcus*, and *Legionella* species and gram-negative organisms.

In the preantibiotic era, *Streptococcus pneumoniae* (pneumococcus) caused more than 90% of cases of pneumonia in adults. After 1950, the proportion of pneumonia caused by pneumococcus began to decline. Pneumococcus has continued to decline; at present, this organism is identified in fewer than 10% to 15% of CAP cases. Gram-negative bacilli, *Staphylococcus aureus, Chlamydia, Mycoplasma,* and *Legionella* are each identified in 2% to 5% of patients with pneumonia who require hospitalization. Viruses are found in 25% of patients, and up to one-third of these have bacterial coinfection. Recent studies demonstrate that there is failure to identify a causative organism in more than 50% of cases (Musher et al., 2017).

Aspiration pneumonia is commonly caused by anaerobic bacteria swallowed from the oropharynx. Some pathogens, particularly *Staphylococcus* species, may be spread via the bloodstream to the lungs. *Staphylococcus* usually enters the bloodstream via an IV route from a central vein catheter or IV drug abuse. *Staphylococcus* is also the microorganism most commonly involved in HAP and VAP; specifically, methicillin-resistant *Staphylococcus aureus* (MRSA). In addition to MRSA, *Enterococcus* is commonly involved in VAP, specifically vancomycin-resistant enterococcus (VRE). Other microorganisms frequently involved in HAP and VAP are *Pseudomonas, Klebsiella,* and *Acinetobacter. Legionella* causes a unique kind of pneumonia, which is spread via water systems such as air conditioning, mists sprayed on produce in grocery stores, and hot tubs. *Legionella* pneumonia commonly affects small clusters of individuals living together in hotels, dormitories, or cruise ships. *Mycoplasma* is a small bacteria-like organism that can cause a syndrome called walking pneumonia. In this mild form of pneumonia, the patient may not appear very ill but has persistent cough and commonly headache and earache.

One of the major risk factors for pneumonia is influenza infection. Viruses commonly alter the pulmonary immune defenses and make the lungs vulnerable to bacterial infection, referred to as secondary pneumonia. Although influenza virus is the most common agent, other respiratory viruses, such as respiratory syncytial virus, parainfluenza viruses, SARS-CoV2 (coronavirus) adenovirus, and rhinoviruses, may also predispose individuals to pneumonia as a secondary bacterial infection. Immunosuppression can predispose patients to pneumonia. In HIV infection and AIDS, pneumonia is commonly caused by *Pneumocystis jirovecii. Pneumocystis* is a yeast-like fungal organism formerly known as *Pneumocystis carinii. Pneumocystis* pneumonia is often referred to as PCP.

Aspiration can also predispose the patient to pneumonia caused by accidental inhalation of substances refluxed from the stomach. Comatose patients and those with impaired gag reflex are at highest risk for aspiration pneumonia. Chronic gingivitis and periodontitis increase the risk of aspiration pneumonia and lung abscess.

Other risk factors for pneumonia include lung cancer or tumors, COPD, and bronchiectasis. Smoking impairs resistance to infection. Alcohol or drug intoxication increases the risk of aspiration pneumonia with asphyxiation. Pneumonia is the second most common cause of nursing home–associated infection after urinary tract infection. Postviral, aspiration, and bacterial pneumonias are major causes of death in nursing home residents.

Emerging infections are often the cause of pneumonia. Avian influenza virus, severe acute respiratory system coronavirus (SARS-CoV2), and Middle Eastern respiratory syndrome (MERS) virus are among the causes of these pneumonias. In 2020, approximately 15% to 20% of SARS-CoV2 (also called COVID-19) infections caused pneumonia, with 5% of people requiring mechanical ventilation (Alipoor et al., 2020; Mason, 2020). Environmental sources of pathogens can cause clusters of infection in the population, such as *Legionella pneumophila* (referred to as Legionnaire's disease). Bioterrorism pathogens can cause pneumonia, particularly *Bacillus anthracis*—the cause of anthrax.

Pathophysiology

Pneumonia is most commonly caused by inhalation of droplets containing bacteria or other pathogens. The droplets enter the upper airways and then enter the lung tissue. Pathogens adhere to respiratory epithelium and stimulate an inflammatory reaction. The acute inflammation spreads to the lower respiratory tract and alveoli. At the sites of inflammation, vasodilation occurs, and neutrophils travel out of capillaries into the air spaces. The neutrophils phagocytize microbes and kill them using reactive oxygen species, antimicrobial proteins, and degradative enzymes. There is an excessive stimulation of respiratory goblet cells that secrete mucus. Mucous and exudative edema accumulate between the alveoli and capillaries. The alveoli attempt to open and close against the purulent exudate; however, some cannot open. The sounds heard with the stethoscope over the alveoli opening against the exudative fluid are crackles. A layer of edema and infectious exudate at the capillary–alveoli interface hinders optimal gas exchange. The patient can become hypoxic and hypercapnic, with obstructed exchange of O_2 and CO_2 at the pulmonary capillaries.

Clinical Presentation

The clinical presentation of bacterial pneumonia usually starts with a sudden onset of symptoms. Cough, which may or may not be productive of sputum; fever; and chills are usually initial manifestations. Pleuritic chest pain, which is pain with deep breaths; dyspnea; hemoptysis; and decreased exercise tolerance develop as the disorder continues. Other nonspecific symptoms that may be seen with pneumonia include myalgias, headache, abdominal pain, nausea, and vomiting. Headache and earache, with less cough and fever, are the symptoms that occur with *Mycoplasma* pneumonia.

On physical examination, the patient is likely to demonstrate fever, tachypnea, use of accessory muscles with breathing, tachycardia, and possibly cyanosis. Crackles are pathognomonic of pneumonia, and the clinician can elicit egophony, bronchophony, and whispered pectoriloquy. There may be dullness to percussion and increased fremitus over the site of pneumonia. The patient may have periodontal disease, which can increase susceptibility to aspiration pneumonia with anaerobic infection. Poor cough and gag reflex increases the risk of aspiration pneumonia. Otitis media (middle ear infection) and myringitis (inflammation of the tympanic membrane) typically occur in *Mycoplasma pneumoniae* infection.

When interviewing the patient, it is important to assess exposure to any other persons who are ill and evaluate if the patient has any aspiration risks or immunosuppression factors. The clinician should ask the patient about current medications, allergies, and past medical history. Conditions such as influenza, asthma, or COPD increase susceptibility to pneumonia. Social habits, such as smoking and use of alcohol or illicit drugs, are also factors that increase risk for pneumonia.

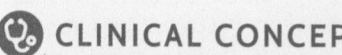

CLINICAL CONCEPT

Cough, crackles, and fever are the characteristic signs of pneumonia. In older adult patients, hypothermia may present instead of fever.

Diagnosis

A chest x-ray is the most important diagnostic study in the diagnosis of pneumonia (see Fig. 20-6). CBC with differential will suggest either a bacterial or viral infection. Pulse oximetry can demonstrate oxygenation. Sputum culture and sensitivity can exhibit the

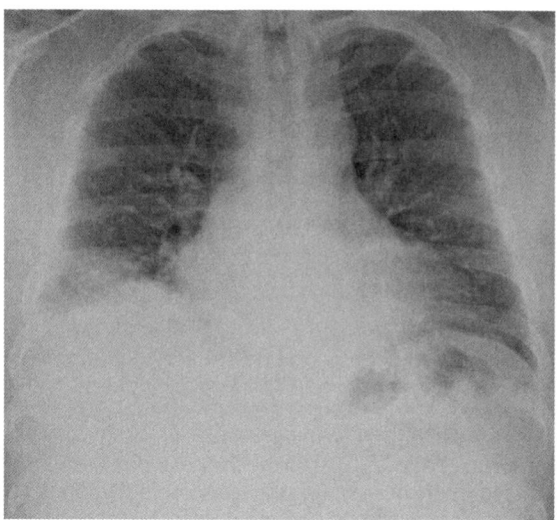

FIGURE 20-6. Chest x-ray showing pneumonia.

organism and antibiotic susceptibility. Ultrasound and thoracocentesis are useful if pleural effusion is suspected. Sputum, serum, and urinary antigen tests are available for *S. pneumoniae* and *Legionella*.

Treatment

Antibiotic therapy and oxygenation of the patient are key priorities in the treatment of pneumonia. Fowler's position and oxygen via nasal cannula or mask are recommended. The patient may require IV fluids if dehydrated. Analgesia, antipyretics, and bronchodilators may be needed. To prevent pneumonia in older adults, infants, and children with risk factors, the pneumococcal vaccine is recommended.

 CLINICAL CONCEPT

In primary care, it is sometimes difficult to evaluate the need for hospitalization for the patient with pneumonia. The clinician can use the pneumonia severity index (PSI) as a guide for inpatient care and mortality risk (see Fig. 20-7).

Patient characteristic*	Score
Nursing home resident	+10
Cancer	+30
Heart failure	+10
Stroke	+10
Kidney disease	+10
Altered level of consciousness	+20
Respiratory rate greater than 30/min	+20
Systolic BP lower than 90	+20
Fever	+15
Pulse greater than 125	+10
Blood ph lower than 7.35	+30
PO₂ lower than 60 mm Hg	+10
SaO₂ lower than 90%	+10
*Incomplete list **Risk score**	

0–90	**Low risk**
91–130	**Moderate risk**
Greater than 130	**High risk**

FIGURE 20-7. The pneumonia severity index (PSI). Some patients can recover from pneumonia with outpatient antibiotics. However, there are situations where pneumonia requires hospitalization. To determine whether the patient with pneumonia requires inpatient care, the PSI is often used. This can categorize the patient into classes according to risk. A score can be calculated using numerical values for different patient characteristics. This table is a modified example of how the PSI is scored.

Lung Abscess

A lung abscess is a localized area of purulent exudate that results in tissue necrosis and a central area of liquefaction. A common cause of a lung abscess is the aspiration of oral contents containing anaerobic bacteria into the lungs.

Epidemiology

Lung abscess accounts for up to 4 to 5.5 per 10,000 hospital admissions each year in the United States. They occur at any age, but most frequently from the sixth to eighth decades, and are seen predominantly in men. Immunosuppression is increasing the incidence of lung abscess in younger adults; however, specific statistics are unclear.

Etiology and Risk Factors

Lung abscess can develop as a complication of bacterial pneumonia. The exudate can form a walled-off, localized collection of infectious material. However, aspiration of anaerobic bacteria from the oral cavity is more often the etiology of lung abscess. Patients who aspirate anaerobic bacteria and develop a lung abscess are usually debilitated from other health problems or are immunosuppressed. Risk factors include advanced age, alcoholism, debilitation, malnutrition, HIV infection or other forms of immunosuppression, and malignancy. IV drug abuse is a risk factor specifically for staphylococcal lung abscesses. Puncture of the skin allows entry of staphylococcal organisms into the bloodstream. Staphylococcal endocarditis usually occurs initially. It is often caused by tricuspid valve endocarditis with staphylococcal organisms. This is followed by the development of septic emboli, which commonly develop from right-sided endocarditis, that travel into the lungs to form abscesses. An abscess may also develop secondary to carcinoma of the bronchus; bronchial obstruction can cause an obstructive pneumonia, which may lead to abscess formation.

Pathophysiology

An abscess occurs after the alveoli have filled with fluid, purulent exudate, and microorganisms, causing the tissue to become necrotic. This process continues until the abscess ruptures and leaves a cavity filled with air and fluid. The purulent material that is released can obstruct bronchioles and the alveolar–capillary transfer of oxygen, which can eventually cause acute respiratory distress. Complications can occur if bacteria enter the bloodstream and cause sepsis. Bloodstream infection can lead to cerebral infection and meningitis.

Clinical Presentation

The major symptom of a lung abscess is copious amounts of foul-smelling sputum. Other symptoms include a productive cough, chills and fever, chest pain, malaise, and anorexia. Breath sounds are diminished, and crackles may be heard in the region of the abscess.

Diagnosis

A CBC may indicate leukocytosis, and a chest x-ray may show a thick solitary cavity with surrounding consolidation. A CT scan may demonstrate a better image of the abscess than an x-ray. The causative organism is usually identified by a sputum culture after the cavity has ruptured.

Treatment

Treatment for a lung abscess includes IV antibiotic therapy. Surgical drainage or lobectomy may be required. Bronchoscopy may be used to drain the abscess; if the pleural space is involved, a chest tube may be inserted. Postural drainage is often helpful in relieving the obstruction and promoting drainage.

Tuberculosis

TB is an infection caused by the **Mycobacterium tuberculosis** bacterial organism. Although most commonly occurring in the lungs, TB can infect other parts of the body, such as the adrenal gland, vertebrae, meninges, and lymph nodes. It can also spread within the bloodstream and cause multisystem disease. There are two forms of TB: TB disease and latent TB infection (LTBI) (see Fig. 20-8). In TB disease, the infected individual has

symptoms and clinical evidence of active disease. They are usually severely ill, infectious to others, and can die if not treated. In LTBI, the individual has been infected with the *M. tuberculosis* organism but the disease is dormant. The individual has no clinical symptoms and is noninfectious. Both forms require treatment, as LTBI can convert to active TB disease at any point during the individual's lifetime if not treated.

Epidemiology

TB is one of the top 10 causes of death in the world. HIV infection and TB are among the most lethal infectious diseases. It is estimated that globally, 2 billion people—one-fourth of the world's population—are infected with *M. tuberculosis*. The majority, 1.7 billion persons, have latent TB infection. Approximately 10% of these persons are speculated to progress to active TB disease in their lifetime.

The prevalence of TB is particularly high in Africa, India, and Asia. In 2019, the incidence of TB in the United States was 2.7 per 100,000 persons, which was considered the lowest on record. However, during 2021, the U.S. TB incidence increased by 9.4%. The increased incidence is believed to be due to delayed detection of cases in 2020 that were not diagnosed until 2021 because of the COVID-19 pandemic. During the pandemic, many persons delayed seeking health care and there were interruptions in health-care services.

African Americans, Hispanic Americans, and immigrants have the highest incidence of TB in the United States. Persons with immunosuppression, particularly persons with HIV, those receiving cancer chemotherapy, or those receiving biological agents for autoimmune disease, have the highest susceptibility to TB.

According to the World Health Organization (WHO), due to an effective international treatment campaign to eradicate TB, the incidence has been declining globally by approximately 1.5% per year. Currently, there are two sets of goals put forth by the WHO for the elimination of TB: a 90% reduction in incidence by 2035 and fewer than one case per million population per year by 2050. According to experts, this is a formidable challenge. In the United States, the CDC is working to raise awareness of TB among communities at risk through the new "Think. Test. Treat TB" campaign.

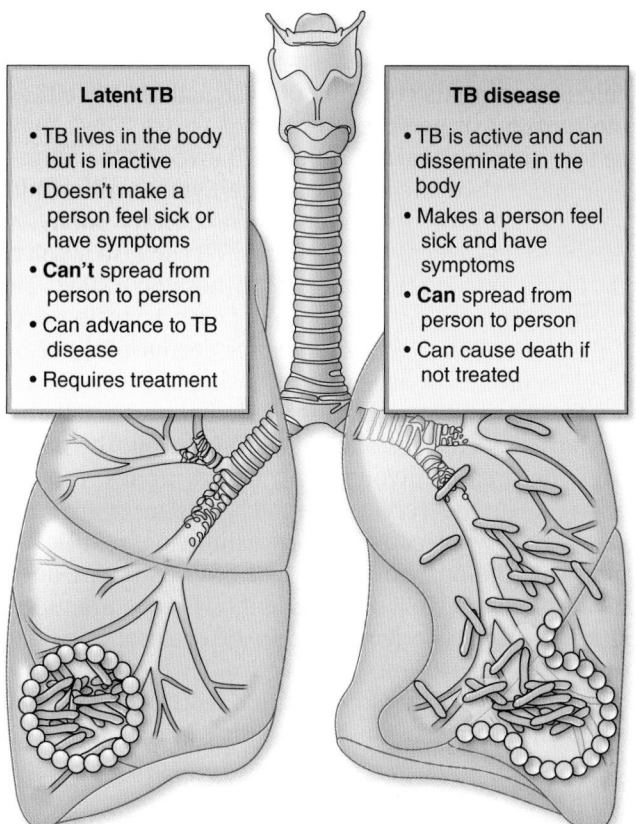

Latent TB
- TB lives in the body but is inactive
- Doesn't make a person feel sick or have symptoms
- **Can't** spread from person to person
- Can advance to TB disease
- Requires treatment

TB disease
- TB is active and can disseminate in the body
- Makes a person feel sick and have symptoms
- **Can** spread from person to person
- Can cause death if not treated

FIGURE 20-8. Latent TB infection versus TB disease. *(From U.S. Dept. of Health and Human Services [2018]. HIV opportunistic infection, coinfections, and conditions. https://clinicalinfo.hiv.gov/en/news/hiv-and-opportunistic-infections-coinfections-and-conditions)*

 CLINICAL CONCEPT

Persons with AIDS are 20 to 40 times more likely than persons who are immunocompetent to develop active TB. TB is a leading cause of mortality among persons infected with HIV.

Etiology

TB is spread by the inhalation of airborne droplets containing *M. tuberculosis* bacteria. Persons at high risk for contracting TB are those who are immunosuppressed.

Persons living in crowded environments are at risk when living with an infected person. Inhalation is the main route for transmission; approximately 20% of people in household contact with a TB patient develop infection. Populations at high risk for acquiring the infection include health-care personnel, urban residents, nursing home residents, and prisoners. Infection with HIV, IV drug abuse, alcoholism, silicosis, immunosuppressive therapy, cancer of the head and neck, hematological malignancies, end-stage renal disease, intestinal bypass surgery or gastrectomy, chronic malabsorption syndromes, and low body weight also increase the risk for disease. Persons with diabetes have three times the risk of developing TB compared with individuals without diabetes. Travel to an area of the world where TB is endemic, such as China or India, is a risk factor.

 CLINICAL CONCEPT

Biological agents used for the treatment of autoimmune disease will immunosuppress the patient and increase the risk for TB.

Tumor necrosis factor-alpha (TNF-α) antagonists, used in the treatment of rheumatoid arthritis, psoriasis, and several other autoimmune disorders, have been associated with a significantly increased risk for TB. Patients taking a TNF-α antagonist should be screened for latent TB and counseled regarding the risk of contracting the disease. Patients on systemic or inhaled steroids are also at increased risk. Persons who regularly use inhaled steroids have 1¼ times the risk. Smoking is a risk factor for relapse of TB in those who have inactive TB.

Pathophysiology

M. tuberculosis is inhaled from another person's cough or sneeze, and droplets pass down the airway, eventually settling in the bronchial tree. A person who contracts the *M. tuberculosis* bacteria can either develop active TB disease or LTBI. After contracting the bacteria, an individual is at highest risk for developing active TB disease within 2 years. The risk of active disease then declines; however, the individual remains at risk for their lifetime.

The TB organism is aerobic and prefers areas of lung tissue with high O_2 levels, such as the apex. Tissue inflammation occurs as the bacteria multiply and pulmonary macrophages and white blood cells (WBCs) migrate to the infected area. Although WBCs cannot kill the organism, a cell-mediated immune response occurs that eventually walls off the infection. The lesion, called a tubercle, is a granulomatous accumulation of WBCs, bacteria, and fibrotic tissue. Scar tissue eventually grows around the tubercle, and the bacteria become inactive. Histologically, the lesion in TB is referred to as Ghon's focus; when calcified, it is called a Ranke complex.

The bacteria continue to multiply, and macrophages and T cells degrade the bacteria. The macrophages and T cells continue to be stimulated, secrete enzymes, and kill bacteria. The enzymes, however, also damage lung tissue. Necrotic lung tissue takes on a cheese-like appearance; histologically, it is called caseous necrosis. In this tissue, the bacteria remain dormant, though any impairment of the patient's immune response allows reactivation of TB infection. The bacteria reinfect the bronchial tree, allowing the patient to spread the disease.

 CLINICAL CONCEPT

LTBI is a state of persistent immune reaction to *M. tuberculosis* without clinical manifestations of active TB disease. The person cannot transmit the infection to others; however, they can develop active TB disease any time in their life.

Clinical Presentation

The signs and symptoms of active pulmonary TB disease are chronic cough, which produces purulent sputum; hemoptysis; weight loss; anorexia; chest pain; and a low-grade fever with night sweats. Older adults usually do not exhibit all the classic signs because they cannot mount a strong immune response.

Persons can present with TB of the bones, lymph nodes, meninges, or adrenal gland. Patients with tuberculous meningitis complain of headache that is either intermittent or persistent for 2 to 3 weeks. Fever may be low-grade or absent. Skeletal TB involves the vertebrae and is also called Pott's disease. Symptoms include back pain or stiffness, and lower-extremity paralysis occurs in up to half of the patients. TB can also involve the joints, causing swelling and stiffness. Scrofula is TB of the lymph nodes, which usually occurs in the neck. TB of the adrenal gland can cause decreased cortisol levels exhibited by severe hypotension and weakness.

On physical examination, pulmonary TB will be exhibited by crackles or bronchial sounds in the lungs over the area of involvement. Lymph nodes may be enlarged in the cervical, supraclavicular, or axillary areas. However, many persons exhibit no significant physical findings, so absence of physical signs does not exclude active TB. In patients who are immunosuppressed, classic symptoms are often absent. In fact, up to 20% of patients with active TB may not have any symptoms. Therefore, sputum testing is essential when chest x-ray is consistent with TB.

 CLINICAL CONCEPT

Classic signs of TB are chronic cough, weight loss, night sweats, and hemoptysis.

Diagnosis

The **Mantoux tuberculin skin test** is a screening test for TB. The test can indicate only if an individual has had prior exposure and sensitization to the organism *M. tuberculosis*. It does not differentiate LTBI from active TB disease. In the Mantoux tuberculin test, a small amount of purified protein derivative (PPD), which is an extract of the tubercle bacteria, is injected intradermally into the forearm. For this reason, the Mantoux test is sometimes referred to as a **PPD test**. After 48 hours, the injection site should be checked for a reaction of induration, which appears as elevated and hardened. If there is no induration at the site, the test is negative and the individual is considered uninfected. An induration of 5 to 15 mm may be positive, depending on the person's risk factors and susceptibility to TB. A reaction greater than 15 mm of induration is interpreted as positive in all persons.

 CLINICAL CONCEPT

Persons with a positive reaction on the Mantoux test require a chest x-ray.

In some countries of Europe, the Middle East, Africa, and Asia, individuals commonly receive the Bacillus Calmette–Guérin (BCG) TB vaccine. This vaccine protects the individual from contracting TB. These individuals will test positive on the Mantoux test, an indication of previous sensitization with PPD. The positive reaction does not necessarily mean that the individual is infected with TB. However, most individuals who test positive are required to get a chest x-ray to check for active disease.

The **interferon gamma release assay (IGRA)** is a blood test also used to screen for TB. This test demonstrates whether the immune system has been exposed to TB bacteria. A positive IGRA test requires further testing of the individual to decipher if there is latent TB infection or active TB disease. A chest x-ray or CT scan can rule out active TB. The IGRA result is not affected by a previous BCG vaccine.

The WHO recommends the rapid test called Xpert MTB/RIF to expedite the diagnosis of TB. The test diagnoses TB and detects resistance to rifampicin, a first-line TB medication. Diagnosis can be made within 2 hours, and the test is recommended as the initial diagnostic test for all persons with signs and symptoms of TB. If positive, it is followed by additional testing.

A sputum smear for acid-fast culture and sensitivity of *M. tuberculosis* is the most reliable test for diagnosis of TB. This test also can determine which antibiotic will be most effective against the bacteria. NAAT also can be used to detect *M. tuberculosis* in sputum and infected tissue. Although it is used to support the diagnosis of TB, acid-fast culture is the primary laboratory test. Chest x-ray, as well as HIV testing, is important. If

chest x-ray findings suggest TB and the sputum smear is positive for acid-fast bacteria, treatment is initiated.

The classic chest x-ray exhibits a round granuloma, called a "tubercle," usually toward the apex of the lung (see Fig. 20-9). CT scan or MRI can also demonstrate the granulomatous mass in TB.

Treatment

Antimicrobial medications, including isoniazid, rifampicin, pyrazinamide, ethambutol, and streptomycin, are used in combination therapy to treat patients with active TB and as prophylactic therapy for those who have had exposure to and are at risk for developing active TB. Isoniazid and rifampicin are the first-line drugs within the regimen.

TB bacteria mutate rapidly and easily acquire resistance to any one drug; therefore, usually a combination of four different drugs is used. Multidrug therapy is required for a long time, usually 6 to 12 months, and may need to continue longer in patients with an HIV infection or those with drug-resistant strains of TB. Treatment protocols are based on the health of the patient and the type of TB strain.

Because the bacteria travel through the air, patients are placed in respiratory isolation until they are no longer considered contagious. Adequate hydration and nutrition are necessary to aid in recovery from the disease. TB is considered chronic in nature, as there is a potential for reactivation of active disease if a patient becomes immunosuppressed. Patient teaching is needed about the possibility of recurrence and spread of the disease. Because drug therapy extends over a prolonged period, the proper use of prescribed medications needs

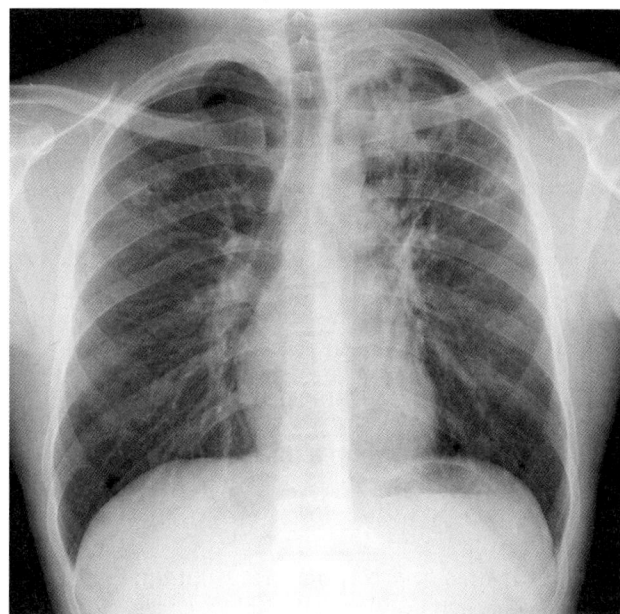

FIGURE 20-9. Chest x-ray showing TB. A round granuloma is highlighted by surrounding inflammatory tissue in the upper-left apical region. Interior of lesion has tissue necrosis. *(From Du Cane Medical Imaging Ltd./Science Source.)*

to be reinforced. Many patients fail to maintain the full regimen, which can lead to the development of resistant TB bacteria. Multidrug-resistant (MDR) TB is an increasing problem. This most often occurs when patients fail to take the complete medication regimen. TB organisms mutate and possess genetic mechanisms that can endow them with resistance when exposed to medication. Currently, resistance to isoniazid and rifampicin, the two most powerful first-line drugs, is increasing in the population, which is becoming a public health crisis.

Chapter Summary

- URIs are among the most common reasons for patients to seek health care.
- Rhinitis can be caused by infection or allergy; infection is mainly caused by rhinovirus or adenovirus.
- GABHS is a common cause of pharyngitis; it can lead to rheumatic fever, rheumatic heart disease, glomerulonephritis, and other disorders.
- Epiglottitis, a condition that can occur as a complication of laryngitis and tracheitis, is a medical emergency that can cause asphyxiation.
- The right bronchus is vertical and wider than the left bronchus, making aspiration pneumonia more common in the right lung.
- Aspiration pneumonia can occur in debilitated persons, those with decreased level of consciousness, and persons with a weak gag or cough reflex.
- Acute bronchitis is a common complication of URI and influenza infection.
- Chronic bronchitis is diagnosed if the patient suffers bronchitis for 3 months out of the year for 2 years.
- Atelectasis commonly occurs in the postoperative period and predisposes individuals to pneumonia.
- Patients with atelectasis should be encouraged to cough and deep-breath and use an incentive spirometer.
- Impending respiratory failure occurs when the patient's PO_2 decreases toward 60 mm Hg and PCO_2 increases toward 50 mm Hg.
- The most common cause of CAP is *S. pneumoniae*.
- HIV-related pneumonia is caused by *Pneumocystis jirovecii*.

- Cough, fever, and crackles are classic signs of pneumonia.
- Septic emboli, which commonly develop from right-sided endocarditis, can form lung abscesses in IV drug abusers.
- Bronchial tumor obstruction of mucus and secretions can cause a lung abscess.
- There are two forms of TB: TB disease and LTBI.
- TB disease consists of actively growing *M. tuberculosis* bacteria, symptoms, and infectious potential.
- LTBI consists of inactive *M. tuberculosis* bacteria, no symptoms, and no infectious potential. However, LTBI can progress to TB disease at any point during a person's lifetime.
- Persistent cough, weight loss, night sweats, and hemoptysis are classic signs of TB.
- Immunosuppression caused by infection with HIV increases susceptibility to TB.
- TB is an opportunistic infection that can occur in HIV infection.
- The Mantoux tuberculin skin test is positive for active TB if the individual develops 15 mm or more of erythematous induration at the site of intradermal injection of PPD after 48 to 72 hours. Reactions of less than 15 mm need to be interpreted in terms of certain conditions.
- Treatment of TB requires a long-term, multidrug regimen; isoniazid and rifampicin are the most powerful first-line drugs used.

Making the Connections

Pathophysiology

Signs and Symptoms	Physical Assessment Findings	Diagnostic Testing	Treatment
Rhinitis | Inflammation of nasal mucosa and pharynx, commonly caused by viral infection or allergy.			
Stuffed nose, nasal discharge, sneezing. Sore throat.	Nasal mucosa and turbinates red, nasal discharge, conjunctivitis possible. Pharyngeal erythema. Allergic rhinitis shows gray-colored nasal mucosa and turbinates.	CBC shows neutrophils in bacterial infection, lymphocytes in viral infection, and eosinophils in allergy.	Symptomatic treatment, antihistamines, and antipyretics. Acetaminophen. Corticosteroid anti-inflammatory nasal spray for allergic rhinitis.
Pharyngitis | Inflammation of pharynx, usually caused by a virus. It is important to test for GABHS as a bacterial cause of pharyngitis. Patients with pharyngitis and enlarged cervical lymph nodes should be tested for EBV with a heterophile antibody test.			
Malaise, fever, and sore throat.	Red, swollen pharyngeal membrane and tonsils. Lymphoid follicles swollen and covered with white exudate. Cervical lymph nodes tender.	Rapid strep test. Throat culture and sensitivity show GABHS if present. Heterophile antibody test to rule out EBV may be necessary.	If throat culture is positive for GABHS, antibiotic such as penicillin, erythromycin, or a cephalosporin. If viral pharyngitis, symptomatic relief, antipyretics, NSAIDs, and antihistamines. Warm saltwater gargle.
Sinusitis | Infection of facial maxillary and frontal sinuses, causing inflammation and the obstruction of the sinus cavity.			
Headache, malaise, fever, stuffy, runny nose. Sore throat. Earache.	Facial pain or pressure over sinus area. Pain in sinuses that worsens with leaning forward, head-down position. Nasal obstruction and nasal discharge. Fever, headache, and ear pain. Decreased sense of smell. Sore throat.	Visual inspection and palpation of frontal and maxillary sinuses. No visualization of transmaxillary sinus light. Sinus x-rays.	Antibiotics if bacterial infection. Decongestants. Antihistamines. Saline sprays. Heated mist. Mucolytic agents. NSAIDs or acetaminophen.
Tonsillitis | Infection and inflammation of tonsils may be caused by GABHS. Patients with tonsillitis and enlarged cervical lymph nodes should be tested for EBV.			
Sore throat. Fever, malaise, anorexia, and pain with swallowing. May have earache with sore throat.	Red inflamed pharynx. Tonsillar tissues edematous and erythematous. White exudate over tonsillar tissue. Cervical lymphadenopathy.	Throat culture and sensitivity testing for GABHS. Heterophile antibody test for EBV may be necessary.	Antibiotics if GABHS is etiology. Tonsillectomy if recurrent infections or severe tissue hypertrophy occurs.
Epiglottitis | Infection and inflammation of epiglottis caused by bacteria, viruses, or fungi. Swelling between the base of the tongue and epiglottis, which, if untreated, may lead to airway obstruction, which is an emergency.			
Severe sore throat with inability to speak and difficulty breathing. Drooling of saliva caused by difficulty swallowing.	Red, swollen inflamed pharynx and tonsils. Swollen epiglottis.	Laryngoscopic examination. Neck x-rays. Increased WBC count. Arterial blood gas may show respiratory acidosis. Culture and sensitivity indicates causative organism.	Antibiotics. Humidified oxygen. IV fluids. Maintenance of the airway. Tracheostomy equipment at bedside to be used if airway is obstructed.

Continued

Making the Connections–cont'd

Signs and Symptoms	Physical Assessment Findings	Diagnostic Testing	Treatment
Laryngitis and Tracheitis | Infection and inflammation of larynx or trachea; usually caused by a virus, but may be bacterial in nature.			
Sore throat and difficulty speaking.	Hoarseness or complete loss of voice. Stridor may be heard. Irritating high-pitched, brassy cough. Yellow, green, or mucoid sputum. Wheezing mainly upon exertion.	Throat culture and sensitivity.	Resting of the voice. Bronchodilators. Antibiotics. Treatment of symptoms. NSAIDs. Acetaminophen.
Acute Bronchitis | Infection and inflammation of the bronchi caused by either bacteria or a virus. Loss of cilia from the respiratory cells lining the trachea and bronchi, resulting in impairment of mucociliary movement.			
Cough, fever, sore throat, general malaise.	Fever possible. Cough. Mucus production. Rhonchi heard over lungs.	Chest x-ray to rule out pneumonia. CBC with differential: High neutrophils usually indicate bacteria. Lymphocytes indicate virus. Sputum culture and sensitivity.	Expectorants. Cough suppressants. Antibiotics. Bronchodilator. Antipyretics. Acetaminophen.
Pneumonia | Infection and inflammation process in the lobes of the lungs caused by bacteria, viruses, fungi, parasites, mycoplasma, or chemicals. Exudates fill the alveolar air spaces, creating consolidation and impaired air exchange, resulting in hypoxia.			
Difficulty breathing. Fever, cough, chills, malaise, myalgias. Pleuritic chest pain. Sputum production.	Fever. Dyspnea. Diminished breath sounds. Crackles. Increased sputum, blood tinged to purulent. Tachycardia. Increased tactile fremitus over areas of pneumonia. Egophony, bronchophony, and whispered pectorilo-quy elicited.	Chest x-ray. Sputum culture and sensitivity. Arterial blood gases. Pulse oximetry. Urine antigen test.	Antibiotics. Bronchodilators. Expectorants. Humidified oxygen. Antipyretics. Acetaminophen.
Lung Abscess | Localized area of infection and purulent inflammation, resulting in tissue necrosis. Usually caused by bacteria.			
Fever, chills, productive cough. Pleuritic chest pain. Anorexia, cachexia.	Fever. Copious amounts of foul-smelling sputum. Productive cough. Decreased breath sounds in area of abscess.	Arterial blood gases. CBC (leukocytosis). Chest x-ray (solitary cavity with consolidation). Sputum culture.	Antibiotics. Surgical treatment may be needed. Bronchoscopy to drain abscess. Chest tube may be needed. Postural drainage. Humidified oxygen. Treatment of symptoms. Antipyretics.

Making the Connections—cont'd

Signs and Symptoms	Physical Assessment Findings	Diagnostic Testing	Treatment
Tuberculosis | Infection and inflammation of lung(s) caused by *M. tuberculosis*.			
Chronic cough, weight loss, night sweats, and hemoptysis. Fever, malaise, dyspnea, pleuritic chest pain.	Cough with purulent sputum or hemoptysis. Weight loss. Fever.	Chest x-ray, positive Mantoux test showing greater than 15 mm, red, indurated area over intradermal injection site after 48 hours. PPD test similar to Mantoux test. Positive IGRA. Sputum culture; acid-fast bacteria. NAAT.	Antimicrobial medications in combination therapy for long term. Adequate hydration and nutrition. Antipyretics.

Bibliography

Available online at fadavis.com

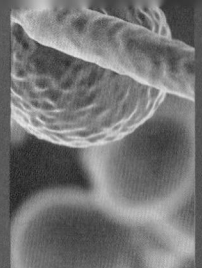

Restrictive and Obstructive Pulmonary Disorders

Learning Objectives

Upon completion of this chapter, the student will be able to:

- Discuss basic concepts of the structure and function of the respiratory system.
- Differentiate between the pathological mechanisms in obstructive versus restrictive pulmonary disease.
- Describe the pathological mechanisms that occur in COPD, which include those of chronic bronchitis, asthma, and emphysema.
- Discuss common causes of obstructive versus restrictive pulmonary disease.

- Identify signs, symptoms, and clinical manifestations that characterize asthma and COPD.
- Compare and contrast signs, symptoms, and clinical manifestations of obstructive versus restrictive pulmonary disease.
- Recognize laboratory procedures used to diagnose obstructive versus restrictive pulmonary disease.
- Discuss treatment modalities used in obstructive and restrictive pulmonary disease.

Key Terms

Acute respiratory distress syndrome (ARDS)

Asthma

Blue bloater

BODE index

Bronchial thermoplasty (BT)

Bronchiectasis

Chronic bronchitis

Chronic obstructive pulmonary disease (COPD)

COPD assessment test (CAT)

Compliance

Cor pulmonale

Emphysema

Endotype-phenotype classification of asthma

Forced expiratory volume (FEV)

Forced expiratory volume in 1 second (FEV_1)

Forced vital capacity (FVC)

Fractional exhaled nitric oxide (FeNO)

Global Initiative for Asthma (GINA)

Global Initiative for Chronic Obstructive Lung Disease (GOLD)

Hypercapnia

Hypoxia

Leukotriene receptor antagonist (LTRA)

Long-acting beta-2 adrenergic agonist (LABA)

Long-acting muscarinic antagonist (LAMA)

Lung volume reduction procedures

Medical Research Council (MRC) Dyspnea Scale

Methacholine bronchoprovocation test

Obstructive disease

Peak expiratory flow (PEF)

Pink puffer

Pleural effusion

Pleuritis (pleurisy)

Pneumothorax

Pulmonary function test (PFT)

Pulmonary hypertension

Restrictive disease

Short-acting beta-2 adrenergic agonist (SABA)

Short-acting muscarinic antagonist (SAMA)

Spirometry

T2 High asthma (T2 asthma)

T2 Low asthma (non-T2 asthma)

Total lung capacity (TLC)

Most lung disease can be clinically classified according to results on a **pulmonary function test (PFT)** (also called **spirometry**). Based on the results of these tests, pulmonary disorders can be categorized as obstructive or restrictive lung disease. **Obstructive disease** is characterized by an increase in resistance to airflow from the trachea and larger bronchi to the terminal and respiratory bronchioles. **Restrictive disease** is characterized by reduced expansion of lung tissue, with decreased **total lung capacity (TLC).** Lungs are stiff and noncompliant in restrictive disease.

Major obstructive lung diseases include emphysema, chronic bronchitis, bronchiectasis, and asthma. Major restrictive lung diseases include hypersensitivity pneumonitis, pneumothorax, pleural effusion, pulmonary fibrosis, pneumoconiosis, and thoracic cage deformities.

Epidemiology

More than 37 million Americans are living with chronic lung disease such as asthma and chronic obstructive pulmonary disease (COPD). Long-term cigarette smoking is the primary cause of COPD, and great attention has been given to the effects of secondhand smoke. There is an increased prevalence of respiratory illness and reduced levels of pulmonary function in nonsmokers who reside with smokers. Nonsmokers exposed to secondhand smoke at home or work increase their risk of developing lung cancer by 20% to 30%. Secondhand smoke exposure also increases risk of heart disease by 25% to 30%.

Asthma rates have been surging around the globe over the past three decades. Around 300 million people have asthma worldwide, and it is likely that by 2025, a further 100 million may be affected. In the United States, 1 in 12 people (about 25 million, or 8% of the population) have asthma, compared with 1 in 14 (about 20 million, or 7%) in 2001. Some researchers believe the rise in allergies and asthma is due to increased airborne pollens, the energy-proofing of our indoor living environments, urban air pollution, and antibiotics overuse. In 2020, 4,145 people died from asthma, which is more than in any other year in the past 2 decades. Nearly all of these deaths are avoidable with the right treatment and care.

Many individuals are also at risk for developing serious respiratory disorders as a result of occupational or environmental exposures. Approximately 2.4 million workers in the United States have been exposed to environmental causes of lung disease such as coal, silica, and asbestos. A 2018 study found that the national prevalence of pneumoconiosis, which is black lung from coal exposure, in long-tenured coal miners still exceeds 10% today. In central Appalachia, 21% of long-tenured miners have radiographic evidence of pneumoconiosis. Asbestos exposure, long recognized as a cause of lung cancer, is estimated to affect approximately 1.3 million workers in construction still today. Mainly this is occurring during maintenance activities or remediation of buildings containing asbestos. Radon gas, which is emitted from natural radium in earth materials and can be trapped indoors, is a risk factor for lung cancer. Levels of radon gas associated with lung cancer risk may be present in as many as 8% to 12% of households in the United States. Smokers who reside in households contaminated by radon have a potentially greater risk of lung cancer.

Respiratory illnesses have also been attributed to indoor chemical agents emitted from various kinds of synthetic fibers and building materials. Chemical agents such as formaldehyde, diisocyanates, and latex particles that circulate within the air of poorly ventilated buildings have been implicated as the cause of various respiratory complaints. Exact numbers are not available, but millions of workers inhale chemical agents and synthetic particles in unventilated workplaces daily.

Basic Concepts of Pulmonary Structure and Function

The lungs are sponge-like organs that have the unique property of compliance—the flexibility to expand and contract. With inhalation, the lung tissue expands to bring in a large volume of oxygen for transfer into the bloodstream. With exhalation, the elastic lung tissue contracts to push out carbon dioxide. The bronchioles also have the ability to dilate and constrict. Bronchodilation allows enhanced filling of the lungs with oxygen, whereas bronchoconstriction diminishes ventilation.

Bronchodilation and Bronchoconstriction

The trachea divides into two main bronchi, which further divide into smaller-diameter airways called bronchioles. The bronchi and bronchioles are laced with smooth muscle controlled by the autonomic nervous system. The coordinated contraction and relaxation of the smooth muscle layer control the diameter of these airways. During inspiration, the smooth muscle of the airways relaxes, causing bronchodilation, or widening of the airways. Conversely, during exhalation, the smooth muscle of the airways contracts, stimulating bronchoconstriction, or narrowing of the airways.

Both types of autonomic nerves—sympathetic and parasympathetic—innervate the bronchiole smooth muscle. Sympathetic nerves dilate the bronchioles, whereas the parasympathetic nerves constrict the bronchioles. Sympathetic nerve endings in the bronchioles are also referred to as adrenergic nerve endings. The sympathetic nerves within the bronchioles specifically act on beta-2 adrenergic receptors within the walls of the airways. These receptors are similar to the beta-1 adrenergic receptors within heart tissue. Stimulation of beta-2 adrenergic receptors dilates the bronchioles and amplifies the ventilatory capacity of the lungs. During times of high stress, the fight-or-flight response causes stimulation of the sympathetic nerves, which causes the bronchioles to dilate; this allows for maximal ventilation into the lungs. Stimulation of the sympathetic nervous system also causes blood vessel vasoconstriction and inhibition of bronchial secretions. Conversely, parasympathetic nervous system stimulation causes bronchoconstriction, blood vessel vasodilation, and an increase in bronchial secretions. The parasympathetic nerves are also referred to as cholinergic or muscarinic nerve endings within the bronchioles. Inflammatory mediators such as leukotrienes, which are secreted by white blood cells (WBCs), and histamine, which is released from mast cells, also stimulate bronchoconstriction.

Compliance

During the process of respiration, the lungs expand and contract. On inspiration, lungs expand and increase their total volume. On expiration, the lungs recoil based on their elasticity. The change in lung volume during this process is described as **compliance**, which is the flexibility of the lungs. Compliance is reduced by illness that makes the lungs stiffer, thereby increasing the work of breathing, as seen in bronchitis and pneumonia when the lungs are congested with fluid.

Compliance is also reduced by inflammatory conditions such as pulmonary fibrosis and sarcoidosis.

The Pleural Membrane

The pleural membrane lines the thoracic cavity and envelops the lungs. The outer layer lies on the chest wall, and the inner layer adheres to the lung tissue. The inner and outer layers of the pleural membrane form a cavity known as the pleural space. A thin film of fluid called surfactant is contained within the pleural space to keep the membrane layers separated and lubricated. Other than surfactant, there is no air or fluid within the pleural space; it is a vacuum. Because it is a vacuum, the pleural space has negative intrathoracic pressure. When lung tissue fills with air during inspiration, the lung tissue develops positive intrathoracic pressure and expands into the vacuous pleural space. The lungs easily expand and retract during inhalation and exhalation within the empty pleural space. However, if air or fluid is contained within the pleural space, the positive pressure of the air or fluid pushes against the lung tissue and prevents its full expansion. Therefore, it is critical that the pleural space be completely devoid of air or fluid.

 CLINICAL CONCEPT

The lungs are composed of spongy, compressible tissue, which is why they easily collapse when pressure is placed against them by fluid in the pleural space (termed a pleural effusion) or if air accumulates in the pleural space (termed a pneumothorax).

Basic Pathophysiological Concepts of Pulmonary Disorders

Pathological conditions that occur in lung disease include hypoxia, hypercapnia, and inflammation. Chronic hypoxia and chronic hypercapnia can occur gradually over years of disease. Inflammation can be due to immune hyperactivity and can lead to remodeling of the airways, particularly apparent in asthma and COPD.

Hypoxia is the lack of oxygen that is available to the body tissues. Hypoxemia is a term that specifically means lack of oxygen in the bloodstream. **Hypoxia** occurs when the lungs cannot fully ventilate or acquire maximal oxygenation. In turn, if lungs cannot acquire oxygenation, the bloodstream develops hypoxemia. **Hypercapnia** is a high level of carbon dioxide in the body or bloodstream. Hypercapnia develops when the lungs cannot fully expel carbon dioxide. Hypoxia and hypercapnia often occur together when the lungs cannot adequately ventilate. Inadequate ventilation occurs when the lungs cannot

bring in oxygen (O_2) via inhalation or expel carbon dioxide (CO_2) via exhalation.

Chronic Hypercapnia

The pressure of CO_2 gas in the bloodstream is measurable and termed the partial pressure of CO_2 (P_{CO_2}). CO_2 accumulation in the bloodstream stimulates the medulla and drives normal breathing. The ideal P_{CO_2} is between 35 mm Hg and 45 mm Hg. When breathing rate slows down (referred to as bradypnea), CO_2 accumulates in the bloodstream. When P_{CO_2} exceeds the upper limit of normal in the bloodstream (greater than 45 mm Hg), the condition is known as hypercapnia. Hypercapnia can develop because of bradypnea, which is an abnormally slow breathing rate. Slowed breathing allows accumulation of CO_2 in the bloodstream. The accumulation of CO_2 in the blood causes stimulation of the brain's respiratory center, found in the medulla, to increase breathing rate.

 CLINICAL CONCEPT

The healthy person is stimulated to breathe when CO_2 accumulates in the bloodstream and activates the respiratory center in the brain. If breathing slows down, CO_2 accumulates in the bloodstream (termed hypercapnia) and activates the respiratory center, which in turn sends impulses to the body to breathe.

Inadequate ventilation or any cause of obstructed gas exchange leads to insufficient exhalation of CO_2 and hypercapnia. Causes of inadequate ventilation include asphyxiation, aspiration, asthma, COPD, pneumonia, pulmonary edema, thoracic muscle paralysis, and opiate toxicity. Some of the clinical symptoms of chronic hypercapnia include headache, drowsiness, intellectual impairment, and disorientation, all of which may progress to stupor and coma.

Hypercapnia and hypoxia commonly occur simultaneously. Chronic hypercapnia is a common finding in patients with progressive hypoxic lung disease. When chronic hypercapnia develops over a number of years, the central chemoreceptors in the medulla eventually become insensitive to CO_2 levels. The stimulus for breathing shifts to the chemoreceptors in the carotid and aortic bodies, which are triggered by low oxygen in the bloodstream. Patients with chronic hypercapnia incur a distinct change in their stimulus to breathe. Instead of CO_2 accumulation being the stimulus to breathe, hypoxia becomes the impetus for the patient to take another breath. This is a significant change in physiological response, which commonly occurs in severe COPD.

Chronic Hypoxia

The pressure of O_2 gas in the bloodstream is measurable and termed the partial pressure of O_2 (PO_2). The ideal PO_2 ranges from 90 mm Hg to 100 mm Hg. Chronic hypoxia is a chronic lack of oxygen that occurs in respiratory dysfunction. The term is often used interchangeably with hypoxemia, which refers to diminished O_2 levels in the blood. Body tissues vary in their vulnerability to hypoxia; some, such as bone, can withstand episodes of hypoxia for much longer periods than others, such as the heart, kidney, and brain. For example, the brain can tolerate hypoxia for only 5 to 6 minutes before brain cells die. The kidney can sustain hypoxia for 20 minutes before nephrons die.

If the PO_2 of tissues falls below a critical level (60 mm Hg), cellular aerobic metabolism ceases and anaerobic metabolism takes over with formation of lactic acid. Mild hypoxemia causes few symptoms because hemoglobin (Hgb) saturation remains high, at approximately 90%, with PO_2 levels as low as 70 mm Hg. However, there is a dramatic drop in Hgb saturation of oxygen at a PO_2 of 60 mm Hg. At a PO_2 of 60 mm Hg, Hgb starts to release all its oxygen molecules, placing the patient in a state of severe hypoxemia. Severe hypoxemia causes behavioral changes, restlessness, uncoordinated movements, impaired judgment, delirium, and eventually stupor and coma.

ALERT! At a PO_2 of approximately 60 mm Hg, oxygen saturation of Hgb dramatically falls. The patient will develop severe hypoxia with lack of tissue oxygenation.

The body compensates for hypoxia by increasing ventilation, stimulating pulmonary arteriole vasoconstriction, and having the kidney release erythropoietin (see Fig. 21-1). Erythropoietin stimulates the bone marrow to synthesize red blood cells (RBCs). Chronic hypoxia causes constant synthesis of RBCs, a condition called erythropoiesis. Chronic hypoxia also causes pulmonary arterial vasoconstriction; this leads to **pulmonary hypertension**, a condition of high blood pressure within the pulmonary arterial system. Pulmonary hypertension develops because in lung regions where there is lack of oxygen, the arterioles vasoconstrict to

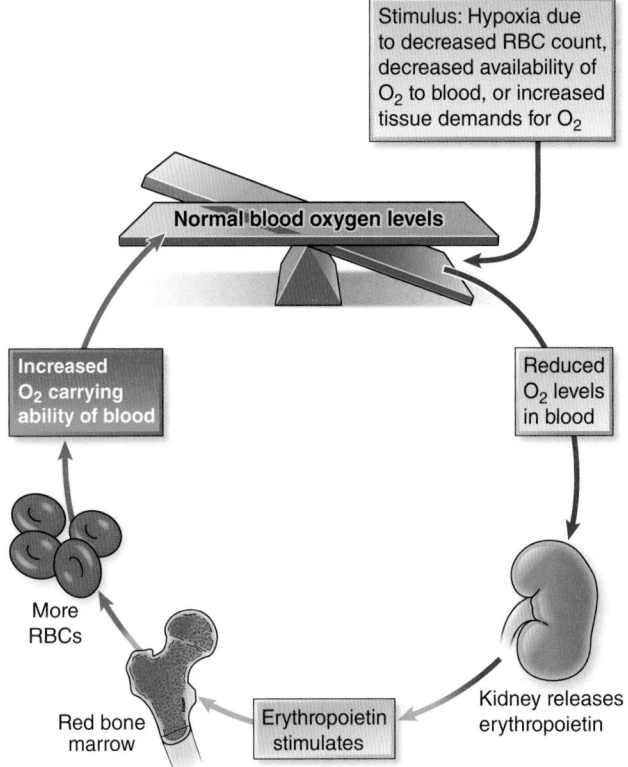

FIGURE 21-1. Erythropoiesis. When the blood develops hypoxia, the kidney secretes erythropoietin. Erythropoietin then stimulates bone marrow to synthesize RBCs.

limit blood flow to those deoxygenated areas. If there are a large number of lung areas with chronic hypoxia, then the large areas of vasoconstriction of pulmonary arterioles cause the pulmonary artery to increase in pressure; this is termed pulmonary hypertension. High pulmonary artery pressure places high resistance against the right ventricle of the heart, which can lead to right ventricular hypertrophy and eventually excessive strain that leads to right ventricular failure.

Immune Responses, Chronic Inflammation, and Remodeling

Other pathological processes that are important in respiratory disease, particularly asthma and COPD, include immune hyperactivity, chronic inflammation, and remodeling of airways. Type 1 and type 2 describe distinct immune responses that are mainly regulated by subpopulations of CD4+ T cells known as T helper 1 (Th1) and Th2 cells, respectively. In diseases such as asthma, Th2 cells are activated and secrete cytokines termed interleukins: IL-4, IL-5, and IL-13. Also, the inflammatory response involves B cell–produced IgE antibodies and eosinophils.

Respiratory disease such as asthma and COPD are chronic inflammatory diseases that show structural remodeling with time. Remodeling features include hyperplasia of goblet cells that increasingly secrete mucus. Also, subepithelial collagen proliferation and fibrosis stiffen airway walls, and smooth muscle hypertrophy within the airways decreases elasticity and reduces bronchodilation ability.

Pulmonary Assessment

To thoroughly assess the patient with pulmonary disease, a detailed history and physical examination should be completed. When taking a history, the clinician should review all the risk factors for lung disease. Smoking and occupational exposure are key risk factors to explore. If the patient is exposed to occupational inhalants, the clinician should inquire if the patient wears a protective mask at work. After completion of a thorough history, all the components of physical examination—inspection, palpation, percussion, and auscultation—are used during pulmonary assessment.

Risk Factors

A history of current and past smoking habits should be sought from all patients. If the patient has smoked, the clinician should ask the patient the number of years they have smoked and multiply that number by the number of packs of cigarettes smoked per day; this yields a smoking history in pack-years. For example, a 76-year-old patient who has smoked two packs per day since age 16 years has a 120 pack-year smoking history (2 packs per day × 60 years). If the patient has no smoking history, the clinician should ask about exposure to secondhand smoke.

Occupational exposure to toxic agents should be investigated. Common occupational exposures linked to lung disease include mineral dust, coal, asbestos, silica, farming and landscaping materials, and reactive chemicals such as toluene. Asbestos exposure is a particularly significant risk factor for pulmonary disease. Asbestos was used as a building material before 1980; therefore, construction workers, firefighters, shipyard and power plant workers, mechanics, and others may have been exposed. The patient should be asked about exposure to animals, pet dander, molds, pollen, ragweed, household dust, and cockroaches. Illicit drug use, particularly marijuana, cocaine, and IV drugs, needs to be discussed. The patient should be asked about possible contact with individuals with respiratory infections and exposure to infectious agents such as tuberculosis (TB).

A history of any respiratory or nonrespiratory disorder should be sought, particularly cardiac disease, HIV infection, immunosuppressive conditions, cancer, and autoimmune disease such as systemic lupus erythematosus, scleroderma, or sarcoidosis. A complete list of the patient's current medications and treatments is needed, particularly radiation therapy, immunosuppressive agents, steroids, chemotherapeutic agents, beta blockers, and angiotensin-converting enzyme (ACE) inhibitors. A family history of pulmonary and nonpulmonary disease should be investigated, particularly TB, asthma, cystic fibrosis, alpha-1 antitrypsin (AAT) deficiency, and heart disease.

Signs and Symptoms

The clinician should use the physical examination techniques of inspection, palpation, percussion, and auscultation when assessing the patient's pulmonary system. On inspection, note the patient's rate, rhythm, and depth of breathing. Observe the use of intercostal and accessory muscles, symmetrical or asymmetrical expansion of the chest, and structural abnormalities of the thoracic cage and spine. Observe the patient for dyspnea, which is breathing difficulty, and orthopnea, which is difficulty breathing when lying flat. The patient may cough while being examined. A cough is described as productive if sputum is expectorated with the cough; if blood is expectorated with the cough, this is called hemoptysis. Check the patient's hands for clubbing of the fingers (see Fig. 21-2), as this is a finding consistent with chronic hypoxia. Cyanosis, a bluish discoloration of the skin and mucous membranes, occurs with hypoxia; this is caused by the excessive concentration of deoxygenated Hgb in the small blood vessels.

The thoracic cage should be examined. In healthy persons, the width of the chest should be twice the size of the depth of the chest (2:1 ratio of width to depth). In patients with long-term COPD, the width of the chest and depth are equal, with a characteristic 1:1 ratio of the width to the lateral diameter of the chest, creating a "barrel-shaped" chest (see Fig. 21-3).

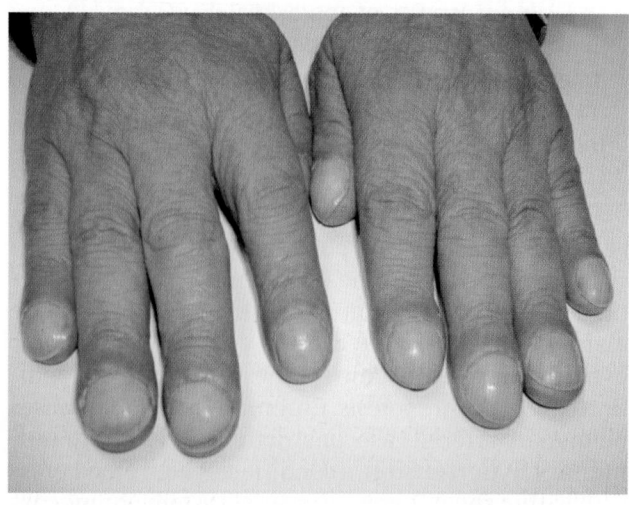

FIGURE 21-2. Clubbing of fingers occurs in chronic hypoxia. (Courtesy of Desherinka.)

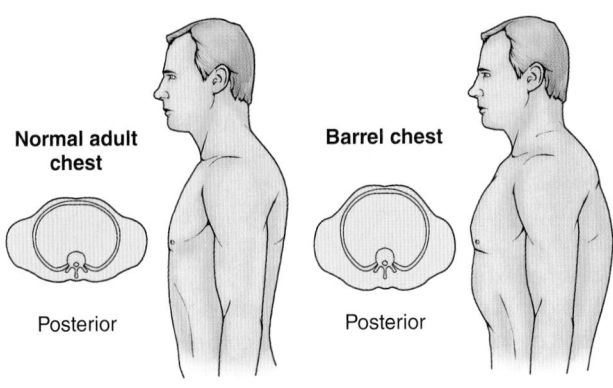

FIGURE 21-3. Barrel chest.

The clinician should palpate the bony structures of the thoracic cage, such as the clavicles and ribs, for tenderness or fracture. Also, the lymph nodes should be palpated for tenderness or enlargement. It is important to focus on the cervical, supraclavicular, infraclavicular, and axillary nodes. The clinician should also inspect and palpate the oral cavity for lesions.

A unique palpation technique can be used when assessing the lungs. Tactile fremitus is a vibration in the lungs caused by vocalization that a clinician can detect using the palms. The patient is asked to repeat the words "ninety-nine" as the examiner palpates the vibrations transmitted though the posterior chest. Transmission of vibrations increases over areas of pulmonary consolidation, such as pneumonia or neoplasm. Transmission of vibrations is decreased or absent over areas of pleural fluid.

The clinician can use percussion in physical examination of the chest. The normal sound percussed over lung tissue is called resonance. Percussion is performed with the index and middle finger of one hand tapping on the middle finger of the other hand over the posterior chest. Percussion of dull sounds is heard over consolidated areas of lung tissue or pleural fluid. Hyperresonance, a low, drumlike sound, is percussed over areas of emphysema or air in the pleural cavity.

On auscultation, the examiner should listen to the quality of breath sounds and for any adventitious sounds. Adventitious sounds include stridor, bronchial sounds, crackles (also called rales), wheezes, and rhonchi.

The clinician should ask the patient to breathe in through the nose and out slowly through the mouth. Breath sounds are diminished by bronchial obstruction or by air or fluid in the pleural cavity. Stridor is a high-pitched sound that occurs when the trachea is obstructed. Tubular breath sounds, also called bronchial sounds, are heard over consolidated areas of the lung, as in pneumonia. Whistling sounds, termed wheezes, can be heard in the lungs when bronchioles are constricted as air attempts to pass through narrowed airways. Rhonchi are lower-toned snoring-type sounds that can be heard over the bronchioles when they are obstructed by mucus. Crackles (also called rales) are sounds that occur due to alveoli opening and closing against fluid as in pulmonary edema or pneumonia.

Sound transmission can also be assessed by listening with the stethoscope to the vocal sounds of the patient transmitted through the lung and chest wall. The clinician may be able to elicit sounds referred to as bronchophony, egophony, and whispered pectoriloquy (see Chapter 20). These vocal sounds can be used to assess regions of pneumonia in the lungs.

 CLINICAL CONCEPT

Crackles are commonly heard in pneumonia and pulmonary edema.

Diagnosis

Chest x-ray is commonly the initial diagnostic study performed to evaluate patients with pulmonary signs and symptoms by assessing heart size, diaphragm borders, pulmonary tissue and vascularity, mediastinal lymph nodes, and pleural membranes (see Fig. 21-4). Anteroposterior and lateral views of the lungs are usually indicated. Increased opacity on chest x-ray usually indicates a solid mass or fluid. Increased radiolucency usually indicates air-filled or cystic conditions.

Further information about pulmonary health can be obtained from computed tomography (CT) scans, magnetic resonance imaging (MRI), ultrasonography, bronchoscopy, angiography, thoracocentesis, positron emission tomographic (PET) scans, arterial blood gas (ABG) analysis, pulse oximetry, and ventilation-perfusion (V-Q) scans.

Pulmonary disease can be categorized as obstructive or restrictive using **pulmonary function tests (PFTs)** (also called **spirometry**), which measure different lung volumes as the patient exhales into a specialized pulmonary spirometry device (see Box 21-1). A specific type of pulmonary function test called fractional exhaled nitric oxide (FeNO) is a noninvasive test that can be used to assist in the diagnosis of asthma.

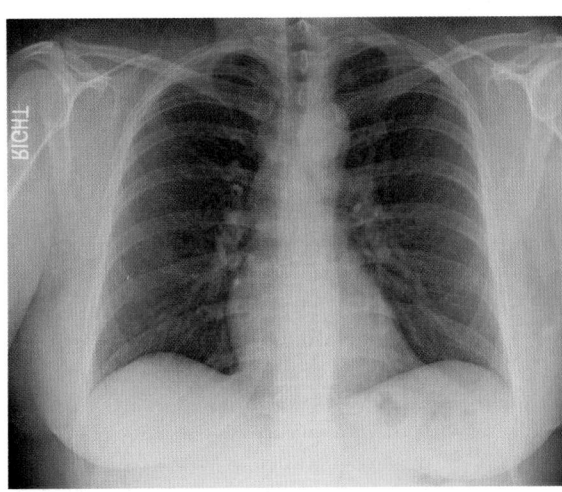

FIGURE 21-4. Normal chest x-ray.

BOX 21-1. (A) and (B). Lung Volumes Measured by a Pulmonary Function Test

(A)

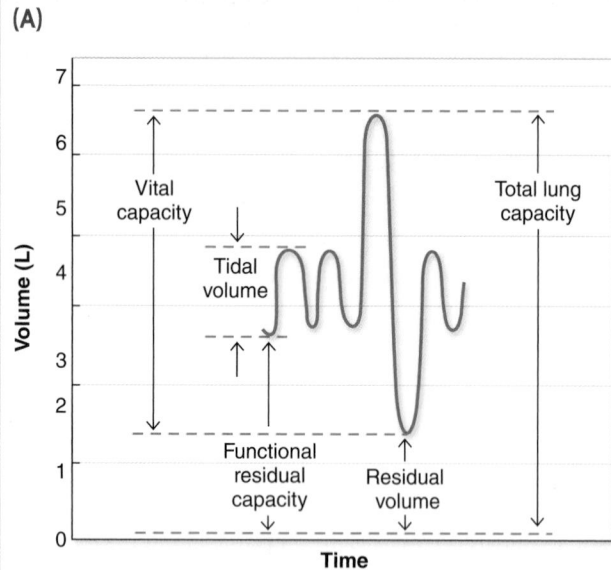

- **Total lung capacity (TLC):** This measures the amount of air in an individual's lungs after inhaling as deeply as possible.
- **Functional residual capacity (FRC):** This measures the amount of air in an individual's lungs at the end of a normal exhaled breath.
- **Residual volume (RV):** This measures the amount of air in an individual's lungs after a complete exhalation. It can be done by breathing in helium or nitrogen gas and seeing how much is exhaled.
- **Tidal volume (TV):** This shows an individual's usual relaxed breathing volumes in inhalation and exhalation.

(B) Normal Forced Expiratory Volume in First Second (FEV_1) of Exhalation.

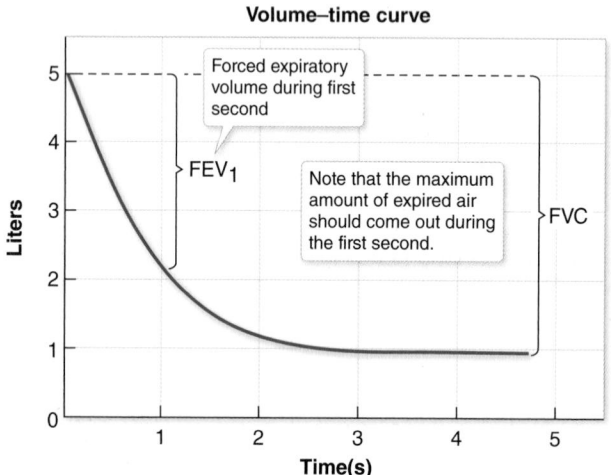

The more common lung function values measured with spirometry are:

- **Forced vital capacity (FVC):** This measures the amount of air an individual can exhale with force after inhaling as deeply as possible.
- **Forced expiratory volume (FEV):** This measures the amount of air an individual can exhale with force in one breath. The amount of air exhaled may be measured at 1 second (FEV_1), 2 seconds (FEV2), or 3 seconds (FEV3). FEV_1 divided by FVC can also be determined.
- **Forced expiratory flow 25% to 75% (FEV25%-75%):** This measures the airflow halfway through an exhale.
- **Peak expiratory flow (PEF):** This measures how quickly an individual can exhale. It is usually measured at the same time as the FVC.

The FEV_1 is the amount of air exhaled in the first second of expiration. Normally, approximately 80% of air in the lungs should be exhaled in the first second.

Treatment

Bronchodilators are commonly used to treat the obstructive lung diseases asthma and COPD to counteract bronchoconstriction. Since these diseases also cause chronic inflammation, anti-inflammatory agents are used as well. Bronchodilators are available as beta-2 adrenergic agonist inhalers and anticholinergic (also called antimuscarinic) inhaler agents. Asthma and COPD treatment regimens commonly require a long-acting bronchodilator inhaled medication for maintenance or daily use; this is also referred to as controller therapy. Short-acting bronchodilator, inhaled medication, referred to as rescue or reliever medication, is used for acute attacks of bronchoconstriction. Maintenance (controller) therapy is prescribed for once- or twice-daily use to control asthma or COPD. Rescue (reliever) therapy is used to resolve acute episodes of bronchospasm that may "break through" the maintenance therapy.

Beta-2 adrenergic agonists are sympathetic stimulants that directly enhance dilation of the bronchioles. Beta-2 adrenergic agonists can be long acting as daily maintenance medication (**long-acting beta-2 adrenergic agonists [LABAs]**) or short acting (**short-acting beta-2 adrenergic agonists [SABAs]**) for sudden attacks of bronchospasm in asthma or COPD. Albuterol is a commonly prescribed SABA used as a rescue bronchodilator to counteract sudden attacks of acute bronchospasm. Formoterol is a commonly prescribed LABA that is used once or twice daily as a maintenance medication. **Short-acting muscarinic antagonists (SAMAs),** which inhibit parasympathetic bronchoconstriction, can also be used for some persons with asthma or COPD. Ipratropium is the most commonly used SAMA. **Long-acting muscarinic antagonists (LAMAs)** can be used for long-term control in some persons with asthma or COPD. A commonly used LAMA is tiotropium.

Anti-inflammatory agents are also available as **inhaled corticosteroids (ICS)**, oral corticosteroids, and oral leukotriene antagonists. An example of a commonly used ICS is budesonide. A commonly used oral corticosteroid is prednisone, and an oral leukotriene receptor antagonist (LTRA) is montelukast. Oral corticosteroids are usually prescribed only during exacerbations of asthma or COPD to control inflammation for a short period. Oral corticosteroids, if used for prolonged periods, have numerous side effects; therefore,

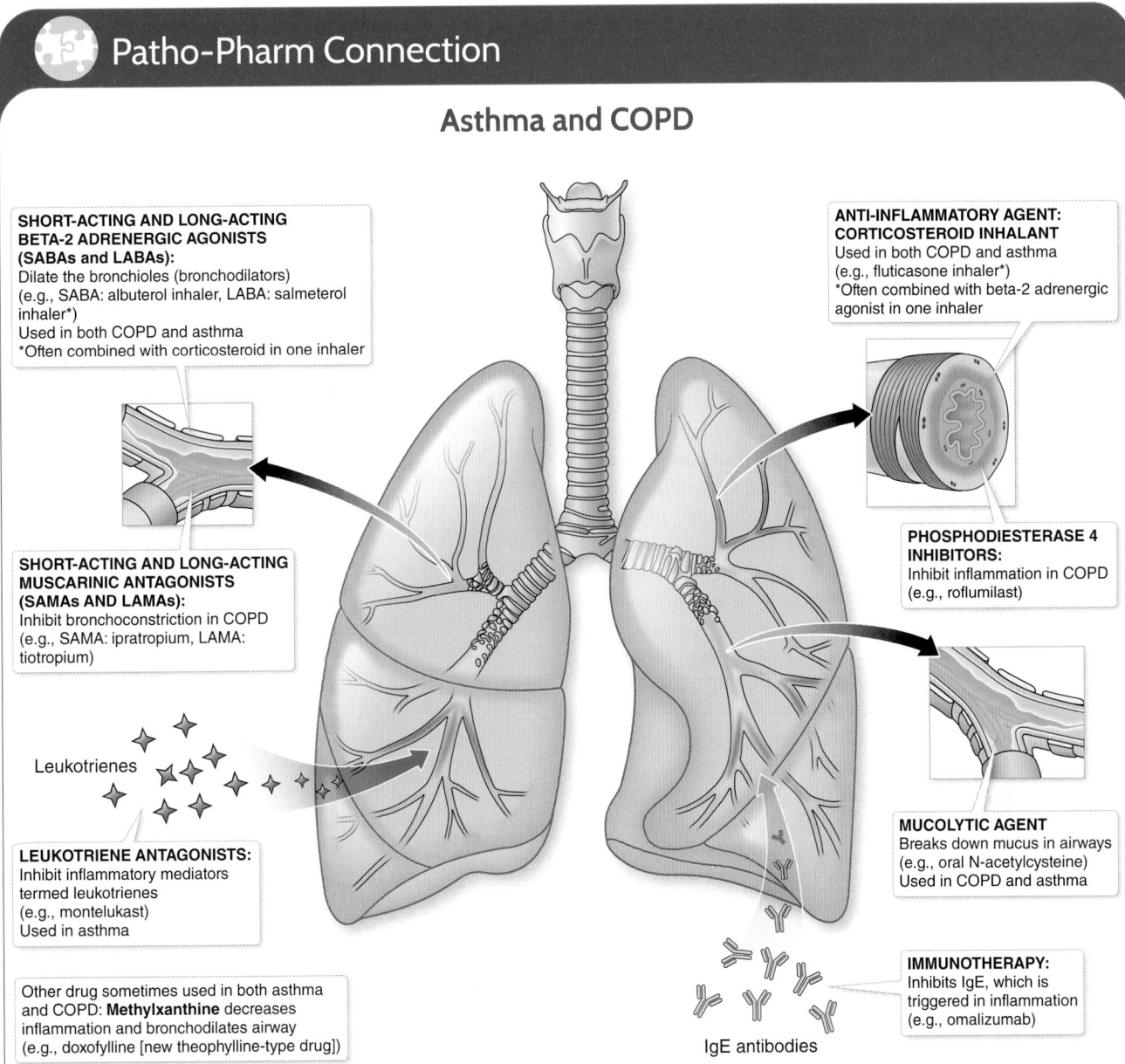

Patho-Pharm Connection

Asthma and COPD

Treatment of asthma and COPD involves beta-2 adrenergic agonist inhalers that stimulate bronchiole smooth muscle, leading to direct bronchodilation, and anticholinergic (also called antimuscarinic) inhaler agents that counteract bronchoconstriction. Inhaled beta-2 adrenergic bronchodilators are either short-acting beta-2 adrenergic agents (SABAs) or long-acting beta-2 adrenergic agents (LABAs). Albuterol is a commonly used SABA that directly bronchodilates airways rapidly. Salmeterol is a LABA commonly in maintenance inhalers, which are used daily. Short-acting muscarinic antagonists (SAMAs) such as ipratropium and long-acting muscarinic antagonists (LAMAs) such as tiotropium counteract bronchoconstriction of airways. Inhaled corticosteroids (ICSs) such as flucatisone are also used in addition to LABAs or LAMAs, as these are anti-inflammatory agents. ICSs are often used in combination inhalers with LABAs or LAMAs.

Phosphodiesterase 4 inhibitors such as roflumilast can be added to the regimen, particularly in patients with chronic bronchitis, as these are anti-inflammatory drugs. Methylxanthines, theophylline-like drugs, are oral agents that enhance bronchodilation. Doxofylline is a new methylxanthine. Oral leukotriene antagonists are anti-inflammatory agents that can be added to the daily regimen in patients with asthma. Mucolytics such as oral N-acetylcysteine can decrease viscosity of mucus and enhance lung function. Omalizumab is an immunomodulator, a monoclonal antibody, that is particularly effective in refractory cases of asthma.

they are only prescribed for a limited time. **Leukotriene receptor antagonists (LTRAs)** inhibit inflammatory mediators called leukotrienes, which cause bronchial inflammation and bronchoconstriction. LTRAs are prescribed for daily maintenance to control bronchial inflammation with few side effects.

Some inhalers contain a combination of a LABA and an ICS, as a dual kind of maintenance medication. The bronchodilator portion of the inhaler prevents bronchospasm, and the corticosteroid portion controls inflammation. An example of this kind of dual-acting drug is a formoterol/budesonide combination inhaler. During periods of exacerbations of asthma or COPD, patients require a short period of a low-dose oral corticosteroid such as prednisone. Also, many patients with allergy-triggered asthma carry a prefilled syringe of epinephrine (a potent adrenergic agonist) for emergencies.

In some cases, patients may require a nebulizer for better absorption of medication. Nebulized adrenergic agonists deliver the medication in an easily absorbed mist that can get into the lower bronchial airways. Theophylline and aminophylline are phosphodiesterase inhibitors that can be used to enhance bronchodilation. Pleural disorders such as pleural effusion or pneumothorax require chest tube insertion and suction or thoracotomy. Surgical procedures are often needed to remove lung masses or highly distended alveoli.

Bronchial thermoplasty (BT) is a nonpharmacological intervention for asthma that applies thermal energy to the smooth muscle in the airways via a bronchoscope. It aims to reduce hypertrophied airway smooth muscle that causes bronchoconstriction.

A specific type of surgical procedure termed lung volume reduction surgery (LVRS) (also called reduction pneumoplasty) is used in the treatment of COPD with emphysematous changes. In this procedure, the most damaged alveoli are excised from the lung. Less invasive endoscopic lung volume reduction procedures insert endobronchial coils or endobronchial valves via a bronchoscope with fluoroscopic guidance. These are also currently used for emphysema. Placement of biologically inert nitinol coils within the bronchioles can increase lung recoil in patients with emphysema. Insertion of valves in bronchioles can prevent hyperinflation of alveoli in patients with emphysema. Endoscopic thermal vapor ablation is another procedure that reduces the emphysematous portions of the lungs via the bronchoscope. Heated water vapor induces inflammatory tissue changes that are followed by healing with fibrosis.

Endotracheal intubation and mechanical ventilation are used in patients who endure critical illness and respiratory failure due to lung disease. Lung transplant is considered for those patients with severe end-stage pulmonary disease. There are eligibility requirements, and patients must wait for an appropriately matched donor.

Pathophysiology of Selected Obstructive Disorders

Obstructive disease is characterized by an increase in resistance to airflow from the trachea and larger bronchi to the terminal and respiratory bronchioles. The major obstructive lung diseases are asthma, COPD, and bronchiectasis.

Asthma

Asthma, also called hyperreactive airway disease, is a chronic inflammatory disorder that causes reversible airway constriction because of bronchial hyperreactivity. With each acute attack, remodeling and inflammatory changes develop in the bronchioles, so the aim of treatment is to prevent acute asthma attacks.

Epidemiology

Asthma is a common disease affecting more than 300 million persons worldwide, including 25 million Americans. According to the CDC in 2020, approximately 8% of persons in the United States have asthma. In adults, the prevalence is 8.4%, and in children, prevalence is 5.8%. In children, asthma is more prevalent in boys. However, in adults, asthma is significantly more prevalent in women (10.4%) than in men (6.2%). It affects almost 12% of those who experience poverty and in those who report being an ethnic or racial minority, especially Black race (10.2%) and Puerto Rican Hispanic ethnicity (14.9%). More than 4,000 people die of asthma each year, one-third of whom are age 65 or older. More than 40% of persons with asthma report one or more asthma attacks in the past 12 months. Poor clinical control of the disorder among patients is the major cause of nearly 1.3 million emergency department visits and 439,000 hospitalizations per year. The mortality rate is nearly 3 times higher in African American males than in European American males and 2½ times greater in African American females than in European American females.

Etiology

Asthma has many different etiologies and is considered a multifactorial disorder. It is caused by a combination of environmental factors, hypersensitivity, genomic and biome influences, and social determinants of health.

Allergy (also termed atopy) is the most common etiology of asthma. It is believed that many persons with asthma are hypersensitive to different allergens in the environment. Allergens include exhaust fumes, perfumes, pollen, grasses, flowers, dust, cigarette smoke, animal dander, molds, and spores. Tobacco smoke is particularly known for triggering bronchospasm. Dust mites, common microscopic household organisms, are some of the most common allergens implicated in asthma. Dog and cat dander are also common indoor allergens. About 25% to 65% of children with persistent asthma are sensitive to allergens found in the saliva, skin, and hair follicles of cats and dogs. These pet allergens are airborne and adhere to surfaces, carpets, and clothing. Cockroach allergen and mouse allergen, common in many urban indoor settings, have been shown to trigger and exacerbate asthma. Some molds found in the indoor and outdoor environments have been linked to asthma and allergies. Occupational exposure to chemical agents can also trigger asthma. More than 300 agents are known to stimulate bronchoconstriction. Employment settings with the highest risk for these chemical triggers include farming, painting, construction, landscaping, and janitorial work. Occupation-associated asthma can occur immediately after exposure to the chemical agent or as an immune-mediated disorder that occurs months to years after exposure.

Air pollution due to urbanization has been attributed to asthma exacerbations, as well as the development of asthma. Ozone, sulfur dioxide, nitrogen oxide, and particulate matter have been implicated as the likely causative agents. These pollutants typically come from vehicles and power generation, including the use of fossil fuels. This is especially true among minority and low-income children, who have been shown to be at increased risk of air pollution effects.

Some particular genes have been implicated in the development of asthma. These include *ADAM33, DPP10, PHF11, NPSR1, HLA-G, CYFIP2, IRAK3,* and *OPN3.* One of the most studied loci in asthma genetics is the 17q21 locus, which contains several genes associated with early onset asthma.

Viral infections, such as those caused by rhinovirus and respiratory syncytial virus, are common triggers for asthma in children. Between 80% and 85% of asthma attacks in children are preceded by viral infection. In addition, viral infection commonly causes acute bronchitis with bronchospasm in adults. Adults with COPD are particularly at risk for viral respiratory infection with bronchospasm. Sinusitis is also a known stimulant of asthma; 50% of asthma patients have a concurrent sinus infection.

There is a clinical syndrome that includes asthma, nasal polyps with chronic sinusitis, and aspirin or NSAID sensitivity. The mechanism of this reaction is not well understood but is likely caused by some abnormality in the cyclooxygenase pathway of inflammation. This is commonly referred to as aspirin-exacerbated respiratory disease (AERD).

Also, those persons who suffer from gastroesophageal reflux disease (GERD) can experience asthma when gastric secretions reflux into the bronchi and act as a bronchospastic trigger. GERD is a common trigger of nocturnal asthma attacks that awaken patients from sleep.

Nocturnal asthma may also be caused by sleep-related circadian rhythm changes; these cause respiratory function to decrease during early morning hours. Concurrently, during the early morning hours, cortisol level, a natural anti-inflammatory substance, is low and eosinophil activity is increased.

Asthma can be silent in individuals and only present during exercise. Exercise-induced bronchospasm occurs during vigorous physical activity in some individuals with airway hyperreactivity. Exposure to cold air often worsens exercise-induced asthma.

Pathophysiology

Asthma is a chronic inflammatory disease that causes episodes of spastic reactivity in the bronchioles. With each bout of acute bronchospasm in asthma, deleterious bronchial remodeling occurs. Prevention of asthma attacks is critical to avert bronchial airway alterations.

Allergy is a common stimulus of asthma. Allergens trigger the immune system, causing bronchial constriction, inflammation, and an increase in the size and number of goblet cells that secrete mucus. There is bronchoconstriction, bronchial edema, viscous mucus, and thickening of the bronchial basement membrane.

T lymphocytes in particular are involved in the pathophysiology of asthma. It is theorized that T2 helper cells (Th2) are highly active during asthma. Th2 cells are stimulated by allergens and assist B cells to transform into plasma cells that produce immunoglobulin E (IgE). Th2 cells attract mast cells, eosinophils, and basophils, which promote inflammation. IgE binds to mast cells and provokes their degranulation, which releases mediators such as histamine and leukotrienes. Leukotrienes are inflammatory mediators that are responsible for the development of bronchoconstriction, bronchial hyperreactivity, edema, and eosinophilia. Mast cells release histamine that contributes to bronchospasm and inflammation. T cells release cytokines called interleukins that maintain the damaging effects of the asthma attack. Eosinophils migrate to the reactive airway, compounding cell damage and airway edema. A cholinergic effect maintains the bronchoconstriction, increased mucus production, and vasodilation.

Asthma is also commonly triggered by viral respiratory infections that stimulate the production of IgE directed toward the viral antigens. Viral and bacterial upper respiratory infections commonly cause bronchospasm and copious mucus production.

Exercise can induce asthma by provoking loss of heat and water from the tracheobronchial tree; it is particularly exaggerated by cold air.

Inhaled chemicals, such as those contained in strong exhaust fumes, induce bronchospasm by irritating receptors that stimulate a vagal reflex. Chemicals that trigger asthma include sulfur dioxide, nitrogen dioxide, ozone, toluene, epoxy resins, and formaldehyde commonly found in the workplace, as well as sulfites used in food processing.

Multiple episodes of asthma promote the process of airway remodeling, which involves proliferation of respiratory epithelium and hypertrophy of respiratory smooth muscle; they can also lead to a relatively fixed airway obstruction. Additionally, epithelial cell injury exposes the airway to triggers for hyperreactivity, resulting in more frequent episodes of bronchospasms.

Clinical Presentation

The clinician should assess the severity of the patient's asthma through a variety of important questions. A history of childhood asthma and family history are important. Questions to ask include:

- Are you experiencing dyspnea, wheeze, or cough?
- Are symptoms worse at night or after exercise?
- How often do you experience symptoms?
- Does exposure to certain environmental allergens such as dust or pet dander provoke symptoms? How about episodes of respiratory infection or GERD?
- What is your occupation? What kind of materials do you handle? Do you wear a protective mask when using inhalants?

The history regarding the severity of asthma can be augmented by asking the patient to complete the Asthma Control Questionnaire (ACQ). This is a simple 7-item self-administered questionnaire to measure the adequacy of asthma control or change in asthma control that has occurred spontaneously or as a result of treatment. There is also a more extensive Asthma Quality of Life questionnaire, which is a more detailed, 32-question survey.

Comorbidities should be investigated as these can contribute to asthma flare-ups and complicate asthma management. These include allergic rhinitis, chronic rhinosinusitis, GERD, obesity, obstructive sleep apnea, depression, and anxiety.

Signs and Symptoms. Asthma is characterized by wheezing, cough, dyspnea, and chest tightness. The severity of the symptoms depends on the degree of bronchial hyperresponsiveness and reversibility of the bronchial obstruction (see Fig. 21-5). Prolonged exhalations are commonly an early sign of airway obstruction. Severe attacks are accompanied by use of accessory muscles, distant breath sounds, and diaphoresis. The patient may be able to speak only one or two words before taking a breath. Patients going into respiratory failure caused by marked airway constriction have inaudible breath sounds and a repetitive, hacking cough. Rhonchi may be present if larger bronchial airways are involved. If the asthma is related to allergies, signs of chronic rhinitis may be present, including nasal edema, nasal polyps, rhinorrhea, and oropharyngeal erythema. Eczema, which indicates allergy, may be present on the patient's skin, particularly the neck and the antecubital or popliteal spaces.

Diagnosis

Asthma can be difficult to diagnose as there is no gold standard test. Diagnosis of asthma is based on a thorough history and physical examination, laboratory findings, and PFTs. The history regarding the severity of asthma can be enhanced by asking the patient to complete an asthma control questionnaire (ACQ). Sputum and blood eosinophil levels can be measured as these are biomarkers that can indicate certain treatment. Blood levels of IgE are also useful in the overall assessment as the presence of high antibody titers can indicate allergen-induced asthma.

The PFT (also called spirometry) measures of **forced expiratory volume at 1 second (FEV$_1$)** and **forced vital capacity (FVC)** are used to diagnose and evaluate the severity of an asthma attack. During an acute asthma attack, FEV$_1$ decreases, which diminishes the overall FEV$_1$/FVC ratio. This ratio should then be reassessed after a bronchodilator is administered to diagnose and evaluate the severity of asthma. The diagnosis of asthma should be considered if there is an increase of 12% or greater and 200 mL in FEV$_1$ after inhaling a short-acting bronchodilator.

The **methacholine bronchoprovocation test** can be useful in the diagnosis of asthma. Methacholine is an inhaled drug that causes mild narrowing of the airways in the lungs. The test starts with a baseline PFT including an FEV$_1$ to assess basic lung function. Progressively larger doses of inhaled methacholine are given by a nebulizer. PFTs are performed before and after each dose of inhaled methacholine to measure the amount of airway narrowing. A methacholine challenge test is considered positive if methacholine causes the lung function (FEV$_1$) to drop by 20% or more compared with the baseline.

In individuals age 5 years and older for whom the diagnosis of asthma is uncertain using history, clinical findings, PFTs, and bronchodilator responsiveness testing, or in whom PFTs cannot be performed, the NHLBI Expert Panel recommends the addition of **fractional exhaled nitric oxide (FeNO)** measurement as an adjunct to the evaluation process. Nitric oxide can be measured in exhaled breath and can serve as a measure of the level of airway inflammation. When airway inflammation is present, fractional exhalation of

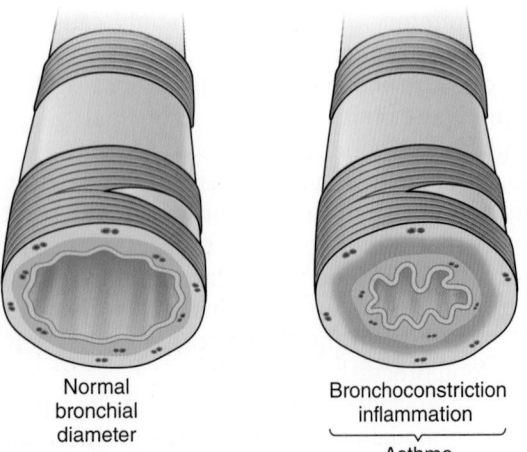

Normal bronchial diameter

Bronchoconstriction inflammation

Asthma

FIGURE 21-5. Bronchoconstriction in asthma.

nitric oxide increases. FeNO testing requires an expiratory maneuver into a device designed for this purpose. FeNO testing enhances the accuracy of asthma diagnosis in individuals ages 5 years and older.

Classification of Asthma: Evolving Terminology.

In 2007, the National Heart, Lung, and Blood Institute Expert Panel Report 3 classified asthma as intermittent or persistent, and further subdivided persistent asthma as mild, moderate, or severe. These classifications have remained the same in the updated 2020 National Heart, Lung, and Blood Institute Expert Panel Report 4 (see Box 21-2).

However, asthma is increasingly being classified in distinct ways by different professional societies and experts in pulmonary medicine, immunology, and allergy. There are various ways of classifying asthma according to etiology, clinical presentation, or difficulty to treat. These classifications are evolving and clinicians need to understand the various terms used to classify asthma as it has implications for diagnosis, prognosis, and treatment.

The 2020 American Thoracic Society/European Respiratory Society (ATS/ERS) Task Force classified asthma in terms of difficulty to treat. The categories include mild, moderate, or severe asthma depending on how it responds to specific treatments (GINA Report, 2022; see Box 21-3).

The American Academy of Allergy, Asthma, and Immunology (AAAAI) recognizes there are differences in the types of underlying inflammation observed in asthma and differences in the clinical features of the disease between different patients. They assert these differences in asthma are called "phenotypes." The AAAAI (2022) asserts that identifying the specific asthma phenotype of an individual patient helps clinicians better manage the disease. The current treatment of asthma is now moving toward treating the more specific phenotype of asthma for individual patients rather than using the same treatment regimen for all patients. This has led to another classification system that asserts "asthma" is an umbrella term for different disease processes with distinct pathophysiological mechanisms (termed **endotypes**) and variable clinical presentations (termed **phenotypes**). The **endotype-phenotype classification of asthma** recognizes that the basic pathological mechanism in asthma involves T2 helper cells as the principal drivers of eosinophilic airway inflammation and release of the cytokines, interleukins IL-4, IL-5, and IL-13. The endotype-phenotype classification system of asthma is more precise in terms of the etiology, clinical manifestations, associated biomarkers, laboratory test findings, and treatments. Experts find this classification system lends itself to the new age of precision medicine.

Asthma endotypes are broadly divided into two subgroups depending on the involvement of allergy, T helper cells, and eosinophilic inflammation. The two main endotypes are called **T2 high asthma** associated with allergy and eosinophilia, and **T2 low** or **non-T2 asthma**, which does not involve atopy or eosinophilia. The nomenclature is increasingly abbreviated in the literature as **T2 asthma and non-T2 asthma**.

BOX 21-2. Classification of Asthma According to NIH/NHLBI 2007 and 2020

According to the *2007 NIH/NHLBI Expert Panel Report 3 (EPR3): Guidelines for the Diagnosis and Management of Asthma*, asthma categories are based on frequency and severity of asthma symptoms, FEV_1, and FEV_1/FVC measurements (updated 2020, EPR 4).

MILD INTERMITTENT

In mild intermittent asthma, symptoms occur less than two times a week during waking hours and less than twice a month during the night. In between asthma attacks, no symptoms occur at all, and the attacks themselves are generally brief, though their intensity can vary. The FEV_1 is greater than 80% of normal during asthma attacks. The FEV_1/FVC ratio is normal.

MILD PERSISTENT

In mild persistent asthma, symptoms occur more than twice a week but less than daily. They may occasionally wake the patient up at night, but that happens less than two times a month. Asthma attacks may interfere with activity temporarily. The FEV_1 is greater than or equal to 80% of normal during asthma attacks. The FEV_1/FVC ratio is normal.

MODERATE PERSISTENT

In moderate persistent asthma, the disorder is starting to interfere more with daily living. Symptoms occur every single day, and the patient needs to use a quick-relief inhaler daily. Asthma attacks occur at least twice a week, often interfere with activity, and may last for days at a time. The patient is probably also waking up one or more times a week with symptoms. FEV_1 is between 60% and 80% of normal. The FEV_1/FVC ratio is reduced by 5%.

SEVERE PERSISTENT

In severe persistent asthma, the most severe form of the disorder, symptoms are basically continuous. Activity is severely limited, and asthma attacks and night symptoms are frequent. The FEV_1 is lower than 60% of normal. The FEV_1/FVC ratio is reduced by more than 5%.

National Asthma Education and Prevention Program Expert Panel Report 3: Guidelines for the Diagnosis and Management of Asthma, 2007. U.S. Department of Health and Human Services, National Institutes of Health (NIH), National Heart, Lung, and Blood Institute (NHLBI). Also in accordance with 2020 Focused Updates to the Asthma Management Guidelines: A Report from the National Asthma Education and Prevention Program Coordinating Committee Expert Panel Working Group.

BOX 21-3. Asthma Classification According to American Thoracic Society/European Respiratory Society (ATR/ERS)

The currently accepted definition of asthma severity is based on "difficulty to treat." The current definition of asthma severity, recommended by an ATS/ERS Task Force and included in most asthma guidelines, is that severity should be assessed retrospectively from the level of treatment required to control the patient's symptoms and exacerbations; i.e., after at least several months of treatment.

Mild asthma is currently defined as asthma that is well controlled with as-needed ICS-formoterol, or with low-dose ICS plus as-needed SABA.

Moderate asthma is currently defined as asthma that is well controlled with low- or medium-dose ICS-LABA.

Severe asthma is defined as asthma that remains uncontrolled despite optimized treatment with high-dose ICS-LABA, or that requires high-dose ICS-LABA to prevent it from becoming uncontrolled. Severe asthma must be distinguished from asthma that is difficult to treat due to inadequate or inappropriate treatment, or persistent problems with adherence or comorbidities such as chronic rhinosinusitis or obesity. There are very different treatment implications compared with asthma that is relatively refractory to high-dose ICS-LABA or even OCS.

By this retrospective definition, asthma severity can only be assessed after good asthma control has been achieved and treatment stepped down to find the patient's minimum effective dose or if asthma remains uncontrolled.

Abbreviations: ATS, American Thoracic Society; ERS, European Respiratory Society; ICS, inhaled corticosteroid; LABA, long-acting beta-2 adrenergic agonist; OCS, oral corticosteroids; SABA, short-acting beta-2 adrenergic agonist.
Adapted from: 2022 Global Initiative for Asthma (GINA) Main Report. 2022 GINA Report, Global Strategy for Asthma Management and Prevention. https://ginasthma.org/gina-reports/

T2-high (T2) phenotypes are further classified into three groups: early onset allergic asthma, late-onset eosinophilic asthma, and aspirin-exacerbated respiratory disease (AERD). T2-low (non-T2) phenotypes are further classified according to nonatopic clinical characteristics that include obesity, smoking, and age. Obesity-associated asthma, smoking-associated asthma, and very late–onset asthma (occurring after age 50) are the three phenotypes of non-T2 asthma (see Box 21-4). Phenotype overlap is extremely common in patients with asthma and can make treatment decisions more challenging. Patients can also have phenotype overlap between asthma and COPD.

Treatment

The goal of treatment is to control asthma and prevent acute episodic exacerbations of bronchospasm. Preventing acute episodes can diminish the remodeling that occurs in the bronchioles and decrease the severity of asthma.

Treatment guidelines have been developed by the 2022 Global Initiative for Asthma. Each step of treatment includes patient education, environmental control, and management of comorbidities, as well as medication. In the stepwise approach, the clinician escalates treatment as needed (by moving to a higher step) or, if possible, de-escalates treatment (by moving to a lower step) once the individual's asthma is well controlled for at least 3 consecutive months (see Figure 21-6).

One specific update relates to individuals with allergy-induced asthma. For those who have symptoms related to exposure to identified allergens, confirmed by history taking or allergy testing, the Expert Panel recommends a multicomponent allergen-specific mitigation intervention. Allergen mitigation involves allergen testing, patient education regarding environmental and lifestyle changes to prevent exposure, and allergen immunotherapy (AIT). AIT involves administering minute amounts of allergen by injection to the patient over a course of several visits to desensitize the individual. An alternative allergen immunotherapy treatment is sublingual immunotherapy (SLIT) without injections.

In the stepwise treatment of asthma, medications fall into two general classes: maintenance (also called controller) medication for daily use and rescue (also called reliever) medication for acute bronchospastic episodes.

Maintenance medication commonly consists of an inhaler that contains a LABA in combination with an ICS. A commonly recommended long-acting maintenance inhaler medication is formoterol, a long-acting **adrenergic beta-2 agonist (LABA)**. Budesonide is a commonly recommended ICS. There are inhalers that contain a combination of a LABA and ICS that are often used for maintenance therapy; an example is formoterol/budesonide (Symbicort).

Alternatively, anticholinergic (also called antimuscarinic) inhaler agent can be administered if adrenergic agonist is not effective. A common long-acting muscarinic antagonist (LAMA) agent is tiotropium.

The **Global Initiative for Asthma (GINA)** 2022 treatment recommendations are described in terms of two tracks. Track 1 recommends low-dose ICS-formoterol as the rescue/reliever medication, which is the preferred strategy (see Figure 21-6). Track 2, with SABA as the rescue/reliever medication, is an alternative, but not preferred, strategy. Experts assert it is less effective than Track 1 for reducing severe

BOX 21-4. Endotype-Phenotype Classification of Asthma

ENDOTYPE	PHENOTYPE	CLINICAL MANIFESTATIONS	BIOMARKERS/ LABORATORY TESTS
T2 High asthma (T2 asthma)	Early onset allergic asthma	Positive allergy tests	High eosinophils, high IgE, high FeNO
	Late-onset eosinophilic asthma	Chronic rhinosinusitis, nasal polyps	High eosinophils, high FeNO, high or normal IgE, high interleukins
	Aspirin-exacerbated respiratory disease (AERD)	Chronic rhinosinusitis, nasal polyps, COX-1 inhibitor-induced respiratory reactions	
T2 Low asthma (non-T2 asthma)	Obesity-associated	Commonly female, middle-aged, nonatopic	High neutrophils (not eosinophils), high interleukins
	Smoking-associated	Asthma-COPD overlap, at least 10 pack-year smoking history, older than age 40	High neutrophils
	Very late onset	Age older than 50, decreased elastic recoil of alveoli, immunosenescence	High neutrophils

Adapted from: Kuruvilla, M. E., Lee, F. E., & Lee, G. B. (2019). Understanding asthma phenotypes, endotypes, and mechanisms of disease. *Clin Rev Allergy Immunol, 56*(2), 219–233. doi: 10.1007/s12016-018-8712-1

exacerbations. However, Track 2 is recommended if Track 1 is not possible or if a patient has good treatment results with their controller, and has had no exacerbations in the last 12 months. SABA-only treatment is not recommended any longer in asthma treatment. It has been found that SABA-only treatment can lead to reduced bronchodilator response, increased allergic responses, and increased eosinophilia.

In individuals with uncontrolled persistent asthma, a LAMA can be added to ICS controller therapy or a LAMA can be added to ICS-LABA therapy for a triple-therapy approach.

Clinicians need to ensure that patients are using inhalers correctly through patient education materials. A demonstration of the proper inhaler technique is recommended. A return demonstration by the patient with clinician observation is advised. Improper inhaler technique is common and reduces medication lung deposition, and thus reduces its effectiveness. Spacer devices are often necessary to ensure proper drug delivery in children with asthma.

If additional maintenance control is needed, an oral leukotriene antagonist (LTRA) can be added to the daily regimen. Furthermore, a phosphodiesterase inhibitor, theophylline or aminophylline, can be used to enhance bronchodilation.

For severe exacerbations of acute asthma, an oral corticosteroid, usually prednisone, is added to the regimen for a short time. A short course of oral prednisone in a tapered dose regimen is prescribed. An injection of epinephrine can also be administered if the acute exacerbation is severe.

In addition to AIT for allergic individuals, immunomodulator-type medications are recommended. Immunomodulators are monoclonal antibody medications that prevent binding of IgE to basophils and mast cells. Immunomodulators include omalizumab, dupilumab, mepolizumab, benralizumab, and reslizumab.

In patients with severe persistent asthma that is refractory to medications, bronchial thermoplasty is recommended. Bronchial thermoplasty, performed with a bronchoscope, uses a wire probe to deliver heat to the airway wall to decrease the mass of smooth muscle that constricts the airway.

Complications

Status asthmaticus is defined as persistent bronchoconstriction that endures despite attempts to treat the attack with medications. In this severe asthma attack, pulmonary gas exchange is diminished by the uneven distribution of ventilation resulting from generalized bronchoconstriction. The major physiological abnormality is a grossly uneven V-Q distribution, leading to a dramatic fall in arterial oxygenation; this is referred to as ventilation-perfusion (V-Q) mismatching. In ventilation-perfusion mismatching, areas are ventilated in the lung that do not have adequate circulation; therefore, inadequate oxygenation of the

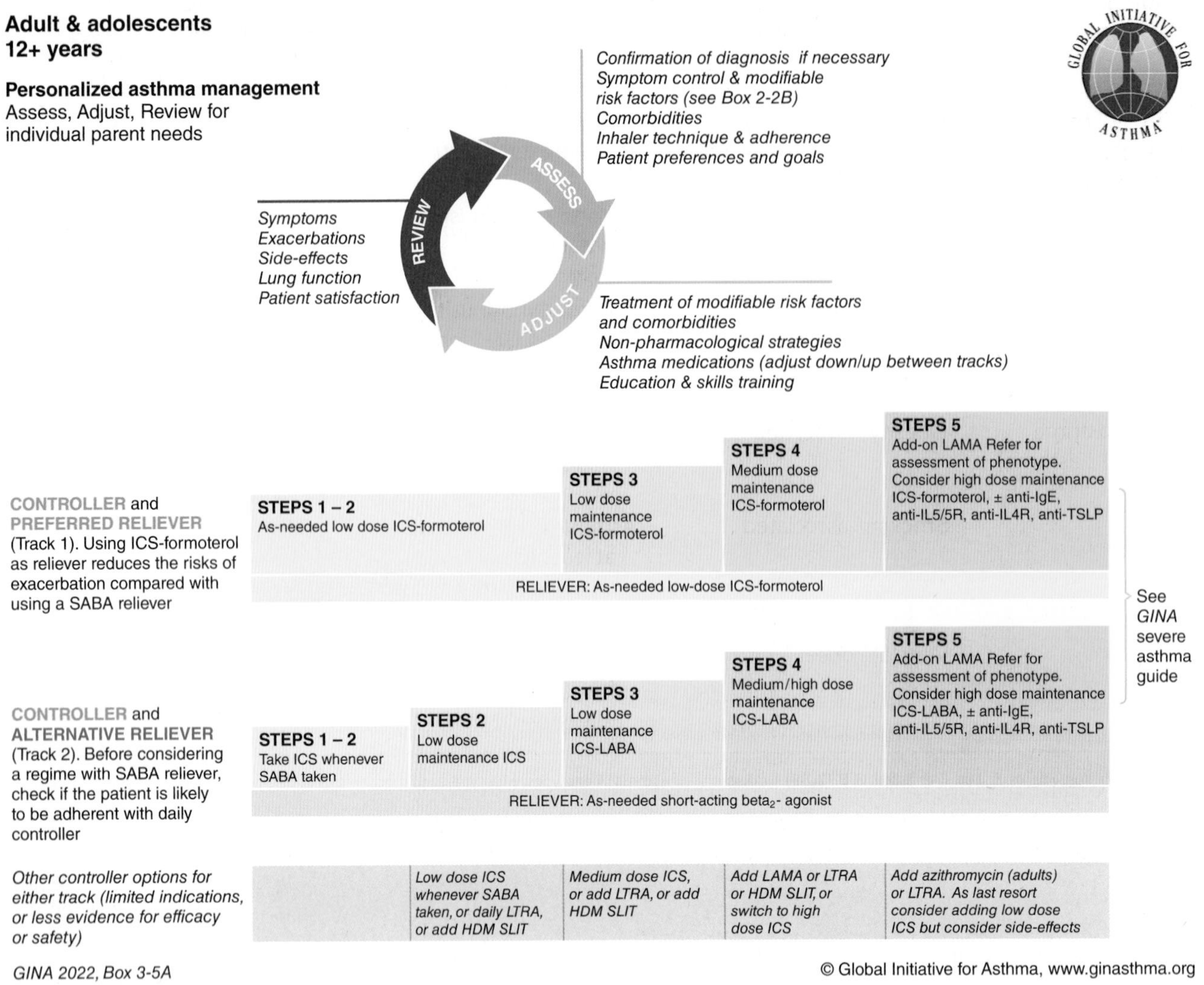

**Adult & adolescents
12+ years**

Personalized asthma management
Assess, Adjust, Review for
individual parent needs

Confirmation of diagnosis if necessary
Symptom control & modifiable
risk factors (see Box 2-2B)
Comorbidities
Inhaler technique & adherence
Patient preferences and goals

ASSESS
REVIEW
ADJUST

Symptoms
Exacerbations
Side-effects
Lung function
Patient satisfaction

Treatment of modifiable risk factors
and comorbidities
Non-pharmacological strategies
Asthma medications (adjust down/up between tracks)
Education & skills training

GLOBAL INITIATIVE FOR ASTHMA

CONTROLLER and **PREFERRED RELIEVER** (Track 1). Using ICS-formoterol as reliever reduces the risks of exacerbation compared with using a SABA reliever	**STEPS 1 – 2** As-needed low dose ICS-formoterol		**STEPS 3** Low dose maintenance ICS-formoterol	**STEPS 4** Medium dose maintenance ICS-formoterol	**STEPS 5** Add-on LAMA Refer for assessment of phenotype. Consider high dose maintenance ICS-formoterol, ± anti-IgE, anti-IL5/5R, anti-IL4R, anti-TSLP
	RELIEVER: As-needed low-dose ICS-formoterol				

See GINA severe asthma guide

CONTROLLER and **ALTERNATIVE RELIEVER** (Track 2). Before considering a regime with SABA reliever, check if the patient is likely to be adherent with daily controller	**STEPS 1 – 2** Take ICS whenever SABA taken	**STEPS 2** Low dose maintenance ICS	**STEPS 3** Low dose maintenance ICS-LABA	**STEPS 4** Medium/high dose maintenance ICS-LABA	**STEPS 5** Add-on LAMA Refer for assessment of phenotype. Consider high dose maintenance ICS-LABA, ± anti-IgE, anti-IL5/5R, anti-IL4R, anti-TSLP
	RELIEVER: As-needed short-acting beta$_2$- agonist				

Other controller options for either track (limited indications, or less evidence for efficacy or safety)	Low dose ICS whenever SABA taken, or daily LTRA, or add HDM SLIT	Medium dose ICS, or add LTRA, or add HDM SLIT	Add LAMA or LTRA or HDM SLIT, or switch to high dose ICS	Add azithromycin (adults) or LTRA. As last resort consider adding low dose ICS but consider side-effects	

GINA 2022, Box 3-5A

© Global Initiative for Asthma, www.ginasthma.org

FIGURE 21-6. Stepwise treatment of asthma from GINA 2022 Report, including both preferred and alternate treatment guidance.

bloodstream occurs. Conversely, there are areas of the lung that have circulation but no ventilation. In status asthmaticus, if bronchoconstriction is not relieved and the patient becomes exhausted and dehydrated, total alveolar ventilation fails, leading to cyanosis and carbon dioxide retention, a potentially fatal condition.

Chronic Obstructive Pulmonary Disease

Chronic obstructive pulmonary disease (COPD) is a combination of chronic bronchitis, emphysema, and hyperreactive airway disease. It is characterized by the features of these three disorders.

Epidemiology
COPD is the fourth leading cause of death in the United States and a leading cause of disability. It is estimated that there are 16 million persons with COPD; most are older than age 45. However, the prevalence is believed to be up to twice that number because of underreporting of individuals who do not seek health care. In the past, COPD had a higher prevalence in men, but from 1980 to 2000, the mortality rate from COPD increased dramatically in women. Today, more women than men die of COPD. In the United States, the economic burden of this disease, estimated at $24 billion annually, is caused by the cost of medical care and days lost from work.

Etiology
Smoking is the major cause of COPD; however, as many as 25% of persons with COPD have never smoked. Occupational and environmental exposures to chemicals, dusts, and secondhand smoke are also causes. Fumes from unventilated wood-burning stoves causes COPD in many persons in underdeveloped countries. COPD is caused by a combination of genetic susceptibility and environmental factors. One such genetic predisposition to COPD is caused by alpha 1 antitrypsin (AAT) deficiency. This rare genetic variant accounts for less than 1% of all COPD cases. AAT, a serum protein normally found in the lungs, inhibits elastase, a proteolytic enzyme released by WBCs. AAT deficiency allows elastase to destroy lung tissue unchecked. The genetic mutation causing AAT deficiency is found on chromosome 14. AAT deficiency leads to premature

development of emphysema in young adults, often with chronic bronchitis and bronchiectasis.

IV drug abuse has been associated with emphysema. This is caused by some of the components of the illicit drug that are injected into the bloodstream. Components such as talc enter the venous system and can travel to the right side of the heart and then into the pulmonary circulation and lung tissue.

Pneumocystis jiroveci infection in individuals with AIDS is associated with emphysematous changes in the lungs. Bullous cysts called pneumoceles are commonly found within lung tissue in AIDS sufferers.

Connective tissue diseases, which include Marfan syndrome and Ehlers–Danlos syndrome, also predispose individuals to emphysema. Connective tissue changes in the walls of the alveoli cause decreased elasticity and recoil of lung tissue.

Pathophysiology

COPD is characterized by poorly reversible airflow limitation caused by a combination of chronic bronchitis, emphysema, and hyperreactive airway disease. The characteristic features of **chronic bronchitis** are hypersecretion of mucus in the large and small airways, hypoxia, and cyanosis. Excessive mucus creates obstruction to inspiratory airflow, which inhibits optimal oxygenation. To be diagnosed with chronic bronchitis, the individual has to have had a cough for 3 months out of the year for 2 consecutive years.

In **emphysema**, the characteristic finding is overdistention of alveoli with trapped air, which creates obstruction to expiratory airflow, loss of elastic recoil of the alveoli, and high residual volume of carbon dioxide in the lung. The airways are also hyperreactive to irritants, and episodes of bronchoconstriction are common in COPD.

The pathological changes leading to airflow limitation in COPD include narrowing, excessive mucus and fibrosis in the bronchioles, loss of alveolar elastic recoil, and smooth muscle hypertrophy. Inflammatory changes of chronic bronchitis cause permanent remodeling of the pulmonary structure (see Fig. 21-7). The remodeled bronchioles demonstrate chronic inflammatory changes, thickening of the walls, and constriction of the lumens. Inflammation causes stimulation of macrophages followed by accumulation of neutrophils, T lymphocytes, and cytokines. Leukotrienes, interleukins, and tumor necrosis factor are among the inflammatory mediators that act in a proteolytic manner, chronically damaging lung structures. There is a proteolytic-antiproteolytic enzyme imbalance in the lungs of patients with COPD that leads to alveolar membrane damage in emphysema. Neutrophils and macrophages secrete proteases, elastases, and metalloproteinases, which are all proteolytic enzymes. Smoking activates proteolytic enzymes, which are released from neutrophils and macrophages. Cigarette smoke also contains free radicals that damage respiratory cell membranes and arterial endothelial cells.

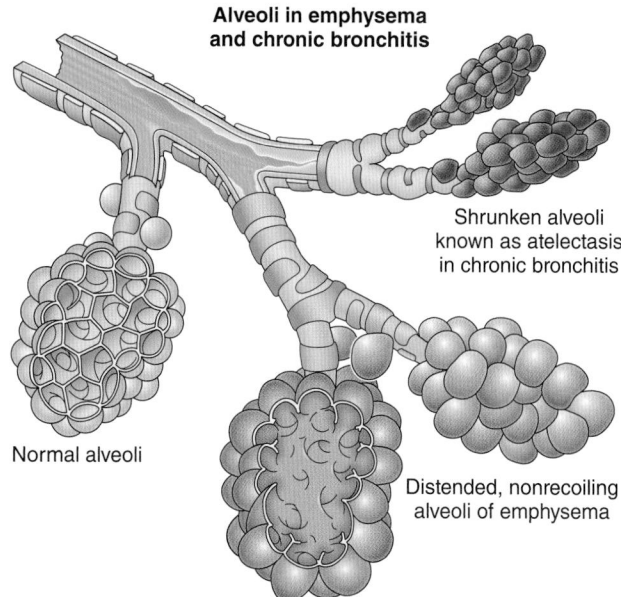

Alveoli in emphysema and chronic bronchitis

Normal alveoli

Shrunken alveoli known as atelectasis in chronic bronchitis

Distended, nonrecoiling alveoli of emphysema

FIGURE 21-7. The bronchioles and alveoli in COPD. COPD is a combination of chronic bronchitis and emphysema. In chronic bronchitis, there is inflammation, edema, and excess mucus production within the airways. In emphysema, there is an excess of air in the alveoli. The alveolar walls are weakened, distended, and cannot recoil. Some alveoli shown here are also atelectatic from lack of ventilation caused by chronic bronchitis.

Concurrently, smoking inactivates the body's natural antioxidants and antiproteolytic enzymes.

In severe COPD, particularly in those areas demonstrating changes consistent with chronic bronchitis, there is poor ventilation in the lungs and hypoxia. In areas of poor ventilation, chronic hypoxia develops. Chronic hypoxia stimulates pulmonary arterial vasoconstriction. Pulmonary arterial vasoconstriction, which is called **pulmonary hypertension**, causes increased resistance in the main pulmonary artery and, in turn, increased resistance against the right ventricle. Chronic pulmonary hypertension causes right ventricular hypertrophy and eventual right ventricular failure. Right ventricular failure caused by pulmonary disease is called **cor pulmonale**. In cor pulmonale, the patient suffers all the signs and symptoms consistent with right ventricular failure, including jugular venous distention, ascites, hepatomegaly, splenomegaly, and ankle or sacral edema.

In severe COPD, increased levels of CO_2 become chronic and the arterial chemoreceptors and respiratory center in the medulla become insensitive to high CO_2 levels. The normal respiratory drive stimulus changes from P_{CO_2} accumulation to low levels of P_{O_2}. In severe COPD, hypoxia becomes the stimulus for breathing. In other words, the patient needs to be hypoxic to stimulate independent breathing. Administering high doses of oxygen can depress the patient's independent drive to breathe and cause respiratory arrest. Careful, slow upward titration of oxygen is necessary when the patient requires oxygen therapy. Any agents that depress respiratory drive, such as tranquilizers, sedatives, and opiates, should be used with caution.

Clinical Presentation

Patient age and smoking history are important features in establishing a pattern of obstructive disease. Whereas asthma occurs in all age groups, COPD is generally a disease of older persons. The mean age of patients with emphysema is 65. Patients with COPD caused by AAT deficiency are usually younger adults aged 40 to 50 years. Commonly, the patient with COPD complains of dyspnea and cough. It is important to ask what precipitates the dyspnea, such as climbing a flight of stairs, lifting heavy objects, walking several blocks, or the performance of activities of daily living such as bathing and dressing. This gives the examiner an idea of the severity of airflow limitation. Other questions to ask include:

- What is the frequency and quality of the cough? Is it productive of sputum? Is hemoptysis present? If so, how much?
- Has there been any wheezing?
- Is there a history of smoking? If so, what is the pack-year history?
- Is secondhand smoke a problem at work or home?
- Has there been any weight loss? What is the patient's pattern of exercise?
- Is there a history of alcohol use? Illicit drugs?
- Is there a family history of respiratory illness?

Along with these questions, ask about the patient's past and present occupations, particularly focusing on possible exposure to toxins such as asbestos, silica, hydrogen sulfide, lead, mercury, coal, cotton dust, and diisocyanates. Also obtain the patient's complete list of current medications, including herbal and over-the-counter medications, as well as information about allergies. The COPD assessment test (CAT) and/ or the MRC Dyspnea Scale can be used to augment the history of patients with COPD. These are self-administered questionnaires that can assess the impact of COPD on the patient's quality of life.

Signs and Symptoms. Signs and symptoms of COPD include those of chronic bronchitis, emphysema, and asthma. Dyspnea is usually the first symptom, initially occurring with heavy exertion. As the disease progresses, dyspnea becomes increasingly worse with less and less vigorous exertion. Cough or wheezing may be a chief complaint. The cough may be productive, and sputum should be expectorated for culture. Productive cough, hypoxia, and cyanosis are classic signs of chronic bronchitis. The hypoxia of chronic bronchitis stimulates pulmonary arterial vasoconstriction. Over time, because of the high resistance against the right ventricle, right ventricular failure occurs. The signs and symptoms of right-sided heart failure, such as jugular venous distention, ascites, hepatosplenomegaly, and ankle edema, develop after long-term chronic bronchitis.

Observe the patient for signs of respiratory distress, use of intercostal muscles or accessory muscles with breathing, and clubbing of the fingers (see Fig. 21-2).

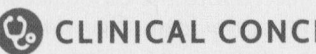

CLINICAL CONCEPT

Clubbing of fingers indicates chronic hypoxia.

Examine the thoracic cage structure. A barrel-shaped chest is commonly present in emphysema; this is a shape that has an equal diameter of the width and depth of the chest. In healthy persons the width of the chest should be double the depth of the chest. In emphysema, there is an accumulation of air in the alveoli, which over time increases the width and depth of the thoracic cage.

Observe the patient's complexion. Cyanosis, commonly visible around the lips, indicates hypoxia. In those with a lengthy smoking history, the teeth or fingertips may be tobacco stained. Examine the jugular veins, abdomen, and ankles. Distended jugular veins, ascites, and ankle edema indicate cor pulmonale (right ventricular failure).

With regard to vital signs, focus particularly on respiratory rate, rhythm, and depth. Patients with COPD often have prolonged exhalation and purse the lips when exhaling. The examiner can palpate the posterior lung fields bilaterally for tactile fremitus. Vibrations over lung fields should be equal as the patient vocalizes "ninety-nine." The posterior lung fields can also be percussed bilaterally for resonance. In severe emphysema, hyperresonance may be percussed because of the extra air retained in the lungs. Auscultate the heart and note any abnormal sounds. Commonly, wheezing is heard over the lung fields in COPD. Diminished breath sounds may suggest severe disease. Identify the location of any adventitious sounds.

CLINICAL CONCEPT

Individuals with chronic bronchitis are known as **blue bloaters**—blue because of hypoxia and cyanosis, and bloater because of the edema that occurs as a result of right ventricular failure. Individuals with emphysema are known as **pink puffers**—pink because they remain well-oxygenated until late in their disease, and puffer because they have a characteristic manner of exhalation using pursed-lip breathing.

Diagnosis

The **COPD Assessment Test (CAT)** is a patient questionnaire that asks specific questions about the patient's breathing ability and activity limitations due to their pulmonary symptoms. There are eight questions that ask about breathlessness, cough, chest tightness, sputum, and activity level. Each item is scored on a scale of 0 to 5, with a higher total score indicating more severe disease.

Another questionnaire, the **Medical Research Council (MRC) Dyspnea Scale** is simple to administer as it allows the patients to indicate the extent to which their breathlessness affects their mobility. The 1–5 stage scale is used alongside questions to establish clinical grades of breathlessness.

PFTs (also called spirometry) are a key part of the diagnosis of COPD (see Box 21-1). Common parameters measured in PFT s include FVC and FEV_1. FVC is the total volume of air that can be exhaled with maximum effort. FEV_1 is the volume of air expelled during the first second of exhalation of air from the lungs. Airflow limitation of COPD is identified by a FEV_1/FVC ratio of less than 70%. FEV_1 significantly diminishes in COPD because the patient's exhalation phase is slow and prolonged (see Fig. 21-8).

The **BODE index** is a multidimensional 10-point scale that is used to evaluate the severity of COPD. It includes body mass index, airflow obstruction, dyspnea score, and exercise capacity by using the 6-min walk distance. A 6-minute walk test on a treadmill should be ordered in patients with progressively worsening dyspnea or lung function. It can assess for hypoxia with exertion and candidacy for long-term oxygen therapy. This is usually accomplished in a pulmonary rehabilitation department of a health-care facility.

A complete blood count (CBC), blood chemistry panel, chest x-ray, electrocardiogram (ECG), and ABGs should be analyzed. In individuals with mild to moderate disease, all laboratory data should be normal except for the PFTs. In severe COPD, the chest x-ray may show characteristics consistent with emphysema: flattened, low diaphragm borders and hyperinflation of both lung fields caused by retained air. The ECG commonly demonstrates a right axis deviation caused by right ventricular hypertrophy. Also in severe COPD, an enlarged heart may be visible because of right ventricular failure. The pulmonary vasculature may be constricted if pulmonary hypertension exists because of chronic bronchitis. In those with severe hypoxia, the CBC will indicate erythrocytosis (high number of erythrocytes) caused by the constant secretion of erythropoietin from the kidney. The eosinophil count on a CBC can help guide the decision to initiate or discontinue inhaled corticosteroids (ICSs) because patients with higher eosinophil counts generally respond better to this class of inhalers. Eosinophilia will be present if allergy exists.

An ABG test is helpful in diagnosis as it can reveal chronic hypercapnia and hypoxia, which may be used to evaluate the patient for supplemental oxygen treatment.

Obtaining a chest CT scan may be needed in patients with COPD exacerbations to rule out pulmonary embolism and assess for the presence of other coexisting pulmonary abnormalities, such as bronchiectasis, interstitial lung disease, or lung mass.

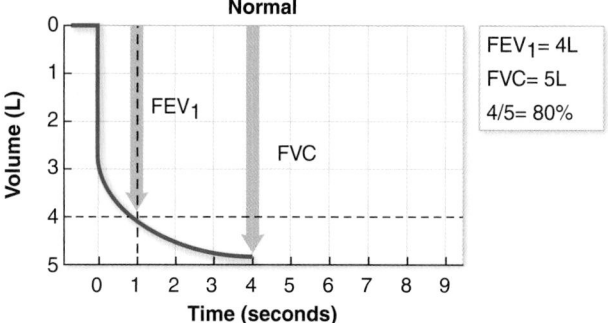

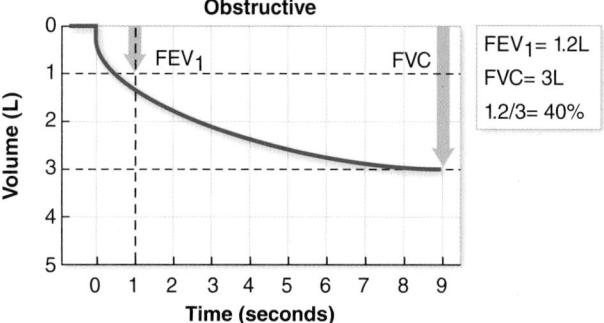

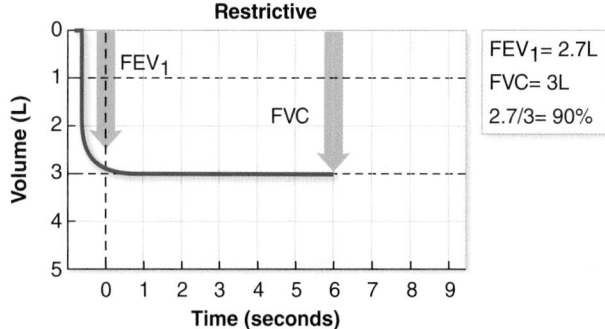

FIGURE 21-8. Spirometry measures in obstructive versus restrictive pulmonary disease. Forced expiration over 1 second (FEV_1) is a simple PFT. A person inhales to total lung capacity and then exhales as completely as possible into a spirometer. The spirometer then prints out a curve on a graph. The graph will show total FVC and the amount of exhaled air in the first second of expiration. The FEV_1 is compared with the FVC to diagnose an obstructive versus a restrictive pulmonary disease. (A) In a normal forced expiration curve, the total FEV that the healthy subject can expire in 1 second (FEV_1) is about 80% of the total FVC. The FVC is approximately 5 liters. In a healthy subject, almost all of the air can be exhaled within the first second. (B) In an obstructive pulmonary condition, such as asthma, bronchitis, or emphysema, the FVC is reduced and the rate of expiratory flow is also reduced. The subject takes a prolonged time to exhale all the air from the lungs. Thus, an individual with an obstructive defect might have an FVC of only 3.0 liters, and in the first second of forced expiration, exhale only 1.2 liters, giving an FEV_1/FVC ratio of 40%. (C) With a restrictive disease, such as interstitial pulmonary fibrosis, FVC is also reduced. However, because of the stiffness of the lung, there is a high recoil and the FEV_1/FVC ratio may be normal or even greater than normal. For example, a patient with a restrictive condition might have an FVC of 3.0 liters, but the FEV_1 might be as high as 2.7 liters, giving an FEV_1/FVC ratio of 90%. The patient exhales the air rapidly in the first second.

Clinicians should also consider measuring the 1-antitrypsin level particularly in those with early onset COPD; those with a family history of 1-antitrypsin deficiency; and those with emphysema, bronchiectasis, and liver disease.

 CLINICAL CONCEPT

Expiratory airflow limitation, demonstrated by a low FEV_1, is the hallmark of COPD.

Classification of COPD

Once the diagnosis of COPD is established, the PFT results can be used to categorize the severity of pulmonary impairment. The forced expiratory volume in 1 second (FEV_1) is the major criterion for classifying the severity of COPD. There are four classifications including mild, moderate, severe, and very severe COPD established by the 2022 **Global Initiative for Chronic Obstructive Lung Disease (GOLD)** (see Table 21-1).

The 2022 GOLD further categorizes COPD into an ABCD classification of four groups based on symptom severity, exacerbation history, and MRC and CAT scores (see Box 21-5).

Treatment

Treatment of COPD involves beta-2 adrenergic agonist inhalers that stimulate bronchiole smooth muscle, leading to direct bronchodilation and anticholinergic (also called antimuscarinic) inhaler agents that counteract bronchoconstriction. Inhaled beta-2 adrenergic bronchodilators are either SABAs or LABAs. LAMAs can be used instead of LABAs or added to the LABA-ICS regimen (see Box 21-5). Similar to asthma, a combination inhaler that contains a LABA and ICS is commonly prescribed for daily maintenance treatment.

The GOLD recommendations for COPD treatment are based on the classification of patients into groups of A, B, C, D according to MRC and CAT scores and patient symptoms. They include indications for LABA, LAMA, and ICS (see Box 21-5).

Phosphodiesterase inhibitors, such as theophylline, can be added to the regimen, particularly in patients with chronic bronchitis. These oral agents can enhance bronchodilation in patients on LABA/ICS combination inhalers. Oral corticosteroids may be used when the patient has an acute exacerbation and does not respond adequately to bronchodilators. The patient needs to use oral corticosteroids in low doses for a short time and be weaned off them slowly.

Antibiotics such as erythromycin or azithromycin can be added to the treatment regimen when patients have exacerbations. Mucolytics such as erdosteine or carbocysteine can decrease viscosity of mucus and enhance lung function.

ALERT! Tranquilizers, sedatives, and opiates can depress respiratory drive and cause respiratory failure in patients with severe COPD.

Nonpharmacological interventions include smoking cessation, pneumococcal and influenza vaccines, pulmonary rehabilitation, and oxygen therapy. Pulmonary rehabilitation involves a slowly progressive program of aerobic exercise and endurance training with supervision. Ventilatory muscle training is used with patients who have decreased respiratory muscle strength and debilitating breathlessness. Pulmonary rehabilitation should be used for symptomatic patients who demonstrate an FEV_1 less than 50% of normal on PFTs.

Continuous oxygen therapy is indicated when arterial PO_2 is lower than or equal to 55 mm Hg or the saturation of oxygen in the blood is less than or equal to 88%. Oxygen is also indicated if there is evidence of pulmonary hypertension, cor pulmonale, cognitive impairment caused by hypoxia, or polycythemia and a PO_2 of 56 to 59 mm Hg. Oxygen should be used in the lowest doses that can enhance the patient's oxygenation. Oxygen therapy requires slow upward titration to the level that assists the patient's oxygenation

GOLD level	Classification of COPD	Pulmonary Function Test (PFT) Result
GOLD 1	Mild COPD	FEV_1 >80 % of predicted value
GOLD 2	Moderate COPD	FEV_1 = 50% to 70% of predicted value
GOLD 3	Severe COPD	FEV_1 = 30% to 49% of predicted value
GOLD 4	Very Severe COPD	FEV_1 <30% of predicted value

TABLE 21-1. Classification of COPD According to Global Initiative for Chronic Obstructive Lung Disease (GOLD) (based on postbronchodilator use)

Abbreviations: FEV_1, forced expiratory volume in 1 second.
Adapted from: Global Initiative for Chronic Obstructive Lung Disease. (2022). Global Strategy for the Diagnosis, Management and Prevention of Chronic Obstructive Pulmonary Disease: 2022 Report.

BOX 21-5 Global Initiative for Chronic Obstructive Lung Disease Group Classification System for Treatment Recommendations

	GROUP A	GROUP B	GROUP C	GROUP D
For patients with 2 or more moderate exacerbations or 1 or more hospitalizations			LAMA (mMRC 0-1, CAT <10)	LAMA or LAMA + LABA (highly symptomatic; e.g., CAT >20) or ICS + LABA (if eos ≥ 300) (mMRC ≥ 2, CAT ≥ 10) *Consider roflumilast if FEV₁ <50% predicted and patient has chronic bronchitis *Consider macrolide (in former smokers)
For patients with 1 or 0 moderate exacerbations (no hospitalizations)	Bronchodilator (mMRC 0-1, CAT <10)	Long-acting bronchodilator (LABA or LAMA) (mMRC ≥ 2, CAT ≥ 10)		

In Group D row, the roflumilast note references $FEV_1 < 50\%$ predicted.

Adapted from: Global Initiative for Chronic Obstructive Lung Disease (2022), https://goldcopd.org/2022-gold-reports-2/

while still maintaining the patient's independent respiratory drive.

> **ALERT!** When oxygen is administered to a patient with severe COPD, the lowest dose of oxygen that relieves the patient is recommended. It is important to recognize that the patient's stimulus to breathe is hypoxia, and high oxygen levels can decrease the patient's independent drive to breathe. Oxygen administration higher than 2 liters per minute will decrease or interrupt the stimulus for breathing and can result in respiratory arrest.

Mechanical ventilator support via an endotracheal tube is indicated for patients with severe respiratory distress unrelieved by other therapies, life-threatening hypoxemia, severe hypercapnia, respiratory acidosis, or respiratory arrest. There is a 17% to 30% mortality rate for patients with COPD requiring mechanical ventilatory support. For patients older than 65 years who require critical care for COPD, the mortality rate doubles to 60%, regardless of the need for mechanical ventilation.

There are a number of pulmonary nonsurgical and surgical treatments that can be used to improve lung function in patients with COPD that show large emphysematous changes. These are referred to as **lung volume reduction procedures**. Endoscopic lung reduction procedures are completed via a bronchoscope and anesthesia. These include insertion of endobronchial coils or valves. In endobronchial coil treatment, under fluoroscopic guidance, nitinol coils are inserted that can enhance the flexibility of bronchioles. In endobronchial valve treatment, removable, one-way valves are inserted that reduce lung hyperinflation by allowing trapped air to escape. Bronchoscopic thermal vapor ablation is another procedure that can eliminate hyperinflated areas in the patient with emphysematous changes. A catheter is inserted into the lungs to occlude the target area using heated water vapor.

Lung volume reduction surgery (LVRS), also called pneumoplasty or bilateral pneumectomy, is indicated in severe emphysema when nonsurgical therapies are limited in effectiveness. The goals of LVRS are to remove the most severely diseased areas of emphysematous lung and decrease the degree of lung hyperinflation. The procedure removes the severely damaged alveoli that act as dead spaces that do not allow diffusion of oxygen into the circulation. A thoracic surgeon removes small wedges of damaged lung tissue, usually about 20% to 30% of each lung, to allow the remaining tissue to function better.

Bronchiectasis

Bronchiectasis is a disease caused by untreated infections, immune dysregulation, and ciliary dyskinesia that lead to chronic inflammation and dilation of bronchi. The relationship between asthma, COPD, and bronchiectasis is unclear. Bronchiectasis can be seen in the setting of both asthma and COPD and has been associated with more advanced stages of these diseases. Conversely, as bronchiectasis progresses, increasing degrees of chronic airway obstruction can be seen and labeled as COPD. Some patients with bronchiectasis may have features of asthma such as eosinophilia, elevated IgE, and at least partially reversible airway obstruction.

The diagnosis of bronchiectasis is increasing worldwide. Previously classified as a rare or orphan disease, bronchiectasis has now been reported at rates up to 566 per 100,000 population with a prevalence that has increased 40% in the past 10 years.

Chronic infections that lead to bronchiectasis are frequently caused by *Bordetella pertussis, Pseudomonas aeruginosa, Haemophilus influenzae, Staphylococcus aureus,* TB, *Mycobacterium avium,* and *Klebsiella.* Adenovirus, measles, and influenza virus are the main viruses that cause bronchiectasis. *Aspergillus* fungal organisms that cause allergic bronchopulmonary aspergillosis can also lead to the disorder. Cystic fibrosis is the most common congenital cause of bronchiectasis.

In bronchiectasis, the structural components of the bronchiole wall, including cartilage, muscle, and elastic tissue, are destroyed and replaced by fibrous tissue. Because of multiple infections over time, the bronchioles become irreversibly dilated. The permanently dilated airways commonly contain static, thick, purulent secretions, and the peripheral airways are often obstructed or obliterated by secretions and replaced by fibrous tissue.

Patients typically present with persistent or recurrent cough and purulent sputum production. Hemoptysis caused by bleeding from inflamed airway mucosa occurs in 50% to 70% of patients. Dyspnea or wheezing indicates widespread bronchiectasis or underlying COPD. Chest x-ray may not reveal significant changes to diagnose bronchiectasis. Bronchography, which involves coating the airways with a radiopaque dye through a bronchoscope, can provide visualization of the dilated airways. A CT scan can also provide a view of the dilated airways. Examination of sputum reveals a high number of neutrophils and the infectious agent. Bronchoscopy may be necessary to investigate endobronchial obstruction and rule out neoplasm. PFTs demonstrate airflow obstruction similar to COPD and hyperreactive airways. A slow, prolonged FEV_1 and decreased FEV_1/FVC ratio are common findings.

Treatment involves elimination of the underlying problem such as infection. The choice of antibiotic should be guided by clinical severity, airway microorganisms and their antibiotic susceptibility (obtained from sputum or bronchoscopy samples), prior antibiotic response, and allergies and drug interactions. Inhaled antibiotics (e.g., gentamicin, tobramycin, colistin, ciprofloxacin) may be used in selected patients with bacterial colonization and recurrent exacerbations. Inhaled antibiotics have the ability to deliver a high concentration of drug to the airway while markedly reducing systemic absorption and toxicity. Studies also show that long-term use of oral macrolide antibiotics in selected patients can reduce exacerbation frequency.

The routine use of long-term inhaled corticosteroids and/or long-acting bronchodilators should be avoided unless concomitant chronic obstructive pulmonary disease or asthma exists. Mucolytic agents can decrease viscosity of mucus. Nebulized agents including hypertonic saline and mannitol enhance mucociliary clearance. Smokers should be supported to quit. All patients should receive influenza and pneumococcal vaccination. Patients with impaired exercise capacity should receive pulmonary rehabilitation.

Sleep-Disordered Breathing

Sleep-disordered breathing (SDB) comprises three types of disorders: obstructive sleep apnea (OSA), central sleep apnea (CSA), or a combination of the two. Apnea is defined as a reduction in airflow by 90% for at least 10 seconds. U.S. data show that SDB is present in 20% of the adult population aged 30 to 70 years and approximately one-third of those aged between 50 and 70 years. SDB can be due to upper airway obstruction caused by intermittent collapse of the upper airway tissues, called OSA. Alternatively, SDB can be caused by an episodic loss of respiratory drive that originates in the brainstem, called CSA. In both of these disorders, the patient endures sleep disturbances, daytime sleepiness, hypoxemia, reduced immunity, depression, and hemodynamic changes that increase cardiovascular disease. OSA has a clearly defined etiology, whereas the cause of CSA is less evident and under study.

In OSA, the upper airway closes repeatedly during sleep. Symptoms include loud snoring, choking or gasping during sleep, and unrestful sleep. Basic factors, such as airway anatomy (e.g., large tonsils), nasal blockage, presence and distribution of body fat, and muscle tone, contribute to the severity of this disorder. Obesity is the most common risk factor. A specific form of OSA, Pickwickian syndrome, is caused by a short, thick neck circumference. OSA is worsened by the use of alcohol and sedative-hypnotic medications.

Severe OSA increases the risk of arrhythmias including atrial fibrillation, influences risk management in stroke, and is highly prevalent in patients with type 2 diabetes. Patients with coronary artery disease also have a high prevalence of SDB, which is independently associated with worse outcomes. Of those patients referred for coronary artery bypass surgery, 87% have OSA. There is a strong bidirectional relationship between OSA and arterial hypertension, with about 30% to 40% of patients with arterial hypertension having clinically relevant OSA and approximately half of all patients with OSA having hypertension. The prevalence of OSA is as high as 80% in patients with severe drug-resistant hypertension, and the prevalence of arterial hypertension increases as OSA severity increases. In heart failure, both heart failure with preserved ejection fraction and heart failure with reduced ejection fraction, 75% of patients are found to have OSA and tend to have worse prognosis. Sleep apnea is highly prevalent in patients with atrial fibrillation. More than 50% of patients with paroxysmal or persistent artial fibrillation have been shown to have clinically relevant SDB. The coexistence of COPD and OSA (termed overlap syndrome) is relatively common in patients with either disease (3% to 66%).

Diagnosis of OSA requires a sleep study, also called polysomnography. Patients are clinically observed overnight in a sleep laboratory and have various body functions measured. Home sleep apnea tests are also available. The presence and severity of OSA are measured by the apnea-hypopnea index (AHI), defined as the number of apnea episodes plus hypopnea episodes per hour of sleep (or hour of recording for home tests). Hypopnea is defined as at least a 4% decline in blood oxygen saturation. The Epworth Sleepiness Scale is a commonly used questionnaire to assess self-reported daytime sleepiness.

Treatment includes behavioral changes such as abstinence from alcohol, smoking cessation, avoidance of the use of sedatives, weight loss, and continuous positive airway pressure (CPAP). Nasal CPAP prevents the airways from closing by delivering air through a mask that forces the air through the nasal passages. CPAP should be used for the entire sleep duration every night. Supplemental oxygen is not recommended for individuals with OSA because it may prolong respiratory pauses and worsen hypercapnia. Other treatment modalities include mandibular repositioning devices or upper airway hypoglossal nerve stimulation therapy. Mandibular repositioning devices consist of plates made to fit the upper and lower teeth. Hypoglossal nerve stimulation is a surgical procedure that increases pharyngeal dilator muscle tone during sleep. It involves unilateral placement of an electrode on a branch of the hypoglossal nerve to enhance tongue protrusion. A pressure sensor is placed between internal and external intercostal muscles to detect inspiratory effort. A small neurostimulator is implanted in the chest wall that triggers the hypoglossal electrode in response to respiratory effort. Surgery may be done to increase the size of the pharyngeal opening and upper airway. The most extensively studied procedure is uvulopalatopharyngoplasty, which involves resection of the uvula and part of the soft palate.

Pathophysiology of Selected Restrictive Disorders

Restrictive pulmonary diseases are those that prevent complete ventilation, diminish total lung capacity, and impede the opening of all the alveoli. Pneumothorax and pleural effusion are the most common causes of restrictive respiratory diseases. Lung diseases that damage the lung tissue directly, such as pulmonary

fibrosis and environmental lung disorders, can also cause restrictive disease, as can musculoskeletal disorders that cause structural alterations of the thoracic cage. Vertebral abnormalities such as kyphosis and scoliosis can restrict pulmonary function. Immunological-mediated disorders, such as sarcoidosis, cause restrictive lung disease. Neurological disorders such as muscular dystrophy, myasthenia gravis, and Guillain–Barré syndrome, all of which can impair full thoracic cage expansion, can also cause a restrictive pulmonary disorder.

Pneumothorax

A **pneumothorax**, also known as a collapsed lung, is the presence of air in the pleural cavity that causes collapse of a large section or whole lobe of lung tissue (see Fig. 21-9). Air can enter the pleural cavity because of chest trauma or rupture of alveoli. There are five types of pneumothorax:

1. Primary spontaneous pneumothorax (PSP)
2. Secondary spontaneous pneumothorax (SSP)
3. Traumatic pneumothorax
4. Tension pneumothorax
5. Iatrogenic pneumothorax

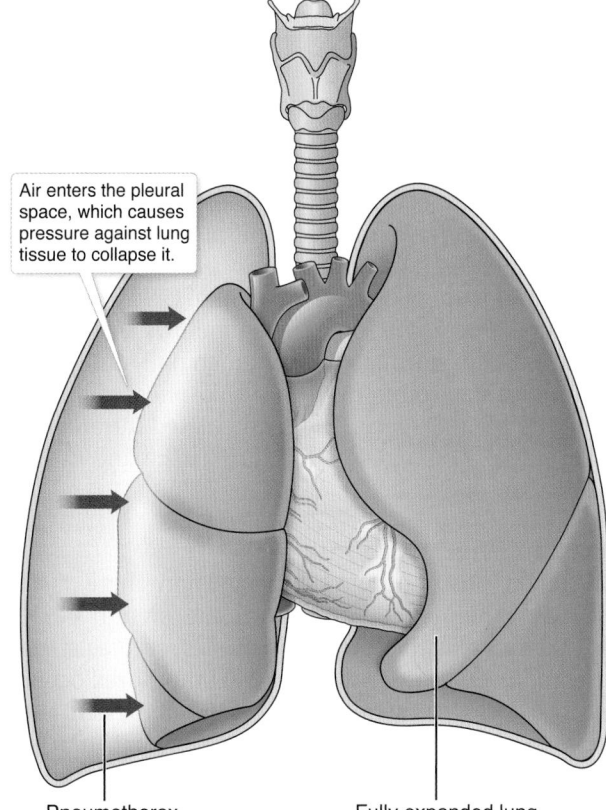

Air enters the pleural space, which causes pressure against lung tissue to collapse it.

Pneumothorax   Fully expanded lung

FIGURE 21-9. Pneumothorax is a collection of air in the pleural space that causes part or all of a lung to collapse. Normally, the pleural space is a vacuum with no air or fluid. The pressure in the lungs is greater than the pressure in the pleural space. However, if air enters the pleural space, the air presses against the lung tissue, causing the lung to collapse partially or completely. Pneumothorax can be either spontaneous or caused by trauma.

Primary Spontaneous Pneumothorax

PSP occurs in people without underlying lung disease and in the absence of an inciting event. Air is present in the intrapleural space without preceding trauma and without underlying clinical or radiological evidence of lung disease. The incidence of PSP is 7.4 to 18 cases per 100,000 persons per year for men and 1.2 to 6 cases per 100,000 persons per year for women. It is more common in tall young males between the ages of 10 and 30 years old; it is rarely seen in people older than 40 years. The etiology is unclear, but ruptured alveoli are theorized to be the cause. Some individuals who suffer PSP have a genetic predisposition. For example, PSP frequently occurs in persons with the genetic disorder Marfan syndrome. Cigarette smokers also have an increased risk of PSP.

Secondary Spontaneous Pneumothorax

SSP occurs in people with a wide variety of lung diseases. In SSP, an underlying pathological process occurs in the lung. Air enters the pleural space via ruptured blebs, which are overly distended and damaged alveoli. Patients with long-term emphysema often suffer SSP caused by ruptured alveoli. Other diseases that may be present when SSPs occur include TB, sarcoidosis, cystic fibrosis, malignancy, and idiopathic pulmonary fibrosis (IPF). *P. jirovecii* pneumonia is a common cause of SSP in patients with AIDS.

Traumatic Pneumothorax

A traumatic pneumothorax is commonly caused by a penetrating wound of the thoracic cage and underlying pleural membrane. Commonly, a thoracic injury causes a rib fracture that punctures the pleural membrane. The punctured thoracic cage and pleural membrane create an opening between the pleural cavity and outside atmosphere. The open wound allows the pleural cavity, which is normally a vacuum, to pull air into the opening of the wound from the atmosphere and build up in the pleural space. The accumulated intrapleural air eventually compresses the lung tissue and causes lung collapse.

Tension Pneumothorax

A tension pneumothorax occurs when there is an escalating buildup of air within the pleural cavity that compresses the lung, bronchioles, cardiac structures, and vena cava. A tension pneumothorax occurs because a closed, penetrating wound allows air into the pleural cavity but will not allow air out. Increasing air accumulation causes a rapid rise in intrathoracic pressure, which inhibits venous return and optimal function of the heart and lungs. This is a life-threatening disorder.

Iatrogenic Pneumothorax

Iatrogenic pneumothorax is a complication of medical or surgical procedures. It most commonly results from transthoracic needle aspiration but can be caused by therapeutic thoracentesis, pleural biopsy, central venous catheter insertion, transbronchial biopsy, positive pressure mechanical ventilation, and inadvertent intubation of the right mainstem bronchus. Therapeutic thoracentesis is complicated by pneumothorax 30% of the time when performed by inexperienced clinicians, in contrast to only 4% of the time when performed by experienced clinicians.

Clinical Presentation

The clinical signs and symptoms of a pneumothorax include chest pain, dyspnea, and increased respiratory rate. On inspection, there may be an obvious asymmetry of the chest, as well as intercostal muscle retractions. Percussion may reveal chest hyperresonance, whereas auscultation may reveal a lack of breath sounds on the affected side.

Diagnosis

Chest radiography, ultrasonography, or CT can be used for diagnosis, although diagnosis from a chest x-ray is most common. Radiographic findings of 2.5 cm air space are equivalent to a 30% pneumothorax. On chest x-ray, a linear shadow of visceral pleura with lack of lung markings peripheral to the shadow may be observed, indicating a collapsed lung (see Fig. 21-10). A mediastinal shift toward the contralateral, undamaged lung may be apparent. Pulse oximetry and ABG analysis demonstrate hypoxemia; ABG analysis can also show varying degrees of acidosis and hypercapnia, the occurrence of which depends on the extent of cardiopulmonary compromise at the time of collection.

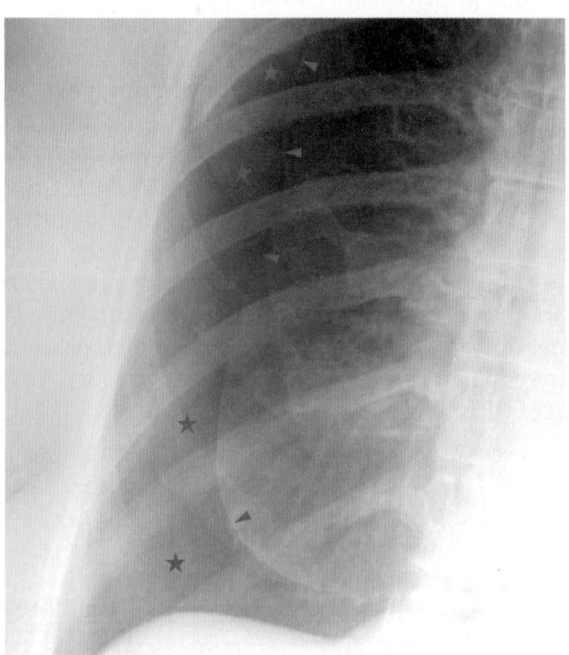

FIGURE 21-10. Chest x-ray showing pneumothorax. Stars indicate lack of lung tissue due to air in the pleural space; arrows indicate the border of the collapsed lung. *(From Weber, E. C. [2013]. Practical radiology. Philadelphia: F.A. Davis Company, with permission.)*

Treatment

If a patient is hemodynamically unstable with suspected tension pneumothorax, intervention is not withheld to await imaging. Needle decompression can be performed emergently. In secondary spontaneous pneumothorax, if size/depth of pneumothorax is less than 1 cm and there is no dyspnea, then the patient is admitted and high-flow oxygen is given, and the patient is observed for 24 hours. Air can reabsorb from the pleural space at a rate of 1.5%/day. Using supplemental oxygen can increase this reabsorption rate.

Treatment of an open traumatic pneumothorax requires a chest tube with suction on the affected side and supplemental oxygen. The chest tube apparatus pulls the air out of the pleural cavity and allows the collapsed lung to reexpand.

In some cases of spontaneous pneumothorax, a procedure called pleurodesis is performed to prevent recurrence. Pleurodesis intentionally causes chemical or surgical irritation of the layers of the pleural membrane. The irritation causes the visceral and parietal pleural membrane layers to adhere to each other and close off the pleural space. Those who are susceptible to a spontaneous pneumothorax should be cautioned to avoid cigarette smoking, high altitudes, unpressurized aircraft, and scuba diving.

Pleural Effusion

A **pleural effusion** is an abnormal collection of fluid within the pleural cavity that compresses lung tissue and inhibits lung inflation (see Fig. 21-11). It is commonly edematous fluid that accumulates within the pleural space because of heart failure, severe pulmonary infection, or neoplasm. The fluid may be an exudate or transudate, purulent, lymph, or sanguineous (bloody). **Pleuritis** (also called **pleurisy**) is inflammation of the pleural membrane. This condition is common in infections that extend to the pleura.

Epidemiology

The estimated incidence of pleural effusion is 1.5 million cases per year, with most effusions caused by heart failure, malignancy, infections, and pulmonary emboli.

Etiology

Transudates are filtrates of the blood that accumulate within the pleural space because of an imbalance in the capillary forces: hydrostatic and oncotic pressure. Elevated hydrostatic pressure causes fluid to leak out of capillaries into the pleural space. Major etiologies of transudates are listed in Box 21-6.

In contrast, exudates are mainly caused by pleural or lung inflammation or infection. Less commonly, exudates come from impaired lymphatic drainage of the pleural space or from extension of inflammatory fluid from the peritoneal space. Common causes of exudates are listed in Box 21-7.

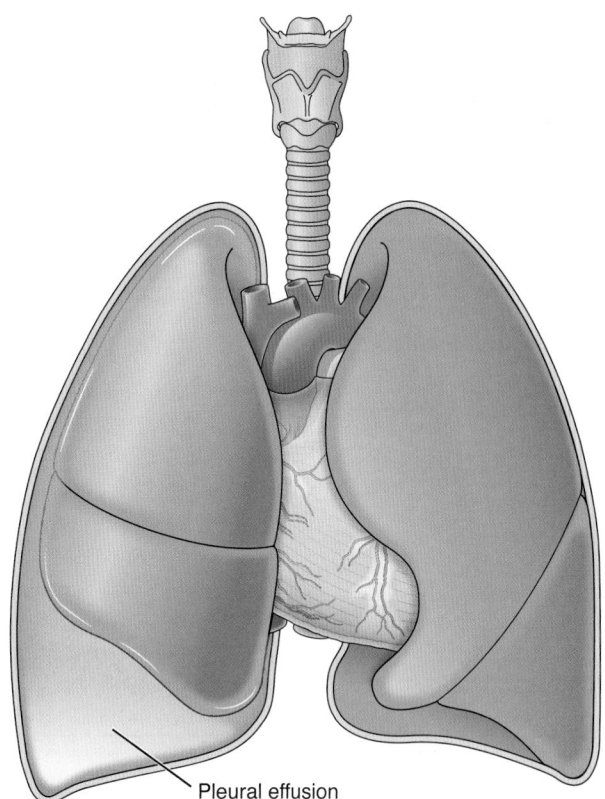

FIGURE 21-11. Pleural effusion is an accumulation of fluid within the pleural space. A pleural effusion presses against the lung tissue, inhibiting the lung's full expansion. The midline of the chest cavity deviates to the side opposite of the pleural effusion.

Pathophysiology

The pleural space normally contains approximately 1 mL of fluid that lubricates the visceral and parietal pleural membranes. The pleural cavity should be free of any additional fluid or air. Pleural effusions result from disruption of the balance between hydrostatic and oncotic forces in the lung tissue. When hydrostatic pressure in the lung tissue greatly exceeds oncotic pressure, fluid leaks out of the pulmonary

---

BOX 21-6. Transudative Pleural Effusion Etiologies

A transudate is a filtrate of the bloodstream that is noninfectious, clear, and low in protein content. Transudates develop because of high hydrostatic pressure within the capillaries and consequent fluid accumulation in the involved tissues. Etiologies include:

- Atelectasis
- Cirrhosis
- Congestive heart failure
- Constrictive pericarditis
- Hypoalbuminemia
- Myxedema
- Nephrotic syndrome
- Peritoneal dialysis

BOX 21-7. Exudative Pleural Effusion Etiologies

An exudate is a cloudy, edematous fluid with high protein content. It is most commonly caused by an infectious, immunological, or inflammatory process. Etiologies include:

- Asbestos exposure
- Chylothorax
- Collagen-vascular conditions
- Drug use
- Esophageal perforation
- Malignancy
- Meigs syndrome
- Pancreatitis
- Parapneumonic causes
- Postcardiac injury syndrome
- Radiation pleuritis
- Sarcoidosis
- Trauma
- Tuberculosis

capillaries and cells into the pleural space, causing a pleural effusion.

Clinical Presentation

The most common signs of a pleural effusion are dyspnea, tachypnea, sharp pleuritic chest pain, dullness to percussion, and diminished breath sounds on the affected side. Percussion over the area demonstrates a flat, dull sound that indicates fluid blocking the normally resonant lung tissue. Tactile fremitus is decreased over a pleural effusion.

Diagnosis

Chest x-ray, CT scan, and ultrasound can all detect the presence of a pleural effusion. With large pleural effusions, mediastinal structures are pushed away from the side of the pleural effusion. Alternatively, if mediastinal structures are pushed toward the side of the effusion, it may indicate an obstruction within the bronchus caused by malignancy or, less commonly, a foreign body.

Thoracentesis should be performed to relieve pressure on the lungs and provide fluid for analysis. Laboratory testing helps distinguish pleural fluid transudates from exudates. The fluid is analyzed for blood, glucose, infectious material, WBCs, tumor markers, and other constituents that assist in the diagnosis.

CT angiography should be ordered if pulmonary embolism (PE) is suspected. If TB or a malignancy is suspected, biopsy of the lesion is necessary. Bronchoscopy is necessary if a lesion is suspected within a bronchiole. Thoracoscopy and thoracotomy are other diagnostic procedures that can allow biopsy of the pleural membrane.

Treatment

Treatment is aimed at the cause of the pleural effusion. Suction and drainage of a pleural effusion are usually necessary. Surgical intervention is most often required for effusions that cannot be drained adequately by needle or small-bore catheters.

Environmental Lung Disorders

Environmental lung diseases, known as pneumoconioses, result from occupational exposure to specific airborne agents or particulate air pollution. The most dangerous particles are those that reach the terminal small airways. Normally, inhaled particulate matter is phagocytosed by pulmonary macrophages. However, in pneumoconioses, macrophages are overwhelmed by a large quantity of dust or particles deposited because of environmental exposures. Also, large particles may resist dissolution by macrophages and persist within the lung tissue. Some of the most common environmental exposures are coal worker's pneumoconiosis, asbestosis, and silicosis.

Coal Worker's Pneumoconiosis

In coal worker's pneumoconiosis, also called anthracosis, the findings in the lung depend on the amount of exposure to coal dust. The disorder ranges from asymptomatic with little pulmonary dysfunction to complicated pneumoconiosis with progressive massive pulmonary fibrosis.

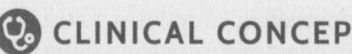

CLINICAL CONCEPT

Coal worker's pneumoconiosis is not limited to coal workers, as it is also present in the lungs of urban dwellers because of air pollution.

Coal worker's pneumoconiosis is characterized by coal particles of 1 to 2 mm in diameter and larger coal nodules in the lungs. Coal dust that enters the lungs can neither be destroyed nor removed by the body. The particles are engulfed by alveolar macrophages and remain in the lungs, residing in the connective tissue or pulmonary lymph nodes. Macrophages release various products, including enzymes, cytokines, free radicals, and fibroblast growth factors, that cause inflammation and fibrosis. These lesions are scattered throughout the lung fields and develop over the course of many years. Autopsy will show intensely blackened lung tissue consisting of coal dust and collagen with necrotic centers.

The patient exhibits cough with gray sputum, wheezes, and dyspnea on exertion. Diagnosis involves chest x-ray, CT scan, sputum culture, and PFTs. Chest x-ray and CT scan demonstrate round, dark opacities throughout the lungs. PFTs demonstrate hypoxemia, decreased FEV, and decreased TLC as in obstructive disease. Treatment involves an occupational change that limits contact with coal dust, if possible, as well as oxygen, bronchodilators, and pneumococcal and influenza vaccine. Smoking cessation is critical.

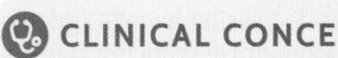

CLINICAL CONCEPT

Coal worker's pneumoconiosis can be considered both a fibrotic and obstructive lung disorder because it is associated with chronic bronchitis and emphysema.

Asbestosis

Asbestos is a mineral crystal that was previously used extensively in industries such as welding, construction, shipbuilding, and mining. It is largely recognized as a carcinogen, and specific types of full-face respirator masks are required of workers who are exposed to asbestos. Asbestos causes pulmonary fibrosis that is related to the intensity and duration of exposure. This restrictive disease causes a decrease in all lung volumes. Asbestos exposure also increases susceptibility to lung cancer, particularly in smokers, with squamous cell carcinoma and adenocarcinoma being the most frequent types of cancer associated with asbestos. Mesothelioma, a type of tumor specifically associated with asbestos, is often present within the pleural membrane, but can also metastasize.

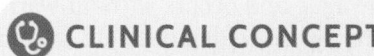

CLINICAL CONCEPT

Cancers related to asbestos can develop decades after exposure.

Silicosis

Silica is a quartz crystal that, if inhaled, can cause pulmonary fibrosis. The major occupational exposures occur in mining; stonecutting; industries using abrasives such as stone, clay, glass, and cement; packing of silica flour; and quarrying, particularly of granite. The disease can occur after as little as 2 years of exposure to silica. Silicosis increases susceptibility to TB, and all patients exposed to silica should receive a Mantoux test. Talc dust, a type of silica, can also cause pulmonary fibrosis. Pleural and lung cancer have also been associated with exposure to talc dust.

Thoracic Cage Deformity

Thoracic cage deformity is a deviation in the vertebral column related to either structural changes or postural defects. The term *kyphoscoliosis* is used to describe the combination of a curve of the cervical spine (kyphosis) and twisting of the thoracic vertebral column (scoliosis).

A thoracic cage deformity such as kyphoscoliosis causes restrictive lung disease. The deformity causes rigidity of the chest wall and limited chest expansion that results in breathing difficulty, breathlessness on exertion, and hypoventilation. The ventilation of the lungs is diminished because of the distorted thoracic cage.

Clinical manifestations of kyphoscoliosis include a noticeable deformity, with one shoulder or hip higher than the other and hunched posture. Diagnosis is made by a physical examination and confirmed by x-rays, CT scan, or MRI. With advancing age, the chest wall stiffens and degenerative changes in ligaments and joints aggravate the spinal deformity. Decreased ventilation leads to carbon dioxide retention and hypoxemia. Chronic hypoxia leads to pulmonary hypertension and right ventricular failure. Treatment of a thoracic cage deformity requires an orthopedic brace or surgical intervention. Early correction of spinal deformity can reverse the decreased lung capacity.

Idiopathic Pulmonary Fibrosis

IPF is a restrictive lung disease caused by repeated injury of lung tissue by an unidentified agent. The alveoli undergo repeated episodes of inflammation, also called alveolitis, that eventually involve fibroblastic proliferation and fibrotic changes. In IPF, an exaggerated fibrotic response occurs with consequent stiffening of lung tissue. According to recent findings, p53 is believed to play a pivotal role in the development and progression of pulmonary fibrosis. The p53 gene is an important tumor suppressor gene, located on human chromosome 17p13.1. Studies show that excessive alveolar epithelial cell apoptosis occurs during the development and progression of pulmonary fibrosis. Lung fibroblasts in IPF have shortened telomeres, which indicate aging of these cells, and tissue shows excessive oxidative stress.

Patients with IPF present with dyspnea, tachypnea, crackles, and eventual cyanosis. Currently, the diagnosis and assessment of pulmonary fibrosis rely mainly on a comprehensive analysis of the patient's medical history, clinical manifestations, chest x-ray, high-resolution computed tomography (HRCT), and pulmonary function tests, as well as bronchoscopy or lung biopsy if necessary. The chest x-ray reveals a pattern of diffuse markings called a "ground glass" appearance in the lower lung fields. Later in the disease, nodules and a honeycomb lung pattern can be observed. Erythrocyte sedimentation rate is usually elevated, indicating inflammation. PFTs demonstrate restrictive lung disease changes, including reduced vital capacity, residual volume, increased FEV_1, and decreased compliance. Evidence of airway obstruction is minimal. Hypoxemia is present, but PCO_2 is usually normal. Bronchoscopy is performed to obtain lung tissue biopsies and confirm the diagnosis. Collagen vascular disease, such as sarcoidosis and pneumoconiosis, must be ruled out because these diseases often have a similar presentation.

Treatment for IPF aims to reduce inflammatory and fibrotic changes in the lungs. Oxygen, bronchodilators, and corticosteroids are used to counteract bronchospasm and inflammation. Pulmonary vasodilators counteract pulmonary hypertension. Treatment of right ventricular failure with diuretics may be necessary. Many treatments tend to fail, and lung transplantation is commonly necessary.

Hypersensitivity Pneumonitis

Hypersensitivity pneumonitis is an immunologically mediated lung disorder caused by prolonged, intense exposure to inhaled organic dusts that act as antigens. Commonly, the organic dusts are made of bacterial spores, fungi, or animal proteins. Affected persons have an abnormally heightened sensitivity to the antigen that causes alveolar inflammation.

Signs and symptoms include acute attacks of dyspnea, cough, fever, and an elevated WBC count. Symptoms appear 4 to 6 hours after exposure, and prolonged exposure can lead to pulmonary fibrosis. PFTs demonstrate restrictive disease, and chest x-rays show nodular infiltrates. Farmer's lung, pigeon-breeder's lung, and air conditioner lung are specific forms of hypersensitivity pneumonitis. Corticosteroids are standard treatment for severely ill patients with all varieties of hypersensitivity pneumonitis.

Pathophysiology of Selected Pulmonary Vascular Disorders

Pulmonary edema, PE, and pulmonary hypertension are disorders caused by a vascular problem in the lungs. Pulmonary edema is the manifestation of heart failure. PE is most commonly caused by venous thrombosis of the lower extremities. Chronic hypoxia stimulates pulmonary hypertension.

Pulmonary Edema

Pulmonary edema is the accumulation of fluid around the alveoli that inhibits oxygen transfer at the alveolar–capillary interface. It occurs when there is an increase in hydrostatic pressure in the capillary bed of the lungs. The most common cause of pulmonary edema is left ventricular heart failure (LVF). In LVF, the weakened left ventricle cannot eject all the blood within the chamber, causing blood to accumulate in the left ventricle. As a result, hydrostatic pressure builds backward into the left atrium, pulmonary veins, and, eventually, the pulmonary capillaries. The high hydrostatic pressure within the pulmonary capillaries causes fluid from the blood to diffuse into the interstitial tissues.

The main symptom of pulmonary edema is severe respiratory distress. The patient exhibits extreme shortness of breath, which may be accompanied by pink, frothy sputum. As pulmonary edema worsens, the lack of oxygen to the brain causes confusion and stupor. Coarse, loud crackles are heard on auscultation. Diagnosis is made by clinical presentation, and a chest x-ray demonstrates congested pulmonary vasculature and infiltrates.

Treatment is aimed at decreasing hydrostatic pressure in the pulmonary capillaries, reducing the fluid in the pulmonary interstitium, and increasing oxygen content in the blood. Diuretic medications, oxygen administration, digitalis, and ACE inhibitors are prescribed. Diuretics enhance water loss from the bloodstream and thereby lessen edema in the lungs. Digitalis is used to enhance left ventricular function. ACE inhibitors can reduce the constant cycling of the renin–angiotensin–aldosterone system (RAAS) that occurs in left ventricular failure.

Pulmonary Embolism

A PE is a clot that has traveled to the pulmonary arterial circulation and caused obstruction of arterial blood flow through the lungs. Usually, the embolism has originated in the venous circulation as a deep vein thrombus in the leg or in the right side of the heart as an atrial thrombus. The most common precursor to PE is deep venous thromboembolism (DVT) (see Chapter 19). Thrombi also often form around central venous catheters and travel to the right side of the heart into the pulmonary artery, causing a PE.

PE is a leading cause of death because the clinical presentation is often vague and occurs without warning. The patient with PE may demonstrate cough, dyspnea, and chest pain. However, most cases are diagnosed at autopsy because the patient did not demonstrate symptoms. Diagnostic tests include a D-dimer test and CT pulmonary angiography. The D-dimer test measures the amount of fibrin degradation products in the blood. If the D-dimer test is normal, there is little chance that the patient is enduring a PE.

Direct oral anticoagulants (DOACs) (e.g., rivaroxaban, apixaban) are first-line treatment options for venous thromboembolism. DOACs are preferred over the vitamin K antagonist warfarin because they are associated with a lower risk of bleeding than warfarin and do not require frequent laboratory testing. Thrombolytic agents (e.g., tissue plasminogen activator [tPA]) are used if PE is associated with hemodynamic instability. Anticoagulant treatment should be continued for at least 3 months to prevent early recurrences. Surgical implantation of an inferior vena cava filter may be necessary with multiple PE formation.

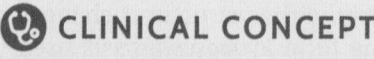 **CLINICAL CONCEPT**

At autopsy, 60% of hospitalized patients demonstrate existence of a PE, with 70% of these cases undiagnosed.

Pulmonary Hypertension

Pulmonary hypertension is abnormally high pressure within the pulmonary arteries. Normal pulmonary artery pressure is approximately 25 mm Hg. Pulmonary hypertension is present when pulmonary arterial pressure is greater than 25 mm Hg at rest or 30 mm Hg with exercise.

Etiology

There are two types of pulmonary hypertension. Primary pulmonary hypertension is a genetic disorder caused by abnormal structure of the pulmonary blood vessels. Secondary pulmonary hypertension is an increase in pulmonary artery pressure as a result of elevated pulmonary venous pressure, increased pulmonary blood flow, pulmonary vascular obstruction, or hypoxemia. COPD, collagen vascular disease, and recurrent pulmonary thromboemboli may be causes of secondary pulmonary hypertension.

Chronic hypoxia is a common cause of pulmonary hypertension because the lung response to decreased ventilation or hypoxia is pulmonary arterial vasoconstriction. Pulmonary arterial vasoconstriction causes increased pulmonary vascular resistance and increased workload of the right ventricle. Prolonged pulmonary hypertension causes the right ventricle to hypertrophy and fail. Failure of the right side of the heart caused by a pulmonary disorder is known as cor pulmonale.

As pulmonary hypertension progresses, right ventricular failure causes diminished cardiac output. The decreased cardiac output is particularly apparent during exercise. Symptoms include syncope, dyspnea on exertion, and fatigue.

Diagnosis

Pulmonary hypertension is diagnosed through x-rays, echocardiography, and Doppler ultrasonography. A right heart cardiac catheterization is done to obtain pulmonary arterial pressure. Transthoracic echocardiogram is the preferred test for screening for pulmonary hypertension. Complete PFTs should be obtained for any person with pulmonary hypertension. A CT scan of the lungs is also performed on those with abnormal PFTs. Individuals with a history of excessive daytime somnolence or witnessed apneas should be tested with overnight oximetry or polysomnogram to rule out pulmonary hypertension related to SDB.

Treatment

Treatment for pulmonary hypertension focuses on vasodilation of the pulmonary arterial vessels, improving function of the right ventricle, and enhancing oxygenation. Supplemental oxygen and calcium channel blockers may be effective in the early stages of the disease. As pulmonary hypertension worsens, epoprostenol, a pulmonary vasodilator, and bosentan, a vasoconstriction antagonist, are frequently used. Tadalafil, a vasodilator, is also used to decrease pulmonary artery pressure in patients with right-sided heart failure and pulmonary hypertension. Macitentan, an endothelin receptor antagonist, and selexipag, a prostacyclin receptor agonist, are newer agents that are also demonstrating effective results. In a recent investigation called the AMBITION study, the combination of ambrisentan, an endothelial antagonist, with tadalafil showed superior results.

Acute Respiratory Distress Syndrome

Acute respiratory distress syndrome (ARDS) is pulmonary dysfunction characterized by diffuse alveolar injury, pulmonary capillary damage, bilateral pulmonary infiltrates, and severe hypoxemia. It occurs in critically ill patients and is commonly a sequela to trauma, sepsis, drug overdose, massive transfusion, acute pancreatitis, or aspiration. Patients developing ARDS are critically ill, often with multisystem organ failure, and they may not be capable of providing historical information. Typically, the illness develops within 12 to 48 hours after an inciting event, although in rare instances it may take up to a few days. ARDS is responsible for 1 in 10 admissions to intensive care units and 1 in 4 mechanical ventilations. In-hospital mortality for patients with severe ARDS ranges from 46% to 60%.

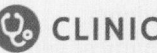

CLINICAL CONCEPT

The most common risk factor for ARDS is sepsis, but multiple other risk factors exist, including direct lung injury, most commonly aspiration of gastric contents; systemic illnesses; and injuries.

One of the characteristics of ARDS is sudden progressive pulmonary edema. An inflammatory trigger initiates the release of cellular and chemical mediators. The mediators damage the alveolar–capillary membrane, and fluid leaks into the alveolar interstitial spaces. Intravascular coagulation in the alveolar capillaries leads to microthrombi. Alveoli collapse, small airways are narrowed, and lung compliance decreases. The lungs lose the ability to ventilate, and perfusion is diminished at the alveolar–capillary level, resulting in severe hypoxemia and hypercapnia. As hypoxemia progresses, there is a decreased level of consciousness, compensatory tachycardia, diminished peripheral circulation, diaphoresis, restlessness, and anxiety. As hypoxemia continues, the alveoli become fibrotic, and lungs become stiff with dead air space. Crackles are a sign of fluid leaking into the pulmonary interstitium. A fibrotic phase that occurs in some patients is characterized by ongoing inflammation, extensive basement membrane damage, persistent edema, intra-alveolar and interstitial fibrosis, and microvascular damage. Progression to the fibrotic phase is associated with prolonged mechanical ventilation and increased mortality.

Diagnosis is based on clinical presentation and diagnostic studies. A defining feature of ARDS is arterial hypoxemia that does not improve with administration of oxygen. The Berlin criteria lists diagnostic conditions that include the following:

- Respiratory symptoms must have begun within 1 week of a known clinical insult, or the patient must have new or worsening symptoms during the past week.
- Bilateral opacities must be present on a chest x-ray or CT scan. These opacities must not be fully explained by pleural effusions, lobar collapse, lung collapse, or pulmonary nodules.
- The patient's respiratory failure must not be fully explained by cardiac failure or fluid overload. An objective assessment (e.g., echocardiography) to exclude hydrostatic pulmonary edema is required if no risk factors for ARDS are present.
- A moderate to severe impairment of oxygenation must be present, as defined by the ratio of arterial oxygen tension to fraction of inspired oxygen (PaO_2/FIO_2). The severity of the hypoxemia defines the severity of the ARDS.

ABG levels demonstrating a PO_2 of 50 mm Hg or less and PCO_2 of 50 mm Hg or above are diagnostic; these values are also consistent with respiratory failure. Chest x-rays demonstrate pulmonary edema.

Supportive treatment includes mechanical ventilation to facilitate oxygenation of tissues. The patient requires sedation and neuromuscular blockade when on mechanical ventilation. Nutritional support via enteral feedings or total parenteral nutrition (TPN) may be needed. Conservative fluid management using a central venous catheter may be necessary. DVT and gastrointestinal ulcer preventive measures are needed. Low molecular weight heparin, low-dose unfractionated heparin, or fondaparinux are recommended to prevent DVT. Intravenous pantoprazole can decrease GI ulcers and gastrointestinal bleeding.

Prone positioning is recommended for patients with moderate or severe ARDS. Prone positioning requires moving a patient from the traditional supine position while maintaining the integrity of the patient-ventilator circuit and all venous, arterial, urinary, and other access lines. When this technique is used, the position should be maintained for at least 12 to 16 hours per day. It is thought to improve ventilation-perfusion matching by recruiting more lung and allowing each inspired breath to be more uniformly distributed over a greater surface. Inhaled nitric oxide is a vasodilator that may be used to improve oxygenation. Inhaled prostacyclin has also shown to improve oxygenation. Intravenous corticosteroids may be used. Extracorporeal membrane oxygenation (ECMO) should be considered. ECMO involves using a venoarterial or venovenous circuit to remove blood from the body, introduce oxygen and remove carbon dioxide, then return the blood to the body. Health-care–associated pneumonia can occur, and patients must be vigilantly monitored for infection.

Patients with ARDS spend an average of 16 days in the ICU and a total of 26 days in the hospital. Patients with an anticipated ventilation requirement of more than 10 days may benefit from tracheostomy. Patients on mechanical ventilation for more than 24 hours require a ventilator weaning protocol with spontaneous breathing trials as they recover.

After discharge from the ICU, patients with ARDS may have a lower quality of life, significant weakness from neuropathy or myopathy, persistent cognitive impairment, and delayed return to work. Mental health challenges after ARDS survival include depression, post-traumatic stress disorder, and anxiety. Not all of the deleterious health effects of ARDS resolve over time. After hospitalization, multidimensional health care (e.g., physical and occupational therapy, rehabilitation and home health care, subspecialists) is used to promote optimal health and function. Although lung function approaches normal at 5 years, 6-minute walking distance, physical function, and quality of life measures often remain decreased.

Chapter Summary

- Pulmonary disorders can be categorized according to the results of a PFT as obstructive or restrictive disease.

- A pneumothorax, also called a collapsed lung, occurs when air enters the pleural space and presses on lung tissue so that it cannot expand. A chest tube inserted to provide suction is the treatment of pneumothorax.

- A pleural effusion occurs when fluid enters the pleural space and hinders lung tissue from fully expanding. An effusion can be a transudate or an exudate. Thoracotomy is the treatment for pleural effusion.

- Major obstructive diseases include asthma and COPD, which are two of the most common diseases worldwide.

- Asthma is a chronic inflammatory disease with acute episodes of bronchospasm.

- T2 helper cells, interleukins, and eosinophils are involved in the pathological mechanism of allergy-induced asthma, which is termed T2 high asthma or T2 asthma.

- Non-T2 asthma is the term used for asthma that does not involve allergies or eosinophils.

- Pulmonary function tests (also called spirometry), particularly the FEV_1 measurement, are used to diagnose asthma and COPD.

- Pulmonary forced exhalation of nitric oxide (FeNO), which is an indicator of airway inflammation, can augment diagnostic accuracy of asthma.

- Asthma and COPD are both bronchospastic and chronic inflammatory diseases. Medication regimens commonly consist of inhalers that contain long-acting beta-2 adrenergic agonists (LABAs), long-acting muscarinic antagonists (LAMAs), and inhaled corticosteroids (ICSs).

- In asthma and COPD, LABAs and ICSs are commonly prescribed for daily maintenance therapy.

- Alternatively, in asthma and COPD, LAMAs, which counteract bronchoconstriction, can be prescribed.

- In asthma and COPD, commonly prescribed combination inhalers contain a LABA or LAMA plus an ICS for daily maintenance therapy use. A LAMA can be added to a LABA/ICS regimen in severe asthma for a triple therapy approach.

- Leukotriene receptor antagonists (LTRAs), mucolytic agents, and immunomodulator therapy can be added to the asthma treatment regimen.

- Each acute attack of asthma remodels the bronchioles to make them more susceptible to acute bronchospasm and inflammation.

- Bronchial thermoplasty, which decreases smooth muscle hypertrophy in the airways, is recommended for persistent asthma that is refractory to medication.

- Persons with asthma due to allergy-induced bronchospasms are recommended to undergo allergy immunotherapy treatment (AIT).

- Status asthmaticus occurs when an asthma attack resists treatment and is potentially fatal.

- COPD is a combination of emphysema, chronic bronchitis, and asthma. Individuals can have COPD that has more features of emphysema or chronic bronchitis.

- Long-term cigarette smoking and exposure to secondhand smoke are primary causes of COPD.

- Smoking history is defined in terms of packs of cigarettes per day multiplied by how many years the patient smoked.

- In emphysema, the alveoli are injured, cannot recoil, and become enlarged because they accumulate excessive carbon dioxide.

- In chronic bronchitis, the bronchioles are edematous and full of mucus, which prevents oxygen from entering the alveoli.

- Individuals with emphysema classically have a high amount of residual air in the lungs, which causes expansion of the thoracic cage called a barrel-shaped chest. Because of this retained air, they have chronic hypercapnia.

- Individuals with chronic bronchitis classically have cyanosis, cough, chronic hypoxia, and susceptibility to right ventricular failure.

- Patients with chronic bronchitis are nicknamed "blue bloaters" because of cyanosis caused by hypoxia and edema caused by their susceptibility to right-sided heart failure.

- Patients with emphysema are nicknamed "pink puffers" because they usually remain oxygenated and "pink" until late in the disease. They are nicknamed "puffers" because they have a characteristic prolonged phase of exhalation during breathing.

- Chronic bronchitis commonly leads to right-sided heart failure (also called cor pulmonale). This is because chronic hypoxia causes pulmonary arterioles to vasoconstrict. This often leads to high pressure within the pulmonary artery, termed pulmonary hypertension. Pulmonary hypertension leads to high resistance against the right ventricle, which leads to right ventricular failure.

- Patients with COPD commonly have a prolonged exhalation phase of breathing. They use pursed-lip breathing to expel their air.

- COPD is characterized by a decreased FEV during the FEV_1. FVC is the total volume of exhaled air expelled from the lungs when the patient uses maximal effort. The diagnosis of COPD is based on the FEV_1:FVC ratio. The condition is diagnosed if the ratio of FEV_1 to FVC is less than 70%.

- In patients with long-term COPD, the respiratory center becomes insensitive to carbon dioxide. The patient's drive to breathe is stimulated by hypoxia.

- High oxygen concentration can shut down the hypoxic drive to breathe for a patient with severe COPD. Sedatives, narcotics, and any drugs that suppress respiratory rate should be used with caution in patients with long-term COPD.

- Mucolytics, macrolide antibiotics, and low-dose prednisone in a tapered regimen can be used in COPD exacerbations.

- SDB is the episodic cessation of breathing during sleep and includes OSA and CSA. OSA is associated with obesity and excess pharyngeal tissue mass that inhibits airflow. OSA is associated with hypertension, arrhythmias, heart failure, diabetes, and stroke.

- Types of treatments available for SDB including CPAP, oral appliance devices, oropharyngeal surgery, and hypoglossal nerve stimulators.

- Most disorders caused by environmental exposures such as asbestosis, silicosis, and hypersensitivity pneumonitis cause restrictive lung disease.

- Coal worker's pneumoconiosis can be considered both a fibrotic and obstructive lung disorder because it is associated with chronic bronchitis and emphysema.

- Asbestosis increases susceptibility to lung cancer decades after initial exposure.

- Restrictive lung disease causes increased FEV_1 because of the compressive forces of the stiffened lung tissue, whereas obstructive lung disease causes decreased FEV_1.

- Collagen vascular diseases such as sarcoidosis cause fibrotic changes in the lungs.
- DVT can cause a PE that obstructs perfusion of the lungs. Direct oral anticoagulant medications are used to prevent PE.

- Pulmonary edema is a consequence of left-sided heart failure.
- Sepsis is a risk factor for ARDS. Mechanical ventilation is required in ARDS. ARDS is a critical illness with high mortality rate.

 Making the Connections

Pathophysiology

Signs and Symptoms	Assessment Findings	Diagnosis	Treatment
Asthma | Chronic inflammatory disorder that causes reversible bronchospasm because of bronchial hyperreactivity. It often referred to as T2 asthma if allergy and eosinophilia are involved, or non-T2 asthma if there is no allergic component.			
Wheezes, cough, dyspnea, chest tightness.	Wheezes, prolonged exhalations, rhonchi, retractions, and use of accessory muscles during breathing.	During an acute asthma attack, PFTs reveal slow, prolonged FEV_1, decreased FEV_1/FVC ratio, and decreased **peak expiratory flow (PEF)** on peak flow meter caused by bronchoconstriction, which decreases ability to inhale and exhale. Most apparent by measuring expiratory volume. FeNO test can confirm presence of inflammation in diagnosis.	For allergic individuals, AIT or SLIT is recommended. A stepwise approach is recommended that includes LABA bronchodilator (e.g., formoterol) and ICS to counteract bronchospasms and inflammation for maintenance/controller treatment. Alternative treatment is SABA plus ICS. LAMA can be added to ICS-LABA treatment. If severe bronchospasm, add epinephrine and oral corticosteroid (prednisone) for short time. Other types of medications include leukotriene antagonists used daily, mucolytics, theophylline, and immunomodulator agents such as omalizumab. Bronchial thermoplasty is recommended for severe, persistent, refractory asthma.
Chronic Obstructive Pulmonary Disease | A combination of emphysema, chronic bronchitis, and asthma. Bronchospasm, excessive mucus, edema, and fibrosis in the bronchioles. Also loss of lung elastic recoil, alveolar membrane injury, and smooth muscle hypertrophy.			
Dyspnea, cough, and wheezes.	Wheezes, prolonged exhalations, rhonchi, barrel-shaped chest, and cyanosis. Right ventricular failure findings such as jugular venous distention, ascites, ankle edema, hepatosplenomegaly possible.	PFTs reveal slow, prolonged FEV_1, FEV_1/FVC ratio lower than 70%. Chest x-ray reveals hyperinflation of lungs and flattened diaphragm. Hyperinflation of lungs is caused by alveolar accumulation of CO_2.	LABA bronchodilators and ICS via combination inhaler for maintenance treatment. Alternatively, long-acting anticholinergic agent (also called LAMA) bronchodilator and ICS via combination inhaler. SABAs can be used for acute bronchospasm in mild COPD. Careful administration and titration of oxygen is included in treatment, pulmonary rehabilitation. COPD exacerbations require inhaled LABA-ICS, mucolytics, macrolide antibiotics, and short course tapered dosage of oral prednisone. Pulmonary rehabilitation program recommended. Pneumonia, influenza, and COVID vaccinations are recommended. Mechanical ventilation, if severe exacerbation causes critical illness. Lung reduction surgery that removes excessively distended alveoli. Bronchoscopic lung reduction, which inserts bronchiole coils or valves to improve ventilation and exhalation of CO_2. Bronchial thermal ablation technique also via bronchoscope.

Making the Connections–cont'd

Signs and Symptoms	Assessment Findings	Diagnosis	Treatment
Bronchiectasis | Abnormal and permanent dilation of bronchi, fibrotic changes of bronchioles, and static, thick purulent secretions.			
Dyspnea, cough, wheezes, sputum production, and hemoptysis.	Dyspnea, cough, and wheezes throughout lung fields.	CT scan; bronchography shows dilated, fibrotic airways. Difficulty with inhalation and exhalation of air shown by decreased FEV_1/FEV. Sputum culture may show infectious agent.	Mucolytic agents; bronchodilators; oxygen, if needed; antibiotics, if needed; surgical excision of dilated airways may give relief; lung transplantation may be necessary.
Sleep-Disordered Breathing | Intermittent cessation of airflow during sleep that causes a 90% drop in oxygenation over 10 seconds. SBD can be either OSA or CSA. In OSA, the upper airway closes repeatedly during sleep.			
Daytime sleepiness, snoring.	Snoring or apneic episodes during sleep. Obesity is common.	Polysomnography shows recurrent episodes of sleep apnea of 2 to 3 minutes in duration.	CPAP keeps airway open during sleep. Surgery may be needed to reduce pharyngeal tissues.
Pneumothorax | Presence of air in the pleural cavity that presses against an area of lung tissue and causes collapse of a large section or whole lobe of lung tissue.			
Dyspnea, chest pain, increased respiratory rate.	Lack of breath sounds over area of pneumothorax, asymmetric chest expansion with inhalation, percussion of hyperresonance over area of pneumothorax.	Chest x-ray shows collapsed lung and air in the pleural space.	Chest tube attached to suction to pull air from pleural space and allow reexpansion of lung.
Pleural Effusion | Abnormal collection of fluid within the pleural cavity that can be either transudate or exudate. Fluid accumulation within the pleural space can be caused by heart failure, severe pulmonary infection, or neoplasm.			
Dyspnea, increased rate of breathing, pleuritic chest pain.	Lack of breath sounds over area of effusion, asymmetric chest expansion with inhalation, percussion of dullness over area of effusion.	Chest x-ray, ultrasound, or CT scan shows fluid in the pleural space that compresses lung tissue. Thoracocentesis allows fluid extraction for analysis.	Thoracotomy and chest tube attached to suction.
Coal Miner's Pneumoconiosis | Coal dust stimulates an inflammatory reaction in the lungs. The particles are engulfed by alveolar macrophages and remain in the lungs. Chronic bronchitis develops. The lungs eventually become fibrotic because of chronic inflammation.			
Cough, dyspnea on exertion, wheezes.	Cough, dyspnea, and wheezes heard throughout lung fields. Gray sputum.	Chest x-ray or CT scan reveals dark opacities caused by coal dust and macrophages within the lungs. PFTs reveal decreased FEV and TLC. ABGs show hypoxemia. Patient can develop right ventricular failure caused by pulmonary hypertension that develops because of chronic hypoxia.	Oxygen and bronchodilators to enhance ventilation. Smoking cessation. Pneumococcal and influenza vaccine to prevent lung infections.

Continued

Making the Connections–cont'd

Signs and Symptoms	Assessment Findings	Diagnosis	Treatment
Asbestosis | Inhalation of fine asbestos crystals from different types of manufacturing and inhaled in different occupations. Crystals stimulate a chronic inflammatory reaction with eventual fibrotic changes in the lungs.			
Dyspnea, cough. Symptoms occur decades after exposure.	Dyspnea, cough, crackles, wheezes across lung fields. Patient may have signs of right ventricular failure such as jugular venous distention and hepatosplenomegaly. Finger clubbing.	Chest x-ray may show abnormalities such as areas of plaques of foreign matter. CT scanning is better to visualize areas of plaque. PFTs reveal a restrictive lung disease pattern. Susceptibility to malignancy is increased; may show on chest x-ray or CT scan.	Cease exposure. Treatment of symptoms. Oxygen. Surgery, if malignancy present. Smoking cessation.
Silicosis | Inhalation of fine quartz crystals from different types of manufacturing and inhaled in different occupations. Crystals stimulate a chronic inflammatory reaction with eventual fibrotic changes in the lungs.			
Dyspnea, cough. Symptoms occur decades after exposure.	Dyspnea, cough, crackles, wheezes across lung fields. Patient may have signs of right ventricular failure such as jugular venous distention and hepatosplenomegaly. Finger clubbing.	Chest x-ray may show abnormalities such as areas of plaques or foreign matter. CT scanning is better to visualize areas of plaque. PFTs reveal a restrictive lung disease pattern. Susceptibility to TB and malignancy is increased; may show on chest x-ray or CT scan. Mantoux test used for TB.	Cease exposure. Treatment of symptoms. Oxygen. Surgery, if malignancy present. Smoking cessation. Antitubercular drugs, if TB present.
Thoracic Cage Deformity | Severe deviation in the vertebral column related to either structural changes or defects.			
Postural abnormality.	Kyphoscoliosis or scoliosis. One hip higher than other or one shoulder higher than other. Decreased thoracic expansion.	Chest, neck, and thoracic x-ray. PFTs show restrictive lung disease. ABGs show hypoxemia and hypercapnia caused by poor gas exchange in restricted lungs.	Orthopedic bracing or surgery.
Idiopathic Pulmonary Fibrosis | A restrictive lung disease caused by repeated injury of lung tissue by some unidentified agent. The alveoli undergo repeated episodes of inflammation that eventually involves fibroblastic proliferation and fibrotic changes in lungs.			
Dyspnea, tachypnea, cough, and cyanosis.	Dyspnea, cough, tachypnea, crackles, and cyanosis.	Elevated erythrocyte sedimentation rate (ESR). Serology tests are negative for immunological collagen vascular diseases. Hypoxemia on ABG. Chest x-ray shows "ground glass" appearance of lungs. PFTs demonstrate restrictive disease.	Oxygen, bronchodilators, corticosteroids. Pulmonary vasodilators to treat pulmonary hypertension. Treatment of right ventricular failure with diuretics may be necessary. Many treatments tend to fail, and lung transplantation may be necessary.
Hypersensitivity Pneumonitis | An immunologically mediated lung disorder caused by prolonged, intense exposure to inhaled organic dusts that act as antigens. There is widespread alveolar inflammation.			
Acute attacks of cough, dyspnea, and fever.	Dyspnea, cough, fever, and an elevated WBC count.	PFTs demonstrate restrictive disease. Chest x-rays show nodular infiltrates.	Corticosteroid treatment.

Making the Connections–cont'd

Signs and Symptoms	Assessment Findings	Diagnosis	Treatment
Pulmonary Edema	Accumulation of fluid around the alveoli that inhibits oxygen transfer at the alveolar–capillary interface. An increase in hydrostatic pressure in the capillary bed of the lungs is caused by backward effects of left ventricular failure (LVF).		
Cough, dyspnea, or stridor may occur.	Cough; dyspnea; stridor; pink, frothy sputum. Coarse, loud crackles in both lung fields.	Chest x-ray. Cardiac catheter can show poor left ventricular (LV) ejection fraction lower than 40%. High pulmonary capillary wedge pressure is caused by backward pressure from left ventricle.	Oxygen. Diuretics to decrease fluid in lungs. Digitalis to enhance cardiac contractility; ACE inhibitors to decrease RAAS effects in heart failure.
Pulmonary Embolus	A clot that has traveled to the pulmonary arterial circulation and caused obstruction of arterial blood flow through the lungs.		
Dyspnea, chest pain, increased respiratory rate.	Sudden respiratory distress, tachycardia.	V-Q scan shows decreased perfusion in area of embolism blocking circulation.	DOACs are most common treatment. If a PE is causing hemodynamic compromise, a thrombolytic agent is used. Pain medication; inferior vena cava filter can inhibit clot travel into the right heart and pulmonary artery.
Pulmonary Hypertension	Abnormally high pressure within the pulmonary arteries.		
Syncope, dyspnea on exertion, and fatigue.	Dyspnea on exertion; dizziness on exertion.	Transthoracic echocardiogram, CT scan, Doppler ultrasound, or cardiac catheterization can show evidence of high pulmonary artery pressure, right ventricular hypertrophy, or right ventricular failure.	Vasodilators, calcium channel blockers, oxygen. Epoprostenol, a pulmonary vasodilator, and bosentan, a vasoconstriction antagonist, are frequently used. Tadalafil, a vasodilator, is also used to decrease pulmonary artery pressure. Newer drugs; ambrisentan, an endothelin receptor antagonist, and selexipag, a prostacyclin receptor agonist, have shown effective treatment results. Combination tadalafil plus ambrisentan has been superior to other agents.
Acute Respiratory Distress Syndrome	Pulmonary dysfunction characterized by diffuse alveolar injury, pulmonary capillary damage, and bilateral pulmonary infiltrates in critically ill patients. Commonly a sequela to trauma, sepsis, drug overdose, massive transfusion, acute pancreatitis, or aspiration.		
Critically ill patient commonly in intensive care for another diagnosis.	Severe respiratory distress; coarse, loud crackles across lungs. Tachycardia, elevated blood pressure.	ABGs show hypoxemia and hypercapnia. Chest x-ray shows pulmonary edema. Berlin criteria are used to diagnose ARDS.	Supportive treatment should focus on major etiological disorders. Intubation and mechanical ventilation with sedation and neuromuscular blockade. DVT and gastric ulcer prophylaxis. Inhaled nitric oxide or prostacyclin may be used to improve oxygenation. Prone positioning has been shown to improve oxygenation. ECMO may be used instead of mechanical ventilation.

Bibliography

Available online at fadavis.com

Renal Disorders

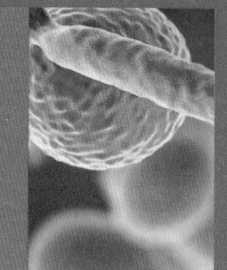

Learning Objectives

After completion of this chapter, the student will be able to:

- Describe the various actions of the kidney and how these actions are affected in renal dysfunction.
- Identify causes of prerenal, intrarenal, and postrenal dysfunction of the kidney.
- Explain the signs and symptoms of major causes of kidney dysfunction.

- Recognize assessment modalities and laboratory tests used to diagnose kidney dysfunction.
- Differentiate between acute kidney injury and chronic kidney disease.
- Discuss pharmacological and nonpharmacological treatment modalities used in renal dysfunction.

Key Terms

Acute kidney injury (AKI)

Acute tubular necrosis (ATN)

Albuminuria

Aldosterone

Antiglomerular basement membrane (anti-GBM) disease

Azotemia

Continuous renal replacement therapy (CRRT)

Costovertebral angle (CVA) tenderness

Creatinine clearance (CrCl)

End-stage renal disease (ESRD)

Erythropoietin

Glomerular filtration rate (GFR)

Goodpasture's syndrome

Hematuria

Hemodialysis

Hydronephrosis

Intrarenal dysfunction

Nephrolithiasis

Nephrotic syndrome

Obstructive uropathy

Oliguria

Peritoneal dialysis (PD)

Postrenal dysfunction

Prerenal dysfunction

Proteinuria

Pyelonephritis

Renal osteodystrophy

Renin-angiotensin-aldosterone system (RAAS)

Urea

Vesicoureteral reflux

The kidneys are commonly recognized as the organs of excretion because they filter the bloodstream of waste products and excrete urine. However, they also perform many other functions essential for life. The kidneys play a major role in controlling blood pressure, regulating red blood cell (RBC) production, breaking down drugs, metabolizing hormones, synthesizing vitamin D, managing electrolytes, conserving and excreting water, and balancing the pH of the bloodstream. The kidneys influence every system of the body from brain to bone, and it is only in their failure that we can appreciate the kidneys' multiple actions and far-reaching effects on the body.

Epidemiology

The incidence of kidney disease continues to grow in the United States. As of 2021, according to the Centers for Disease Control (CDC), one in seven—15% or 37 million—adults in the United States have chronic kidney disease (CKD). Also, as many as 9 in 10 adults with CKD do not know they have this disorder. It is most common in persons over age 65. Adults with diabetes mellitus (DM), hypertension (HTN), or both have a high risk of developing kidney disease. One in three adults with DM and one in five adults with

HTN have kidney disease. African Americans have the greatest incidence of CKD. African Americans make up 13% of the U.S. population but constitute 35% of persons with kidney failure. Between 1990 and 2015, the incidence of **end-stage renal disease (ESRD)** increased by almost 100% within the population. Nearly 786,000 Americans have kidney failure, 558,000 (71%) are on dialysis, and approximately 228,000 (29%) live with a functioning kidney transplant.

Basic Concepts of Renal Function

Renal function begins with blood flow to the renal vasculature. The kidneys receive 20% to 25% of the body's cardiac output. It is filtered at a rate of approximately 90 to 120 mL/min. The renal blood filtered per unit of time, known as the **glomerular filtration rate (GFR)**, is directly related to renal perfusion (see Fig. 22-1). Disease processes that decrease blood pressure and renal perfusion result in a decreased GFR. As an individual ages, the normal GFR rate of 90 to 120 mL/minute diminishes. Peak function of the kidneys occurs at age 30 years; for each year after, GFR decreases by 1 mL/minute until by age 70 years, normal GFR is 70 mL/min. This reduction in GFR in the older adult can cause accumulation of toxins, particularly drug metabolites, in the blood.

Excretory Functions

The basic unit of the kidney is the nephron, a sequence of tubes that filters the blood of waste and conserves the fluid and electrolytes that the body needs. Each nephron is surrounded by blood vessels, where the exchange of water and electrolytes between the blood and the tubule fluid occurs. At the glomerular capillaries, the major mechanisms of the nephron—waste removal and water recycling—begin. The different sections of the nephron perform various functions to form the final product, which is concentrated urine. Urine must contain all the waste products, electrolytes, metabolites, and nitrogenous compounds for excretion. At the same time, urine needs to be sparing of water; the kidney needs to conserve the water the body needs.

The Nephron

Renal blood flow through the glomerulus, a tuft of capillaries within Bowman's capsule, requires high hydrostatic pressure to push blood through the filtration process. The kidneys autoregulate renal blood flow to maintain sufficient pressure to push blood through the glomeruli, regardless of whether blood volume is high or low.

As blood flows through the glomerulus and a membranous cap called Bowman's capsule, water and

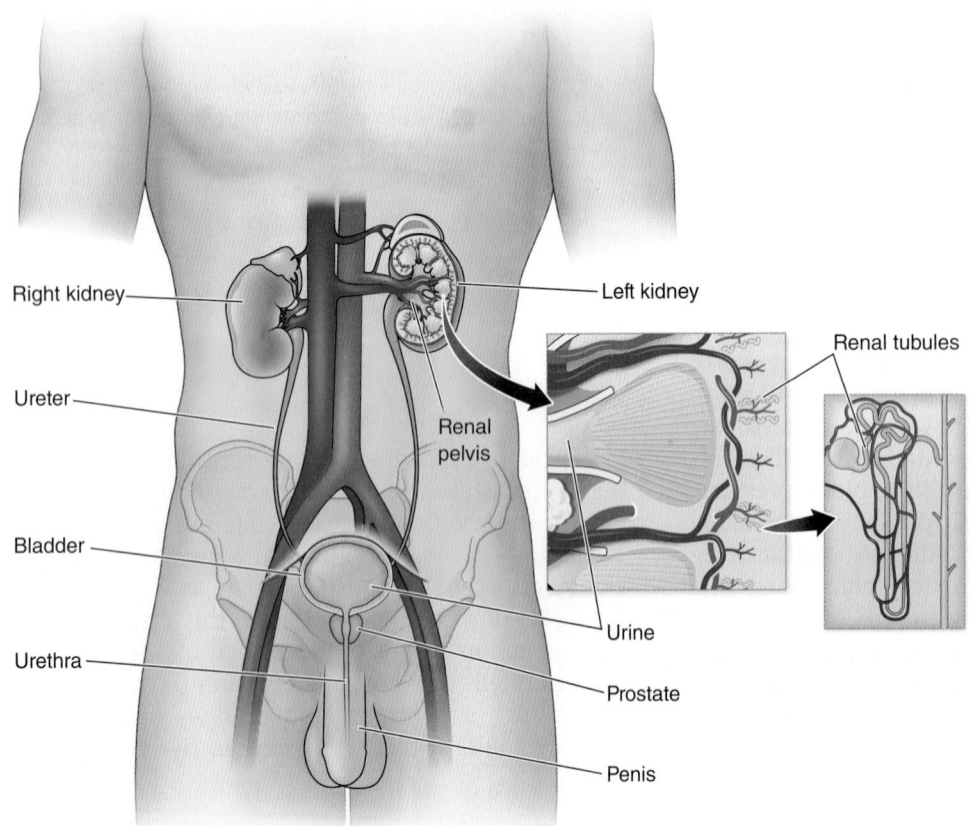

Right kidney
Ureter
Bladder
Urethra
Left kidney
Renal pelvis
Renal tubules
Urine
Prostate
Penis

FIGURE 22-1. Kidney and urological anatomy.

electrolytes leave the blood and pass into the proximal tubule. At this point, the glomerular filtrate is very dilute and contains a high amount of electrolytes, glucose, and metabolic waste products.

At the proximal tubule, approximately 60% of water is reabsorbed back into the bloodstream. As the tubule fluid travels through the various parts of the nephron, water and electrolytes such as sodium and potassium move to and from tubule fluid and blood. Within the next section of the nephron, called the loop of Henle, **urea**, a composite of nitrogenous waste that needs to be excreted, is secreted into the tubule fluid. At this juncture within the nephron, the tubule fluid, which contains urea, starts to resemble the finished product: urine. Overall, the loop of Henle reabsorbs about 25% of filtered electrolytes, such as sodium, chlorine, potassium, calcium, and bicarbonate, and 15% of the filtered water. At the distal tubule, **aldosterone** acts to reabsorb more sodium and water into the bloodstream and secrete potassium into the tubule fluid. Here again, tubule fluid is further concentrated and the body saves water. Finally, at the collecting duct, under the influence of antidiuretic hormone, the last amount of water needed by the body is reabsorbed from the tubule fluid back into the bloodstream. At this last stage, the highly concentrated tubule fluid is urine (see Fig. 22-2).

Acid–Base Balance

Normal body function is dependent on acid–base balance, and the kidneys play a major role in this through the regulation of bicarbonate and hydrogen reabsorption or secretion. Acids are produced during normal metabolic processes, requiring the physiological response of buffering to maintain the physiological pH of 7.35 to 7.45. The kidneys' role in maintaining acid–base balance involves excretion or conservation of hydrogen ions [H^+] and bicarbonate ions [HCO_3^-].

Waste Elimination

During the cell's metabolic activity, waste products are accumulated. These waste products include such substances as urea, uric acid, creatinine, and drug metabolites. If not excreted in the urine, waste products become toxic to body tissues, particularly breakdown products of drugs. A reduction in renal function can prolong the effect of some medications, which can lead to adverse effects or toxicity.

Secretory Functions

The kidney has several unique secretory functions that are triggered by certain conditions in the body. Hypoxia and low blood volume are two such conditions. Hypoxia stimulates erythropoietin secretion by the kidney. Low blood volume stimulates renin secretion by the kidney.

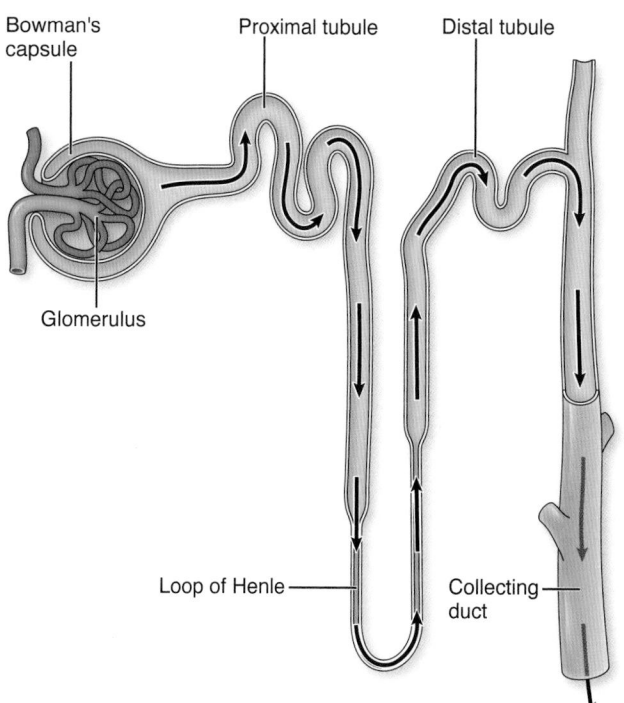

FIGURE 22-2. Basic functions of the nephron. The nephron's basic goal is to yield a concentrated urine that contains waste products. The blood and tubule fluid undergo a great deal of exchange before the tubule fluid becomes urine. The glomerulus is a tuft of capillaries from which blood is filtered at the Bowman's capsule. The glomerulus allows substances such as water, sodium, bicarbonate, acids, and urea out of the blood. However, the glomerulus does not allow large proteins such as albumin out of the blood. At the proximal tubule, a large amount of water, sodium, and potassium are reabsorbed into the bloodstream. At the descending loop of Henle, a high amount of sodium is reabsorbed, and urea is secreted from the blood into the tubule. Aldosterone, a hormone secreted by the adrenal gland, increases sodium and water reabsorption. In the distal tubule, sodium and water are reabsorbed from the tubule fluid into the bloodstream and urine is formed. If the body needs more water, antidiuretic hormone (ADH) from the posterior pituitary works at the collecting duct to increase water reabsorption into the bloodstream for a more concentrated urine.

Control of Blood Pressure

The major mechanism whereby the kidneys influence systemic blood pressure and blood volume is the **renin–angiotensin–aldosterone system (RAAS)**. The RAAS contributes to sodium and water reabsorption into the bloodstream and potassium excretion at the renal tubules. A specialized region of the nephron called the juxtaglomerular apparatus is sensitive to sodium. This is the specific region around the glomerulus in each nephron. These cells sense low sodium and, in response, secrete renin. Other triggers for renin secretion include decreased renal perfusion and increased sympathetic nervous system activity. The net effects of the RAAS activity are sodium and water reabsorption, potassium excretion, and arterial vasoconstriction.

Red Blood Cell Production

The kidney secretes **erythropoietin**, which stimulates synthesis of RBCs in the bone marrow. Erythropoietin is released in response to low oxygen levels in arterial blood. The kidney also secretes erythropoietin in response to anemia and cellular hypoxia.

 CLINICAL CONCEPT

Individuals who have chronic hypoxia, such as those with chronic obstructive lung disease, often have higher-than-normal hemoglobin and hematocrit levels because of constant secretion of erythropoietin. Conversely, patients with renal failure have lower hemoglobin and hematocrit levels because of deficient erythropoietin.

Vitamin D Synthesis and Calcium Balance

The kidneys synthesize components that comprise vitamin D. Without kidney function, vitamin D is inactive, which affects calcium absorption. In the gastrointestinal tract, calcium is absorbed with the facilitation of vitamin D. Without vitamin D, calcium absorption is diminished, which disrupts calcium balance in the bloodstream.

Glucose Homeostasis

The renal tubules reabsorb glucose from the glomerular filtrate up to the renal threshold of a blood glucose level of 180 mg/dL. If the blood glucose level is greater than the renal threshold, the excess glucose is excreted in the urine. Additionally, in states of prolonged fasting or starvation, the kidneys can create glucose from amino acids in a process known as gluconeogenesis. The kidneys are also responsible for the degradation of insulin. Patients with renal failure have decreased insulin clearance, which affects glucose metabolism.

Basic Pathophysiological Concepts of Renal Disorders

The kidneys are at risk for injury because they require a large blood flow to function and because they process potentially toxic waste products. For the nephrons to function properly, the blood entering at the glomerulus must be at high hydrostatic pressure. The kidneys are susceptible to ischemic injury if not provided with high blood flow. All tubule fluid from the nephrons must travel toward the renal pelvis and out the ureter. The nephrons need high pressure to push tubule fluid out of the kidney without any stasis or backflow. The tubule fluid contains waste products that can be toxic to the fragile nephron cells. The nephron cells are at risk if urine outflow is not maintained. Any obstruction to urine outflow, also called **obstructive uropathy**, can cause urine to back up from the ureter into the renal pelvis and cause cellular injury.

The causes of kidney dysfunction are divided into three categories based upon the mechanism of injury:

1. **Prerenal dysfunction**: caused by decreased blood flow and perfusion to the kidney.
2. **Intrarenal dysfunction**: develops secondary to actual injuries to the kidney itself.
3. **Postrenal dysfunction**: related to obstruction of urine outflow from the kidneys.

Prerenal Dysfunction

Prerenal dysfunction of the kidney describes pathophysiological processes that affect GFR and are directly related to blood flow and renal perfusion (see Fig. 22-3). Any condition that directly or indirectly decreases renal perfusion may lead to prerenal dysfunction. Prerenal dysfunction occurs because of reduced cardiac output or severe hypovolemia (low blood volume). In any type of shock, the patient is vulnerable to prerenal dysfunction. Maintenance of a

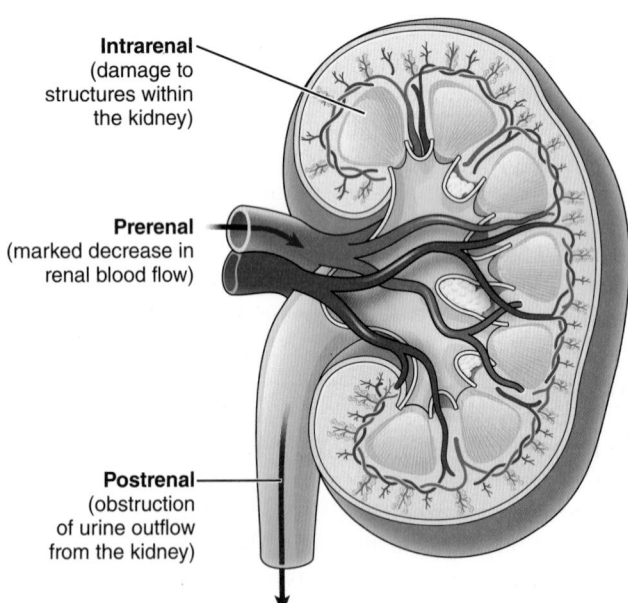

FIGURE 22-3. The three basic categories of renal dysfunction are prerenal, intrarenal, and postrenal. These are sometimes referred to as prerenal, intrarenal, or postrenal azotemia. Prerenal azotemia occurs in severe dehydration or hemorrhage; there is inadequate blood flow to optimally perfuse the kidney. The kidney is not the cause of prenatal azotemia; rather, a circumstance that decreases perfusion of the kidney is the source of the problem. In intrarenal azotemia, there is a problem intrinsically with the kidney, such as trauma to the kidney, infection, or nephrotoxic drugs. Postrenal azotemia occurs when urine outflow is obstructed. Urine needs to flow freely out of the kidney; if backed up, it is toxic to the nephrons. Prostate enlargement, kidney stones, a kinked ureter, or tumors can cause postrenal azotemia.

sufficiently high blood pressure is necessary for kidney function because glomerular filtration requires high hydrostatic pressure. Large blood loss from the body, as in hemorrhage, is a common cause of prerenal kidney injury caused by ischemia.

Intrarenal Dysfunction

Direct damage to renal tissue, as in trauma or toxic injury, causes nephron damage within the kidney itself, known as intrarenal dysfunction. This is most commonly caused by nephrotoxic medications, renal infections, or systemic illnesses that affect the kidney. Common examples include nephrotoxicity caused by NSAIDs and poststreptococcal glomerulonephritis (PSGN). Both of these conditions cause direct injury to the kidney. Autoimmune diseases, untreated HTN, and uncontrolled DM also directly harm the kidney, causing intrarenal dysfunction.

Postrenal Dysfunction

Postrenal dysfunction is caused by obstructive uropathy, a problem that prevents urine outflow from the kidney. Conditions that can cause obstruction include kidney stones in the ureter, prostate gland enlargement, and bladder cancer. In postrenal kidney dysfunction, urine backs up within the ureter and into the kidney, which can lead to **hydronephrosis**, a fluid-filled, swollen kidney. Urine is toxic to the nephron cells, and urine stagnation increases the risk of infection.

Acute Tubular Necrosis

Ischemia and hypoxia can damage the renal tubules and result in **acute tubular necrosis (ATN)**, the most common cause of **acute kidney injury (AKI)**. With ischemia, cells of the nephron tubules slough into the tubular lumen. The lumen becomes blocked, preventing fluid from flowing through them, thereby reducing urine formation. The blocked lumen further contributes to ischemic injury to cells lining the tubules, causing additional intrarenal injury. Unless this process is reversed, renal failure with permanent injury to the kidney will occur.

Assessment

The history and physical assessment for patients with renal disease includes determining exposure to any medications or nephrotoxic substances. Additionally, any systemic illnesses or infections associated with renal damage need to be identified. Illnesses such as HTN and DM are important causes of renal damage.

Patients need to be asked about their pattern of urine excretion and the character of their urine. Typical questions would include the following:

- Does the urine have an unusual odor or color?
- Is the urine foamy?
- Is the urine very dark or tea-colored?
- Is there blood in the urine?
- Is there pain or burning on urination? Is there abdominal or flank pain on urination?
- Have you noticed any change in the amount of urine or the frequency of urination?

Risk Factors

Exposure to nephrotoxic agents is one of the greatest risks for the development of renal disorders. A list of current medications is needed, as many drug metabolites are particularly nephrotoxic. Specific questions concerning HTN and DM are important. The patient needs to describe the duration of the disorder, medications involved, and management of the disorders.

> **ALERT!** Long-term DM and HTN often lead to renal failure.

The patient should be asked about a recent streptococcal infection because poststreptococcal glomerulonephritis (PSGN) can occur. Patients who have had major surgery are at risk for altered renal function, as major surgery can reduce renal blood flow and lead to kidney injury. A reduction in renal blood flow is also a concern for patients who have had an acute myocardial infarction or heart failure. Renal ischemia is a common complication of severe heart failure.

Signs and Symptoms

The patient with renal failure generally has a variety of multisystemic symptoms, which are the result of reduced secretory and excretory functions of the kidney. The symptoms can include fatigue, weakness, nausea, constipation, abdominal pain, and confusion. Patients with renal calculi may have abdominal or flank pain in addition to hematuria. **Costovertebral angle (CVA) tenderness** is a classic sign of a kidney disorder, particularly infection (see Fig. 22-4).

The presence of blood (**hematuria**) or protein (**proteinuria**) in urine is often readily apparent to the patient. Urine looks pink or red when blood is present and foamy when it contains high levels of protein. Tea-colored urine often indicates bilirubin is in the urine, as occurs in jaundice. All these signs are an indication for further study.

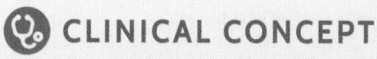

CLINICAL CONCEPT

Hematuria is most often a sign of renal calculi or an infection.

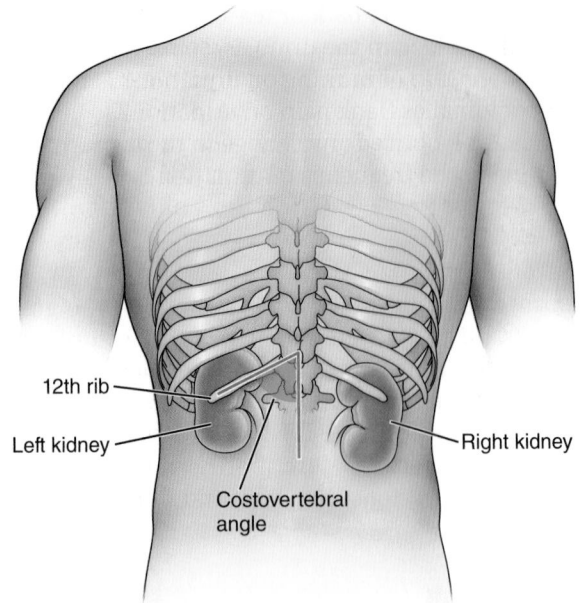

FIGURE 22-4. The kidney is located in the costovertebral angle (CVA) region. In physical examination, the examiner should firmly tap the CVA to assess its pain of kidney disorder. The pain of nephrolithiasis and pyelonephritis is commonly in the CVA region.

Proteinuria, also called microalbuminuria, indicates that the urine contains proteins. Normal total protein excretion does not usually exceed more than 150 mg/day. Excess protein in the urine is abnormal and is usually an indication of glomerular injury. The glomerular capillaries should not filter out blood proteins; however, when injured, they develop excessive permeability that allows escape of albumin into the nephron tubule. Glomerular injury can occur in such disorders as glomerulonephritis, DM, and HTN.

Diagnosis

Renal function can be evaluated through examination of the urine and blood. Imaging studies can be performed to evaluate the anatomy of the kidneys and renal blood flow and visualize renal calculi, tumors, or cysts.

Urinalysis

Urinalysis is a basic examination of urine that includes a description of the character of the urine, as well as biochemical and microscopic analysis. Normally, urine is odorless and clear or slightly hazy with a color ranging from yellow to amber. The color varies according to the concentration of solutes and water content of the urine. For example, a dehydrated person has amber-colored urine, whereas a well-hydrated person has light yellow urine, although urine color can vary with some medications or certain disorders. For example, hepatitis will cause a dark-brown, tea-colored urine caused by bile pigments.

Reagent strips, also called dipsticks, are used for analysis of the urine. Urinary pH should be close to a neutral pH of 7, but it does vary from acidic to basic. The specific gravity should be between 1.001 when dilute and 1.030 when highly concentrated. All of the biochemical tests that are measured by reagent strips should be negative in healthy individuals. If any of these tests are positive, they are suggestive of a variety of illness states (see Table 22-1).

The presence of glucose and ketones is indicative of diabetic ketoacidosis. Leukocyte esterase measures the amount of enzyme secreted by white blood cells (WBCs); a high amount (positive result) is indicative of either a bladder or kidney infection. Crystals are often seen in the urine of patients with renal calculi. Casts are substances that are secreted into the nephron tubules and retain the shape of the tubules. They are

TABLE 22-1. Urine Analysis Using Reagent Strips		
Test	**Normal Value**	**Common Etiology**
Glucose	Negative	If positive: hyperglycemia, diabetes
Ketones	Negative	If positive: starvation or diabetic ketoacidosis
Protein	Negative or trace	Minimal: exercise or infection Moderate: polycystic kidney disease (PKD), infection, heart failure, diabetic kidney disease Marked: PKD, glomerulonephritis, diabetic kidney disease, nephrosis, lupus nephritis
Blood	Negative	If positive: infection, kidney stone, or bladder cancer
Bilirubin	Negative	If positive: hemolysis or liver disease
Urobilinogen	Minimal	If high: liver disease
Nitrite	Negative	If positive: urinary tract infection
Leukocyte esterase	Negative	If positive: urinary tract infection

made of protein or fats and can either be benign or signify kidney disease.

Blood Urea Nitrogen

Azotemia is the increase of blood urea nitrogen (BUN) within the bloodstream. The normal level for BUN is 5 to 20 mg/dL. An elevated BUN can occur when there is a decrease in the GFR, which leads to accumulation of nitrogenous waste products in the blood. However, a high BUN level is not always an indicator of kidney dysfunction; it can result from dehydration, which highly concentrates the urea in the urine. A high BUN level can also occur in any condition that elevates the amount of nitrogen waste in the bloodstream. Extremely muscular individuals will have a high nitrogen level in the bloodstream because of high muscle breakdown. The muscle cell proteins break down into amino acids, which are nitrogen compounds. High BUN levels also occur in persons on high-protein diets, as the large load of protein breakdown into amino acids raises nitrogen in the bloodstream.

 CLINICAL CONCEPT

Because of the possible elevation of BUN with nonrenal conditions such as dehydration, the clinician should not rely on BUN alone as an indicator of renal dysfunction.

Serum Creatinine

Creatinine is a muscle breakdown product that is filtered almost completely at the glomerulus. The normal range of serum creatinine is approximately 0.5 to 1.5 mg/dL. After being filtered out of the bloodstream, it is not reabsorbed by the nephron tubules.

 CLINICAL CONCEPT

Serum creatinine is a reliable indicator of kidney function.

Accumulation of serum creatinine indicates decreased filtering of creatinine at the glomerulus. There are exceptions to this rule in extremely muscular individuals and very frail individuals. Because serum creatinine is based on muscle tissue breakdown, serum creatinine can vary depending on the patient's muscle mass. A person who has an increased amount of muscle breakdown daily may have an abnormally high serum creatinine, whereas a frail individual will have a low amount of serum creatinine daily.

ALERT! Nephrotoxic antibiotics include aminoglycosides. Whenever these are administered, serum levels of the medication and serum creatinine levels must be monitored.

Creatinine Clearance

Creatinine clearance (CrCl) is sometimes used to assess the GFR. The test requires measurement of both blood and urine creatinine and 24-hour urine volume. CrCl can also be estimated using a mathematical formula. The amount of creatinine filtered at the glomerulus is the total amount of creatinine that appears in the urine. A decreased creatinine clearance indicates decreased GFR and impaired renal function. This can be caused by conditions such as renal disease or can result from lack of circulation to the kidney, which occurs in hypotension, heart failure, and shock. Increased creatinine clearance indicates there is more creatinine in the urine than normal. This can be seen in pregnant women, patients with DM, patients with large muscle mass, or those with high protein intake.

Imaging Studies

Visualization of the kidneys through various imaging studies can provide valuable information about renal size and function. Renal ultrasound is used to determine the size of both kidneys. It can also be used in the diagnosis of hydronephrosis, renal cysts, tumors, and kidney stones. Abdominal x-rays can sometimes visualize radio-opaque stones or nephrocalcinosis. Computed tomography (CT) scan or magnetic resonance imaging (MRI) can also visualize kidney stones and abnormalities. Renal biopsy can be performed if imaging tests do not reveal sufficient information.

ALERT! IV contrast-enhanced imaging studies should be avoided in patients with renal impairment because radiopaque dye can cause renal failure. Dehydration markedly increases this risk.

Treatment

Regardless of the etiology, all of the functions regulated by the kidney must be maintained when treating renal disease. It is important to maintain fluid, electrolyte, and acid–base levels; to control blood glucose; to control blood pressure; and to monitor RBC production. To accomplish this, patients usually need multiple medications to maintain physiological homeostasis; sodium bicarbonate can help control metabolic acidosis, whereas beta blocker medications can control blood pressure. Epogen is a synthetic form of erythropoietin that can be used to stimulate RBC production. Diuretics can be used to stimulate water loss from the body. However, when these medications cannot reverse the imbalances of renal failure, dialysis is necessary. Indications for dialysis include persistent hyperkalemia, uncompensated metabolic acidosis, and fluid volume excess that is unresponsive to diuresis.

There are two types of dialysis: hemodialysis and peritoneal dialysis. One functioning kidney can perform all functions and maintain homeostasis. When both kidneys are no longer functioning and the patient is in relatively good health, renal transplant may be considered.

Peritoneal Dialysis

In **peritoneal dialysis (PD)**, the patient's peritoneum is filled with a dialysis solution that pulls wastes and extra fluid from the blood into the abdominal cavity. The dialysis solution, called the dialysate, contains certain electrolytes that cause diffusion of solutes and ultrafiltration of fluid from the blood to cross the peritoneal membrane. The process works based on the principle that diffusion of substances in water tends to move from an area of high concentration to an area of low concentration. After the fluid is instilled, it sits in the peritoneal cavity for a period, called a dwell time, of approximately 4 hours. After the dwell time, the solution is drained from the peritoneal cavity and discarded. PD is uncommon, but at times it is used as an alternative to hemodialysis. The process of draining and filling takes about 30 to 40 minutes. A typical schedule of PD requires approximately four exchanges a day, each with a dwell time of 4 to 6 hours (see Fig. 22-5).

Hemodialysis

Hemodialysis is a treatment during which the patient's blood is drawn out of the body at a rate of 200 to 400 mL/minute and passed through a device called a dialyzer. There are two sections in the dialyzer: the section for dialysate and the section for the blood. The two sections are divided by a semipermeable membrane, which has microscopic perforations that allow only some substances to cross. Because it is semipermeable, the membrane allows water and waste to pass through, but does not allow blood cells to pass through. Commonly, a patient has an arteriovenous fistula created in the arm that can facilitate this process. For example, a tubular connection between the brachiocephalic artery and cephalic vein is often surgically implanted. Blood is drained from the brachiocephalic artery and pumped into a dialyzer, which removes excess solutes and fluid from the blood. The blood is then returned to the body via the cephalic vein. The dialysis solution is a sterile solution of electrolytes. Urea and other waste products, such as potassium and phosphate, diffuse into the dialysis solution. During the treatment, the patient's entire blood volume (about 5000 mL) circulates through the machine every 15 minutes. Electrolytes, serum albumin, BUN, and serum creatinine are normalized during the dialysis procedure. The procedure is usually required at least three times a week, and each session lasts 4 to 6 hours (see Fig. 22-6).

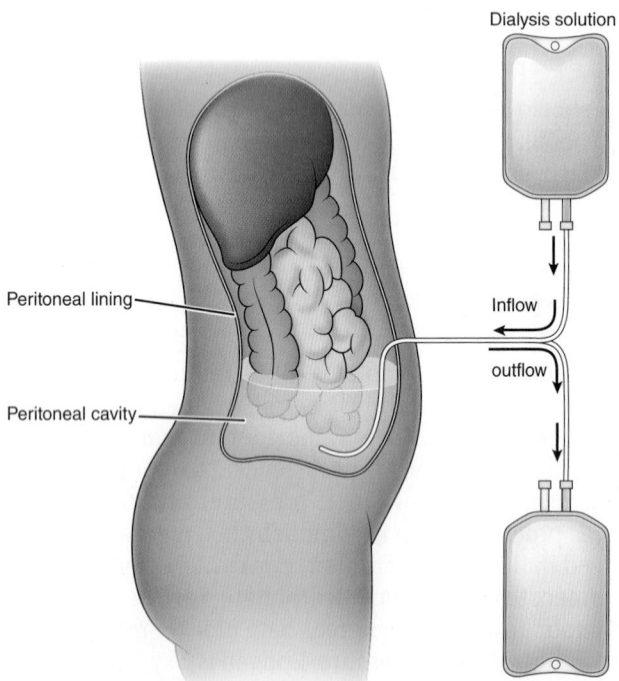

FIGURE 22-5. Peritoneal Dialysis: In peritoneal dialysis, dialysate solution is instilled into and removed from the peritoneal cavity at regular intervals to achieve clearance of solutes. The dialysate solution has a high concentration of dextrose. Ultrafiltration of water is achieved by the creation of an osmotic gradient across the peritoneal membrane. It is a slow process that is sometimes better tolerated by hypotensive patients than hemodialysis.

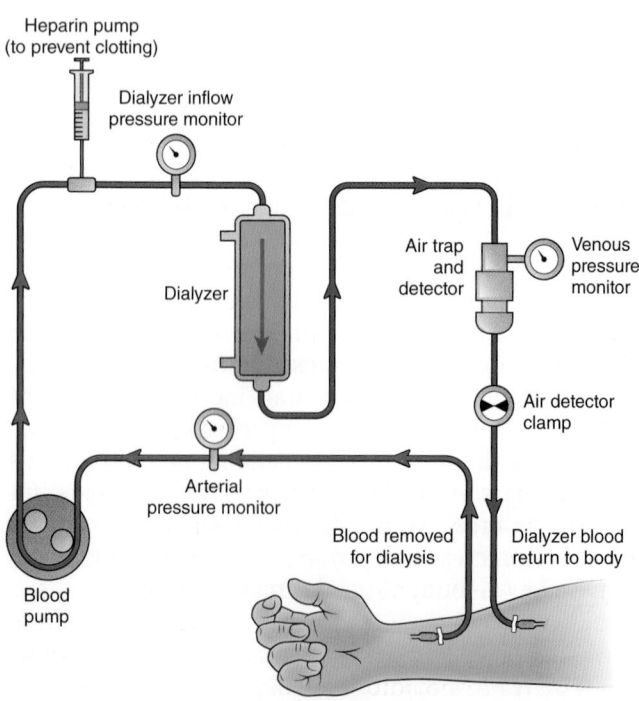

FIGURE 22-6. Hemodialysis: In hemodialysis, blood is removed from the body and filtered through a man-made membrane called a dialyzer, and then the filtered blood is returned to the body.

Continuous Renal Replacement Therapy

Continuous renal replacement therapy (CRRT) is similar to hemodialysis; however, it is a slower process used for patients who are hemodynamically unstable and fluid overloaded. This continuous process takes smaller volumes of blood from the patient and filters it through a dialyzer over 24 hours. It is most commonly used in patients with acute kidney injury.

Pathophysiology of Selected Disorders

Major pathophysiological conditions of the kidney include acute glomerulonephritis, nephrotic syndrome, nephrolithiasis, pyelonephritis, polycystic kidney disease, Goodpasture's syndrome, acute kidney injury, and chronic kidney disease.

Acute Glomerulonephritis

Acute glomerulonephritis (AGN) is a renal disorder that is due to inflammation of the glomerulus. In most cases, AGN is due to an immunological mechanism that triggers inflammation that damages the membranes of the glomerulus. It can lead to significant illness because the glomerulus is the critical, initial region of every nephron unit that filters the blood. Damage to the glomerular capillaries causes a loss of vital substances, such as albumin, from the blood into the tubule fluid, which becomes urine. Glomerular injury increases glomerular permeability, which allows albumin to leave the capillaries and enter the tubules.

Epidemiology

Glomerulonephritis may be an acute, mild disease or a rapidly progressive disease that can lead to renal dysfunction. AGN is the cause of 25% to 30% of all cases of ESRD. In cases that progress to ESRD, the disease course is fairly rapid. In severe disease, end-stage renal failure may occur within weeks or months of the onset of AGN. Most cases of AGN occur in patients aged 5 to 15 years; only 10% occur in patients older than 40 years. It predominantly affects males with a 2:1 male-to-female ratio.

Etiology

Poststreptococcal glomerulonephritis (PSGN) is the most common cause of acute glomerulonephritis. Acute infection with group A beta-hemolytic streptococcus (GABHS) usually begins as pharyngitis and then causes a secondary immunological reaction at the glomeruli. PSGN can also occur after a skin infection with GABHS, known as impetigo. Although AGN most commonly develops because of streptococcal infection, it can also arise because of other types of bacterial, viral, fungal, or parasitic infections. AGN can follow infections such as rubella, mumps, Epstein–Barr virus, hepatitis B or C, or cytomegalovirus. Autoimmune and immunological diseases such as systemic lupus erythematosus (SLE) frequently cause AGN. Glomerulonephritis can also occur as part of an active infectious process. This type of AGN includes staphylococcus-associated glomerulonephritis (SAGN) that develops in people with an infection with methicillin-sensitive or methicillin-resistant *Staphylococcus aureus*. It can also occur in persons with bacterial endocarditis and central venous catheter infections.

AGN of any type can progress to chronic disease, particularly in patients with other risk factors. The course of chronic glomerulonephritis is often gradual and silent. By the time of diagnosis, the patient is commonly already in the early stages of ESRD.

Pathophysiology

Postinfectious glomerulonephritis, the most common type of AGN, begins with an antigen–antibody reaction. An antigen, such as streptococcus, enters the body and stimulates antibody synthesis. There are two theoretical explanations for the mechanism of disease. One theory claims that the antibodies attack the antigen, but also form antigen–antibody complexes that float freely in the bloodstream until they deposit within glomerular membranes. The other theory asserts that molecular mimicry occurs, where the antibodies that are stimulated attack the antigen and mistakenly attack the glomerular membranes as well (see Fig. 22-7).

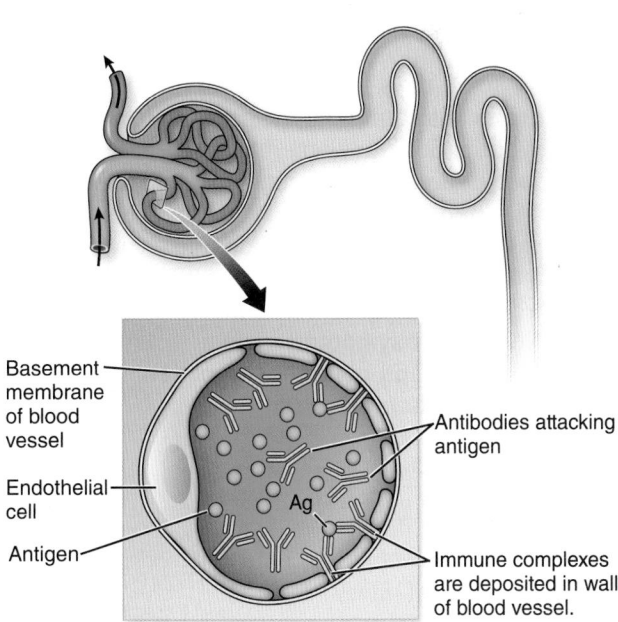

FIGURE 22-7. Glomerular damage in glomerulonephritis. The damage to glomerular membranes in glomerulonephritis is caused by antibodies. These antibodies are commonly activated by *Streptococcus* bacteria. The antibodies combine with antigen and deposit as immune complexes within the kidney that are normally eliminated in the circulation. However, in glomerulonephritis, the immune complexes accumulate and cause inflammation and membrane damage.

Regardless of mechanism, the antigen–antibody complexes damage the structure of the glomeruli and cause nephron dysfunction throughout the kidneys. Glomerular injury causes hyperpermeability of the capillaries, which allows loss of albumin and RBCs in the urine. The large loss of albumin from the bloodstream causes proteinuria, also called microalbuminuria. Because albumin content of the bloodstream decreases, diminished colloid oncotic pressure (COP) occurs throughout the body. According to Starling's Law of Capillary Forces, the decrease of COP causes an imbalance in hydrostatic and oncotic pressure. The low COP is overcome by hydrostatic pressure, which causes edema.

Also, because glomerular filtration of the blood is diminished, urine production is also diminished. As GFR decreases, **oliguria**, which is lack of sufficient urine production, develops. The patient becomes hypervolemic and edematous, and blood pressure rises.

 CLINICAL CONCEPT

A certain amount of urine production is necessary to excrete waste products. An inadequate amount of urine is termed oliguria. Oliguria is defined as less than 400 mL of urine output per day or less than 20 mL of urine per hour.

Clinical Presentation

Acute glomerulonephritis has a classic presentation of sudden edema (most prevalent in the periorbital region), hematuria, proteinuria, oliguria, and HTN. The onset of clinical manifestations occurs approximately 7 to 21 days following a streptococcal infection. This is consistent with the time frame needed for antibody formation. As glomerular function decreases, urinary output decreases. As glomerular injury increases, hematuria and proteinuria increase. The patient develops puffiness of the eyelids and facial edema. The urine is dark because it contains RBCs; it has been described as cola-colored. Blood pressure is often elevated. Nonspecific symptoms include weakness, fever, abdominal pain, and malaise. The patient may complain of CVA tenderness.

 CLINICAL CONCEPT

Point tenderness over the flank and CVA tenderness is a classic symptom of kidney infection.

Diagnosis

The gold standard for diagnosing glomerulonephritis is a kidney biopsy, with hallmark glomerular inflammation characterized by increased glomerular cellularity. However, the diagnosis is most often made on a clinical basis without biopsy. CBC and complete metabolic panel are necessary. Serum creatinine and BUN will be modestly elevated in PSGN. Mild anemia is common in the early stages due to decreased erythropoietin secretion. Serum complement levels C3 and C4 are low as they are used up by the formation of immune complexes deposited in the glomerular membranes. Hypoproteinemia is often present due to loss of protein in the urine (proteinuria). A 24-hour urine protein quantification is necessary. Serum electrolytes are usually normal. Urine studies will show a large amount of protein, WBCs, and blood in the urine with hyaline or cellular casts. Urine creatinine clearance will be low because dysfunctional kidneys do not excrete nitrogenous wastes. Creatinine accumulates in the blood. Serum albumin will be low as it is filtered out of the permeable, inflamed glomerulus. Hepatitis B and C and HIV serology testing are necessary. The streptozyme test is used to measure five different types of antistreptococcal antibodies: antistreptolysin O, antihyaluronidase (AHase), antistreptokinase (ASKase), antinicotinamide–adenine dinucleotidase (anti-NAD), and antiDNAse B antibodies. Blood tests for antineutrophil cytoplasmic antibodies (ANCA), anti–double-stranded DNA antibody, and antiglomerular basement membrane (GBM) serology are done to rule out causes of rapidly progressing AGN. Imaging studies do not provide valuable diagnostic information.

Treatment

The management of AGN is based largely upon clinical presentation and symptoms. Antibiotics are necessary if the etiology is poststreptococcal infection. The treatment of glomerulonephritis associated with an active infection is aimed at eradication of the current infection. Antipyretics and analgesics are also needed. If HTN is present, antihypertensive medication is necessary. If edema is present, diuretics may be indicated. Dietary restrictions of sodium and protein are also advised.

IgA Nephropathy

IgA nephropathy is one of the most common forms of glomerulonephritis. There are geographical differences in the incidence of this disease across the world. There is a 30% prevalence in Asia and the Pacific Rim, 20% prevalence in Southern Europe, and much lower prevalence in Northern Europe and North America. There is a male preponderance with peak incidence in the second and third decade of life. The most common clinical presentation includes hematuria, often after a respiratory infection accompanied by proteinuria. The majority of patients have benign disease with complete remission. However, IgA nephropathy can have a rapidly progressive course to renal failure. Deposits of IgA, either alone or with IgG, IgM, and complement protein, are found in the glomerular region of the nephrons. There is an inflammatory type of hypercellularity with destruction of capillaries and fibrosis of the nephron tubules. Angiotensin-converting enzyme inhibitors, corticosteroids, and immunosuppressants have been effective in some patients. Plasmapheresis, a procedure that removes the antibodies from the plasma portion of the bloodstream, has also been used for some patients.

Nephrotic Syndrome

Nephrotic syndrome is a combination of clinical findings that occurs when the glomeruli are damaged. When glomeruli are injured, they become hyperpermeable to proteins and other substances in the bloodstream. The blood becomes depleted of albumin and other large molecules as they enter into the nephron tubules and become excreted with the urine.

Epidemiology

Diabetic nephropathy is the most common type of nephrotic syndrome, with an incidence of 50 to 100 cases per million population per year. Native Americans, Latino Americans, and African Americans have a higher incidence than do European Americans. There is a male predominance in the occurrence of nephrotic syndrome, as there is for CKD in general. However, nephrotic syndrome secondary to SLE is more common in women.

Etiology

Three systemic diseases—DM, amyloidosis, and SLE—are implicated in more than 90% of all cases of nephrotic syndrome in adults. Other causes include immune-complex deposition disease, vasculitis, allergies, preeclampsia, morbid obesity, malignant HTN, and infections such as bacterial endocarditis and tuberculosis. In children, 70% to 90% of cases of nephrotic syndrome are caused by minimal change disease (MCD) which is associated with edema, severe hypoalbuminemia, and massive proteinuria. The cause of MCD is unknown.

Pathophysiology

Glomerular damage occurs either as a primary insult or secondary to one of the causes described. Structural changes that occur in the glomerulus include injury to the endothelial cells, derangement of the basement membrane, and damage to the epithelium. Massive **albuminuria** (also called **proteinuria**) is a consequence of the glomerular damage. As albumin is lost in the vascular space, edema forms because of decreased colloidal osmotic pressure.

Clinical Presentation

Patients have albuminuria with consequent edema. Facial edema is common, especially in the periorbital region. With severe albumin loss, edema of the lower extremities, pleural effusion, and ascites can develop. Patients also often present with hematuria and HTN.

Diagnosis

The work-up for nephrotic syndrome includes urinalysis and blood tests for albumin, BUN, and serum creatinine. Urinalysis usually shows proteinuria and hematuria. Elevations in BUN and serum creatinine occur and are followed to assess renal function. The serum albumin level is classically low in nephrotic syndrome, below its normal range of 3.5 to 4.5 g/dL. Tests for hepatitis B and C, HIV, and lupus, including antinuclear antibody (ANA), anti–double-stranded DNA (antidsDNA) antibodies, and complement, are commonly done when the etiology of nephrotic syndrome is unclear. In immunological etiologies of nephrotic syndrome, complement in the bloodstream is decreased.

A 24-hour urine sample is collected for analysis. The urine can contain up to 3 grams of protein over 24 hours (normal is fewer than 150 mg/day). The urine also contains fatty casts caused by loss of lipoproteins at the glomerulus, which take on the shape of the tubules before excretion into urine. Renal ultrasonography and renal biopsy may be done when etiology is unclear.

Treatment

The patient with nephrotic syndrome needs to be vigilant of nutritional needs. The diet should provide adequate energy (caloric) intake and adequate protein (1 to 2 g/kg/d). However, supplemental dietary protein is of no proven value because it will be excreted. A low-sodium diet (fewer than 1500 g/day) will help to limit fluid overload. Adequate fluid intake is essential, but overhydration should be avoided.

Because albumin levels are low, it is important to recognize that there are fewer binding sites for drugs. This will increase the amount of free active drug in the bloodstream. Also in nephrotic syndrome, immunoglobulins are lost to the urine. This increases susceptibility to infection. Pneumococcal and influenza vaccines should be administered to protect the patient from infection. Angiotensin-converting enzyme (ACE) inhibitors or angiotensin II receptor blockers (ARBs) are used to lower blood pressure. They also slow the progression of kidney disease.

Complications

As nephrotic syndrome progresses, hyperlipidemia may develop secondary to increased lipoprotein synthesis in the liver. As the liver increases synthesis of albumin to replenish the lost albumin in the urine, it also hypersynthesizes lipids. There is commonly an elevation in low-density lipoprotein (LDL) and triglycerides. Hyperlipidemia requires drugs such as statins that decrease liver synthesis of lipids. With increased loss of protein in the urine, there is loss of antithrombin III and plasminogen, the body's natural thrombolytic substances. This increases the risk of thromboembolism, and patients may require anticoagulants (see Fig. 22-8).

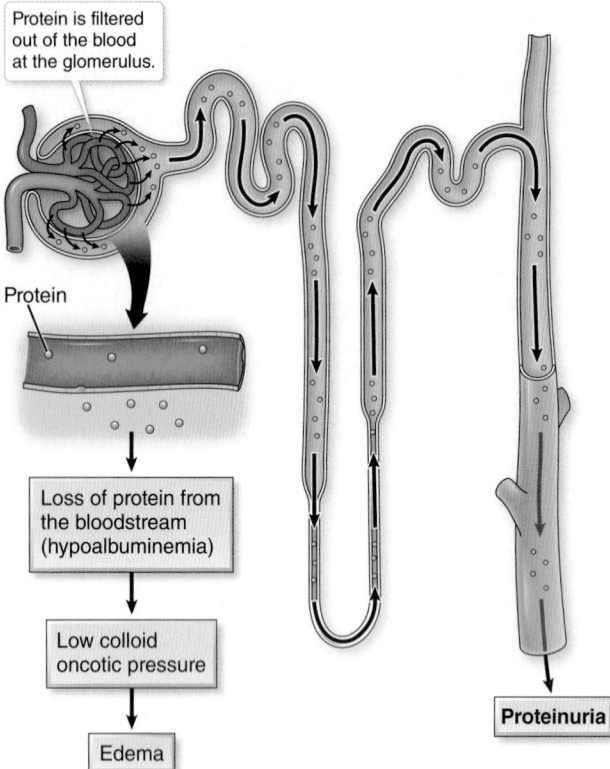

Protein is filtered out of the blood at the glomerulus.

Protein

Loss of protein from the bloodstream (hypoalbuminemia)

Low colloid oncotic pressure

Edema

Proteinuria

FIGURE 22-8. Nephrotic syndrome. In nephrotic syndrome, the glomerulus is damaged, allowing proteins to be filtered out of the bloodstream. The major protein from the bloodstream that is lost is albumin; thus, hypoalbuminemia results. The loss of protein (albumin) from the bloodstream causes decreased colloid oncotic pressure, which leads to edema. Therefore, the signs of nephrotic syndrome are hypoalbuminemia, proteinuria, and edema.

CLINICAL CONCEPT

Hypoalbuminemia, edema, and proteinuria are the three distinguishing features of nephrotic syndrome. Hyperlipidemia and HTN are also associated with nephrotic syndrome.

Nephrolithiasis

Nephrolithiasis is the formation of stones, also called calculi, in the kidney. Calculi can form in the kidney and travel into the ureter, when it is then referred to as urolithiasis. Although pain is a presenting sign with all types of renal calculi, characteristics vary based upon the stone's location.

Epidemiology

In the United States, the lifetime risk of developing nephrolithiasis is approximately 11% for men and 7% for women. Approximately 2 million patients seek health care for kidney stones each year. Dehydration increases susceptibility to kidney stone formation. For this reason, people living in the south and southwest United States have higher incidences of kidney stones than people living in other parts of the country because the hot, dry climate predisposes them to develop dehydration.

Nephrolithiasis is more common in European Americans than in African Americans, and the disease is predominately found in males. Kidney stones most commonly develop in adults aged 20 to 49 years, with a peak incidence at age 35 to 45 years old. The mean age is 44.8 years in men and 40.9 years in women. A family history doubles the risk of kidney stones. Recurrence of nephrolithiasis is common. After suffering a kidney stone, individuals have a 52% chance of suffering another stone within 10 years.

Etiology

The exact cause of nephrolithiasis is unknown, but about 90% of patients who present with clinical manifestations have at least one metabolic risk factor: hypercalcemia, hyperoxaluria, hyperuricemia, hyperparathyroidism, or gout. In addition, low fluid intake is a significant risk factor because dehydration enhances kidney stone formation. There is a genetic predisposition, with more than 30 genetic variations associated with renal calculi development. Differences in intestinal calcium absorption, renal calcium transport, and renal phosphate transport have all been attributed to genetic variation. In patients without specific metabolic or genetic risk factors, nephrolithiasis is attributed to dietary habits, such as excessive calcium supplements and low fluid intake. Hypercalciuria and low fluid content of the urine are the most common predisposing factors that lead to nephrolithiasis (see Box 22-1).

BOX 22-1. Predisposing Factors of Nephrolithiasis

There are many predisposing factors for nephrolithiasis. Nephrolithiasis is usually caused by a number of different conditions that act together to cause precipitation of calculi in the kidney.

- Age greater than 40 years
- Male gender
- Certain medications (e.g., sulfonamides, indinavir, acetazolamides)
- Dietary factors (e.g., purines, calcium, oxalate)
- Gastric bypass surgery
- Geographic location (hot, arid climates)
- Hypercalciuria
- Hyperparathyroidism
- Hyperuricemia
- High-sodium diet
- Inflammatory bowel disease
- Inherited conditions (e.g., polycystic kidney disease, renal tubular acidosis)
- Low hydration/low urine volume
- Obesity
- *Proteus* urinary tract infection

Excessive bone resorption caused by immobility, bone disease, hyperparathyroidism, and renal tubular acidosis are all predisposing risk factors to calcium stone formation. Gout predisposes persons to uric acid stone formation. Gastrointestinal malabsorption due to inflammatory bowel disease or bariatric surgery also predisposes persons to nephrolithiasis. Indinavir, a drug used for HIV infection, predisposes individuals to calcium stones. Urinary tract infection (UTI) and alkaline urine can predispose individuals to struvite (magnesium ammonium phosphate) stones, which are usually large.

 CLINICAL CONCEPT

Struvite stones commonly cause staghorn calculi, which can fill the entire renal pelvis (see Fig. 22-9).

Pathophysiology

The formation of renal calculi involves many different factors that include dietary and intestinal absorption factors, endocrine abnormalities, crystalline components in the blood, constituents of urine, pH of urine, urinary tract structures, and heredity.

The most common renal calculi are:

- Calcium stones
- Struvite stones
- Uric acid stones
- Cystine stones

Seventy-five percent of renal calculi consist of calcium; most are composed of calcium oxalate. The cause for these stones is attributed to hyperabsorption of calcium and oxalate from the gastrointestinal tract.

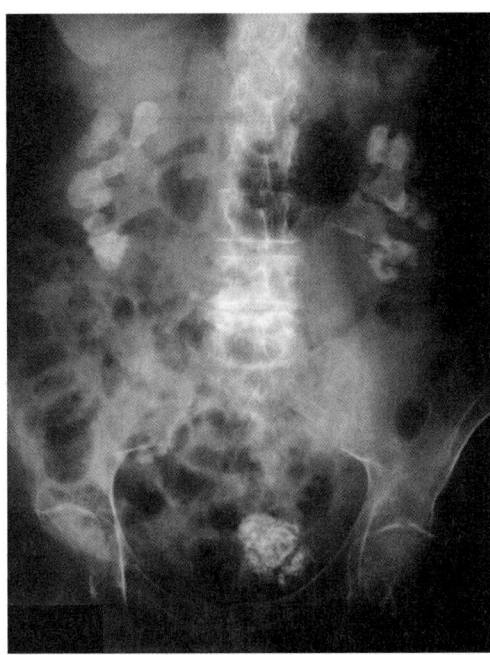

FIGURE 22-9. X-ray showing staghorn calculus. A staghorn calculus is a large calcification that occupies the renal pelvis. *(From Scott Camazine/Science Source.)*

Struvite stones account for 15% of cases and are associated with chronic UTI and specific urine pH. Usual organisms include *Proteus, Pseudomonas,* and *Klebsiella* species; urine pH is typically alkaline, greater than 7. The bacteria possess the enzyme urease, which can react with urea in the urine to form ammonia and carbon dioxide. Ammonia makes the urine alkaline.

Uric acid stones account for 6% of renal calculi and are associated with high purine intake, malignancy, and gout. Purines are derived from the DNA of animal cells or cancer cells. High purine levels in the bloodstream occur with high ingestion of meats or whenever there is high cellular breakdown, as in treatment of malignancy. Approximately 25% of patients with uric acid stones have gout, which is caused by hyperuricemia.

Cystine stones account for 2% of renal calculi and arise because of failure of renal tubular reabsorption of cystine, an amino acid, into the blood. Urine becomes supersaturated with cystine, with resultant crystal deposition.

There are three main theories regarding the formation of renal calculi. The first theory proposes that there is supersaturation of the urine by stone-forming crystalline constituents. Crystals can act as a nucleus, upon which more crystalline constituents settle and build into a calculus. Depending on where it is formed, in the renal pelvis or ureter, the calculus becomes impacted in a site in the ureter as it passes along with urine toward the urinary bladder.

The second theory proposes that there is a deposition of calcium phosphate, a normal compound from breakdown of bone, onto an area of tubule cell membranes in the renal papilla, an area of kidney that empties into the minor calyx. The calcium phosphate compound collects layers of collagenous material and cellular debris, at which point it is called a Randall plaque, within the subepithelial membrane. The plaque collects layers of crystalline elements, becomes a calculus, and eventually erodes through the urothelium of the renal pelvis to enter the ureter.

The third theory suggests that persons with nephrolithiasis have a deficiency of one or all proteins that inhibit stone formation. The kidney is supposed to secrete three types of stone-inhibitors: nephrocalcin, Tamm–Horsfall mucoprotein, and uropontin.

Regardless of etiology or composition, a renal calculus flows into the ureter, becomes impacted, and causes an obstruction. As the stone travels down the ureter, it scrapes against the ureter's membrane, causing minor bleeding into the urine and intense pain. The ureter spasms around the stone, causing a colicky type of pain. Obstruction of urine can lead to increased pressure within the kidney. Based upon the degree of obstruction, the stone can cause backpressure into the renal pelvis, a condition called hydronephrosis. Hydronephrosis occurs when edema and distention of the renal pelvis interfere with renal blood flow and function (see Fig. 22-10). Prolonged hydronephrosis

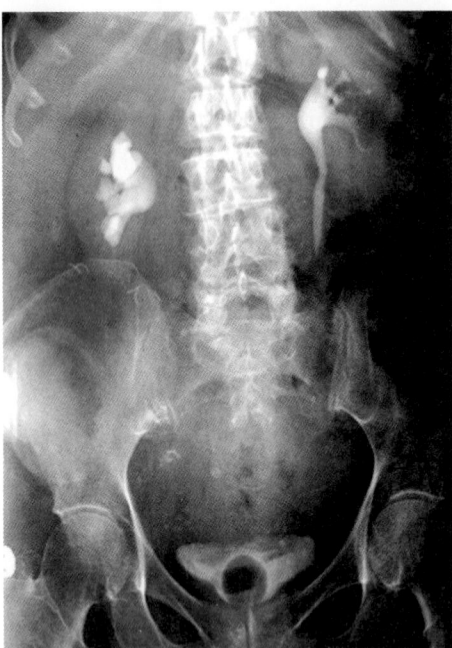

FIGURE 22-10. X-ray showing swelling of the renal pelvis termed hydronephrosis. It can develop in cases of severe obstruction of urine outflow. *(From Living Art Enterprises, LLC/Science Source.)*

causes compression of the kidney tissue, ischemia, and irreversible kidney damage.

Clinical Presentation

Pain is the major symptom of nephrolithiasis. The pain is described as renal or ureteral colic because it occurs in waves. It is also described as acute, excruciating pain in the flank and upper outer quadrant of the abdomen on the affected side, and it is often accompanied by radiating pain into the lower abdomen and groin (see Fig. 22-11). The patient is commonly bent over. They may writhe in pain or pace in an attempt to change their position to try to find one that is comfortable. Pain related to distention of the renal pelvis and calyx causes a dull, deep ache in the flank or back that may

vary in intensity. This type of pain is often associated with increased intake of fluids that distends the calyx. Because of the intensity of the pain, the patient often presents with cool, clammy skin; nausea; and vomiting. Hematuria is noted because of damage caused by obstruction or movement of the stone.

 CLINICAL CONCEPT

Flank pain with radiation into the groin, hematuria, and crystalluria are classic signs of nephrolithiasis.

Diagnosis

The clinical presentation may be similar with varying types of stones; therefore, a definitive diagnosis requires stone analysis. The patient should strain their urine during the course of passing the stone. Kidney stones can vary from the size of the head of a pin to the size of a piece of gravel or larger (see Fig. 22-12). Serum electrolytes, creatinine, calcium, and uric acid should be measured in the blood. Routine urinalyses are conducted, along with analysis of any stone fragments. Urinalysis is done to check for key signs of nephrolithiasis or urolithiasis (stone in the ureter): hematuria, infection, and crystalluria. Two collections of 24-hour urine that analyze volume, calcium oxalate, citrate, uric acid, sodium, potassium, phosphorus, pH and creatinine are recommended. Serum PTH level and vitamin D levels should be measured if there are high urine calcium levels. The gold standard diagnostic test is a helical noncontrast CT scan. Renal ultrasound is also useful as an alternative imaging study.

Treatment

The approach to definitive treatment is based upon symptom management, as well as the type and composition of the renal calculi. Pain relief is a priority because of the excruciating nature of the pain that interferes with activities of daily living. Antibiotics may be necessary if UTI is present. Most renal stones

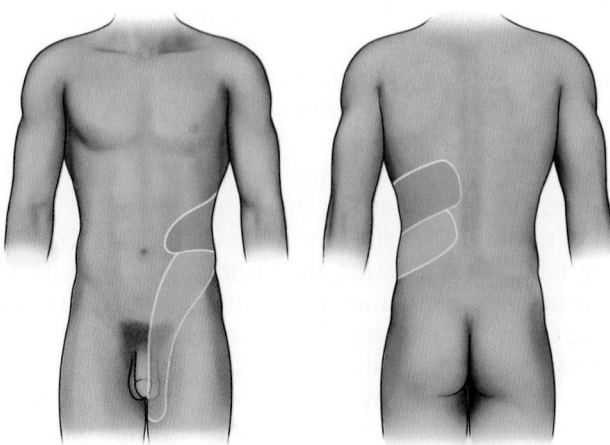

FIGURE 22-11. Pain of nephrolithiasis usually begins in the costovertebral angle region of the back and radiates around into the abdomen and down into the groin.

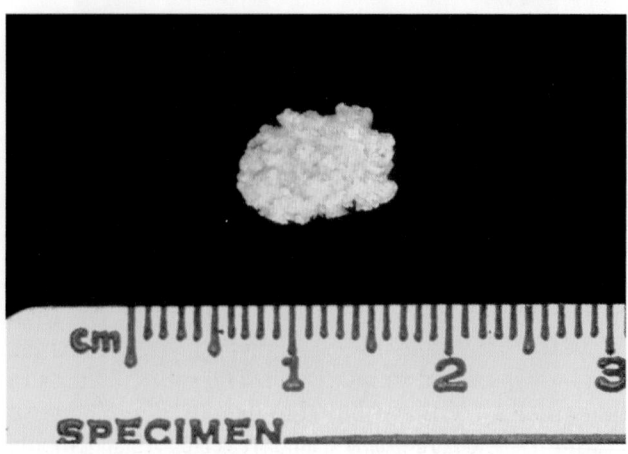

FIGURE 22-12. Kidney stone. *(From Southern Illinois University/Science Source.)*

will pass spontaneously with administration of large amounts of fluid to increase urine volume. Patients are instructed to drink at least 3 liters of fluid a day and strain all urine. If the patient cannot pass the stone, extracorporeal shock wave lithotripsy (ESWL) is often used. Lithotripsy utilizes sound waves to break up the stone into smaller particles to facilitate passage. If lithotripsy is unsuccessful, ureterocystoscopic surgery may be necessary.

A major treatment goal in the patient with nephrolithiasis is to prevent recurrence, and this is largely dependent on determining the stone composition. Dietary changes may be necessary. High doses of thiazide diuretics can reduce the risk of calcium stone formation. Allopurinol can also prevent formation of calcium stones. Citrate supplementation in the form of potassium citrate can prevent calcium, uric acid, and cystine stone formation.

Calcium phosphate, calcium carbonate, and magnesium phosphate stones develop in alkaline urine; when this occurs, the urine is kept acidic. Uric acid, cystine, and calcium oxalate stones precipitate in acidic urine; in this situation, the urine should be kept alkaline or less acidic than normal. Meat and cranberry juice can keep the pH of urine acidic. A diet rich in citrus fruits, legumes, and vegetables raises the pH and produces urine that is more alkaline.

Complications

Infection is one complication that may develop related to damage to renal tissue and urinary stasis. With a UTI, there is a risk for pyelonephritis or urosepsis. Although uncommon, with bilateral stones, renal damage caused by scarring from stone formation may lead to acute or chronic kidney disease. Hydronephrosis is a serious complication that occurs because of complete obstruction of urine outflow that causes urine to back up into the renal pelvis and destroy kidney tissue.

Pyelonephritis

Pyelonephritis is an infection of the renal pelvis and interstitium. It can be either acute or chronic and is most often caused by bacteria that ascend from the lower urinary tract.

Epidemiology

The estimated annual incidence of pyelonephritis is 459,000 to 1,138,000 cases in the United States. Generally, the percentage of patients who are hospitalized is lower than 20% among young women but higher among young children and adults older than 65 years. The incidence is higher in young women, commonly related to lower UTI. The rate increases in older males and is attributed to increased incidence of prostate enlargement, which can obstruct urine outflow. Approximately 20% to 30% of pregnant women develop pyelonephritis.

Etiology

Risk factors for lower urinary tract infection such as sexual activity, new sexual partner, spermicide exposure, and history of UTI also confer a predisposition to pyelonephritis. However, less than 3% of cases of cystitis and asymptomatic bacteriuria progress to pyelonephritis. Pyelonephritis usually occurs when bacteria from the GI tract enter the bladder and ascend to the kidneys. The anatomical proximity of the anus and urethra in women increases risk of urinary tract infection.

Pyelonephritis also commonly occurs if there is obstruction somewhere in the renal system, also referred to as obstructive uropathy. Obstructive uropathy can be caused by calculi in the ureter, tumor, or pregnancy. Whenever there is obstructed outflow of urine, the stagnant urine acts as a medium for bacterial growth, which can ascend into the kidney to cause pyelonephritis.

An anatomical abnormality called **vesicoureteral reflux** is a common predisposing factor for pyelonephritis. Reflux of urine occurs from the bladder into the ureter. The refluxed urine acts as a medium for bacterial growth, which leads to ascending bacterial infection (see Fig. 22-13). Neurogenic bladder is another condition that predisposes individuals to ascending bacterial infection and pyelonephritis. Neurogenic bladder occurs in patients with conditions such as multiple sclerosis, spinal cord injury, or transection of pelvic parasympathetic nerves. Because of the lack of neurological control of the bladder, the patient is unable to empty the bladder completely, and urine retention is common. The retained urine acts as a medium for bacterial growth, and ascending infection leads to pyelonephritis.

Another risk factor for pyelonephritis is urological instrumentation with catheters or cystoscopes.

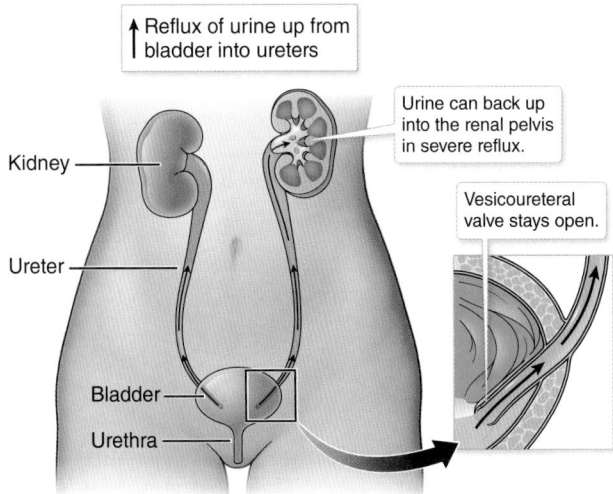

FIGURE 22-13. Vesicoureteral reflux (VUR). Urine should flow in one direction—down from the kidneys, through the ureters, to the bladder. VUR is the abnormal flow of urine from the bladder back up into the ureters.

Instruments can introduce pathogens into the bladder during procedures. Lastly, pregnancy increases the risk of pyelonephritis, partly because of obstruction by the enlarged uterus and partly because of ureteral relaxation secondary to elevated progesterone levels.

Pathophysiology

The pathophysiology of pyelonephritis varies based upon whether the condition is acute or chronic. With acute pyelonephritis, an inflammatory process develops, usually secondary to infection. Most often the infection ascends from the lower urinary tract and is associated with gram-negative bacteria. Less frequently, the infection is from the bloodstream and is most often secondary to a *Staphylococcus aureus* infection.

Chronic pyelonephritis occurs because of repeated kidney infection. Because of recurrent infections and inflammatory processes, permanent changes develop in the renal tissue that increase susceptibility to infection. Any deformity, scar, or fibrotic tissue can cause reflux of urine or stagnant urine that leads to growth of microorganisms and an infectious process.

Clinical Presentation

The clinical presentation of acute pyelonephritis includes fever, chills, flank or groin pain, CVA tenderness, urinary frequency, and dysuria. Flank or CVA pain can be mild or severe, but the patient usually feels a general malaise. Nausea and vomiting commonly accompany this disorder. Hematuria is present in 30% to 40% of patients. The patient may or may not present with signs of lower UTI such as dysuria, urgency, and frequency. Symptoms can develop gradually and can be present for weeks before the patient seeks health care. In patients with chronic pyelonephritis, the clinical manifestations may be more subtle; patients present with urinary frequency, dysuria, and flank pain, with HTN possibly accompanying these symptoms. Chronic pyelonephritis may present more insidiously, particularly with unilateral involvement. As renal function declines because of this disorder, polyuria, nocturia, and proteinuria are common.

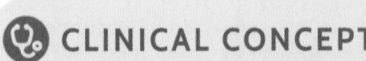

CLINICAL CONCEPT

Costovertebral tenderness, fever, chills, and pyuria are classic signs of pyelonephritis.

Diagnosis

In both acute and chronic processes, urine cultures are important diagnostic tools. The most common bacteria that cause acute pyelonephritis are uropathogenic *Escherichia coli.* Others include *S. saprophyticus, Proteus mirabilis,* and *Klebsiella pneumoniae.* On dipstick urinalysis, almost all patients with acute pyelonephritis

have significant pyuria, which is defined as more than 20 WBCs per high power field (hpf).

A positive leukocyte esterase test is found with presence of WBCs in the urine. The nitrite test can be used for bacteriuria and is usually positive, though it may be falsely negative in the presence of diuretic use, low dietary nitrate, or organisms that do not produce nitrate reductase, such as *Enterococcus, Pseudomonas,* or *Staphylococcus.* The cardinal confirmatory test is the urine culture, which typically yields 10,000 or more colony-forming units of a uropathogen per milliliter of urine. Gross hematuria usually does not occur in pyelonephritis but is more common with cystitis, calculi, cancer, glomerulonephritis, tuberculosis, trauma, and vasculitis. Microscopic hematuria may be present in patients with uncomplicated acute pyelonephritis, but other causes also should be considered, particularly calculi. Proteinuria is expected (up to 2 g/day). When it exceeds 3 g/day, glomerulonephritis should be considered.

Blood cultures to rule out sepsis may be necessary in ambiguous cases (e.g., in populations with a high prevalence of asymptomatic bacteriuria or in patients who have received previous antimicrobial therapy). Imaging studies are reserved for patients with suspected obstruction or a new decrease in the glomerular filtration rate to 40 mL/minute or lower (which is suggestive of obstruction). Noncontrast, helical CT scan or renal ultrasound are recommended.

Treatment

Acute pyelonephritis is usually treated with antibiotic therapy; antibiotic selection depends on the specific microorganism identified by urine culture. Antipyretic medications and analgesics may be necessary. The patient is advised to drink large amounts of water (e.g., 3 L per day). If symptoms recur, repeat urine cultures are recommended at 1 and 4 weeks after completion of the antibiotic regimen. For patients with hypovolemia, extended care in the emergency department or observation unit for more extensive resuscitation and initial intravenous antimicrobial therapy may be necessary. Hospital admission is warranted for patients who have severe illness, unstable coexisting medical conditions, an unreliable psychosocial situation, or no acceptable oral therapy option.

Treatment of chronic pyelonephritis includes management of an infectious process and prevention of further renal function deterioration. During exacerbations of chronic pyelonephritis, antibiotics are administered. If an obstruction is found to be the underlying cause of the recurrent infections, the obstruction must be relieved for cure.

Complications

With appropriate treatment of acute pyelonephritis, long-term complications are infrequent. Bacteremia can occur in 20% to 30% cases of pyelonephritis. Emphysematous pyelonephritis can occur if there are gas-excreting pathogens. This almost exclusively occurs in patients with preexisting DM. Pyelonephritis can also be complicated by abscess formation, which should be suspected if there is continual fever or bacteremia despite antibacterial treatment. Xanthogranulomatous pyelonephritis is an aggressive, rare form of chronic pyelonephritis. Chronic renal insufficiency deteriorating to renal failure may develop in the patient with chronic pyelonephritis. It is estimated that 10% to 20% of ESRD is secondary to chronic pyelonephritis.

Polycystic Kidney Disease

Polycystic kidney disease (PKD) is a genetic disorder that affects the kidneys and other organs. Because of the development of cysts in the renal tissue, renal function is impaired. Typically discovered in affected subjects during young adulthood, the progressive formation of cysts can number in the hundreds to thousands by age 50. Kidney enlargement occurs due to cysts. Kidneys can increase to four times normal size and weigh up to 20 times normal weight. Cysts also develop in other organs of the body, such as the liver.

Epidemiology

PKD affects approximately 600,000 people in the United States. It is the fourth leading cause of renal failure. The most common type of PKD is autosomal-dominant polycystic kidney disease (ADPKD), one of the most common inherited disorders. It is the most common hereditary cause of renal disease in adults and accounts for 6% to 8% of patients on dialysis in the United States. It is the most common cause of ESRD in the United States. Almost all people who inherit the ADPKD gene develop renal cysts by the age of 30 years.

The disease can also be inherited because of a recessive gene; this form is referred to as autosomal-recessive polycystic kidney disease (ARPKD). This is a much less common form because both parents must carry the gene in order for an individual to develop the disorder. There is a 5% to 10% incidence of ARPKD with no family history, and this is attributed to a sporadic type of genetic mutation. ARPKD is generally diagnosed in utero or within the neonatal period. HTN and lack of complete formation of the biliary tract and liver are also involved. Pulmonary hypoplasia, characteristic facies, and spine and limb abnormalities can be present in severe neonatal cases, with death from respiratory distress. About 30% of affected newborns die shortly after birth.

Etiology

ADPKD is categorized as either ADPKD 1 or ADPKD 2, depending on the mutation of either of two genes. The majority of cases are ADPKD 1 caused by the *PKD1* genetic mutation located at 16p13.3, which encodes for a protein called polycystin 1. The less common type is ADPKD 2, which involves a mutation at 4q21-22 of the *PKD2* gene, which encodes for a protein called polycystin 2.

Both polycystin 1 and 2 are involved in renal epithelial cell cycle regulation and intracellular transport of calcium. ADPKD 1 is a more severe disease than ADPKD 2.

Pathophysiology

ADPKD leads to formation of fluid-filled cysts in both kidneys. The renal epithelial cell cycle becomes dysfunctional, leading to hyperplasia of renal epithelial cells. The hyperplastic cells cause an outpocketing of the nephron tubule walls, with the formation of cysts that fill with fluid derived from glomerular filtrate. The cystic structures have continual hyperplastic growth and proliferate within the kidney. Glomerular filtrate accumulates in the cysts, and the surrounding normal renal tissue is compressed and damaged. As cysts increase in number and size, the kidneys enlarge. Fibrotic changes occur in the kidneys with time. The cystic structures also develop blood vessels. The blood vessels are extremely fragile and susceptible to rupture, which causes leakage of blood into the cysts. With the entry of blood, the cystic walls stretch, causing excruciating pain. Cysts often rupture into the renal calyces, causing gross hematuria.

Aside from cystic kidneys, patients with ADPKD are also susceptible to disorders of other organs. Cysts can form in the liver, pancreas, and spleen. Diverticula, which are saccular structures that form in the intestinal wall, often occur in the colon. Heart valve problems such as mitral valve prolapse commonly develop, causing heart murmur. Cerebral aneurysms occur four to five times more frequently in ADPKD patients than the general population. Cerebral aneurysms are weakened areas of a cerebral artery that are prone to rupture, which can lead to hemorrhagic stroke. Thoracic aortic aneurysm is also a common problem in patients with ADPKD. ADPKD also increases susceptibility to renal carcinoma.

Clinical Presentation

Patients with ADPKD usually present with pain caused by the pressure associated with fluid accumulation in the cysts. Because of stagnation of fluid within the cysts, uric acid and calcium crystals can precipitate and renal calculi can develop, which cause obstruction. In these cases, the patient presents with the pain of renal colic and hematuria. The kidneys cannot concentrate the urine; therefore, urine concentration defects occur with polyuria. Proteinuria, the loss of proteins into the urine, is a prognostic indicator in ADPKD. Stagnation of fluid within the cysts also increases susceptibility to kidney infection. CVA tenderness, fever, and pyuria occur if pyelonephritis develops. In addition, cysts place pressure on kidney blood vessels, which activates the RAAS. If this occurs, the patient will present with hypervolemia and HTN. The patient with ADPKD can demonstrate various symptoms, depending on the involvement of other organs, such as the heart, colon, cerebral arteries, thoracic aorta, liver, spleen, or pancreas. By age 60, 50% of persons with ADPKD develop renal failure.

Diagnosis

Ultrasonography and abdominal CT scans are used in diagnosis. In 80% to 90% of people with ADPKD, cysts are detectable by the age of 20 years via CT scanning. MRI is the best diagnostic study that can visualize cysts in the kidneys and extrarenal organs. The number of MRI-detected cysts considered to be diagnostic is more than 10 in those aged 16 to 40 years. MRI can also rule out renal carcinoma. Genetic testing can be used to determine the type of disease. Serum chemistry profiles should include calcium and uric acid levels. Urinalysis shows microalbuminuria. Magnetic resonance angiography should be used to investigate the possibility of cerebral aneurysms.

Treatment

Treatment consists of controlling HTN, preventing UTIs, and tolvaptan, a recently approved drug. Tolvaptan is a vasopressin receptor 2 antagonist that can decrease formation of cysts in the kidney. ACE inhibitors or ARBs are commonly used to control blood pressure. A low-sodium diet and increased fluid intake of greater than 3 L/day are recommended. Acute flank pain is often associated with kidney cyst hemorrhage, infection, or kidney stones. Chronic pain is usually attributable to cyst enlargement that causes kidney capsule stretching or marked enlargement of the kidneys. Smoking cessation, maintenance of normal body weight, and daily physical activity are also recommended. Reversing metabolic imbalances associated with ESRD is necessary. Conditions such as hyperkalemia, hypocalcemia, and metabolic acidosis require treatment. UTIs are common in ADPKD, and antibiotic treatment is needed. Large cysts of the kidney can be surgically decompressed if they cause severe pain. Hemodialysis is necessary if the disease progresses to ESRD. Patients are usually eligible for kidney transplant. Development of cysts in the liver, hepatomegaly, and liver failure can occur in ADPKD. Patients may require liver transplant.

Goodpasture's Syndrome

Antiglomerular basement membrane (anti-GBM) disease is an immunological disease of the kidney. The disorder is an acute, rapidly progressive type of glomerulonephritis caused by circulating autoantibodies. These antibodies are directed against an antigen intrinsic to the collagen in the glomerular basement membrane (GBM). When this disease includes lung involvement, usually in the form of pulmonary hemorrhage, it is considered a pulmonary-renal syndrome called **Goodpasture's syndrome**.

Epidemiology

Goodpasture's syndrome is an uncommon disorder that affects 1% to 2% of the U.S. population annually. This autoimmune disease affects the kidney and lungs. It is more common in European Americans than African Americans. Most commonly, young adults from age 20 to 30 years, as well as older adults aged 60 to 70 years, develop the disease. Among young adults, men are more likely to develop the disease. Among older adults, women are predominately affected compared with men. Between 60% and 80% of patients have clinically apparent manifestations of pulmonary and renal disease, 20% to 40% have renal disease alone, and fewer than 10% have disease that is limited to the lungs.

Etiology

Goodpasture's syndrome is an autoimmune disease of unknown etiology. Autoantibodies develop against the collagen in renal glomerular membranes and pulmonary alveolar membranes. There is a strong genetic predisposition in Goodpasture's syndrome, and persons with the specific tissue type HLA-DR15 are more susceptible than others. Pulmonary involvement is influenced by factors that increase the permeability of the alveolar–capillary membrane such as smoking, infection, or exposure to solvents.

Pathophysiology

In Goodpasture's syndrome, autoantibodies develop against a specific type of collagen within the glomerular and alveolar membranes and initiate an inflammatory process. Direct immunofluorescence techniques demonstrate linear deposition of immunoglobulins in the glomerular and alveolar membranes. Persons with tissue type HLA-DR15, HLA DRB1*1501, and HLA-B7 are at high risk for the disorder in the kidney and lungs. T cells play a key role in the initiation of the disorder. T cells assist B cells to secrete immunoglobulins that attack kidney and lung membranes. Glomerular inflammation causes decreased nephron function. The ability of the kidneys to filter blood and excrete urine is impaired. Autoantibody attacks on alveolar membranes cause diminished gas exchange and inflammatory changes in the lungs.

Clinical Presentation

The patient with Goodpasture's syndrome presents with nonspecific symptoms of malaise, chills, and fever. Renal manifestations include hematuria, edema, high blood pressure, and eventually renal failure. Along with pulmonary involvement, dyspnea, pleuritic chest pain, cough, and hemoptysis are common initial signs. Massive pulmonary hemorrhage is possible, which is a medical emergency. Physical examination reveals tachypnea, tachycardia, cyanosis, pulmonary crackles, and HTN.

Diagnosis

Blood tests can determine the presence of anti-GBM antibodies. Radioimmunoassays or enzyme-linked immunosorbent assays for anti-GBM antibodies should be performed. Positive results should be confirmed by a Western blot test. The titer of anti-GBM antibodies can be used to monitor the severity of disease and efficacy of treatment. Antineutrophilic cytoplasmic antibodies (ANCAs) can also develop, and a titer for this antibody is commonly done. Urinalysis demonstrates proteinuria, hematuria, and RBC casts. The complete blood count (CBC) may show anemia secondary to pulmonary bleeding. There is leukocytosis, elevated BUN, and serum creatinine. Kidney biopsy may be necessary, but is preferably avoided because the kidney is a highly vascular organ and severe bleeding is common. Renal biopsy show focal or segmental necrosis and crescent formations in the Bowman's capsule region. Immunofluorescent staining shows IgG antibodies and complement proteins. Chest x-ray shows bilateral hilar lymphadenopathy and consolidations throughout both lung fields. Pulmonary function testing will reveal a restrictive disease pattern.

Treatment

Plasmapheresis is a process of filtering the blood that can remove anti-GBM and other antibodies. Oral prednisone and cyclophosphamide are used with plasmapheresis. Maintenance treatment with immunosuppressants such as rituximab or azathioprine can be used to stop further production of antibodies. Various pulmonary treatments may be needed, depending on the disorder. Dialysis or kidney transplantation may be indicated if disease deteriorates to ESRD. However, anti-GBM disease can occur in the newly transplanted kidney as well.

Acute Kidney Injury

AKI, previously called acute renal failure, is related to an abrupt insult to the kidney that causes a rapid decrease in renal filtration function. It usually occurs in the setting of acute or chronic illness. It is a sudden decrease in glomerular filtration rate manifested by an increase in serum creatinine and oliguria. Because of this decline in function, nitrogenous waste products accumulate in the body. AKI is staged based on the magnitude of rise in serum creatinine and duration of oliguria. With appropriate interventions, normal renal function can return, usually within 2 weeks to 3 months of the initial precipitating event.

Epidemiology

AKI occurs in 20% of hospitalized patients yearly in the United States. In critical care units, up to 67% of patients have AKI. AKI also develops postoperatively in approximately 1% of general surgery cases. Because of an aging population and increasing prevalence of HTN and DM, from 2005 to 2014, the number of hospitalizations with a principal diagnosis of acute kidney injury increased from 281,500 to 504,600, and the number of hospitalizations with a secondary diagnosis of acute kidney injury increased from 1 million to 2.3 million. Morbidity of AKI in those admitted to the ICU exceeds 50%. AKI increases risk for development of CKD and development of dialysis-requiring ESRD.

Etiology

There are various causes of AKI, but the major cause is reduced renal blood flow that in turn reduces GFR. Acute illness, complications of medications, and medical procedures are the most common causes of AKI. Older age and preexisting CKD are the main susceptibility factors. As renal function decreases, there is an accumulation of nitrogenous wastes and impairment of fluid and electrolyte balance. AKI is frequently superimposed on other conditions affecting the patient. There are three classifications of AKI:

1. Prerenal azotemia
2. Intrinsic renal disease
3. Postrenal obstruction

Approximately 60% of patients suffer AKI because of prerenal azotemia disorders. The prefix "azo" means nitrogen, the suffix "emia" means in the blood. It is the designation for a rise in serum creatinine and BUN concentration due to inadequate renal blood flow to support the hydrostatic pressure needed for glomerular filtration. Decreased blood flow is the major cause of prerenal AKI and is usually reversible with timely treatment. This type of AKI can occur any time there is an extreme drop in blood volume. Various shock states, including hypovolemic, cardiogenic, and septic shock, which result in decreased renal perfusion, lead to prerenal AKI. Ischemia associated with prolonged blood loss due to hemorrhage from trauma or surgery can also cause AKI. Severe burns over the body can also cause extensive fluid loss, which causes lack of blood flow to the kidney. Prolonged renal hypoperfusion will cause damage of the nephron tubule epithelial cells, a condition known as **acute tubular necrosis (ATN)**.

Intrinsic renal disease as a cause of AKI is due to actual damage to kidney tissue often associated with nephrotoxic agents, infectious processes, trauma, or obstruction of nephron tubules. A common cause of AKI is ATN caused by nephrotoxic agents. Common nephrotoxic agents include NSAIDs, aminoglycoside antibiotics, chemotherapeutic agents, and radiopaque dye used in imaging studies. Angiotensin-converting enzyme inhibitors (ACEi) and angiotensin II receptor blockers (ARBs) can also cause changes in the vasoregulatory mechanisms of the kidney and can decrease perfusion leading to AKI. Infectious processes such as glomerulonephritis or pyelonephritis can cause intrinsic AKI. Obstruction of nephron tubules can occur in disorders that cause excretion of a large amount of breakdown products from hemoglobin, myoglobin, or purines. These breakdown products in need of excretion can overwhelm the nephron tubules. For example, hemoglobinuria is seen in transfusion reactions and other hemolytic disorders. Myoglobinuria can occur in severe muscle trauma or extreme exertion. Excessive purines within the bloodstream occur when there is a massive tumor or cellular destruction. For example, in chemotherapy, a large amount of cellular deterioration occurs; tumor cell breakdown releases purines, which are DNA breakdown products. These can overwhelm the nephron tubules.

Postrenal AKI develops secondary to obstruction of urine outflow. Obstruction of urine outflow leads to retrograde pressure and interference with glomerular filtration in the involved kidney. There is an abrupt increase in intratubular pressure within the nephrons that can cause AKI. Obstruction can occur in nephrolithiasis, ureteral stricture, prostatic enlargement, or obstructive bladder disorders. Approximately 5% of AKI cases are caused by postrenal etiologies.

Pathophysiology

Decreased glomerular filtration of the blood in AKI leads to azotemia, high serum creatinine, and fluid retention. AKI can be divided into four phases:

1. Initial
2. Oliguria
3. Diuresis
4. Recovery

The initial phase usually last hours or days and is determined as the time from the precipitating insult until the time of initial manifestations of AKI. The oliguric phase is associated with a significant decrease in GFR, as well as retention of urea, potassium, sulfate, and creatinine. Urine formation is usually decreased during this time and is accompanied by signs of fluid overload. The nephrons are filled with WBCs, and inflammation occurs. In the diuretic phase, the kidneys are beginning to recover from the initial insult. Healing occurs, and fibrotic tissue may begin to form in regions of damaged nephrons. The urine output is high; however, it may not be sufficiently concentrated or diluted. Urine may have the same osmolarity as the bloodstream. This indicates that the kidney is excreting urine that does not contain all waste products from the bloodstream. The recovery phase is the time needed for final repair of renal damage and usually starts with the onset of increased urine output. During this phase, nephrons that are healthy compensate for those nephrons that are damaged. The undamaged nephrons demonstrate hyperfiltration and hypertrophic

changes and can perform normal clearance of solutes from the bloodstream. During the recovery phase, urine is appropriately concentrated, inflammation is diminished, and renal function returns to normal. This stage can last months, and scar tissue is apparent in regions of kidney damage.

Clinical Presentation

The patient's clinical presentation is influenced by the cause of AKI. For example, AKI caused by autoimmune disease will present with different symptoms than AKI due to renal trauma. However, regardless of etiology, AKI causes oliguria and fluid overload. Nitrogenous waste builds up in the blood, and signs and symptoms of uremia, such as encephalopathy, anemia, hyperkalemia, metabolic acidosis, thrombocytopenia, and neuromuscular irritability, occur. Encephalopathy can be manifested as confusion, disorientation, to a stuporous mental change depending on the severity of the kidney dysfunction. Hyperkalemia can cause cardiac rhythm changes and requires continuous ECG monitoring. Thrombocytopenia can cause spontaneous bleeding or bruising. As urine output decreases, signs of fluid overload, such as edema of the face and extremities, occur. Pulmonary edema can develop, causing respiratory distress. Arterial blood gases should be monitored. As renal function returns, the patient demonstrates a diuresis phase, with urine output increasing to 1 to 2 liters per day and resolution of hypervolemia.

Diagnosis

The presence of AKI is defined by an elevation in the serum creatinine or reduction in urine output. AKI is confirmed by a rise in serum creatinine by at least 0.3 mg/mL within 48 hours or at least 50% higher than baseline within 1 week, or a reduction in urine output greater than 0.5 mL/kg/hr longer than 6 hours. The stage of AKI is determined using these parameters (see Table 22.2). Anuria usually does not occur in AKI; whereas oliguria (less than 400 mL/24 hours) is common.

Urinalysis, serum electrolytes, serum creatinine, BUN, arterial blood gases, protein biomarkers, and CBC

TABLE 22-2. Stages of AKI

KIDNEY DISEASE: IMPROVING GLOBAL OUTCOMES STAGING OF AKI IN ADULTS		
Stage	Serum Creatinine	Urine Output
Stage 1	1.5–1.9 times baseline (or ≥0.3 mg increase)	<0.5 mg/kg/h for 6–12 hrs
Stage 2	2.0–2.9 times baseline	<0.5 mg/kg/h for ≥12 hrs
Stage 3	>3 times baseline or >4 mg/dL or initiation of renal replacement treatment	<0.3 mg/kg/h for ≥24 hrs or anuria ≥12 hrs

From: Acute Kidney Injury Work Group (2012). Kidney disease: Improving global outcome (KDIGO). KDIGO clinical practice guidelines for acute kidney injury. *Kidney Int Suppl, 2* (suppl 1), 19.

are used in the diagnosis of AKI. Buildup of nitrogenous wastes in the blood, manifested as an elevated BUN, is a hallmark of AKI. When BUN rises >100 mg/dL, mental status changes and thrombocytopenia can occur.

Analysis of the urinary sediment by a nephrologist can lead to confirmation of the cause of AKI. For example, prerenal azotemia usually presents with unremarkable urinary sediment. Proteinuria suggests damage to the glomerulus. AKI due to ATN usually yields pigmented "muddy brown" casts. Glomerulonephritis can yield red blood cells or red blood cell casts in the urine.

The CBC will commonly reveal anemia. AKI often leads to hyperkalemia, hyperphosphatemia, hypocalcemia, and metabolic acidosis. Other recommended laboratory blood tests that can indicate glomerulonephritis and vasculitis include low complement levels, antinuclear antibodies, antineutrophil cytoplasmic antibodies (ANCAs), and anti-GBM antibodies.

There are biomarkers for AKI including kidney injury molecule (KIM-1), which can be detected in the urine and blood after ischemic or nephrotoxic injury. Neutrophil gelatinase associated lipocalin (NGAL) is present in blood and urine in inflammatory conditions of the kidney.

Radiographic imaging may be used to assess for any type of obstructive process or changes in the kidneys' size and structure. Findings of obstruction include dilation of the kidney pelvis and hydronephrosis. Vascular imaging may be useful if venous or arterial obstruction is suspected, but the risks of contrast dye administration should be kept in mind. MRI with gadolinium-based contrast agents should be avoided. A renal biopsy may be used to evaluate for intrarenal etiology of AKI.

Treatment

In 2012, Kidney Disease: Improving Global Outcomes (KDIGO) published a guideline on the classification and management of AKI. Since then, some new evidence has arisen that has implications for clinical practice. In general, management principles for AKI include determination of volume status, fluid resuscitation with isotonic crystalloid, treatment of volume overload with diuretics, discontinuation of nephrotoxic medications, and adjustment of prescribed drugs according to renal function. Additional supportive care measures include optimizing nutritional status and glycemic control.

Treatment of AKI depends on the underlying cause. With prerenal AKI, fluid administration is indicated. Crystalloid solutions such as lactated Ringer's solution are recommended. Once the patient develops oliguria, diuretics such as furosemide (Lasix) may be used cautiously. Electrolytes are monitored; with hyperkalemia, cardiac monitoring is necessary. Discontinuation of renin-angiotensin-aldosterone inhibitors and NSAIDs is recommended. Pharmacist consultation on the effect of patient medications on renal function is recommended. In patients who do not have rapid resolution of AKI, continuous renal replacement therapy (CRRT) or hemodialysis may be indicated. Patients with AKI requiring renal dialysis and other forms of renal replacement therapy are 50 times more likely to progress to CKD than those not requiring renal replacement therapy. CRRT is a blood purification process that occurs over 24 hours within a critical care setting, whereas hemodialysis is an intermittent process occurring a few times a week. CRRT is preferred in patients with hemodynamic instability, cerebral edema, or severe hypovolemia. Peritoneal dialysis can be used alternatively, which may be better tolerated in some patients.

Nutrition should provide adequate calories with restricted potassium and phosphate. KDIGO guidelines for patients with AKI recommends a total energy intake of 20–30 kcal/kg per day. Minimal nitrogenous waste production is desirable in AKI; however, protein restriction is not recommended.

Chronic Kidney Disease

CDK is an irreversible, progressive disease process. Gradual in onset, the disease may develop over months to years, with 90% to 95% of the nephrons affected. CKD can progress to ESRD. In ESRD, kidney function deteriorates to the point that the kidney is unable to excrete waste products or control volume status, making dialysis or a kidney transplant the only options to support life.

Epidemiology

The incidence of CKD continues to increase in the United States. This increase is partially explained by the increase in the prevalence of DM and HTN, the two most common causes of CKD. It is estimated that almost 8% of adults 20 years old and older have some evidence of CKD based upon a severely reduced GFR. The highest incidence rate of ESRD occurs in older adults. The prevalence of CKD is 38% among patients older than 70 years. The incidence of CRF is significantly greater in the African American population, which may be attributed to increased HTN in this population. A great number of genetic mutations have been discovered that correlate with increased predisposition to CKD. Genetic predisposition, secondary illness, lifestyle, and environmental factors all contribute to the development of CKD. In the United States 37 million persons have CKD, which is approximately 7% of the population. Forty-eight percent of persons with severely reduced kidney function are unaware of their kidney disease. The mortality rate for patients with CKD is high; patients with late-stage CKD have more than a 75% mortality rate.

Etiology

There are numerous causes of CKD, with DM, HTN, glomerulonephritis, and ADPKD the leading etiologies (see Box 22-2).

> ## BOX 22-2. Causes of Chronic Kidney Disease
>
> There are many different etiologies and risk factors for CKD. Many different conditions can lead to CKD. The two most common are DM and HTN.
> - Family history of kidney disease
> - Age greater than 60 years
> - Atherosclerosis
> - Bladder obstruction
> - Chronic glomerulonephritis
> - Congenital kidney disease
> - Diabetes
> - HTN
> - Systemic lupus erythematosus
> - Overexposure to some toxins
> - Sickle cell disease
> - Nephrotoxic medications

Pathophysiology

The pathological changes that occur in CKD are due to significant deterioration of nephrons. CKD is defined as abnormal kidney structure or function lasting more than 3 months with associated health implications. Indicators of CKD include albuminuria, urine sediment abnormalities, abnormal renal imaging findings, serum electrolyte or acid–base imbalances, and GFR less than 60 mL/minute per 1.73 m^2. The patient's GFR needs to be calculated using age, sex, and serum creatinine of the individual. To calculate GFR, clinicians commonly use the Chronic Kidney Disease Epidemiology Collaboration equation (http://www.kidney.org/professionals/kdoqi/gfr_calculator.cfm). CKD can have an insidious onset based upon etiology. The rate of nephron deterioration differs according to etiology and can range from several months to many years. According to the National Kidney Foundation, the progression of CKD usually occurs in five stages:

- Stage 1: kidney damage with normal GFR (greater than 90 mL/min)
- Stage 2: mild reduction in GFR (60 to 89 mL/min)
- Stage 3: moderate reduction in GFR (30 to 59 mL/min)
- Stage 4: severe reduction in GFR (15 to 29 mL/min)
- Stage 5: kidney failure (GFR lower than 15 mL/min)

Glomerular filtration of the bloodstream is accomplished by approximately 1 million nephrons in each kidney. The kidney is a resilient organ because of its huge number of nephrons, more than double the number necessary for maintenance of normal GFR (90 to 120 mL/min). Thus, normal filtration of the blood is possible with only one kidney. With mild kidney damage, which occurs in stages 1 and 2, filtration problems usually do not occur. The patient is usually asymptomatic, and blood and urine tests may appear normal because the functioning nephrons compensate for the damaged nephrons. Hyperfiltration and hypertrophy of the functioning nephrons maintain normal kidney function.

In stage 3, there is diminished renal function, and symptoms start to become apparent because less than 50% of nephrons are functioning. In this stage, there is moderate reduction in GFR, serum creatinine and BUN begin to rise, and creatinine clearance starts to decrease. The functioning nephrons start to become unable to compensate for the lost nephrons. The damaged nephrons start to undergo fibrosis, and glomerulosclerosis is apparent on renal biopsy. In stage 4, a state of renal insufficiency becomes apparent. Nephrons start to become overwhelmed, and GFR is lower than 20% of normal. The kidney's health is precarious in this stage. The patient must restrict dietary protein because remaining healthy nephrons have difficulty removing nitrogenous wastes from the bloodstream. Finally, in stage 5, renal failure develops and GFR falls to less than 5% of normal. At this stage, nephrons cannot accomplish complete filtration of the bloodstream. The kidney's varied functions, such as erythropoietin synthesis, blood pressure maintenance, and acid–base balance, are lost. As a consequence, fluid, electrolyte, and acid–base imbalances occur, and effects on other organ systems become apparent. ESRD occurs with widespread effects of uremia. The term "uremia" actually means urine in the bloodstream. Uremia leads to disturbances in the function of virtually every organ system. The kidneys deteriorate in function and begin to atrophy. Dialysis and renal transplant are the only options for survival.

Clinical Presentation

In CKD, accumulation of nitrogenous wastes causes systemwide symptoms. The brain cannot function in a high nitrogenous environment and encephalopathy occurs—confusion, disorientation, or stupor and coma. Platelets and RBCs lyse because of the blood's high nitrogen content, resulting in thrombocytopenia and anemia. Thrombocytopenia causes bruising and spontaneous bleeding, whereas anemia causes severe fatigue, weakness, and dyspnea. Metabolic acidosis and electrolyte imbalances have varying effects. Hyperkalemia can cause life-threatening cardiac dysrhythmias and extreme muscle weakness. Because the kidneys cannot synthesize vitamin D, calcium absorption from the gastrointestinal tract decreases, causing hypocalcemia, which in turn can cause neuromuscular irritability, tetany, and seizures. Hypocalcemia also stimulates the parathyroid glands to release parathyroid hormone (PTH), which causes bone breakdown. This bone demineralization process is referred to as **renal osteodystrophy**. Bone mineral density is diminished, and fracture susceptibility increases. Peripheral and autonomic neuropathy occur that cause paresthesias and burning in the legs and feet. Restless leg syndrome can occur, which is characterized by ill-defined sensations in the legs that are relieved by movement. Hiccups, abdominal cramps, and muscular twitching can occur. Gastritis, peptic ulcer disease, constipation, and mucosal ulcerations of the GI tract often occur. Uremic fetor, a urine-like odor on the breath, from the breakdown of urea to ammonia in saliva, can occur. Anorexia, nausea, and vomiting due to the retention of toxins is common. Pruritus is very common in CKD, and hyperpigmentation of the skin can occur due to retained metabolites and toxins.

Glucose metabolism is impaired in CKD. Serum glucose and serum insulin levels can be elevated. In women with CKD, estrogen levels are low and menstrual abnormalities, infertility, and inability to carry pregnancies to term are common. Pregnancy can worsen kidney function in women with CKD, and spontaneous abortion is common. Men with CKD have diminished testosterone levels with decreased sperm count and sexual dysfunction.

Diagnosis

A CBC with differential, serum electrolytes, serum creatinine, total albumin, BUN, and urinalysis will demonstrate abnormalities of renal failure. Normochromic normocytic anemia is seen in CKD caused by lack of erythropoietin. Sodium, potassium, bicarbonate, and other electrolytes will be elevated in the bloodstream. Hyperkalemia may cause cardiac dysrhythmias, requiring electrocardiogram (ECG) monitoring. BUN and creatinine levels will be elevated because all nitrogenous wastes are accumulating in the bloodstream. When 50% of nephrons are dysfunctional, serum creatinine rises to approximately double the normal blood level. Patients will have hypoalbuminemia caused by glomerular damage, which causes loss of protein into the urine. Proteinuria is a classic sign of renal dysfunction. Serum calcium and vitamin D levels are low and PTH levels are elevated. CKD causes secondary hyperparathyroidism, which leads to decreased bone density and fragility. Hyperphosphatemia occurs because of hypocalcemia. Renal ultrasound and other imaging studies may be indicated. Other more disease-specific blood tests may be done according to etiology of renal failure.

Urinalysis will likely show protein, RBCs, and WBCs, as these will all be lost in the urine. A 24-hour urine collection for protein and creatinine clearance will show excessive loss of protein. However, a single urine specimen can be used to calculate the protein-to-creatinine ratio, which allows reliable approximation of total 24-hour urinary protein excretion. The calculation usually shows protein loss greater than 2 grams in the urine.

Noninvasive renal imaging studies such as x-ray, ultrasound, CT, and MRI can show any intrarenal masses, cysts, or calcium stones. IV contrast-enhanced studies should be avoided in renal failure.

Treatment

Fluid and electrolyte management is critical to the management of patients with CKD. Excess fluid can lead to heart failure and pulmonary edema. Salt restriction and loop diuretics (e.g., furosemide) are commonly necessary. HTN due to renin hypersecretion and anemia due to lack of erythropoietin develop early during the course of CKD. Blood pressure management is indicated with cautious use of ACE inhibitors or angiotensin receptor blockers. These agents can raise potassium; therefore, potassium levels must be monitored. Erythropoietin-stimulating medications (e.g., epoetin alfa) are also usually administered. Iron supplements are needed when erythropoietin-stimulating agents are administered because of active RBC production. Hyperphosphatemia can be treated with dietary phosphate binders (e.g., PhosLo) and dietary phosphate restriction. Dysfunctioning kidneys do not produce portions of vitamin D; therefore, calcium is not absorbed from the GI tract. This causes hypocalcemia, which stimulates parathyroid hyperfunction. Hypocalcemia can be treated with calcium supplements that contain vitamin D. Calcitriol is synthetic vitamin D. Calcimimetic agents are used to counteract the hyperparathyroid activity. Hyperkalemia can be reduced with potassium-lowering agents, such as patiromer or sodium polystyrene, and low-potassium diet. Dietary salt substitutes should not be used as these are potassium-based. Intractable hyperkalemia is an indication to start dialysis in a CKD patient. Metabolic acidosis can be reversed with sodium bicarbonate administration. Blood glucose levels and serum insulin levels can become abnormal. Certain antidiabetic medications such as metformin and sulfonylureas are contraindicated in CKD. However, the gliflozin antidiabetes medications that inhibit sodium-glucose transport in the nephron (also called SGLT2 inhibitors) are considered renal-protective. SGLT2 inhibitors (e.g., dapagliflozin) can lower blood glucose and stabilize GFR in kidney disease. They have been shown to decrease cellular injury in the proximal tubules of the nephrons in patients with CKD. These medications are currently under study to see if they confer kidney protection in other renal diseases (Wheeler et al., 2020). To counteract pruritus, topical corticosteroids and antihistamines can be used (see Patho-Pharm Connection).

Complications

CKD can progress to ESRD. In ESRD, there are body-wide adverse effects (see Fig. 22-14). As the disease progresses and other systems are involved, the patient may develop respiratory compromise related to fluid overload, HTN, and uremic coma. In ESRD, treatment options include hemodialysis (in clinical setting or

Patho-Pharm Connection

Renal Failure

Continual secretion of renin-angiotensin-aldosterone system - - -> hypertension:
ACE inhibitors (ACEi) or angiotensin receptor blockers (ARBS)

Oliguria - - -> hypervolemia:
Loop diuretics (e.g., furosemide)

Lack of erythropoietin - - -> anemia
Erythropoiesis stimulating agent (e.g., epoetin-alfa)
Iron supplements

Lack of vitamin D - - -> lack of GI absorption of calcium - - -> hypocalcemia - - -> stimulation of parathyroid glands - - ->PTH - - -> bone breakdown:
Calcitriol (vitamin D)
Calcimimetic (e.g., cinacalcet) lowers PTH

Glucose metabolism dysfunction:
Gliflozins (SGLT2 inhibitors)—antidiabetic agents (e.g., dapagliflozin) that are renoprotective

Lack of acid-base balance - - -> metabolic acidosis:
Sodium bicarbonate

Electrolyte imbalances:
Hyperkalemia: patiromer
Hyperphosphatemia: phosphate binders (e.g., PhosLo)
Hypocalcemia: calcium supplement

Dermatologic pruritus:
Topical corticosteroids
Antihistamines

Renal failure causes multiple systemic complications. Pharmacological agents are used to counteract the potential adverse effects. With the kidneys not functioning, fluid balance is disturbed and hypervolemia can occur. Loop diuretics can enhance water loss from the body. The failing kidney does not secrete erythropoietin; therefore, epoetin-alfa (synthetic erythropoietin) is administered. This stimulates RBC production, which requires iron supplementation. Blood pressure (BP) is not controlled when the kidneys fail; HTN occurs due to constant secretion of renin. Therefore, antihypertensive medications such as ACE inhibitors or angiotensin receptor blockers are commonly used to control BP. Vitamin D is not produced when the kidneys fail; therefore, Calcitriol (vitamin D supplement) is

necessary. There is constant stimulation of the parathyroid glands in kidney failure; therefore, calcimimetic medications can decrease parathyroid hormone (PTH). Glucose metabolism is disrupted with kidney failure; therefore, glifozin-type antidiabetic agents are used. Electrolyte disturbances occur such as hyperkalemia, hypocalcemia, and hyperphosphatemia. Patiromer lowers blood potassium level, phosphate binders lower PO_4^-, and calcium supplements can be given. Acid-base balance is not maintained when the kidneys fail and metabolic acidosis occurs. Sodium bicarbonate can counteract acidosis. The nerve endings become hypersensitive due to excess urea in the bloodstream causing pruritus (itching). Topical corticosteroids and antihistamines can be used.

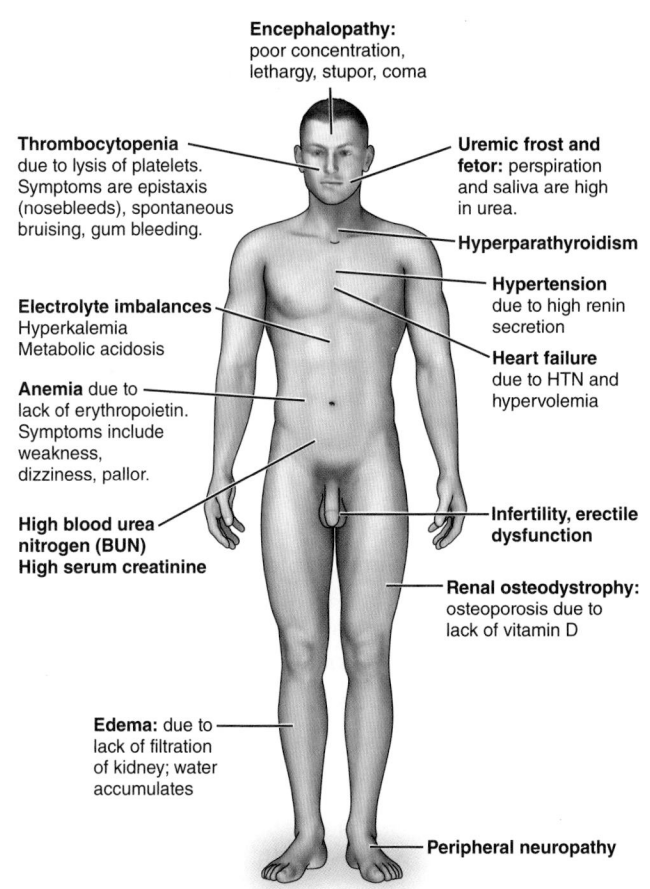

Encephalopathy: poor concentration, lethargy, stupor, coma

Thrombocytopenia due to lysis of platelets. Symptoms are epistaxis (nosebleeds), spontaneous bruising, gum bleeding.

Uremic frost and fetor: perspiration and saliva are high in urea.

Hyperparathyroidism

Hypertension due to high renin secretion

Electrolyte imbalances Hyperkalemia Metabolic acidosis

Heart failure due to HTN and hypervolemia

Anemia due to lack of erythropoietin. Symptoms include weakness, dizziness, pallor.

High blood urea nitrogen (BUN) High serum creatinine

Infertility, erectile dysfunction

Renal osteodystrophy: osteoporosis due to lack of vitamin D

Edema: due to lack of filtration of kidney; water accumulates

Peripheral neuropathy

FIGURE 22-14. Widespread complications of ESRD.

home setting), peritoneal dialysis, or renal transplant. In contrast to hemodialysis, peritoneal dialysis is much less efficient in terms of solute clearance. Greater than 85% of CKD patients utilize hemodialysis in a clinical setting. Commonly accepted criteria for initiating patients on dialysis include:

- The presence of uremic symptoms
- The presence of hyperkalemia unresponsive to conservative measures
- Persistent hypervolemia despite diuretic treatment
- Acidosis refractory to medical therapy
- Tendency to spontaneously bleed or bruise
- Creatinine clearance or estimated GFR less than 10 mL/min per 1.73 m^2

Once the GFR is lower than 10 mL/min (normal 90 to 120 mL/min), dialysis is initiated, and the patient will be evaluated for a kidney transplant. Kidney transplantation offers the best potential for complete rehabilitation because dialysis replaces only a fraction of the kidney's filtration function and none of the other vital functions of the kidney.

Chapter Summary

- Between 1990 and 2015, the prevalence of ESRD has increased almost 100% within the population. Aging of the population and increased prevalence of DM and HTN are reasons for increased kidney disease in the United States.
- As of 2021, one in seven adults in the United States have chronic kidney disease (CKD). Also, as many as 9 in 10 adults with CKD do not know they have this disorder.
- African Americans have the greatest incidence of kidney disease.
- The renal blood filtered per unit of time is known as the GFR. Normal GFR is 90 to 120 mL/min.
- To calculate accurate GFR, clinicians need to use a specific formula that involves age and sex of the patient and serum creatinine.
- The GFR decreases as a physiological change of aging. Because older adults take the greatest number of prescription drugs, decreased GFR raises risk of medication toxicity.
- AKI is divided into three categories based upon the mechanism of injury: prerenal azotemia, intrinsic renal disease, and postrenal obstruction.

- Prerenal azotemia is caused by lack of circulation to the kidney due to hypovolemia, excessive blood loss, or severe dehydration.
- Intrinsic renal disease is commonly due to nephrotoxic drugs, infection, autoimmune disease of the kidney, or trauma of the kidney.
- Postrenal obstruction is caused by obstruction of urinary outflow, which is commonly caused by nephrolithiasis, prostate enlargement (BPH or cancer), neurogenic bladder, or bladder tumor.
- Postrenal obstruction can lead to hydronephrosis, swelling of the renal pelvis, and compression of nephrons.
- ADPKD is the most common hereditary cause of renal disease in adults.
- ATN occurs when there is ischemia of the kidney. It is the most common cause of AKI.
- Azotemia is the increased amount of urea in the bloodstream.
- Serum creatinine is the best parameter used to indicate kidney function.

- Creatinine clearance, the volume of blood plasma cleared of creatinine per unit time, can also be used to gauge kidney function.
- BUN should not be used alone to gauge kidney function as it rises in dehydration and high-protein diets.
- Oliguria is less than 400 mL of urine output per day.
- In acute postinfectious glomerulonephritis, an immunological reaction triggers inflammation that damages the membranes of the glomerulus.
- Nephrotic syndrome is caused by glomerular injury and causes hypoalbuminemia, edema, and proteinuria. Hyperlipidemia and HTN are also associated with the syndrome.
- Anti-GBM disease is autoimmune destruction of the glomerulus and is commonly part of Goodpasture's syndrome, which also involves autoimmune disease of the lungs.
- Pyelonephritis is an infection of the kidney that causes fever, chills, and CVA tenderness.
- An anatomical abnormality called vesicoureteral reflux is a common predisposing factor for pyelonephritis. Reflux of urine occurs from the bladder into the ureter.

- Nephrolithiasis causes colicky pain in the back radiating to the groin, hematuria, and crystalluria.
- The most common type of kidney stone is made of calcium oxalate.
- Hydronephrosis is swelling of the renal pelvis that can occur with obstructive uropathy.
- AKI is most often caused by ischemia of the kidney, which is reversible.
- DM and HTN are the most common causes of CKD.
- CKD is irreversible and categorized into five stages according to serum creatinine and GFR.
- CKD causes widespread systemic symptoms such as hypervolemia, encephalopathy, thrombocytopenia, anemia, HTN, metabolic acidosis, hyperparathyroidism with renal osteodystrophy, peripheral and autonomic neuropathy, hyperkalemia, azotemia, impaired glucose metabolism, hypocalcemia, and hyperphosphatemia. CKD can lead to heart failure, left ventricular hypertrophy, pulmonary edema, and uremic pericarditis.
- ESRD occurs when there is 5% to 10% nephron function.
- Hemodialysis is most often used to treat ESRD. Kidney transplant is the only treatment that leads to complete rehabilitation.

Making the Connections

Pathophysiology

Signs and Symptoms	Assessment Findings	Diagnostic Tests	Treatment
Glomerulonephritis | Most commonly caused by GABHS antibodies that develop against the antigen (strep); for unknown reasons, antibodies attack glomerular membranes (molecular mimicry theory). Another theory asserts that antigen–antibody complexes develop and deposit in glomerular membranes, causing inflammation.			
Back pain (CVA tenderness). Edema (commonly periorbital). Fever. Cola-colored urine. Malaise.	HTN. Proteinuria. Hematuria. Edema (periorbital region common).	Elevated serum creatinine and elevated BUN. Urinalysis shows a large amount of protein and blood. Urine 24-hour creatinine clearance is low because creatinine is not being filtered by dysfunctional kidneys. Streptolysin antibody titer demonstrates antibodies are present against GABHS. Cryoglobulin titer indicates antigen–antibody complexes are present. Complement in the blood is low and is depleted because immune reaction uses up complement. Blood tests for antineutrophil cytoplasmic antibodies (ANCA), antidouble stranded DNA antibody, and antiglomerular basement membrane (GBM) serology are done to rule out causes of rapidly progressive AGN.	Antibiotics, antipyretics, and analgesics are needed. With systematic manifestations such as edema and elevated blood pressure, diuretics and antihypertensive agents may be indicated. Dietary restrictions of sodium and protein are also advised.

Making the Connections–cont'd

Signs and Symptoms	Assessment Findings	Diagnostic Tests	Treatment
Nephrotic Syndrome | Any disorder that causes glomerular injury. When glomeruli are injured, they become highly permeable and allow proteins to filter out of blood. Albumin leaves the blood and is excreted in the urine, called proteinuria or albuminuria. Hypoalbuminemia causes edema. Glomerulonephritis caused by infection and immunological inflammatory disease is a cause of nephrotic syndrome.			
Edema, especially of periorbital region and face.	Edema of the face is common, especially in the periorbital region. HTN. With severe albumin loss, edema of lower extremities, pleural effusion, and ascites can develop.	Albuminuria. Hypoalbuminemia. Hematuria. Hyperlipidemia. Hypertriglyceridemia. Elevated serum creatinine and BUN. 24-hour urine collection shows more than 3 grams of protein /dL. ANAs may be positive if etiology is an autoimmune disease.	Diet low in sodium. Adequate protein and fluid. ACE inhibitors or ARBs may be used.
Nephrolithiasis | The formation of calculi in the kidney, which can cause obstructive uropathy. Calculi are commonly composed of calcium.			
Severe back pain with radiation into the groin. Severe abdominal pain. Chills.	CVA tenderness. Hematuria. Crystalluria.	Blood may show high calcium, uric acid, or purines, depending on the etiology of nephrolithiasis. Elevated blood pressure and tachycardia are caused by pain. Urinalysis shows RBCs and crystals. Abdominal x-ray, CT, or ultrasound can show calculi.	IV fluid. Analgesics. Strain urine. Urinalysis needed. Increase oral fluid intake to more than 3 liters/day. Lithotripsy. Ureterocystoscopic surgery.
Pyelonephritis | Infection of the upper urinary tract, commonly caused by an ascending lower UTI.			
Back pain. Fever. Malaise. Chills. Dysuria. Frequency.	CVA tenderness. Fever.	Elevated WBC count. Microscopic hematuria. Pyuria. Bacteriuria. Proteinuria.	Antibiotics. Antipyretics and analgesics may be necessary.
Polycystic Kidney Disease | Disease causing multiple cysts in the kidneys and dysfunction caused by genetic mutation at 16p13.3 or 4q21-22.			
Back pain. Fever (if infection).	CVA tenderness, if infection. Hematuria.	Hematuria. Crystalluria. Bacteriuria. Ultrasound or CT scan can show cysts within kidneys.	Supportive treatment: low-sodium diet, physical activity, smoking cessation, and normal body weight maintenance. Tolvaptan. ACE inhibitors or ARBs to treat HTN. Prevention and treatment of UTIs. Hemodialysis if necessary. Renal transplant.

Continued

Making the Connections–cont'd

Signs and Symptoms	Assessment Findings	Diagnostic Tests	Treatment

Goodpasture's Syndrome (anti-GBM disease) | An autoimmune disease where the kidney nephrons and pulmonary alveolar membranes are attacked as an antigen.

Signs and Symptoms	Assessment Findings	Diagnostic Tests	Treatment
Malaise, chills, fever, dyspnea, pleuritic chest pain, cough, and hemoptysis. Massive pulmonary hemorrhage possible.	Renal manifestations include hematuria, edema, and high blood pressure. Pulmonary symptoms include tachypnea, cyanosis, and pulmonary crackles.	Elevated serum creatinine, BUN, WBC count. Anti-GBM antibody titer (immunoassay and Western blot). ANCA titer. Chest x-ray shows bilateral hilar lymphadenopathy and diffuse consolidations. Urinalysis shows hematuria, proteinuria, and RBC casts. Pulmonary function test reveals restrictive disease.	Immunosuppressants. Plasmapheresis. Dialysis. Renal transplant.

Acute Kidney Injury | Reversible failure of the kidneys caused by prerenal, intrinsic, or postrenal disorders. Prerenal AKI is most commonly renal ischemia caused by decreased blood volume. Intrinsic AKI is most commonly caused by nephrotoxic drugs, immune disorder, or infection. Postrenal AKI is most commonly caused by obstructive uropathy, as with nephrolithiasis, prostate enlargement, or bladder disorders.

Signs and Symptoms	Assessment Findings	Diagnostic Tests	Treatment
Edema of the face and extremities. Lack of urine output initially. Dyspnea if pulmonary edema present. Confusion, sleepiness, stupor, or coma if nitrogenous wastes are high. Easy bruising if thrombocytopenia develops. Fatigue, weakness, palpitations if anemia present. Muscle spasms possible if hypocalcemia present.	Oliguria. Fluid overload. Edema in the face and extremities. Pulmonary edema can develop, causing respiratory distress. Hypervolemia leads to HTN. Signs of uremia can develop, such as encephalopathy, hyperkalemia, metabolic acidosis, thrombocytopenia, and neuromuscular irritability. As renal function returns, the patient demonstrates a diuresis phase, with urine output increasing to 1 to 2 liters per day and resolution of hypervolemia.	Urinalysis, serum electrolytes, serum creatinine, BUN, arterial blood gases, and CBC. Calculate GFR. Radiographic imaging may be used to assess for any type of obstructive process or changes in size and structure of the kidneys. Renal biopsy may be used to evaluate for intrarenal etiology.	Diuretics. Cardiac monitor. Hemodialysis or CRRT in unstable patients.

Making the Connections—cont'd

Signs and Symptoms	Assessment Findings	Diagnostic Tests	Treatment

Chronic Kidney Disease | Deterioration of 90% to 95% of nephrons. ESRD. Kidneys cannot filter nitrogenous wastes or excrete fluid. All kidney functions diminished.

Signs and Symptoms	Assessment Findings	Diagnostic Tests	Treatment
Confusion, stupor, or coma caused by high nitrogenous wastes affecting brain. Bruising caused by thrombocytopenia. Fatigue and dyspnea on exertion caused by anemia. Edema caused by fluid overload, which can lead to heart failure. Lack of urine output. Muscle spasms or seizures caused by hypocalcemia. Bone breakdown. Amenorrhea, male and female infertility caused by lack of excretion of sex hormones. Sex hormones negatively feed back to organs.	High blood pressure. Oliguria. Edema. Pallor. Dyspnea. Muscle spasms or seizure. GI disturbances. Peripheral and autonomic neuropathy. Uremic fetor. Extreme pruritus.	Calculate GFR. Laboratory tests will show: Hyperkalemia. Hypoalbuminemia. Hyperphosphatemia. Hypocalcemia. Secondary hyperparathyroidism. Urinalysis shows proteinuria, RBCs, and WBCs. Elevated serum creatinine and BUN. Arterial blood gases show metabolic acidosis. CBC shows anemia. Ultrasound, x-ray, CT, MRI can show kidney size, masses, stones, or cysts. A renal biopsy may be used to evaluate for intrarenal etiology.	Hemodialysis. Medications to counteract complications such as diuretics, antihypertensives, erythropoietin-stimulating agents and iron supplements, calcitriol, calcimimetic agents, sodium bicarbonate, sodium polystyrene or patiromer, phosphate binders, SGLT2 inhibitors. Pruritus can be relieved with topical corticosteroids and antihistamines. Salt restriction and nutritional guidance. Do not use salt substitutes. Renal transplant can provide complete recovery.

Bibliography

Available online at fadavis.com

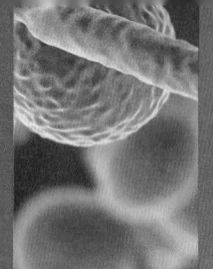

Urological Disorders

Learning Objectives

Upon completion of this chapter, the student will be able to:

- Differentiate between normal urological function and urological dysfunction.
- Recognize the common etiologies of urological dysfunction.
- Identify signs, symptoms, and clinical manifestations of urological disorders.

- Recognize laboratory tests, procedures, and imaging studies used in the diagnosis of disorders that cause urological dysfunction.
- Discuss nonpharmacological and pharmacological treatment modalities used in urological dysfunction.

Key Terms

Cystitis
Hydronephrosis
Hydroureter
Interstitial cystitis (IC)
Lower urinary tract symptoms (LUTS)
Micturition reflex

Obstructive uropathy
Oliguria
Overactive bladder (OAB)
Painful bladder syndrome (PBS)
Proteinuria
Pyelonephritis

Pyuria
Urinary casts
Urolithiasis
Urosepsis
Vesicoureteral reflux

Urological disorders are those pathophysiological conditions that affect the lower urinary tract, specifically the ureters, bladder, and urethra. In males, the prostate is also considered part of the urological system. Normal urological function is integral to healthy renal function. Healthy kidneys require the free, unencumbered flow of urine out of the body—**obstructive uropathy** refers to any condition that blocks such free flow of urine from the body. A severe obstructive uropathy can cause backflow of urine into the kidney, which leads to **hydronephrosis,** a condition that potentially causes kidney failure. Early recognition and treatment of urological disorders are keys to preventing renal dysfunction.

Epidemiology

Lower urinary tract infection (UTI) is the most common urological disorder. Approximately 6 million visits to primary care clinicians each year are for UTI. Lower UTI, also referred to as **cystitis,** is a common condition in women. Up to 40% of women in the United States aged 20 to 40 years have endured a lower UTI. Young adult women, particularly those in the childbearing years, are 30 times more likely to suffer a lower UTI compared with young adult men. Although lower UTI is a frequent condition among

women, it is rare in males. The incidence of UTI in males is approximately 5 to 8 per 10,000 population in the United States. A lower UTI in a young adult male should prompt the clinician to investigate the urological system further.

Another common urological problem is urinary obstruction. The most common causes of urinary obstruction are **urolithiasis** and benign prostatic hyperplasia (BPH). Both of these conditions are more common in males. The lifetime prevalence of urolithiasis is approximately 12% for men and 7% for women in the United States. BPH occurs in up to 14 million men per year, with most instances in men older than age 50.

Basic Concepts of Urological Function

As discussed in the previous chapter, the nephron, the basic unit of the kidney, acts to filter the blood at the glomerulus, reabsorb water at the tubules, secrete urea into the tubule fluid, reabsorb water at the collecting duct, and form a concentrated urine that passes out into the renal pelvis and ureter. Normal urine production in an adult depends on hydration. Adequate hydration is essential for optimal kidney function. The kidney must excrete at least 400 mL of urine per day to rid the body of wastes; any amount less than 400 mL per day is termed **oliguria.**

Adequate urine volume and unimpeded urine outflow from the body are essential for kidney health. Urine outflow depends on adequate pressure from the glomerulus into the nephron tubules, peristalsis of the ureters, and the effects of gravity. Adequate hydration enhances the volume of the blood filtered at the glomerular capillaries; this, in turn, increases flow of tubule fluid through the nephrons. Ureteral peristalsis moves urine from the renal pelvis down into the urinary bladder, where it is collected before urination (also called micturition). Passing urine, emptying the bladder, and urination involve involuntary and voluntary neuromuscular control of the structures in the lower urinary tract (see Fig. 23-1).

Neuromuscular Control of the Bladder

The detrusor muscle is the major muscle of the bladder; its fibers are arranged in spiral, longitudinal, and circular layers. This arrangement of muscle fibers allows the bladder to expand as it fills and to expel urine when it contracts. The sympathetic (adrenergic) and parasympathetic (cholinergic) autonomic nerves innervate the detrusor muscle. Sympathetic nerves, specifically alpha-adrenergic fibers, relax the detrusor muscle while they tighten the internal sphincter of the bladder neck; these actions allow filling of the bladder. The stretching of the bladder signals the parasympathetic nervous system to contract the detrusor muscle and relax the internal sphincter, actions that enable the bladder to expel urine through the urethra. The urethral sphincter, a voluntarily controlled muscle, must be relaxed for urine to exit the bladder. Urination is controlled both autonomically and voluntarily.

The urinary bladder usually holds 300 to 400 mL of urine. As urine accumulates, the bladder wall thins as it stretches, allowing the bladder to contain increasing amounts of urine without a significant rise in interior pressure. The urge to urinate usually starts when the stretched bladder reaches approximately 25% of its volume. When the amount of urine reaches 100% of the urinary bladder's capacity, the voluntary external urethral sphincter cannot remain closed and urine is expelled.

The Micturition Reflex

Micturition is a term that is synonymous with urination. The **micturition reflex,** a reflex involving the spinal cord and cortex of the brain, controls voiding. It involves nerve impulses traveling from the urinary bladder to the spinal cord and impulses passing from the spinal cord to the bladder. Neurons in the spinal cord coordinate this reflex, but the cerebral cortex can override it, thereby enabling conscious control of micturition. When the bladder wall stretches to accommodate the increasing volume of urine, the parasympathetic nerves in the reflex arc respond by stimulating the detrusor muscle in the bladder wall to contract. At the same time, the spinal cord sends nerve impulses up to the cerebral cortex, thereby allowing a conscious decision about whether it is appropriate to void. If voiding is not appropriate, the cerebral cortex initiates impulses that travel back down the spinal cord to inhibit the reflex arc, thereby preventing micturition. These impulses play a significant role in inhibiting micturition by keeping the external urinary sphincter contracted. When micturition is appropriate, impulses from the cerebral cortex stimulate the micturition reflex. The spinal cord nerves allow the external urinary sphincter to relax, thereby allowing urine to be expelled through the urethra.

Basic Pathophysiological Concepts of Urological Function

To understand the pathophysiology of urological disorders, certain terminology and urinary functions first need to be described.

Obstructive Uropathy

Obstruction is one of the most common pathophysiological problems that occur in the urinary tract. Renal calculi, also known as kidney stones, are the most common cause of urinary obstruction in young and middle-aged men. After age 60 years, urinary obstruction is most common in men secondary to benign prostatic hyperplasia (BPH). In young and middle-aged women, kidney stones, gynecological surgery, pregnancy, and cancers of pelvic organs are important etiologies of obstruction.

Obstruction of the urinary tract at any level eventually results in elevation of intraluminal ureteral pressure. With prolonged obstruction, ureteral peristalsis is overcome and increased hydrostatic pressures are transmitted directly to the nephron tubules. As pressures in the proximal tubule and Bowman's capsule

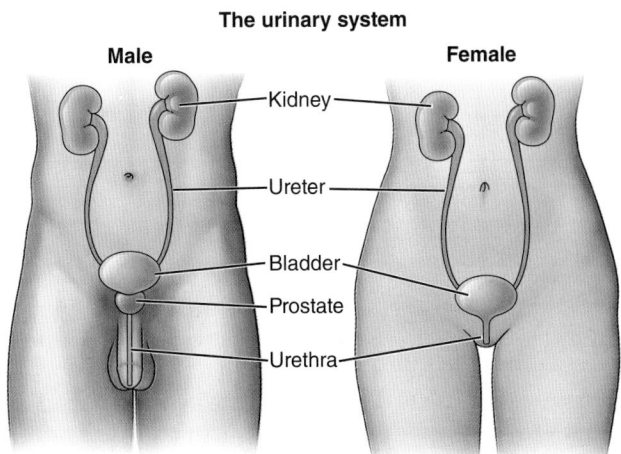

FIGURE 23-1. Anatomy of the urological system.

increase, glomerular filtration rate (GFR) decreases. After 12 to 24 hours, if complete obstruction is not relieved, a depressed GFR is maintained and renal blood flow decreases. With continued obstruction, renal blood flow progressively falls, resulting in ischemia and incremental nephron loss. Obstructive uropathy can lead to obstruction of urine at the kidney, backup of urine into the kidney, and kidney failure. Recovery of GFR depends on the duration and level of obstruction, preobstruction blood flow, and coexisting medical illness or infection.

Hydronephrosis and Hydroureter

Hydronephrosis is the distention of the renal calyces and pelvis as a result of obstruction of the outflow of urine distal to the renal pelvis, whereas **hydroureter** is the dilation of the ureter caused by obstruction. Hydronephrosis can cause kidney tissue damage; microscopic changes consist of dilation of the nephron tubules and flattening of the tubular epithelium. The renal calyces become enlarged and edematous. In children, the major causes of obstructed urine flow are anatomical abnormalities such as vesicoureteral reflux, urethral stricture, or stenosis. In comparison, calculi are the most common cause of obstruction in young adults, whereas BPH or pelvic neoplasms are primary causes in older patients.

> ### ⚕ CLINICAL CONCEPT
>
> Acute hydronephrosis is a short-term condition, and when corrected, allows full recovery of renal function. Chronic hydronephrosis, however, is a situation in which the loss of function is irreversible even with correction of the obstruction.

Assessment

A complete history regarding the patient's present illness, past illnesses and surgeries, current medications, allergies, environmental exposures, and family history is necessary. The patient's daily diet, exercise routine, and occupation should also be noted. If a urological problem is suspected, the clinician should focus on symptoms concerning the patient's urinary frequency; pain quality, location, and duration; urine control; nocturia; and the color and amount of urine per day.

Signs and Symptoms

Disorders of urological function present with similar signs and symptoms, including dysuria, frequency, urgency, and hesitancy. Table 23-1 provides a description and common causes of these signs and symptoms.

Diagnosis

The diagnostic studies used to investigate urological conditions include macroscopic or dipstick urinalysis, microscopic urinalysis, urine culture and sensitivity, serum electrolytes, and complete blood count (CBC) with differential. Specific procedures such as cystoscopy, CT scan, and urodynamic testing are used when diseases such as bladder cancer, urolithiasis, or **interstitial cystitis (IC)** are suspected.

Urinalysis

In addition to the history and physical examination, a urinalysis is needed if a urological disorder is suspected. Proper collection of the urine is necessary to decrease the possible contaminants that could alter the results. A clean-catch midstream urine specimen is used for macroscopic and microscopic urinalysis.

> ### ⚕ CLINICAL CONCEPT
>
> A clean-catch midstream urine specimen limits the number of contaminants; it is not a sterile specimen. The challenge of the midstream clean-catch procedure is to obtain a patient-collected sample without contamination by vaginal, epidermal, or perianal flora. The patient should be given specific instructions on how to cleanse the urethral region then collect urine during the middle of urine flow.

TABLE 23-1. Common Signs and Symptoms of Urological Dysfunction

Sign or Symptom	Description	Common Cause
Dysuria	Pain and burning on urination	UTI
Frequency	An abnormally high number of times that the patient needs to urinate	UTI, BPH, urological obstruction, IC/PBS
Hesitancy	Interrupted flow of a urinary stream	BPH
Urgency	A feeling that urination will occur imminently	UTI, BPH, IC/PBS

A macroscopic observation of the urine refers to that which is visible with the naked eye and apparent on a dipstick analysis. The physical appearance of the urine is inspected. The examiner notes the amount, color, clarity, odor, and cloudiness of the urine, as well as any other visible characteristics, such as the presence of blood or sediments. Abnormalities in color, clarity, and cloudiness may suggest conditions such as dehydration, infection, liver disease, protein loss, or muscle breakdown (rhabdomyolysis). Medications can change the color of urine.

A quick analysis can be accomplished using a chemical-coated dipstick on the urine sample. The dipstick can grossly detect glucose, ketones, blood, bilirubin, protein, leukocyte esterase, and nitrites. A microscopic laboratory analysis of urine takes longer but is more accurate than the dipstick method.

Table 23-2 lists the constituents of a laboratory urinalysis.

Urine Culture and Sensitivity

A urine culture reveals whether bacteria is growing in the urine. For clean-catch samples that have been properly collected, cultures with greater than 100,000 colony-forming units (CFU) per mL of one type of bacteria usually indicate infection. For samples collected using a technique that minimizes contamination, such as a sample collected with a urinary catheter, results as low as 1,000 microorganisms CFU/mL may be considered significant. In such cases, additional tests will often be performed to identify the specific strain of bacteria, as well as susceptibility testing to determine the most appropriate antibiotic treatment. A culture that is reported as "no growth in 24 or 48 hours" usually indicates that there is no infection.

TABLE 23-2. Abnormal Laboratory Findings on Urinalysis

Urinalysis Finding	Description	Common Cause
Bacteriuria	Bacteria in the urine that can be visualized on microscopy	UTI or asymptomatic bacteriuria (ASB)
Bilirubinuria	Bilirubin in the urine	Liver disorders Excessive hemolysis
Crystalluria	Crystals or pieces of a kidney stone in the urine; commonly calcium or uric acid	Nephrolithiasis or urolithiasis
Glucosuria	Glucose in the urine	Uncontrolled diabetes mellitus (DM)
Hematuria	Blood in the urine	UTI Nephrolithiasis or urolithiasis Urological malignancy
Ketonuria	Ketones in the urine	Fasting Starvation Uncontrolled DM
Leukocyte esterase	WBCs in the urine	UTI or ASB
Nitrites	Bacteria in the urine	UTI or ASB
Proteinuria (microalbuminuria)	A condition in which urine contains an abnormal amount of protein. Normally, urine should contain no more than 200 mg of protein per liter.	Glomerular injury Kidney dysfunction caused by diabetes Kidney dysfunction caused by high blood pressure Inflammation of the kidneys
Pyuria **Urinary casts**	WBCs (neutrophils) in the urine Cylindrical mucoprotein structures produced by the nephron tubules that appear in the urine. Various casts found in urine sediment include hyaline, waxy, granular, fatty, crystal, RBC, WBC, bacterial, and epithelial.	UTI or ASB Nephrotic syndrome Dehydration Vigorous exercise Diuretics Tubular necrosis Autoimmune disorders Pyelonephritis Other kidney diseases

CLINICAL CONCEPT

A clean-catch urine sample may contain contaminants if not performed correctly by the patient. A clinical laboratory will describe a urine sample as contaminated with descriptors such as mixed flora, skin flora, vaginal flora, or multiple isolates. Most laboratories use a urine contamination threshold of equal to or greater than 10,000 CFU/mL, with equal to or greater than two isolates.

Serum Electrolytes

Serum levels of sodium, potassium, chloride, bicarbonate ion, calcium, and phosphate need to be reviewed when urological problems are present. A urological problem can cause abnormalities in nephron function, and this can alter electrolyte excretion and reabsorption.

CBC With Differential

To diagnose infection, a white blood cell (WBC) count is necessary. An elevated WBC count is present with upper UTI or **pyelonephritis.** A lower UTI is a confined, localized infection and should not raise the WBC count.

Imaging Studies

Imaging studies of the urological system can include a plain x-ray of the abdomen called a kidney–ureter–bladder (KUB) x-ray. This can exclude masses in the pelvis or abdomen, or can discern stones in the urological system. A computed tomography (CT) scan with or without contrast is commonly used to investigate the tissue of the kidney, masses, or stones in the urological system. Magnetic resonance imaging (MRI) is also used to obtain a three-dimensional picture of the renal and urological system. A magnetic resonance angiogram (MRA) can provide views of the arterial system of the kidneys. Radionuclide scans involve injection of radioactive chemicals that can highlight renal circulation. An intravenous pyelogram (IVP) can also be used to study the function of the urological system and highlight areas of the kidney and ureter; however, a CT scan is preferable.

Ultrasound studies can be used to examine the kidneys and bladder. For example, small, portable ultrasound devices can help determine the extent of bladder overfilling or distention. Cystoscopy, an invasive study that uses a scope inserted into the urethra and bladder, can provide direct visualization of the bladder. During this procedure, dye can be injected into the bladder and ureters to highlight the anatomy. Cystoscopy can also be used to biopsy bladder tumors, and cystoscopic surgical procedures can also be performed.

Urodynamic studies help to evaluate the bladder's neuromuscular status. Studies are done during both bladder filling and emptying. This testing can determine whether the bladder can fully expand and the actual process of voiding to determine whether the bladder can contract properly. An example of a urodynamic study is a voiding cystourethrogram (VCUG), which can demonstrate bladder function as a person is urinating.

Treatment

Treatment of urological disorders depends on the etiology of the particular disorder. For example, antibiotics will be used for an infection. For renal calculi, treatment involves pain medication, increased fluid intake (more than 3 liters/day of water), and straining of the urine. Lithotripsy, the application of sound waves to break up ureteral calculi, may be necessary. Cystoscopic surgery may be required for urolithiasis or tumors of the bladder. Surgical procedures are commonly used for BPH and bladder cancer. Medication, surgery, and Kegel's exercises are most commonly used to treat urinary incontinence.

Pathophysiology of Selected Urological Disorders

The major urological disorders include lower UTI; asymptomatic bacteriuria (ASB); interstitial cystitis (IC); urolithiasis, also commonly called nephrolithiasis; bladder cancer; and urinary incontinence.

Lower Urinary Tract Infections

Lower UTIs account for 1% to 3% of all visits to family clinicians. The patient commonly presents with pain and burning on urination, as well as urinary frequency and urgency. If the infection persists, the symptoms can progress to cloudy, strong-smelling urine and hematuria. An untreated lower UTI can put the patient at risk for an ascending UTI that can result in pyelonephritis, which is kidney infection.

Epidemiology

Lower UTI is the reason for 6 to 7 million primary care visits per year. Lower UTIs are more prevalent in women than men. In women, a lower UTI is commonly referred to as cystitis. The majority of women with lower UTI are young adults aged 20 to 40 years old. It is estimated that approximately 50% of all women will have a UTI at some point in their lifetime. Conversely, men have a much lower prevalence of UTI. A lower UTI is rare in young adult males and requires further investigation of the urological system. However, after age 60, BPH is a common cause of UTI in men.

CLINICAL CONCEPT

Women are at higher risk for lower UTI than men because of the anatomical proximity of the rectum to the female urethra.

Risk Factors

Factors that increase susceptibility to UTI in women include improper perineal hygiene; wearing tight, restrictive clothing; and use of irritating bath products. Sexual intercourse increases a woman's risk of UTI, and use of contraceptive diaphragms and spermicides are also known to increase susceptibility. Pregnancy commonly causes ASB, which is defined as bacteria in the urine with no symptoms. Pregnancy and ASB increase a woman's risk for pyelonephritis, especially at the end of the second trimester and the beginning of the third trimester.

UTIs in older males are generally associated with urinary tract obstruction caused by enlargement of the prostate gland. The prostate gland anatomically surrounds the urethra, and with hyperplasia, cell growth can constrict the urethra. Benign prostatic hyperplasia (BPH) is the overgrowth of cells in the prostate gland that surround the urethra. This is a normal physical change in older adult males. This causes urine retention in the bladder, which is a medium for bacterial growth. BPH also causes specifically related **lower urinary tract symptoms (LUTS)** that include weak urinary stream, hesitancy, frequency, dribbling after urination, and feeling of incomplete bladder emptying. Lower UTI in men before the age of 50 years is uncommon. With prostate enlargement and UTI in males, the clinician should rule out possibility of prostate cancer. (For more information about prostate disorders, see Chapter 27.)

In both males and females, other risk factors for UTI include dehydration, urinary catheterization, diabetes, bladder cancer, cancer in tissues adjacent to the bladder, and cancer treatments.

Etiology

The etiological organism that most commonly causes lower UTI is *Escherichia coli,* which originates from the bowel. This organism causes approximately 75% to 90% of all UTIs. *Proteus, Pseudomonas, Streptococci, Enterococci, Staphylococcus epidermidis, S. saprophyticus,* and *Klebsiella* are other organisms of etiological significance. In hospital-acquired infections, multidrug-resistant bacterial organisms often cause UTI.

 CLINICAL CONCEPT

E. coli is commonly transmitted from the rectum to the urethra in women due to the anatomical proximity of the anus to the urethra.

Pathophysiology

A healthy urinary tract is sterile, and bacterial flora are normally confined to the urethral opening. In women, the anatomical proximity of the rectum and urinary tract enable bacteria to easily colonize the urethra. However, urine contains high osmolarity, urea, and organic acids that diminish bacterial viability in the bladder. Any obstruction of urinary outflow decreases the bladder's resistance to bacterial infection. Stagnant urine is a good medium for bacterial growth. Continual free outflow of urine clears bacteria from the body. Immunoglobulin A (IgA), secreted by WBCs in the urinary tract, also prevents adherence of bacteria to the bladder wall. However, many women are nonsecretors of IgA, which decreases their ability to combat bacterial invasion of the bladder.

When host defenses are overcome, urine can act as a medium for bacterial growth. Uropathogenic bacteria can adhere, proliferate, and resist host defenses when in the bladder. The bacteria frequently have resistant outer capsules that can resist the acid in the urine. The bacteria can also secrete hemolysins and cytotoxic necrotizing factor (CNF), which can enhance their migration up to the bladder.

Proteus mirabilis, another bacterium from the bowel, secretes urease, which decreases the acidity of urine and enhances its ability to invade the bladder. The bacteria are flagellated and swarm in large groups when migrating up to the bladder. The bacteria also change the pH of the urine, which enhances formation of struvite staghorn calculi in the kidney. *Proteus* UTI is most commonly associated with the use of urinary instrumentation or catheterization.

Interference with urinary outflow occurs in such conditions as chronic voluntary suppression of urination, sexual intercourse, urinary tract obstruction, instrumentation of the urinary tract, use of catheters not drained to gravity, and vesicoureteral reflux. Frequent emptying of the bladder is necessary for the health of the urinary tract. Visualization of the urinary tract with a cystoscope or catheter increases the risk of bacterial contamination into the bladder. Sexual intercourse and use of a contraceptive diaphragm increase the urethra's exposure to bacteria. **Vesicoureteral reflux** commonly occurs in young female children. The condition is caused by an anatomical abnormality at the junction where the ureter enters the bladder. This anatomical anomaly allows urine to reflux up toward the kidney, which increases the risk of UTI. *Candida albicans,* a fungal pathogen that colonizes the vaginal area, can also cause UTI. Risk factors for *Candida* UTI are diabetes mellitus, antibiotic use, and urinary catheters.

Although common, UTIs in women are not a serious disease unless they are associated with urinary obstruction or pregnancy. In males, UTIs are very uncommon and the cause should be thoroughly investigated. Prostatitis and epididymitis are associated with lower UTI in young adult males. In young men, risk factors for lower UTI include anal intercourse, intercourse with an infected female, lack of circumcision, and HIV infection. The most common reason for infection in older males is stasis of urine caused by obstruction of the urethra because of BPH.

Hospital-acquired UTI is often associated with urinary catheterization and multidrug-resistant pathogens. Polymicrobial infections that are resistant to antibiotics are common hospital-acquired UTIs. Urosepsis, bacterial invasion of the bloodstream, can be a complication of UTI in older adults, particularly those with long-term indwelling urinary catheterization.

Clinical Presentation

Most of the time, the history reveals the classic lower urinary tract infection symptoms of frequency, pain or burning on urination (dysuria), urgency, and occasionally hematuria. UTI symptoms are caused by the inflammation and edema of the urethra and bladder. Commonly in UTI, the bladder does not completely empty and urinary retention causes frequent small amounts of urine flow. Urgency is the sensation that urination is imminent and can cause frequent trips to the bathroom only to yield small amounts of urine. Rarely, there might be suprapubic tenderness. Severe infections can cause bladder spasms; in men, these spasms can produce severe referred pain in the glans penis. Usually, no changes are noted in the physical examination.

> **CLINICAL CONCEPT**
>
> Lower UTI does not cause fever. Fever should prompt the clinician to suspect pyelonephritis.

Diagnosis

Urinalysis and urine culture are used to diagnose lower UTI. A urinalysis using a dipstick usually shows some red blood cells (RBCs); positive leukocyte esterase, which indicates WBCs; and nitrates, which indicate bacteria. On microscopic urinalysis, neutrophils, RBCs, and bacteria are present in a clean-catch midstream specimen of urine. On a urine culture, infection is indicated by a colony count of bacteria greater than 10^5/mL. However, a colony count of bacteria as low as 1,000/mL may be a cause of significant infection.

Treatment

The usual treatment for lower UTI is an antibiotic. The appropriate antibiotic can be determined by culture and sensitivity testing. Nitrofurantoin and/or trimethoprim–sulfamethoxazole are commonly prescribed. Fluoroquinolones may also be used. Phenazopyridine (Pyridium) may be prescribed for urinary tract pain relief. Hydration to accentuate the unidirectional clearance of bacteriuria is also part of recommended treatment. Some studies have shown that cranberry juice can decrease the risk of UTI because it lessens the adherence of bacteria to the bladder wall.

> **ALERT!** If a patient is ordered phenazopyridine, let the patient know that one of the side effects of the medication is that it can turn urine red and alter the color of contact lenses.

Complications

Urosepsis, a condition caused by bacteremia, is a serious complication of UTI. Patients with urosepsis are acutely and severely ill with symptoms of fever, chills, confusion, disorientation, and hypotension. Bacterial endotoxins are responsible for the clinically observable effects of the bacteremia in the host. Older adults, catheterized patients, and those who are immunocompromised are particularly susceptible to urosepsis. Obstruction within the urinary tract increases an individual's susceptibility. Older males with BPH are at increased risk.

Asymptomatic Bacteriuria

ASB refers to two consecutive urine cultures growing more than a colony count of 100,000/mL of bacteria in a patient lacking symptoms of a UTI. It is a common disorder, with prevalence varying by age, sex, sexual activity, and the presence of genitourinary abnormalities. It is more common in women than in men. In healthy women, the prevalence of bacteriuria increases with age, from about 1% in females 5 to 14 years of age to more than 20% in women at least 80 years of age.

E. coli is the most common organism isolated from patients with ASB. Other infecting organisms include *Enterobacteriaceae, Pseudomonas aeruginosa, Enterococcus* species, and group B streptococcus. Organisms isolated in patients with ASB are influenced by patient variables: healthy persons commonly have *E. coli,* whereas nursing home residents with a urinary catheter are more likely to have multidrug-resistant bacteria. *Enterococcus* species and gram-negative bacilli are common in men.

Among patients with ASB, treatment with antibiotics has not been found to improve patient outcomes. For this reason, as well as increased antimicrobial resistance, it is important to refrain from treating patients with ASB unless there is evidence of potential benefit. Women who are pregnant should be screened for ASB in the first trimester and, if positive, treated to reduce the risk of pyelonephritis.

Interstitial Cystitis

IC is a syndrome characterized by urgency and frequency of urination, a feeling of bladder fullness, and pain. **Painful bladder syndrome (PBS)** is a term often used synonymously with IC. The pathophysiology of this disorder is based on different theories. This syndrome is diagnosed primarily on the basis of symptoms, as there is currently no certain etiology and pathophysiology is unclear.

Epidemiology

The latest research suggests two different types of IC based on etiology: ulcerative and nonulcerative. Nonulcerative IC is more prevalent and accounts for approximately 90% of all cases, whereas ulcerative IC occurs in 10% of affected individuals. Ninety percent of those affected with IC are women, and the average age of onset is 40 years; most are of European ancestry. In the United States, there are conflicting studies regarding the prevalence of IC. Current studies estimate that 2.7% to 6.5% of women in the United States have symptoms consistent with a diagnosis of interstitial cystitis/bladder pain syndrome (IC/BPS). However, many investigators assert IC/PBS is underreported and therefore underdiagnosed, particularly in males.

Etiology/Risk Factors

The etiology of IC is uncertain, but proposed causes include (a) diminished glucosaminoglycan (GAG) layer of the bladder, (b) altered permeability of the bladder epithelium, (c) uroinflammation, and (d) neural upregulation. A history of physical trauma to the bladder and coexisting chronic pain disorders, such as irritable bowel syndrome (IBS) and fibromyalgia, are risk factors for developing interstitial cystitis and can co-occur in as many as 50% of patients with IC. Previous use of ketamine is also considered a risk factor. Ketamine can be used as an anesthetic or antidepressant clinically or as an illicit hallucinogen.

Pathophysiology

In nonulcerative IC, the bladder wall is basically intact but shows small tears and hemorrhages when the bladder is distended. In ulcerative IC, a lesion called a Hunner's ulcer is present on histological examination of the bladder wall. These ulcers become apparent only after overdistention of the bladder on urodynamic testing.

One theoretical cause of IC/PBS is a thinning of the GAG layer of the bladder. The GAG layer acts as a barrier that aids in protecting the bladder epithelium from harmful substances. In patients with IC, this GAG layer is rendered dysfunctional and therefore allows the entry of electrolytes, bacteria, and solutes into the bladder wall. Damage to the GAG layer can arise from infection, inflammation, and damage from infiltration of urine solutes. Once the GAG layer is impaired, an imbalance in urine storage and concentration can result, causing pain and both urinary urgency and frequency. The altered permeability theory asserts that the bladder epithelium (urothelium) has increased permeability that causes dysfunction of the detrusor muscle. Another theory claims there is uroinflammation with activation of mast cells. Mast cells release

histamine, which in turn stimulates afferent pain nerves in the bladder. Lastly, the sympathetic nervous system and hypothalamo-pituitary-adrenal (HPA) axis may be contributory to the pathogenesis of IC. In patients with IC, one or both of these pathways may become dysfunctional, resulting in neuronal dysregulation.

Clinical Presentation

Patients with IC report chronic pelvic pain, perineal pain, dysuria, a sense of fullness of the bladder, urinary urgency, and frequency. In severe IC, a patient may feel the need to urinate more than 50 times a day and endure many episodes of nocturia. The bladder usually has normal size and capacity. The pain begins during bladder filling and is relieved by emptying the bladder. Symptoms may occur daily or weekly, or may be constant and unrelenting for months or years and then resolve spontaneously with or without therapy. The disorder commonly occurs in a pattern of remissions and exacerbations.

Diagnosis

To diagnosis a patient with IC, they must present with symptoms persisting longer than 6 weeks. The Interstitial Cystitis Symptom Index (ICSI), is an eight-question assessment tool that asks patients to define both the frequency of their symptoms and the interference of these symptoms on quality of life. The clinician must first rule out an infectious cause of symptoms through urinalysis and urine culture. In women, endometriosis needs to be ruled out, which requires hysteroscopy and laparoscopy. In men, prostate disease should be ruled out. Patients require cystoscopy, urine cytology, and biopsy of any suspicious bladder lesions to rule out bladder cancer. Cystoscopy can confirm the inflammation or ulcerations of the bladder walls. A cystoscopy examination with bladder hydrodistention is done under local anesthesia. The cystoscope can facilitate bladder biopsy if necessary. Urodynamic studies can evaluate bladder sensation and neuromuscular function. Urodynamic studies measure how well the bladder, sphincters, and urethra store and release urine. Most urodynamics testing focuses on the bladder's ability to hold and empty urine using a specialized pressure-sensing urinary catheter. Ultrasound, videography, and electromyography may also be utilized during the testing.

Treatment

There is no single treatment for all cases of IC. Pelvic floor rehabilitation and bladder training programs are usually attempted first. Kegel exercises are recommended, and the patient is advised to gradually increase voiding intervals over a course of weeks. Certain foods have been known to aggravate symptoms of IC. The patient is advised to avoid tomatoes, chocolate, spicy foods, alcohol, coffee, and vinegar.

If dietary and behavioral therapies are ineffective, the clinician usually attempts drug therapy. Anticholinergic agents such as oxybutynin and tolterodine can be used to treat the urinary frequency component of the condition, but these agents can cause urinary retention, can impair bladder emptying, and may exacerbate pelvic pain.

The tricyclic antidepressant amitriptyline has also been effective in the treatment of pain associated with IC. Amitriptyline can produce pain relief by modulating the descending pain pathway through norepinephrine, and, to a lesser extent, serotonin reuptake inhibition. Amitriptyline also has anticholinergic and antihistaminergic effects, which could theoretically ameliorate urinary urgency and inflammatory symptoms associated with IC. In addition, an oral medication called pentosan polysulfate sodium (Elmiron) has been shown to be effective in some persons with IC. It is thought that this compound adheres to the damaged GAG layer of the bladder epithelium, protecting it from noxious substances in the urine. Multiple immunosuppressive drugs have been evaluated as potential treatment options for IC if other measures are ineffective. Cyclosporine A and the tumor necrosis factor inhibitor adalimumab have also been effective.

At times, patients report relief of IC after hydrodistention of the bladder, which is done during diagnostic evaluation and intravesical therapy. In intravesical therapy, the clinician instills medication directly into the bladder using a catheter. This therapy may require several episodes of instillation before it is effective. There are various intravesical agents that are intended to replenish the urothelial GAG layer such as hyaluronic acid, chondroitin sulfate, and pentosan polysulfate. Intravesical instillation therapy with dimethyl sulfoxide (DMSO) has been effective, particularly in patients with ulcerative IC. In patients with Hunner's lesions, the injection of the corticosteroid triamcinolone into the submucosal layer directly under the lesion has also been effective. Intravesical capsaicin has also been used for IC. Capsaicin works by stimulating sensory receptors in the uroepithelium and detrusor muscle. Another intravesical treatment is instillation of resiniferatoxin (RTX), an ultrapotent capsaicin analog.

Transurethral intradetrusor muscle injection of botulinum toxin in conjunction with hydrodistention of the bladder has proven effective in some cases. Acupuncture and transcutaneous electrical nerve stimulation (TENS) have also shown some success. Electrodes or acupuncture needles can be placed over the sacral nerve region or suprapubic area. If all treatments fail to provide relief, surgical techniques may be attempted. Surgical fulguration, laser treatment, and resection of ulcerations in the bladder can be attempted.

Urolithiasis

Urolithiasis is the condition of calculi that are formed or located anywhere in the urinary system. The term *nephrolithiasis* (renal calculus) refers to stones that are in the kidney, whereas *ureterolithiasis* refers to stones that are in the ureter. Cystolithiasis (vesical calculi) refers to stones that form in or have passed into the bladder.

Epidemiology

Urolithiasis affects an estimated 10% of Americans annually. This estimate consists of persons who have suffered more than one incident of stones in the urinary system. A history of stone disease is more common in European Americans than African Americans and is more common in males than females. Incidence increases among men in their 20s and peaks in the late 50s. In women, the incidence rate is approximately equal across all age groups. Recurrence of the formation of calculi is common, with 35% at 5 years and 52% at 10 years after the initial incident.

Etiology/Risk Factors

Genetics, diet, metabolic abnormalities, and structural abnormalities in the urinary tract can lead to urolithiasis (see Box 23-1). Having a family member with kidney stones is a strong risk factor. Lack of adequate hydration also contributes to stone formation. A low fluid intake, with a subsequent low volume of urine production, produces high concentrations of stone-forming solutes in the urine.

Another contributing factor to the formation of stones is diet. Diets that are high in animal protein, sodium, and calcium can lead to urolithiasis. Stones can be a result of excessive consumption of certain minerals or faulty metabolism of minerals. The following are the four main types of renal calculi:

1. Calcium stones
2. Struvite (magnesium ammonium phosphate) stones
3. Uric acid stones
4. Cystine stones

BOX 23-1. Conditions Leading to Urolithiasis

Various conditions increase susceptibility to kidney stone formation. A condition involving kidney stones is referred to as urolithiasis, in which a stone is impacted within the ureter or bladder.

- Biliary cirrhosis
- Chronic dehydration
- Cystinuria
- Distal renal tubular acidosis
- Ehlers–Danlos syndrome
- Hypercalciuria
- Hyperoxaluria
- Hyperparathyroidism (hypercalcemia)
- Lesch–Nyhan syndrome
- Marfan's syndrome
- Multiendocrine neoplasm
- Polycystic kidney disease
- Sjögren's syndrome

Calcium Stones. Calcium is the most common component of urological stones, and hypercalciuria is the most common metabolic abnormality found in urolithiasis. Some cases of hypercalciuria are related to increased intestinal absorption of calcium, which is associated with excess dietary calcium and overactive calcium absorption mechanisms; some are related to excess resorption of calcium from bone, such as in hyperparathyroidism; and some are related to an inability of the renal tubules to properly reabsorb calcium in the glomerular filtrate, such as in renal-leak hypercalciuria.

Struvite Stones. Struvite stones are composed of a combination of magnesium, ammonium phosphate, and carbonate apatite and can grow to occupy the entire pelvis of the kidney, called a staghorn calculus. Struvite stones occur when urea is split into ammonia, bicarbonate, and carbonate ions by urease-producing organisms, especially *P. mirabilis.* Other organisms that cause struvite stones include *Haemophilus influenzae, Staphylococcus aureus,* and *Yersinia enterocolitica.* Factors that predispose individuals to struvite stone formation include anatomical abnormalities in the urinary tract, neurological disorders of the bladder, and indwelling catheters.

CLINICAL CONCEPT

Patients with spinal cord injuries are particularly vulnerable to the formation of struvite stones; 8% of these patients form stones, 98% of which are struvite stones.

Uric Acid Stones. Foods high in animal proteins contain a high amount of purines, which break down into uric acid. Meats increase the amount of uric acid in the bloodstream, which can then precipitate out of solution at the kidney and form uric acid stones.

Cystine Stones. Cystine stones are uncommon. They are associated with a genetic disorder associated with the faulty metabolism of the amino acid cystine.

Pathophysiology

Urolithiasis occurs because of supersaturation of the urine with stone-forming salts as a result of chemical, metabolic, or genetic causes. Stones in the bladder can also occur as a result of stasis of urine, repeated UTIs, urinary obstruction, or neurogenic bladder. Intraureteral stones cause pressure proximal to the stone in the ureter, which causes spasm. Spasms of the ureter occur because of obstruction at one of four sites:

1. The ureteropelvic junction, the point where the ureter attaches to the kidney
2. Midureter at the level of the iliac vessels
3. The posterior aspect of the pelvis in women, at the point the ureter crosses the broad ligament
4. The ureterovesical junction, the point where the ureters connect with the bladder

After a stone forms, it travels slowly down the ureter, pushed by urine flow. It shears off some of the ureteral mucosa, which causes superficial bleeding of the membrane. The stone causes a buildup of pressure and spasms proximally within the ureter, causing intense pain. Low urine flow slows the passage of the stone, which is why increased hydration is recommended to increase urine volume. Lack of urine passage can cause backward accumulation of pressure into the renal pelvis, causing hydronephrosis, or swelling of the renal pelvis. Backward accumulation of urine is toxic to nephrons and can result in kidney failure.

CLINICAL CONCEPT

Dehydration is a significant contributor to urolithiasis, and incidence of the disorder is greater in regions with hot climates.

Clinical Presentation

Diagnosis of urolithiasis is most often based on the patient's history because there are distinct symptoms. The physical examination frequently does not reveal significant findings.

History. The patient suspected of urolithiasis should fully describe their pain. The characteristics of the pain in urolithiasis are distinctive and often the basis of diagnosis. Pain should be assessed completely, including location, onset, duration, characteristics, radiation, and aggravating factors. The patient should also be asked about treatment that relieves the pain. Current medications, including over-the-counter medications and herbal supplements, should be assessed because some drugs can predispose individuals to stone formation. Past medical history and family history of kidney stones are key because there is a strong genetic predisposition, and repeat episodes of kidney stones are common. Any disorders that increase susceptibility to hypercalcemia or hyperuricemia are important, as calcium and uric acid are common components of stones. Patients with hyperparathyroidism or malignancy often have hypercalcemia and hypercalciuria, whereas patients with gout have hyperuricemia. Frequent UTIs or any possible cause of urinary stasis should be investigated because these are risk factors.

Signs and Symptoms. Patients typically present with costovertebral angle pain, also called flank pain, or abdominal pain when the kidney stone is high in the urinary tract in the ureter. The pain of urolithiasis is regarded as severe and intermittent. Rather than lying still, patients usually constantly move in an effort to control the pain. The distinctive pain, referred to as renal colic, can be associated with nausea, vomiting, fever, hematuria, pyuria, crystalluria, and painful urination. Renal colic typically comes in waves lasting 20 to 60 minutes, beginning in the flank or lower back and often radiating to the groin or genitals. The patient usually describes the pain as severe. The patient may be able to painfully pass a kidney stone or stone particles with high urine flow. The stone should be analyzed for composition.

Diagnosis

The diagnosis of urolithiasis is made on the basis of information obtained from the history and physical examination, as well as urinalysis and imaging studies. The patient's description of the pain is key in the diagnosis because renal colic is distinctive. Urinalysis will be positive for blood and will often show crystals. Serum analysis for electrolytes, calcium, and uric acid is important. Ultrasound may be more sensitive in detecting urolithiasis than abdominal x-rays of the KUB. X-rays can miss stones that are not opaque calcifications. CT scans with and without contrast can visualize stones. MRI may be necessary if CT does not reveal the calculus.

A confirmation of urolithiasis is made on passing of the stone, surgical recovery of the stone, or by radiological imaging. Stone analysis, together with serum and 24-hour urine metabolic evaluation, can identify the cause of the stone in more than 95% of patients.

Treatment

Patients are advised to increase hydration (more than 3 liters of water/day) in order to attempt to pass the stone in the urine. Patients should also strain urine to catch the stone for analysis. Pain medications such as intravenous ketorolac or opioids are usually necessary. Pharmacological intervention is specific to the type of stone. Diuretics such as hydrochlorothiazide can limit calcium excretion into urine. The patient may require extracorporeal shock wave lithotripsy to enable passing of the stone. Lithotripsy uses sound waves to break up a stone into smaller pieces so they may be passed more easily. Cystoscopic surgery may be needed if the stone does not pass. Ureterorenoscopy (URS) is used if the stone is high in the upper ureter and is routinely performed under general anesthesia. Local anesthetic flexible URS is another option for those who cannot tolerate general anesthesia.

Bladder Cancer

Although not a common disorder, cancer of the bladder is the most common type of urological cancer. Urothelial cancer (UC) is the predominant type of bladder cancer in the United States and Europe. UC is categorized as muscle invasive bladder cancer (MIBC) or nonmuscle invasive bladder cancer (NMIBC). NMIBCs account for approximately 75% of new bladder cancer diagnoses. MIBC represents approximately 18% of newly diagnosed cases of bladder cancer. MIBCs extend into the detrusor muscle of the bladder and have a greater propensity to spread to lymph nodes and other organs.

Epidemiology

Bladder cancer comprises 5% of new cancer diagnoses in the United States and is the sixth most prevalent malignancy. Approximately 80,400 persons had bladder cancer in 2019 and more than 17,000 died from the disorder. Bladder cancer is three times more common in males than in females. It affects Whites about twice as often as Blacks or Hispanics, but it is more likely to be diagnosed at an advanced stage in Black patients. Approximately 90% of those diagnosed are older than 55 years with the average age of 73.

Etiology

Up to 80% of bladder cancers are related to environmental exposure, with cigarette smoking the major risk factor. The degree of risk is directly proportional to the number of pack-years of the patient. A smoker's risk of bladder cancer is up to six times higher than that of nonsmokers. This is due to the high levels of carcinogenic toxins present in cigarette smoke.

Occupational exposure is another major risk factor. Use of various organic chemicals, such as naphthalene, benzidine, and aniline, which are present in industrial dyes, are associated with bladder cancer. Hair dyes and hair sprays used by hairdressers have been suspected carcinogenic causes of bladder cancer. Chronic exposure to diesel exhaust, rubber, and petroleum products have also been associated with bladder cancer. The chemotherapeutic agent cyclophosphamide is also a risk factor, as is radiotherapy to the pelvis. Additional associations with bladder cancer include diabetes mellitus, obesity, and human papillomavirus. Use of pioglitazone (Actos) for more than 1 year is independently associated with a slightly increased risk of bladder cancer. Consuming large amounts of processed red meat may also slightly increase risk.

In developing countries, particularly the Middle East, bladder cancer is commonly caused by a parasitic infection caused by *Schistosoma haematobium*. The eggs of the parasite are found within the bladder wall.

Patients with spinal cord injuries who require a long-term indwelling urinary catheter have 16 to 20 times greater risk of developing bladder cancer than the general population.

Certain genetic mutations are also associated with bladder cancer. Loss of portions of chromosome 9 is found to be an early molecular change. Mutations of the tumor suppressor gene *p53* found on chromosome 17 are associated with high-grade invasive bladder cancer. The retinoblastoma (*Rb1*) tumor suppressor gene located on chromosome 13 at 13q14.1-q14.2 is also associated with bladder cancer. Persons who possess the Rb oncogene have predisposition to cancers of the retina, lung, bone, and bladder. Genomic alterations are found in the *FGFR3* gene, which provides instructions for making a protein called fibroblast growth factor receptor 3. Recent studies show that this mutation enhances the tumor's sensitivity to tyrosine kinase inhibitor therapy (Roskoski, 2020; Jing et al., 2022). Another mutation found in 70% to 80% of urothelial cancers is the gene that codes for the enzyme telomerase reverse transcriptase (TERT). This mutation allows for enhanced growth and cyclical proliferation of the cancer cells. Genomic and molecular research continues regarding bladder cancer and has allowed clinicians to determine prognosis and prescribe specific targeted treatments.

Pathophysiology

Bladder cancer, also called urothelial cancer, is divided into two types based on the depth of invasion within the bladder wall. Nonmuscle invasive bladder cancer (NMIBC) and muscle invasive bladder cancer (MIBC) are the two major categories of urothelial cancer. NMIBC are tumors that affect only the uroepithelium; the inner epithelial layer of bladder cells or the connective tissue layer below the uroepithelium. This is sometimes referred to as carcinoma in situ. MIBC are tumors that invade the muscle wall of the bladder, surrounding serosal tissue, and may spread to other pelvic organs including rectum, vagina, prostate, or cervix. Approximately 75% of bladder cancer is NMIBC, 18% is MIBC, and 3% presents with metastasis to distant organs.

Clinical outcomes of patients with bladder cancer are associated with the stage at diagnosis. Disease confined to the bladder epithelium is considered stage I–II and has a 70% to 90% 5-year survival rate. Disease that has penetrated the muscle wall or spread to lymph nodes is considered stage III with a 36% to 50% 5-year survival rate. Bladder cancer that has metastasized to other organs is stage IV with a 5% survival rate.

Clinical Presentation

The cardinal feature of bladder cancer is painless, intermittent, gross hematuria. Other symptoms include frequency, pain, and burning on urination, as well as the sensation of incomplete bladder emptying. Some types of bladder cancer present similarly to a UTI with urgency, frequency, and dysuria. Usually located deep within the bladder, bladder cancer rarely presents as a palpable mass. Patients can present with flank pain when significant urinary obstruction has occurred, causing hydronephrosis of the kidney.

Diagnosis

Often the first suspicion of bladder cancer occurs because a urinalysis using a standard dipstick or microscopic evaluation shows RBCs in the urine. A microscopic urinalysis should be repeated to confirm the presence of RBCs and exclude other causes of hematuria. Urine cytology, which uses microscopy to identify cancer cells in the urine, has high false negative and false positive rates. In urine cytology tests, low-grade malignancies are often missed and benign inflammatory conditions can result in false positive results. The bladder tumour antigen (BTA stat) test is a rapid, noninvasive, qualitative urine test that detects bladder tumor–associated antigen in urine. Due to a high false positive rate, the BTA test should be used in addition to urine cytology testing.

Cystoscopy is the gold standard for evaluating unexplained hematuria. It is the best diagnostic procedure for detecting bladder lesions and is definitive when combined with transurethral biopsy. Abdominal CT scan with contrast is the preferred imaging investigation when evaluating high-risk patients with gross painless hematuria and patients suspected of having invasive tumors. Abdominal and pelvic ultrasound combined with cystoscopy may be used in lower-risk patients, such as young women with unexplained hematuria. A magnetic resonance urogram can be used in patients with poor renal function.

There are some specific proteins secreted by urothelial cancer cells that act as biomarkers and have emerged as new therapeutic targets in bladder cancer treatment. Nectin-4 is a tumor-associated antigen found on the surface of most urothelial carcinoma cells. It is a protein involved in cellular adhesion and intercellular communication. High nectin-4 expression is associated with increased tumor size, severe grade, and invasiveness. Another protein called Programmed Cell Death Protein 1 (PD-1) is overexpressed in malignant bladder cancer cells. These proteins allow cancer cells to evade the immune mechanisms of the body. These tumor proteins are being used as new targets in treatments for bladder cancers that are resistant to traditional chemotherapeutic agents. This research is in its beginning stages and emerging with regard to bladder cancer.

> **ALERT!** Painless hematuria is usually the only sign of bladder cancer. Because of this, any amount of hematuria–no matter how small–requires further investigation.

Treatment

In patients with NMIBC (also called carcinoma in situ), the disease has not invaded the muscle wall and can be treated via intravesical instillations of medication,

> **CLINICAL CONCEPT**
>
> Assumption of a UTI, especially in women, is a common cause of a delayed diagnosis of bladder cancer.

meaning the agent is administered directly into the bladder. The most commonly used therapeutic agent is bacillus Calmette–Guérin (BCG). How BCG exerts its effect on bladder cancer is not fully understood but it stimulates a local immune response in the lumen of the bladder against the cancer cells. Repeated BCG treatments are possible with recurrences. Other conservative treatment involves transurethral resection of bladder tumor (TURBT), combined with adjuvant intravesical therapy, such as mitomycin. For muscle invasive bladder cancer, more aggressive treatment is necessary. TURBT plus cisplatin-based chemotherapy and radiation treatment can be attempted (cisplatin chemotherapy is often referred to as platinum-based therapy).

Recently investigated treatments are based on genetic mutations or tumor markers found in cancer cells. Agents inhibiting the programmed cell death protein 1 (PD 1 and PD-L1) have become additional options for treatment. These agents, such as pembrolizumab, avelumab, and atezolizumab, utilize the patient's own immune system to recognize and eliminate the cancer cells. In patients with FGFR factor mutations, the oral tyrosine kinase inhibitor erdafitinib is an optional treatment. Additionally, the nectin-4 targeting antibody drug enfortumab vedotin targets the nectin-4 protein on bladder cancer cells.

In the most severe cases, partial cystectomy with reconstruction is possible. However, in many patients with severe muscle invasive disease, radical cystectomy, which is surgical removal of the entire bladder, is necessary.

Urinary Incontinence and Overactive Bladder

Many persons endure urinary incontinence silently and do not seek medical attention. The majority are women. Many are reticent to admit to the disorder because of embarrassment; therefore, prevalence is difficult to determine.

Epidemiology

In the United States, it is estimated that 10 million persons endure urinary incontinence, the majority of whom are women. Female incontinence in the United States increases with age, from 20% to 30% during young adulthood to almost 50% in older women. The prevalence of daily incontinence in older men is 2% to 11%. Urinary incontinence occurs in 30% of men who have had surgery for prostate disease. Urinary incontinence affects 50% to 84% of older adults in long-term care facilities.

Etiology/Risk Factors

There are various risk factors for incontinence, which include increasing age, pregnancy, childbirth, obesity, diabetes, stroke, and neurological impairment. Prostate disease and its treatments are significant risk factors in men.

Pathophysiology

Types of incontinence are summarized in Table 23-3. The most common type of urinary incontinence is stress incontinence, and it is more common in women than in men. This occurs because of loss of muscle

---

TABLE 23-3. Types of Incontinence

Type of Incontinence	Description
Stress incontinence	Involuntary leakage of urine as abdominal pressure rises, which typically occurs during coughing and sneezing. The leakage occurs because of either poor pelvic support or weakness in the urethral sphincter.
Urge incontinence, also called overactive bladder (OAB)	Detrusor muscle overactivity is the cause of the urine leakage. The cause is unclear, but IC is thought to be the etiology in some patients. The patient complains of feelings of urgency and frequency of urination many times a day.
Overflow incontinence	Chronic overdistention and urinary retention in the bladder results in overflow incontinence. BPH, which obstructs urine outflow, is the most frequent cause in men. Failure of the detrusor muscle caused by damage of the pelvic spinal nerves can also cause this type of incontinence.
Neurogenic bladder	This disorder is the result of an interruption of the sensory nerve fibers between the bladder and the spinal cord or the afferent nerve tracts to the brain. Chronic overdistention of the bladder occurs.
Functional incontinence	Inability to hold urine caused by CNS problems such as stroke, psychiatric disorders, prolonged immobility, dementia, or delirium.
Mixed incontinence	Combination of stress incontinence and OAB.

support in the pelvic floor. Menopause, multiple episodes of childbirth, aging of the musculature, immobility, and surgery such as hysterectomy can cause weakness of the pelvic muscles. Low estrogen levels of menopause contribute to the pelvic muscle weakness.

Overactive bladder (OAB) (also called urge incontinence) is another type of urinary incontinence that is mainly caused by detrusor muscle overactivity. The exact mechanism for OAB is unclear. Proposed etiologies include neurological impairment, urothelium and suburothelium dysfunction, and IC. Obesity and chronic obstructive pulmonary disease (COPD) can also contribute to OAB. In men, the most common cause is prostate surgery. Bladder sphincter dysfunction occurs after nerves are disrupted in surgery.

Overflow incontinence results from chronic over-distention and urinary retention in the bladder. The detrusor muscle of the bladder wall loses strength and elasticity. BPH is the most frequent cause in men. Failure of the detrusor muscle caused by damage of the pelvic spinal nerves can also cause this type of incontinence. Pelvic surgery, trauma, compression of spinal nerves, tumor, or infection can be the cause.

Another type of incontinence referred to as neurogenic bladder is associated with spinal cord disorders that cause peripheral nerve weakness, as well as sympathetic and parasympathetic nerve dysfunction. The spinal cord nerves are insensitive to bladder filling and muscles cannot contract to release the urine.

Functional incontinence is the inability to hold urine because of prolonged immobility, central nervous system (CNS) lesions such as stroke, delirium, or psychiatric disorders such as dementia.

A type of incontinence categorized as mixed incontinence is a combination of stress incontinence and OAB.

Clinical Presentation

Patients with incontinence should be assessed with a thorough history, physical examination, and urinalysis. Women should also have a gynecological examination.

History. A thorough health history is necessary regarding any systemic illnesses, past surgeries, UTIs, or other urinary problems. Male patients should be asked about history of prostate surgery. They should also be questioned about symptoms of prostate disorders, such as weak urinary stream, hesitancy of stream, postvoid dribbling of urine. The patient may report loss of urine with straining or coughing. Alternatively, the patient can report an inability to hold urine and/or repetitive feelings of urinary urgency throughout the day. It is important to ask about the use of absorbent pads or sanitary napkins because these are useful to quantify urine loss. It is important for the clinician to review all the medications and supplements that the patient takes on a regular basis, as some medications can contribute to incontinence (see Table 23-4). A simple three-item questionnaire can assist in distinguishing between the most common types of incontinence (see Box 23-2). A

TABLE 23-4. Medications and Substances That Can Contribute to Urinary Incontinence

Medications that cause decreased bladder contractility (can cause urinary retention and overflow of urine)	ACE inhibitors Antidepressants Antihistamines Antimuscarinic (anticholinergic drugs) Anti-Parkinson's agents Antipsychotic agents Beta-adrenergic agonists Calcium channel blockers Opioids Sedatives Skeletal muscle relaxants
Substances that increase detrusor muscle irritability or creatinine clearance (can cause urge incontinence/OAB)	Caffeine Alcohol Diuretics
Medications that increase urethral sphincter tone (can cause urinary retention and overflow of urine)	Alpha-adrenergic agonists Amphetamines Tricyclic antidepressants
Medications that decrease urethral sphincter tone (can cause stress incontinence)	Alpha-adrenergic antagonists

From Khandelwal, C., & Kistler, C. (2013). Diagnosis of urinary incontinence. *Am Fam Physician, 87*(8):543–550. https://www.aafp.org/afp/2013/0415/p543.html

3-day voiding diary may be helpful in clarifying fluid intake, symptoms, and situations in which urinary incontinence occurs.

Signs and Symptoms. The patient's report of urinary loss should prompt further investigation. Physical examination may or may not reveal signs of a disorder that is causative of urinary incontinence. A complete neurological examination is particularly important. All possible causes and contributing factors need to be ruled out, such as CNS problems, diabetes, spinal cord compression, urinary tract anomalies, UTI, cystocele, and nephrolithiasis. The patient may be asked to keep a voiding diary or complete a specific questionnaire regarding urinary symptoms.

Diagnosis

A simple urinary cough test may be diagnostic. Asking the patient to forcefully cough with a full bladder

BOX 23-2. The Three Incontinence Questions (3IQ) Assessment Tool

This assessment tool can help distinguish between stress incontinence and urge incontinence.
1. During the last 3 months, have you leaked urine (even a small amount)?
   Yes
   No --→ Questionnaire completed.
2. During the last 3 months, did you leak urine (check all that apply):
   a. When you were performing some physical activity, such as coughing, sneezing, lifting, or exercise?
   b. When you had the urge or feeling that you needed to empty your bladder, but you could not get to the toilet fast enough?
   c. Without physical activity and without a sense of urgency?
3. During the last 3 months, did you leak urine most often (check only one):
   a. When you are performing some physical activities, such as coughing, sneezing, lifting, or exercise?
   b. When you had the urge or feeling that you needed to empty your bladder, but you could not get to the toilet fast enough?
   c. Without physical activity or a sense of urgency?
   d. About equally as often with physical activities as with a sense of urgency?

Definitions of the type of urinary incontinence are based on responses to Question 3

Response to Question 3.	Type of Incontinence
Most often with physical activity	*Stress incontinence*
Most often due to urge to empty bladder	*Urge incontinence*
Without physical activity or urgent sensation	*Other cause of incontinence*
About equally with physical activity and urgent sensation	*Mixed*

in the standing position can demonstrate urinary incontinence. Mobility and strength of the bladder sphincter can be assessed with a cotton swab test. A sterile cotton swab lubricated with lidocaine is inserted transurethrally into the bladder with the patient in the supine position. The patient is asked to cough or perform the Valsalva maneuver, and the angle of the cotton swab can indicate if stress incontinence is present. A change in cotton swab angle of more than 30 degrees from resting position is considered positive, indicating urethral hypermobility and stress incontinence.

X-ray of the KUB is essential. Ultrasound and CT scan can rule out kidney stones or urological anatomic anomalies. However, urodynamic testing and cystoscopy may be necessary. Measurement of postvoid residual volume in the bladder is needed.

Treatment

Nonsurgical treatments for incontinence in women include electrostimulation, medical devices, and local estrogen therapy, though the effectiveness of these treatments is inconclusive. Kegel's exercises can improve pelvic muscle strength, and bladder training can reduce urge incontinence and stress incontinence. Some women may require urological surgery for stress incontinence due to pelvic muscle weakness and bladder prolapse. Surgery may include urethral sling procedure and urethropexy to support urethral constriction or to stabilize the bladder neck and urethra.

Anticholinergic drugs such as oxybutynin or tolterodine can be used; however, avoid these in older adults due to potential cognitive effects. Selective antimuscarinic agents darifenacin or solifenacin are preferred to treat stress or urge incontinence (OAB syndrome). These drugs diminish bladder activity and allow retention of urine. In some patients, the antidepressant duloxetine has been effective because it has alpha-agonist properties. The beta-3 adrenergic agent mirabegron, which relaxes the detrusor muscle, has also been effective. Intradetrusor muscle injection of botulinum toxin is being used when all pharmacological agents fail.

Chapter Summary

- Lower UTI is one of the most common problems presented to primary care clinicians.

- The classic symptoms of a lower UTI include dysuria, frequency, and urgency.

- Lower UTI is common in young adult women but rare in young adult men.

- In males over age 60, BPH frequently causes lower UTI.

- In older adults, particularly those in long-term care facilities, lower UTI can lead to urosepsis.

- *E. coli* is the most common pathogen that causes lower UTI.

- Urinalysis is the diagnostic test used most often to determine the presence of infection, blood, or crystals in the urine.

- An abdominal x-ray of the area encompassing the KUB can be used to diagnose many conditions.

- Classic signs and symptoms of nephrolithiasis and urolithiasis include flank pain that radiates into the groin, hematuria, and crystalluria.

- The most common type of calculi in urolithiasis is calcium oxalate. Other types of calculi are uric acid, struvite, and cystine.

- Asymptomatic bacteriuria (ASB) refers to two consecutive urine cultures growing more than a bacterial colony count of 100,000/mL in a patient lacking symptoms of a UTI. ASB is common in older adult women. Antibiotic therapy is not recommended for ASB.

- Interstitial Cystitis (IC) (also called painful bladder syndrome) is a urological disorder with an unclear etiology (see theories of etiology) that causes chronic pelvic pain, perineal pain, dysuria, a sense of fullness of the bladder, urgency, and urinary frequency.

- Cystoscopic investigation is often the most definitive diagnostic procedure for urological disorders.

- Urodynamic studies obtain information about the bladder as it fills and empties.

- Painless, gross hematuria is frequently the only sign of bladder cancer.

- Nonmuscle invasive bladder cancer (NMIBC) is the most common type of bladder cancer.

- There are different types of urinary incontinence: stress, overflow, urge (OAB), neurogenic, functional, and mixed.

Making the Connections

Pathophysiology

Signs and Symptoms	Assessment Findings	Diagnostic Testing	Treatment
Lower UTI | Invasion of the bladder mucosa by bacteria, typically *E. coli,* which usually inhabits the bowel.			
Dysuria, frequency, urgency, general fatigue, and malaise. Urine often has a cloudy appearance and can have a foul odor.	No physical examination findings.	Dipstick urine shows + leukocyte esterase and + nitrites. Urinalysis and culture and sensitivity tests will reveal the bacterial etiology and appropriate antibiotic.	Antibiotics used to eradicate the organism. Increase fluids to enhance flushing out infectious material from the bladder. Phenazopyridine (Pyridium) may be used for urinary tract pain.
Asymptomatic Bacteriuria | A chronic condition of a bacterial count of more than 100,000/mL in the urine without patient symptoms.			
No symptoms.	No physical findings.	Urinalysis and culture and sensitivity tests will reveal the bacterial etiology.	No antibiotics recommended if no symptoms are present.

Making the Connections–cont'd

Signs and Symptoms	Assessment Findings	Diagnostic Testing	Treatment
Interstitial Cystitis/Painful Bladder Syndrome | The pathology of IC is not well understood. Two different types: nonulcerative and ulcerative. In nonulcerative IC, the bladder wall shows thinning, small tears, and hemorrhages. In ulcerative IC, a Hunner's ulcer, erythema, and inflammation are found on the inner bladder wall.			
Urgency, frequency, and discomfort. Pelvic pain.	No physical findings.	Filling cystometry used to assess detrusor muscle function when bladder is full.	Dietary changes and Kegel's exercises. Bladder training. Tricyclic antidepressants, selective anticholinergic agents, or oral pentosan polysulfate sodium. Hydro-distention of the bladder may be therapeutic. DMSO or pentosan polysulfate intravesical therapy is effective. Alternatively, surgery may be required.
Urolithiasis | Kidney stone formation in the urinary tract. Stones occur because of supersaturation of the urine with stone-forming salts. Anatomical abnormalities in the urinary tract predispose to stone formation. Urease-producing bacteria can increase susceptibility to formation of struvite stones.			
Severe back and flank pain radiating into the groin. Severe abdominal pain occurs if stone is high in ureter. Frequency, urgency, and dysuria may or may not be present.	Low-grade fever may be present, as well as costo-vertebral angle tenderness, hematuria, crystalluria.	Microscopic hematuria and crystalluria. CT scan or ultrasound useful to visualize stones.	Conservative management includes analgesics, high fluid intake, low-animal-protein diet, and low sodium intake. Extracorporeal shock wave lithotripsy or surgery may be necessary. Straining of urine necessary.
Bladder Cancer | Uroepithelial cancer; nonmuscle invasive or muscle invasive bladder cancer are two types. Muscle invasive bladder cancer is the more severe disease.			
Microscopic to frank hematuria.	No physical assessment findings. Painless hematuria.	Urinalysis and urine cytology may show cancer cells; cystoscopy shows bladder tumor. Biomarkers on tumor cells may assist in distinguishing the target treatment.	Transurethral resection of bladder tumor combined with chemotherapy or adjuvant intravesical therapy and possible radiation. Immunotherapy agents and targeted cancer agents may also be attempted. Radical cystectomy in refractory cases.
Urinary Incontinence | Several different types. (1) Stress incontinence caused by pelvic muscle weakening. (2) Urge incontinence (overactive bladder [OAB]) caused by spasms of detrusor muscle. (3) Overflow incontinence caused by obstructive uropathy. (4) Neurogenic incontinence caused by loss of spinal nerve function. (5) Functional incontinence caused by dementia, delirium, immobility, stroke, or psychiatric problems. (6) Mixed urinary incontinence has features of stress incontinence and OAB.			
Leakage of urine or complete inability to hold urine.	Inability to suppress urination with leakage of urine.	Full serum metabolic panel; CBC, electrolytes, blood urea nitrogen (BUN), creatinine. Urinalysis, urine culture. Urinary cough test. Cotton swab test.	Pelvic floor exercises (Kegel exercises), bladder training, estrogen treatment are used for stress incontinence. Vaginal ring pessaries for pelvic organ prolapse may be tried for stress incontinence.

Making the Connections—cont'd

Signs and Symptoms	Assessment Findings	Diagnostic Testing	Treatment
		Urodynamic evaluation of bladder filling or voiding phase. Some patients may require cystoscopy.	Urological surgery for stress incontinence in women includes sling procedures and urethropexy to support urethral constriction or to stabilize the bladder neck and urethra. Selective antimuscarinic agents (darifenacin, solifenacin) are preferred over nonselective agents (oxybutynin, tolterodine). Mirabegron is a beta-adrenergic agonist that relaxes the detrusor muscle. Patients with neurogenic bladder often require urinary catheterization

Bibliography

Available online at fadavis.com

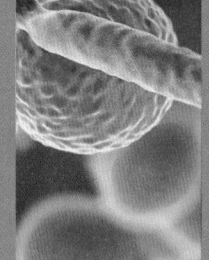

Endocrine Disorders

Learning Objectives

Upon completion of this chapter, the student will be able to:

- Explain the hypothalamus–pituitary–hormone axis and feedback system.
- Recognize the multiple hormones that originate in the anterior and posterior pituitary glands.
- Differentiate among diseases associated with hyperfunction versus hypofunction of the pituitary, thyroid, and adrenal glands.

- Compare and contrast the signs and symptoms associated with hyperfunction versus hypofunction of the pituitary, thyroid, and adrenal glands.
- Recognize laboratory tests involved in the diagnosis of hyperfunction and hypofunction of the pituitary, thyroid, and adrenal glands.
- Discuss treatments for hyperfunction and hypofunction of the pituitary, thyroid, and adrenal glands.

Key Terms

Acromegaly

Adenohypophysis

Addison's disease

Adrenal insufficiency

Adrenocorticotropic hormone (ACTH)

Antidiuretic hormone (ADH)

Arginine vasopressin (AVP)

Cortisol

Cushing's disease

Cushing's syndrome

Diabetes insipidus (DI)

Exophthalmos

Goiter

Goitrogen

Graves' disease

Growth hormone (GH)

Hypophysis

Hypothalamic–pituitary–hormone axis

Hypothalamus–hypophyseal portal system

Mineralocorticoid

Myxedema

Neurohypophysis

Pheochromocytoma

Pituitary adenoma (pituitary neuroendocrine tumor)

Prolactin (PRL)

Prolactinoma

Somatotropin

Syndrome of inappropriate antidiuretic hormone (SIADH)

Thyroid-stimulating hormone (TSH)

Thyroxine (T_4)

Tropic hormone

The endocrine glands are a unique group of organs that secrete chemical messengers known as hormones. In the endocrine system, there is a set sequence of hormone secretion from organ to organ. In most sequences, the hypothalamic portion of the brain secretes a releasing factor that stimulates the pituitary gland. The pituitary, also called the master gland, has widespread effects throughout the body. With effects on growth, reproduction, fluid balance, and metabolism, the pituitary is involved in all endocrine organ sequences.

After the pituitary is stimulated, it releases a substance referred to as a **tropic hormone** that targets a specific endocrine organ. The target endocrine organ then secretes a hormone that acts on the body and causes a physiological effect. The sequence of endocrine organ function is termed the hypothalamic–pituitary–hormone axis.

Endocrine gland hormones include thyroxine, **cortisol,** epinephrine, growth hormone (GH), parathyroid hormone (PTH), and **antidiuretic hormone (ADH).** These well-known hormones keep the body in homeostatic balance and are kept in check by a unique endocrine feedback system. After the appropriate physiological action by the target organ is achieved, the endocrine system can shut off the effect. Conversely, if the target organ action is not achieved, the endocrine system keeps the sequence cycling.

When the endocrine system dysfunctions, there is an imbalance of hormones that can cause hyperfunction or hypofunction of the target organs. Dysfunction can occur at the hypothalamus, the pituitary, or the individual endocrine gland itself. In this chapter, dysfunction of the pituitary, thyroid, adrenal, and parathyroid glands will be discussed. For dysfunction of the pancreas, ovaries, and testes, see the chapters on diabetes (see Chapter 25), female reproductive systems (see Chapter 26), and male reproductive systems (see Chapter 27), respectively.

Epidemiology

Some endocrine diseases, such as diabetes mellitus (DM), are common (see Chapter 25), whereas others, such as pheochromocytoma, are rare. Thyroid disease is another prevalent endocrine disorder, particularly among middle-aged women. The thyroid is in control of the body's metabolism and has widespread effects on multiple body systems. Hypothyroidism occurs in 4.6% of the population in the United States. Iodine is an integral constituent of thyroid hormone. In areas of the world where iodine deficiency is prevalent, the number of individuals with thyroid disease is much higher. Worldwide, approximately 1 billion people are at risk for hypothyroidism because of iodine deficiency.

Like the thyroid, the adrenal gland, which secretes cortisol, has widespread effects on the body. Cushing's syndrome, a disorder caused by an excess of cortisol, has been estimated at 13 cases per 1 million individuals per year in the United States. Of these cases, approximately 70% are caused by a pituitary adrenocorticotropic hormone (ACTH)–secreting tumor, 15% by an adrenal gland tumor, and another 15% caused by administered corticosteroids or a cancerous lesion that secretes ACTH. Females are affected more often than males, with an incidence of 5:1. The average age of those affected is between 25 and 40 years old.

In contrast, Addison's disease, a hypofunction of the adrenal gland, is rare. The reported incidence of Addison's disease is 5 or 6 cases per million per year in the United States. More females are affected with Addison's disease, with a female-to-male ratio of 3:1. There are numerous causes of hypoadrenalism, including malignancy and infectious disease. It can occur in persons of any age, but is most common in people aged 30 to 50 years old.

Pituitary dysfunction is uncommon, and symptoms can be gradual and subtle. Because the pituitary is the master gland that controls all other endocrine functions, its dysfunction sets off multiple endocrine abnormalities. The annual incidence of pituitary neoplasms varies from 1 to 7 cases per 100,000 population worldwide. A pituitary neoplasm is the most common type of intracranial tumor.

Basic Concepts of Endocrine Function

There is a unique relationship between the hypothalamus, pituitary, and endocrine glands. The hypothalamus, the coordinating center of the endocrine system, consolidates signals derived from thoughts, feelings, autonomic function, environmental cues, and peripheral endocrine feedback. The hypothalamus secretes a releasing factor that delivers precise signals to the pituitary gland. In turn, the pituitary gland releases a specific tropic hormone that stimulates a specific endocrine target organ. The regulatory link between the hypothalamus, pituitary gland, and endocrine target organ is the **hypothalamic–pituitary–hormone axis;** this fundamental control system exists with all endocrine organs. The pituitary, also called the **hypophysis,** has two distinct sections: The anterior pituitary is called the **adenohypophysis,** and the posterior pituitary is referred to as the **neurohypophysis.** The hypothalamus and pituitary gland are in communication with each other via specialized neurovascular tissue called the **hypothalamus–hypophyseal portal system.**

The Pituitary as Master Gland

The pituitary, a pea-sized organ located in the center of the brain, is called the master gland because it regulates all the body's endocrine glands. It can be compared with a dispatcher because in response to a signal from the hypothalamus, it releases one of its many tropic hormones (see Fig. 24-1). The anterior pituitary secretes **growth hormone (GH), prolactin (PRL), adrenocorticotropic hormone (ACTH), thyroid-stimulating hormone (TSH),** follicle-stimulating hormone (FSH), and luteinizing hormone (LH). The hypothalamus synthesizes ADH and oxytocin (OXT), which are stored and released by the posterior pituitary. ADH is also called **arginine vasopressin (AVP)** and GH is also called **somatotropin.**

The Feedback System

As a result of pituitary stimulus, an endocrine gland secretes a specific hormone. After the hormone is secreted, the pituitary senses its level in the bloodstream. This unique feature of the endocrine gland is called a feedback system (see Fig. 24-2). The pituitary interprets the level of hormone as normal, high, or low and then responds by either rereleasing the tropic hormone or ceasing tropic hormone release, thereby maintaining a normal hormone level from the target organ. Feedback control, both negative and positive, is a fundamental feature of the endocrine system. Negative feedback regulates each of the hypothalamic–pituitary–hormone axes, a process that maintains hormone levels within a narrow range.

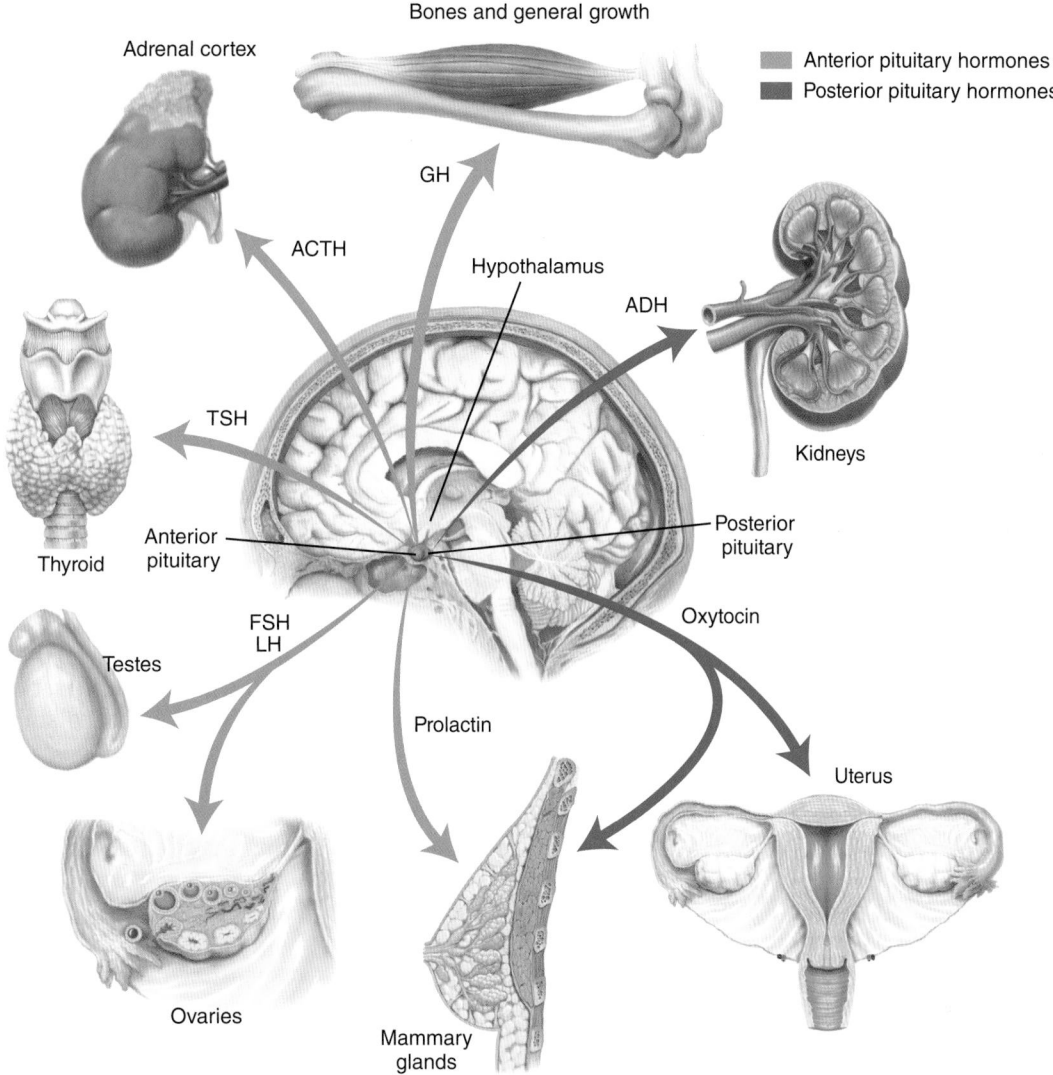

FIGURE 24-1. The hypothalamus–pituitary hormone pathway. The hypothalamus stimulates the anterior and posterior sections of the pituitary gland. The pituitary is the master gland of the endocrine system, which secretes different types of tropic hormones.

For example, when an individual is running in a marathon, the hypothalamus receives signals from the body that the muscles and organs have extra metabolic needs. The hypothalamus secretes corticotropin-releasing factor (CRF), which stimulates the pituitary gland. The pituitary gland secretes ACTH, which, in turn, stimulates the adrenal gland to secrete the hormone cortisol. As cortisol levels in the bloodstream rise, the pituitary senses the increased level and shuts off the stimulus to the adrenal gland; this is an example of the endocrine negative feedback system.

The Regulation of Endocrine Gland Receptors

Pituitary hormones act on receptors located on endocrine glands to secrete hormones. The reactions of the receptors on endocrine glands vary depending on the amount of stimulation by these pituitary hormones. For instance, prolonged, excessive stimulation of an endocrine gland often results in receptor insensitivity and may decrease its number of receptors in a process known as a downregulation of receptors. Conversely, upregulation of receptors is an increase in the number of receptors and their sensitivity. The most common reason for upregulation is a reduction in the receptor stimulation by hormones. An example of downregulation occurs when an individual takes an excessive, prolonged dose of glucocorticoid drugs. The pituitary senses the high blood level of glucocorticoids and, as a result, it does not need to secrete ACTH. There is no need to stimulate the adrenal gland because natural glucocorticoids are unnecessary; the body is receiving more than enough exogenous glucocorticoids. As a result, the adrenal gland downregulates its receptors and becomes less sensitive to ACTH stimulation.

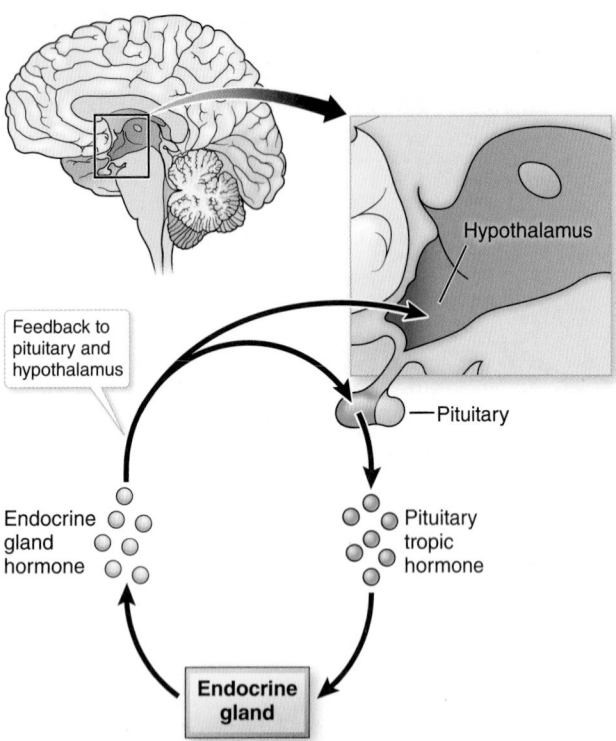

FIGURE 24-2. The hypothalamic–pituitary–endocrine gland axis feedback mechanism.

Basic Pathophysiological Concepts of Endocrine Dysfunction

Endocrine dysfunction occurs when the hypothalamus–pituitary–hormone axis is disrupted. Endocrine disease can be divided into three major types of conditions:

1. Hormone deficiency
2. Hormone excess
3. Hormone resistance

Most examples of hormone deficiency occur because of glandular destruction caused by autoimmunity, infection, inflammation, infarction, or tumor infiltration. The endocrine cells are damaged and cannot synthesize any hormone. An example is autoimmune destruction of the pancreatic islet cells in type 1 DM. Damaging autoantibodies render pancreatic cells nonfunctional, which results in complete insulin deficiency.

Syndromes of hormone excess are caused mainly by tumor growth, autoimmune disorders, or genetic mutations that cause excessive function of endocrine cells. For example, Graves' disease is an autoimmune disease that causes overproduction of thyroid hormone. In this disease, autoantibodies form that mimic TSH. These autoantibodies excessively stimulate the thyroid gland to release elevated levels of thyroxine. Elevated thyroxine causes multiple systemic effects, such as atrial fibrillation, tremulousness, hot flashes, and muscle weakness.

Hormone resistance syndromes are caused mainly by genetically inherited defects that produce dysfunctional membrane receptors. These disorders are characterized by defective hormone action at the receptor despite the presence of elevated hormone levels. A common example of resistance to a hormone is type 2 DM. Despite the pancreatic secretion of high levels of insulin, cells throughout the body are insensitive to insulin in this type of diabetes.

Types of Endocrine Dysfunction

Endocrine gland dysfunction can be divided into two categories: hypofunction and hyperfunction. Hypofunction of an endocrine gland occurs when there is an inadequate amount of hormone secreted by the gland. Hyperfunction of an endocrine gland occurs when there is an excessive amount of hormone secreted by the gland.

Dysfunction of an endocrine gland can be caused by any of the organs in the hypothalamus–pituitary–hormone axis. Endocrine gland hypofunction or hyperfunction can be caused by the hypothalamus, the pituitary, or the endocrine gland itself. Hypothalamic or pituitary origin of endocrine dysfunction is uncommon. When the endocrine dysfunction is caused by the pituitary, it means that the pituitary is either secreting its tropic hormone excessively or releasing insufficient tropic hormone. If the etiology of the disorder lies with the endocrine gland itself, then the gland is secreting either excessive or insufficient amounts of hormone. Endocrine gland disorders are commonly caused by an autoimmune, inflammatory, neoplastic, or vascular disease of the gland.

Endocrine dysfunction can also be referred to as a primary, secondary, or tertiary disorder:

- Primary disorder: dysfunction caused by the endocrine gland itself
- Secondary disorder: dysfunction caused by abnormal pituitary activity
- Tertiary disorder: dysfunction caused by a hypothalamic origin

For example, hypothyroidism due to autoimmune destruction of the thyroid gland itself is primary hypothyroidism. Hypothyroidism occurring because of lack of secretion of TSH by the pituitary gland is secondary hypothyroidism. Hypothyroidism occurring because of lack of secretion of releasing factor by the hypothalamus is tertiary hypothyroidism.

Role of Autoimmunity in Endocrine Dysfunction

Many endocrine disorders occur because of autoimmunity, which itself occurs when the body manufactures antibodies against its own tissues. The cause for these autoantibodies is unknown, but they trigger inflammation in the organs they target. In the endocrine system, autoimmunity can cause either hypofunction or hyperfunction of the gland.

Role of Neoplasia in Endocrine Dysfunction

Another common cause of endocrine dysfunction is neoplasia, or tumor formation. Tumors can be a source of excess hormones and cause hyperfunction of the gland. They can also interfere with hormone production and cause hypofunction. A pituitary tumor can cause dysfunction in multiple organs because of the wide array of endocrine glands under its control.

 CLINICAL CONCEPT

Pituitary tumors can cause such problems as growth disturbances, electrolyte imbalances, and infertility. They classically cause visual disturbances because of their proximity to the optic chiasm in the brain.

Some cancers cause development of paraneoplastic disorders. These are disorders where, for an unknown reason, the cancer cells have the ability to secrete an endocrine hormone. For example, specific types of lung cancer often secrete ACTH.

Endocrine-Disrupting Compounds in the Environment

Endocrine-disrupting compounds (EDCs) are chemicals in the environment that have the potential to mimic, block, or alter the synthesis, transport, binding, or metabolism of endogenous hormones. These chemicals can have adverse effects on the health of humans, animals, and their offspring. The most compelling evidence for the health effects of EDCs comes from research on some wildlife species. Some studies have found the following well-established examples of adverse health effects:

- Poor reproductive success and egg abnormalities in bird species exposed to high levels of DDT
- Male genitalia development in female species of marine mollusks that have been exposed to paints on ships that contain organotin compounds
- Feminization of male freshwater fish in rivers or lakes exposed to sewage effluents
- Impaired reproduction in alligators and turtles in polluted lakes of Florida and the Great Lakes of the United States

A growing body of evidence suggests that many synthetic chemicals once considered safe can be harmful to the developing fetus, infant, and child. There is particular concern about the developmental effects of EDCs in the environment. Research studies have shown the following EDCs are of particular concern:

- Polybrominated diphenyl ethers added as flame-retardants to computers, televisions, and furniture
- Phthalates added to soften plastics (e.g., toys) and vinyl products or to carry fragrances in cosmetics and household cleaners
- Bisphenol A, a component of hard plastics that leaches from some plastic containers and the linings of cans
- Perfluorooctanoic acid, which forms nonstick, stain repellant, or waterproof coatings on cookware, carpets, and clothing
- Organochlorines (e.g., polychlorinated diphenyl ethers), many of which are banned but are still found in the environment

All of the EDCs listed have been detected in the blood and urine of most U.S. children and adults in representative samples of the National Health and Nutrition Examination Survey cohort. They, along with more than 100 other environmental contaminants, have also been detected in breast milk and umbilical cord blood. Research studies have linked them to neurodevelopmental effects, including lowered IQ and attention deficits; reproductive effects, such as hypospadias, cryptorchidism, decreased fertility, and accelerated puberty; immune dysfunction causing asthma and allergies; and hormonally mediated cancers (see Box 24-1).

BOX 24-1. Endocrine Gland Disruptors

Endocrine disruptors, also referred to as hormonally active agents, are man-made substances in the environment that interfere with the natural hormones in the body. These agents are widely dispersed in the environment and are shown to accumulate in the body. One endocrine disruptor under intense investigation is bisphenol A (BPA), which is commonly found in plastic bottles such as water bottles and baby bottles, dental materials, and the linings of metal food cans. Studies have found that BPA can exert estrogen-like effects on both males and females. Laboratory animals exposed to low levels of BPA have elevated rates of diabetes, mammary and prostate cancers, decreased sperm count, reproductive problems, early puberty, obesity, and neurological problems.

Phthalates (PAEs) are industrial chemicals that are listed as the most widespread pollutant in water and soil. PAEs are plasticizers that increase the flexibility and softness of plastic. They are constituents of personal care products, automotive parts, children's toys, food packaging, and building materials. As an endocrine disruptor, phthalates act like estrogen and have been associated with harmful effects in pregnant women, such as higher rates of miscarriage, preterm delivery, low-birth-weight infants, and reproductive system abnormalities in newborns.

The research into the health effects of EDCs is in the early stages. Currently, no clear-cut relationships have been established between adverse health effects and exposure to specific endocrine disruptors in humans. Large-scale human epidemiological studies are still needed to correlate definite health effects with exposure to specific EDCs.

Assessment

To evaluate a patient for an endocrine disorder, the clinician needs to perform a complete history and physical examination, as well as specific types of diagnostic studies. The patient's risk factors, present symptomatology, and physical signs of disease are key parts of the complete assessment. Symptoms commonly involve multiple body systems, and a high index of suspicion is needed.

The patient's complaints regarding the present illness are most important in the history, as endocrine disorders often cause a change in metabolic function that may present in subtle ways. Also, endocrine symptoms overlap with signs of other diseases that can confound the clinical picture. For example, in hyperthyroidism, the patient's chief complaint may be heart palpitations, which can lead to multiple cardiovascular diagnostic procedures versus thyroid investigation.

When symptoms are multisystemic, the clinician should look at the whole patient picture and recognize that an endocrine disorder may cause a syndrome, a constellation of symptoms from different systems. Symptoms reported by the patient from different body systems are often part of one endocrine gland dysfunction syndrome. Thyroid diseases, for example, are exhibited by abnormalities of the cardiovascular, musculoskeletal, and reproductive systems. Atrial fibrillation, nervousness, hot flashes, muscle weakness, and menstrual irregularities constitute some of the changes that occur in hyperthyroidism. These symptoms arise from dysfunction of different body systems and may be mistakenly treated separately instead of as one syndrome.

Endocrine dysfunction commonly has an effect on mood and behavior as well. Often, the presenting symptoms are misinterpreted as emotional or psychological distress. For example, the patient with hypothyroidism may describe a lack of energy and excessive sleepiness, which is often misinterpreted as depression.

Family history is also very important because many endocrine disorders are genetic in origin. Thyroid disease, for example, is often seen among members of the same family. Diabetes is also familial.

Occupational and environmental exposures are also key pieces of information. Many chemical compounds are endocrine disruptors that interfere with pathways within the endocrine system. Over-the-counter and prescription medications, as well as possible toxic exposures, should be reviewed.

Risk Factors

Each endocrine gland has different risk factors for dysfunction, but major risk factors for endocrine disease include genetic predisposition, radiation exposure, medications, and pollutants.

Genetic predisposition is a known risk factor for many endocrine disorders, particularly thyroid disorders. For example, Graves' disease, hyperfunction of the thyroid, is more common in individuals with 6p and 20q mutations.

Radiation exposure has been strongly linked to endocrine disorders. Radiation can trigger cancerous transformation of cells in the body; for example, irradiation of the head and neck, particularly in childhood, increases the susceptibility to thyroid cancer later in life.

Many medications can increase an individual's susceptibility to endocrine dysfunction. Lithium, phenothiazines, and glucocorticoids are some examples that affect the pituitary and adrenal glands.

Pollutants in the environment that cause endocrine gland dysfunction are increasingly being recognized. These substances, called endocrine disruptors, include environmental contaminants such as heavy metals, drug metabolites, and organic hydrocarbon compounds.

Signs and Symptoms

To diagnose an endocrine disorder, the clinician needs to be vigilant of physical manifestations of hormone deficiency or excess. Most endocrine organs are not easily accessible on physical examination. The most accessible endocrine gland is the thyroid, and commonly a small lesion is nonpalpable. Astute clinical skills and knowledge of the patient's baseline level of health are important because endocrine abnormalities can be difficult to distinguish from nonspecific physical findings. For example, a patient with the hyperadrenalism of Cushing's disease may present with excessive body fat, striae, hypertension, and muscle weakness. These findings on physical examination may not be distinguished as signs of a single endocrine disorder.

Diagnosis

Immunoassays, or blood levels of hormones, are the most important diagnostic tool in endocrine disorders. Most hormone measurements are based on samples of blood plasma.

Urinary hormone levels are useful for some conditions. Urinary collection over 24 hours often can provide useful information in the analysis of metabolic function. With any urinary collection, a measurement of urine creatinine is needed to provide information about the patient's renal function. A 24-hour urine cortisol level is an example of a test that provides a measurement of biologically active hormones.

The normal ranges of hormones are commonly affected by gender, age, or circadian rhythm. Cortisol values increase fivefold between midnight and dawn, female reproductive hormones vary with the menstrual cycle, and estrogen and testosterone levels vary according to age.

Suppression tests are used when endocrine hyperfunction is suspected. One example is the dexamethasone suppression test to diagnose Cushing's syndrome. Dexamethasone, a potent corticosteroid, is administered and should decrease the adrenal gland's activity. If the dexamethasone does not suppress adrenal secretion of cortisol, the adrenal gland is hyperactive.

Stimulation tests such as the ACTH stimulation test are commonly used to assess endocrine hypofunction. The ACTH stimulation test assesses the adrenal gland response in patients suspected of adrenal insufficiency.

 CLINICAL CONCEPT

Normally, the adrenal gland should be stimulated by ACTH, but a hypofunctioning adrenal gland will not be stimulated by administration of ACTH.

Ultrasound is commonly used to investigate thyroid masses. The thyroid specifically binds to iodine for synthesis of thyroxine, and radioactive iodine uptake is used for thyroid imaging. Fine needle aspiration biopsy is commonly used when investigating thyroid nodules. Computed tomography (CT) and magnetic resonance imaging (MRI) are used to investigate tumors or masses in all endocrine organs.

Treatment

Hormone replacement therapy is used to treat hormone deficiency. The most common replacement treatments include glucocorticoids, thyroid hormone, sex steroids, GH, and vasopressin (also called ADH). Dosage schedules attempt to mimic physiological hormone production.

Suppression of hormone overproduction is accomplished medically or surgically. An example of medical suppression involves the use of bromocriptine, a dopamine agonist, in pituitary prolactinomas. Surgical procedures are used to excise growths or tumors of endocrine organs. Transsphenoidal surgery, a procedure that uses the sphenoid sinus to gain access to the pituitary gland, is used in removal of pituitary tumors. Radiation is used either as a primary therapy or as an adjunct treatment in endocrine tumors. Radioactive iodine ablation therapy is commonly used in hyperfunctioning thyroid disease. For specific information on diagnostic studies and treatment, see the sections on specific disorders as they are covered in this chapter.

Pathophysiology of Selected Endocrine Disorders

Each endocrine gland disorder can be categorized according to its hypoactivity or hyperactivity. Epidemiology, etiology, pathophysiology, clinical presentation, and treatment all differ according to which gland is dysfunctioning and whether the gland is secreting either a low amount or excessive amount of hormone.

Pituitary Gland Disorders

The pituitary gland, as the master gland, affects many different organ systems when it is dysfunctional. The side effects of the gland's dysfunction vary according to the individual's age. Growth defects are the major problem in children, whereas in adults there is a wide number of organ disorders.

Hypopituitarism

Hypopituitarism, also known as pituitary insufficiency, is the hyposecretion of one or more of the pituitary hormones.

It is difficult to estimate the incidence and prevalence of hypopituitarism as there are few epidemiological studies and widely diverse etiologies. For example, epidemiological studies of the postpartum population find an incidence of Sheehan's syndrome, which causes hypopituitarism, in up to 3% of women annually (Reale et al., 2020). Alternatively, congenital hypopituitarism in neonates is cited as 1 in 4,000 to 10,000 infants annually in the United States (Bosch et al., 2021). The population that seems most commonly affected are those with traumatic brain injury (TBI). Hypopituitarism is found in up to 50% of patients after TBI (Tanriverdi et al., 2015). Another study regarding hypopituitarism due to pituitary adenomas shows an increasing incidence (between 3.9 and 7.4 cases per 100,000 per year) and prevalence (76 to 116 cases per 100,000 population) in the general population (Daly & Beckers, 2020).

Etiology. There are many possible etiologies for hypopituitarism, including pituitary tumor, complications following brain surgery, or radiation of a brain tumor. Complete and sudden loss of pituitary function is most often caused by trauma, ischemia, infarction, or hemorrhage. Sheehan's syndrome is pituitary ischemia and infarction that develop after childbirth because of severe hemorrhage. Empty sella syndrome, a condition caused by compression of the pituitary gland by brain tissue herniation, is also a cause of hypopituitarism. Panhypopituitarism, a rare disorder, is the complete loss of all the pituitary hormones.

Pathophysiology. Many different tropic hormones are secreted by the pituitary gland; therefore, dysfunction of the gland can cause multisystemic problems.

Hormones secreted by the anterior pituitary include the following:

- Thyrotropin, or TSH
- Gonadotropins, or FSH and LH
- Somatotropin, or GH
- Corticotropin, or ACTH
- Prolactin, or PRL

The posterior pituitary does not produce its own hormones; it stores hormones. The hypothalamus produces ADH (also referred to as AVP) and oxytocin (OXT). These two hormones are released into the hypothalamic–hypophyseal tract to the posterior pituitary, where they are stored. They are released from the posterior pituitary into the circulation when needed.

In hypopituitarism, tropic hormone production is reduced and, in turn, target gland hormone production is decreased. Normally, low levels of target gland hormone feedback to the pituitary gland increase tropic hormone production. However, in hypopituitarism, the pituitary gland is dysfunctional and the response is absent or inadequate. This results in secondary failure of the target endocrine glands.

Some cases of congenital hypopituitarism are associated with mutations in the *POU1F1, PROP1, LHX3, LHX4,* and *HESX1* genes. The prevalence of genetic mutations varies worldwide, such that *PROP1* mutations account for the majority of genetic multiple pituitary hormone deficiency in Europe, but are much less common in Asia. Mutations in these genes cause multiple pituitary hormone deficiencies, leading to lack of GH, PRL, and TSH. The lack of these hormones causes body-wide effects, such as growth failure, weakness, diminished muscle mass, poor bone density, poor memory, and depression. In females, amenorrhea, infertility, and deficient lactation also occur.

The most common causes of hypopituitarism include tumors, cranial radiation, TBI, subarachnoid hemorrhage, infectious and inflammatory disorders, and postpartum pituitary necrosis (Sheehan's syndrome). The **pituitary adenoma (pituitary neuroendocrine tumor)**, a benign, epithelial neoplasm, is the most common tumor of the pituitary gland. It can compress pituitary tissue or interfere with the delivery of hypotalamic hormones to the pituitary gland. The etiology of the adenoma is unknown.

Another intracranial tumor associated with hypopituitarism is a craniopharyngioma. This is a benign neoplasm that can develop close to the pituitary gland or in the pituitary stalk. It causes pressure on the pituitary gland, which renders the gland nonfunctional.

Sheehan's syndrome, which can occur after childbirth, is another cause of hypopituitarism. During pregnancy, the pituitary gland enlarges because of hyperplasia and hypertrophy of the cells that produce PRL, the hormone that stimulates lactation in the postpartum period. When there is a large loss of blood during childbirth or afterward in the postpartum period, blood supply to the pituitary is severely reduced, causing ischemia, infarction, and necrosis of the gland. The degree of necrosis correlates with the severity of the hemorrhage. Women who suffer from Sheehan's syndrome develop widespread endocrine gland failure because of the many tropic hormones that originate in the pituitary. Because ACTH, TSH, FSH, LH, ADH, and PRL are diminished, the effects of Sheehan's syndrome include adrenal insufficiency, hypothyroidism, amenorrhea, diabetes insipidus (DI), and inadequate lactation.

Pituitary apoplexy is the sudden destruction of the pituitary tissue caused by infarction or hemorrhage into the gland. TBI is the most common cause, but it can occur in patients with DM, pregnancy, sickle cell anemia, anticoagulation, or increased intracranial pressure.

Empty sella syndrome, another cause of hypopituitarism, occurs when the meningeal membrane that surrounds the brain herniates into the sella turcica, a bony area where the pituitary gland sits in the brain. The herniation of this membrane flattens the pituitary against bone, and pituitary insufficiency results. Empty sella syndrome can be caused by increased intracranial pressure, radiation, or trauma.

TBI due to a motor vehicle accident, fall, blast injury, or projectile such as a gunshot can directly harm the pituitary or its stalk or hypothalamus. Hypopituitarism can develop immediately or several months or years later. Recovery can occur in some cases by regeneration of tissue.

In some physiological or psychological conditions, hypothalamic function can be impaired, thereby decreasing stimulation of the pituitary. Poor nutrition can reduce the hypothalamic secretion of gonadotropin-releasing hormone (GnRH), which, in turn, decreases stimulation of pituitary secretion of FSH and LH. Other causes of hypothalamic dysfunction include excessive stress, emotional disorders, changes in body weight, excessive exercise, anorexia, bulimia, heart failure, renal failure, and certain medications.

Clinical Presentation. The signs and symptoms of pituitary insufficiency are dependent on which tropic hormones are not secreted. The symptoms are secondary endocrine gland deficiencies. For example, if a pituitary adenoma interferes with ACTH secretion, secondary adrenal insufficiency symptoms develop. These symptoms include severe hypotension, weakness, and weight loss. The onset of hypopituitarism is often gradual over a period of years, but rapid onset can occur. The most serious concerns are adrenal insufficiency, hypothyroidism, and **diabetes insipidus (DI),** the last of which occurs because of a lack of posterior pituitary secretion of ADH.

The problems that arise because of hypopituitarism depend on the age of onset. The infant mainly exhibits growth failure. Clinical presentation in the neonate and infant include dwarfism, developmental delay, various visual and neurological symptoms, seizure disorder, and a number of congenital malformations.

Adults with hypopituitarism have different clinical manifestations according to the specific hormones that are deficient. Adults often exhibit gradual symptoms of hypothyroidism, adrenal insufficiency, and ADH deficiency. The clinical presentation may be weakness, weight loss, and hypotension caused by adrenal insufficiency, or weight gain, sluggishness, and depression caused by hypothyroidism. Lack of ADH causes excessive urination and dehydration, a syndrome known as DI.

Patients in whom hypopituitarism is due to a pituitary tumor may have symptoms related to the pressure of the mass on the optic chiasm, which is adjacent to the gland. Symptoms include headache, visual loss, and/or diplopia.

When hypopituitarism is acute, the patient presents in a rapidly deteriorating state of hypotension; severe dehydration; neurological deficits; and abnormalities in electrolyte levels, glucose levels, body temperature, and heart rate.

Diagnosis. Hypopituitarism causes low tropic hormone levels and, as a result, low corresponding endocrine organ hormone levels in the bloodstream. Hypothalamic releasing factors normally stimulate the pituitary to secrete tropic hormones; however, in hypopituitarism, there is no response from the pituitary. The diagnosis is made by finding low serum levels of pituitary tropic hormones, such as TSH, ACTH, FSH, LH, GH, PRL, and ADH, and low corresponding endocrine organ hormones, such as thyroxine (T_4), cortisol, and estrogen. Each pituitary hormone must be tested separately because there is a variable pattern of hormone deficiency among patients with hypopituitarism. For example, low free thyroxine in the setting of low TSH level suggests secondary hypothyroidism, which is due to hypopituitarism or dysfunction of the hypothalamus. Similarly, low testosterone without elevation of gonadotropins, LH, or FSH suggests hypopituitarism.

According to Snyder (2020), testing of basal ACTH secretion is recommended to diagnose hypopituitarism. A morning serum cortisol (8 a.m. to 9 a.m.) should be measured and the results should be interpreted as follows: A low serum cortisol value of less than or equal to 3 mcg/dL (normal range 5 to 25 mcg/dL) confirmed by a repeated test is strong evidence of cortisol deficiency due to hypopituitarism.

Another recommended diagnostic test is the metapyrone test. Metyrapone blocks 11-beta-hydroxylase, which is the enzyme that catalyzes the conversion of 11-deoxycortisol to cortisol. Therefore, metapyrone reduces cortisol secretion. The ensuing fall in serum cortisol should, if the hypothalamic-pituitary-adrenal axis is normal, cause an increase in ACTH secretion and an increase in adrenal release of cortisol. In patients who have decreased ACTH due to hypothalamic or pituitary disease, the serum 11-deoxycortisol concentration will be low and the serum cortisol less than normal at the end of 24 hours.

CT and MRI scans are also used, particularly when pituitary tumor or empty sella syndrome is suspected. Imaging studies are interpreted in combination with serum levels of tropic hormones.

Treatment. Treatment for hypopituitarism varies depending on which tropic hormones are lacking. The treatments for corticotropin (ACTH), thyroid-stimulating hormone (TSH), luteinizing hormone (LH), and follicle-stimulating hormone (FSH) deficiencies are in many ways the same as the treatments for primary deficiencies of the respective target glands. Treatment of ACTH deficiency consists of the administration of hydrocortisone in an amount and timing to mimic the normal pattern of cortisol secretion. Treatment of TSH deficiency is treated with T_4 (levothyroxine). Treatment of luteinizing hormone (LH) and follicle-stimulating hormone (FSH) deficiency depends on sex and whether fertility is desired. Testosterone replacement is indicated in men who have secondary hypogonadism and are not interested in fertility. Men with hypogonadism due to hypopituitarism who wish to become fertile can be treated with gonadotropins if they have pituitary disease or with gonadotropin-releasing hormone (GnRH) if they have hypothalamic disease. Women with hypogonadism due to pituitary disease who are not interested in fertility should be treated with estradiol-progestin replacement therapy. Women with secondary hypogonadism who wish to become fertile should be offered ovulation induction with gonadotropins. In adult patients with growth hormone deficiency, recombinant growth hormone once daily subcutaneously can serve as treatment. Snyder (2020) recommends somapacitan, which is a long-acting formulation of GH linked to albumin that is given once weekly. The only known presentation of prolactin deficiency is the inability to lactate after delivery, for which there is currently no available treatment. Recombinant human prolactin (r-hPRL), although not commercially available, has been used experimentally.

For pituitary tumors, transsphenoidal resection or transcranial surgery is necessary. Radiation is often used as either primary therapy or as an adjunct to surgery.

Diabetes Insipidus

DI is a disorder of hypopituitarism that originates in the posterior pituitary, also called the neurohypophysis. The disorder involves ADH, and there are two categories of disease: central DI, which occurs because of a lack of secretion of ADH from the posterior pituitary, and nephrogenic DI, which occurs when the kidney fails to respond to ADH.

Central DI is uncommon in the United States, with a prevalence of 4 cases per 100,000 population. Nephrogenic DI is less common, with a prevalence of 0.4 per 100,000 persons, and can be inherited as an X-linked disorder. It can also be acquired because of medications or renal disease.

Etiology. The etiology of central DI includes tumors such as craniopharyngiomas or head trauma that causes injury of the posterior pituitary or the hypothalamic–hypophyseal tract. Other causes include pituitary surgery, inflammatory disorders, infection, or exposure to chemical toxins. Nephrogenic DI (NDI) is often caused by nephrotoxic drugs such as lithium, obstructive uropathy, ischemia of the kidney, hypokalemia, or hypocalcemia. The genetic causes, which are rare, commonly present in childhood. Congenital X-linked NDI results from an inactivating gene mutation that codes for the vasopressin V2 receptor in the kidney and accounts for 90% of inherited NDI.

Pathophysiology. Whether there is decreased ADH secretion from the posterior pituitary gland or an insensitive ADH receptor in the kidney, the same pathophysiological process occurs. The nephron does not perform antidiuresis, meaning that the nephron does not reabsorb water from the tubule fluid. As a consequence, the body loses high amounts of water in the urine, causing polyuria and highly dilute urine. The bloodstream loses water, which concentrates its sodium content, causing hypernatremia, polyuria, dilute urine, and dehydration.

CLINICAL CONCEPT

A syndrome known as psychogenic polydipsia can present similarly to DI. In psychogenic polydipsia, the patient drinks excessive amounts of water and therefore has excessive, very dilute urine.

Clinical Presentation. The symptoms associated with DI, regardless of etiology, are those of dehydration and hypernatremia. The patient will report frequent urination (polyuria) and thirst (polydipsia). In addition, because of dehydration, neurological problems can occur, including confusion, disorientation, myoclonus, seizures, and, in severe cases, coma. These neurological changes are potentially reversible with adequate hydration and hormone replacement.

Diagnosis. Differentiating DI from other causes of polyuria requires blood glucose testing, as well as analyzing urine for glucose, specific gravity, osmolality, and sodium. Serum osmolality and sodium levels should be obtained at the same time that urinary testing is performed. A serum osmolality greater than 300 mOsm/kg with a urine osmolality less than 300 mOsm/kg confirms a diagnosis of DI. Central DI can be distinguished from nephrogenic DI by the administration of ADH (also referred to as AVP). If the kidney responds to ADH, then the problem is lack of secretion of ADH by the posterior pituitary, and the

diagnosis is central DI. If administration of ADH does not concentrate the urine, then the kidney is resistant to ADH, and the diagnosis is nephrogenic DI. AVP has a short half-life and may be difficult to measure. The precursor of AVP, copeptin, has proved to be more stable than AVP, and it can be used to measure AVP levels.

To distinguish psychogenic polydipsia from DI, patients must be put on fluid restriction. If urine osmolality increases after fluid restriction, the disorder is psychogenic polydipsia; however, if polyuria and a dilute urine still occur following fluid restriction, the diagnosis is DI, either central or nephrogenic.

For patients with central DI, magnetic resonance imaging is recommended to examine the pituitary stalk for structural causes.

Patients diagnosed with central DI should also be screened for deficits in other anterior pituitary hormones, including TSH, ACTH, FSH, LH, and GH.

> **ALERT!** Because polyuria and dehydration occur in both DM and DI, it is important to measure serum glucose to differentiate DM from DI. Serum glucose is elevated in DM, but not in DI.

Treatment. Treatment of DI depends on whether the patient has CDI or NDI. For CDI, oral desmopressin (DDAVP) is typically used. It is available as intranasal therapy; however, it is more difficult to titrate and can lead to eye irritation, headaches, rhinitis, epistaxis, coughing, and flushing. Caution should be taken when giving DDAVP to young children and postoperative patients as there is a risk of hyponatremia and water intoxication. Infants with CDI can be managed with thiazide diuretics, which have a paradoxical antidiuretic effect in DI, until they make the transition to a solid diet. They should be monitored for hypokalemia or be given amiloride to preserve potassium. Nephrogenic DI is difficult to treat, other than by eliminating its underlying cause. Congenital nephrogenic DI is treated with foods with a high ratio of calories to osmotic load. In consultation with nephrology, thiazide diuretics, possibly in combination with amiloride or indomethacin, may also be used to reduce urine output.

Hyperpituitarism

Hyperpituitarism, or primary hypersecretion of pituitary hormones, is rare in both children and adults. Pituitary adenoma is the most common cause. The prevalence of pituitary adenomas has increased to 115 cases per 100,000 population over the past several decades, probably as a result of enhanced awareness and improved diagnostic imaging. Distinct hyperpituitary disorders depend on the cell of origin: corticotropin-secreting corticotroph adenomas result in Cushing's disease, growth hormone–secreting somatotroph adenomas result in acromegaly, prolactin-secreting lactotroph adenomas result in hyperprolactinemia, and thyrotropin-secreting thyrotroph adenomas result in hyperthyroidism. Gonadotroph adenomas, which are typically nonsecreting, lead to hypogonadism.

A PRL-producing pituitary adenoma, also called **prolactinoma,** is the most common cause of hyperpituitarism. The incidence of prolactinoma is 54 cases per 100,000 population. In some research studies, the tumor accounts for approximately 25% to 30% of all pituitary adenomas, with the highest incidence in females younger than 20 years old.

A GH-secreting pituitary adenoma is rare. Incidence is estimated to be 3 to 4 cases per million population per year in the United States. In children, a GH-secreting tumor causes gigantism, whereas in adults, it causes acromegaly.

Pathophysiology. Pituitary adenomas may occur in association with several genetic syndromes. Multiple endocrine neoplasia type 1 is associated with pituitary adenomas; parathyroid and pancreatic-islet tumors; and less commonly, carcinoid, thyroid, and adrenal tumors. McCune–Albright syndrome is characterized by polyostotic fibrous dysplasia and cutaneous pigmentation, with sexual precocity, hyperthyroidism, hypercortisolism, hyperprolactinemia, and acromegaly. The Carney complex includes pituitary adenomas with benign cardiac myxomas, schwannomas, thyroid adenomas, and pigmented skin spots.

Most pituitary adenomas secrete a specific hormone that produces a characteristic clinical presentation. Overall, prolactinomas are the most common pituitary adenoma encountered in childhood; they cause symptoms secondary to excess PRL, which causes antiestrogenic and antiandrogenic effects. In females, menstrual abnormalities, amenorrhea, galactorrhea, vaginal dryness, and osteopenia occur. In males, hypogonadism, decreased libido, erectile dysfunction, and infertility occur. The prolactinoma can also cause symptoms secondary to the space-occupying effects of the tumor itself. Large tumors can cause headache, dizziness, and visual disturbances because of proximity to the optic nerve chiasm. The tumor can also compress pituitary tissue, reducing the gland's ability to secrete other hormones.

In children, ACTH-producing adenomas, also called corticotropinomas, are commonly observed before puberty, although they occur in people of all ages. They are more prevalent in females. The tumor secretes excessive ACTH that stimulates excess cortisol secretion from the adrenal gland. The affected individual has all the features of Cushing's syndrome, which is covered later in this chapter.

GH-secreting adenomas, also called somatotropinomas, are uncommon but can cause gigantism in children (see Fig. 24-3). In children, GH stimulates the growth plates of long bones, which results in excessive

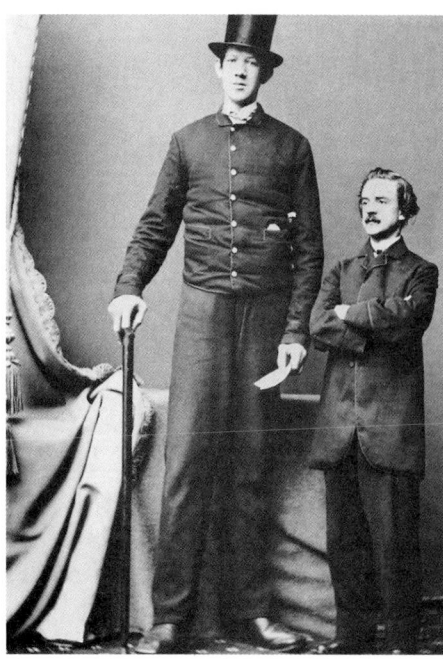

FIGURE 24-3. Gigantism of hyperpituitary function. *(From Science Source.)*

longitudinal growth. The affected individual grows to a height of 7 feet or more. The individual often suffers from other endocrine or genetic conditions that negatively affect overall health.

In adults, excessive GH stimulates a gradual growth of certain bones such as the jaw, hands, and feet, a condition called **acromegaly**.

Clinical Presentation. Prolactinoma is the most common type of pituitary adenoma. Most pediatric cases occur in adolescence, predominately in females. Females with these tumors present with amenorrhea and galactorrhea, whereas males present with gynecomastia and hypogonadism. Somatotropinomas are rare but cause gigantism in children. Individuals exhibit tall stature; moderate obesity; large hands and feet; coarse facial features; cardiac hypertrophy; and endocrine disorders such as hypogonadism, diabetes, and hyperprolactinemia.

In adults, excess GH results in acromegaly. Symptoms of acromegaly develop slowly and gradually, taking years to decades to become apparent (see Fig. 24-4). Signs include overgrowth of the jaw and facial bones; enlarged hands and feet; organ overgrowth, including tongue enlargement (macroglossia) and hypertrophy of the heart, thyroid, liver, and kidneys; insulin resistance; and increased risk of colon polyps. The patient may also suffer the effects of the pressure of the pituitary tumor against brain tissue, which can result in headaches and visual impairment.

ACTH-secreting adenomas often present in prepubescent children. ACTH stimulates the adrenal gland to produce excess cortisol, and the presentation is called Cushingoid appearance. The signs include obesity; stunted growth; swollen face, called moon facies;

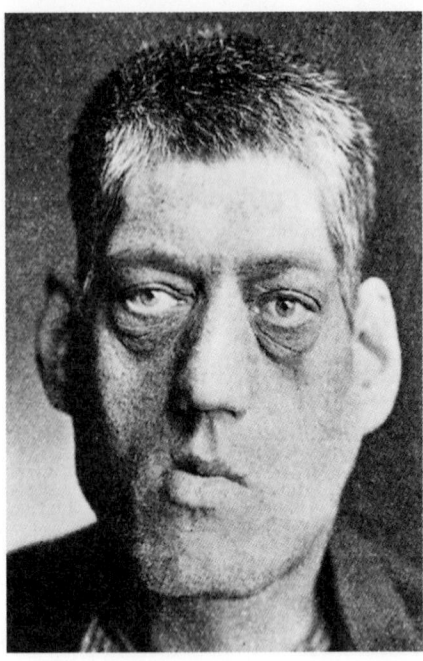

FIGURE 24-4. Acromegaly from hyperpituitary function. *(From SPL/Science Source.)*

acne; ruddy complexion; hirsutism; fat in the posterior neck area, called buffalo hump; and striae, also known as stretch marks. TSH-secreting adenomas are rare but can present with signs and symptoms of hyperthyroidism, including nervousness, tremulousness, palpitations, weight loss, visual disturbances, headaches, and hypersensitivity to heat.

Diagnosis. Hyperpituitarism causes high tropic hormone levels and, as a result, high corresponding endocrine organ hormone levels in the bloodstream. The diagnosis is made by finding high serum levels of pituitary tropic hormones, particularly GH and PRL. Other tropic hormones, such as ACTH and TSH, and corresponding endocrine organ hormone levels can also be high. Urine hormone levels, such as urinary free cortisol, can be measured as well. The thyrotropin-releasing hormone (TRH) stimulation and dexamethasone suppression tests can be used in the diagnosis. Measurement of the serum insulin-like growth factor-1 (IGF-1) and serum IGF binding protein-3 are used for diagnosis of acromegaly. An oral glucose tolerance test (OGTT) can also be used to determine whether it suppresses growth hormone. CT and MRI scans are used when pituitary tumor is suspected. Imaging studies are interpreted in combination with serum levels of tropic hormones.

Treatment. Treatment requires medications that block GH and surgical excision of any pituitary tumor. In prolactinoma, oral dopamine agonists, cabergoline and bromocriptine, block secretion of PRL and can shrink tumors. For treatment of corticotropin-secreting pituitary tumors, transsphenoidal surgery is usually required in addition to medication. A number of steroidogenic inhibitor medications are available to counteract the consequences of the corticotropin-secreting tumor. Adrenal enzyme inhibitors, such as ketoconazole, are prescribed to block formation of adrenal hormones. Alternatively, pasireotide LAR can lower ACTH levels. Osilodrostat, an oral hydroxylase inhibitor, can block cortisol secreted by the adrenal gland. Metyrapone and mitotane, other hydroxylase inhibitors, can also normalize cortisol levels. Mifepristone is a glucocorticoid receptor antagonist that blocks peripheral cortisol action. Other agents include cyproheptadine, trilostane, and IV etomidate.

In somatotropin-secreting tumors, somatotropin receptor ligands, octreotide or lanreotide, are used as long-acting depot formulations to suppress excessive GH secretion. Patients who do not get effective treatment can try another medication, pasireotide LAR. Cabergoline and octreotide used in combination have been able to shrink tumors. Alternatively, a GH receptor antagonist, pegvisomant, can normalize growth hormone levels when used for 3 months. External radiation treatment may be used as adjuvant therapy for GH-secreting tumors.

Syndrome of Inappropriate Antidiuretic Hormone

Syndrome of inappropriate antidiuretic hormone (SIADH) secretion is a common condition in patients who sustain brain injury or those who undergo neurosurgery for brain disorders. It can also occur as a paraneoplastic disorder in many different types of cancer, particularly small cell lung cancer. Many different drugs can induce SIADH. Some vascular and infectious diseases have also been found to cause SIADH. The syndrome is characterized by hyponatremia and hypo-osmolality of the blood that result from excessive secretion or action of ADH.

Epidemiology. Acute brain injury is one of the most common triggers of SIADH, though few studies have demonstrated the exact incidence or prevalence of the disorder. However, in one investigation of patients with traumatic brain injury and subarachnoid hemorrhage, 5% of patients demonstrated SIADH after surgery. SIADH is commonly found in patients with lung cancer, in particular small-cell lung cancer (SCLC). The prevalence in this group is estimated to be 7% to 16% and it seems that 70% of all SIADH due to malignancy is attributable to SCLC. In head and neck tumors, SIADH incidence is 3%. SIADH is the most important cause of hyponatremia in oncological and hospitalized patients.

Etiology. There are numerous causes of SIADH, including nervous system disorders such as stroke and meningitis, neoplastic causes such as lung and colon cancer, and pulmonary diseases such as emphysema and pneumonia. SIADH can be a side effect of brain injury, brain surgery, or may be secreted by tumors; particularly lung cancer. Pain, stress, and some medications have also been associated with it. Chemotherapeutic agents are particularly associated with risk of SIADH.

Pathophysiology. ADH is synthesized by the hypothalamus and transmitted via nerve tracts to the posterior pituitary, where it is stored and secreted. Essential for fluid balance in the body, ADH stimulates reabsorption of water into the bloodstream at the collecting duct of the nephron. SIADH causes excess water reabsorption into the bloodstream. This excess water creates hypervolemia, dilutional hyponatremia, and highly concentrated urine. SIADH is particularly significant if it occurs rapidly. There is an increase in water in the brain that causes cerebral edema. The edema causes brain expansion that exceeds skull capacity and downward pressure on the brain occurs. This can cause brain herniation, pressure on the brainstem, and consequent death from respiratory arrest and/or vascular cerebral injury. This usually happens when hyponatremia develops quickly and the brain has too little time to readjust to this hypotonic environment.

Clinical Presentation. Patients with SIADH may complain of symptoms related to fluid volume overload and dilutional hyponatremia, including fatigue, weakness, confusion, and headache. Neurological symptoms can be found in patients with hyponatremia: with sodium value between 135 mEq/L and 125 mEq/L (mild hyponatremia), patients can be asymptomatic or complain nausea, vomiting, dizziness. The physical examination of the hyponatremic patient may be normal, but if hyponatremia is severe or rapid in onset, findings include myoclonus, slowed reflexes, seizures, problems with gait and balance, nystagmus, dysarthria, dysphagia, and coma.

Diagnosis. To diagnose SIADH, measurements of sodium, electrolytes, and water of the blood and urine are most important. Diagnostic tests include urine specific gravity, urine osmolality, hematocrit, and plasma osmolality. SIADH causes dilutional hyponatremia, elevated urine osmolality, excessive urine sodium, and decreased serum osmolality.

A normal blood sodium level is between 135 and 145 mEq/L. Hyponatremia occurs when the sodium in blood falls below 135 mEq/L. Determining plasma osmolality is the first step in hyponatremia diagnostic work-up. If not available on laboratory results, it can be calculated using this formula: $2 \times Na$ (mmol/L) + glucose (mg/dL)/18 + urea (mg/dL)/2.8. Effective serum osmolarity is less than 275mg/dL. If high osmolality (greater than 280 mOsm/kg) is found, excessive concentration of osmotically active solutes in plasma must be identified. The blood should be checked for hyperglycemia and high concentration of mannitol should be ruled out: glucose and mannitol are the most important effective osmoles. Urine osmolarity should be checked on a spot urine sample: if it is less

than 100 mOsm/kg H_2O, that means maximum urine dilution, primarily caused by excessive water intake. If urine osmolality is greater than or equal to 100 mOsm/kg H_2O, SIADH should be considered.

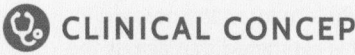

CLINICAL CONCEPT

SIADH causes dilutional hyponatremia, elevated urine osmolality, excessive urine sodium, and decreased serum osmolality.

Treatment. Elimination of the underlying disorder or drug responsible for SIADH is of primary importance. To ensure optimal management of SIADH, factors such as etiology, onset timing, severity, symptoms, and extracellular volume status should guide correction measures. Fluid restriction is a first-line treatment that can resolve hyponatremia. Fluid restriction should be 500 to 800 mL per day for a gradual normalization of sodium levels. Slow correction of hyponatremia by 1 to 2 mEq/L per hour over 24 hours using 3% hypertonic saline is recommended if fluid restriction does not raise sodium. Conivaptan or tolvaptan, both ADH receptor antagonists, may be necessary. Furosemide may be used to increase excretion of water. The tetracycline medication demeclocycline can also be used as treatment because it reduces nephron sensitivity to ADH.

Thyroid Disorders

The thyroid gland is a 2-inch, butterfly-shaped gland located in the neck. The hormones of the thyroid gland, triiodothyronine (T_3) and **thyroxine (T_4),** have a wide range of physiological effects. Thyroxine is the regulator of body metabolism, which influences almost every body system. Thyroid dysfunction presents as either hypothyroidism or hyperthyroidism, both of which are more common in women than men. The thyroid is easily examined but normally should not be palpable in the neck. An enlarged thyroid can occur in hypofunction or hyperfunction. Primary thyroid disorders, where the thyroid gland itself is dysfunctional, are the most common type of disease. The frequency of hypothyroidism, goiters, and thyroid nodules increases with age.

Goiter

A **goiter** is an enlargement of the thyroid gland with or without symptoms of thyroid dysfunction. When there are no symptoms of thyroid disease, the enlargement is referred to as a nontoxic goiter. Excess pituitary TSH can stimulate enlargement of the thyroid gland and cause goiter formation. Alternatively, if iodine levels are decreased in the body, thyroid hormone synthesis is diminished, as iodine is a necessary component in the synthesis of thyroid hormone. Low iodine levels cause low thyroid hormone manufacture, which the pituitary senses and then attempts to compensate for by increasing TSH, which incites goiter formation.

Enlargement of the thyroid gland can also occur from **goitrogens.** Goitrogens are foods and medications that interfere with thyroid hormone action. This lack of thyroid hormone action, in turn, can lead to elevated TSH and growth of the thyroid gland. Certain foods such as cruciferous vegetables (e.g., cauliflower, broccoli) and medications (e.g., lithium, phenytoin, and rifampin) are considered goitrogenic. Individuals on these medications need to have thyroid hormone levels monitored.

Hypothyroidism

Hypothyroidism occurs when there are insufficient levels of the thyroid hormones T_3 and T_4. Primary hypothyroidism, where the thyroid gland itself is not secreting T_3 and T_4, is the predominant type of hypothyroidism, affecting approximately 95% of patients. In a minority of individuals, secondary hypothyroidism is the cause, where the pituitary is not secreting sufficient TSH; this, in turn, causes low T_3 or T_4 synthesis.

Epidemiology. Hypothyroidism affects up to 5% of the general population, with a further estimated 5% being undiagnosed. Over 99% of affected patients suffer from primary hypothyroidism. Worldwide, environmental iodine deficiency is the most common cause of all thyroid disorders, including hypothyroidism, but in areas of iodine sufficiency, Hashimoto's disease (chronic autoimmune thyroiditis) is the most common cause of hypothyroidism. Primary hypothyroidism is up to 8 to 9 times more common in women than in men, and the prevalence increases with age, with a peak incidence between the ages of 30 and 50 years. In the United States, hypothyroidism affects an estimated 4% of women aged 18 to 24 years and 21% of women older than 74 years; respective values in men are 3% and 16%. European Americans have a higher incidence of hypothyroidism than African Americans. The postpartum period is particularly a time of high incidence of thyroiditis, with 10% of women suffering the disorder in the 2 to 12 months after pregnancy. Hypothyroidism may also occur as a congenital condition in children causing cretinism. The incidence of this is 1 in 5,000 in the European American population and 1 in 32,000 in the African American population.

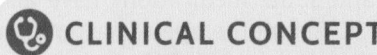
Etiology. Hypothyroidism is a common endocrine disorder resulting from deficiency of thyroid hormone. It usually is a primary process in which the thyroid gland produces insufficient amounts of thyroid hormone. Several syndromes, genetic mutations, and medications can cause hypothyroidism. Risk factors include age older than 50 years; female gender; pregnancy; autoimmune disease; radiation to the neck; family history; and certain drugs, including radioactive iodine, amiodarone, interferon alpha, interleukin, and lithium.

Subacute granulomatous thyroiditis (also known as de Quervain disease) is an inflammatory condition of the thyroid. It occurs mainly in middle-aged women and causes transient hyperthyroidism followed by transient hypothyroidism.

Numerous drugs have the potential to cause hypothyroidism, including amiodarone, lithium, interferon-alfa, phenobarbital, and phenytoin. Radioactive iodine (I-131) used for the treatment of Graves' disease causes permanent hypothyroidism. External neck radiation can cause hypothyroidism as well.

There are several genetic etiologies of hypothyroidism. Genome-wide association studies have shown that persons with a single nucleotide polymorphism located near the *FOXE1* gene tend to have hypothyroidism. Congenital hypothyroidism, called cretinism, is associated with mutations in the *FOXE, NKX2-1, PAX8,* and *NKX2-5* genes and others. Pendred's syndrome is caused by a mutation in the *SLC26A4* gene that results in defective iodine incorporation into thyroid hormone. Autoimmune polyendocrinopathy type 1 is caused by a mutation in the *AIRE* gene.

Pathophysiology. A negative feedback loop regulates the thyroid hormone in conjunction with the pituitary and hypothalamus. The hypothalamus produces thyrotropin-releasing hormone that controls anterior pituitary gland secretion of TSH, regulating the secretion of thyroid hormone (triiodothyronine [T_3] and thyroxine [T_4]) by the thyroid gland.

In Hashimoto's thyroiditis, biopsy of thyroid tissue reveals a high number of lymphocytes in the thyroid gland. TSH receptor antibodies are present as well. When these antibodies bind to the TSH receptor, there is an absence of the normal response of T_3 and T_4 synthesis and secretion. Other antibodies associated with this condition include antithyroglobulin antibody and antithyroperoxidase (anti-TPO) antibody.

CLINICAL CONCEPT

Anti-TPO antibodies are the hallmark of Hashimoto's thyroiditis.

Clinical Presentation. Adult patients with hypothyroidism take on an altered appearance because of a combination of factors. Reduction in the conversion of carotene to vitamin A causes hypercarotenemia, which gives skin a yellow-orange tint. A puffy face occurs because of accumulation of sodium and water from protein/polysaccharide complex deposits. A characteristic hoarse voice also develops.

Lack of thyroid hormone causes a decrease in the body's various metabolic activities. Reduced levels of low-density lipoprotein (LDL) receptors in the liver lead to elevations in cholesterol and triglycerides. Anemia occurs from decreased hematopoiesis. Reduced kidney function causes decreased clearance of medications and increased susceptibility to drug toxicity. Alterations in pulmonary function lead to hypercapnia and hypoxia. Over time, an increased risk of cardiomegaly develops. The longer the hypothyroid condition lasts, the more profound the effects.

The effects of the reduced levels of T_3 and T_4 are seen in all body systems (see Fig. 24-5). Constitutional symptoms include cold intolerance, weight gain, lethargy, and fatigue. Other symptoms include memory deficits, poor attention span, muscle cramps, constipation, decreased fertility, puffy face, hair loss, and brittle nails. In the adult, severe hypothyroidism is called **myxedema**.

Subacute granulomatous thyroiditis (de Quervain's thyroiditis) can present with thyroid tenderness, fever, and dysphagia. This is an inflammatory condition of the thyroid that can be transient, however 50% of patients develop hyperthyroidism. Females are affected more than males.

Cretinism is the result of thyroid hormone deficiency during embryonic development and early neonatal life. The child exhibits short stature, intellectual disability, and other metabolic disorders.

Pendred's syndrome results from defective iodine incorporation into thyroid hormone. It is associated with sensorineural hearing loss and an enlarged thyroid gland.

Autoimmune polyendocrinopathy is a rare disorder where the body develops antibodies against a number of endocrine organs. It is associated with Addison's disease, hypoparathyroidism, mucocutaneous candidiasis, and hypothyroidism.

Subclinical hypothyroidism, which is common in older adults, can cause subtle neuropsychiatric problems such as disorientation, depression, and pseudodementia (see Box 24-2 for more details).

Screening for Thyroid Disorders. The American Thyroid Association recommends thyroid screening tests in women at age 35 and every 5 years thereafter; however, other organizations differ in their recommendations. The American College of Physicians recommends screening women aged 50 and older who have one or more clinical features of the disorder. The U.S. Preventive Services Task Force concludes that there is insufficient evidence to screen for thyroid dysfunction in nonpregnant, asymptomatic adults. However, in certain patients, screening is recommended. These include patients with Down syndrome; Turner syndrome; subtotal thyroidectomy; type 1 diabetes; autoimmune adrenal insufficiency (Addison disease); radioiodine treatment; radiation therapy of the neck; and use of medications such as amiodarone, lithium, interferons, and rifampin. Other medications that may prompt screening include tyrosine kinase inhibitors, phenobarbital, interleukin-2, and immune checkpoint inhibitors.

At birth, currently, neonatal screening mainly detects elevated levels of TSH that increase in response to the reduction in thyroid hormone. This screening identifies 90% of cases of congenital hypothyroidism.

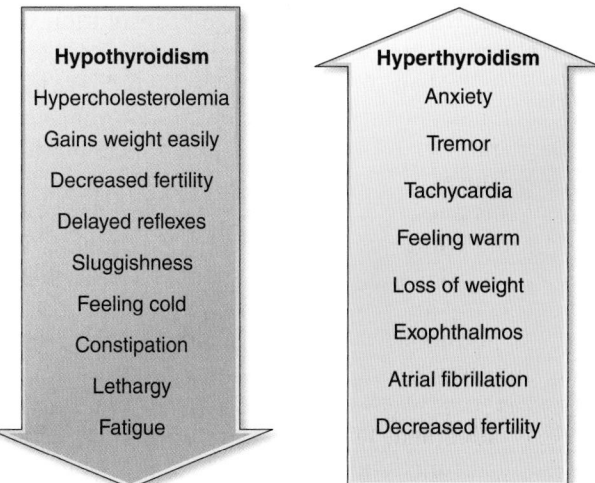

FIGURE 24-5. Signs and symptoms of thyroid disorder.

Hypothyroidism	Hyperthyroidism
Hypercholesterolemia	Anxiety
Gains weight easily	Tremor
Decreased fertility	Tachycardia
Delayed reflexes	Feeling warm
Sluggishness	Loss of weight
Feeling cold	Exophthalmos
Constipation	Atrial fibrillation
Lethargy	Decreased fertility
Fatigue	

BOX 24-2. Subclinical Hypothyroidism

Subclinical hypothyroidism is a disorder in which thyroid function is only mildly low, so that the blood level of thyroxine (T_4) remains within the normal range, but the blood level of TSH is elevated, indicating mild thyroid failure. Individuals can suffer mild symptoms of hypothyroidism, such as fatigue, difficulty losing weight, and depression. Subclinical hypothyroidism can be treated with a single daily dose of thyroxine; however, treatment is controversial. This treatment requires monitoring of the thyroid hormone levels in the blood over several months. Recent studies suggest that treatment is warranted, especially if the blood TSH level is greater than 10 mU/L.

Diagnosis. Diagnosis of hypothyroidism requires testing of the TSH blood level, as well as free T_3 and T_4 levels. A high TSH level with low T_3 and T_4 is diagnostic of primary hypothyroidism, as low hormone secretion by the thyroid gland constantly signals the pituitary to secrete TSH. Early in hypothyroidism, T_3 may be normal; however, free T_4 level is low. Blood is also tested for the presence of thyroid autoantibodies referred to as antithyroglobulin (anti-Tg) and anti-TPO antibodies. These antibodies indicate autoimmune destruction of the thyroid gland. A high TSH level with normal T_3 and T_4 levels indicates mild or subclinical hypothyroidism. In secondary hypothyroidism, TSH and T_4 will be low because the pituitary gland is the cause of inadequate thyroid function. Most likely, if the pituitary is not secreting TSH, other tropic hormones will also be deficient. A complete blood count, serum metabolic profile, serum creatinine, and liver enzymes are needed. Anemia, hyponatremia, and hyperlipidemia are commonly found in hypothyroidism. A PRL level is sometimes elevated in the setting of increased TRH and TSH.

Ultrasound is used to visualize any nodules in the thyroid along with a fine needle biopsy to take tissue samples. However, in hypothyroidism, thyroiditis is usually the etiology without the presence of nodules. The use of color Doppler flow ultrasound will demonstrate decreased vascular flow in hypothyroidism.

Treatment. Treatment for primary hypothyroidism includes replacement hormone therapy with levothyroxine and surgical intervention, if necessary. In adult patients who are not pregnant, TSH should be monitored every 6 to 8 weeks until within normal range, then every 6 to 12 months, barring a change in clinical status.

ALERT! When hypothyroidism is untreated, it can progress to myxedema coma, a serious illness with a high mortality rate. There are severe hypothyroid symptoms, as well as susceptibility to SIADH, hypoglycemia, and hyponatremia. If left untreated, the symptoms will progress to confusion and coma.

Hyperthyroidism

Hyperthyroidism, sometimes referred to as thyrotoxicosis, is an excessive secretion of the thyroid hormones T_3 and T_4. The most common etiology is **Graves' disease,** an autoimmune stimulation of the thyroid gland. Other common causes include toxic multinodular goiter, and thyroid adenoma (also called toxic adenoma). There is a familial susceptibility to Graves' disease, with 15% of patients reporting a relative with this same disease. The overall incidence of hyperthyroidism is 1.3%, which increases to up to 5% in older women. Most persons with Graves' disease are in the 40- to 60-year-old age range. More women than men are affected with thyroid disease. Graves' disease has a male-to-female ratio of 1.5:10. Toxic multinodular goiter and thyroid adenoma have a male-to-female ratio of 1.2:4. European Americans are affected by hyperthyroidism more than African Americans. Interestingly, Graves' disease often affects spouses simultaneously.

Risk Factors. Persons at increased risk for hyperthyroidism include those with goiters, type 1 diabetes, other autoimmune diseases, and a family history of thyroid disease. Medications that increase risk include amiodarone, interferon, interleukin-2, lithium, iodide, iodinated contrast agents, immune checkpoint inhibitors, and alemtuzumab. There is a higher prevalence of Graves' disease in patients with specific HLA tissue types such as HLA-DR3, HLA-C, and HLA-B8, HLA-B*46, and HLA-B27. It is also more common in persons with polymorphisms in immunoregulatory genes *CTLA-4, CD25, PTPN22, FCRL3, CD226,* and the gene encoding for the thyroid-stimulating hormone receptor.

Etiology. The most common cause of hyperthyroidism is Graves' disease, which occurs in 60% to 80% of cases. Graves' disease is an autoimmune disorder caused by thyroid-stimulating immunoglobulins (TSIs) that are synthesized by lymphocytes in the thyroid gland. These immunoglobulins are detected by immunoassay TSH receptor antibody (TRAb). Other antibodies found include anti-TPO and anti-Tg antibodies in 80% of cases.

The next most common cause of hyperthyroidism is subacute thyroiditis, an inflammation of the thyroid gland that causes release of excessive thyroid hormone. It occurs in approximately 15% to 20% of cases of hyperthyroidism, often following extreme stress or infection. Subacute thyroiditis, commonly a self-limited disorder that occurs over a number of months, often presents as a triphasic disorder. There is a first stage of hyperthyroidism, a second stage of hypothyroid function, and a third stage of resolution with normal thyroid function. A specific type of subacute thyroiditis, called de Quervain's thyroiditis, often causes pain of the inflamed thyroid.

Toxic multinodular goiter, also called Plummer's disease, causes 15% to 20% of cases of hyperthyroidism. This is a form of primary hyperthyroidism where the thyroid contains autonomously hyperfunctioning nodules. It occurs more commonly in older individuals, especially in patients with a long-standing goiter. Thyroid hormone excess develops very slowly over time and often is only mildly elevated at the time of diagnosis.

Toxic adenoma, another etiology, is caused by a single hyperfunctioning thyroid tumor. Patients with a toxic thyroid adenoma account for approximately 3% to 5% of patients who are hyperthyroid.

Iodide-induced thyrotoxicosis, also known as Jod–Basedow phenomenon, occurs in patients with excessive iodine intake, such as after an iodinated radiocontrast study. Patients can also endure hyperthyroidism secondary to administration of amiodarone, a cardiac antiarrhythmic agent. Amiodarone contains iodine and is structurally similar to thyroid hormone.

Patients can develop hyperthyroidism secondary to pregnancy. Placental human chorionic gonadotropin (hCG) is structurally similar to TSH, and the increase in hCG during pregnancy can stimulate TSH receptors.

Sometimes difficult to identify, self-medication with excessive synthetic thyroxine hormone can also cause hyperthyroidism. Patients often do this to lose weight; however, it has detrimental side effects.

Struma ovarii is an uncommon syndrome where thyroid tissue develops within specific types of tumors of the ovary: dermoid tumors, or ovarian teratomas. The thyroid tissue can secrete excessive amounts of thyroid hormone and produce thyrotoxicosis.

McCune–Albright syndrome is a disorder caused by a mutation in the *GNAS* gene. The syndrome includes facial asymmetry, Cushing's disease, acromegaly, and hyperthyroidism. Other syndromes that also include hyperthyroidism due to a mutation in the *TSHR* gene include familial gestational hyperthyroidism, congenital thyrotoxicosis, and toxic thyroid adenoma. Type II autoimmune polyendocrine syndrome also includes hyperthyroidism, type 1 diabetes, adrenal insufficiency, and mucocutaneous candidiasis.

Pathophysiology. The most common mechanism of hyperthyroidism occurs when the thyroid gland secretes an excessive amount of thyroid hormone. This typical mechanism is demonstrated in Graves' disease. In Graves' disease, there are excess levels of T_3 and T_4 because of thyroid-stimulating autoantibodies. Thyroid-stimulating antibodies bind to and activate thyrotropin receptors within the thyroid gland, causing the gland to enlarge and continually synthesize thyroid hormones. This is termed a primary hyperthyroid disease process, meaning the thyroid gland itself is secreting T_3 and T_4 excessively. The high levels of T_3 and T_4 exert a negative feedback inhibition of pituitary TSH. However, in the presence of low TSH, the thyroid gland continually secretes hormones. In secondary hyperthyroidism, there is an increase in pituitary TSH secretion that stimulates the excess release of T_3 and T_4. In tertiary hyperthyroidism, there is an excessive secretion of hypothalamic TRH, which causes excess secretion of TSH, T_3, and T_4. Both secondary and tertiary hyperthyroidism are uncommon.

Clinical Presentation. Because the thyroid hormones regulate many physiological processes, the effects of hyperthyroidism are seen in all body systems. Generally, all metabolic activities are accelerated, and energy expenditure increases with a concomitant rise in heat production. The typical patient presents with nervousness, insomnia, sensitivity to heat, and weight loss. The gland is usually enlarged and palpable, and an audible bruit may be heard because of high glandular blood flow.

In Graves' disease, there is an enhanced sensitivity to the activity of the sympathetic nervous system neurotransmitters (catecholamines). Patients are at risk for cardiac arrhythmias, such as atrial fibrillation, and the development of heart failure. **Exophthalmos,** a wide-eyed stare that is often present, is associated with increased sympathetic tone and infiltration of the extraocular area with lymphocytes and mucopolysaccharides. These deposits push the eyes forward and produce periorbital edema and bulging of the eyes, which is termed Graves' ophthalmopathy (see Fig. 24-6). Visual impairment can result if Graves' ophthalmopathy is present for a prolonged period. Women are more often affected with Graves' ophthalmopathy than men.

Thyroid dermopathy, also called pretibial myxedema, refers to skin changes in the lower legs. Because of accumulation of glycosaminoglycans, the skin becomes thickened and develops a nonpitting edema. Myxedema can be seen in hypothyroidism or hyperthyroidism.

Diagnosis. The most reliable screening test for hyperthyroidism or Graves' disease is TSH level. The suppression of TSH is found with high thyroid hormone levels (total T_3 and free T_4).

Measurement of serum thyrotropin receptor antibodies (TRAbs) is recommended. If TRAb levels are

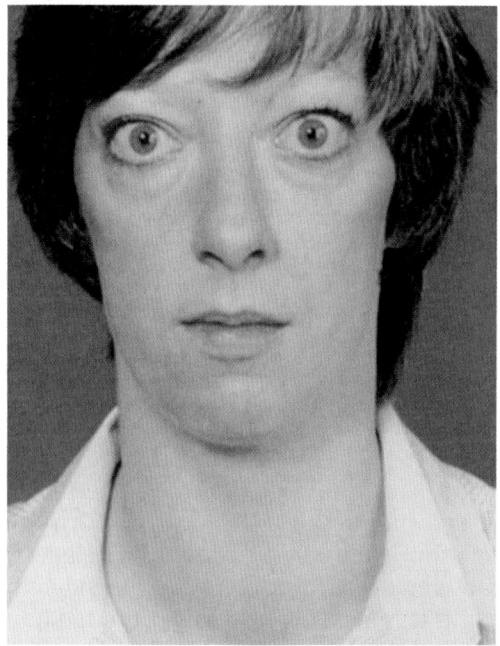

FIGURE 24-6. Graves' ophthalmopathy, also called exophthalmos. Graves' disease is an autoimmune disorder causing hyperthyroidism. The eyes develop an inflammatory disorder that affects the orbit around the eye, characterized by upper eyelid retraction, edema, conjunctivitis, and bulging eyes. *(From Biophoto Associates/Science Source.)*

positive, the diagnosis is usually Graves' disease and no further tests are needed. TRAbs have sensitivity of 96% to 97% and specificity of 99% for Graves' disease but can be weakly positive in subacute thyroiditis. If thyroid nodules are present or if TRAb levels are negative or borderline positive, a radioactive iodine uptake (RAIU) test and a thyroid scan should be ordered. Hyperthyroidism (thyrotoxicosis with high or normal RAIU) usually results from one of three disorders: Graves' disease, toxic multinodular goiter, or toxic thyroid adenoma.

Ultrasound with color Doppler evaluation should be performed as a first step in all patients who are hyperthyroid. Radioactive iodine scanning and measurements of iodine uptake are useful in differentiating the causes of hyperthyroidism. The terms "hot," "warm," and "cold" nodules are used in radioactive uptake scans, which is related to their concentration of isotope in tissue. Thyroid tissue that is producing excessive thyroid hormone is considered "hot" and appears darker on the scan compared with normal thyroid tissue. Thyroid tissue that is not producing thyroid hormone is considered "cold." Diffuse uptake by the thyroid gland tissue of radioactive isotope commonly occurs in Graves' disease, patchy uptake (multiple nodules) is seen with toxic multinodular goiter, and uptake in a single nodule with suppression of the remainder of the thyroid gland is seen with toxic adenoma.

Biotin supplements can interfere with accuracy of thyroid tests. Biotin is a common supplement in over-the-counter preparations for treatment of hair loss and brittle nails. At the high doses used in these products, biotin can produce false results. Patients who are taking biotin supplements should stop 2 to 3 days before having hormone measurements.

Treatment. Treatment involves ablation of the hyperactive thyroid through the use of antithyroid hormone medication such as propylthiouracil (PTU), carbimazole, methimazole, or radioactive iodine treatment. Radioactive iodine (I-131) or antithyroid medications are taken up by the gland and suppress its activity. Pregnancy is an absolute contraindication for radioactive I-131 ablation because this radioisotope can destroy the developing fetal thyroid gland. Therefore, women of childbearing potential should always have a documented negative pregnancy test result before receiving I-131. Other contraindications to I-131 therapy include lactation, diagnosed or suspected thyroid cancer, and the presence of significant Graves' ophthalmopathy. Alternatively, the thyroid gland can be surgically removed. After the gland is rendered inactive or if it is removed, replacement thyroid hormone (levothyroxine) is needed for life.

Thyrotoxic Crisis

Thyrotoxic crisis, also called a thyroid storm, is an intense, overwhelming release of thyroid hormones that exerts an intense stimulus on the metabolism. This is a life-threatening condition most commonly precipitated by surgery, trauma, or infection. Thyrotoxic crisis is a rare disorder. Approximately 1% to 2% of patients with hyperthyroidism progress to thyrotoxic crisis. Patients typically have high fever, tachycardia, nausea and vomiting, tremulousness, agitation, and psychosis. Serum-free T_4 and total T_3 levels are often highly elevated, and the TSH level is usually undetectable. Late in the progression of the disease, patients may become stuporous or comatose with hypotension. The immediate goals of therapy for thyroid storm are:

1. Decrease thyroid hormone synthesis with an antithyroid drug (e.g., methimazole or PTU).
2. Inhibit thyroid hormone secretion with oral potassium iodide or intravenous sodium iodide.
3. Reduce the heart rate with a beta blocker (e.g., esmolol) and/or a calcium-channel blocker.
4. Support the circulation with stress doses of intravenous glucocorticoids. (Plasmapheresis can be used in patients who have experienced previous significant toxicity to antithyroid drugs.)

> **ALERT!** Thyrotoxic crisis is a medical emergency. Heart failure and pulmonary edema can develop rapidly and cause death.

Thyroid Nodules

Most thyroid nodules are asymptomatic, but they can cause hypothyroidism or hyperthyroidism. Individuals with thyroid nodules will occasionally report complaints of dysphagia, dysphonia, and pain caused by the structural pressure created by the nodule.

A single thyroid nodule is associated with an increased risk of malignancy, whereas multiple nodules are often benign, though the presence of any nodule must be carefully evaluated to rule out neoplastic disease (see Box 24-3). A TSH assay and T_3 and T_4 levels are needed. Anti-TPO antibody and anti-Tg antibody tests are needed.

Ultrasound-guided fine needle aspiration biopsy is the most useful diagnostic test to rule out a malignant thyroid nodule. A technetium scan, using a radioactive isotope, is also used to differentiate malignant from benign nodules. The technetium scan identifies nodules as hot, warm, or cold according to their uptake of radioactive isotope. A hot nodule is a hyperfunctioning tumor, a warm nodule indicates normal tissue, and a cold nodule is hypofunctional tissue that is sometimes malignant. Surgical intervention is the treatment for a thyroid nodule that is malignant or obstructive.

Parathyroid Gland Disorders

The parathyroid glands are four pea-sized glands nestled within the thyroid tissue of the neck. The glands

> **BOX 24-3. Characteristics Associated With Malignant Thyroid Nodule**
>
> Factors suggesting a malignant thyroid nodule include the following:
> - Age younger than 20 years or older than 70 years
> - Male sex
> - Associated symptoms of dysphagia or dysphonia
> - History of neck irradiation
> - Firm, hard, or immobile nodule
> - Presence of cervical lymphadenopathy

produce and secrete parathyroid hormone (PTH) in response to low calcium levels in the blood. PTH promotes calcium reabsorption in the renal tubules and the release of calcium from bone. It also promotes vitamin D production by the kidney, which helps maintain normal calcium levels within the body. Many of the effects seen in parathyroid disorders are related to alterations in calcium levels.

Hypoparathyroidism

Hypoparathyroidism is an uncommon disorder. The etiology of primary hypoparathyroidism most often is trauma or inadvertent damage or removal of the parathyroid glands during thyroid surgery. It most commonly occurs as a complication of anterior neck surgery (in approximately 78% of cases). It is therefore seen more frequently in older adult women, who are more likely than others in the general population to undergo thyroid surgery. Neck irradiation, autoimmune disease, many different genetic disorders, and metal toxicity can cause primary parathyroid gland insufficiency. Fetal alcohol syndrome and many other congenital disorders can also cause diminished parathyroid gland function. Secondary hypoparathyroidism, which is the lack of pituitary parathyroid-stimulating hormone, can occur because of any primary disease that causes hypercalcemia. The high calcium levels send feedback to the pituitary gland to diminish parathyroid-stimulating hormone.

PTH is required for normal skeletal remodeling, allowing the replacement of mature bone by newly formed bone. In states of chronic hypoparathyroidism, bone metabolism is affected, with low bone turnover being a key feature. Due to reduced bone turnover, bone mineral density is typically greater in hypoparathyroidism than in normal subjects of the same age and sex. However, some studies show that microarchitectural changes in bone that may increase susceptibility to fracture. Fracture risk in hypoparathyroidism is still unclear and needs more research (Cusano et al., 2020; Starr et al., 2020).

The symptoms associated with hypoparathyroidism are the result of insufficient PTH secretion and the resultant decrease in serum calcium levels. There is often a concomitant increase in blood phosphate levels because low PTH lessens phosphate excretion by the kidney.

The most serious symptoms of primary hypoparathyroidism are the result of low levels of calcium. The patient can present with muscle cramps, irritability, tetany, and convulsions. Hypocalcemia also causes a carpal spasm known as Trousseau's sign and facial muscle twitch called Chvostek's sign. Diagnostic tests include serum PTH, calcium, phosphate, and vitamin D levels. Treatment includes replacement of PTH and normalizing serum calcium and vitamin D levels. If urgent treatment is necessary, calcium gluconate is preferred because it can be administered in a peripheral vein, whereas other preparations must be administered by means of a central venous catheter. Given the arrhythmogenic effects of acute calcium alterations, cardiac monitoring during calcium infusions is recommended. During maintenance treatment, oral calcium supplements and calcitriol or alfacalcidol (vitamin D) are recommended. Some patients may need magnesium supplements. Recombinant human PTH 1–84 or teriparatide (PTH 1–34 fragment) are the types of PTH that can be prescribed. Phosphate binders may be necessary depending on blood levels. Frequent monitoring of blood calcium, phosphate, magnesium, serum creatinine levels, and urinary calcium excretion is essential to avoid over- or undertreatment.

Hyperparathyroidism

Hyperparathyroidism is excessive secretion of PTH that affects calcium homeostasis in the body. Primary hyperparathyroidism occurs when the parathyroid glands themselves are the cause of the excessive secretion of PTH. Secondary hyperparathyroidism occurs when the parathyroid glands are constantly stimulated by another disorder such as vitamin D deficiency, chronic kidney disease, or use of certain diuretics. Hypersecretion of PTH leads to bone breakdown that causes release of calcium into the bloodstream, leading to hypercalcemia.

The prevalence has been reported to be approximately 21 cases per 100,000 persons annually. The average age of those affected is between 52 and 56 years, and women are affected more often than men.

Pathophysiology.

In approximately 85% of cases, primary hyperparathyroidism is caused by an adenoma of the parathyroid gland. The growth in the parathyroid gland causes excessive secretion of PTH. Primary hyperparathyroidism is frequently a progressive disease; approximately a quarter of patients without initial evidence of disease or symptoms develop end-organ manifestations within 5 years.

Clinical Presentation.

The systemic effects of hyperparathyroidism are related to bone breakdown and excessive levels of blood calcium. The most common effects of hypercalcemia include muscle weakness, poor concentration, neuropathies, hypertension, kidney stones, metabolic acidosis, and constipation. Bone breakdown causes osteopenia or osteoporosis and can lead to pathological fractures. Neuropsychiatric manifestations are also common and may include depression, confusion, or subtle cognitive deficits. Increased calcium can increase gastric acid secretion, and persons with hyperparathyroidism may have a higher prevalence of peptic ulcer disease. Physical examination findings are usually insignificant. Examination may reveal muscle weakness and depression. A palpable neck mass is not commonly found.

Diagnosis.

Blood testing for PTH levels is required for diagnosis. An elevated PTH level with an elevated ionized serum calcium level is diagnostic of primary hyperparathyroidism. However, hyperparathyroidism can develop gradually, with elevated serum calcium levels and inappropriately normal (nonsuppressed) serum PTH levels. The biochemical profile in primary hyperparathyroidism can change over time; up to three-quarters of patients with classic primary hyperparathyroidism can take up to 5 years to establish a definite diagnosis. A radiolabeled sestamibi scan and ultrasound are also used to detect parathyroid tumors. If a kidney stone is suspected, renal ultrasound and CT scan are recommended. Other recommended laboratory tests include bone density DEXA scan, serum vitamin D, serum phosphorus, and 24-hour urine for creatinine and calcium.

Treatment.

Parathyroidectomy is the definitive treatment for primary hyperparathyroidism and is indicated for patients with symptomatic disease. Treatment also involves reducing elevated serum calcium levels through the use of diuretics, calcitonin, and bisphosphonates. Calcitonin and bisphosphonates can cease bone breakdown and improve bone density. Vitamin D should also be administered. Annual laboratory testing and bone densitometry every 1 to 2 years are recommended.

Adrenal Gland Disorders

The adrenal gland consists of two parts: the cortex and medulla. The cortex secretes corticosteroids, also called glucocorticoids; androgens; and mineralocorticoids, mainly aldosterone. The medulla secretes epinephrine and norepinephrine—referred to as catecholamines. Corticosteroids, mainly cortisol, assist the body in dealing with stress; they stimulate gluconeogenesis to increase blood sugar, mobilize fat stores, and break down proteins. During an acute stressful event in the fight-or-flight reaction, cortisol gives the body great strength and vigor for a temporary period. However, long-term secretion of corticosteroids has negative effects on the body, such as suppression of the immune system and breakdown of bone. White blood cells (WBCs) do not function well in the presence of prolonged elevated blood cortisol levels, so immune defenses diminish.

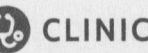

> ### CLINICAL CONCEPT
>
> Chronic stress, which causes high cortisol levels, diminishes efficiency of WBCs, leading to immunosuppression.

Mineralocorticoids from the adrenal gland, mainly aldosterone, assist in fluid and electrolyte balance. Aldosterone increases sodium and water reabsorption into the blood at the nephron. It also causes secretion of K+ into the nephron tubule, which eventually causes loss of K+ in the urine. It is particularly active in the renin–angiotensin–aldosterone system (RAAS).

As in other endocrine feedback systems, the hypothalamus secretes corticotropin-releasing factor (CRF), which stimulates the pituitary gland to release adrenocorticotropic hormone (ACTH). This, in turn, stimulates the adrenal gland to release its hormones: cortisol, epinephrine, norepinephrine, androgens, and aldosterone.

Disorders of the adrenal gland mainly consist of adrenal gland insufficiency or overactivity. The most common disorder of adrenal insufficiency is Addison's disease, caused by disorders of the adrenal gland. The major disorder of adrenal gland overactivity or exposure to excess corticosteroids is termed **Cushing's syndrome.** If adrenal gland overactivity is caused by the pituitary's release of excess ACTH, this is termed **Cushing's disease**.

Adrenal Insufficiency (Hypoadrenalism)

Adrenal insufficiency can occur because of decreased ACTH from the pituitary gland or dysfunction of the adrenal gland, both of which cause decreased cortisol secretion. Primary adrenal insufficiency, which is failure of the adrenal glands, is also called **Addison's disease.** Primary adrenal insufficiency (PAI) or Addison's disease causes glucocorticoid- and/or mineralocorticoid deficiency due to failure of the adrenal cortex. This disorder has a prevalence of 100 to 140 cases per million people in the Western world. Today, 80% of PAI cases are caused by autoimmune disease of the adrenal gland, followed by tuberculosis or other infectious diseases (e.g., HIV/AIDS, CMV, candidiasis, histoplasmosis, syphilis, and others) and malignant diseases (e.g., lung, breast, and colon cancer, among others) in about 10% of cases. More than half of autoimmune adrenal disease occurs in combination with other autoimmune disorders. Autoimmune causes of adrenal insufficiency occur more frequently in women and most often develop between 30 and 50 years of age. About two-thirds of patients go on to develop other autoimmune diseases in the context of an autoimmune polyendocrine syndrome (APS), including autoimmune thyroid disease (AITD), autoimmune gastritis, type 1 diabetes, premature ovarian failure (POF), vitiligo, or celiac disease.

Ten percent of PAI is caused by (bilateral) adrenalectomy (e.g., for Cushing's syndrome or adrenal tumors), genetic diseases (e.g., congenital adrenal hyperplasia [CAH], adrenal hypoplasia congenita, and adrenoleukodystrophy in males), and adrenal hemorrhage (e.g., Waterhouse-Friderichsen syndrome in sepsis).

Secondary adrenal insufficiency due to suppression of the HPA axis can occur as a consequence of pituitary dysfunction or chronic corticosteroid drug use (termed exogenous corticosteroids). Exogenous corticosteroid suppression of the HPA axis due to drug use is a disorder occurring in up to 2% of the population. Due to the increasing age in our population with chronic illness often requiring complex medical treatment and polypharmacy, pharmacological adverse effects of other drugs affecting the adrenal gland also occur. Adrenal hemorrhage associated with anticoagulants, drugs affecting glucocorticoid synthesis, action, or metabolism like specific antimycotics and other compounds are becoming more relevant as potential predisposing factors to secondary adrenal insufficiency. It is also increasingly important that novel drugs such as immune checkpoint inhibitors and monoclonal antibody therapeutic regimens may induce the manifestation of immune-mediated endocrine disorders including PAI.

Etiology. PAI is most commonly caused by autoimmune destruction of the adrenal gland as an isolated glandular disorder or as part of autoimmune polyglandular syndromes. Isolated primary adrenal insufficiency is most commonly caused by autoimmune destruction of the adrenal gland, which is caused by two types of antibodies: adrenal cortex antibodies and antibodies to the steroid enzymes. These antienzyme antibodies prevent the conversion of precursor hormones to the adrenal hormones, potentially leading to adrenocortical failure.

Pathophysiology. Gradual autoimmune destruction of the adrenal gland leads to a decreased cortisol response to stress and reduced cortisol reserve. As the glandular destruction increases, less cortisol is available, and this can lead to adrenal crisis (see Box 24-4).

BOX 24-4. Adrenal Crisis

Lack of sufficient levels of corticosteroids in conjunction with increased need because of stress, trauma, infection, or surgery increases the risk of developing an adrenal crisis. Patients will present with severe abdominal pain, high fever, weakness, confusion, nausea, and vomiting. Diagnostic studies will show hyponatremia, hyperkalemia, leukocytosis, and hypoglycemia. This is a life-threatening condition. If not treated appropriately, profound hypotension, organ failure, and coma can occur.

Hypoadrenalism can also be caused by excessive administration of exogenous glucocorticoids, such as prednisone. When patients are administered prolonged corticosteroid treatment beyond 4 to 5 weeks, negative feedback suppression of CRF and ACTH occurs. As a result, the adrenal gland can downregulate its receptors and undergo glandular atrophy. With atrophy, the ability to secrete natural cortisol decreases. When corticosteroid therapy is abruptly stopped or there is an episode of severe trauma or stress, the hypothalamic–pituitary–adrenal axis is not able to respond appropriately. The patient will then develop symptoms of adrenal insufficiency, and in the case of high stress, surgery, or infection, the patient may develop adrenal crisis (see Fig. 24-7).

> **ALERT!** When administering corticosteroids to patients, the smallest dose should be used for a short period. Long-term corticosteroid administration can cause decreased secretion of natural cortisol and atrophy of the adrenal gland.

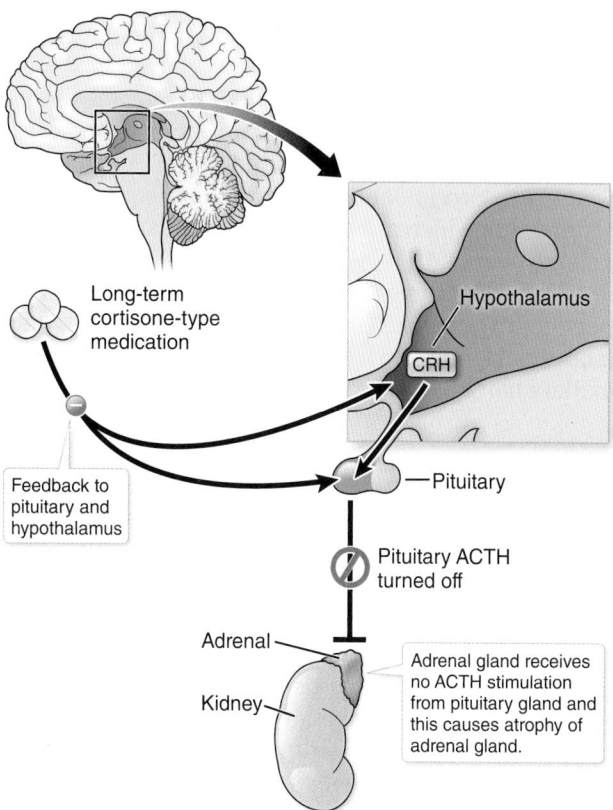

FIGURE 24-7. Effects of excess corticosteroid medications on the adrenal gland. Long-term use of corticosteroids can cause adrenal gland atrophy. (1) Excess corticosteroid medications in the bloodstream will be sensed by the hypothalamus and pituitary gland. (2) The hypothalamus will cease release of corticotropin-releasing hormone (CRH). (3) The pituitary will then not be stimulated by CRH and cease secreting ACTH. (4) The adrenal gland will not receive sufficient stimulation from the pituitary, and eventually cells will atrophy.

Clinical Presentation. In PAI, the adrenal cortex secretes deficient amounts of hormones. The adrenal cortex secretes diminished glucocorticoids, mainly cortisol, and diminished mineralocorticoids, mainly aldosterone. As in other endocrine feedback mechanisms, the pituitary gland senses the low hormone level. The pituitary, in response, secretes ACTH. Uniquely, when ACTH is secreted excessively, melanocyte-stimulating hormone (MSH) is triggered as well because both ACTH and MSH have the same precursor. The adrenal gland is provoked, ACTH is released, and MSH stimulates melanocytes. The stimulated melanocytes give patients a tanned appearance. However, in primary adrenal insufficiency, the stimulated adrenal gland cannot yield sufficient amounts of corticosteroids or mineralocorticoids.

The development of adrenal insufficiency is often gradual. The initial symptoms are nonspecific symptoms of weakness, hypotension, lethargy, easy fatigue, anorexia, nausea, and vomiting. Some patients have episodes of hypoglycemia.

Electrolyte imbalances occur from mineralocorticoid (aldosterone) deficiency. Aldosterone normally functions to stimulate the nephron to reabsorb sodium and water into the bloodstream and excrete potassium. In the absence of aldosterone, these functions do not occur. Sodium and water are lost and potassium is retained. Patients experience hyponatremia, hyperkalemia, and dehydration. The physiological response to this electrolyte imbalance is an increase in secretion of ADH by the posterior pituitary. ADH stimulates water reabsorption at the nephron; consequently, this water volume increase predisposes the patient to fluid volume overload.

Other symptoms of adrenal insufficiency include personality changes, inability to concentrate, and emotional lability. In women, there is loss of pubic and axillary hair and amenorrhea.

Diagnosis. Measurements of concentrations of ACTH, cortisol, and plasma renin and aldosterone in blood samples collected in the morning (at 8:00 a.m.) are required to confirm the diagnosis of adrenal insufficiency. An increase of ACTH levels (more than twofold over the upper limit of the normal range) together with low levels of cortisol are diagnostic for primary adrenal insufficiency. Low cortisol levels with normal/low ACTH levels denote secondary adrenal insufficiency.

The conventional ACTH test (an intravenous injection of 250 µg of synthetic corticotropin) in adults is the gold standard for assessing adrenal function. A peak cortisol concentration of less than 500 nmol/L (18 µg/dL) at 30 to 60 min after ACTH administration is considered diagnostic for primary adrenal insufficiency. The simultaneous measurements of plasma renin and aldosterone levels confirm the presence of mineral corticoid deficiency.

Abdominal CT scan may be normal or may show bilateral enlargement of the adrenal glands in patients with Addison's disease because of tuberculosis, fungal infections, adrenal hemorrhage, or infiltrating diseases involving the adrenal glands. CT-guided fine needle biopsy may be necessary to define the diagnosis. Alternatively, adrenal atrophy may be the cause of adrenal insufficiency; this will be apparent on CT scan.

Treatment. Natural glucocorticoids and mineralocorticoids are secreted in a circadian fashion, with a peak at 8:00 a.m. and a nadir at 12:00 a.m. The patient needs replacement doses of glucocorticoid and mineralocorticoid daily. This is commonly achieved with 100 mg or more of hydrocortisone per day and 9-alpha-fludrocortisone in doses of 0.05 to 0.10 mg per day or every other day. Patients may need to be advised to increase salt intake in hot weather. Surgery may be necessary if there is an adrenal tumor or mass.

Parenteral steroid coverage should be used in times of major stress, trauma, or surgery, and during any major procedure. In stress situations, the normal adrenal gland output of cortisol is approximately 250 to 300 mg in 24 hours. This amount of hydrocortisone should be given, preferably by continuous infusion.

Cushing's Syndrome (Hyperadrenalism)

Cushing's syndrome, also called hyperadrenalism or hypercortisolism, is an endocrine disorder caused by high levels of cortisol in the blood. There are two terms that connote different sources of hyperadrenalism: Cushing's syndrome and Cushing's disease. Cushing's disease refers to a tumor of the pituitary gland that produces large amounts of ACTH that results in excessive cortisol production. Cushing's syndrome is hyperadrenalism caused by a hyperactive adrenal gland that secretes excessive cortisol. Alternatively, excessive cortisol can occur because of certain cancers that secrete inappropriate ACTH or prolonged use of corticosteroid drugs such as prednisone or dexamethasone. Cushing's syndrome is more common than Cushing's disease; the most common source of the syndrome is excessive use of corticosteroid drugs.

Epidemiology. Cushing's syndrome is diagnosed in an estimated 10 to 15 persons per million each year. It is more common in women than in men, with a female-to-male ratio of 8:1. Although it can occur at any age, it is most often seen in people between the ages of 20 and 50 years. It is characterized by excessive levels of glucocorticoids and their physiological effects.

Etiology. Pituitary adenomas are the most common cause of Cushing's disease. Pituitary adenomas cause excessive secretion of ACTH from the anterior pituitary gland. ACTH then stimulates the adrenal cortex to produce excessive adrenal corticosteroids. If large, the adenoma can put pressure on the pituitary and cause decreased production of other anterior pituitary hormones (TSH, FSH, LH, GH, and PRL) and the posterior pituitary hormone ADH.

Nelson's syndrome can occur in patients who have had an adrenalectomy due to Cushing's disease. This is caused by a large ACTH-secreting pituitary tumor; the pituitary secretes excessive ACTH in an attempt to raise corticosteroids; however, there is no adrenal gland. Without an adrenal gland, there is no feedback to the pituitary from the adrenal gland to shut off the ACTH secretion.

Cushing's syndrome can occur because of a few different etiologies. The syndrome can be caused by adrenal neoplasms, which include adrenal adenoma, adrenal carcinoma, and adrenal hyperplasia. The Carney complex is a genetic disorder that includes hyperplasia of the adrenal gland, which causes Cushing's syndrome. McCune–Albright syndrome is a rare cause of hyperfunction of the adrenal glands that leads to Cushing's syndrome and precocious puberty. Cushing's syndrome can also be caused by secretion of ACTH from tumors of the lung or other cancers. Ectopic ACTH is commonly secreted by oat cell or small-cell carcinoma of the lung or by carcinoid tumors.

Administration of exogenous corticosteroids can lead to the development of Cushing's syndrome. Cushing's syndrome symptoms can occur with the administration of oral, injected, or inhaled corticosteroids. This is likely the most common cause of the disease; however, many cases are not reported, and the prevalence is unknown.

Pathophysiology. Patients with Cushing's disease have diffuse hyperplasia of the cells of the anterior pituitary, which is responsible for the production and secretion of ACTH. The hyperplasia may be caused by excess secretion of CRF by the hypothalamus or an adenoma of the pituitary. The constant secretion of ACTH stimulates hyperplasia of the adrenal glands. Interestingly, the precursor of ACTH is also the precursor of MSH, which causes melanin pigmentation of the skin.

> ### 🔬 CLINICAL CONCEPT
>
> When ACTH is secreted in excess, melanocyte-stimulating hormone (MSH) is also secreted, which gives the skin a tan appearance.

Under normal conditions, there is a circadian rhythm of ACTH secretion; throughout the day, ACTH and cortisol rise and fall in a predictable pattern. However, this pattern is absent in Cushing's disease. Instead, ACTH secretion is excessively released in a random pattern. Also, the negative feedback signal to the pituitary is blunted with persistently high ACTH levels.

Normally in times of stress, ACTH is released; this stimulates adrenal secretion of cortisol. In response to stress, there should be a spike in the level of ACTH. However, in Cushing's disease, ACTH is excessive, yet there is no rise in ACTH level in response to stress. Therefore, patients with Cushing's disease need to be carefully monitored for complications associated with lack of appropriate ACTH secretion in response to stressors such as trauma, surgery, or infection. For example, the patient with Cushing's disease undergoing surgery may need to have ACTH or cortisol administered preoperatively.

In Cushing's syndrome caused by an adrenal tumor, cortisol secretion is also random and episodic. However, there is an intact negative feedback response by the pituitary. The pituitary gland senses excessive levels of cortisol, leading to reduced ACTH production. The reduced ACTH stimulus of the adrenal gland often causes atrophy of the adrenal gland.

Clinical Presentation. The clinical features of cortisol excess are initially subtle, but easily recognizable when the patient's pictures from several years earlier are compared with the patient at present (see Fig. 24-8). Weight gain is evident, with a redistribution of body fat to the face, trunk, and abdomen. Patients develop a characteristic rose-colored, puffy face called

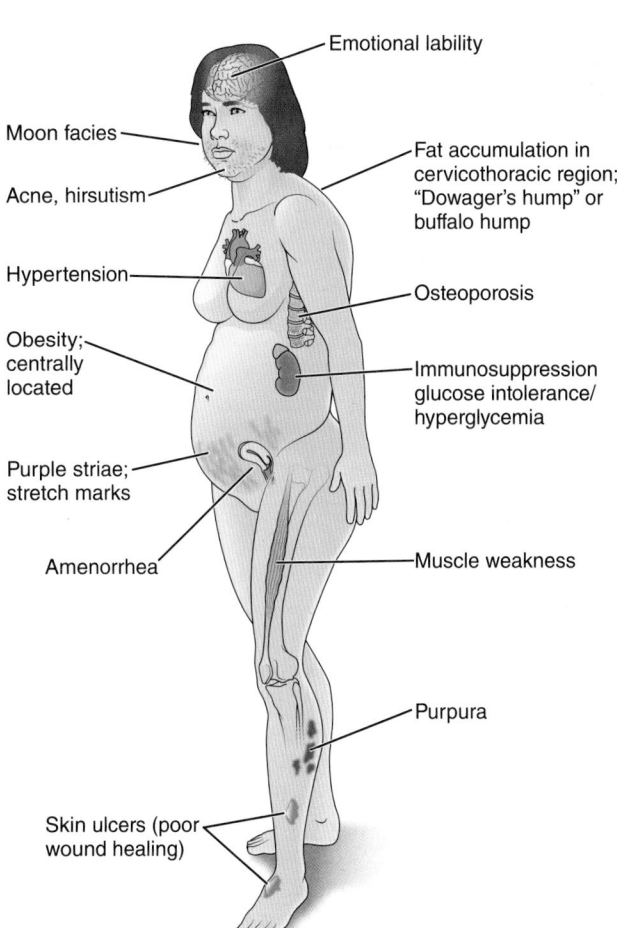

Emotional lability
Moon facies
Acne, hirsutism
Hypertension
Obesity; centrally located
Purple striae; stretch marks
Amenorrhea
Skin ulcers (poor wound healing)
Fat accumulation in cervicothoracic region; "Dowager's hump" or buffalo hump
Osteoporosis
Immunosuppression glucose intolerance/ hyperglycemia
Muscle weakness
Purpura

FIGURE 24-8. The widespread effects of Cushing's syndrome.

"moon facies," as well as extra subcutaneous fat in the cervicothoracic area called "buffalo hump." There is an increase in the waist-to-hip circumference ratio, with apple-shaped fat distribution. Over time, the patient develops acanthosis nigricans, or a darkening of the skin at friction sites such as under the breasts, the belt line, and the neck. Increased subcutaneous fat deposits, particularly in the abdomen, lead to the development of purple stretch marks called striae. There is easy bruising and poor wound healing. Women will also demonstrate hirsutism, which is male-pattern hair growth.

Elevated cortisol levels are associated with enhanced gluconeogenesis, which is glucose production by the liver. Cortisol also blocks the action of insulin, decreasing the body's utilization of glucose, which means that the patient will have hyperglycemia. Additionally, excess cortisol inhibits bone formation and accelerates bone reabsorption, which leads to the development of osteopenia, osteoporosis, and an increased risk of bone fracture.

Cortisol's anti-inflammatory effects suppress the normal response to infection and injury. This occurs from reduced formation of inflammatory mediators such as thromboxanes, prostaglandins, and prostacyclins. Cortisol also suppresses the formation of antibodies and inhibits the migration of WBCs to sites of inflammation. Therefore, WBCs function less efficiently when blood cortisol levels are high. These effects immunosuppress the patient with Cushing's syndrome.

Patients with elevated cortisol levels often have elevated blood pressure, though the mechanism is unclear. It may be caused by excess sodium and water retention or increased vascular responsiveness to catecholamines.

CLINICAL CONCEPT

High cortisol levels counteract insulin leading to hyperglycemia; accelerate bone breakdown, leading to osteoporosis; elevate blood pressure, causing hypertension; and diminish efficiency of WBCs, leading to immunosuppression.

Diagnosis. The laboratory abnormalities associated with Cushing's syndrome include elevated WBC count greater than 11,000/mm³, hyperglycemia, and hypokalemia. High cortisol levels cause elevated WBCs, glucose release from the liver, and a mineralocorticoid effect at the kidney, causing potassium excretion. The diagnosis of Cushing's syndrome caused by overproduction of cortisol requires the demonstration of inappropriately high blood or urine cortisol levels. An 11 p.m. measurement of salivary cortisol is a simple screening test. If salivary cortisol level is elevated, this is followed by 24-hour urinary free cortisol test and a dexamethasone suppression test.

The dexamethasone suppression test is administered to test the interactions of the hypothalamic–pituitary–adrenal axis and to find the cause of excessive blood cortisol levels. Dexamethasone is a synthetic glucocorticoid medication that can suppress hypothalamus–pituitary–adrenal (HPA) function in healthy individuals. However in Cushing's syndrome dexamethasone fails to suppress HPA function. There are two major types of dexamethasone suppression tests based on administration of low-dose or high-dose dexamethasone:

- Overnight low-dose 1-mg dexamethasone suppression test
- Overnight high-dose 8-mg dexamethasone suppression test

High blood cortisol levels can be due to excessive secretion by the adrenal gland itself, excessive secretion of pituitary ACTH, or an ACTH-secreting tumor in the body external to the pituitary gland. The low-dose dexamethasone suppression test assesses if excessive cortisol production is caused by the adrenal gland itself. The high-dose dexamethasone suppression test distinguishes Cushing's disease (caused by pituitary hypersecretion of ACTH) from Cushing's syndrome caused by nonpituitary ACTH-secreting tumors.

Once the diagnosis of Cushing's disease is established with the laboratory tests, the next step is to determine the etiology using imaging studies. Abdominal CT scan of the adrenal glands and a contrast-enhanced MRI of the pituitary may reveal the presence of a tumor. Chest x-ray is necessary to rule out an ACTH-secreting pulmonary tumor. F-FDG-PET (fluorodeoxyglucose-positron emission tomography) scan, 8Ga-DOTATATE PET/CT scan, and octreotide scintigraphy can rule out ectopic ACTH-secreting tumors in the body.

Inferior petrosal sinus sampling (IPSS) has been considered the gold standard test for differentiating Cushing's disease from ectopic ACTH syndrome. However, this test is highly invasive and requires highly skilled clinicians. As a standard method, serum ACTH levels are measured simultaneously in the catheterized bilateral inferior petrosal sinus before and after CRH administration. A baseline ACTH central to peripheral ratio greater than 2:1 or a CRH-stimulated ratio greater than 3:1 is indicative of Cushing's disease.

Treatment. Treatment of Cushing's syndrome is directed by the cause. In general, therapy should reduce the cortisol secretion to normal to reduce the risks associated with hypercortisolism. The treatment of choice for Cushing's syndrome is surgical resection of the causative tumor. The surgical procedure for Cushing's disease is transsphenoidal surgery to reduce a pituitary tumor. The surgical procedure for adrenal tumors is adrenalectomy.

Medical treatment can be considered a valuable alternative to pituitary surgery for patients with Cushing's disease with contraindications to surgery or with disease persistence or recurrence. Medical treatment agents can be categorized as follows: tumor-directed drugs, adrenal steroidogenesis inhibitors, and glucocorticoid receptor antagonists. Tumor-directed drugs target the pituitary tumor and suppress release of hormone and shrink the tumor. Tumors usually express somatostatin and dopamine receptors. Pasireotide and cabergoline bind to these receptors and inhibit the ACTH-secreting tumor. Adrenal steroidogenesis inhibitors include metyrapone, ketoconazole, mitotane, and etomidate. Currently, mifepristone is the only available glucocorticoid receptor antagonist.

Pheochromocytoma and Paraganglioma

Pheochromocytoma and paraganglioma are rare catecholamine-secreting tumors derived from the sympathetic or parasympathetic nervous system. These tumors may arise sporadically or be inherited in association with multiple endocrine neoplasia type 2 (MEN 2), von Hippel-Lindau disease, or other syndromes.

Pheochromocytoma is commonly located within the adrenal medulla and secretes norepinephrine and epinephrine. It is estimated to occur in 2 to 8 out of 1 million persons. Mean age at diagnosis is 40 years, although these tumors can arise from childhood to old age.

The etiology of pheochromocytoma is often unknown; however, it causes excessive stimulation of alpha-adrenergic and beta-adrenergic receptors in the body. The symptoms caused by overstimulation of adrenergic receptors include severe hypertension, tremors, increased cardiac contractility, cardiac arrhythmias, and elevated heart rate. The classic triad of symptoms of pheochromocytoma are palpitations, headache, and profuse sweating. The dominant sign is hypertension. A pheochromocytoma is associated with a hypertensive or catecholamine crisis that is characterized by severely elevated blood pressure, tachycardia, anxiety, altered mental status, focal neurological signs and symptoms, and seizures. Possible neurological complications include stroke caused by cerebral infarction or intracerebral hemorrhage. Patients can develop heart failure and pulmonary edema. Collection of a 24-hour urine sample that is analyzed for an excessive amount of catecholamine metabolites is the most useful diagnostic test. An MRI with contrast of the abdomen to visualize the adrenal gland is also necessary. Tumors can also be localized by procedures using radioactive tracers including I-MIBG scintigraphy, somatostatin analogue scintigraphy, or specific types of positron emission tomography (PET) scans. Surgical removal of the tumor and adrenergic blocker medications are treatment measures. Preoperatively, use of alpha-adrenergic receptor blockade and volume expansion followed by beta blockade is mandatory to reduce intraoperative intravascular instability and blood pressure fluctuation due to tumor manipulation. Other antihypertensive agents such as calcium channel antagonists and angiotensin-converting enzyme inhibitors are also effective.

Multiple Endocrine Neoplasia

Multiple endocrine neoplasia (MEN) is characterized by tumors involving two or more endocrine glands. There are four major types of MEN, referred to as MEN types 1-4. In addition to MEN types 1-4, there are other syndromes associated with multiple endocrine and other organ neoplasia (MEON). MEONs include Carney complex, von Hippel-Landau disease, neurofibromatosis type I, Cowden's syndrome, and McCune–Albright syndrome. The most common type of multiple endocrine neoplasia is MEN type 1 (MEN-1), also referred to as Werner's syndrome. MEN-1 is caused by a defective tumor suppressor gene at 11q13 that allows tumor growth in several different endocrine glands. The endocrine glands most frequently involved are the parathyroid gland, anterior pituitary gland, and pancreas. There can be involvement of adrenal cortical tumors, GI carcinoid tumors, meningiomas, lipomas, facial angiomas, and collagenomas. The prevalence of MEN-1 is 1% to 18% of patients with primary hyperparathyroidism, 16% to 38% among patients with pancreatic islet tumors, and 3% among patients with pituitary tumors. MEN-1 occurs in all age groups.

Primary hyperparathyroidism caused by tumor is the most common disorder associated with MEN-1, occurring in 90% of patients. Parathyroid tumors cause excessive bone breakdown with resulting hypercalcemia and osteopenia. Nephrolithiasis is also associated with hyperparathyroidism. Pancreatic islet cell tumors called insulinomas and gastrinomas occur in 75% of patients with MEN-1. These tumors lead to disturbed glucose metabolism, gastric hyperacidity (Zollinger–Ellison syndrome), peptic ulcer disease, and diarrhea. The effects seen from pituitary adenomas are related to excessive secretion of GH, PRL, and ACTH. The clinical presentation of MEN depends on the specific hormone that is secreted excessively. Although the symptoms do not often appear until the patient is about 40 years of age, abnormal hormone levels may be seen as early as age 14 years. Surgical removal of tumors, medical antagonists of the excess hormones, and supportive therapies are treatment measures.

Pineal Gland Dysfunction

The pineal gland is a neuroendocrine gland located in the brain near the hypothalamus. This gland contains sympathetic neurons that travel to the retina. Upon stimulation, the pineal gland converts sympathetic input into hormonal output by producing melatonin with the phases of the light–dark cycle. The gland releases melatonin with darkness, which facilitates sleep. Pineal tumors represent about 1% of all brain tumors in adults. A pineal tumor is problematic mainly because of the pressure it places on adjacent brain tissue. They often compress parts of the brain that drain cerebrospinal fluid (CSF), causing a buildup of pressure called hydrocephalus. Symptoms include headache, nausea and vomiting, seizures, memory disturbances, and visual changes. Hydrocephalus can be treated by placement of a ventriculoperitoneal shunt, which is a long tube placed within one of the CSF-containing spaces of the brain; it is then passed under the skin to the abdominal cavity to provide a pathway for CSF drainage and absorption in the abdomen.

The pineal gland has been under-researched; however, investigators have found that in addition to its secretion of melatonin in relation to light and dark, it may have roles in aging, Alzheimer's disease, precocious puberty, and some headache syndromes.

Chapter Summary

- The endocrine system is made up of glands that produce and secrete hormones.
- The endocrine feedback mechanism is the most important and unique property of the system.
- The regulatory link among the hypothalamus, pituitary gland, and endocrine target organ is the hypothalamic–pituitary–hormone axis; this fundamental control system exists with all endocrine organs.
- Hormones are regulated by the pituitary gland and hypothalamus. The hypothalamus secretes releasing factors that stimulate the pituitary. The pituitary secretes tropic hormones that stimulate a target endocrine gland to secrete its hormone. As the level of this hormone rises in the circulation, the hypothalamus and the pituitary gland shut down secretion of their hormones, which in turn slows the secretion by the target gland. This mechanism is disrupted in endocrine disorders and results in either hyperfunction or hypofunction of the gland.
- EDCs are chemicals found in the environment that can cause disruption of hormone synthesis, transport, action, and metabolism. There is currently a growing body of evidence linking EDCs to possible adverse health effects in animals and humans.
- The pituitary gland is called the master gland because it controls all the endocrine glands.
- The pituitary is divided into anterior pituitary (adenohypophysis) and posterior pituitary (neurohypophysis).
- The anterior pituitary gland secretes GH, TSH, ACTH, PRL, FSH, and LH. The posterior pituitary secretes oxytocin and ADH.
- When an endocrine gland dysfunctions, the condition is a primary disease. For example, a tumor of the thyroid gland that secretes excessive hormone is a primary disorder of the thyroid gland.
- When the pituitary gland dysfunctions, the problem is a secondary disease. For example, ACTH deficiency causes adrenal insufficiency secondary to pituitary dysfunction, termed secondary adrenal insufficiency.
- Hyperpituitarism of the child will cause gigantism and excessive growth of the long bones and organs, whereas hyperpituitarism of the adult causes acromegaly, which results in coarsening of facial features; enlarged jaw, hands, and feet; and organ dysfunction.
- A pituitary adenoma that secretes PRL is the most common type of pituitary tumor.
- Pituitary tumors often present with visual problems due to the pressure on the optic chiasm, which is in close proximity to the pituitary gland.
- Hypopituitarism of the posterior pituitary causes DI, which is a lack of ADH that causes polyuria, dehydration, and thirst. ADH is also referred to as AVP.
- Excessive secretion of ADH by the posterior pituitary causes SIADH, which causes hypervolemia, dilutional hyponatremia, and edema.
- Hypothyroidism, commonly caused by Hashimoto's thyroiditis, causes classic signs of cold sensitivity, sluggishness, excessive fatigue, weakness, weight gain, constipation, slowed mentation, and depression.
- Myxedema coma occurs because of long-standing, untreated hypothyroidism and has an associated mortality rate of 30% to 40%.
- Hyperthyroidism, commonly caused by Graves' disease, causes classic signs of heat sensitivity, weight loss, tremulousness, palpitations, insomnia, and exophthalmus.
- Thyroid storm, also called thyrotoxic crisis, is a severe discharge of thyroid hormone triggered by infection or stress, which can cause hypertension, heart failure, and pulmonary edema.
- Adrenal gland hyperactivity causes high cortisol levels, which presents as Cushing's syndrome—a classic presentation of moon facies, buffalo hump, obesity, hirsutism, and striae. It also causes hypertension, hyperglycemia (glucose intolerance), osteoporosis, and immunosuppression.
- Adrenal insufficiency causes Addison's disease, which classically presents with weight loss, weakness, and severe hypotension.

- Adrenal crisis is a life-threatening condition that causes profound weakness, severe abdominal pain, fever, and shock.
- Pheochromocytoma is a rare tumor of the adrenal medulla that secretes epinephrine and causes hypertensive crisis and cardiac arrhythmias.

- MEN-1 is a disorder caused by tumor growth in the parathyroid, pancreas, and pituitary glands.
- Pineal gland tumors compress adjacent brain tissue, causing buildup of CSF, visual disturbances, seizures, and headache.

 ## Making the Connections

Disorder and Pathophysiology

Signs and Symptoms	Physical Assessment Findings	Diagnostic Testing	Treatment
Hypopituitarism | Low pituitary hormones such as ACTH, GH, TSH, FSH, or LH, commonly caused by a pituitary adenoma.			
In child: dwarfism and small stature. In adult: deficiency of many tropic hormones causes a wide variety of endocrine gland deficiency symptoms.	In child: short stature or intellectual disability. In adult: a variety of findings, depending on tropic hormone deficit.	Each pituitary hormone must be tested separately because there is a variable pattern of hormone deficiency among patients with hypopituitarism. Testing of basal ACTH secretion or the metapyrone test is recommended for pituitary malfunction. CT and MRI may show mass or pituitary enlargement.	GH replacement and other tropic hormones are used, if deficient. Replacement needed for life.
Diabetes Insipidus | Lack of ADH from the posterior pituitary, which causes lack of water reabsorption at the nephron and consequent water loss.			
Polydipsia (thirst). Polyuria.	Signs of dehydration: poor skin turgor, low blood pressure (BP), concentrated urine, and dry mucous membranes.	Low ADH level. CT/MRI scan of head looks for pituitary tumor.	Replacement hormone treatment is given with oral desmopressin (DDAVP).
Hyperpituitarism | High pituitary hormones, often caused by tumor, commonly prolactinoma, which secretes excess PRL; this hormone stimulates lactation.			
In child: gigantism and organomegaly. In adult: acromegaly, which has subtle symptoms of coarsening of facial features; if prolactinoma is present, symptoms include gynecomastia, galactorrhea, amenorrhea, headache, or visual disturbances caused by tumor near the optic chiasm.	If tumor is prolactinoma: galactorrhea, amenorrhea, visual impairment, may have high BP, arrhythmias, and thyroid or adrenal enlargement, depending on the hormone excess.	Measurements of tropic hormones such as ACTH, PRL, FSH, LH, or TSH to look for elevations of levels of any pituitary hormones. Urine hormone levels, such as urinary free cortisol, can be measured. The thyrotropin-releasing hormone (TRH) stimulation and dexamethasone suppression tests can be used. Measurement of the serum insulin-like growth factor-1 (IGF-1) and serum IGF binding protein-3 are used for diagnosis of acromegaly. An oral glucose tolerance test (OGTT) can also be used to determine whether it suppresses growth hormone.	In prolactinoma, oral dopamine agonists, cabergoline and bromocriptine, block secretion of PRL and shrink tumors. For treatment of corticotropin-secreting pituitary tumors, transsphenoidal surgery in addition to steroidogenic inhibitor medications ketoconazole or pasireotide LAR can lower ACTH levels. Osilodrostat, an oral hydroxylase inhibitor, metapyrone, or mitotane can block cortisol. Mifepristone blocks cortisol action. Other agents include cyproheptadine, trilostane, and IV etomidate.

Continued

Making the Connections–cont'd

Signs and Symptoms	Physical Assessment Findings	Diagnostic Testing	Treatment
		CT and MRI scans of the head are provided to look for pituitary tumor.	In somatotropin-secreting tumors, octreotide, lanreotide, or pasireotide to suppress excessive GH secretion. Cabergoline and octreotide combination can shrink tumors. GH receptor antagonist, pegvisomant, can normalize growth hormone. External radiation treatment may be adjuvant therapy for GH-secreting tumors.

Syndrome of Inappropriate Antidiuretic Hormone (SIADH) | Excess ADH is caused by brain trauma or a variety of other etiologies. It causes excess water reabsorption at the nephron and consequent dilution of electrolytes, such as dilutional hyponatremia.

Signs and Symptoms	Physical Assessment Findings	Diagnostic Testing	Treatment
Confusion, seizures, nausea, vomiting.	Patient may have no significant physical findings.	Dilutional hyponatremia is caused by excess water in the bloodstream. Highly concentrated urine is caused by excess reabsorption of water from the nephrons. High ADH level is present. Low serum osmolarity (dilute blood) is present. High urine osmolality (concentrated urine) is present. CT/MRI may show pituitary mass.	ADH antagonists; conivaptan or tolvaptan are used. Furosemide is used to diminish the water content of blood. Tetracyclines can decrease the ADH effect on the kidney. Surgery performed, if warranted.

Hypothyroidism | There is a lack of sufficient thyroid hormone released by the thyroid gland.

Signs and Symptoms	Physical Assessment Findings	Diagnostic Testing	Treatment
In child: cretinism. In adult: sluggishness, weight gain, sensitivity to cold, constipation, depression.	Enlarged thyroid or nodule. If myxedema present: puffy face, periorbital edema, interstitial tibial edema.	In primary hypothyroidism, TSH level is high. T_3 and T_4 are low. There may be thyroid antibodies causing autoimmune disease (called Hashimoto's thyroiditis). Antithyroid peroxidase antibodies are present. Antithyroglobulin antibodies are present. Ultrasound may show mass or cyst. Radioactive iodine scan shows slow function of gland.	Levothyroxine (replacement thyroid hormone). Surgery to remove thyroid if nodule present.

Hyperthyroidism | Excess secretion of thyroid hormone by thyroid gland occurs.

Signs and Symptoms	Physical Assessment Findings	Diagnostic Testing	Treatment
Weight loss, sensitivity to heat, palpitations, tremor, nervousness, restlessness, diaphoresis.	Enlarged thyroid or nodule, exophthalmos, tremor, lower limb weakness, atrial fibrillation, audible bruit over thyroid gland caused by high blood flow over gland.	In primary hyperthyroidism, TSH level is low. T_3, T_4 will be elevated because of hyperactive gland.	Surgery is used to remove thyroid, or radioactive iodine medication is used to ablate the gland.

Making the Connections—cont'd

Signs and Symptoms	Physical Assessment Findings	Diagnostic Testing	Treatment
		Thyroid antibodies often cause hyperthyroidism (called Graves' disease). Measurement of serum thyrotropin receptor antibodies (TRAbs) is recommended. Radioactive iodine uptake (RAIU) test and a thyroid scan should be ordered. Antithyroid peroxidase antibodies. Antithyroglobulin antibodies. Ultrasound may show mass or cyst.	Antithyroid medications PTU, methimazole, or carbimazole can suppress gland activity.

Adrenal Insufficiency | This condition causes lack of cortisol, which is often caused by autoimmune destruction of the adrenal gland, called Addison's disease.

Signs and Symptoms	Physical Assessment Findings	Diagnostic Testing	Treatment
Feeling faint when standing from seated position; weight loss, weakness.	Orthostatic hypotension, tanned appearance.	Measurements of ACTH, cortisol, and plasma renin and aldosterone in blood samples collected in the morning (at 8:00 a.m.). The conventional ACTH test (an intravenous injection of 250 mcg of synthetic corticotropin) in adults is the gold standard for assessing adrenal function. Abdominal CT scan to visualize adrenal glands.	Replacement of ACTH or cortisol (hydrocortisone) depending on cause of hypoadrenal function. Replacement of mineralocorticoid (alpha-fludrocortisone). Extra corticosteroid administration in times of stress.

Cushing's Syndrome | Excess cortisol causes characteristic bodily changes.

Signs and Symptoms	Physical Assessment Findings	Diagnostic Testing	Treatment
Weight gain in central region of body, puffy face called "moon facies," easy bruising, striae, hirsutism, fat in cervicothoracic region called "buffalo hump."	Moon facies, buffalo hump, hirsutism, striae, central obesity, high blood pressure, low bone density.	Low ACTH and high cortisol, androgen, and aldosterone levels occur in primary hyperadrenalism. Dexamethasone suppression test shows high natural cortisol levels are nonsuppressible. An 11:00 p.m. saliva cortisol level followed by 24-hour urine free cortisol level and dexamethasone suppression test. Abdominal CT scan may show tumor or enlarged adrenal gland. Contrast-enhanced MRI of the pituitary. Specialized scintigraphy scans to find ectopic ACTH-secreting tissue. Chest x-ray is necessary to rule out an ACTH-secreting pulmonary tumor.	Surgery performed if adrenal tumor is present. Administration of ketoconazole suppresses cortisol (mechanism unclear).

Continued

Making the Connections–cont'd

Signs and Symptoms	Physical Assessment Findings	Diagnostic Testing	Treatment
		Inferior petrosal sinus sampling (IPSS) for differentiating Cushing's disease from ectopic ACTH syndrome. However, this test is highly invasive.	

Hyperparathyroidism | Excess PTH is secreted by the parathyroid, often caused by adenoma.

Bone demineralization causing pain, increased fracture risk. Muscle weakness. Hypercalcemia causes constipation.	May not show any physical findings.	High PTH level, hypercalcemia, low bone density, sestamibi scan of parathyroid glands to rule out adenoma. Ultrasound of parathyroid glands to check for cysts, masses, gland enlargement.	Calcium and vitamin D for bone building. Bisphosphonates, which inhibit osteoclast activity. Calcitonin, which inhibits bone breakdown. Increased water intake to prevent kidney stones.

Hypoparathyroidism | There is a lack of PTH secreted by parathyroid glands.

Muscle spasms, tetany, seizures.	Chvostek's and Trousseau's signs, which are present in hypocalcemia.	Hypocalcemia caused by lack of PTH. Sestamibi scan and ultrasound to look for masses or cysts of parathyroid glands.	If urgent treatment is necessary, calcium gluconate IV with cardiac monitoring. Maintenance treatment includes oral calcium supplements, calcitriol (vitamin D). Recombinant human PTH 1–84 or teriparatide (PTH 1–34 fragment) prescribed. Magnesium and phosphate binders may be needed.

Pheochromocytoma | Tumor of the adrenal medulla that secretes excess catecholamines: norepinephrine and epinephrine.

Palpitations, tremor, altered mental status, seizure, and possible focal neurological signs of stroke such as slurred speech or weakness.	Severe hypertension, tachycardia, cardiac arrhythmias. May have signs of stroke: weakness of an extremity, facial droop, slurred speech.	24-hour urine for catecholamines. CT or MRI scan of abdomen to look for adrenal tumor. Tumors can also be localized by specialized scintigraphy scans or specific types of PET scans.	Adrenergic blockers. Surgery to remove tumor.

Multiple Endocrine Neoplasia (MEN)-1 | Tumors are found within endocrine glands, particularly pancreas, parathyroid, and pituitary. Pancreatic insulinoma and gastrinoma are common.

Symptoms depend on the endocrine gland affected. Parathyroid tumor causes osteopenia, bone pain, or susceptibility to fractures. Pancreatic tumors can cause excessive gastric acid production, causing ulcer pain or diarrhea.	Physical findings depend on the endocrine gland affected. Parathyroid tumor causes bone pain and a susceptibility to fractures. Pituitary tumors can cause visual disturbances and may oversecrete PRL, causing galactorrhea or gynecomastia in the male.	Blood levels of hormones commonly involved: PTH, PRL, GH, ACTH. Blood level of gastrin and insulin.	Hormone antagonists, depending on which hormone is oversecreted. Surgery to remove tumors.

Making the Connections—cont'd

Signs and Symptoms	Physical Assessment Findings	Diagnostic Testing	Treatment
Pituitary tumors cause visual disturbances resulting from pressure on the optic chiasm and may oversecrete PRL, causing galactorrhea or gynecomastia in the male.			

Pineal Tumor | A neuroendocrine gland that secretes melatonin located near hypothalamus. Enlargement of the gland or tumor places pressure on adjacent brain tissue.

Headache, nausea and vomiting, seizures, memory disturbances, and visual changes.	Often there are no physical findings. Disturbed vision may be present.	CT/MRI of head is used to look for tumor.	Surgical removal of tumor. Ventriculoperitoneal shunt to decrease blockage of CSF.

Bibliography

Available online at fadavis.com

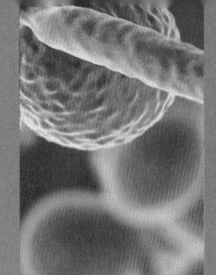

Diabetes Mellitus and the Metabolic Syndrome

Learning Objectives

Upon completion of this chapter, the student will be able to:

- Identify the risk factors for type 1 diabetes, type 2 diabetes, and metabolic syndrome.
- Recognize the signs, symptoms, and clinical manifestations of type 1 diabetes, type 2 diabetes, and metabolic syndrome.
- Describe the pathological mechanisms that cause type 1 diabetes, type 2 diabetes, and metabolic syndrome.

- List the laboratory tests that are used in the diagnosis of type 1 diabetes, type 2 diabetes, and metabolic syndrome.
- Discuss the different treatments used in the management of diabetes and metabolic syndrome.
- Recognize the potential complications of uncontrolled diabetes and untreated metabolic syndrome.

Key Terms

Alpha-glucosidase inhibitors
Amylin
Biguanides
Diabetic ketoacidosis (DKA)
Estimated average glucose (**eAG**)
Gestational diabetes mellitus (GDM)
Glucagon
Glucagon-like peptide 1
Gluconeogenesis
Glucosuria
Glycated hemoglobin (A1c)
Glycemic index
Glycogenesis

Glycogenolysis
Hyperglycemia
Hyperinsulinism
Hyperosmolar hyperglycemic syndrome (HHS)
Hypoglycemia
Impaired glucose tolerance (IGT)
Incretin
Insulin
Islets of Langerhans
Ketonemia
Ketonuria
Meglitinides

Metabolic syndrome
Metformin (Glucophage)
Oral glucose tolerance test (OGTT)
Polydipsia
Polyphagia
Polyuria
Postprandial
Postprandial glucose
Prediabetes
Preprandial blood glucose
Sulfonylureas
Thiazolidinediones

Diabetes mellitus (DM), a disorder of carbohydrate metabolism, is characterized by high levels of blood glucose resulting from the body's inability to produce or utilize insulin. The chronic high levels of blood glucose that occur in diabetes predispose the affected individual to cardiovascular disease (CVD), renal damage, peripheral vascular disease, and disorders of the eyes and nervous system. Diabetes is a leading cause of ischemic heart disease, blindness, renal failure, peripheral neuropathy, and lower extremity amputation.

Because of an increased susceptibility to these long-term complications, there is increased morbidity and mortality among diabetic individuals. The risk of death in persons with diabetes is approximately twice that of individuals who do not have diabetes.

According to the American Diabetes Association (ADA), diabetes can be classified into the following general categories (see Table 25-1):

1. Type 1 diabetes (T1DM)
2. Type 2 diabetes (T2DM)
3. Gestational diabetes mellitus (GDM)
4. Specific types of diabetes due to other causes

The classification of diabetes has changed many times over the years as research has revealed more about the underlying pathological processes involved in this disorder. Each type of diabetes is caused by a different pathophysiological mechanism, and every individual who is diabetic requires an individualized treatment regimen.

The incidence of diabetes has reached epidemic proportions in the United States and is continuing

TABLE 25-1. Classification of Diabetes Mellitus

Classification	Etiology
Type 1 diabetes	Autoimmune beta-cell destruction, usually leading to absolute insulin deficiency
Type 2 diabetes	Progressive loss of beta-cell insulin secretion commonly due to cellular insulin resistance
Gestational diabetes mellitus (GDM)	Diabetes diagnosed in the second or third trimester of pregnancy that was not clearly overt diabetes before gestation
Specific types of diabetes due to other causes	Examples are monogenic diabetes syndromes (such as neonatal diabetes and maturity-onset diabetes of the young [MODY]), diseases of the exocrine pancreas (such as cystic fibrosis and pancreatitis), and drug- or chemical-induced diabetes (such as with glucocorticoid use, in the treatment of HIV/AIDS, or after organ transplantation).

From American Diabetes Association Professional Practice Committee (2022). 2. Classification and diagnosis of diabetes: Standards of medical care in diabetes–2022. *Diabetes Care, 45*(Suppl 1), S17–S38. doi: 10.2337/dc22-S002

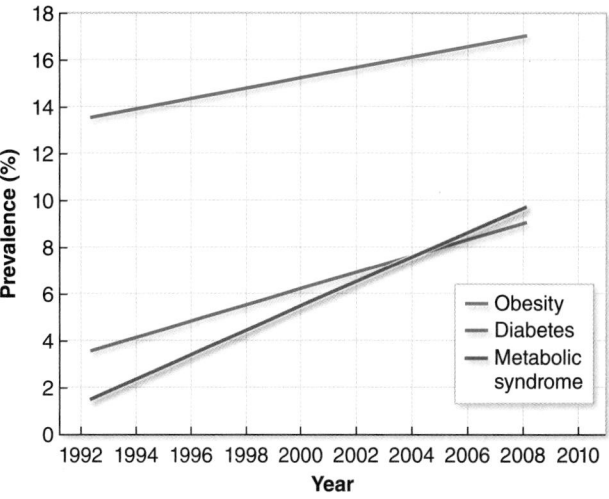

FIGURE 25-1. The prevalence of obesity has paralleled the rise in the diagnosis of diabetes and metabolic syndrome.

to increase within the population. It is essential that clinicians across all health-care settings understand the pathophysiology of diabetes, because they will undoubtedly encounter patients with this disorder.

Epidemiology

In the United States, diabetes affects an estimated 37.3 million people, or approximately 11.3% of the population. Among those affected, approximately 90% have type 2 diabetes (T2DM), 5% have type 1 diabetes (T1DM), and 5% have some other cause of diabetes. Prevalence increases with age; of persons 65 years or older, 29.2% (16 million) have diabetes. The incidence of diabetes is increasing worldwide, a trend that has paralleled a rise in obesity within the population (Fig. 25-1). Obesity and sedentary behavior, which have steadily increased in incidence in the last decade, are major risk factors for diabetes.

The age-sex–adjusted percentage of adults living with diagnosed or undiagnosed diabetes is 22% in Hispanics, 20% in non-Hispanic Blacks, 19% for non-Hispanic Asians, and 12% for non-Hispanic Whites.

The Centers for Disease Control and Prevention (CDC) estimates that diabetes affects more than one in four people older than age 65 years in the United States; at current rates of diagnosis, prevalence will increase 165% by 2050.

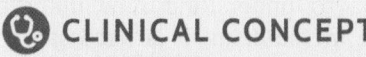 **CLINICAL CONCEPT**

Risk of death in persons with diabetes is approximately twice that of individuals who do not have diabetes.

Etiology of Diabetes

The most common forms of diabetes are T1DM and T2DM. These are polygenic disorders, meaning they occur due to mutations in multiple genes. Environmental factors also play a role in development of both forms. Common environmental factors include diet, endocrine disruptors, and other environmental polluters and gut microbiome composition. Obesity, sedentary behavior, and insulin resistance are accelerators of T1DM and T2DM.

Autoimmune mechanisms are the major cause of T1DM. In T1DM, deficient insulin results from T-cell–mediated autoimmune destruction of the insulin-secreting beta cells of the pancreas. The person has circulating autoantibodies to islet cells, insulin, and enzymes involved in insulin production. In T1DM, there is an absence of insulin. T2DM develops more gradually than T1DM. It is believed to be due to cellular insulin resistance that develops over time. Sedentary behavior and obesity are major risk factors for T2DM. Also, eventually, it is possible for the pancreatic reserve of insulin to become exhausted in T2DM. There is some evidence that a small percentage of persons with T2DM undergo autoimmune destruction of pancreatic islet cells, possibly due to environmental triggers (e.g., diet, infection).

Gestational diabetes mellitus (GDM) develops only during pregnancy. It is believed to be due to hormonal changes that make the cells less responsive to insulin. GDM can be harmful to mother and fetus and requires treatment.

Some other causes of diabetes include diseases of the exocrine pancreas, such as cystic fibrosis and pancreatitis, and chemically induced diabetes due to toxic drug treatment, such as prolonged glucocorticoid use. Also in this category are monogenic (single-gene mutation) forms of diabetes, which account for only 1% to 4% of cases. Neonatal diabetes mellitus (NDM) and maturity-onset diabetes of the young (MODY) are the two main forms of monogenic diabetes. NDM occurs in newborns and young infants. MODY is much more common than NDM and usually occurs first in adolescence or early adulthood.

Basic Concepts of Carbohydrate Metabolism

Dysfunctional carbohydrate metabolism is the major pathophysiological process and cause of complications in diabetes. To understand how diabetes affects carbohydrate metabolism, it is necessary to have basic knowledge of normal and impaired glucose regulation, as well as action of insulin and other glucose-regulating hormones.

Normal Blood Glucose Regulation

Ingested carbohydrates, which are broken down into monosaccharides in the intestine, are the major source of glucose in the bloodstream. Glucose is a major energy source for cell function. Before glucose can be utilized for energy, it must be transported through the plasma membrane into the cytoplasm of the cells. However, glucose is a large molecule that cannot diffuse freely across the plasma membrane; it requires a process termed *facilitated diffusion,* which is an insulin-supported process that occurs at the cell's plasma membrane.

Insulin is a hormone produced by the beta cells of the **islets of Langerhans**—specialized tissue within the pancreas. After eating, glucose is absorbed into the bloodstream at the intestine. The rise in blood glucose stimulates the pancreas to release insulin; this, in turn, causes rapid uptake, storage, and use of glucose by almost all cells of the body (Fig. 25-2).

After eating, there is a synchronous physiological rise and fall of insulin and glucose in the bloodstream. The rate of cellular uptake of glucose is controlled by the rate of insulin secretion by the pancreas (Fig. 25-3).

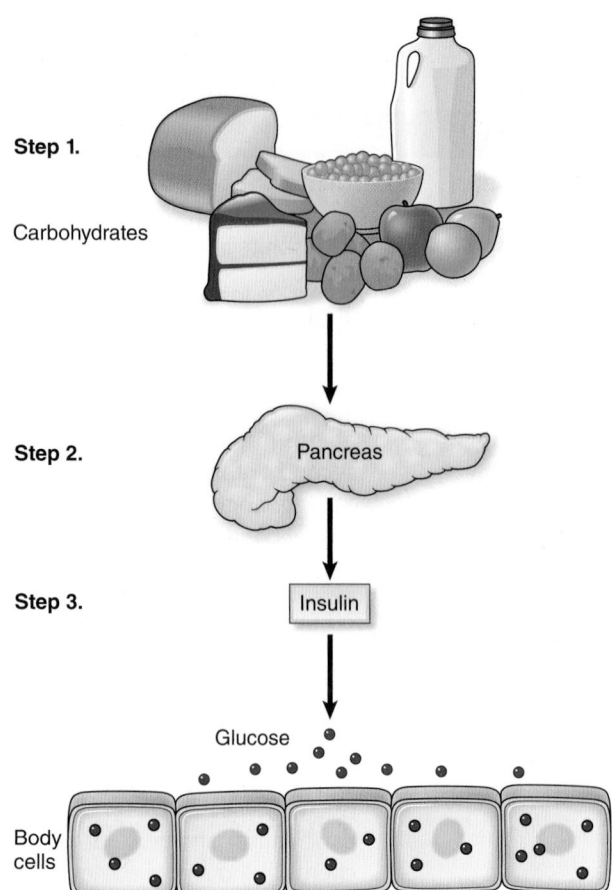

FIGURE 25-2. Glucose stimulation of normal pancreatic insulin secretion. (1) Carbohydrate ingestion leads to glucose absorption from the gastrointestinal system. (2) Glucose in the bloodstream stimulates the pancreatic islet beta cells to secrete insulin. (3) Insulin facilitates cellular uptake of glucose.

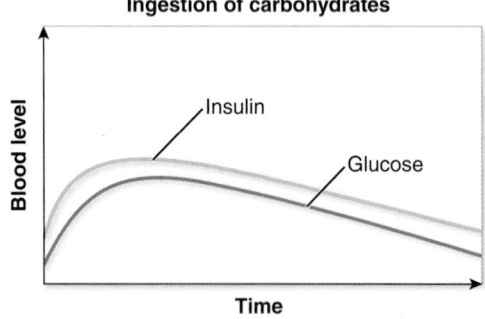

FIGURE 25-3. Synchronous physiological rise and fall of insulin and glucose in the bloodstream after carbohydrate ingestion.

After absorption into cells, glucose can be used for energy production, stored in the form of glycogen, or converted into fat. All cells can store some glucose in the form of glycogen, but the liver and muscle cells can store the largest amounts.

Glycogenesis is the process of glycogen formation. In cells, glucose is stored as glycogen to a saturation point—an amount sufficient to supply cells with energy for 12 to 24 hours. Cells require glucose for energy; during periods of starvation, the body is capable of producing glucose through the processes termed *glycogenolysis* and *gluconeogenesis*.

Glycogenolysis is the breakdown of the body's stored glycogen to yield glucose (Fig. 25-4). This process occurs when the body does not have sufficient circulating blood glucose from carbohydrate ingestion. The hormones epinephrine, released from the adrenal gland, and glucagon, released from the pancreas, can activate the enzymatic breakdown of glycogen. A well-nourished person who is fasting can rely on the breakdown of glycogen stores for 12 to 24 hours. *Fasting* is defined as an 8-hour lapse of eating or drinking.

Blood Glucose Maintenance in Starvation

During times when fasting is prolonged or starvation occurs, glycogen stores in the liver will be depleted. The liver can then synthesize glucose by another process: **gluconeogenesis** (Fig. 25-4). In gluconeogenesis, amino acids and fats are converted into glucose. Fats are mobilized from stored adipose tissue and broken down into two components: fatty acids and glycerol. The glycerol is used in gluconeogenesis, but fatty acids are not; instead, the fatty acids accumulate in the bloodstream.

As fatty acids accumulate, they are converted into acetoacetic acid, beta-hydroxybutyric acid, and acetone, three substances referred to as *ketoacids* or *ketones* (Fig. 25-4). Ketone accumulation in the bloodstream is known as *ketosis* or *ketoacidosis*. Ketones in the bloodstream cause the breath, saliva, and sweat to take on a fruity odor. High levels of ketones affect the brain, causing poor concentration and, at times, confusion and disorientation. **Diabetic ketoacidosis (DKA)** is a condition that develops in persons with no insulin reserves.

> ### 🔬 CLINICAL CONCEPT
>
> One-third of children with T1DM present with DKA when first diagnosed with the disease. Some persons with T2DM, particularly people of color, also present with DKA. DKA is a critical condition requiring immediate treatment.

Along with fats, proteins are used to manufacture glucose in gluconeogenesis. Proteins are mobilized mainly from muscle tissue by cortisol, a hormone produced by the adrenal gland. Proteins are broken down into amino acids, which the liver depletes of nitrogen. Therefore, during periods of starvation, adipose tissue and muscle tissue are utilized to manufacture glucose (see Fig. 25-4). Consequently, prolonged starvation causes depletion of fat stores and muscle mass.

Impaired Blood Glucose Maintenance

In a healthy person, blood glucose concentration is narrowly controlled and must be maintained at sufficiently high levels for cellular nutrition. Normal blood

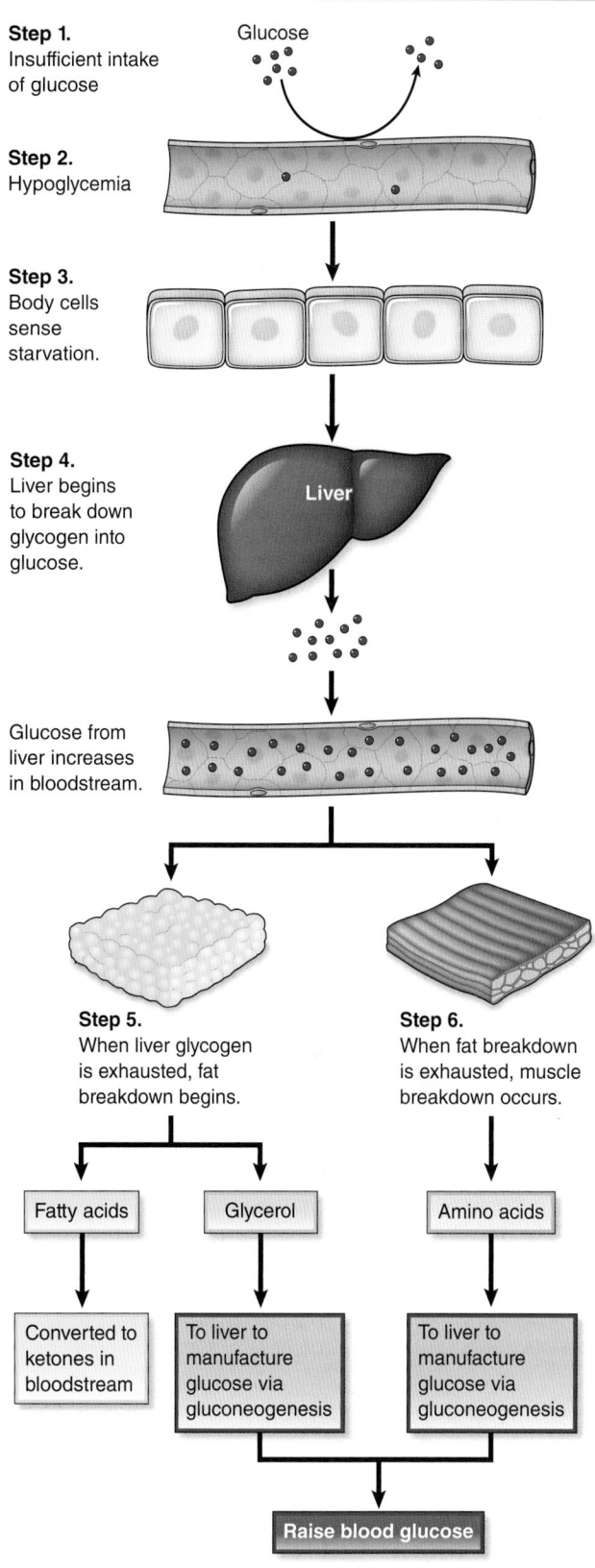

FIGURE 25-4. Glucose regulation during prolonged fasting or starvation. (1) Insufficient intake of glucose. (2) Hypoglycemia develops in the bloodstream. (3) Body cells sense starvation. (4) Liver is activated to break down its storage form of glucose called glycogen. (5) When glycogen is exhausted, fat breakdown occurs. Fat breaks down into fatty acids and glycerol. Fatty acids are converted to ketones, whereas glycerol goes to the liver for manufacture of glucose via hepatic gluconeogenesis. (6) When fat sources are depleted, muscle breakdown begins. Muscle proteins break down into amino acids, which go to the liver and manufacture glucose via gluconeogenesis. The process of hepatic gluconeogenesis raises blood glucose.

glucose concentration in a fasting person is approximately 70 mg/dL with an upper limit of 100 mg/dL.

Brain function relies solely on glucose; therefore, blood glucose levels must not decline to very low levels, a condition termed **hypoglycemia.** Hypoglycemia occurs when blood glucose levels fall to lower than 70 mg/dL. Most cells can utilize proteins or fats for energy if carbohydrates are unavailable, but glucose is the only nutrient utilized by the brain.

Although it is vital that blood glucose levels are sufficient for cellular nutrition, it is also important that blood glucose levels do not rise to extremely high levels. A blood glucose level greater than or equal to 200 mg/dL is referred to as **hyperglycemia.** Blood glucose values corresponding to hyperglycemia are diagnostic of DM.

After a meal containing carbohydrates, blood glucose normally rises to a maximum level of approximately 200 mg/dL. A fasting blood glucose level of 100 mg/dL to 125 mg/dL is referred to as **impaired glucose tolerance (IGT)** or a condition called **prediabetes** (Table 25-2). Persons with prediabetes have blood glucose levels higher than normal but not high enough to be classified as diabetes. A fasting blood glucose level greater than or equal to 126 mg/dL is considered diabetes.

A blood glucose level measured after eating is termed a **postprandial** glucose level. A postprandial blood glucose level greater than 140 mg/dL and lower than 200 mg/dL is also considered IGT or prediabetes. Postprandial blood glucose levels greater than or equal to 200 mg/dL are consistent with diabetes (Box 25-1).

Role of Insulin in Regulation of Blood Glucose

Immediately after ingestion of a carbohydrate meal, the glucose that is absorbed into the blood stimulates the pancreas to release insulin. Within seconds, circulating insulin binds to cell surface membrane receptors, making cells permeable to glucose. Insulin causes rapid uptake, storage, and use of glucose by almost all tissues of the body, particularly muscle, adipose tissue, and liver cells. In nonexercising muscle, the glucose that enters is stored as glycogen. Exercising muscle, however, does not require much insulin, because the contractile tissue is highly permeable to glucose. Brain cells, highly reliant on glucose for function, also do not require insulin for glucose entry.

Insulin has several effects on the liver. One of insulin's most important effects is to facilitate glucose storage in the liver in the form of glycogen. Insulin promotes glycogen formation and inactivates the enzymes that break down glycogen. When the quantity of glucose entering the liver cells is more than can be stored as glycogen, insulin promotes the conversion of excess

TABLE 25-2. Values in the Diagnosis and Management of Diabetes

	A1c Test	Fasting Plasma Glucose	Oral Glucose Tolerance Test
Normal	<5.7%	<100 mg/dL	<140 mg/dL
Prediabetes	5.7% to <6.5%	100 mg/dL to <126 mg/dL	140 mg/dL to <200 mg/dL
Diabetes	6.5%	126 mg/dL	200 mg/dL

From American Diabetes Association Professional Practice Committee. (2022). 2. Classification and diagnosis of diabetes: Standards of medical care in diabetes–2022. *Diabetes Care, 45*(Suppl 1), S17–S38. doi: 10.2337/dc22-S002

BOX 25-1. Diagnostic Criteria for Diabetes Mellitus

FASTING BLOOD GLUCOSE
- **Prediabetes:** 100 to 125 mg/dL
- **Diabetes:** 126 mg/dL or greater

TWO-HOUR PLASMA GLUCOSE DURING OGTT (ORAL GLUCOSE TOLERANCE TEST)*
- **Prediabetes:** 140 to 199 mg/dL
- **Diabetes:** 200 mg/dL or greater

RANDOM PLASMA GLUCOSE
- **Diabetes:** 200 mg/dL or greater

A1c (USED FOR DIAGNOSIS OR TRACKING GLUCOSE CONTROL)
- **Prediabetes:** 5.7% to 6.4%
- **Diabetes:** 6.5% or greater

These values can be used as categories when repeated on two different days of venous blood drawn (except for random sample of plasma glucose). Fasting glucose and A1c test can be paired on the same day; if both are in the diabetes range, diagnosis is confirmed.

*OGTT based on loading dose of 75 g. To convert values to millimoles, multiply by 0.05551.
Adapted from American Diabetes Association Professional Practice Committee (2022). Classification and diagnosis of diabetes: Standards of medical care in diabetes-2022. *Diabetes Care, 45* (suppl 1), S17–S38. https://doi.org/10.2337/dc22-S002

glucose into fatty acids, which in turn become stored as adipose tissue.

In many ways, insulin decreases the utilization of fat stores by the body and is considered a "fat sparer." First, insulin inhibits the body's use of fats for energy by enhancing the body's use of glucose. Second, insulin inhibits the action of lipase, the enzyme that causes hydrolysis of fat. Insulin also inhibits liver enzymes that activate gluconeogenesis and inhibits the breakdown of body proteins. In addition to increasing cellular permeability to glucose, insulin enhances cellular permeability to amino acids. It inhibits muscle tissue from breaking down and promotes the building of muscle, storage of fat, and formation of glycogen. Because of its bodybuilding functions, insulin is referred to as an anabolic hormone.

At the normal fasting blood glucose level of 70 to 90 mg/dL, the rate of insulin secretion is minimal. Ideally, when blood glucose levels remain within the normal range, the rise and fall of blood insulin concentration is proportional to the rise and fall in blood glucose. However, if blood glucose concentration suddenly increases by two to three times the normal level and remains at this level for a prolonged time, insulin secretion increases dramatically. Insulin concentration increases almost 10-fold within 3 to 5 minutes after the sudden elevation of blood glucose. However, this initial high rate of secretion is not maintained, and in 5 to 10 minutes, insulin concentration drops. After 15 minutes of a high blood glucose level, insulin secretion rises a second time and reaches a new plateau in 2 to 3 hours at a rate of secretion greater than the initial phase (Fig. 25-5).

A condition termed **hyperinsulinism** can occur when body cells are resistant to insulin. In this disorder, the pancreas attempts to compensate for the body's cellular resistance to insulin by overworking

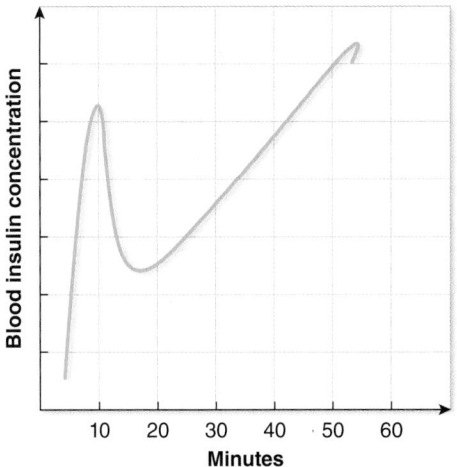

FIGURE 25-5. After a sudden increase in blood glucose to two to three times normal, plasma insulin concentration increases. There is an initial rapid surge in insulin concentration and then a delayed, but higher and continuing, increase in concentration beginning 15 to 20 minutes later. *(Adapted from Guyton, A. C., & Hall, J. E. [2020]. Textbook of medical physiology [14th ed.]. Philadelphia, PA: W. B. Saunders.)*

and increasing secretion, which increases the level of insulin in the blood to high levels. This increased secretion of insulin can compensate for cellular resistance for many years, with maintenance of normal glucose levels. However, with time, cellular insulin resistance usually worsens or pancreatic secretion ability declines; blood glucose levels then begin to rise.

Alternatively, excessive pancreatic secretion of insulin without any body cell insulin resistance can cause hyperinsulinism. The excessive insulin causes severely low blood glucose levels, a condition referred to as hyperinsulinemic hypoglycemia. Congenital hyperinsulinism can occur in infants and young children. In adults, severe hyperinsulinemic hypoglycemia is often caused by an insulinoma, an insulin-secreting tumor of the pancreas.

Other Major Glucose-Regulating Hormones

The pancreas and other organs moderate blood glucose levels by responding to states of hyperglycemia or hypoglycemia. The pancreas does not only respond to high blood glucose levels; it is also stimulated by hypoglycemia. Glucagon and somatostatin are other hormones secreted by the pancreas that regulate blood glucose levels. Endocrine glands such as the adrenal gland can also secrete glucose-regulating hormones. Cortisol and epinephrine can stimulate pancreatic secretion of insulin or provoke the breakdown of glycogen in the liver, thereby lowering or raising blood glucose levels. The gastrointestinal (GI) tract secretes hormones called incretins, which slow the GI absorption of carbohydrates. In response to a meal, incretins slow the rise of blood glucose.

Glucagon. **Glucagon,** a hormone secreted by the alpha cells of the pancreatic islets of Langerhans, has several functions that counteract insulin action. It can be referred to as a hyperglycemic hormone because it works to increase the concentration of glucose in the bloodstream. The major effects of glucagon include breakdown of glycogen stores in the liver (glycogenolysis) and activation of gluconeogenesis in the liver. In gluconeogenesis, glucagon enhances the rate of amino acid uptake by the liver and their conversion to glucose. Both of these processes increase blood glucose concentration and make more glucose available to the body cells. Glucagon also activates lipase, the enzyme that breaks down adipose tissue into fatty acids and inhibits storage of fat in the liver.

Glucagon secretion is regulated by blood glucose concentration. A rise in blood glucose concentration inhibits glucagon secretion, and a fall in blood glucose stimulates its secretion (Fig. 25-6). Severely low levels of blood glucose, as in hypoglycemia, increase glucagon secretion several-fold. This high amount of glucagon then greatly increases the output of glucose from the liver through glycogenolysis and gluconeogenesis, making more glucose available to body tissues (Fig. 25-7).

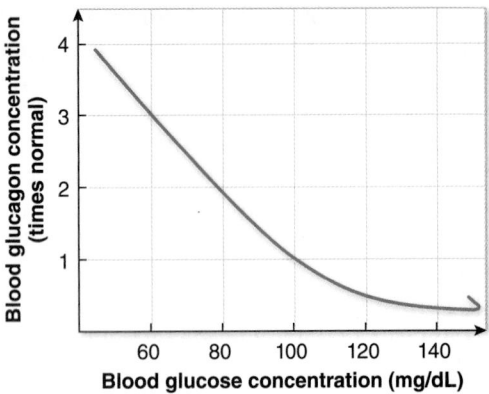

FIGURE 25-6. Approximate blood glucagon concentration at different blood glucose levels. When blood glucose levels are severely low, glucagon levels are high. When blood glucose levels are normal or high, glucagon levels are low. *(Adapted from Guyton, A. C., & Hall, J. E. [2020]. Textbook of medical physiology [14th ed.]. Philadelphia, PA: W. B. Saunders.)*

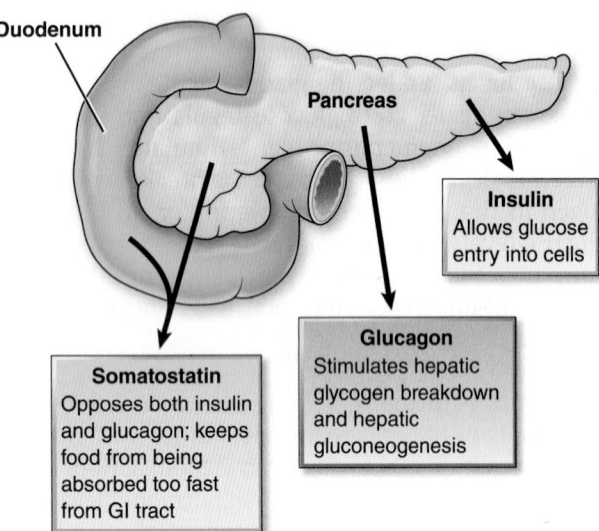

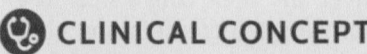

FIGURE 25-7. Major hormones involved in regulation of blood glucose concentrations.

> **⊘ CLINICAL CONCEPT**
>
> In severe hypoglycemia, glucagon can be administered as an injectable medication to raise blood glucose levels.

Somatostatin. The delta cells of the islets of Langerhans within the pancreas secrete the hormone somatostatin. After ingestion of food, the secretion of somatostatin is stimulated by the increase in glucose, amino acids, and fatty acids within the bloodstream. Somatostatin diminishes the secretion of insulin and glucagon and decreases the activity of the GI tract. Diminished insulin and glucagon decrease cellular uptake of glucose, amino acids, and fatty acids. Slowing the activity of the GI tract prolongs the period of time over which food nutrients are absorbed into the bloodstream. Through these activities, somatostatin prevents rapid exhaustion of nutrients and extends the period of time that ingested nutrients are available.

Gastrointestinal Glucose-Regulating Hormones. Several GI hormones stimulate insulin secretion, including gastrin, secretin, cholecystokinin, gastric inhibitory peptide (GIP), and **glucagon-like peptide-1 (GLP-1).** GIP and GLP-1 are also called **incretins.** All of these hormones are released in the GI tract after ingestion of a meal. They cause an anticipatory increase in the blood insulin in preparation for the glucose, amino acids, and fatty acids to be absorbed from the meal. In addition to stimulating insulin, GLP-1 suppresses glucagon secretion during hyperglycemia, delays gastric emptying, slows gut motility, and enhances satiety. All these activities of GLP-1 attempt to bring high levels of glucose down to normal.

Endocrine Glucose-Regulating Hormones. The other hormones that either directly increase insulin secretion or enhance the glucose stimulus for insulin secretion include growth hormone, cortisol, epinephrine, progesterone, and estrogen. Prolonged secretion of any one of these hormones can lead to prolonged stimulation of insulin-secreting pancreatic beta cells and eventual pancreatic beta cell exhaustion. Diabetes often occurs as a secondary condition in endocrine disorders that cause hypersecretion of hormones. For example, diabetes occurs in individuals affected by Cushing's disease, which is caused by a hyperfunctioning adrenal gland that secretes extremely high levels of cortisol.

Classification of Diabetes

Diabetes mellitus (DM) is classified according to the etiological process that causes the disorder. Assigning a type of diabetes to an individual often depends on the clinical signs and symptoms at diagnosis. Many diabetic individuals do not fit easily into a single category.

The classification of diabetes has changed numerous times over the years. Many classifications used in the past are now obsolete, including juvenile-onset DM, insulin-dependent DM, noninsulin-dependent DM, adult-onset DM, and maturity-onset DM. As our knowledge base has broadened regarding the pathology of diabetes, the classifications have changed.

> **⊘ CLINICAL CONCEPT**
>
> For the clinician, it is more important to understand the pathogenesis of the disease process than to categorize the patient.

According to the ADA, the majority of cases of DM fall into T1DM, T2DM, GDM, and other specific types (Table 25-1). In addition, some experts describe an intermediate form of diabetes termed latent autoimmune diabetes of adults (LADA), or type 1.5 diabetes. LADA is a slowly progressing form of diabetes with features of both T1DM and T2DM.

It is also important for the clinician to be familiar with the classification of prediabetes, which describes IGT that develops before diabetes. Despite the many different classifications, most experts focus on the two major classifications: T1DM and T2DM.

T1DM accounts for only 5% to 10% of all cases of diabetes and is caused by autoimmune destruction of pancreatic beta cells within the islets of Langerhans, which leads to insulin deficiency. T2DM is mainly characterized by cellular resistance to insulin, which can eventually cause pancreatic beta cell exhaustion. For unknown reasons, in T2DM, body cells are insensitive to the effects of insulin and therefore do not allow entry of glucose. T2DM accounts for 90% to 95% of all cases of diabetes. This form of diabetes often goes undiagnosed for many years because hyperglycemia develops slowly and individuals do not exhibit the classic symptoms in the early stages. T2DM can affect children, adolescents, and adults.

Gestational diabetes mellitus (GDM) is defined as any degree of glucose intolerance that occurs during pregnancy. It complicates approximately 4% of all pregnancies in the United States and can cause maternal and fetal complications.

Some other causes of diabetes include diseases of the exocrine pancreas, such as cystic fibrosis and pancreatitis, and chemically induced diabetes due to toxic drug treatment, such as prolonged glucocorticoid use. This "other causes" category also includes monogenic forms of diabetes, which are due to a single genetic mutation. Only 1% to 4% of cases of diabetes are due to this rare form. Neonatal diabetes mellitus (NDM) and maturity-onset diabetes of the young (MODY) are the two main forms of monogenic diabetes. NDM occurs in newborns and young infants. MODY is much more common than NDM and usually first occurs in adolescence or early adulthood.

Pathological Mechanism of Type 1 Diabetes

T1DM is caused by deficient insulin resulting from T-cell–mediated autoimmune destruction of the insulin-secreting beta cells of the pancreas. The individual has circulating autoantibodies to islet cells, insulin, and enzymes involved in insulin production. This form of the disease has a strong genetic influence based on multiple genetic variants. Among affected individuals, the rate of beta cell damage is variable, being rapid mainly in infants and children and slow mainly in adults. The presenting sign of T1DM is often ketoacidosis, particularly in children. Many affected adults retain some beta cell function that prevents ketoacidosis for many years, but they eventually become dependent on exogenous insulin for survival. Often, individuals with this immune-mediated type of diabetes are susceptible to other autoimmune disorders.

Clinical Manifestations of Type 1 Diabetes

Initial symptoms of T1DM include the classic triad (three "Ps"): **polydipsia** (constant thirst), **polyuria** (excessive urination), and **polyphagia** (increased appetite). The individual may also complain of visual disturbances. Inability to concentrate, fatigue, weakness, and a general feeling of malaise may be experienced before the initial diagnosis. A history of chronic *Candida* infection of the genital tract may also be the male or female patient's initial complaint. Physical examination in the patient with new-onset T1DM may be unremarkable unless an infection is present. Often, DKA is the presenting sign of those with T1DM.

Pathological Mechanism of Type 2 Diabetes

Cellular insulin resistance is the major pathophysiological process that causes T2DM. Cellular insulin resistance is the decreased ability of insulin to act effectively on target tissues (particularly skeletal muscle, liver, and fat). The precise pathophysiology of insulin resistance is not clear; however, molecular-level mechanisms involving oxidative stress, inflammation, insulin receptor mutation, and mitochondrial dysfunction are thought to contribute.

Pancreatic insulin deficiency, to a lesser degree, is also involved in the pathogenesis of T2DM. The insensitivity of body cells to insulin causes the pancreas to attempt to compensate by secreting increasing amounts of insulin. Greater-than-normal amounts of pancreatic insulin are required to produce a normal biological response, causing the pancreas to overwork. Eventually, the pancreas becomes exhausted and cannot continue to secrete insulin in amounts commensurate with glycemic levels. Blood glucose levels climb as the pancreas becomes dysfunctional and cells continually resist insulin. There is no immunological damage of the pancreas and the exact cause for insulin resistance is unknown.

The risk of developing this form of diabetes increases with age, obesity, and lack of physical activity. It also occurs frequently in women who endured gestational diabetes when pregnant and in individuals affected by hypertension and dyslipidemia.

> ## 🔬 CLINICAL CONCEPT
>
> Obesity is a major contributing factor to the development of T2DM. Fat cells are particularly resistant to insulin; the greater the adiposity of an individual, the greater the insulin resistance.

Glucose intolerance, or T2DM, is also part of a constellation of disorders termed **metabolic syndrome.** Persons with metabolic syndrome have hypertension, dyslipidemia, hyperinsulinism, centralized or "apple-shaped" obesity, glucose intolerance, and a predisposition to T2DM. Metabolic syndrome increases the risk of coronary artery disease and other diseases related to arteriosclerosis, such as stroke and peripheral vascular disease. The syndrome has become increasingly common in the United States, with 50 million Americans affected by the disorder (see Box 25-2).

In T2DM, insulin resistance frequently improves with weight reduction, increased physical activity, and pharmacological treatment of hyperglycemia. Many individuals affected by T2DM do not require exogenous insulin and are adequately treated with oral antidiabetic medications.

There is a strong genetic predisposition associated with T2DM, more so than with T1DM. Ketoacidosis seldom occurs in T2DM, but a similar disorder termed **hyperosmolar hyperglycemic syndrome (HHS)** can develop. In HHS, there are extremely high glucose levels, causing severely high osmolarity of the bloodstream, but no ketacidosis.

> ## BOX 25-2. What Is Metabolic Syndrome?
>
> The American Heart Association (AHA) and the National Heart, Lung, and Blood Institute (NHLBI) recommend that metabolic syndrome be identified as the presence of three or more of these components:
> - **Elevated waist circumference:**
>   - Men: equal to or greater than 40 in. (102 cm)
>   - Women: equal to or greater than 35 in. (88 cm)
> - **Elevated triglycerides:** equal to or greater than 150 mg/dL
> - **Reduced HDL cholesterol:**
>   - Men: lower than 40 mg/dL
>   - Women: lower than 50 mg/dL
> - **Elevated blood pressure:** equal to or greater than 130/85 mm Hg
> - **Elevated fasting glucose (IGT):** equal to or greater than 100 mg/dL.
>
> Adapted from American Heart Association (2022). Symptoms and diagnosis of metabolic syndrome. https://www.heart.org/en/health-topics/metabolic-syndrome/symptoms-and-diagnosis-of-metabolic-syndrome

Clinical Manifestations of Type 2 Diabetes

The clinical manifestations of T2DM are similar to those of T1DM: polyuria, polydipsia, and polyphagia. These three classic symptoms occur because of the same pathological process as in T1DM—the development of hyperglycemia caused by deficient insulin action. Hyperglycemia causes intracellular fluid shifts, resulting in polydipsia and excessive diuresis at the kidney that causes polyuria. With lack of glucose entry, cells sense starvation, resulting in polyphagia.

DKA is not typically a feature of T2DM because of the presence of some insulin. However, it can occur in T2DM as pancreatic insulin secretion capacity dwindles. The pancreas is able to secrete insulin, albeit erratically, in most individuals with T2DM. The presence of insulin allows for some glucose uptake by the cells and inhibits breakdown of fat, thereby preventing the development of ketoacids. Insulin protects the individual from developing overt DKA; however, the acute complication of HHS can develop if blood glucose climbs to high levels.

> **ALERT!** HHS causes severe dehydration, confusion, stupor, and possibly coma.

Gestational Diabetes Mellitus

Diabetes or any degree of glucose intolerance that develops during pregnancy is considered GDM, which is diagnosed, regardless of whether the patient requires insulin or only diet modification. It affects approximately 4% of all pregnant women in the United States and occurs more frequently in African Americans, Hispanics, and Native Americans. GDM requires treatment to normalize maternal blood glucose levels in order to avoid complications in the infant. In the absence of treatment, GDM can cause fetal defects, premature delivery, hypoglycemia in the newborn, and large-for-gestational-age infants.

The etiology of GDM is unclear, but the high hormone levels secreted during pregnancy create cellular insulin resistance. Women are at high risk for GDM if they are obese, hypertensive, had GDM in a previous pregnancy, gave birth to a large infant (heavier than 9 lbs) or an infant with a birth defect, or had a stillbirth in the past. Also, pregnant women with glucose in the urine during their prenatal checkup require screening for GDM (see Box 25-3). Commonly, pregnant women are screened for GDM with an oral glucose tolerance test (OGTT) during the second trimester, and ultrasounds are performed more frequently to assess the size of the fetus in GDM.

BOX 25-3. Maternal Risk Factors for Gestational Diabetes Mellitus

According to the ADA, a pregnant woman is considered at high risk for GDM if any of the following conditions exist:

- Hypertension
- Obesity (BMI greater than 30)
- History of GDM in a previous pregnancy
- Strong family history of diabetes
- Urine is positive for glucose at the prenatal visit
- Previous birth of a large-for-gestational-age infant (greater than 9 lbs)
- Unexplained stillbirth in the past
- Previous delivery of an infant with a birth defect

Keep in mind that many women who develop GDM don't have any risk factors.

High levels of estrogen, the major hormone that sustains pregnancy, can cause cellular insensitivity to insulin and consequent hyperglycemia. Hyperglycemia and insulin resistance make the maternal pancreas overwork to secrete more insulin to compensate. A pregnant woman with GDM may need three times the normal amount of insulin secretion from her pancreas. Insulin is a large molecule and does not cross the placenta; however, glucose does cross the placenta. Because the mother has hyperglycemia, the fetus develops high blood glucose levels. This glucose stimulates the fetus's pancreas to synthesize extra insulin to bring down blood glucose levels.

In uncontrolled GDM, the constant high maternal blood glucose levels cause high fetal blood glucose levels. Because these glucose levels exceed what the fetus needs for normal growth, extra glucose is stored as fat in the fetus. The extra fat synthesized in the fetus often leads to large-for-gestational-age newborns, known as macrosomia. Macrosomia increases the risk for the maternal complication of cephalopelvic disproportion, where the neonate is too large to naturally pass through the birth canal. The infant can also suffer shoulder dystocia at delivery, where the infant's shoulders are too large to pass through the birth canal. Nerve damage or fracture can occur in these cases, but most deliveries are accomplished by caesarean section. Also, because of the extra insulin made by the fetus's pancreas, newborns may develop very low blood glucose levels. Neonatal hypoglycemia often occurs shortly after birth in GDM. Lastly, studies show newborns who are born with excess insulin are at risk for obesity and T2DM as they become older.

GDM is usually transient and resolves after pregnancy. However, about two-thirds of women with GDM are at high risk for the disorder in future pregnancies as well. In some women, the stress of pregnancy provokes the development of a permanent condition of diabetes. Studies show that about 50% of women who endure GDM will develop T2DM within the first 5 years after delivery.

Diagnosis of Diabetes Mellitus

Blood Glucose Levels in Diabetes

Diagnosis of all types of diabetes is based on the same venous blood glucose parameters.

The **oral glucose tolerance test (OGTT)** is also a procedure used to diagnose diabetes. It evaluates how efficiently the body utilizes glucose from carbohydrates that are ingested. During an OGTT, an individual ingests a specific amount of carbohydrate-rich soda (75 g glucose load) and then has blood glucose measured 2 hours later. After 2 hours, if the patient registers a postprandial blood glucose level of 140 to 199 mg/dL, prediabetes is diagnosed. If the measurement is greater than or equal to 200 mg/dL, diabetes is diagnosed.

The **glycated hemoglobin (A1c)** (also called hemoglobin A1c or Hb A1c) test can be used to diagnose diabetes and assess blood glucose control over the preceding 3 months. Glycated hemoglobin (A1c) is chemically linked with glucose. An A1c value of greater than 6.5% is diagnostic of diabetes and a value between 5.7% and 6.4% is considered prediabetes. The ADA allows A1c testing paired with fasting plasma glucose on the same day. If the values of both are in the diabetic range, the diagnosis is confirmed. Recent data indicate that the A1c test may be of limited use in certain individuals because of interference from factors such as hemoglobin variants (e.g., sickle cell anemia), race (African American patients), ethnicity, or conditions linked to high red blood cell turnover (e.g., anemia, renal failure). Significant differences between plasma glucose and A1c results indicate that the A1c test may not be reliable. Another test, called the **estimated average glucose (eAG),** is the average glucose over the last few months measured in mg/dL. The ADA recommends an eAG of lower than 154 mg/dL.

In the general population, screening for diabetes is recommended every 3 years beginning at age 45. However, it is important for clinicians to recognize that T2DM is increasingly diagnosed in young adults, children, and adolescents.

CLINICAL CONCEPT

The gold standard laboratory test used to diagnose diabetes is a fasting plasma glucose level. A fasting plasma glucose level greater than 126 mg/dL on 2 separate days confirms the diagnosis. A random plasma glucose greater than 200 mg/dL that is repeated more than once is also diagnostic of the disorder.

Urine Testing in Diabetes

During hyperglycemia of uncontrolled diabetes, blood filtered by the kidney contains a high level of blood glucose. At the nephrons of the kidney, glucose is reabsorbed back into the bloodstream to a certain threshold, and the remaining unreabsorbed glucose remains within the tubule fluid. The tubule fluid continues farther onward within the nephron to become urine containing residual glucose. Glucose in the urine is termed **glucosuria**.

A urine dipstick test or urinalysis will reveal glucosuria, which is indicative of uncontrolled diabetes. Also, ketones in the blood, which are filtered at the kidney, can appear in the urine. Urine that contains ketones is termed **ketonuria.** If ketonuria exists, a urine dipstick or urinalysis will reveal positive ketones, which can be indicative of prolonged fasting or uncontrolled diabetes. Urine testing can also be used to monitor treatment effectiveness, but should not be relied upon for diagnostic purposes.

Islet Cell Autoantibodies

Several types of autoantibodies can be detected at the onset of immune-mediated T1DM. Islet cell, insulin, and insulin receptor autoantibodies are immunological markers that can be used for diagnostic purposes. The most commonly measured autoantibody level is that of islet cell autoantibodies (ICAs). The presence of this autoantibody can assist in the diagnosis of T1DM and can be used to differentiate T1DM from T2DM. In nondiabetics, the presence of ICAs indicates increased risk for subsequent development of T1DM.

C-Peptide Test

The C-peptide test is used to detect if there is natural insulin secretion from the pancreas. When the pancreas secretes insulin, it also releases C-peptide. A C-peptide test can differentiate between T1DM and T2DM.

In T1DM, C-peptide levels can evaluate if an individual has residual pancreatic beta cell function. Low or absent C-peptide levels are consistent with T1DM. With T2DM, the test may be ordered to monitor the status of the pancreatic beta cells and insulin production over time. A high C-peptide level indicates high insulin production by the pancreas, which occurs in T2DM, when the pancreas overworks to compensate for cellular insulin resistance.

C-peptide measurements also can be used in conjunction with blood insulin and glucose levels to help diagnose the cause of hypoglycemia and monitor its treatment. It can distinguish between excessive natural insulin production and excessive exogenous insulin administration as the cause for hypoglycemia. Administration of excessive exogenous insulin suppresses natural insulin released from the pancreas. If excessive exogenous insulin is administered, the blood will contain a high insulin level and low or absent C-peptide level.

In cases of pancreatectomy (removal of part of the pancreas) or pancreatic islet cell transplants, C-peptide levels may be monitored to verify natural insulin production and function of the pancreas.

Complications of Diabetes Mellitus

In all types of diabetes, acute and long-term complications are possible. Acute complications occur early in the course of the disease and are often the first sign of the disorder. Long-term complications occur mainly because of chronic episodes of hyperglycemia, which can occur in poorly controlled diabetes.

Acute complications result from either extreme hyperglycemia or severe hypoglycemia. In any type of diabetes, lack of insulin or insensitivity to insulin hinders cellular uptake of glucose and can result in severe hyperglycemia. Individuals with severe hyperglycemia develop a constellation of symptoms and require emergency treatment and hospitalization.

One of the most serious acute complications caused by severe hyperglycemia is DKA, which occurs mainly in T1DM and is not common in T2DM. In T2DM, severe hyperglycemia usually causes HHS. Both DKA and HHS can be life-threatening disorders and are often the first sign of diabetes for many individuals.

The other serious acute complication of all types of diabetes is hypoglycemia. Hypoglycemia causes a constellation of symptoms, can be life threatening, and requires emergency treatment. Both acute hyperglycemia- and hypoglycemia-provoked complications of diabetes are short-term systemic effects that are reversible with treatment.

There are also long-term systemic complications from prolonged uncontrolled diabetes. Most of these complications are caused by chronic hyperglycemia and the damaging effect that glucose has on the arteries and arterioles. The retina, kidney, cardiovascular, peripheral vascular, and nervous systems are affected. These complications are usually irreversible and are the cause of much of the increased morbidity and mortality that accompany diabetes.

Hypoglycemia

Hypoglycemia can occur because of excessive exogenous insulin, inadequate food intake, stress, excessive physical activity, infection, illness, alcohol use disorder, drug interactions, surgery, and excess insulin or oral antidiabetic medication.

A fall in blood glucose triggers a cascade of compensatory mechanisms that attempt to return the body to a state of normoglycemia, which is normal glucose level in the bloodstream. When blood glucose levels fall to hypoglycemic levels (lower than 70 mg/dL), the hypothalamic region of the brain and portal vein of the liver sense the drop in glucose. These glycemic sensors initiate a compensatory response, mainly involving the adrenal gland, pancreas, and liver. Epinephrine and glucagon are released, causing activation of the sympathetic nervous system and rise in blood glucose. Activation of the sympathetic nervous system is responsible for most of the initial signs and symptoms of hypoglycemia, which include sweating, hunger, dizziness, nervousness, tremulousness, irritability, headache, and heart palpitations. In addition, confusion, disorientation, inability to concentrate, seizures, and loss of consciousness can occur (see Box 25-4).

As hypoglycemia continues, epinephrine and glucagon promote glycogenolysis and gluconeogenesis in the liver. Usually, the liver can sustain blood glucose levels for 12 hours or more, unless glucose demand is increased by strenuous exercise, illness, or starvation. In times of extreme need, the kidney can also act as a source of glucose through gluconeogenesis. Muscle protein, triglycerides, and fat tissue are broken down to supply the liver and kidney with amino acids and glycerol as sources for gluconeogenesis. As hypoglycemia progresses, cortisol and growth hormone are released to further stimulate the liver and sustain glucose output.

Hypoglycemia can also present as unexplained night sweats or a clouded mental state upon arising in the morning. Nocturnal hypoglycemia can present as sleep disturbances, vivid nightmares, morning headache, chronic fatigue, or depression.

Those with long-term diabetes need to understand that they may be affected by autonomic dysfunction that causes unawareness of hypoglycemia.

 CLINICAL CONCEPT

Autonomic neuropathy, a possible side effect of diabetes, can cause dysfunction of the compensatory sympathetic response to low blood glucose. The patient fails to experience the warning signs of hypoglycemia, such as tachycardia and nervousness, and can unknowingly endure the condition until suffering loss of consciousness.

Managing Hypoglycemia

Individuals with diabetes need to be educated about the possible signs and symptoms of hypoglycemia and develop an action plan. Ingestion of fast-acting carbohydrates such as commercially available glucose tablets or gels, juices, soft drinks, or candy will remedy an acute episode of hypoglycemia. The suggested amount of carbohydrate consumption in hypoglycemia is 15 g. Five grams of carbohydrate will increase blood glucose by approximately 15 mg/dL. Foods rich in fat will delay carbohydrate absorption and should be avoided. If after 15 minutes, blood glucose is still less than 70 mg/dL and symptoms have not diminished, an additional dose of 15 g is recommended. The glycemic response to hypoglycemia is transient; therefore, a snack or meal is advised after correction of hypoglycemia (see Box 25-5).

Intravenous (IV) glucose (25 g) may be necessary if hypoglycemia is severe or if the individual is unable to take oral carbohydrates. A 1-mg dose of glucagon by subcutaneous injection is an alternative; however, IV injection of 50 mL of 50% dextrose is a more rapid—and preferred—remedy.

BOX 25-4. Signs and Symptoms of Hypoglycemia

- Sweating
- Hunger
- Dizziness
- Nervousness
- Tremulousness
- Irritability
- Headache
- Heart palpitations
- Confusion
- Disorientation
- Inability to concentrate
- Seizures
- Stupor or loss of consciousness

BOX 25-5. "Quick-Fix" Snacks for Counteracting Hypoglycemia

- 4 glucose tablets
- 15 g of carbohydrate gel (1 tube)
- ½ cup (4 ounces) of any fruit juice
- ½ cup (4 ounces) of a regular (not diet) soft drink
- 1 cup (8 ounces) of milk
- 5 or 6 pieces of hard candy
- 1 or 2 teaspoons of sugar or honey
- 2 tablespoons of raisins

PATIENT ADVICE

After ingesting one of these snacks, wait 15 minutes and check the blood glucose level again to make sure that it is no longer too low. If it is still too low, repeat these steps until blood glucose is at least 70 mg/dL. Then, if it will be an hour or more before your next meal, have a snack.

Adapted from NIH/NIDDK (2016). Low blood glucose (hypoglycemia). https://www.niddk.nih.gov/health-information/diabetes/overview/preventing-problems/low-blood-glucose-hypoglycemia

Frequent episodes of hypoglycemia can eventually blunt the compensatory responses and hormone counterregulation of low blood glucose levels. If an individual endures repetitive episodes of hypoglycemia, the clinician should reassess the patient's dietary intake, dosage, and timing of insulin or antidiabetic medication administration, as well as the blood glucose testing procedure. The bedtime glucose level is usually predictive of subsequent hypoglycemia developing during sleep.

> **ALERT!** Hypoglycemia is a life-threatening medical emergency that requires urgent treatment.

Somogyi Effect and Dawn Phenomenon

Individuals on insulin therapy can experience nocturnal hypoglycemia, which is usually a consequence of excessive insulin dosage or peaking of insulin action during sleep. During the night while the patient is asleep, hypoglycemia stimulates hepatic breakdown of glycogen and gluconeogenesis, which raise blood glucose. Epinephrine, growth hormone, cortisol, and glucagon are all released in response to hypoglycemia, which raise blood glucose further. This results in a raised blood glucose level, allowing for the development of hyperglycemia by early morning.

Upon arising, the patient's fasting blood glucose measurement is within the hyperglycemic range. A hyperglycemic fasting morning glucose measurement may be confusing to the patient and clinician. Therefore, morning hyperglycemia should raise suspicion of nighttime hypoglycemia. This syndrome of nocturnal hypoglycemia with rebound morning fasting hyperglycemia is known as the Somogyi effect, named after the physician who investigated the phenomenon.

A bedtime glucose measurement is usually predictive of the possibility of subsequent hypoglycemia developing during sleep. Reduction of insulin dosage, rescheduling of insulin administration, or changing the type of insulin should rectify the nocturnal hypoglycemia and resultant fasting morning hyperglycemia.

Morning fasting hyperglycemia can also be related to nocturnal elevations of growth hormone, which raises blood glucose. This syndrome occurs without nocturnal hypoglycemia and is known as the dawn phenomenon. Patients with diabetes who have little endogenous insulin, and therefore limited capacity to bring glucose into the cells, are mainly affected by this phenomenon. During the night, peaks of growth hormone slow the cellular utilization of glucose, allowing the glucose level to rise in the bloodstream. These effects result in a morning fasting hyperglycemic blood glucose measurement.

Individuals with serious fluctuations in blood glucose should be advised to test bedtime and early morning blood glucose to detect either the dawn phenomenon or the Somogyi effect. If the blood glucose level is low between 2 a.m. and 4 a.m., nocturnal hypoglycemia is present and the Somogyi effect should be suspected. If the blood glucose level is normal or high between 2 a.m. and 4 a.m., it is likely the dawn phenomenon.

To remedy the Somogyi effect or dawn phenomenon, the clinician needs to reevaluate the patient's insulin or antidiabetic medication regimen, mealtimes, and exercise patterns.

Short-Term Acute Complications of Type 1 Diabetes

As discussed earlier in the chapter, the classic signs of T1DM are excessive thirst (polydipsia), frequent urination (polyuria), and increased appetite (polyphagia).

Polydipsia and Polyuria

Hyperglycemia in all types of diabetes causes multiple adverse short-term systemic effects. High numbers of glucose molecules are solutes that raise the osmolarity of the bloodstream. The bloodstream is the extracellular fluid compartment that requires specific osmolarity to limit fluid from shifting out of the compartment. Hyperglycemia raises osmotic pressure within the extracellular compartment and alters fluid balance at the capillary–cell interfaces throughout the body. As osmotic pressure rises within the extracellular compartment, a gradient develops that moves intracellular fluid into the bloodstream. High osmolarity in the bloodstream causes a shift of water out of the cells and interstitial compartments into the extracellular fluid compartment (see Fig. 25-8). The result is cellular dehydration, which causes the individual to perceive thirst. This constant fluid shift from cells into the bloodstream creates polydipsia and polyuria (Fig. 25-9).

Polyuria also occurs because of the effect of hyperglycemia at the kidney nephrons. When the kidney filters hyperglycemic blood, high glucose levels develop within the fluid of nephron tubules. At the nephron, fluid within the tubules is reabsorbed into

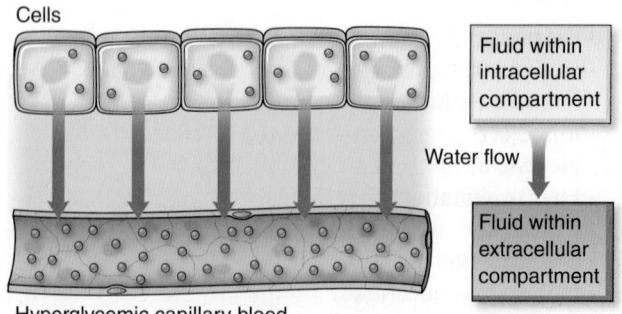

Cells

Water flow

Fluid within intracellular compartment

Fluid within extracellular compartment

Hyperglycemic capillary blood

FIGURE 25-8. Osmotic gradient that causes fluid shifts in hyperglycemia from intracellular to extracellular compartment.

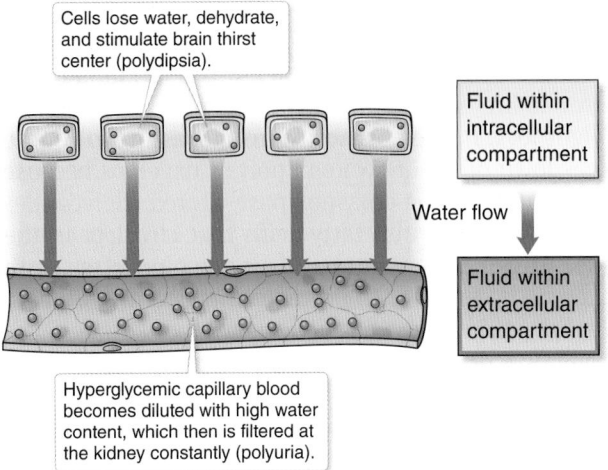

FIGURE 25-9. Cellular dehydration from hyperglycemia. In hyperglycemia, fluid from the body cells moves into the capillaries. The cellular dehydration causes thirst, called polydipsia. The water that moves into the bloodstream causes high water content that has to be eliminated; this causes excessive urination, called polyuria.

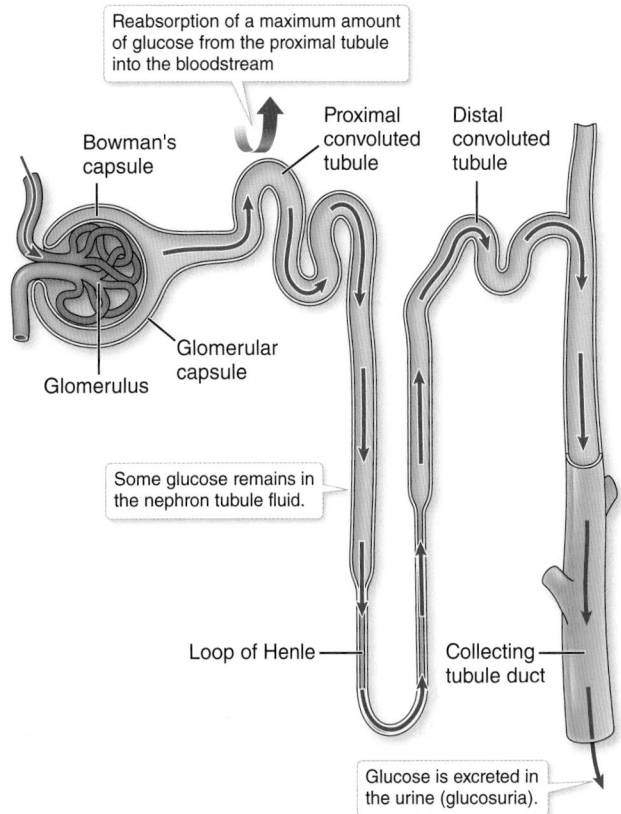

FIGURE 25-10. Acute effects of hyperglycemia at the nephron. Glucose is filtered out of the blood at the glomerulus. Glucose is then reabsorbed back into the bloodstream at the proximal tubule to a maximum threshold. Some glucose is left in the nephron tubule because the blood cannot reabsorb all of it. Glucose remains in the tubule fluid and is then eliminated in the urine, called glucosuria.

the bloodstream to concentrate the urine. However, nephron tubules have a threshold for the amount of glucose they can reabsorb back into the bloodstream. Reabsorption of glucose occurs to a maximum level and then excess glucose remains within the tubule fluid. When blood glucose reaches between 300 and 500 mg/dL, glucosuria often develops. High glucose in the tubule fluid sets up an osmotic gradient that pulls water from the cells lining the tubules into the urine. The nephron tubule cells lose water to the tubule fluid, which becomes urine. The osmotic gradient creates excess water in the urine, increasing the amounts and frequency of urination, as well as glucosuria (see Fig. 25-10).

Blurred Vision
Blurring of vision can occur because of the accumulation of glucose in the aqueous fluid of the eye. Aqueous fluid is a filtrate of blood; in uncontrolled diabetes, blood is hyperglycemic. The high glucose changes the osmolarity of the aqueous fluid that bathes the cornea, which changes the refraction of light coming into the eye.

Electrolyte Imbalances
Electrolyte imbalances can occur with fluid shifts in uncontrolled diabetes. Water shifting from the intracellular fluid compartment into the bloodstream can dilute the blood, causing dilutional hyponatremia. Potassium within the cells also moves out with the fluid into the bloodstream, creating an intracellular depletion of potassium and a *false* level of either normokalemia or hyperkalemia in the blood. With insulin treatment, these false levels may become true hypokalemia after potassium ions move back into the cells.

Polyphagia
Another classic symptom of T1DM and T2DM is polyphagia. In uncontrolled T1DM, the individual typically has increased appetite with an incongruous loss of weight. Because insulin is deficient, the body's cells are not receiving glucose. As a response, the body cells perceive that starvation is occurring, which has several physiological consequences.

When the body senses starvation, compensatory processes are activated to increase blood glucose levels (Fig. 25-11). Glycogen stores within the organs, mainly the liver, are broken down to release glucose into the bloodstream. However, this "assistive" glucose release by the liver is detrimental because the blood is already high in glucose related to the lack of insulin. The liver will also attempt to compensate for the cellular starvation by synthesizing glucose from noncarbohydrate sources. Hepatic glucose is manufactured through the process of gluconeogenesis. In gluconeogenesis, the liver can synthesize glucose from proteins and fats. Breakdown of muscle, fat, and triglycerides supply the liver with amino acids and fatty acids for gluconeogenesis.

As a consequence of hepatic glycogenolysis and gluconeogenesis, blood glucose levels rise higher. Therefore, in diabetes, the liver attempts to assist the body

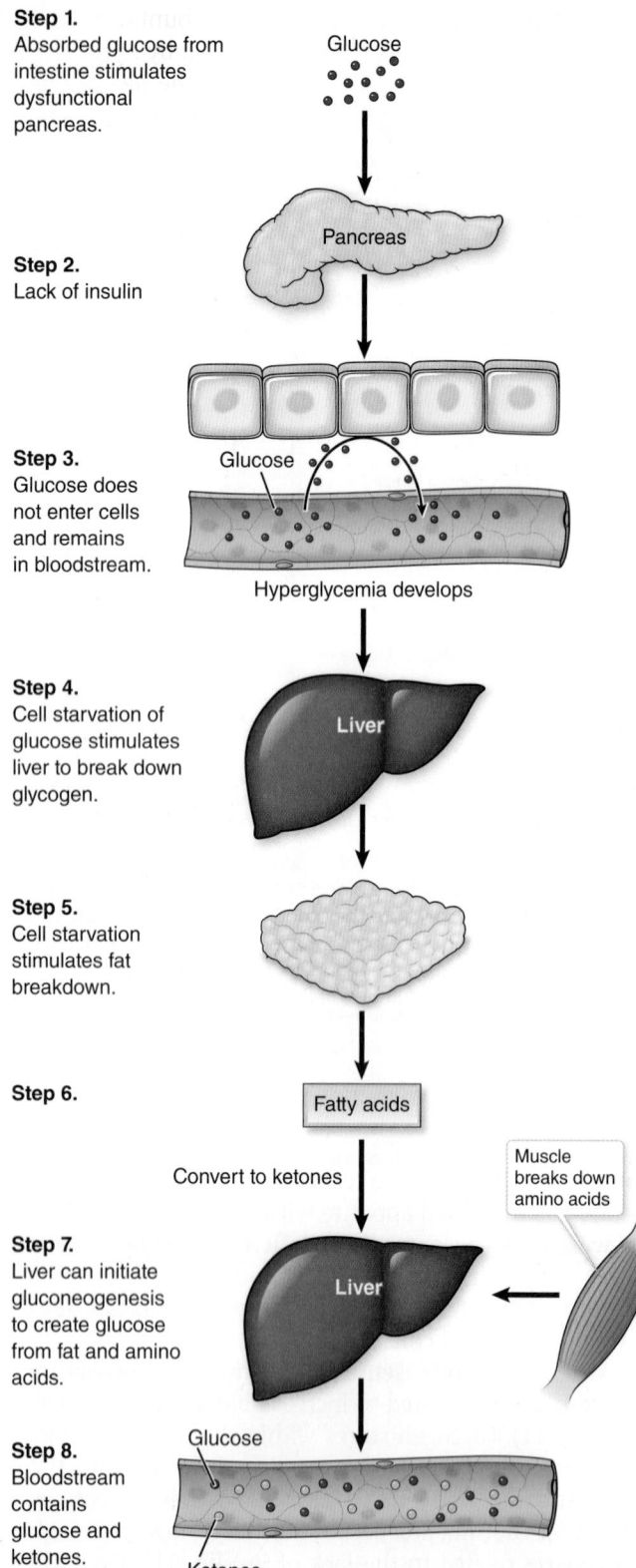

Step 1.
Absorbed glucose from intestine stimulates dysfunctional pancreas.

Glucose

Pancreas

Step 2.
Lack of insulin

Step 3.
Glucose does not enter cells and remains in bloodstream.

Glucose

Hyperglycemia develops

Step 4.
Cell starvation of glucose stimulates liver to break down glycogen.

Liver

Step 5.
Cell starvation stimulates fat breakdown.

Step 6.

Fatty acids

Convert to ketones

Muscle breaks down amino acids

Step 7.
Liver can initiate gluconeogenesis to create glucose from fat and amino acids.

Liver

Step 8.
Bloodstream contains glucose and ketones.

Glucose

Ketones

FIGURE 25-11. Basic process of the development of hyperglycemia and ketones in DM. (1) Ingestion of glucose causes a rise in blood glucose, which stimulates the dysfunctional pancreas. (2) The pancreas does not secrete insulin. (3) Glucose cannot enter body cells, hyperglycemia develops, and cells stimulate the body to go into starvation mode. (4) The liver starts to break down its storage of glycogen. (5) Fat starts to break down after glycogen storage is exhausted. (6). Fats break down into fatty acids, which are converted into ketones. (7) Liver initiates gluconeogenesis, making glucose from amino acids and fats, which raises blood glucose. (8) Finally, blood contains high glucose and ketones.

to deal with the cellular lack of glucose; however, its actions add to the existing problem of hyperglycemia.

As the body continues to sense starvation, adipose tissue is broken down and the individual experiences weight loss. In the absence of insulin, as in T1DM, the breakdown of fat known as lipolysis develops because of activation of the enzyme lipase. Stored triglycerides are broken down into fatty acids that circulate in the bloodstream. Excess fatty acids in the bloodstream are taken up by the liver to promote cholesterol synthesis, glucose production, and the formation of ketones. The promotion of cholesterol synthesis contributes to the enhanced development of atherosclerosis in diabetes. Hepatic glucose production further increases hyperglycemia, and the formation of ketones begins when fatty acids are taken up by liver cell mitochondria. Mitochondria oxidize the fatty acids to yield large amounts of acetoacetic acid, some of which is used by body cells, with the excess converted into beta-hydroxybutyric acid and acetone, which are ketones.

Ketones accumulate in the bloodstream, as well as in other body fluids such as urine, saliva, and sweat. The individual with uncontrolled diabetes can develop **ketonemia,** ketonuria, ketone breath, and ketone body odor, which can be identified as a fruity odor. If ketones accumulate to high levels, DKA can occur.

Diabetic Ketoacidosis

It is important to note that ketone formation is a consequence of lipolysis, which occurs in the absence of endogenous insulin; therefore, it mainly occurs in T1DM. Ketone formation seldom occurs in T2DM because, in most cases, there is some endogenous insulin available that prevents lipolysis. However, if pancreatic beta cell failure occurs in T2DM, ketone formation and DKA can occur.

Ketones are strong acids that accumulate in the blood, alter blood pH, and cause metabolic acidosis, specifically DKA. Severe nausea, vomiting, and profound dehydration can occur in DKA. The severe hyperosmolarity of the blood and the consequent loss of intracellular fluid in the brain can cause coma. Diagnostic criteria for DKA include a blood glucose level greater than or equal to 250 mg/dL, arterial pH lower than 7.3, serum bicarbonate (HCO_3^-) lower than 15 mEq/L, and ketonuria and ketonemia (see Box 25-6). Often, individuals with T1DM do not recognize their symptoms until they experience DKA and seek health care in this emergency state.

In DKA, the lungs attempt to rid the body of acid by hyperventilating to release carbon dioxide (CO_2). Hyperventilation decreases the CO_2 content of blood, which in turn lessens the hydrogen (H^+) concentration of the bloodstream (see Fig. 25-12).

🔬 CLINICAL CONCEPT

The characteristic rapid, deep respirations exhibited by the patient in DKA are called Kussmaul's respirations.

BOX 25-6. Diagnostic Criteria for Diabetic Ketoacidosis

- **Blood glucose level:** 250 mg/dL or greater
- **Arterial pH:** lower than 7.3
- **Serum bicarbonate:** lower than 18 mEq/L
- Ketonuria
- Ketonemia

Adapted from Karslioglu French, E., Donihi, A. C., & Korytkowski, M. T. (2019). Diabetic ketoacidosis and hyperosmolar hyperglycemic syndrome: Review of acute decompensated diabetes in adult patients. *BMJ, 365,* 1114. doi: 10.1136/bmj.l1114./

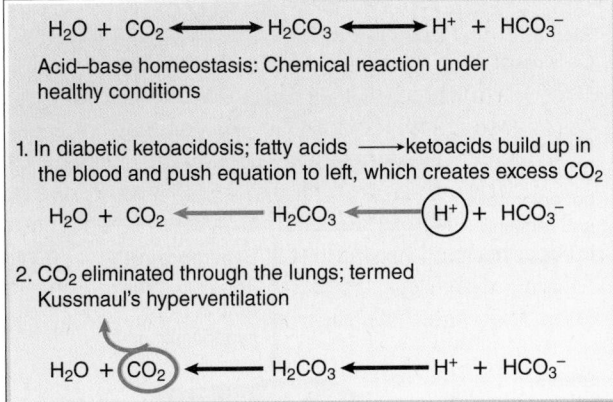

$$H_2O + CO_2 \leftrightarrow H_2CO_3 \leftrightarrow H^+ + HCO_3^-$$

Acid–base homeostasis: Chemical reaction under healthy conditions

1. In diabetic ketoacidosis; fatty acids $\longrightarrow$ ketoacids build up in the blood and push equation to left, which creates excess CO_2

$$H_2O + CO_2 \leftarrow H_2CO_3 \leftarrow \text{(}H^+\text{)} + HCO_3^-$$

2. CO_2 eliminated through the lungs; termed Kussmaul's hyperventilation

$$H_2O + \text{(}CO_2\text{)} \leftarrow H_2CO_3 \leftarrow H^+ + HCO_3^-$$

FIGURE 25-12. The chemistry of hyperventilation in DKA. DKA causes acid (H^+) to build up in the blood. The excess H^+ causes production of excess carbon dioxide (CO_2). The CO_2 is eliminated via the lungs in Kussmaul's respirations.

Managing DKA. Many patients with diabetes die of DKA each year. Most patients with DKA present with polyuria, polydipsia, polyphagia, weakness, abdominal pain, Kussmaul's respirations, nausea, and vomiting. The patient may be lethargic, stuporous, or comatose. Signs of dehydration, such as dry mucous membranes, tachycardia, and hypotension, are found. Often the patient has ketone breath, ketonuria, and ketone body odor. Common causative factors of DKA include new onset of diabetes, noncompliance with insulin treatment, the stress of infection, myocardial infarction, or alcohol use disorder.

Selected patients with mild DKA who are alert and able to take oral fluids may be treated in the emergency department and discharged after stabilization. Patients in DKA should have blood glucose evaluated every 1 to 2 hours until stabilized. Blood urea nitrogen (BUN), serum creatinine, serum sodium, potassium, and bicarbonate levels also should be monitored frequently. Urine should be checked for ketones and glucose periodically. Cardiac monitoring is necessary with significant electrolyte imbalances. Patients with severe DKA should be admitted to an intensive care clinical setting.

Fluid replacement is essential to counteract the dehydration and hyperosmolarity caused by hyperglycemia. IV insulin is administered until the blood glucose diminishes to lower than 250 mg/dL. The patient can be switched to subcutaneous insulin to maintain blood glucose in the range of 150 to 200 mg/dL.

Before treatment, serum potassium levels may appear normal or elevated. This is usually a falsely high potassium level, because intracellular potassium moves into the extracellular compartment in acidosis. H^+ ions replace the intracellular potassium (K^+), which displaces K^+ into the bloodstream. As insulin is administered and acidosis is diminished, K^+ moves back into the cellular compartment, which then reveals the true blood levels of potassium as hypokalemia, which is why potassium supplementation is necessary in DKA.

Serum sodium levels may appear falsely low because of dilution of excess fluid in the bloodstream, a condition known as dilutional hyponatremia. Sodium levels usually normalize with correction of blood glucose levels.

Cerebral edema is a severe complication that can develop in DKA. The patient may present to the emergency department in this severe state or may develop this during treatment of DKA. Early signs are headache, confusion, and lethargy. Papilledema, which is swelling of the optic disc; hypertension; and hyperpyrexia may also occur. In more severe cases, seizures, pupillary changes, and respiratory arrest from brainstem pressure may occur. There is a 70% mortality rate once severe symptoms of cerebral edema develop. To prevent this potentially fatal event, the clinician needs to be careful to not overhydrate the patient, and the blood glucose level should be decreased slowly during treatment.

🩺 CLINICAL CONCEPT

During treatment for DKA, IV insulin is administered until the blood glucose diminishes to lower than 250 mg/dL.

Short-Term Acute Complications of Type 2 Diabetes

Patients with T2DM usually do not exhibit DKA; however, a disorder called HHS can occur. Cells resist insulin, causing critically high plasma glucose levels.

Hyperosmolar Hyperglycemic Syndrome

The major short-term complication of T2DM is HHS, characterized by severe hyperglycemia, hyperosmolarity, and dehydration. In some cases, mild ketonemia and ketonuria can be present.

In T2DM, because of cellular insulin resistance, glucose is not absorbed into the cells. Hyperglycemia develops as a result and sets up an osmotic gradient as it does in T1DM. The hyperosmolarity of the blood causes intracellular fluid to move into the extracellular compartment. Extracellular fluid volume increases and cellular dehydration occurs.

Simultaneously, the cells are not absorbing glucose and begin to sense starvation. As in T1DM, the body enters starvation mode with hepatic glycogen breakdown and activation of gluconeogenesis. These mechanisms attempt to compensate for cellular starvation. As a result, with cells continually resisting the glucose, blood glucose levels rise higher (Fig. 25-13).

Because insulin is present in T2DM, ketones are not commonly formed. Ketone formation is a result of fat breakdown, and insulin counteracts lipolysis. Therefore, the presence of insulin in T2DM can block fat breakdown and the consequent formation of ketones. However, when the pancreas is exhausted in T2DM and there is no insulin reserve, ketones can form in T2DM.

An early event in HHS is glucosuric diuresis. At the nephron, the glucose-rich blood is filtered and the glucose reabsorption threshold is exceeded, causing high levels of glucose to remain in the tubule fluid. The high osmolarity created by the glucose in the tubule fluid pulls water into the tubule. This is an osmotic diuresis resulting in extra water excreted in the urine. As in T1DM, glucosuria and dehydration occur.

Thirst and polyuria are the initial complaints caused by these pathological processes. If water intake is insufficient to counteract the water loss, hypovolemia, dehydration, and hyperosmolarity of the bloodstream develop. A mild metabolic acidosis can be present in some individuals with nonketotic HHS. The laboratory parameters include blood glucose greater than 600 mg/dL, arterial pH greater than 7.3, serum bicarbonate level greater than 18 mEq/L, and blood osmolarity greater than 320 mOsm/L (see Box 25-7). Although there is metabolic acidosis in HHS, it is less severe than the acidosis in DKA. Severe hyperosmolarity of the bloodstream is the major disturbance in HHS.

This syndrome can develop insidiously over days to weeks. Anorexia, weight loss, weakness, visual disturbances, poor tissue turgor, tachycardia, and confusion are common complaints. Seizure and neurological disturbances can occur. Approximately 25% of patients present in coma because of the effect of blood hyperosmolarity on the brain.

Clinical Manifestations of HHS. HHS is manifested by blood glucose levels greater than 600 mg/dL and extremely high blood osmolarity levels in patients with T2DM. Common precipitating factors include infection, noncompliance with diet or medication, new-onset T2DM, substance abuse disorder involving alcohol or cocaine, or coexisting diseases. In T2DM, the most common cause of HHS is infection: pneumonia, urinary tract infection, or sepsis. Severe stresses such as myocardial infarction, stroke, or pulmonary embolus can also precipitate poor glycemic control. Although some insulin is present in T2DM, it is not sufficient to control extremely high levels of blood glucose.

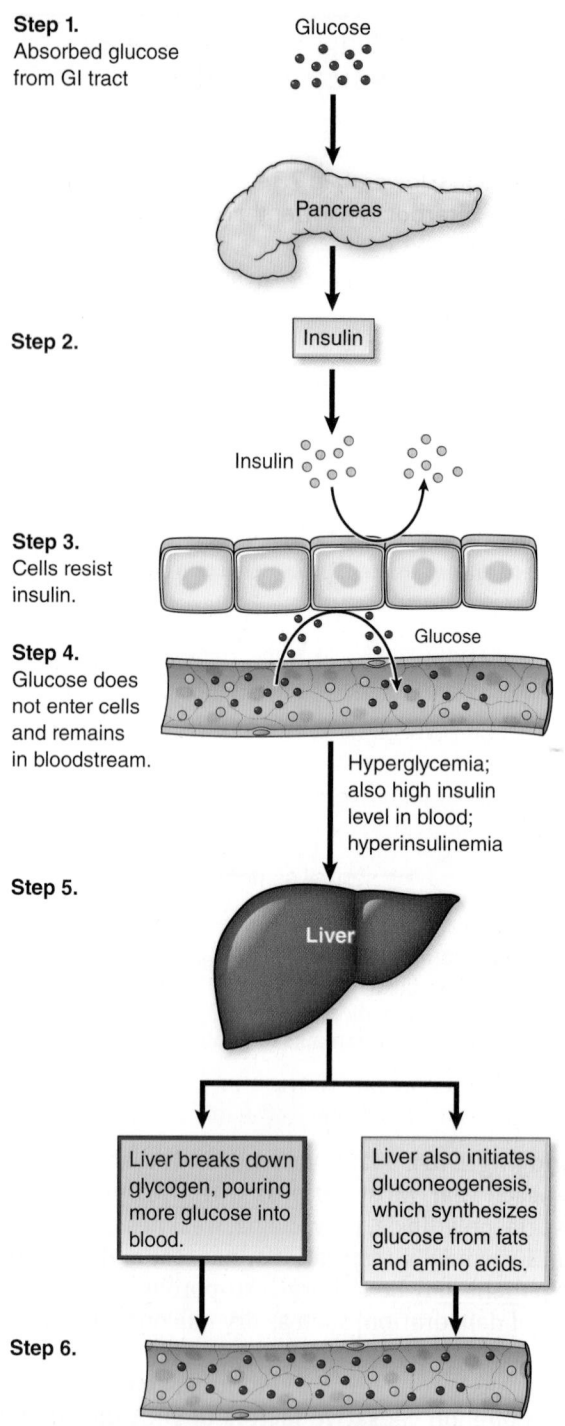

FIGURE 25-13. Development of hyperglycemia and hyperosmolarity in type 2 diabetes. (1) Glucose is absorbed from the gastrointestinal tract. (2) The pancreas is stimulated to secrete insulin. (3) Body cells resist insulin and glucose cannot enter cells. (4) Glucose accumulates in the blood (hyperglycemia) and insulin builds up in the blood, called hyperinsulinemia. (5) Cell starvation stimulates the liver to break down glycogen storage and initiate gluconeogenesis. (6) The blood develops hyperglycemia and hyperosmolarity. Fat is not broken down in the presence of insulin; therefore, ketone formation is minimal.

> **BOX 25-7. Laboratory Values in Hyperosmolar Hyperglycemic Syndrome of Type 2 Diabetes**
>
> - **Blood glucose:** greater than 600 mg/dL
> - **Arterial pH:** mild acidosis; pH greater than 7.3
> - **Serum bicarbonate level:** greater than 18 mEq/L
> - **Blood osmolarity:** greater than 320 mOsm/L
> - **Urine ketone:** small
> - **Blood ketone:** small

Adapted from Karslioglu French, E., Donihi, A. C., & Korytkowski, M. T. (2019). Diabetic ketoacidosis and hyperosmolar hyperglycemic syndrome: Review of acute decompensated diabetes in adult patients. *BMJ, 365*, 1114. doi: 10.1136/bmj.l1114./

> **BOX 25-8. Symptoms of Hyperosmolar Hyperglycemic Syndrome in Type 2 Diabetes**
>
> - Extreme hyperglycemia
> - Rapid, thready pulse
> - Hypotension
> - Profound dehydration
> - Polydipsia
> - Polyuria
> - Confusion, disorientation, stupor, possible seizures, or coma

Adapted from Karslioglu French, E., Donihi, A. C., & Korytkowski, M. T. (2019). Diabetic ketoacidosis and hyperosmolar hyperglycemic syndrome: Review of acute decompensated diabetes in adult patients. *BMJ, 365*, 1114. doi: 10.1136/bmj.l1114

Dehydration is the major pathophysiological mechanism that causes complications in HHS. When blood glucose rises to a high level, blood osmolarity rises. Osmotic diuresis causes constant loss of water in the urine, which concentrates the electrolytes in the bloodstream, resulting in increased serum osmolarity that can be calculated using the following equation:

$$2 \times Na^+ \, (mEq/L) + \frac{plasma \, glucose \, (mg/dL)}{18} = serum \, osmolarity$$

Serum osmolarity levels greater than 320 mOsm/kg are associated with HHS.

As in DKA, serum potassium levels may appear normal or falsely high because of the shift of K^+ from the intracellular compartment into the extracellular compartment. As rehydration and insulin treatment ensue, potassium returns to the intracellular compartment. Serum potassium levels then decrease as the K^+ ions move back into the cells. Therefore, hypokalemia results from HHS, and K^+ replacement is usually necessary in the treatment plan.

HHS presents with signs of profound dehydration; hypotension; rapid, thready pulse; and changes in mental status, from lethargy to coma. Abdominal distention can occur because of gastroparesis, which resolves with rehydration. Seizures are possible if blood osmolarity reaches severely high levels (see Box 25-8).

Management of HHS. Treatment of HHS includes IV rehydration, electrolyte replacement, and IV insulin. Adequate fluids should be administered first. If insulin is administered before fluids, extracellular water will move intracellularly, worsening hypotension and possible hypovolemic shock. IV insulin should be given after rehydration stabilizes the patient's osmolarity; it can be administered until blood glucose reaches 300 mg/dL, at which time subcutaneous insulin can be initiated. The precipitating cause of HHS should be corrected, and patients should be cared for in an intensive care setting.

Long-Term Complications of Diabetes

Long-term DM of any type can lead to multiple serious complications (see Table 25-3 and Fig. 25-14). Chronic hyperglycemia is the major pathophysiological mechanism that causes most of the complications. In treating diabetes, it is difficult to mimic the physiological control of blood glucose achieved by endogenous, natural insulin. Episodic elevation of blood glucose commonly occurs despite the most stringent treatment regimens.

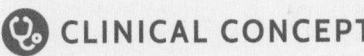

CLINICAL CONCEPT

Postprandial hyperglycemia has been found to be the most damaging of all blood glucose fluctuations.

The risk of complications increases in relation to duration of chronic hyperglycemia, usually becoming apparent after years of this disorder. There is also a probable genetic susceptibility for the development of certain complications because there is variability in individual development of complications despite comparable levels of glycemic control.

Chronic hyperglycemia is the major cause of damage to the small and large arterial vessels. Vascular damage, termed angiopathy, is a major cause of the long-term complications in diabetes.

The pathological mechanism of hyperglycemia involves glycosylation of the endothelial cells causing damage of the lining of the arterioles and arteries. Hyperglycemic damage to the smallest arterial blood vessels occurs initially, with arterial vessels of the retina, nutrient arterial vessels of the neurons, and arterial vessels surrounding the nephrons primarily demonstrating this endothelial damage. Eventually, diabetic retinopathy, neuropathy, and nephropathy develop. Injury of retinal arteries can be seen on dilated

TABLE 25-3. Systemic Long-Term Complications of Diabetes

Body System	Complication	Pathological Process	Signs and Symptoms
Arterial	Accelerated atherosclerosis	Arterial plaque buildup, narrowing of arteries, with possible plaque disruption and thrombotic or embolic obstruction of arterial blood flow	Pain caused by ischemia of any organ system that results from blockage of arterial circulation Hypertension
Cardiac	Coronary artery disease	Coronary artery plaque buildup, narrowing of arteries, with plaque disruption and emboli, resulting in angina pectoris or myocardial infarction	Chest pain due to ischemia (angina) Dyspnea Myocardial infarction (often silent; without classic signs and symptoms) Sudden death possible because of cardiac arrest
Cerebrovascular	Stroke Transient ischemic attack	Atherosclerosis of cerebral arteries or carotid arteries causing emboli or thrombi to block circulation to brain	Dizziness, disorientation, hemiparesis or hemiparalysis, cranial nerve dysfunction, possible aphasia
Peripheral vascular	Peripheral arterial disease of lower extremities	Arterial plaque buildup, narrowing of arteries, and obstruction of arterial blood flow in lower extremities	Pain of lower extremity due to ischemia (intermittent claudication) Weak or absent pulses Paresthesias in feet Pallor of lower extremity Coolness to palpation of lower extremity Poor wound healing that may lead to amputation
Retina	Retinopathy	Narrowing of retinal arteries, hemorrhages, exudates	Vision impairment with possible blindness
Kidneys	Nephropathy	Damage to glomeruli and renal arterial circulation	Microalbuminuria Renal insufficiency Possible renal failure
Peripheral nervous system	Peripheral neuropathy; mainly sensory/motor to lesser extent	Damage to endoneurial arterial circulation that decreases blood flow to nerves, particularly sensory nerves of lower extremity	Loss of sensation in feet, paresthesias of feet, foot deformities (Charcot joint), gait disturbance
Autonomic nervous system	Autonomic neuropathy	Damage to endoneurial arterial circulation, which decreases blood flow to autonomic nerves; dysfunction of sympathetic and parasympathetic nervous systems	Postural hypotension Gastroparesis Bladder and bowel dysfunction Anhidrosis (sweat gland dysfunction) Lack of sympathetic nervous symptoms in hypoglycemia ("hypoglycemia unawareness")

TABLE 25-3. Systemic Long-Term Complications of Diabetes—cont'd

Body System	Complication	Pathological Process	Signs and Symptoms
Immune system	Immunosuppression	WBC dysfunction in high glucose environment	Susceptibility to infections, gangrene Poor wound healing (particularly lower extremities)
Reproductive system	*Candida* vaginitis *Candida* balanitis Gestational diabetes	Glycogen accumulation within vaginal cells Susceptibility to infection IGT in pregnancy	*Candida* vulvovaginitis; pruritus, vaginal discharge *Candida* balanitis; pruritic rash in uncircumcised males Fetal defects, premature delivery, large-for-gestational-age newborn
Dermatological system	Skin ulceration, susceptibility to staphylococcal infection, and poor wound healing Necrobiosis lipoidica diabeticorum Acanthosis nigricans Lipoatrophy and lipohypertrophy Intertriginous *Candida* infection	Skin ulceration: anhidrosis, dry skin, prolonged wound healing caused by immunosuppression Necrobiosis lipoidica diabeticorum: unknown etiology Acanthosis nigricans: unknown etiology Lipoatrophy and lipohypertrophy can occur at sites of repeated insulin injection	Skin breakdown with susceptibility to infection caused by staphylococcal colonization of skin, immunosuppression, and poor wound healing Necrobiosis lipoidica diabeticorum: ulcerated lesions commonly on legs Acanthosis nigricans: hyperpigmented, velvety macular lesions usually located on the neck, axilla, or extensor surfaces of arms Lipoatrophy and lipohypertrophy: soft tissue damage at injection sites Intertriginous *Candida* infection: pruritic papular or macular rash between folds of skin
Psychological/emotional effects	Anxiety Depression Eating disorders "Insulin purging" Denial of the disorder termed "psychological insulin resistance"	Stress, misinterpretation of the disease process, and lack of appropriate coping skills	Excessive worrying Feelings of sadness Feelings of loss Anhedonia Withdrawal "Insulin purging" (underdosing or omitting doses of insulin) Weight loss and excessive concern about weight gain Frequent episodes of poor glycemic control Excessive exercising Noncompliance with recommended insulin injection administration

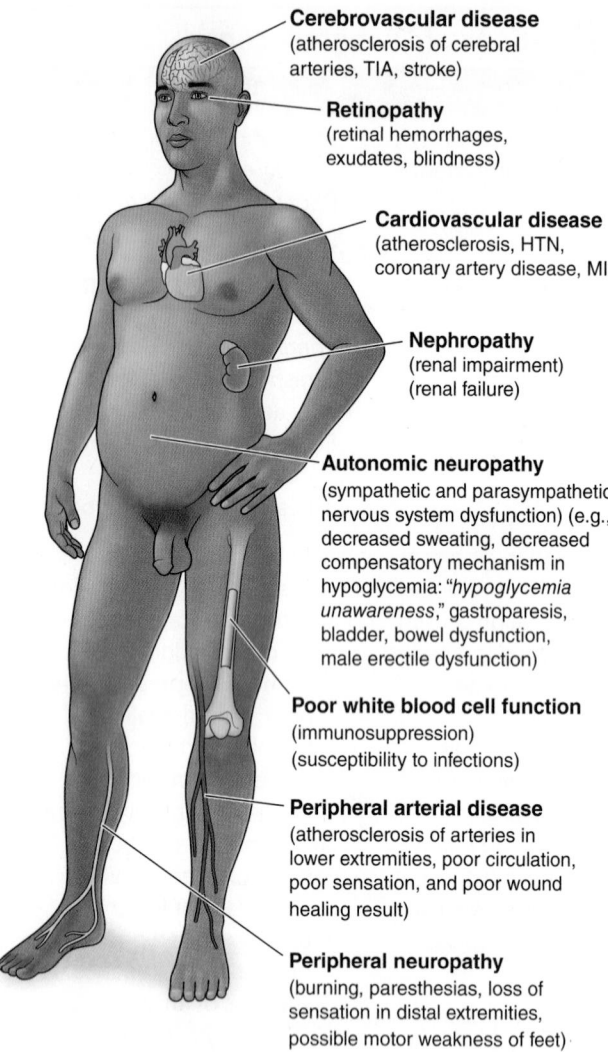

Cerebrovascular disease
(atherosclerosis of cerebral arteries, TIA, stroke)

Retinopathy
(retinal hemorrhages, exudates, blindness)

Cardiovascular disease
(atherosclerosis, HTN, coronary artery disease, MI)

Nephropathy
(renal impairment)
(renal failure)

Autonomic neuropathy
(sympathetic and parasympathetic nervous system dysfunction) (e.g., decreased sweating, decreased compensatory mechanism in hypoglycemia: "*hypoglycemia unawareness*," gastroparesis, bladder, bowel dysfunction, male erectile dysfunction)

Poor white blood cell function
(immunosuppression)
(susceptibility to infections)

Peripheral arterial disease
(atherosclerosis of arteries in lower extremities, poor circulation, poor sensation, and poor wound healing result)

Peripheral neuropathy
(burning, paresthesias, loss of sensation in distal extremities, possible motor weakness of feet)

FIGURE 25-14. Systemic long-term complications of diabetes.

fundoscopic examination. Neuron damage causes sensory and motor peripheral nerve dysfunction. Injured autonomic nerves, also called autonomic neuropathy, cause dysfunction of the parasympathetic and sympathetic nervous system. Impaired arterial vessels of the nephron cause renal insufficiency and failure. Injury to larger-diameter arterial vessels, termed macrovascular angiopathy, may be demonstrated by coronary artery disease, cerebrovascular disease, and peripheral vascular disease. In addition to arterial vessel damage, hyperglycemia causes white blood cells (WBCs) to function less efficiently. This negative effect on WBCs causes immunosuppression, poor wound healing, and increased susceptibility to infection.

Diabetes as an Atherosclerosis Accelerator

CVD is the number-one cause of mortality, and acute cardiac events occur two to four times more often in diabetic individuals than in the general population. One of the major reasons for this high mortality rate in individuals with diabetes is that chronic hyperglycemia causes damage to the endothelial lining of artery walls. Endothelial injury is the initiating event

of atherosclerosis. Macrovascular and microvascular angiopathy are terms used for the injury to large arterial vessels and small arterial vessels, respectively.

The exact pathological mechanism of vascular injury in diabetes is yet to be explained, but several theories exist. Each theory describes how a specific biochemical change caused by hyperglycemia affects the endothelium.

Four major biochemical abnormalities result in vascular damage:

- Activation of the polyol pathway
- Increased formation of advanced glycation end-products (AGEs)
- Activation of protein kinase C (PKC)
- Activation of reactive oxygen species (ROS)

Although each plays a role in the vascular injury of diabetes in a distinctive manner, these pathways have an underlying commonality. All the biochemical abnormalities caused by hyperglycemia of diabetes result in oxidative stress caused by overproduction of mitochondrial reactive oxygen species (ROS), also called free radicals.

Polyol Pathway Theory. The polyol pathway theory asserts that in cells that do not require insulin for entry of glucose, such as brain and exercising muscle cells, intracellular hyperglycemia activates an enzyme called aldose reductase. An enzymatic reaction ensues, which transforms glucose into polyol sorbitol. Intracellular sorbitol causes osmotic cellular damage of endothelial cells and consequent vascular dysfunction. Also, constant activation of the enzymatic reaction of aldose reductase to form sorbitol causes oxidative stress and the overproduction of damaging ROS.

Glycation Theory. The pathogenesis of vascular injury also involves the advanced glycation end-product (AGE) theory. During episodes of hyperglycemia, glucose damages the endothelial cell membranes through the process of glycation. In glycation (also called glycosylation), glucose chemically attaches to the amino acids of the proteins that make up the endothelial membranes. The degree of glycation is directly related to the level of blood glucose. There are a variety of harmful extracellular and intracellular products of glycation that have been termed AGEs. Extracellular AGEs alter endothelial cell protein function, whereas intracellular AGEs alter endothelial cell gene expression. As a result of damage, endothelial permeability increases, coagulation activity is enhanced, cytokines and growth factors are released, and fibroblast and smooth muscle cells proliferate within the walls of arteries. The net result of these AGE-induced changes is oxidative stress and abnormal vascular function of the endothelium.

Protein Kinase C Theory. The PKC theory describes PKC as an important intracellular signaling molecule that regulates many vascular functions, including endothelial permeability, endothelial activation, and growth factor signaling. In the PKC theory, pathological activation of PKC occurs in diabetes, specifically in blood vessels from the retina, kidney, and nerves. The activation of PKC has several effects, including production of vascular endothelial growth factor (VEGF), which is implicated in diabetic retinopathy. PKC also stimulates endothelin, a potent vasoconstrictor, and inhibits nitric oxide, a potent vasodilator. PKC enhances production of coagulant molecules and proinflammatory cytokines. Oxidative stress, coagulation of blood, vascular damage, and disordered vascular proliferation are the end results of PKC activation.

Reactive Oxidation Theory. All the pathways involved in the pathogenesis of vascular injury have a common denominator: the activation of ROS, or free radicals. The ROS theory asserts that regardless of the biochemical pathways involved, hyperglycemia of diabetes causes oxidative stress on the endothelium. The oxidation of glucose releases free radicals that damage the endothelial cell membranes; this causes extensive vascular injury and blood vessel dysfunction.

Resultant Endothelial Injury

Regardless of the etiological mechanism, chronic hyperglycemia in diabetes is known to cause endothelial injury; this, in turn, activates inflammation. Inflammation brings WBCs, inflammatory mediators, and platelets to the site of endothelial injury. Lipid and macrophage deposition within the injured area causes the eventual formation of foam cells, precursors to atherosclerotic plaque. Simultaneously, in response to injury, endothelial membranes secrete endothelin. Endothelin inhibits arterial vasodilation and promotes vascular smooth muscle proliferation. This narrows the diameters of arterial vessels, increasing the risk of hypertension in individuals with diabetes (Fig. 25-15). Every arterial blood vessel is susceptible to injury, and the sequelae are most evident in coronary, cerebral, and retinal arteries; glomerular capillaries; and arteries of the lower extremity.

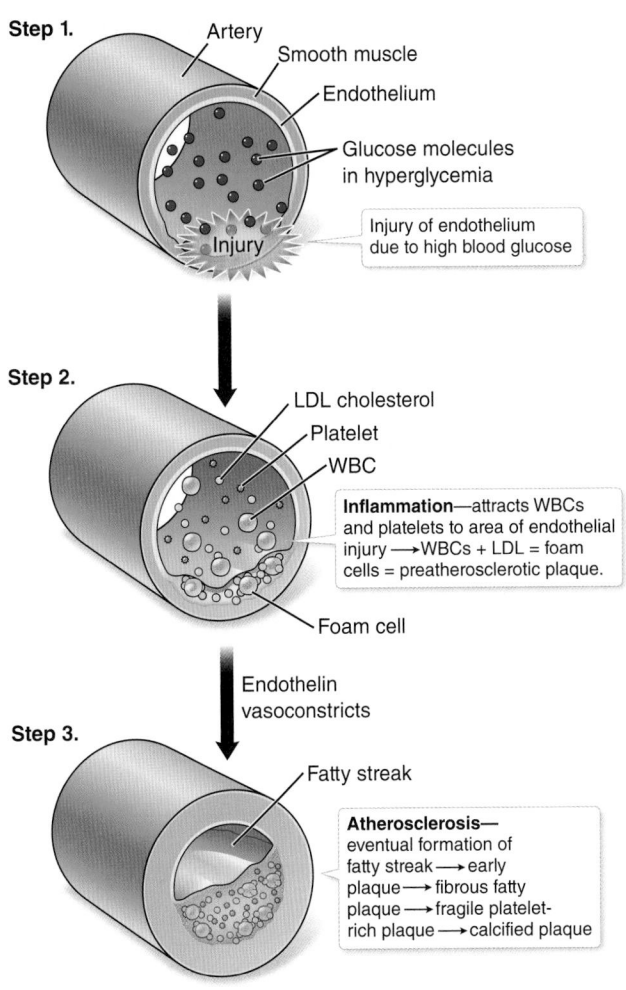

FIGURE 25-15. Diabetes as an atherosclerosis accelerator. (1) High glucose in the bloodstream damages the endothelial lining of the artery. (2) Inflammation of the artery lining attracts WBCs, platelets, and inflammatory mediators to the site. WBCs take in LDLs, which are in the bloodstream and form foam cells. Endothelial cells secrete endothelin, which is a potent vasoconstrictor. (3) Foam cells eventually form a fatty streak, which is early atherosclerotic plaque. Atherosclerotic plaque eventually matures into calcified plaque. The results of high glucose in the bloodstream are atherosclerotic plaque formation and vasoconstriction.

🦠 CLINICAL CONCEPT

Compared with nondiabetic individuals, persons with diabetes have a greater susceptibility to myocardial ischemia, myocardial infarction, stroke, visual impairment, renal impairment, and peripheral vascular disease caused by the endothelial injury of hyperglycemia.

Peripheral Neuropathy of Diabetes

Distal symmetric polyneuropathy, a neural dysfunction of the sensorimotor nerves in the lower extremities, is one of the most common complications of diabetes. It is theorized that hyperglycemia damages the endoneurial arterioles, the small-nutrient arterioles that supply the nerves with blood. As a result of the lack of blood flow, the nerves undergo demyelination and axonal degeneration. The fragile small-caliber sensory nerve fibers of the lower extremities usually demonstrate this damage first. Peripheral neuropathy of diabetes most commonly presents as sensory loss in the feet and progresses proximally up the lower extremity. Symptoms of burning, pain, and paresthesias of the feet may be reported by individuals. A motor neuropathy can also present as pain accompanied by motor weakness. Individuals may develop a gait disturbance from the lack of sensorimotor capacity in the feet.

The sensory and motor neuronal disruption can also lead to abnormal muscle mechanics and structural changes in the foot, including hammer toe, claw toe deformity, prominent metatarsal heads, and neuropathic joint disease or Charcot joint. Charcot joint is demonstrated by instability of joints and deformity, commonly occurring in the metatarsal and tarsal joints of the feet. This complication usually occurs in older adults with many years of long-standing diabetes.

Peripheral neuropathy also blunts pain sensation for the individual with diabetes. The pain associated with serious inflammatory conditions and myocardial ischemia or infarction may not be perceived. Silent myocardial ischemia is particularly common in those with diabetes and concomitant coronary artery disease. Because pain may not be a chief complaint, individuals with diabetes have atypical presentations of disease processes.

> **ALERT!** Silent, painless myocardial ischemia can occur in persons with diabetes due to sensory nerve impairment.

Individuals with long-standing diabetes can develop autonomic neuropathy. This involves dysfunction of the sympathetic and parasympathetic nervous systems. The mechanism of injury likely involves the endoneurial arterioles, which supply the nerves, similar to peripheral neuropathy. The dysfunction of these two major involuntary nervous systems has system-wide effects. Autonomic neuropathy affecting the cardiovascular system may cause resting tachycardia and postural hypotension. The GI system demonstrates parasympathetic dysfunction by gastroparesis, a gastric-emptying abnormality. The individual with gastroparesis suffers anorexia, nausea, vomiting, early satiety, and abdominal bloating. Bowel dysfunction can occur, presenting as alternating bouts of diarrhea and constipation.

Bladder problems can develop as a result of parasympathetic dysfunction, including autonomic bladder complications such as the inability to sense a full bladder and diminishing bladder contractility. As bladder contractility decreases, urine retention occurs, which increases the risk of urinary tract infection. Bladder and bowel incontinence can also result from sympathetic neuropathy. Erectile dysfunction and female sexual dysfunction are also side effects of autonomic neuropathy.

In addition, autonomic neuropathy can mask the signals of hypoglycemia in the patient who is diabetic. In hypoglycemia, a nondiabetic individual receives symptoms signaling blood sugar is dangerously low, including sweating, tachycardia, headache, lack of concentration ability, irritability, pallor, and tremors. These symptoms occur because of the sympathetic stress response and the brain cells' lack of glucose. However, these warning signals of hypoglycemia may

not occur in persons with diabetes because of autonomic dysfunction. Autonomic neuropathy blunts the individual's ability to perspire, which is a necessary mechanism of heat regulation. Tachycardia and tremors may not occur because of the lack of sympathetic neuron discharge. The diabetic patient may suffer from episodes of hypoglycemia unawareness to the point of loss of consciousness.

In addition, lack of sweating can cause:

- Heat intolerance in warm weather
- Problems during exercise, as heat release from the body is blocked
- Anhidrosis leading to dry skin, which increases the risk of skin breakdown in the feet

> **ALERT!** Anhidrosis, decreased blood flow, and lack of sensation in the feet together dramatically increase the susceptibility to foot ulcers.

CLINICAL CONCEPT

Older adults are particularly susceptible to hyperthermia and heat stroke because of autonomic neuropathy.

Lack of appropriate sympathetic and parasympathetic nervous system responses also contributes to atypical clinical presentation of disease processes. The individual with diabetes who is experiencing a concomitant condition such as acute abdomen, myocardial infarction, inflammatory disease, or infection may not present with expected symptoms. Autonomic neuropathy alters cardiovascular, bronchial, GI, and genitourinary responses to illness.

Susceptibility to Infection

Individuals with diabetes have a greater susceptibility to infection than the general population. T cells and WBC phagocytic function are detrimentally affected by the hyperglycemic environment of the bloodstream. WBCs become less able to fight infection, resulting in a level of immunosuppression.

Hyperglycemia caused by poor glycemic control is a factor for the colonization of certain microorganisms. Individuals with poor glycemic control have an increased colonization of *Staphylococcus aureus* on the skin, which increases susceptibility to wound infection. Pneumonia, urinary tract infection, and skin and soft tissue infections are more common in the diabetic population, as are tuberculosis and fungal infections.

Candida (yeast) is a frequent cause of infection of the genital tract and also commonly develops within intertriginous skinfolds. Chronic *Candida* vaginitis may be a presenting feature of diabetes before other signs. *Candida* infection is common in diabetes because with hyperglycemia, the vaginal cells become glycogen-rich. High glucose changes the pH of the vaginal canal, making it more conducive to proliferation of *Candida* organisms.

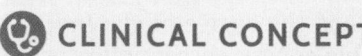

CLINICAL CONCEPT

Both males and females can have *Candida* infection of the genital tract caused by diabetes.

Diabetes as a Cause of Lower Extremity Amputation

Diabetic foot complications are the most common cause of nontraumatic lower extremity amputation both in the United States and worldwide. Foot complications are also the most frequent cause of hospitalization in patients with diabetes. With long-term exposure to hyperglycemia, the nerves and arterial vessels of the lower extremity are damaged, with the most distal nerves and arterial vessels affected initially.

Peripheral neuropathy and microvascular injury lead to a loss of sensation and poor circulation in the feet. In addition, the inhibitory effects of hyperglycemia on WBCs cause increased risk of infection in the lower extremities. All of these factors contribute to the risk of nonhealing wounds and infections in the lower extremities of patients with diabetes.

It is important to understand that individuals with diabetes can sustain a minor foot injury without sensory perception of the wound. However, minor skin injury can rapidly develop into an infected foot ulcer caused by peripheral neuropathy, poor circulation, and WBC dysfunction, which decrease the efficiency of wound healing (Fig. 25-16). Poorly healing wounds can lead to deeper tissue infection and the complication

of gangrene, a bacterial infection that can develop in wounds with poor circulation. In gangrene, *Clostridium,* a gas-producing bacterium, invades the ischemic tissue of the foot and causes tissue necrosis. The infection can spread upward into the more proximal regions of the lower extremity.

Osteomyelitis, infection of the bone, can develop if an infection such as *S. aureus,* a common bacterial inhabitant of the skin, extends deep into lower-level tissue. Osteomyelitis and gangrene are often the complications that necessitate amputation in the individual with diabetes (see Fig. 25-17).

Careful examination of the diabetic foot is the most effective measure to prevent lower extremity amputation. Meticulous neurological and vascular assessment of the feet is needed on a regular basis. Examination of foot sensation using light touch over noncallused areas is recommended (see Fig. 25-18). During the examination, it is important to have the patient close their eyes so as not to visually detect the regions the examiner is testing. The neurological examination of the lower extremities should include testing the Achilles tendon reflex, light sensation, sense of toe position, and vibration sense. Regular podiatric care is also

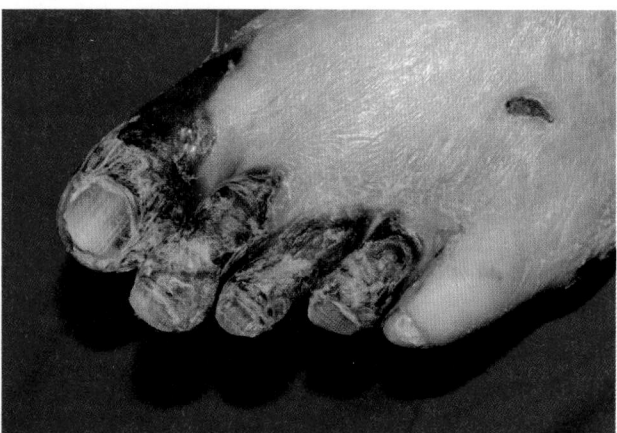

FIGURE 25-17. Osteomyelitis and gangrene of the diabetic foot. *(From Scott Camazine/Science Source.)*

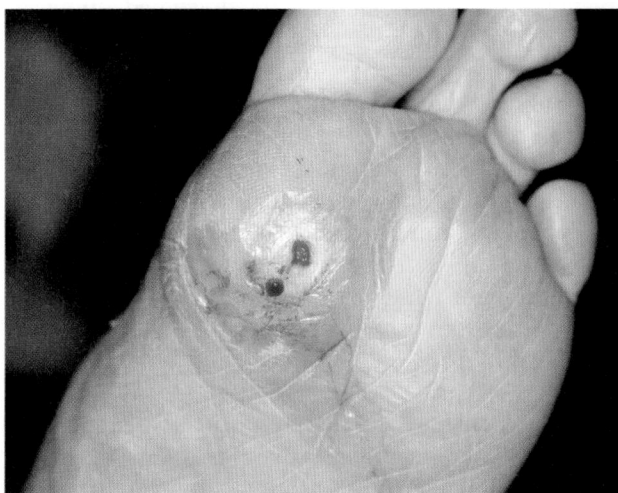

FIGURE 25-16. Diabetic foot ulcer. *(From Roberto A. Penne-Casanova/ Science Source.)*

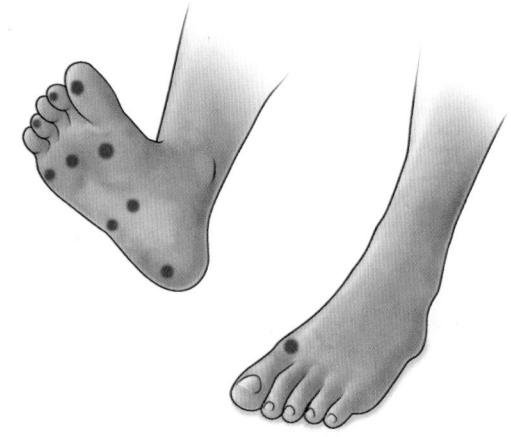

FIGURE 25-18. Sensory testing of the feet in diabetes.

recommended, because sensory loss may prevent the individual with diabetes from performing safe care.

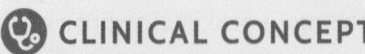

CLINICAL CONCEPT

Because of sensory loss in the feet, individuals with diabetes need specialized foot care by a podiatrist.

Diabetic Retinopathy as a Cause of Blindness

Diabetes is one of the leading causes of blindness in adults. The hyperglycemia of poorly controlled diabetes damages the fragile retinal artery endothelium. Endothelial injury incites inflammation, which attracts WBCs and platelets to the sites. Products of inflammation eventually occlude the small-caliber retinal arterioles and capillaries, causing retinal ischemia. Injured endothelium becomes hyperpermeable, allowing fluid to leak into the tissue, resulting in edema. Blindness is the end result of years of retinal circulatory damage caused by exposure to high blood glucose. Concomitant hypertension accelerates damage to the retina. Clinical signs of retinopathy are microaneurysms, hemorrhages, macular edema, exudates, and "cotton wool spots" (infarcted regions of the retina from prolonged ischemia) evident on fundoscopic examination. Later in the course of the disease, during the stage called proliferative retinopathy, proliferation of new retinal artery branches emerge from the optic disc region (see Fig. 25-19). It is theorized that hypoxia of the retinal tissue stimulates endothelial secretion of VEGF, which causes the proliferation of new blood vessels in a process called neovascularization. These new fragile arterial branches grow in between the internal surface of the retina and vitreous gel. Rupture

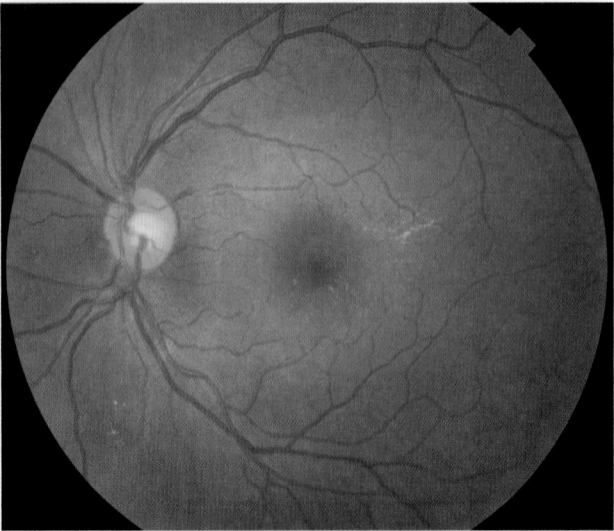

FIGURE 25-19. Changes of the retina in diabetic retinopathy. *(From Paul Whitten/Science Source.)*

of these vessels pulls the retinal layer away from the aqueous gel, which causes the patient to see floaters and flashes of light, as well as experience visual disturbances. Proliferative retinopathy increases the risk of retinal detachment.

The development of retinopathy depends on the duration of diabetes and the degree of glycemic control. There is a probable genetic susceptibility as well. After initial signs and symptoms of retinopathy are detected, progression to a more advanced form of the disease occurs within 5 years if untreated. Routine nondilated eye examinations are inadequate to detect diabetic retinopathy. Periodic, regular fundoscopic and complete ophthalmological examinations are advised. Laser photocoagulation therapy, used to treat retinopathy, has decreased the development of blindness among individuals with diabetes.

Diabetic Nephropathy as a Cause of Renal Failure

Diabetes is the leading cause of end-stage renal disease in adults. Microscopic glomerular injury is the initial mechanism that causes kidney dysfunction in diabetes. Hyperglycemia of poorly controlled diabetes damages the glomerular capillaries, causing them to become hyperpermeable, allowing albumin to be filtered out of the blood. Under healthy conditions, the glomerulus should not filter any significant amount of protein out of the blood. Glomerular injury becomes apparent when small amounts of albumin from the bloodstream leak into the urine in microalbuminuria. Standard urinalysis dipstick tests cannot detect this minute amount of albumin in the urine, and frank proteinuria develops after glomerular damage is sustained for years. Proteinuria typically increases as renal function decreases.

In diabetic nephropathy, the glomerular basement membrane (GBM) thickens and the renal vasculature demonstrates atherosclerotic changes. Factors that trigger thickening of the GBM include glycosylation end-products, angiotensin II, growth hormone, and insulin-like growth factor. The thickened glomerular walls eventually cause glomerular hypertension and obliteration of the glomerular capillary lumens. If enough glomeruli are affected, glomerulosclerosis, a cause of renal dysfunction, results. Renal dysfunction leads to constant renin secretion, which increases blood pressure. The renal impairment is a source of hypertension, which further damages glomeruli and worsens renal function; the damage then continues in a cyclical manner. Diabetic retinopathy, also worsened by hypertension, usually precedes the complication of nephropathy.

Dermatological Complications of Diabetes

The most significant skin manifestations of diabetes are prolonged wound healing and skin ulceration, but less serious skin lesions are also common. Pigmented pretibial papules known as diabetic skin spots are hyperpigmented areas on the legs that develop because of minor trauma in the tibial region. Necrobiosis lipoidica diabeticorum is a rare disorder that develops in a similar manner; however, atrophy and ulceration also occur within the lesions. Acanthosis nigricans is a conglomeration of tiny, hyperpigmented, velvety, macular lesions usually located on the neck, axilla, or extensor surfaces in individuals with insulin resistance and diabetes. Lipoatrophy and lipohypertrophy can occur at sites of insulin injection but are not common with the use of human insulin. Dry skin and pruritus are common complaints of individuals with diabetes because of the anhidrosis of autonomic neuropathy.

 CLINICAL CONCEPT

To prevent lipoatrophy and lipohypertrophy, rotation of insulin injection sites between the abdomen, deltoid, and thigh is recommended.

Psychological and Emotional Aspects of Diabetes

Depression is twice as common in persons with diabetes than in the general population. Guilt and discouragement are emotions frequently expressed by individuals with diabetes, despite their best efforts to manage the condition. Many patients tend to view their blood glucose measurements, weight, and A1c values as a report card of their ability to control the disease. Individuals with poor glycemic control often blame themselves and feel powerless and angry about their inability to manage the disease process.

Anxiety is also a common emotional response of patients affected by diabetes. Many patients find it stressful to manage a chronic disease because it requires planning of diet and exercise, precautions with traveling, and self-administration of scheduled medication. Unlike other diseases, the responsibility for management of diabetes lies with the patient. Patients are often worried about their ability to maintain adequate glycemic control and fear long-term complications. Some patients cite specific concerns, such as fear of hypoglycemia, needles, problems with pregnancy, complications, or weight gain. Anxiety particularly affects those suffering infection and poor circulation of the lower extremity. Inadequate wound healing increases the diabetic individual's risk for gangrene and amputation. Many patients in this situation worry about the prospect of amputation.

Denial is common among many individuals with diabetes. Many affected individuals refuse to comply with insulin administration. Clinicians refer to this as psychological insulin resistance. This is particularly common in persons with T2DM, who initially obtain good glycemic control with oral medications and later in the course of the disease require insulin. Many patients in this situation view taking insulin as a loss of control and refuse to comply with medical advice. Some patients worry that taking insulin will rob their lives of spontaneity, make travel and dining out difficult, and place restrictions on their lifestyle. Others refuse to take insulin because they worry about the threat of hypoglycemia and weight gain. The clinician should not imply that the addition of insulin is because of the patient's inability to control glucose or failure of oral medication. Insulin treatment should not be depicted in negative terms or as punishment for poor glycemic control. At the time of diagnosis, the clinician should discuss the likelihood that insulin will be needed for optimal control of blood glucose as the disease progresses. In addition, clinicians should periodically assess the patient's psychosocial needs and provide emotional support as part of a holistic treatment plan.

Eating Disorders and Diabetes. Eating disorders are pervasive among adolescents, particularly females. Studies have shown that many young women with T1DM have a heightened risk for food bingeing and bulimia (vomiting or using laxatives to avoid weight gain).

Often, upon initial diagnosis of T1DM, an individual presents with symptoms that include weight loss. This occurs because of the deficiency of insulin, lack of cellular glucose uptake, and consequent breakdown of fats. Among some individuals, this weight loss may be perceived as a desirable effect of diabetes.

After diagnosis, to obtain optimal glycemic control, the individual with T1DM must adhere to strict dietary, exercise, and insulin regimens. After optimal glycemic control is established, weight gain often occurs because of the anabolic effects of insulin. Insulin inhibits fat breakdown, enhances cellular uptake of glucose, and blocks hepatic glucose production.

Individuals with diabetes often find this weight gain undesirable and associate it with insulin administration. To initiate weight loss, the diabetic individual with an eating disorder administers less insulin despite glycemic needs. Studies show that one-third to one-half of young women with T1DM may engage in this practice, known as insulin purging. These individuals often completely omit dosages of insulin, endure frequent episodes of hyperglycemia, and allow the body to enter starvation mode to enhance fat breakdown.

ALERT! Eating disorders should be suspected in patients with recurrent DKA or chronically poor glycemic control.

These individuals are at increased risk for DKA or HHS. Ultimately, the prolonged exposure to hyperglycemia damages organs and increases the risk of long-term complications in these patients.

Treatment of Diabetes

Managing diabetes requires an understanding of the extremes of poor glycemic control—hypoglycemia versus hyperglycemia (see Fig. 25-20). In both types of diabetes, individuals on insulin are susceptible to hypoglycemic episodes; blood glucose should be maintained within a narrow range of 70 to 140 mg/dL, regardless of food intake or physical activity. In mild hypoglycemia with a blood glucose level lower than 60 mg/dL, the individual experiences hunger, irritability, palpitations, pallor, nervousness, headache, and an inability to concentrate. As hypoglycemia worsens, tachycardia, hypertension or hypotension, diaphoresis, slurred speech, blurred vision, and syncope can occur. If blood glucose falls to extremely low levels, such as 30 mg/dL or lower, seizure and coma are possible.

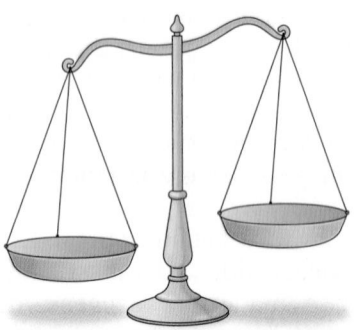

Diabetes

Hypoglycemia	Hyperglycemia
Blood glucose too low; symptoms: nervousness or tremors, diaphoresis, pallor, weakness, inability to concentrate, irritability, headache, tachycardia, syncope, coma	Blood glucose too high; symptoms: blurry vision, polyuria, polydipsia, polyphagia, weight loss, confusion, weakness, nausea, vomiting, ketone breath, coma, *DKA or hyperosmolar hyperglycemic syndrome*
Possible etiologies: too much insulin or antidiabetic medication excessive exercise lack of eating drug interactions alcohol use extreme stress illness infection	**Possible etiologies:** inadequate insulin (endogenous or exogenous) insulin resistance infection ingestion of excess carbohydrates low physical activity drug interactions "Somogyi effect"

FIGURE 25-20. The extremes of poor glycemic control in diabetes.

Insulin excess is the most common cause of hypoglycemia; however, other causative factors are misuse of alcohol, drug interactions, strenuous physical activity, inadequate dietary intake, or carbohydrate malabsorption. Beta-adrenergic blockers and sulfonylureas are drugs that increase the risk of hypoglycemia.

> **ALERT!** Beta-adrenergic blockers will mask the symptoms of hypoglycemia in patients with diabetes.

Beta-adrenergic blockers blunt the process of hepatic glycogenolysis and mask the symptoms of hypoglycemia. Beta-adrenergic blockers counteract the hypoglycemia warning signs of tremor, tachycardia, and other symptoms of sympathetic nervous system activation.

Individuals with T1DM or T2DM can delay or prevent complications by maintaining near-normal blood glucose levels. Strict glycemic control is the goal of all forms of treatment. Aggressive control of lipids and blood pressure also assists to counteract the development of complications. The individual with diabetes should try to avoid large fluctuations in blood glucose levels. The clinician uses three major indices to guide and evaluate treatment efficacy:

- A1c level
- Fasting blood glucose level
- Postprandial blood glucose level

Diabetes involves a delicate balancing act in blood glucose control: prevention of hypoglycemia versus hyperglycemia.

Glucose Control During Hospitalization

In diabetes, any major stress, including emotional, can cause erratic variations in blood glucose and necessitate altered glycemic control measures. Critical illnesses such as liver, renal, or heart failure; serious infection; and sepsis increase the risk of hypoglycemia or hyperglycemia. Hospitalization is a stressor that can change the patient's usual pattern of glycemic control. During hospitalization, there are less stringent guidelines for glycemic control than in the outpatient setting. The main goals for hospitalized patients are prevention of hypoglycemia and hyperglycemia, as these states are associated with increased morbidity and mortality. Hyperglycemia is defined as greater than 140 mg/dL, and the hypoglycemia alert value is less than or equal to 70 mg/dL. Insulin therapy is commonly recommended if blood glucose is difficult to regulate or if blood glucose is greater than or equal to 180 mg/dL. Once insulin therapy is initiated, a target glucose range of 140 to 180 mg/dL is recommended for most hospitalized patients. After discharge, the patient can resume their usual method of glucose control.

Lifestyle Modifications

A diagnosis of diabetes often provokes a patient to review their lifestyle. Diet, exercise, and habits such as use of alcohol or smoking need to be assessed to find areas where the patient needs modification. Often diet and exercise alone can control diabetes.

Diet

Maintaining ideal body weight is an important factor in diabetes because obesity causes insulin resistance. Patients with newly diagnosed diabetes should consult with a nutritionist or diabetes educator to identify individualized daily calorie recommendations, preferred food choices, daily menus, cooking recommendations, and exercise regimens. Although numerous studies have attempted to identify the optimal mix of macronutrients for the meal plans of people with diabetes, a systematic review found that there is no ideal mix that applies broadly and that macronutrient proportions should be individualized. In general, a diet low in sugar and carbohydrates is advised, with carbohydrates comprising about 40% to 50% of daily caloric intake. Each gram of carbohydrate contains 4 calories.

To achieve optimal glycemic control, carbohydrate counting is one method that is advised. For example, an individual who is diabetic on a 1600-calorie diet can aim to consume approximately 50% of total calories from carbohydrates. This would be a total of 800 calories of carbohydrate. To calculate how many grams of carbohydrate this is equal to, take 800 calories divided by 4 calories/gram. This is equal to 200 grams of carbohydrate spread out over the day. For examples of how many grams of carbohydrates are in some common foods, see Table 25-4.

The individual's recommended total daily calorie intake is determined based on the patient's gender, body mass index (BMI), goal weight, physical activity level, and body build. A schedule for meals and snacks can be determined based on the patient's medication regimen and daily routine. A nutritionist or diabetes educator can advise which foods and how many servings per day are recommended.

Because the patient who is diabetic is at increased risk of CVD, a low-fat, low-sodium diet is also recommended. In general, fats and sodium should be limited as follows:

- Total fats: 25% to 30% of total calories
  - Saturated fats: less than 7% of total calories
  - Monounsaturated fats: less than 10% of total calories
  - Polyunsaturated fats: less than 10% of total calories
- Cholesterol: less than 200 mg daily
- Sodium: less than 2300 mg per day (1500 mg if hypertension present)

Fats are categorized as being saturated or unsaturated (monounsaturated or polyunsaturated). Trans fats may be unsaturated, but they are structurally different and have negative health effects. The type of fat consumed is more important than total fat in the diet in terms of supporting metabolic goals and influencing the risk of CVD. Nutritional guidelines recommend replacing foods high in saturated fat (i.e., full-fat dairy products, butter, marbled meats and bacon, and tropical oils such as coconut and palm) with items that are rich in monounsaturated and polyunsaturated fat (i.e., vegetable and nut oils, including canola, corn, safflower, soy, and sunflower; vegetable oil spreads; whole nuts and nut butters; and avocado).

A variety of diets have shown efficacy in managing diabetes. These include a Mediterranean-style, Dietary Approaches to Stop Hypertension (DASH)–style, plant-based (vegan or vegetarian), and low-fat and low-carbohydrate diets. There is no standard meal plan or eating pattern that works universally for all

TABLE 25-4. Different Carbohydrate Sources and Gram Count

Food	Amount	Carb Grams	Food	Amount	Carb Grams
1% fat milk	1 cup	12	Yogurt, fruited	1 cup	40
Bran Chex	²/₃ cup	23	Yogurt, plain	1 cup	9
Frosted Flakes	³/₄ cup	26	Raisin Bran	³/₄ cup	28
Fruit juice	1¹/₂ cup	15	White bread/toast	1 slice	15
Banana	¹/₂	15	Cane sugar	1 tsp.	4
Pancake syrup	2 Tbsp.	30	Pancakes	2	22
Low-fat granola	¹/₂ cup	30	Sugar-free syrup	2 Tbsp.	4

From Norman J. Treatment of diabetes: The diabetic diet. Table of carb-containing foods.
Available at www.endocrineweb.com/conditions/diabetes/treatment-diabetes. With permission.

people with diabetes. However, it is prudent to recommend a diabetic diet consisting of approximately 45% carbohydrates, 25% to 30% fats (subdivided as previously categorized), and 25% to 30% protein. Carbohydrate intake from vegetables, fruits, whole grains, legumes, and milk should be encouraged over other sources of carbohydrates, or sources with added fats, sugars, or sodium, in order to obtain the best nutrient intake. People with diabetes should limit or avoid intake of sugar-sweetened beverages (SSBs) (from any caloric sweetener, including high-fructose corn syrup and sucrose) to reduce the risk for weight gain and worsening of cardiometabolic risk profile. Fiber is also an important component of the diet, with 25 g/day recommended for women and 38 g/day for men.

The total calorie count is calculated according to how much weight loss is desired or if weight maintenance is the goal. To maintain weight, patients with diabetes should follow a diet that has approximately 35 calories per kg of body weight per day (or approximately 16 calories per pound of body weight per day). To lose weight, nutritionists would recommend a lower total daily calorie count, depending on the individual patient's goal.

Glycemic Index

A diet can also be devised that takes glycemic index into consideration. The **glycemic index** measures how a carbohydrate-containing food raises blood glucose. Carbohydrate-containing foods with a low glycemic index include dried beans and legumes, most vegetables, most fruit, and whole-grain breads and cereals. As a general rule, the more processed a food is, the higher the glycemic index. A low-glycemic-index diet combines low-glycemic-index foods with high-glycemic-index foods. Some nutritionists can be consulted about this strategy. Portion sizes are still relevant for managing blood glucose, as well as for losing or maintaining weight. Research shows that both the amount and type of carbohydrate in food affect blood glucose levels. Studies also show that the total amount of carbohydrate in food, in general, is a stronger predictor of blood glucose response than the glycemic index.

Exercise

Exercise is beneficial for individuals with diabetes because contractile muscle activity enhances cellular uptake of glucose, and contracting muscle cells do not require insulin for glucose entry, which is why individuals with diabetes can lower their blood glucose levels with vigorous physical activity. In addition, exercise builds collateral blood vessels in the heart and large muscle groups, raises high-density lipoprotein (HDL) cholesterol, reduces obesity, and lowers blood pressure. Collateral blood vessel growth, elevated HDL cholesterol levels, and reduced blood pressure are advantageous cardiovascular effects that counteract coronary artery and peripheral vascular disease, which are major complications of diabetes. Exercise also counteracts obesity, which is a major cause of insulin resistance.

ALERT! Strenuous muscle activity lowers blood glucose, which can lead to hypoglycemia.

However, individuals with diabetes must remember that strenuous muscle activity will reduce blood glucose levels, which can lead to hypoglycemia. To reduce the risk for hypoglycemia, insulin doses should be reduced before vigorous physical activity. Exercise should be scheduled 1 to 2 hours after a meal or when insulin is not at peak levels. The individual should ingest carbohydrate snacks during sustained exercise and vigilantly monitor blood glucose. Delayed hypoglycemia can occur for 6 to 15 hours, or as long as 24 hours, after strenuous exercise. Postexercise delayed hypoglycemia is a result of increased glucose uptake of skeletal muscle, heightened insulin sensitivity of skeletal muscle, and depletion of hepatic glycogen stores. The replenishment of hepatic glycogen stores may require higher carbohydrate intake in the hours following exercise.

The individual who performs vigorous exercise should carry glucose tablets or gel and a diabetic identification bracelet or card. They should also exercise with a partner who is aware of the possibility of hypoglycemia. A glucagon kit may be necessary to keep as a precaution for episodes of hypoglycemia.

Proper foot care is essential for athletic individuals with diabetes. Vigilant inspection of foot surfaces is important after exercise because peripheral neuropathy can hinder the sensation of lesions. Autonomic neuropathy can cause heat intolerance, lack of perspiration, dependent edema, orthostatic hypotension, and hypoglycemic unawareness with exercise. Because individuals with diabetes are at increased risk for coronary artery and peripheral vascular disease, a periodic cardiology consultation is advisable before beginning a regular vigorous exercise routine.

Aerobic exercise activities benefit individuals with diabetes. Strength training with light weights and high repetitions is recommended for young persons, but not for older patients or those with long-standing diabetes. Both clinicians and patients need to be aware of the risks of strenuous exercise. Meticulous attention to blood glucose monitoring, diet, insulin, and medication are particularly important for athletic individuals with diabetes.

Health Maintenance

Diabetes increases the risk of CVD, so periodic measurement of serum lipids and blood pressure is advised. The ideal goals to prevent CVD in diabetes include maintaining the following:

- Most patients with T2DM can be advised to keep BP less than or equal to 140/90 Hg; however, individualization is important. Those with CVD risk factors or chronic kidney disease should keep BP less than 130/80 mm Hg

- Low-density lipoprotein (LDL) cholesterol: lower than or equal to 100 mg/dL or lower than 70 mg/dL if at high risk for CVD or if CVD is present
- HDL cholesterol: greater than or equal to 60 mg/dL
- Triglycerides: lower than or equal to 150 mg/dL
- Sodium in diet: less than 2300 mg, increase fruits and vegetables to 8 to 10 servings/day, and 2 to 3 servings/day of low-fat dairy products
- Weight loss if BMI is greater than 25
- Limit alcohol to one serving/day for women and two servings/day for men
- Cessation of smoking
- Daily exercise = 150 minutes/week

Periodic cardiac assessment should include exercise testing and identification of risk for autonomic neuropathy. Exercise tolerance testing, also known as stress testing, is key because silent myocardial ischemia and infarction can occur in diabetes. Smoking increases susceptibility to cardiac and peripheral vascular disease, and cessation methods should be advised. Diabetic individuals should aim for an ideal body weight and learn how to maintain it.

Because an increased risk of infection is present with diabetes, individuals should receive the flu vaccine annually and, depending on age, a pneumococcal vaccine every 5 years. Patients need to understand that infection can cause changes in glycemic levels. The possibility of blood glucose fluctuations requires more frequent blood glucose monitoring during illness.

> **ALERT!** Infection can cause significant fluctuations in blood glucose. Frequent blood glucose monitoring is important during illness.

Foot care is a key element in the prevention of complications. Individuals need to understand the possible loss of sensation and their vulnerability to foot ulcers. Well-fitting shoes, dry socks, and daily foot inspection are essential. Those with long-term diabetes should have regular podiatric care.

Older patients with diabetes and those with long-term disease need to be aware of the possibility of visual problems and complications of the eye. Annual ophthalmological examination, including a dilated fundoscopic examination, is recommended.

Urine glucose and ketones should be checked during periodic physical examinations. Clinicians also need to check for microalbuminuria, which may be an early warning sign of nephropathy.

Patient Self-Monitoring of Blood Glucose

All individuals with diabetes need to have a blood glucose measuring device known as a glucometer. Use of a glucometer requires thorough patient education so that lifetime blood glucose testing becomes part of the patient's daily routine. Clinicians should demonstrate use of the device and have the patient give a demonstration in response to ensure understanding. These devices require a drop of blood obtained by a lancet. The sample of blood obtained from a finger or forearm is placed on a clinical testing strip and inserted into the glucometer. The device then evaluates the glucose level within the blood droplet. Blood glucose levels should be evaluated twice to several times per day, depending on the clinician's recommendation. Commonly, clinicians recommend measurement of blood glucose before eating, known as **preprandial blood glucose;** 2 hours after eating, known as **postprandial glucose;** and at bedtime. The following are parameters that indicate adequate control of blood glucose as recommended by the ADA:

- A1c less than or equal to 7%
- Preprandial glucose level: 80 to 130 mg/dL
- Postprandial glucose level less than or equal to 180 mg/dL

The clinician may use their discretion with these guidelines, depending on specific patient conditions. More rigorous glucose control, such as A1c levels less than or equal to 6.5%, may be applicable to pregnant women or those at low risk of hypoglycemia. Less rigorous A1c levels, such as less than 8%, may be considered if the patient has a history of severe hypoglycemia; advanced microvascular or macrovascular complications; certain comorbidities; or long-standing, difficult-to-control diabetes.

Many types of glucometers have memory of daily glucose values, and the patient can have the clinician review the glucometer readings for periodic assessment of glucose control.

Basics of Insulin Therapy

The goal of insulin therapy is to mimic physiological control of blood glucose levels through basal and postprandial levels of insulin. Basal insulin levels occur during fasting, whereas postprandial insulin levels occur after eating a meal. To mimic physiological control of glucose, insulin regimens must closely mimic pancreatic secretory patterns without causing hypoglycemia. Conventional insulins and insulin analogues are the two types of insulin available. There are short-, intermediate-, and long-acting forms of both types of insulin. The combined use of these types of insulin can be used to simulate fasting and postprandial pancreatic insulin release.

Currently, in the literature, several different insulin regimens are under investigation and being compared for optimal glycemic control.

Conventional Insulins. Used for many years, conventional insulins are synthetic human insulins. These include:

- **Regular:** rapid-acting, short duration
- **NPH:** intermediate-acting, longer duration

- **Lente:** intermediate-acting, longer duration
- **Ultra lente:** long-acting, long duration

For an in-depth comparison of the different insulins, see Table 25-5.

Insulin Analogues. Although fairly effective in reducing blood glucose levels, conventional insulins cannot mimic normal physiological insulin secretion. Insulin analogues, synthetic preparations with a structure that is slightly different from human insulin, have pharmacokinetic profiles that closely approximate physiological endogenous insulin secretion. The analogues and their activity considerations include:

- **Insulin lispro (Humalog)**—rapid-acting: Compared with regular insulin, insulin lispro has a more rapid onset of action, an earlier peak effect, and a shorter duration of action. It reaches peak activity 0.5 to 2.5 hours after injection. Therefore, insulin lispro should be injected 15 minutes before a meal compared with regular insulin, which is injected 30 to 60 minutes before a meal.

- **Insulin aspart (NovoLog)**—rapid-acting: Insulin aspart has a rapid onset of action (20 minutes) and a shorter duration of action (3 to 5 hours) than regular human insulin. It reaches peak activity 1 to 3 hours after injection.
- **Insulin glulisine (Apidra)**—rapid-acting: Insulin glulisine has onset of action in 5 to 15 minutes and duration of 3 to 5 hours.
- **Inhaled insulin (Afrezza)**—rapid-acting: The powdered form of insulin for inhalation acts within 12 to 15 minutes and has a duration of 180 minutes.
- **Insulin glargine (Lantus, Toujeo)**—long-acting: Insulin glargine has a slower onset of action (70 minutes) and a longer duration of action (24 hours) than regular human insulin. Its activity does not peak.
- **Insulin detemir (Levemir)**—long-acting: Insulin detemir also has a duration of action of 24 hours and slow onset of action.
- **Insulin degludec (Tresiba)**—ultra–long-acting: Insulin degludec has a long, depot kind of effect

TABLE 25-5. Pharmacokinetics of Conventional Insulins and Insulin Analogues

Insulin	Classification	Onset of Action	Peak of Activity	Duration
Regular insulin (Novolin R) (Humulin R)	Rapid-acting conventional insulin	½ to 1 hour	2 to 6 hours	3 to 8 hours
Aspart insulin (NovoLog)	Rapid-acting analogue insulin	Less than ½ hour	1 hour	3 to 4 hours
Lispro insulin (Humalog)				
Glulisine (Apidra)				
Insulin inhalation powder (Afrezza)	Rapid-acting analogue insulin	15 to 20 minutes	1 hour	2 to 3 hours
NPH (Novolin N) (Humulin N)	Intermediate-acting conventional insulin	2 to 4 hours	4 to 10 hours	10 to 20 hours
Lente (Novolin L) (Humulin L)	Intermediate-acting conventional insulin	3 to 4 hours	4 to 12 hours	10 to 20 hours
Ultra lente (Humulin U)	Long-acting conventional insulin	6 to 10 hours	Dose dependent	16 to 20 hours
Glargine insulin (Lantus, Basaglar, Toujeo)	Long-acting analogue insulin	2 to 3 hours 6 to 8 hours	None (steady level)	24 hours 6 to 24 hours depending on dosage
Detemir insulin (Levemir)				
Degludec insulin (Tresiba)	Ultra–long-acting	1 to 4 hours	25 hours	42 hours

A mixture of 70% NPH human insulin and 30% regular human insulin (Novolin 70/30, Humulin 70/30) is available in vials, cartridges, and prefilled syringes.

From American Diabetes Association. (2018). Pharmacological approaches to glycemic treatment–Standards of medical care in diabetes–2018. *Diabetes Care, 41*(Suppl 1), S73–S85.

that has a peak of 24 hours and duration of up to 42 hours.

Individualized Insulin Regimens. An individualized insulin regimen is devised according to the patient's specific needs for glucose control. The basal–bolus insulin regimen is a common type of treatment for optimal glycemic control. This regimen uses a once-daily injection of a long-acting insulin to control the fasting plasma glucose level (basal insulin) and boluses of a rapid-acting insulin for postmeal glucose elevations (prandial insulin). A commonly used regimen in the past combined NPH, which is an intermediate-acting insulin, with regular insulin, a short-acting preparation. The NPH would be administered once daily, and the regular insulin was administered before mealtime. Currently, different short-acting and intermediate- or long-acting insulin analogues are commonly combined in daily regimens. For example, the long-acting insulin analogue, glargine, can be administered once daily with boluses of lispro, a short-acting insulin analogue, administered around mealtimes. The clinician prescribes the dosages and approximate times when the patient should administer insulin in the basal–bolus regimen. Alternatively, there are premixed combinations of short-acting and longer-acting insulins that can be administered once or twice daily. For example, there is 70% NPH human insulin and 30% regular human insulin (called Novolin 70/30 or Humulin 70/30) available for this type of regimen. There is also a combination preparation of an ultra–long-acting insulin analogue, degludec, and the short-acting insulin, aspart (called IDegAsp), which can be administered once daily. Currently, the basal–bolus insulin regimen has been found to closely approximate normal physiological insulin patterns and is preferred by many clinicians. However, there are many research studies that compare different kinds of insulin regimens to find the most effective method for optimal glycemic control.

Clinicians individualize insulin treatment regimens based on the patient's age, lifestyle, self-reported symptoms, existence of concomitant conditions, and history of glycemic control. Insulin dosage, route of administration, and times for administration need to be tailored to patient needs. Commonly, insulin is injected subcutaneously using a syringe or pen-like device. However, there are some alternative methods for administering insulin that include insertion aids, infusers, jet injectors, and inhalable powder (see Box 25-9). Also, insulin can be administered at a steady rate via a programmable pump. The subcutaneous tissues of the abdomen, upper arm, or thigh are recommended injection sites and should be rotated. Some insulin suspensions require refrigeration.

Patient education regarding proper insulin administration is required. Family members or significant others should ideally be taught the technique as well.

Early in insulin treatment, the clinician and patient must closely monitor daily preprandial, postprandial, bedtime, and possibly early morning blood glucose levels. The clinician reviews the various blood glucose values, evaluates the patient's condition, and tailors the insulin dosage to obtain optimal glycemic control.

Inhalable Insulin/Pulmonary Insulin. Inhalable insulin is in powdered form delivered to the lungs. Currently, Afrezza, developed by Mannkind, uses a technology called technosphere to deliver bolus insulin via an inhaler. Approved by the FDA in 2014 for treatment of T1DM or T2DM, it has rapid onset and should be used just before meals. It peaks after 12 minutes and its duration is up to 2 hours. It is contraindicated in patients with asthma, lung cancer, or COPD. It should not be used in DKA or in persons who smoke. Potential side effects are bronchospasm and cough. Before use of this type of inhalable insulin, spirometry testing is necessary to ensure lung function is adequate to allow delivery of sufficient insulin. McGill et al. (2021) demonstrated that technosphere-type inhaled insulin (Afrezza) added to a basal insulin regimen achieved comparable efficacy to insulin lispro in patients with T1DM. Inhaled insulin has a similar onset of action to lispro but a more rapid postprandial glycemic response. Hypoglycemia event rates were also significantly lower with Afrezza compared with lispro. Thus far, inhalable insulin has not been a commercial success and more studies are needed.

Antidiabetic Noninsulin Agents in the Management of Type 2 Diabetes

Treatment of T2DM is a stepwise approach that begins with lifestyle modification. Antidiabetic noninsulin agents are initiated when lifestyle modifications prove insufficient to maintain glycemic control. **Metformin (Glucophage)** is the recommended initial pharmacological agent in T2DM when lifestyle changes alone are not controlling blood glucose. If metformin with lifestyle modifications cannot control blood glucose levels, another medication is added to the regimen. Combinations of medications are commonly effective, and numerous presynthesized combination pharmacological agents are available. If this strategy does not control blood glucose, insulin is added to the medication regimen.

There is a wide array of different types of oral and injectable noninsulin antidiabetic agents. Different categories of drugs have different mechanisms of action and pharmacokinetics. The following are the categories of available oral and injectable antidiabetic agents:

- Insulinotropic agents, also called insulin secretagogues
  - Subcategories: sulfonylureas, meglitinides
- Biguanides

BOX 25-9. Different Methods Used to Administer Insulin

VIAL AND SYRINGE

A conventional method using a disposable tuberculin syringe, 28-gauge needle (subcutaneous), and reusable vial of insulin.

INSULIN PEN

Disposable, prefilled pen-like instrument with a dial for choosing the correct dosage; complete with 28-gauge needle.

INJECTION AIDS

These include devices that can stabilize the vial or shield syringes to hide the needle and devices that can assist patients with impaired vision to hear clicks as the syringe draws up the insulin. Syringe magnifiers and colored syringe caps can differentiate between types of insulin. An injection port with adhesive that attaches to the skin via an introducer needle attached to a flexible cannula, both inserted under the skin, can be used for 3 days to administer insulin.

INSULIN PATCH

A penny-sized patch that contains many microfine needles that are packed with storage units of insulin and glucose sensors. Insulin is released when the patch senses high glucose levels.

JET INJECTORS

A needleless system that uses a pressurized fine spray of insulin that penetrates the pores of the skin. The patient has to insert the correct dosage of insulin.

INHALABLE INSULIN POWDER

Powdered insulin in an inhaler with single cartridges that contain a single dose of insulin.

INSULIN PUMP

Open-Loop System

An insulin pump is an external device that continuously delivers rapid-acting insulin through a small cannula placed under the skin. Insulin pumps are programmed by the user to continuously deliver small doses of rapid-acting insulin between meals or overnight during fasting. This dose is called a basal insulin level. At meals, the user programs an extra dose of insulin, called a bolus, to cover the increase in blood glucose. This is called an open-loop insulin delivery system. An open-loop delivery system requires some level of patient or clinician involvement in insulin administration. This will require a blood glucose measurement, an estimate of the meal to be consumed, and an estimate of the insulin requirement. The open-loop method requires a patient to live a predictable lifestyle, one in which meals are prepared according to the given insulin bolus and exercise is performed only in accordance with the insulin received.

Closed-Loop System

The closed-loop insulin delivery pump (also called the artificial pancreas) does not require the patient's active participation. The pump is programmed to sense and control blood glucose levels. It consists of three connected devices: a glucose sensor, a patch insulin pump, and a smartphone-like terminal device. The continuous glucose sensor monitors the user's blood glucose level and sends data to the terminal, which is preprogrammed with an algorithm. The terminal controls the connected insulin pump by calculating and ordering the optimal amount of insulin in accordance with the blood glucose level. The patient does not have to monitor their blood glucose or control the insulin dosage. For maximum accuracy, patients can enter food intake and physical activity information.

- Thiazolidinediones
- Alpha-glucosidase inhibitors
- GLP-1 agonists (incretin mimetics)
- Amylin mimetics
- DPP-4 inhibitors
- SGLT-2 inhibitors

See Table 25-6 for a detailed breakdown of the different categories of noninsulin antidiabetic agents.

Insulinotropic Agents

Insulinotropic agents stimulate pancreatic beta cells to secrete insulin and are used in T2DM. These agents require that individuals have some endogenous pancreatic insulin reserve. Sulfonylureas and meglitinides are the two types of medications in this category.

Sulfonylureas are the oldest oral antidiabetic medications and have long been the cornerstone of T2DM treatment. Chlorpropamide (Diabinese) is the only first generation drug still used. There are four second generation drugs:

- Glipizide (Glucotrol)
- Glyburide (Micronase, Glynase, DiaBeta)
- Glimepiride (Amaryl)
- Gliclazide (Diamicron)

Sulfonylureas are generally taken once or twice daily before meals. They have similar effects in reducing blood glucose but differ in side effects, duration of action, and interactions with other drugs. Hypoglycemia and weight gain are two common side effects. Allergy to sulfa is a contraindication to use of these drugs. Alcohol use is also contraindicated with some sulfonylureas. Sulfonylureas have no effect on triglycerides or cholesterol.

The majority of sulfonylureas undergo renal elimination. For example, chlorpropamide should not be

TABLE 25-6. Noninsulin Antidiabetic Agents

Noninsulin Antidiabetic Agent Generic and (Brand) Name	Classification	Action	Indications/Usage
Glimepiride (Amaryl) Glipizide (Glucotrol) Glyburide (DiaBeta) Chlorpropamide (Diabinese)	Sulfonylureas (insulinotropic)	Stimulates pancreas to secrete insulin	T2DM; patient must have the ability to secrete natural endogenous insulin
Metformin (Glucophage or Fortamet)	Biguanide	Sensitizes cells to insulin; inhibits hepatic glucose production; lowers cholesterol, triglycerides, and LDLs; raises HDLs	T2DM; patient with mainly insulin resistance; hyperinsulinism; patients with metabolic syndrome
Acarbose (Precose or Miglitol)	Alpha-glucosidase inhibitor	Blocks enzyme that assists in intestinal absorption of carbohydrates	T2DM; patient with insulin resistance, metabolic syndrome, or pancreatic beta cell dysfunction
Pioglitazone (Actos) Rosiglitazone (Avandia)	Thiazolidinedione (also called glitazones)	Counteracts insulin resistance by sensitizing cells to insulin, reduces glucose production by liver	T2DM; patient with mainly insulin resistance; hyperinsulinism; patients with metabolic syndrome
Repaglinide (Prandin) Nateglinide (Starlix)	Meglitinides (insulinotropic)	Stimulates pancreas to secrete insulin	T2DM; patient must have the ability to secrete natural endogenous insulin
Sitagliptin (Januvia) Linagliptin (Trajenta) Alogliptin (Nesina) Saxagliptin (Onglyza)	DPP-4 inhibitor (also called gliptins)	Inhibits the enzyme dipeptidyl peptidase-4 that destroys GLP-1 and GIP and thereby increases the levels and activity of both hormones; as a result, blood glucose levels fall	T2DM
Canagliflozin (Invokana) Dapagliflozin (Farxiga) Empaglifozin (Jardiance) Ertugliflozin (Steglatro)	SGLT-2 inhibitor	Inhibits reabsorption of glucose at the kidney	T2DM
Exenatide (Byetta) Liraglutide (Victoza) Dulaglutide (Trulicity) Lixisenatide Albiglutide (Tanzeum) Semaglutide (Ozempic)	GLP-1 receptor agonists (incretin mimetics)	Stimulates insulin secretion when glucose rises, suppresses postprandial glucagon levels, and delays gastric emptying	T2DM

From American Diabetes Association (2021). 9. Pharmacologic approaches to glycemic treatment: Standards of medical care in diabetes–2021. *Diabetes Care, 44*(Suppl 1), S111–S124. doi: 10.2337/dc21-S009

used in patients with renal dysfunction (20% is excreted unchanged in the urine), and the active metabolites of glyburide can accumulate in patients with a creatinine clearance lower than 30 mL/min. Glipizide is preferred in patients with moderate to severe renal dysfunction. Compared with other oral antidiabetic medications, the sulfonylureas are the least expensive.

Meglitinides, like sulfonylureas, stimulate the pancreatic beta cells to secrete insulin. Repaglinide (Prandin, Gluconorm) and nateglinide (Starlix) are rapid-acting drugs with short durations of action that are taken before each meal. Meglitinides lower postprandial hyperglycemia. A possible side effect is hypoglycemia.

Biguanides

Biguanides are insulin sensitizers that make body tissues less resistant to endogenous insulin and inhibit hepatic synthesis of glucose. Metformin (Glucophage, Fortamet, Glumetza) is the only biguanide approved for use in the United States by the U.S. Food and Drug Administration (FDA). It mainly lowers blood glucose by making body cells more sensitive to insulin and decreases the amount of glucose produced by the liver. Metformin decreases triglyceride concentrations, LDL cholesterol, total cholesterol, and body weight. It also increases HDL cholesterol. It can be taken once or twice a day. Metformin is recommended by both the ADA and the American Association of Clinical Endocrinologists as the first-line oral agent for the management of T2DM.

When used as monotherapy, metformin has not been associated with hypoglycemia. However, GI disturbances such as nausea, abdominal pain, bloating, anorexia, metallic taste, and diarrhea are common side effects. Additionally, asymptomatic subnormal vitamin B$_{12}$ levels may occur. A rare condition termed lactic acidosis can occur with the use of metformin; therefore, patients presenting with vague, flu-like illness should be assessed for the presence of lactic acidosis. Metformin is contraindicated in patients with renal or hepatic dysfunction, congestive heart failure, or history of alcohol use disorder. Additionally, patients undergoing procedures requiring radiographic contrast media should have metformin discontinued before the procedure, withheld 48 hours postprocedure, and should not be restarted until the patient's renal function has been evaluated as normal.

Thiazolidinediones

Rosiglitazone (Avandia) and pioglitazone (Actos) are the two thiazolidinediones that are FDA-approved for use in the United States. **Thiazolidinediones** act by sensitizing skeletal muscle and adipose tissue to insulin and blocking hepatic gluconeogenesis. When used as monotherapy, both rosiglitazone and pioglitazone have not been associated with hypoglycemia but can cause weight gain and raise blood lipid levels. Rosiglitazone raises HDL, but it may also slightly raise LDL cholesterol with minimal effect on triglyceride concentrations. In comparison, pioglitazone raises HDLs, has minimal effect on LDLs, and decreases triglyceride concentrations.

Rosiglitazone and pioglitazone should be used with caution in patients with advanced congestive heart failure. It is also important to note that pioglitazone may decrease the concentration of oral contraceptives, so patients taking pioglitazone and oral contraceptives should be informed of this potential interaction. Additionally, thiazolidinediones may cause resumption of ovulation in premenopausal anovulatory women.

The clearance of rosiglitazone and pioglitazone is decreased in patients with moderate to severe liver disease. Thus, liver function should be monitored every 2 months for 1 year, then periodically thereafter.

Alpha-Glucosidase Inhibitors

The alpha-glucosidase inhibitors are acarbose (Precose) and miglitol (Glyset). **Alpha-glucosidase inhibitors** block the action of alpha-glucosidase enzymes at the brush border of the intestine. The inhibition slows the breakdown of dietary carbohydrates, which decreases postprandial glucose concentrations.

Acarbose, a prototypical alpha-glucosidase inhibitor, has minimal effect on cholesterol and body weight. GI adverse events are common, including abdominal pain, diarrhea, and flatulence. Acarbose, eliminated by the liver, may cause elevations in liver function tests; it is recommended to monitor hepatic enzymes every 3 months for 1 year, then periodically thereafter.

It is important to note that pancreatic enzyme tablets will reduce the effectiveness of acarbose. Also, patients taking alpha-glucosidase inhibitors should not use table sugar or soft drinks (sucrose) to raise blood glucose during hypoglycemic events because these will be ineffective. Milk, apple juice, orange juice, or glucose tablets should be used to reverse hypoglycemia instead, because the absorption rates of sucrose and other complex carbohydrates are drastically reduced with the administration of alpha-glucosidase inhibitors.

Incretin Mimetics (GLP Agonist, GIP Agonist)

The term *incretin* refers to an insulin-stimulating factor found in the GI tract. In response to food, incretin factors are produced by the GI tract and stimulate pancreatic insulin secretion. Incretins include glucagon-like peptide 1 (GLP-1) and glucose-dependent insulinotropic peptide (GIP). Incretins also preserve pancreatic cell mass and enhance the proliferation of pancreatic cells.

Incretin dysfunction results in significant postprandial hyperglycemia as manifested in IGT and T2DM. Studies show that GLP-1 is reduced in patients who are obese with insulin-resistant T2DM. Standard meal tests in patients with T2DM have decreased GLP-1 responses and decreased insulin secretion compared with patients without diabetes. These lower GLP-1 levels are thought to be caused by impaired secretion and decreased response of the incretin. Incretin mimetics (also called GLP-1 agonists) include exenatide (Byetta), liraglutide (Victoza), dulaglutide (Trulicity), albiglutide (Tanzeum), semaglutide (Ozempic), and lixisenatide (Adlyxine). Semaglutide (Ozempic) has been recommended for weight loss as well as glycemic control.

Exenatide. Exenatide (Byetta) is a prototypical incretin mimetic agent (also called GLP-1 agonist) that has multiple mechanisms of action resulting in better glycemic control in diabetics. There are advantageous immediate and delayed effects of the incretin mimetic drugs. The immediate effects include glucose-dependent insulin secretion, suppression of postprandial high glucagon levels, and delayed gastric emptying. The delayed effects include weight loss and improved beta cell mass and function.

The most striking feature of this drug is glucose-dependent insulin secretion, meaning that it stimulates insulin secretion mainly in the postprandial period. Because its insulin-stimulating action is glucose dependent, insulin secretion rises and falls in synchrony with blood glucose. This is similar to the physiological rise and fall of insulin in response to glucose.

In addition, exenatide decreases postprandial glucagon secretion, which further augments its antidiabetic effect. Blocking postprandial glucagon decreases hepatic glucose production, which reduces the patient's insulin requirements. It does not impair normal glucagon response to hypoglycemia. Additionally, exenatide slows gastric emptying, thereby delaying absorption of carbohydrates into the bloodstream. This leads to a feeling of satiety and fullness, resulting in decreased appetite, which may manifest as loss of weight. Exenatide also reduces postprandial triglyceride levels.

At the cellular level, exenatide promotes the growth and development of pancreatic beta cells and improves their life span and function. In addition, it promotes nerve growth factor and may rejuvenate degenerating neurons, which is valuable in diabetic neuropathy.

Adverse drug reactions are few and mild to moderate in severity. These include dizziness, jitteriness, headache, uneasiness, nausea, vomiting, diarrhea, dyspepsia, and a decrease in appetite. When combined with a sulfonylurea, hypoglycemia can occur. Because exenatide is available only as an injectable, allergic reactions at the injection site are possible.

Exenatide is recommended as an adjunct to metformin or sulfonylureas in the dose of 5 mcg subcutaneously twice a day within 60 minutes of morning and evening meals. It is important to remember that it is not indicated in T1DM or DKA and that it is not an insulin substitute. It is not recommended for diabetics with end-stage renal disease (creatinine clearance lower than 30 mL/min) and severe GI disease like gastroparesis. It is yet to be studied in pregnant or lactating mothers.

Amylin Mimetics

Pramlintide (Symlin) is an injectable antidiabetic medication indicated for patients with T2DM or T1DM using insulin who have not achieved desired glucose control. It is a synthetic form of human **amylin,** a naturally occurring pancreatic hormone that, with insulin, helps to control glucose during the postprandial period. Naturally occurring amylin slows gastric emptying and suppresses glucagon secretion, which diminishes hepatic glucose production and controls appetite. In patients with diabetes, amylin, much like insulin, is absent or deficient.

Pramlintide slows nutrient absorption in the GI tract, inhibits glucose synthesis by the liver, promotes a feeling of satiety and fullness, and suppresses appetite. It limits postprandial rise in blood glucose and can lead to weight loss. Most adverse events are GI in nature, such as nausea and vomiting. The drug is administered by subcutaneous injection at mealtimes and eliminated by the kidney.

Pramlintide and insulin should be administered as separate injections and should never be mixed. Adverse events associated with pramlintide include an increased risk of insulin-induced severe hypoglycemia. Proper patient selection and an initial 50% reduction in mealtime insulin are critical to safe and effective use of pramlintide.

DPP-4 Inhibitors

Sitagliptin (Januvia) is a prototypical oral dipeptidyl peptidase-4 (DDP-4) inhibitor that reduces blood glucose levels in patients with T2DM. Other DPP-4 inhibitors include saxagliptin (Onglyza), linagliptin (Trajenta), and alogliptin (Nesina). These drugs inhibit dipeptidyl peptidase-4 (DPP-4), which is an enzyme that destroys the GI incretin hormones GLP-1 and GIP. In response to food, the incretin hormones GLP-1 and GIP are released from the intestine, and their levels increase in the blood. GLP-1 and GIP stimulate the pancreas to secrete insulin and block the release of glucagon. Drugs that inhibit DPP-4, in turn, block enzymatic breakdown of GLP-1 and GIP, allowing these hormones to remain in circulation for a longer amount of time.

The net effect of increased release of GLP-1 and GIP is to reduce blood glucose levels. Therefore, DPP-4 inhibitors, by increasing the amounts of GLP-1 and GIP, reduce blood glucose levels. Hypoglycemia and GI disturbances are the possible adverse side effects.

SGLT2 Inhibitors

Sodium glucose cotransporter 2 (SGLT-2) inhibitors are another class of oral antidiabetic medications for T2DM. SGLT-2 is a protein that enhances glucose reabsorption in the proximal tubule of the nephron. SGLT-2 inhibitors block glucose reabsorption into the bloodstream at the kidney, enhance glucose excreted in the urine, and diminish levels of glucose in the bloodstream. Drugs in this class include canagliflozin (Invokana), dapagliflozin (Farxiga), empagliflozin (Jardiance), and ertugliflozin (Steglatro). This class of drug is informally referred to as a "glucoretic" medication (see Patho-Pharm Connection).

Patho-Pharm Connection

Type 2 Diabetes Mellitus

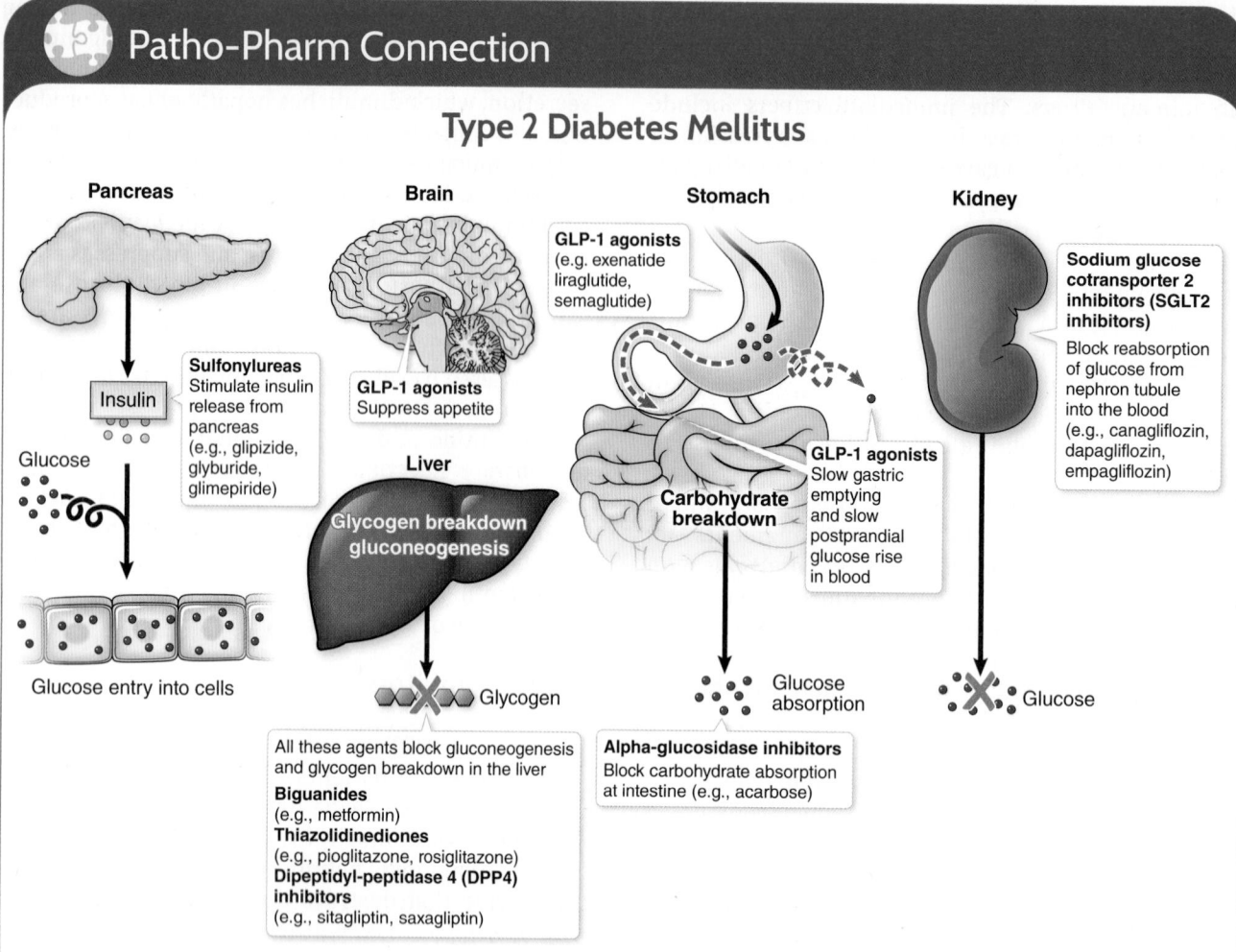

T2DM can be treated with a variety of pharmacological agents that have different actions. The goal of all pharmacological agents used in T2DM is to decrease glucose level in the bloodstream.

In T2DM, the patient has pancreatic insulin reserves that can be stimulated. Some pharmacological agents stimulate the pancreas to release that insulin. These include insulin secretagogues, sulfonylureas (e.g., glibenclamide, glyburide, glipizide, and gliclazide), and meglitinide analogues (nateglinide and repaglinide).

Because in T2DM the cells are not absorbing glucose, the body senses that there is starvation. Therefore, the body goes into starvation mode, which activates the liver to release its glucose stores. The liver releases large volumes of glucose from breakdown of glycogen (glycogenolysis) and a process called gluconeogenesis (synthesis of glucose from protein and fats). Therefore, it is necessary to block glucose release from the liver in T2DM. Glucose release from the liver can be inhibited by a number of pharmacological agents including the biguanide agent metformin and thiazolidinediones called pioglitazone and rosiglitazone. Metformin is one of the most commonly prescribed medications in T2DM.

After eating, the gastrointestinal hormone glucagon-like peptide-1 (GLP-1), called an incretin, stimulates insulin secretion. After eating, GLP-1 slows gastric emptying and suppresses appetite. These are helpful actions in T2DM; therefore, agents that stimulate GLP-1, termed GLP-1 agonists, are used. GLP-1 agonists include exenatide, dulaglutide, liraglutide, and semaglutide. These are commonly added to the antidiabetes treatment regimen. Some are orally administered and some are injectables.

Dipeptidyl peptidase 4 (DPP-4) is an enzyme that breaks down GLP-1. As explained previously, GLP-1 is a helpful hormone in T2DM. Therefore, allowing GLP-1 to function for a longer period of time is helpful. DPP-4 inhibitors block the enzyme DPP-4 from breaking down GLP-1 and allow it to act for a longer period of time. DPP-4 inhibitors (called gliptins) include sitagliptin, saxagliptin, linagliptin, and alogliptin.

Alpha-glucosidase is an enzyme in the intestinal border that breaks down sugars that are ingested. Alpha glucosidase inhibitors block the breakdown of sugar and therefore decrease the glucose that gets into the bloodstream. The alpha-glucosidase inhibitor most used is acarbose.

Sodium-glucose cotransporter 2 (SGLT-2) is a substance that increases glucose reabsorption from the nephron tubule fluid into the bloodstream in the kidney. SGLT-2 inhibitors (also called flozins) block this substance from reabsorbing glucose into the bloodstream, thereby lowering blood glucose. SGLT-2 inhibitors include canagliflozin, dapagliflozin, and empagliflozin.

Combination Medications for Type 2 Diabetes

Because more than one drug is often necessary to control blood glucose in T2DM, there are presynthesized combination drugs, which combine two different classes of the following antidiabetic drugs:

- Thiazolidinedione + biguanide (Avandamet)
- DPP-4 inhibitors + biguanide (Janumet, Janumet XR, Jentadueto, Komboglyze)
- SGLT2 inhibitor + biguanide (Xigduo, Invokamet, Synjardy, Stegluromet)
- DPP-4 inhibitor + SGLT-2 inhibitor (Glyxambi, QTERN, Steglujan)
- GLP-1 agonist + insulin degludec (Xultophy)
- GLP-1 agonist + insulin glargine (Soliqua)
- Alternative agents that can exert glycemic control

In addition to lifestyle modifications, there are alternative kinds of pharmacological treatments that can be effective. The bile acid sequestrant colesevelam (Welchol) has been shown to improve glycemic control. The exact mechanism by which it lowers blood glucose is unclear. Also, the dopamine agonist bromocriptine can effectively lower blood glucose as an adjunct to diet and exercise. Bromocriptine is a rapid-acting drug that acts at the brain. It resets the hypothalamic stimulation of elevated glucose, triglycerides, and free fatty acid levels in fasting and postprandial states in patients with insulin resistance.

Surgical Treatment of Diabetes Mellitus

Pancreas and islet cell transplantation have been shown to effectively control blood glucose; however, the patient must be on lifelong immunosuppressant treatment to prevent rejection and autoimmune islet cell destruction. This type of surgery has been reserved for patients with T1DM who are also undergoing renal transplant or those who endure frequent DKA or hypoglycemia despite intensive glycemic control.

Chapter Summary

- DM is a complex metabolic disease that causes decreased glucose absorption into body cells.

- The disease has reached epidemic proportions in the United States. There are mainly two types of diabetes: T1DM and T2DM.

- In T1DM, there is a deficiency of insulin. In T2DM, body cells resist insulin. Both types result in glucose accumulation in the bloodstream.

- Metabolic syndrome is a constellation of disorders that increase the risk of CVD and DM: apple-shaped obesity, hypertension, insulin resistance (prediabetes), and hyperlipidemia.

- In uncontrolled DM, hyperglycemia has a wide range of acute and long-term effects on the body.

- The classic acute symptoms of DM are polydipsia, polyuria, and polyphagia.

- As glucose is prevented from entering body cells, hyperglycemia develops.

- A fasting plasma glucose of 126 mg/dL or greater is diagnostic of DM.

- An A1c of 6.5% or greater or a random glucose of 200 mg/dL or greater are also diagnostic of DM.

- In T1DM, cells "sense" starvation and the body goes into starvation mode, where the liver and fat tissue liberate glucose and fatty acids, respectively, causing development of DKA—a life-threatening complication that requires emergency treatment.

- In T2DM, hyperosmolar hyperglycemic syndrome (HHS) requires emergency treatment.

- With chronic hyperglycemia, the arteries throughout the body are damaged. Arterial injury incites a cascade of effects that lead to widespread arteriosclerosis. Coronary arteriosclerosis leads to early myocardial infarction. Retinal artery damage leads to blindness. Damage to the fragile glomerular capillaries causes kidney failure. Peripheral arteriosclerosis leads to ischemic stroke and ischemic necrosis of the lower extremities.

- The lower extremities suffer lack of circulation, decreased sensation, and increased susceptibility to infection, all of which increase the risk of gangrene and amputation.

- In the management of DM, the patient must carefully monitor blood glucose, diet, and exercise daily.

- Metformin (Glucophage) is a commonly used oral anti-diabetic agent in persons with T2DM.

- The GLP-1 agonist, Semiglutide (Ozempic) is also commonly prescribed for weight loss as well as glycemic control.

- There are various types of insulin, oral, and injectable antidiabetic agents that can stave off the harmful effects of diabetes.

Making the Connections

Signs and Symptoms	Physical Assessment Findings	Diagnostic Testing	Treatment
Type 1 Diabetes: Immune-Mediated Type 1 Diabetes | Autoimmune destruction of insulin-secreting pancreatic islet beta cells occurs. Without insulin, glucose cannot enter cells. Cells "sense" starvation, and complications such as liver synthesis of glucose and fat breakdown into fatty acids are set in motion. Cellular dehydration occurs. Fatty acids become ketones and hyperglycemia worsens.			
Type 1 Diabetes: Idiopathic Type 1 Diabetes | No autoimmune aspect is present; pancreatic beta cell dysfunction occurs for an unknown reason. Same pathophysiological mechanism occurs as with the previous condition.			
Polydipsia. Polyuria. Polyphagia. Weight loss. Weakness. Fatigue. Vision disturbances. Infection possible.	No significant findings except in cases of infection or DKA. Possible visual impairment. If in DKA: fever, abdominal pain, nausea, vomiting, dehydration, possible decreased level of consciousness.	Fasting blood glucose: 126 mg/dL or greater. Random blood glucose: 200 mg/dL or greater. A1c: 6.5% or greater. Glucosuria: excess glucose cannot be reabsorbed by the kidney and it spills into urine. Ketonuria: ketones in urine are caused by a high amount of fatty acids (ketoacids) in the bloodstream.	Insulin replacement.
Type 2 Diabetes | Insulin resistance of body cells and pancreatic dysfunction occurs.			
Polydipsia. Polyuria. Polyphagia. Weight loss. Weakness. Fatigue. Vision disturbances. Infection possible.	Obesity and hypertension common findings.	Fasting blood glucose: 126 mg/dL or greater. Random blood glucose: 200 mg/dL or greater. A1c: 6.5% or greater. Glucosuria: excess glucose cannot be reabsorbed by the kidney and it spills into urine. Hyperlipidemia common. Metabolic syndrome common. Hyperinsulinemia.	Oral antidiabetic medications, injectable diabetic medications, or insulin.

Bibliography

Available online at fadavis.com

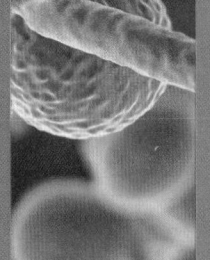

Learning Objectives

Upon completion of this chapter, the student will be able to:

- Recognize the normal hormone fluctuations and changes that occur in the ovary and endometrium during the menstrual cycle.
- List common signs, symptoms, and changes in the reproductive tract that occur during menopause.
- Explain important aspects of assessment of the female regarding reproductive disorders.

- Discuss common laboratory tests and imaging studies used in the diagnosis of pregnancy and female reproductive disorders.
- Identify common disorders that affect the female menstrual cycle and reproductive tract.
- Describe common disorders that affect breast tissue.
- Discuss common treatment modalities used in female reproductive disorders.

Key Terms

Amenorrhea

Beta-human chorionic gonadotropin (b-hCG)

Carcinoembryonic antigen 125 (CA-125)

Colposcopy

Corpus luteum

Culdoscopy

Dysfunctional uterine bleeding (DUB)

Dysmenorrhea

Dyspareunia

Ectopic pregnancy

Endometrium

Follicle-stimulating hormone (FSH)

Gonadotropic hormone

GPAL

Gravidity

Hormone replacement therapy (HRT)

Human papillomavirus

Hysteroscopy

In vitro fertilization (IVF)

Infertility

Laparoscopy

Last menstrual period (LMP)

Liquid-based cytology (LBC)

Luteinizing hormone (LH)

Mammoplasty

Mastopexy

Menarche

Menopause

Menorrhagia

Menstrual cycle

Mittelschmerz

Myometrium

Nabothian cyst

Naegele's rule

Papanicolaou test

Parity

Pelvic inflammatory disease (PID)

Polycystic ovarian syndrome (PCOS)

Precocious puberty

Premenstrual dysphoric disorder (PMDD)

Premenstrual syndrome (PMS)

Thelarche

Vulvovaginitis

Disorders of the female reproductive system can have broad effects on a patient's overall health. Hormonal fluctuations influence the way females manifest disease, and distinct changes occur in the body at puberty, childbearing, and menopause. These changes endow females with the potential for different types of disorders than those experienced by males. Menstrual disorders are the most common reason females seek the attention of a healthcare provider, whereas childbirth is the most common reason females seek emergency medical treatment.

Epidemiology

During the reproductive years of a female's life, there are many reasons to seek the attention of a health-care provider. Common disorders include painful menstrual periods, termed dysmenorrhea, and **dysfunctional uterine bleeding (DUB).** Dysmenorrhea affects 25% of adult females and up to 90% of adolescents. DUB, which can cause excessive uterine blood loss **(menorrhagia)** or excessive uterine bleeding outside of the normal menstrual cycle, occurs in approximately 5% of females aged 30 to 49 years annually. Premenstrual syndrome (PMS), which causes headache, mood swings, insomnia, and other symptoms, occurs in 90% of all females at some time during their reproductive years. Nearly 100% of females will experience a disorder of the menstrual cycle at some point during their lifetime.

Menopause is the natural physiological cessation of ovulation and menstrual cycles later in a patient's life. This condition is a normal part of the aging process that begins on average at age 51. It can be associated with a wide range of symptoms due to hormonal fluctuations. Patients may experience hot flashes, night sweats, vaginal dryness, mood changes, and insomnia. It is estimated that as many as 85% of post-menopausal females have experienced a menopause-related symptom in their lifetime.

Basic Concepts of Female Reproduction

The female reproductive organs consist of the ovaries, uterus, fallopian tubes, vagina, and breasts (see Fig. 26-1). The ovaries produce estrogen and progesterone; at puberty, the female begins to secrete these hormones in cyclical phases that trigger ovulation and confer fertility. Estrogen and progesterone make the uterus suitable for the growth of a fertilized egg in pregnancy. Each month the female reproductive system undergoes a series of changes called the **menstrual cycle.** The cycle consists of distinct hormonal, ovarian,

and uterine changes. Each month, the female body readies the uterus for pregnancy through proliferation of the endometrial layer. When pregnancy does not occur, the uterus sheds the endometrial tissue and yields blood during menstruation. The menstrual cycle usually occurs monthly from approximately age 13 years to age 55 years. At menopause, the ovary degenerates and no longer undergoes ovulation, and fertility wanes.

Breast tissue is also somewhat affected by female monthly hormonal changes. However, it is during pregnancy that the breast undergoes the greatest transformation. Because the pituitary releases prolactin (PRL), the mammary glands become active and lactation occurs.

The Menstrual Cycle

Female reproductive potential comes to fruition at puberty, with the activation of the hypothalamic–pituitary–ovarian axis. The hypothalamus secretes

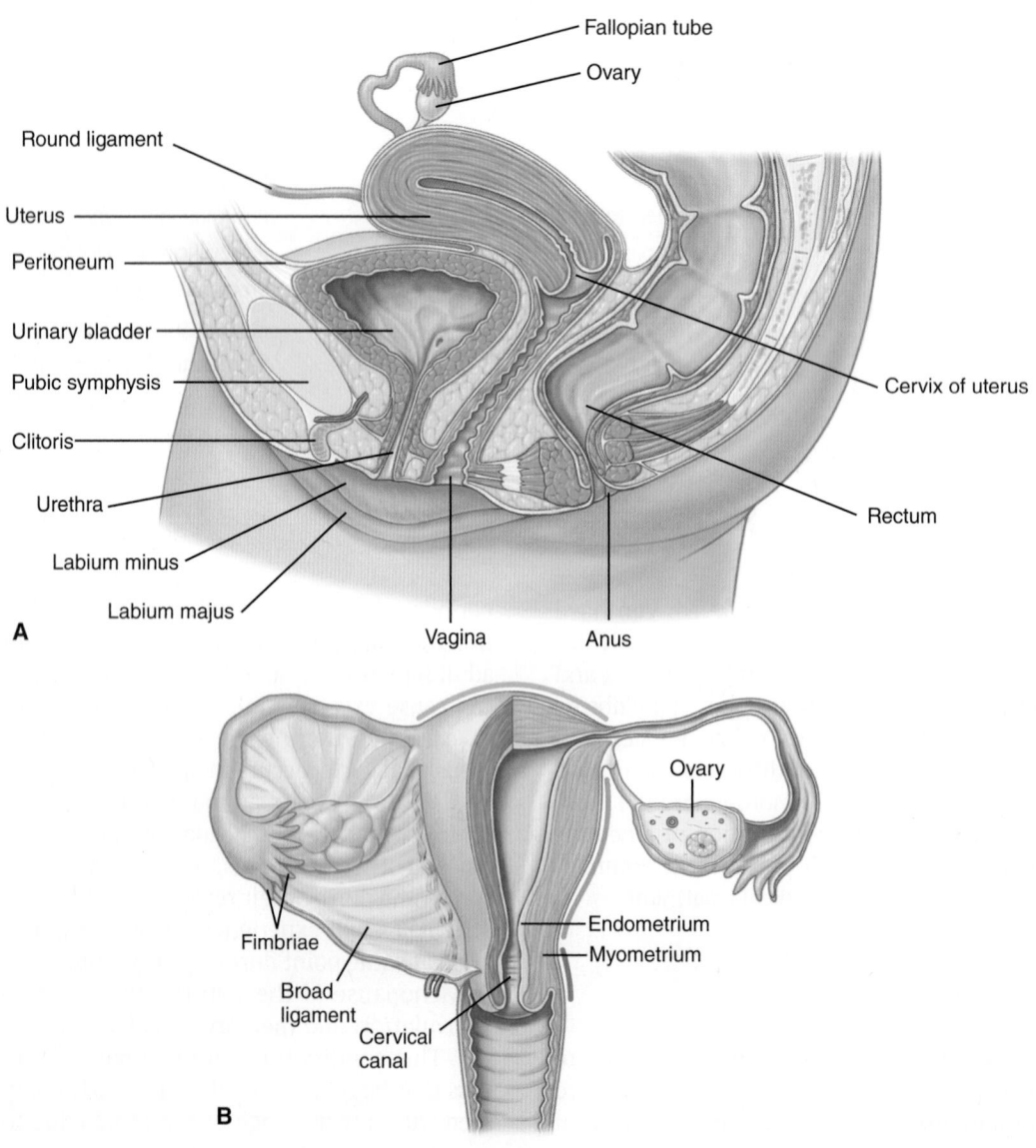

FIGURE 26-1. (A and B) The female reproductive system.

gonadotropin-releasing hormone (GnRH), that in turn stimulates the pituitary to release two gonadotropic hormones: **follicle-stimulating hormone (FSH)** and **luteinizing hormone (LH).** These **gonadotropic hormones** activate ovarian secretion of estrogen and progesterone, which leads to maturation of the reproductive organs.

Female reproductive function begins at **menarche,** the first episode of menstrual bleeding. This bleeding, which occurs on a monthly basis, can last anywhere from 2 to 7 days. At menarche, the ovary starts to release an ovum and the menstrual cycle is initiated. At about the same time, the female also experiences **thelarche,** the development of breast buds. The female adolescent experiences puberty at this time, with accelerated skeletal growth and pubic and axillary hair development.

The menstrual cycle consists of a natural rise and fall of estrogen and progesterone with corresponding changes in the ovary and uterus. During the cycle, an ovum is released from the ovary, and the uterine lining proliferates to prepare for implantation of a fertilized egg. If fertilization does not occur, the uterine lining is shed, causing menses.

The menstrual cycle lasts approximately 28 days, beginning with the first day of menstrual bleeding and ending just before the next menstrual period (see Fig. 26-2). The first part of the cycle is termed the follicular phase and is characterized by increased pituitary gland production of FSH. FSH stimulates estrogen secretion by the ovary and initiates development of an ovum that rises to the surface at a region called the Graafian follicle (mature follicle). At a peak level of FSH, the pituitary releases LH, resulting in ovulation, which is defined as the release of an ovum from the ovary. The ovum travels from the ovary to the uterus via the fallopian tube. Some patients experience mittelschmerz during ovulation. **Mittelschmerz** is one-sided, lower abdominal pain associated with ovulation. German for "middle pain," mittelschmerz occurs midway through a menstrual cycle, at ovulation, about 14 days before the next menstrual period.

After ovulation, remnants of the Graafian follicle on the ovary surface form a region referred to as the **corpus luteum,** which produces progesterone (see Fig. 26-3). This hormone supports the ovum's implantation in the uterine wall and inhibits FSH

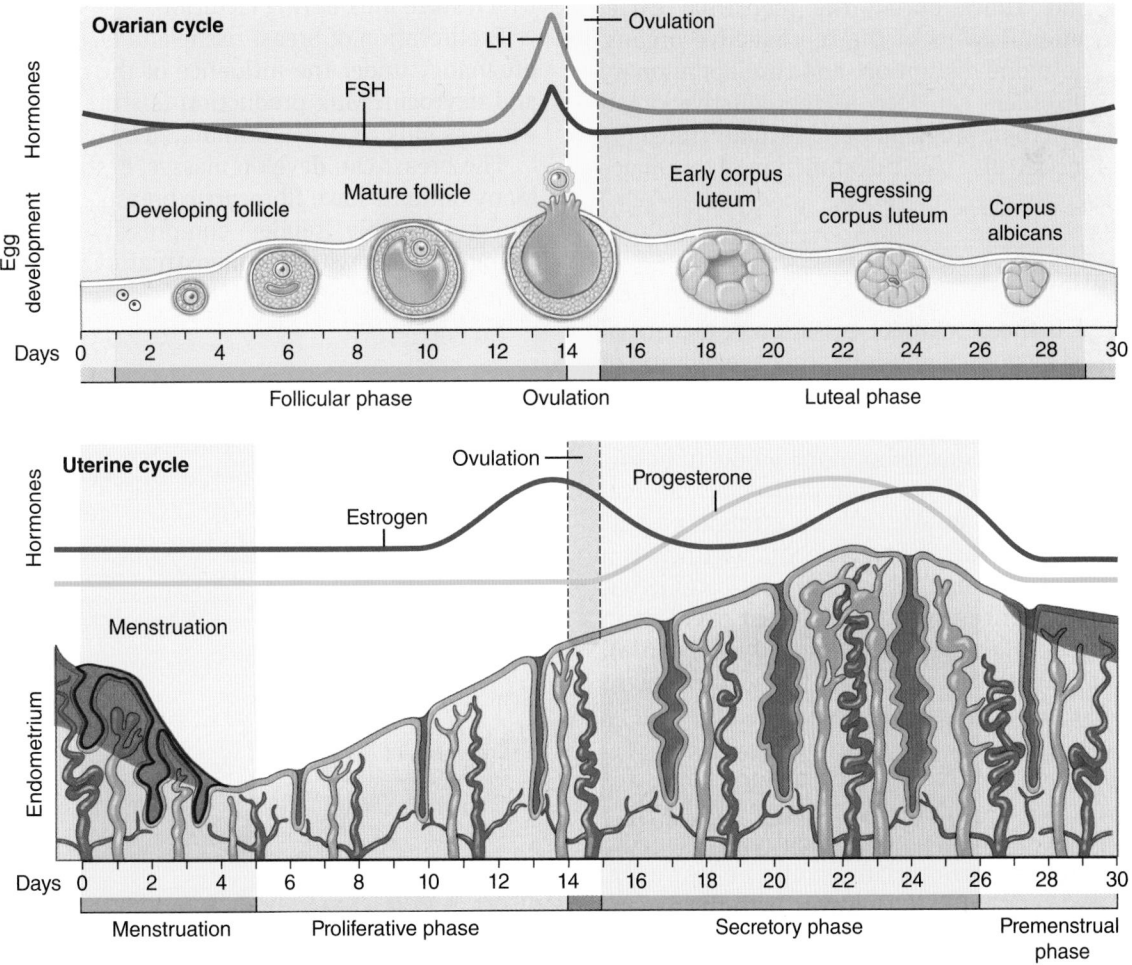

FIGURE 26-2. Hormonal, ovarian, and uterine changes of the menstrual cycle.

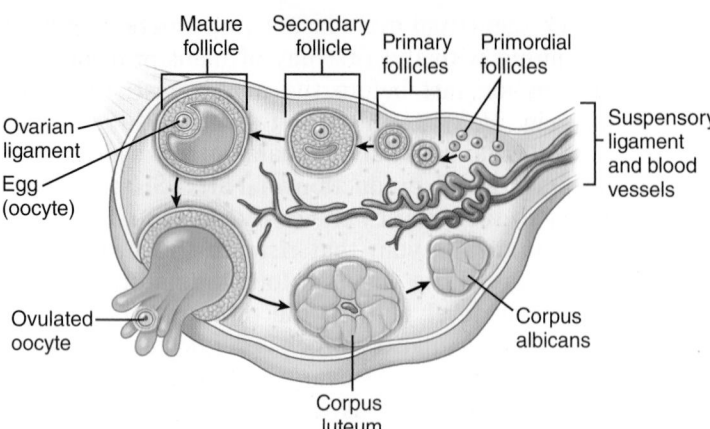

FIGURE 26-3. The corpus luteum.

and LH production. After 14 days, the corpus luteum degenerates if fertilization does not occur and progesterone levels decline. Following progesterone decline, FSH and LH levels begin to rise before the onset of the next menstrual period. If the ovum is fertilized, the corpus luteum continues to secrete progesterone for 5 to 9 weeks to support the pregnancy.

Female fertility requires health of the ovaries, fallopian tubes, uterus, vagina, and external genitalia. In addition, the endocrine hormones, particularly estrogen and progesterone, must be secreted and released at appropriate times during the menstrual cycle. Stress, infection, lesions of the reproductive organs, endocrine hormone disruption, and cardiopulmonary and renal disorders can lead to reproductive organ dysfunction. Ectopic pregnancy and sexually transmitted infections can also cause dysfunction of reproductive organs.

Menopause

Menopause is the permanent cessation of menstrual cycles caused by normal physiological degeneration of the ovaries and the decline of estrogen levels. In the time frame before menopause, called perimenopause, there is a gradual decline in hormone production; this decline can last several years and cause physiological changes that include erratic menses, atrophic vaginitis, and vasomotor instability. Atrophic vaginitis is a marked decrease in natural vaginal lubrication that can cause pH changes, resulting in yeast overgrowth and painful sexual intercourse (termed **dyspareunia).** Vasomotor instability causes hot flashes and night sweats. Mild depressive symptoms, irritability, anxiety, insomnia, and memory problems are also associated with the hormonal changes of perimenopause. Estrogen declines sharply during this time, which causes feedback to the pituitary gland. The pituitary gland, in an attempt to increase ovarian secretion of estrogen, secretes high levels of FSH. However, with the degeneration of the ovaries, estrogen is no longer secreted. The stage of perimenopause can be confirmed by an elevated FSH level.

The Breast

Thelarche, the onset of the development of breast tissue, is stimulated by the pituitary and ovarian hormones at puberty. Each breast, also called a mammary gland, contains approximately 15 to 25 glandular sections called breast lobules, which are separated by Cooper ligaments. Each lobule is composed of a tubuloalveolar gland and adipose tissue. Each lobule drains into a lactiferous duct, which empties onto the nipple's surface (see Fig. 26-4). Lactiferous ducts form large dilated regions called the lactiferous sinuses, which store milk during lactation.

Proliferation of breast tissue and lactation occur in pregnancy under the influence of the hormones PRL and oxytocin. Milk production is stimulated by PRL, whereas milk release is stimulated by oxytocin.

The breast can develop masses, cysts, or infection. Many patients have fibrocystic breasts, which contain benign movable, tender, compressible masses that change in size with the menstrual cycle. Fibrocystic

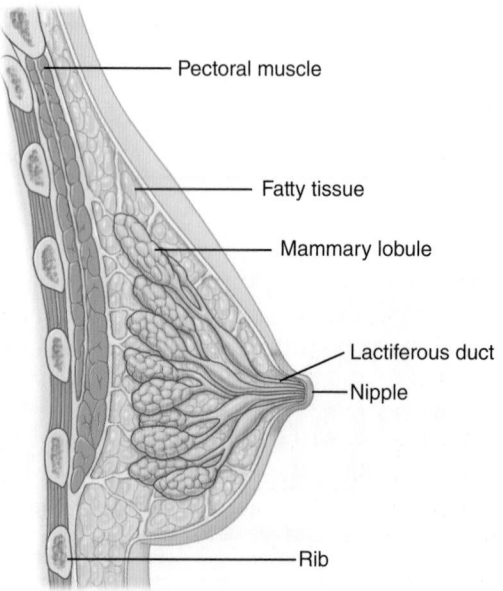

FIGURE 26-4. Anatomy of the breast.

breast changes do not increase the susceptibility to breast cancer.

Basic Pathophysiological Concepts of Female Reproductive Disorders

Puberty is the stage of development when the female body undergoes physical changes that allow for fertility and reproduction. Developmental changes in females during puberty occur over a period of 3 to 5 years, usually between 10 and 15 years of age. They include the occurrence of secondary characteristics that include breast development, the adolescent growth spurt, the onset of menarche, and the beginning of fertility. Early development of these reproductive changes is known as precocious puberty, whereas late development is known as delayed puberty. Menstrual disorders including amenorrhea, dysmenorrhea, menorrhagia, and PMS affect a large percentage of the female population.

Precocious Puberty

Precocious puberty occurs when physical and hormonal signs of puberty occur at an age earlier than what is considered normal. Recent studies indicate that normal puberty is occurring in children earlier than in the past. Studies from 1977 to 2010 show that there has been a steady decrease in the age of puberty in females, particularly in African American females, with some reaching puberty as early as age 6 years. Puberty is considered early, or precocious, if it commences younger than age 8 in European American and 7½ in Hispanic and African American females, and earlier than age 9 in males. The incidence of precocious puberty is estimated to be 1 per 5,000 to 10,000 children in the United States per year. The female-to-male ratio is approximately 10:1.

There are two types of precocious puberty: central precocious puberty and peripheral precocious puberty. Central precocious puberty is the early maturation of the hypothalamic–pituitary–ovarian axis; children with the disorder demonstrate the full range of physical and hormonal changes of puberty that are gonadotropin dependent. Specific genetic mutations have been identified in patients with central precocious puberty. These include mutations in the Kisspeptin 1 (*KISS1*) gene, and its receptor, *KISS1R,* the Makorin RING-finger protein 3 (*MKRN3*) gene, and Delta-like homolog 1 (*DLK1*) gene. Peripheral precocious puberty, less common than central precocious puberty, is gonadotropin independent. The cause is the release of estrogen because of problems with the ovaries, adrenal glands, or pituitary gland.

When evaluating children with premature development of secondary sexual characteristics, precocious pseudopuberty should be excluded. Precocious pseudopuberty is a gonadotropin-independent disorder in which there is an increased production of sex hormones independent of the pituitary secretion of gonadotropin. Excess circulating estrogen from the adrenal gland or ingested sources of estrogen cause the secondary sexual development in precocious pseudopuberty.

Delayed Puberty

Delayed puberty is diagnosed in females when secondary sex characteristics have not appeared by age 13 years. Short stature commonly accompanies delayed puberty. In 95% of cases, delayed puberty is inherited; in these cases, delayed puberty is called constitutional growth delay (CGD). In CGD, the onset of puberty occurs later than average, but the individual reaches normal stature and sexual maturity by adulthood. Other common causes of delayed puberty include chronic illness, eating disorders, strenuous exercise, and drug or alcohol use disorder.

Infertility

Female infertility, male infertility, or a combination of the two affect millions of couples in the United States, with an estimated 10% to 15% of couples classified as infertile. **Infertility** is defined as failure to achieve pregnancy within 12 months of unprotected intercourse or therapeutic donor insemination in females younger than 35 years or within 6 months in females older than 35 years. Females older than 35 years should receive an expedited evaluation and undergo treatment after 6 months of failed attempts to become pregnant, or earlier if clinically indicated. In females older than 40 years, more immediate evaluation and treatment are warranted. Studies suggest that after 1 year of having unprotected sex, 15% of couples are unable to conceive, and after 2 years, 10% of couples still have not had a successful pregnancy. In 40% to 50% of infertility cases, female infertility is the cause, and a male factor is a cause of infertility in 40% to 50% of cases. Factors that can disrupt female fertility include hormonal disorders, polycystic ovarian syndrome (PCOS), primary ovarian insufficiency, fallopian tube disorders, endometriosis, cervical disorders, and uterine tumors or adhesions. In addition to female factors that can cause infertility, male factors include varicocele of the testicle, abnormalities in function or number of sperm, hormonal imbalances, genetic diseases, environmental exposures to toxins or radiation, certain medications, and lifestyle factors (see Box 26-1).

Ovulation disorders account for female infertility in 25% of infertile couples. These can be caused by disruptions in the regulation of reproductive hormones by the hypothalamus or the pituitary gland or by problems in the ovary itself. The pituitary gland produces the two hormones responsible for stimulating ovulation each

BOX 26-1. Most Common Risk Factors for Female and Male Infertility

FEMALE RISK FACTORS FOR INFERTILITY

Older age: After age 32 years, the quantity and quality of a female's eggs begin to decline.

Polycystic ovary syndrome (PCOS)

Anovulation

Uterine fibroids, polyps, or scarring or structural problems of uterus

Endometriosis

Smoking: Tobacco smoking ages ovaries prematurely and increases the risk of miscarriage and ectopic pregnancy.

Excessive use of caffeine: Excessive use is considered consumption of more than 900 mg/day (more than 6 cups coffee/day).

Excessive use of alcohol: Excessive use (more than one drink/day for females) increases the risk of ovulation disorders and endometriosis.

Autoimmune disorders: E.g., Hashimoto's thyroiditis, systemic lupus erythematosus, rheumatoid arthritis.

Sexually transmitted infection: STIs can cause fallopian tube damage.

Obesity: Obesity can cause disruption of the hypothalamic–pituitary–ovarian axis.

Underweight: Being underweight can cause disruption of the hypothalamic–pituitary–ovarian axis.

MALE RISK FACTORS FOR INFERTILITY

Sperm abnormalities: Low sperm production, abnormal shape or poor motility of sperm.

Anatomical abnormalities: Involving the testicles; particularly varicocele.

Blockage: In ducts that carry sperm.

Hormonal problems: Such as low testosterone or hyperprolactinemia.

Sexually transmitted infection or mumps as an adult

Testicular trauma
Immunological conditions: Some persons produce antibodies to sperm.

Genetic disorders: Cystic fibrosis, Klinefelter's syndrome, and hematochromatosis are examples.
Excessive use of alcohol or marijuana: Excessive use of alcohol is more than two drinks/day for males.

Testicular heat exposure: Such as frequent use of hot tubs.

Radiation or toxin exposure

Certain medications: Testosterone replacement therapy, long-term anabolic steroid use, cancer medications (chemotherapy), some ulcer drugs, some arthritis drugs, and certain other medications can impair sperm production and decrease male fertility.

Erectile dysfunction or retrograde ejaculation

Undescended testicles

---

month, FSH and LH, in a specific pattern during the menstrual cycle. Excess physical or emotional stress or a very high or very low body weight can disrupt this pattern and affect ovulation. The main sign of this problem is irregular or absent periods.

Specific diseases of the pituitary may be the cause of infertility, although these are less common. In PCOS, complex changes occur in the hypothalamus, pituitary, and ovary, resulting in overproduction of androgens and causing the ovary to not release ova or produce insufficient progesterone, both of which are needed for pregnancy.

Premature ovarian failure (POF) is a disorder usually caused by an autoimmune response, where the body develops antibodies against ovarian tissue. It results in the loss of ova and decreased estrogen production.

Fallopian tube damage can also prevent pregnancy. When fallopian tubes become damaged or blocked, they keep sperm from getting to the egg or close off the passage of the fertilized egg into the uterus. Causes of fallopian tube damage or blockage can include inflammation of the fallopian tubes (salpingitis); previous **ectopic pregnancy,** in which a fertilized egg becomes implanted and starts to develop in a fallopian tube instead of in the uterus; or previous abdominal or pelvic surgery.

Endometriosis and its treatment can put a patient at risk for infertility because the extra tissue growth—and subsequent surgical removal of it—can cause scarring, which impairs fertility.

Cervical obstruction, also called cervical stenosis, can be caused by an inherited malformation or damage to the cervix. In cervical obstruction, the malformed or damaged cervix cannot produce adequate mucus for sperm mobility and fertilization. In addition, the cervical opening may be closed, preventing any sperm from reaching the egg.

Benign polyps or tumors (fibroids or leiomyomas) in the uterus, common in patients aged 30 to 45 years, can impair fertility by blocking the fallopian tubes or by disrupting implantation.

Scarring or adhesions within the uterus also can disrupt implantation, and some patients born with uterine abnormalities, such as an abnormally shaped uterus, can have problems becoming or remaining pregnant.

Menstrual Disorders

Common menstrual disorders include amenorrhea, dysmenorrhea, and PMS. Dysmenorrhea and PMS are two of the most common reasons that females seek gynecological care.

Amenorrhea

Amenorrhea is the absence of menstrual periods. Primary amenorrhea is diagnosed if the onset of menses does not occur by age 15. Secondary amenorrhea is diagnosed, if after menses has occurred, there is an absence of menses for more than 3 months. Pregnancy is the most common cause of amenorrhea; therefore, the patient should be tested for pregnancy whenever there is a missed menstrual period. Anovulation and irregular menstrual periods are common for up to 2 years after menarche and for 1 to 2 years before menopause. There are many causes of menstrual disorders (see Table 26-1).

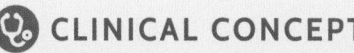

CLINICAL CONCEPT

The etiology of amenorrhea is considered pregnancy until proven otherwise. The **beta-human chorionic gonadotropin (b-hCG)** blood test confirms pregnancy. It should be done on any patient who has missed a menstrual period.

TABLE 26-1. Possible Causes of Menstrual Disorders

Menstrual disorders vary according to the age at menarche, regularity of menstrual cycles, duration and volume of bleeding, and presence of pain.

Menstrual Disorder	Possible Causes
PRIMARY AMENORRHEA	
Lack of development of menses by age 15	• Delay that may be normal if puberty characteristics, such as breast development, are present by age 13 years • Birth defects of the female reproductive system • Genetic disorder • Lack of an opening in the membrane at the entrance of the vagina (imperforate hymen) • Problem with the hypothalamus or pituitary gland • Ovarian failure
SECONDARY AMENORRHEA	
Lack of menses for more than 3 months	• Drastic weight loss • Eating disorders • Pregnancy • Stress and anxiety • Significant weight gain or obesity • Hormonal imbalance, such as with polycystic ovarian syndrome • Endocrine disorders such as thyroid disease or pituitary disease/tumor • IUD • Excessive exercise • Primary ovarian insufficiency (POI) • Menopause, which is normal for females older than age 45 years • Use of birth control pills and other contraceptives • Uterine scarring, usually from procedures such as D&C

Continued

TABLE 26-1. Possible Causes of Menstrual Disorders—cont'd

Menstrual Disorder	Possible Causes
MENORRHAGIA	
Excessive menstrual bleeding; total loss of greater than 80 mL of blood; menses that last longer than 7 days	• Hormonal imbalance • Leiomyoma of uterus • Adenomyosis of uterus • Uterine polyp • Endometriosis • Ovarian disorder • IUD • Pregnancy (miscarriage) • Cancer • Inherited bleeding disorder • Medications (such as anticoagulant)
METRORRHAGIA	
Excessive uterine bleeding, both at the usual time of menstrual periods and at more frequent intervals	• Hormonal imbalance • Leiomyoma of uterus • Adenomyosis of uterus • Uterine polyp • Endometriosis • Ovarian disorder • IUD • Pregnancy (miscarriage) • Cancer • Inherited bleeding disorder • Medications (such as anticoagulant)
OLIGOMENORRHEA	
Irregular periods with long spans of time between periods	• Hormonal imbalance • Leiomyoma of uterus • Adenomyosis of uterus • Uterine polyp • Endometriosis • Ovarian disorder • Pregnancy (miscarriage) • Cancer
DYSMENORRHEA	
Painful menstrual periods	• Hormonal imbalance • IUD • Leiomyoma of uterus • Adenomyosis of uterus • Ovarian cyst • Pelvic inflammatory disease or infection • Cancer • Endometriosis

Amenorrhea can be caused by disorders of the uterus or vagina, or the ovary's lack of ovulation. Many causes of primary amenorrhea are congenital and go unrecognized until puberty. An imperforated hymen, which is an obstructive membrane that exists within the vagina, can also be a cause of amenorrhea. Often, genital tract anomalies or the absence of reproductive organs become apparent at puberty.

Mayer–Rokitansky–Kuster–Hauser (MRKH) syndrome is an anomaly of the genital tract where the uterus is absent and the vagina is foreshortened. Because the ovaries function normally and produce estrogen, breasts are normal in shape and contour. MKRH syndrome accounts for 15% of primary amenorrhea cases and is second to Turner's syndrome as the most common cause of primary amenorrhea.

Asherman's syndrome, which is a lack of the uterine endometrial lining, can be a cause of secondary amenorrhea. This syndrome can occur after a surgical procedure called a dilation and curettage (D&C), which is performed after a miscarriage, delivery, or medical abortion. The endometrium can become scarred with adhesion formations within the uterine cavity. In the extreme, the whole uterine cavity can become occluded by scar tissue. Scarred endometrium fails to respond to estrogen, does not regenerate monthly, and cannot support a pregnancy.

Alternatively, disorders of ovulation can be the cause of amenorrhea. Hypothalamic or pituitary dysfunction can prevent the ovary from releasing an egg. Stress can commonly cause disturbance of the hypothalamic–pituitary–ovarian axis.

 CLINICAL CONCEPT

A patient can miss several menstrual periods because of stress. Menstrual periods can also be lost for several months following dysfunction of the hypothalamic-pituitary-ovarian axis, which can occur after discontinuation of hormonal contraceptives.

Primary ovarian insufficiency (POI) can be idiopathic, secondary to chemotherapy or radiation therapy, or autoimmune in origin. Hypergonadotropic hypogonadism is another ovarian disorder that causes amenorrhea. Elevated levels of FSH and LH characterize this syndrome with low estrogen production. The most common example of hypergonadotropic hypogonadism is found in Turner's syndrome, which is caused by a 45X karyotype. Clinical manifestations of Turner's syndrome include a webbed neck; short stature; broad, shield-like chest; anomalous auricles; and hypoestrogenemia, resulting in sexual immaturity. Gonadal dysgenesis, the lack of development of the ovaries, also causes high FSH and LH and low estrogen levels; it is caused by a mosaic karyotype with an abnormal X chromosome, with loss of part of an X chromosome or translocation, or with a normal karyotype (46,XX) and undeveloped, streak ovaries.

In the postpartum period, hemorrhage can cause pituitary necrosis, also known as Sheehan's syndrome. This syndrome causes lack of pituitary function, which can cause amenorrhea and decreased lactation.

Polycystic ovarian syndrome (PCOS) is a common condition that can cause amenorrhea. In this disease, the ovary cannot release an egg each month. The follicles develop to the point of releasing an egg, but the egg remains under the ovary's surface. This causes the formation of multiple regions of unreleased egg on the ovarian surface, which appear as multiple fluid-filled cysts. PCOS patients are commonly obese with high androgen levels and abnormally high insulin levels.

Functional hypothalamic amenorrhea is caused by excessive exercise, eating disorders, or chronic disease. The hypothalamus does not liberate gonadotropic-releasing factor, and in turn the pituitary does not release FSH or LH. As a result, the ovaries fail to produce estrogen or to release ova.

Hyperprolactinemia (elevated PRL in the blood) can cause amenorrhea in the presence of normal puberty. Often caused by a PRL-secreting pituitary adenoma (prolactinoma), hyperprolactinemia inhibits estrogen release by the ovaries. Aside from prolactinoma, high PRL can occur as a consequence of breastfeeding or psychoactive medications, such as haloperidol, phenothiazines, amitriptyline, benzodiazepines, cocaine, and marijuana.

Dysmenorrhea

Dysmenorrhea is painful menstruation associated with release of prostaglandins in ovulatory cycles. The severity of pain is related to the duration and amount of menstrual flow. Up to 75% of 15- to 25-year-old females experience dysmenorrhea. The chief symptom is cramping pelvic pain with radiation into the groin, back, and legs. Anorexia, nausea, diarrhea, headache, and syncope may accompany painful menstruation. The pain usually begins when prostaglandins are released, usually within the first 48 hours of menstruation; the pain rarely persists more than 2 days.

Patients with dysmenorrhea produce a greater amount of prostaglandin F, which is a uterine muscle stimulant and vasoconstrictor. To diagnose dysmenorrhea, all possible pelvic pathological conditions must be excluded. Primary dysmenorrhea is the diagnosis if there is no associated pathology in the reproductive tract. Secondary dysmenorrhea is diagnosed if there is a pathological cause for painful menstruation, such as fibroid tumor. A thorough medical history and pelvic examination are required. Oral contraceptives, which stop ovulation and decrease prostaglandin synthesis and myometrial contractility, can relieve dysmenorrhea. NSAIDs, such as ibuprofen, counteract prostaglandins and are particularly effective in dysmenorrhea. Low-fat diets, regular exercise, local application of heat, massage, and relaxation techniques are other recommended measures.

Premenstrual Syndrome and Premenstrual Dysphoric Disorder

Premenstrual syndrome (PMS) is the occurrence of distressing physical, emotional, and behavioral changes that interfere with activities of daily living during the luteal phase of the menstrual cycle. It is estimated that 50% or more of females experience mild to moderate PMS, with 5% to 10% experiencing severe to disabling symptoms.

PMS is thought to result from an abnormal tissue response to levels of neurotransmitters that exist during the time before the menses. Because treatment with selective serotonin receptor inhibitors (SSRIs) has been successful, it is thought that PMS is a disorder of decreased synaptic serotonin levels. Fluctuating levels of endorphins, estrogen, and progesterone have been implicated as triggers as well. Alternatively, nutritional deficiency of magnesium or calcium may be causative of PMS.

Emotional symptoms such as depression, anger, irritability, and fatigue have been reported as the most prominent signs, with physical symptoms such as bloating, water retention, and headache also occurring.

 CLINICAL CONCEPT

A more severe form of PMS is **premenstrual dysphoric disorder (PMDD).** The symptoms of PMDD include markedly depressed mood, marked anxiety, tension, marked affective lability, persistent irritability or anger, difficulty concentrating, easy fatigability, food cravings, hypersomnia or insomnia, and a subjective sense of being overwhelmed. PMDD interferes with work or school, social activities, and relationships.

Diagnosis of PMS is based on health history. Treatment focuses on education and self-help techniques. Dietary changes, such as increased intake of complex carbohydrates, fiber, and water, as well as decreased intake of caffeine, alcohol, sugar, and animal fat, are suggested. Medications such as SSRIs are frequently prescribed.

Assessment

The assessment of females for reproductive disorders requires a thorough history and physical examination. The patient should be asked about any history of disease, such as diabetes and endocrine, hematologic, cardiovascular, pulmonary, or renal disorders. Systemic disorders can have an effect on the female's reproductive organs. For example, diabetes increases susceptibility to vaginal *Candida* infection, von Willebrand's disease increases menstrual blood loss, and thyroid problems can cause amenorrhea or excessive menstrual blood loss. Questions regarding abdominal and pelvic pain are essential. Ask the patient to identify the site of pain and its quality. Is it sharp, dull, or cramping? Continuous or intermittent? Ask when the pain occurs and if anything relieves or worsens it. Ask about breast masses, pain, tenderness, or galactorrhea (milk discharge).

Ask the patient about the last menstrual period (LMP), duration of each menstrual period, and how often periods occur. Other questions include:

- Do you have pain with menstruation?
- How much blood loss occurs with each period?

 CLINICAL CONCEPT

The volume of blood loss is a difficult estimation, but you can ask the patient to identify the number of tampons or pads used per day to roughly gauge blood loss. Saturation of a tampon or pad per hour is excessive menstrual blood loss.

Pregnancies are dated in weeks, starting from the first day of the **last menstrual period (LMP).** If menstrual periods are regular and ovulation occurs on day 14 of the menstrual cycle, conception takes place about 2 weeks after the LMP. A patient is therefore considered to be 6 weeks pregnant 2 weeks after the first missed period. The estimated date of childbirth can be calculated using **Naegele's rule:** add 1 year to the LMP, subtract 3 months, and add 7 days. Childbirth occurs approximately 40 weeks after the LMP.

The history of pregnancy and childbirth is integral to the assessment of reproductive organs. Has the patient been pregnant before and, if so, what type of delivery occurred: vaginal or cesarean section? Identifying the patient's gravidity and parity are important to note. **Gravidity** is the number of times a patient has been pregnant. **Parity** is the number of times a patient has given birth to a fetus past 24 weeks of gestation.

CLINICAL CONCEPT

The adult female patient who has not had a pregnancy is referred to as nulliparous, whereas the adult female who has had multiple pregnancies is referred to as multiparous. A patient carrying a first pregnancy is called a primigravida. After delivery, the patient would be called primiparous.

In a patient history, a patient may be described in terms of gravidity and parity. For example, a patient described as "gravida 2, para 2" (sometimes abbreviated to G2 P2) has had two pregnancies and two deliveries after 24 weeks, and a patient who is described as "gravida 2, para 0" (G2 P0) has had two pregnancies, neither of which survived to a gestational age of 24 weeks. **GPAL** is a common acronym used in medical records, indicating G, gravidity; P, para; A, abortion (spontaneous or therapeutic); and L, number of living children.

Sexual history is also an important part of a female patient's health assessment. The patient should be asked about their gender identity. Depending on the patient's age, the age of menarche or menopause is important. Also, it is critical to ask if safe sex is practiced and if birth control is used. If so, what type of birth control is used? The patient should be asked about sexual orientation and number of sexual partners. The number of sexual partners is significant, as having multiple partners increases susceptibility to sexually transmitted infections (STI). According to the Centers for Disease Control (CDC), the following are the 5 Ps of sexual assessment that should be asked of all patients (STIs will be discussed in Chapter 28):

- Partners
- Practices
- Prevention of STIs
- Past history of STIs
- Prevention of pregnancy

Past history of sexually transmitted infections (STIs) is an important aspect of the sexual assessment. The patient should be asked about past STIs such as gonorrhea, chlamydia, genital herpes, **human papillomavirus,** syphilis, and HIV. The patient should be asked about past history of **pelvic inflammatory disease (PID)**. PID is an infection of the female reproductive organs. It usually occurs when sexually transmitted bacteria spread up from the vagina to the uterus, fallopian tubes, or ovaries. Common symptoms include pelvic pain and fever.

The patient should also be asked if there is pain with intercourse, also called dyspareunia. Also, is there bleeding after intercourse? If the patient is perimenopausal, questions about hot flashes, night sweats, and vaginal dryness are indicated.

Family history is significant, as some reproductive disorders are genetic. A history of breast cancer in a first-degree relative is particularly important. The *BRCA* gene is an inherited genetic mutation that increases the risk of breast, ovarian, and other cancers. The number of patients being tested for the mutation is rising. Social habits such as smoking and the use of alcohol, drugs, and caffeine are important to document. Behaviors such as exercise regimen and diet should also be assessed. Females who exercise excessively, underweight athletes, and those with eating disorders frequently report amenorrhea. In addition, current medications, particularly hormonal drugs and oral contraceptives, are important to note in the history. Ask about over-the-counter medications, as well as vitamins and herbal supplements.

A thorough physical examination of females older than age 18 years or sexually active younger females includes a pelvic and breast examination, **Papanicolaou test** (Pap test) and human papillomavirus (HPV) test, and digital rectal examination. The cervical cytology (Pap test) looks for precancerous and cancerous cells. The HPV test looks for the DNA or RNA of strains of the HPV virus (16 and 18) that can cause cancerous cellular changes. The U.S. Preventive Services Task Force (USPSTF), American College of Obstetricians and Gynecology (ACOG), CDC, and the American Cancer Society (ACA) each publish cervical cancer screening guidelines. Each has slightly different recommendations that are updated periodically. For the most up-to-date guidelines, go to the USPSTF, ACOG, CDC, and ACA websites to find the recommendations for cervical cancer screening.

The adolescent needs specific assessments for childhood growth and development, including height, weight, and stage of thelarche and menarche. Assessment of the patient's Tanner stage by inspection of the breast tissue and pubic hair (see Fig. 26-5) is indicated. In adolescents, ascertaining the age of the patient's mother and sisters at menarche is recommended because the age at menarche in family members can occur within a year of the age in others. Also, currently the HPV vaccine (HPV 9-valent vaccine recombinant [Gardasil 9]) is recommended for children as young as age 9 to prevent infection before sexual activity. Currently, most experts recommend the HPV vaccine for persons aged 9 through 26. Persons over 26 may be vaccinated depending on their exposure to HPV and risk of HPV infection.

Diagnosis

Diagnostic studies performed for assessment of female reproductive disorders depend on the patient's symptoms and suspected condition. Some common diagnostic studies include bone age, bone density, thyroid function, PRL levels, adrenal function, and sex hormones, as well as estrogen and progesterone levels. Serum levels of FSH, LH, estradiol, testosterone, thyroid-stimulating hormone, thyroxine, and hCG are also commonly measured. At times, a karyotype needs to be performed, as well as magnetic resonance imaging (MRI) of the pituitary gland.

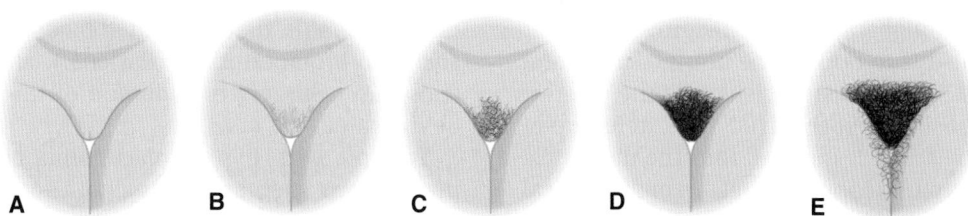

FIGURE 26-5. Tanner stages of female development. (A) Preadolescent. No pubic hair, just fine body hair similar to hair on abdomen. (B) Sparse growth of long, downy hair; straight or slightly curled mainly along labia. (C) Darker, coarser, curlier hair that spreads over pubic symphysis. (D) Hair is coarse, curly, and covers more area. (E) Adult. Hair may spread over medial surfaces of thighs, but not over abdomen.

The **Papanicolaou test,** also called Pap smear or cervical smear, is a common screening test used in gynecology to detect cellular changes associated with cervical cancer. An anal Pap smear is an adaptation of the procedure to screen and detect anal cancers. In performing a Pap smear, a pelvic examination using a speculum is required. Cells from the outer opening of the cervix (exocervix) and the inner surface of the cervix (endocervix) are sampled. The cells are then examined microscopically to look for abnormalities. Another method that is used, called **liquid-based cytology (LBC),** can detect cervical cell changes, cervical cancer, and the presence of HPV.

A clinician performing a **colposcopy** examines the cervix using a colposcope, which provides an illuminated, magnified view of the cervix and the tissues of the vagina and vulva. The main goal of colposcopy is to detect early signs of cervical cancer and allow for a biopsy of the tissue.

Culdoscopy visualizes the fallopian tubes and ovaries using a type of endoscope with a light that can be inserted into the vaginal canal. In an ectopic pregnancy, bleeding commonly occurs into the cul-de-sac, which is a region of the peritoneal cavity behind the uterus. The culdoscope can be inserted into the vagina and then into the region posterior to the cervix to reach this area. In a culdocentesis, the culdoscope is used to search for blood in the cul-de sac. Blood found in this region can diagnose ectopic pregnancy.

Beta-hCG is a hormone produced during pregnancy that is made by the developing placenta. Measurement of this hormone in the bloodstream is the most accurate test used to diagnose pregnancy.

Carcinoembryonic antigen 125 (CA-125) is a biomarker associated with various disorders, including uterine fibroids, endometriosis, pelvic inflammatory disease, and cirrhosis, as well as pregnancy and normal menstruation. Certain cancers, including ovarian, endometrial, peritoneal, and fallopian tube, also can cause CA-125 to be released into the bloodstream. A CA-125 blood level is often used to rule out ovarian cancer.

Common pelvic diagnostic procedures include a transabdominal or transvaginal ultrasound, hysterosalpingography, hysteroscopy, and laparoscopy. Transvaginal ultrasound visualizes the ovaries, fallopian tubes, and uterus using sound waves. This test is commonly used to evaluate the ovaries for masses or cysts. Hysterosalpingography is an imaging study that uses radiopaque dye to outline the uterine cavity and fallopian tubes. **Hysteroscopy** visualizes the interior of the uterus using a specialized thin, telescopic-type device. The scope is inserted into the uterus via the vagina. A **laparoscopy** requires a small surgical incision in the abdominal surface for insertion of a specialized scope that allows internal visualization of the reproductive organs. A surgeon can visualize endometriosis, scarring, masses, cysts, or anatomical abnormalities of the organs.

Proctoscopy is a procedure in which an instrument called a proctoscope is used to examine the anal cavity, rectum, or sigmoid colon. These areas of the body may contain metastatic lesions from the female genital tract. The proctoscope has a hollow barrel through which another instrument may be inserted to take a biopsy of a small amount of tissue. Air may be injected through the proctoscope to help make viewing easier. Similar instruments—the sigmoidoscope and colonoscope—may be used to visualize more proximal parts of the bowel.

Mammography is a specialized x-ray that visualizes breast tissue and is used as a screening tool. The goal of mammography is the early detection of breast cancer, typically through detection of characteristic masses or microcalcifications. Digital mammography and ultrasound-guided fine needle biopsy of breast masses are procedures used when breast cancer is suspected.

Treatment

The treatment for reproductive disorders depends on the cause of the condition. For the adolescent with constitutional delay and anovulation, the goal is stimulation of ovulatory cycles. Estrogen–progestin therapy, which is commonly available in oral contraceptives, can stimulate ovulation. Commonly, oral contraceptives are prescribed to induce ovulation and regulate menstruation in a female of any age with oligomenorrhea.

Hormone replacement therapy (HRT) or estrogen therapy alone is also used to alleviate severe menopausal symptoms such as hot flashes, night sweats, and vaginal dryness. HRT is reserved for those who have severe symptoms or those with hysterectomy-induced menopause. Risks associated with HRT include cardiac disease; stroke; venous thrombus; and breast, ovarian, and uterine cancer. Therefore, health-care providers must weigh the risk and benefits when prescribing HRT.

Hypothalamic amenorrhea is most common in patients who exercise to excess or have eating disorders, caloric restriction, and psychogenic stress. Hypothalamic amenorrhea is best treated using behavioral modification and a multidisciplinary team approach, depending on the root cause.

Symptomatic hyperprolactinemia from a pituitary disorder should first be treated by dopamine agonists such as bromocriptine (Parlodel) and cabergoline (Dostinex). Surgery or radiation of the pituitary may be indicated.

Patients with hyperprolactinemia associated with medications such as antipsychotics and metoclopramide should consider discontinuation or switching of the causative medication.

POI after puberty occurs in 1% of adult females. Treatment should be decided on an individual basis. Some patients may require estrogen replacement therapy (ERT) for hot flashes and other symptomatic menopausal issues. No medications or therapies have been found to induce normal cycling; its occurrence is sporadic, spontaneous, and not inducible.

Fertility drugs, which regulate or induce ovulation, are the main treatment for females who are infertile because of ovulation disorders. In general, they work like the natural hormones FSH and LH to trigger ovulation. Using fertility drugs increases the chances of multiple pregnancies. There are several fertility drugs for abnormal LH and FSH production. These drugs include clomiphene citrate, gonadotropins, human menopausal gonadotropin, FSH, hCG, metformin, and aromatase inhibitors.

Reproductive assistance, or **in vitro fertilization (IVF),** is a highly effective technique that involves retrieving mature eggs from the female, fertilizing them with sperm in a petri dish in a laboratory, and implanting the embryos in the uterus 3 to 5 days after fertilization. IVF is recommended for a number of disorders that cause infertility, including bilateral salpingitis, endometriosis, unexplained infertility, cervical factor infertility, and ovulation disorders. IVF increases the chances of multiple births because multiple fertilized eggs are implanted into the uterus to increase the chances that at least one will develop into an embryo.

Dilation and curettage (D&C) is a common surgical procedure that refers to the dilation of the cervix and surgical removal of the lining of the uterus or contents of the uterus by scraping (curettage). A D&C can be used for diagnostic purposes as well as treatment.

A hysterectomy is the surgical excision of the uterus. This procedure can be done via an abdominal incision or via the vaginal canal. A total hysterectomy is the removal of the ovaries, fallopian tubes, and uterus. A partial hysterectomy usually leaves the ovaries in place.

Endometrial ablation is a procedure that uses a hysteroscope and curettage device to remove the uterine endometrial lining. It eliminates hyperplastic layers of endometrium and menstrual bleeding. This procedure is often used instead of a hysterectomy.

Several surgical procedures use a laparotomy approach, which is a small abdominal or pelvic incision and insertion of a scope to visualize and operate on the reproductive organs. Many reproductive disorders involve use of the laparotomy, such as tissue removal of endometriosis or pelvic adhesions with laser or ablation procedures, tubal ligation, tubal reversal surgery (microscopic) to reconnect fallopian tube integrity, dilation of a fallopian tube, or creation of a new tubal opening.

Cryosurgery (cryotherapy) is the application of extreme cold to destroy abnormal or diseased tissue. Cryosurgery is done after a colposcopy confirms the presence of abnormal cervical cells. It is most commonly used for treatment of cervical lesions such as precancerous cells or cervicitis.

Conization of the cervix is the excision of a cone-shaped or cylindrical wedge from the cervix that includes all or a portion of the endocervical canal. It is used for the definitive diagnosis of squamous or glandular intraepithelial lesions, for excluding microinvasive carcinomas, and for conservative treatment of cervical intraepithelial neoplasia (CIN).

Uterine artery embolization is a procedure mainly used to suppress growth of uterine fibroid tumors. It involves use of a specialized x-ray called a fluoroscope to guide the delivery of small particles into the uterine artery via a catheter. The procedure cuts off blood flow to areas of the uterus where there are fibroid tumors; it is effective in 90% of patients.

Pathophysiology of Selected Female Reproductive Disorders

The common female reproductive disorders encountered in the clinical setting will be discussed in the next sections. For uterine, cervical, ovarian, and breast cancer, see Chapter 40.

Disorders of the Uterus

Endometritis

The **endometrium** is the inner lining of the uterus. It varies in thickness throughout the menstrual cycle. The uterus is a sterile environment, with the cervix acting as a barrier to keep out ascending infection. Infection of the endometrium, called endometritis, can occur in association with instrumentation of the uterus, abortion, childbirth, pelvic inflammatory disease, or an implanted intrauterine device (IUD). Endometritis often occurs in conjunction with inflammation of the fallopian tubes (salpingitis), ovaries (oophoritis), and pelvic peritoneum (pelvic peritonitis).

Endometritis is usually caused by more than one microorganism; it is most commonly caused by an infection ascending from the vagina. It also occurs in 70% to 90% of cases of salpingitis. Endometritis is an uncommon occurrence after vaginal childbirth, occurring at a rate of 1% to 3%, but is more common with cesarean section, depending on the circumstances necessitating surgery. Microorganisms such as *Gonococcus, Chlamydia trachomatis, Enterococcus,* and several strains of anaerobic bacteria are the most common causes of endometritis. The endometrium can be acutely or chronically affected by infection. In acute infection, white blood cells and bacterial organisms invade the endometrial layer. In chronic infection, plasma cells and T lymphocytes are found in the endometrial layer and beneath the endometrium. Symptoms usually include abnormal vaginal bleeding, uterine tenderness, fever, and malodorous discharge. Endocervical cultures should be obtained for gonorrhea and chlamydia when appropriate.

Blood cultures and urinalysis are necessary to rule out extension of the infection into the blood or urinary tract. Ultrasound and computed tomography (CT) scans may be needed if retained tissue of pregnancy is the cause of the infection. Antibiotic therapy is indicated and usually can thoroughly eradicate the condition.

Endometriosis and Adenomyosis

Endometriosis is the growth of endometrial tissue outside the uterus. The most common sites are the ovaries, uterine ligaments, rectovaginal septum, pelvic peritoneum, umbilicus, vagina, vulva, and appendix (see Fig. 26-6). Endometrial tissue in these sites responds to hormone fluctuations in the same way as uterine endometrium. Bleeding can occur at these sites monthly. Endometriosis commonly causes infertility, dysmenorrhea, and pelvic pain.

A related disorder, adenomyosis, occurs when the endometrial tissue grows inside the muscular layer of the uterus. In adenomyosis, the endometrium, in response to hormone fluctuations, bleeds within the muscle wall of the uterus, causing menorrhagia, dysmenorrhea, dyspareunia (pain with sexual intercourse), and pelvic pain.

Approximately 10% to 15% of females have endometriosis; in addition, 80% of females with pelvic pain have endometriosis. There may be a genetic cause of endometriosis, because first-degree relatives frequently have the disease. However, no distinct inheritance pattern has been established for endometriosis. Patients with endometriosis are also six times more likely to have a history of infertility than those without endometriosis.

The cause of endometriosis is unclear, but there are several theories:

- **Regurgitation/implantation theory:** This suggests that menstrual blood containing fragments of endometrium is forced up through the fallopian tubes and into the peritoneal cavity.
- **Metaplastic theory:** This suggests that during embryonic development, immature endometrial tissue spreads over a wider area than normal; during adulthood, it matures and functions like misplaced endometrium.

- **Vascular or lymphatic theory:** This suggests that some endometrial tissue breaks away and metastasizes to other locations in the pelvis.
- **Immunological dysfunction:** This suggests displaced endometrial tissue may trigger an autoimmune reaction. Immunoglobulins attack the endometrial tissue and cause inflammation.
- **Environmental toxicity:** Some studies have shown an association between dioxin (an herbicide) exposure and endometriosis.

Inflammation is a key pathological feature of endometriosis; however, whether inflammation triggers the disease or is a factor that is caused by the disease is not yet known. Estradiol activates the cyclooxygenase 2 pathway in inflammation, which creates prostaglandins. Prostaglandins stimulate endometrial and myometrial cells. There is upregulation of proinflammatory cytokine concentrations including interleukins and tumor necrosis factor alpha. Recent research shows that the effects of endometriosis are not limited to the pelvis. The increased presence of proinflammatory cytokines and immune cells creates widespread inflammation extending outside the pelvis. Data from animal models have shown that cells from endometriotic lesions can migrate into other organs, including the lung, liver, spleen, and brain. Additionally, antibodies to endometrial and ovarian antigens have also been detected in patients affected by the disease. These results suggest endometriosis has features similar to autoimmune diseases.

Pelvic pain in the reproductive years is a common presentation of endometriosis. Cyclic pelvic pain—particularly worsening, progressive dysmenorrhea—is commonly reported. Physical examination findings may be evident on pelvic and rectal examination. Tender uterosacral ligaments and posterior cul de sac, pain or palpable nodules on rectovaginal examination, or adnexal mass or fullness are suggestive of endometriosis. However, commonly there are no physical examination findings. Definitive diagnosis of endometriosis can be accomplished only through laparoscopy. Other helpful tools are transvaginal ultrasonography, MRI, and serum CA-125. Treatment involves pain relief, endometrial tissue suppression, and surgery. First-line treatment consists of NSAIDs, typically in combination with progestin-based therapy. NSAIDs inhibit the function of cyclooxygenase enzymes, thus reducing prostaglandin concentrations and inflammation. Combined oral contraceptives and oral progestins are effective and well tolerated in at least two-thirds of symptomatic patients, especially when used continuously. Progestin-only therapies include medroxyprogesterone, norethisterone, and dienogest. Progestins, such as natural progesterone, can inhibit inflammation and induce apoptosis in endometriotic cells. Both oral and intramuscular medroxyprogesterone have been shown to effectively treat endometriosis-associated pain.

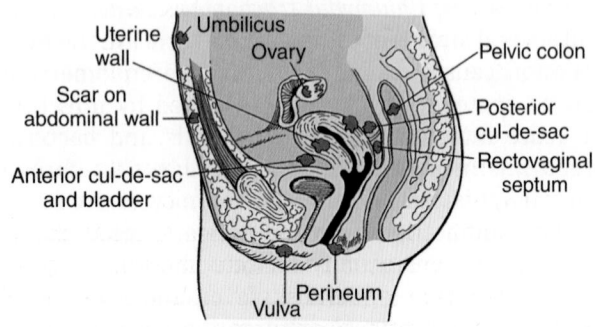

FIGURE 26-6. Sites of endometriosis.

Long-term use of gonadotropin-releasing hormone (GnRH) agonists (e.g., leuprolide) is highly effective. Treatment with GnRH agonists initially stimulates the release of gonadotropins, but after 2 weeks, release is suppressed due to the negative endocrine feedback. GnRH receptor downregulation and desensitization occur. Gonadotropin suppression then causes estradiol concentrations to decrease, which reduces endometrial cell stimulation. Studies show approximately 85% of patients with endometriosis-associated pain obtain relief with GnRH agonists.

GnRH antagonists are also effective. Elagolix is the first oral GnRH antagonist available for the treatment of moderate to severe endometriosis-associated pain. Elagolix prevents the release of FSH and LH, which in turn decreases estradiol stimulation of endometrial tissue.

Aromatase inhibitors (e.g., anastrazole or letrozole) also decrease local estradiol production in endometriosis, thereby minimizing endometrial growth. Recent studies show these effectively manage endometriosis-associated pain.

Other potential therapeutic agents for the management of endometriosis-associated pain include selective progesterone receptor modulators and selective estrogen receptor modulators (SERMs). Mifepristone is the most commonly studied selective progesterone receptor modulator which induces endometrial atrophy, reduces prostaglandin production, induces amenorrhea, and decreases endometriosis-associated pain. Bazedoxifene is a selective estrogen receptor modulator that acts as an endometrial estrogen receptor antagonist. Studies show bazedoxifene in conjunction with conjugated estrogen decreases endometriosis-associated pain in patients with no adverse effects on the reproductive tract. Bazedoxifene plus conjugated estrogen has also been used successfully as an add-on therapy with GnRH agonists.

Laparoscopic surgery involving cautery, laser ablation, and excision techniques is used to treat endometriosis. Laparoscopic surgery is not curative, and 40% to 45% of patients have pain recurrence. Therefore, medical therapy is recommended following surgery to minimize the risk of disease recurrence and to control the widespread systemic effects of endometriosis.

Infertility occurs in 30% to 50% of patients with endometriosis. Chronic inflammation can impair ovarian, tubal, or endometrial function, leading to disorders of ovulation, fertilization, or implantation. Because medical therapies for endometriosis-associated pain inhibit ovulation, their use should not be considered before attempting conception. Unlike medical therapy, surgical treatment can be considered in endometriosis-related infertility. Surgical removal of displaced endometrial tissue has been shown to increase pregnancy rates in females with mild to moderate forms of the disease. If natural conception does not occur, in-vitro fertilization is the most effective treatment of endometriosis-associated infertility.

Patients with endometriosis are at risk for several obstetric-related complications, independent of the use of assisted reproductive technology. These complications include a higher risk of ectopic pregnancy, miscarriage, abnormal placenta location, hypertensive disorders, preterm birth, and intrauterine growth restriction.

Endometrial Polyps

An endometrial polyp is a mass that protrudes into the endometrial cavity. These polyps can be of varying size, from as small as a pencil eraser to as large as a golf ball. They are neoplastic growths of the endometrium of unknown etiology. They are usually benign, but coexistence of atypical endometrial hyperplasia or adenocarcinoma is common. Growth of endometrial polyps has been associated with tamoxifen, a drug used to prevent breast cancer in some females. Polyps may be asymptomatic or cause abnormal bleeding if they ulcerate or undergo necrosis. They most often develop in females between the ages of 40 and 60 years and are a frequent cause of intermenstrual or excessive menstrual bleeding. Studies show that postmenopausal patients with vaginal bleeding have the highest risk of endometrial polyp malignancy. Diagnosis is made by 3D color Doppler transvaginal ultrasound, hysteroscopy, and biopsy. Hysteroscopic surgical polypectomy is the treatment of choice. Histological examination studies reveal that approximately 3% to 5% of endometrial polyps are cancerous. If the endometrial polyp shows atypical hyperplasia or carcinoma, hysterectomy is recommended in all postmenopausal patients and in premenopausal patients without desire for future fertility. Asymptomatic endometrial polyps in postmenopausal patients should be removed if large in diameter (greater than 2 cm) or in patients with risk factors for endometrial carcinoma.

Leiomyomas

Uterine leiomyomas are commonly referred to as fibroid tumors and are the most common benign tumors in humans. As many as three out of four females have uterine fibroid tumors sometime during their lives; however, the majority are asymptomatic and undiagnosed. The etiology of fibroid tumors is unknown, but they tend to be familial, and those who take oral contraceptives have a lesser rate of fibroid tumor than those who do not take them. Fibroid tumors can be small or large enough to distort the shape of the uterus. The tumors are sharply circumscribed, firm growths that are most commonly found in the **myometrium** (see Fig. 26-7). They are composed of smooth muscle and connective tissue in a distinctive swirled pattern when seen on biopsy.

Leiomyomas can be asymptomatic or cause abnormal vaginal bleeding, bladder compression, dysmenorrhea, back pain, or infertility. Excessive menstrual bleeding that causes anemia can occur. Malignant transformation of leiomyoma to leiomyosarcoma is

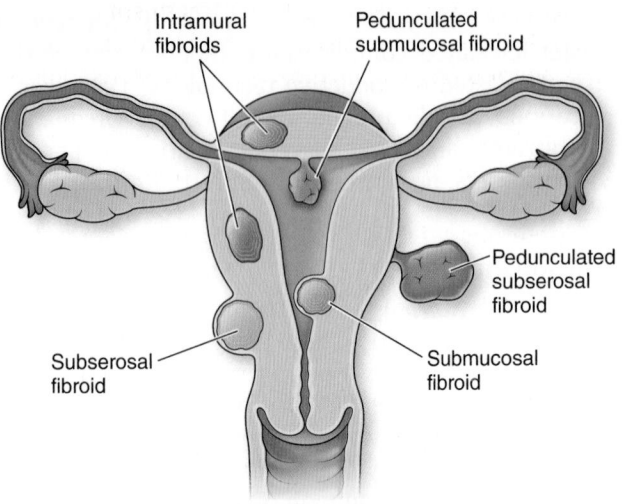

FIGURE 26-7. Sites of leiomyomas of the uterus.

rare, at a rate of less than 1%. There is usually more than one fibroid tumor, and they can increase in size because of estrogen stimulation and with pregnancy. Transabdominal and transvaginal ultrasound are the diagnostic procedures most commonly used to diagnose uterine fibroids. MRI can be used to visualize the tumors. CT scan can also be used, but cannot sharply visualize these tumors unless they are calcified.

Most leiomyomas regress with menopause, but if the tumor causes intolerable pain or bladder compression, surgical excision of the tumor, called myomectomy, can be performed. Hypothalamic GnRH can be given to suppress growth of fibroid tumors. Alternatively, a procedure called uterine artery embolization can obstruct blood supply to a fibroid tumor and diminish its growth.

Abnormal Uterine Bleeding

Abnormal uterine bleeding is a common condition, with a prevalence of 10% to 30% among females of reproductive age. Abnormal uterine bleeding is considered chronic when it has occurred for most of the previous 6 months, or acute when an episode of heavy bleeding warrants immediate intervention. Intermenstrual bleeding occurs between otherwise normal menstrual periods. The prevalence of conditions that cause abnormal bleeding varies according to age. For example, anovulation is more common in adolescents and perimenopausal females, whereas the prevalence of structural lesions and malignancy increases with age. In adolescence, abnormal uterine bleeding is most often due to an immature hypothalamic–pituitary–ovarian axis. There is usually an imbalance in hormone levels.

Anovulatory cycles (failure to ovulate) are a common cause of abnormal uterine bleeding in adolescents and young adult females. Anovulatory cycles can present as a condition of missed periods, prolonged intervals between menses, more frequent periods than normal, or excessive menstrual blood loss. This is not usually caused by a pathological condition, but due to progesterone deficiency or estrogen excess. In the absence of progesterone, unopposed estrogen causes the uterine endometrial layer to proliferate with increased vascularity and glandular development. A lack of ovulation and absence of progesterone allow for excessive uterine endometrial accumulation without menstrual shedding of the tissue. A thick layer of endometrium accumulates with no stimulus for menstruation; consequently, amenorrhea occurs. Eventually, the excessive endometrial layer breaks down and the patient experiences an irregular menstrual cycle and flow irregularities, such as menorrhagia, metrorrhagia, menometrorrhagia, intermenstrual spotting, and oligomenorrhea.

The most common causes of abnormal uterine bleeding can be described using the acronym PALM-COEIN. The etiologies in the PALM group (polyp, adenomyosis, leiomyoma, malignancy, and hyperplasia) are structural and can be diagnosed through imaging or biopsy. The etiologies in the COEIN group (coagulopathy, ovulatory dysfunction, endometrial, iatrogenic, not otherwise classified) are nonstructural causes of abnormal uterine bleeding. These etiologies are not mutually exclusive, and patients may have more than one cause (see Box 26-2).

BOX 26-2. Possible Causes of Abnormal Uterine Bleeding

Coagulopathies
Iatrogenic: medications, hormonal agents, copper IUD
Infection; endometritis, PID
Ovulatory dysfunction
    Hyperprolactinemia
    Immature hypothalamic-pituitary-adrenal axis (adolescence)
    Intense exercise
    Stress
    Ovarian follicle decline (perimenopause)
    Polycystic ovary syndrome
    Eating disorders
    Thyroid disorders
    Adrenal disorders
    Pituitary disorders
Pregnancy
Structural conditions
    Adenomyosis
    Endometriosis
    Leiomyoma
    Malignancy
    Polyp
    Endometrial hyperplasia

In ovulatory cycles, excessive uterine bleeding can occur due to defects in the control mechanisms of menstruation. In patients with ovulatory abnormal uterine bleeding, there is an increased rate of blood loss resulting from endometrial vascular vasodilation, decreased vascular or uterine tone, and excessive prostaglandins. Patients suffer heavy menstrual blood loss, up to three times normal. Large menstrual blood loss often causes anemia and interferes with daily activity.

The approach to patients presenting with abnormal uterine bleeding includes assessing for hemodynamic instability and anemia, identifying the source of bleeding, pregnancy testing, and determining whether evaluation for endometrial carcinoma is indicated. Diagnosis is made by history and clinical examination. Pregnancy must first be ruled out by serum b-hCG. A complete blood count is necessary to rule out anemia caused by gynecological blood loss. Because bleeding can always be caused by coagulation disorders, blood samples for platelet and coagulation factors are drawn. If any endocrine disorders are suspected, blood tests for those are also performed. Disorders of thyroid, pituitary, or adrenal function, primary ovarian insufficiency, ovarian tumor, perimenopause, and PCOS should be ruled out. Eating disorders and lack of sufficient fat tissue in female athletes can also cause abnormal menstrual cycles. Certain medications such as antipsychotic, anticoagulant, or hormonal agents can increase risk of abnormal menstrual cycles. Heavy menstrual bleeding is described as passing blood clots or changing pads/tampons at least hourly. A history of postcoital bleeding (bleeding after vaginal sexual activity) may indicate cervicitis, ectropion, or rarely cervical cancer, whereas abdominopelvic pain may suggest infection, structural lesions, or endometriosis.

An examination of the pelvis, including speculum and bimanual examinations, is an important aspect of the evaluation of abnormal uterine bleeding. The clinician should examine all potential bleeding sites, including the urethra, perineum, and anus. Cervical cancer screening should be performed if it is not up to date. Transabdominal and transvaginal ultrasound can rule out uterine masses or lesions. Hysteroscopy can be used if uterine lesions are suspected. Saline infusion sonohysterography (the infusion of sterile saline into the endometrial cavity while transvaginal ultrasonography is performed) is best at detecting intrauterine lesions. CT scan and endometrial biopsy are sometimes needed. Because older age is an important risk factor for endometrial cancer, all patients with abnormal uterine bleeding who are 45 years or older should undergo endometrial biopsy.

For hemodynamically unstable patients who need immediate cessation of bleeding, uterine tamponade using a Foley catheter or gauze packing can achieve rapid but temporary control of blood loss. Further emergency interventions for hemodynamically unstable patients include intravenous tranexamic acid. Tranexamic acid is an antifibrinolytic drug that inhibits plasminogen and prevents excessive bleeding. Other treatment considerations include intravenous estrogen, dilation and curettage, uterine artery embolization, and hysterectomy as last resort.

For those who do not need emergency treatment, goals involve control of bleeding and hormonal regulation with either progestin–estrogen therapy or progesterone-only treatment. To decrease excessive menstrual bleeding, the 20 mcg per day formulation of the levonorgestrel-releasing intrauterine system (Mirena) is most effective. If the patient has not had a menstrual period for 3 months or more, most clinicians will administer progesterone. This will stimulate endometrial breakdown and menses will occur.

For leiomyoma (fibroid tumor) or endometrial polyps, myomectomy, polypectomy, or uterine artery embolization are treatment options. Total or partial ablation of the endometrium or hysterectomy are surgical procedures used for patients who are older than reproductive age.

Uterine and Pelvic Organ Prolapse

Uterine prolapse is the protrusion of the uterus into the vaginal canal that occurs when supportive ligaments of the pelvic floor are stretched (see Fig. 26-8). Anatomical uterine prolapse affects 14.2% of postmenopausal patients; however, this number is assumed to be low as many patients with uterine or any pelvic organ prolapse may be asymptomatic. Pelvic organs that can potentially prolapse into the vaginal wall include the uterus, bladder, rectum, or intestine. Pelvic organ prolapse occurs more commonly in multiparous patients because childbirth is accompanied by pelvic wall distention and ligament relaxation. Injury to the levator ani muscle or local nerves, especially the pudendal nerve, during childbirth may be responsible for the anatomical abnormality. It may also occur with pelvic masses, obesity, chronic constipation, connective tissue disorders, or neurological conditions. Prolapse of pelvic organs is most common in postmenopausal patients due to lack of estrogen. Estrogen strengthens the pelvic floor musculature. Postmenopausal patients have significantly lower concentrations of

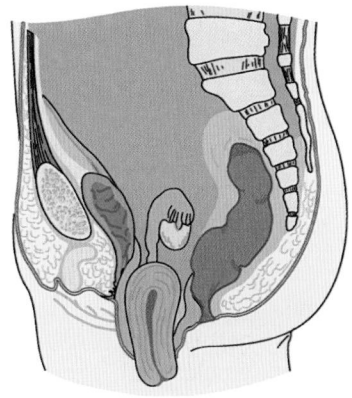

FIGURE 26-8. Uterine prolapse.

serum estrogen and lower numbers of estrogen receptors in the levator ani muscle and uterine ligaments.

Uterine prolapse can be categorized as first, second, or third degree, depending on how far into the vaginal canal the uterus protrudes. In first-degree prolapse, the cervix protrudes into the vaginal canal slightly, whereas in third-degree prolapse, the prolapsed cervix can be seen protruding through the exterior of the vaginal opening. Perineal irritation, dyspareunia, urinary symptoms, bowel symptoms, and pelvic discomfort are the symptoms of uterine prolapse.

Treatment of uterine prolapse consists of vaginal pessary insertion or surgery. Vaginal pessaries are mechanical devices composed of polyvinyl chloride, silicone, or latex that support the vagina and hold the prolapsed organs back in the anatomically correct position. Aside from the uterus, other prolapsed organs can include the bladder and bowel. In uterine prolapse, the pessary device prevents the uterus from descending downward into the vaginal canal. Support pessaries (often called ring pessaries) are positioned between the pubic bone and posterior vaginal fornix, providing support to descending organs. Space-filling pessaries provide support by filling the vaginal space to prevent descent of the uterus.

Surgical repair strategies vary but are often used to treat uterine prolapse. Transvaginal hysterectomy has been used to remove the uterus as a remedy for uterine prolapse for many years. However, the Manchester-Fothergill surgical procedure, which is a uterine-preserving technique, has also been used for many years. Studies show that the Manchester-Fothergill procedure causes less recurrence of pelvic organ prolapse, less postsurgical complications, less bleeding, and shorter recovery time.

Cystocele, Rectocele, and Enterocele

A cystocele is the herniation of the urinary bladder into the vaginal canal. It occurs when muscle support for the bladder is weakened and the bladder sinks below the uterus. It appears as a bulge through the vaginal canal, commonly leading to symptoms of frequency, urgency, and perineal pressure. Stress incontinence can occur at times of lifting, coughing, straining, sneezing, and laughing.

A rectocele is the herniation of the rectum into the vaginal canal. This also occurs because of perineal muscle weakening and appears as a bulge in the vaginal canal.

An enterocele is a herniation of intestine within the area between the uterosacral ligaments posterior to the cervix; these can weaken and form a hernia sac in which the small bowel protrudes. It can cause a feeling of pressure in the perineum, a dull aching sensation, and low backache.

For each of these herniations, surgical intervention is necessary. Most females with symptomatic pelvic organ prolapse are treated with a reconstructive surgical procedure. Hysterectomy is often performed at the time of pelvic organ repair; however, increasing numbers of patients prefer a uterine-preserving procedure. A surgical intervention using a transvaginal mesh material to repair pelvic organ prolapse has been used in the past. Some patients have experienced adverse side effects, such as pelvic pain and inflammation, from this procedure. In general, native tissue repair without synthetic mesh is the preferred approach for transvaginal pelvic organ prolapse surgery because of the higher risk of complications and repeat surgery with mesh-based repairs. Native tissue repair utilizes autograft or allograft material, which is tissue from the patient or cadaveric tissue to reinforce the weakened vaginal region. In addition to surgery, Kegel exercises are recommended to strengthen and maintain the integrity of the perineal musculature.

Disorders of the Cervix

The visible portion of the cervix, or exocervix, is composed of stratified squamous epithelium that is continuous with the vaginal wall. The endocervix, the canal that leads into the uterine cavity, is composed of columnar epithelium that contains mucus-secreting glands. Blockage of a mucus-secreting gland in the endocervix can cause a **nabothian cyst,** a common benign cyst requiring no treatment (see Fig. 26-9).

The junction of the exocervix squamous epithelium and mucus-secreting glandular endocervix cells is called the transformation zone. This zone is the area that is sampled during a Papanicolaou smear and examined during colposcopy to rule out cervical cancer. The Papanicolaou test, also called a Pap test or Pap smear, is a screening test used to detect potentially precancerous and cancerous processes of the cervix.

In performing a Pap test, a speculum is used to open the vaginal canal and allow the collection of cells from the outer region of the cervix and the endocervix. The test is used for early detection of precancerous changes and cervical cancer. The test may also detect infections and abnormalities in the endocervix and endometrium. The cells are examined under a microscope to look for cervical intraepithelial neoplasia (CIN; also called cervical dysplasia). CIN is classified on a

Normal cervix   Nabothian cysts on the cervix

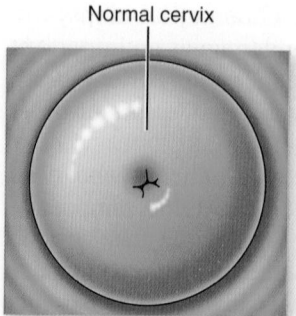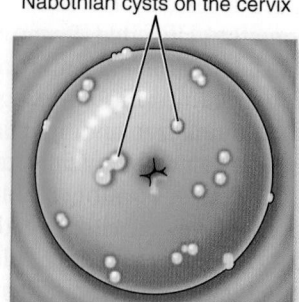

FIGURE 26-9. Nabothian cyst.

scale from one to three. CIN 2 and 3 are more likely to require treatment to prevent cancer. In females who are 30 years and older, a HPV test should be combined with the Pap test. Both cervical cancer and HPV can be detected by a procedure called liquid-based cytology (LBC; ThinPrep).

Prevention of Cervical Cancer

A large body of evidence indicates that infection with high-risk types of human papillomavirus (hrHPV) causes cervical cancer. HPV infections are common, occurring in the majority of sexually active females over their lifetime. Most HPV infections resolve without clinical consequence over a period of several years. The most common types of HPV strains that lead to cancerous changes in the cervix include HPV 16 and HPV 18. HPV 16 is the most carcinogenic and accounts for 55% to 60% of cervical cancers worldwide. HPV 18 is the second most carcinogenic and accounts for 10% to 15% of cervical cancer. Risk factors such as smoking, immunocompromised state, or HIV infection likely lead to persistent HPV infection and increased risk for the development of CIN.

Persistent hrHPV infections can lead to high-grade precancerous cervical lesions (such as CIN grades 2 and 3) that can progress to cervical cancer. Approximately 30% of CIN grade 3 lesions progress to invasive cancer over a 30-year period. During this slow progression, patients have many opportunities for pelvic examination and testing to detect and treat these lesions, thereby disrupting the transformation into cervical cancer.

In 2018, the USPSTF updated its screening guidelines for females of different age groups. In females ages 30 to 65 years, the USPSTF recommends screening for cervical cancer every 3 years with cervical cytology (Pap test) alone, every 5 years with hrHPV testing alone, or every 5 years with hrHPV testing in combination with cytology (Pap test; cotesting).

In females ages 21 to 29, the USPSTF recommends screening for cervical cancer every 3 years with cervical cytology (Pap test) alone. When testing females of this age group, the finding of HPV infection is common and most infections resolve spontaneously without consequences. Therefore, primary hrHPV testing has been found to result in high rates of positive tests in females younger than 30 years and the HPV infection resolves on its own. The high frequency of transient HPV infection among females younger than 30 years can lead to unnecessary follow-up diagnostic and treatment interventions. Therefore, the USPSTF confirmed that testing for hrHPV should begin at age 30 and repeat every 5 years.

In females younger than age 21, the USPSTF confirms that screening for HPV does not reduce cervical cancer incidence or mortality. Cervical cancer is rare in patients younger than 21 years.

For females age 65 and older, evidence suggests that screening beyond 65 years of age in patients with adequate screening history would not have significant benefit. The current guidelines define adequate screening in females older than age 65 as three consecutive negative cytology results or two consecutive negative hrHPV results within 10 years before stopping screening, with the most recent test performed within 5 years. The decision to stop screening at 65 years of age should be made only after confirming that the patient has received adequate prior screening.

To report Pap test results, most laboratories in the United States use a set of categories called the Bethesda system. HPV results are reported as simply positive or negative. The Bethesda system categories range from benign inflammatory changes to malignant cancer (see Box 26-3) (For further detail on cervical cancer, see Chapter 40.)

In addition to screening, clinicians can further the goal of cervical cancer prevention by recommending appropriate HPV vaccination. A two-dose schedule is recommended for patients initiating vaccination at ages 9 to 14 years. Three doses are recommended for those initiating the series at ages 15 to 26 years and for those who are immunocompromised. Until additional evidence emerges regarding the population effect of vaccination, all guideline groups recommend that vaccinated females be screened the same as those who are unvaccinated. New research is frequently emerging in the field of cervical cancer prevention. Clinicians should expect additional changes to clinical guidelines as new evidence develops.

Cervicitis

The cervix is exposed to endogenous vaginal aerobic and anaerobic organisms, such as *Streptococcus, Enterococcus, Escherichia coli,* and *Staphylococcus.* Some degree of cervical inflammation is found in most females and is of little clinical significance. However, clinically important organisms include HIV, gonococci, *Trichomonas vaginalis,* Chlamydiae, HPV, and herpes simplex virus. These organisms are dangerous because of the potential for ascending endometrial infection, systemic infection, pregnancy-related complications, cancer predisposition, or sexual transmission. *Chlamydia trachomatis* is the organism most commonly associated with cervicitis.

Cervicitis is characterized by inflammatory cells, erosion, and epithelial changes, and may be culture positive or culture negative for a specific microorganism. Some inflammatory changes can resemble precancerous lesions, which is why a Pap test is important. Signs of cervicitis include an erythematous, edematous cervix with a large amount of purulent discharge. Diagnosis is based on clinical pelvic examination, colposcopy, Pap test, and biopsy if necessary. Antibiotics may be necessary for treatment of infection. Periodic observation of the cervix is necessary to check for dysplastic development.

BOX 26-3. Interpretation of Pap Test Terminology: The 2014 Bethesda System

In 2014, a task force updated the classification system for reporting Pap test or smear results.

SPECIMEN TYPE

Indicate conventional smear (Pap smear), liquid-based preparation (Pap test) vs. other.

SPECIMEN ADEQUACY

Each laboratory must report if the cervical sample obtained for the test was adequate and if the quality of the smear was satisfactory for examining under the microscope. The smear is marked "satisfactory" or "unsatisfactory." If unsatisfactory, the reasons will be given and the smear will have to be repeated in 2 or 3 months.

INTERPRETATION/RESULT

Negative for Intraepithelial Lesion or Malignancy

This is the desired result and where a "normal" result is reported. There are two important subcategories, where abnormal findings not related to the risk of cancer are reported. These are:

- Organisms: This is where evidence of *Trichomonas*, a fungal (yeast) infection, herpes, or some other infection is reported.
- Other nonneoplastic findings: This is where evidence of injury and response to injury, previously termed "benign cellular changes," is reported.

Other: Endometrial Cells Present (in a female 45 years and older)

This interpretation/result alerts the health practitioner that endometrial cells (cells from the lining of the uterus) are present when they normally should not be. This is a check on the status of the uterus and endometrium, not the cervix. When a patient is having monthly periods, endometrial cells are often present near the time of a period. After menopause, however, they should not be present.

Epithelial Cell Abnormalities

This interpretation/result is where abnormalities that are associated with the risk of developing cancer are reported. The abnormalities range from changes that are only slightly abnormal to definite cancer. There is a spectrum of change. There are two types of epithelial cells in the cervix: squamous and glandular.

Squamous abnormalities (cells that cover most of the external part of the cervix)

The potential for malignancy increases as one moves down the list to the last diagnosis of squamous cell carcinoma, which is an invasive cancer.

- Atypical squamous cells: unknown significance (**ASC-US**) or cannot exclude HSIL or high-grade changes (**ASC-H**)
- Low-grade squamous intraepithelial lesion (**LSIL**)
- High-grade squamous intraepithelial lesion (**HSIL**); one subcategory: "with features suspicious for malignancy"
- Squamous cell carcinoma

Glandular abnormalities (cover the lining of the uterus opening and canal)

Glandular abnormalities are much less common than squamous abnormalities. The list is arranged so that the potential for malignancy increases as one moves down the list. A diagnosis like adenocarcinoma in situ (a cancer limited to the surface that has not invaded) is one of the rarest diagnoses made on a Pap smear and frequently requires consultation among pathologists.

- Atypical cells, not otherwise specified
- Atypical cells, favor neoplastic
- Adenocarcinoma in situ
- Adenocarcinoma (can be endometrial [uterus], endocervical [cervix], extrauterine [origin from outside uterus and cervix], or the site of the malignancy cannot be determined based on the Pap smear)

Other Malignancies

Malignant tumors other than primary squamous carcinoma and glandular adenocarcinoma are occasionally seen on a Pap smear. Patients with abnormal Pap test results are usually examined further for cervical problems. This may involve a colposcopy and biopsy or repeat Pap test. If the Pap result is "ASC-US," then an HPV-DNA test is commonly done in the laboratory to see whether HPV is causing this borderline "normal-abnormal" Pap result.

From Nayar, R., & Wilbur, D. C. (2015). The Pap test and Bethesda 2014. *Cancer cytopathology, 123*(5), 271–281. http://onlinelibrary.wiley.com/doi/10.1002/cncy.21521/full

---

Colposcopically guided laser treatment of abnormal epithelium is common. If squamous cell carcinoma is present, cancer treatments are instituted. See Chapter 40 for content regarding cervical cancer.

Cervical Polyps

Polyps are erythematous lesions that protrude through the cervical os. They are usually a result of benign, inflammatory changes of the endocervix. They are usually asymptomatic but may cause postcoital bleeding. Most are benign, but they should nevertheless be removed and biopsied.

Disorders of the Vagina and External Genitalia

One of the most common disorders of the female reproductive tract is vulvovaginitis. *Candida albicans* is a common cause of inflammation of the vulva and vaginal tract. Inflammation is common, whereas cancer of the vulva is a very rare condition.

Vulvodynia

Vulvodynia is pain of the vulva characterized as burning, irritation, or stinging. Causes of vulvodynia include chronic yeast infection, chemical irritation, or drug effects (particularly prolonged use of topical steroids), irritation from elevated levels of urine calcium oxalate, immunoglobulin A deficiency, genital herpes, and dermatoses such as lichen planus. Diagnosis is made by history and physical examination. Treatment is aimed at symptom relief and elimination of the suspected cause.

Vulvar Cancer

Vulvar cancer is a rare disease in which malignant cancer cells form in the tissues of the vulva over many years. A precancerous condition called vulvar intraepithelial neoplasia can progress to vulvar cancer. Risk factors include human papillomavirus infection and older age. Possible signs of vulvar cancer include bleeding, itching, palpable mass, and tenderness in the vulvar area. Diagnostic tests and procedures include pelvic examination, biopsy, cystoscopy, proctoscopy (visualization of the anus and rectum), IV pyelogram, CT scan, and MRI. The four types of treatment are laser therapy, surgery, radiation, and chemotherapy.

Vaginitis

Vaginitis, also called **vulvovaginitis,** is inflammation of the vagina characterized by discharge, burning, itching, redness, and edema of vaginal tissue. Pain often occurs with urination or sexual intercourse. The disorder can be caused by many different agents, depending on the patient's age. Before menarche, vaginitis is most often caused by poor hygiene, intestinal parasites, or presence of foreign bodies. The most common causes of vaginitis in patients of childbearing age are bacterial vaginosis (40% to 45%), vaginal candidiasis (20% to 25%), and trichomoniasis (15% to 20%). Vaginitis in postmenopausal patients often occurs because of vaginal atrophy resulting from diminishing estrogen levels.

Bacterial vaginosis is the most common cause of vaginitis, accounting for 50% of cases. It is a polymicrobial disorder of the vaginal microbiome that is characterized by the absence of vaginal lactobacilli. This lack of lactobacilli upsets the vaginal ecosystem and there is a subsequent increase in the growth of *Prevotella bivia, Gardnerella vaginalis, Atopobium vaginae,* and megasphaera type 1 organisms. Most organisms are anaerobic bacteria that inhabit the bowel as normal flora. The organisms spread from the rectum into the vaginal canal. It causes a characteristic odor due to the anaerobic metabolism of the involved microorganisms.

Candida, also referred to as yeast, is natural flora within the vagina in as many as 50% of females. However, in vaginal candidiasis, there is an overgrowth of the organism caused by a disruption in the vaginal pH, glycogen content of vaginal cells, or other vaginal environmental changes. *Candida albicans* is the most common organism found in vaginal yeast infections. However, other species include *Candida glabrata,*

Candida krusei, Candida africana, and *Candida dubliniensis.* Factors that can disrupt vaginal conditions and increase risk of infection include oral contraceptive use, IUD use, first intercourse at a young age, increased frequency of intercourse, receptive cunnilingus, diabetes, HIV or other immunocompromised states, long-term antibiotic use, and pregnancy.

Trichomonas vaginalis is an oval-shaped, flagellated protozoan called a trichomonad. These organisms primarily infect vaginal epithelium; less commonly, they infect the endocervix, urethra, and Bartholin's glands. Trichomonads are transmitted sexually and can be found in as many as 80% of male partners of infected females.

Because symptoms of burning, discharge, and itching are common for many different kinds of vaginal infections, precise identification of the pathogen is essential for treatment. Specific culture and sensitivity testing is required. Studies that may be performed in cases of suspected vaginitis include saline wet mount (also called whiff test), pH testing, culture, nucleic acid amplification testing, and a number of other second-line tests.

C. albicans, a common cause of vaginitis, requires a specific diagnostic procedure called a potassium hydroxide (KOH) saline wet mount smear. A small amount of vaginal mucus is placed on a slide with two drops of saline and a small amount of KOH. KOH destroys the vaginal epithelial cells, allowing for visualization of the buds and hyphae that are characteristic of *Candida.*

Trichomonas infection and bacterial vaginosis can be diagnosed using the whiff test. Vaginal discharge is placed on a slide with 10% KOH solution. A positive test result is the release of an amine (fishy) odor after the addition of KOH to the discharge.

The pH of vaginal secretions can also be tested using litmus paper. In bacterial vaginosis, the vaginal pH is 5.0 to 6.0; in vaginal candidiasis, pH is lower than 4.5; and in *T. vaginalis* infection, pH is 5.0 to 7.0. Other tests using the polymerase chain reaction to identify the specific organism are performed by using swabs of the cervix or vagina or by collecting a urine sample.

Candida infections are commonly treated with azole intravaginal medications. Fluconazole or terconazole vaginal applicator cream/suppository is effective for most candida species. Alternative treatment options for nonpregnant patients are oral triazoles (i.e., fluconazole, itraconazole, posaconazole, voriconazole), or polyenes (i.e., nystatin). Probiotics are considered a natural approach for the prevention and treatment of vaginal infections. *Trichomonas* is treated with oral metronidazole, and sex partners of the infected patient should be treated as well. Bacterial vaginosis is treated with the oral or applicator gel form of metronidazole. A recent study showed that oral lactobacilli combined with metronidazole was more effective than metronidazole alone in resolving bacterial vaginosis (Paavonen & Brunham, 2018).

Measures to prevent future vaginal infections include proper perineal hygiene, avoidance of feminine deodorants and douches, and avoidance of tight undergarments.

Atrophic Vaginitis. Genitourinary syndrome of menopause (GSM), previously known as atrophic vaginitis or vulvovaginal atrophy, affects more than half of postmenopausal patients. Caused by low estrogen levels after menopause, it results in vaginal dryness, itching, dyspareunia, urinary urgency and increased frequency, and urinary tract infections. Atrophic vaginitis (or GSM) commonly occurs after menopause or after removal of the ovaries. Estrogen deficiency causes diminished growth of vaginal epithelium, making the tissue susceptible to irritation. Patients with GSM often do not report symptoms of painful vaginal intercourse due to embarrassment, and healthcare professionals do not always actively screen for GSM. As a result, GSM remains underdiagnosed and undertreated. Several effective treatments exist, but low-dose vaginal estrogen therapy is the standard. It is effective for most patients, but should not be used in survivors of hormone-sensitive cancers. Newer treatment options include selective estrogen receptor modulators, vaginal dehydroepiandrosterone, and laser therapy. Nonprescription treatments include vaginal lubricants and moisturizers. Aloe vera vaginal cream has been effective as a natural remedy.

Bartholin's Cyst and Abscess

Bartholin's glands—small, spherical structures at the entry to the vagina—release secretions that enhance lubrication and mobility of sperm. When the ducts of these glands become obstructed, the glandular fluid accumulates and becomes infected. Abscesses can form and cause extremely tender cysts. Treatment includes antibiotics, local application of moist heat, and surgical incision and drainage. Asymptomatic cysts require no treatment.

Disorders of the Ovary

The most common ovarian disorder is a follicular cyst. Each month, females are at risk for a follicular cyst when an ovum comes to the surface of the ovary but is not ejected. In PCOS, many cysts form on the ovary's surface, but anovulation occurs each month. Cancer must be ruled out when any type of ovarian mass is present, whether cystic or solid.

Premature Ovarian Insufficiency

POI is the cessation of ovarian function in a female younger than age 40 years. The condition, also known as primary ovarian insufficiency and hypergonadotropic hypogonadism, results from underfunctioning ovaries or a deficiency in the number of follicles in the ovaries. POI occurs in approximately 4% of the female population. Approximately 10% to 28% of patients with primary amenorrhea and 4% to 18% of those with secondary amenorrhea have POI. At puberty, there are 300,000 to 400,000 follicles within the ovary available for ovulation. During the monthly menstrual cycle, several ova come to the ovary's surface for ovulation; however, only one is released. The degeneration of those that did not release an egg plays an important role in the hypothalamic–pituitary–ovarian axis by secreting regulatory hormones such as estradiol. In POI, there is a reduced number of follicles that leads to disruption of the process of follicular growth and ovulation. Nearly 3 out of 4 patients with POI have some ovarian follicles remaining in the ovary. It is clear that POI in most cases is not a "failure" of the ovary, but rather intermittent and unpredictable ovarian function that can persist for decades.

There are multiple etiologies for POI, including genetic, autoimmune, iatrogenic related to chemotherapy or radiation, surgical, and spontaneous presentation. Many different genetic mutations cause diminished numbers of follicles. Autoimmunity and enzyme deficiencies also cause POI. The most common symptoms of POI are infertility, irregular menstrual cycles, hot flashes, night sweats, irritability, poor concentration, decreased libido, dyspareunia, and vaginal dryness.

Patients with POI may suffer from an endocrine or congenital disorder such as Turner's syndrome, hypothyroidism, or Addison's disease. Physical examination may demonstrate atrophic vaginitis resulting from an estrogen deficiency. A pelvic examination may be normal; however, some may have ovarian enlargement. Patients with Turner's syndrome have characteristic physical signs such as short stature, webbed neck, and shield-like chest. Patients with Addison's disease may have premature gray hair, vitiligo, or increased pigmentation of the gums or the skinfolds. They might also have loss of axillary and pubic hair because of reduced ovarian and adrenal androgen production. Thyroid enlargement may be present resulting from Hashimoto's thyroiditis. To diagnose POI, an FSH level is most important, as this will be elevated. LH, estradiol, and serum levels of endocrine hormones; cortisol; thyroid hormone; and PRL levels may be abnormal. A karyotype and ovarian ultrasound are needed. CT scan and an MRI of the brain are also necessary to rule out pituitary tumor. POI results in adverse effects on the skeleton that increase risk of osteoporosis. There are disturbances of metabolism that predispose to a major increased risk of cardiovascular disease (CVD). Evidence suggests that estrogen is neuro-protective, and thus estrogen deficiency at an early age can increase risk for cognitive decline and dementia.

To decrease complications associated with POI, treatment consists of hormone replacement therapy (HRT) formulations that most closely mimic normal ovarian hormone production and continuing HRT until the normal age of natural menopause, ~50 years. According to the Women's Health Study, oral HRT is associated with increased risks of cardiovascular disease, stroke, and thromboembolism. Therefore, transdermal or transvaginal estradiol therapy is the recommended treatment of HRT for young females with POI or early menopause. Oral HRT has been associated with increased risks of cardiovascular disease, stroke, and thromboembolism. Studies show unlike oral estrogens, transdermal HRT does not adversely alter cardiovascular disease or thromboembolic risk. Most patients with POI have an intact uterus; thus, the recommended hormone replacement is both estrogen and progestin. Cyclical progestin is needed to allow for endometrial sloughing; therefore oral medroxyprogesterone acetate is recommended.

Young patients with POI who desire pregnancy commonly do not respond to traditional fertility treatments. Their options for child-raising include adoption, a small potential for spontaneous pregnancy, donor embryo, or egg donation using in-vitro fertilization. Spontaneous pregnancy will occur in about 5% to 10% of females with 46,XX POI. However, treatment with physiological HRT, such as transdermal estradiol, plus cyclic medroxyprogesterone may enhance the ability of ovarian follicles to mature and respond to an endogenous or exogenous stimulus from gonadotropins, undergo follicular maturation, and ovulate.

For young patients with POI who have a successful pregnancy and want to breastfeed, neither estradiol in oral or transdermal forms, nor hormonal contraceptives, are recommended. Small amounts of hormone are transmitted via breast milk. Additionally, estrogen use may interfere with lactation by decreasing the quantity and quality of breast milk. A nursing mother with POI should be advised not to use HRT, including oral contraceptives, until the child has been completely weaned.

In females who have history of breast cancer or ovarian cancer, HRT is considered unsafe and alternative measures should be used to reduce the risks and symptoms associated with POI. These may include (1) low-dose vaginal estrogens or selective estrogen receptor modulators (SERMS), (2) healthy lifestyle changes to reduce cardiometabolic risk, (3) calcium and vitamin D supplementation and regular weight-bearing exercise to promote bone health, and (4) possibly antidepressants and/or psychotherapy if indicated for depressed mood.

Benign Ovarian Cysts

Benign ovarian cysts are commonly functional cysts, meaning that they are caused by normal physiological events (see Fig. 26-10). In ovulating patients, these cysts are commonly follicular or corpus luteum cysts. For ovulation to occur, the ovary must develop a follicle that matures and contains an ovum. The mature follicle, called a Graafian follicle, is located on the ovary's surface and resembles a small cyst. The Graafian follicle containing the ovum normally ruptures and ejects the ovum in a process known as ovulation.

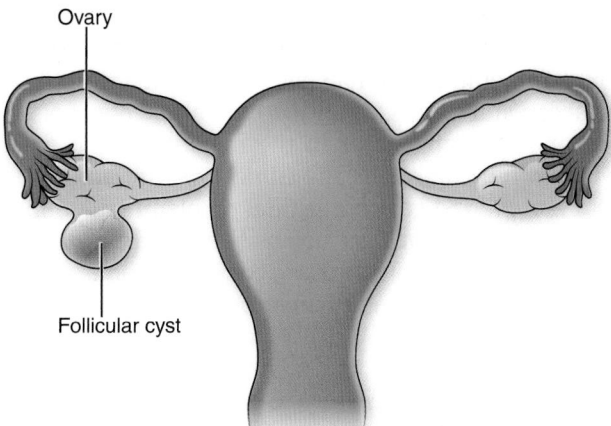

FIGURE 26-10. Ovarian cyst. A follicular cyst can form from an unreleased ovum from the ovarian surface.

When the follicle does not eject the ovum, the result is a follicular cyst. These cysts are usually asymptomatic and require no treatment, as they regress or rupture spontaneously within a few months. However, at times a follicular cyst, although benign, can become large and cause back pain, painful intercourse, chronic abdominal pain, and menstrual irregularities.

A corpus luteum cyst is another type of functional cyst that can occur after ovulation. The corpus luteum is the structure formed by the empty Graafian follicle after ovulation. Under normal conditions, the corpus luteum degenerates. However, a corpus luteum cyst can form because of bleeding inside the corpus luteum 2 to 4 days postovulation. These cysts typically cause symptoms, particularly if they rupture. Symptoms include dull pelvic pain and amenorrhea, followed by irregular or heavy bleeding. Rupture of the cyst occurs during days 20 to 26 of the menstrual cycle. A negative b-hCG blood test is needed to exclude the possibility of pregnancy, and ultrasound confirms the diagnosis. Laparotomy may be necessary to remove the cyst.

Ovarian Torsion

In ovarian torsion, also known as adnexal torsion, the ovary is twisted and blood flow is obstructed. An enlarged ovary caused by a mass or cyst is most susceptible to torsion. Ovarian torsion is usually unilateral, occurring more frequently on the right side. The enlarged ovary will weigh more than normal and dangle lower from the fallopian tube. The ovary can then twist and pinch off arterial and venous vessels. With obstructed blood flow, the ovary can undergo ischemia and infarction.

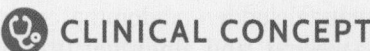

🩺 CLINICAL CONCEPT

Approximately 50% to 60% of cases of torsion of the ovary are associated with an ovarian mass.

The patient with ovarian torsion has unilateral, sudden, severe abdominal pain radiating to the pelvis, groin, and thigh. It is most commonly described as sharp and occurs when the patient is active. Nausea and vomiting occur in the majority of patients, which often confounds the clinical picture and leads to a search for a gastrointestinal problem. Abdominal tenderness may or may not be present. In addition, an ovarian mass may or may not be palpable. Clinical examination must exclude possible diagnoses of appendicitis, gastroenteritis, ectopic pregnancy, pelvic inflammatory disease, and ruptured corpus luteum. A pregnancy test is necessary to rule out ectopic pregnancy. Ultrasound with color Doppler analysis is the best diagnostic procedure because it can show structural and vascular changes of the ovary. Laparotomy, detorsion, or surgical removal of the involved ovary are the common treatments. Evidence supports ovarian detorsion rather than oopherectomy for the management of ovarian torsion. Ovarian salvage is safe and is the preferred treatment. Most salvaged ovaries will maintain viability after detorsion. In females with an ovarian mass, torsion is not always associated with an increased risk of malignancy, and ovarian preservation should still be considered.

> **ALERT!** Ovarian torsion is a gynecological emergency that can present similarly to appendicitis. A pregnancy test is necessary to rule out ectopic pregnancy.

Teratoma of the Ovary

Teratoma of the ovary (also called dermoid cyst) is a cystic mass that has a characteristic composition. Teratomas are made up of various types of embryonic tissue, including epidermal, dermal, bone, and glandular tissue. The interior of the cystic mass is often lined with squamous epithelium and usually contains many sebaceous and sweat glands. Hair and teeth are commonly present within the cyst. Occasionally, the cyst wall may be lined with bronchial or gastrointestinal cells.

Most teratomas are benign and form in the peritoneum or ovaries. They account for 10% to 20% of all ovarian tumors and are bilateral in 8% to 14% of cases.

Teratomas become symptomatic when a complication is present; otherwise, they can be silent. Complications include ovarian torsion, ovarian rupture, infection, hemolytic anemia, and malignant degeneration. Torsion of the ovarian teratoma is the most significant complication, occurring in 3% to 11% of cases. Symptoms include sudden abdominal pain, abdominal mass or swelling, and abnormal uterine bleeding. Imaging studies such as ultrasound, CT scan, and MRI are frequently used to diagnose teratomas. Blood tests include tumor markers alpha fetoprotein

(AFP) and cancer antigen 125 (CA125), beta subunit of human chorionic gonadotropin (beta-hCG), and lactate dehydrogenase (LDH) to determine prognosis. Surgical excision is the most common treatment; however, under particular conditions, ovarian-sparing surgery might be successfully applied. Adjuvant chemotherapy may be indicated.

Polycystic Ovary Syndrome

PCOS is the most common endocrine disturbance affecting young females and is the leading cause of infertility in the United States. The incidence of PCOS has been increasing in the United States, occurring in 18% of young females. This autosomal-dominant genetic disorder is often associated with other endocrine disorders. PCOS most commonly affects females between puberty and 30 years of age.

The etiology of PCOS involves a dysfunctional hypothalamic–pituitary–ovary axis. High serum concentrations of androgenic hormones, such as testosterone, androstenedione, and dehydroepiandrosterone sulfate, are found in these patients. In PCOS, multiple cysts develop on the ovary because of multiple areas of follicular cyst formation. Ova develop within the ovary, come to the ovary's surface, and form a follicular cyst. However, ovulation does not occur, and thus there is no release of eggs from the ovarian surface. The ovarian surface develops multiple areas of unreleased ova that resemble multiple cysts.

Clinical manifestations include amenorrhea or dysfunctional uterine bleeding, hirsutism, acne, and infertility. Approximately 38% of patients with PCOS are obese. Patients with PCOS often have androgen excess, anovulation, and hyperinsulinemia caused by cellular resistance to insulin. Possible sequelae of the disorder include dyslipidemia, diabetes, hypertension, and endometrial hyperplasia, which can lead to endometrial carcinoma.

PCOS can be part of metabolic syndrome. Prevalence of metabolic syndrome in patients with PCOS is twice that of the general population. Different specialty societies have varying criteria for diagnosis of PCOS. Most advise that the following factors be present for diagnosis: biochemical or clinical hyperandrogenism and ovulatory dysfunction such as chronic delayed ovulation with menstrual irregularities, or anovulation. The American College of Obstetrics and Gynecology currently recommends screening for biochemical hyperandrogenism with either total testosterone (T) and sex hormone–binding globulin (SHBG) or bioavailable and free T with exclusion of other causes of hyperandrogenism. Testing of thyroid-stimulating hormone (TSH), prolactin (PRL), and 17-hydroxyprogestone (17-OHP), antimullerian hormone (AMH), and screening for metabolic abnormalities with a 2-hour oral glucose tolerance test as well as fasting lipid levels are also recommended. Transvaginal ultrasonography should be used for the evaluation of the ovaries. Treatment involves reversal of androgen excess, stimulating cyclic menstruation, restoring fertility, and ameliorating endocrine disturbances. For patients with PCOS presenting with menstrual irregularities not seeking fertility, oral contraceptive agents should be the first-line therapy, as they effectively restore cyclic bleeding, reduce hyperandrogenism, and reduce the risk of endometrial hyperplasia. Insulin sensitizers and lipid-lowering agents may be recommended to decrease the insulin resistance and prevent diabetes and heart disease.

Patients with PCOS who seek pregnancy often struggle with infertility. Treatment for these patients centers around fertility enhancement. Traditionally, weight loss and lifestyle modification have been the recommended first-line therapy. To stimulate ovulation, clomiphene citrate (Clomid) or letrozole (Femara) are recommended. Clomiphene citrate binds to estrogen receptors to inhibit negative feedback to the hypothalamus, thereby increasing gonadotropin secretion to trigger ovulation. Unlike clomiphene, letrozole induces ovulation by blocking the conversion of androgens into estrogen, lowering the estrogen levels to reduce negative feedback and increasing gonadotropin production. Some studies show that letrozole is more effective than clomiphene. Letrozole lacks the antiestrogenic properties and is less detrimental to the endometrial lining and cervical mucus, which has in turn led to more pregnancies.

 CLINICAL CONCEPT

Because PCOS may be associated with metabolic syndrome, patients with the disorder should be checked for hypertension, hyperlipidemia, hyperinsulinemia, and glucose intolerance.

Ectopic Pregnancy

Ectopic pregnancy occurs when a fertilized ovum implants outside the uterus. Although 98% of ectopic pregnancies occur within the fallopian tube, implantation can also occur in the cervix, ovary, upper uterus, or peritoneum (see Fig. 26-11). The prevalence is estimated at 25 cases per 1,000 pregnancies. The cause of ectopic pregnancy is slow ovum transport, which may result from decreased fallopian tube motility or distorted tubal structure. Past infection and scarring of the fallopian tube are the most common predisposing conditions for ectopic pregnancy. Risk factors for ectopic pregnancy include pelvic inflammatory disease; therapeutic abortion; tubal ligation; previous ectopic pregnancy; intrauterine exposure to diethylstilbestrol (DES); infertility; and use of fertility drugs, progestin-only oral contraceptives, or levonorgestrel (also called the morning-after pill).

In an ectopic pregnancy, the embryo implants in the wrong place, eventually grows to a size that cannot be accommodated by the region, and then ruptures the

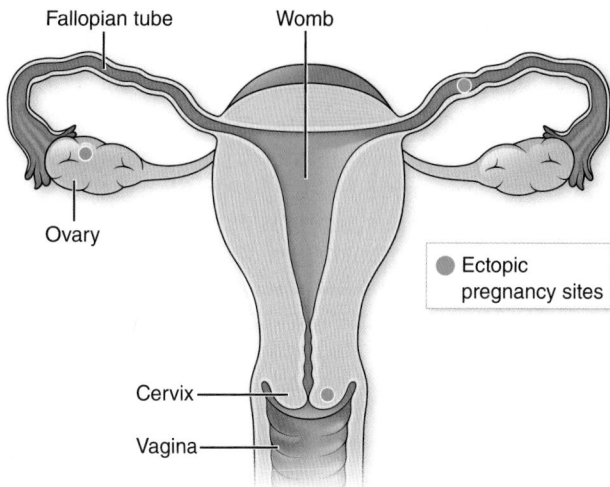

FIGURE 26-11. Possible sites of ectopic pregnancy.

surrounding tissue. The most common site for implantation is in a fallopian tube. The embryo develops until it cannot be accommodated by the tubule diameter and ruptures the fallopian tube.

The classic signs of ectopic pregnancy are pain, vaginal bleeding, and amenorrhea. Rupture of the fallopian tube causes intense lower abdominal pain, bleeding into the abdomen, and referred shoulder pain from bleeding into the abdominal cavity. It is frequently misdiagnosed as an acute abdominal disorder such as appendicitis. Physical examination may reveal adnexal tenderness or adnexal mass. Culdocentesis, extraction of fluid in the area called the cul-de-sac behind the vaginal canal, reveals blood if rupture has occurred. Low levels of hCG are found. Pelvic ultrasound demonstrates an empty uterine cavity and gestational sac outside the uterus.

Treatment requires a laparoscopic salpingostomy to remove the ectopic pregnancy if rupture has not occurred and a salpingectomy if rupture has occurred. This is followed by a course of methotrexate, a chemotherapeutic agent, to eliminate residual pregnancy tissue. Close monitoring of hCG levels is necessary until pregnancy is completely resolved.

ALERT! A diagnosis of ectopic pregnancy should be considered whenever a female of reproductive age complains of abdominal or pelvic pain. It is a gynecological emergency and the leading cause of maternal mortality in the first trimester.

Disorders of the Breast

The majority of breast masses are benign; fibrocystic breast disease is the most common condition of the breasts. Frequently, a singular breast cyst, called a fibroadenoma, develops that has to be differentiated from cancer.

Fibrocystic Breast Disease

Fibrocystic breast disease, the most common disorder of the breast, is present in up to 50% of females older than age 30 in the United States. It presents as benign, nodular, granular breast masses that are most prominent during the progesterone-dominant phase of the menstrual cycle. The symptoms during this phase are tenderness, vascular engorgement, and cystic distention. Minor cyclical breast discomfort is normal and dissipates with the onset of menses. Cyclical breast pain can also be associated with pharmacological hormonal agents (e.g., postmenopausal hormone therapy or oral contraceptive pills). If this is the case, modifications in pharmacological treatment are needed.

Fibrocystic breast disease is largely benign, but certain variants of the disease—including proliferative, epithelial cysts with atypical cells—can increase the risk of breast cancer. The key point in examining a patient with breast pain is to look for signs suggestive of breast malignancy such as a mass, skin changes, or bloody nipple discharge. The four breast quadrants should be systematically examined with the patient both lying supine and sitting with hands on the hips and then above the head. The axillary lymph nodes should be checked and nonpalpable. Diagnostic studies include ultrasound, mammogram, and if necessary, needle biopsy of a cyst for histological examination. Use of a supportive bra and avoidance of foods containing methylxanthines such as coffee, cola, tea, and chocolate are recommended. Acetaminophen, an NSAID, or both, can be used to relieve breast pain.

Fibroadenoma

Fibroadenoma, a benign breast mass, is commonly found in premenopausal females 25 to 45 years old (see Fig. 26-12). Fibroadenomas are benign tumors

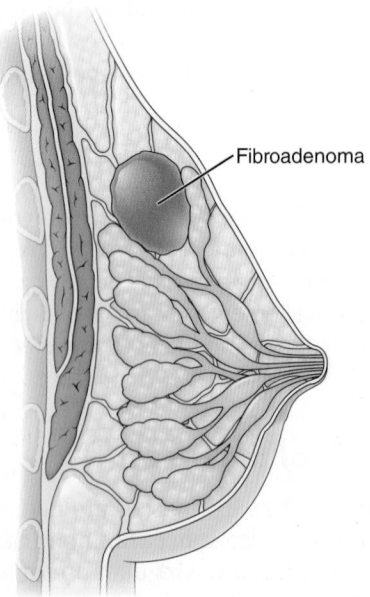

FIGURE 26-12. A fibroadenoma is a benign mass of the breast.

composed of fibrotic tissue and epithelial cells. Fibroadenomas are the most common benign tumor in the breast, accounting for one-half of all breast biopsies. In 20% of cases, multiple fibroadenomas occur in the same breast or bilaterally.

A fibroadenoma is a singular, rubbery, round, movable mass. A small percentage of females have multiple fibroadenomas. It is important to note that the histological features of the fibroadenoma influence the risk of breast cancer. Therefore, all breast masses require biopsy. For the majority of patients with simple fibroadenomas, there is no increased risk of developing breast cancer. The risk of breast cancer is elevated if there are proliferative changes in the tissue or if there is a significant family history of breast cancer. Proliferative changes include sclerosing adenosis, duct epithelial hyperplasia, epithelial calcification, or papillary apocrine changes.

In any patient with a breast lesion, the four quadrants of the breast should be systematically examined with the patient both lying supine and sitting with hands on the hips and then above the head. The axillary lymph nodes should be checked and nonpalpable. Diagnostic studies include ultrasound, mammogram, and needle biopsy of the lesion for histological examination. Surgical excision of the breast mass and biopsy of the mass is necessary.

Mastitis

Mastitis, inflammation of the breast, most frequently occurs during the postpartum period with lactation. It is most often caused by an ascending infection from the nipple to interior ductal structures. The most common pathogens are *Staphylococcus* and *Streptococcus*. Mastitis infection usually occurs during the early weeks of breastfeeding and is manifested by the breast becoming hard, inflamed, and tender. Without treatment, a breast abscess can form, which requires incision and drainage. Treatment of mastitis includes application of hot or cold compresses, analgesics, antibiotics, and a supportive bra.

Galactorrhea

Galactorrhea is the secretion of breast milk in a nonlactating breast, which can result from vigorous nipple stimulation, exogenous hormones, internal hormone imbalance, local chest infection, or trauma. Galactorrhea is usually manifested as bilateral milky nipple discharge involving multiple ducts. The nipple discharge, although usually bilateral and white or clear, may also be unilateral and a variety of other colors, including yellow (straw-colored), green, brown, or gray, but not bloody. Galactorrhea is often caused by hyperprolactinemia, which may be secondary to certain medications, pituitary tumors, endocrine abnormalities, or other medical conditions.

A pituitary tumor that produces large amounts of PRL will cause galactorrhea (see Chapter 24). A complete physical examination, including breast examination is necessary. For patients with bilateral discharge, the physical examination should include checking for a chiasmal syndrome (e.g., bitemporal field loss) and signs of hypothyroidism or hypogonadism. Laboratory evaluation should include a pregnancy test, prolactin levels, renal and thyroid function tests, and appropriate follow-up with an endocrinologist. Diagnosis includes investigating hormone levels and performing mammogram and ultrasound of the breast. Patients with pathological nipple discharge but negative mammogram and ultrasound may undergo breast magnetic resonance imaging (MRI). Galactography or mammary ductography may be necessary. CT scan or MRI of the head may be indicated.

Mammary Duct Ectasia

Mammary duct ectasia is an inflammatory disorder that occurs within the terminal subareolar ducts of the breast. It is common in postmenopausal females. For unclear reasons, the ducts become filled with cellular debris that irritates the duct walls. A small, calcified, palpable mass forms in the central area of the nipple. Fibrous thickening of the surrounding breast tissue can cause dimpling of the breast with nipple inversion. Nipple discharge may be present. A biopsy is usually performed to rule out malignancy. Surgical excision of the affected, dilated subareolar ducts is indicated.

Aesthetic Surgery of the Breast: Mammoplasty

Aesthetic surgery of the breast, or **mammoplasty,** encompasses a spectrum of options from mastopexy to mammoplasty-augmentation or reduction. **Mastopexy** primarily addresses shape of the breast and lifts the breast. Mammoplasty-augmentation or mammoplasty-reduction primarily alters the size of the breast. Before surgery, consultation is necessary to establish the patient's goals. A complete history and physical examination are necessary. History should include a summary of previous surgeries, breast health evaluation, history of breast cancer, abnormal mammograms, and desire for future breastfeeding. Mammogram is necessary before surgery. Informed consent is a critical portion of any mammoplasty consultation and includes a discussion of risks of the procedure including possible need for revisions. Photodocumentation of the breasts are key aspects of the presurgical consultation.

Mammoplasty and mastopexy surgical procedures involve the use of various surgical materials. Mastopexy involves mesh materials or fat grafting. There are four general types of breast implants, defined by their filler material: saline solution, silicone gel, structured, and composite filler.

Complications of breast implants may include breast pain, rashes, skin changes, infection, rupture of implant material, cosmetic changes to the breasts such as asymmetry and hardness, and a fluid collection around the breast. Some investigators have found that silicone-based implants are associated with complications of autoimmune disease and breast implant illness (Cohen Tervaert et al., 2022). The biofilm (microorganisms) that attach to the surface of the implant may be the cause of the problem—it is unclear. However, more investigations are emerging regarding the exact cause of these diseases (Suh et al., 2022). Studies show that incidence of autoimmune diseases such as Sjögren's syndrome, multiple sclerosis (MS), and sarcoidosis are 58% to 98% higher in patients with silicone breast implants (Watad et al., 2018). Another recent study showed an 800% increase in Sjögren's syndrome, 700% increase in scleroderma, and almost 600% increase in rheumatoid arthritis among patients with silicone breast implants compared with the general population of patients of the same age and demographics (Coroneos et al., 2019). Another study showed that a high number of patients who underwent removal of implants reported a significant improvement in their health within a month after their surgery (Wee et al., 2020).

The most serious complication of breast implants is a type of lymphoma (cancer of the immune system) known as breast-implant–associated anaplastic large cell lymphoma (BIA-ALCL). Breast implants with textured surfaces seem to be associated with nearly all cases of BIA-ALCL. The current lifetime risk of BIA-ALCL in the United States is unknown, but estimates have ranged between 1 in 70,000 and 1 in 500,000 females with breast implants (Skelly & Guo, 2021).

The presence of radiologically opaque breast implants (either saline or silicone) might interfere with the radiographic sensitivity of the mammogram; that is, the image might not show any tumor(s) present. In this case, an Eklund view mammogram is required to ascertain either the presence or the absence of a cancerous tumor, wherein the breast implant is manually displaced against the chest wall and the breast is pulled forward, so that the mammogram can visualize a greater volume of the internal tissues. Nonetheless, approximately one-third of the breast tissue remains inadequately visualized, resulting in an increased incidence of mammograms with false-negative results.

Prophylactic Mastectomy for Prevention of Breast Cancer

Currently, it is known that hereditary breast cancer can be due to mutations in *BRCA1* (17q31) and/or *BRCA2* (13q12) genes. Less than 15% of all breast cancers are associated with inherited genetic mutations. The risk estimates are extremely heterogeneous with a mean cumulative lifetime breast cancer risk of approximately 72% in *BRCA1* and 69% in *BRCA2* mutation carriers by age 80. *BRCA1* carriers have earlier-onset, bilateral disease, particularly before age 50 and are more likely to develop aggressive breast cancer than *BRCA2* carriers or those who are *BRCA* mutation negative.

Multiple strategies are effective in managing the risk of breast cancer in patients with *BRCA* genetic mutations, including surveillance, chemoprevention, bilateral salpingo-oophorectomy, and risk-reducing mastectomy. More intensive surveillance, including annual mammography and breast MRI screening (commonly alternated every 6 months) beginning at age 25 or individualized based upon the earliest age of onset in the family, have significantly improved early detection of breast cancer among patients with *BRCA* mutations.

Chemoprevention to reduce the risk of breast cancer is exclusively for patients with high risk and involves the use of selective estrogen receptor modulators (SERMs) (e.g., raloxifene) and aromatase inhibitors (e.g., letrozole).

Risk-reducing bilateral salpingo-oophorectomy (surgical removal of fallopian tubes and ovaries) is recommended for *BRCA* mutation carriers by age 35 to 40 or when childbearing is completed, or individualized based on age of onset of ovarian cancer in the family. Bilateral salpingo-oophorectomy decreases the risk of both breast cancer and ovarian cancer in *BRCA1* and *BRCA2* mutation carriers. Risk-reducing bilateral salpingo-oophorectomy offers an approximate 50% relative reduction in breast cancer risk.

Prophylactic mastectomy provides the greatest reduction in risk of breast cancer development. In both retrospective and prospective observational studies, bilateral prophylactic mastectomy decreases the incidence of breast cancer by 90% or more in patients with *BRCA* mutation (Franceschini et al., 2019). After mastectomy, many patients choose to have immediate breast implant reconstruction with subpectoral muscle implant placement. Subpectoral placement avoids implant exposure and has a very low rate of complications.

Chapter Summary

- The female reproductive system includes the uterus, cervix, ovaries, fallopian tubes, and breasts. Estrogen and progesterone cause monthly menstrual cyclical changes in these tissues. Estrogen increases cellular growth of the endometrium, whereas progesterone enhances the shedding of endometrium, called menstruation.

- Menarche is the time of the first menstrual period. Thelarche is the time of the development of breast tissue. Menopause is the end of menstrual cycles.

- Amenorrhea, regardless of the cause, requires a b-hCG pregnancy blood test.

- Tanner stages depict the phases of development in puberty.

- Puberty is considered early, or precocious, if it commences younger than age 8 in European American and 7½ in Hispanic and African American females.

- There are several different kinds of menstrual dysfunction: amenorrhea is the absence of menstruation, dysmenorrhea is painful menstruation, menorrhagia is the loss of excess blood during menstruation, and oligomenorrhea indicates there is a lengthy amount of time between periods.

- An ovum is developed and brought to the ovary's surface within a follicle. When the ovum is not released, a benign, follicular ovarian cyst can develop. It usually resolves on its own.

- Mittleschmerz is one-sided lower abdominal pain that can occur during ovulation.

- The corpus luteum, which is the empty follicle on the ovary's surface after the egg is released, can develop a cyst that causes abdominal pain. It usually resolves on its own.

- Premenstrual syndrome is the occurrence of distressing physical, emotional, and behavioral changes that interfere with activities of daily living during the luteal phase of the menstrual cycle.

- Infertility is defined as failure to achieve pregnancy within 12 months of unprotected intercourse or therapeutic donor insemination in females younger than 35 years or within 6 months in females older than 35 years.

- GPAL is a common acronym used in medical records, indicating G, gravida; P, para; A, abortion (spontaneous or therapeutic); and L, number of living children. LMP is the acronym for last menstrual period used in medical records. These are important data for the health history.

- Endometritis can occur from an ascending sexually transmitted infection.

- PID is pelvic inflammatory disease; usually an STI that ascends from the vagina into the uterus and fallopian tubes.

- Endometriosis is a common disorder in which endometrial tissue grows in regions outside the uterus.

- Abnormal uterine bleeding can be caused by a disturbance of the menstrual cycle. Anovulatory cycles are the most common cause.

- Leiomyomas, also known as fibroid tumors, are common benign growths within the uterus.

- Uterine prolapse, cystocele, rectocele, and enterocele can occur with weakening of the pelvic muscles.

- Cervicitis, found in most females because of ascending vaginal aerobic and anaerobic bacteria, is benign.

- Cervical cancer is squamous cell carcinoma.

- Certain types of HPV can cause cervical cancer. However, HPV infection can also spontaneously resolve.

- A Pap test and HPV testing are the screening tests recommended for sexually active females. There are different guidelines depending on patient age and risk factors. A standard set of terms, called the Bethesda system, is used to report Pap test results.
- Vaginitis is most commonly caused by *C. albicans, Trichomonas,* or bacterial vaginosis. Each requires different types of medication.
- Vaginal atrophy after menopause can cause vaginitis.
- An ovarian cyst can cause torsion of the ovary, which causes acute abdominal pain and requires surgery.
- Polycystic ovarian syndrome (PCOS) is a common cause of amenorrhea. In PCOS, the ovary cannot release an egg each month. The follicles develop to the point of releasing an egg, but the egg remains under the ovary's surface causing formation of multiple fluid-filled cysts. Patients may develop metabolic syndrome and infertility as well.
- A teratoma is a tumor of the ovary that contains distinctive tissue: teeth, hair, skin, and different glandular tissue.
- Ectopic pregnancy most commonly occurs in the fallopian tube, causes acute abdominal pain, and requires immediate surgical treatment.
- Fibrocystic breasts are common, change in size with a patient's menstrual cycle, and are not a precursor to cancer.
- Fibroadenoma is a singular, benign, movable, discrete breast mass.
- Mammogram, ultrasound, and needle biopsy are commonly used to differentiate benign breast masses from cancerous masses.
- Mastitis is infection of the breast, which is common in the postpartum period.
- Mammoplasty and mastopexy are common aesthetic surgical procedures to reconfigure the breast tissue.
- Silicone breast implants have been associated with autoimmune disease and breast implant illness. This phenomenon is under investigation.
- Females who carry the *BRCA1* or *BRCA2* gene mutation may opt to have bilateral mastectomy and bilateral salpingo-oophorectomy to decrease their risk of breast cancer.

Making the Connections

Disorder and Pathophysiology

Signs and Symptoms	Physical Assessment Findings	Diagnosis	Treatment
Endometritis | An infection of the endometrial layer of the uterus caused by an ascending infection from the vagina.			
Fever, malaise, pelvic pain, and malodorous vaginal discharge.	Fever. Abdominal and pelvic tenderness. Abnormal vaginal discharge.	Culture of the discharge will determine microorganism. Blood cultures will show if infection has entered the bloodstream. Urinalysis is used to look for infection.	Antibiotic treatment.
Endometriosis | A growth of endometrial tissue outside the uterus.			
Painful menstruation.	No physical assessment findings.	Laparoscopy is the standard procedure used for visualizing the endometrial tissue in inappropriate locations.	Combined oral contraceptives and oral progestins may be effective. GnRH agonists and antagonists may be effective. Aromatase inhibitors and selective progesterone receptor modulators or selective estrogen receptor modulators may be effective. Laparoscopic surgical excision of endometrial tissue.

Continued

Making the Connections—cont'd

Signs and Symptoms	Physical Assessment Findings	Diagnosis	Treatment
Leiomyoma of Uterus	A benign, smooth muscle tumor within the uterine muscle wall.			
Painful menstruation.	May be able to palpate mass on pelvic examination.	Ultrasonography, laparoscopy, and hysteroscopy are can visualize leiomyomas.	Surgical excision of tumor. Uterine artery embolization to diminish circulation to the tumor.
Abnormal Uterine Bleeding	Abnormal uterine bleeding is often caused by a disturbance of the menstrual cycle.			
Excessive vaginal bleeding or missed periods or prolonged intervals between menses.	No physical assessment abnormalities.	Hysteroscopy can visualize if there are any lesions inside the uterus that could cause irregular menses. FSH, LH, estrogen, and progesterone levels may be drawn to assess the hormonal cycle. Blood tests to rule out other endocrine disorder or coagulopathy.	If rapid, severe blood loss is occurring, emergency treatment includes uterine tamponade using a Foley catheter or gauze packing. Tranexamic acid can decrease bleeding. Progesterone or HRT is the most common treatment that resets the regularity of the menstrual cycle. Levonorgestrel-releasing intrauterine system (Mirena) has been effective. Endometrial ablation or hysterectomy.
Uterine Prolapse	Protrusion of the uterus into the vaginal canal that occurs when supportive ligaments of the perineum are stretched and there is loss of pelvic muscle strength.			
May feel back pain or pressure in vaginal canal or on bladder or toward rectum.	On pelvic examination, visualization of a protrusion of the uterus into the vaginal canal.	Laparoscopy can visualize uterus, bladder, or rectum displacement.	Vaginal pessary can be used to reinforce tissue. Surgical reinforcement of the ligaments and pelvic muscles.
Cervicitis	A disorder that is commonly caused by infection or inflammation of the cervix.			
Patient may have no symptoms.	Abnormal cervical discharge.	Culture of cervical discharge is taken. Pap smear and HPV testing occur. Colposcopy directly inspects the cervical surface.	Antibiotics, if necessary. Periodic observation to check for dysplastic development. If squamous cell carcinoma is present, cancer treatments are instituted.
Vaginitis	An infection of the vaginal canal with *Candida, Trichomonas,* or bacterial vaginosis.			
Itching and vaginal discharge. Can be a white, thick discharge or fishy odor of discharge.	Vaginal erythema and discharge.	Potassium hydroxide wet mount, whiff test, vaginal pH.	Antibiotic, metronidazole for *Trichomonas* or antifungal agent for *Candida* treatment.

Making the Connections—cont'd

Signs and Symptoms	Physical Assessment Findings	Diagnosis	Treatment
Premature Ovarian Insufficiency | Dysfunction of the hypothalamic–pituitary–ovarian axis. Lack of development of follicles for ovulation.			
Amenorrhea. Infertility. May have other endocrine or congenital disorder such as Turner's syndrome (45,XO), hypothyroidism, or Addison's disease. Turner's syndrome symptoms are webbed neck, short stature, and shield-like chest.	May or may not have physical examination findings. Depends on etiology of disorder.	FSH will be elevated because of a lack of ovarian production of estrogen, which feeds back to pituitary-stimulating FSH. Other hormones may be abnormal, depending on the etiology of POI. Thyroid, cortisol, and PRL hormones may be abnormal. CT and MRI of the brain are used to look for a pituitary tumor. Karyotype is used to check for Turner's syndrome (45,XO) or other genetic disorder.	Hormone treatment to stimulate ovulation.
Ectopic Pregnancy | This is growth of an embryo outside the uterus, most commonly in the fallopian tube.			
Acute abdominal pain, nausea, vomiting.	Abdominal tenderness, abdominal rigidity, abdominal mass palpation possible.	Laboratory test: b-hCG. Transvaginal or pelvic ultrasound is the best test to visualize an ectopic pregnancy. Laparoscopy may be necessary if ultrasound does not show the ectopic pregnancy.	Methotrexate. Surgical excision. Removal of the fallopian tube common.
Benign Ovarian Cyst | Growth composed of the remains of a Graafian follicle that has not ejected the ovum, or remains of the corpus luteum that did not degenerate.			
Abdominal pain.	Abdominal or pelvic mass palpable.	Transvaginal or pelvic ultrasound is the best test to visualize an ovarian cyst. Laparoscopy may be necessary.	Surgical excision.
Torsion of the Ovary | A twisting of the ovary that obstructs arterial flow. Usually occurs only if the ovary is enlarged or if a large cyst is present.			
Intense abdominal pain, nausea, vomiting.	Abdominal or pelvic mass palpable.	Transvaginal or pelvic ultrasound is the best test to visualize an ovarian cyst. Laparoscopy may be necessary.	Surgical excision.

Continued

Making the Connections—cont'd

Signs and Symptoms	Physical Assessment Findings	Diagnosis	Treatment
Polycystic Ovary Syndrome | A hormonal imbalance of androgen and estrogen that causes amenorrhea and infertility. Ova can develop and come to the ovary's surface but are not released. Multiple ova under the surface resemble multiple cysts.			
Amenorrhea. Infertility. Hirsutism. Obesity.	Patient commonly has metabolic syndrome; hypertension, glucose intolerance, hyperlipidemia, and central obesity.	Laparoscopy to visualize ovaries and hormone levels; androgens, FSH, LH, estrogen, and progesterone are performed. Patient has high androgens and an imbalance of other hormones.	Progesterone therapy is recommended to oppose estrogen's effects on the endometrium. Insulin sensitizers and lipid-lowering medications may be needed to decrease the insulin resistance and prevent diabetes and heart disease. Clomiphene or letrozol can be used when pregnancy is desired.
Teratoma of the Ovary | Ovary develops large cystic growth containing embryonic tissue that forms hair, teeth, and other kinds of tissue.			
Abdominal and pelvic pain. Back pain.	Abdominal or pelvic mass may be palpable.	Transvaginal or pelvic ultrasound can visualize the growth. Laparoscopy also can visualize growth.	Surgical excision.
Fibrocystic Breasts | This is not a pathological condition; breasts have multiple, mobile, tender cysts that change in size with menstrual cycle.			
Patient has breast tenderness during menstruation.	Clinical breast examination reveals multiple, movable, compressible cysts throughout breast tissue bilaterally.	Mammogram and ultrasound to rule out any cancerous growths. Needle biopsy may be needed.	NSAIDs. Advise decreased coffee, tea, chocolate, or cola. Supportive bra.
Fibroadenoma of Breast | A singular mass that develops within the breast tissue, which is usually benign.			
Discrete, movable, rubbery mass.	Discrete, movable, rubbery mass on clinical breast examination.	Mammogram, ultrasound. Needle biopsy can demonstrate the lesion as benign or malignant.	Surgical excision.
Mastitis | Infection of the breast caused by *Staphylococcus* or *Streptococcus* ascending from the skin to the duct and glands.			
Tender, erythematous nipple area, usually during breastfeeding.	Tender, erythematous nipple area in a breastfeeding mother.	Mammogram can visualize malignancy. Clinical examination is usually sufficient.	Hot or cold compresses. Analgesics. Antibiotic.

Bibliography

Available online at fadavis.com

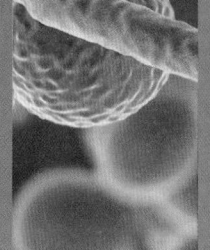

Male Reproductive System Disorders

Learning Objectives

Upon completion of this chapter, the student will be able to:

- Recognize normal physiological processes of the male reproductive tract.
- Identify major risk factors and causes of male reproductive tract disorders.
- Describe the mechanisms of major male reproductive disorders.

- Discuss signs, symptoms, and clinical manifestations of male reproductive disorders.
- Identify methods of assessment needed to diagnose male reproductive disorders.
- Explain treatment modalities used to treat male reproductive disorders.

Key Terms

Benign prostatic hyperplasia (BPH)
Benign prostatic obstruction (BPO)
Bladder outlet obstruction (BOO)
Cryptorchidism
Digital rectal examination (DRE)
Erectile dysfunction (ED)
Hematocele
Hydrocele

Hypospadias
Low testosterone syndrome (low T)
Lower urinary tract symptoms (LUTS)
Orchiectomy
Orchitis
Paraphimosis
Peyronie's disease
Phimosis

Priapism
Prostate surface antigen (PSA)
Spermatic cord
Teratogens
Varicocele
Vas deferens
Vasectomy

The male reproductive system can be divided into its external organs and internal organs. External organs are the penis, scrotum, and urethra, whereas internal organs are the testis, epididymis, vas deferens, seminal vesicles, ejaculatory ducts, prostate, and bulbourethral glands (see Fig. 27-1).

The testes are the male's sex-determining organs because of their essential functions. Each testicle contained within the scrotum produces testosterone, the hormone that endows humans with male characteristics and allows synthesis of spermatozoa. The duct system of the male reproductive system, which includes the ejaculatory ducts, epididymis, vas deferens, and penis, works to mobilize and eject sperm. The glands, which include the seminal vesicles, prostate, and bulbourethral glands, add fluid to the sperm, which is necessary to transport them in the fertilization process. To deliver sperm for fertilization, the penis has the ability to modify its structure to become erect. This is accomplished through vascular dilation and engorgement of erectile tissue, which includes the corpus cavernosum and corpus spongiosum. Dysfunction of any of the hormonal, glandular, ductile organs, or erectile tissue of the male reproductive system can cause problems for sexuality and fertility.

Epidemiology

Disorders of reproductive organs can occur throughout the whole life span of a male. At birth, cryptorchidism and hypospadias are two of the most common congenital abnormalities of the male newborn. **Cryptorchidism,** or undescended testes, is a condition in which the testicle remains within the abdomen or inguinal canal. **Hypospadias** is a disorder in which the urethral orifice of the penis is positioned abnormally. Cryptorchidism affects 2% to 9% of all newborn males and 1% to 3% of males at 3 months of age. Prematurely born males have a higher prevalence of cryptorchidism. For unknown reasons, there has been an increase in the frequency of hypospadias by 100% to 200% over the past 20 years. It occurs in 1 in 200 newborn males, making it one of the most common birth defects. In young adult males, testicular cell tumors are the most common neoplasm, whereas prostate cancer is the overall leading cancer in older males. Among White males, there has been a significant increase in the incidence of testicular cancer, with 2 to 3 times as many cases today compared with 30 to 40 years ago. In 2022, the American Cancer Society estimated 9,900 new cases of testicular cancer were diagnosed in the

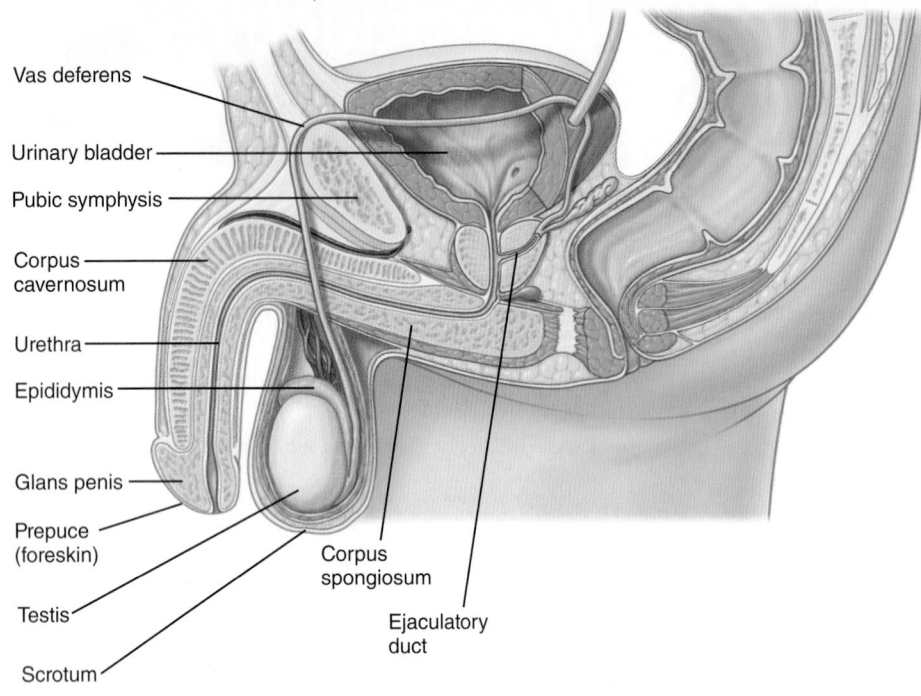

Vas deferens

Urinary bladder

Pubic symphysis

Corpus
cavernosum

Urethra

Epididymis

Glans penis

Prepuce
(foreskin)

Corpus
spongiosum

Testis

Ejaculatory
duct

Scrotum

FIGURE 27-1. The male reproductive system.

United States. Testicular cancer is highly treatable when detected early in young males. The death rate is very low; approximately 0.3 per 100,000 males per year. About 1 male in 8 will be diagnosed with prostate cancer during their lifetime. Prostate cancer is more likely to develop in older males and in non-Hispanic Black males. About 6 cases in 10 are diagnosed in males who are 65 or older. Prostate cancer is rare in males younger than 40. The American Cancer Society estimated that in 2022, there were 268,490 new cases of prostate cancer. Prostate cancer is not a cause of death in most patients who are diagnosed with it. In 2022, more than 3.1 million males in the United States had been diagnosed with prostate cancer and were living after treatment.

In Western societies, as many as 15% of all couples experience infertility problems, with rough estimates indicating that male reproductive dysfunction is responsible in at least 50% of these cases. Failure of the reproductive system affects a significant proportion of males and is of concern not only on an individual basis but also for society, where the financial burden of medical management is substantial.

Basic Concepts of Male Reproductive Function

Male sexuality, spermatogenesis, fertilization ability, and hormonal regulation are the major functions of the male reproductive organs. The most important organs that determine male sexuality are the testes, which synthesize testosterone and generate spermatozoa. Genes on the Y chromosome enable male gonads to become testes. Therefore, the father determines the gender of the fetus. The development of

testes occurs during the first trimester of gestation of the male fetus. The testes develop within the abdomen and descend into the inguinal canal by the time of birth. The descent of the testes into the scrotum occurs within the first few months of the newborn's life. The testes should completely descend into the scrotal sac by the end of the first year.

Testosterone levels remain steady through childhood until puberty, when a surge in testosterone occurs between ages 10 and 13. When a male reaches puberty, the hypothalamus begins to secrete gonadotropin-releasing hormone (GnRH), which affects the pituitary gland. The anterior pituitary is stimulated to secrete luteinizing hormone (LH) and follicle-stimulating hormone (FSH); these hormones are part of a hypothalamic–pituitary–endocrine gland feedback system (see Fig. 27-2). LH stimulates the Leydig cells of the testes to secrete testosterone, enabling the development of male secondary sexual characteristics and spermatogenesis. In this negative feedback system, high levels of testosterone inhibit LH secretion and low levels of testosterone stimulate LH. The FSH secreted by the pituitary stimulates the Sertoli cells of the seminiferous tubules to synthesize spermatozoa. The Sertoli cells also secrete a hormone called inhibin. High inhibin levels send feedback to the pituitary to decrease FSH levels. In contrast, low inhibin levels send feedback to the pituitary to increase FSH secretion by the pituitary.

A gradual, physiological, age-associated decline in serum total testosterone levels begins in males in their mid-30s and continues at an average rate of 1.6% per year.

During spermatogenesis in the testes, the process of meiosis causes each sperm cell to contain 23 chromosomes. Each spermatozoa is a gamete with half the

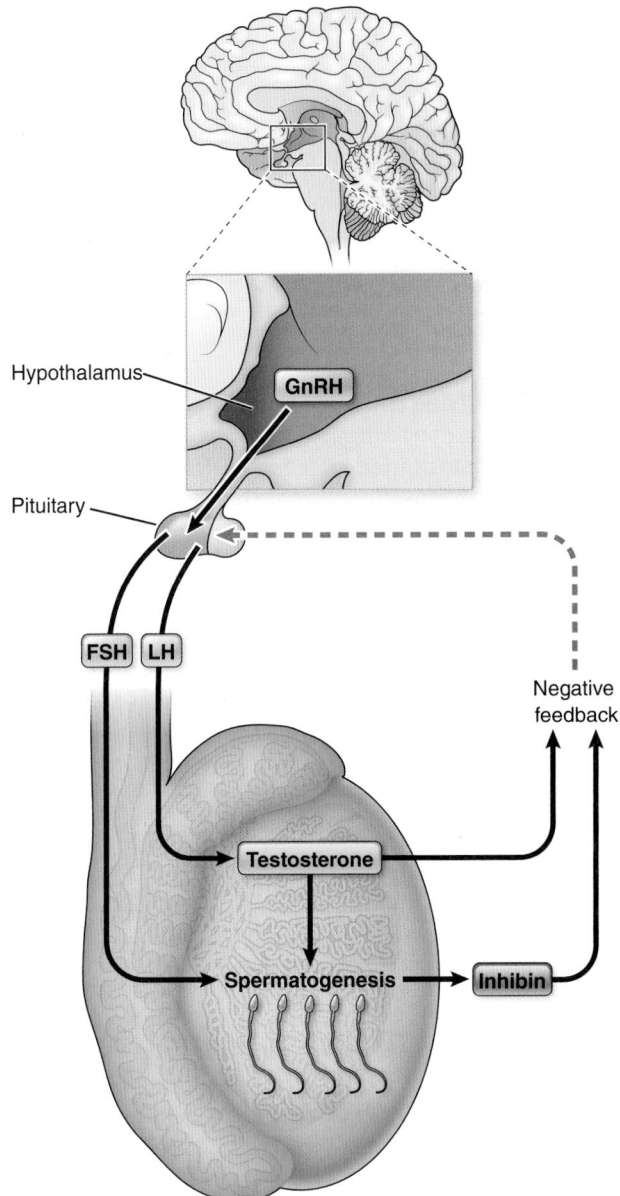

FIGURE 27-2. Endocrine control of testicular function. The hypothalamus secretes GnRH, which stimulates the pituitary to secrete LH and FSH. LH promotes testosterone secretion by the Leydig cells of the testes. Testosterone (T) is used in the synthesis of sperm. FSH promotes spermatogenesis by the Sertoli cells. Inhibin is a hormone that sends feedback to the pituitary to turn off spermatogenesis. Testosterone sends feedback to the pituitary and hypothalamus to turn off LH and GnRH. In the epididymis, spermatids mature into sperm cells.

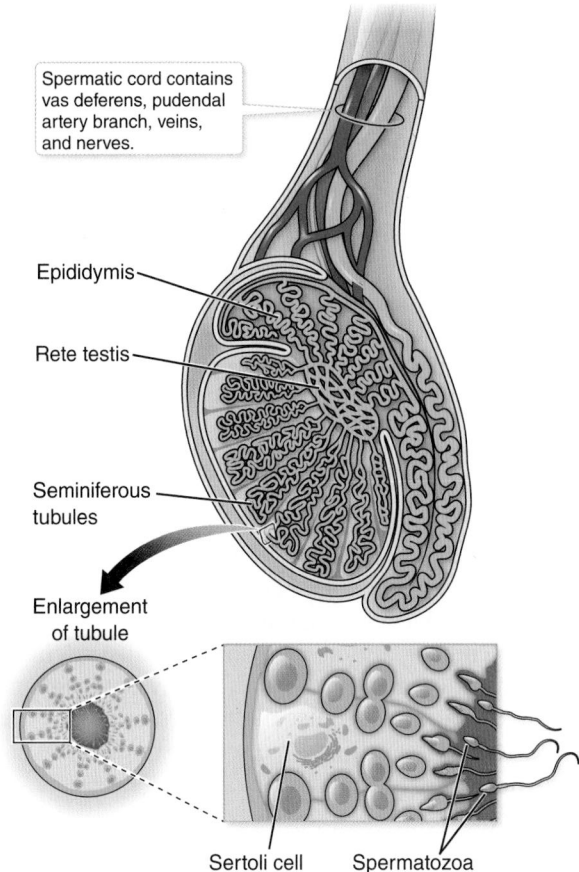

FIGURE 27-3. The testicular sac.

number of human chromosomes. When the sperm fertilizes the female's ovum, a full set of chromosomes is attained in the fertilized egg.

Millions of sperm travel daily from the seminiferous tubules to the epididymis, an organ that sits atop each testis within the testicular sac (see Fig. 27-3). Within the epididymis, sperm undergo maturation and are stored for weeks. The seminiferous tubules also produce the seminal fluid used for sperm motility.

The **vas deferens** is a tubule that ascends from the epididymis on top of each testicle and passes into the urinary bladder. The vas deferens is part of the **spermatic cord** that suspends the testicle from the abdomen into the inguinal region. The vas deferens and seminal vesicle combine to form the ejaculatory duct, which passes into the penis. The structure and function of these tubules need to be normal for male fertility. A **vasectomy** is a procedure in which the vas deferens tubule is cut and consequently blocks sperm delivery to the penis for fertilization. Vasectomy is the most popular form of surgical birth control in the United States; 7% of males aged 15 to 44 and 16% of males aged 36 to 45 undergo the procedure.

The prostate is a gland that sits below the urinary bladder and encircles the urethra. The prostate secretes an alkaline fluid that combines with seminal fluid to form the semen that promotes sperm motility. In addition, the prostate secretes **prostate surface antigen (PSA),** which can be used in the assessment of prostatic structure and function. The prostate gland enlarges naturally with age.

The bulbourethral glands, also called Cowper's glands, are two pea-sized glands located below the prostate that secrete a lubricating fluid that coats the urethra during sexual arousal. Semen, needed for sperm motility, is a combination of fluids secreted by the seminal vesicle, prostate, and bulbourethral glands.

Erectile function of the penis requires adequate circulation and autonomic neurological control. The penis consists of spongy tissue called the corpus spongiosum and corpus cavernosum. Vasodilation of the pudendal branches of the hypogastric artery allows for penile erection and ejaculation. The penile artery is a branch of the pudendal artery that vasodilates with sexual stimulation. The dorsal artery, a branch off the penile artery, provides for engorgement of the glans during erection, whereas the bulbourethral artery supplies the bulb and corpus spongiosum. The cavernous artery causes swelling of the corpus cavernosum and is principally responsible for erection. Neural control is provided by both the sympathetic and parasympathetic nervous systems. Parasympathetic nerves transmitted via the sacral spinal cord allow for penile erection. Sympathetic innervation, which arrives via the lumbar spinal cord to the penis, allows for ejaculation.

Male fertility depends on the quantity of semen, sperm count, morphology of sperm, motility of sperm, adequate circulation, intact hormonal regulation, neurological control, and normal anatomical structure of the male sex organs. Inadequacy of any of these qualities or functions can cause male reproductive system disorders.

Basic Concepts of Male Reproductive Dysfunction

Anatomical anomalies, urinary tract problems, sexually transmitted infections (STIs), trauma, injury, erectile dysfunction, and infertility are the major causes for males to seek health care for the reproductive system.

Infertility

Infertility is defined as the inability to achieve pregnancy after 1 year of unprotected intercourse. An estimated 15% of couples meet this criterion and are considered infertile, with approximately 50% due to female factors alone, 50% due to male factors alone, 20% due to a combination of female and male factors, and 15% unexplained. Fertility problems often provide the impetus for investigation into male reproductive disorders (see Box 27-1). In the assessment of the male, nearly 70% of conditions that cause infertility in males can be diagnosed through history, physical examination, and hormonal and semen analysis alone.

Causes of infertility in males can be categorized as obstructive or nonobstructive. Obstructive causes of infertility include repeated infections, vasectomy, swelling, or defects that cause blockage of sperm from entering the ejaculate. Nonobstructive causes include deficiencies in sperm formation, motility, or concentration (e.g., oligospermia [too few sperm], azoospermia [no sperm in the ejaculate]). Low sperm count, poor semen quality, or both are found to be the cause of 90% of cases of male infertility.

BOX 27-1. Causes of Male Infertility

The most common causes of male infertility include abnormal sperm production or function, impaired delivery of sperm, general health and lifestyle issues, overexposure to environmental elements, other medical conditions, and age.

ABNORMAL PRODUCTION OR FUNCTION OF SPERM
- Cryptorchidism (undescended testicles)
- Genetic defects
- Impaired shape and movement of sperm
- Low sperm concentration
- Sexually transmitted infections (STIs)
- Testosterone deficiency (male hypogonadism)
- Varicocele

IMPAIRED DELIVERY OF SPERM
- Antisperm antibodies
- Blockage of epididymis or ejaculatory ducts
- Cystic fibrosis
- Abnormal placement of urinary meatus
- No semen (ejaculate)
- Psychological issues
- Retrograde ejaculation

GENERAL HEALTH AND LIFESTYLE ISSUES
- Alcohol or substance use disorder
- Cancer and its treatment
- Emotional stress
- Malnutrition
- Obesity

OVEREXPOSURE TO ENVIRONMENTAL ELEMENTS
- Overheating the testicles
- Pesticides and other chemicals
- Substance abuse
- Tobacco smoking

OTHER MEDICAL CONDITIONS
- Severe injury
- Major surgery
- Diabetes
- Thyroid disease
- Cushing's syndrome
- Anemia

In addition to these causes, age plays a factor, as a male older than age 50 years produces about 75% less sperm than a younger male.

It is believed that in many males a genetic cause is responsible for poor spermatogenesis. Microdeletions of the Y chromosome are genetic mutations that are associated with a significant proportion of male infertility cases. Androgens, mainly testosterone, dihydrotestosterone, and a functional androgen receptor (AR), are crucial for male sexual differentiation, secondary sex characteristics at puberty, and sperm maturation. The gene for the AR is on the X chromosome at Xq11-12. An absent or dysfunctional AR gene in otherwise healthy 46,XY individuals causes androgen insensitivity syndrome, undermasculinization, and decreased spermatogenesis. Presently, over 300 different AR gene mutations have been discovered. Treatment options are based on the underlying etiology. Medical therapy or surgical procedures can optimize semen production. Assistive reproductive technologies can aid in conception with as little as one viable sperm and one egg

Erectile dysfunction (ED), also called impotence, is another cause of male infertility. There are many underlying physical and psychological causes of ED. Physiological conditions that reduce blood flow to the penis or those that cause nerve damage are etiological factors of ED.

Anatomical Abnormalities

Cryptorchidism is a condition of undescended testicles, where the testes remain high in the inguinal canal or abdominal cavity. Full descent of the testes into the scrotal sac should occur by age 1 year. The testes need to be in the scrotal sac, which is anatomically located external to the body's core. The distance from the body results in a temperature that is below normal body temperature, which is required for healthy sperm production.

Another common anatomical abnormality that can cause infertility is hypospadias. In hypospadias, the urethral orifice is located on the ventral or underside of the penis instead of the glans. When the urethral orifice is on the dorsal or anterior side of the penis, this is called epispadias.

Other anatomical disorders involve the foreskin of the penis. **Phimosis** occurs when the foreskin is too constricted and cannot easily retract from the penis. **Paraphimosis** occurs when the foreskin is in a permanently retracted position behind the tip of the penis.

Peyronie's disease is an inflammatory vasculitis of unknown etiology where the penis takes on a curvature. It occurs primarily in middle-aged and older males. Those with severe Peyronie's disease may develop scar tissue in the corpora cavernosum that impedes blood flow.

Traumatic injury of the testicles can cause disorders known as varicocele, hematocele, or hydrocele. These conditions can cause swelling of the scrotum, overheating of the testes, lack of blood flow, and interruption of sperm production. If untreated, these disorders can cause permanent male reproductive dysfunction.

Torsion of the testes can occur as a consequence of trauma to the groin; it can also arise without history of injury. In this disorder, the spermatic cord, which suspends the testes, twists and disrupts circulation to the testicle. Torsion of the testes is common in children and adolescents and is considered a urological emergency.

Testicular atrophy is observed as small, intrascrotal testes on clinical examination of the male genitalia.

When atrophy is bilateral, sterility results. Klinefelter's syndrome is a chromosomal disorder that causes a constellation of abnormalities that includes testicular atrophy.

Inflammation and Infection

STIs of the male commonly present with lesions on the penis as well as discharge. Urination is often painful, and there are signs of disease on the genitalia. The chancre of syphilis is an inflammatory ulcer-like lesion on the male genitalia. Condyloma are wartlike lesions that can be signs of syphilis or human papillomavirus (HPV). Herpes genitalis presents as small, tender vesicular lesions. STIs often ascend into organs above the testes and cause prostatitis and epididymitis (see Chapter 28). **Orchitis,** or inflammation of the testes, may be bilateral or unilateral. It is most commonly caused by a bacterial infection or mumps virus.

Precocious Puberty

Precocious puberty is considered to exist if secondary male sexual characteristics are evident before the age of 9 years. In the healthy male, growth during puberty accounts for about 15% to 20% of adult height. This growth occurs before the fusion of the bone growth plates. In precocious puberty, bone growth plate fusion occurs early and results in a reduced adult height. In addition, there is apparent adult development of the male genitalia and the presence of axillary and pubic hair. Evaluation of puberty development is done through use of Tanner staging (see Fig. 27-4).

Delayed Puberty

A teenage male who lacks testicular enlargement and has little or no pubic hair at age 14 years is considered to have delayed puberty. One of the most common causes of delayed puberty is lack of hormonal secretion by the anterior pituitary. However, systemic illnesses such as inflammatory bowel disease and chronic renal failure can also contribute to delayed puberty.

Clinical presentation in delayed puberty includes a small penis and testes, scant pubic and axillary hair, persistent high-pitched voice, gynecomastia, and long arms and legs caused by delayed bone growth plate closure.

Other Common Causes of Male Reproductive Dysfunction

Prostate gland dysfunction can cause male reproductive and urological problems. The prostate gland can be palpated through the rectal wall in the male. Prostatitis is often caused by an STI, and prostatic hyperplasia is a normal consequence of aging. Prostate cancer, the second-most common type of cancer

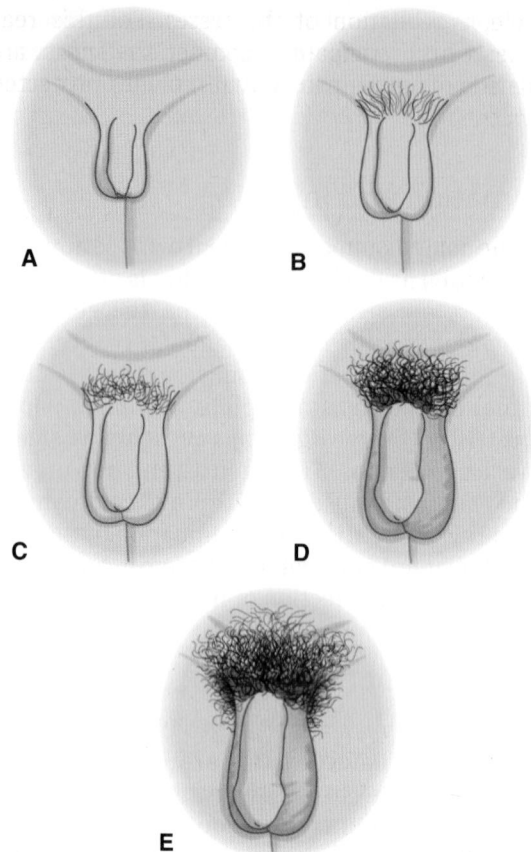

FIGURE 27-4. Male Tanner stages. (A) No pubic hair except for fine body hair similar to that on the abdomen. Penis, testes, and scrotum are the same size and proportions as in childhood. (B) Sparse growth of long, slightly pigmented, downy hair, straight or only slightly curled, chiefly at the base of the penis. Slight or no enlargement of the penis. Testes larger, scrotum larger, somewhat reddened and altered in texture. (C) Darker, coarser, curlier hair spreading sparsely over the pubic symphysis. Larger penis, especially in length. Testes and scrotum further enlarged. (D) Coarse and curly hair, as in adult; area covered greater than in stage 3 but not as great as in adult. Penis further enlarged in length and breadth, with development of glans. Testes and scrotum further enlarged; scrotal skin darkened. (E) Hair same as adult in quantity and quality, spreading to medial surfaces of thighs but not up over abdomen. Penis now adult in size and shape. Testes and scrotum now adult in size and color.

in males, can be lethal if not discovered early in the course of the disease.

Priapism is an abnormally prolonged erection of the penis in the absence of stimulation. It can be extremely painful and may last several hours. Among the known causes of priapism are the drug sildenafil, spinal cord trauma, and the vaso-occlusive crisis of sickle cell anemia.

A physiological, age-related decline in testosterone occurs in males after age 30. With aging, many patients complain of symptoms such as sexual dysfunction, low energy, weakness, and depression that in combination are referred to as **low testosterone syndrome (low T).** Currently, the role of testosterone treatment in managing age-related low testosterone is controversial.

Assessment of Male Reproductive Disorders

To diagnose male reproductive disorders, the clinician needs to inquire about risk factors, present symptoms, lifestyle, and past health history. Inquiry regarding the practice of safe sex is significant. Present and past health history are also important because systemic diseases often affect male reproductive function. A complete physical assessment is necessary and should include prostate, testicular, and rectal examination, as well as tests to rule out hernia.

Risk Factors

A number of risk factors predispose the male to reproductive disorders. Some of the most important risk factors involve fetal exposure to teratogens during gestation. **Teratogens** are toxic substances that cause the development of abnormal cell masses during fetal growth, resulting in physical defects in the fetus. Formation of the male genitalia, which is dependent on male sex hormones, occurs at about 8 to 12 weeks gestation. During this early time of pregnancy, a female can be exposed to any number of teratogens. From the late 1940s to early 1970s, an estrogenic compound, diethylstilbestrol (DES), was used to prevent miscarriages in pregnant patients. Later on, it was found that exposure to this estrogen compound during gestation caused reproductive disorders for male and female offspring. Sons of DES-treated mothers had increased risk of several male reproductive disorders, such as cryptorchidism, urethral abnormalities, epididymal cysts, and testicular hypoplasia. Potential adverse effects of estrogenic compounds on male reproductive function have been reinforced by the fact that several compounds used in industry, agriculture, or the home act as estrogen-like compounds and cause male hormone disruption. Polychlorinated biphenyl compounds found in plastics are examples of these estrogen-like compounds. Growing evidence indicates that in recent years, there has been an increased incidence in male reproductive disorders, including hypospadias and cryptorchidism in newborns, and testicular cancer and lower sperm quality in young adult males. In addition, the timing of puberty has also changed over time. Currently, the cause of these reproductive effects is a matter of intense scientific debate. However, many investigators assert there is a link between male reproductive problems and the presence of estrogenic compounds in the environment and the exposure to these compounds during fetal life.

Other than endocrine disruptors, radiation is known to cause abnormal male sexual development and lack of spermatogenesis. For this reason, the testes should be covered with a lead apron during x-ray procedures. Recent data also show that cigarette smoking has a negative effect on sperm count, as well as seminal fluid volume. Studies show that decreased sperm counts are found among sons of mothers who smoked more than 10 cigarettes per day during pregnancy. Spermatogenesis can also be negatively affected by overheating of the testes. Tight undergarments or hot baths can diminish sperm production.

Many studies focus on ED as a predominant male reproductive health disorder. Evidence suggests that lifestyle risk factors for ED are similar to those for cardiovascular disease and diabetes. These conditions include atherosclerosis, hypertension, obesity, metabolic syndrome, and smoking. Other risk factors for ED include low testosterone levels, Peyronie's disease, enlarged prostate, certain medications, alcohol use disorder and other substance use disorders, and neurological disorders. The brain also plays a key role in triggering the series of physical events that cause an erection, starting with feelings of sexual excitement. A number of psychological disorders can interfere with sexual feelings and cause ED. These include depression, anxiety, high stress, fatigue, or relationship problems.

Age is consistently associated with increased risk of male reproductive health problems, including ED and prostatic hyperplasia. Although some older males may consider poorer reproductive health a consequence of the aging process, changes caused by age are treatable. Decline in testosterone with aging is a physiological phenomenon; however, emerging evidence describes low testosterone (low T) among older males. Many describe sexual dysfunction, low energy, decreased muscle mass, decreased bone density, and other distressing symptoms. Although a controversial diagnosis, some clinicians treat this syndrome with testosterone.

Risk of male reproduction problems occurs with malformations of the male genitalia. The most common malformation, cryptorchidism, can predispose patients to testicular cancer. The exact cause of testicular cancer is unknown. Factors that increase risk include genetic predisposition, abnormal testicle development, and Klinefelter's syndrome. Other possible causes of male reproductive system cancers include exposure to certain chemicals, radiation, HIV, and HPV.

HPV is a prevalent oncogenic virus transmitted through sexual contact by all contact points in all genders. The link between cervical cancer and HPV is well established and screening of females during gynecological examination is common. However, HPV can induce anogenital, oropharyngeal, and penile cancer in males. Also, studies are emerging that show HPV infection affects health of spermatozoa and may cause male infertility. Currently, there are no HPV screening tests recommended for males. More research is needed to characterize HPV natural history at each anatomical site where HPV causes cancer in both males and females.

Trauma can also predispose individuals to reproductive disorders, such as hydrocele, hematocele, varicocele, and torsion of the testes. For this reason, males who participate in competitive sports are encouraged to wear protective gear. Unprotected sexual activity can also increase the risk of infection, which leads to male reproductive dysfunction. Urethritis, prostatitis, and epididymitis can be caused by STIs such as syphilis, gonorrhea, and herpes genitalis. Mumps virus predisposes the male to orchitis, which can lead to infertility.

Signs and Symptoms

The male patient with suspected reproductive disorders should have a complete physical examination with a focus on the lower pelvis, inguinal, and scrotal regions. When examining the male infant, the clinician should inspect and palpate the scrotal sac. The scrotum should contain palpable testes by the end of the first year of life.

In childhood, torsion of the testes is a common disorder. It causes intense unilateral scrotal pain and is a surgical emergency. Testicular torsion is seen most frequently in the 12- to 18-year-old age group, but it can occur at any age, including newborns.

During adolescence, males usually go through puberty from approximately age 11 years through 15 years. Patients age 9 years or younger may exhibit signs of precocious puberty, whereas patients aged 14 years or older may demonstrate delayed puberty. To determine the patient's stage of puberty, the patient's pelvic and inguinal region should be assessed using the Tanner stages.

Klinefelter's syndrome is a genetic disorder in which patients have a karyotype that demonstrates an extra X chromosome as XXY. Signs include small penis; small testicles; diminished pubic, axillary, and facial hair; sexual dysfunction; enlarged breast tissue; tall stature; abnormal body proportions (long legs, short trunk); learning disabilities; and a single crease in the palm.

In older males, swelling of the scrotum often indicates hydrocele, hematocele, or varicocele. The patient may complain of heaviness in the scrotal area.

Painless enlargement of a testicle is diagnostic of testicular cancer. Swollen inguinal lymph nodes, a palpable lump, and a scrotal sac that does not transilluminate are signs of cancer.

To assess the prostate gland, a **digital rectal examination (DRE)** is necessary. The prostate gland is palpable through the rectal tissue. In prostatitis, which is commonly due to infection, the gland feels boggy and is tender. In **benign prostatic hyperplasia (BPH),** the enlargement is firm, painless, and generalized. Lesions of prostate cancer are hard, painless, and unmovable. The patient with an enlarged prostate will commonly complain of **lower urinary tract symptoms (LUTS),** such as difficulty starting urinary stream, frequency, urgency, hesitancy, and weak urine stream. Urethritis, prostatitis, and epididymitis can occur in an STI.

The patient may demonstrate swollen inguinal lymph nodes and a lesion on the external genitalia or penile discharge.

Diagnosis

Because the testes are endocrine glands, diagnostic testing often involves a hormonal analysis for FSH, LH, and testosterone levels. Provocative testing of the hypothalamic–pituitary–gonadal axis can be done with a GnRH stimulation test. A normal response to this test would be elevated levels of FSH and LH. A lack of response to GnRH stimulation indicates pituitary failure; in contrast, a marked elevation in FSH and LH suggests a lack of responsiveness of the testes to produce testosterone.

When a hereditary disorder is suspected, genetic testing can be done. A karyotype can confirm disorders such as Klinefelter's syndrome, which is caused by an extra X chromosome. If cancer is suspected, the biomarkers alpha-fetoprotein and beta-human chorionic gonadotropin (b-hCG) are frequently elevated in testicular cancer. A DRE and the PSA blood test are used when prostate cancer is suspected. However, the PSA has to be carefully evaluated in conjunction with other diagnostic tests because its elevation does not always indicate cancer. Analysis of biomarkers indicative of prostate cancer is also necessary. Computed tomography (CT) scan, magnetic resonance imaging (MRI), and ultrasound-guided biopsy can be used to confirm the diagnosis of cancer. The clinician also performs a DRE with suspected prostate enlargement. Urine flow studies, ultrasound, or cystoscopy may be needed to differentiate prostate cancer from BPH. Squamous cell carcinoma of the penis, associated with HPV, is a rare cancer found mainly in uncircumcised males.

Males with STIs will often present with inflammatory, vesicular, or wartlike lesions of the genitalia and penile discharge. Swollen inguinal lymph nodes often can be palpated. Culture of the lesions and discharge can reveal such pathogens as gonorrhea, syphilis, herpes genitalis, HPV, or *Chlamydia*. Urinalysis and urine culture may also identify the infecting microorganism. Because STIs increase one's susceptibility to HIV infection, HIV testing should be done.

Certain laboratory tests are necessary to diagnose infertility. Semen analysis is the cornerstone of the male infertility work-up. A specimen is collected into a clean, dry, sterile container or during coitus using special condoms containing no spermicidal lubricants. The normal quantity of semen is 1.5 to 5 mL; optimally, it should contain 50 to 250 million sperm per mL. The patient should be abstinent for 2 to 3 days prior to collection of the sample to maximize sperm number and quality. Each day of abstinence is typically associated with an increase in semen volume of 0.4 mL and an increase in sperm density by 10 to 15 million sperm/mL for up to 7 days. The sample should be processed within 1 hour, and two to three samples (at a minimum of 2 to 3 days apart) should be evaluated because of daily variations in sperm number and quality. Various parameters are measured, such as ejaculate volume and sperm density, quality, motility, and morphology.

Common Treatments for Male Reproductive Disorders

Anatomical anomalies such as cryptorchidism, phimosis, hypospadias, and epispadias require surgical treatment. Hydrocele, varicocele, and torsion of the testes also require surgical intervention.

Treatment of STI depends on the microorganism involved. Some STIs are asymptomatic in males but cause symptoms in the female. Antibiotic medication and patient education regarding safe sex are the interventions for the STIs causing urethritis, prostatitis, and epididymitis. Importantly, the patient should be advised to inform sexual partners of the need for treatment as well.

Surgical intervention is often needed for prostate disorders. BPH often causes hyperplastic cell growth around the urethra, which interferes with urination. There are various minimally invasive surgical procedures to remove the hyperplastic tissue of BPH. However, medications can also be used to relieve the pressure of the prostate on the urethra.

Surgical excision of the prostate may be required if cancer is present. When radical prostatectomy is done, pelvic lymph nodes are removed and examined. Radiation in the form of an implant or external beam delivery is commonly necessary. Antiandrogenic hormone chemotherapy may also be required.

When testicular cancer is diagnosed, **orchiectomy**, which is removal of the testicle, and radiation are the common treatment procedures. Chemotherapy or bone marrow transplant may be required. Because treatment causes sterility, freezing of sperm before treatment is commonly done for future procreation.

Disorders of the Male Reproductive System

The common disorders of the male reproductive system include BPH, ED, and prostate cancer. These problems mainly occur in older males. Also, in older males, age-related deficiency of testosterone can cause distressing symptoms referred to as low T. Testicular cancer is a disorder of young adult males, as are testicular torsion, varicocele, hydrocele, and hematocele.

Benign Prostatic Hyperplasia

BPH is characterized by excessive cell growth of the prostate gland, a physiological change of aging. Approximately 14 million males annually have symptoms associated with BPH. The prevalence of BPH in European American and African American males is similar, though the disorder tends to be more severe and progressive in African American males. Males older than age 50 have roughly a 50% chance of developing BPH, and by age 80, 80% to 90% of males are diagnosed with it. The etiology of BPH is testosterone-sensitive cellular proliferation and lack of cellular apoptosis in the prostate gland.

The prostate is a walnut-sized gland that is located anterior to the rectum and below the urinary bladder. The urethra runs through its middle and connects with the penile urethra (see Fig. 27-5). The gland is composed of different kinds of cellular sections called the peripheral, central, anterior, and transition zones. BPH originates in the transition zone, which surrounds the urethra. Cellular proliferation encroaches on the urethra and causes obstruction of urine flow from the bladder, known as **bladder outlet obstruction (BOO).**

The main function of the prostate gland is secretion of an alkaline fluid that comprises approximately 70% of the seminal volume. The secretions produce lubrication and nutrition for the sperm, and the alkaline fluid in the ejaculate helps neutralize the acidic vaginal environment. The prostatic urethra is a conduit for semen and closes off the bladder neck during sexual climax in order to prevent retrograde ejaculation (ejaculation resulting in semen being forced backward into the bladder).

The diagnosis of BPH is often based on the patient signs and symptoms (see Box 27-2). The patient is commonly asked to complete a survey called the International Prostate Symptom Score/American Urological Association Symptom Index (IPSS/AUA-SI). This survey asks the patient questions regarding common

---

BOX 27-2. Signs and Symptoms of Benign Prostatic Hyperplasia

Several symptoms are characteristic of BPH. Usually, these occur in males older than age 50.
- Dribbling of urine
- Frequency
- Hesitancy
- Retention of urine in bladder
- Straining to urinate
- Weak urinary stream
- Urgency

---

symptoms of BPH. Signs and symptoms include lower urinary tract symptoms (LUTS) due to **benign prostate obstruction (BPO).** These include the need to urinate frequently during the day or night but voiding only small amounts of urine with each episode, termed frequency. Also, the patient reports the sudden urge to urinate (urgency), incomplete emptying of the bladder (urine retention in bladder), interruptions in the flow of urine (hesitancy), and the loss of small amounts of urine (urinary incontinence). In addition, the patient with BPH is susceptible to lower urinary tract infection because of retained urine in the bladder, which provides a medium for bacterial growth.

To physically assess the patient for BPH, the clinician performs a DRE. The posterior wall of the prostate can be palpated through the anterior wall of the rectal vault (see Fig. 27-6). On physical examination, the hyperplastic prostate is enlarged, smooth, firm, and nontender. A PSA blood test should be done to

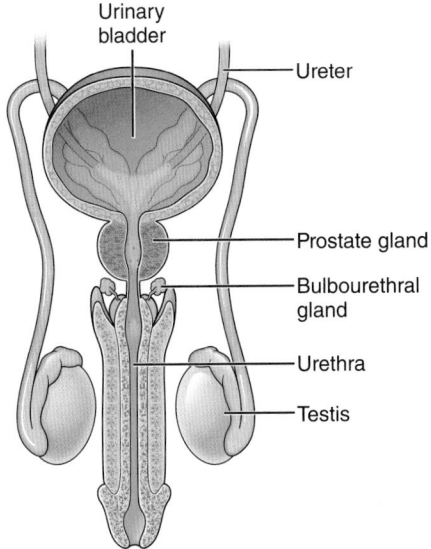

FIGURE 27-5. Cross-section of the prostate gland, urinary bladder, and urethra. The prostate gland surrounds the male urethra; with hyperplasia, the prostate can encroach on the urethra, causing obstruction to urinary flow.

Urinary bladder
Ureter
Prostate gland
Bulbourethral gland
Urethra
Testis

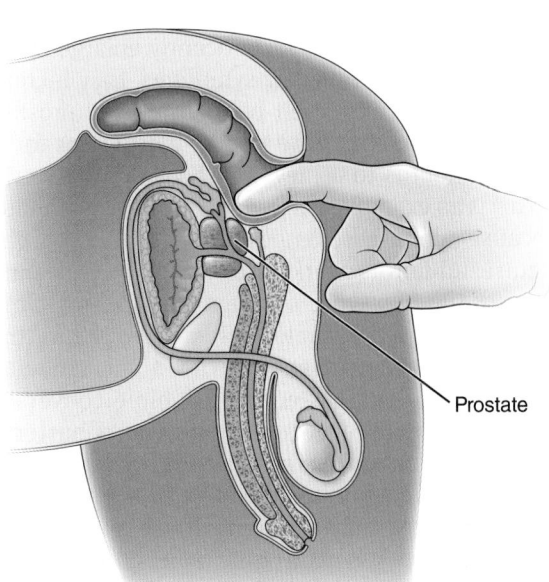

Prostate

FIGURE 27-6. DRE. The clinician can use DRE to assess the prostate gland, which can be palpated through the rectal wall.

rule out prostate cancer. However, a diagnosis of prostate cancer cannot be based solely on PSA testing because the test has a high false-positive rate. The Prostate Health Index (PHI), PSA antigen3, and the 4Kscore, which use total PSA, free PSA, p2PSA to estimate risk, have shown greater predictive values for cancer detection than the PSA test alone. The 4Kscore test is a blood test that assesses a patient's probability for aggressive prostate cancer after an abnormal PSA or DRE result. In addition, MRI with or without transrectal ultrasonography (TRUS) targeted biopsy has shown high detection rates. Urine flow studies, ultrasound, and cystoscopy are other diagnostic tests that may be done.

> **CLINICAL CONCEPT**
>
> At age 50, males should begin having yearly examinations for BPH and prostate cancer, which include DRE and PSA testing. PSA test alone cannot be used to diagnose prostate cancer.

Medical and surgical treatments are available for BPH. The two primary drug classes used for BPH are alpha-adrenergic blockers and 5-alpha-reductase inhibitors. Alpha-blocker drugs relax smooth muscles, especially in the bladder neck and prostate. Alpha-adrenergic blockers help relieve BPH symptoms, but they do not reduce the size of the prostate. However, they can help improve urine flow and reduce the risk of bladder obstruction. They are often the first choice, especially for patients with smaller prostates. A typical alpha-adrenergic blocker is tamsulosin (Flomax).

The 5-alpha-reductase inhibitors are drugs that block the conversion of testosterone to dihydrotestosterone, the male hormone that stimulates the prostate. These drugs are for patients with significantly enlarged prostates. In addition to relieving symptoms, they increase urinary flow and may even help shrink the prostate. However, patients may have to take these drugs for up to 6 to 12 months to achieve full benefits. Finasteride (Proscar) is an example of a 5-alpha-reductase inhibitor.

Because alpha-adrenergic blockers and 5-alpha-reductase inhibitors work in different ways, combinations of the two types of drugs may control symptoms in select patients more effectively than either drug alone. Because of the ability of 5-alpha-reductase inhibitors such as finasteride to inhibit conversion of testosterone to dihydrotestosterone, finasteride may cause abnormalities of the external genitalia of a male fetus when administered to a pregnant female. Females who are or may be pregnant should not handle crushed or broken finasteride tablets.

In addition to alpha-adrenergic blockers and 5-alpha-reductase inhibitors, phosphodiesterase-5 (PDE5) inhibitors are known to stimulate smooth muscle relaxation in the lower urinary tract. The long-acting PDE5 inhibitor tadalafil (Cialis) has commonly been used to improve the symptoms of BPH. Anticholinergic agents can be used in some patients with BPH to limit frequent urination. Herbal agents, such as extracts of saw palmetto and pumpkin seeds, have also been used to relieve urinary symptoms associated with BPH.

> **CLINICAL CONCEPT**
>
> 5-alpha-reductase inhibitor drugs decrease PSA levels, which may mask the presence of prostate cancer.

> **ALERT!** Females should not handle finasteride tablets when they are or may become pregnant.

Several different kinds of surgical procedures can be used to reduce prostatic obstruction of the urethra. These include transurethral needle ablation (TUNA), transurethral microwave or laser treatment, transurethral resection of the prostate (TURP), and transurethral incision of the prostate (TUIP). In all of these procedures, the obstructive prostatic tissue is excised so that the urethra can allow free flow of urine. Prostatic stents and a prostatic implant called the UroLift can be inserted to mechanically reduce the prostatic cellular obstruction. Another procedure, radiofrequency-generated water thermotherapy, uses steam to diminish the prostatic cellular obstruction of the urethra. Other minimally invasive surgical procedures include temporary implantable nitinol device (iTIND), prostate artery embolization (PAE), aquablation, and anatomical endoscopic enucleation of the prostate (AEEP). Aquablation utilizes machine-controlled water jets to ablate the soft tissue of the prostate. Open prostatectomy may be required for large prostatic obstructions of the urethra. This procedure requires hospitalization and involves the use of general/regional anesthesia and a lower abdominal incision. The inner core of the prostate is removed, leaving the peripheral zone intact. Laparoscopic simple prostatectomy is similar to open prostatectomy but is less invasive, involving only a small pelvic incision.

Erectile Dysfunction

Disorders such as ED and female sexual dysfunction are receiving more attention as a result of the aging of the population, direct-to-consumer mass marketing of pharmaceuticals, and new therapies. Sexual dysfunction is highly prevalent in males and females. Complete ED is defined as (1) the total inability to obtain or maintain an erection during sexual stimulation and (2) the absence of nocturnal erections. In the landmark Massachusetts Male Aging Study (MMAS) of 1987–2004, a community-based survey of males aged 40 to 70 years, 52% of the respondents reported some degree of erectile difficulty. However, complete ED was reported by only 10% of the respondents. Extrapolating the MMAS data to the American population, an estimated 18 to 30 million males are affected by ED annually.

ED is essentially a vascular disease. It is often associated with other vascular diseases and conditions such as diabetes, hypertension, and coronary artery disease. Diabetes is a well-recognized cause of ED, affecting approximately 50% of males with diabetes. Diabetes causes endothelial damage and neurological impairment, which leads to circulatory and structural changes in penile tissues. For erection to occur, dilation and engorgement of the penis are required. Arterial insufficiency, defective smooth muscle relaxation, inadequate pudendal neurological control, and lack of engorgement of the corpora cavernosum and spongiosum tissues are effects of diabetes, and these conditions together cause dysfunction of the penis.

Additionally, ED is often an adverse effect of many commonly prescribed medications. Some drugs such as antidepressants, antipsychotic agents, and beta blockers can cause ED. Males with sleep disorders commonly experience ED. Another important consideration is the patient's hormonal status. Low testosterone syndrome, also called low T, can cause low libido and erectile function. There is a wide array of possible causes of ED (see Box 27-3).

Most patients with ED have multiple etiological factors, so assessing how much each is contributing to the problem is difficult. Because of the various possible causes of ED, a thorough general health and sexual history is necessary to correctly identify the specific etiology in an individual. It is difficult to assess the prevalence of ED. Often, clinicians do not complete a sexual history; therefore, it is believed that ED is underdiagnosed. Conversely, it is believed that ED is overdiagnosed as a result of intense mass-media marketing efforts directed toward the public regarding sexual expectations. To diagnose ED, patients may be submitted to laboratory studies; however, in many cases, treatment is based on the patient's subjective symptoms.

Laboratory diagnostic tests include an evaluation of the patient's hormone status, particularly if the symptom is diminished or absent libido. Patients who demonstrate any signs of diminished secondary sexual characteristics should have an endocrine evaluation that consists of measuring morning serum testosterone levels. A measurement of LH and, in some instances, prolactin is obtained if the patient has evidence of pituitary dysfunction or cases of low serum testosterone levels. Hemoglobin A1c, serum chemistry studies, lipid profiles, thyroid hormones,

> ### BOX 27-3. Causes of Erectile Dysfunction
>
> The following are common causes of ED, which most commonly occurs in middle-aged and older adult males.
> - Alcohol and other substance use disorders
> - Atherosclerosis
> - Certain prescription medications
> - Diabetes
> - Fatigue
> - Heart disease
> - High blood pressure
> - Low testosterone
> - Mental health conditions such as depression and anxiety
> - Metabolic syndrome
> - Multiple sclerosis
> - Obesity
> - Parkinson's disease
> - Peyronie's disease; development of scar tissue inside the penis
> - Stress
> - Surgeries or injuries that affect the pelvic area or spinal cord
> - Tobacco use
> - Treatments for prostate cancer or enlarged prostate

and prostate-specific antigen levels should be obtained to assess general health. A urinalysis looking for red blood cells, white blood cells, protein, and glucose is also important. Following completion of this phase, the clinician should be able to determine the patient's medical status; to identify and characterize the type of dysfunction; and to determine the need for additional testing, such as penile or pelvic blood flow studies, nocturnal penile tumescence testing, or other blood tests. Many imaging studies can be used to diagnose ED, but these are rarely performed.

Mechanical devices, implants, and injectable medications are available for ED; however, oral PDE inhibitor medication is the most commonly prescribed treatment. Sildenafil (Viagra), tadalafil (Cialis), and vardenafil (Levitra) are PDE inhibitors. These drugs block the release of PDE in the corpus cavernosum of the penis. Blocking the enzyme PDE enhances the effects of nitric oxide, the natural chemical that produces vasodilation and relaxation of smooth muscles in the penis.

ALERT! PDE inhibitors, such as sildenafil, are absolutely contraindicated in patients taking nitrates. PDE inhibitors potentiate the vasodilatory effects of the nitrate-based medication, resulting in a severe drop in blood pressure.

Low Testosterone Syndrome (Low T)

Low testosterone syndrome (low T) is age-related low testosterone that is accompanied by clinical symptoms associated with androgen deficiency. Currently, there is no well-defined, universally accepted low level of testosterone level that is correlated with adverse health outcomes. However, clinicians define testosterone deficiency in older males as at least three sexual symptoms with a total testosterone level less than 11.1 nanomole/L (320 ng/dL). Sexual symptoms include low libido, erectile dysfunction, and decreased volume of ejaculate. Using these criteria, the incidence of low T in the United States is reported to be approximately 20% in males older than 60, 30% in those older than 70, and 50% in those older than 80 years. Diagnosis and treatment of this condition is controversial. Other symptoms that males with low T find distressing include low energy, weakness, decreased muscle mass, decreased bone density, emotional depressive symptoms, and loss of body and facial hair.

The American College of Physicians (ACP) suggests treating males with low T who have symptoms of sexual dysfunction and seek to improve sexual function. Patients should be counseled about potential benefits, harms, and costs of testosterone treatment. However, the ACP recommends that clinicians not initiate testosterone treatment in patients to improve energy, vitality, physical function, or cognition. The ACP recommends intramuscular rather than transdermal formulations of testosterone as costs are considerably lower for the intramuscular formulation and clinical effectiveness and risks are similar. Also, clinicians should reevaluate symptoms within 12 months and periodically thereafter. Clinicians should discontinue testosterone treatment in males who have been treated but show no improvement in sexual function.

Testicular Torsion

Testicular torsion most commonly occurs in adolescents, although it can occur at any age in the male, even prenatally. Anatomically, the testicle is covered by a fibrous tissue called the tunica vaginalis, which is contained—along with the vas deferens—in a spermatic cord that attaches to the anterior two-thirds of the testicle (see Fig. 27-7). In some patients, there is a congenital anatomical anomaly of high attachment of the tunica vaginalis that allows the testicle to rotate freely. This congenital abnormality is present in approximately 12% of males. Testicular torsion occurs when the testis rotates around the axis of the spermatic cord. Testicular torsion can obstruct blood flow to the testicle, which can lead to ischemia and infarction of the testicle. For this reason, testicular torsion is a urological emergency, as a delay in diagnosis and treatment can lead to loss of the testicle.

Symptoms include sudden onset of severe unilateral scrotal pain. Torsion can occur during activity or

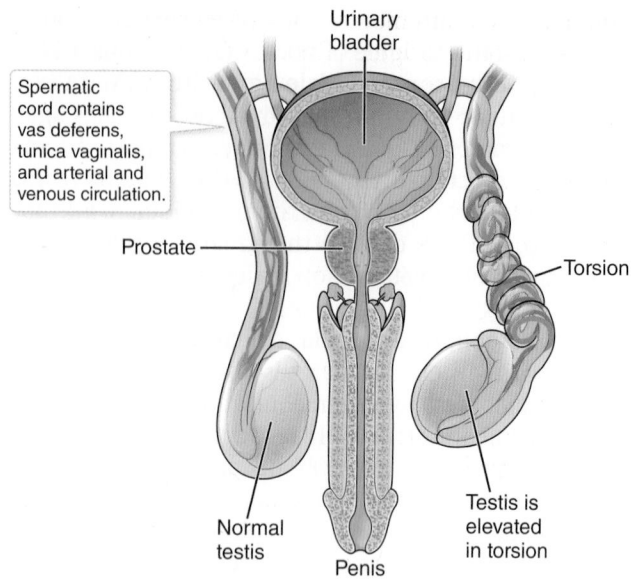

FIGURE 27-7. Testicular torsion is an acute, painful disorder where the spermatic cord twists and cuts off circulation to the testicle. Upon examination, the affected testicle will be elevated up toward the abdomen because of shortening of the spermatic cord.

rest; it is related to trauma in 4% to 8% of cases. Scrotal swelling, erythema, abdominal pain, nausea, and vomiting are other symptoms. The diagnosis of testicular torsion is based on symptoms and clinical presentation. Laboratory tests and imaging studies usually are not necessary. The patient should go directly to surgery without any delay to perform diagnostic studies. If there is uncertainty regarding the diagnosis, radionuclide scan of the testicles or ultrasonography can be helpful to assess blood flow and to differentiate torsion from other conditions. Emergency detorsion surgery is the treatment. There are few complications if detorsion surgery is implemented within 6 hours of pain; however, loss of the testicle can occur if surgery is delayed for 12 to 24 hours.

Testicular Cancer

Testicular cancer is rare, representing 0.5% of cancers in the population. It is the most common cancer in males between the ages of 15 and 35 years in the United States; 50% occur in males aged 20 to 34. Approximately 10,000 new cases are diagnosed annually. The lifetime chance of developing testicular cancer is about 1 in 270, and the risk of dying is very low—about 1 in 5,000. The incidence of testicular cancer is fivefold higher in European Americans than in African Americans; however, African Americans tend to present with more severe disease and have a much worse prognosis. The risk for the disease is higher in first-degree relatives of cancer patients than in the general population.

The most common type of testicular cancer is a germ cell tumor, which is a cellular neoplasm inside the testes. Germ cell tumors are classified as either a seminoma or nonseminoma, based on cellular derivation. Seminomas originate in the germinal epithelium of the seminiferous tubules. About half of germ cell tumors of the testis are seminomas.

In patients with cryptorchidism, the risk of developing a testicular germ cell tumor is increased fourfold to eightfold. Other risk factors include family history, infertility, prior testicular cancer, HIV infection, and environmental exposures. Exposure to DES in utero, Agent Orange, and numerous industrial chemicals increase cancer risk. Persons with Klinefelter's syndrome (47,XXY) and Down syndrome (trisomy 21) have an increased risk of testicular cancer. Also, studies have shown a genetic risk of testicular cancer; 80% of testicular tumors have one or more copies of the short arm of chromosome 12. There is an overexpression of the oncogene *CCDN2* at 12p13, which causes excessive cellular proliferation.

The most common presenting symptom is painless swelling, nodule, or mass lesion of one testicle. On physical examination, the mass cannot be separated from the testis. Dull ache or heavy sensation in the lower abdomen also could be presenting symptoms. Patients who experience a hematoma with trauma should undergo evaluation to rule out testicular cancer.

A complete history and physical examination is needed for diagnosis. On physical examination, a cancer is palpable as a solid, immobile, nontender mass in the scrotum. Diagnostic tests include a chemistry profile, complete blood count, and the serum tumor markers alpha-fetoprotein (AFP) and b-hCG. Ultrasound, CT scan, and lymph node examination are usually done, and biopsy of the testicular mass is necessary. Staging of testicular cancer follows the tumor, node, metastasis system (see Chapter 40). Treatment involves orchiectomy; radiation and chemotherapy also may be necessary. Because 45% to 55% of testicular cancer patients are infertile after therapy, those patients who wish to preserve fertility are offered semen cryopreservation before treatment.

Testicular cancer has one of the highest cure rates of all cancers: greater than 90%; that rate increases to essentially 100% if it has not metastasized. Even for the relatively few cases in which malignant cancer has spread widely, chemotherapy offers a cure rate of at least 85%.

Varicocele, Hematocele, and Hydrocele

A **varicocele** is a dilation of the veins within the scrotum. Approximately 15% to 20% of the healthy fertile male population is estimated to have asymptomatic varicoceles. However, varicoceles are often the cause of infertility and are discovered when the male patient is unable to conceive. Alternatively, the patient may report scrotal pain or heaviness. Careful physical examination remains the primary method of varicocele detection. An obvious varicocele is often demonstrated by a swollen scrotum and palpated by the examiner as a "bag of worms." If physical examination findings are uncertain, high-resolution color flow Doppler ultrasonography is the diagnostic method of choice. Acute problems such as torsion of the testes or hernia need to be ruled out because they also cause a swollen scrotum. Also, abdominal or pelvic mass lesions should be ruled out because they can obstruct testicular blood flow and present as a varicocele. Microsurgical repair is the treatment.

Hydrocele is a collection of serous fluid in the scrotum that causes swelling and a feeling of heaviness. **Hematocele** is a collection of blood in the scrotum that causes the same symptoms. Hydrocele and hematocele are often caused by trauma or infection of the testes. Edema fluid or ruptured blood vessels, respectively, cause each. The scrotum can be transilluminated with a penlight to aid in diagnosis. Ultrasound of the scrotum is also used. Allowing the body to reabsorb the fluid or blood requires watchful waiting as treatment. If absorption does not occur, surgical evacuation of fluid may be necessary.

Chapter Summary

- The male reproductive system is an endocrine feedback system of the hypothalamus that produces GnRH, which stimulates the anterior pituitary to secrete FSH and LH. FSH stimulates spermatozoa production by the testes. LH stimulates testosterone secretion by the testes.

- The most important organs that determine male sexuality are the testes, which synthesize testosterone and generate spermatozoa. The testes need to lie away from the body because optimal spermatogenesis requires temperatures cooler than the core body temperature.

- Puberty can be assessed using criteria set forth by the Tanner stages. Precocious puberty in males occurs when secondary sexual characteristics develop before age 9 years. Delayed puberty in males occurs when sexual development is not occurring by age 14 years.

- Phthalates, bisphenol A, pesticides, and environmental contaminants such as polychlorinated biphenyls and dioxins are known endocrine-disrupting chemicals that have been shown to negatively affect both male and female reproduction.

- Cryptorchidism is the disorder where the testes remain in the abdomen or high in the inguinal canal and do not descend into the scrotum. The testes should lie within the scrotum by the end of the first year of life. Untreated cryptorchidism is a risk factor for testicular cancer.

- Hypospadias and epispadias are anatomical anomalies of the penis. The urethral opening is on the posterior side of the penis in hypospadias and on the anterior side of the penis in epispadias.

- Hydrocele, varicocele, and hematocele are disorders of the scrotum that can occur with trauma.

- Torsion of the testes is an acute condition caused by twisting of the testicle on the spermatic cord. It is extremely painful and a medical emergency.

- BPH is common in males older than 50 years. Physiologically, the prostate enlarges with age, which causes bladder outlet obstruction (BOO).

- BPH can obstruct the urethra and cause urinary symptoms that include urgency, frequency, hesitancy, weak urinary stream, and urinary tract infection. These symptoms are referred to as lower urinary tract symptoms (LUTS) due to benign prostatic obstruction (BPO).

- BPH can be treated with medication or various types of minimally invasive transurethral surgical procedures.

- Testicular cancer, although rare, is the most common cancer in males between ages 15 and 35 years. It is highly treatable.

- Prostate cancer is the most common cancer in males older than age 50. DRE and PSA testing are two screening procedures that can be used to prevent this cancer. Males older than age 50 years should have a prostate examination yearly.

- The PSA test has a high rate of false-positive results for prostate cancer. The diagnosis cannot be based solely on PSA test results. Biomarker tests that include the prostate antigen 3 test, Prostate Health Index (PHI), and the 4Kscore are necessary. MRI-targeted, transrectal ultrasound–guided tissue biopsy is commonly performed.

- From adolescence to middle age, STIs cause significant acute and chronic pain, infertility, and contagious disease. Many STIs are often silent in the male but symptomatic in the female. Prostatitis is most often due to an STI.

- HPV is an oncogenic sexually transmitted virus associated with anogenital, oropharyngeal, and penile cancer in males. It is also emerging as a potential cause of infertility in males.

- ED is common in males with atherosclerosis or diabetes, which impede blood flow to the penis. Medications such as beta blockers, antidepressants, and antipsychotic agents can also cause ED. Phosphodiesterase inhibitors can treat ED. Nitrates are contraindicated with use of medications for ED.

- Older adult males with sexual dysfunction and other symptoms may suffer from low testosterone syndrome (low T), which may require testosterone treatment.

Making the Connections

Disorder and Pathophysiology

Signs and Symptoms	Physical Assessment Findings	Diagnostic Testing	Treatment
Cryptorchidism | Undescended testes that remain in the abdomen or within the inguinal canal.			
Infertility.	Lack of palpable testes in the scrotum.	CT scan of pelvis and abdomen.	Surgery to bring testes down into scrotum.
Hypospadias/Epispadias | Penile orifice misplaced either above or below the glans penis.			
Difficult urination.	Penile orifice apparently misplaced.	Clinical examination.	Surgery to place urethral opening in the tip of the penis.
Testicular Torsion | Testicular tunica vaginalis twisted and obstructing blood flow to testes.			
Acute pain in the scrotum.	Erythema, swelling, and tenderness of scrotum.	Clinical examination.	Surgery; testicular removal may be necessary.
ED | Inability of the penis to achieve erection.			
Infertility.	None.	Patient history.	PDE inhibitor medications such as sildenafil cause vascular vasodilation in the penis. Implants and other devices available.

Making the Connections–cont'd

Signs and Symptoms	Physical Assessment Findings	Diagnostic Testing	Treatment
BPH | Increased cellular growth and size of prostate gland with urethral obstruction; this is a normal physiological change of aging.			
Urinary frequency, urgency, hesitancy, straining to urinate, weak stream, nocturia, susceptibility to urinary tract infection.	Enlarged prostate palpable on DRE.	DRE; clinician palpates enlarged prostate. PSA blood test shows elevated PSA level. Biomarker testing is necessary along with PSA test. PSA antigen 3, Prostate Health Index, and 4Kscore to rule out prostate cancer. CT scan shows enlarged prostate. MRI/transrectal ultrasound-guided biopsy.	Alpha-adrenergic blocker medications, 5-alpha-reductase inhibitors. Various surgical procedures include prostatic urethral lift (Urolift), convective radiofrequency water vapor thermal therapy (Rezum), temporary implantable nitinol device (iTIND), prostate artery embolization (PAE), transurethral resection of the prostate (TURP), photoselective vaporization of the prostate (PVP), aquablation, and anatomical endoscopic enucleation of the prostate (AEEP).
Testicular Cancer | Most common cancer type is germ cell seminoma; neoplastic growth of the seminiferous tubule cells.			
Swelling or mass in testes within scrotum.	Swelling or mass in testes within scrotum.	Elevated AFP and beta-hCG. Biopsy.	Surgery. Cryopreservation of sperm. Radiation. Chemotherapy.
Hydrocele, Hematocele, Varicocele | Hydrocele is fluid in the scrotal sac, causing swelling of the scrotum. Hematocele is a collection of blood in the scrotal sac. Varicocele is a condition of distended veins and lack of blood drainage of the testes.			
Heaviness and swelling in scrotum.	Swelling in scrotum.	Ultrasound shows fluid or enlarged vessels in the scrotum.	Surgery to drain fluid from scrotum.

Bibliography

Available online at fadavis.com

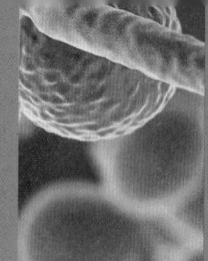

Sexually Transmitted Infections

Learning Objectives

Upon completion of this chapter, the student will be able to:

- Identify the common sexually transmitted infections (STIs) within the population.
- Recognize the signs, symptoms, and clinical manifestations of STIs within the population.
- Discuss risk factors and modes of transmission of STIs within the population.

- Describe the screening tests and laboratory procedures used to diagnose STIs within the population.
- Explain the potential complications of undiagnosed or untreated STIs in affected patients.
- Discuss pharmacological, nonpharmacological, and preventive modalities used in the treatment and prevention of STIs in the population.

Key Terms

Bacterial vaginosis (BV)

Buboes

Chancroid

Chancre

Chandelier sign

Chlamydia trachomatis

Chronic respiratory papillomatosis

Condyloma acuminata

Condyloma lata

Donovanosis

Granuloma inguinale

Gummas

Herpes simplex virus

Human papillomavirus (HPV)

Hutchinson teeth

Jarisch–Herxheimer reaction

Lesbian, gay, bisexual, transgender, and queer+ (LGBTQ+)

Lymphogranuloma venereum (LGV)

Men who have sex with men (MSM)

Mycoplasma genitalium

Neisseria gonorrhoeae

Nucleic acid amplification test (NAAT)

Ophthalmia neonatorum

Pelvic inflammatory disease (PID)

Polymerase chain reaction (PCR)

Sexually transmitted infection (STI)

Syphilis

Tabes dorsalis

Treponema pallidum

Trichomoniasis

Urethritis

Women who have sex with women (WSW)

Zika virus (ZIKV)

A **sexually transmitted infection (STI),** also termed *sexually transmitted disease* or *venereal disease,* is an infection that is transmitted between humans by means of sexual behavior, including vaginal intercourse, oral sex, and anal sex. A person with an STI is infected and may potentially infect others, with or without showing signs of disease. Some STIs can also be transmitted via blood, reuse of IV drug needles, pregnancy, childbirth, and breastfeeding.

STIs affect both males and females. In pregnant females, STIs can have adverse effects on the fetus. In terms of transmission, STIs are highly contagious, so prevention and screening are important interventions, particularly in the teen and young adult populations.

Most STIs are treated with antibiotics and behavior modification. However, some STIs, such as HIV infection, can cause significant morbidity and mortality (see Chapter 11 for information on HIV infection).

Epidemiology

STIs are a major public health challenge in the United States, with approximately 26 million new cases annually. Approximately 50% of STIs occur in persons ages 15 to 24 years. Although older teens and young adults have the highest rate of STIs, within the past 5 years, STI rates among those age 55 and older have more than doubled. In 2014, older adults had an average population rate of chlamydia, gonorrhea, and syphilis of 11.8 per 100,000 people. In 2019, the average rate of these STIs in older adults was 24.8 per 100,000.

According to the Centers for Disease Control and Prevention (CDC), as of 2021, there are nine common STIs in the United States, including human papillomavirus (HPV), chlamydia, gonorrhea, syphilis, trichomoniasis, bacterial vaginosis, genital herpes, hepatitis B virus (HBV), and HIV. There are five nationally reportable STIs: chlamydia, gonorrhea, syphilis, HIV, and chancroid.

In the United States, there are large disparities in the incidence of STIs by race, age, and sexual orientation. Men who have sex with men (MSM), considered a sexual minority, have the highest incidence of STIs. MSM are disproportionately at risk for HIV infection. In the United States, the estimated lifetime risk for HIV infection among MSM is 1 in 6, compared with heterosexual males at 1 in 524 and heterosexual females at 1 in 253. It is important to recognize that STIs can occur in various anatomical sites depending on sexual activity. Studies have demonstrated that among MSM, prevalence of rectal gonorrhea and chlamydia ranges from 0.2% to 24% and 2.1% to 23%, respectively, and prevalence of pharyngeal gonorrhea and chlamydia ranges from 0.5% to 16.5% and 0% to 3.6%, respectively.

Individuals who are members of racial and ethnic minority groups continue to face a disproportionate share of new and chronic cases of STIs. Due to barriers such as poverty, decreased access to health care, perceived stigma of STIs, and limited trust in health care providers, incidence and prevalence rates of STIs have consistently remained higher among members of racial and ethnic minority populations. For example, gonorrhea rates among Blacks are several times higher than those of Whites and Hispanics. The gonorrhea rate among Hispanics is twice that of Whites, while American Indians/Alaska natives have STI rates four times that of Whites. These statistics not only highlight the importance of providing culturally tailored patient education to each population whenever possible, but creating a "safe space" for individuals to seek health care in a nonjudgmental, therapeutic atmosphere.

The CDC estimates that HPV accounts for the majority of newly contracted STIs; however, these infections are not reportable. Primary care clinicians are urged to screen young adults for STIs when possible. Undetected and untreated STIs increase a person's risk for HIV infection, which can be present with no symptoms for a lengthy period.

CLINICAL CONCEPT

Untreated gonorrhea and chlamydia often cause **pelvic inflammatory disease (PID)** in females, a condition that can cause infertility. At least 1 million females contract PID annually. Each year, 1 in 10 females with PID become infertile in the United States.

Untreated syphilis can lead to serious long-term complications, including brain, cardiovascular, and organ damage. Syphilis in pregnant females can also result in congenital syphilis (syphilis among infants), which can cause stillbirth, death soon after birth, and, in children who survive, physical deformity and neurological complications. Untreated syphilis in pregnant females results in infant death in up to 40% of cases. Studies suggest that individuals with gonorrhea, chlamydia, or syphilis are at increased risk for HIV. Frequently, individuals are infected with more than one STI at the same time.

Basic Concepts of Sexual Disease and Dysfunction

Common STIs include chlamydia and gonorrhea, which are easily treatable. Early diagnosis and treatment are important to prevent complications. For example, gonorrhea can cause PID, which can lead to infertility. Chlamydia can cause conjunctivitis in the newborn that is delivered vaginally. It is also important to recognize that an individual with an STI should be tested for other STIs. For example, syphilis is often found with HIV infection, and gonorrhea is often found with chlamydia infection. Some STIs are completely curable and have no complications. However, STIs such as HIV, syphilis, and HBV are associated with widespread systemic complications that include cardiac and neurological problems, immunosuppression, and liver failure.

Etiology

STIs can be caused by bacteria, viruses, fungi, or parasites. There are more than 20 types of STIs (see Box 28-1). Each organism causes different signs and symptoms, and each type of infection requires specific diagnostic and treatment interventions.

Obtaining a Sexual History

Sexual activity is the risk factor for STIs, as STIs can be transmitted during any type of sexual exposure,

---

BOX 28-1. Common STIs

- Bacterial vaginosis
- Chancroid
- Chlamydia
- Genital herpes (herpes simplex virus [HSV])
- Gonorrhea
- Granuloma inguinale (donovanosis)
- Hepatitis A, B, C
- HIV/AIDS
- Human papillomavirus (HPV)
- Lymphogranuloma venereum (LGV)
- *Mycoplasma genitalium*
- Syphilis
- Trichomoniasis

Adapted from CDC (2019).

including vaginal, anal, and oral sexual practices. Adolescents and young adults are at highest risk for contraction of STIs. In addition, persons with multiple sex partners and **men who have sex with men (MSM)** are at high risk for STIs. **Women who have sex with women (WSW)** are often not asked about their sexual activity, as many clinicians assume heterosexuality. It is important for clinicians to be aware that many persons have sexual activity with persons of both genders.

It is well known that the **lesbian, gay, bisexual, transgender, and queer+ (LGBTQ+)** population faces health disparities in terms of STIs. It is also clear that this population perceives discrimination in the health-care environment. Commonly, there is an implicit heterosexual bias in medicine, and many clinicians admit to ignorance about sexual-minority health issues. LGBTQ+ persons often face stigma, discrimination, and gaps in provider competence when attempting to access health care. They may therefore postpone, avoid, or be denied adequate health care.

To obtain a thorough sexual history and deliver effective prevention counseling, interviewing skills characterized by respect, compassion, and a nonjudgmental attitude toward all patients are essential. Some patients may not be comfortable talking about their sexual history, sex partners, or sexual practices. The clinician should try to put patients at ease and let them know that taking a sexual history is an important part of a regular physical examination. It is important to provide privacy and assure patient confidentiality. It is important for the clinician to inquire about specific sexual behaviors in order to assess the specific risk factors of the patient. All patients should be asked about risk of HIV and past history of HIV testing. It is important to recognize that the CDC recommends all adolescents and adults ages 13 to 64 get tested for HIV at least once as part of routine medical care. The patient has the right to opt out of HIV testing; however, if the clinician deems HIV testing is necessary, this should be discussed. Persons should be informed about all STIs for which they are being tested and notified about tests for common STIs that are available but not being performed. All patients should also be asked about exposure to violence from a partner or others. Clinicians should assess the mental health of the patient at each encounter. Most STIs require the patient to notify their partner(s) about the infection and advise them to seek health care as well.

According to the CDC, the following are the 5 Ps of sexual assessment that should be asked of all patients:

- Partners: number, gender, and partner risk factors
- Practices: specific behaviors
- Prevention of STIs
- Past history of STIs
- Prevention of pregnancy

Some STIs can be prevented with the use of a condom during sexual activity, although others, such as HSV2 (also known as genital herpes), merely require close skin-to-skin contact for transmission. It is important to ask about specific sexual practices in order to assess risk for certain STIs, counsel about risk reduction strategies, and identify anatomical sites from which to take specimens. Blood-to-blood transmission is also a risk factor; STIs can be transmitted from person to person during sharing of unsterile needles used for IV drug use. Patients should be asked about use of illicit drugs, particularly injectable drugs. Patients should also be asked if their partner(s) use illicit drugs. Some practices such as tattooing and piercing can transmit HIV or hepatitis if needles are unsterile. Female patients should be asked about pregnancy and last menstrual period. The patient should be tested for pregnancy if suspected. STIs are commonly transplacentally transmitted from mother to child during gestation or passed to the newborn during childbirth or breastfeeding.

Pathophysiology

There are different pathological mechanisms for each type of STI. Organisms that cause STIs may have localized effects, systemic effects, or both. An organism such as herpes simplex may exert an effect mainly on the reproductive tract, or as in the case of syphilis, an organism may cause multiple organ pathology. It is important to note that the presence of an STI increases an individual's susceptibility to HIV. Organisms that cause genital tract ulcers such as herpes simplex virus (HSV) or syphilis are highly associated with the transmission of HIV. HIV causes a decreased immune response, which in turn allows the STI to flourish. STIs that cause a vaginal or urethral discharge, such as chlamydia or gonorrhea, are also associated with higher transmission rates of HIV. There is a synergistic effect noted in the combined exposure to certain STIs along with exposure to HIV (see Chapter 11 for information on HIV infection).

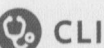 **CLINICAL CONCEPT**

The presence of an STI should alert the clinician to test for HIV. HIV increases susceptibility to other STIs.

Clinical Presentation

In females, STIs can be classified as either lower tract infections—those that affect the vulva, vagina, and cervix—or upper tract infections—those that affect the uterus, fallopian tubes, and the ovaries. Purulent vaginal discharge or bleeding and pelvic or abdominal pain and tenderness are commonly signs of an STI in females. Some STIs can cause external lesions that are apparent during pelvic examination, whereas others can remain dormant and unobservable. STIs can lead to occlusion of the fallopian tubes, which can cause ectopic pregnancy or infertility. Some STIs can be transmitted to the fetus during pregnancy or the intrapartum period, causing perinatal loss, neonatal infection, low birth weight of the newborn, or preterm labor.

In males, STIs commonly cause inflammation of the urethra, termed **urethritis,** which consists of burning upon urination and a thick or watery discharge leaking from the meatus of the penis. The infectious process can ascend to the testicles (orchitis), prostate (prostatitis), or epididymis (epididymitis), causing tenderness and pain.

In both males and females, STIs can affect the anogenital or oropharyngeal regions as a result of transmission through oral or anal sexual activity. HPV is the most prevalent STI in the world. HPV infection is an oncogenic viral infection that can lead to cervical, vulvar, penile, anal, or oropharyngeal cancer.

Diagnosis

The diagnosis of an STI requires a laboratory procedure that can demonstrate growth of the suspected etiological organism. These laboratory procedures vary according to the suspected organism. For example, HIV infection requires antibody testing or viral ribonucleic acid (RNA) levels, which require a blood sample and specific immunoassay procedures.

In lieu of cultures, the diagnostic test called **polymerase chain reaction (PCR)** is increasingly being used to detect microorganisms in sample tissue, blood, or body fluid. PCR is a type of **nucleic acid amplification test (NAAT).** In the diagnosis of STIs, PCR is used to detect the DNA or RNA of a microorganism in a cell sample. PCR is highly sensitive and can detect minute quantities of microorganism DNA or RNA. PCR can also reveal the number of microorganisms in a cell sample. For example, the number of HIV viral particles can be quantified by PCR early after contraction of the virus. PCR can reveal the presence of viral RNA before antibody appears in the blood. Other diagnostic techniques will be discussed in subsequent sections of this chapter.

Treatment

Treatments for different STIs vary; however, most require an antimicrobial drug. In addition, education regarding contagion, transmission, and prevention of the infection is necessary. Different therapies will be discussed in subsequent sections of this chapter.

Pathophysiology of Sexually Transmitted Infections

STIs can be caused by a number of different bacteria, viruses, and parasites. Each type of infection presents differently and causes distinct symptoms.

Bacterial Infections

The most common bacterial microorganisms that cause STIs include chlamydia, gonococcus, and syphilis. Chlamydia is often a silent infection, whereas gonorrhea and syphilis have evident symptoms.

Chlamydia

Chlamydia trachomatis infection is a widespread disease that does not cause many signs or symptoms. Often this infection is present along with other STIs, particularly gonorrhea. *C. trachomatis* infection can affect the cervix, urethra, fallopian tubes, uterus, rectum, nasopharynx, and epididymis; it is the most commonly reported bacterial STI in the United States and a leading cause of infertility in females. *C. trachomatis* also causes conjunctivitis or pneumonia in neonates born vaginally to infected mothers.

Epidemiology. Chlamydia is one of the most common STIs in the United States. Females have higher rates of infection than males. It is difficult to estimate prevalence of chlamydia infection as it is often asymptomatic and persons do not obtain routine testing for chlamydia. Approximately 4 million cases of chlamydial infection are reported per year in the United States, with an overall prevalence of 5% in the population. Two-thirds of new chlamydial infections occur among youth aged 15 to 24 years. Estimates show that 1 in 20 sexually active young females aged 14 to 24 years has chlamydia. Disparities persist among racial and ethnic minority groups. In 2020, chlamydia rates for African Americans/Blacks were six times that of European Americans/Whites. Chlamydia is also common among MSM. Among MSM screened for rectal chlamydial infection, positivity ranges from 3.0% to 10.5%. Among MSM screened for pharyngeal chlamydial infection, positivity has ranges from 0.5% to 2.3%. Approximately 100,000 neonates are exposed to chlamydia at childbirth each year. This can cause ophthalmia neonatorum (conjunctivitis) or pneumonia in some infants. Rectal or genital infection can persist 1 year or longer in infants infected at birth. However, sexual abuse should be a consideration among young children with vaginal, urethral, or rectal infection beyond the neonatal period.

Risk Factors. Unprotected sexual activity is the major risk factor for chlamydial infection. Vaginal, anal, or oral sexual practices can transmit this bacterial infection. In addition, contraction of neonatal infection can occur as an infant is delivered vaginally from an infected mother. Two-thirds of infants born to mothers with chlamydia develop conjunctivitis or pneumonia. Specific risk factors for chlamydial infection include multiple sexual partners, a new sexual partner, lack of barrier contraceptive, and coinfection with another STI. Oral and anal sexual activity increase risk of chlamydia infection. MSM are at high risk for rectal and oropharyngeal chlamydia infection. Cervical ectopy, when endocervical cells are present in the ectocervix, increases susceptibility to chlamydial infection in females.

Etiology. *C. trachomatis* is a gram-negative, obligate intracellular bacteria that can live only inside a host's cells. Obligate intracellular bacteria cannot reproduce outside their host cell, meaning that the organism's life cycle is entirely dependent on host cell resources (see Fig. 28-1).

Pathophysiology. *C. trachomatis* causes cervicitis, urethritis, PID, and a type of conjunctivitis known as *inclusion conjunctivitis*. The bacterium invades mucosal epithelium, and its incubation period is 1 to 3 weeks. The most common initial infection affects the columnar epithelial cells present on the cervix. Upon infection, the initial inflammation reaction attracts neutrophils, followed by lymphocytes, macrophages, plasma cells, and eosinophils. The release of cytokines and interferon by white blood cells maintains the inflammation reaction. Infection stimulates both antibody-mediated and cellular immune responses, demonstrated by the presence of secretory immunoglobulin A (IgA), circulatory immunoglobulin M (IgM), immunoglobulin G (IgG) antibodies, and T cells.

C. trachomatis is an intracellular bacterium that has a propensity for columnar epithelial cells of the host. Adolescent and young adult females are particularly susceptible to infection because the external surface of the cervix in this age group contains squamocolumnar epithelial cells. The bacterium has a biphasic life cycle, with two types of presentation depending on whether

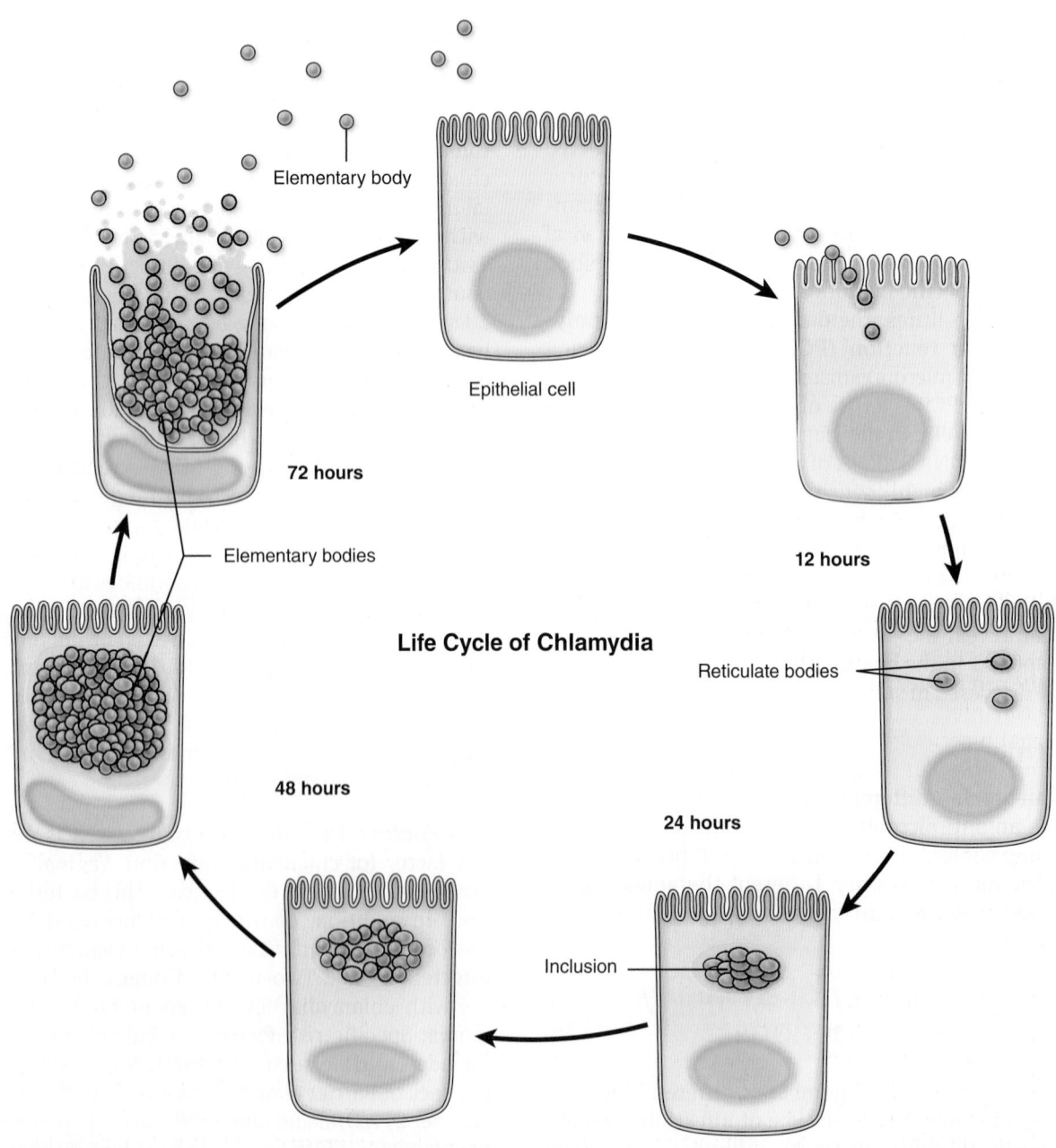

Life Cycle of Chlamydia

FIGURE 28-1. Life cycle of *Chlamydia trachomatis*.

the organism is located inside or outside the host epithelial cell. The bacterium needs to live inside a host cell and uses the host cell's energy for replication. Chlamydia alternates between two forms: the extracellular infectious elementary body and the intracellular noninfectious reticulate body. Elementary bodies are similar to infectious spores. Elementary bodies enter the host epithelial cells and differentiate into noninfectious reticulate bodies. The reticulate bodies undergo several rounds of replication within a membrane-bound compartment called an *inclusion*. After replication is over within the inclusion, the reticulate bodies redifferentiate into elementary bodies and are released. The elementary bodies leave the host cell and go on to continually infect neighboring cells (see Fig. 28-1).

Clinical Presentation. Chlamydia is a silent infection without symptoms in approximately 50% of infected males and 80% of infected females. In females, it can present as inflammation of the cervix on pelvic examination. The infection sometimes causes a mucopurulent cervicitis in females and urethritis in males, which alerts the patient of the need for treatment. Males with symptoms typically have a mucoid or watery urethral discharge and dysuria. Some males develop epididymitis with unilateral testicular pain, tenderness, and swelling.

In females, the bacteria can easily ascend upward from the cervix into the uterus and infect the fallopian tubes, causing salpingitis, which can cause obstruction and scarring of the fallopian tubes and lead to infertility. Without early diagnosis, ascending infection can result in PID in females and is the most common cause of epididymitis in males younger than 35 years. Of females with PID, 5% to 10% develop peritonitis and perihepatitis, also called Fitz–Hugh–Curtis syndrome. Fibrotic adhesions develop around the liver and cause right upper quadrant tenderness of the abdomen.

In males, up to 50% of nongonococcal urethritis can be attributed to chlamydia. Aside from infecting the cervix in the female and urethra in the male, chlamydia can infect the rectum or the pharynx, depending on sexual practices. Rectal pain, discharge, and rectal bleeding can occur. There are no typical symptoms of oropharyngeal chlamydia. Conjunctivitis can occur in both males and females through contact with infected genital secretions.

Chlamydia infection can also cause an acute or insidious reactive arthritis termed *Reiter's syndrome* that is an autoimmune-mediated inflammatory disorder occurring 1 week to 1 month after genitourinary chlamydia infection. It usually affects the knees, ankles, or feet. Persons with genotype HLA-B27 are highly susceptible to Reiter's syndrome.

Chlamydial infection develops in 60% of newborns who are delivered vaginally to infected mothers. Newborns can develop inclusion conjunctivitis, which presents as mucopurulent discharge of the eyes and can lead to blindness. The inflammation of the conjunctiva begins between 7 and 12 days after birth. *C. trachomatis* is one of the most common causes of pneumonia in the newborn.

Diagnosis. The lack of reported symptoms caused by silent infection makes clinical assessment difficult. It also contributes to the delay in treatment. Because the disease is prevalent among adolescents and young adults, raising awareness and screening in this population is important.

Chlamydial infection causes inflammation of the cervix with fragile epithelial lesions that bleed easily. Frequently, a mucopurulent discharge can be visualized at the cervical opening (cervical os) on pelvic examination. External signs are usually not visible to the infected female; however, many times, slight vaginal bleeding after intercourse can be indicative of the infection.

NAATs are the most sensitive tests for detecting *C. trachomatis* infection. Endocervical, rectal, urethral, and oropharyngeal secretions should be obtained for NAAT. It is important to be sure to sample cells from the endocervix in females and 1 to 2 cm deep into the urethra in males. A DNA probe on a urine sample will also reveal the microorganism. To diagnose genital chlamydia in females using a NAAT, vaginal swabs are the optimal specimen. Urine is the specimen of choice for males. Urine is an effective alternative specimen type for females. Alternative diagnostic testing may include tissue culture, enzyme-linked immunosorbent assay (ELISA), or direct fluorescent antibody (DFA) testing. Culture is necessary if there are legal implications or suspicion of sexual abuse. An HIV test should be performed, and in females, a Pap test should be done. An RNA test can be used on liquid cytology Pap test samples. Females should also be given a pregnancy test because certain treatments for chlamydia are contraindicated in pregnancy.

In the newborn with *C. trachomatis* conjunctivitis, discharge from the eye can be sampled and cultured. Chlamydial inclusion bodies found in the cells of the sample are diagnostic.

Treatment. The CDC recommendations for treatment of chlamydia STI include antibiotics and patient education. Amoxicillin, erythromycin, or doxycycline are commonly used for chlamydia infection. Noncompliance is common in adolescents. A single 1 g dose of azithromycin can be offered to those who may not adhere to longer-term treatment. It is important to educate the patient that treatment is necessary to prevent PID, which can lead to infertility or sepsis. For assurance of cure, a repeat NAAT diagnostic test should be done 3 weeks after initial treatment. A positive test is usually not a failure of treatment, but a sign of noncompliance or reinfection. Reinfection often occurs if the sexual partner is not treated. It is important that the infected person make sexual partners aware of the diagnosis and need for treatment. Newborns are treated with erythromycin ophthalmic ointment at birth to prevent chlamydia conjunctivitis.

Gonorrhea

Neisseria gonorrhoeae is a bacterial organism that infects mucous membranes by sexual transmission. Infections can cause cervicitis, proctitis, urethritis, PID, conjunctivitis, and pharyngitis. Complications include ectopic pregnancy, infertility, and increased susceptibility to HIV. During vaginal delivery, newborns can contract gonorrhea and develop conjunctivitis, which may lead to blindness.

Epidemiology. *N. gonorrhoeae* infection is a prevalent STI, with an estimated 200 million new cases annually worldwide. The CDC estimates that approximately 1.6 million new gonococcal infections occurred in the United States in 2018, and more than half occur among young people aged 15 to 24 years. Gonorrhea is the second most commonly reported bacterial STI in the United States. Because it is an underdiagnosed disease, prevalence may be as much as 50% higher than reported. The rate of gonorrhea is eight times higher in African Americans compared with European Americans. There is a high prevalence of infection in the rural southeastern United States, as well as in urban areas.

Incidence of gonorrhea is greater in males than in females, at 202 cases per 100,000. The major age group affected consists of individuals who are 19 to 24 years old. It is transmitted through sexual contact; however, infected untreated mothers can also transmit the disease to their newborns. Incidence of gonorrhea in children usually indicates sexual abuse and should be reported.

Risk Factors. The major risk factor associated with gonorrheal infection is sexual contact. Multiple sex partners, MSM, and lack of condom protection are also risk factors. Perinatal transmission to the newborn during vaginal childbirth can cause an eye infection. Gonorrhea commonly causes neonatal conjunctivitis, a mucopurulent eye infection called **ophthalmia neonatorum,** which is treatable with antibiotics. Sepsis is also possible in the infected newborn. MSM have the highest rate of carrier status and frequently contract antibiotic-resistant strains of gonococcus. Untreated gonorrhea can result in epididymitis in males and PID in females. *N. gonorrhoeae* and *C. trachomatis* account for most cases of epididymitis in males younger than 35 years. In females, infection can be followed by salpingitis, resulting in scarring of the fallopian tubes, infertility, or ectopic pregnancy.

Pathophysiology. *N. gonorrhoeae* is a gram-negative, diplococcal bacterium. It is spread by sexual contact, including vaginal, anal, and oral sex, or through vertical transmission during childbirth. It mainly affects human columnar epithelium, making any mucous membrane susceptible to infection. It is commonly transmitted to individuals in combination with HIV and chlamydia.

The gonococcal organism has unique characteristics that enhance its virulence. The gonococcal surface has pili, which are hairlike appendages that allow the bacteria's attachment to mucosal surfaces. They are adherent to mucosal membranes, particularly the cervix, urethra, and conjunctiva of the eye.

The gonococcal organisms are resistant to many of the body's defense mechanisms because of their genetic mutation ability. Gonococcal organisms carry antibiotic-resistance genes, most notably penicillinase-coding genes; therefore, gonococcal organisms can resist penicillin. The gonococcal organism also has frequent mutation of surface protein–coding genes that allows transformation in its appearance to the immune system. The surface antigens change, elude host immune processes, and easily result in reinfection of the host. Most strains have become resistant to multiple antibiotics, and effective gonorrhea treatment has become a public health challenge.

Retrograde spread of gonorrhea from the cervix into the uterus, fallopian tubes, and abdomen can lead to PID, gonococcal peritonitis, and Fitz–Hugh–Curtis syndrome. *N. gonorrhoeae,* like *C. trachomatis,* can cause Reiter's syndrome. Gonococcal conjunctivitis can occur in adults and children following direct transfer of organisms by hand–eye contact. Gonococcal conjunctivitis can lead to blindness. Ophthalmia neonatorum can occur at childbirth.

Uniquely, changes in the vaginal pH that occur during menses, pregnancy, and the postpartum period make the vaginal environment more suitable for the growth of gonococcus and provide increased access to the bloodstream. This allows disseminated gonococcal infection that can affect the skin, joints, heart, and meninges.

Clinical Presentation. Ninety percent of infected males and 50% of infected females complain of symptoms with gonococcal infection. Males develop dysuria 2 to 5 days after exposure, often followed by copious purulent discharge. Unilateral epididymitis with penile edema can be present. Females will often be asymptomatic or report a purulent vaginal discharge, dysuria, genital pruritus, and occasional vaginal spotting. Rectal pain, pruritus, and discharge can be involved in both males and females. Abdominal pain usually indicates PID in females. PID is also characterized by cervical motion tenderness on bimanual pelvic examination. Disseminated gonococcal infection often starts with fever, rash, joint pain, and tendonitis, which can become septic arthritis. The knee is often involved in a purulent gonococcal joint infection. Gonococcal infection of the bloodstream can lead to arthritis, meningitis, endocarditis, or myocarditis. In newborns, gonococcal infection of the conjunctiva can cause erythema, eye pain, and discharge. Without treatment, it can lead to blindness.

Diagnosis. Purulent exudate can be sampled and cultured for identification of the microorganism and antibiotic sensitivity. In the female, it is very important to collect the specimen from the endocervix with a large swab. In the male, the swab should be inserted 1 to 2 cm into the urethra. Urine culture can demonstrate urethral gonococcus in males. With cervical or urethral infection, anal culture should also be sampled. If pharyngeal gonococcus infection is suspected, a throat culture is also necessary. Gram stain and culture are commonly used, but molecular testing that includes DNA probe and PCR methods are simpler screening methods. One swab can test for more than one STI. Patients suspected of having gonorrhea should also be checked for HIV, chlamydia, HBV, herpes simplex, and syphilis. In addition, females should receive a pregnancy test.

Treatment. Treatment should be based on analysis of the microorganism's specific antibiotic sensitivity. Dual drug therapy with a cephalosporin and azithromycin are currently the treatment of choice. However, increasing numbers of antibiotic-resistant cases, including treatment failures, are growing concerns. It is highly recommended that the patient be retested after treatment for cure to ensure eradication of infection and identify resistance. New antimicrobials for treatment of gonorrhea are in clinical development; the antibiotic zoliflodacin appears promising.

If the patient has not been tested for chlamydia, the CDC recommends treating for chlamydia at the same time as gonorrhea. As with all STIs, persons infected with gonorrhea are advised to notify sexual partners of the need for treatment. Infants can become infected from cervical or vaginal exudates during delivery. The infection manifests itself after 2 to 5 days as sepsis or ophthalmia neonatorum. Sepsis can include meningitis and rhinitis. Symptoms improve with prompt antibiotic treatment.

> ### 🔎 CLINICAL CONCEPT
>
> To prevent gonorrheal ophthalmia neonatorum, most states mandate use of erythromycin or tetracycline ointment in the eye of the newborn at birth as prophylaxis. The antibiotics also prevent chlamydial eye infection.

Syphilis

Syphilis is an infectious disease caused by the bacterial organism ***Treponema pallidum***, a spirochete. Syphilis is transmissible by sexual contact, transplacentally from mother to fetus in utero, via blood product transfusion, and occasionally through breaks in the skin that come into contact with infectious lesions. Syphilis has many different presentations; in advanced stages, it affects almost every body system. It can mimic several different infections and autoimmune diseases, making it known as "the great impostor."

Epidemiology. Syphilis was a common infection before the invention of penicillin in the 1940s. Following the introduction of penicillin, syphilis incidence greatly declined, reaching its lowest point in the year 2000, with 2.1 cases per 100,000. During 2020, there were 133,945 new cases of syphilis (all stages). Men who have sex with men (MSM) are at highest risk for syphilis. They accounted for 43% of all primary and secondary syphilis cases in 2020. Males are affected more frequently than females, with a male-to-female incidence ratio of approximately 8:1. Although rates of syphilis are lower among females, rates have increased 147% during 2016 to 2020, suggesting that the heterosexual syphilis epidemic continues to rapidly increase in the United States.

Since 2013, the rate of congenital syphilis has increased each year. In 2020, 2,148 cases of congenital syphilis were reported, including 149 congenital syphilis-related stillbirths and infant deaths. The national congenital syphilis rate of 57.3 cases per 100,000 live births in 2020 represents a 254% increase relative to 2016.

African Americans are affected 4.5 times more frequently than European Americans. There is a high rate of syphilis and HIV coinfection, with 45% of MSM infected with both diseases.

Etiology. Syphilis is caused by *T. pallidum,* which is a long, spiral-shaped bacterium called a spirochete. The bacterium enters the body via mucous membranes, transplacentally to a fetus, or through blood-to-blood transfer. The organism can survive only briefly outside of the body; transmission almost always requires direct contact with the infectious lesion.

Risk Factors. People considered at high risk for syphilis include persons who engage in high-risk sexual behavior, persons diagnosed with other STIs, those who exchange sex for drugs, people engaging in prostitution, people who use IV drugs, and incarcerated adults. In addition, a fetus can be infected transplacentally in pregnant females.

> ### 🔎 CLINICAL CONCEPT
>
> Patients who have syphilis should be tested for HIV, hepatitis B, gonorrhea, HPV, herpes simplex, chlamydia, *Haemophilus ducreyi,* and hepatitis C. There is an estimated two- to fivefold increased risk of acquiring HIV when syphilis is present.

Pathophysiology. *T. pallidum* penetrates intact mucous membranes, and within a few hours, enters the lymphatics and bloodstream. The incubation period from time of exposure to development of a primary lesion can range from 10 to 90 days.

There are four specific phases of syphilis infection: primary, secondary, latent, and tertiary. In the primary phase, syphilis bacteria enter the host through mucous membranes or a break in the skin. At the point of contact, treponema organisms multiply. Two to 10 weeks after contact, the primary manifestation becomes apparent: a sore known as a **chancre** (see Fig. 28-2). The chancre is usually on the external genitalia, and it heals within about a week. As it heals, *T. pallidum* organisms enter the bloodstream.

After 2 to 10 weeks, the secondary stage develops, in which a rash appears all over the body. Bacteria disseminate throughout the lymphatics and bloodstream, and tissue injury occurs. Invasion of the tissues occurs with cellular changes that include endothelial injury, called endarteritis, and infiltrates that contain numerous plasma cells, macrophages, and T cells.

Both primary and secondary syphilis are highly infectious states, during which spirochetes can be recovered from lesions and the bloodstream. After the lesions of secondary syphilis heal, there is a latent period, during which time one-third of infected persons heal spontaneously, another third remain asymptomatic, and another third progress to tertiary syphilis. During latent disease, granulomas called **gummas,** which consist of macrophages, plasma cells, and T cells, form in many different organs. The granulomatous lesions interfere with organ function and can be found in the skin, bones, liver, heart, and brain. Aortic valve deformity and aortic aneurysm are common forms of cardiovascular syphilis. Some of the granulomatous lesions cause ulceration and necrosis of tissue.

Tertiary syphilis is the stage of degenerative changes in various organs of the body. Lesions in the neurological system commonly cause mental status changes, as well as vision and hearing disorders. Neurosyphilis can cause meningitis, stroke, paresis, and dementia. Aortic arteritis and neurological degeneration are disorders characteristic of tertiary syphilis.

CLINICAL CONCEPT

The *T. pallidum* microorganism is evident in the bloodstream throughout the infection, which can span decades. A low level of antibodies stay in the blood for months to years after the disease has been treated.

Clinical Presentation. The primary stage of syphilis, demonstrated by a skin lesion called a chancre, is the most clinically observable sign of the infection. The chancre, usually located in the genital area weeks after sexual contact, starts as a papule and becomes an ulcerlike lesion. This lesion often goes unnoticed by the infected person because it is painless. The primary lesion usually is associated with regional lymphadenopathy that may be unilateral or bilateral. Inguinal lymph nodes are enlarged, firm, mobile, and painless, without overlying skin changes.

After this chancre heals, a rash, appearing as erythematous maculopapular lesions over all areas of the body, becomes observable in some individuals. Uniquely, the rash can appear on the palms of the hands and soles of the feet. This nonpruritic rash is often the first visible sign of illness to the patient. The rash can also present as pustular or mixed lesions. Patchy areas of alopecia may occur. Systemic symptoms of secondary syphilis include malaise, sore throat, headache, fever, anorexia, and, rarely, the stiff neck of meningitis. Gastrointestinal dysfunction, arteritis, hepatitis, proctitis, arthritis, and optic neuritis can also occur. Commonly, **condyloma lata,** a wartlike lesion, can be found in the genital region.

After the body rash fades, there is a latent asymptomatic period that can last for years. Gradual damage to organs with formation of granulomas (gummas) develops during latent syphilis. Tertiary syphilis occurs when there are granulomatous lesions in the neurological system. These lesions commonly cause mental status changes, as well as vision and hearing disorders. Neurosyphilis can cause meningitis, stroke, paresis, and dementia. Cerebral atrophy can occur in late neurosyphilis. **Tabes dorsalis** is the term used for syphilitic involvement of the posterior columns of the spinal cord that causes ataxia and sensory changes in the limbs. The Argyll Robertson pupil is a neurological phenomenon in syphilis that causes a nonreactive pupil.

Syphilis can also be transmitted by mother to fetus. This transmission occurs when the placenta is beginning to function, at 10 to 15 weeks' gestation. *T. pallidum* crosses the placenta, where it can cause miscarriage or stillbirth. Even if the fetus is born alive, there are often signs of congenital syphilis, such as

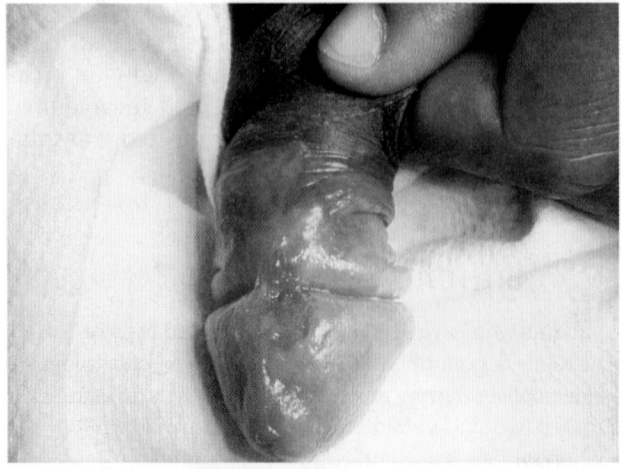

FIGURE 28-2. Chancre lesion of primary syphilis. *(Courtesy of CDC.)*

Hutchinson teeth, saddle nose, and various neurological manifestations. There is a 100% chance of transmission if the mother has early syphilis, because it is at that time that the spirochetes can pass through the placenta. If the mother has been infected for a long time, transmission is less likely.

Diagnosis. Various tests are available for the diagnosis of syphilis. Serological tests are most commonly used and search for treponemal antigen or antibodies in the blood. The serological tests used are the Venereal Disease Research Laboratory (VDRL), rapid plasma reagin (RPR), immune-capture enzyme immunoassay (ICE) syphilis recombinant antigen test, and fluorescent treponemal antibody absorption (FTA-ABS) test. The results are expressed in terms of antibody levels, or titers. It is recommended that all pregnant females be tested for syphilis at the first prenatal visit. All patients tested for syphilis should also be tested for HIV infection.

Unlike other infections, which show a decline in titers or become nonreactive with effective treatment, syphilis antibody–specific tests usually remain reactive for life. Therefore, treponemal-specific test titers are not useful for assessing treatment efficacy.

> **CLINICAL CONCEPT**
>
> The FTA-ABS is a first test that becomes positive in early syphilis. When this test is positive in the newborn, it provides good evidence of congenital syphilis.

The enzyme immunoassay (EIA) test is used to screen large numbers of individuals and can be used at any stage during syphilis.

PCR testing for syphilis can be used for diagnosis during the primary syphilis stage, but it displays only moderate sensitivity in blood from secondary syphilis.

Lumbar puncture for analysis of cerebrospinal fluid (CSF) should be done in patients suspected of suffering from neurosyphilis.

Chest x-ray is necessary to look for aortic dilation or calcifications that are present in syphilitic aortitis or aneurysm. Computed tomography (CT) scanning and magnetic resonance imaging (MRI) of the head and body may be used to document the complications of tertiary syphilis.

> **CLINICAL CONCEPT**
>
> An antibody titer against syphilis remains reactive for life.

Treatment. The treatment of syphilis depends on whether the infection is in the primary, secondary, latent, or tertiary stage. Often, a patient is being treated because of a positive screening test and has no history of an infection and no signs and symptoms of syphilis. Usually, the clinician chooses to err on the side of caution by treating for a higher level of involvement. Benzathine penicillin, administered intramuscularly, is the single drug of choice in the treatment of syphilis. The patient should notify sexual partners that they need testing and possible treatment. There are high rates of reinfection among MSM. Patient education is necessary with treatment. The clinician should discuss safe sexual practices and advise people who use IV drugs to not share needles.

A phenomenon called the **Jarisch–Herxheimer reaction** can occur during treatment. This occurs when large numbers of bacteria are killed by antibiotic all at once, causing a large release of bacterial endotoxins. Fever, chills, myalgias, and exacerbation of skin lesions occur. Patients who are treated should have repeat testing at 6 and 12 months to ensure treatment efficacy. Pregnant patients should have testing monthly throughout the pregnancy.

Lymphogranuloma Venereum, Chancroid, and Granuloma Inguinale

Lymphogranuloma venereum (LGV), chancroid, and granuloma inguinale, once uncommon in the United States, are increasingly diagnosed in HIV-infected individuals. All these diseases cause genital ulcerations and inguinal lymphadenopathy. Chancroid is thought to be transmitted through casual sexual contact, mostly by people engaged in prostitution. Uncircumcised males are most vulnerable. Recently, the incidence of LGV has been increasing among MSM.

Pathophysiology. **Chancroid** is caused by a short, compact, gram-negative, streptobacillary rod, *Haemophilus ducreyi.* LGV is caused by *C. trachomatis,* and granuloma inguinale by *Klebsiella granulomatis* (previously called *Calymmatobacterium granulomatis*). *C. trachomatis* is an obligate, intracellular bacterial organism that can only live and reproduce within the cells of the host (see section on *C. trachomatis* infection). *K. granulomatis* is a gram-negative bacterium that contains cytoplasmic granules called *Donovan bodies;* thus, **granuloma inguinale** is also called **donovanosis.**

Clinical Presentation. Chancroid features a chancre-like lesion that is soft in contrast to the more solid chancre of syphilis. The microorganism of chancroid, *H. ducreyi,* enters through a break in the skin in the genital area. Incubation of 3 to 10 days produces a papule that soon ulcerates. The ulcer of chancroid is painful, as opposed to the painless chancre of syphilis. Lymphadenopathy of the inguinal lymph nodes is common. These enlarged lymph nodes are called **buboes.**

LGV presents in three stages, similar to syphilis. The first stage is a painless induration at the point of entry of the microorganism, *C. trachomatis.* After this resolves, the second stage of painful inguinal lymphadenopathy occurs. The enlarged lymph nodes (buboes) develop ulceration and sinuses that yield drainage of purulent discharge. Oral ulceration associated with cervical lymphadenopathy can occur. The third stage consists of anogenitorectal syndrome where proctocolitis, perirectal abscesses, and fistulas develop. Hemorrhagic proctitis can mimic inflammatory bowel disease. Systemic symptoms, such as fever, malaise, and arthralgia, are often present.

Granuloma inguinale begins as a painless, indurated papule that develops into a wide ulceration up to 20 cm in diameter. Repeated exposure to the organism is necessary to become infected. Without treatment, these ulcerations can evolve into squamous cell or basal cell carcinoma.

Diagnosis. All patients who have genital ulcers should be evaluated with a serological test for syphilis and a diagnostic evaluation for genital herpes. In settings where chancroid is prevalent, a test for HIV should also be performed. Other laboratory tests that should be done include VDRL test or RPR for syphilis and PCR assays for *H. ducreyi,* HSV2, HSV, gonorrhea, chlamydia, and HIV antibodies because patients with LGV commonly have contracted other STIs.

Specific tests for evaluation of genital ulcers include syphilis serology and either a dark-field examination or direct immunofluorescence test for *T. pallidum,* culture or antigen test for HSV, and culture for *H. ducreyi.* Diagnosis of LGV is made with identification of *C. trachomatis.* Laboratory diagnosis for granuloma inguinale is made by scraping the lesion and examining scraped cells under a microscope; stained *K. granulomatis* are observed and identified. Intracellular *K. granulomatis* organisms within white blood cells are referred to as Donovan bodies.

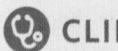 **CLINICAL CONCEPT**

Nucleic acid amplification tests (NAAT) and PCR tests are increasingly used in lieu of cultures for an accurate and rapid diagnosis of STIs.

Treatment. Antibiotic treatment is used for all three of these infections. Ulcerated lesions usually improve symptomatically within 3 days. If no clinical improvement is evident, the clinician must consider whether the diagnosis is correct, the patient is coinfected with another STI, the patient is infected with HIV, the patient was noncompliant with treatment, or the bacterial strain is resistant to the antibiotic. The time required for complete healing depends on the size of the ulcer; large ulcers might require more than 2 weeks. Clinical resolution of the fluctuant lymphadenopathy lesions (buboes) is slower than resolution for ulcers and might require needle aspiration or incision and drainage.

Bacterial Vaginosis

Bacterial vaginosis (BV) is a common infection prevalent in 29% of females ages 15 to 44 years. It occurs because of changes in the vaginal bacterial flora from *Lactobacillus* to a mixture of gram-negative and anaerobic bacterial organisms, largely *Gardnerella vaginalis, Prevotella* species, and *Mobiluncus* species. The new bacterial organisms produce large amounts of proteolytic enzymes that break down vaginal peptides, causing a change in pH and accumulation of volatile, malodorous compounds. There is vulvar and vaginal pruritus and an associated thin, off-white vaginal discharge that has a "fishy odor." Discharge contains clue cells, which are vaginal epithelial cells with adherent coccobacilli that can be detected on microscopic examination. Diagnosis is based on clinical findings, positive whiff–amine test, and Gram stain. The whiff-amine test is based on an amine odor when potassium hydroxide 10% solution is added to a drop of vaginal secretions. BV is highly prevalent in WSW, particularly those who have multiple partners. BV can increase the risk of contracting many STIs such as HIV, human papillomavirus (HPV), *Neisseria gonorrhea* (NG), *Chlamydia trachomatis* (CT), *Trichomonas vaginalis* (TV), and herpes simplex virus-2 (HSV2). It can be asymptomatic, and pregnant females with the disease have an increased risk of preterm delivery. Male partners are not affected by BV. Antibiotic treatment with metronidazole or clindamycin is effective orally or intravaginally.

Mycoplasma Genitalium

Mycoplasma genitalium is the smallest known self-replicating bacterium and is related to the organism *Mycoplasma pneumoniae* that causes atypical pneumonia. *Mycoplasma genitalium* is a sexually transmitted bacterium associated with a number of urogenital conditions in females such as cervicitis, endometritis, pelvic inflammatory disease, infertility, and susceptibility to HIV. It is a common coinfection with chlamydia. In females, it can be asymptomatic. It is a cause of nongonoccocal urethritis in males, which includes dysuria, urethral discharge, pruritus, and inflammation of the glans penis. However, it can be asymptomatic and resolve without causing disease. Its prevalence varies among different groups, with the average being 0.5% to 10% in the general population and 20% to 40% in females with STIs. Having multiple sexual partners increases the risk of *M. genitalium* infection. Diagnosis involves NAAT of the urethral discharge, first-void urine, or vaginal discharge. The antibiotic azithromycin is the recommended treatment. Sexual partners should be treated as well. However, antibiotic resistance has increased in recent years, which is significantly lowering the cure rate. New treatment regimens need to be investigated due to increasing drug resistance.

Protozoan Infection

Trichomoniasis

Trichomoniasis is a common protozoan vaginal infection in females and the most common nonviral STI worldwide. Coinfection of *Trichomonas vaginalis* and BV is common. Females can acquire the disease from sexual contact with both females and males. Males generally do not transmit the disease to other males. Females can be asymptomatic or complain of pruritus; burning on urination; and a greenish-yellow, malodorous vaginal discharge. Males usually can have urethritis or no symptoms. Microscopic analysis and/or NAAT of vaginal discharge can diagnose the infection. Rapid antigen identification tests are also available. Testing for HIV and other STIs should be done in patients with *Trichomonas* infection. Oral metronidazole or tinidazole is recommended treatment, and sexual partners should be treated as well.

Viral Infections

Common viral STIs include HPV, genital herpes, viral hepatitis (see Chapter 31), and HIV (see Chapter 11). Zika virus, most harmful to the fetus, can be transmitted by sexual activity.

Human Papillomavirus

Human papillomavirus (HPV) is a DNA virus in which approximately 70 distinct genetic types have been identified. Several types of these are considered cancer-causing (oncogenic) viruses (see Box 28-2). Not all cases of HPV go on to become cancer; however, the following have been associated with the virus:

- Cancers of the cervix, vagina, and vulva in females
- Cancers of the penis in males
- Cancers of the anus, rectum, and oropharyngeal region; back of the throat, including the base of the tongue and tonsils in both females and males
- Chronic respiratory papillomatosis; lesions in larynx, airways, lung tissue, esophagus

In the United States approximately 45,000 human papillomavirus (HPV)–associated cancers are diagnosed annually, with nearly 60% detected in females and 40% in males. HPV-related cervical cancer is highly preventable in females with gynecological screening tests. However, other HPV-associated cancers do not have any screening guidelines. Currently in the United States, the HPV vaccine is recommended for males and females ages 9 to 26 years. The vaccine is also approved for prevention of anal, vulvar, and oropharyngeal cancers in males and females.

Epidemiology. HPV infection is the most common STI in the world. The incidence of infection has dramatically increased during the past 20 years. In the United States, about 42% of adults ages 18 to 59 years have genital HPV infections and about 7% have oral HPV. Experts estimate 80% of sexually active people are infected. Approximately half of HPV cases occur in females ages 15 to 24, with the highest incidence in the 20- to 24-year-old age group. Anogenital warts, also called condylomata acuminata, are the characteristic external manifestations of HPV infection. The annual incidence of anogenital warts is estimated between 500,000 and 1 million cases, with similar rates in males and females. Approximately two-thirds of individuals who have sexual contact with an infected partner develop genital warts.

About 99.7% of cervical cancer cases are caused by persistent genital high-risk HPV infection. In the United States, 2.5 million females are estimated to have a cytological diagnosis of low-grade cervical cancer precursor annually. HPV has also been implicated in anorectal, vulvar, vaginal, penile, rectal, oropharyngeal, and laryngeal cancers. There is also a chronic disease called recurrent respiratory papillomatosis (RRP) that can occur. In this disorder, HPV lesions can be found on the larynx, trachea, bronchioles, lung tissue, and esophagus.

Etiology/Risk Factors. Several types of HPV affect humans. HPV types 6 and 11 account for the genital wart infection condylomata acuminata. Types 16, 18, 31, 33, and 51 are more commonly found in cervical cancer. According to some sources, when the most sensitive detecting tests are used, it shows that 80% of young females are infected with HPV. Some infections can be transient and cleared by the host's immune responses. Infection rate correlates with multiple partners, early onset of sexual activity, and high frequency of different sexual partners. Sexual activity is the most common risk factor for HPV infection; this includes oral, anal, penile, and vaginal sexual activity. HPV infection can lead to oropharyngeal, anorectal, penile, and cervical cancer. HPV can also cause respiratory papillomatosis, which causes lesions on the larynx, trachea, bronchi, bronchioles, lung tissue, and esophagus. MSM are at highest risk for anorectal HPV-induced cancer. Patients who are immunosuppressed and those with HIV infection are at higher risk for HPV infection.

BOX 28-2. Cancers Caused by Human Papillomavirus

The percentages of cancers caused by oncogenic HPV are as follows:
- Cervical cancer: 100%
- Anal cancer: 90%
- Vulvar cancer: 40%
- Vaginal cancer: 40%
- Oropharyngeal cancer: 12%
- Oral cancer: 3%

Pathophysiology. HPV integrates its DNA into the genetic material of the host cell. Humans are the only carriers of HPV, and the virus can live outside the body for many months. HPV reproduction occurs in keratinocytes found at the skin surface and mucous membranes. Cells containing the virus are ultimately shed into the environment. Infection occurs when mucosal epithelial cells in the host are exposed to HPV through a break in the epithelial barrier, as would occur during sexual intercourse or after minor skin abrasions. Viral genes transform the mucosal cells into benign genital warts or preneoplastic types of warts. HPV proteins inactivate the host's tumor suppressor proteins, thereby resulting in unregulated host cell proliferation and malignant transformation. HPV particles are released as a result of degeneration of desquamating cells. Although HPV is highly contagious and can lead to cancer, the immune system is capable of clearing the virus. Therefore, not all cases of HPV lead to cancer. High-risk HPVs can cause several types of cancer. There are about 14 high-risk HPV types; two of these, HPV16 and HPV18, are responsible for most HPV-related cancers.

Clinical Presentation. The classic skin manifestations of HPV are small wartlike lesions that are raised, flat, or shaped like cauliflower, termed **condyloma acuminata.** These are single or multiple clusters of papular lesions most commonly seen around the vagina or anus or on the penis (see Fig. 28-3). They are easily visible with the naked eye.

Signs of HPV-induced cervical cancer include pain and bleeding after vaginal sexual activity, bleeding between menstrual periods, abnormal vaginal discharge,

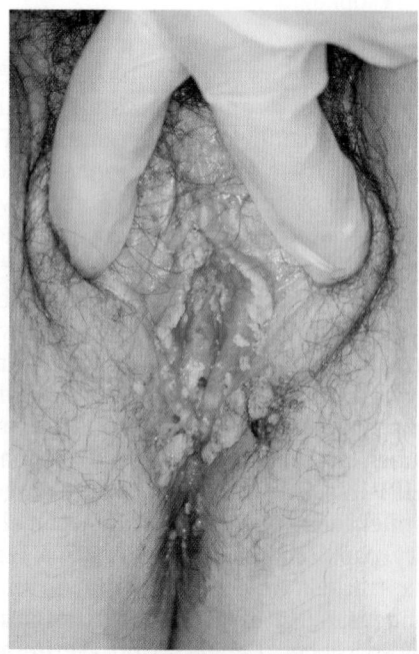

FIGURE 28-3. Genital warts caused by HPV. *(Courtesy of CDC/Joe Millar.)*

and swollen lymph nodes. Signs and symptoms of HPV-induced anal cancer include rectal bleeding, mass at the anal opening, pain or feeling of fullness in the anal area, changes in bowel movements, abnormal anal discharge, and swollen lymph nodes of the anal and perineal region. Oropharyngeal HPV can cause oropharyngeal squamous cell carcinoma (OPSCC). Symptoms include hoarseness, throat irritation, difficulty swallowing, hemoptysis, chronic pharyngitis, and enlarged lymph nodes. HPV can also cause pulmonary lesions, referred to as **chronic respiratory papillomatosis.** The HPV lesions are found on the larynx, trachea, bronchi, bronchioles, lung tissue, and esophagus. Progressive hoarseness, stridor, dyspnea, acute respiratory distress, and chronic cough are the most frequent symptoms. This disease is easily misdiagnosed as asthma, croup, chronic bronchitis, and vocal nodules, which often delays its definitive diagnosis and treatment.

Diagnosis. Condyloma acuminata diagnosis can be made by clinical observation. For cervical HPV diagnosis, cervical cytology (Papanicoulou test [Pap test]) and HPV testing should be done on cervical cells during a gynecological examination. Colposcopy should be done on females who test positive for HPV types 16 or 18. Cone biopsy can sample cells for histological evaluation. For anatomical locations such as penile, anorectal, vulvar, vaginal, and oropharyngeal, a biopsy of suspicious lesions is necessary for diagnosis. Biopsy of the lesions and DNA identification techniques can be used to detect the viral genome. Nuclear amplification HPV-DNA detection techniques are standard tests capable of detecting several high-risk HPV types. Because HPV infection is often associated with other STIs, other diagnostic tests for HIV, HBV, hepatitis C, herpes virus, chlamydia, syphilis, and gonococcus should be done. Digital rectal examination and anal Pap test should be done annually on MSM.

Treatment. There is no cure for HPV because it is a viral infection. Condyloma acuminata can be cosmetically removed using podofilox or imiquimod. Alternatively, trichloroacetic acid or bichloroacetic acid, intralesional interferon, or fluorouracil can be used. Condyloma can also be removed via cautery or laser treatment. Although these treatments can reduce the appearance of the warts, the virus remains in the person's body, so most persons need multiple treatments. HPV infection often recurs and spreads easily between sexual partners. Patients must notify their sexual partners that they need to be examined and possibly treated.

Cervical dysplasia and cancer caused by HPV are treated according to the level of invasion. Current standard-of-care treatments for cervical cancer include radiotherapy, chemotherapy, and/or surgical resection; however, they have significant side effects and limited efficacy against advanced disease.

There are a few treatment options for recurrent or metastatic cases.

Immunotherapy agents are under investigation. HPV-related malignancies have unique viral antigens that can be targeted by novel immunotherapeutic approaches. One such immunotherapeutic agent is pembrolizumab for certain kinds of HPV-induced metastatic or recurrent cervical cancer.

For HPV-induced oropharyngeal cancer, cisplatin-based chemoradiotherapy is considered the standard of care. Multimodal therapy remains the mainstay of treatment for HPV-induced anorectal cancer. For most patients, chemotherapy with mitomycin and 5-fluorouracil and radiation remain the primary treatment modalities. For patients with metastatic disease, cisplatin-based chemotherapy combined with 5-FU has been established as optimal treatment. As with many other malignancies, immunotherapy has become a promising area of research in anorectal cancer. Currently nivolumab and pembrolizumab are tried for refractory metastatic anorectal cancer. Surgery in combination with radiotherapy is the standard treatment for vulvar cancer. Surgery is recommended for penile cancer. Some lesions may be treated with radiation or brachytherapy. Immunotherapeutic agents are currently under clinical investigation for application in penile cancer. Cidofovir is an antiviral agent that has been effective for HPV-induced chronic respiratory papillomatosis.

Prevention of HPV Infection. HPV vaccine is most effective in persons who have not had exposure to HPV. For this reason, HPV vaccine (Gardasil) is recommended for routine vaccination in children, before sexual activity, at age 11 or 12 years. However, vaccination can be started as early as age 9. The Advisory Council on Immunization Policies (ACIP) also recommends vaccination for everyone through age 26 years if not adequately vaccinated when younger. Vaccination is not recommended for those older than age 26 years as commonly there has been exposure to HPV by that age. However, some adults ages 27 through 45 years might decide to get the HPV vaccine based on discussion with their clinician, if they did not get adequately vaccinated when they were younger. HPV vaccination of people in this age range provides less benefit, for several reasons, including that more people in this age range have already been exposed to HPV. HPV vaccination prevents new HPV infections but does not treat existing HPV infections or diseases. For adults ages 27 through 45 years, clinicians can consider discussing HPV vaccination with people who are most likely to benefit. HPV vaccine is not recommended for use during pregnancy.

Two doses of HPV vaccine are recommended for most persons starting the series before their 15th birthday. The second dose of HPV vaccine should be given 6 to 12 months after the first dose. Adolescents who receive two doses less than 5 months apart will require a third dose of HPV vaccine. Three doses of HPV vaccine are recommended for teens and young adults who start the series at ages 15 through 26 years and for immunocompromised persons. The recommended three-dose schedule is 0, 1 to 2 months, and 6 months. Three doses are recommended for immunocompromised persons (including those with HIV infection) aged 9 through 26 years. For more information, see https://www.cdc.gov/vaccines/vpd/hpv/hcp/recommendations.html.

> **CLINICAL CONCEPT**
>
> A vaccine, Gardasil, is available that offers protection against HPV. The vaccine has demonstrated nearly 100% efficacy in preventing precancerous lesions of the cervix and vagina. Vaccination of preteen girls and boys is recommended. Adolescents and young adults up to age 26 can also be vaccinated.

Herpes Simplex Virus

Herpes simplex virus (HSV) causes genital herpes. Genital herpes is an STI caused by the herpes simplex virus type 1 (HSV1) or type 2 (HSV2). Most cases of genital herpes are caused by HSV2. These viruses are capable of causing both acute and latent viral infections. During the acute phase, the virus is highly proliferative and symptomatic, causing vesicular lesions on the skin. However, during the latent phase of the infection, the viral DNA remains in the neuron's nucleus in a dormant state, when no viral proteins are produced. During this dormant state, the immune system does not detect the virus; however, the virus can reactivate at a later time, causing symptoms. At times of immunosuppression, the virus commonly reactivates.

Epidemiology. The prevalence of genital HSV infection worldwide has increased over the last several decades, making it a major public health concern. It is estimated that 50 million persons are infected annually. The CDC estimated that there were 572,000 new genital herpes infections in the United States in 2022. Nationwide, 11.9% of persons aged 14 to 49 years have HSV2 infection. However, the prevalence of genital herpes infection is higher than that because an increasing number of genital herpes infections are caused by HSV1.

Most persons have had exposure to HSV1 by adulthood, as it is readily transmitted via oral secretions. However, exposure to HSV2 infection usually begins at puberty and is correlated with level of sexual activity. HSV2 infection is more common in females than males. This is possibly because genital infection is more easily transmitted from males to females than from females to males during penile-vaginal sex. HSV2 infection is more common among non-Hispanic Blacks (34.6%) than among non-Hispanic Whites (8.1%).

Most infected persons may be unaware of their infection; in the United States, an estimated 87.4% of 14- to 49-year-olds infected with HSV2 have never received a clinical diagnosis. HSV2 can be transmitted to the neonate at childbirth because of contact with maternal genital lesions. It is important to recognize that the presence of HSV2 infection in children can be a sign of sexual abuse. Most persons who have HSV2 infection are not aware that they are infected, so they can transmit the virus during sexual contact. Genital herpes is a lifelong viral illness, with exacerbations when symptoms are present and remissions when symptoms are absent.

Risk of HIV infection is increased in persons with genital herpes disease. There is an estimated two- to fourfold increased risk of acquiring HIV, if individuals with genital herpes infection are genitally exposed to HIV. Ulcerations in mucous membranes of the mouth, vagina, or rectum from a herpes infection increase a person's vulnerability to HIV. The breaks in the skin or mucous membranes are potential areas of entry for HIV. In addition, genital herpes increases the number of CD4 cells in the mucous membranes. CD4 cells are the target cells for HIV. In persons with both HIV and genital herpes, there is activation of HIV replication at the site of genital herpes ulcerations. This can increase the risk that HIV will be transmitted to a noninfected sexual partner during contact with the mouth, vagina, or rectum.

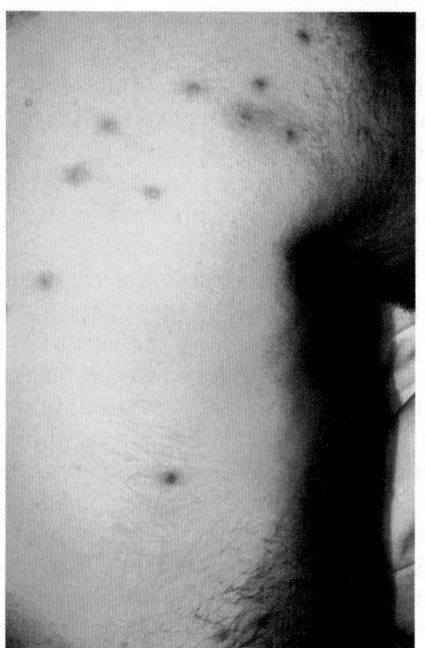

FIGURE 28-4. Genital herpes. *(Courtesy of CDC.)*

> ### 🔎 CLINICAL CONCEPT
>
> HSV2 can be transmitted during symptomatic and asymptomatic periods.

Pathophysiology. Humans are the only carriers of HSV, which is a DNA virus. The features of HSV infection are skin invasion, neurological involvement, dormancy, and reactivation. HSV1 or HSV2 virus enters the mucosa or injured epithelium at the site of contact. Close skin contact, mucosa secretions, or saliva can transmit HSV. The virus reproduces within the skin, causing blisters and ulceration, but travels rapidly to the dorsal ganglion of sensory nerves. In the neurons, the virus either (1) replicates and travels back to the skin, where it produces blisters, or (2) becomes dormant until later reactivation. The time from initial contraction to infection is 6 to 7 days. The virus usually remains dormant within the trigeminal or sacral spinal nerves. During times of low immunity or stress, reactivation often occurs.

Clinical Presentation. Classic manifestations of HSV infection include local tenderness, burning, and erythema, followed by eruption of vesicles that rupture into painful ulcers covered with yellow exudates (see Fig. 28-4). The patient may have fever and

lymphadenopathy in the region of the lesions. Crusting of ulcerative lesions occurs after several days. New lesions appear through the first week, peaking between 8 and 10 days. Dysuria, urethritis, meningitis, and pharyngitis can be the symptoms, depending on the site of infection. Lesions are commonly observable on the external genitalia and perineal area of both males and females. However, lesions can be occult within the vaginal canal and cervix. Recurrences of herpes infection are usually similar in symptomatology but have a much shorter duration.

Diagnosis. Culture of HSV is the diagnostic test of choice. Serological testing, which demonstrates HSV antibody levels in the blood, can also be used. However, a rise in antibody titer does not occur during recurrences of HSV infection. Therefore, the test is generally not useful for the diagnosis of HSV relapse. Detection of HSV DNA in clinical specimens is possible with PCR techniques. PCR can detect viral shedding during symptomatic or asymptomatic phases. Currently, there is no recommendation for universal screening of the population for HSV infection.

Treatment. There is no cure for HSV. The oral antiviral medications acyclovir, valacyclovir, or famciclovir can be used to treat the infection. Treatment is aimed at reducing symptoms and the extent of outbreak. Importantly, treatment can prevent infection from mother to fetus. The CDC recommends treatment with antiviral medication three times a day for 7 to 10 days.

Persons with herpes should abstain from sexual activity with partners when herpes lesions or other symptoms of herpes are present. It is important to know that even if a person does not have any symptoms, they can still infect sex partners. Sex partners of infected persons should be advised that they may become infected and they should use condoms to reduce the risk. Daily treatment with valacyclovir decreases the rate of HSV2 transmission in discordant, heterosexual couples in which the source partner has a history of genital HSV2 infection. Such couples should be encouraged to consider suppressive antiviral therapy as part of a strategy to prevent transmission, in addition to consistent condom use and avoidance of sexual activity during recurrences.

Herpes infection is usually self-limited, except in pregnancy, when a fetus is involved. In females, during a herpetic attack, the cervix is almost always involved. Neonatal HSV-2 infection can occur transplacentally to the fetus. More often, however, the mother transmits the infection during delivery as the neonate passes through the birth canal. Maternal transmission of HSV-2 to the neonate can occur whether the mother is symptomatic or asymptomatic at the time of birth. Herpes encephalitis or meningitis is the feared complication in the newborn. Females with active recurrent genital herpes should be offered suppressive acyclovir, valacyclovir, or famciclovir therapy at or beyond 36 weeks of gestation. Cesarean delivery is indicated in females with active genital lesions or prodromal symptoms (e.g., vulvar pain or burning) at the time of delivery because these symptoms may indicate an impending outbreak.

Zika Virus

Zika virus (ZIKV) is an RNA flavivirus related to dengue, yellow fever, and West Nile virus. It is transmitted via the *Aedes* mosquito. The virus was first identified in the African regions in Kampala, Uganda, in the Zika forest in 1947 in a rhesus monkey. The spread of ZIKV infection around the world caused panic, especially in Latin American and Caribbean nations, with approximately 440,000 to 1,300,000 cases in Brazil during the 2016 outbreak. Currently, ZIKV virus outbreaks have declined in the America regions from 2017 through 2019.

ZIKV RNA has been detected in the semen of ZIKV-infected patients. The virus can be transmitted between both sexes; however, the highest transmission frequency is from male to female. ZIKV is also vertically transmitted from mothers to their fetuses during pregnancy.

The majority of persons with ZIKV are asymptomatic. About 20% to 25% of infected patients develop skin rashes, headache, fever, joint pains, and conjunctivitis, with an incubation period of about 1 week. Some patients also vomit and have diarrhea, redness of eyes, weakness, edema, abdominal pain, loss of appetite, and experience hematospermia. In pregnant females, ZIKV can lead to neurological complications in the fetus, most commonly underdevelopment of the brain and microcephaly.

ZIKV is transmitted to persons via mosquito bite, sexual activity (oral, vaginal, or anal), blood products, maternal–fetal transmission, or organ transplantation. It is diagnosed mainly by PCR of ZIKV RNA testing of serum, whole blood, or urine. There is currently no antiviral treatment for ZIKV infection and no vaccine. Supportive care and use of condoms for sexual activity are recommended. Aspirin and NSAIDs should be avoided due to the risk of bleeding from possible coinfection with dengue fever and Reye's syndrome in children. Prevention involves personal protection and environmental control measures against mosquitoes. Sexual transmission is a particular risk because the virus can remain viable in semen and vaginal secretions for long periods. The WHO recommends abstaining from unprotected sexual activity for at least 6 months after infection. Pregnant females should abstain from unprotected sexual activity for the duration of pregnancy.

Monkeypox

Monkeypox (MPX) is an emerging zoonotic disease caused by *monkeypox virus* (MPXV), a member of the *Orthopoxvirus* genus, which is similar to smallpox. At the time of writing this textbook in 2022, monkeypox outbreaks have occurred globally. In the United States, the total number of cases numbered 9,492. The MPXV is transmitted mainly by close intimate contact. The highest-risk population is MSM. Monkeypox can spread to anyone through close, skin-to-skin contact, particularly if in contact with rash lesions, body fluids, or respiratory secretions. Also the virus can spread from objects or surfaces in close contact with the person with MPXV. It can be transmitted through oral, anal, or vaginal sexual activity. Prolonged face-to-face contact and kissing can also transmit the virus. A pregnant person can spread the virus to their fetus through the placenta.

The clinical presentation closely resembles smallpox; however, there is early lymph node enlargement at the onset of fever. A rash usually appears 1 to 3 days after onset of fever with lesions appearing simultaneously. The distribution of the rash is mainly peripheral but can occur anywhere on the body. The infection lasts approximately 4 weeks as the lesions desquamate. Patients can suffer from a range of complications including secondary bacterial infections, respiratory distress, bronchopneumonia, gastrointestinal involvement, dehydration, sepsis, encephalitis, and corneal infection with ensuing loss of vision.

No specific treatment for a MPXV infection currently exists, and patients are managed with supportive care and symptomatic treatment. Smallpox vaccine is administered as prevention for those at high risk.

Pelvic Inflammatory Disease (PID)

PID is the most serious STI in females, and 85% of the cases occur in females of childbearing age. Any infection ascending from the vagina and cervix to the internal upper reproductive organs, including the uterus, fallopian tubes, or ovaries, is considered PID. Females who are most at risk include those who have a history of multiple sex partners, past STIs, intrauterine device use, or failure to use contraceptive methods. Females who have had a dilation and curettage (D&C), abortion by vacuum curettage, or hysterosalpingogram are at increased risk.

Pathophysiology

The majority of cases of PID are caused by *N. gonorrhoeae* or *C. trachomatis*. Less commonly, PID is caused by aerobic and anaerobic organisms such as *G. vaginalis, Prevotella* sp., *Haemophilus influenzae, Escherichia coli, Streptococcus agalactiae, S. pyogenes, S. pneumoniae,* Cytomegalovirus, *Mycoplasma hominis,* and *Ureaplasma urealyticum.*

The two phases involved in PID are (1) infection of vagina or cervix and (2) upward ascent of the infection into the uterus, fallopian tubes, and ovary. Inflammation of the vaginal canal, sexual activity, and disruption of the balance of flora in the vagina allow the microorganisms to reach the internal organs. Inflammation resulting from *N. gonorrhoeae* and *C. trachomatis* infections makes the fallopian tubes susceptible to invasion by anaerobic organisms. When the causative organism is *N. gonorrhoeae,* exudates from the fallopian tubes may enter the peritoneum, causing pelvic peritonitis. The uterus, fallopian tubes, and ovaries can become fixed by pelvic inflammatory adhesions. Fallopian tubes and ovaries often adhere to the posterior uterus or are prolapsed in the cul-de-sac; this disrupts the position of the uterus, causing dyspareunia, chronic pelvic pain, and infertility. Peritoneal involvement may result in Fitz–Hugh–Curtis syndrome, a disorder that causes adhesions of the outer liver.

C. trachomatis salpingitis is usually asymptomatic, which is why universal screening has been recommended for females younger than age 25 years. The organism can attach to sperm, which ascend to the fallopian tube and cause cell injury and scarring of the tube by destroying the cilia. The ciliated cells of the fallopian tubes are very important in moving an ovum into the uterus; interference with their function can lead to infertility.

Clinical Presentation

When a female of childbearing age presents with such symptoms as lower abdominal pain, pelvic tenderness, or possible genital tract infection or inflammation, further investigation is necessary (see Box 28-3). If uterine and adnexal tenderness are present and if pain with cervical motion exists, the diagnosis of PID should be considered.

PID presents as an acute, chronic, or silent infection. The acute presentation, which is characterized by the classic pelvic pain and possibly fever or chills, is the more common presentation and is more likely to be treated. The causative organism in the acute type of PID is most often *N. gonorrhoeae*. The silent

---

BOX 28-3. Diagnoses to Exclude When PID Is Suspected

When pelvic or abdominal pain is part of the clinical presentation, PID and the following conditions must be ruled out:

- Ectopic pregnancy
- Acute appendicitis
- Ruptured ovarian cyst
- Endometritis
- Endometriosis
- Septic abortion
- Tubo-ovarian abscess

---

type, which is usually caused by chlamydia, has a more insidious presentation and is often misdiagnosed as mild salpingitis; thus, it is not treated as aggressively. Because of its unrecognized silent presentation, it may account for up to 40% of infertility cases involving tubal dysfunction. In chronic PID, inflammation of the walls of the fallopian tubes leaves scars, which then create problems for egg transport. Scarred fallopian tubes can lead to infertility or ectopic pregnancy.

 CLINICAL CONCEPT

If there is exquisite tenderness of the cervix on a pelvic examination, this is often called **Chandelier sign**, which is pathognomonic for PID.

Diagnosis

PID can be difficult to diagnose. A general health and sexual history is essential, as are a physical examination and pelvic examination. A pregnancy test is also required because ectopic pregnancy is possible. Specific symptoms and laboratory test findings are usually the sources used to diagnose PID (see Box 28-4).

BOX 28-4. Diagnosing Pelvic Inflammatory Disease

Pelvic or lower abdominal pain in combination with the following signs and symptoms strengthen the diagnosis of PID:

- Oral temperature of 101° F
- Abnormal vaginal or cervical mucopurulent discharge
- Presence of white blood cells (on microscopic survey of vaginal secretions)
- Elevated erythrocyte sedimentation rate
- Elevated C-reactive protein
- Laboratory documentation of gonococcus or chlamydia

Imaging studies usually do not contribute much to the diagnosis. MRI may visualize thickened, inflamed fallopian tubes, uterus, and ovaries. Transvaginal ultrasound might visualize some inflammation of the ovaries, uterus, and fallopian tubes. Laparoscopic examination of the abdomen and pelvic region may be necessary.

> **ALERT!** Any female presenting with abdominal or pelvic pain should have a pregnancy test to rule out ectopic pregnancy.

Treatment

According to CDC guidelines, clinicians may treat a patient with PID as an outpatient or an inpatient. The decision to hospitalize the patient depends on certain criteria (see Box 28-5). Regardless of the place of treatment, the patient with PID is treated with high-dose antibiotics.

Sexual Health Care Needs and the LGBTQ+ Patient Population

Sexuality is a human dimension that can best be described on a continuum; not all persons feel that they can be singularly categorized as heterosexual, homosexual, or bisexual. These are societal constructs that are not applicable to all patients. At birth, an individual's biological sex of male or female is based on genetic, physiological, anatomical, and hormonal characteristics. However, a person's gender identity does not always correspond to their biological sex at birth. A person's gender identity is their internal sense of being male, female, both, or neither. Gender dysphoria is distress associated with biological sex when it differs from a person's preferred gender identity and expression.

BOX 28-5. Criteria for Hospitalization in PID

The following criteria can be used when deciding whether to hospitalize a patient with suspected PID:
- When diagnosis is uncertain
- If surgical emergencies cannot be excluded
- If a pelvic abscess is suspected
- If the patient is pregnant
- If the patient is a minor
- If the patient's condition is severe, such as high fever, nausea, or vomiting
- If the patient is unable to follow or tolerate an outpatient regimen, or if clinical follow-up is not possible within 72 hours of starting treatment

---

In health care and the media, the acronym **LGBTQ** stands for lesbian, gay, bisexual, transgender, and queer (or questioning). Another acronym used in the media is LGBTQIA2S+, which stands for lesbian, gay, bisexual, transgender, queer and/or questioning, intersex, asexual, two-spirit, and others. Sexual orientation is how a person describes their physical and/or emotional attraction to others; this is distinct from biological sex or gender identity. LGB refers to sexual orientation: lesbian, gay, or bisexual. Persons who are gender nonconforming sometimes use the umbrella terms queer or questioning to describe themselves. According to studies of sexuality within the population, many persons do not describe their gender or sexual orientation in terms of these distinct categories. Some people do not identify with any gender. People whose gender is neither male nor female use many different terms to describe themselves, with "nonbinary" being one of the most common. In July 2021, the Census Bureau began collecting information on the sexual orientation and gender identity of respondents to its Household Pulse Survey. For adults over age 18, self-report surveys revealed that 88.3% of respondents identified as straight, 3.3% identified as gay or lesbian, 4.4% identified as bisexual, 2.1% reported "I don't know," and 1.9% reported "something else."

Persons of the LGBTQ+ community are identified as underrepresented sexual groups and are a growing medically underserved population in the United States. In the health-care setting, commonly used terminology includes MSM (men who have sex with men) and WSW (women who have sex with women). These categories are used to identify specific risk factors associated with behaviors, understand diseases related to sexuality, and treat patients according to their specific health-care needs. Understanding the patient's sexual behavior is critical in order to assess risk of disease. The clinician needs to inquire about oral, anal, and vaginal sexual activity. Patients should be asked if they practice safe sex using condoms or dental dams and about the number and gender of their sexual partners. In addition, they should be asked if they know of any specific risk factors of their sexual partners. Use of contraceptives or desire for pregnancy should be discussed. Females should be asked about last menstrual period and history of pregnancy, and both males and females should be asked about history of STIs. The clinician also needs to ask if the patient has had hormone or sexual reassignment surgery and ascertain what types of disorders the patient is susceptible to according to their reproductive tract anatomy.

Specific STIs Affecting MSM

MSM are at high risk for STIs that affect the rectum, genitalia, urethra, and oropharynx, as well as some systemic diseases such as viral hepatitis, syphilis, and HIV (see Box 28-6). It is important to ask the patient about rectal pain and anal discharge, which occur in

---

BOX 28-6. Most Common STIs in MSM

- HIV infection
- Viral hepatitis A, B, or C
- HPV infection (genital, rectal, or oropharyngeal)
- *Neisseria gonorrhoeae* (genital, rectal, or oropharyngeal)
- Chlamydia (genital, rectal, or oropharyngeal)
- Herpes (genital, rectal, or oropharyngeal)
- Shigella infection*
- Meningococcal meningitis*

---

*Sporadic outbreaks have been reported.
Adapted from Wilkin, T. (2015). Primary care for men who have sex with men. *N Engl J Med, 373*(9), 854–862.

proctitis. The presence of these symptoms should prompt testing for syphilis, *N. gonorrhoeae,* HPV, HIV, and *C. trachomatis,* which require a rectal swab for NAAT. Certain strains of *Chlamydia* can cause LGV, which causes bloody discharge and ulcerative anal lesions. LGV is often a coinfection with HIV. Even in the absence of symptoms, screening for STIs—including serological testing for HIV and syphilis and oral, rectal, and urinary testing for *N. gonorrhoeae* and *C. trachomatis*—is recommended for MSM once a year or twice a year for those at high risk.

Risk of HIV Among MSM

According to the CDC, in all regions of the United States, gay and bisexual males are the group most affected by HIV. In the United States, the estimated lifetime risk for HIV infection among MSM is one in six, compared with heterosexual males at one in 524 and heterosexual females at one in 253.

In 2019, about 70% of new HIV infections were among gay and bisexual males, even though they make up only 2% of the population, with the highest burden among Black and Hispanic/Latino males. By age group, people ages 25 to 34 years have the highest rate of annual HIV infections. In 2019, youth ages 13 to 24 years accounted for 21% of new HIV infections and are the least likely of any age group to have a suppressed viral load. Furthermore, just 23% of the estimated more than one million Americans who could benefit from pre-exposure prophylaxis (PrEP) are using it, and some of the largest gaps are among gay and bisexual males of color and transgender females. Over the past decade, HIV incidence in young MSM of color has increased by 87%. Patient education is vital to protect MSM from contracting HIV. Health-care professionals should teach MSM the importance of practicing safe sex: using condoms and nonpetroleum-based lubricants. Preventive primary care for MSM includes PrEP and postexposure prophylaxis for HIV (see Chapter 11 for information on HIV infection).

Risk of HPV Among MSM

A prominent health issue in the MSM community is HPV, which can cause anal papillomavirus and/or anal cancer. Human papillomavirus (HPV) is the most common STI globally. Studies have found HPV infection of the anal canal in up to 80% of MSM, compared with 15% in heterosexual males. Notably, prevalence of HPV anal infection has been found in almost 100% of HIV-seropositive MSM. HIV-infected MSM also have an increased risk of anal, penile, and oropharyngeal cancer, compared with males without HIV (see information on HPV infection previously in this chapter).

Risk of Viral Hepatitis in MSM

MSM are at high risk for contracting hepatitis A, B, and C. Hepatitis A virus (HAV) is spread primarily through the fecal–oral route, either from person to person or through exposure to contaminated food or water. Most acute infections (85%) are asymptomatic. In all types of hepatitis, the patient may present with low-grade fever, anorexia, gastrointestinal symptoms, abdominal pain in the upper right quadrant, fatigue, pale stools, dark urine, and jaundice. HAV causes a self-limited infection of less than 2 months' duration and confers immunity when resolved. A vaccine is available for HAV and should be recommended to MSM.

HBV is transmitted via blood or mucosal exposure to body fluids of an infected person. In the United States, the most common mode of transmission is by sexual contact and injection drug use. HBV can lead to chronic hepatitis, hepatitis fibrosis, cirrhosis, or liver cancer. According to the CDC, an estimated 24% of new HBV infections occur in MSM. Immunization against HBV is recommended for all MSM. Hepatitis B immunoglobulin (HBIg) can also be administered to impart temporary immunity to those exposed to HBV. Clinicians should educate patients regarding the necessity of three doses of HBV vaccine and the availability of postexposure HBIg that can reduce the risk in close contacts.

Hepatitis C virus (HCV) is transmitted by exposure to infected blood, most commonly through injection drug use. Sexual transmission occurs in rare cases; however, in both MSM and heterosexuals, the likelihood of sexual transmission rises with increase in number of sex partners and when sex partners are infected with HIV. Acute HCV infection progresses to chronic liver disease in 75% to 85% of cases. Infection commonly causes no symptoms, and the incubation period lasts several months to years. Mild to moderate liver disease may produce vague symptoms, such as chronic fatigue, for years. Due to an immune complex component of HCV infection, extrahepatic manifestations are possible. These include arthralgias, purpura, glomerular dysfunction, peripheral neuropathy, central nervous system vasculitis, and reduced complement levels. Chronic HCV infection is the leading cause of liver-related death and hepatocellular carcinoma in the Western world. It is estimated that only 50% of those chronically infected persons have been diagnosed.

Other STIs in MSM

Shigella Infection

MSM are at high risk for *Shigella* infection, also known as shigellosis or gay bowel syndrome. *Shigella* is transmitted via the fecal–oral route or from contaminated food or water. One to 2 days after exposure, *Shigella* infection causes fever, diarrhea, abdominal pain, and tenesmus. Immunosuppression increases the risk for *Shigella,* and there is a high prevalence in HIV-positive MSM. *Shigella* infection can resolve after 5 to 7 days; severe cases may require antibiotic treatment. Some strains of *Shigella* are resistant to antibiotics.

Meningococcal Meningitis

Outbreaks of meningococcal meningitis have been reported among MSM. This population is reported to have an increased prevalence of oropharyngeal colonization with *N. meningitides* compared with the general population. Current guidelines from the Advisory Committee on Immunization Practices (ACIP) do not include MSM as a group that is at high risk for meningococcal meningitis and do not recommend routine vaccination. However, outbreaks of meningococcal meningitis are increasingly being reported. It is prudent for MSM who are living in areas of outbreaks to obtain the meningitis vaccine.

Underuse of Preventive Health Care in WSW

WSW are not a homogeneous group who exclusively have sex with females. It is common for WSW to also engage in sexual activity with males. Studies show that up to 87% of females who self-identify as lesbians have also engaged in sexual activity with males. Many clinicians assume heterosexual behavior of their female patients and do not ask females about sexual activity with females. Studies also show that WSW are commonly uncomfortable sharing information about their same-sex sexual activity; thus, females are commonly not given advice on how to engage in safe sex with other females.

Also, there is an unfounded belief among WSW that they have a lesser chance of acquiring STIs; however, WSW are at risk of acquiring STIs from both females and males. It is important to educate WSW that there are various modes of transmission of STIs (see Box 28-7).

Many WSW also believe they have less need for Pap tests and cervical cancer screening. WSW are 10 times more likely not to have received timely Pap tests and 10 times more likely not to have received timely

---

> ### BOX 28-7. Modes of Transmission of STIs Among WSW
>
> - Skin-to-skin contact
> - Mucous membrane contact
> - Vaginal fluid
> - Menstrual blood
> - Sex toys
> - Semen from male donor for pregnancy

mammograms compared with women who have sex with men (WSM). Recommendations for cervical cancer, HPV, and breast cancer screening in lesbians and bisexual females, regardless of their sexual history with males, should not differ from screening recommendations for females in general. Findings from the National Health Interview Survey revealed that females in same-sex relationships experience greater odds of breast and cervical cancer mortality compared with heterosexual females because of nulliparity, more common in WSW, and underuse of Pap tests and mammography screening.

STIs in WSW

C. trachomatis and *N. gonorrhoeae* are the two most common bacterial STIs in the general population. Both of these STIs are reported to be less common in females who have sex exclusively with females. However, these STIs are higher in prevalence among bisexual females than the general population; therefore, it is prudent to screen for *C. trachomatis* and *N. gonorrhoeae* in WSW. Untreated chlamydia and gonorrhea can lead to PID, tubal infertility, and chronic pelvic pain (see previous information in chapter on chlamydia and gonorrhea).

HPV, an STI that can cause cervical and anal cancer, can be transmitted through sexual activity between females. HPV-associated squamous intraepithelial lesions have occurred in lesbians who have never had sex with males. Up to 30% of females who report having sex with females test positive for HPV infection. Also, HPV infection is common in females who are seropositive for HIV; therefore, screening for HPV should be the same in WSW as for WSM (see previous information on HPV in this chapter).

Genital herpes caused by HSV1 or HSV2 is common in WSW and bisexual females. It is important to educate females that HSV can be transmitted by skin-to-skin and mouth-to-genital contact. HSV infection is often asymptomatic, and subclinical infection is highly contagious. Shedding of the virus among those who are asymptomatic is exceedingly common, accounting for the majority of transmission events (see previous information in chapter on genital herpes).

Bacterial vaginosis (BV) is particularly common in WSW, with an estimated prevalence of 25% to 52%. Having a history of female sex partners confers a twofold increase in risk of BV (see previous information in chapter on BV infection). Exchange of vaginal fluid among female partners contributes to the initiation of BV. Susceptibility to BV among WSW increases with an increased number of different female sexual partners.

Syphilis, HAV, HBV, and HIV are uncommon STIs in WSW; however, WSW who engage in high-risk behaviors are susceptible to HIV. These behaviors include unprotected sex with males, unprotected sharing of sex toys with females, and injection drug use (see Box 28-8). WSW are also uniquely at risk for HIV through the use of unscreened semen donation from sources other than a sperm bank (see Chapter 11 for information on HIV infection).

Transgender Individuals

Transgender is a term for individuals who are "gender nonconforming" and have a gender identity or gender expression that differs from their biological sex. A transgender individual whose gender identity is male despite a female biological sex at birth is termed a transgender man, trans man, or FtM (female to male). A transgender individual whose gender identity is female despite a biological male sex at birth is termed a transgender woman, trans woman, or MtF (male to female). Cisgender describes a person whose gender identity corresponds to their sex assigned at birth. The word cisgender is the antonym of transgender.

BOX 28-8. Common Health Problems in WSW and Bisexual Females

- HPV infection (genital, rectal, and oropharyngeal)
- Genital herpes
- Bacterial vaginosis
- Chlamydia
- *Neisseria gonorrhoeae*
- Trichomoniasis
- HIV
- Lack of regular Pap tests increases risk of cervical cancer
- Lack of regular mammograms increases risk of breast cancer
- Violence
- Depression and suicide
- Anxiety
- Substance abuse
- Smoking (increases risk of heart disease)
- Overweight/obesity (increases risk of heart disease)

From Centers for Disease Control and Prevention (CDC). (2017). Lesbian, gay, bisexual and transgender health. http://www.cdc.gov/lgbthealth; ACOG (2012, reaffirmed 2018). Committee opinion: Health care for lesbians and bisexual females. https://www.acog.org/Clinical-Guidance-and-Publications/Committee-Opinions/Committee-on-Health-Care-for-Underserved-Women/Health-Care-for-Lesbians-and-Bisexual-Women

---

The prevalence of adult transgenderism is difficult to estimate. A commonly quoted estimate puts the number of U.S. transgender adults at about 1.3 million, or 0.5% of the population. Research has consistently shown that transgender individuals are medically underserved and experience stigma, discrimination, and socioeconomic disadvantages, leading to myriad poor health outcomes and high rates of disease burden. Transgender individuals experience major challenges accessing health care because of a lack of transgender-competent and inclusive health services, and systemic discrimination in primary health services and hospitals.

Transgender patients may have extreme discomfort with their bodies, and they may find some elements of a physical examination traumatic. It is recommended that provider/patient trust be established before examining sensitive areas (e.g., genital, rectal, and vaginal), unless there is an immediate, urgent need to proceed. The provider should ascertain the patient's comfort/discomfort and take the time to discuss the plan for the examination before beginning. The provider should assure confidentiality and ensure privacy. An understanding of transgender terminology and the experience of gender dysphoria is key. Developing an understanding of potential gender-affirming treatments and surgeries also optimizes patient care. However, it is important to recognize that not all transgender individuals will choose gender-affirming treatments and/or surgeries.

Hormonal Treatment

Transitioning to the opposite sex can include hormone therapy, psychological therapy, and surgery. The aim of hormonal treatment is to stimulate the development of the secondary sex characteristics of the new sex and to diminish those of the natal sex. The clinician must provide care for the anatomy that is present, but also recognize that there will be some health needs due to the remaining anatomic features from birth. For example, although a transgender MtF patient may have had gender-confirming surgery, they may still need to have prostate-specific antigen levels checked as they age.

MtF Transgender Individuals. For MtF transition, androgenic hormones need to be counteracted by estrogen. Estrogen hormone therapy is prescribed to induce breast formation, atrophy of the testicles, and female distribution of fat, and reduce male-pattern hair growth. When providing health care for transgender patients, the clinician needs to ask about the details of the sexual reassignment surgery in order to consider the anatomy of the patient. For example, the patient should be asked if orchiectomy had been performed. If not, testicular cancer may be a risk. The prostate gland is usually left in place and can develop benign hyperplasia or cancer. The enlarged breast tissue can develop cancer, and thus mammography may be necessary. Hormonal treatment with ethinyl estradiol, although efficacious, should be avoided. When taken at the dosages required for sex reassignment, there is increased risk of deep venous thrombosis and death from cardiovascular causes compared with 17ß-estradiol. Smoking should be discouraged, as this increases the risk of thrombus formation in estrogen therapy. Studies assessing the metabolic effects of androgen deprivation and estrogen therapy in MtF individuals have shown that increases in visceral fat are associated with increases in triglyceride levels, insulin resistance, and blood pressure. Also, estrogen treatment can cause metabolic syndrome. Therefore, lipid and serum glucose levels should be periodically checked.

FtM Transgender Individuals. Treatment is intended to virilize the FtM individual with testosterone administration. Changes due to testosterone include male-pattern hair growth, degeneration of ovaries and uterus, enlargement of the clitoris, and the cessation of uterine bleeding. Depending on the sexual reassignment surgery, a hysterectomy and oophorectomy may be involved, or the ovaries may be left in place. Because androgens are partially metabolized into estradiols, there may be estrogenic stimulation of the remaining breast tissue, which increases the risk of cancer. FtM patients are particularly at risk if they have the *BRCA1* or *BRCA2* genetic mutation. FtM patients who have not had oophorectomy can develop polycystic ovaries or cancer. FtM patients who have not had a hysterectomy can develop proliferation of the endometrium, and cervical tissue can undergo cancerous changes. Therefore, a periodic Pap smear is necessary. The clinician needs to completely understand the anatomy of the FtM patient in order to make clinical decisions about screening and treating disease.

Long-Term Treatment. After sex-reassignment surgery, including gonadectomy, hormonal therapy must be continued. Some MtF individuals continue to have male-pattern hair growth; continued administration of antiandrogens, typically at approximately half the preoperative dose, reduces male-pattern hair growth. Continued administration of estradiol is required to avoid symptoms and signs of hormone deficiency, such as vasomotor symptoms and osteoporosis in MtF transgender individuals. Observational studies have shown that bone mass is generally maintained with estrogen alone in MtF individuals and with testosterone alone in FtM individuals when prescribed at the doses typically used to treat hypogonadism.

Cancer. Long-term administration of cross-sex hormones may increase risk of hormone-dependent cancer. In both MtF and FtM, estrogen-dependent cancers can develop because in MtF patients, estrogen is administered, and in FtM patients, testosterone is partially converted into estradiol.

STIs. Transgender patients may have sex with males, females, or both. Because of the diverse nature of sexual partners among transgender persons, providers must recognize symptoms of common STIs and screen for asymptomatic STIs on the basis of individual sexual practices.

Transgender individuals have high rates of HIV and AIDS. Studies have found approximately 28% of transgender persons are HIV positive. Higher rates, up to 56%, are found among African American MtF patients. Studies have found that the rate of HIV infection is more than four times the national average, with highest rates among MtF persons. Early sexual experiences, having multiple partners, needle sharing, and random sexual contacts increase the risk for HIV/AIDS, especially for MtFs. HBV, HCV, syphilis, and HPV coinfections are common in transgender people with HIV who are engaged in prostitution. HPV is particularly common in transgender people engaged in prostitution, with up to a 97% prevalence rate that puts them at high risk for anogenital cancer. Periodic Pap tests, HIV and STI testing, and HPV vaccination are advised.

Chapter Summary

- Female adolescents and young adult females are at increased risk of infection with HPV, chlamydia, gonorrhea, HIV, and syphilis. MSM are also at high risk for these STIs.

- Children with STIs should be assessed for child abuse.

- Chlamydia, gonorrhea, chancroid, HIV, and syphilis are reportable diseases.

- *C. trachomatis* is one of the most common causes of STIs, such as cervicitis, urethritis, PID, and a type of conjunctivitis known as inclusion conjunctivitis. It is usually a silent, asymptomatic disease.

- BV is due to a change in normal vaginal flora to anaerobes and *G. vaginalis*. Vaginal discharge is thin, white, and has a "fishy odor." Whiff–amine test is positive.

- Gonorrheal infections can cause cervicitis, proctitis, urethritis, PID, conjunctivitis, and pharyngitis. Complications include ectopic pregnancy, infertility, and increased susceptibility to HIV. Strains are becoming increasingly resistant to antibiotics.

- *M. genitalium* causes cervicitis and urethritis, discharge, and penile inflammation in males. Multiple sex partners and chlamydia increase the risk of infection.

- Syphilis infection occurs in four stages: primary, secondary, latent, and tertiary. Syphilis has many different presentations, and in advanced stages it can appear as many other diseases, making it known as "the great impostor." The classic lesion of syphilis is the painless chancre, rash on palms and soles, and condylomata lata. Granulomas, called gummas, develop in different organs. Syphilis infection can span several decades. It increases susceptibility to HIV infection.

- Chancroid is a reportable disease caused by *H. ducreyi*. It causes a painful ulceration with inguinal lymphadenopathy (buboes).

- LGV is an STI that is increasing incidence among MSM. Classic signs of disease are buboes, which are enlarged inguinal lymph nodes.

- Granuloma inguinale (donovanosis) demonstrates intracellular *K. granulomatis* organisms within white blood cells called Donovan bodies.

- Patients with LGV, chancroid, or granuloma inguinale should have testing for syphilis, gonorrhea, chlamydia, genital herpes, hepatitis, and HIV.

- Trichomoniasis is a vaginitis that can also affect males, causing urethritis. Greenish vaginal malodorous discharge is common in females. Metronidazole is the treatment.

- HPV infection is a precursor to cervical, anal, rectal, oropharyngeal, penile, and laryngeal cancer. Condyloma acuminata are the genital warts that occur in HPV infection. There is no cure, but a vaccine is available.

- HPV vaccination is most effective before exposure to HPV and therefore is recommended for preteens and adults up to age 26. However, adults can receive HPV vaccine depending on their risk factors.

- Genital herpes, commonly referred to as HSV2, is a lifelong viral illness, with periods of exacerbations when symptoms are present and remissions when symptoms are absent. It is important to understand that HSV2 can be transmitted during symptomatic and asymptomatic periods.

- Genital herpes HSV2 can cause neurological problems in newborns born to infected mothers.

- Zika virus is transmitted to persons via mosquito bite, sexual activity (oral, vaginal, or anal), blood products, maternal–fetal transmission, or organ transplantation.

- The majority of cases of PID are caused by *N. gonorrhoeae* or *C. trachomatis*. Females with abdominal or pelvic pain should have a pregnancy test to rule out ectopic pregnancy. Complications associated with PID are ectopic pregnancy and infertility.

- Gender dysphoria is distress associated with one's biological sex because it differs from the preferred gender identity and expression.

- Gender identity is the internal sense of being male, female, both, or neither.

- Persons of the LGBTQ+ community are identified as underrepresented sexual groups and are a growing medically underserved population in the United States.

- Understanding the patient's sexual behavior is critical in order to assess the risk of disease. The clinician needs to inquire about oral, anal, penile, and vaginal sexual activity.

- HPV, an STI that can cause cervical, penile, oropharyngeal, throat, and anorectal cancer, can be transmitted through the sexual activity. It can also cause respiratory papillomatosis.

- MSM who are HIV seropositive are at risk for HPV and other STIs.

- WSW are 10 times more likely not to have received timely Pap tests and 10 times more likely not to have received timely mammograms compared with WSM.

- The clinician needs to treat the transgender patient according to the anatomy that is present or that may be still existent from birth. For example, MtF patients need prostate surface antigen testing after age 50.

- Long-term administration of cross-sex hormones in transgender patients may increase the risk of hormone-dependent cancer.

Making the Connections

Disorder and Pathophysiology

Signs and Symptoms	Physical Assessment Findings	Diagnostic Testing	Treatment
Bacterial Infections			
Bacterial Vaginosis | Change in the vaginal bacterial flora from *Lactobacillus* to a mixture of gram-negative and anaerobic bacterial organisms (largely *Gardnerella vaginalis*) that cause breakdown of vaginal peptides.			
Vulvar and vaginal pruritus. Thin, off-white vaginal discharge that has a "fishy odor."	Female: pelvic examination shows vaginal malodorous discharge.	Characteristic clue cells found in vaginal secretions. Positive whiff–amine test and Gram stain.	Metronidazole or clindamycin. Treatment of female sex partners. Testing for other STIs advisable.

Making the Connections–cont'd

Signs and Symptoms	Physical Assessment Findings	Diagnostic Testing	Treatment
Chlamydia | An obligate, intracellular microorganism that reproduces in the cells of the host. *Chlamydia* can protect itself from the host's immune system by converting into a sporelike inclusion body.			
Often asymptomatic in both males and females. Female: possible vaginal bleeding/discharge. Male: possible urethritis.	Female: pelvic examination shows friable cervix and discharge. Male: painful urination and discharge from meatus.	Culture in special medium. Characteristic inclusion body found in cervical cells.	Antibiotics.
Gonorrhea | *Gonococcus* is a gram-negative, diplococcal microorganism that invades mucosal epithelium. It is highly virulent because of pili that attach to mucosa. Organism has a high mutation ability.			
Often asymptomatic in both males and females. Females: purulent vaginal discharge can occur. Males: urethritis can occur.	If symptomatic, purulent discharge. Female: inflamed cervix. Male: painful urination, discharge from penile meatus.	Culture on special medium. Gram stain slide on microscope. PCR testing can identify organism DNA.	Antibiotics are curative.
Mycoplasma genitalium | *Mycoplasma* bacterial organism that causes nongonoccocal urethritis in males and cervicitis and PID in females.			
Females often have asymptomatic cervicitis, whereas males usually present with dysuria, urethral discharge, pruritus, and inflammation of the glans penis.	Pelvic examination shows cervicitis; male urethritis, discharge.	Diagnosis involves NAAT of the urethral discharge, first-void urine, or vaginal discharge.	Azithromycin. Sexual partners should be treated. Other STI testing should be done.
Syphilis | A bacterial spirochete, *T. pallidum,* that can infect the body and remain dormant for decades. It invades mucous membranes or can be transferred to the fetus through the placenta. It forms granulomas called gummas that disrupt body organs.			
Primary stage: painless chancre on the external genitalia often not readily apparent. Secondary stage: rash appears on body, palms, and soles of feet. Tertiary stage: neurological and cardiovascular complications become apparent.	Painless, ulcerated lesion at site of inoculation. Maculopapular rash all over body, including palms of hands and soles of feet. Late stages cause neurological problems such as ataxia, stroke, and dementia.	Dark-field microscope (observe spirochetes). VDRL: positive. RPR: positive. Fluorescent treponemal antibodies: absorbed. PCR testing can detect organism DNA.	Benzathine penicillin intramuscular injection.
LGV, Chancroid, Granuloma Inguinale | LGV is caused by *C. trachomatis;* chancroid is caused by *H. ducreyi;* and granuloma inguinale by *K. granulomatis.* Granuloma inguinale is also called donovanosis.			
Soft chancre; enlarged inguinal nodes called buboes.	Ulcer at site of inoculation. Enlarged inguinal lymph nodes called buboes.	Microorganisms are found via culture. Scraping the lesion and examining scraped cells under microscope; stained bacteria are observed and identified. Nucleic acid amplification and PCR testing used. Donovan bodies in granuloma inguinale.	Antibiotics are curative. Other laboratory tests should be done: VDRL, RPR, PCR assays for *H. ducreyi* and HSV2 and HIV antibodies.

Continued

Making the Connections—cont'd

Signs and Symptoms	Physical Assessment Findings	Diagnostic Testing	Treatment
Trichomoniasis | Protozoan infection that is common in females and can be transmitted to males.			
Urethritis, vaginitis, greenish, malodorous discharge.	Female pelvic examination shows greenish, malodorous discharge.	Microscopic analysis and/or NAAT of vaginal discharge. Rapid antigen identification test.	Metronidazole or tinidazole. Testing for other STIs advised. Treatment of sexual partners.
Viral Infections **Herpes Simplex Virus** | Genital herpes can be caused by HSV1 or HSV2. Viruses invade skin and remain dormant in neurological tissue. Remissions and exacerbations of lesions can occur.			
May be asymptomatic or painful recurrent blisters.	Blisters in pelvic area.	Viral culture of scrapings of blisters.	Antivirals such as acyclovir can only diminish symptoms; they are not curative. They can also be taken as prophylactic treatment.
HPV | These genital warts can increase the risk of cervical cancer. HPV infection can occur in other areas predisposing to cancer: anal, rectal, oropharyngeal, penile, or laryngeal cancer.			
Fleshy, warty growths, usually in pelvic area.	Painless, fleshy papules in and around genitalia or anal region.	Clinical evaluation. HPV: Pap tests to identify types.	Podophyllin, laser ablation. Trichloroacetic acid application. Not curative but can decrease appearance of warts. Frequent Pap test is needed to prevent cervical cancer.
PID | Most common causes are *N. gonorrhoeae* and *C. trachomatis*. The microorganisms ascend from the vagina into the uterus, fallopian tubes, and ovaries.			
Lower abdominal pain, fever, chills, myalgias.	Cervical motion tenderness Abdominal or pelvic tenderness on palpation.	Pelvic examination shows tenderness of cervix. Specific criteria for PID.	Oral or IV antibiotics.

Bibliography

Available online at fadavis.com

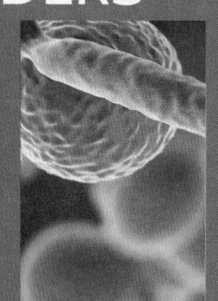

CHAPTER

29

Esophagus, Stomach, and Small Intestine Disorders

Learning Objectives

Upon completion of this chapter, the student will be able to:

- Describe normal anatomy and physiology of the esophagus, stomach, and small intestine.
- Recognize common disorders of the esophagus, stomach, and small intestine.
- Identify signs, symptoms, and clinical manifestations of disorders of the esophagus, stomach, and small intestine.

- Recognize assessment techniques, laboratory tests, and imaging studies used in the diagnosis of disorders of the esophagus, stomach, and small intestine.
- Discuss pharmacological and nonpharmacological treatment modalities used for disorders of the esophagus, stomach, and small intestine.

Key Terms

Achalasia
Barrett's esophagus
Borborygmi
Celiac disease
Dyspepsia
Dysphagia
Emesis
Endoscopy
Enterohepatic circulation
Eructation

Functional heartburn
Gastroesophageal reflux disease (GERD)
Gastroparesis
Helicobacter pylori
Hematemesis
Hiatal hernia
Laparoscopy
Laparotomy
Melena
Odynophagia

Paralytic ileus
Peptic ulcer disease (PUD)
Peritoneal lavage
Peritonitis
Reflux hypersensitivity
Steatorrhea
Thrush
Upper gastrointestinal bleed (UGIB)
Villi

Gastrointestinal (GI) disease takes many forms and affects people across the world in both industrialized and undeveloped countries. GI disorders are among the most common disorders encountered within the U.S. population; however, because many individuals self-medicate using over-the-counter medications, many disorders go unreported and undiagnosed.

The GI tract can be divided into upper and lower segments. This chapter focuses on the upper GI segment. The esophagus, stomach, and small intestine comprise the upper GI tract (see Fig. 29-1). These organs have the primary role of food and fluid digestion and absorption of essential nutrients, vitamins, and minerals. Any alteration in upper GI organ function can cause indigestion, malabsorption,

malnutrition, or dehydration, all of which have profound effects on the whole body.

Epidemiology

One of the major disorders of the upper GI tract is **gastroesophageal reflux disease (GERD).** This disorder is diagnosed if a person has esophagitis more than a few times a week. GERD occurs in all ages, most commonly in infants and in persons older than 40 years. Approximately 25% to 40% of Americans experience GERD at some point in their lives.

A disorder that can be associated with esophagitis and GERD is **peptic ulcer disease (PUD).** In the United States, PUD affects approximately 4.5

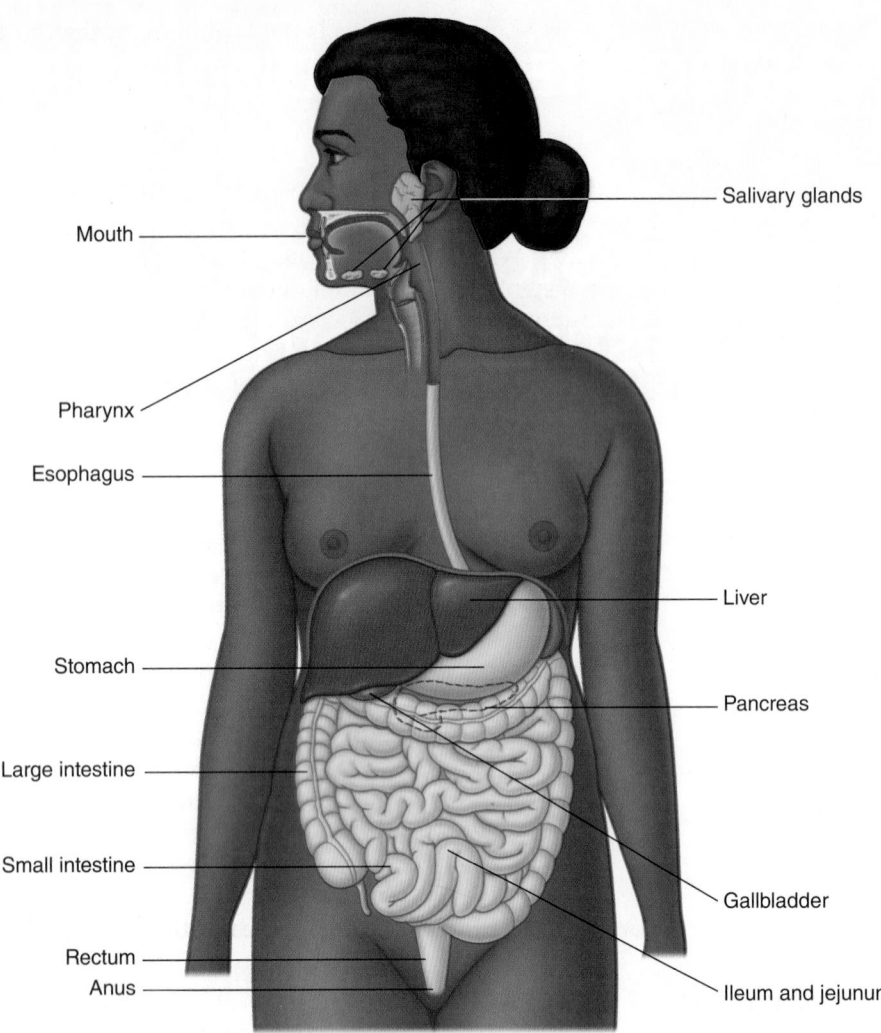

Mouth

Pharynx

Esophagus

Stomach

Large intestine

Small intestine

Rectum

Anus

Salivary glands

Liver

Pancreas

Gallbladder

Ileum and jejunum

FIGURE 29-1. The GI system.

million people annually. Approximately 10% of the U.S. population has evidence of a duodenal ulcer. If PUD goes untreated, there is the possibility of acute GI bleeding. This potentially life-threatening abdominal emergency is a common cause of hospitalization, affecting 100,000 individuals annually in the United States.

The most common GI disorder across the world is gastroenteritis, although most cases are undiagnosed, unreported, and treated by affected individuals themselves. Most cases are caused by a virus that lasts 1 to 2 days. However, in many parts of the world, gastroenteritis is a potentially lethal condition.

Basic Concepts of Esophageal, Stomach, and Small Intestine Function

The upper GI tract consists of the esophagus, stomach, and small intestine. These organs are responsible for the major digestion and absorption of vital nutrients. Dysfunction of any of the upper GI organs can lead to malnutrition and dehydration.

Esophagus

The esophagus is a tubelike structure that lies behind the trachea in the thorax and extends from the pharynx to the stomach. A sphincter is located at each end of the esophagus: the upper esophageal sphincter (UES) and the lower esophageal sphincter (LES), also known as the cardiac sphincter. Both are contracted in their resting state and open in response to nerve stimulation. The UES directs food and liquids into the esophagus and prevents their aspiration into the airway. The epiglottis is a membrane that closes over the trachea during eating to prevent food from entering the respiratory system.

In the esophagus, ingested food moves down by peristalsis. Peristalsis occurs by the contraction and relaxation of the muscle of the esophagus, innervations by the sensory neurons, and moisture from the mucosal membranes. The peristaltic waves continue to the LES, where the vagus nerve stimulates the opening of the sphincter and the bolus is pushed into the stomach cavity.

Stomach

The stomach is located in the upper part of the abdomen and consists of three portions: the fundus, the uppermost portion of the stomach; the body, the center and largest part of the stomach; and the pylorus, the lower portion of the stomach. Two sphincters help regulate the inflow and outflow of stomach contents—the LES, located between the lower esophagus and the stomach, and the pyloric sphincter, which separates the stomach from the duodenum.

The digestive process in the stomach consists of three phases:

1. Cephalic phase
2. Gastric phase
3. Intestinal phase

The cephalic phase occurs in response to a sensory stimulus, such as the sight, smell, or taste of food. It consists of activation of the vagal nerve, secretion of acetylcholine, and parasympathetic motor response. To follow this, cells prepare for the second phase of digestion, the gastric phase. As part of this preparation, histamine and gastrin are released from stomach cells. The gastric phase starts as food or fluids enter the stomach, stimulating the activity of mucus and gastric acid from stomach secretory cells. Types of stomach cells include gastric goblet cells, parietal cells, chief cells, and G cells. Gastric goblet cells secrete mucus, and parietal cells secrete hydrochloric acid (HCl) and intrinsic factor. HCl sterilizes and breaks down food, mainly proteins and carbohydrates. Intrinsic factor is necessary for the absorption of vitamin B_{12} in the small intestine.

Within the parietal cells the proton pump regulates synthesis of acid. Acid is stimulated by acetylcholine, histamine, or gastrin. Acetylcholine, histamine, and gastrin bind to receptors on the parietal cells; this triggers the action of the proton pump, which elevates the stomach's hydrogen (H+) ion concentration.

Chief cells secrete pepsinogen, which in the acidic environment converts to pepsin, an enzyme utilized for protein digestion. The stomach's cells are capable of secreting 1500 mL of gastric secretions a day while maintaining an acidic pH of 1.5 to 2.0 because of HCl. To counteract the acid in the stomach, gastric mucosal cells secrete prostaglandin E2 (PGE2), a lipid-rich molecule, which exerts a strong protective effect. PGE2 stimulates gastric mucus production and pancreatic bicarbonate secretion, which reduce the effects of HCl.

To digest proteins, G cells, located in the pylorus, secrete gastrin. G cells are endocrine-like cells that increase gastric motility, stimulate secretions from parietal and chief cells, and trigger the release of bile from the gallbladder and enzymes from the pancreas. The bile and pancreatic enzymes enter the digestive system via the common bile duct into the duodenum.

The stomach's peristaltic function enables the mixing of food and digestive enzymes. Food is broken down into small particles and enzymatically liquefied to form chyme. Chyme is then propelled toward the pyloric sphincter and into the duodenum for the final stages of digestion. This is the beginning of the third stage of digestion, the intestinal phase.

Small Intestine

The small intestine is the largest GI organ, measuring approximately 20 feet long, and its primary function is absorption and digestion. The duodenum marks the beginning of the small intestine, followed by the jejunum, ileum, and ileocecal valve.

The mucosal lining of the small intestine is covered with thousands of tiny fingerlike projections known as **villi;** each villus contains goblet cells, whose functions are to release digestive enzymes, secrete mucus, and absorb nutrients. A unique characteristic of the small intestine is the presence of microvilli, located on the villi's epithelial cells. This double set of villi is known as the brush border. The combination of the villi and microvilli double the surface area, significantly increasing the small intestine's absorptive capacity (see Fig. 29-2).

The final phase of the digestive process, the intestinal phase, includes neural and hormonal responses. The neural response, the enterogastric reflex, is responsible for the opening of the pyloric sphincter. This reflex is stimulated by intestinal distention and decreases gastric motility and acid production.

In the duodenum, bile from the liver, enzymes from the pancreas, and chyme from the stomach come together to complete the digestive process. Both the duodenum and jejunum contain receptors that sense acidity, osmotic pressure, and such products of digestion as fats and peptides. Secretin, a hormone secreted by the intestine, inhibits gastric secretion. Gastric emptying into the duodenum is decreased if the duodenal pH is lower than 3.5. Acidic stomach contents enter the duodenum gradually at a rate that allows for neutralization by pancreatic bicarbonate.

The primary function of the middle section of the intestine, the jejunum, is absorption. Nutrients such as amino acids; glucose; iron; calcium; and the fat-soluble vitamins A, D, E, and K are absorbed in the jejunum.

The primary function of the ileum—the last and longest segment of the small intestine—is the reabsorption of vitamin B_{12} and the return of bile acids to the liver. The return of bile acids to the liver from the ileum is termed the **enterohepatic circulation** process. Bile acids are recycled by this process. The gastroileal reflex stimulates the opening of the ileocecal valve, which controls the release of digestive contents into the large intestine.

Basic Pathophysiological Concepts of the Esophagus, Stomach, and Small Intestine

The functions of the GI tract are to ingest, digest, absorb, and eliminate. Normal movement of gastric contents through the digestive tract is necessary for

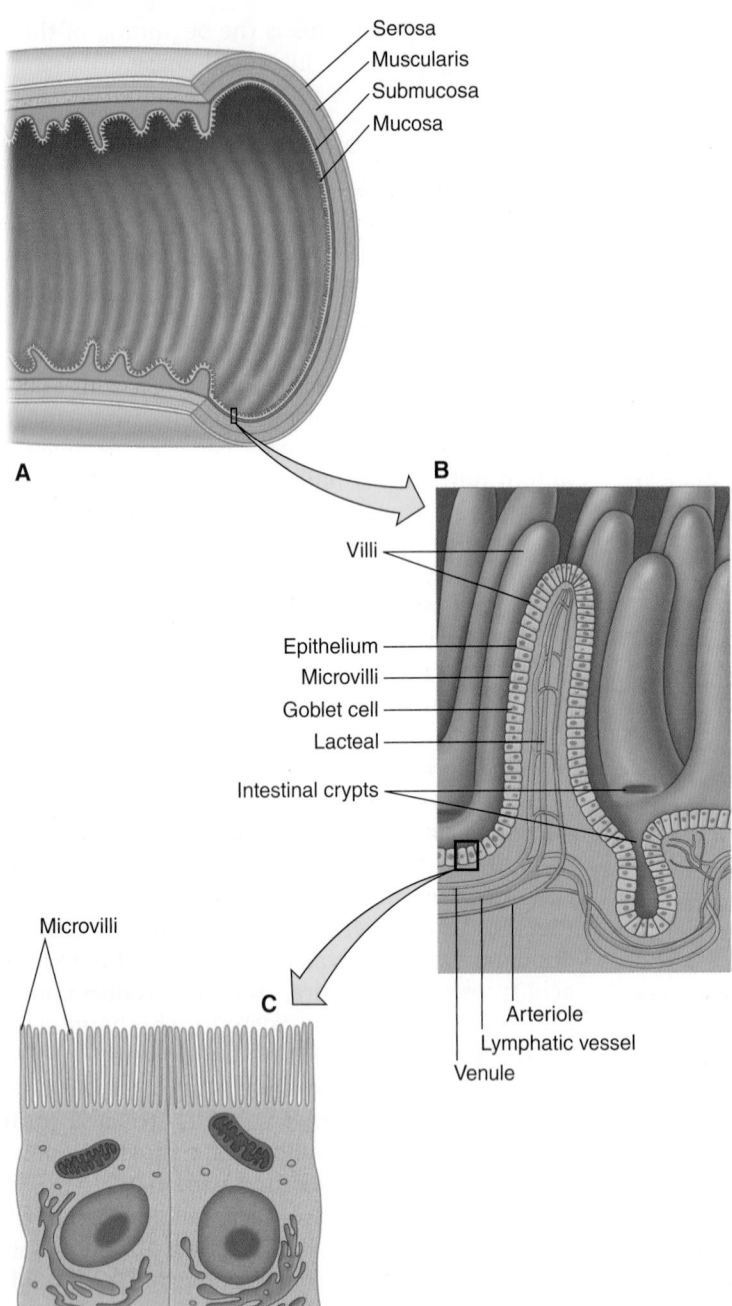

Serosa
Muscularis
Submucosa
Mucosa

A

B

Villi

Epithelium
Microvilli
Goblet cell
Lacteal

Intestinal crypts

Microvilli

C

Arteriole
Lymphatic vessel
Venule

FIGURE 29-2. (A) The intestinal lining contains circular folds that slow the progress of chyme and its contact with the mucosa. On top of the circular folds are projections called villi. **(B)** The villi are covered by absorptive epithelial cells as well as mucus-secreting goblet cells. An arteriole, a venule, and a lymph vessel called a lacteal fill the core of each villus. Pores at the base of the villi, called intestinal crypts, contain goblet cells that secrete mucus that helps the passage of food. They also serve as sites for rapid cellular growth, producing new cells to replace those shed from the cell. **(C)** Epithelial cells covering the villi have a brush border of ultrafine microvilli. Besides further increasing the absorptive area, the microvilli produce digestive enzymes. *(From Thompson, G. S. [2020]. Understanding anatomy and physiology [3rd ed.]. Philadelphia, PA: F. A. Davis Company, with permission.)*

digestion and absorption of nutrients. An alteration in the ingestion process where contents cannot progress from one area of the GI tract to subsequent areas creates motility dysfunction. Contents that progress too quickly fail to be adequately broken down, which results in malabsorption; in contrast, contents that move too slowly often cause nausea and vomiting. Inflammation, as well as structural and cellular abnormalities, in any of the GI structures will also have a direct effect on motility and absorption.

Assessment

The history and physical examination of the patient provide information for initial evaluation of an upper GI disorder. In general, with regard to the GI tract, the patient should be questioned about swallowing, indigestion, **eructation** (belching), and abdominal pain. If swallowing pain is present, it needs to be fully explored regarding onset, location, and duration. Is the pain a burning, gnawing feeling, as occurs in esophagitis? Does the pain occur with or between meals? Is the pain relieved by food, as in PUD? Are there nocturnal symptoms, as in GERD? Is there any swallowing difficulty? Which is more difficult to swallow: solids or liquids? Is there a problem with regurgitation? Swallowing difficulty and regurgitation can be due to esophageal cancer, Zenker's diverticulum, or Plummer–Vinson syndrome. The patient should also be asked about weight loss or anorexia. How much weight loss has occurred over what length of time? Unintentional weight loss of 10 lbs over 1 month should be investigated.

If nausea or vomiting is a problem, the clinician should review the onset of nausea, triggering factors, the time frame in regard to eating, and whether vomiting occurs. Does the **emesis** (vomitus) contain blood, mucus, or bile? Does it have a coffee-ground appearance, as occurs in upper GI bleeding? Is blood visible in the vomitus? Does the patient take NSAIDs or aspirin? How much coffee does the patient drink? What other medications are taken? Does the patient take antacids, proton pump inhibitors (PPIs) such as lansoprazole (Prevacid), or histamine-2 receptor antagonists (H2RAs) such as famotidine (Pepcid), and how often? The patient's medication list can often be responsible for GI symptoms or reveal information about symptoms. Questioning the patient about alcohol use and smoking is also important, as these often cause GI irritation. The clinician needs to ask about bowel movements. Has there been any diarrhea, as in malabsorptive diseases? Is there any bleeding or dark stools, as in GI bleeding? Black, tarry stools indicate GI blood loss.

One of the major risk factors for upper GI problems is the use of NSAIDs, including aspirin. These medications are often associated with gastric irritation and erosion and can be the cause of PUD. Alcohol use and smoking are associated with esophagitis, PUD, and esophageal cancer. Alcohol use disorder, the etiology of cirrhosis of the liver, can also cause problems for the upper digestive tract. Upper GI bleeding is often caused by esophageal varices, which occur in cirrhosis. Frequent heartburn can cause GERD, which is a precursor of Barrett's esophagus, a precancerous change of the esophagus. Upper GI tract bleeding can also be due to a bleeding or perforated peptic ulcer. Patients who are bulimic have frequent vomiting episodes that can cause esophageal tears, called Mallory–Weiss syndrome or Boerhaave syndrome. Both cause upper GI bleeding. Immunosuppressed individuals are susceptible to esophagitis caused by *Candida* infection, also called **thrush.** *Candida*-related esophagitis causes a white exudate over the oral cavity and tongue and painful swallowing. Other possible infectious agents include herpes virus, cytomegalovirus, and human papillomavirus (HPV). HPV is increasingly becoming a causative factor of oral and esophageal cancer.

The patient's family history is also significant. The patient should be asked about any GI disorders in the family. Disorders with genetic predisposition include celiac disease, inflammatory bowel disease (Crohn's disease or ulcerative colitis), esophageal or stomach cancer, Lynch syndrome, Peutz-Jeghers syndrome, liver disorders, hematochromatosis, and neuroendocrine disease.

Diagnosis

Often, esophageal or upper GI pain cannot be immediately distinguished from cardiac chest pain, so an acute coronary event needs to be ruled out before exploration of a GI disorder. If the patient has upper GI bleeding, hemodynamic stabilization of the patient is necessary; a nasogastric aspirate can be used to investigate the source of bleeding. If the stomach contains bile but no blood, upper GI bleeding is less likely. If the aspirate reveals clear gastric fluid, a duodenal site of bleeding may be possible.

The most accurate method of diagnosing upper GI tract disorders is upper **endoscopy.** The endoscope can be used to diagnose, take a biopsy of tissue, and treat upper GI problems. Videocapsule endoscopy is an alternative if conventional endoscopy cannot be used. This vitamin-sized capsule contains a camera; when swallowed, it travels through the digestive tract, taking pictures of the internal GI tract.

Upper GI barium x-rays, also called an upper GI series, may be done to highlight the anatomy of the upper GI tract. The patient is instructed to swallow barium, a radiopaque substance, which allows visualization of the esophagus, stomach, and duodenum. If perforation of the GI tract is suspected, a water-soluble, iodinated contrast agent, gastrografin, is used instead of barium. Clinicians can also visualize the patient's ability to swallow by using fluoroscopic x-ray procedures. Esophageal manometry studies are often performed to measure the strength of the esophageal sphincter muscles. Manometry is performed using a special nasogastric tube that is passed from the nostril to the stomach. Esophageal acidity can be monitored using 24-hour ambulatory pH. Multichannel intraluminal impedance and pH monitoring (MII-pH) is considered the most accurate test to detect gastroesophageal reflux.

Helicobacter pylori studies are done when peptic ulcer is suspected. Antibodies to *H. pylori* can be measured in the blood. Using an endoscope, a gastric mucosal biopsy can be sampled and tested for *H. pylori*. Fecal antigen testing identifies active *H. pylori* infection in the stool. Urea breath tests detect active *H. pylori* infection by analyzing the breath.

If there is bleeding, type and crossmatch of the patient's blood are necessary. Other laboratory tests that are commonly performed include complete blood count (CBC), electrolytes, blood urea nitrogen (BUN), serum creatinine, liver function tests, prothrombin time/partial thromboplastin time, and international normalized ratio (INR). A gastrin level is done to rule out Zollinger–Ellison syndrome (ZES), which causes peptic ulcers. Amylase and lipase levels are also checked to exclude a pancreatic disorder or perforation of an organ.

Treatment

Any disorder that includes bleeding, such as esophageal varices and perforated ulcer, requires primary

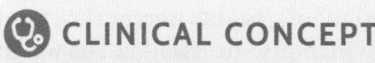

CLINICAL CONCEPT

Chronic use of NSAIDs often causes PUD and GI bleeding.

hemodynamic stabilization. Patients with occasional indigestion should take antacids and make lifestyle modifications such as weight loss if obese, decreased alcohol and coffee intake, and smoking cessation, if appropriate. Esophagitis that occurs more often can be treated with PPIs such as lansoprazole (Prevacid) for 4 to 8 weeks. Some clinicians suggest PPIs or histamine-2 receptor antagonists such as famotidine (Pepcid) for patients with ulcer-like symptoms. These agents decrease gastric acid production by inhibiting the proton pump mechanism and blocking histamine-2 receptors in gastric parietal cells.

Patients with upper GI bleeding caused by esophageal varices often require esophagogastric balloon tamponade, which is the insertion of a catheter with an inflatable balloon on the tip. The esophagogastric tube can be used as a temporary measure to exert pressure on the esophageal veins to stave off bleeding. Endoscopy can be used in diagnosis and treatment. Endoscopic sclerotherapy, endoscopic band ligation, and other types of endoscopic ablation are used to treat esophageal varices and esophageal cancer. Another procedure, insertion of a transjugular intrahepatic portosystemic shunt (TIPS), can be used to permanently treat esophageal varices due to portal hypertension. Surgery is needed in patients with a perforated viscus, such as in perforated duodenal ulcer, perforated gastric ulcer, and Boerhaave syndrome (esophageal rupture). Surgery may involve a laparoscopic procedure to suture bleeding vessels in the esophagus, stomach, or duodenum; it might also involve cutting the vagus nerve to the stomach to cease acid stimulation.

Disorders of the Esophagus, Stomach, and Small Intestine

Disorders of each organ within the upper GI tract are different because of their distinct composition and function. The esophagus mainly undergoes inflammation. Although tumor growth is uncommon, stricture, spasm, or diverticula can occur. The stomach commonly undergoes inflammation or ulceration. Tumor growth is rare in the stomach. The small intestine disorders are mainly those of inflammation or obstruction, which can cause severe malabsorption, dehydration, and malnutrition. Crohn's disease, an inflammatory bowel disease, can affect any segment of the upper or lower gastrointestinal tract (see Chapter 30 for more information).

Disorders of the Esophagus

The initial section of the GI tract, the esophagus, can undergo specific types of defects and alterations. The purpose of the esophagus is to propel food and fluid from the mouth to the stomach. A series of contractions and relaxations within the esophageal tract creates peristalsis, which facilitates the movement of food to the stomach. Alterations of esophageal motility, inflammation, or obstruction within the esophagus will result in the person's inability to effectively swallow.

Dysphagia

Dysphagia, or swallowing difficulty, is a term that is widely used with disorders of the esophagus. A wide range of causes result in dysphagia, making incidence difficult to report. Dysphagia is associated with the lack of a gag reflex, as occurs in degenerative neurological diseases and stroke. Between 50% and 70% of individuals affected by stroke have a decreased gag reflex and dysphagia. In diseases such as myasthenia gravis or amyotrophic lateral sclerosis, dysphagia and loss of gag reflex occur late in the disease and can cause death.

Etiology. Dysphagia most often occurs because of neuromuscular dysfunction; however, structural abnormalities of the esophagus are causes as well. Zenker's diverticulum is a weakening in the wall of the esophagus that causes an outpouching or sac where food can accumulate. Food accumulates within the sac and fills to create an obstructive mass in the esophagus that interferes with swallowing. Esophageal strictures, rings, or tumors can also cause dysphagia. A Schatzki ring is a constrictive muscular band of esophageal tissue. This congenital abnormality is often found in the distal esophagus. Thin membranous webs of tissue can also form in the esophagus and cause dysphagia. In Plummer–Vinson syndrome, patients have trouble swallowing because of congenital or acquired webs of tissue in the upper esophagus. Another cause of dysphagia is an esophageal stricture, which is an abnormal thinning or narrowing of the esophagus. Strictures can occur as a result of chronic esophagitis, GERD, tumors, Barrett's esophagus, inflammatory disorders such as scleroderma, or congenital abnormality. **Achalasia** is an esophageal motility problem that involves the smooth muscle of the esophagus. There is incomplete relaxation of the LES, as well as increased muscular tone. It is characterized by lack of peristalsis of the esophagus.

Pathophysiology. Dysphagia frequently begins with difficulty swallowing solid foods and progresses to the inability to swallow liquids. An individual may complain of feeling as though the food gets stuck, and frequent attempts to swallow are necessary for movement of food. Structural abnormalities of the esophagus such as diverticula, stricture, webs, and rings cause mechanical problems of swallowing. Food becomes obstructed because of the anatomical abnormality. Damage or dysfunction of cranial nerves IX, X, or XII can also cause inability to swallow solids or liquids. These nerves can become dysfunctional in stroke, spinal cord injury, degenerative neurological diseases, and trauma.

The esophagus lies posterior to the trachea, creating a high risk for aspiration. Any time there is altered motility of the esophagus, there is an increased risk of food or fluids entering the trachea rather than the esophagus, known as aspiration. The inhaled contents will follow the path of the trachea and eventually lodge within the sterile environment of the respiratory system, leading to an infection called aspiration pneumonia. Individuals with the greatest risk for aspiration pneumonia are those with a history of a stroke, trauma to the upper spinal cord, brain injury, or a patient who is receiving enteral feedings.

> ### 🔍 CLINICAL CONCEPT
>
> Aspiration pneumonia is demonstrated by the presence of pulmonary crackles, an elevated white blood cell (WBC) count, and fever. It most commonly occurs in the right lung.

Clinical Presentation. The patient with dysphagia may exhibit evidence of cranial nerve dysfunction. A unilateral facial droop indicates that cranial nerve VII is dysfunctional. In a patient with an absent gag reflex, the tongue and uvula may be deviated to one side, which indicates dysfunction of cranial nerves IX, X, and XII. Regurgitation of food or fluids is associated with esophageal impairment; patients will have pooling of food or liquid in the back of the throat, and individuals may have drooling of food from one side of the mouth. Frequent coughing while eating is indicative of dysphagia and places the person at high risk for aspiration. Painful swallowing, or **odynophagia,** may occur as efforts to swallow are ineffective and necessitate repeated attempts to swallow.

> ### 🔍 CLINICAL CONCEPT
>
> To assess the gag reflex, ask the patient to open the mouth and say "ah." The uvula and soft palate should rise as the patient vocalizes. In addition, the uvula should be in the midline position.

Diagnosis and Treatment. A barium swallow test, also called a video fluoroscopy swallow study, is a specialized x-ray used to diagnose dysphagia. This procedure demonstrates the patient's ability to swallow. If esophageal abnormalities are suspected, endoscopy is a necessary diagnostic procedure. Another diagnostic test is high-resolution esophageal manometry. This test uses a nasogastric tube to measure the pressures generated by the esophageal muscle when the muscle is at rest and during swallows. The presence of aspiration pneumonia can be confirmed with a conventional chest x-ray. An individual with dysphagia can be trained to swallow during rehabilitation. Often the patient requires puréed foods and thickened fluids. Individuals with a neurological impairment of the esophagus will require enteral nutrition, which is composed entirely of liquid and has a high caloric content. This form of nutrition is given through a tube that transports the food into the stomach or intestine (see Fig. 29-3).

Esophagitis

Esophagitis is an acute or chronic inflammation of the esophagus. This condition most commonly arises from an irritation to the mucosa of the esophageal lining by refluxed acid. It can also be caused by the fungal organism *C. albicans* in immunosuppressed individuals.

Esophagitis is a disorder that can occur occasionally or it can be a more serious condition that occurs frequently and is diagnosed as gastroesophageal reflux disease (GERD). Generally, 33% to 44% of the population has esophageal reflux symptoms at some time during a month. However, up to 10% of people have daily symptoms, which indicates a diagnosis of GERD. candidal esophagitis, also called thrush, is the most common type of infectious esophagitis.

Etiology. Acute esophagitis occurs from an infection, chemical ingestion, medications, excessive vomiting, or occasional episodes of acid reflux. Obesity, pregnancy, smoking, alcohol, fatty foods, and coffee increase susceptibility to esophagitis. Some medications, such as

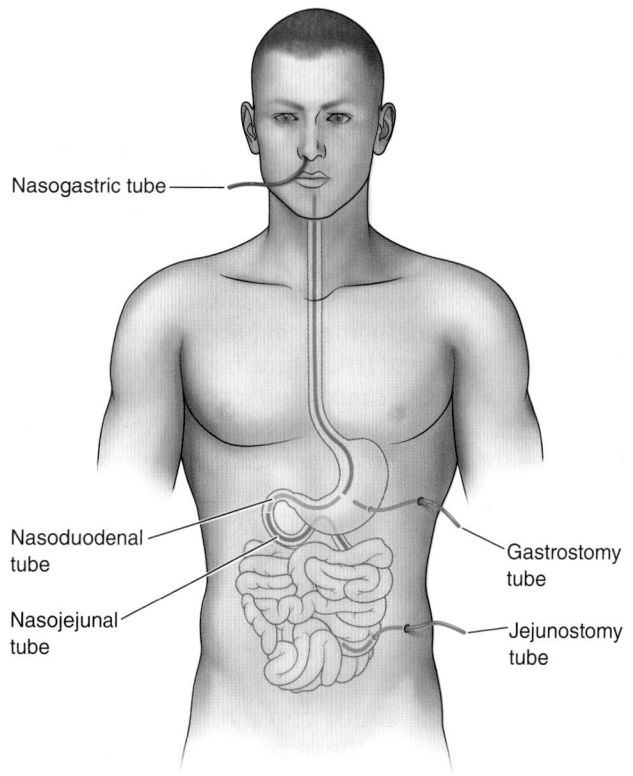

Nasogastric tube

Nasoduodenal tube

Nasojejunal tube

Gastrostomy tube

Jejunostomy tube

FIGURE 29-3. Types of enteral feedings.

calcium antagonists, anticholinergics, NSAIDs, and bisphosphonates, increase susceptibility to esophagitis. Chronic esophagitis is most often associated with the presence of poorly controlled GERD. Major predisposing factors for candidal esophagitis include antibiotic use, radiation therapy or chemotherapy, hematological malignancies, and AIDS. Other conditions associated with an increased incidence of candidal esophagitis include esophageal stasis, alcohol use disorder, malnutrition, and advanced age.

Pathophysiology. Esophagitis occurs as a result of an irritation to the squamous epithelium, the protective lining of the esophagus. The body responds to the injury by initiating the inflammatory process. Edema will occur as a result of vasodilation. Pain is associated with the erosion, or destruction, of the epithelium. The area of injury is repeatedly irritated as the contractions of peristalsis and the progression of food or fluids move through the esophagus. A risk for esophageal obstruction exists with severe esophageal inflammation because the edema and inflammation can block foods from being swallowed. In addition, chronic irritation to the esophagus can lead to ulcerations, scarring, or strictures.

Thrush often begins as an infection in the mouth. *Candida* is yeast that is considered part of the normal flora of the oral cavity. When a person is immunosuppressed, overgrowth of *Candida* in the mouth is common. This condition is commonly found in neonates; individuals with AIDS; and those receiving chemotherapy, immunomodulators, or long-term antibiotic therapy. If thrush is not quickly identified or properly treated, the infection can progress into the esophagus, causing candidal esophagitis.

H. pylori are aggressive bacteria that invade the lining of the stomach, leading to peptic ulcer disease (PUD). *H. pylori* resists acid and burrows under the stomach mucosa. In GERD, acid and *H. pylori* constantly reflux upward into the esophagus. The esophageal epithelial mucosa becomes severely irritated by acid, and *H. pylori* can cause ulceration in the lower esophageal cells. Other organisms that can cause esophagitis include herpes simplex, varicella zoster, cytomegalovirus, and HIV. A growing body of evidence is showing that HPV can also infect the esophagus.

Chemical or corrosive esophagitis can occur with ingestion of household chemicals. Many chemicals consist of strong alkali or acid components that are corrosive to the esophagus's lining. The caustic action of the ingested chemicals often leads to perforation and bleeding of the esophageal lumen. Vomiting should not be induced because of the risk for additional injury to the esophagus as the corrosive agents are expelled.

Chronic use of NSAIDs or aspirin can cause drug-induced ulcerations of the esophagus. Additional medications that may be irritating to the esophageal lining include antibiotics, chemotherapy, bisphosphonates,

and potassium. As these medications dissolve, they may become corrosive to the esophageal lining. Individuals should be encouraged to drink adequate amounts of water with these medications to ensure that the pills have not lodged against the wall of the esophagus.

 CLINICAL CONCEPT

Persons taking bisphosphonates should sit upright or stand for 30 minutes after swallowing the drug to prevent esophagitis.

The process of vomiting causes irritation to the epithelium of the esophagus as acidic gastric contents are forcefully expelled. The combination of the pressure of the expulsion and the acidity of gastric contents can lead to erosion of the esophagus and deterioration of the LES. Recurrent vomiting, as seen with eating disorders or pregnancy, can lead to esophagitis.

Mallory–Weiss syndrome, which is a vertical tear in the lower esophagus, can occur with forceful, frequent bouts of vomiting as occurs in persons with bulimia. This may lead to esophageal bleeding and hematemesis. Boerhaave syndrome, a transmural rupture of the esophagus, can occur because of excessive, forceful vomiting as occurs in persons with bulimia or because of instrumentation of the esophagus. Severe hematemesis occurs with loss of an extensive amount of blood.

Clinical Presentation. In esophagitis, the most common complaint is a burning sensation in the throat or midsternal chest. Dysphagia, odynophagia, and heartburn are other symptoms associated with esophagitis. A complaint of a sore throat or tongue and white patches on the tongue, palate, or buccal mucosa are hallmark signs of thrush. Hematemesis, nausea, and vomiting can also occur.

Diagnosis and Treatment. The diagnosis and severity of esophagitis can be ascertained with endoscopy, which allows for visualization of ulcerations or perforations and provides the option to obtain a biopsy of the affected area. Barium studies can also be used in the diagnosis. Treatment of esophagitis is primarily focused on treating the inflammation and relieving symptoms. The clinician should advise lifestyle changes, such as smoking cessation, alcohol limitation, reduced caffeine intake, and avoidance of NSAIDs and aspirin. Pharmacological treatment includes H2RAs such as famotidine or PPIs such as omeprazole for 4 to 8 weeks. Sucralfate is a viscous adhesive substance that can augment the stomach's protective lining. In *Candida* infection, antifungal agents such as fluconazole can be used. Surgery can be done when lifestyle and pharmacological management has been ineffective.

Gastroesophageal Reflux Disease

GERD is the most common and most costly GI disorder in the United States. Over 700,000 persons are hospitalized with GERD per year. However, many persons with GERD self-medicate with over-the-counter drugs, so there are many unreported cases. Approximately 20% of the U.S. population experiences GERD at least once per week. GERD is most common in infants and those older than age 40 years. Most patients with typical symptoms of GERD receive empiric treatment with a proton pump inhibitor (PPI) and do not undergo diagnostic testing. However, in patients with alarm symptoms such as dysphagia, odynophagia, anorexia, weight loss, and upper gastrointestinal bleed, investigation with an upper endoscopy is warranted. The use of other diagnostic tests, such as catheter-based pH test, wireless pH capsule, impedance + pH, and others, are reserved for specific clinical scenarios when further management is needed in patients who showed partial or complete lack of response to PPI treatment.

Etiology. The most common cause of GERD is a functional or mechanical problem that decreases muscular tone of the lower esophageal sphincter (LES). Relaxation of the LES allows for regurgitation of stomach contents into the esophagus. Different conditions, foods, and medications can cause decreased strength of the LES (see Box 29-1).

Pathophysiology. In GERD, the LES is weak and allows the contents of the stomach to reflux up into the esophagus. The stomach contents are acidic, so when refluxed upward, they irritate the esophageal squamous epithelium. Although the LES is dysfunctional in GERD, **gastroparesis,** the delayed emptying of gastric contents into the duodenum, is also a problem. Gastroparesis causes increased gastric distention that leads to increased pressure within the stomach against the LES. Any cause of increased gastric or intra-abdominal pressure can place tension on the LES. Obesity and pregnancy, for example, commonly

cause GERD. A hiatal hernia also interferes with the closure of the LES, resulting in a reflux of gastric secretions into the esophagus.

In GERD, the esophageal epithelial cells are not able to withstand the acidity of the refluxed stomach contents. The gastric acid can quickly erode the protective mucosal epithelial layer and lead to ulceration of the esophagus. Repeated injury to the epithelial layer commonly causes metaplasia, the change of esophageal epithelial cells into stomachlike columnar epithelium. The metaplastic cellular change at the gastroesophageal junction, called **Barrett's esophagus,** is a precancerous change of cells (see Fig. 29-4).

🔍 CLINICAL CONCEPT

Barrett's esophagus requires periodic endoscopic examination to check for dysplastic cell changes.

Clinical Presentation. The most frequent symptoms associated with GERD are dysphagia, heartburn, epigastric pain, and regurgitation. Frequent heartburn may also be described as acid indigestion, or **dyspepsia.** Individuals often describe regurgitation as a bitter taste in their mouth. Respiratory complaints, such as chronic dry cough, asthma, and aspiration pneumonia, are also associated with the presence of GERD. Individuals frequently complain of increased pain following the ingestion of certain foods, such as those that have a high fat content and take longer to digest, thereby causing delayed gastric emptying and increased gastric distention. Postural positioning, such as lying flat or

BOX 29-1. Causes of LES Dysfunction

Certain conditions, substances, foods, or medications can weaken or hinder closure of the lower esophageal sphincter:
- Alcohol
- Chocolate
- Coffee
- Fatty meals
- Medications, including anticholinergics, beta-agonists, calcium channel blockers, nitrates, and hormones such as progesterone
- Nicotine
- Obesity
- Pregnancy

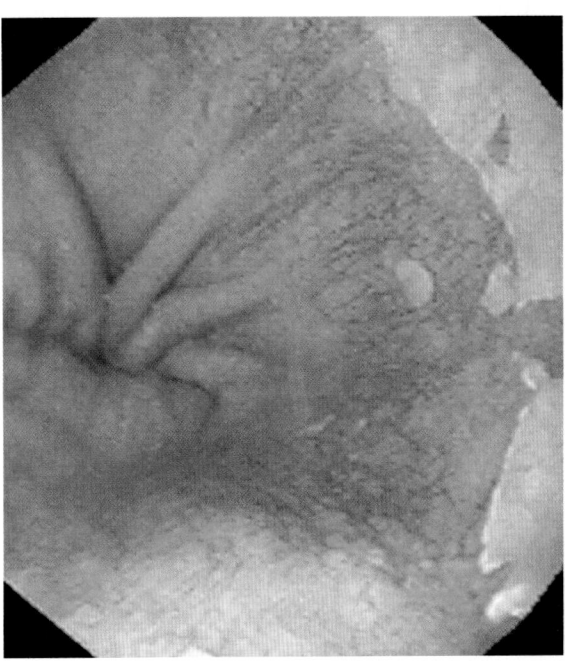

FIGURE 29-4. Endoscopic view of Barrett's esophagus. *(Courtesy of H. Worth Boyce, MD.)*

bending over, will also aggravate GERD. These positions will cause increased pressure from the stomach to the LES, forcing the LES to weaken and resulting in reflux of gastric contents.

In severe cases of GERD, an individual may present with complaints of weight loss, frequent cough, aspiration pneumonia, GI bleeding, or anemia. Any of these symptoms carry an increased cause for concern because they represent a progression of the disease. The GI bleeding is related to chronic irritation of the mucosal tract and erosion into the cellular layer. Anemia may be related to blood loss or nutritional deficits. A frequent cough and repeated episodes of aspiration pneumonia are indicative of the progression of GERD further up the esophageal tract. GERD with aspiration can occur while the patient is asleep; the regurgitation of acidic contents into the lungs can often stimulate nocturnal asthma attacks.

Diagnosis and Treatment. In the initial evaluation, the patient can complete the GERD questionnaire (GERDQ). GERDQ is a six-item, easy-to-use questionnaire based on symptoms experienced by the patient. The most effective diagnostic tools for GERD are endoscopy and manometry. Through an endoscope, the clinician can visualize the esophageal mucosa and perform manometry and pH testing. Manometry can determine the pressure at the LES. Ambulatory 24-hour pH testing can be done to confirm acid reflux in patients with atypical presentations or when endoscopy fails to reveal reflux. Multichannel intraluminal pH-impedance (MII-pH) is another investigation for assessing esophageal function in patients who are refractory to treatment. This investigation is useful in differentiating between acid and nonacid reflux. Ambulatory esophageal pH and MII-pH monitoring are done using nasogastric catheter or with a wireless pH probe (a small, capsule-like device) inserted during endoscopy. The capsule measures pH levels in the esophagus and transmits readings to a receiver worn by the patient.

If GERD has been present for 5 years or more, an endoscopic biopsy should be done to screen for the presence of Barrett's esophagus.

Treatment for GERD is focused on lifestyle changes. These include eating small, frequent meals to prevent abdominal distention; not lying down for 2 to 3 hours following a meal; losing weight if obese; and smoking cessation. The clinician should also review the patient's medications because the side effects of some are LES dysfunction.

Pharmacological treatments of GERD focus on decreasing the acidity levels of gastric secretions and improving the function of the LES. PPIs, H2RAs, and antacids are commonly prescribed. PPIs are the most effective medical therapy in controlling symptoms of the various presentations of GERD. Currently in the United States, four PPIs are available over the counter (omeprazole, lansoprazole, esomeprazole, and

omeprazole-sodium bicarbonate) and three can be obtained by a prescription (dexlansoprazole, pantoprazole, and rabeprazole). The value of continuous treatment with a PPI versus an on-demand or intermittent therapy remains controversial. Studies report that continuous treatment yields greater patient satisfaction than on-demand therapy. However, others have demonstrated that on-demand therapy is superior to continuous treatment in patients with mild GERD because it is less costly and relieves concern about chronic use of PPIs. Studies show that patients who are refractory to PPI are commonly not consuming the PPI optimally (30 minutes before a meal). Instead, they were consuming it more than an hour before a meal, during a meal, and at bedtime. Thus, it is important to explain to patients about proper timing of PPI consumption for maximum effect. Another important step in optimizing PPI treatment is the need to follow lifestyle modifications related to GERD. Patients need to avoid large, spicy, fatty meals; lose weight; and follow nighttime recommendations, which include elevating the head of the bed and avoiding eating at least 3 hours before bedtime.

In patients who continue to demonstrate GERD despite treatment, twice-daily PPI can be attempted. Also, the addition of an H2RA such as famotidine at bedtime can be tried. Another medication, baclofen, a gamma-aminobutyric acid-B agonist, has been effective in refractory GERD by reducing the rate of transient lower esophageal sphincter relaxations, and thus gastroesophageal reflux.

Reflux hypersensitivity and **functional heartburn** are possible causes for heartburn that is refractory to PPI treatment. These are newly discovered disorders caused by sensitivity to physiological amounts of gastroesophageal reflux. In these patients, there is normal esophageal motility, pH, normal pH impedance, and biopsy. The etiology is unclear. However, there are highly active sensory receptors to substance P and neurokinin in the esophagus. Also factors such as stress, hypervigilance psychological disorders, and poor sleep play an important role in enhancing perception of intraesophageal stimuli. These patients are commonly managed with neuromodulators including tricyclic antidepressants, selective serotonin reuptake inhibitors, serotonin-norepinephrine reuptake inhibitors, and trazodone.

Endoluminal therapies for the management of GERD are procedures done via the endoscope. Transoral incisionless fundoplication (TIF) is used to restore the angle of His by creating a valve at the esophagogastric junction. The Stretta procedure reinforces the strength of the LES by applying radiofrequency waves to stimulate growth of fibrotic tissue around the sphincter.

Laparoscopic antireflux surgery (also called fundoplication) is the surgical procedure used when other treatments have failed. During fundoplication surgery, the fundus, which is the upper curve of the stomach, is wrapped around the esophagus and sutured into place. This surgery strengthens the LES to block acids from refluxing up into the esophagus. Another esophageal sphincter–strengthening device composed of magnets is called the LINXR Reflux Management System. This is a minimally invasive procedure that can also alleviate reflux in many patients. Bariatric surgery is the mainstay surgical option for patients with GERD and obesity. Gastric bypass surgery leads to a decreased size of the stomach cavity, which reduces the number of acid-producing parietal cells and decreases intra-abdominal pressure by promoting weight loss.

Upper Gastrointestinal Bleed

The presence of bleeding in the esophagus, stomach, or duodenum is classified as an **upper gastrointestinal bleed (UGIB).** The bleeding can occur from a lesion, erosion, ulceration, varicosed vein, or tear in the GI lining. The incidence of UGIB is approximately 100 cases per 100,000 population per year. Bleeding from the upper GI tract is four times more common than bleeding from the lower GI tract, and mortality rates from UGIB are 6% to 10% overall.

Etiology. Several disorders, such as PUD, esophageal varices, Mallory–Weiss syndrome, Boerhaave syndrome, esophageal cancer, and hemorrhagic gastritis, can cause UGIB. The morbidity of GI bleeding is directly associated with the amount of blood loss.

Pathophysiology. UGIB can be classified as chronic or acute. An acute bleed is associated with a rupture, tear, or perforation in the esophageal or gastric lining, resulting in blood loss. The severity of clinical symptoms is associated with the amount of blood lost; for example, a large blood loss causes sudden hypotension and hypovolemia. An acute UGIB can quickly develop into hypovolemic shock. A chronic bleed is the result of a small tear or opening in the GI tract that causes a gradual, small amount of blood loss. A chronic bleed causes complaints of fatigue, low hemoglobin, and low iron levels. Slow UGIB often leads to iron-deficiency anemia. The stool contains blood in chronic blood loss, a condition referred to as **melena.**

Clinical Presentation. Classic symptoms of UGIB include hematemesis, melena, and occult blood. **Hematemesis** is vomitus with bright-red, bloody streaks or a dark, coffee-ground appearance. The presence of bright-red blood indicates a current bleed. Melena is occult blood in the stool that causes a black, tarry appearance. Occult blood is the presence of blood in the stool that is not visible. Individuals experiencing a slow, chronic GI bleed may have vague symptoms of fatigue and lethargy. Pain may or may not be present.

A sudden or massive UGIB may present with rapid onset of anxiety, dizziness, weakness, shortness of breath, or change in mental status. Tachycardia and tachypnea will occur because of decreased cardiac output. The skin will be pale and clammy as a result of the body's effort to shut down peripheral blood flow.

 CLINICAL CONCEPT

In hematemesis, blood that has a coffee-ground appearance indicates the blood has mixed with the stomach's acid. If bright-red blood is apparent, bleeding is currently occurring from a blood vessel.

Diagnosis and Treatment. A slow GI bleed may reveal low hemoglobin and low iron levels, which confirm the presence of anemia. A stool guaiac test, also known as a fecal occult blood test (FOBT), can determine the presence of blood in a stool sample. BUN levels will be elevated secondary to decreased fluid volume and the absorption of blood proteins into the small intestine. Diagnostic tests include endoscopy, CBC, and stool samples for occult blood. A videocapsule endoscopy can visualize the entire GI tract, including the walls of the small intestine. However, it does not offer the option to obtain biopsy or perform any surgical repair, compared with traditional endoscopic procedures.

 CLINICAL CONCEPT

A positive FOBT occurs when there is blood in the stool (melena). For increased accuracy, three tests should be done on 3 different days.

Treatment for an acute GI bleed includes rapid fluid replacement, insertion of a nasogastric tube to prevent abdominal distention from accumulation of blood, and administration of blood transfusions. Numerous therapeutic endoscopic strategies can be used for hemostasis of an UGIB. These include injection of sclerosing agents or fibrin glue, electrocoagulation, laser and argon coagulation, band ligation, and application of hemoclips. Insertion of a TIPS is recommended for some patients with esophageal varices. Transcatheter angiographic embolization is recommended for patients with bleeding peptic ulcers who are poor surgical candidates. **Laparoscopy** and surgical repair at the site of the bleeding are often done for acute episodes with large amounts of blood loss. A chronic UGIB is treated primarily with PPIs such as omeprazole (Prilosec) for 4 to 8 weeks. Sucralfate is a viscous adhesive medication that can be used to augment the gastric lining if ulceration is present.

Esophageal Varices

Esophageal varices are engorged varicose veins that develop in the lower third of the esophagus because of portal vein hypertension in the liver. Cirrhosis of the liver is the major cause of esophageal varices.

Etiology. Portal vein hypertension, which occurs in liver disease, is the cause for the development of esophageal varices. Alcohol-related and viral cirrhosis of the liver are the major diseases associated with esophageal varices.

> ### 🩺 CLINICAL CONCEPT
>
> Individuals with long-term alcohol use disorder often have hematemesis from esophageal varices.

Pathophysiology. The portal vein of the liver drains all the venous blood from the GI system before the blood enters the inferior vena cava. Liver disease, most often cirrhosis, causes congestion and high pressure within the portal vein (portal hypertension). The pressurized portal vein develops backup pressure into the veins of the GI system. In an attempt to decrease pressure within the portal vein, collateral veins develop, particularly around the lower esophagus. The esophageal veins, in turn, take on the pressure of the portal vein and gradually take on more pressure as conditions in the liver worsen. The pressurized, engorged esophageal veins eventually become enlarged and protrude into the esophageal lumen. The venous pressure weakens the esophageal venous walls, creating the risk for rupture. When rupture occurs, bleeding into the esophagus, hematemesis, and hemorrhage occurs (see Fig. 29-5).

Clinical Presentation. The patient with esophageal varices usually presents with symptoms of cirrhosis of the liver. The patient will have jaundice, nausea,

vomiting, weight loss, dark urine, and abdominal distention because of liver dysfunction. The primary clinical symptoms of esophageal varices include hematemesis and melena if there is a slow leak of blood from the veins. However, the esophageal veins often rupture and cause major hemorrhage. In the event of hemorrhage, the patient will present with bright red blood in the vomitus, hypotension, tachycardia, abdominal pain, and confusion. The clinical presentation is an acute UGIB with massive blood loss.

> ### 🩺 CLINICAL CONCEPT
>
> Ten percent of episodes of UGIB are caused by bleeding from esophageal varices. Esophageal varices have fragile membranes, so rupture with hemorrhage is common. In patients with long-term cirrhosis, there is a 60% to 70% chance of esophageal variceal bleeding.

Diagnosis and Treatment. Ultrasound can be used to diagnose portal hypertension in cases of esophageal varices. In addition, computed tomography (CT) and magnetic resonance imaging (MRI) can be used if ultrasound findings are inconclusive. Diagnosis of esophageal varices is confirmed with endoscopy. Treatment is focused on the prevention of a rupture. Beta-adrenergic blockers and isosorbide mononitrate will help decrease blood pressure, thereby decreasing portal hypertension. Ruptured esophageal veins require immediate surgical treatment and often carry a poor prognosis.

Esophageal balloon tamponade can be used as a temporary measure to stop bleeding. This involves insertion of a specialized tube with an inflatable tip that is placed against the area of an acute bleed. Vasopressin, somatostatin, and octreotide are strong vasoconstrictors that can be administered intravenously to control the bleeding. Sclerotherapy, vein ligation, or banding of the esophageal veins are common treatments. Other procedures include the surgical portal decompression shunt or TIPS.

> **ALERT!** UGIB caused by esophageal varices requires emergency medical treatment.

Esophageal Cancer

Esophageal cancer is a disease with a poor prognosis and high mortality rate. In 2016, approximately 17,000 patients were diagnosed with esophageal cancer and 16,000 died of the disease. Squamous cell carcinoma and adenocarcinoma are the major causes of esophageal cancer, together accounting for 95% of cases. The incidence of squamous cell carcinoma is approximately 3 to 6 cases per 100,000 persons and

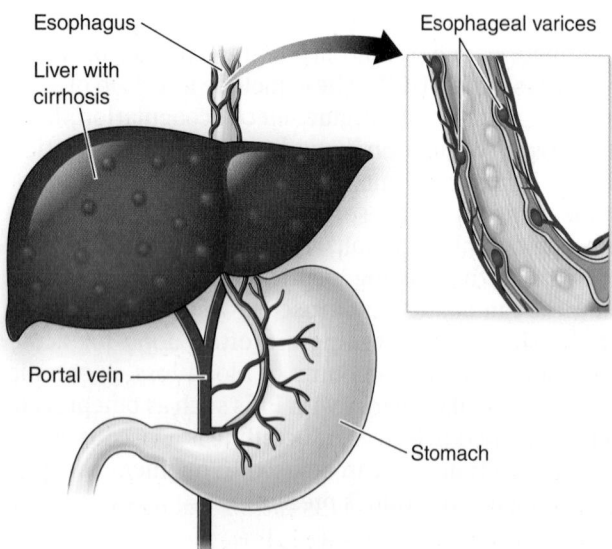

FIGURE 29-5. Esophageal varices. In portal hypertension, which is high pressure within the portal vein, backup or venous pressure occurs, causing the veins at the base of the esophagus to become dilated and fragile. The veins are termed *esophageal varices,* and they are susceptible to rupture and bleeding.

is most common in China, other Asian countries, and Africa. Males and females are affected equally, with most persons between 60 and 70 years of age. Higher numbers of African Americans are affected than European Americans. However, adenocarcinoma of the esophagus affects more persons in the United States and Europe, with an incidence of 12 to 16 per 100,000 persons. Males are affected eight times more than females; African Americans are affected five times more than European Americans.

Etiology. Currently, adenocarcinoma accounts for more than 70% of all new cases of esophageal cancer in the United States. The cancer most often arises in the distal esophagus and gastroesophageal junction. Tobacco use, GERD, and Barrett's esophagus, a complication of GERD, are the primary risk factors for adenocarcinoma of the esophagus. Obesity is also a risk factor for esophageal adenocarcinoma. Both high body mass index and increased abdominal obesity are associated with cancer risk.

In squamous cell carcinoma, cancer cells invade the lining of the esophagus. Chronic alcohol consumption and tobacco use are risk factors for esophageal squamous cell carcinoma. Recent studies also show that HPV infection increases incidence of esophageal papilloma and esophageal squamous cell carcinoma (ESCC). HPV is a common sexually transmitted infection that is a leading cause of oropharyngeal, cervical, and anal cancer.

A genome study has identified susceptible gene loci on chromosomes 3p13, 5q11, 6p21, 10q23, 12q24, and 21q22. Persons with mutations of the tumor suppressor gene *TP53* and Barrett's esophagus develop adenocarcinoma. The findings suggest that there is involvement of both genes and environment in the development of esophageal cancer.

> ### 🔍 CLINICAL CONCEPT
>
> The risk of esophageal adenocarcinoma among patients with Barrett's esophagus has been estimated to be 30 to 60 times that of the general population.

Pathophysiology. Chronic irritation of the epithelial cells that line the esophagus causes chronic cellular injury. Commonly, the irritation is caused by acid from GERD. In GERD, a metaplastic change often occurs at the lower esophagus, called Barrett's esophagus. From metaplasia, over time, the cells become dysplastic and gradually turn into adenocarcinoma. Almost all cases of esophageal adenocarcinoma are preceded by Barrett's esophagus. The proliferation of cancerous cells is apparent with alterations in the size, shape, function, and density of cells. The reproduction of multiple abnormal cells leads to the development of tumor growth and the potential for metastasis of cancerous cells to other parts of the body.

Clinical Presentation. The clinical symptoms of esophageal cancer appear late in the course of the disease. Dysphagia is the most common complaint that occurs when the disease is in advanced stages. The inability to swallow is initially noted with solids and eventually progresses to liquids and saliva. Weight loss and change of eating patterns frequently occur in response to dysphagia. The inability to swallow effectively increases the risk of aspiration pneumonia. Additional complaints include chest pain or a burning sensation behind the sternum. The area and size of the cancer can cause pressure on nerves, leading to such symptoms as hiccups, hoarse voice, pain at the back of the throat, chronic cough, and odynophagia (painful swallowing). Difficulty breathing can arise if the pressure on nerves limits the rise and fall of the diaphragm.

Diagnosis and Treatment. Diagnosis is confirmed with endoscopy and tissue biopsy. Chromoendoscopy (application of stains to mucosal tissue to improve visualization of growths) and narrow-band imaging (use of blue and green light to improve visualization of blood vessels and other features of tumor growths) are often used during endoscopy to improve identification of suspicious lesions. An endoscopic ultrasound is commonly done to visualize the depth of the tumor. Chest and abdominal CT scan with and without contrast is usually done. Bronchoscopy may be performed to identify areas of metastasis. Tumors are staged according to the tumor size, lymph node involvement, and existence of metastasis. Positron emission tomography (PET) scans are used to detect distant metastasis sites.

Treatment involves surgical resection, chemotherapy, and chemoradiotherapy. Endoscopic surgical procedures can be used with techniques such as radiofrequency ablation to remove the cancerous tissue. If more extensive surgery is needed, an esophagectomy can be done via endoscope or open abdominal surgery. In an attempt to improve outcomes for patients after surgery, some patients are given neoadjuvant therapy concurrently. Esophageal stents and brachytherapy (local radiotherapy) can be used in treatment of advanced cancer. The use of chemotherapy before and after surgical treatment for individuals with adenocarcinoma has shown an increase in survival rates. Over 75% of adenocarcinomas of the esophagus are at an advanced stage upon diagnosis. Overall, the 5-year survival rate ranges between 5% and 47%. When esophageal cancer is found early and when it is small, the 5-year survival rate is higher. When it is already large or has spread to other parts of the body, treatment is more difficult and the 5-year survival rate is lower.

Disorders of the Stomach

Gastric dysfunction can be caused by structural problems, inflammatory disorders, or neoplasms of the stomach. Structural problems include hiatal hernia and pyloric stenosis. Inflammatory disorders of the stomach include gastritis and PUD. Stomach cancer is rare in the United States, but its incidence is rising for unclear reasons.

Hiatal Hernia

A hernia is a protrusion of an organ into surrounding tissue as the result of an anatomical defect in the barrier that normally contains it. A **hiatal hernia** occurs when part of the stomach pushes up through the opening in the diaphragm and protrudes into the thoracic cavity (see Fig. 29-6). Hiatal hernia is a very common disorder; however, many are undiagnosed, asymptomatic, and discovered incidentally. They become more

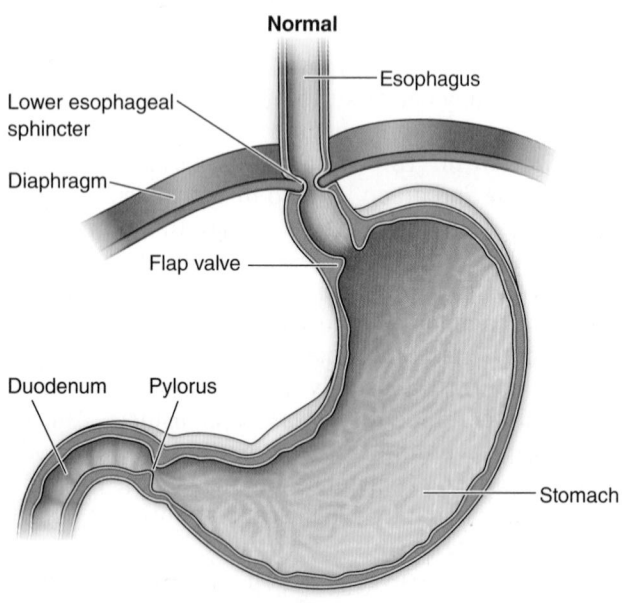

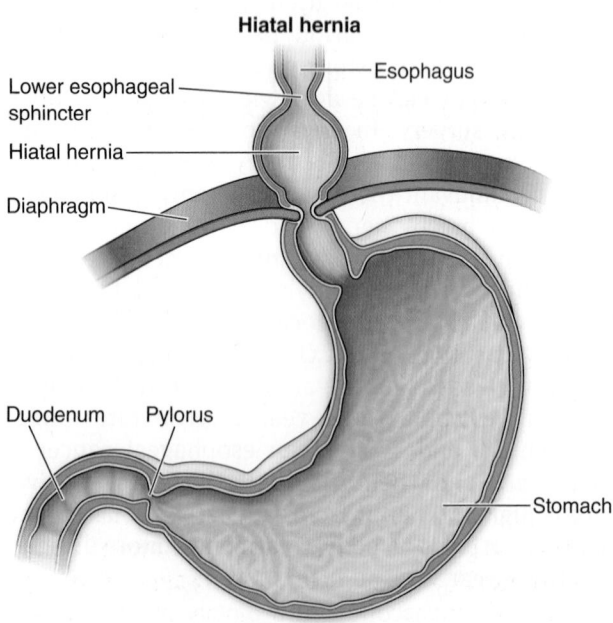

FIGURE 29-6. Hiatal hernia. A hiatal hernia occurs when part of the stomach protrudes up through the diaphragmatic opening in the chest. This allows acid from the stomach to reflux back up into the esophagus.

common with advanced age, and incidence increases significantly after age 60 years. Seventy percent of cases occur in persons over age 70.

Etiology. There are two types of hiatal hernias: a sliding hiatal hernia, also referred to as a direct hernia, and a paraesophageal hernia, or rolling hiatal hernia. The sliding type of hernia is the most common, accounting for 90% to 95% of cases. Any cause of increased intra-abdominal pressure can cause hiatal hernia; for example, obesity and pregnancy are major risk factors for the condition.

Pathophysiology. The esophageal hiatus is the opening in the diaphragm that allows the esophagus and vagus nerve to connect with the stomach. This opening weakens and widens with age, and the stomach is able to protrude upward through the aperture into the thorax. The fundus of the stomach pushes upward into the thoracic cavity, which prevents the LES from properly closing, thereby allowing reflux of gastric contents into the esophagus; this creates esophagitis or GERD.

A sliding hiatal hernia can easily protrude above the diaphragm when the person is lying supine. When the person stands, the hernia slides back into the abdominal cavity. A paraesophageal hernia is the protrusion of only the fundus part of the stomach into the thorax while the gastroesophageal junction stays below the diaphragm. This type of hernia is less common and has a higher risk for complications because the fundus of the stomach pushes into the thorax cavity and remains above the diaphragm. This leads to the potential for gastritis, ulcer formation, or strangulation of the herniated portion of the stomach.

Clinical Presentation. Clinical symptoms of sliding hiatal hernia usually occur as a result of esophagitis or GERD, which include dysphagia, substernal burning, belching, and epigastric discomfort. A paraesophageal hernia rarely has symptoms associated with reflux because the gastroesophageal junction remains below the diaphragm. The pain is associated with strangulation of the hernia and presents as acute chest pain or dysphagia.

Diagnosis and Treatment. The diagnosis of a hiatal hernia is easily confirmed with endoscopy or an upper GI barium x-ray. Treatment aims to prevent reflux and accumulation of acid contents in the esophagus. Lifestyle changes that assist in treatment include weight loss, small meals, coffee limitation, and smoking cessation. Individuals should also refrain from lying down after eating. Sleeping with the head of the bed elevated or the use of two pillows will help decrease gastric reflux. Pharmacological agents such as histamine-2 blockers (e.g., famotidine) or PPIs (e.g., omeprazole) relieve symptoms of hiatal hernia associated with GERD. Surgical repair called laparoscopic fundoplication can decrease episodes of reflux and may be needed if symptoms do not respond to other treatments.

Pyloric Stenosis

Pyloric stenosis is a constriction of the pyloric sphincter, the muscular valve that connects the stomach to the duodenum. The narrowing of this region impairs the movement of gastric contents into the small intestine. In infants, this is a congenital abnormality. The incidence of infantile pyloric stenosis is 2 to 4 per 1000 live births. It occurs most commonly in White newborns and has a 4:1 incidence in males compared with females. This is an uncommon condition in the adult but may develop secondary to an ulceration or fibrosis of tissue surrounding the pyloric sphincter.

The role of the pyloric sphincter is to control the release of gastric contents from the stomach into the duodenum. The stenosis, or inadequate opening, of the pyloric sphincter delays the emptying of the gastric contents, causing gastroparesis (distended stomach). Pyloric stenosis can develop into pyloric obstruction, which occurs when the stenosis becomes severe and the passage through the sphincter is blocked. The accumulation of food and fluids in the stomach leads to abdominal pain and distention. Nausea and vomiting are common symptoms. Weight loss, dehydration, and electrolyte imbalances also can occur. The abdomen will be firm upon palpation, particularly over the pylorus, and visible peristalsis may be noted. Projectile vomiting of undigested food eaten a few hours earlier is associated with a pyloric obstruction. Diagnosis is confirmed with x-ray, upper GI series, and ultrasound. Surgical repair is necessary, with a resulting good prognosis.

Acute Gastritis

Acute gastritis, also known as erosive gastritis, is an inflammation in the lining of the stomach. It can be caused by a number of medications and factors such as infection, allergy, acute stress, bile reflux, alcohol use disorder, radiation, and direct trauma. Chronic use of aspirin, NSAIDs, or corticosteroids commonly causes gastritis. These medications suppress the inflammatory response and irritate the stomach lining by blocking gastric mucus production. They are known to frequently cause GI bleeding or PUD.

The wall of the stomach consists of three layers: an inner mucosal lining, a middle muscle layer, and an outer serous coat. Inflammation associated with acute gastritis is limited to the mucosa layer. An irritant to the mucosa, such as an NSAID, triggers an inflammatory response. With inflammation, WBCs rush to the area and increase the blood supply, causing edema. The swelling creates increased pressure within the tissue layers, causing pain. NSAIDs are prostaglandin inhibitors; prostaglandins cause the pain in inflammation, but also stimulate the production of gastric mucus. Although NSAIDs relieve the inflammation, they deplete the gastric mucus. By eradicating prostaglandins, NSAIDs impair the stomach's protective mechanism. Without mucus, the gastric lining is exposed to acidic contents that increase the pain.

Clinical symptoms include complaints of heartburn, nausea, and epigastric pain. Diagnosis is based on history, physical examination, and endoscopy; treatment is focused on the cause of injury. Acute gastritis will typically heal within a few days when causative agents are removed. Antacids, H2RAs, or PPIs are prescribed for gastritis.

CLINICAL CONCEPT

Chronic use of NSAIDs will diminish the formation of gastric mucus, which can lead to gastritis and PUD.

Chronic Gastritis

Chronic gastritis, also known as nonerosive gastritis, is associated with an underlying disease or severe infection. It is different from acute gastritis because it causes atrophy of the glandular stomach lining, a condition called atrophic gastritis. The presence of the *H. pylori* bacterium, which usually affects the fundus of the stomach, is the most common cause.

H. pylori bacterium attacks the mucosal layer of the stomach wall. If the mucosal wall is eroded, it is unable to repair or regenerate cells. The death of chief cells and parietal cells diminishes the production of pepsin, HCl, and intrinsic factor. With low HCl levels, gastrin is repeatedly secreted in efforts to increase acid production. HCl is constantly stimulated and destroys mucosal cells. Erosion of the mucosa occurs, which enhances the environment for replication of *H. pylori*. A vicious cycle of bacterial replication and cellular tissue death occurs. The total destruction of parietal cells eventually leads to achlorhydria, which is a marked reduction in acid secretion. Atrophy of the gastric wall and loss of HCl results. Additionally, there is an insufficient level of intrinsic factor, which decreases the body's ability to absorb vitamin B_{12}, causing pernicious anemia.

CLINICAL CONCEPT

Chronic gastritis is a precursor for the development of stomach cancer.

Symptoms associated with chronic gastritis include burning or gnawing epigastric pain, nausea, weight loss, anorexia, and hematemesis. Diagnosis is confirmed with endoscopy and a biopsy of the affected tissue. Antibiotics will be prescribed to eradicate the *H. pylori*. Antacids, PPIs, or histamine-2 antagonists may be indicated to decrease the acid level in the stomach. Replacement of vitamin B_{12} will be required.

Peptic Ulcer Disease

PUD is an inflammatory erosion in the stomach (gastric ulcer) or duodenal lining (duodenal ulcer). Duodenal ulceration is four times more common than gastric ulceration. Duodenal ulcers commonly occur in the region termed the duodenal bulb, the upper portion of the duodenum near the pyloric sphincter, because of its proximity to the highly acidic gastric contents of the stomach. Approximately 4.5 million persons are affected annually in the United States, and approximately 10% of the U.S. population has evidence of a duodenal ulcer at some time in their lives. The hospitalization rate for PUD is approximately 30 patients per 100,000 cases. The incidence of PUD is equal in males and females.

Etiology. The most frequent causes of PUD are the bacterium *H. pylori* and the use of NSAIDs or aspirin. Low-dose aspirin for the prevention of cardiovascular disease has become an important cause of symptomatic ulcer, as well as the complications of bleeding and perforation of peptic ulcer. Cotherapy of NSAIDs with steroids, anticoagulants, other NSAIDs, low-dose aspirin, selective serotonin reuptake inhibitors (SSRIs), and bisphophonates dramatically increase the risk of ulcer complications. Though most adults are colonized with the *H. pylori* bacteria, it is unclear exactly how the bacterium is contracted or transmitted. However, not all persons colonized by *H. pylori* develop ulcer disease.

Genetic susceptibility is believed to play a role in PUD development. A genetic polymorphism of the hepatic cytochrome P450 system delays the metabolism of several NSAIDs, which prolongs duration of the drugs and enhances their ulcerogenic effect. Individuals who have a first-degree relative diagnosed with a duodenal ulcer are three times more likely to develop one.

Additional risk factors include stress, alcohol-related cirrhosis, excessive caffeine, smoking, pancreatitis, hyperthyroidism, and chronic obstructive pulmonary disease. Stressful conditions such as severe burns, sepsis, central nervous system (CNS) trauma, and severe hypotension can also cause peptic ulcers. NSAIDs and aspirin cause PUD because they counteract prostaglandin E secretion, the major stimulant of gastric mucus production, and diminish the stomach's protective layer. However, the most significant risk factor is the presence of *H. pylori*.

ALERT! Persons have a high risk of ulcer when NSAIDs and/or aspirin are used frequently and *H. pylori* is present.

Pathophysiology. The underlying pathophysiology of PUD is hypersecretion of HCl, ineffective GI mucus production, and poor cellular repair. These abnormalities lead to the erosion of the mucous membrane in the stomach or duodenum. In PUD, the protective mechanisms of the intestinal mucosal barrier are damaged by *H. pylori,* which are helically shaped, gram-negative bacteria that secrete the enzyme urease. Urease breaks down urea, which is a normal component of stomach mucus, into carbon dioxide and ammonia (NH_3). The ammonia is converted to ammonium (NH_4) by accepting a proton ($H+$) from HCl; the acid is then neutralized. This neutralization of acid protects the integrity of the *H. pylori* colony. The ammonia produced by the breakdown of urea is toxic to the epithelial cells of the stomach and duodenum. Intestinal cell damage also occurs because of other products of *H. pylori,* such as proteases, cytotoxins, and phospholipases.

The erosion in the mucosal lining of the stomach or duodenum permits the diffusion of HCl into the stomach wall and blood vessels. This stimulates an inflammatory response with the release of prostaglandins and histamine. Prostaglandins trigger the stomach cells to release additional mucus and bicarbonate in an attempt to neutralize the acid. However, the parietal cells keep releasing histamine and HCl, substances that are required for normal digestion. The HCl irritates and destroys the stomach lining as it continues to trigger inflammation. Histamine causes vasodilation and stimulates the release of pepsin, a proteolytic enzyme, and gastrin, a hormone that stimulates acid, which together damage the unprotected stomach lining. Cellular repair can occur, but repeated episodes of elevated gastric acidity will cause scarring and fibrosis of the GI lining. Fibrosis prevents the reproduction of healthy cells, thereby decreasing the mucus and bicarbonate production to protect the gastric lining.

Ulcers can vary in size from millimeters to centimeters; depending on the depth of penetration into the cellular layer, the worn area may be classified as an erosion or ulcer (see Fig. 29-7). If the superficial layer of the gastric mucosa is affected and does not extend into the muscularis layer, it is considered an

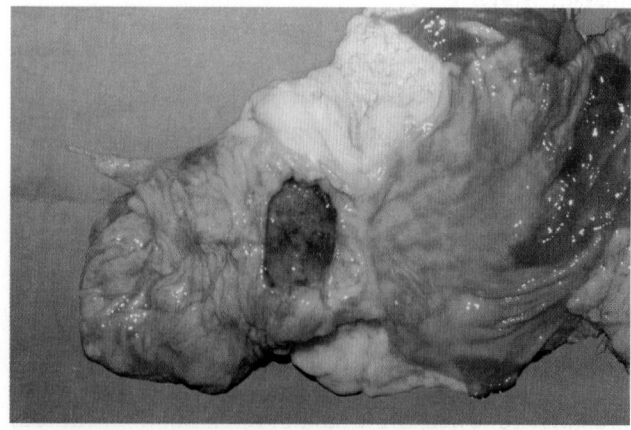

FIGURE 29-7. A peptic ulcer is an area of severe irritation, inflammation, and erosion in the duodenum. A gastric ulcer is a similar lesion in the stomach. *(From Biophoto Associates/Science Source.)*

erosion. An ulcer extends beyond the mucosa and into the muscularis layer.

Clinical Presentation. The main symptom of gastric and duodenal ulcers is epigastric abdominal pain. Episodes of pain occur between meals, about 2 to 3 hours after eating. The pain is described as an intense, burning, and gnawing sensation that can be relieved slightly by food and can be strong enough to awaken a person from sleep. Approximately 70% of peptic ulcers are asymptomatic.

Bleeding peptic ulcer presents with nausea, hematemesis (bright-red or coffee-ground emesis), and melena (black, tarry stools). Between 43% and 87% of patients with bleeding peptic ulcers present without prior symptoms. If the ulceration progresses to perforation of the stomach or intestinal wall, symptoms include sudden, excruciating abdominal pain that radiates to the back, abdominal rigidity, pale skin, hematemesis, and cold sweat.

Complications of peptic ulcer include bleeding and perforation. Older adults and individuals on NSAIDs or aspirin are more likely to endure ulcer complications.

Diagnosis. Identifying the characteristics, region, and timing of the abdominal pain is important in determining the diagnosis. The pain of PUD is distinct because it occurs when the stomach is empty.

Patients with suspected cases of PUD are tested for the presence of *H. pylori;* a blood sample is analyzed for the presence of antibodies to *H. pylori.* This is the most common method of preliminary diagnosis in PUD. Upper endoscopy is the most accurate diagnostic procedure for confirming PUD. It is done to visualize the location and severity of the ulceration, obtain a biopsy specimen, check for the presence of *H. pylori,* and rule out cancer. Although cancer is uncommon, it is found more often with gastric ulceration than with duodenal ulcer.

A rapid urease test is the endoscopic diagnostic test of choice for detection of *H. pylori.* The biopsy specimen is tested for the presence of the bacterial product urease, which confirms *H. pylori* infection. Alternatively, a fecal *H. pylori* antigen test can be performed on a stool sample to identify active *H. pylori* infection. An upper GI series (also called barium radiography) is used less frequently, but can visualize the ulceration on x-ray.

Another diagnostic test that is available but seldom used is the urea breath test. Patients swallow urea with radiolabeled carbon 14. After 10 to 30 minutes, the detection of radioactive carbon dioxide in the patient's exhaled breath indicates that the urea was split, indicating the presence of *H. pylori* bacteria.

Treatment. Once the underlying cause is identified, the focus of treatment is to reduce acid levels and protect the gastric mucosal lining. Triple or quadruple drug therapy for 10 to 14 days is a common treatment regimen. Healing the ulcer requires interrupting acid secretion and eradicating *H. pylori* bacteria. An antibiotic, a H2RA, and a PPI are commonly prescribed. The choice of antibiotic is influenced by the patient's genotype and strain of *H. pylori.* Polymorphisms in the patient's CYP2C19 gene and antibiotic susceptibility of the *H. pylori* influence the choice of antibiotic. H2RAs inhibit the release of histamine, which in turn decreases the production of gastric acid. PPIs block the generation of gastric acid. Bismuth is sometimes added to the medication regimen to coat the gastric mucosa.

Lifestyle changes are necessary to decrease the risk of relapse during the healing process. Individuals should try to avoid caffeine, alcohol, and tobacco because they stimulate acid production. Foods that are spicy, high in fat, or are acidic in nature should also be avoided. NSAIDs and aspirin should be avoided, as they block prostaglandins that stimulate gastric mucus production. For patients who must continue using aspirin or NSAIDs, cotherapy with a PPI or misoprostol is recommended. Alternatively, changing to a cyclooxygenase (COX)-2 selective inhibitor is an option.

Complications. Complications of peptic ulcer include bleeding, penetration, and perforation through the gastric or intestinal wall and gastric outlet obstruction. IV high-dose PPI therapy is necessary in bleeding ulcer. Somatostatin and octreotide reduce intestinal blood flow, inhibit gastric acid secretion, and may protect the gastric mucosa. Prokinetic agents such as metoclopromide or erythromycin may be given to push blood forward and enhance endoscopy efficacy.

Therapeutic endoscopic treatment is used to promote hemostasis if there is active bleeding or high risk of bleeding from the ulcer. Treatments include epinephrine injection therapy, thermal coagulation therapy, hemostatic clips, fibrin sealant, or hemostatic nanopowder spray. For persistent or recurrent peptic ulcer bleeding, angiography with transarterial embolization (TAE) is another treatment modality.

In refractory cases of bleeding peptic ulcer, vagotomy, surgical resection with gastric drainage, and suturing of the bleeding tissue may be necessary. Vagotomy decreases the stomach's ability to produce acid. Certain types of surgical procedures may also be performed. A gastroduodenostomy, also known as Billroth I, is the removal of the distal portion of the stomach; the remainder of the stomach is then directly connected to the duodenum. The benefit of surgery is the removal of the parietal cells, which are responsible for release of HCl.

A gastrojejunostomy, also known as Billroth II, is the removal of the lower stomach, with the remaining portion of the stomach connected to the jejunum. This surgery eliminates the gastrin-producing properties of the lower stomach and the duodenum.

Perforated duodenal ulcers can generally be treated by closure with a piece of omentum, which is called a Graham patch. For perforated ulcers close to the pylorus, vagotomy with pyloroplasty (widening of the pyloric sphincter) is performed.

 CLINICAL CONCEPT

There is a 90% chance that an ulcer with *H. pylori* can be cured if patients take the full dose of recommended antibiotics. However, patients need to continue taking the medication even when symptoms may have subsided.

Zollinger–Ellison Syndrome

ZES is a rare disorder that accounts for fewer than 1% of duodenal or gastric ulcers. It is most commonly caused by a gastrin-secreting tumor (gastrinoma) of the pancreas. The tumor may alternatively be located in the duodenum, lymph nodes, or another site.

In ZES, there is constant secretion of gastrin from a tumor. Gastrin stimulates the proliferation of parietal cells, which yield excessive HCl. The high level of HCl eventually leads to ulceration of the GI mucosa. ZES may occur sporadically or as part of an autosomal-dominant familial syndrome called multiple endocrine neoplasia type 1 (MEN type 1). The pathophysiology of cellular destruction is similar to that of PUD, with erosion of the mucosa and constant HCl secretion.

Clinical symptoms are similar to those of a peptic ulcer, although more severe. Common complaints include abdominal pain, diarrhea, nausea, vomiting, weight loss, fatigue, and GI bleeding. Complications include hemorrhage secondary to ulcer perforation and obstruction related to inflammation.

Hypergastrinemia can be detected in serum blood tests and through a fasting serum gastrin level. CT scan or MRI scan can visualize the tumor. PPIs also can be used because these medications inhibit the activity of the parietal cells and decrease their ability to manufacture acid. Surgical removal of the pancreatic tumor or a gastrectomy, which is the removal of all or a portion of the stomach, is frequently required.

Bariatric Surgery

Obesity is a public health problem that has reached epidemic proportions in the United States. Up to two-thirds of the U.S. population is overweight, and half of the people in this group can be classified as obese. Obesity is defined as a body mass index (BMI) greater than 30 (for more information about obesity, see Chapter 5). Obesity is associated with increased risk of many disorders, including cardiovascular disease, diabetes, cancer, sleep apnea, and arthritis. For those who are morbidly obese, with a BMI of greater than 40, diet and exercise are recommended as primary treatment. However, when conservative treatment has proven unsuccessful, bariatric surgery can significantly reduce morbidity and mortality associated with obesity. Indications for bariatric surgery include a BMI of greater than or equal to 40, a BMI of 35 to 39.9 with an obesity-related comorbidity (e.g., diabetes, hypertension, GERD, osteoarthritis), or a BMI of 30 to 34.9 with difficult-to-control type 2 diabetes mellitus or dysmetabolic syndrome X.

Bariatric surgery induces weight loss through two basic mechanisms: malabsorption and restriction. Procedures have restrictive and/or malabsorptive components. There is also growing recognition that bariatric surgical procedures contribute to neurohormonal effects on metabolism and hunger control.

Types of Bariatric Procedures

Sleeve Gastrectomy. This is the surgical procedure most commonly performed for obesity in the United States. The greater curvature of the stomach is largely removed, leaving a smaller, tubular stomach (see Fig. 29-8). Sleeve gastrectomy is mainly a restrictive procedure, but gastric motility changes and ghrelin-producing cells are largely removed. This cellular change causes less hunger, less insulin resistance, and enhanced glycemic control. At 2 years postsurgery, patients can expect 60% weight loss.

Roux-en-Y Gastric Bypass (RYGB). This is another procedure that reduces stomach size and attaches it to a section of jejunum. The duodenum and part of the jejunum are left as blind tracts. RYGB creates a stomach with a capacity of approximately 20 mL, which gives the patient a feeling of fullness after eating a small meal. There is intentional malabsorption because it detours around the distal stomach, the entire duodenum, and part of the jejunum (see Fig. 29-9). In addition, RYGB induces physiological and hormonal responses; ghrelin levels are reduced and leptin levels are enhanced, which results in decreased hunger and increased satiety, respectively.

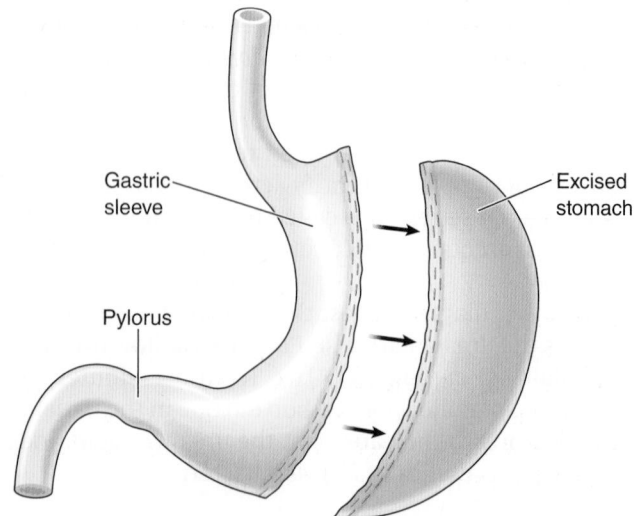

FIGURE 29-8. A vertical sleeve gastrectomy requires vertical stapling of the stomach and reduces its size to 15% of normal. The remaining 85% is removed from the abdomen at the time of surgery.

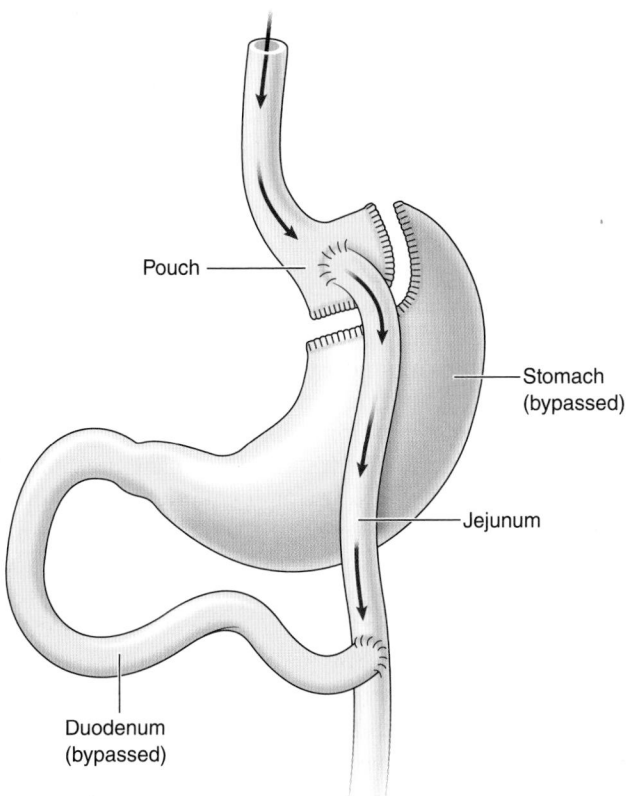

FIGURE 29-9. Gastric bypass surgery, also called Roux-en-Y bypass, is a procedure that decreases the size of the stomach and attaches a small portion of small intestine directly to the stomach. The major portion of the stomach is bypassed, and some small intestinal length is unused.

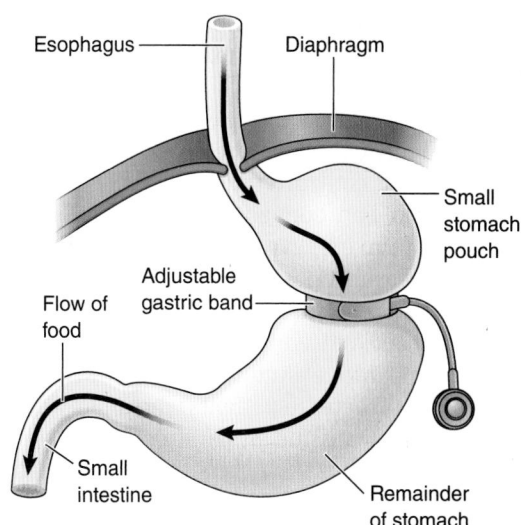

FIGURE 29-10. In gastric band surgery, a band is placed around the upper stomach to decrease its size and capacity. The volume of food allowed in the small stomach is restricted. The band can be adjusted according to the patient's needs.

Gastric Banding. Gastric banding involves placing an inflatable band around the upper portion of the stomach to restrict the amount of food the individual can consume (see Fig. 29-10). The inflatable gastric band is connected to a tube that is brought out through the skin to a port. Using the port, the band can be gradually tightened during a slow period of treatment, which is about 1 to 2 years for weight loss. Patients are advised about dietary changes to accommodate the smaller stomach.

Biliopancreatic Diversion. Biliopancreatic diversion with duodenal switch involves a 75% gastrectomy, resulting in a tubular stomach. The distal end of the ileum is attached to the duodenum (see Fig. 29-11). Weight loss occurs from both restriction and malabsorption: restriction of feedings because of the small stomach, and malabsorption because the procedure detours around the jejunum. There is an optional appendectomy and cholecystectomy. Compared with other bariatric surgery, this procedure causes less malabsorption of fats and proteins.

Results of Bariatric Surgery

Results of studies of gastric bypass procedures demonstrate that patients lose an average of 69% of their excess weight by 12 months and 83% at 24 months

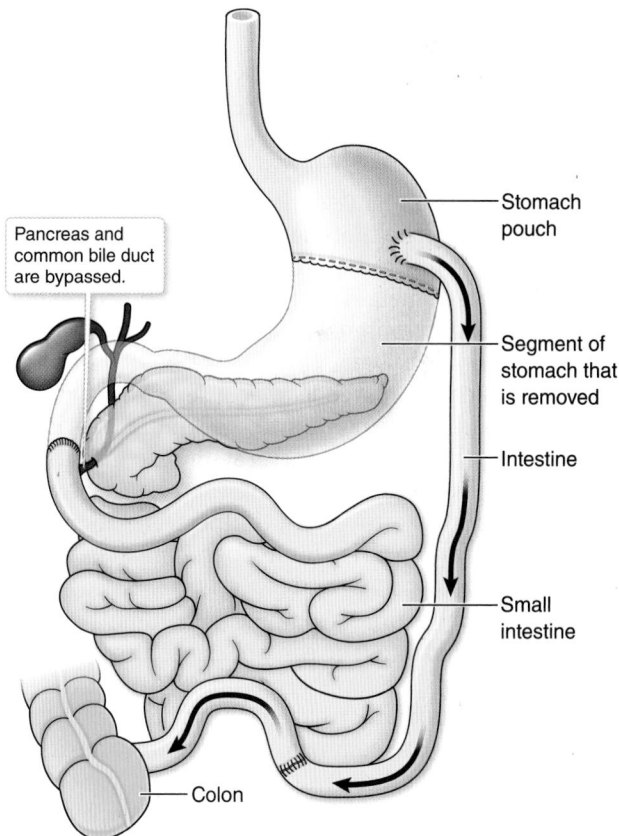

FIGURE 29-11. In biliopancreatic diversion, the stomach size is decreased and the intestine is attached to the segment of stomach. The procedure bypasses the pancreas and common bile duct.

postsurgery. Studies show weight loss after gastric banding has been 50% to 60% of excess body weight over approximately 2 years. Patients followed after sleeve gastrectomy have been found to lose 33% to 83% of their excess weight after a period of 6 months to 3 years. In contrast, biliopancreatic diversion has resulted in 75% to 85% of excess body weight loss by 18 months.

The Swedish Obese Subjects (SOS) study compared 2,000 morbidly obese subjects who underwent bariatric surgery with a control group of 2,000 morbidly obese patients who had conventional weight loss methods used in the primary health-care system. Compared with the control group, obese adults who underwent surgery experienced a reduced number of cardiovascular deaths and a lower incidence of heart attack and stroke. Other similar comparative studies have shown an 11-year remission of diabetes in patients who underwent surgery versus 2-year remission in patients who received conventional treatment. A Cochrane review from 2014 that included 22 trials with 1,798 participants concluded that surgical treatment of obesity yielded greater improvement in weight loss and weight-associated comorbidities than nonsurgical interventions did, regardless of the type of procedure. The RYGB and sleeve gastrectomy had comparable outcomes, and both had better outcomes than adjustable gastric banding.

Dumping Syndrome

Dumping syndrome is caused by rapid gastric emptying. This is a common complication following any surgical procedure that removes part or all of the stomach, such as bariatric surgery. Poorly digested material enters the intestine before its breakdown in the stomach. The material tends to be hypertonic, causing a shift of fluid out of the intestinal cells into the intestinal lumen. The fluid shift reduces blood volume, creates hypotension, and stimulates the sympathetic nervous system to increase heart rate. The abdomen becomes distended because of the ingested contents and the fluid shift into the jejunum. Peristalsis and intestinal motility increase in response to the abdominal distention. The pancreas releases excess insulin in response to gastric fullness and increased peristalsis, creating a risk for hypoglycemia.

Clinical Presentation. Dumping syndrome has two phases: early and late. The early phase occurs within 30 minutes of eating. Abdominal cramping, nausea, hyperactive bowel sounds, diarrhea, tachycardia, diaphoresis, and palpitations are common symptoms and are associated with the fluid shift that occurs from the bloodstream into the small intestine and the decrease in blood volume. The late phase occurs 2 to 3 hours after eating and includes epigastric fullness, syncope, palpitations, and symptoms associated with hypoglycemia.

The epigastric discomfort of dumping syndrome is the result of excess fluid volume in the stomach pushing upward upon the diaphragm. The risk for hypoglycemia is related to the pancreatic release of excessive amounts of insulin stimulated by gastric fullness.

Diagnosis and Treatment. Endoscopy and upper GI series will show a partial stomach. Treatment focuses on dietary management. Frequent, small feedings are recommended to decrease the volume ingested at one time. The patient should be prescribed a low-carbohydrate, high-protein, high-fat diet. Simple carbohydrates should be eliminated, as they increase intestinal osmolarity. Drinking fluids in between meals rather than with food consumption is an alternative to reduce rapid filling of the intestine. Medications that delay gastric emptying may be prescribed. Patients should supplement their diet with multivitamins, iron, and calcium, usually on a twice-daily basis. Ursodiol may be given to minimize the risk of developing gallstones during the period of acute weight loss. Patients must modify their eating habits by avoiding chewy meats and other foods that inhibit normal emptying of their stomach pouch. Nutritional and metabolic blood tests must be performed on a periodic basis.

Disorders of the Small Intestine

The small intestine is the main part of the intestinal tract that absorbs nutrients. A long length and distinctive villous mucosal epithelium provide a large amount of surface area. Different kinds of disorders affect the small intestine, including a congenital disorder called Meckel's diverticulum. A loop of intestine can herniate through a weak muscle in the abdominal wall. Inflammation of the intestine can occur because of ingestion of pathogens. Autoimmune and allergic reactions can cause inflammation of the mucosal lining of the small intestine, leading to malabsorption.

Meckel's Diverticulum

Meckel's diverticulum is the most common congenital abnormality of the gastrointestinal tract. The reported incidence is 1% to 4% in the general population. It is an outpouching of the small intestine formed from incomplete obliteration of the omphalomesenteric canal. This is a remnant of embryological development of the intestine. It can contain stomach or pancreatic tissue. Meckel's diverticula are often asymptomatic, particularly in adults, but can present problems in childhood. An asymptomatic Meckel's diverticulum is often discovered during abdominal exploration for the evaluation of another unrelated pathology. They are sometimes found incidentally on diagnostic imaging. Meckel's diverticulum can become inflamed or cause small intestine obstruction. When symptomatic, Meckel's diverticulum may present with abdominal pain or symptoms of gastrointestinal bleeding or bowel obstruction. The symptoms can resemble symptoms of other gastrointestinal disorders such as inflammatory bowel disease, acute appendicitis, or peptic ulcer disease. Diagnosis can be made on laparoscopy, abdominal x-ray, ultrasound, or CT scan. Technetium-99m pertechnetate scanning is the best noninvasive procedure for diagnosing Meckel's diverticulum. The main treatment for Meckel's diverticulum is surgical removal. Elective surgery is not recommended for cases where the diverticulum is asymptomatic and discovered incidentally on radiological imaging.

Hernia

A hernia is a protrusion of a section of the small intestine through a weakened abdominal wall muscle. As much as 10% of the population develops some type of hernia during their lifetime. More than a half-million hernia operations are performed in the United States each year. Males have a higher rate than females.

Etiology. There are several different types of hernia: umbilical, inguinal, obturator, femoral, or incisional (see Fig. 29-12). The most common is an inguinal hernia, which occurs when a loop of the small intestine protrudes down into the inguinal canal in the groin. Its occurrence is significantly higher in males because of the anatomical location of the scrotal sac. Between the scrotum and abdominal cavity there is a gap in the membranes that allows displacement of the intestines. It is most likely to occur before the first year of life or in the later stages of puberty. Inguinal hernias can also develop with advanced age as abdominal muscles weaken. Risk factors include positive family history for inguinal hernia, obesity, ascites, pregnancy, heavy lifting, chronic cough, or chronic constipation.

Pathophysiology. The pathophysiological processes are similar for all types of hernias. They differ based on the location of the protrusion of the loop of bowel. An inguinal hernia is directly related to the anatomical location of the scrotum and weak abdominal muscle wall. The pressure within the intestines pushes against the lower abdominal wall, eventually forcing the weakened area to separate, permitting protrusion of the intestine into the inguinal canal. It is possible that a severe herniation could extend into the entire scrotal sac. Hernias can be reducible, incarcerated, or strangulated. A reducible hernia is one in which the loop of bowel can be pushed back into normal position with manual pressure. Incarceration occurs when the loop of intestine becomes trapped in between muscle fibers. Strangulation of a hernia occurs when blood supply to the incarcerated loop of intestine is obstructed and at risk for ischemia.

Clinical Presentation. Clinical symptoms and severity will depend on the location and degree of the protrusion of intestine. The patient may be asymptomatic or have pain near the hernia site. Coughing or straining can cause the herniation to protrude and induce pain. If the hernia is pressing toward the bladder, urinary frequency or incomplete bladder emptying can occur. Pain occurs if strangulation of the hernia occurs with intestinal ischemia.

Diagnosis and Treatment. Diagnosis is based on the patient's history and the physical examination. The patient can usually demonstrate the bulging of the hernia in the abdomen. During the examination, the clinician will instruct the patient to cough or strain; this will raise intra-abdominal pressure, which will make the hernia protrude, thus confirming diagnosis. Some hernias can be manually reduced with gentle pressure while the patient is placed in the supine position, whereas others require surgical repair. A surgical hernia repair, called a herniorrhaphy, involves reinforcement of the weakened muscle with synthetic surgical material.

Gastroenteritis

Gastroenteritis occurs from an irritation to the lining of the stomach, small intestine, or large intestine by a pathogen or toxin. The disease can occur from a virus, bacteria, parasite, or chemical toxin. Gastroenteritis is transmitted from person to person or can be a waterborne or foodborne illness.

The incidence of gastroenteritis is difficult to estimate because most cases are not reported. In the United States, as many as 100 million cases occur per year, accounting for several million health-care visits and thousands of hospitalizations. Children account for more than 1.5 million outpatient visits. According to the Centers for Disease Control and Prevention, probably more than 21 million cases a year and nearly 50% of foodborne outbreaks in adults are caused by norovirus, the most common etiological agent of gastroenteritis.

Etiology. Norovirus is highly contagious and transmitted through the fecal–oral route or through close contact.

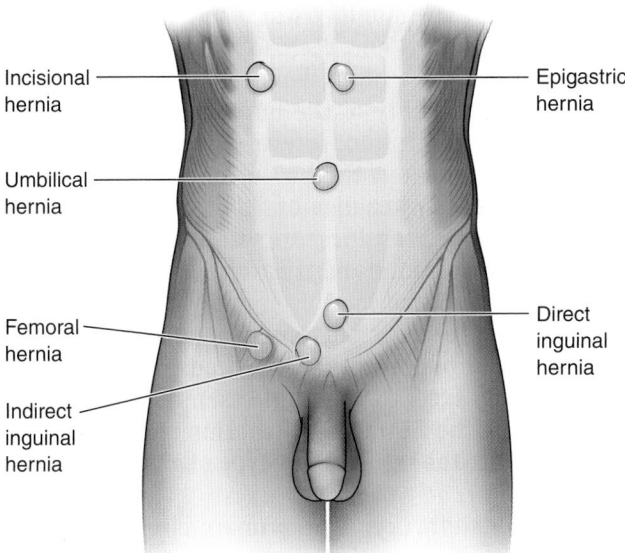

Incisional hernia

Umbilical hernia

Femoral hernia

Indirect inguinal hernia

Epigastric hernia

Direct inguinal hernia

FIGURE 29-12. There are several types of hernias. These weakened areas in the abdominal muscle wall allow protrusion of intestine just under the skin. On physical examination, there is a bulge in the abdominal or inguinal region. A hernia can become incarcerated when a section of intestine is strangled or squeezed by the abdominal muscle wall. Intestinal contents cannot move forward in an incarcerated hernia, which requires immediate treatment.

In children, rotavirus is a common etiological agent that is also transmitted via the fecal–oral route. Some bacterial organisms, such as enterotoxigenic *Escherichia coli,* Salmonella, Shigella, and Campylobacter, can cause severe illness with bloody diarrhea. Recent antibiotic use or hospitalization can predispose the patient to *Clostridium difficile* infection. Parasites such as amoeba and giardia can cause dysentery, which is a severe diarrheal condition with dehydration. Box 29-2 lists organisms that cause gastroenteritis. Individuals who are in close contact with others, such as those in nursing homes, day-care centers, cruise ships, and dormitories, are at increased risk for viral or bacterial gastroenteritis.

Pathophysiology. Infectious microorganisms are usually responsible for acute gastroenteritis and are often contracted via the oral route. These microorganisms cause diarrhea by adherence to the mucosa, invasion into the mucosal layer, or toxin production. The end result of most microbial infections is increased fluid to shift into the lumen of the intestine, to a point where the excessive fluid cannot be adequately reabsorbed. This fluid shift results in watery, small intestinal contents that pass into the large intestine and are then excreted as diarrhea. The fluid shift also can cause dehydration and loss of electrolytes and nutrients. Gastroenteritis diarrheal illness can occur by different mechanisms:

- Osmotic diarrhea occurs because of an increase in the osmotic load presented to the intestinal lumen because of diminished absorption.
- Inflammatory diarrhea occurs when the mucosal lining of the intestine is inflamed, edematous, and unable to reabsorb fluid or nutrients.
- Secretory diarrhea occurs when an organism stimulates the intestine to secrete fluid and mucus.
- Motility diarrhea is caused by intestinal neuromuscular disorders.

Pathogens or toxins either act directly on the intestinal epithelium, causing inflammation and malabsorption, or stimulate secretory mechanisms that produce watery diarrhea. The epithelium of the microvilli, which provides the surface area of the small intestine, is often the target of the infectious agent. The virus or bacteria attaches to the epithelium and impairs the small intestine's ability to absorb carbohydrates, fats, fluids, or electrolytes. Sometimes the infectious agent secretes a toxin that irritates the intestinal membrane. The infectious agent or its toxin stimulates inflammation of the GI tract and destruction of the epithelial lining. The villi are often damaged, which decreases the absorptive ability of the intestinal brush border. With lack of absorption, intestinal contents become hypertonic compared to the surrounding intestinal cells. An osmotic exchange of fluids and salts occurs at the intestine, resulting in water entry into the intestine. An osmotic diarrhea also occurs, producing watery stool and loss of electrolytes. A secretory diarrhea can result if microorganisms stimulate the intestine to produce mucus and fluids. In any of the mechanisms, excess water and essential electrolytes are lost from the GI tract. Dehydration and electrolyte imbalance are the result of any type of gastroenteritis.

BOX 29-2. Common Organisms That Cause Gastroenteritis

Viral, bacterial, and parasitic microorganisms most commonly cause gastroenteritis.

VIRAL (APPROXIMATELY 70% OF CASES)
- Adenovirus
- Coronavirus
- Norovirus
- Parvovirus
- Rotavirus

BACTERIAL (15% TO 20% OF CASES)
- *Bacillus cereus*
- *Campylobacter jejuni*
- *Clostridium difficile*
- *Clostridium perfringens*
- *Escherichia coli*–Enterohemorrhagic O157:H7, enterotoxigenic, enteroadherent, enteroinvasive
- *Listeria*
- *Mycobacterium avium-intracellulare,* immunocompromised
- *Providencia*
- *Salmonella*
- *Shigella*
- *Vibrio cholera*
- *Vibrio parahaemolyticus*
- *Vibrio vulnificus*
- *Yersinia enterocolitica*

PARASITIC (10% TO 15% OF CASES)
- Amebiasis
- *Cryptosporidium*
- *Cyclospora*
- *Giardialamblia*

FOODBORNE TOXIGENIC DIARRHEA
- Preformed toxin: *Staphylococcus aureus, Bacillus cereus*
- Postcolonization: *Vibrio cholera, Clostridium perfringens,* enterotoxigenic *E. coli, Aeromonas*

Clinical Presentation. The primary clinical presentation is nausea, vomiting, abdominal cramping, and diarrhea. If the gastroenteritis is associated with a virus, symptoms can usually persist between 12 and 72 hours. A bacterial form of gastroenteritis will produce symptoms until the causative agent is eradicated. Hyperactivity of the intestine produces intestinal cramping as well as high-pitched bowel sounds, known as **borborygmi.** Hyponatremia and hypokalemia can occur as a result of fluid loss, as well as acid–base imbalances of metabolic acidosis or alkalosis. Individuals must be closely monitored for dehydration.

> **ALERT!** Clinical signs or "red flags" that may indicate a need for hospitalization in patients with acute gastroenteritis include:
>
> - Severe volume depletion/dehydration
> - Abnormal electrolytes or renal function
> - Bloody stool/rectal bleeding
> - Weight loss
> - Severe abdominal pain
> - Prolonged symptoms (more than 1 week)
> - Hospitalization or antibiotic use in the past 3 to 6 months
> - Age 65 or older
> - Comorbidities (e.g., diabetes mellitus, immunocompromised)
> - Pregnancy

Diagnosis and Treatment. Diagnosis is aimed at identifying the causative factor. Stool cultures can be tested for WBCs, parasites, ova, or bacteria. Nucleic acid amplification tests can be done that identify the microorganism causing the gastroenteritis. Most times, gastroenteritis is diagnosed and treated based on clinical presentation.

Treatment is aimed at relieving symptoms and preventing transmission. Medical management is focused on resting the bowel and providing fluid replacement. Fluid replacement should be accomplished with broths and sports drinks or oral rehydration products that contain electrolytes. For patients with severe hypovolemia or inability to tolerate oral rehydration, IV normal saline or Ringer's lactate is required. Medications to suppress the vomiting and diarrhea may be indicated. Antibiotics are routinely ordered if gastroenteritis is identified as bacterial. Many of the bacterial pathogens associated with gastroenteritis have become increasingly resistant to antibiotics. Judicious use of antibiotics is advised as antibiotics exert negative effects on the natural microbiome in the GI tract. It is important to recognize that most cases of acute gastroenteritis, both viral and bacterial, resolve without specific antimicrobial therapy.

After fluids and broths are tolerated, the patient can move to a bland diet that can include cereals, potatoes, noodles, rice, toast, and crackers. Milk products should be avoided until symptoms resolve. Probiotics may augment the immune response through interaction with the gut-associated microorganisms. Some research has demonstrated a modest reduction in the duration of infectious diarrhea with the use of probiotics. Individuals with acute gastroenteritis should maintain diligent hand hygiene to help prevent spread of

infection to their family and contacts. Chlorine-based products can be used for disinfection of surfaces.

> **ALERT!** Children and older adults are at high risk of dehydration in gastroenteritis. Often hospitalization is needed to administer IV fluids to replace losses.

Celiac Disease

Celiac disease, also known as sprue and gluten-sensitive enteropathy, is a condition that occurs from a hypersensitivity reaction to gluten, a by-product of wheat, barley, and rye. The cause is unknown, but it is considered an autoimmune disease. It occurs in 1% of the American population; however, many individuals with the disorder go undiagnosed, as another 3 million people in the United States are estimated to be affected. Onset of celiac disease can appear in young children as foods are being introduced into the diet. In adults, celiac disease can occur between the ages of 20 and 50 years.

Etiology. In celiac disease, a gluten-derived peptide called gliadin damages the intestinal mucosa in persons with genetic predisposition to this disease. The exact etiology is unknown, but T cells predominate in an autoimmune inflammatory reaction against intestinal villi. There is a higher prevalence in those with a first-degree relative, such as a parent or sibling, with celiac disease, type 1 diabetes, or Down syndrome. More than 90% of affected persons have the cell surface marker HLA-DQ2.5 or HLA-DQ8.

Pathophysiology. The pathophysiology of celiac disease is related to an autoimmune, inflammatory process that destroys the intestinal villi. This destruction leads to a decreased surface area, causing atrophy of the intestinal wall. The atrophy creates a flattened appearance of the intestinal villi, greatly reducing the absorptive and transport properties of the small intestine. The decreased surface area impairs the absorption of all nutrients, vitamins, minerals, electrolytes, and bile salts.

The inability to digest carbohydrates leads to a buildup of gases within the intestinal system, causing abdominal bloating and diarrhea. The inability to absorb proteins impairs the body's ability to build and maintain muscle tone, causing muscle wasting. When fats are not absorbed, vitamins A, D, E, and K are not absorbed, causing fat to be excreted in the stool. **Steatorrhea** is the loss of fat in the stool; with steatorrhea, stool is light colored and soft. Deficiency of vitamin A will cause visual disturbances, particularly difficulty with vision in diminished light, a condition called night blindness. Vitamin D is necessary for the absorption of calcium. With vitamin D deficiency, calcium absorption is diminished and hypocalcemia occurs. Hypocalcemia causes symptoms such as muscle spasms and tetany; it also stimulates parathyroid hormone (PTH). PTH causes breakdown of bone with resulting osteomalacia and susceptibility to fractures. Vitamin E, which protects cellular membranes, is also not absorbed. Red blood cells and platelet membranes become excessively fragile, leading to hemolysis, anemia, and thrombocytopenia. Deficiency of vitamin K causes defective clotting mechanisms, leading to spontaneous bleeding and bruising. In addition, iron is not absorbed, causing iron-deficiency anemia.

Clinical Presentation. Numerous clinical symptoms are associated with celiac disease, mainly caused by malabsorption of essential nutrients, vitamins, and minerals. Weight loss occurs early in the disease, and if diarrheal illness occurs, dehydration is also common. Initial symptoms are fatigue, abdominal pain, bloating, and steatorrhea. As the disease progresses, symptoms associated with vitamin deficiencies will present, including anemia, high incident of fractures or bone pain, abnormal growth, bruising, poor skin turgor, and dehydration.

Diagnosis and Treatment. A serology celiac panel can determine whether an immune reaction to gluten is present. Affected individuals show a positive antibody titer of IgA antitissue transglutaminase (IgA TTG). If the results of this test are positive, a biopsy of the duodenum or jejunum is necessary. Treatment of celiac disease is aimed at making dietary changes. A consultation with a nutritionist is recommended to identify and eliminate gluten products in the diet. The patient frequently needs vitamin replacement. If the immune response is extreme, corticosteroids may be prescribed.

Short-Bowel Syndrome

The average length of the small intestine is 600 cm. Short-bowel syndrome is a result of any disease, traumatic injury, vascular accident, or other pathology that leaves less than 200 cm of small intestine, which is approximately one-third of the size of the normal small intestine. Studies show that, in the United States, approximately 10,000 to 20,000 patients receive total parenteral nutrition for short-bowel syndrome per year.

Etiology. Intestinal abnormalities that may require a partial removal of the small intestine include Crohn's disease, trauma to the bowel, strictures, tumors, radiation enteritis, mesenteric ischemia, strangulated hernia, and volvulus. Short-bowel syndrome can also occur because of congenital defects.

Pathophysiology. Short-bowel syndrome is directly associated with the amount of bowel that is remaining, the segment of the intestine that was removed, the health of the remaining intestine, and the functioning ability of the ileocecal valve. The ileum is the largest segment of the small intestine; it is responsible for absorption of fluids, electrolytes, fats, carbohydrates, proteins, vitamin B_{12}, and the return of bile to the liver. Removing any part of the ileum reduces the GI absorptive surface and can lead to nutritional deficiencies.

In short-bowel syndrome, the remaining intestine gradually adapts to the changes. The remaining intestinal villi increase in number and enlarge to accommodate the need for increased absorption. It is necessary for individuals with small-bowel syndrome to receive enteral nutrition during the postoperative period until the intestine adapts sufficiently to adjust to oral feedings.

Clinical Presentation. Short-bowel syndrome is divided into three phases:

1. Acute phase
2. Adaptation phase
3. Maintenance phase

The acute phase presents with symptoms of dehydration; electrolyte imbalance; weight loss; loss of folic acid; and loss of fat-soluble vitamins A, D, E, and K and vitamin B_{12}. These signs and symptoms are related to the small intestine's inability to absorb nutrients because of lost surface area and length. Fluid loss can be 6 to 8 liters per day. Malnutrition can rapidly develop, leading to muscle wasting, fatigue, skin irritation, and anemia. The acute phase lasts up to 3 months, followed by the adaptation phase, which may last 12 to 18 months. During this phase, the body begins to adjust by lengthening the microvilli, which creates an increased surface area for reabsorption. During the maintenance phase, the patient accommodates diet to the changed intestine, focusing on what amount of oral intake can be consumed without causing nausea, vomiting, or diarrhea.

Diagnosis and Treatment. The most definitive diagnostic test for short-bowel syndrome is a barium-contrast x-ray series. This allows for visualization and measurement of the small intestine. Abdominal CT scan with contrast and ultrasound may also be done. If the length of the bowel is less than 200 cm, short-bowel syndrome is confirmed. Treatment goals are to slowly increase fluid and nutrient intake. The need for enteral or total parenteral nutritional replacement to meet caloric and nutritional demands may be required. Oral intake should be encouraged with a trial-and-error approach of slowly adding new foods into the diet. Medications such as somatropin, which is a synthetic form of growth hormone, can stimulate intestinal cell proliferation. Teduglutide, an analog of glucagon-like peptide (GLP), can be used to enhance the absorptive ability of the remaining intestinal mucosa. GLP-2 analogs are recommended by the European Society of Parenteral and Enteral Nutrition (ESPEN). GLP-2 analogs have been shown to decrease the patient's dependence on parenteral nutrition. PPIs and histamine-2 blockers can reduce the effect of acid on the intestine. Diphenoxylate/atropine (Lomotil), codeine, and loperamide hydrochloride (Imodium) are used to reduce diarrhea. Octreotide, a somatostatin analog, is used in cases of severe diarrhea. Surgical procedures that can decrease patient dependence on parenteral nutrition include surgical lengthening of the remaining small intestine, insertion of a reversed intestinal loop to slow intestinal transport, or intestinal transplantation.

Small Bowel Obstruction

A small bowel obstruction (SBO) can be acute or chronic and partial or complete. An acute obstruction has a sudden onset that can occur with adhesions or a herniation of the bowel, whereas a chronic obstruction is often seen with inflammatory disease or tumors. A partial obstruction decreases the flow of intestinal contents through the bowel, whereas a complete obstruction prevents passage of all contents and fluid through the bowel and is considered a surgical emergency.

Etiology. The major cause of SBO is postsurgical adhesions (60%), followed by malignancy, Crohn's disease, and hernias. Postoperatively, surgeries that most often cause adhesions are appendectomy, colorectal surgery, and gynecological and upper GI procedures.

Pathophysiology. Adhesions are bands of connective tissue that form between tissues and organs, often as a result of injury during surgery. In the abdomen, adhesions commonly bond sections of intestine together. The adhesions cause obstruction and interfere with the intestine's normal function. Intestinal contents cannot move forward through the bowel. At the point of obstruction, there is increased peristalsis and mucus accumulation that worsen the blockage.

Clinical Presentation. The presentation of intestinal symptoms is directly related to the severity of the obstruction. The larger the obstruction, the more dramatic the symptoms. Abdominal distention, pain, nausea, vomiting, and hyperactive bowel sounds occur. Abdominal distention occurs proximal to the site of obstruction from the accumulation of chyme and intestinal gases. Pain is sharp, cramping, and intermittent, occurring with the contractions of hyperactive peristalsis. Pain that is continuous and steadily increases in severity is associated with a strangulation of the intestine. This indicates ischemia or necrosis of the intestinal lumen and requires emergency surgery. Nausea and vomiting can cause fluid and electrolyte depletion, which could potentially lead to dehydration, hypotension, or hypovolemic shock. Diarrhea is present with a partial obstruction because liquid intestinal contents can leak around an obstruction in the lumen.

Diagnosis and Treatment. Abdominal x-ray provides visualization of the area of obstruction and severity of the blockage (see Fig. 29-13). X-ray will show excessive gas in the area of intestine proximal to the obstruction. Multiphasic CT and ultrasound can also be used to identify the obstruction. CT with intravenous contrast can reliably diagnose SBO and bowel perfusion. A nasogastric tube is inserted to decompress the bowel and remove the accumulation of fluid within the bowel. IV fluids are given to ensure adequate fluid and electrolyte balance. The majority of partial SBOs can resolve with medical treatment. Pain management, antiemetic medications, and antibiotics are frequently necessary. Complete obstructions usually require surgical intervention.

Peritonitis

The peritoneal membrane is the serous membrane that surrounds the abdominal cavity and covers the organs. The peritoneal cavity is a sterile environment and can become contaminated with intestinal or organ rupture. **Peritonitis** is the inflammation of the peritoneal membrane caused by bacterial infection or leakage of intestinal contents into the peritoneal cavity. The overall incidence of peritonitis is unclear because it often occurs as a complication of another condition or surgical complication and is diagnosed as part of that disorder.

Etiology. Peritonitis most often occurs when organ rupture introduces bacteria, bile, acids, or enzymes into the sterile peritoneal environment. Less often, peritonitis is caused by hematogenous spread of infection from bacteremia. Most often, intestinal perforation allows *E. coli,* anaerobic bacteria, and other microorganisms to spill into the peritoneal cavity and cause

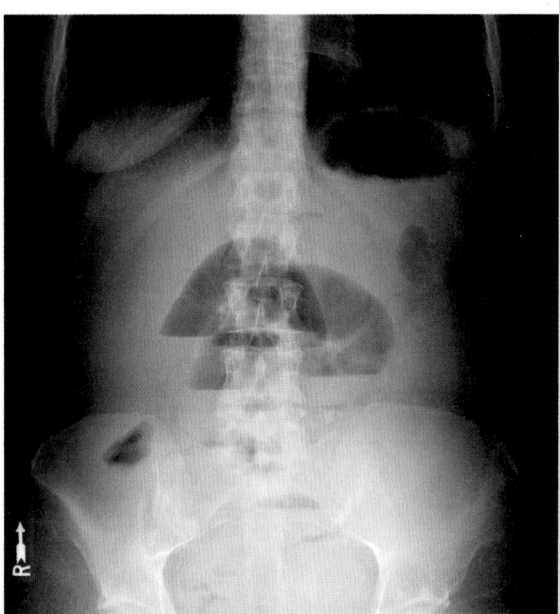

FIGURE 29-13. In SBO, there are specific findings on an abdominal x-ray. Areas that are filled with air or gas will appear black and fluid lines will be gray in color. Areas the x-ray cannot penetrate, such as an obstruction, will appear white.

abdominal sepsis. A perforated gallbladder or a lacerated liver can cause bile to enter the peritoneal cavity; gastric acid from a perforated ulcer can also leak into the peritoneal cavity. Peritonitis can also result from traumatic injury. Females can develop peritonitis from an infected fallopian tube or a ruptured ovarian cyst. Spontaneous bacterial peritonitis is a main infectious complication in patients with end-stage liver disease. Peritonitis is also a common and severe complication in peritoneal dialysis (PD).

Pathophysiology. Peritonitis is classified according to whether perforation of an organ has occurred. Primary peritonitis is limited to the inflammation of the peritoneum; there is no perforation of any organ. Secondary peritonitis is associated with trauma or is secondary to an infection from surrounding organs, such as appendicitis, pancreatitis, bowel obstruction, ischemic bowel disease, or the perforation of a peptic ulcer. A rupture from these areas will release bacteria into the peritoneal cavity. The contamination of the bacteria into the peritoneum causes a movement of fluid from intravascular spaces into the peritoneal cavity, called a peritoneal fluid shift. The excess fluid creates peritoneal edema but decreases blood volume and increases the risk of hypovolemic shock. In addition, these fluid shifts can lead to electrolyte imbalances.

Secondary complications of peritonitis include paralytic ileus, abdominal abscess, cardiac arrhythmias, and shock. An abdominal abscess is an area of purulent exudate that accumulates in a small cavity surrounded by inflammation. A **paralytic ileus** is the decrease or absence of intestinal motility that occurs during peritonitis. The body responds to peritonitis by decreasing peristalsis and shifting blood flow to the area of injury. Blood is shifted to the bowel or abdomen, causing a decrease in circulating blood volume, resulting in hypotension. Cardiac arrhythmias can occur because of electrolyte imbalances, which result from the fluid shift or from the loss of absorption because of reduced GI motility. The decrease or absence of peristalsis stops the movement of undigested material through the intestinal tract. As this content lies in the intestine, it continues to ferment, producing gas and swelling within the intestine. There is a high risk for intestinal perforation, septicemia (bloodstream infection), and shock if emergency treatment is not provided.

Clinical Presentation. The classic triad of symptoms in peritonitis is abdominal pain, abdominal rigidity, and rebound tenderness. Abdominal pain occurs with any movement of inflamed tissues. The patient wants to remain still with peritoneal inflammation so as not to disturb any peritoneal contents, because even a cough will usually cause abdominal pain. The patient's abdominal musculature is contracted in peritonitis; when palpated, the abdomen is rigid, a sign called involuntary guarding. Rebound tenderness occurs as the clinician palpates the abdomen.

Fluid shifts occur in peritonitis, with fluid moving into the peritoneum from the bloodstream. As the infection and fluid shifts progress, the patient will present with symptoms associated with severe hypotension or shock—tachycardia, tachypnea, clammy skin, decreased or absent bowel sounds, and oliguria. Electrolyte imbalances will occur because of the shift of intravascular fluid into the peritoneum. Fever occurs if the peritonitis is related to an infection.

CLINICAL CONCEPT

Assess for rebound tenderness by having the patient lie supine with knees slightly flexed. Place one hand with fingers pointing down into the right lower quadrant of the abdomen. Apply a gradual and deep pressure, followed by a quick release of the hand. If the patient experiences pain upon the release of the pressure, it indicates rebound tenderness.

Diagnosis and Treatment. Diagnosis is initially based upon physical examination, laboratory findings, and an x-ray. A WBC count will be markedly elevated (greater than 11,000 cells/mcL) with a high neutrophil count, whereas an x-ray will show air or fluid in the abdominal cavity. A paracentesis is a procedure where a sample of peritoneal fluid is withdrawn and analyzed; ultrasound can be used to guide the paracentesis. In patients undergoing peritoneal dialysis, cloudy effluent should be presumed to indicate peritonitis and treated as such until the diagnosis is confirmed or excluded. Peritoneal fluid with neutrophil count greater than 500 cells/mcL is an indicator of peritonitis. Bacterial count, Gram stain, and culture of peritoneal fluid are necessary. The diagnosis can be confirmed with CT scan or emergency surgical **laparotomy,** which is a surgical incision through the abdomen into the peritoneal cavity. On abdominal x-ray, free air under the diaphragm may be present if there is perforation of the intestine or organ. Treatment consists of **peritoneal lavage,** which is a sterile cleansing of the peritoneum. In patients on peritoneal dialysis, intraperitoneal administration of antibiotics is the preferred route unless there are features of systemic sepsis. The basic principle is to provide adequate coverage of both gram-positive and gram-negative organisms, including *Pseudomonas* species. IV fluids are necessary to replace fluids and electrolytes, as well as prevent cardiac arrhythmias and dehydration. Large doses of IV antibiotics should be administered to limit the spread of infection. Decompression of the GI tract occurs with the insertion of a nasogastric tube. Intestinal abscesses can be drained percutaneously or surgically removed.

Chapter Summary

- The upper GI tract consists of the esophagus, stomach, and small intestine. These organs are responsible for the major digestion and absorption of vital nutrients.
- Endoscopy is the standard diagnostic test used for upper GI disorders.
- The procedure most commonly used to cease upper GI bleeding is endoscopic hemostatic treatment.
- Dysphagia is a risk factor for aspiration pneumonia. It can be caused by disorders such as achalasia, Zenker's diverticulum, esophageal stricture, stroke, and neuromuscular disease.
- Assessment for dysphagia includes checking the patient's gag reflex, tongue, and uvula position.
- GERD is a common disorder that can lead to metaplasia of the lower esophageal epithelium and Barrett's esophagus.
- Fundoplication is antireflux surgery performed to treat GERD.
- Esophageal varices are commonly due to portal hypertension, as occurs in cirrhosis of the liver.
- Surgery is needed in patients with a perforated viscus, such as in perforated duodenal ulcer, perforated gastric ulcer, and Boerhaave syndrome (esophageal rupture).
- Esophageal cancer is commonly adenocarcinoma. It has a poor prognosis and a high mortality rate.
- Meckel's diverticulum, a common congenital abnormality of the gastrointestinal tract, is an outpouching of the small intestine that is a remnant of embryological development. It can contain stomach or pancreatic tissue, and may be asymptomatic or cause inflammation or obstruction of the small intestine.
- Hiatal hernia is a common disorder that increases susceptibility to acid reflux and esophagitis.
- Chronic gastritis causes achlorhydria and is a risk factor for stomach cancer.
- PUD is an inflammatory erosion in the stomach or duodenal lining that is most commonly caused by H. pylori and use of NSAIDs or aspirin.

- Diagnostic tests to confirm the presence of H. pylori include a serological test for antibodies to H. pylori, fecal antigen test, endoscopic tissue biopsy, and urease breath test.
- PPIs are drugs used to treat GERD and PUD.
- PUD requires triple or quadruple drug therapy that includes antibiotics, histamine-2 receptor antagonists, PPIs, and bismuth.
- Bariatric surgery can effectively decrease susceptibility to hypertension, diabetes, coronary artery disease, sleep apnea, and arthritis.
- Four major types of bariatric surgery have been successful in treating morbid obesity. Sleeve gastrectomy is the most common procedure.
- Dumping syndrome is caused by rapid gastric emptying. This is a common complication following any surgical procedure that removes part or all of the stomach.
- Abdominal hernia is the protrusion of a loop of intestine through the abdominal muscle wall. It can become strangulated, which causes ischemia of the intestine.
- Gastroenteritis is commonly caused by pathogens contracted via the oral route or through waterborne or foodborne illness. This diarrheal illness can cause dehydration. Norovirus is the most common cause of gastroenteritis.
- Celiac disease is a condition that occurs from a hypersensitivity reaction to gluten, a by-product of wheat, barley, and rye. Although the cause is unknown, it is considered an autoimmune disease.
- Individuals with celiac disease show a positive antibody titer of IgA TTG.
- Short-bowel syndrome, which causes malabsorption, is a result of any disease, traumatic injury, vascular accident, or other pathology that removes a large segment of the intestine.
- Adhesions are the most common cause of SBO. There are characteristic patterns on the abdominal x-ray that indicate bowel obstruction.
- Peritonitis causes extreme abdominal pain, guarding, and rebound tenderness. It can cause a paralytic ileus, which is a lack of peristaltic activity in the intestine.

Making the Connections

Signs and Symptoms	Physical Assessment Findings	Diagnostic Testing	Treatment
Dysphagia | Difficulty swallowing related to structural or neurological impairment.			
Pooling of liquids in the back of the throat. Frequent coughing while eating. Repeated attempts to swallow.	Assess gag reflex, tongue, and uvula to check for dysphagia. Poor gag and deviated tongue and uvula indicate dysphagia. Drooling of food or liquids may be a sign of dysphagia. Abnormal lung sounds, such as crackles, are indicative of aspiration pneumonia. Elevated temperature indicates aspiration pneumonia.	Elevated WBC count is present with aspiration pneumonia. Swallow test, barium swallow, and esophagography show the patient's swallowing ability.	Keep head elevated greater than 60 degrees while eating. Provide small, frequent meals. Puréed and thick liquids are necessary because these are easiest to swallow. A powder called Thick-It should be added to fluids.
Esophagitis | Inflammation of the esophagus caused by reflux of gastric acid that injures the esophageal squamous epithelium.			
Patient complains of burning sensation in the throat, painful swallowing, or substernal or epigastric pain.	No significant physical assessment signs.	If chronic esophagitis, endoscopy is used to determine the cause.	Instruct the patient to avoid eating or drinking items that have an extreme temperature or spiciness. Decrease inflammation and relieve symptoms through antacids such as PPIs.
GERD | Inability of the LES to completely close; the opening permits the reflux (backflow) of acid contents from the stomach up into the esophagus. The epithelium of the esophagus can become metaplastic; this condition is called Barrett's esophagus.			
Patient complains of burning sensation in the throat, painful swallowing, or substernal or epigastric pain. Increased pain is present after eating acidic or spicy foods. Dry cough is present. Nocturnal asthma can be caused by GERD.	No particular physical assessment findings.	Endoscopy. Barium swallow (upper GI series). Esophageal manometry will show pressure within the LES. Ambulatory 24-hour pH testing. Biopsy of lower esophageal cells to look for metaplastic changes if suspect Barrett's esophagus or to check for dysplasia.	Keep head elevated greater than 60 degrees while eating. Provide small, frequent meals. Encourage weight loss. Encourage smoking cessation. Administer PPIs to decrease stomach acid and give esophagus time to heal. Periodic endoscopic examination is necessary to check for development of Barrett's esophagus.
Upper Gastrointestinal Bleed (UGIB) | An area in the esophagus, stomach, or duodenum that is bleeding small, moderate, or large amounts. Most common causes of UGIB are esophageal varices and PUD.			
Fatigue. Anemia. Abdominal pain. Rapid pulse. Syncope. Shortness of breath. Decreased urine output.	Hematemesis; blood in vomitus, sometimes referred to as "coffee-ground" emesis. Melena; tarry, dark stool caused by blood in stool. Hypotension.	Decreased hemoglobin and hematocrit caused by bleeding. Decreased plasma volume because of fluid loss with bleeding. Increased BUN caused by dehydration. Positive FOBT.	Treatment is specific to the cause of bleeding. Surgical repair is performed of esophageal varices or perforated ulcer in the stomach or duodenum. Endoscopic sclerotherapy, endoscopic band ligation, and other types of endoscopic ablation; insertion of a TIPS can be used to permanently treat esophageal varices due to portal hypertension. Blood transfusions. Rapid IV fluid infusion.

Making the Connections–cont'd

Signs and Symptoms	Physical Assessment Findings	Diagnostic Testing	Treatment
Esophageal Varices | Distended, fragile veins located at the lower esophagus that expand because of portal hypertension, usually caused by liver disease.			
No symptoms if unruptured; however, other signs of portal hypertension are frequently present, such as ascites and enlarged liver. If the varices rupture, hematemesis results. Other concerns are hypotension, tachycardia, pallor, and dizziness caused by blood loss.	Hematemesis; blood in vomitus, sometimes referred to as "coffee-ground" emesis. Melena; tarry, dark stool caused by blood in stool. Hypotension, pallor, tachycardia, syncope if large blood loss.	Decreased hemoglobin and hematocrit caused by bleeding. Decreased plasma volume caused by fluid loss with bleeding. Increased BUN because of dehydration. Positive FOBT. Endoscopy best demonstrates varices. Ultrasound, CT, or MRI may be done.	Temporary tamponade of the lower esophageal veins. Endoscopic sclerotherapy, endoscopic band ligation, and other types of endoscopic ablation, insertion of a TIPS. Vasopressin, somatostatin, and octreotide are strong vasoconstrictors that can be administered intravenously to control the bleeding. Beta blockers or nitrate may be needed to reduce blood pressure. Blood transfusion may be needed. Rapid IV fluid infusion may be needed.
Esophageal Cancer | Neoplastic cellular replication of esophageal cells.			
Difficulty swallowing. Heartburn. Weight loss. Change in eating pattern. Sore throat.	Weight loss. Cough.	Endoscopy will reveal cancer tumor. Biopsy of esophageal tumor. CT scan to locate tumor.	Encourage smoking cessation and avoidance of alcohol ingestion. Educate the patient about proper nutrition. Surgical removal of cancer tumor. Chemotherapy following surgery.
Hiatal Hernia | A protrusion of part of the stomach upward into the chest. It can occur when the diaphragm opening for the esophagus and vagus nerve is stretched out.			
Heartburn, particularly when lying flat.	No physical findings.	Chest x-ray, upper GI series (barium swallow) highlights the abnormal position of stomach above the diaphragm.	Encourage smoking cessation and avoidance of alcohol ingestion. PPIs or histamine-2 blockers are used to reduce acid. Surgical procedure called fundoplication is used to reinforce stomach in the correct position.
Pyloric Stenosis | Narrowing and hypertrophy of the pyloric sphincter, which causes backup of contents of the stomach.			
Projectile vomiting. Abdominal pain and distention.	A palpable mass may be felt at the pyloric area of the stomach.	Ultrasound, upper GI series (barium) are used to demonstrate the narrowing at the pylorus.	Surgical dilation of the pyloric sphincter.
Acute Gastritis | Inflammation of the gastric mucosa.			
Epigastric, burning pain.	No physical assessment findings.	Endoscopy if no success with conservative treatment.	Lifestyle changes related to smoking, food intake, caffeine, and stress. PPIs to allow healing of stomach.

Continued

Making the Connections–cont'd

Signs and Symptoms	Physical Assessment Findings	Diagnostic Testing	Treatment
Chronic Gastritis | Atrophy of the gastric mucosa and achlorhydria, most commonly caused by *H. pylori* infection that attacks the mucosal layer of the stomach wall. Lack of HCl decreases absorption of iron and vitamin B_{12}. Achlorhydria increases risk of stomach cancer.			
Epigastric pain, nausea, vomiting. Hematemesis.	Hematemesis.	Endoscopic examination with biopsy if no success with conservative treatment.	Lifestyle changes related to smoking, food intake, caffeine, and stress. Antacids or PPIs or histamine-2 blockers.
Peptic Ulcer Disease (PUD) | Multiple small erosions into the mucosa or submucosa layer related to an overproduction of acid and pepsin in the stomach.			
Epigastric, gnawing, burning pain in between meals. Nausea. Weight loss. Nocturnal epigastric pain.	Abdominal pain and tenderness.	Presence of *H. pylori* antibodies in the blood. Low hemoglobin and hematocrit if it is a bleeding ulcer. *H. pylori* fecal antigen test. Endoscopic urease test indicating presence of *H. pylori*. Endoscopy with biopsy to visualize *H. pylori* or any cancerous cells.	Lifestyle changes related to smoking, food intake, caffeine, and stress. Antibiotics administered to eradicate *H. pylori*. Histamine-2 receptor blockers to diminish acid. PPIs to diminish stomach acid to allow ulcer to heal.
Duodenal Ulcer | Single erosion near the duodenal bulb, with a punched-out appearance.			
Pain relief when eating. Pain increases in stomach 2 to 3 hours after eating. Epigastric or upper abdominal pain. Nocturnal epigastric pain.	Fatigue. Abdominal pain and tenderness. Hematemesis. Melena.	Presence of *H. pylori* antibodies in the blood. *H. pylori* fecal antigen test. Endoscopic urease test indicating presence of *H. pylori*. Low hemoglobin and hematocrit if it is a bleeding ulcer. Endoscopy with biopsy to visualize *H. pylori* or any cancerous cells.	Antibiotics to eradicate *H. pylori*. PPIs to decrease acid to allow ulcer to heal. Histamine-2 receptor blockers to diminish acid. Instruct the patient to avoid spicy foods that increase gastric acid. Endoscopic hemostasis treatments if bleeding peptic ulcer or angiographic transarterial embolization.
Zollinger–Ellison Syndrome (ZES) | Rare disorder most commonly caused by a gastrin-secreting tumor (gastrinoma) of the pancreas. The tumor may alternatively be located in the duodenum, lymph nodes, or another site. Gastrinoma stimulates excessive acid in the stomach.			
Abdominal pain, diarrhea, nausea, vomiting, weight loss, fatigue.	Often does not show any physical findings.	Fasting serum blood test may show excessive gastrin. CT scan or MRI may show tumor. FOBT may show blood in stool.	PPIs to reduce acid. Histamine-2 receptor blockers to diminish acid. Surgical removal of tumor.
Dumping Syndrome | Rapid gastric emptying because of removal of part of the stomach.			
Phase 1: abdominal pain, diarrhea, diaphoresis. Phase 2: gastric fullness, symptoms of hypoglycemia.	Diaphoresis, tachycardia, hyperactive bowel sounds.	Endoscopy, upper GI series.	Frequent, small feedings; fluids only between meals. Medications that slow peristalsis. Diet supplementation with multivitamins, iron, and calcium.

Making the Connections–cont'd

Signs and Symptoms	Physical Assessment Findings	Diagnostic Testing	Treatment
Hernia | Protrusion of loop of bowel through the muscle layers of the abdominal wall. It can become incarcerated or strangulated, causing ischemia of the bowel.			
With increased abdominal pressure, a protrusion of intestine under the skin is demonstrated.	Ask the patient to cough or exert the Valsalva maneuver to demonstrate herniation of intestine through the abdomen wall. Severe abdominal pain is present if a hernia is incarcerated or strangulated.	Physical examination usually demonstrates the problem. Loop of intestine is commonly palpable in the inguinal region.	If reducible, manual pressure can return the intestine to the proper position. If incarcerated or strangulated, immediate surgical repair of the hernia is required.
Gastroenteritis | Inflammation of the GI lining caused by a pathogen.			
Frequent episodes of watery diarrhea. Weight loss. Fatigue. Fever possible. Colicky cramping.	Auscultation of borborygmi. Dehydration. Fever.	Presence of bacteria or virus in serum or stools. Dehydration and electrolyte imbalance caused by fluid loss and fluid shifts. Decreased albumin caused by malabsorption.	Fluid and electrolyte replacement to treat dehydration. Antibiotics to eradicate bacteria. Antidiarrheal medications. Antiemetic medications to stop vomiting.
Celiac Disease | Autoimmune disorder triggered by gluten, which causes malabsorption.			
Abdominal pain and bloating. Diarrhea. Weight loss. Steatorrhea. Weakness. Fatigue.	Steatorrhea. Abdominal distention. Muscle wasting.	Low hemoglobin and hematocrit levels caused by malabsorption of iron, vitamin B_{12}, and vitamin K. Abnormal electrolytes caused by malabsorption. Positive celiac disease antibodies in blood. Tissue biopsy to confirm celiac disease.	Removal of gluten from diet. Vitamin A, D, E, K replacement. Corticosteroids.
Short-Bowel Syndrome | A result of any disease, traumatic injury, vascular accident, or other pathology that leaves less than 200 cm (less than one-third) of the small intestine.			
Diarrhea, dehydration, weight loss, muscle wasting, fatigue, skin irritations, weakness.	Poor skin turgor, hypotension, pallor, muscle wasting, weakness.	Upper GI series/barium study or CT scan to show shortened bowel. Low hemoglobin and hematocrit levels caused by malabsorption of iron, vitamin B_{12}, and vitamin K. Abnormal electrolytes caused by malabsorption.	Vitamin replacement. Parenteral or enteral nutrition. Slowly increase oral feedings until bowel regenerates enough absorptive surface for total oral nutrition.
Small Bowel Obstruction | Tumor, adhesions, hernia, or inflammation can cause obstruction. A partial obstruction decreases the flow of intestinal contents through the bowel. A complete obstruction prevents passage of all contents and fluid through the bowel.			
Abdominal pain, abdominal distention, nausea, vomiting. Diarrhea, if partial obstruction.	Abdominal distention, vomiting, and hyperactive bowel sounds. Diarrhea, if partial obstruction.	Abdominal x-ray shows excessive intestinal gas proximal to the obstruction. CT scan or ultrasound can show area of obstruction.	Nasogastric tube to decompress intestine. IV fluids. Pain management, antiemetic medications, and antibiotics are frequently necessary. May require surgical intervention.

Continued

Making the Connections–cont'd

Signs and Symptoms	Physical Assessment Findings	Diagnostic Testing	Treatment
Peritonitis | Inflammation of the peritoneal membrane. Infection of peritoneum commonly caused by rupture of organs into the peritoneal cavity.			
Abdominal pain and rigidity. Anxiety. Increased heart rate and respirations. Fever.	Abdominal tenderness on palpation and guarding of abdomen. Rebound tenderness. Hypoactive or absent bowel sounds. Tachycardia. Fever. Tachypnea.	Elevated WBC count caused by inflammation. Electrolyte imbalance caused by fluid shifts into the peritoneum. CT scan to find source of peritoneal inflammation, such as ruptured organ.	Fluid and electrolyte replacement caused by fluid shifts into peritoneal cavity. Antibiotics to eradicate bacteria entering peritoneum. Peritoneal lavage to cleanse the peritoneal cavity. Nasogastric tube to decompress GI system.

Bibliography

Available online at fadavis.com

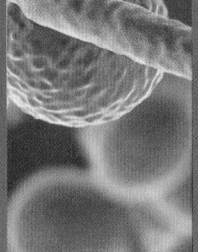

CHAPTER 30

Large Intestine Disorders

Learning Objectives

Upon completion of this chapter, the student will be able to:

- Describe normal anatomy and physiology of the large intestine.
- Recognize inflammatory, obstructive, and motility disorders that affect the large intestine.
- Recognize common causes, signs, and symptoms of an acute abdomen.

- Identify signs, symptoms, and clinical manifestations of disorders of the large intestine.
- Recognize assessment techniques, laboratory tests, and imaging studies used in the diagnosis of disorders of the large intestine.
- Discuss pharmacological and nonpharmacological treatment modalities used for disorders of the large intestine.

Key Terms

Acute abdomen
Acute colonic pseudoobstruction (ACPO)
Anastomosis
Appendicitis
Borborygmi
Cathartic colon
Colectomy
Colostomy
Diverticula
Diverticulitis

Diverticulosis
Dysbiosis
Fecal impaction
Fecal occult blood test (FOBT)
GI microbiome
Hematochezia
Hemorrhoids
Ileostomy
Inflammatory bowel disease (IBD)
Irritable bowel syndrome (IBS)

McBurney's point
Melena
Murphy's sign
Obstipation
Peritonitis
Pseudopolyp
Skip lesions
Stoma
Toxic megacolon
Volvulus

The normal functions of the intestinal tract are to propel digested food forward, absorb nutrients and water, and finally to excrete waste and indigestible contents. Inflammation, irritation, infection, obstruction, and certain medications can all interfere with these normal functions. Inflammatory bowel disease (IBD) hinders adequate absorption of nutrients and causes pain in the affected individual throughout life. IBD produces extremely painful intestinal lesions visible on colonoscopy; in contrast, irritable bowel syndrome (IBS) causes similar abdominal pain but has no clear etiology or apparent pathology.

Obstruction of the large bowel can occur abruptly and cause sudden, severe abdominal pain; this condition requires prompt intervention. Inflammation of the intestine commonly causes a tender abdomen, intense pain, and fever, a syndrome known as **acute abdomen,** which is a surgical emergency. Obstructive neoplasms, diverticulitis, and twisting of the intestine can lead to a serious, potentially lethal complication known as peritonitis. **Appendicitis** can lead to perforation if not diagnosed promptly. Perforation of the

bowel and peritonitis are the major concerns of clinicians treating disorders of the large intestine.

Epidemiology

Disorders of the large intestine can be classified as either alterations in the integrity of the gastrointestinal (GI) wall or alterations in motility. Alterations in the integrity of the GI wall can occur anywhere along the large bowel; they can be caused by IBD, such as Crohn's disease and ulcerative colitis (UC), and inflammatory conditions, such as appendicitis and diverticulitis. IBD affects an estimated 1 to 2 million people in the United States, with a prevalence of approximately 200 cases per 100,000 adults.

Common disorders that cause alterations in motility include IBS, bowel obstruction, and intestinal herniation. Between 30% and 45% of all GI conditions are caused by intestinal motility disorders, with up to 30 million Americans affected per year. Colonic motility dysfunction caused by malignancy occurs most commonly in older adults. Approximately 60% of large bowel obstructions (LBOs) are caused by malignancies, 20% are caused by diverticular disease, and 5% are the result of colonic volvulus. There is no clear pathological cause of IBS, but it is prevalent in people aged 20 to 40 years, affecting females three times more often than males. Dysfunctional colonic motility may be caused by diet, changes in the GI microbiome, or autonomic imbalance.

Basic Concepts Regarding Function of the Large Intestine

There are a number of different kinds of large intestine disorders. To understand the pathophysiology of intestinal dysfunction, knowledge of the normal functions of the intestine is required.

Structure of the Large Intestine

The large intestine is a hollow tube approximately 1.5 m in length and 6 to 7 cm in diameter. It works to absorb water and salt and to store feces until defecation. The large intestine is made up of the cecum; ascending, transverse, descending, and sigmoid colon; rectum; and anal canal (see Fig. 30-1).

The cecum is a blind pouch that projects downward at the junction of the ileum portion of the small intestine and the colon. The appendix, which is approximately 2.5 cm in length, arises from the cecum and has no apparent function. The ileocecal and rectosigmoid

sphincters control the flow of contents through the large intestine. The ileocecal sphincter, also called the ileocecal valve, located at the junction of the ileum and the cecum, allows approximately 500 to 700 mL of fluid waste to flow through it every day. The ascending colon arises from the cecum on the right side of the abdomen and curves to the left just under the liver, where it becomes the transverse colon. The transverse colon, the largest portion of the bowel, lies beneath the stomach and spleen. The portion under the liver is called the hepatic flexure, whereas the portion beneath the spleen is called the splenic flexure. Throughout the ascending and transverse colon, a large amount of water and electrolytes is absorbed from the intestinal contents. The descending colon passes down through the upper back portion of the abdomen and along the side of the left kidney. A large amount of water is also reabsorbed within the descending colon.

The large intestine continues into the S-shaped sigmoid colon that sits in the pelvis. By the time the mass gets to the sigmoid colon, it consists entirely of wastes and is now called feces. Feces is made up of water, food residue, unabsorbed GI secretions, shed epithelial cells, bile pigments, and bacteria. At the sigmoid, intestinal contents are solid and are slowed up in their forward progress by the rectosigmoid sphincter, which controls the movement of wastes from the sigmoid colon into the rectum. The rectum is a 6- to 8-inch length of bowel that functions as a holding site for feces until excretion through the anal canal.

The large intestine is composed of longitudinal and circular muscle layers. The longitudinal layer is made up of three long muscle bands called taenia coli. These muscle bands are shorter than the colon, producing a gathered appearance, much like the way a skirt is gathered at the waist. The circular muscle layer separates the colon into segments termed *haustra,* which gives the large intestine its characteristic appearance (see Fig. 30-2).

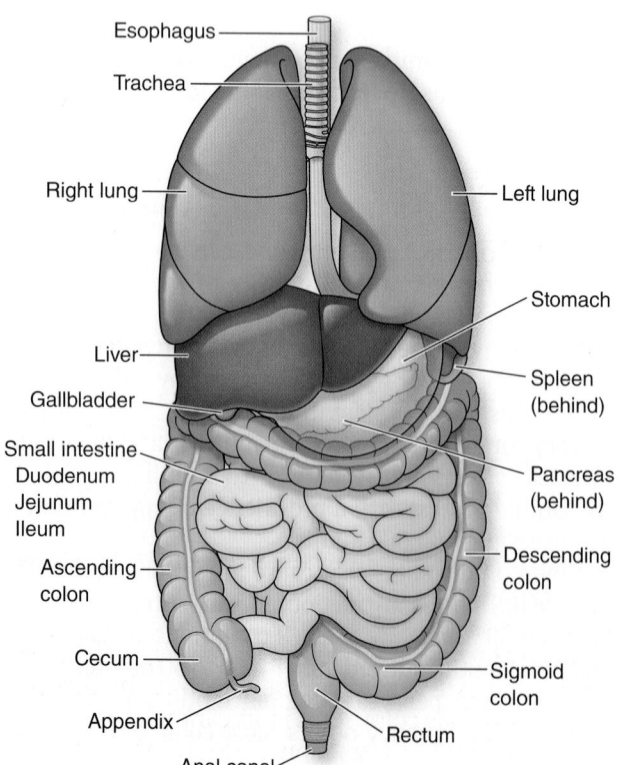

FIGURE 30-1. Anatomy of the GI system.

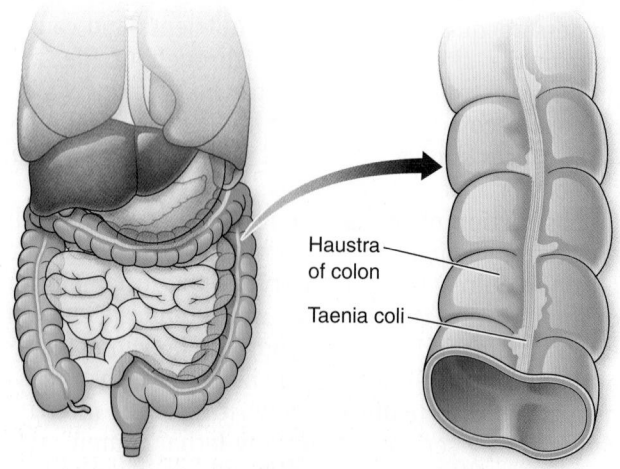

FIGURE 30-2. Haustra and taenia coli of the large intestine. Haustra, pouchlike formations of the wall of the large intestine, are formed by circular muscle fibers called taenia coli that are 1 to 2 cm apart.

Structure of the GI Wall

The GI wall begins below the upper one-third of the esophagus and has five layers:

1. Inner
2. Middle
3. Circular
4. Longitudinal
5. Outer

The inner layer, also known as the mucosa, is composed mainly of goblet cells and columnar epithelial cells. Goblet cells produce mucus to lubricate the intestine and protect it from injury. Columnar epithelial cells absorb fluid and electrolytes. The mucosal layer constantly replicates, and approximately 250 grams of mucosal epithelial cells are shed every day in the stool.

The middle layer, also known as the submucosal layer, contains connective tissue, blood vessels, nerves, and cellular structures responsible for secreting digestive enzymes. Beneath the submucosa are muscle layers. The circular and longitudinal muscle layers facilitate the forward peristaltic movement of intestinal contents along the colon. Finally, the outer layer, also known as the peritoneal serosa, is loosely attached to the entire outer wall of the intestine; it is the largest serous membrane in the body (see Fig. 30-3).

Colonic Motility

The movements in the large intestine can be classified as two types: haustrations and propulsions. Haustrations are segmental mixing or kneading movements that shuffle the contents back and forth among the haustra. This increases the contact time with the mucosa to facilitate the absorption of water and electrolytes and allow time for bacteria to accumulate. The circular muscles contract and relax at different sites, creating a shuffling effect. This is the primary type of movement in the colon, which is initiated by the autonomic nerves within the smooth muscle cells.

Propulsions, or propulsive mass movements, generally occur after meals. A large segment of the colon (longer than 20 cm) contracts as one unit, moving fecal contents forward. A series of these movements lasts approximately 10 to 30 minutes and occurs several times per day. After contents arrive at the rectum, defecation is initiated by one of these movements. Within the anal canal, there are voluntary muscles that allow self-control of defecation.

The gastrocolic reflex initiates propulsion of the entire colon, usually during or after eating. This causes the fecal mass to pass rapidly into the sigmoid colon and the rectum, which stimulates defecation. The hormones gastrin and cholecystokinin participate in the stimulation of this reflex. Epinephrine is an inhibitor of this reflex, as can be seen in the fact that during the fight-or-flight response, when levels of epinephrine are high, the urge to defecate is suppressed.

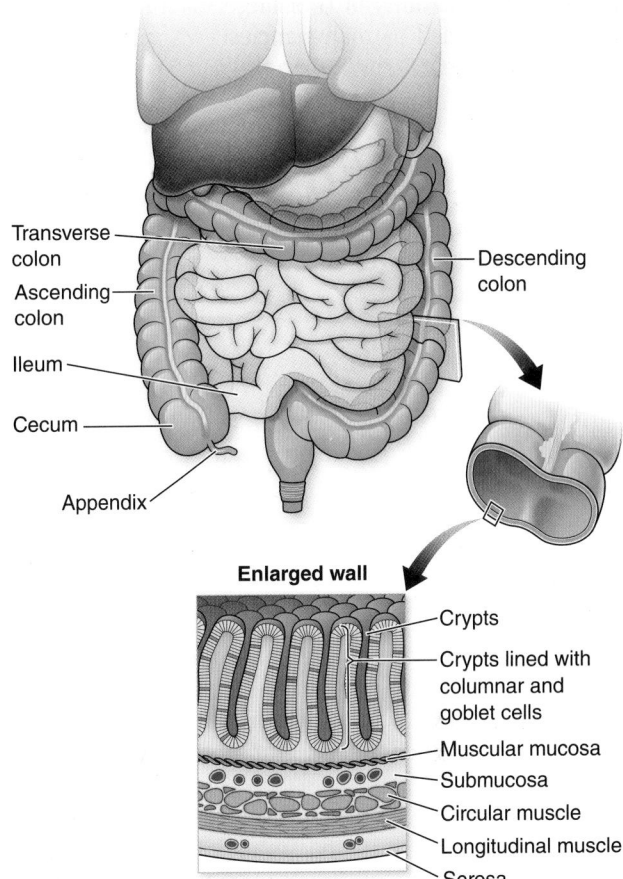

FIGURE 30-3. The mucosal lining of the large intestine is a large surface area that can absorb water and nutrients. There is a large presence of goblet cells that secrete mucus. Smooth muscles within the wall perform peristalsis to keep intestinal contents moving forward.

Neural Control of the GI Tract

Neural control of the large intestine is generally directed by the autonomic nervous system, as well as the nerves that compose the enteric nervous system, which lies entirely in the wall of the GI tract. Neurons in the wall of the GI tract consist of two networks: the myenteric and the submucosal plexuses. Both are aggregates of ganglionic cells that extend along the length of the GI wall.

The myenteric plexus controls the motility of the entire gut, as it extends all the way down the intestinal wall. The submucosal plexus innervates each segment of the GI tract separately and controls local motility and secretory functions as well as absorption. The myenteric plexus regulates both motor and secretory activity.

Extrinsic parasympathetic innervation occurs through the vagus nerve, passing through the pelvic nerves and extending from the cecum to the first part of the transverse colon. This innervation is responsible for the rhythmic contraction of the colon. The internal anal sphincter is usually maintained in a state of contraction; however, when the rectum is distended, the reflex is stimulated to relax. The intrinsic nerve plexuses provide the major innervation to the internal anal sphincter, which also receives sympathetic stimulation to maintain contraction and then parasympathetic stimulation, which stimulates relaxation when the rectum is full and stretched.

The external anal sphincter is innervated by branches of nerves from the sacral division of the spinal cord. This is sympathetic stimulation from the celiac and the superior mesenteric ganglia. The sympathetic stimulation of the large intestine is responsible for modulating reflexes, conveying somatic sensations of fullness and pain, participating in the defecation reflex, and constricting blood vessels. The blood supply to the large intestine is provided through branches of the superior and inferior mesenteric arteries.

Absorption Within the Large Intestine

The surface of the large intestine is smooth, and one of its main functions is the absorption of water and electrolytes—mainly sodium and chloride. Sodium is actively absorbed, whereas chloride follows passively down an electrochemical gradient. Water follows osmotically.

Most of the digestion and absorption of food and nutrients take place in the small intestine. As such, the large intestine does not secrete any digestive enzymes. It secretes alkaline mucus, which coats and protects the mucosa from chemical and mechanical injury. This alkalinity neutralizes acids produced by local bacteria fermentation. Less absorption takes place in the large intestine than the small intestine, because of the smaller amount of surface area in the large intestine.

The electrochemical gradient established by sodium movement enhances the diffusion of serum potassium from the capillaries in the lumen. As more sodium is absorbed, more potassium is lost.

Aldosterone responds when sodium is low or potassium is high. Aldosterone increases the membrane permeability to sodium, and it increases both the diffusion of sodium into cells and its active transport into interstitial fluid.

Microorganisms in the colon, termed the **GI microbiome,** are responsible for the breakdown of proteins that were not digested or absorbed in the small intestine. Proteins break down into amino acids, which are further broken down to yield ammonia. This ammonia is carried to the liver and is converted to urea. The majority (95%) of the bacteria in the large intestine are anaerobes. The most common organisms are bacteroides, *Clostridia, Anaerobic lactobacilli,* and *Escherichia coli.* Bacteria contribute to one-third of the bulk of solid feces.

At birth, the large intestine is sterile. There are no *E. coli* bacteria in the newborn intestine, which are integral to the production of vitamin K. For this reason, at birth, vitamin K is administered. By 3 to 4 weeks after birth, normal flora are established. The microorganisms of the colon do not have any digestive or absorptive function. However, they do play a part in the metabolism of bile salts by helping to absorb bile and remove toxic metabolites. Microorganisms also function in the metabolism of estrogens, androgens, and lipids. They convert unabsorbed carbohydrates into absorbable organic acids. They are also integral in the production of vitamin K and vitamin B_{12}. Finally, microorganisms in the large intestine aid in the metabolism of various nitrogenous substances and drugs and also protect against infection.

Defecation

Defecation is controlled by the internal and external anal sphincters. The urge to defecate occurs with the movement of feces into the sigmoid colon and the rectum. When food enters the stomach, the gastrocolic reflex causes mass movements to occur in the colon. This is most evident after the first meal of the day. The reflex center for defecation is in the sacral portion of the spinal cord, which contains parasympathetic nerve fibers. These nerves produce contraction of the rectum and relaxation of the internal anal sphincter. Nerve endings in the rectum become stretched, sending a signal to the sacral cord, which then reflexively sends them back to the descending and sigmoid colon, rectum, and anus. The internal anal sphincter is innervated to relax, which creates the urge to defecate.

This reflex can be overridden by voluntary contraction of the external anal sphincter, which then reduces the urge to defecate. Stress or pain can inhibit defecations and, possibly, lead to constipation. Defecation is facilitated by squatting or sitting, because this straightens out the angle between the rectum and the anal canal and increases the efficiency of straining.

At times, instead of feces, intestinal gas, or flatus, passes through the intestine. The gas that is passed originates from either of two sources: swallowed air (can be up to 500 mL per meal) and the gas that is produced from bacterial fermentation in the colon. Rushing of fluids and gurgling sounds, known as **borborygmi,** can be heard as the gas percolates through the lumen of the large intestine. Eructation, or burping, removes most of the gas that is swallowed, but some of it passes into the intestine. Most of the gas in the colon is a result of the bacterial activity, but the quantity and the nature of the gas depend on the food eaten.

Basic Concepts of Pathophysiology of Large Intestine Dysfunction

Pathophysiological conditions that affect the large intestine are caused by alterations in the integrity of the intestinal wall or disruptions of intestinal motility. Intestinal motility disorders range from frequent, spasmodic, repetitive, abnormal intestinal contractions to loss of intestinal motility called paralytic ileus. The major inflammatory conditions include appendicitis, diverticulitis, and IBD.

Intestinal Motility Dysfunction

Any alteration in the transit of foods and secretions in the digestive tube may be considered an intestinal motility disorder. These would include an obstructive lesion, intestinal pseudoobstruction (Ogilvie syndrome), IBS, fecal incontinence, and constipation.

An obstructive lesion in the large intestine causes ineffective intestinal propulsion. Common causes of obstruction include a cancerous mass, benign polyps, diverticular disease, adhesions, volvulus, incarcerated hernia, or intussusception. Signs characteristic of dilated tubular loops of intestine related to the obstruction are seen on imaging studies, such as abdominal x-ray.

In a condition referred to as **acute colonic pseudoobstruction (ACPO)**, the patient experiences the same symptoms of intestinal nonpropulsion—abdominal distention and cramping caused by gas collection in the bowel. However, there is no obstructive lesion. The etiology of pseudoobstruction is thought to involve dysfunctional changes in the neuromuscular system of the intestine.

Commonly used drugs, particularly those with anticholinergic side effects, can interfere with intestinal motility. Specific drugs that cause constipation include tricyclic antidepressants, benzodiazepines, lithium salts, and diuretics. Narcotic bowel syndrome, which causes decreased intestinal motility, is commonly observed in patients who abuse opiates for chronic pain. Endocrine disorders such as myxedema can also cause slowed colonic motility or pseudoobstruction.

Laxatives, including purgatives and cathartic agents, are agents taken to induce bowel movements or to loosen the stool. They are most often taken to treat constipation. Laxatives work to increase the movement of fecal matter along the colon. Certain stimulant, lubricant, and saline laxatives are used to evacuate the colon for rectal or bowel examinations and may be supplemented by enemas under certain circumstances.

Sufficiently high doses of laxatives cause diarrhea. Some laxatives combine more than one active ingredient to produce a combination of the effects. Laxatives may be oral or in suppository form. Chronic use of laxatives is not recommended because it can lead to lack of natural colonic motility. Excessive laxative use is defined as more than three times per week for at least 1 year. **Cathartic colon** is the anatomical and physiological change in the colon that occurs with chronic use of stimulant laxatives. Signs and symptoms of cathartic colon include bloating, a feeling of fullness, abdominal pain, and incomplete fecal evacuation.

Radiological studies show an atonic and redundant colon. Chronic use of stimulant laxatives can lead to serious medical consequences, such as fluid and electrolyte imbalance, steatorrhea, protein-losing gastroenteropathy, osteomalacia, and vitamin and mineral deficiencies. When the drug is discontinued, radiographic and functional changes in the colon may only partially return to normal because of drug-induced neuromuscular damage to the colon.

Constipation is a common problem, especially in older adults. Problems occur when severe constipation causes fecal impaction and obstipation. **Fecal impaction** occurs when hard stool that cannot be passed is lodged in the sigmoid colon and rectum. Commonly, a patient can develop liquid stools that pass around a fecal impaction. **Obstipation** is the urge to defecate but there is no passage of stool, liquid, or gas from the colon.

Inflammation of the Bowel

Aside from motility disorders, inflammation of the colon's interior can occur. Appendicitis is one of the most common inflammatory conditions of the GI tract. The appendix, a small, tubular appendage off the cecum that has no function, can become filled with indigestible contents and become inflamed. Appendicitis causes intense abdominal pain and requires surgery.

Abdominal pain also occurs in **irritable bowel syndrome (IBS).** Patients experience frequent episodes of abdominal pain, bloating, and abdominal distention. There are also bouts of constipation and diarrhea; however, there is no pathological change within the interior of the bowel, and etiology is unclear.

Inflammatory bowel disease (IBD), in contrast, is caused by pathological changes in the wall of the colon. Ulcerative colitis (UC) and Crohn's disease (CD), both types of IBD, cause severe abdominal pain, diarrhea, bloody stools, and weight loss. The bowel mucosa is friable, edematous, ulcerated, scarred, and bleeding. There are some extraintestinal symptoms such as fever, dermatological lesions, weight loss, and arthralgias.

Diverticulitis is another inflammatory disorder of the colon. Diverticuli are weak areas that form pouches off the wall of the large intestine. Commonly, these pouches become filled with stagnant intestinal contents, leading to obstruction and inflammation of the bowel wall.

Assessment

The clinician should obtain a complete patient history, with particular attention to the following:

- Abdominal pain, cramping, nausea or vomiting, excessive gas, and rectal fullness
- Frequency, amount, and timing of normal defecation and any recent change

- Any change in stool color, consistency, any black stool, or any blood in stool
- Type of diet, amount of daily fiber, use of laxatives or enemas
- Amount of activity or exercise daily
- Past medical and surgical history, including current medications

With a large bowel obstruction (LBO), the patient may complain of abdominal distention, nausea, vomiting, cramping, and colicky abdominal pains. It is important to distinguish complete bowel obstruction from partial obstruction, which is associated with the passage of some gas or stools. Partial obstruction is a less urgent condition than complete obstruction. An abrupt onset of symptoms makes an acute obstructive event, such as volvulus, a likely diagnosis. Obstruction that dilates the colon causes vague, abdominal cramps; anorexia; and, late in the disorder, vomiting. LBO may be accompanied by fever or leukocytosis. A history of chronic constipation, long-term laxative use, and straining at stools implies diverticulitis or malignancy. Changes in the patient's caliber of stool and dark color can suggest malignancy as well. Dark stools may contain blood, a condition called **melena.** When weight loss accompanies changes in stool, the likelihood of malignancy increases. A history of recurrent left lower quadrant (LLQ) abdominal pain over several years is consistent with diverticulitis, diverticular stricture, or similar disorder. Intense abdominal pain may indicate peritonitis. In **peritonitis,** the inflamed peritoneum is highly sensitive and any movement of the abdominal contents causes pain.

CLINICAL CONCEPT

Colicky pain, intense abdominal pain that occurs in waves, is often a characteristic of large bowel disorders.

Physical Examination

The physical examination of the abdomen should be done in the order of inspection, auscultation, percussion, and palpation. The abdomen may appear distended if filled with gas because of obstruction. When auscultating the abdomen, bowel sounds may be normal early in the course of the disorder, but may become quiet or rushing as time passes. If the bowel is filled with gas, percussion of the abdomen may reveal tympany, a high-pitched sound. Palpation of the abdomen may reveal tenderness, rigidity, and involuntary guarding, which are signs of peritoneal membrane inflammation. An abdomen that is tender and showing signs of peritoneal membrane inflammation is referred to as an acute abdomen. Signs of acute abdomen include involuntary guarding and rebound tenderness (see Table 30-1).

During the physical examination, it is important that the clinician palpate the tender area of the abdomen

TABLE 30-1. Signs of Acute Abdomen on Physical Examination

Abdominal pain	Waves of sharp constricting pain that take the breath away. Pain is worsened by movement.
Involuntary guarding	The patient's abdominal muscles contract with palpation.
Abdominal rigidity	The abdomen is stiff to the touch.
Rebound tenderness	When the examiner deeply palpates the abdomen, the patient feels pain as the examiner releases the pressure.

last. Any disruption of abdominal contents will cause pain in peritonitis. Patients want to lie as still as possible when being examined because movement causes pain. Right lower quadrant (RLQ) tenderness is commonly caused by appendicitis, whereas LLQ tenderness is commonly associated with diverticulitis. Upper right quadrant (URQ) tenderness elicited by palpation is called **Murphy's sign,** which is commonly caused by cholecystitis, an inflammation of the gallbladder (see Fig. 30-4). A rectal examination may elicit pain in disorders such as appendicitis. A digital examination may also demonstrate hard stool in the rectum with fecal impaction. A stool sample should be obtained for fecal occult blood testing (FOBT). In female patients, a pelvic examination is needed to rule out a gynecological source of pain; for example, ectopic pregnancy or ovarian cysts can cause abdominal pain that appears similar to GI pain.

ALERT! Females with acute abdomen require a pelvic examination and pregnancy test to rule out ectopic pregnancy.

Evaluation of the inguinal and femoral regions should be an integral part of the examination in a patient with suspected LBO. Incarcerated hernias represent a frequently missed cause of bowel obstruction. In particular, colonic obstruction is often caused by a left-sided inguinal hernia with the sigmoid colon incarcerated in the hernia.

Diagnosis

One of the simplest diagnostic studies that can be performed is a **fecal occult blood test (FOBT).**

define the cause of the obstruction. Flexible colonoscopy can visualize the large bowel up to the cecum.

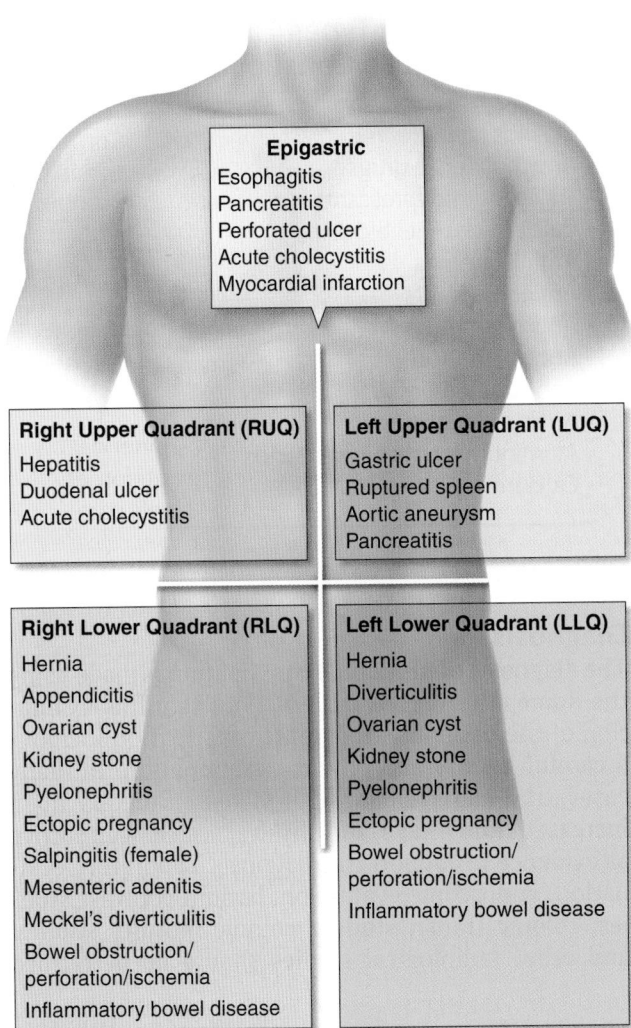

Epigastric
Esophagitis
Pancreatitis
Perforated ulcer
Acute cholecystitis
Myocardial infarction

Right Upper Quadrant (RUQ)
Hepatitis
Duodenal ulcer
Acute cholecystitis

Left Upper Quadrant (LUQ)
Gastric ulcer
Ruptured spleen
Aortic aneurysm
Pancreatitis

Right Lower Quadrant (RLQ)
Hernia
Appendicitis
Ovarian cyst
Kidney stone
Pyelonephritis
Ectopic pregnancy
Salpingitis (female)
Mesenteric adenitis
Meckel's diverticulitis
Bowel obstruction/
perforation/ischemia
Inflammatory bowel disease

Left Lower Quadrant (LLQ)
Hernia
Diverticulitis
Ovarian cyst
Kidney stone
Pyelonephritis
Ectopic pregnancy
Bowel obstruction/
perforation/ischemia
Inflammatory bowel disease

FIGURE 30-4. Causes of acute abdomen by abdominal quadrant in which pain is felt.

Blood in the stool, termed melena, can be detected in such disorders as bleeding peptic ulcer or bowel malignancy using a FOBT. Laboratory studies can demonstrate dehydration and electrolyte imbalance. A complete blood count (CBC), serum chemistry, and urinalysis should also be conducted. A decreased hemoglobin (Hgb) and hematocrit (Hct) can indicate iron-deficiency anemia, which often develops with chronic GI bleeding. An elevated serum amylase can indicate a perforated organ or pancreatitis. A chest x-ray can demonstrate free air under the diaphragm, which indicates perforation of the intestine or a hollow organ. Abdominal x-rays can clearly show shadows of the dilated, obstructed bowel. Contrast studies using barium or gastrografin can highlight the bowel anatomy. Radiological signs of bowel obstruction include bowel distention and the presence of multiple gas–fluid levels on supine and erect abdominal x-rays. Contrast barium enema, GI series, or computed tomography (CT) scan can be used to define the level of obstruction, determine whether the obstruction is partial or complete, and help

CLINICAL CONCEPT

- FOBT or stool guaiac tests can detect blood in the stool. Accuracy is highest after completion of three tests at three different times.
- A chest x-ray can show free air under the diaphragm when there is perforation of the bowel or abdominal organ. Air under the diaphragm from perforation of the bowel commonly causes shoulder pain.

Until a diagnosis, is made it is important to withhold opioid medications for pain in disorders of the abdomen. The patient's pain is important in the assessment of the disorder; the pattern, location, and intensity of the pain all need to be taken into account when making a diagnosis. Opioids relieve pain but they also decrease the peristalsis of the bowel, which may be harmful until a diagnosis is made.

Treatment of Large Intestine Disorders

In general, a diet high in fiber is recommended for bowel health. However, when there is an obstructive lesion or acute inflammation, resting the bowel is necessary. IV fluid, nothing-by-mouth (NPO) orders, analgesics, and antipyretics are used in appendicitis, diverticulitis, and inflammatory bowel disease (IBD). Antibiotics, corticosteroids, and immunomodulators are used in IBD.

Surgical intervention is commonly used to relieve a bowel obstruction. In most patients, the obstructing lesion is surgically excised; if necessary, a colostomy or ileostomy is then performed. An **ileostomy** or **colostomy** is a surgical procedure in which the healthy end of the intestine is brought out of the abdomen through an incision in the anterior abdominal wall. In ileostomy, the ileum of the small intestine is surgically brought out to the exterior abdominal wall. In colostomy, the colon is similarly brought out to the anterior abdomen. The opening, called a **stoma,** allows for excretion of intestinal contents into an attached collection appliance. An ileostomy or colostomy may be either reversible or irreversible. Alternatively, endoscopically placed expandable stents can be used to relieve LBO.

Pathophysiology of Specific Disorders of the Large Intestine

The large intestine can undergo many different kinds of pathophysiological conditions. Inflammation, perforation, structural problems, and acute abdominal processes all present in different ways and require various kinds of medical or surgical treatment.

Constipation

Constipation is the most common GI complaint of the adult population. Prevalence increases with age, with 25% to 35% of adults over age 65 reporting chronic constipation. Although a subjective complaint with varying meanings to different patients, constipation is defined as frequency of fewer than three stools per week.

There are many different causes of chronic constipation (see Table 30-2). Idiopathic constipation is diagnosed if there is no organic cause for the disorder. However, constipation can be secondary to metabolic (diabetes mellitus, hypothyroidism, hypercalcemia, heavy metal intoxication), neurological, or obstructive intestinal disease. Hirschsprung's disease is an example of a neurological disorder of the bowel caused by a congenital defect. Usually diagnosed in childhood, it is also referred to as aganglionic megacolon. The intestinal wall lacks development of the enteric nerves, which in turn causes absence of the contractions of peristalsis. Severe constipation is a prominent feature of the patient history. Constipation can also be a side effect of many medications (see Box 30-1).

BOX 30-1. Drug Types That Commonly Cause Constipation

- Opioids
- Anticholinergic drugs
- Tricyclic antidepressants
- Calcium channel blockers
- Antihistamines
- Anticonvulsants
- Antispasmodics
- Antipsychotics
- Iron supplements
- Antihypertensives
- Aluminum-containing antacids
- Calcium supplements

Diagnosis

The diagnosis of functional constipation is made using the Rome criteria (see Table 30-3). The initial evaluation of the patient with chronic constipation includes a careful history and physical examination. In many cases, trial management with increased dietary fiber, increased fluid intake, and physical activity can suffice as evidence to support the diagnosis. Laboratory evaluation, endoscopic evaluation, barium contrast studies, colonic transit studies, colonic motility studies, and other radiological studies should be performed

---

TABLE 30-2. Causes of Chronic Constipation

Functional Disorders	Irritable bowel syndrome Normal colonic transit Slow transit constipation Dyssynergic defecation
Peripheral Neurological Disorders	Autonomic neuropathy Hirschsprung disease Chagas disease Intestinal pseudoobstruction
Central Neurological Disorders	Multiple sclerosis Spinal cord injury Parkinson disease
Metabolic Disorders	Diabetes mellitus Hypothyroidism Hypokalemia Pregnancy
Systemic Disorders	Systemic sclerosis Myotonic dystrophy
Other factors	Anorexia nervosa Dietary/lifestyle Obstruction (masses or strictures)
Drugs	See Box 30-1.

TABLE 30-3. ROME IV Criteria for Diagnosis of Constipation

ROME IV CRITERIA FOR FUNCTIONAL CONSTIPATION (MUST HAVE AT LEAST 2 OF 6):

- Fewer than three bowel movements per week
- Straining during bowel movements more than 25% of the time
- Lumpy or hard stools more than 25% of the time
- Sensation of anorectal obstruction more than 25% of the time
- Sensation of incomplete evacuation more than 25% of the time
- Manual maneuvers required to aid defecation more than 25% of the time

In addition to the items listed here, the following three criteria should also be met to diagnose functional constipation: (1) Loose stools should rarely be present without the use of laxatives. (2) Insufficient criteria for IBS. (3) Present for at least 3 months during a period of 6 months.

Adapted from Drossman, D. A. (2016). Functional gastrointestinal disorders: History, pathophysiology, clinical features, and Rome IV. *Gastroenterology*, S0016-5085(16)00223-7. doi: 10.1053/j.gastro.2016.02.032

only in selected individuals; for instance, those with irritable bowel syndrome, bowel obstruction, diverticular disease, or inflammatory bowel disease.

Treatment

Dietary fiber and bulk-forming laxatives such as psyllium or methylcellulose are the most natural and effective approach to treatment. Taken together with adequate fluids, these can often alleviate constipation. The recommended amount of dietary fiber is 20 to 35 g/day. In addition to consuming foods high in fiber, patients may add raw bran (2 to 6 tablespoons with each meal) followed by a glass of water or another beverage to achieve the fiber intake goal.

An osmotic laxative polyethylene glycol (PEG) (MiraLAX) increases intestinal water secretion and stool frequency. Stool softeners can increase water entering stool, but are not as effective as fiber or PEG. Saline laxatives such as milk of magnesia, magnesium citrate, or water containing high amounts of magnesium sulfate are poorly absorbed and act as hyperosmolar solutions that increase water in the intestine. Hypermagnesemia, seen primarily in patients with renal failure, is a potential complication.

Stimulant laxatives such as bisacodyl (e.g., some forms of Dulcolax), senna (e.g., Senokot), and sodium picosulfate (e.g., Dulcolax drops) exert their effects primarily via alteration of electrolyte transport by the intestinal mucosa. They also increase intestinal motor activity. However, daily ingestion of these agents may be associated with hypokalemia, protein-losing enteropathy, and salt depletion. Thus, these drugs should be used with caution if needed on a long-term basis.

For treatment of defecatory dysfunction, an initial trial of suppositories (glycerin or bisacodyl) is recommended, because suppositories can be effective in liquefying stool and thereby overcoming obstructive defecation.

Patients with a fecal impaction (a solid immobile bulk of stool in the rectum) should initially be disimpacted starting with manual fragmentation if necessary. After this is accomplished, an enema with mineral oil can be administered to soften the stool and provide lubrication.

For chronic idiopathic constipation, some newer agents have been approved by the Food and Drug Administration (FDA). Linaclotide and plecanatide are minimally absorbed peptide agonists of the guanylate cyclase-C receptor that stimulate intestinal fluid secretion and colonic transit. Lubiprostone is a locally acting chloride channel activator that enhances chloride-rich intestinal fluid secretion.

Inflammatory Bowel Disease

IBD includes Crohn's disease, also called regional enteritis, and ulcerative colitis (UC). Both Crohn's disease and UC are chronic, incurable diseases that can occur at any age, but they are more prevalent in the young adult. Prevalence is approximately 200 cases per 100,000 adults in the United States. Urban areas have a higher prevalence of IBD than rural areas, and individuals of greater socioeconomic status have a higher prevalence than persons of lesser socioeconomic resources.

Crohn's Disease

Crohn's disease is a chronic, transmural, inflammatory process of the bowel that often leads to fibrosis and obstructive symptoms; it can affect any part of the GI tract from the mouth to the anus. The most common location is the terminal ileum and ascending right colon. The rate of Crohn's disease in women is 1.1 to 1.8 times higher than that in men. The peak of onset occurs between age 15 and 30 years, and a second peak occurs between age 60 and 80 years. However, most cases begin before age 30 years, and approximately 20% to 30% of all patients with Crohn's disease are diagnosed before age 20 years.

Etiology. *The exact cause of Crohn's disease is unclear.* It is believed to occur because of interplay among genetic susceptibility, immunological factors, environmental influences, and intestinal microflora, resulting in an abnormal mucosal immune response and compromised epithelial barrier function. When both parents have Crohn's, there is a 50% chance that their children will have the disease. Although an association has been established between Crohn's disease and high consumption of refined sugars and saturated fats, no conclusive dietary etiology has been identified. Also, smoking has been strongly linked to the development of the disorder.

The GI microbiome in patients with IBD is different from that of unaffected individuals. The presence of enteroinvasive and adherent *E. coli* and lack of some anaerobic bacteria causes a state of imbalance, termed **dysbiosis.** It is uncertain if these changes drive the disease or are a consequence of inflammation.

Psychological and psychosocial stress factors can precipitate exacerbations. It has also been proposed that infection with *Mycobacterium paratuberculosis, Pseudomonas,* or *Listeria* may be causative of Crohn's disease. A diet high in fatty foods has also been implicated as an etiological agent.

Risk factors include genetic predisposition, ethnicity, and cigarette smoking. An individual has a high risk of Crohn's disease if a family member has it. European Americans are affected more often than African Americans. Those of Ashkenazi Jewish ethnic background are particularly at high risk. Urban living has also been associated with Crohn's disease. There is an increasing amount of information about Crohn's disease and mutated genes on several different chromosomes. Mutations within the *NOD2* gene have been shown to confer susceptibility to Crohn's disease. The *NOD2* gene, which is found on chromosome 16, regulates intracellular immune responses to bacterial products. Approximately 25% of European American children have the *NOD2* gene, compared with only 2% of African American and Hispanic children. Other regions linked to IBD are the *CCR6* gene on chromosome 6 and the *IL12B* gene on chromosome 5. A protective gene, termed the *IL23R* gene, has recently been discovered. Individuals with a mutated *IL23R* gene have a susceptibility to Crohn's disease. Another recent discovery is a single nucleotide polymorphism in the *ATG16L1* gene on chromosome 2, which predisposes individuals to Crohn's disease. Research regarding genetic mutations and susceptibility to IBD continues to evolve. It is most likely a disorder caused by a combination of genetic and immunological factors.

Pathophysiology. In IBD, the intestinal epithelial layer has excessive permeability that allows pathogens to leak through to the underlying mucosal layers. It is believed that this triggers an autoimmune reaction with persistent activation of immune cells. Neutrophils, lymphocytes, and lymphoid tissue produce proinflammatory cytokines such as tumor necrosis factor-α (TNF-α) and interleukins (ILs) that perpetuate the inflammatory response and continual tissue destruction. Approximately one-third of patients with CD have an increased amount of mucosa-associated, adherent-invasive *E. coli*. These bacteria cross the mucosal barrier, adhere to and invade intestinal epithelial cells, and replicate within macrophages, which provokes the secretion of high amounts of TNF-α. The intestinal inflammatory infiltrate in CD contains T cells and antibodies that act against the intestinal bacteria. The lesions are visible as edematous, reddish-purple areas in a segmental pattern. There are areas of disease separated by healthy areas, referred to as **skip lesions**.

Lymph nodes in the submucosa are enlarged. Small superficial ulcerations with deep fissures penetrate the bowel and lead to fistulas and abscesses. Anal fissures are common; ulceration of the perianal area can result from chronic diarrhea. Characteristic lesions, known as crypt abscesses, are composed of polymorphonuclear leukocytes, lymphocytes, red blood cells, and cellular debris. The bowel mucosa develops granulomas; this is exhibited as an effect called cobblestoning (see Fig. 30-5). Secondary infections occur, leaving scarred and fibrotic tissue, narrowing of the lumen, thickening of the bowel wall, and shortening of the colon.

Toxic megacolon occasionally occurs in Crohn's disease. **Toxic megacolon** is the extreme dilation of a segment of the diseased colon, commonly the transverse colon. It causes complete obstruction and impaired absorption of fluids and electrolytes. Life-threatening perforation and peritonitis can result.

Clinical Presentation. The typical presentation of Crohn's disease occurs in remissions and exacerbations. The patient usually demonstrates episodes

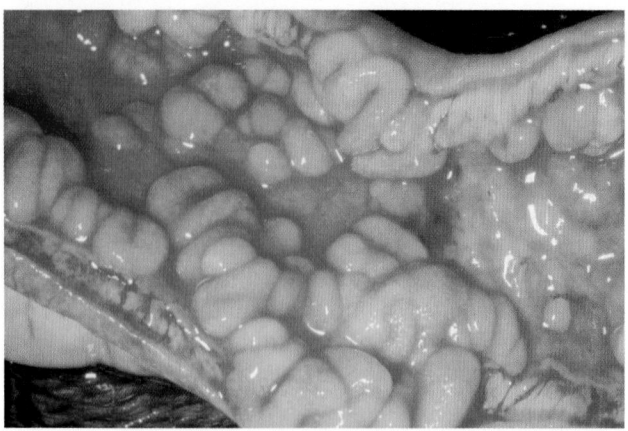

FIGURE 30-5. Inflammatory cobblestoning found in Crohn's disease. *(From Biophoto Associates/Science Source.)*

of fever, fatigue, weight loss, diarrhea, and abdominal pain. The clinician should focus on associated GI symptoms, such as appearance of stool, blood in the stool, number of stools per day, and aggravating or alleviating factors.

Malabsorption and nutritional deficiencies are a prominent sign of Crohn's disease with resultant anemia and fatigue. Absorption of fats; folic acid; iron; calcium; and vitamins A, B_{12}, C, D, E, and K are impaired. Electrolytes, trace elements, and minerals, including sodium, potassium, magnesium, zinc, and copper, are lost through diarrhea. The patient can become anemic from loss of blood in the stool, as well as dehydrated from loss of fluid in the stool. The patient's weight is important, as many affected by Crohn's disease suffer malabsorption. Laxative or antibiotic use, dietary intake of certain foods, and emotional stress can stimulate an exacerbation.

Signs and Symptoms. The signs and symptoms of Crohn's disease include abdominal tenderness, increased bowel sounds, steady progressive weight loss, anorexia, nausea, vomiting, diarrhea, pallor, and, in acute exacerbations, fever. Severe bouts can cause intestinal obstruction with accompanying signs of borborygmi (hyperactive bowel sounds), abdominal distention, and tympany on percussion.

Aside from intestinal symptoms, Crohn's disease can cause arthritis, uveitis, cheilitis, and dermatological problems. Ankylosing spondylitis and sacroiliitis are common musculoskeletal conditions that cause back pain. Cheilitis is an inflammatory lesion of the lips, commonly in the corners of the mouth. Canker sores, also called aphthous ulcers, may develop as well. Uveitis is the inflammation of the middle layer of the eye where circulation is provided to the retina. Retinal detachment can result from uveitis. Dermatological lesions, referred to as erythema nodosum, can develop; they are tender, red nodules commonly occurring on the shins. Hepatic or bile duct inflammation can also occur.

Diagnosis. A diagnosis of IBD is based on clinical signs and symptoms and endoscopic, radiological, and histological criteria. Distinguishing between Crohn's disease and UC can be a challenge because of their similar presenting symptoms; however, a colonoscopy can differentiate the disorders (see Table 30-4).

Colonoscopy with terminal ileoscopy and biopsy is central to the diagnosis of Crohn's disease. Chromoendoscopy, which uses dye or narrow band color imaging to enhance features of the mucosal surface, can be used to provide details. Biopsies should be taken of both the inflamed and normal tissues for pathological analysis. Capsule endoscopy can be used to study the whole length of the GI tract. Otherwise, upper GI and lower GI studies need to be performed as well as upper endoscopy and colonoscopy. Upper and lower GI contrast studies are used in diagnosis. Gastrografin is the contrast medium used because it is nontoxic if the intestine is perforated. CT enterography and magnetic resonance imaging (MRI) enterography are the procedures used in diagnosis.

Laboratory tests should include CBC; complete metabolic panel; pregnancy test before treatment; C-reactive protein level; erythrocyte sedimentation rate; and stool studies for *Clostridium difficile,* ova and parasites, and stool culture. Fecal lactoferrin and calprotectin are proteins released from white blood cells (WBCs) that increase when there is active inflammation in the bowel. Both of these are biomarkers that are becoming an integral part of diagnosis and management of IBD.

Anemia and malabsorption are common in patients with CD. Hemoglobin and hematocrit should be monitored periodically along with folate, iron, vitamin B_{12}, and 25-hydroxyvitamin D levels. The most common etiologies for anemia in CD include iron deficiency, anemia of chronic disease, and vitamin B_{12} deficiency. Involvement of the terminal ileum is particularly associated with vitamin B_{12} deficiency. Holotranscobalamin (holoTC) combined with methylmalonic acid (MMA) is the most accurate method to identify impaired B_{12} status. Renal and hepatic function testing should be performed before treatment. Tuberculosis screening and hepatitis B serological testing should be completed before prescribing biological agents.

A grading system, called the Crohn's Disease Activity Index (CDAI) that is based on patient-reported symptoms, has been used to assess disease activity and determine treatment. Patients are considered to be in one of four disease states: clinical remission, mild, moderate, or severe-to-fulminant Crohn's disease. Patients are also stratified into American Gastroenterology Association high- or low-risk categories according to endoscopy, colonoscopy, and laboratory test results.

Treatment. In Crohn's disease, medications with different mechanisms of action are used to suppress the disease and induce and maintain remission. Combinations of medications act synergistically and include the following:

- Oral 5-aminosalicylates (e.g., sulfasalazine, mesalamine)
- Glucocorticoids (e.g., prednisone, budesonide)
- Immunomodulators (e.g., azathioprine, 6-mercaptopurine, methotrexate)
- Biological therapies (e.g., infliximab, adalimumab, certolizumab pegol, natalizumab, vedolizumab, ustekinumab)

Two different treatment strategies can be used: step-up or top-down therapy. Step-up therapy typically starts with less potent medications, such as aminosalicylates, that are often associated with fewer side effects. More potent and potentially more toxic medications are used only if the initial therapies are ineffective. Top-down therapy starts with more potent therapies, such as biological therapy and immunomodulator therapy, relatively early in the course of the disease before glucocorticoid use.

Patients are also advised to consume adequate fluids, a balanced diet, and multivitamins. Patients are commonly lactose-intolerant and therefore are advised to take calcium/vitamin D supplements. Chronic diarrhea in Crohn's disease responds well to antidiarrheals, such as loperamide. Patients with terminal ileal

TABLE 30-4. Differences Between Ulcerative Colitis and Crohn's Disease

Ulcerative Colitis	Crohn's Disease
Only affects the large intestine	Can affect any part of the GI tract, from mouth to anus (terminal ileum common)
Affects from rectum continually upward into colon	Affects GI tract with skip lesions; healthy tissue interrupted by areas of diseased tissue
Affects only upper layers of intestinal wall (mucosa and submucosa)	Affects the whole thickness of the intestinal wall (transmural)
Pseudopolyps seen on examination of the colon	Cobblestoning seen on examination of the colon
No fistula or anal fissure formation	Anal fistula and anal fissure formation
Predisposes to colon cancer	Extraintestinal clinical manifestations; e.g., musculoskeletal, ocular, dermatological, hepatic conditions
	Does not characteristically predispose to cancer

disease may not absorb bile acids normally, which can lead to secretory diarrhea in the colon. These patients may benefit from bile acid sequestrants, such as cholestyramine.

Although most patients with Crohn's disease require surgical intervention during their lifetime, surgery does not cure the disorder. Between 75% and 80% of persons with Crohn's disease require surgery within 20 years of the onset of symptoms. Many require multiple procedures. Within 1 year after surgery, 20% to 30% of patients experience a recurrence of disease. Every attempt at conserving the bowel is made in the surgical approach to Crohn's disease. However, repeated intestinal resection is common, and its complication, short-bowel syndrome, can occur.

Advances in the study of genetics have fueled research into the composition and function of the intestinal microbiome in health and disease. Investigators are studying the interplay between the GI bacterial flora and the immune system. Current research for IBD is focusing on treatment strategies that manipulate the microbiome through diet, probiotics, antibiotics, or fecal bacterial transplantation. Future studies are needed to investigate if alterations in the GI microbiome can potentially modulate IBD activity.

Patients with CD are at increased risk for cancer, osteoporosis, anemia, nutritional deficiencies, depression, and infection. There is a risk for opportunistic infection with use of biological agents and immunomodulators. Patients often have anxiety about pregnancy and medication use. Persons with CD should be up to date on all immunizations, undergo vigilant cancer screening, and should receive bone mineral density testing for osteoporosis. Persons of childbearing age should be counseled about family planning. Laboratory testing is necessary because of potential anemia and myelosuppression associated with specific medications. Smoking cessation is necessary as smokers have more complicated disease (e.g., increased flareups). Patient education, nutritional counseling, and emotional support are necessary.

Complications. Small bowel obstruction can be a complication of long-standing CD. Obstruction often results from improper healing processes that occur in chronic intestinal inflammation. Chronic inflammation can cause formation of a stricture or spasm of the intestine, which narrows the lumen. Alternatively, undigested food can become impacted, or adhesions can develop in patients who have had prior surgery. Other complications include microperforations with localized peritonitis or abscess. These often require antibiotic treatment and surgical intervention. Patients with IBD are also at high risk for venous thromboembolism and pulmonary embolism. Prophylaxis with low molecular weight heparin is advised. Patients on immunomodulators and/or corticosteroids are at increased risk for osteoporosis, anemia, skin cancer, and cervical cancer and therefore should be periodically screened

for these disorders. Due to increased risk of infection, patient immunizations such as pneumonia and flu vaccine should be kept up to date.

Ulcerative Colitis

Like Crohn's disease, UC is an IBD, and they each present with similar symptoms and pathophysiological changes of the intestine. However, UC affects only the mucosal layer of the large intestine, whereas CD has transmural involvement anywhere within the GI system. UC can also lead to colon cancer.

The prevalence of UC in the United States is 238 cases per 100,000 people per year. It is three times more common than CD, and it is more frequent in European Americans than in African Americans or Hispanics. Incidence is reported to be two to four times higher in Ashkenazi Jews and slightly more common in women than in men. There is a peak age of onset at age 15 to 25 years and another peak at age 55 to 65 years, although the disease can occur in people of any age. Approximately 20% to 25% of all cases of UC occur in people aged 20 years or younger.

Etiology. There is no known cause of UC; however, like Crohn's disease, etiological theories involve genetic, immunological, and environmental influences that contribute to an overactive inflammatory response to unknown triggers. It is thought that genetically susceptible individuals produce an immune reaction against intestinal bacteria that predisposes them to colonic inflammation. Serum and mucosal autoantibodies against intestinal epithelial cells are found in UC. Sulfate-reducing bacteria, which produce sulfides, are found in large numbers in patients with UC. There is also a decreased amount of *Klebsiella* bacteria in the ileum of patients with UC compared with people who do not have UC. NSAID use is higher in patients with UC compared with people without the condition, and one-third of patients with an exacerbation of UC report recent NSAID use. Milk consumption has also been found to exacerbate the disorder. Psychological and psychosocial stress factors also precipitate exacerbations.

Risk factors include genetic predisposition, family history, and ethnic background. An individual has a high risk of developing UC if a family member has suffered the disease. Those of Ashkenazi Jewish ethnic background have a particularly high risk. There is conflicting information as to whether use of the acne medication isotretinoin (Accutane) can increase the risk of IBD. Some research has suggested a link, whereas other studies have found no such evidence. Studies are complicated by the fact that individuals treated with acne are also treated with tetracycline-class antibiotics. There is controversy as to whether tetracyclines also play a part in the development of UC. IBD is a multifactorial disease that involves a combination of different genetic mutations. Some of the same genes that are involved with UC are also associated with Crohn's disease. Like CD, in patients with UC, the GI microbiome is different from that of unaffected individuals. The presence of enteroinvasive and adherent *E. coli* and lack of some anaerobic bacteria causes a state of dysbiosis. Also similar to CD, in UC there is uncontrolled immune activity and overactivity of proinflammatory mediators and T cells, causing inflammation of the bowel.

Pathophysiology. A variety of immunological changes have been documented in UC. Cytotoxic T cells accumulate in the wall of the diseased colonic segment. Also, there is an increased number of B cells and plasma cells, with increased production of immunoglobulin G and immunoglobulin E. Microscopically, there is an acute and chronic inflammatory infiltrate of the intestinal wall with formation of crypt abscesses. These findings are accompanied by a discharge of mucus from the goblet cells, the number of which is reduced as the disease progresses. The ulcerated areas become covered by connective tissue, leading to the formation of inflammatory areas of protruding growths termed **pseudopolyps.** Pseudopolyps and continuous areas of inflammation in the large intestine are characteristic of UC (see Fig. 30-6).

In severe cases of UC, there can be damage to the nerves in the intestinal wall, resulting in colonic dysmotility, dilation, and eventual infarction and gangrene. This condition causes toxic megacolon, which predisposes the area to perforation. Chronic and severe cases of UC can be associated with areas of precancerous changes. Colon cancer develops in 3% to 5% of patients with the disorder, and the risk increases as the duration of disease increases. The risk of colonic malignancy is higher in cases in which onset of the disease occurs before the age of 15 years.

Clinical Presentation. As in Crohn's disease, the patient affected by UC usually describes episodes of diarrhea and abdominal pain. The disease has a pattern of remissions and exacerbations, with approximately 15% of patients requiring hospitalization. The clinician should focus on associated GI symptoms,

such as the characteristics of pain, appearance of stool, blood in the stool, number of stools per day, and aggravating or alleviating factors. Colicky abdominal pain is usually described. The patient with UC can have more than 20 stools per day and a fluid loss of 500 to 2,000 mL over 24 hours. The patient's weight is important, as many affected by UC suffer malabsorption. Severe dehydration and anemia can occur, especially in the older adult population. Emotional stress, laxative or antibiotic use, or dietary intake of certain foods can incite an exacerbation.

Physical Examination. An exacerbation of UC is marked by severe abdominal pain and tenderness, abdominal guarding, fever, leukocytosis, and abdominal distention. Aside from intestinal symptoms, UC is associated with various other manifestations. These include ocular problems, such as uveitis, as well as the dermatological disorders pyoderma gangrenosum and erythema nodosum. Arthritis and pleuritis are common. Inflammation of the liver and bile ducts can also occur.

Diagnosis. It is important to distinguish UC from Crohn's disease. Although both have the same symptomatology, there are some specific characteristic features of each (see Table 30-4). For example, pseudopolyps are involved in UC but not Crohn's disease. Crohn's disease affects the whole thickness of the intestinal wall, whereas UC invades only the mucosal surface. Fecal lactoferrin and calprotectin are proteins released from WBCs that increase when there is active inflammation in the bowel. Both of these are biomarkers that are becoming an integral part of diagnosis and management of IBD. Stool *C. difficile* toxin assay is also needed to rule out infection.

Colonoscopy and biopsy are the most significant diagnostic studies. Chromo-colonoscopy, which uses dye or narrow band color imaging to enhance features of the mucosal surface, can be used to provide more detail of sites for biopsy.

Treatment. Topical 5-aminosalicylic acid (5-ASA) is an NSAID that is recommended as first-line treatment for UC. 5-ASA suppositories and/or enemas given rectally induce remission in more than 90% of patients with mild to moderate UC. Mesalamine enema is a similar medication that can induce remission. Topical therapies can induce more rapid response than oral preparations and typically require less frequent dosing. Patients who are unwilling or unable to tolerate rectal medications can be treated with oral 5-ASA. Topical and oral glucocorticoids are also used in severe cases of UC. Glucocorticoid therapy should be used as a temporary intervention and tapered to avoid side effects. After an adequate clinical response and/or remission has been achieved, usually in 6 to 8 weeks, oral 5-ASAs should be continued to maintain remission, Severe episodes of UC may require antibiotics and/or

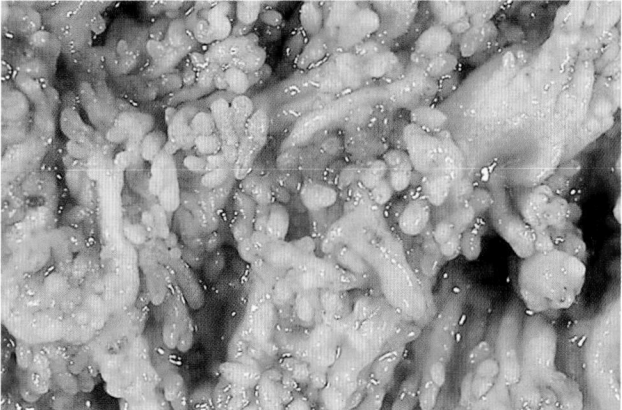

FIGURE 30-6. Pseudopolyps in UC. *(Photograph by Ed Uthman, MD: http://web2.airmail.net/uthman/index.html.)*

immunomodulators such as cyclosporine, azathioprine, and anti–tumor necrosis factor agents. Adequate diet, fluids, antidiarrheal agents, and multivitamins are also recommended. Because patients with IBD are at increased risk for infection, immunizations should be kept current. Patients with UC are at increased risk for colon cancer and should be screened with colonoscopy more frequently than the general population as advised by a gastroenterologist. The stool marker calprotectin can be used to monitor disease activity in patients with IBD. Patients with UC are at increased risk for venous thromboembolism and should receive low molecular weight heparin.

When medical treatment alone is ineffective, surgery is performed. Surgical options include colostomy and ileostomy. As with Crohn's disease, current research is focusing on how the GI microbiome and immune system interact in IBD. Treatment strategies that manipulate the microbiome through diet, probiotics, antibiotics, or fecal bacterial transplantation are under investigation.

> **ALERT!** Severe UC or Crohn's disease can cause toxic megacolon, which is a medical emergency.

Large Bowel Obstruction

The inability of intestinal contents to move through the large intestine is referred to as an intestinal obstruction or LBO. Obstructions may be partial or complete, acute or chronic, and reversible or irreversible. Approximately 10% to 15% of bowel obstructions occur in the large intestine, with the majority occurring in the sigmoid section of the bowel. LBO has a high mortality rate if diagnosis and treatment are not commenced within the first 24 hours.

Epidemiology
Approximately 20% of patients who present to the hospital with abdominal pain are suffering from bowel obstruction. The epidemiology of LBO depends on the cause of the disorder. Approximately 50% to 60% of all cases of LBO in the United States are caused by cancer of the colon or rectum, 20% are caused by diverticular disease, and up to 5% result from a volvulus. The prevalence of LBO increases with age. Sigmoid and cecal volvulus most commonly occur in individuals aged 60 years and older. Individuals older than age 60 are also at increased risk for acute colonic pseudoobstruction of the large intestine, especially following surgery or severe medical illness.

Etiology
The etiology of an LBO can be classified as mechanical or nonmechanical. A mechanical obstruction physically blocks the movement of material through the intestines. Mechanical blockage may be caused by scar tissue from prior surgery (adhesions), benign or malignant tumors, abdominal hernia, a swallowed foreign body, a gallstone that migrated into the intestine, bolus of undigested food, intussusception, volvulus, stricture, fecal impaction, or diverticula.

Nonmechanical causes stem from certain intestinal conditions, such as a disruption of the peristalsis caused by weakness of muscles of the intestinal wall (dysmotility syndrome or pseudoobstruction) or paralysis of the bowel wall (paralytic ileus). Also in older adults, peristaltic contractions can cease, causing air and secretions to collect in the bowel. The bowel appears to be obstructed but is actually dilated. The condition is called acute colonic pseudoobstruction or Ogilvie syndrome.

Abdominal surgery, appendectomy, gynecological surgery, hernia, bowel tumors, diverticular disease, and digestive disturbances put individuals at higher risk for intestinal obstruction. Adhesions that form after these surgeries account for a high number of LBOs. A mass lesion in the bowel and diverticular disease obstruct the intestine more than any other disorder. Diverticula, which are pouches formed in a weak bowel wall, can fill with intestinal contents and become a mass obstruction.

Pathophysiology
Mechanical LBO refers to an obstruction that causes the bowel to become dilated proximal to the obstruction. The main result of an obstruction is abdominal distention, intestinal mucosa inflammation, and the loss of fluids and electrolytes.

Distention is aggravated by the swallowing of gases such as air. This distention of the bowel results in an increase in peristalsis in an effort to excrete intestinal contents through the obstruction. As the distention progresses and pressure rises within the bowel, the bowel's ability to absorb fluids is impaired, and blood flow to the bowel is decreased, causing ischemia. If the obstruction is not resolved, perforation of the bowel wall may occur. Perforation of the bowel leads to the spilling of fecal material into the peritoneal cavity, causing peritonitis. Bowel inflammation and ischemia can result in increased permeability of the bowel's mucosa that facilitates bacterial invasion, infection, and fluid and electrolyte imbalances. Endotoxins released by invading bacteria can cause circulatory shock that may result in death.

With nonmechanical obstruction, motility through the intestine is impaired. This can be caused by weakness of intestinal peristalsis, also known as paralytic ileus. Ileus can result from neurological disease, acute colonic pseudoobstruction, metabolic disturbances, ischemia of the bowel, or infection of an abdominal organ.

Clinical Presentation
The patient's symptoms will depend on whether a complete or a partial bowel obstruction has occurred.

With a complete intestinal obstruction, the individual will report an inability to produce a bowel movement or pass gas. Abdominal pain is the major complaint. Nausea and vomiting usually accompany small intestinal obstruction but are not usually present in LBO. For those with a partial obstruction, gas or bowel movements are possible, but abdominal pain and distention are consistently present. The clinician should focus on questions regarding the characteristic of stool; the quality of pain, which may be colicky and cramping; and the ability to pass gas. With a complete obstruction, a rectal examination will find no feces in the rectum, unless the obstruction is caused by fecal impaction. In that case, diarrhea may occur if the intestinal contents pass around the obstruction. If the obstruction enlarges, the abdominal pain can become more continuous. Sweating, anxiety, and restlessness also occur.

Signs and Symptoms. Clinical manifestations of LBO depend on the position and amount of bowel involved in the obstruction, as well as the interference with the blood supply. Cardinal manifestations of an LBO are abdominal pain, abdominal distention, tenderness, and rigidity upon examination.

With a partial obstruction, bowel sounds are high pitched or tympanic; patients may continue to have flatus or diarrhea. With a complete obstruction, bowels sounds are absent. In the presence of bowel perforation, signs of infection and shock become evident as the bowel contents contaminate the peritoneal cavity.

> ### CLINICAL CONCEPT
>
> In a partial obstruction, auscultation of the abdomen reveals high-pitched bowel sounds. In a complete obstruction or paralytic ileus, bowel sounds are absent.

Diagnosis. Radiological studies such as abdominal x-ray and CT or MRI scan are most commonly used to diagnose LBO. The abdominal x-ray can reveal a distended colon, with loops of dilated bowel readily apparent. If a perforation has occurred, free air is commonly visualized under the diaphragm. The CT scan with contrast dye is useful to confirm a mechanical obstruction and its extent. A colonoscopy may be needed if other tests are inconclusive. Diagnostic laboratory results include elevated WBC count and electrolyte imbalance.

> ### CLINICAL CONCEPT
>
> Serum amylase levels are elevated with perforation of the bowel or organ.

Treatment

Treatment of LBO depends on the cause and type of obstruction, as well as whether it is acute or chronic. The overall management of LBO includes fluid replacement, prophylactic antibiotic therapy, intestinal decompression, and surgical consultation. For intestinal decompression, a nasogastric tube is inserted into the stomach or a colorectal tube through the rectum to relieve pressure from the obstruction.

With acute obstruction, medical management is focused on maintaining fluid and electrolyte balance and preventing shock. Resting the bowel and using pharmacological agents, such as high doses of dexamethasone, are methods to treat inflammation, nausea, and pain.

A complete obstruction usually requires surgical intervention to remove the diseased or nonfunctioning segment of intestine. Some surgical procedures remove the dysfunctional area of large intestine and then reattach the healthy ends together. The connection between the two ends is called an **anastomosis.** Alternatively, an endoscopic stent may be inserted to expand a blocked area of bowel. In some cases, surgical resection of the bowel, known as a **colectomy,** and a colostomy are necessary. If obstruction is the result of adhesions, laparoscopic surgery can be performed.

> ### CLINICAL CONCEPT
>
> A colostomy is a surgical procedure that brings one end of the large intestine out through the abdominal wall, where a stoma is created.

> ALERT! Laxative or motility agents are contra-indicated in complete bowel obstruction. These agents can worsen symptoms, as they stimulate the bowel to propel contents forward against an obstruction in the bowel.

Appendicitis

Appendicitis is an inflammation of the vermiform appendix, which is a blind-ended, pouchlike area that protrudes from the cecum, where the small intestine meets the large intestine. In humans, the appendix is a nonfunctional organ—a structure that is a remnant rendered unnecessary through the process of evolution. It is believed that the appendix once contained important bacterial flora that helped digest cellulose. Appendicitis is one of the most common causes of acute abdomen. If left untreated, the appendix can rupture, causing peritonitis.

Appendicitis usually develops between childhood and young adulthood, but it can occur at any age. In the United States, the incidence is 10 cases per 100,000 population per year. The median age of appendectomy is 22 years. Perforation of the appendix happens most often in children and older adults. There is a low mortality rate of 0.2% to 0.8%, which is caused by the complications of the disease rather than the surgery. The mortality rate in children ranges from 0.1% to 1%; in patients older than age 70 years, the rate rises above 20%, primarily because of a delay in diagnosis.

Etiology

It is hypothesized that appendicitis results from a nearby blockage, commonly caused by stool or fecalith (calcified feces). Blockage of the appendix often occurs when neighboring mesenteric lymph nodes become inflamed in response to a viral or bacterial infection and compress the appendix. Abdominal trauma can initiate an inflammatory response that results in inflammation of the appendix. Alternatively, appendicitis can occur if the appendix becomes twisted or occluded by bowel adhesions.

The incidence of appendicitis is lower in cultures that consume a diet high in dietary fiber. Dietary fiber is thought to decrease the viscosity of feces, decrease bowel transit time, and discourage formation of fecaliths, which predispose individuals to obstructions of the appendiceal lumen. Having a family history of appendicitis increases risk for the disorder, especially in males, and having cystic fibrosis also seems to put a child at higher risk.

Pathophysiology

There are two major initiating events for appendicitis:

1. Narrowing of the appendix lumen because of an obstruction that results in ischemia and a compromised blood supply to the region.
2. Development of a medium for bacterial growth as normal mucus secretions remain trapped behind the lumen because of narrowing. These trapped secretions add to the increasing intraluminal pressure and distention.

As a result of these two events, the protective mucosa layer of the appendix becomes compromised as luminal bacteria multiply and attack the wall of the appendix, causing inflammation. This inflammation, in combination with tissue ischemia, leads to necrosis and perforation of the appendix. With perforation, the contents of the appendix, which include bacteria, WBCs, and mucus, spill into the peritoneal cavity, leading to peritonitis.

Clinical Presentation

The individual with appendicitis complains of vague pain in the abdomen, which usually starts in the umbilical or epigastric region. The pain usually increases in severity over time and localizes to the RLQ of the abdomen. The pain increases with any jarring movements, coughing, or taking deep breaths. Nausea, vomiting, anorexia, fever, and chills are reported. Constipation or diarrhea and abdominal bloating are usually present.

CLINICAL CONCEPT

On average, the period from onset of vague umbilical pain to the localized RLQ pain of acute appendicitis takes 1 to 3 days.

Signs and Symptoms. Typical manifestations of appendicitis include abdominal pain that originates in the umbilical region radiating to the RLQ, also known as **McBurney's point.** The pain becomes more severe and localized as the appendix becomes more inflamed. Rebound tenderness in the RLQ of the abdomen is apparent on physical examination (see Table 30-5). Positive psoas sign, Rovsing's sign, and obturator sign are indicative of appendicitis, which can be elicited on physical examination (see Fig. 30-7). As the pain increases, the affected individual often guards the RLQ by being immobile and drawing the legs up in the fetal position to relieve tension on the abdominal muscles. Abdominal distention and low-grade fever are usually present.

TABLE 30-5. Signs of Appendicitis on Physical Examination	
Sign	**How Elicited**
Rebound tenderness	The examiner deeply palpates the abdomen; upon release of the hand, the patient feels intense pain.
Psoas sign	Examiner asks the supine patient to actively flex the right thigh at the hip. If abdominal pain results, this is positive for psoas sign.
Rovsing's sign	The examiner palpates the LLQ of the abdomen. If pain in the patient's RLQ develops, this is positive for Rovsing's sign.
Obturator sign	Internal and external rotation of the patient's flexed right hip causes pain in the RLQ.

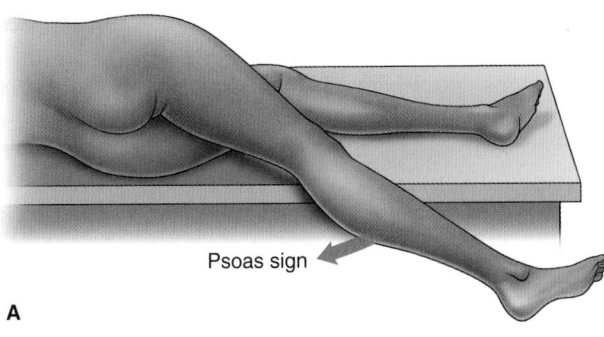

Psoas sign

A

Obturator sign

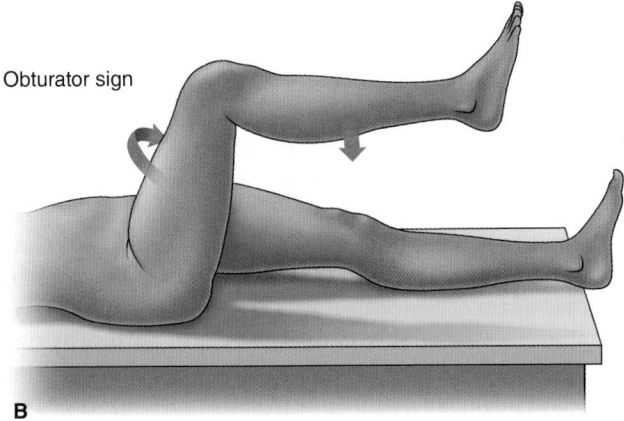

B

FIGURE 30-7. Signs indicative of appendicitis. **(A)** Psoas sign indicates irritation to the iliopsoas group of hip muscles and indicates an inflamed appendix, which lies within the region. It is elicited by passively extending the thigh of a patient lying on the side with knees extended. If abdominal pain results, it is a positive psoas sign. **(B)** To elicit an obturator sign, the patient lies on the back with the hip and knee both flexed at 90 degrees. The clinician holds the patient's ankle with one hand and knee with the other hand. The clinician rotates the hip by moving the patient's ankle away from the body while allowing the knee to move only inward. This is flexion and internal rotation of the hip. Pain in the RLQ that radiates into the groin occurs if appendicitis is present.

ALERT! It is important for females with abdominal pain to have a qualitative beta-human chorionic gonadotropin (hCG) blood test and pelvic examination to rule out pregnancy. Ectopic pregnancy causes acute abdominal pain that can be mistaken for a gastrointestinal disorder.

Diagnosis

A clinical diagnosis of appendicitis is based on a combination of physical examination findings, abdominal x-ray, CT scan, abdominal ultrasound, elevated C-reactive protein, and elevated WBC count. An ultrasound will not visualize a normal appendix, only one that is inflamed and edematous. An abdominal x-ray is usually not informative unless a calcium stone is present within the appendix. Urinalysis is necessary to rule out a kidney stone or pyelonephritis, which

can present similarly to appendicitis. High 5-HIAA, a breakdown product of serotonin, may be evident in the urine in appendicitis. The appendix contains many serotonin-producing cells. A pelvic examination and hCG blood test should be done on all females of childbearing age to rule out pregnancy or other gynecological disorder.

 CLINICAL CONCEPT

The CT scan yields the most accurate information in the diagnosis of appendicitis.

Treatment

Early treatment with antibiotics that are effective against gram-negative bacteria should be initiated preoperatively and administered up to at least 48 hours postoperatively. Laxatives should be avoided; in addition, pain medications should be avoided before diagnosis of appendicitis, as these can mask diagnostic signs. Continuous monitoring for peritonitis and IV therapy to restore or maintain fluid and electrolyte balance is essential. In acute appendicitis, effective pain management in conjunction with surgical removal of the appendix through laparoscopic surgery is the primary treatment. The surgeon's goal is to selectively operate on patients with true appendicitis and to minimize performing surgery on patients without an inflamed appendix. The surgeon wants to avoid performing unnecessary surgery; however, waiting to perform surgery can allow perforation to occur. A 10% to 15% negative appendectomy rate has been accepted to minimize the incidence of perforated appendicitis, with its increased morbidity.

Some patients with nonperforated appendicitis can be treated with antibiotics alone. Compared with those who underwent immediate appendectomy, patients treated with antibiotics have lower or similar pain scores, require fewer doses of narcotics, have a quicker return to work, and do not have a higher perforation rate. Approximately 70% of those successfully treated with antibiotics during the initial admission are able to avoid surgery during the first year. The other 30% eventually require appendectomy for recurrent appendicitis or symptoms of abdominal pain. Often patients who have mesenteric adenitis, defined as swollen mesenteric lymph nodes, present with signs and symptoms exactly like appendicitis; these patients undergo negative appendectomies.

Irritable Bowel Syndrome

IBS is a GI disorder characterized by abdominal pain and altered bowel activity in the absence of specific pathology. No specific motility or structural disorders of the intestine or bowel are seen. The lay terms for IBS are colitis, irritable colon, or spastic colon. This chronic and relapsing motility disorder affects the intestinal tract. Common findings related to IBS include abdominal discomfort and alterations in elimination, such as diarrhea and constipation, or a combination of the two. IBS is not linked to long-term mortality, but does negatively affect one's quality of life. IBS should not be confused with IBD.

As much as 20% of the adult population, or one in five Americans, has symptoms of IBS, making it one of the most common disorders seen in primary care. It occurs more often in women than in men, and it usually begins before the age of 35 years. In the United States, there is a lower prevalence of IBS in Hispanics and Asians. The role of different cultural influences is unclear.

Etiology

The cause of IBS is unclear. Altered gastrointestinal motility, microbiome alterations, visceral hypersensitivity, postinfectious reactivity, food sensitivity, and disrupted brain-gut interactions have all been implicated in the pathogenesis of IBS.

Risk factors for IBS include female gender, age under 40 years, family history, stress, and possibly history of traveler's diarrhea. Sedentary work, lack of exercise, and Western high-carbohydrate diet and processed food are well-established risk factors. IBS is almost twice as prevalent in women, pointing toward a possible hormonal relationship. IBS may also be related to consumption of dairy, wheat, fructose, or sorbitol. Although there is no definitive proof that any of these dietary items cause IBS, they may trigger symptoms. Acute bacterial gastroenteritis is the strongest risk factor known for IBS and highly dependent on the infecting organism. In 36% of individuals having suffered from infection with both *Campylobacter jejuni* and *E. coli* O157:H7 still have IBS symptoms after 2 years caused by a persistent elevation in gut permeability. This is termed postinfectious IBS (IBS-PI).

Pathophysiology

Despite unclear etiology, an alteration in GI motility is linked to central nervous system–directed motor functions of the bowel. Peristaltic waves are either slowed or increased in intensity as they push food through the intestine. There is no evidence of inflammation or pathological changes in the intestinal mucosa. The intestine appears normal in all diagnostic studies.

IBS is caused by a combination of gastrointestinal (GI) dysmotility, hypersensitivity, immune activation, and changes in composition and function of the GI microbiome and the GI mucosal barrier. The integrated actions and communication between the microbiota and the autonomous nervous system are referred to as the gut-brain axis (GBA). Disruption of the physiological relationship between the human host and the microbiota is called dysbiosis and is regarded a basic factor for initiating and maintaining IBS. The common

dysbiotic finding in IBS is an increase in Streptococcus species, reduced Lactobacillus species, and reduced Bacteroides species, constituting an overall reduction in beneficial bacteria and an increase in pathogeneic species. An increase in the Clostridiae group may also play a significant role, as well as a decrease in the probiotic Bifidobacterium. Some cases of IBS are thought to result from disruption of the entero-hepatic circulation of bile acids. It is estimated that up to 50% of IBS patients have bile acid malabsorption.

Clinical Presentation

The main manifestations of IBS are chronic abdominal pain lasting for at least 6 months and a change in normal bowel patterns to constipation, diarrhea, or both. IBS associated with mainly diarrhea, is referred to as IBS-D, whereas those cases related to constipation are referred to as IBS-C; mixed type is termed IBS-M.

The abdominal pain is often caused by eating and relieved by bowel movement. Other associated manifestations may include anxiety, flatulence, mucus in stools, nausea and vomiting, and abdominal distention. Patients also have greater visceral pain sensitivity. The patient commonly reports a stressor in their life. The physical examination is normal in IBS.

Certain signs of IBS are referred to as "alarm" symptoms; these require specific diagnostic testing such as colonoscopy (see Table 30-6). These alarm symptoms include weight loss, iron-deficiency anemia, and family history of GI illness such as colon cancer or celiac sprue.

Diagnosis

The diagnosis of IBS is commonly made by the patient's description of signs and symptoms. For some patients, such as those with rectal bleeding, more in-depth diagnostic studies are completed. The diagnostic tests that are commonly performed to rule out other underlying disease processes or structural abnormalities include

---

TABLE 30-6. Alarm Symptoms That Suggest Organic Intestinal Disease vs. IBS

- A change in bowel habit to looser and/or more frequent stools persisting for more than 6 weeks in an individual
- Family history of bowel or ovarian cancer
- Rectal bleeding
- Rectal masses
- Abdominal masses
- Anemia
- Unintentional and unexplained weight loss
- Increased inflammatory markers

Adapted from National Institute for Health and Care Excellence (2015). Developing NICE guidelines: the manual [Internet]. London: National Institute for Health and Care Excellence (NICE).https://www.nice.org.uk/process/pmg20/chapter/introduction

stool samples for ova and parasites, occult blood, and culture and sensitivity to assess for inflammation or infection.

The Rome Criteria IV is the current gold standard for the diagnoses of IBS (see Table 30-7). A CBC with differential and erythrocyte sedimentation rate are performed routinely to rule out anemia, infection, or inflammation. Transglutaminase antibody testing should be completed to rule out celiac sprue. Thyroid hormone testing is needed to rule out hypothyroidism or hyperthyroidism. Hydrogen breath testing can exclude the possibility of lactose or fructose intolerance. An upper endoscopy and colonoscopy can identify any structural or functional abnormalities, although none are usually present. Abdominal CT scan can exclude the possibility of tumor, obstruction, or pancreatic disease. Finally, GI motility is evaluated through either an upper GI series or a barium enema. Rarely, manometry or an electromyogram may be used to measure pressure changes in the intestinal lumen caused by spasms. All diagnostic studies are usually negative.

Treatment

The primary goals of management are to regulate bowel movements, relieve abdominal pain, and decrease stress. These goals are achieved through pharmacological interventions, dietary alterations, and lifestyle changes to manage the symptoms.

Dietary management for IBS includes modification of dietary intake to reduce the incidence of diarrhea and constipation. Patients should keep a food diary to keep track of symptoms in relation to foods. The avoidance of gas-producing foods and beverages that contain caffeine is recommended. Although IBS is not regarded as a gluten enteropathy, a gluten-free diet does reduce symptoms in many patients with IBS.

A diet low in fermentable oligosaccharides, disaccharides, monosaccharides, and polyols (FODMAPs) is also recommended. This includes eliminating foods high in fructose, lactose, and the polyols: sorbitol, mannitol, maltitol, and xylitol. These short-chain carbohydrates are poorly absorbed and are osmotically active in the intestinal lumen, where they are rapidly fermented, resulting in symptoms of abdominal bloating and pain.

In patients with persistent constipation, PEG, lubiprostone, or linaclotide are recommended. Lubiprostone and linaclotide activate mechanisms that increase the amount of fluid secreted into the intestine. Loperamide and aldosterone can also slow bowel motility in IBS patients with persistent diarrhea. Antispasmodic agents, dicyclomine and hyoscyamine, can also be used to decrease bowel irritability in diarrhea. Rifaximin (Xifaxan) is an oral antibiotic used for the treatment of IBS with diarrhea. Rifaximin acts mainly within the GI tract without systemic absorption. It has activity against anaerobic, gram-positive, and gram-negative bacteria, including *C. difficile*. It may also reduce bacterial overgrowth in the small intestine and reduce bacterial by-products, such as ammonia. Tricyclic antidepressants can also be used in IBS-D, as they slow bowel motility. Other medications include eluxadoline, an opioid receptor agonist-antagonist, and alosetron, a serotonin antagonist. These can be used in IBS-D in patients who have been refractory to other medications. Lifestyle changes, such as regular exercise, stress management, and relaxation techniques, can decrease stress and facilitate coping with IBS. Nutritional consultation regarding recommended dietary changes is necessary.

Diverticular Disease

The two disorders associated with diverticular disease are diverticulosis and diverticulitis. In **diverticulosis,** the bowel wall has multiple weakened areas that form small outpouchings called **diverticula.** Most diverticula are found in the sigmoid and descending colon. Diverticula can collect intestinal contents and form a colonic obstruction. Diverticula often become inflamed, at which point the condition becomes **diverticulitis**.

Epidemiology

Asymptomatic diverticulosis is a common condition that increases with age. Of patients with diverticulosis, 80% to 85% remain asymptomatic. The risk of developing diverticulosis before age 40 years is lower than 5%; however, this percentage rises to greater than 65% by age 85 years. Approximately 15% to 20% of those with diverticulosis develop diverticulitis, and 15% to 25% of those with diverticulitis develop complications leading to surgery; these complications include abscess formation, intestinal rupture, peritonitis, and fistula formation. Patients with diverticulitis who do not undergo surgery have a recurrence rate of 20% to 35%. The disease occurs equally in males and females. The mean age at presentation with diverticulitis appears to be about age 60 years.

TABLE 30-7. Rome IV Criteria for Diagnosing IBS

Recurrent abdominal pain at least 1 day/week in the last 3 months, with at least two of the following criteria:
- Related to defecation
- Associated with a change in frequency of stool
- Associated with a change in form (appearance) of stool

The criteria should be met for the past 3 months and the symptoms begin at least 6 months before diagnosis.

Adapted from Schmulson, M. J., & Drossman, D. A. (2017). What is new in Rome IV. *Neurogastroenterol Motil, 23*(2), 151–163.

Etiology

The etiology of diverticular disease is associated with two main factors: weakness of the bowel wall and increased intraluminal pressure. Diverticulitis occurs when intestinal contents block the diverticulum, thus cutting off the blood supply and providing an environment conducive to the formation of infection.

The most significant risk factor for diverticular formation is a diet low in fiber. Diverticulosis is very common in Western countries and is thought to be associated with lack of dietary fiber and obesity. There are also genetic factors, as those with a family history tend to have an increased risk of disease.

Pathophysiology

Weakness in the bowel musculature can occur where branches of the blood vessels enter the colonic wall, thus creating areas for bowel protrusion during periods of increased intra-abdominal pressure. These entry points for blood vessels are the areas where diverticula develop (see Fig. 30-8). When the bowel does not drain effectively, intestinal contents can become trapped, collect and form a mass, and cause obstruction and irritation, thereby leading to diverticulitis. Chronic diverticulitis can cause scarring and narrowing of the bowel lumen.

Clinical Presentation

The signs and symptoms of diverticular disease are dependent on the severity of the inflammation and where in the bowel it occurs. There may be dull, episodic, or steady left quadrant or midabdominal pain. Acute lower abdominal pain, fever, and tachycardia may also be present. There are usually alterations in bowel habits, including constipation, diarrhea, increased flatulence, anorexia, and low-grade fever.

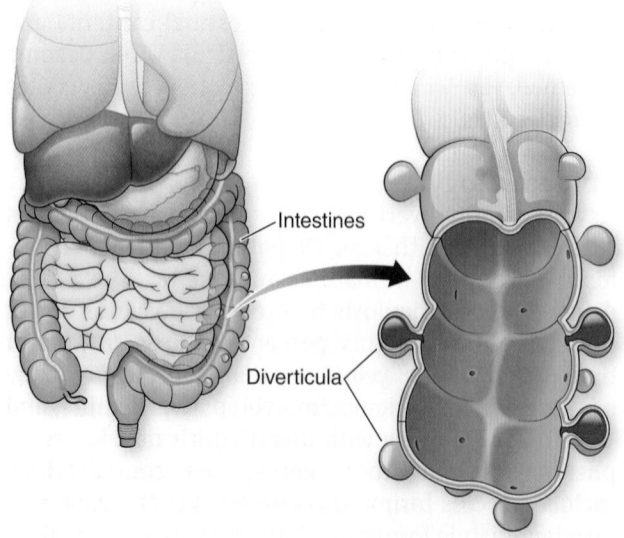

Intestines

Diverticula

FIGURE 30-8. In diverticulosis, there are small, weakened areas in the wall of the colon. The weak areas bulge and create pouches that can become impacted and inflamed. Once inflamed, the condition is called diverticulitis.

The patient with diverticulosis may have no signs of the disorder on physical examination. If diverticulitis exists, the patient classically has LLQ abdominal tenderness, fever, and nausea. Traces of occult blood may be found in the stool. Patients with right-sided diverticular disease can have RLQ tenderness of the abdomen similar to appendicitis. Pain of diverticular disease of the transverse colon can simulate pain of peptic ulcer or pancreatitis. Approximately 20% to 50% of patients endure recurrent bouts of diverticulitis.

Diagnosis

Diagnostic studies include abdominal x-ray, abdominopelvic CT scan, ultrasound, and MRI. Colonoscopy can also visualize the location of diverticula within the colon; however, it should not be done during acute diverticulitis. CT scan with or without contrast is the primary recommended diagnostic procedure for diverticulitis. A pelvic examination for women is recommended to exclude gynecological sources of pain. In women of childbearing age, a pregnancy test is essential. Laboratory testing includes CBC with differential, serum electrolytes, serum amylase, and lipase to exclude perforation of viscera, liver enzymes, and bilirubin. Stool studies may be needed in patients with diarrhea.

Treatment

Outpatient treatment of uncomplicated diverticulitis involves resting the bowel with a liquid diet and gradual reintroduction of a soft diet. Seven to 10 days of antibiotic therapy and pain medications are also used. The majority of patients with diverticulitis do not have complications; however, 15% can develop abscess, perforation, fistula, or colonic obstruction. Recurrent attacks of acute diverticulitis or persistent inflammation may cause progressive fibrosis and scarring, resulting in the formation of a stricture. Patients with a colonic stricture may present with an acute colonic obstruction. Certain conditions such as sepsis, advanced age, immunosuppression, or peritonitis require inpatient treatment.

Inpatient treatment includes administration of IV antibiotics, fluids, and pain medications. Patients who continue to improve are discharged to complete a course of oral antibiotics; those who fail to improve are referred for surgery for complicated diverticulitis.

The aim of surgery is to remove the diseased colonic segment while attempting to preserve the colonic integrity by creating an anastomosis (connection between two segments of bowel). Surgery can be accomplished via an open abdominal or laparotomy procedure. For patients with abscess, a one-stage procedure is performed that involves resection of the diseased colonic segment and a primary anastomosis of the remaining healthy segment of bowel. For patients with peritonitis, a Hartmann's procedure is the most commonly performed procedure. This two-stage procedure involves resecting the diseased colonic segment, creating an end colostomy and a rectal stump, followed by reversal of the colostomy 3 months later.

Volvulus

A **volvulus** is a twisting of the large intestine around a point of attachment in the abdomen. Neonates are most often affected by a volvulus caused by congenital abnormality; however, more than 40% of cases occur at older ages. Sigmoid volvulus, the most common type found in adults, is responsible for 10% to 15% of LBO cases and is mainly a disease of older adult men.

The sigmoid colon is most susceptible to volvulus when it is weighed down from chronic constipation and a high-fiber diet. The weight of the sigmoid colon increases its susceptibility to twisting on the mesentery. Volvulus of the intestine results in bowel obstruction and ischemia of the bowel. Venous and lymphatic vessel obstructions usually occur, causing bowel edema and possible GI bleeding. Lymphatic congestion causes the formation of enlarged mesenteric lymph nodes or ascites caused by accumulation of lymphatic fluid. The intestinal lumen accumulates gas and fluid up to the point of obstruction. The large volume of gas and fluid can place pressure on the intestinal wall, cutting off circulation. This can lead to ischemia and infarction of the intestinal wall. Perforation and necrosis of the affected intestinal wall can occur.

The symptoms of volvulus include bilious vomiting, abdominal pain (colicky at first, then steady), anorexia, blood and mucus in the stool, abdominal tenderness, and, eventually, shock. The most definitive test is an abdominopelvic CT scan. Abdominal x-ray may show distended bowel proximal to the sigmoid colon. When advanced through the twisted segment of the colon, a sigmoidoscope can untwist a sigmoid colon volvulus, thereby restoring the blood supply. The sigmoidoscopy also allows visualization of the viability of the colon. If surgery is necessary, a sigmoid volvulus resection with primary anastomosis or a Hartmann's procedure (see "Diverticulitis") can be done. Surgery can usually be performed through a small LLQ transverse incision. It is most important to recognize the diagnosis early before infarcted bowel occurs.

Hemorrhoids

Hemorrhoids are dilated, swollen venous blood vessels in the lower rectum. They are among the most common causes of lower intestine pathology. The prevalence of symptomatic hemorrhoids is estimated at 4.4% in the general population of the United States. This is a low estimate because only one-third of individuals affected with hemorrhoids seek medical attention. Many affected persons self-medicate with over-the-counter preparations. The prevalence of hemorrhoids increases with age, with a peak in persons aged 45 to 65 years.

Hemorrhoids are mainly caused by decreased venous return and venous pooling in the blood vessels of the rectum. Hemorrhoids can be likened to varicose veins in the perianal region. High venous pressure in the rectal region is commonly caused by constipation and straining during defecation, high pressure within the portal vein of the liver, anal intercourse, pregnancy, prolonged sitting, and aging of support structures in the rectoanal region. In addition, lack of fiber in the diet causes chronic constipation, which leads to hemorrhoids. In pregnancy, the gravid uterus places high pressure on the inferior vena cava, leading to hemorrhoids.

Hemorrhoids generally cause symptoms when they become inflamed, thrombosed, or prolapsed. Hemorrhoid symptoms usually depend on the location, whether they are internal or external blood vessels. Internal hemorrhoids lie inside the rectum. Straining or irritation when passing stool can damage the hemorrhoid's fragile surface and cause it to bleed. Bleeding from hemorrhoids, exhibited as small amounts of bright-red blood from the rectum, is called **hematochezia**. Commonly, straining at defecation pushes an internal hemorrhoid through the anal meatus; this is known as a prolapsed hemorrhoid. External hemorrhoids are more superficial, just under the skin around the anus. When irritated, external hemorrhoids can itch or bleed. Sometimes blood may pool in an external hemorrhoid and form a thrombosed hemorrhoid, resulting in severe pain, swelling, and inflammation.

Diagnosis requires digital rectal examination, anoscopy, flexible sigmoidoscopy, or colonoscopy. External hemorrhoids usually require no specific treatment unless they become acutely thrombosed or cause patient discomfort. Conservative treatments involve use of over-the-counter hemorrhoid cream or a suppository containing hydrocortisone, or use of pads containing witch hazel or a numbing agent. Low-grade internal hemorrhoids can be effectively treated with medication and nonoperative measures such as rubber-band ligation and injection sclerotherapy. Surgery is indicated for high-grade internal hemorrhoids, or when nonoperative approaches have failed, or complications have occurred. Although excisional hemorrhoidectomy remains the mainstay operation for advanced hemorrhoids and complicated hemorrhoids, several minimally invasive operations can be used including ligature hemorrhoidectomy, Doppler-guided hemorrhoidal artery ligation, and stapled hemorrhoidopexy.

Chapter Summary

- The normal functions of the intestinal tract are to propel digested food forward, absorb nutrients and water, and finally to excrete waste and indigestible contents.
- Pathophysiological conditions that affect the large intestine are caused by alterations in the integrity of the intestinal wall or disruptions of intestinal motility.
- The order of physical examination techniques used in abdominal assessment should be inspection, auscultation, percussion, and palpation.
- Any disorder that causes sudden, severe acute abdominal pain and tenderness is referred to as an acute abdomen.
- IBD includes Crohn's disease and UC.
- Crohn's disease can occur anywhere throughout the whole GI tract.
- Crohn's disease causes malabsorption, dehydration, arthritis, uveitis, cheilitis, and dermatological problems. Hepatic and bile duct inflammation can also occur. It is characterized by transmural inflammation with skipped areas of the intestine.
- UC is an inflammatory disease limited to the surface of the large intestine. Pseudopolyps and continuous areas of inflammation in the large intestine are characteristic.
- UC predisposes individuals to colon cancer.
- Severe Crohn's disease or UC can cause toxic megacolon, which is a medical emergency.

- IBS is a condition of abnormal bowel activity with no organic pathology and unknown etiology.
- LBO is most commonly caused by cancer or tumor of the colon.
- A colostomy is a surgical procedure that brings one end of the large intestine out through the abdominal wall, where a stoma is created.
- Appendicitis begins with vague pain in the umbilical region, which increases in severity over time and localizes to the RLQ.
- Appendicitis causes peritoneal inflammation, demonstrated by rebound tenderness at McBurney's point in the RLQ.
- In diverticulosis, the bowel wall has multiple weakened areas that form small outpouchings called diverticula. Diverticulitis occurs when these weakenings in the wall become inflamed, most commonly causing LLQ tenderness.
- A volvulus is a twisting of large intestine that can cause ischemia and infarction of the intestinal wall.
- Hemorrhoids are swollen blood vessels in the lower rectum that can bleed, become thrombosed, or become prolapsed. Treatment involves either conservative topical treatment or minimally invasive surgical procedures.

Making the Connections

Signs and Symptoms	Physical Assessment Findings	Diagnostic Testing	Treatment
Constipation | Although a subjective complaint with varying meanings to different patients, constipation is defined as the infrequent passage of stools or difficulty with evacuation of stools and is diagnosed according to the Rome IV criteria (see the following).			
Diagnosis is based on Rome IV criteria (at least 2 of 6 of the following): <3 bowel movements/wk, straining >25% of time, hard stools >25% of the time, sensation of anorectal obstruction >25% of time, sensation of incomplete evacuation >25% of time, manual maneuvers needed >25% of time. In addition to the previous items, the following three criteria should also be met: (1) Loose stools should rarely be present	Abdominal distention, fullness in LLQ.	None.	Dietary fiber and bulk-forming laxatives such as psyllium or methylcellulose with adequate fluids. The recommended amount of dietary fiber is 20 to 35 g/day. An osmotic laxative (PEG) (MiraLAX). Stool softeners. Saline laxative: milk of magnesia, magnesium citrate. Stimulant laxatives such as bisacodyl (e.g., some forms of Dulcolax), senna (e.g., Senokot), and sodium picosulfate (e.g., Dulcolax drops).

Making the Connections–cont'd

Signs and Symptoms	Physical Assessment Findings	Diagnostic Testing	Treatment
without the use of laxatives. (2) Insufficient criteria for IBS. (3) Present for at least 3 months during a period of 6 months.			For treatment of defecatory dysfunction, suppositories (glycerin or bisacodyl). Linaclotide, plecanatide, or lubiprostone.

Crohn's Disease | Autoimune disorder with inflammation of any part of the GI tract from the mouth to anus; involves the whole thickness of the intestine's wall, characteristic skip lesions, cobblestone mucosa, and anal fistulas.

Signs and Symptoms	Physical Assessment Findings	Diagnostic Testing	Treatment
Abdominal pain. Chronic diarrhea with bleeding or mucus. Malabsorption causes weight loss. Symptoms come in remissions and exacerbations.	Abdominal tenderness, fever, anal fistulas possible. Weight loss. Commonly extraintestinal manifestations of musculoskeletal, dermatological, and ocular systems.	Stool: High fecal calprotectin levels detected. Colonoscopy can visualize the inflamed areas of the intestine. Biopsy will show the inflammation of the whole wall of the intestine.	Combinations of: • Oral 5-aminosalicylates (e.g., sulfasalazine, mesalamine) • Glucocorticoids (e.g., prednisone, budesonide) • Immunomodulators (e.g., azathioprine, 6-mercaptopurine, methotrexate). • Biological therapies (e.g., infliximab, adalimumab). Low molecular weight heparin to prevent deep venous thrombosis (DVT). Surgical resection of the large intestine may be necessary in severe cases.

Ulcerative Colitis (UC) | Inflammation of the large bowel; involves the mucosal layer of intestine. Ulcerated areas become covered by granulation tissue, leading to formation of inflammatory areas of protruding growths termed pseudopolyps. An autoimmune disorder that predisposes individuals to colon cancer.

Signs and Symptoms	Physical Assessment Findings	Diagnostic Testing	Treatment
Abdominal pain. Chronic diarrhea with bleeding or mucus. Malabsorption causes weight loss. Remissions and exacerbations.	Abdominal tenderness, fever; stool may contain blood, pus, and mucus; weight loss.	Stool: High fecal calprotectin levels detected. Colonoscopy can visualize the inflamed areas of the large intestine. Biopsy will show the inflammation of the mucosa of the intestine.	Aminosalicylates: topical or oral. Glucocorticoids. Immunomodulators and antibiotics may be used in severe UC. Low molecular weight heparin to prevent DVT. Surgical resection of the large intestine may be necessary in severe cases.

Large Bowel Obstruction (LBO) | Inability of intestinal contents to move through the large intestine. Can be caused by mechanical, vascular, or neurogenic disorders and can be complete or partial. The bowel dilates proximal to the obstruction. Causes include diverticular disease, volvulus, hernia, and neoplasm.

Signs and Symptoms	Physical Assessment Findings	Diagnostic Testing	Treatment
Acute or chronic colicky lower abdominal pain, distention, tenderness, and rigidity caused by buildup of pressure and gas proximal to obstruction.	Abdominal tenderness, distention. High-pitched bowel sounds auscultated if a partial obstruction. Lack of bowel sounds if a complete obstruction.	Abdominal x-ray shows a classic pattern of gas and bowel distention. X-ray may show free air under the diaphragm if perforation occurs. Elevated WBC count and serum amylase levels occur with inflammation and perforation.	Volume replacement of the bloodstream caused by loss of a large amount of water in fluid shifts intraintestinally. Prophylactic antibiotic therapy is used to prevent bacteremia if perforation allows spill of bacteria into the peritoneum. Gastric decompression allows gas out from the intestine. Insertion of a stent or colectomy may be necessary. Dexamethasone is used to diminish inflammation.

Continued

Making the Connections—cont'd

Signs and Symptoms	Physical Assessment Findings	Diagnostic Testing	Treatment
Appendicitis | Condition caused by narrowing of the appendix lumen from obstruction. Inflammation of the wall of the appendix develops. Inside the appendix, there is development of a medium for bacterial growth.			
Acute abdominal pain, fever, constipation, abdominal pain originating in the umbilicus and radiating to the RLQ.	Abdominal tenderness at McBurney's point. Rebound tenderness caused by peritoneal inflammation. Abdominal rigidity, also called involuntary guarding.	CT scan is the best image study to visualize an inflamed appendix. Abdominal ultrasound can demonstrate an inflamed appendix. Elevated WBC count is caused by inflammation.	IV therapy for fluid replacement. Surgery to remove appendix or antibiotic therapy may be used alone.
Irritable Bowel Syndrome (IBS) | Alteration in GI motility that is linked to alteration in central nervous system–directed motor function of the bowel. Enhanced visceral sensitivity exists; no evidence of inflammation.			
Acute or chronic colicky abdominal pain lasting 6 months or more.	Complaints of abdominal cramping and pain. Chronic constipation or diarrhea. Physical examination is normal.	Stool samples to rule out other causes of pathology. Sigmoidoscopy to visualize large bowel up to sigmoid. CBC shows no WBC elevation. Upper GI studies show no abnormality. Lower GI studies show no abnormality.	A diet low in FODMAPs is recommended. Lubiprostone or linaclotide. Antispasmodic agents, dicyclomine and hyoscyamine. Rifaximin (Xifaxan).
Diverticular Disease | Weakness in bowel wall musculature, which allows protrusion of small outpouchings or sacs called diverticula. Diverticula can become infected (called diverticulitis) or inflamed or can fill with intestinal contents and cause an obstructive mass.			
Chronic dull LLQ episodic or steady pain OR acute pain, fever, constipation, or diarrhea.	Pain and tenderness in LLQ, abdomen, fever.	Elevated WBC count caused by inflammation. Sigmoidoscopy to visualize the lower bowel. CT scan.	Liquid diet followed by gradual reintroduction of a soft diet allows colon to rest. Antibiotics and pain relievers are used. Surgery, if necessary, after acute episode passes. Resection of diseased segment of colon with anastomosis performed immediately or some months later. Encourage increased fiber in diet to prevent diverticulitis.
Volvulus | A twisting of the intestine that cuts off the circulation to the intestinal wall.			
Abdominal pain. Vomiting, abdominal distention.	Abdominal tenderness. Vomiting. Abdominal distention.	Lower GI series can visualize the twisted segment of bowel.	Insertion of sigmoidoscope can unwind the intestine. Alternatively, resection of diseased segment of colon and anastomosis performed immediately or months later.

Making the Connections—cont'd

Signs and Symptoms	Physical Assessment Findings	Diagnostic Testing	Treatment
Hemorrhoids | Enlarged, inflamed blood vessels at the rectal–anal region.			
Rectal pain, loss of small amount of bright-red blood per rectum (hematochezia).	Hematochezia. Thrombosis within a prolapsed vein at the anal meatus.	Digital rectal examination. Sigmoidoscopy or colonoscopy if other pathology suspected.	Topical corticosteroid cream to decrease the inflammation. Minimally invasive procedures that decrease circulation to the veins causing the hemorrhoid.

Bibliography

Available online at fadavis.com

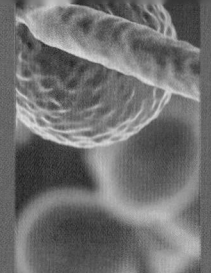

Infection, Inflammation, and Cirrhosis of the Liver

Learning Objectives

Upon completion of this chapter, the student will be able to:

- Describe normal anatomy and physiology of the liver and biliary system.
- Recognize common disorders of the liver and biliary system.
- Identify signs, symptoms, and clinical manifestations of disorders of the liver and biliary system.

- Recognize assessment techniques, laboratory tests, and imaging studies used in the diagnosis of disorders of the liver and biliary system.
- Discuss pharmacological and nonpharmacological treatment modalities used for disorders of the liver and biliary system.

Key Terms

Asterixis
Bilirubin
Caput medusa
Cholestasis
Cirrhosis
Conjugated bilirubin
Conjugation
Deamination
Enterohepatic recycling

Gluconeogenesis
Glycogenesis
Glycogenolysis
Hepatitis
Hepatocytes
Hyperbilirubinemia
Icterus
Intrahepatic jaundice
Jaundice

Non–alcohol-related fatty liver disease (NAFLD)
Non–alcohol-related steatohepatitis (NASH)
Prehepatic jaundice
Portal hypertension
Posthepatic jaundice
Spider angioma
Steatorrhea
Steatosis
Unconjugated bilirubin

The liver is the largest internal organ in the body, weighing 1,500 grams in the average adult. Metabolically complex, it functions simultaneously as an accessory organ of digestion, an endocrine organ, a hematological organ, and an excretory organ. Its cells have a distinctive regenerative capacity that enables it to function until approximately 80% of its cells are destroyed.

Liver disease can be caused by hepatocellular injury, obstructive injury, or both cellular and obstructive injury. Because of the liver's abundant blood reserve and regenerative capability, symptoms of liver dysfunction may not become evident until the hepatocytes are severely damaged or bile outflow is significantly obstructed.

Because of the liver's complex metabolic functions, liver disease often results in systemic, life-threatening complications, regardless of whether the disease is primary or secondary or is manifested by acute or chronic symptoms.

Epidemiology

Worldwide, hepatitis is one of the most common pathological conditions of the liver. Acute hepatitis is commonly the result of infection with one of several types of viral agents, but the clinical presentations of the various types of the illness are similar. In 5% of hepatitis B virus (HBV) cases and 85% of hepatitis C virus (HCV) cases, the patient is unable to produce an immune response to clear the liver of the virus, leading to a chronic infectious condition that may predispose the patient to hepatocellular cancer. In most of the world, HBV and HCV are the common causes of **cirrhosis,** whereas in the United States, alcohol use disorder is a predominant cause. However, there is an increasing prevalence of non–alcohol-related liver disease in the United States and worldwide. Non–alcohol-related fatty liver disease (NAFLD) and non–alcohol-related steatohepatitis (NASH) are fast becoming significant causes of chronic liver disease. NAFLD and NASH represent 75% of all chronic liver disease in the United States, affecting 80 to 100 million people. Persons with obesity, metabolic syndrome, and type 2 diabetes are commonly affected.

Chronic liver disease and cirrhosis result in about 40,500 deaths each year in the United States. Cirrhosis is the 12th leading cause of death in the United States and is responsible for 1.2% of all deaths in the

United States, with many patients dying from the disease in their fifth or sixth decade of life.

Each year, 2,000 additional deaths are attributed to liver failure, which may be caused by viral hepatitis, drugs such as acetaminophen, toxins, autoimmune hepatitis, NAFLD, alcohol-related hepatitis, or a variety of less common etiologies. Patients with liver failure have a 50% to 80% mortality rate unless they have liver transplantation. Approximately 20% of all organ transplants in the United States are liver transplants. Liver transplants can come from a deceased or live donor, with a 72% success rate at 5 years post-transplant.

Basic Concepts of Liver Function

The liver is located in the right upper quadrant (RUQ) of the abdomen, immediately beneath the diaphragm. A thick connective tissue called Glisson's capsule, which contains nerves, lymph, and blood vessels, covers the liver.

The liver is a vascular organ and has a dual blood supply from the hepatic artery, which is a branch of the aorta, and the portal vein, which drains the veins of the gastrointestinal tract. These vessels supply the liver with approximately 1,500 mL of blood per minute. The hepatic artery delivers 25% of the blood, whereas the portal vein supplies 75% of the blood. The liver synthesizes and secretes bile for fat digestion into the hepatic duct. Along with the pancreatic duct, the hepatic duct empties into the common bile duct, which carries bile into the intestine (see Fig. 31-1).

Hepatocytes, the functional cells of the liver that are capable of regeneration, excrete metabolic substances into small channels called canaliculi. These canaliculi are responsible for conduction of bile to the hepatic duct. Sinusoids are vascular spaces located between the hepatocytes that contain a mixture of venous and arterial blood from the hepatic artery and portal vein. Kupffer cells, specific macrophages of the liver, line the sinusoids and protect the body by detoxifying the bloodstream. Kupffer cells engulf and phagocytose foreign matter and pathogens that pass from the gastrointestinal tract into the portal circulation. They also ingest and destroy worn-out RBCs. The liver is histologically divided into lobules; each lobule contains a branch of arterial and venous blood vessel and a portion of bile duct—known as a portal triad (see Fig. 31-2).

Normal Hepatic Physiology

The liver serves as a digestive organ; an organ of metabolism; and a hematological, endocrine, and excretory organ (see Table 31-1). It also plays an important role in filtration and detoxification of the

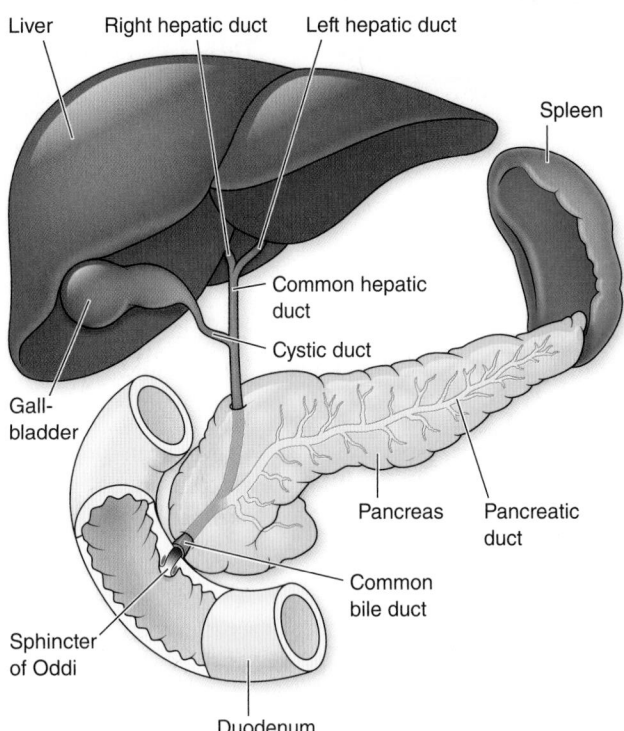

FIGURE 31-1. Gross anatomy of the liver and common bile duct. Note how the hepatic duct, cystic duct, and pancreatic duct come together to form the common bile duct. The common bile duct empties into the small intestine.

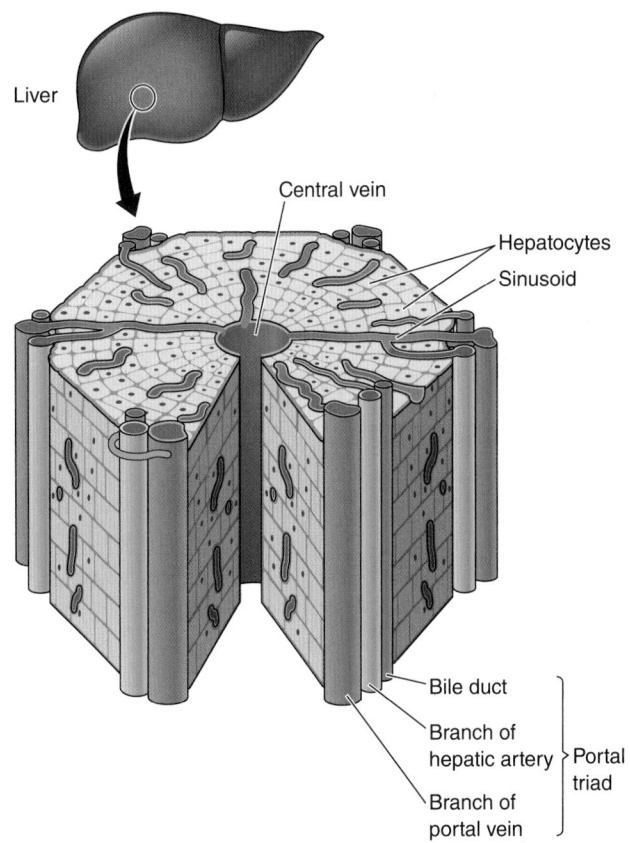

FIGURE 31-2. Cellular anatomy of a liver lobule.

TABLE 31-1. Normal Functions of the Liver

Function	Description
Digestion	The liver manufactures bile and secretes it into the hepatic duct, which enters the common bile duct and, in turn, empties into the intestine for digestion of fats.
Bilirubin conjugation	To convert bilirubin into bile, it has to be made water-soluble (conjugation). In the liver, glucuronic acid is used to conjugate bilirubin.
Fat metabolism	In the intestine, fat is broken down by bile into triglycerides. Triglycerides are then absorbed across the GI mucosa into the bloodstream. All venous blood from the GI tract flows into the liver's portal vein. In the liver, triglycerides are further broken down into fatty acids, cholesterol, and glycerol.
Protein metabolism	The liver both synthesizes and breaks down protein. The liver manufactures most of the body's albumin. Proteins are broken down (referred to as deamination) into ammonia, which is then absorbed into the bloodstream and excreted in urine.
Carbohydrate metabolism	Glucose builds up in the liver, which is stored in the form of glycogen (glycogenesis). There is also breakdown of glycogen by the liver when the body needs it (glycogenolysis). When the body needs more glucose, gluconeogenesis, which is the synthesis of glucose from amino acids and fats, occurs in the liver.
Hematological role	The liver synthesizes coagulation factors using vitamin K.
Endocrine role	Pancreatic glucagon acts at the liver to break down glycogen. Glucagon also stimulates lipolysis. With fat breakdown, there is formation of fatty acids. Fatty acids are converted into ketones in the liver.
Detoxification	The portal vein brings all substances absorbed by the GI system into the liver, which then detoxifies substances through biotransformation and first-pass effects.
Other functions	The liver stores vitamin A, D, B_{12}, iron, and copper. The liver produces B lymphocytes. The liver synthesizes angiotensinogen, which has a role in the renin–angiotensin–aldosterone system (RAAS). The liver synthesizes thrombopoietin, which stimulates platelet production in bone marrow.

bloodstream. Any damage to the liver cells will result in hindrance of these important functions.

Digestion

As an accessory organ of digestion, the liver is responsible for bile salt secretion to aid in fat digestion in the small intestine. Bile, a yellow-green alkaline fluid, is formed in the hepatocytes; some is stored in the gallbladder for later use, whereas other bile salts continue to the ileum and colon for excretion. Some bile salts are reabsorbed from the ileum into the portal vein, return to the liver, and become secreted again in a process called **enterohepatic recycling** (see Fig. 31-3).

CLINICAL CONCEPT

High amounts of bile salts in the bloodstream can cause pruritus.

Bilirubin Metabolism

One of the liver's most important functions is the conversion of bilirubin into bile. **Bilirubin,** a yellow-colored compound, is derived from the breakdown of aged red blood cells (RBCs). Hemoglobin in the RBCs breaks down into heme and globin; heme is then further broken down into iron and porphyrin. The porphyrin fraction is converted into biliverdin, which rapidly changes into free or **unconjugated bilirubin.** Unconjugated bilirubin travels to the liver. For the body to excrete bilirubin in the bile, it must be water-soluble. Through the process of **conjugation** in the liver, bilirubin is transformed into a water-soluble form. **Conjugated bilirubin** goes on to be excreted in the bile. Some conjugated bilirubin in the distal ileum and colon is converted by bacteria to urobilinogen. Most urobilinogen is reabsorbed from the gastrointestinal (GI) tract into the bloodstream and then excreted in urine. Urobilinogen gives urine its yellow color. Some urobilinogen continues on in the GI tract, where bacteria convert it to stercobilinogen, which is then excreted in the feces (see Fig. 31-4).

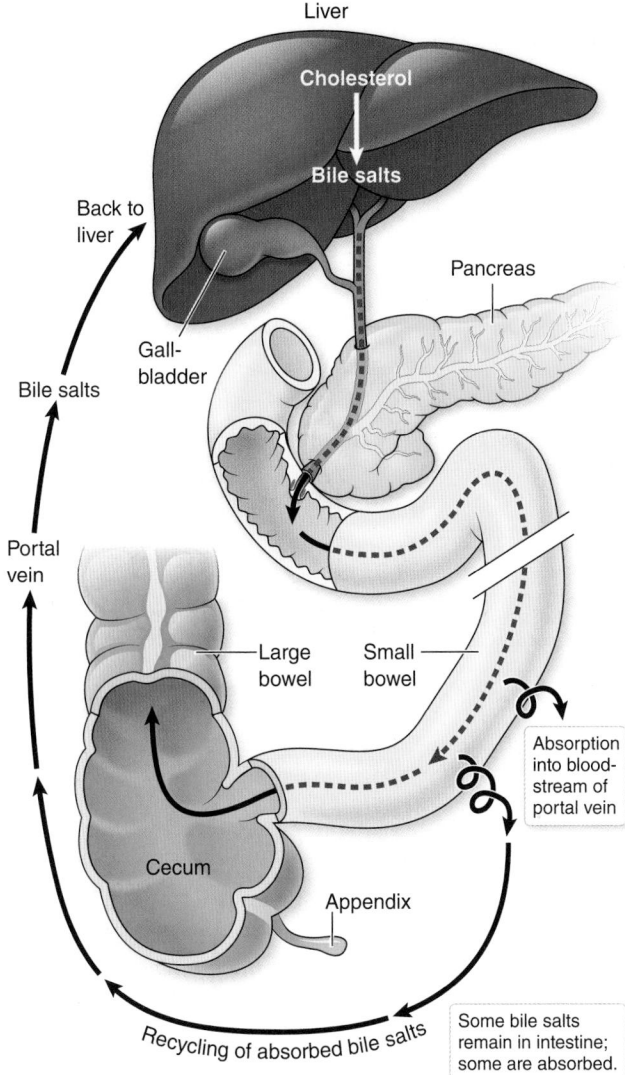

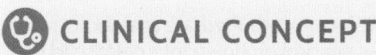

FIGURE 31-3. Bile secretion and enterohepatic recycling of bile salts. Bile salts are formed from cholesterol and secreted into the small intestine to aid fat digestion. Ninety percent of bile salts are reabsorbed into the blood and recycled via enterohepatic circulation.

> ## 🩺 CLINICAL CONCEPT
>
> Unconjugated bilirubin is also referred to as indirect bilirubin in diagnostic studies, whereas conjugated bilirubin is also referred to as direct bilirubin.

Fat and Protein Metabolism

The liver secretes bile into the intestine, which breaks down fats efficiently and rapidly. After bile acts on fats in the intestine, the fats are broken down into triglycerides. These are absorbed into the portal vein and enter the liver, where they are further broken down into fatty acids, cholesterol, and glycerol. The liver is a major producer of cholesterol.

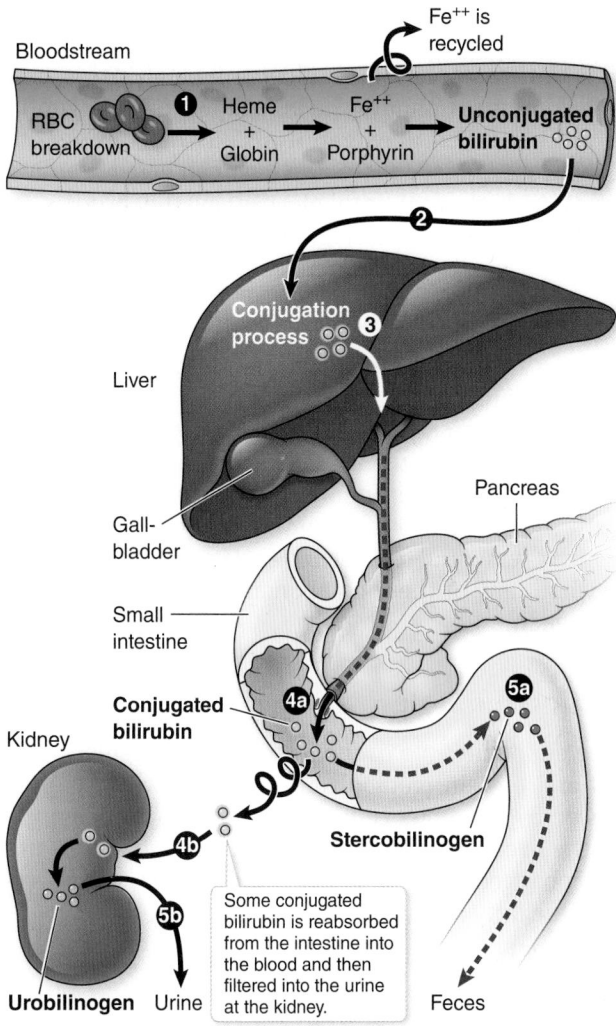

FIGURE 31-4. Conjugation of bilirubin and excretion. (1) RBCs are broken down into iron (Fe ++) and protein called porphyrin. Porphyrin is converted to biliverdin, which is further transformed into bilirubin. Iron becomes recycled. Bilirubin needs to be excreted. (2) Bilirubin in the blood enters the liver. (3) The liver conjugates the bilirubin. (4a) Some conjugated bilirubin enters the intestine, (4b) whereas some continues on in the bloodstream. (5a) Some conjugated bilirubin remains in the intestine and is converted into stercobilinogen, which is then excreted in the feces, (5b) whereas other conjugated bilirubin is absorbed by the kidney and is converted into urobilinogen, which gives urine its yellow color.

The liver is capable of both synthesizing and breaking down protein. In its role as a manufacturer of protein, the liver produces most of the body's albumin, which exerts colloid oncotic pressure within the bloodstream. In breaking down protein, the liver performs **deamination**—a process that removes nitrogen from proteins and converts it to ammonia (NH_3). Ammonia is absorbed into the bloodstream, becomes integrated into urea, and is then excreted by the kidneys in urine.

Carbohydrate Metabolism

The liver stores glucose as glycogen through the function termed **glycogenesis.** Because of glycogenesis, the liver can store large amounts of glucose that can be used when the body needs energy. When the body is enduring starvation or undergoing high stress, catecholamines stimulate the breakdown of glycogen in a process called **glycogenolysis.** If the body's store of glucose is inadequate, the liver can convert amino acids and glycerol into glucose by the process of **gluconeogenesis** (see Fig. 31-5).

Hematological Role

As part of its hematological function, the liver synthesizes fibrinogen and coagulation factors I, II, VI, IX, and X for clotting. With the exception of factor VIII, all of the elements of clotting are made by the hepatocytes. Prothrombin is produced by the liver with the assistance of vitamin K and bile. Vitamin K, which is essential for clotting, is a fat-soluble vitamin. Without any of these components, there is great risk of bleeding.

Endocrine Role

The endocrine role of the liver involves regulation of fat and protein metabolism. Glucagon, which is produced by the alpha cells of the pancreas, acts mainly in the liver and stimulates hepatic glycogenolysis and gluconeogenesis; it also stimulates lipolysis, converting free fatty acids to ketones in the liver.

> 🧬 **CLINICAL CONCEPT**
>
> Administration of glucagon stimulates the liver to secrete glucose from its glycogen stores.

Detoxification

The liver plays an active role in the detoxification of ingested substances and drugs. After a substance is ingested, it is absorbed by the GI system and then passes into the portal vein. The portal vein brings all absorbed substances through the liver, where the detoxification processes called biotransformation and the first-pass effect occur. Through these processes, substances are broken down by the liver into detoxified metabolites before reaching the systemic circulation (see Fig. 31-6). In the metabolism of drugs, the liver enzymatically processes the compounds by the cytochrome P450 system, which is a diverse group of enzymes that catalyze the oxidation of many different organic substances, metabolites, hormones, and toxic chemicals.

Biotransformation and the first pass through the liver greatly reduce the bioavailability or concentration of available drug in the bloodstream. The liver transforms drugs into inert compounds that are excreted into the bile and eliminated via the GI tract.

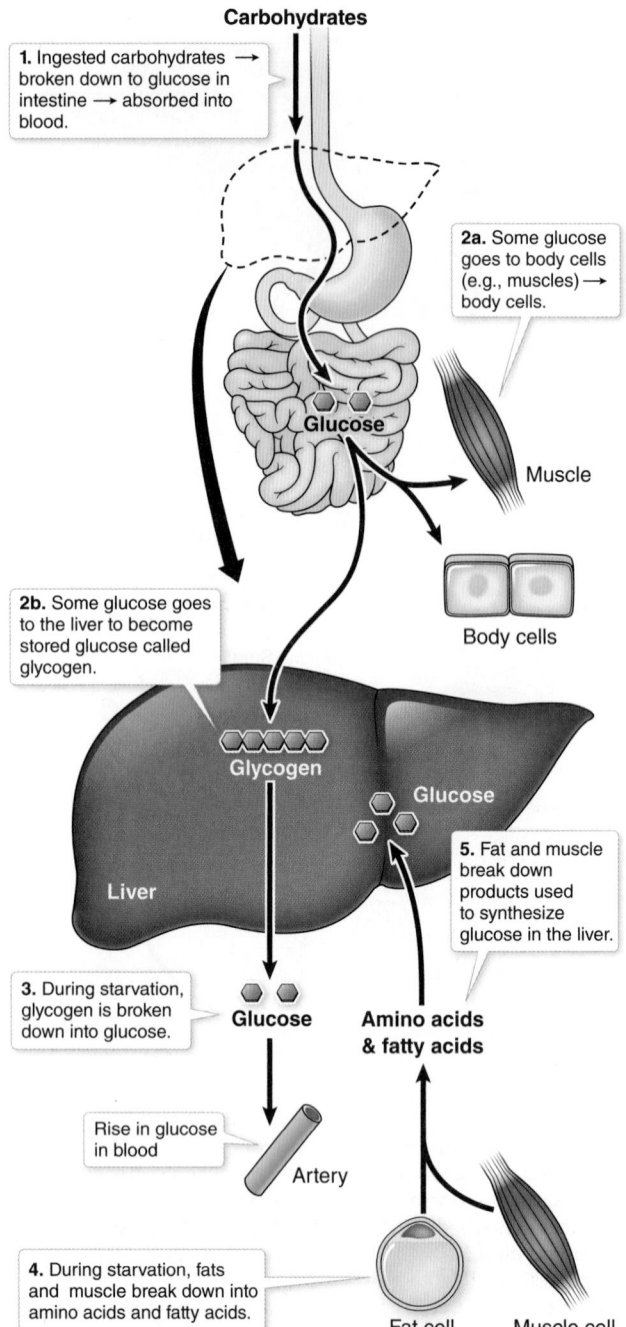

Carbohydrates

1. Ingested carbohydrates → broken down to glucose in intestine → absorbed into blood.

2a. Some glucose goes to body cells (e.g., muscles) → body cells.

Glucose

Muscle

2b. Some glucose goes to the liver to become stored glucose called glycogen.

Body cells

Glycogen

Glucose

Liver

5. Fat and muscle break down products used to synthesize glucose in the liver.

3. During starvation, glycogen is broken down into glucose.

Glucose

Amino acids & fatty acids

Rise in glucose in blood

Artery

4. During starvation, fats and muscle break down into amino acids and fatty acids.

Fat cell   Muscle cell

FIGURE 31-5. Role of the liver in carbohydrate metabolism. (1) Ingested carbohydrates are broken down into glucose in the intestine; glucose is then absorbed into blood. (2a) Some glucose goes to body cells such as muscles, (2b) whereas other glucose goes to the liver to synthesize glycogen, called glycogenesis. (3) During starvation or fasting, glycogen in the liver is broken down in a process called glycogenolysis. (4) When glycogen stores are exhausted, muscle and fat break down to form amino acids and fatty acids. (5) Amino acids and fatty acids are then used by the liver to make glucose in a process called gluconeogenesis.

> 🧬 **CLINICAL CONCEPT**
>
> Hepatocyte injury disrupts the liver's detoxification activity, which results in excess accumulation of drugs, hormones, or metabolites in the blood, tissues, or organs.

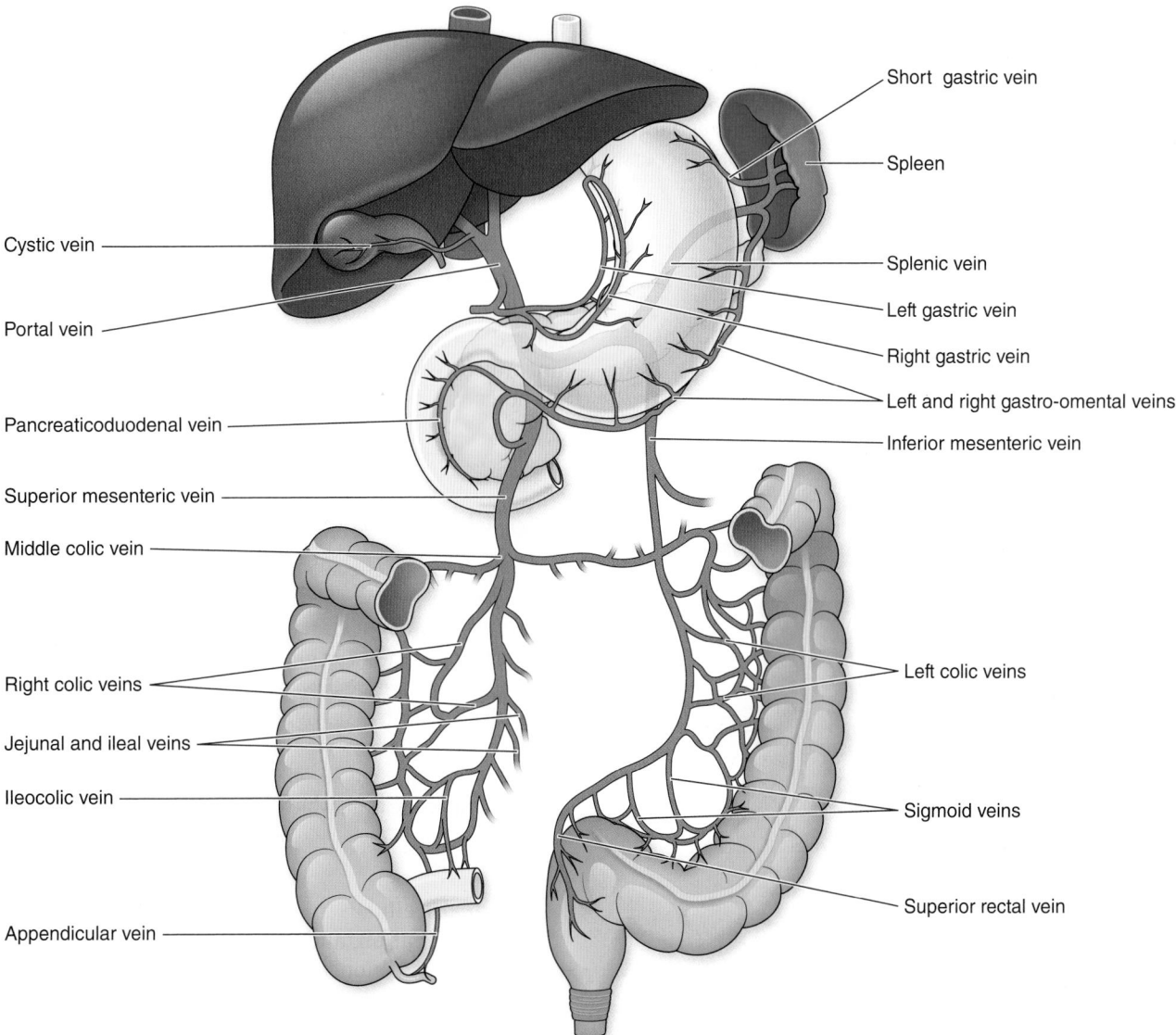

FIGURE 31-6. Detoxification of blood via the portal vein. Drainage of the veins of the gastrointestinal organs enters the portal vein, which carries blood to the liver. The hepatic portal vein is a blood vessel that drains blood from the gastrointestinal tract and spleen and brings it into the liver. This blood is rich in nutrients that were extracted from food, which the liver processes; it also filters toxins that may have been ingested with the food. The liver receives about 75% of its blood through the hepatic portal vein, with the remainder coming from the hepatic artery. The blood leaves the liver and travels to the heart via the hepatic veins and the inferior vena cava.

Other Functions

The liver stores vitamins A, D, and B_{12}; iron-rich ferritin; and copper, all of which are necessary for efficient cellular functions. The liver also produces insulin-like growth factor 1, a polypeptide protein hormone that plays an important role in childhood growth and has anabolic effects in adults. The liver synthesizes thrombopoietin, the hormone that regulates the production of platelets by the bone marrow. The liver also synthesizes angiotensinogen, a hormone that takes part in the renin–angiotensin–aldosterone system, which maintains blood pressure. The liver is responsible for immunological protection; the reticuloendothelial system of the liver contains B lymphocytes and immunoglobulins and also acts as a filter for antigens carried to it via the portal system.

Basic Pathophysiological Concepts of Liver Dysfunction

Liver dysfunction occurs by either cholestasis, which is caused by bile flow obstruction; hepatocellular injury, which is a result of inflammation; or a mixture of both. The consequences of liver disease are related to failure of the liver's main functions: synthesis, metabolism, detoxification, storage, or clearance.

Hyperbilirubinemia and Jaundice

Jaundice, yellowing of the skin and sclera, is the key symptom of liver disease. **Hyperbilirubinemia,** a high amount of bilirubin in the bloodstream, causes jaundice, also called **icterus.** Hyperbilirubinemia occurs because of one of three specific etiologies:

- Excessive RBC hemolysis
- Hepatocellular injury
- Bile duct obstruction

These causes are referred to as prehepatic, intrahepatic, and posthepatic jaundice, respectively (see Fig. 31-7).

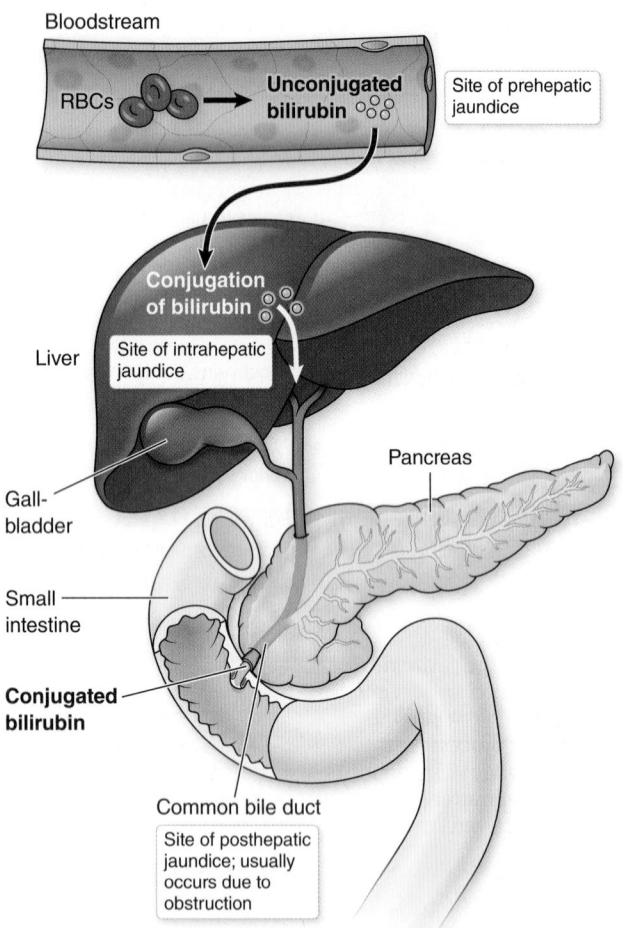

FIGURE 31-7. Causes of jaundice. (1) Prehepatic jaundice occurs when there is an overwhelming amount of hemolysis occurring in the body. With overwhelming hemolysis, there is an abundance of bilirubin, and all bilirubin cannot be processed by the liver. Because the bilirubin is backing up into the bloodstream and has not entered the liver, it is called prehepatic jaundice. (2) Intrahepatic jaundice occurs when the liver is having problems conjugating the bilirubin, resulting in only a portion becoming conjugated. This is referred to as an intrahepatic problem, so it is called intrahepatic jaundice. (3) Posthepatic jaundice occurs when the bilirubin has been conjugated and fully processed by the liver. The bilirubin, however, is not backing up because there is an obstruction in the bile duct–either in the hepatic duct or common bile duct. Bilirubin that has already left the liver cannot get to the bile duct for secretion, so this is called posthepatic jaundice.

Hemolysis of RBCs causes breakdown of hemoglobin into heme and globin. Heme breaks down further into iron and a protein called porphyrin. Porphyrin breaks down into biliverdin, which is then converted to bilirubin in the bloodstream. Therefore, an excessive amount of RBC breakdown leads to hyperbilirubinemia. Through conjugation, the liver processes bilirubin to make it water-soluble. If there is a large amount of hemolysis, bilirubin levels can overwhelm the liver, and some bilirubin can go into the bloodstream without being conjugated, which is why prolonged hemolysis increases both conjugated and unconjugated bilirubin concentrations. This type of jaundice is referred to as **prehepatic jaundice.**

> ### 🩺 CLINICAL CONCEPT
>
> An example of prehepatic jaundice is exhibited in physiological jaundice of the newborn. In this disorder, the breakdown of RBCs causes accumulation of bilirubin in the bloodstream. The newborn develops jaundice because its immature liver cannot effectively conjugate the bilirubin. Both conjugated and unconjugated bilirubin are found in the newborn's bloodstream. The infant becomes temporarily jaundiced until RBCs are processed by the immature liver, which takes a few days.

In hepatocellular injury, the liver cannot conjugate bilirubin at all, and unconjugated bilirubin accumulates in the bloodstream. This type of jaundice, referred to as **intrahepatic jaundice,** is commonly the result of inflammation of the liver.

In bile duct obstruction, the liver can conjugate the bilirubin, but the bile duct does not allow its excretion, resulting in increased levels of conjugated bilirubin circulating in the bloodstream. This is referred to as **posthepatic jaundice,** and it commonly occurs because of gallstones or tumors that obstruct the common bile duct.

Hepatocyte Inflammation and Infection

Inflammation of the liver is most often caused by a virus, drugs or toxic substances, or excessive alcohol use. The most common viruses that infect the liver are hepatitis virus A, B, C, D, and E. Other viruses include cytomegalovirus and Epstein–Barr virus (EBV). Viral hepatitis usually begins as an acute syndrome that involves liver enzyme elevation and hyperbilirubinemia. Acute infection with a hepatitis virus may result in conditions ranging from subclinical disease to self-limited symptomatic disease to fulminant hepatic failure. Common changes in the liver with hepatitis include infiltration of white blood cells (WBCs) and increased permeability of hepatocyte cell membranes. When viral hepatitis lasts longer than 6 months, it can become a chronic, long-term inflammatory condition. Chronic hepatic inflammation increases the risk of hepatocellular cancer.

Toxic hepatitis occurs when the liver is affected by drugs or toxic substances (see Box 31-1). Acetaminophen is one of the most common causes of toxic hepatitis. Specific enzymes in the liver, called the cytochrome P450 system, detoxify substances in the blood. Activation of some enzymes in the cytochrome P450 system can lead to oxidative stress; this injures hepatocytes and bile duct cells, which leads to accumulation of bile acid inside the liver. This accumulation causes liver damage, which involves dysfunction of liver macrophages (also called Kupffer cells) and activation of fat-storage cells within the liver called stellate cells. Activation of stellate cells leads to fat and collagenous tissue accumulation. Alternatively, many chemicals can damage cellular mitochondria. Dysfunctional mitochondria diminish energy production within the liver, thereby slowing its many metabolic functions. Mitochondrial dysfunction also causes release of oxidizing free radicals, further injuring hepatic cells.

Alcohol is a common cause of long-term, chronic liver disease. With chronic inflammation, stellate cells within the liver are stimulated to synthesize collagen and fibrotic tissue. Other classic histological features of the disease include bile duct damage, lymphoid follicles or aggregates, and macrovesicular steatosis. Steatosis is the infiltration of fat in the liver. Fatty liver is a characteristic change in alcohol use disorder.

Non–alcohol-related fatty liver disease (NAFLD) and **non–alcohol-related steatohepatitis (NASH)** are also common pathophysiological conditions of the liver. Although the etiology is unclear, the patient usually has comorbidities of obesity, hypertriglyceridemia, or diabetes. The liver becomes infiltrated with fat and fibrotic tissue. NAFLD is a major cause of cirrhosis.

Severe cases of hepatocellular injury may progress to fulminant hepatic failure, which is acute liver failure complicated by hepatic encephalopathy—involvement of the brain. Hepatic encephalopathy is exhibited by lethargy, confusion, and, in extreme cases, stupor and coma. The encephalopathy of fulminant hepatic failure is attributed to increased permeability of the blood–brain barrier and brain swelling. Cerebral edema is a potentially fatal complication of fulminant hepatic failure.

Bile Duct Obstruction

Biliary obstruction refers to the blockage of any duct that carries bile from the liver to the small intestine (see Fig. 31-8). The major signs and symptoms of biliary obstruction result directly from the failure of bile to be excreted. Failure of bile to reach the ducts for excretion causes a backup of bile, also referred to as **cholestasis.** Intrahepatic cholestasis generally occurs at the level of the hepatocyte or biliary canalicular membrane. Causes include hepatocellular disease, drug-induced cholestasis, biliary cirrhosis, and alcohol-related liver disease.

In hepatocellular disease, interference in the three major steps of bilirubin metabolism—uptake, conjugation, or excretion—usually occurs. Excretion is usually impaired to the greatest extent. As a result, conjugated bilirubin accumulates in the blood. Extrahepatic obstruction to the flow of bile may occur within the ducts or secondary to external compression. Overall, gallstones are the most common cause of biliary obstruction. Other causes include malignancy, infection, and biliary cirrhosis. External compression of the ducts may occur secondary to inflammation and malignancy.

Regardless of the cause, physical obstruction of the bile duct causes conjugated bilirubin to accumulate in the blood and subsequent deposition in the skin, which, in turn, causes jaundice. When bilirubin is filtered by the kidneys, dark-colored urine is seen.

BOX 31-1. Common Causes of Hepatic Inflammation

The following agents can directly injure hepatocytes:

DRUGS
- Acetaminophen
- Acetylsalicylic acid (aspirin)
- Allopurinol
- Captopril
- Carbamazepine
- Diazepam
- Erythromycin
- Estrogen
- Halothane
- Methotrexate
- Methyldopa
- Oral contraceptives
- Phenobarbital
- Phenytoin
- Sulfonamides
- Tetracycline

TOXINS
- Carbon tetrachloride
- Ethyl alcohol
- Kava (herb)
- Trichloroethylene
- Toluene
- Wild mushrooms (some)

VIRUSES
- Coxsackie virus
- Cytomegalovirus
- Epstein–Barr virus
- Hepatitis viruses A, B, C, D, E, and G

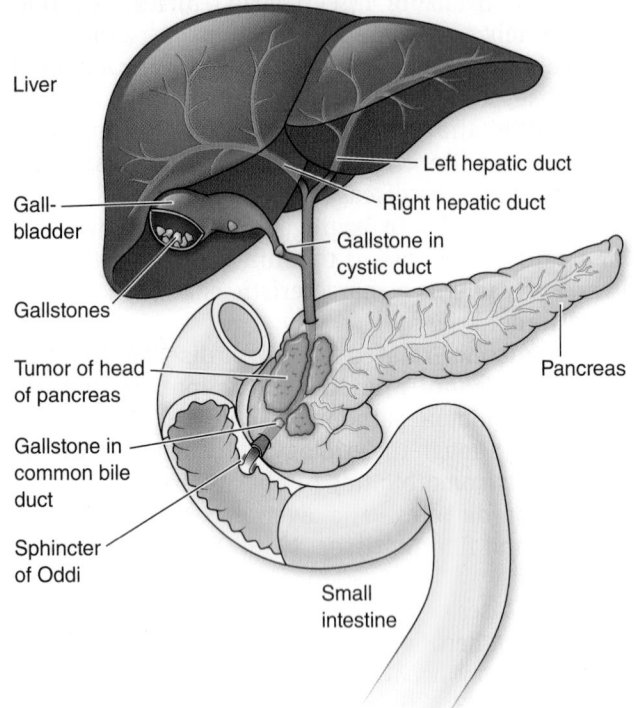

FIGURE 31-8. Common causes of bile obstruction. The most common causes of bile duct obstruction are gallstones and tumor of the head of the pancreas. In cholelithiasis, a gallstone commonly lodges in the cystic duct, which causes backup of pressure and bile in the gallbladder, resulting in cholecystitis. A gallstone can also travel out of the cystic duct and lodge in the common bile duct, which causes backup of bile into the liver and then into the bloodstream, causing jaundice. A tumor of the head of the pancreas also commonly leads to obstruction of the common bile duct. This causes bile to back up into the liver and blood, leading to jaundice.

Assessment

Assessment of the patient with liver dysfunction requires a thorough history, complete physical examination, and use of laboratory tests and diagnostic procedures. Risk factors for liver disease should also be investigated (see Box 31-2).

History

In the history, the clinician should focus on the etiology of disease, along with the patient's appetite, digestion, exercise tolerance, and bowel changes. The patient with liver dysfunction often reports extreme fatigue, abdominal pain, weakness, anorexia, nausea, vomiting, abdominal bloating, changes in bowel habits, and weight loss. Interestingly, smokers often lose their taste for tobacco. Because the liver may not be secreting bile for fat digestion, the patient may complain of **steatorrhea,** which are defined as light-colored, soft stools. Jaundice and dark urine are signs of bilirubin accumulation in the bloodstream. Accumulation of bile salts in the bloodstream often causes pruritus, or itching of the skin.

BOX 31-2. Risk Factors for Liver Disease

The following conditions increase susceptibility to liver disease:
- Alcohol use disorder, excessive
- Certain medications
- Gastric bypass surgery
- HBV or HCV, chronic
- High cholesterol
- High triglycerides
- Iron overload
- Malnutrition
- Metabolic syndrome
- Obesity
- Toxins, chemicals
- Weight loss, rapid
- Wilson disease

Signs and Symptoms

In the physical examination, RUQ tenderness may be present. When Glissom's capsule, which covers the liver, is stretched, the distention gives rise to RUQ pain and allows lymphatics to leak fluid into the peritoneal space. This produces ascites, also known as peritoneal edema. Hepatomegaly may be palpated on abdominal examination. Hyperbilirubinemia occurs and, because of bilirubin's affinity for elastin fibers, the skin and sclera become yellow. The presence of jaundice in the sclera indicates a minimum level of 3.0 mg/dL of serum bilirubin. Other sites to examine for jaundice are under the tongue and, in persons of color, the mucous membranes of the mouth. Examination of the skin may show spider angioma, caput medusa over the abdomen, and palmar erythema. **Spider angioma** are fine capillaries that fan out from a central point on the skin's surface (see Fig. 31-9). Caput medusa are obvious dilated veins over the umbilical area of the abdomen. Ascites

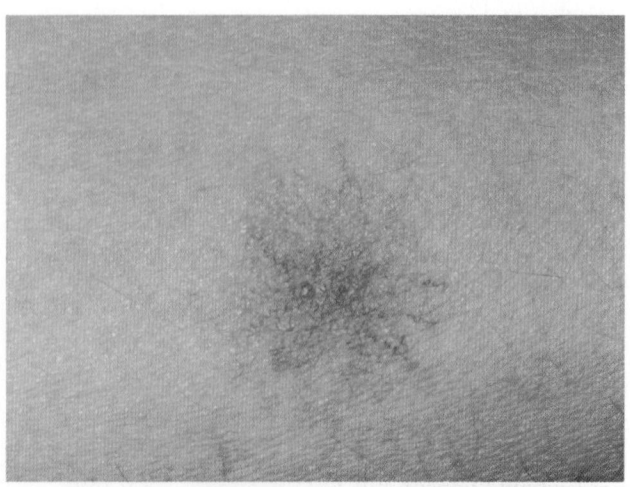

FIGURE 31-9. Spider angioma. *(From SPL/Science Source.)*

is common in liver disease and can be confirmed by eliciting "shifting dullness" in the abdomen. Steatorrhea can occur when bilirubin is not excreted into the intestine. Dark urine can occur in liver disease because of the backup of bilirubin into the bloodstream that is filtered at the kidney. Box 31-3 details classic signs of liver disease.

Diagnostic Tests

The initial battery of tests for liver function include liver enzymes, serum alanine transaminase (ALT), serum aspartate transaminase (AST), alkaline phosphatase, direct and indirect bilirubin, albumin, and prothrombin levels (see Table 31-2). The pattern of abnormalities enables the differentiation between hepatocellular and cholestatic disease and determination of acute or chronic stages. Blood ammonia (NH_3) levels are drawn and are elevated in chronic liver disease and liver failure. A hepatitis serology panel is done that includes specific laboratory data regarding hepatitis A, B, C, D, or E (see Table 31-3). Autoimmune markers help in determining biliary cirrhosis. Diagnostic imaging uses ultrasound tomography, computerized tomography (CT) scans, and magnetic resonance imaging (MRI). Liver biopsy is the gold standard test for diagnosing the stages and severity of liver disease, predicting prognosis, and monitoring therapy.

Treatment

Treatment for liver disorders includes control of symptoms and supportive care with rest and small, high-calorie, high-protein meals. The patient should avoid alcohol or any drugs, unless prescribed. Treatment regimens for hepatitis include interferon, nucleoside analogues, protease inhibitors, and other antiviral agents. Patients with encephalopathy should be monitored in an intensive care setting. As encephalopathy progresses, maintenance of the airway and circulation requires frequent assessment. Careful attention should be paid to fluid management and hemodynamics. Monitoring of metabolic parameters, surveillance for infection, maintenance of nutrition, and prompt recognition of GI bleeding are crucial. Coagulation parameters, complete blood cell count (CBC), and metabolic panel should be checked frequently. Serum aminotransferases and bilirubin are generally measured daily to follow the course of infection. Liver transplantation, in selected cases, is an option if the patient has fulminant hepatic failure.

BOX 31-3. **Classic Signs of Liver Disease**

The following signs and symptoms occur anytime there is hepatocyte injury or obstruction of bile excretion:
- Anorexia
- Ascites
- Dark urine
- Hepatomegaly
- Hyperbilirubinemia
- Jaundice
- RUQ tenderness
- Splenomegaly
- Steatorrhea

Select Pathophysiological Disorders of the Liver

Liver dysfunction is caused by either damage to hepatocytes or blockage of bile flow. Interference with

TABLE 31-2. **Diagnostic Test Results in Different Types of Liver Disease**

Test	Normal Levels	Abnormality
AST	5 to 40 units/mL	Elevated in alcohol-related liver disease
ALT	5 to 35 units/mL	Elevated in liver disease
Alkaline phosphatase	35 to 150 units/mL	Elevated in hepatitis and liver disease
Bilirubin, indirect	Less than 0.8 mg/dL	Elevated unconjugated bilirubin occurs in Gilbert's disease
Bilirubin, total	Less than 1.0 mg/dL	Elevated bilirubin causes jaundice in hepatitis
PT	11.5 to 14 sec	Prolonged suggests hepatic dysfunction
Ammonia (NH_3)	<35 micromoles/L	Elevated in chronic liver disease
Serum albumin	3.5 to 5.5 g/dL	Decreased indicates hepatic dysfunction
Serum globulin	2.5 to 3.5 g/dL	Elevated in autoimmune hepatitis
γ-Glutamyl transpeptidase	10 to 48 Units/mL	Large elevation in alcohol-related liver disease

TABLE 31-3. Viral Hepatitis Diagnostic Tests

After a patient is diagnosed with viral hepatitis, it is important to clarify which kind of hepatitis virus is causing the infection. The following laboratory tests are used to diagnose the different types of hepatitis virus infections.

Test	HAV	HBV	HCV
Alkaline phosphatase	Elevated	Elevated	Elevated
Aminotransferase	Elevated	Elevated	Elevated
Anti-HCV antibodies			Diagnostic of HCV infection
Bilirubin	Elevated	Elevated	Elevated
HBsAg		Diagnostic of HBV infection	
Immunoglobulin M anti-HAV virus antibody	Diagnostic of acute HAV infection		
Immunoglobulin M anti-HBcAg antibodies		Diagnostic of acute HBV infection	
Prothrombin		Prolonged	Prolonged
Viral assay	HAV RNA viral assay	HBV DNA viral assay	HCV RNA viral assay

bile outflow causes backup of bilirubin into the bloodstream, which is manifested as jaundice. Hepatocyte damage commonly leads to fatty degeneration of the liver, which terminates in a fibrotic change of the liver known as cirrhosis.

Hepatitis

Hepatitis is a systemic infection affecting the liver, commonly caused by one of the following agents:

1. Hepatitis A virus (HAV)
2. Hepatitis B virus (HBV)
3. Hepatitis C virus (HCV)
4. Hepatitis D virus (HDV)
5. Hepatitis E virus (HEV)
6. Hepatitis G virus (HGV)

With the exception of HBV, which is caused by a DNA virus, all the others are ribonucleic acid (RNA) viruses. Nonviral hepatitis results from exposure to toxic chemicals or certain drugs. Other viruses that can cause inflammation of the liver are cytomegalovirus and EBV. Generally, all types of hepatitis produce similar clinical manifestations, ranging from mild symptoms to fulminant infections or chronic progressive liver disease.

Hepatitis A Virus

HAV is usually caused by ingestion of contaminated food or water or contracted from person to person by the fecal–oral route. The virus is able to live on surfaces at room temperature, but is killed by cooking food thoroughly. HAV is absorbed by the intestine and travels to the liver, where it damages the hepatocytes. It mainly causes a mild disease with no complications.

In 2018, a total of 12,474 cases of hepatitis A were reported in the United States, but due to underreporting, the actual number of cases is likely around 24,900. The incidence of HAV infection decreased more than 95% between 1995 and 2011 when some states required routine vaccination of children with HAV immunization. In accordance with these findings, in 2006, the Centers for Disease Control and Prevention (CDC) recommended an expansion of routine HAV vaccination to include all children in the United States ages 12 to 23 months. HAV vaccination has made infection uncommon. However, HAV infection is endemic in Asia, Africa, Mexico, and South America. Also men who have sex with men (MSM) have an increased risk of HAV infection. Substantial increases in incident cases of hepatitis A have occurred since late 2016 (3,366, 12,474, and 18,846 reported cases in 2017, 2018, and 2019, respectively) due to ongoing outbreaks reported to CDC among people who use illicit drugs and people experiencing homelessness as well as outbreaks among MSM.

Etiology and Risk Factors. HAV is an RNA virus that uses its own RNA polymerase to achieve replication of its viral parts in the hepatocyte. HAV is contracted through the fecal–oral route, although isolated cases of parenteral transmission have been reported. HAV is most commonly transmitted between people in close contact or via contaminated water or food. It is a self-limited disease that enters the body via the gastrointestinal tract and travels to the liver, where it damages hepatocytes. Boiling water is an effective means of destroying it; chlorine and iodine are similarly effective.

HAV outbreaks commonly occur due to poor sanitary conditions, water contamination, and inadequate sewage disposal. Outbreaks can also occur due to contaminated food or water. Fresh produce can spread HAV infection because the virus is difficult to wash off surfaces of fruits and vegetables. It can occur from food service workers who do not appropriately wash hands and sanitize. Shellfish are particularly associated with HAV transmission because water is highly filtered through these forms of sea life and they concentrate the virus. Transmission can also occur among children in day care centers if sanitation measures are not observed with diaper changes. Sexual practices that result in anal-oral contact can transmit HAV.

Pathophysiology. Uptake of HAV and viral replication occur within hepatocytes. After entry into the cell, viral RNA is converted into DNA by polymerase enzymes. Viral proteins are synthesized, and assembled virus particles are shed into the biliary tree and excreted in the feces. HAV can be found in bile, stool, and blood. Person-to-person contact is the most common means of transmission and is generally limited to close contacts. The period of greatest contagion of HAV is during the first 14 to 21 days after infection, when jaundice has not yet occurred. After exposure to the virus, antibodies to HAV of the immunoglobulin (Ig) M class can be detected in blood. The antibody response persists for several months. After acute illness, anti-HAV antibodies of the IgG class remain detectable. IgG antibodies endow immunity to prevent repeat infection.

🔬 CLINICAL CONCEPT

A very small proportion of patients develop a relapse of HAV weeks to months after acute infection. Rarely, cholestatic hepatitis characterized by jaundice, pruritus, and liver test abnormalities can persist for up to a year postinfection. However, even when these complications occur, HAV infection is self-limited and does not progress to chronic liver disease.

Clinical Presentation. Patients with HAV infection report fever, abdominal pain, mild flu-like symptoms of nausea and vomiting, fatigue, malaise, myalgias, arthralgias, and mild headache. Anorexia and loss of taste for food may also be reported. Smokers often lose their taste for tobacco. The clinician should ask questions regarding the patient's possible exposure to HAV and also inquire about their occupation, living conditions, diet, and recent travel or exposure to others who travel. The patient may have contracted HAV through food eaten weeks in the past; however, a dietary history is difficult to track.

Signs and Symptoms. Flulike symptoms are commonly present, and the physical examination may demonstrate hepatomegaly and jaundice. Jaundice occurs in most (70% to 85%) adults. Stool may have a pale appearance, and dark urine and pruritus may accompany jaundice. Children who acquire HAV usually do not develop jaundice and are mildly symptomatic.

Diagnosis. HAV has an incubation period of 2 to 4 weeks, and liver enzymes will rise after the first 4 weeks (see Fig. 31-10). HAV is apparent in the stool early, within the first 2 to 4 weeks. HAV RNA appears in the blood up to 2 weeks before clinical illness develops. IgM antibodies against HAV appear after the first 4 weeks, and IgG antibodies rise after 8 to 12 weeks. HAV antibodies remain elevated and provide long-term immune protection.

The diagnosis of acute hepatitis A requires clinical and laboratory criteria (see Box 31-4).

Treatment. Treatment is supportive and does not change the course of the disease. Rest and good nutrition are important, along with avoidance of alcohol and acetaminophen. Good hygiene is also necessary. HAV vaccine endows immunity with one dose. Passive immunization with HAV immunoglobulin (Ig) is also available for contacts of patients with HAV infection. This immunization is a short-term, rapid dose of protective antibodies given to family members and close contacts before exposure or during the early incubation period. For postexposure prophylaxis, HAV Ig can be administered as late as 2 weeks after contact. The vaccine is available for all who want or need prevention before exposure.

Prevention of HAV by vaccine is the standard approach across much of the world, and many countries

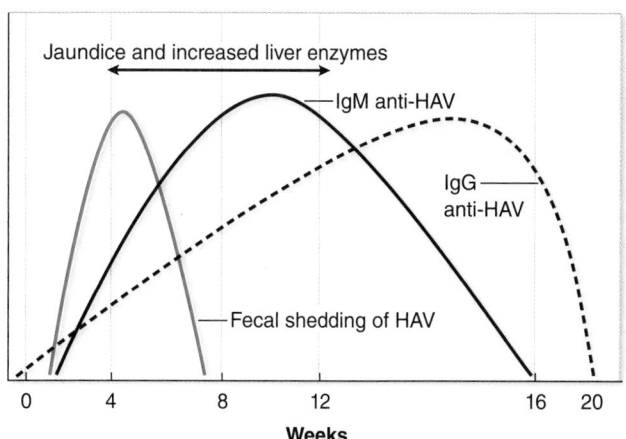

FIGURE 31-10. Timeline of HAV infection. HAV is an infection spread by the fecal–oral route. After contraction of HAV, the virus is shed in the feces. Jaundice and increased liver enzymes become apparent after approximately 2 weeks. The first antibodies to develop against HAV are immunoglobulin (Ig) G antibodies. IgG antibodies against HAV are formed in large amounts later and remain elevated for more than 20 weeks.

BOX 31-4. Diagnosis of Acute Hepatitis A: Clinical and Laboratory Criteria

CLINICAL CRITERIA

An acute illness with a discrete onset of any sign or symptom consistent with acute viral hepatitis (e.g., fever, headache, malaise, anorexia, nausea, vomiting, diarrhea, abdominal pain, or dark urine)

AND

a) Jaundice or elevated total bilirubin levels ≥ 3.0 mg/dL, OR

b) Elevated serum alanine aminotransferase (ALT) levels >200 IU/L

c) The absence of a more likely diagnosis

CONFIRMED LABORATORY CRITERIA

Immunoglobulin M (IgM) antibody to hepatitis A virus (anti-HAV) positive

OR

Nucleic acid amplification test (NAAT; such as polymerase chain reaction [PCR] or genotyping) for hepatitis A virus RNA positive

IgG anti-HAV antibodies remain elevated and provide long-term immune protection.

---

have adopted universal vaccination against HAV in their children. HAV vaccine is also a mainstay of postexposure prophylaxis. Postexposure prophylaxis for HAV is best achieved with either HAV vaccine or immunoglobulin, and both seem to be equally effective. The United States offers two commercially available hepatitis A vaccines and one combination HAV-HBV vaccine. The HAV vaccine is typically administered in two doses, 6 months apart, whereas the HAV-HBV vaccine usually requires three doses.

Hepatitis B Virus

HBV is a stable virus spread by blood products, body fluids, or sexual contact. Once in the bloodstream, the virus produces viral proteins in the hepatocyte. The virus does not directly kill the cell, but the host's own immune system attacks hepatocytes when the viral antigens are encountered on the surface. Individuals carry HBV for life, and hepatocellular carcinoma (HCC) can occur because of the chronic inflammation caused by the virus.

Globally, 2 billion persons have evidence of past or present HBV infection. In 2018, a total of 3,322 cases of acute hepatitis B were reported to the CDC, for an overall incidence rate of 1 case per 100,000 population. However, this is a conservative estimate as many cases of hepatitis B are not reported or diagnosed. After adjusting for underdiagnosis, an estimated 21,600 acute hepatitis B cases occurred in 2018. In some individuals, acute hepatitis B becomes chronic HBV infection. It is estimated that between 880,000 to

1.89 million people are living with chronic HBV infection in the United States, two-thirds of whom may be unaware of their infection. The risk for chronic infection varies according to the age at infection and is greatest among young children. Approximately 90% of infants and 25% to 50% of children aged 1 to 5 years who contract HBV remain chronically infected. However, approximately 95% of adults recover completely from HBV infection and do not become chronically infected. Chronic hepatitis B disproportionately affects people born outside the United States; while accounting for only 14% of the U.S. general population, non–U.S.-born people account for 69% of the U.S. population living with chronic HBV infection. In 2018, a total of 1,649 U.S. death certificates had HBV recorded as an underlying or contributing cause of death. Superinfections with HCV, HDV, and HEV in individuals with HBV are possible and can lead to rapidly progressive liver disease for which treatment options are limited.

Etiology. HBV is an extremely resilient virus capable of withstanding extreme conditions. It can survive when stored for years at temperatures below zero and for weeks at temperatures over 110°F. Certain hepatitis viral antigens are significant when following the progress of the viral infection. Hepatitis surface antigen (HBsAg) is a protein found on its outer surface that can be used to measure the number of viral particles. The antibody to this protein is anti-HBsAg. The protein expressed by the viral DNA is called HBV core antigen (HBcAg), and its corresponding antibody is anti-HBcAg. The e antigen, HBeAg, comes from the core and is a marker of active viral replication. The best indication of active viral replication is the presence of HBV DNA in the serum.

Risk factors include non-Hispanic African American ethnicity, cocaine use, a high number of sexual partners and unprotected sexual activity, sexually transmitted infection, HIV-positive status, handling of blood products, IV drug use and use of unsterile needles, MSM, household contact with someone with HBV, and hemodialysis. Also, travel to regions with high rates of HBV, such as Africa, Central and Southeast Asia, and Eastern Europe, places a person at risk (see Box 31-5). Perinatal transmission is possible, as is oral passage of the virus, but this is uncommon.

Pathophysiology. The pathophysiology of HBV is caused by the interaction of the virus and the human immune system. The immune system attacks HBV and causes liver injury. Activated CD4+ and CD8+ cells react with HBV proteins located on the surface of infected hepatocytes, and an immunological reaction occurs. Four different stages have been identified in the viral life cycle of HBV:

- **Stage 1:** In the first stage, the incubation period, there are no signs or symptoms; however, the patient can pass the virus to others. The duration

BOX 31-5. Populations at High Risk for Development of HBV Infection

- Foreign travelers to countries with endemic hepatitis
- Health-care providers
- Household contacts of persons with HBV
- Men who have sex with men
- Patients on hemodialysis
- Persons who use IV drugs or illicit drugs
- Persons with HCV
- Persons with a history of sexually transmitted infections
- Persons with multiple sex partners
- Persons with HIV
- Prison inmates

of this stage is approximately 2 to 4 weeks. For newborns, the virus can incubate for years. Active viral replication is occurring during this stage without elevation in the liver enzyme (aminotransferase levels).

- **Stage 2:** In the second stage, an inflammatory reaction of the hepatocytes occurs. The patient may experience flu-like symptoms and jaundice begins to develop. HBeAg, HBsAg, and HBV DNA can be detected in the bloodstream. Liver enzymes begin to increase. The duration of this symptomatic stage is approximately 3 to 4 weeks.
- **Stage 3:** In the third stage, the immune system reacts to the infected hepatocytes and HBV. Viral replication slows. The HBV DNA levels are lower or undetectable, and liver enzyme levels decrease to normal.
- **Stage 4:** In the fourth stage, the virus cannot be detected and antibodies to HBsAg, HBcAg, and HBeAg have been produced.

The production of antibodies against HBsAg confers long-term protective immunity and can be detected in patients who have recovered from HBV or in those who have been vaccinated. Antibody to HBcAg is detected only in those with actual previous infection with HBV. Those with vaccination do not obtain the HBcAg in the vaccine. The HBcAg blood test can be used to differentiate persons who have contracted the disease from those who have undergone vaccination. Only those who have endured the disease have circulating HBcAg in the bloodstream.

In the patient's lifetime, HBV antigens and HBV DNA can persist and recur in extrahepatic sites, such as the lymph nodes, bone marrow, spleen, and pancreas. However, the virus does not appear to harm tissue in these organs.

The final stage of HBV disease is cirrhosis. Patients with cirrhosis and HBV are likely to develop HCC. This stage may occur after many years of chronic disease.

Clinical Presentation. The patient with HBV presents to the clinician after a prolonged incubation period of 2 to 6 months, during which the patient is asymptomatic (see Fig. 31-11). When symptomatic, the patient presents with a flu-like syndrome, anorexia, RUQ or epigastric pain, jaundice, pruritus, dark urine, and light-colored stools. Because it is contagious, the clinician should encourage the patient to disclose their HBV status to persons they live with, sexual partners, or anyone with whom they have close contact. Contacts can obtain hepatitis B immunoglobulin (HBIg), which can provide rapid passive immunity against HBV.

During the patient's recovery, symptoms gradually subside. The course is variable and may run from a moderate illness to fulminant hepatitis. Patients with chronic HBV can be healthy carriers without any evidence of active disease.

Signs and Symptoms. The patient presents with fever, flu-like symptoms, jaundice, and hepatomegaly. Splenomegaly, lymphadenopathy, spider angioma, and palmar erythema may be evident. Jaundice can last for months. Patients with severe cases of infection may present with signs of hepatic encephalopathy—somnolence, confusion, stupor, or coma.

Diagnosis. Diagnosis of HBV is usually made by the presence of HBsAg in the bloodstream. However, the level of HBsAg in the bloodstream is not correlated with the severity of disease. Indeed, some with low titers have severe disease, whereas high titers can be present with mild disease. HBeAg blood levels are

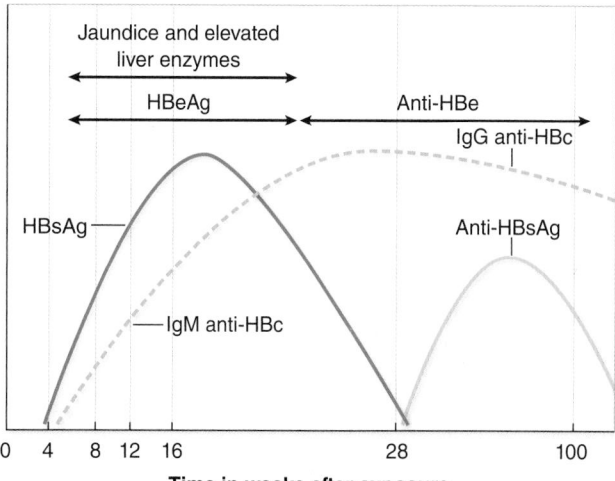

FIGURE 31-11. Timeline of HBV infection. HBV is an infection spread by blood or body fluids. After contraction of HBV, jaundice and increased liver enzymes become apparent after approximately 4 weeks. Hepatitis B surface antigen (HBsAg) and hepatitis B antigen (HBeAg) rise in the blood after approximately 4 weeks. The first antibodies to develop against HBV are immunoglobulin (Ig) M type antibodies against HBcAg. Later in the course of disease, IgG antibodies against HBcAg are formed. Antibodies against HBV antigen and HBV surface antigen develop much later in the course of disease.

present during the time of active replication of the virus. HBeAg is most closely monitored during the convalescent phase. Tests for detection of HBV DNA in the liver and bloodstream are also available. To distinguish between acute and chronic infection, IgM-versus IgG-type antibodies are assessed. Anti-HBc antibodies are IgM-type antibodies that are present in acute infection, whereas IgG-type anti-HBc antibodies are present in chronic infection. Liver enzymes and bilirubin levels are elevated in active disease. Serum albumin, prothrombin time (PT), and coagulation factors also should be monitored over the course of the disease. Diagnosis of HBV infection requires meeting clinical and laboratory criteria (see Box 31-6).

Treatment. Treatment is symptomatic and is usually supportive with rest. The patient should be encouraged to eat small, high-calorie, high-protein meals. Currently, polyethylene glycol (PEG) interferon and drugs that inhibit viral polymerase, such as lamivudine, telbivudine, adefovir, entecavir, and tenofovir, are used to treat HBV. Although currently available antiviral therapies achieve suppression of HBV replication in the majority of patients, complete clearance of the virus is rarely achieved despite long-term antiviral treatment. Various clinical trials of agents that interrupt the HBV life cycle in hepatocytes are under way. Potential treatment strategies such as immunomodulators and other new agents are emerging as an eventual HBV cure.

Prevention is the key to disease control. The HBV vaccine is recommended for all people. During the course of the disease, close contacts of the patient can receive HBIg for short-acting immediate immunity. For unvaccinated individuals who are exposed to HBV, postexposure prophylaxis with a combination of HBIg and the HBV vaccine is recommended.

 CLINICAL CONCEPT

Most individuals with HBV do not recover completely. Patients who are of advanced age and have serious underlying medical conditions may have a prolonged course and suffer severe disease. Some patients with acute HBV go on to develop chronic HBV. This is common in infants, those affected by Down syndrome, patients on long-term hemodialysis, and those who are immunosuppressed and HIV-positive.

BOX 31-6. Diagnosis of HBV Infection: Clinical and Laboratory Criteria

An acute illness with
- a discrete onset of symptoms* **AND**
- jaundice or elevated serum alanine aminotransferase levels (>100 IU/L)

LABORATORY CRITERIA FOR DIAGNOSIS
- HBsAg positive **AND**
- Immunoglobulin M (IgM) antibody to hepatitis B core antigen (IgM anti-HBc) positive (if done)
  Persons with chronic HBV infection may have no evidence of liver disease or may have a spectrum of disease ranging from chronic hepatitis to cirrhosis or liver cancer. Persons with chronic infection may be asymptomatic.

LABORATORY CRITERIA FOR CHRONIC HBV DIAGNOSIS
- IgM anti-HBc negative AND a positive result on one of the following tests: HBsAg, HBeAg, or NAT for HBV DNA (including qualitative, quantitative, and genotype testing) **OR**
- HBsAg positive or NAT for HBV DNA positive (including qualitative, quantitative, and genotype testing) or HBeAg positive 2 times at least 6 months apart (Any combination of these tests performed 6 months apart is acceptable.)

*A documented negative HBsAg laboratory result within 6 months before a positive test (either HBsAg, hepatitis B e antigen [HBeAg], or HBV nucleic acid testing [NAT] including genotype) result does not require an acute clinical presentation to meet the surveillance case definition.

ALERT! Persons who have endured and recovered from HBV infection become carriers of inactive HBV.

Hepatitis C

HCV is a virus that targets hepatocytes and B lymphocytes. Acute HCV infection is usually mild, and chronic hepatitis occurs in at least 75% of patients. The mode of transmission is via blood, as in IV drug use, and sexual transmission is possible. HCV can live dormant in the patient for years before symptoms develop.

HCV is a global public health problem and a major cause of both acute and chronic viral hepatitis. The World Health Organization estimates that 170 million individuals worldwide are infected with HCV. In 2019, a total of 4,136 cases of acute hepatitis C were reported to CDC, which is equivalent to 1.3 persons per 100,000 population. This is a conservative estimate as most cases are unreported or undiagnosed. After adjusting for underdiagnosis, an estimated 57,500 acute hepatitis C cases occurred in 2019. Intravenous drug users are at highest risk. The highest rates of HCV occurred in persons aged 20 to 39 years, consistent with age groups most affected by the nation's opioid crisis. Some persons can go on to develop chronic HCV infection. An estimated 2.4 million people in the United States were living with chronic hepatitis C during 2013 to 2016. Chronic HCV infection can progress to hepatic fibrosis, cirrhosis, and hepatocellular carcinoma (HCC).

Etiology. HCV is an RNA virus that is closely related to hepatitis G, dengue, and yellow fever viruses. It can replicate rapidly and can produce at least 10 trillion new viral particles each day. There are six different genotypes of HCV; each has a different severity, response to therapy, and mode of transmission. Approximately 75% of Americans with HCV have genotype 1 of the virus (which can be subtypes 1a or 1b), and 20% to 25% have genotypes 2 or 3, with small numbers of patients infected with genotypes 4, 5, or 6. Most patients with HCV are found to have only one principal genotype, rather than multiple genotypes. Genotype 4 is much more common in Africa, and genotype 6 is common in Southeast Asia. The major HCV genotype worldwide is genotype 1, which accounts for 40% to 80% of all isolates. Genotype 1 is thought to be associated with severe liver disease and a high risk of HCC. Genotypes 1a and 1b are prevalent in the United States. HCV genotype 1 does not respond to therapy as well as other genotypes. Genotypes 2a and 2b are found in 10% to 15% of affected persons in the United States and have good response to therapy.

 CLINICAL CONCEPT

There are many different genotypes of HCV caused by the virus's great potential to mutate.

Transmission of HCV occurs mainly via blood, or less commonly, body fluids. People who inject illegal drugs with nonsterile needles or who use cocaine with shared straws are at highest risk for HCV. Although not common, sexual transmission is possible, particularly in persons with multiple partners or those who partake in anal sexual activity. The screening of donated blood for HCV antibody has decreased the risk of transfusion-associated HCV to fewer than 1 case in 230,000 donations. Health-care providers can contract HCV via needlestick injuries or other occupational exposures. Needlestick injuries in the health-care setting result in a 3% risk of HCV transmission. Nosocomial patient-to-patient transmission may occur by means of contaminated instruments, such as a colonoscope, dialysis equipment, or surgical tools. HCV may also be transmitted via tattooing, sharing razors, and acupuncture. The use of disposable needles for acupuncture, which is standard practice, has eliminated this transmission route. Maternal-fetal transmission is possible but uncommon. Co-infection with HIV type 1 appears to increase the risk of both sexual and maternal–fetal transmission of HCV. Persons with HCV should be tested for HBV and HIV, as these may be transmitted together. It is uncommon for HCV to be transmitted through casual contact; kissing; touching; or sharing cutlery, cups, or dishes.

Pathophysiology. After contracting HCV, the incubation period can vary from 2 weeks to 8 months (see Fig. 31-12). During this time, the patient is asymptomatic and can spread the virus. Although replication of HCV is rapid, it is imperfect. RNA polymerase, an enzyme critical in HCV replication, allows for inaccurate copying of the virus, generating a large number of mutant viruses known as HCV quasispecies; these pose a major challenge to vaccine development. HCV RNA can be detected weeks to months before antibody development and remains detectable indefinitely. After contracting the virus, there is a strong response by cytotoxic T lymphocytes and helper T cells. In most infected people, viremia is accompanied by hepatic inflammation and fibrosis. Acute HCV becomes chronic in 70% of patients.

Clinical Presentation. The patient history may include apparent risk factors for HCV, such as IV drug use. Patients usually present with low-grade fever, nausea, vomiting, fatigue, malaise, jaundice, anorexia, and weight loss. Physical examination signs are similar to other types of viral hepatitis (see Box 31-7). Some people may be asymptomatic. The course of disease is widely erratic, with wide fluctuations in liver enzymes. Most patients progress to a chronic illness or a carrier state. HCV remains one of the causes of end-stage liver disease.

Diagnosis. Diagnostic testing for HCV involves the recombinant immunoblot assay. A positive immunoblot assay result is defined as the detection of antibodies against two or more antigens. HCV RNA assay and HCV genotyping should be performed as well. Genotyping can predict the likelihood of response and duration of treatment. Patients with genotypes 1 and 4 are generally treated for 12 months, whereas 6 months of treatment is sufficient for other genotypes. Liver

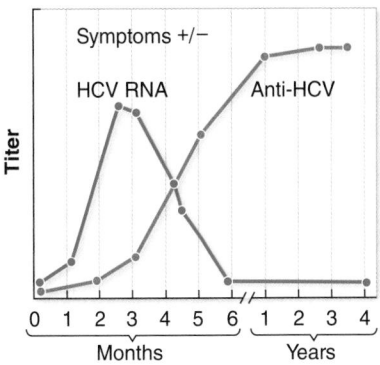

FIGURE 31-12. Timeline of HCV infection. Most patients with chronic HCV infection are asymptomatic or may have nonspecific symptoms for months. The HCV ribonucleic acid (RNA) assay indicates virus particles in the bloodstream. HCV RNA develops within the bloodstream approximately 1 to 2 months after contraction of the virus. Antibodies against HCV develop late in the course of infection, months to years later.

BOX 31-7. Signs and Symptoms of Viral Hepatitis

The following are classic signs and symptoms that occur in viral hepatitis infections:

- Anorexia
- Arthralgias
- Fatigue
- Fever
- Myalgias
- Nausea and vomiting

} Flulike illness

- Dark urine
- Hepatomegaly
- Jaundice
- RUQ tenderness
- Splenomegaly
- Steatorrhea
- Weight loss

BOX 31-8. Diagnosis of HCV Infection: Clinical and Laboratory Criteria

One or more of the following should be present:
- Jaundice, **OR**
- Peak elevated total bilirubin levels ≥ 3.0 mg/dL, **OR**
- Peak elevated serum alanine aminotransferase (ALT) levels >200 IU/L,
  AND

The absence of a more likely diagnosis (which may include evidence of acute liver disease due to other causes or advanced liver disease due to preexisting chronic Hepatitis C virus [HCV] infection or other causes, such as alcohol exposure, other viral hepatitis, hemochromatosis, etc.)

LABORATORY CRITERIA
Confirmatory laboratory evidence:
- Positive hepatitis C virus detection test: Nucleic acid test (NAT) for HCV RNA positive (including qualitative, quantitative, or genotype testing), **OR**
- A positive test indicating presence of hepatitis C viral antigen(s) (HCV antigen)

PRESUMPTIVE LABORATORY EVIDENCE:
- A positive test for antibodies to hepatitis C virus (anti-HCV)

---

biopsy is done when diagnosis is uncertain. In addition, CBC with differential, bilirubin level, liver function tests, thyroid function studies, screening tests for co-infection with HIV or HBV, and screening for alcohol use disorder and substance use disorder should be performed. The CBC demonstrates thrombocytopenia in approximately 10% of patients. Low thyroxine levels are found in approximately 10% of patients as well. (See Box 31-8.)

Treatment. Antiviral drugs are effective for treating HCV infection. Current drug therapy can achieve nondetectable levels of virus in 12 weeks. A sustained virological response is associated with a 99% chance of being HCV RNA negative during long-term follow-up and can therefore be considered cured of the HCV infection. Most drug treatment consists of protease inhibitor combinations, commonly a paritaprevir–ritonavir–ombitasvir-based regimen. A prototype vaccine has not been developed because of rapid HCV viral mutations. Immunoglobulin is ineffective in preventing HCV and is not recommended for postexposure prophylaxis. Health-care personnel who sustain a needle-stick injury involving an HCV-infected patient should undergo HCV RNA assay immediately and then every 2 months for 6 months. If positive, treatment should be commenced.

🩺 CLINICAL CONCEPT

Chronic hepatitis with HCV is common. After acute infection, the persistence of HCV-RNA levels demonstrates chronic infection. Biopsy samples of the liver reveal chronic liver inflammation, and cirrhosis develops in 20% to 50% of patients. Liver failure and HCC can eventually result. HCC occurs in 11% to 19% of patients.

Hepatitis D and Hepatitis E

HDV is a defective RNA virus that requires the helper function of HBV for its replication, expression, and duration. It accelerates the progress of liver disease in those with HBV. HDV can either infect a person simultaneously with HBV or superinfect a person who is already infected with HBV. Similar to HBV, its mode of transmission is parenteral drug use or sexual contact. Because cases of hepatitis D are not clinically distinguishable from other types of acute viral hepatitis, diagnosis can be confirmed only by testing for the presence of antibodies against HDV and/or HDV RNA. HDV infection should be considered in any person with a positive hepatitis B surface antigen (HBsAg) who has severe symptoms of hepatitis or acute exacerbations. No treatment is available for HDV infection specifically. Pegylated interferon alfa has shown some efficacy, but virological response is low (25%). New therapies are being evaluated. In cases of fulminant hepatitis and end-stage liver disease, liver transplantation may be considered. Currently there is no vaccine to prevent hepatitis D. However, prevention of hepatitis B with hepatitis B vaccine also protects against future hepatitis D infection. HEV is clinically similar to HAV, which is spread by the oral–fecal route. The most common source of HEV infection is contaminated drinking water. In developed countries, sporadic cases of HEV have occurred following consumption of uncooked/undercooked pork, deer meat, or shellfish. It is the most common cause of hepatitis in India, Asia, Africa, and Central America, and its actions are similar to those of HAV. Serological testing for HEV infection is not routinely available in the United States. Most people with hepatitis E recover completely with supportive treatment.

Hepatitis G

Hepatitis G virus (HGV) is a rare cause of hepatic inflammation. HGV, also referred to as GB virus type C (GBV-C), is an RNA virus similar to hepatitis C virus. In adults, infection by HGV/GBV-C results in viremia that lasts for months to years, but the virus eventually is cleared by formation of antibody. HGV/GBV-C is transmitted through the same routes as HIV and HCV—blood, injection drug use, sexual activity, and vertical transmission from mother to infant. Active infection is demonstrated by the detection of circulating HGV/GBV-C RNA, and past infection is identified by the presence of antibody to HGV/GBV-C. Coinfection with HGV/GBV-C occurs in greater than 20% of subjects with HCV infection. Ongoing or past infection by HGV/GBV-C is detected in two-thirds or more of IV drug users and patients with HIV. There are no treatments that target HGV specifically. In persons coinfected with HIV and HGV, peginterferon and ribavirin treatment has led to sustained HCV clearance in some patients, with no effect on the course of HIV infection. In patients coinfected with HGV and HCV who were treated with interferon and ribavirin, HGV RNA disappeared from serum during therapy but reappeared in all patients following discontinuation of therapy.

Chronic Hepatitis

Chronic hepatitis occurs as a result of the progression of acute hepatitis. Hepatitis is considered chronic when inflammation and necrosis of hepatic tissue continue for 6 months or longer. Most cases of chronic hepatitis are from autoimmune diseases, drug toxicity, or progression of HBV or HCV. After acute HCV, 85% to 90% of affected individuals suffer chronic infection. Chronic HCV accounts for over 40% of cases of chronic liver disease and patients undergoing liver transplantation. Clinical and laboratory features that suggest progression of acute hepatitis to chronic hepatitis include continual weight loss, anorexia, fatigue, and persistent hepatomegaly. Liver function tests and bilirubin remain elevated for over 6 months.

Chronic hepatitis predisposes a patient to cirrhosis or carcinoma of the liver. Patients with chronic active hepatitis caused by HBV or HCV are considered carriers and can transmit the disease. Treatment for chronic hepatitis is mainly supportive. Patients with end-stage disease may require a liver transplant.

Autoimmune Hepatitis

Autoimmune hepatitis, also called idiopathic hepatitis, is a chronic disorder characterized by inflammation, fibrosis, and necrosis of the liver. In this form of hepatitis, there is no preceding virus or exposure to toxic agents. The hepatic tissue shows evidence of cell-mediated immunological attack with lesions composed of cytotoxic T cells, antinuclear antibodies, and rheumatoid factor. Lymphocytes of patients with this disorder are sensitized to hepatic cell membrane proteins, react against liver cells, and cause hepatocyte destruction. Patients often respond favorably to anti-inflammatory and immunosuppressive agents.

Toxic Hepatitis

Liver injury can follow the inhalation, ingestion, or parenteral administration of some pharmacological and chemical agents. Exposure to certain drugs, such as isoniazid and acetaminophen, or chemicals, such as carbon tetrachloride or vinyl chloride, cause toxic hepatitis. Liver damage may be rapid after contact, depending on the amount of exposure or drug dosage. Most individuals with nonviral hepatitis recover, but some may develop chronic liver damage.

Non–Alcohol-Related Fatty Liver Disease

Non–alcohol-related fatty liver disease (NAFLD) is one the fastest-emerging manifestations of metabolic syndrome worldwide. Non–alcohol-related steatohepatitis (NASH), the progressive form of NAFLD, may culminate in cirrhosis and hepatocellular cancer (HCC), and is presently a leading cause of liver transplant. The number of NAFLD cases in the United States has been increasing from 83.1 million in 2015 and projected to increase to 100.9 million in 2030, a large proportion of which will be persons with NASH. This rise will lead to an increase in the number of patients with cirrhosis and end-stage liver disease, leading to a steep rise in HCC and need for liver transplantation.

Etiology

NAFLD is caused by the build-up of extra fat in liver cells that is not caused by alcohol. It is normal for the liver to contain some fat. However, if more than 5% to 10% percent of the liver's weight is fat, then the condition is called a fatty liver (steatosis).

In some patients, fatty liver is accompanied by hepatic inflammation and scarring. This condition is called non–alcohol-related steatohepatitis (NASH). NASH is the most extreme form of NAFLD, and is regarded as a major cause of cirrhosis of the liver.

The condition most commonly associated with NAFLD is metabolic syndrome, a combination of hyperlipidemia, insulin resistance, and obesity. Other risk factors include diabetes mellitus, protein malnutrition, hypertension, and sleep apnea. Obesity is the most apparent risk factor, with NAFLD risk increasing as individuals' weight increases in the population.

Various drugs, such as amiodarone, tamoxifen, and methotrexate can cause NAFLD (see Box 31-9).

BOX 31-9. Drugs Associated With NAFLD

The following drugs can potentially damage hepato-cytes and initiate the development of NAFLD:
- Amiodarone
- Antiviral drugs (nucleoside analogues)
- Aspirin (as part of Reye's syndrome in children)
- Corticosteroids
- Methotrexate
- Tamoxifen
- Tetracycline

Metabolic abnormalities—such as galactosemia, glycogen storage diseases, homocystinuria, celiac disease, Wilson disease, and tyrosinemia—are also associated with the disorder.

Pathophysiology

Insulin resistance and obesity play important roles in the development of the disease. Under normal conditions, insulin enhances free fatty acid storage in adipose tissue. However, when insulin resistance occurs, fat storage is shifted to nonadipose tissues, such as the liver. Insulin resistance and obesity also result in decreased levels of adiponectin, which inhibits liver gluconeogenesis and suppresses lipogenesis. Therefore, decreased levels of adiponectin increase gluconeogenesis and enhance lipogenesis in the liver. These processes lead to an accumulation of glucose and fat in the liver.

Steatosis is the abnormal accumulation of lipids within a cell. A small amount of fat accumulation within the liver is of no consequence. However, when 5% to 10% of the liver contains fat, this is hepatic steatosis, also called fatty degeneration. The excess lipid accumulates in vesicles that displace the cytoplasm of the hepatocyte. A small amount of fat accumulation within a cell is not detrimental, but large accumulations can disrupt cellular organelles, and in severe cases the cell can rupture. When the vesicles are large enough to distort the nucleus, the condition is known as macrovesicular steatosis; otherwise, the condition is known as microvesicular steatosis. Most patients with NAFLD have microvesicular steatosis and are reported to have a benign clinical course.

A serious complication of NAFLD is NASH. It is theorized that the development of NASH is the result of two types of liver injury, referred to as a two-hit process. With the initial hit, macrovesicular steatosis occurs; this alters the metabolic pathways of uptake, synthesis, degradation, and secretion of free fatty acids within the liver cell. Ultimately, the alteration leads to accumulation of a large amount of lipids in the hepatocytes. Mitochondrial dysfunction occurs because of the large accumulation of fat inside the cell. With mitochondrial dysfunction comes the release of free radicals. These free radicals make the liver susceptible to a second hit, which results in inflammation and progression of liver damage. Proinflammatory cytokines, such as tumor necrosis factor, are believed to play an important role in the progression of liver damage to cirrhosis. NASH cirrhosis is a risk factor for development of HCC.

Clinical Presentation

Individuals with a mild case of NAFLD commonly have no noticeable symptoms, though there has been a correlation with morbid obesity. Most often individuals come to the attention of the clinician because of abnormal liver enzymes on a routine physical examination.

Individuals with NASH usually have obvious liver impairment. Symptoms include fatigue, weakness, loss of appetite, nausea, RUQ abdominal pain, spiderlike blood vessels, yellowing of the skin and eyes (jaundice), ascites, ankle edema, and mental confusion.

Diagnosis

When making the diagnosis of NAFLD, the clinician must rule out all other possible causes of liver disease, such as alcohol use disorder or primary diseases that cause secondary NAFLD. All potentially reversible and treatable causes of fatty liver must be excluded. Serological tests must rule out the possibility of HAV, HBV, or HCV.

There is no one biomarker or blood test yet developed that can diagnose NAFLD with absolute accuracy. The biomarker procollagen C3 can discriminate between patients with or without histological diagnosis of NASH, and it increases with severity of NASH. However, diagnosis of NAFLD is more challenging. Clinicians often assume that the patient with elevated liver enzymes, metabolic syndrome, or type 2 diabetes probably also has NAFLD. However, liver enzymes can be normal in up to 80% of persons with NAFLD. Therefore, biomarkers and noninvasive tests are currently under investigation for diagnosis of NAFLD and NASH.

There are several indices that can be used to determine the presence of NAFLD. The NAFLD Liver Fat Score (NLFS) evaluates the measurement of liver fat content and is calculated based on metabolic syndrome, type 2 diabetes, fasting serum insulin, and fasting serum aspartate aminotransferase/alanine aminotransferase ratio (AAR). The Hepatic Steatosis Index (HSI) is based on liver enzymes AST/ALT ratio, BMI, diabetes, and gender information. The Fatty Liver Index (FLI) includes BMI, waist circumference, and serum levels of triglycerides and the liver enzyme gamma-glutamyltransferase (GGT).

Liver biopsy is the gold standard test in the diagnosis of NASH, but false-negative results are possible if the sample is not obtained from a representative area of the liver with high fat content. Also liver biopsy is highly invasive and can cause pain and bleeding.

Currently, magnetic resonance imaging-derived proton density fat fraction (MRI-PDFF) is the most accurate test for fatty liver diagnosis. However, this test is not available at all medical centers.

The diagnostic test termed transient elastography is an ultrasound-based study that can be used to diagnose NASH. The controlled attenuation parameter (CAP) is a measure of hepatic steatosis using the process of transient elastography. CAP has high diagnostic accuracy in detecting NASH. Another noninvasive test is magnetic resonance elastography (MRE); a technology that combines MRI imaging with low-frequency vibrations to create a visual map (elastogram) that shows stiffness of the liver. Currently, MRE is used to detect liver fibrosis and inflammation in chronic liver disease. At present, not all diagnostic modalities are widely available. However, there is emerging research regarding accurate biomarkers that can be detected in the blood.

Treatment

Treatment is aimed at each component of metabolic syndrome. The patient should be advised about a diet and exercise plan with a goal of that patient's ideal BMI. Physical activity is a key component in alleviating obesity and NAFLD. Low-carbohydrate diets increase high-density lipoprotein (HDL) and reduce serum triglycerides and glucose. Calorie restriction is recommended for improvement of NAFLD and the overall calorie intake is recommended to be 1,200–1,500 kcal/day for females and 1,500–1,800 kcal/day for males. A low fructose diet is recommended. Fructose is a profound lipogenic substrate that stimulates lipogenesis and contributes to the development of NASH. Weight loss of 1 to 2 pounds per week is advisable. In more than 80% of cases, improvements in NASH have been shown with weight loss. Liver enzymes can decrease to normal levels with loss of as little as 4% to 5% of body weight. If a traditional low-calorie diet is unsuccessful, bariatric surgery is recommended for patients with morbid obesity.

Because insulin resistance is a common feature of NAFLD, insulin sensitizers are recommended. Biguanides such as metformin and glitazones such as pioglitazone have been found to lower liver enzymes, enhance cellular insulin sensitivity, and improve NAFLD. Glucagon-like peptide-1 (GLP-1) agonists are also recommended for NAFLD. GLP-1 is an intestinal peptide that stimulates insulin secretion, inhibits glucagon secretion from the pancreas, delays gastric emptying, and suppresses appetite. GLP-1 secretion is reported to be impaired in patients with NAFLD and NASH. Studies suggest that GLP-1 agonists enhance weight loss and reduce fat accumulation in the liver.

Other new medications under investigation include SCD-1 inhibitors. The synthesis of mono-unsaturated fatty acids is catalyzed by the enzyme stearoyl-CoA desaturase 1 (SCD-1) in the liver. Obese patients with NASH have been found to have hyperactivity of SCD-1. Aramchol is an SCD-1 inhibitor that has shown efficacy in decreasing the fat accumulation in NASH. Other new agents under investigation include farsenoid X (FXR) receptor agonists. The farnesoid X receptor is a key regulator of the metabolic pathways of glucose and fat in the liver. Obeticholic acid (OCA) stimulates the FXR and has been shown to decrease the fibrosis of the liver in NASH.

Alcohol-Related Liver Disease

Chronic and excessive ingestion of alcohol is a major cause of liver disease. Alcohol is the most commonly used drug in the United States, and 14 million adults meet the diagnostic criteria for alcohol use disorder.

Alcohol-related hepatitis is an acute disorder that causes a distinct syndrome of reversible and transient symptoms; it can resolve if ingestion of alcohol ceases, but long-term effects often remain. Alcohol-related liver disease, also known as alcohol-related cirrhosis, is a pathological condition that develops over a long period and is permanent. It can be diagnosed by the presence of histopathological changes in the liver.

In the United States, alcohol-related liver disease affects more than 2 million people, or approximately 1% of the population. However, this is believed to be a low estimate because individuals commonly will not admit to heavy alcohol use. Alcohol is directly hepatotoxic; between 10% and 20% of patients with alcohol use disorder develop alcoholic hepatitis. There is no known genetic predisposition, but alcohol abuse tends to run in families. Alcoholism and alcoholic liver disease are more common in minority groups, particularly among Native Americans, than other nationalities. Alcohol-related liver disease is one of the main causes of chronic liver disease worldwide and accounts for up to 48% of cirrhosis-associated deaths in the United States. Alcohol-related cirrhosis of the liver causes severe functional impairment, and the prognosis is poor, with a mortality rate of nearly 60% at 4 years after diagnosis.

Etiology

The time it takes to develop alcohol-related liver disease is dependent on the amount of alcohol consumed. The alcohol content of one beer or 4 ounces of wine is approximately 12 grams. Alcohol-related liver disease usually develops in males who ingest more than 60 to 80 grams of alcohol per day for 10 years, whereas for females this amount is 20 to 40 grams per day for 10 years. Ingestion of 160 grams per day is associated with a 25-fold increased risk of developing alcohol-related liver disease.

Pathophysiology

Alcohol is a potent toxin to hepatocytes. Hepatocytes can sustain injury and regenerate but have a low tolerance for repeated damage. Repeated bouts of alcohol-related hepatitis will lead to alcohol-related liver disease. The initial cellular change that takes place with excessive, chronic alcohol abuse is steatosis. Fatty liver develops in every individual who consumes more than 60 grams of alcohol per day. Chronic ingestion of ethanol inhibits the oxidation of fatty acids in the liver. Fat accumulates in and around hepatocytes as constant alcohol use occurs, and this fat accumulation within the hepatocyte disrupts the integrity of the organelles. Nuclear disruption causes death of the hepatocytes. Disrupting the mitochondria leads to free radical release and inflammation.

 CLINICAL CONCEPT

A distinctive histological sign of alcohol-related hepatitis found on biopsy is the Mallory body—a filamentous structure composed of keratin within a swollen hepatocyte. After fatty liver develops, large areas of hepatocyte injury, necrosis, inflammation, and fibrosis occur. When the liver demonstrates fibrosis and scar tissue, the disorder is referred to as cirrhosis.

About 50% of alcohol-related hepatitis patients will progress to alcohol-related liver disease and cirrhosis, with poor prognosis for recovery. If alcohol use ceases, alcohol-related hepatitis can resolve slowly over weeks to months, sometimes without permanent sequelae but often with residual cirrhosis.

Clinical Presentation

The diagnosis of alcohol-related liver disease requires an accurate history of alcohol amount and duration. The condition is frequently discovered by a primary care provider in a routine examination of a patient for an unrelated matter. It is common for the patient not to admit to an excessive amount of alcohol use. Sensitive inquiry is required by the provider. Alcohol use assessment tools exist that ask standard, validated questions of the patient. Both the health-care provider and patient can review these questions together to assess alcohol use. The primary screening tool to detect alcohol use disorder and dependence is AUDIT, a 10-item questionnaire, which has been validated as a clinical tool for the accurate detection of alcohol consumption.

Clues to the presence of alcohol use disorder include a history of multiple motor vehicle accidents, convictions for driving while intoxicated, and poor interpersonal relationships. Alcohol use disorder exhibits a genetic predisposition, and a history of alcohol use disorder in a close relative may also indicate that a patient is at risk.

Signs and Symptoms. Patients with acute alcohol-related hepatitis typically present with mild, non-specific symptoms of RUQ pain, nausea, malaise, and low-grade fever. Jaundice and darkened urine may be present because of liver dysfunction and bilirubin accumulation in the bloodstream. The liver is usually enlarged, often with mild hepatic tenderness. The short-term prognosis is good, and no specific treatment is required.

In contrast, individuals with severe alcohol-related hepatitis are at high risk of death. The patient may present with signs of severe liver dysfunction, such as hepatic encephalopathy—confusion, disorientation, or stupor. There may be coagulation dysfunction, which causes spontaneous bruising and bleeding. Hyperbilirubinemia may be present and cause jaundice. The patient may exhibit GI bleeding via hematemesis.

Liver disease caused by chronic alcohol use disorder is more common than acute alcohol-related hepatitis. Malnutrition of variable degree and muscle wasting is present in most patients with chronic alcohol use disorder. Other signs include Dupuytren contracture, rhinophyma, spider angioma, palmar erythema, and evidence of portal hypertension. Signs of portal hypertension include splenomegaly, ascites, and esophageal varices. Esophageal varices are apparent on endoscopy. Ascites is demonstrated by abdominal distention. The physical examination of the abdomen demonstrates bulging flanks with shifting abdominal dullness when the patient is in the supine position.

A person who uses alcohol heavily may come to medical attention because of another medical illness that requires abstention of alcohol as part of recovery. The patient may not admit to alcohol use disorder or recognize the problem. Frequently during this time, patients with alcohol use disorder develop withdrawal symptoms of restlessness, mood disturbance, tremors called delirium tremens, and, possibly, seizures.

 CLINICAL CONCEPT

Decreased synthesis of coagulation factors occurs in patients with alcohol use disorder due to effects on the liver. This can lead to increased risk of bleeding esophageal varices and subdural hematoma in head injury.

Diagnosis

Patients with alcohol-related liver disease are often identified through abnormal diagnostic study results. Modest elevation of liver enzymes accompanied by hypertriglyceridemia, hypercholesterolemia, and, at times, hyperbilirubinemia are present. In alcohol-related cirrhosis specifically, aspartate aminotransferase (AST) and alanine aminotransaminase (ALT) liver enzymes are elevated from two- to sevenfold. Hypoalbuminemia and coagulation disturbances indicate severe liver dysfunction. Carbohydrate-deficient transferrin (CDT) combined with gamma-glutamyl transferase (GGT), another liver enzyme, has sensitivity of about 75% to 90% to detect alcohol use disorder. Newer biomarkers using metabolites of alcohol such as ethyl glucuronide can reveal alcohol use up to 3 to 4 days after the last alcoholic drink. However, due to its high sensitivity, it can yield false-positive results. Measurement of ethyl glucuronide in hair samples can detect alcohol use for a longer period of up to 1 month.

Treatment

Alcohol withdrawal syndrome (AWS) can occur in alcohol-dependent patients who abruptly cease alcohol consumption. AWS usually develops within 6 to 24 hours after the last alcoholic drink. Symptoms may include nausea/vomiting, hypertension, tachycardia, tremors, hyperreflexia, irritability, anxiety, and headache. These symptoms may progress to more severe forms of AWS, which is associated with delirium tremens, generalized seizures, and coma. Patients with AWS require close monitoring of vital signs, volume status, and neurological function. Supplemental folate and thiamine are recommended. Vitamin K should be administered parenterally.

After the acute syndrome is resolved, alcohol cessation, psychological support, and nutritional consultation are key aspects of treatment. Many pharmacological agents have been used for treatment of alcohol use disorder including disulfiram, acamprosate, gabapentin, naltrexone, topiramate, sertraline, and baclofen. Of these, only baclofen is safe in patients with alcohol-related liver disease and cirrhosis. Benzodiazepines are the most commonly used drugs to treat AWS to protect against seizures and delirium. Integrated therapy with cognitive behavioral therapy, medical care, rehabilitation, and support group interventions are recommended for alcohol use disorder.

CLINICAL CONCEPT

Cirrhosis of the liver and liver failure may be the outcome of alcohol-related liver disease. Patients with alcohol-related hepatitis may have improvement of liver function if there is 6 months of abstinence from alcohol. If cirrhosis develops, they can be considered for liver transplantation if they remain committed to sustained abstinence.

Cirrhosis and End-Stage Liver Disease

Chronic liver disease and cirrhosis result in about 35,000 deaths each year in the United States. Cirrhosis is the ninth leading cause of death in the United States and is responsible for 1.2% of all U.S. deaths. The majority of cases are currently attributed to excessive alcohol consumption and viral hepatitis. Many patients die of the disease in their fifth or sixth decade

of life. The incidence of non–alcohol-related fatty liver disease (NAFLD) and non–alcohol-related steatohepatitis (NASH) is expected to rise in the near future. Estimates suggest that non–alcohol-related steatohepatitis will become the leading cause of cirrhosis in the United States sometime between 2025 and 2035.

Cirrhosis often is a silent and gradual disease; most patients remain asymptomatic until a late stage of liver impairment marked by ascites, spontaneous bacterial peritonitis, hepatic encephalopathy, or variceal bleeding from portal hypertension. The liver becomes irreversibly damaged with collagen and connective tissue infiltration.

Established cirrhosis has a 10-year mortality of 34% to 66%, largely dependent on the cause of the cirrhosis; alcohol-related cirrhosis has a worse prognosis. The incidence of cirrhosis is higher in males than in females.

Etiology

The most common causes of cirrhosis of the liver are HCV, alcohol-related liver disease, and NAFLD. HCV often causes chronic inflammation, which leads to cirrhosis or liver cancer. Cirrhosis, the final stage of liver injury, can be caused by many different etiologies (see Box 31-10).

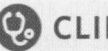 CLINICAL CONCEPT

HCV is the major cause of cirrhosis of the liver in the United States. Alcohol use disorder, the major cause of cirrhosis in years past, is second to HCV.

BOX 31-10. Common Causes of Cirrhosis of the Liver

A wide range of diseases and conditions can damage the liver and lead to cirrhosis.
Some of the causes include:
- Chronic alcohol use disorder
- Chronic viral hepatitis (hepatitis B, C, and D)
- Non–alcohol-related fatty liver disease
- Hemochromatosis
- Cystic fibrosis
- Wilson's disease
- Alpha-1 antitrypsin deficiency
- Inherited disorders of sugar metabolism (galactosemia or glycogen storage disease)
- Autoimmune hepatitis
- Primary biliary cirrhosis (cholangitis)
- Primary sclerosing cholangitis
- Infection, such as syphilis or brucellosis
- Many medications, including methotrexate, acetaminophen, or isoniazid

Pathophysiology

In cirrhosis, the liver undergoes structural changes and fails to function. Stellate cells, which usually comprise the extracellular matrix of the liver, become stimulated by cell injury. The cells produce an abundant amount of collagenous fibrous tissue, which interferes with hepatocyte function. Stellate cells also exert a constrictive effect on the liver's portal venous system. Collagen infiltration increases liver density and changes the liver's structural architecture. On autopsy, the liver is severely scarred and distorted in shape (see Fig. 31-13). The progression of liver injury to cirrhosis usually occurs over years. Portal hypertension, an elevated pressure within the portal vein, is a key pathophysiological change associated with cirrhosis.

Portal Hypertension. A significant pathophysiological occurrence in cirrhosis is the increased resistance within the portal vein termed **portal hypertension** (see Fig. 31-14). The portal vein drains the venous circulation of the GI system. The intestine, spleen, pancreas, stomach, and esophagus have venous networks that drain into the portal vein, which empties into the inferior vena cava. As cirrhosis develops, large veins develop collateral branches that initially decrease pressure within the portal vein. However, as cirrhosis worsens, pressure within the portal vein increases, causing backup of pressure to the GI veins and collaterals. Dilated, superficial veins become visible around the umbilicus, a sign referred to as **caput medusa.** Increased venous pressure builds within the vascular beds of the GI system, producing splenomegaly, esophageal varices, rectal varices, and eventually ascites. The esophageal veins and rectal veins are fragile submucosal veins that are prone to rupture; ruptured esophageal veins can cause vomiting of blood (hematemesis), whereas ruptured rectal veins can cause rectal bleeding.

Decreased Detoxification Capability. Patients on some medications may experience the toxic effects of drugs caused by lack of liver metabolism in cirrhosis.

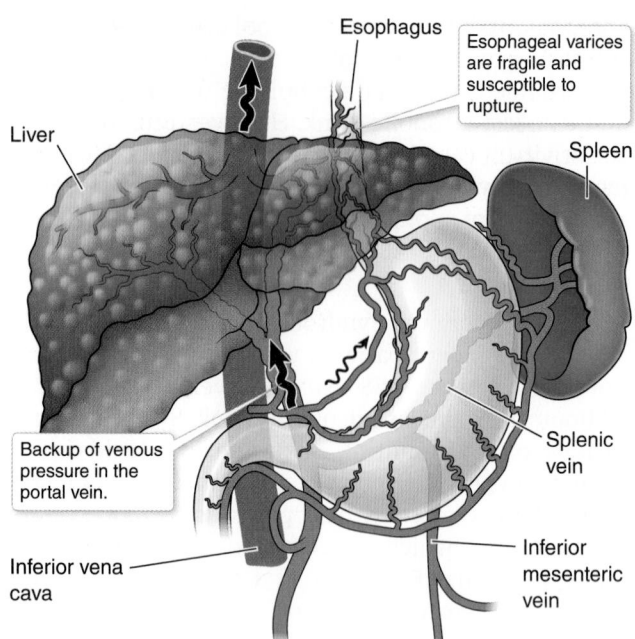

FIGURE 31-14. Portal hypertension. High blood pressure within the portal vein is referred to as portal hypertension. This heightened venous pressure causes backup of pressure within all the veins of the gastrointestinal system. The veins at the lower end of the esophagus become distended and are referred to as esophageal varices. The vein walls become fragile and tend to rupture, causing bleeding in the form of hematemesis.

Nitrogenous wastes accumulate in the blood, causing high ammonia (NH_3) levels; this increases susceptibility to encephalopathy. Lethargy, confusion, and inability to concentrate are initial signs of encephalopathy. Stupor and coma are late signs.

Decreased Bile Synthesis. Diminished synthesis of bile by the cirrhotic liver will cause problems with fat digestion. Undigested fat in the digestive system leads to steatorrhea. Excretion of undigested fat eventually causes decreased stores of fat-soluble vitamins A, D, E, and K.

Decreased Albumin Synthesis. Decreased synthesis of albumin by the liver causes nutritional deficiency and decreased colloid oncotic pressure. According to Starling's Law of Capillary Forces, decreased colloid oncotic pressure will allow hydrostatic pressure to go unbalanced. Hydrostatic pressure causes edema, which is most apparent in the peritoneal cavity as ascites. Edema can occur in the pulmonary system, causing impaired pulmonary function. Pleural effusions and the diaphragmatic elevation caused by massive ascites may alter the ventilation-perfusion ratio.

Hyperbilirubinemia. The liver has a decreased ability to process bilirubin, which is the product of degenerated RBCs. Bilirubin builds within the bloodstream and causes jaundice of skin and sclera. High bilirubin levels can also cause kernicterus, also called bilirubin

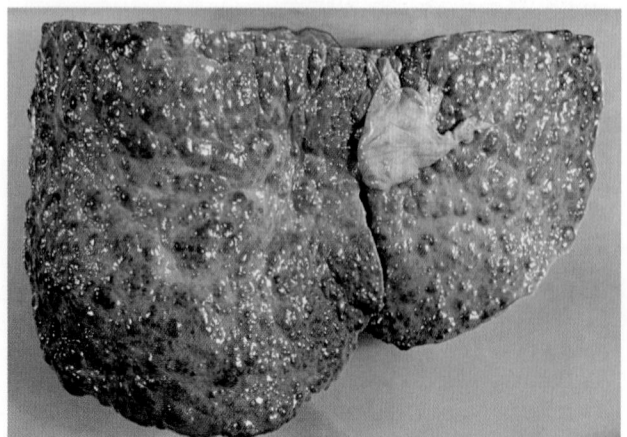

FIGURE 31-13. Cirrhosis of the liver. *(From Biophoto Associates/Science Source.)*

encephalopathy, which can cause confusion, lethargy, and stupor to coma.

Bleeding of Esophageal Varices. In portal hypertension, venous drainage backs up within the GI system; this causes congestion within the spleen, as well as in intestinal, gastric, and esophageal veins. Esophageal veins become distended and evolve into varicose veins. Because of their fragility, they easily rupture, causing bleeding at the gastroesophageal junction; this leads to hematemesis.

 CLINICAL CONCEPT

In hematemesis, blood mixed with gastric fluids and acid is often referred to as "coffee-ground emesis" because of its appearance.

Coagulopathy. As cirrhosis develops, coagulation factors fail to be synthesized. In addition, patients may have thrombocytopenia from hypersplenism caused by portal hypertension. A prolonged PT is a laboratory test that indicates clotting deficiency. The patient can exhibit spontaneous bruising, nosebleeds, and hematemesis. Bleeding of the dilated varices in the esophagus and rectum often occurs.

 CLINICAL CONCEPT

Patients with cirrhosis may have spontaneous bleeding or bruising caused by low coagulation factors.

Osteoporosis Osteoporosis is common in patients with liver disease caused by malabsorption of vitamin D and decreased calcium ingestion. The rate of bone resorption exceeds bone formation in cirrhosis.

 CLINICAL CONCEPT

Low vitamin D causes lack of calcium absorption from the GI tract, leading to bone demineralization.

Hepatic Encephalopathy. Hepatic encephalopathy is an alteration of mental status and cognitive function in the presence of liver failure. Its development in patients with cirrhosis is associated with a grave prognosis. Patients can exhibit confusion, personality change, or stupor. GI toxins and nitrogenous wastes, such as NH_3 (ammonia) that are not removed by the liver, affect the brain. Patients exhibit symptoms from

confusion and disorientation to stupor and coma. **Asterixis,** which is a flapping tremor of the hands, may be present with hepatic encephalopathy. Cerebral edema can occur in severe encephalopathy; in addition, brain herniation is a serious complication.

 CLINICAL CONCEPT

Asterixis is elicited by having the patients extend their arms and bend the wrists backward. In this maneuver, patients with hepatic encephalopathy have a sudden forward movement of the wrist, known as a "liver flap."

Spontaneous Bacterial Peritonitis. Spontaneous bacterial peritonitis may develop in patients with alcohol-related hepatitis and ascites, especially in those with concomitant GI bleeding. Bacterial translocation is the presumed mechanism, with GI bacterial flora traveling from the intestine into the mesenteric lymph nodes, ascitic fluid, and bloodstream. The most common organisms are *Escherichia coli, Streptococcus viridans, Staphylococcus aureus,* and *Enterococcus.*

Iron Overload. As many as 50% of patients with alcohol-related liver disease have increased hepatic iron content. This excess deposition of iron may play a significant role in the progression of alcohol-related liver damage. Occasionally, this excessive iron deposition leads to hemochromatosis.

Anemia and Thrombocytopenia. Anemia may result from folate deficiency, hemolysis, or hypersplenism. Thrombocytopenia usually is secondary to hypersplenism and decreased levels of thrombopoietin.

 CLINICAL CONCEPT

Thiamine and folic acid deficiency are common in alcohol-related cirrhosis of the liver.

Hepatorenal Syndrome. Hepatorenal syndrome (HRS) is a type of renal failure that occurs in approximately 10% of patients with cirrhosis. For unclear reasons, the kidney vessels undergo vasoconstriction; progressive impairment of renal function then occurs. HRS is often seen in patients with a large amount of ascites.

Clinical Presentation

Some patients with cirrhosis are completely asymptomatic and have a normal life expectancy. Others experience many of the most severe symptoms of end-stage liver disease and have a poor prognosis (see Fig. 31-15). Common signs and symptoms of

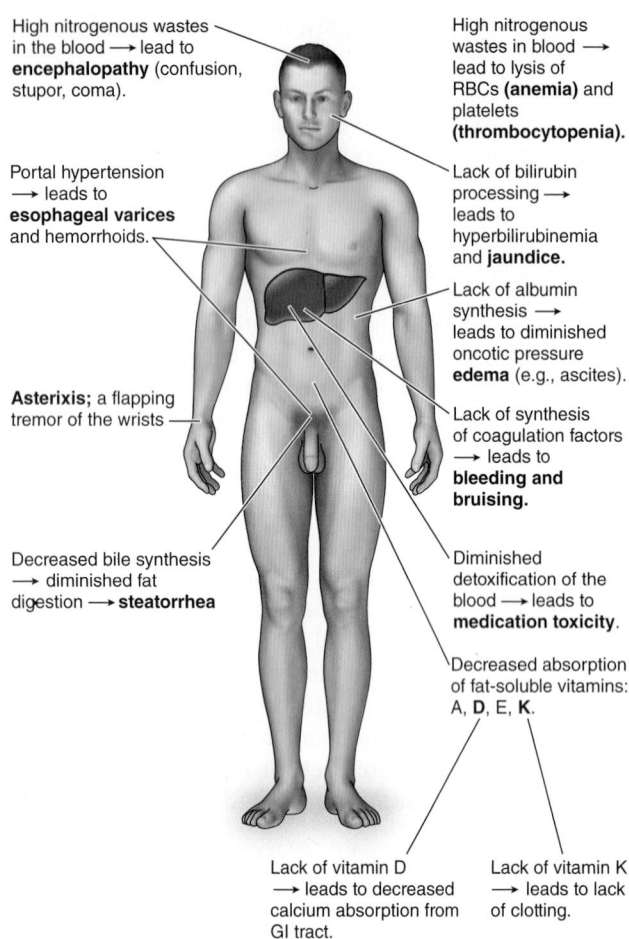

High nitrogenous wastes in the blood → lead to **encephalopathy** (confusion, stupor, coma).

High nitrogenous wastes in blood → lead to lysis of RBCs **(anemia)** and platelets **(thrombocytopenia)**.

Portal hypertension → leads to **esophageal varices** and hemorrhoids.

Lack of bilirubin processing → leads to hyperbilirubinemia and **jaundice**.

Lack of albumin synthesis → leads to diminished oncotic pressure **edema** (e.g., ascites).

Lack of synthesis of coagulation factors → leads to **bleeding and bruising**.

Asterixis; a flapping tremor of the wrists

Decreased bile synthesis → diminished fat digestion → **steatorrhea**

Diminished detoxification of the blood → leads to **medication toxicity**.

Decreased absorption of fat-soluble vitamins: A, **D**, E, **K**.

Lack of vitamin D → leads to decreased calcium absorption from GI tract.

Lack of vitamin K → leads to lack of clotting.

FIGURE 31-15. The widespread effects of liver failure.

cirrhosis are caused by decreased hepatic synthetic function, decreased detoxification capabilities of the liver, or portal hypertension.

In the history, the patient should be asked about risk factors for HBV and HCV, as these infections can lead to chronic hepatitis and cirrhosis. The patient should also be asked about possible exposures to hepatotoxic substances or chronic use of alcohol. Obesity, diabetes, and hypertriglyceridemia are often present in those with NAFLD. The patient may present with symptoms of severe liver dysfunction such as jaundice, steatorrhea, and darkened urine. Some patients may present with symptoms of portal hypertension, such as ascites and hematemesis caused by esophageal varices.

> ### 🩺 CLINICAL CONCEPT
>
> Signs of portal vein hypertension include ascites, splenomegaly, esophageal varies, caput medusa, and hemorrhoids.

Signs and Symptoms. Patients with cirrhosis usually complain of fatigue, anorexia, and weight loss. Dermatological manifestations of cirrhosis include jaundice (yellowing of the sclera), spider angiomata, skin telangiectasias, petechiae, palmar erythema, and finger clubbing. Pruritus often develops because of accumulation of bile salts in the bloodstream. Muscle wasting and ascites are common because of protein loss. Males may develop gynecomastia and impotence. Loss of axillary and pubic hair is noted in both males and females. Signs of portal hypertension, such as ascites and caput medusa, are often present. Dupuytren contracture, a progressive fibrosis of the palmar fascia limiting extension of fingers, can be caused by chronic alcohol use disorder. Fetor hepaticus is a sweet odor of breath due to dimethyl sulfide.

Diagnosis

Early in cirrhosis, laboratory tests can be normal. With progression, however, many different abnormalities become apparent. Low albumin, thrombocytopenia, and elevated liver enzymes AST, ALT, and gamma-glutamyl transferase are common. Platelet count is often reduced early in disease, which is caused by hypersplenism of portal hypertension. Serum bilirubin can be elevated with jaundice exhibited by the patient. PT is often prolonged due to coagulation factor disruption. Patients may be anemic if there is GI blood loss from esophageal varices or bone marrow suppression of RBC synthesis by alcohol. Viral hepatitis serologies, ferritin, and transferrin saturation should be ordered.

Liver biopsy remains the gold standard for assessing fibrosis of the liver; however, use of noninvasive methods has become increasingly common in clinical practice. Transient elastography, an ultrasound technique, is rapidly replacing biopsy as the preferred method for fibrosis staging. A Fibro-scan determines liver stiffness in kilopascals (kPa) by measuring the velocity of low-frequency elastic shear waves propagating through the liver. Liver stiffness greater than 20 kPa, low platelet count, increased spleen size, and/or the presence of portosystemic collaterals on imaging can diagnose portal hypertension and warrant endoscopic screening for esophageal varices. The severity of fibrosis of the liver can be scored using the Metavir Scoring System. There are four grades of liver fibrosis; beginning with no fibrosis as F0, minimal fibrosis as F1, to F4 which is cirrhosis with advanced liver scar tissue.

Staging Cirrhosis

After the diagnosis of cirrhosis is established, Child-Turcotte-Pugh and Model for End-Stage Liver Disease scores should be used to identify the stage of cirrhosis and mortality risk, respectively. The Child-Turcotte-Pugh scoring system was designed to predict mortality in cirrhosis patients. It is based on presence and severity of encephalopathy, ascites, bilirubin level, albumin level, and prothrombin time or INR values. A score is summed for these assessments and parameters (see Table 31-4).

TABLE 31-4. Child-Turcotte-Pugh Score for Staging Cirrhosis

CHILD-TURCOTTE-PUGH CLASSIFICATION FOR SEVERITY OF CIRRHOSIS

Clinical and Laboratory Criteria	Points*		
	1	**2**	**3**
Encephalopathy	None	Mild to moderate (grade 1 or 2)	Severe (grade 3 or 4)
Ascites	None	Mild to moderate (diuretic responsive)	Severe (diuretic refractory)
Bilirubin (mg/dL)	<2	2–3	>3
Albumin (g/dL)	>3.5	2.8–3.5	<2.8
Prothrombin time 　Seconds prolonged 　International normalized ratio	 <4 <1.7	 4–6 1.7–2.3	 >6 >2.3

*CHILD-TURCOTTE-PUGH CLASS OBTAINED BY ADDING SCORE FOR EACH PARAMETER (TOTAL POINTS)

Class A = 5 to 6 points (least severe liver disease)

Class B = 7 to 9 points (moderately severe liver disease)

Class C = 10 to 15 points (most severe liver disease)

The Child-Turcotte-Pugh (CTP) classification system utilizes two clinical parameters (encephalopathy and ascites) and three laboratory values (bilirubin, albumin, and prothrombin time). Patients are classified as class A, B, or C based on their total points.

Sources: D'Amico, G., Garcia-Tsao, G., & Pagliaro, L. (2006). Natural history and prognostic indicators of survival in cirrhosis: A systematic review of 118 studies. *J Hepatol, 44*(1), 217–231. doi: 10.1016/j.jhep.2005.10.013; D'Amico, G., Morabito, A., Pagliaro, L., & Marubini, E. (1986). Survival and prognostic indicators in compensated and decompensated cirrhosis. *Dig Dis Sci, 31*(5), 468–475. doi: 10.1007/BF01320309

Severity of End-Stage Liver Disease

The Model for End-Stage Liver Disease (MELD) score is used as a predictor of survival in patients with cirrhosis, alcohol-related hepatitis, acute liver failure, and in patients with acute hepatitis. The MELD score is often used in the decision regarding which patients warrant liver transplantation. It estimates a patient's chances of surviving their disease during the next 3 months. Organ allocation is determined by the Organ Procurement and Transplantation Network (OPTN). Livers from deceased donors are allocated to the sickest patients first.

The MELD score ranges from 6 to 40 and is based on results from several laboratory tests. The higher the number, the more likely a patient is to receive a liver from a deceased donor when an organ becomes available. The MELD score is based on results from four blood tests:

- INR (internal normalized ratio): indicates whether the liver is manufacturing coagulation factors
- Creatinine: indicates function of the kidneys
- Bilirubin: indicates how well the liver is releasing bile
- Serum sodium: indicates fluid balance

Persons with a MELD score less than 15 are often not listed for a liver transplant because their chance of receiving a liver through traditional allocation is low. However, a living-donor liver transplant is an alternate life-saving option and the opportunity to receive a transplant sooner. By exploring a living donor transplant, patients with a low MELD score can still be considered for a liver transplant.

Treatment of Cirrhosis and End-Stage Liver Disease

The primary goals of treatment of cirrhosis and end-stage liver disease are to prevent complications and death. For patients with cirrhosis, a basic metabolic panel, liver function tests, complete blood count, and PT/INR should be completed every 6 months to recalculate Child-Turcotte-Pugh and MELD scores. Patients with a MELD score of 15 or higher should be referred for liver transplantation evaluation; patients with ascites, hepatic encephalopathy, or variceal hemorrhage should also be referred.

Patients need counseling and therapy to completely abstain from alcohol use. Obesity and diabetes management are necessary. Patients need to avoid bacterial infection. They should abstain from seafood as contaminated water can cause infection which can be

Patho-Pharm Connection

Liver Failure

Diuretic
(spironolactone) and
Alpha-adrenergic agonist
(midodrine, clonidine)

Decreased albumin production leads to hypoalbuminemia, which cause low colloid osmotic pressure ⟶ Edema (ascites). Diuretic decreases edema; alpha-adrenergic agonists enhance diuresis.

Nonselective beta blockers
(propranolol, nadolol)

Decrease blood pressure in the liver; treat portal hypertension

Bile acid sequestrant
(cholestyramine)

Binds to bile salts that cause pruritus

HMG-CoA reductase inhibitors (statins)
(e.g., lovastatin)

In some liver disease, cholesterol excretion is impaired, which causes hypercholesterolemia.

Fibrates (e.g., gemfibrozil)
In some liver disease, triglycerides are elevated; fibrates treat hypertriglyceridemia.

Proton pump inhibitor
(esomeprazole)

Histamine-2 blocker
(famotidine)

Decrease GERD, which can lead to irritation of fragile esophageal varices

Nonabsorbable disaccharides
(lactulose, rifaximin)

Bind high ammonia levels (NH_3) ⟶ hepatic encephalopathy treatment

Liver failure due to acetaminophen toxcity

Treatment: acetylcysteine

Vitamin D
Vitamin K

Due to decreased absorption of fat-soluble vitamins

A number of medications are used in patients with liver failure to counteract the complications due to lack of liver function. Fluid retention is a significant problem in liver failure due to lack of synthesis of albumin. Albumin is the major colloid oncotic protein, which exerts pressure within the bloodstream. With lack of albumin, there is lack of oncotic pressure within the bloodstream allowing hydrostatic pressure to cause edema. Diuretics such as spironolactone enhance diuresis to rid the body of fluid. Alpha adrenergic agonists such as midodrine or clonidine can be used to boost the effect of diuretics to decrease the fluid retention. In liver failure, portal vein blood pressure increases, termed portal hypertension. This pressure can

be decreased using nonselective beta-adrenergic blockers such as propranolol or nadolol. Esophageal varices are common in liver failure due to increased portal vein pressure. These distended veins are fragile and esophageal vein bleeding can occur. Stomach acid is suppressed prophylactically to decrease risk of irritation of the distended veins in the lower esophagus. Proton pump inhibitors such as esomeprazole and histamine-2 blockers such as famotidine are used to suppress acid. Nitrogenous wastes accumulate in liver failure due to the lack of the detoxification function of the liver. The nitrogen combines with hydrogen to create ammonia (NH_3) in the bloodstream. NH_3 accumulation causes hepatic encephalopathy and

Patho-Pharm Connection–cont'd

confusion, which can lead to stupor and coma. To rid the body of this excess blood nitrogen, lactulose or rifaximin enhance loss of NH_3 from the bowel. Bile back-up in the liver causes bile salt accumulation in the bloodstream, which causes extreme pruritus. To decrease this complication, cholestyramine is used, which binds to bile salts. In liver dysfunction, cholesterol and triglyceride excretion can be decreased, which causes accumulation in the bloodstream; hypercholesterolemia and hypertriglyceridemia. HMG-CoA reductase inhibitors (statins) and fibrates can be used to decrease these blood levels of cholesterol and triglycerides. Loss of fat in the stool occurs, which also causes excretion of fat-soluble vitamins D and K. These vitamin supplements are necessary. If liver failure is caused by acetaminophen overdose, acetylcysteine is the antidote.

---

fatal. Also unpasteurized products can contain *Listeria* and must be avoided.

Vaccinations are necessary with yearly flu vaccine, pneumococcal vaccine, and hepatitis A and B vaccine. Pain relievers, particularly acetaminophen, should be limited; NSAIDs should not be used. Benzodiazepines and opiates should be avoided. Iron supplements should also be avoided. Numerous pharmacological agents can be used to manage the symptoms associated with end-stage liver disease (see Patho-Pharm Connection feature).

Studies have demonstrated biopsy-proven fibrosis improvement rates as high as 88% after antiviral treatment in patients with HBV and HCV and as high as 85% after bariatric surgery in patients with NASH.

Esophageal varices, hepatic encephalopathy, spontaneous peritonitis, hepatorenal syndrome, and ascites are complications that require critical care management.

Biliary Cholangitis

Biliary cholangitis is a cholestatic disease in which bile production is dysfunctional. It is caused by prolonged obstruction of the intrahepatic or extrahepatic biliary system that can evolve into cirrhosis. The prevalence ranges from 20 to 40 cases per 100,000 individuals. It occurs more often in females than males, mainly in the fifth or sixth decade of life. It can be a primary disorder with autoimmune etiology or it can occur secondary to another disorder.

Etiology and Pathophysiology

Inflammation and fibrous destruction of the intrahepatic bile ductules are the tissue evidence of primary biliary cholangitis (PBC). It is an autoimmune disease in genetically susceptible people. PBC is associated with HLA complex single nucleotide polymorphisms on chromosome 6p21. The *HLA DRB1*08* is a predisposing allele and *HLADRB1*11* and *DRB1*13* are protective alleles. A mutation located on chromosome 11q23.1 is also related to susceptibility to PBC. Antimitochondrial antibodies and specific antinuclear antibodies are specifically found in the disease. The positivity of these antibodies and a biochemical cholestasis are sufficient for diagnosis, without the need for liver biopsy. There are four developmental stages for PBC:

- **Stage I:** inflammation of the portal triads and destruction of small and medium bile ducts
- **Stage II:** inflammation progresses with a decrease in the number of bile ducts
- **Stage III:** destruction of liver cells, taking over of hepatic cells by fibrotic tissue, and loss of intralobular bile ducts
- **Stage IV:** development of micronodular or macronodular cirrhosis

In secondary biliary cirrhosis, chronic destruction of larger hepatic ducts occurs from prolonged obstruction by postoperative adhesions or gallstones. Unrelieved blockage of the extrahepatic bile ducts will cause bile stasis with areas of necrosis. The portal bile ducts enlarge with infiltration of the surrounding tissue with WBCs. The fibrotic ducts then expand and rupture, with bile exuding into the necrotic tissue, forming "lakes of bile." The liver tissue regenerates into a nodular cirrhosis with loss of metabolic and chemical function.

Clinical Presentation

In the early stages, most patients are asymptomatic; if biliary cirrhosis is found at this stage, it is usually during a routine screening, when the patient's alkaline phosphatase level is elevated. Common signs with advancing stages include jaundice; steatorrhea; pruritus, especially of the palms; and elevated lipid levels that lead to xanthelasmas, which are cholesterol deposits around the eyes. Signs and symptoms of portal hypertension and ascites develop as the disease worsens. Osteomalacia, with accelerated osteoporosis, occurs as the disease progresses because of decreased vitamin D absorption. Raynaud's phenomenon and esophageal motility disorder are common.

Diagnosis

An elevation of liver enzymes is seen in most patients with PBC, but significant elevations of immunoglobulin levels (mainly IgM) are usually the most prominent findings. Lipid levels and cholesterol levels may be increased, with an increased high-density lipoprotein fraction. An increased erythrocyte sedimentation rate is another finding. As the disease progresses to cirrhosis, an elevated bilirubin level, a prolonged PT, and a decreased albumin level can be found. The increased bilirubin level is an ominous sign of disease progression, and liver transplantation must be considered. The hallmark of this disease is the presence of antimitochondrial antibodies (AMAs) in the blood. AMAs can be found in 90% to 95% of patients with PBC.

 CLINICAL CONCEPT

AMAs are key findings in the diagnosis of PBC.

Treatment

Ursodeoxycholic acid (UDCA) is the specific treatment with an excellent response in more than 60% of patients. The use of UDCA in PBC delays progression of liver disease. However, 40% of PBC patients do not respond adequately to UDCA, and these patients are at high risk for serious complications. Obeticholic acid (OCA), a farsenoid X (FXR) agonist, has been studied in PBC patients with inadequate response to UDCA and shown promising results. In combination with UDCA the treatment has led to significant reduction of serum alkaline phosphatase (ALP, an important prognostic marker in PBC).

The goal of therapy should be the normalization of ALP and bilirubin below 0.6, the upper limit of normal. Bezafibrate is another option in patients with inadequate response to UDCA. Triple therapy with UDCA, OCA, and bezafibrate may be considered in patients showing inadequate response to dual therapy. Finally, budesonide may be considered in patients refractory to treatments who have marked portal inflammation. New research shows that a monoclonal antibody that targets B cells, rituximab, is showing promising results in persons with PBC.

Crigler-Najjar Syndrome

Crigler-Najjar syndrome is a disease caused by deficiency of the enzyme glucuronyl transferase, which is used to conjugate bilirubin in the liver. Bilirubin is the normal by-product of the breakdown of hemoglobin. Bilirubin circulates in the blood bound to albumin and is taken up by hepatocytes in the liver. Within hepatocytes, bilirubin is conjugated by glucuronyl transferase. Conjugated (also called direct) bilirubin is secreted into bile. This process is normally highly efficient so plasma unconjugated (indirect) bilirubin concentrations remain low. In Crigler-Najjar syndrome, indirect bilirubin levels increase and can deposit in tissues, particularly neurological tissue.

Type I Crigler-Najjar syndrome is very rare; it is found in neonates who have a complete absence of the enzyme because of inherited genetic mutations from both parents. Crigler-Najjar syndrome is inherited in an autosomal recessive pattern, which means both copies of the UGT1A1 gene in each cell have mutations. A less severe condition called Gilbert syndrome can occur when one copy of the UGT1A1 gene has a mutation.

Infants born with Crigler-Najjar type I syndrome require liver transplant to survive. Type II Crigler-Najjar syndrome is more common; it is caused by a genetic mutation inherited from a parent carrier. The patient has a reduced amount of glucuronyl transferase enzyme. Patients live into adulthood with elevated serum bilirubin levels. Kernicterus encephalopathy caused by excessive bilirubin in the blood can occur when the patient is under stress.

Diagnostic tests used to evaluate liver function include liver enzymes, conjugated bilirubin, total bilirubin, and unconjugated bilirubin in blood and liver biopsy. Treatment includes intensive light therapy, also called phototherapy. In infants, this is done using bilirubin lights (bili or "blue" lights). Phototherapy enhances bilirubin excretion. Plasmapheres is a procedure that can remove bilirubin from blood. Liver transplantation is needed in type I disease. Calcium compounds are sometimes used to bind with and remove bilirubin in the intestine. The drug phenobarbital can also be used to decrease bilirubin in the bloodstream.

 CLINICAL CONCEPT

If bilirubin levels in the blood become too high, brain damage, also called kernicterus, can occur.

Gilbert's Syndrome

Gilbert's syndrome is caused by decreased activity of the enzyme glucuronyl transferase, which conjugates bilirubin in the liver. Because of a genetic mutation, the disease is present in approximately 5% of the population. This is a mild, chronic disorder in which patients have elevated serum bilirubin levels and jaundice during periods of stress, infection, or fasting. Individuals may have problems with liver detoxification of certain drugs. In Gilbert's syndrome, hyperbilirubinemia usually resolves with removal of the stressful event. Treatment is unnecessary.

Hemochromatosis

Hemochromatosis is a genetic disorder that is characterized by an accumulation of iron in the liver caused by excessive absorption of iron from the intestine. Primary hemochromatosis is the most common genetic disorder in the United States, affecting an estimated 1 of every 200 to 300 Americans. Primary hemochromatosis is caused by a reduction in the iron regulatory hormone hepcidin or a reduction in hepcidin-ferroportin binding. Hepcidin regulates the activity of ferroportin, which assists in excretion of iron. The most common form of hemochromatosis is due to homozygous mutations in *HFE,* which encodes for the hereditary hemochromatosis protein. Secondary hemochromatosis is a side effect of excessive RBC breakdown associated with thalassemia, sideroblastic anemia, or multiple blood transfusions. Occasionally, it may be seen with chronic alcohol use disorder.

Primary hemochromatosis is more common in European Americans than African Americans and affects more males than females. Symptoms are often seen in males between the ages of 30 and 50 years and in females older than age 50 years. The liver is the primary site of iron storage; with accumulation of iron, the organ enlarges. Diagnosis includes high serum ferritin, serum transferrin, and free iron levels. Patients often demonstrate fatigue, hepatomegaly, skin hyperpigmentation, arthritis, and erectile dysfunction. Treatment involves phlebotomy and chelation with deferoxamine. If left untreated, cirrhosis can develop.

Wilson Disease

Wilson disease (WD) is a rare, inherited metabolic disorder characterized by excessive copper deposits in the liver, brain, and eye. It occurs in 1 in 300,000 persons due to the gene mutation ATP7 B. Excessive copper in the liver leads to fibrosis and destruction of the hepatocytes. The hepatic presentation of WD can look similar to non–alcohol-related fatty liver disease (NAFLD), resembling mainly steatosis but also steatohepatitis (NASH). Differentiating WD from NAFLD clinically is important because treatment strategies are completely different. The best discriminator appears to be basal 24-hour urinary copper excretion, which is high in WD and low in NAFLD.

The patient may develop hepatitis, fatty deposits in the liver, and encephalopathy. The patient demonstrates symptoms of hepatic dysfunction: jaundice, ascites, prominent abdominal veins, spider nevi, palmar erythema, and hematemesis. Common symptoms are difficulty speaking, tremor, arthritis, excessive salivation, clubbing, ataxia, masklike facies, clumsiness, and personality changes. Diagnosis is made by identification of copper rings in the cornea called Kayser–Fleischer rings, low levels of a serum copper transport protein (ceruloplasmin), and increased levels of hepatic and urinary copper. Treatment involves chelation with penicillamine or trientine. If left untreated, Wilson disease leads to cirrhosis and liver failure.

Chapter Summary

- The liver is a multifunctional organ that synthesizes albumin and coagulation factors, detoxifies the blood, and enables fat digestion. It also stores glucose, vitamins, and minerals.
- The liver conjugates bilirubin to make it water-soluble. Conjugated bilirubin is also called direct bilirubin. Unconjugated bilirubin is also called indirect bilirubin.
- The breakdown of RBCs, hepatocellular dysfunction, and obstructed bile release can lead to bilirubin in the bloodstream. These conditions are referred to as prehepatic, intrahepatic, and posthepatic jaundice.
- Hyperbilirubinemia leads to jaundice, a yellowing of skin and sclera. High bilirubin can also affect the brain causing encephalopathy.
- The most common causes of liver dysfunction are HCV, alcohol use disorder, and NAFLD.
- The hepatitis viruses include hepatitis A, B, C, D, E, and G.
- HAV causes the mildest disease, is spread solely by the fecal–oral route, is self-limiting, and leads to no complications.
- Vaccines are available to prevent HAV and HBV. Presently there is treatment for HCV but no vaccine.

- HBV and HCV cause hepatocellular dysfunction, lead to chronic infection, and are spread by blood and body fluids.
- HBV and HCV are often present with HIV, and both can lead to HCC.
- HCV infection can be treated effectively with combination antiviral protease inhibitor drugs to achieve undetectable levels of virus in the bloodstream, which has been referred to as a "cure" for infection.
- HDV is spread mainly by blood containing HBV, and HEV–similar to HAV–is spread by the fecal–oral route.
- To diagnose hepatitis, a laboratory test can reveal viral antigen and antibody levels.
- Alcohol use disorder is second to HCV as the main cause of cirrhosis of the liver.
- Before cirrhosis, the liver undergoes the process of steatosis, the accumulation of fat.
- The changes of cirrhosis of the liver include hepatocyte necrosis, connective tissue infiltration, fibrosis, and buildup of scar tissue throughout a shrunken liver.
- NAFLD is associated with metabolic syndrome, hyperlipidemia, obesity, and insulin resistance.

- NAFLD, the most common form of liver disease in the United States, can lead to a more severe form of the disease called NASH; this, in turn, can cause cirrhosis and hepatocarcinoma.

- In cirrhosis, the patient exhibits characteristic signs and symptoms, such as jaundice, poor fat digestion, diminished coagulation factor synthesis, and inefficient detoxification of the blood.

- Portal hypertension is a complication of cirrhosis that can lead to life-threatening side effects.

- Esophageal varices caused by portal hypertension result in hematemesis.

- There are very few treatments for liver disease, and liver transplantation is often the only alternative. Live donor transplants are an alternative to traditional liver whole organ transplantation from a deceased donor.

 ## Making the Connections

Signs and Symptoms	Physical Assessment Findings	Diagnostic Testing	Treatment
Hepatitis A Virus | HAV is usually caused by ingestion of contaminated food or water or contracted from person to person by the fecal–oral route. HAV is absorbed by the intestine and travels to the liver, where it damages the hepatocytes.			
Fatigue, nausea, vomiting, anorexia, malaise, abdominal pain, fever, myalgias, headache, jaundice, dark urine, light-colored stools.	RUQ tenderness, hepatomegaly, jaundice.	Fecal HAV is demonstrated in the first 4 weeks. Blood shows IgM anti-HAV antibodies during the first 4 weeks; IgG anti-HAV antibodies at 8 to 12 weeks; elevated liver enzymes in the first 4 weeks; and elevated serum bilirubin, WBC, and prolonged PT for 4 weeks. No chronic disease is present.	Supportive, including rest. Nutrition includes small high-caloric meals, no alcohol. Patient should not take acetaminophen. Patient should be on enteric precautions. HAV Ig can be administered to contacts for temporary immunity. For long-term immunity, administration of HAV vaccine is necessary.
Hepatitis B Virus | HBV is a stable virus spread by blood products, body fluids, or sexual contact. Once in the bloodstream, the virus produces viral proteins in the hepatocyte. The virus does not directly kill the cell, but the host's own immune system attacks hepatocytes when the viral antigens are encountered on the surface.			
Fatigue, vomiting, anorexia, malaise, abdominal pain, fever, myalgias, headache, jaundice, dark urine, light-colored stools.	RUQ tenderness, hepatomegaly, jaundice. More severe signs include splenomegaly, lymphadenopathy, spider angioma, palmar erythema, and encephalopathy.	Blood shows positive HBsAg, HB DNA, HBeAg, HBcAg, and anti-HBc IgM antibodies. Blood shows anti-HBc IgG antibodies in chronic infection. Elevated liver enzymes, serum bilirubin, WBC, and prolonged PT are present. An HBV carrier state is possible, and chronic long-term disease can lead to HCC.	Supportive, including rest. Nutrition includes small high-caloric meals, with no alcohol or acetaminophen. Patient needs to be on blood and body fluid precautions. PEG-interferon and drugs that inhibit viral polymerase, such as lamivudine, telbivudine, adefovir, entecavir, and tenofovir, are used to treat HBV. For temporary immunity for contacts, HBIg can be administered. For long-term immunity, HBV vaccine should be administered.

Making the Connections–cont'd

Signs and Symptoms	Physical Assessment Findings	Diagnostic Testing	Treatment
Hepatitis C Virus | HCV is an RNA virus that can replicate rapidly and can produce at least 10 trillion new viral particles each day. There are six different genotypes of HCV caused by mutation capability, and each has different severity and response to therapy. Symptoms can take 2 weeks to 8 months to appear and can lead to chronic infection and HCC.			
Fatigue, vomiting, anorexia, malaise, abdominal pain, fever, myalgias, headache, jaundice, dark urine, light-colored stools.	RUQ tenderness, hepatomegaly, jaundice. More severe signs include splenomegaly, lymphadenopathy, spider angioma, palmar erythema, and encephalopathy.	HCV can live dormant in the body for lengthy time frames before signs and symptoms develop. Blood shows positive HCV RNA assay, anti-HCV antibodies, elevated liver enzymes, high serum bilirubin, high WBC, and prolonged PT. Low thyroxine is present.	Combination antiviral drug treatment with protease inhibitors can effectively treat the infection. Supportive, including rest. Nutrition includes small high-caloric meals. No alcohol, no acetaminophen. Patient must be on strict blood and body fluid precautions. No vaccine is available.
Non–alcohol-related fatty liver disease | Accumulation of fat in the liver not due to alcohol. It is normal for the liver to contain some fat; however, if more than 5% to 10% percent of the liver's weight is fat, it is called a fatty liver (steatosis). The more severe form of NAFLD is called non–alcohol-related steatohepatitis (NASH).			
Usually associated with metabolic syndrome; obesity, hyperlipidemia, hypertension, and insulin resistance.	Symptoms associated with metabolic syndrome, high BMI. Signs of hypercholesterolemia such as xanthomas or xanthelasma may be present. High blood pressure.	Hyperlipidemia. Hyperglycemia. Elevated liver enzymes possible. The most common abnormal laboratory test results are elevated alanine transaminase (ALT) and aspartate transaminase (AST), usually one to four times the upper limits of normal. Several indices available that use different clinical parameters to diagnose NAFLD. Elastography scans of liver.	Dietary changes; low carbohydrate and calorie restriction and physical activity as lifestyle modifications. Glitazones, metformin, and GLP-1 agonists can assist in weight loss and glucose control. Obeticholic acid (OCA) can decrease fat in liver.
Alcohol-related Liver Disease | Alcohol is a potent toxin to hepatocytes. Repeated misuse of alcohol leads to steatosis, which is the replacement of hepatocytes with fat. Chronic ingestion of ethanol inhibits the oxidation of fatty acids in the liver. Fat accumulates in and around hepatocytes and disrupts the integrity of the organelles. Nuclear disruption causes death of the hepatocytes. With time, large areas of hepatocyte injury, necrosis, inflammation, and fibrosis develop. When the liver demonstrates fibrosis and scar tissue, the disorder is referred to as cirrhosis.			
Fatigue, vomiting, anorexia, malaise, abdominal pain, fever, myalgias, headache, jaundice, dark urine, light-colored stools. Hematemesis possible because of esophageal varices. Hepatic encephalopathy: confusion, lethargy, stupor.	RUQ tenderness, hepatomegaly, and jaundice. Signs of portal hypertension, which include ascites, caput medusa, esophageal varices, and rectal hemorrhoids. Proximal muscle wasting, altered hair distribution, asterixis, and gynecomastia. Hepatic encephalopathy signs. Delirium tremens. Seizure possible.	Blood shows elevated liver enzymes, high serum bilirubin, high WBC, prolonged PT, hypertriglyceridemia, hypercholesterolemia, and hypoalbuminemia. Liver enzymes elevated: serum GGT and transaminases (ALT, AST). Ultrasound of liver. Liver biopsy.	Supportive, including rest. Alcohol withdrawal syndrome requires critical care. Nutrition includes small high-caloric meals with low protein. No alcohol, no acetaminophen. Folate, thiamine, vitamin K. Benzodiazepines may be necessary in AWS. Many agents used to counteract alcohol use such as disulfram, gabapentin, baclofen, and others. If cessation of alcohol, consideration for liver transplant.

Continued

Making the Connections–cont'd

Signs and Symptoms	Physical Assessment Findings	Diagnostic Testing	Treatment
Cirrhosis and Liver Failure | Cirrhosis is the term for fibrotic changes of the liver. Hepatocytes are severely injured, dysfunctional, and replaced by fibrotic tissue. Liver is scarred and shrunken.			
Anorexia, nausea, weight loss, steatorrhea, dull abdominal pain, jaundice, dark urine. Signs of hepatic encephalopathy. Bleeding tendencies, pruritus, osteoporosis, musty odor to breath, ascites, signs of portal hypertension. HRS possible.	Enlarged, firm nodular liver on palpation. Jaundice, palmar erythema, spider angiomas, skin telangiectasia, clubbing of fingers, caput medusa, splenomegaly, testicular atrophy, gynecomastia in males, ascites. Hematemesis possible because of portal hypertension.	Elevated liver enzymes, high serum bilirubin, high WBC, prolonged PT, hypertriglyceridemia, elevated blood ammonia levels, hypercholesterolemia, hypoalbuminemia. Ultrasound of liver. Liver biopsy.	Remove underlying cause of cirrhosis or fibrosis. Good nutrition with vitamins. Rest and avoidance of exposure to toxins/chemicals or infections. No alcohol or sedatives. Low-protein diet for encephalopathy. Diuretics for edema and other pharmacological agents to counteract complications. Paracentesis for ascites. Ligation of bleeding varices.
Biliary Cholangitis | Inflammation of the liver with cholestasis. Bile secretion is disrupted, and hepatocytes become necrotic. Etiology of primary biliary cirrhosis is theorized to be autoimmune disease. Eventually, fibrotic changes develop in the liver; cirrhosis is the end result.			
Asymptomatic early in disease. Later signs include fatigue, anorexia, weight loss, pruritus, xanthelasma, steatorrhea, muscle wasting, ascites, spider angioma, and loss of axillary and pubic hair. Advanced disease shows signs of portal hypertension, jaundice, or ascites.	No signs early. Jaundice, ascites, osteoporosis seen in later stages. Xanthelasma, muscle wasting, ascites, spider angioma, loss of axillary and pubic hair. Advanced disease shows signs of portal hypertension and jaundice.	Elevated liver enzymes, elevated alkaline phosphatase, elevated lipids, high serum bilirubin, high immunoglobulins, high erythrocyte sedimentation rate, prolonged PT, decreased albumin. AMAs are present. Reduction of serum alkaline phosphatase with treatment (ALP, an important prognostic marker in PBC).	Ursodiol. Other pharmacological agents include obeticholic acid, bezafibrate, and budesonide. Rituximab is newest therapeutic agent under study. Liver transplant.
Crigler-Najjar Syndrome Type I and II | Genetic syndrome of a deficiency of the enzyme glucuronyl transferase, which is used to conjugate bilirubin in the liver. Bilirubin accumulates in the blood. Kernicterus (brain damage) caused by excessive bilirubin in the blood can occur when the patient is under stress.			
Type I: severe hyperbilirubinemia and brain damage and death. Type II: no symptoms usually. Jaundice can occur when body is under stress.	Type I: usually fatal. Type II: jaundice.	Blood shows elevated liver enzymes, high unconjugated bilirubin, and high total bilirubin.	Calcium compounds can bind bilirubin and aid in excretion. Phototherapy aids in the breakdown and excretion of bilirubin. Phenobarbital can lower bilirubin levels. Plasmapheresis can decrease bilirubin. Liver transplant performed in severe disease.
Gilbert's Syndrome | Decreased amount of glucuronyl transferase is made by the liver.			
Often asymptomatic. Abdominal cramps, anorexia, fatigue, and jaundice with severe stress on body.	Jaundice with severe stress on body.	High unconjugated bilirubin levels when body is under stress.	No treatment needed.

Making the Connections—cont'd

Signs and Symptoms	Physical Assessment Findings	Diagnostic Testing	Treatment
Hemochromatosis | Primary hemochromatosis is a genetic disorder that is caused by an accumulation of iron in the liver from excessive absorption of iron from the intestine. Secondary hemochromatosis is caused by excessive RBC breakdown in hemolytic anemias and thalassemia.			
May be asymptomatic or may exhibit fatigue, arthralgias, skin hyperpigmentation, or erectile dysfunction.	Hepatomegaly. Hyperpigmentation of skin (bronze). Arthritis.	High iron levels in body. High serum ferritin and transferrin. Genetic testing.	Periodic phlebotomy. Chelation with deferoxamine.
Wilson Disease | Autosomal-recessive genetic disorder of copper metabolism that causes excessive deposition of copper in the liver, brain, and other tissues.			
Signs of hepatic dysfunction: jaundice, ascites, prominent abdominal veins, spider nevi, palmar erythema, digital clubbing, hematemesis. Difficulty speaking, tremor, arthritis, excessive salivation, ataxia, masklike facies, clumsiness, personality changes.	Jaundice, ascites, prominent abdominal veins, clubbing, erythema of palms, Kayser–Fleischer rings of the cornea: green-gold in color. Difficulty speaking, tremor, arthritis, excessive salivation, ataxia, masklike facies, clumsiness, personality changes.	Low ceruloplasmin levels, high levels of urinary copper, liver biopsy shows high copper. CT and MRI of the brain.	Lifelong use of chelation agents such as penicillamine or trientine. Liver transplant.

Bibliography

Available online at fadavis.com

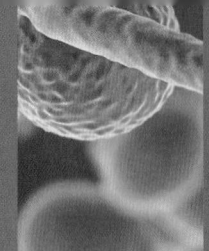

Gallbladder, Pancreatic, and Bile Duct Dysfunction

Learning Objectives

Upon completion of this chapter, the student will be able to:

- Describe normal anatomy and physiological function of the gallbladder, pancreas, and bile duct.
- Recognize common disorders of the gallbladder, pancreas, and bile duct.
- Identify signs, symptoms, and clinical manifestations of disorders of the gallbladder, pancreas, and bile duct.

- Recognize assessment techniques, laboratory tests, and imaging studies used in the diagnosis of disorders of the gallbladder, pancreas, and bile duct.
- Discuss pharmacological and nonpharmacological treatment modalities used for disorders of the gallbladder, pancreas, and bile duct.

Key Terms

Acalculous cholecystitis
Acute pancreatitis
Ampulla of Vater
Biliary colic
Biliary sludge
Biliary stasis
Calculous cholecystitis
Cholangitis
Cholecystectomy

Cholecystitis
Choledocholithiasis
Cholelithiasis
Chronic pancreatitis (CP)
Courvoisier's sign
Cullen sign
Empyema
Endoscopic retrograde cholangiopancrea-
    tography (ERCP)

Grey Turner sign
Hydroxy iminodiacetic acid (HIDA) scan
Jaundice
Laparoscopic cholecystectomy
Murphy's sign
Pancreatitis
Pseudocyst
Sphincter of Oddi
Virchow's node

The gallbladder, pancreas, and biliary tract are key components of the gastrointestinal system (Fig. 32-1). The liver manufactures bile, the major emulsifier of fats, and releases it into the hepatic duct, which leads to the common bile duct. The gallbladder stores and concentrates bile until it is released into the cystic duct, which empties into the common bile duct. The pancreas has both endocrine and exocrine function. The endocrine portion of the pancreas produces insulin, glucagon, and somatostatin and releases them into the vascular system. The exocrine portion of the pancreas secretes the digestive enzymes lipase, amylase, trypsin, chymotrypsin, and bicarbonate and releases them into the pancreatic duct, eventually emptying into the common bile duct. The common bile duct is where the cystic, hepatic, and pancreatic ducts come together and is the major conduit that empties bile and digestive enzymes into the small intestine at the **ampulla of Vater.** The muscular valve at the ampulla of Vater is the **sphincter of Oddi** (Fig. 32-2).

Epidemiology

Gallbladder disease occurs frequently in the United States. **Cholelithiasis,** commonly known as gallstones, is the most frequent type of gallbladder disease. **Cholecystitis,** which is inflammation of the gallbladder caused by cholelithiasis, is a common cause of emergency medical care. Gallbladder disease affects approximately 20 million people in the United States. Acute cholecystitis is diagnosed in approximately 200,000 people in the United States each year. There are approximately 500,000 cholecystectomies done yearly in the United States for gallbladder disease.

Acute pancreatitis, chronic pancreatitis, and pancreatic cancer are the most common pancreatic disorders in the United States. Acute pancreatitis ranges from mild to severe forms of the disease. It has an incidence in the United States of 40 to 50 per 100,000 persons. Approximately 275,000 people in the United States are admitted to hospitals each year

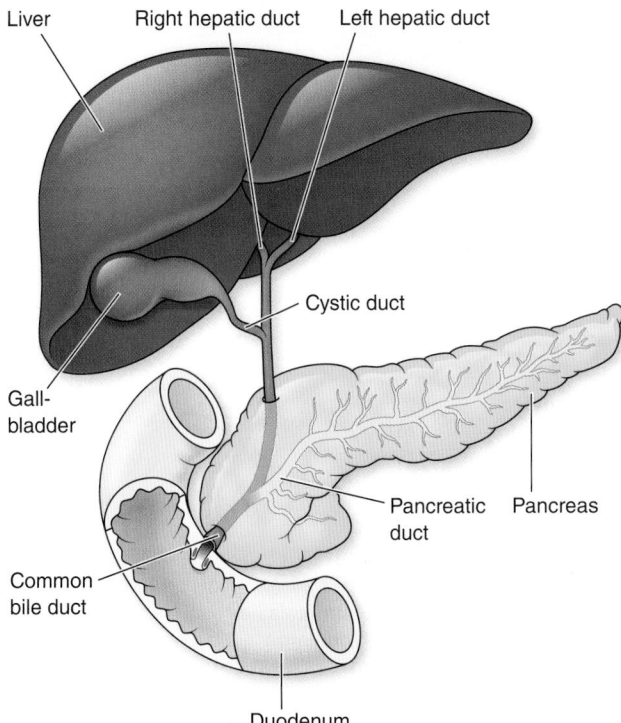

FIGURE 32-1. Anatomy of the gallbladder, pancreas, and biliary tract.

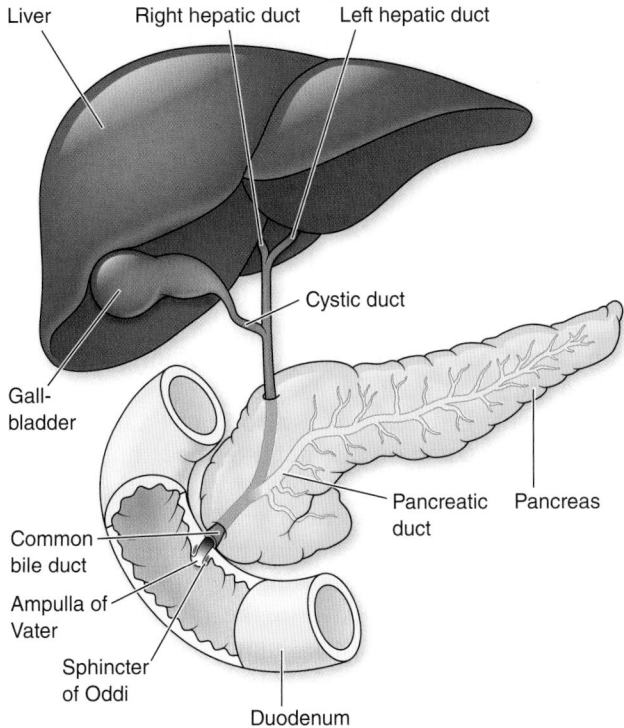

FIGURE 32-2. The common bile duct, ampulla of Vater, and sphincter of Oddi.

with acute pancreatitis. There is a 10% mortality rate associated with severe acute pancreatitis, with gallstones and alcohol use disorder the most common causes. Chronic pancreatitis has a prevalence of 50 persons per 100,000 in the United States, with alcohol use disorder as the most common cause.

Chronic pancreatitis in the United States results in more than 122,000 outpatient visits and more than 56,000 hospitalizations per year. Although the cause of pancreatic cancer is unclear, it is responsible for nearly 30,000 annual deaths and is the third most common cause of cancer death in the United States.

Basic Concepts of Gallbladder, Pancreas, and Biliary Function

Bile is manufactured by the liver and is composed of bile acids (80%), phospholipids (16%), and cholesterol (4%). It has two major functions: digestion and elimination. Bile emulsifies fats and facilitates absorption of fat-soluble vitamins. It also carries waste products for elimination. One of the waste products contained in bile is bilirubin, which is processed by the liver and is a breakdown product of hemoglobin. Some bile is released into the hepatic duct, which travels into the common bile duct. Some bile is stored and concentrated in the gallbladder.

The gallbladder is a hollow organ that sits just beneath the liver and is divided into three sections: fundus, body, and neck. The neck tapers and connects to the biliary tree via the cystic duct, which then joins the common hepatic duct to become the common bile duct. When food containing fat enters the digestive tract, it stimulates the secretion of cholecystokinin (CCK) by the small intestine. In response to CCK, the gallbladder, which stores about 50 milliliters of bile, releases its contents into the duodenum via the common bile duct.

The pancreas produces the digestive enzymes lipase, which digests fats, and amylase, which digests carbohydrates. Trypsin and chymotrypsin, other enzymes also manufactured by the pancreas, digest proteins. The pancreas also produces bicarbonate, which is a natural antacid. The pancreas is located behind the stomach and is surrounded by the duodenum, liver, and spleen. It is about 6 inches long and is shaped like a flat pear. The wide, medial portion, called the head of the pancreas, is located in the epigastric region behind the duodenum. The body and tail of the pancreas extend into the left hypogastric region. When food enters the stomach, pancreatic enzymes are triggered by the hormone secretin, which is produced by the intestine. The enzymes travel from the pancreatic duct into the common bile duct, which enters the small intestine at the ampulla of Vater. In the small intestine, pancreatic enzymes along with bile break down fats, proteins, and carbohydrates.

Basic Pathophysiological Concepts of Gallbladder, Pancreas, and Biliary Dysfunction

Gallbladder, biliary tract, and pancreatic disorders may occur as primary or secondary disorders. The anatomical position and the function of both the gallbladder and pancreas create a situation where one organ's function influences another's function. Patients experiencing gallbladder or pancreatic dysfunction generally present with multiple metabolic disturbances. Nutritional disturbances and pain ranging from mild to severe are common. Disorders of the gallbladder, biliary tract, and pancreas have overlapping symptoms requiring careful assessment and management.

Disorders of the gallbladder and pancreas can be acute or chronic. With acute gallbladder or pancreatic disorders, there is a sudden and short-term dysfunction of the gland with resolution. In contrast, chronic forms of the diseases cause recurring episodes of inflammation that lead to permanent glandular tissue changes and gland dysfunction.

Gallbladder Dysfunction

Gallbladder motility disturbances and stasis of bile are the most common causes of obstruction, inflammation, and infection of the gallbladder. Motility disturbances causing stasis of bile generally precede gallstone formation. In stagnant bile, the constituents, particularly cholesterol, can precipitate out, forming crystals that gradually form stones. Terms used in the discussion of gallbladder disease are cholelithiasis, cholecystitis, cholangitis, and **choledocholithiasis.** Fig. 32-3 shows the differences among these disorders. Cholelithiasis is the presence of gallstones within the gallbladder. **Biliary sludge** is the precursor to gallstones. It is a combination of bile salts, bile acids, bile pigments, lecithin (phospholipid), and cholesterol. These components of bile become highly concentrated in the gallbladder. The concentration of bile and gallbladder motility disturbances cause the formation of biliary sludge. **Biliary stasis,** or delayed emptying of the gallbladder, leads to the precipitation of cholesterol and bile components to form calculi (gallstones). There are three types of gallstones:

1. **Cholesterol stones:** These are the most common stones formed in the gallbladder because of supersaturated cholesterol in bile. Eighty percent of all gallstones are made of cholesterol, whereas 20% are made of pigment stones.
2. **Black pigment stones:** These are small, hard gallstones composed of calcium bilirubinate and inorganic calcium salts. The formation of black pigment stones is related to alcohol-related liver disease, chronic hemolysis, and aging.
3. **Brown pigment stones:** These are composed of calcium salts of unconjugated bilirubin, with small amounts of cholesterol and protein. They are often located in the bile ducts and cause obstruction and inflammation.

Gallstones can remain in the gallbladder for years without any symptoms. However, gallstones and

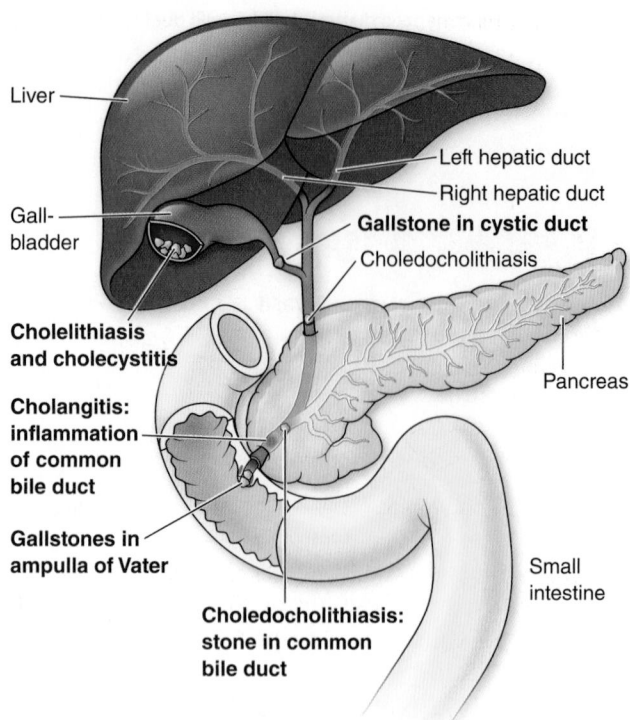

FIGURE 32-3. Locations of common bile duct disorders.

motility dysfunction of the gallbladder often cause inflammation, termed cholecystitis. In cholecystitis, gallstones commonly travel into the cystic duct, which arises from the gallbladder as the outflow tract of bile. A gallstone can cause inflammation of the cystic duct termed **cholangitis.** Inflammation is caused by release of the enzyme phospholipase from the epithelial lining of the gallbladder. Phospholipase disrupts that normal epithelial layer and allows for tissue damage from the concentrated bile salts stored in the gallbladder. Inflammation and obstruction of the cystic duct can cause acute or chronic episodes of inflammation, called acute or chronic cholecystitis.

However, gallstones can also travel farther and obstruct the common bile duct, termed choledocholithiasis. When gallstones lodge in the common bile duct, bile backs up into the liver. The backup allows the constituents of bile, mainly bilirubin, to back up into the bloodstream, causing hyperbilirubinemia. Bile salts also accumulate in the bloodstream and can cause intense pruritus. Complete obstruction of the common bile duct leading to hyperbilirubinemia causes **jaundice.** Jaundice develops because bilirubin has a yellow hue and adheres to elastin components in the skin and sclera. Common bile duct obstruction also restricts bile from entering the small intestine and breaking down fats. This causes fat in the stool, termed steatorrhea. High bilirubin levels in the blood become filtered at the kidney, causing dark, tea-colored urine. Lack of bilirubin pigment in the stool leads to clay-colored stool. This is considered a more critical condition and usually requires emergency care.

Gallstones can also obstruct bile flow in the common bile duct, and bile backup can irritate the pancreas. More critically, gallstones can move into the pancreas and cause pancreatitis, a potentially fatal inflammatory disorder.

 CLINICAL CONCEPT

The most common causes of obstruction of the common bile duct are gallstones and tumor of the head of the pancreas. Obstruction of the common bile duct causes obstructive jaundice.

Biliary Colic

Biliary colic is a syndrome of spasmodic pain associated with irritation of the gallbladder, commonly secondary to gallstones. The pain is steady, intense, and can last from 30 minutes to several hours. Nausea, vomiting, and right upper quadrant (RUQ) pain, right flank pain, or midchest pain can occur. Sharp RUQ pain upon palpation of the abdomen in the region of the gallbladder is called **Murphy's sign.** The pain of cholecystitis commonly radiates to the right shoulder or posterior thoracic region at the scapula. Additionally, although any type of food can precipitate the pain, fatty foods, in particular, incite pain.

Biliary colic is often associated with dilation of the biliary tract, elevation of plasma liver enzyme concentration, and elevation of serum bilirubin. Biliary colic is most frequently caused by obstruction of the free flow of bile from the gallbladder into the cystic duct or common bile duct. A gallstone is the most common cause. However, biliary colic can occur in the absence of gallstones or an identifiable cause. Acalculous biliary colic, which is pain without stones, can occur and be a consequence of dysfunction of the biliary tree and the sphincter of Oddi of the small intestine. Individuals can endure multiple bouts of biliary colic before severe pain and vomiting prompt them to seek health care.

Pancreatic Exocrine Dysfunction

The pancreas is both an endocrine and exocrine gland. As an endocrine gland, the pancreas secretes the hormones insulin, glucagon, and somatostatin, which are involved in glucose metabolism. As an exocrine gland, the pancreas is a major gastrointestinal secretory organ that manufactures and releases key digestive enzymes that break down proteins, carbohydrates, and fats. Pancreatic digestive enzymes include the proteases trypsin and chymotrypsin, which break down proteins; lipase, which breaks down fats; and amylase, which breaks down carbohydrates. The pancreas also secretes bicarbonate, which neutralizes acid. Pancreatic exocrine dysfunction occurs when the pancreas does not secrete sufficient digestive enzymes. Without digestive enzymes, food is not broken down, and malabsorption results. Malabsorption leads to deficiencies of essential nutrients and lack of fat absorption. Severe pancreatic insufficiency occurs in cystic fibrosis, chronic pancreatitis, and surgeries of the gastrointestinal system in which portions of the stomach or pancreas are removed. Certain gastrointestinal diseases, such as stomach ulcers, celiac disease, and Crohn's disease, as well as autoimmune disorders, such as systemic lupus erythematosus, may contribute to the development of pancreatic insufficiency.

Pancreatitis is inflammation of the pancreas that causes pancreatic insufficiency, malabsorption, and diabetes. Pancreatitis can be an acute or a chronic disorder. With acute pancreatitis, there is a sudden, short-term episode of inflammation. With chronic pancreatitis, the gland undergoes repeated episodes of inflammation and gradual deterioration. Acute pancreatitis can be caused by gallstones, excessive alcohol consumption, high blood triglycerides, abdominal injury, and certain medications and toxins. During the inflammatory process, the digestive enzymes attack the pancreatic tissue, which causes autodigestion. In chronic pancreatitis, recurring inflammation occurs, causing gradual destruction of the gland, leaving it nonfunctional, fibrotic, and atrophied.

Assessment of Gallbladder, Pancreatic, and Biliary Tract Disorders

The clinical presentations of gallbladder, pancreatic, and biliary tract disorders are similar. Because of this, the patient's history is important, as it can assist the clinician in differentiating between them.

Risk Factors

Risk factors for gallbladder dysfunction are different from those for pancreatic and biliary tract disorders. Some of the major risk factors include age, female gender, estrogen level, low-calorie diets, fatty foods, and obesity.

Pancreatic disorders affect males and females almost equally. Alcohol use disorder, gallstones, and biliary tract disorders are the most common risk factors for pancreatic dysfunction.

 CLINICAL CONCEPT

Biliary tract disorders are most commonly caused by obstruction of the common bile duct by a pancreatic tumor or gallstone.

Signs and Symptoms

Assessment of the patient for biliary disorders should include a complete history and physical examination. The clinician should focus on the location, timing, intensity, and quality of pain. Relieving and exacerbating factors should be noted. Nausea and vomiting often accompany biliary disorders. The patient may also report a feeling of fullness, and abdominal distention may be present. The timing of nausea and vomiting in relation to the time of eating should be noted, as gallbladder disorders often present with pain after eating fatty foods. The clinician should also inspect the patient for jaundice of the skin and sclera and should monitor temperature and white blood cell (WBC) count as possible signs of infection. Abdominal assessment may reveal RUQ guarding and tenderness, often referred to as Murphy's sign.

In pancreatic disorders, nausea, vomiting, and abdominal pain are common. Patients with biliary or pancreatic disorders may have changes in stool caused by fat malabsorption. Steatorrhea, or fat-containing stool, is soft, and stool that lacks bilirubin is clay colored.

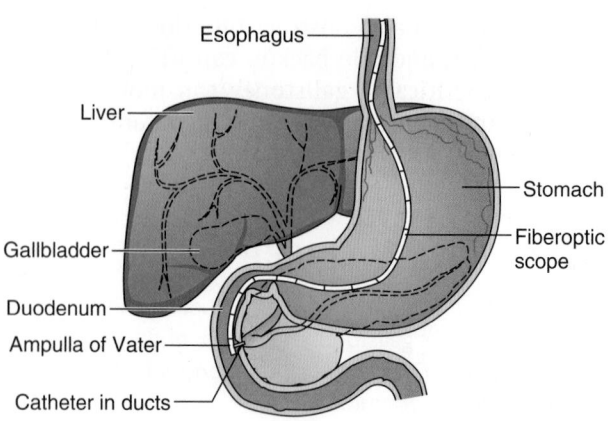

FIGURE 32-4. Endoscopic retrograde cholangiopancreatography (ERCP). This is a procedure where an endoscope is passed through the oral cavity through the esophagus and stomach, into the duodenum, through the sphincter of Oddi, and farther into the common bile duct and pancreatic duct. The clinician can visualize, examine, and perform procedures using this technology.

PTC, dye is directly injected into the liver for x-rays to visualize the biliary tract.

 CLINICAL CONCEPT

Pain caused by pancreatic dysfunction often presents in the epigastric area, which radiates straight into the back.

Diagnosis

Specific laboratory tests and imaging studies are designed to evaluate the gallbladder, pancreas, and biliary tract. Elevated WBC count, erythrocyte sedimentation rate (ESR), and C-reactive protein (CRP) are present in states of gallbladder or pancreatic inflammation. Liver enzymes and bilirubin level may be elevated. Serum amylase and lipase levels are elevated with pancreatic inflammation. Commonly used imaging tests are abdominal ultrasound; computed tomography (CT) scan; and **hydroxy iminodiacetic acid (HIDA) scan,** also called cholescintigraphy/hepatobiliary scintigraphy. **Endoscopic retrograde cholangiopancreatography (ERCP)** is an invasive procedure that uses an endoscope with a camera to inspect the anatomy of the biliary tract (see Fig. 32-4). In addition to visualization, ERCP can be used to remove obstructive gallstones from the common bile duct. It can also be used to perform surgical procedures such as sphincterotomy of the sphincter of Oddi and stent insertion into the sphincter to allow for easier passage of bile sludge. These procedures may be necessary if bile sludge or stone is obstructing bile flow from the bile duct into the intestine. Percutaneous transhepatic cholangiography (PTC) can be performed if results of other tests are equivocal. In

Treatment of Gallbladder, Pancreatic, and Biliary Tract Disorders

Surgery and supportive management are the most common treatments for biliary and gallbladder disorders. Supportive management includes IV fluids, pain management, and antibiotics. For patients who cannot tolerate surgery, medications that attempt to dissolve biliary stones can be administered. Ursodiol and chenodiol are such medications. **Cholecystectomy** is the surgical removal of the gallbladder, which is usually done via laparoscopy. Patients with pancreatitis are usually placed on IV solution, as well as on antibiotics and pain relievers. The goal is to rest the pancreas and gastrointestinal system. The patient's diet should be free of fat, caffeine, and alcohol. Pancreatic enzyme supplementation may be necessary with recovery. Pancreatic cancer commonly requires surgery called the Whipple procedure.

Pathophysiology of Select Disorders of the Gallbladder, Pancreas, and Biliary Tract

Biliary colic describes the typical pain experienced by individuals with gallbladder or pancreatic disease. Cholecystitis, which causes episodes of intense biliary colic, is one of the most common surgically treated disorders. Pancreatic disease is less common but can lead to serious complications.

Cholecystitis

Cholecystitis can occur as an acute or chronic disorder, with gallstones being the most common cause. **Calculous cholecystitis** is the term used for inflammation of the gallbladder plus stones. **Acalculous cholecystitis** is inflammation of the gallbladder without stones.

 CLINICAL CONCEPT

Individuals can have gallstones for many years before they cause gallbladder inflammation.

An estimated 10% to 20% of Americans have gallstones, and as many as one-third of these individuals go on to develop acute cholecystitis. Cholecystectomy for either recurrent biliary colic or acute cholecystitis is the most common major surgical procedure performed by general surgeons, resulting in approximately 500,000 operations annually. Gallstones are two to three times more common in females than in males, resulting in a higher incidence of acute cholecystitis in females.

ALERT! Because epigastric pain with radiation to the shoulder is a common symptom, many patients can mistake an episode of acute cholecystitis for cardiac chest pain.

Etiology

Acute cholecystitis most often occurs because of biliary stasis and gallstones. Cholesterol calculi are the most common type of gallstones formed because of biliary stasis. Pigment stones that contain bilirubin can also develop in the gallbladder. Inflammation and spasms of the gallbladder can also occur without the formation of stones. Highly concentrated bile without calculi can irritate the interior gallbladder mucosa and cause spasms of the gland. Acalculous cholecystitis can occur because of critical illness, major surgery, sickle cell disease, *Salmonella* infections, AIDS, burns, sepsis, total parenteral nutrition, or prolonged fasting.

Individuals older than 40 years, especially females with a family history of cholecystitis, are prone to the disorder. There are several classic risk factors that predispose individuals to cholecystitis (see Box 32-1).

Pathophysiology

Ninety percent of cases of cholecystitis are caused by gallstones that lodge in the cystic duct, called calculous cholecystitis; the other 10% of cases occur because of acalculous cholecystitis. Obstruction of the cystic duct by gallstones causes distention of the gallbladder. As the gallbladder becomes distended, blood flow and lymphatic drainage are compromised,

---

BOX 32-1. Common Risk Factors for Cholecystitis

- Older than 40 years
- Diet, if high-calorie, high-cholesterol
- Estrogen
- Female gender, particularly those who have had multiple pregnancies
- Genetic predisposition
- Obesity
- Oral contraceptives
- Rapid weight loss, particularly after bariatric surgery
- Cholesterol-lowering drugs (e.g., fibrates)
- Other drugs include GLP-1 agonists used to manage type 2 diabetes (e.g., liraglutide), octreotide (synthetic growth hormone), and ceftriaxone (antibiotic)
- Pregnancy
- Congenital hemolytic anemias (e.g., thalassemia)

---

leading to mucosal ischemia and necrosis. The distention of the gallbladder irritates the nerves that innervate the wall, causing intense pain. As distention subsides, the pain wanes, leading to a pattern of spasmodic pain known as biliary colic.

The pathophysiology of acalculous cholecystitis is less clear. One theory suggests that this disorder begins with a noncontracting gallbladder, as bile can become highly concentrated and irritating in a gallbladder that does not contract. A gallbladder that remains noncontractile can be caused by either lack of organ response to CCK or prolonged fasting. Eating stimulates intestinal CCK; if an individual undergoes frequent fasting, the gallbladder lacks the stimulus to contract and does not release bile.

The inflammatory process associated with acute cholecystitis can also occur because of bacterial infection that can progress to a purulent effusion of the gallbladder, called an **empyema.** *Escherichia coli, Streptococci,* and *Salmonella* are the bacteria most commonly involved.

Acalculous cholecystitis caused by infection is more serious than calculous cholecystitis because gangrene of the gallbladder wall, perforation, and empyema can all develop rapidly. In another condition called emphysematous cholecystitis, gas-forming bacterial organisms such as *Clostridia* can infect the gallbladder and cause gangrene and perforation of the gland.

Chronic cholecystitis can occur when the gallbladder becomes thickened, rigid, and fibrotic and functions poorly. This pathological change in the structure of the gallbladder results from repeated attacks of cholecystitis, calculi, or chronic episodes of irritation. Chronic cholecystitis commonly causes episodes of intense heartburn, eructations, flatulence, and indigestion. Repeated attacks of symptoms may occur and resemble acute cholecystitis.

Choledocholithiasis occurs when small gallstones pass from the gallbladder and cystic duct into the common bile duct. Stones remain in the common bile duct, causing obstruction, which causes backup of bile into the liver; this results in backup of bilirubin and bile salts in the bloodstream. Accumulation of bilirubin in the bloodstream results in jaundice, and backup of bile salts into the bloodstream causes pruritus (itching).

Clinical Presentation

The most common presenting symptom of acute cholecystitis is abdominal pain in the RUQ. The patient usually complains of anorexia, nausea, vomiting, eructations, heartburn, feeling full after eating, and perhaps fever. A key sign of cholecystitis with peritoneal inflammation is Murphy's sign, where the patient takes in a quick inspiration as the clinician palpates the RUQ. In some patients, the pain of cholecystitis radiates to the right shoulder or scapula. Although the pain may initially be described as spasmodic or colicky, it becomes constant in many cases.

Although patients with acalculous cholecystitis may present similarly, the condition commonly occurs in severely ill patients without a prior history of biliary colic. Patients with acalculous cholecystitis usually present with fever and sepsis, without history or physical examination findings consistent with acute cholecystitis.

Older adults, especially those with diabetes, may present with vague symptoms and without many classic findings. Pain and fever may be absent, and localized tenderness may be the only presenting sign. Older adults may also rapidly progress to complicated cholecystitis and rupture of the gland without warning.

Diagnosis

The diagnostic criteria for acute cholecystitis are referred to as the Tokyo Guidelines (see Table 32-1). Laboratory tests used in cholecystitis include WBC count, ESR, CRP, liver enzymes, and bilirubin levels. Abdominal ultrasonography is the imaging study of choice for evaluating the gallbladder and biliary tree. Ultrasound reveals the presence of stones, thickening of the gallbladder wall, and distention of the lumen, which are signs of cholecystitis. However, because ultrasound scans often cannot visualize stones in the common bile duct, other diagnostic tests are necessary. A hepatic iminodiacetic acid (HIDA) scan (also called hepatobiliary scintigraphy) can provide an assessment of gallbladder function. CT scan and ERCP are useful for visualizing gallbladder and biliary tract abnormalities when other studies are equivocal.

 CLINICAL CONCEPT

ERCP can be used in both diagnosis and treatment; it may be used to perform ultrasonography, remove stones from the bile duct, or insert a bile duct stent.

Treatment

Laparoscopic cholecystectomy is the treatment of choice for symptomatic cholelithiasis and cholecystitis. This minimally invasive procedure has a low risk of complications and generally requires a hospital stay of less than 24 hours. The procedure is usually performed with four small incisions through which instruments are inserted. The gallbladder is freed either by electrosurgical or laser excision and is then withdrawn through one of the small incisions. Advantages of this technique include less postoperative pain than after laparotomy (open surgical investigation of the abdomen); small incisions; and more rapid return to daily activities. Incision length and the accompanying postoperative pain make open cholecystectomy more difficult for patients in terms of recovery.

 CLINICAL CONCEPT

Not all patients are candidates for laparoscopic cholecystectomy, and there is always the risk that a laparoscopic cholecystectomy may be converted to a laparotomy or open cholecystectomy during the procedure.

TABLE 32-1. Diagnostic Criteria for Acute Cholecystitis According to Tokyo Guidelines

Local Signs	Systemic Symptoms	Imaging Study Findings
Murphy's sign present	Fever	Confirming findings on ultrasound
Some RUQ tenderness	Leukocytosis	Confirming findings on HIDA scan
Mass palpable in RUQ	Elevated C-reactive protein (CRP)	

DIAGNOSIS OF ACUTE CHOLECYSTITIS SHOULD BE MADE IF:

one local sign, one systemic symptom, and one imaging confirmatory finding are present.

From Yokoe, M., Hata, J., Takada, T., Strasberg, S. M., Asbun, H. J., et al. (2018). Tokyo Guidelines 2018: Diagnostic criteria and severity grading of acute cholecystitis (with videos). *J Hepatobiliary Pancreat Sci, 25*(1), 41–54. doi: 10.1002/jhbp.515

When there is concern that stones may have moved into the common bile duct, intraoperative cholangiography and choledochoscopy may also be performed. This allows full exploration of the common bile duct. Occasionally, a transhepatic T tube may need to be placed in the common bile duct to decompress the biliary tree and decrease inflammation. The T tube is inserted to maintain patency of the duct and promote bile passage while the edema decreases. It can also be used in cases of biliary obstruction when obstructive jaundice is present. Excess bile in the common bile duct is collected in a drainage bag secured below the surgical site until bile drainage is complete.

After cholecystectomy, intracorporeal lithotripsy may be used to fragment retained stones in the common bile duct by pulsed laser or hydraulic lithotripsy applied through an endoscope directly to the stones. The stone fragments are removed by irrigation or aspiration. Retained stones may also be removed by basket retrieval through endoscopy or the percutaneous transhepatic biliary approach.

Dietary Management. The dietary management of gallbladder disease involves avoiding eating during an acute attack of cholecystitis. A nasogastric tube may be inserted to relieve nausea and vomiting. For patients who are able to eat, dietary fat intake may need to be limited, especially if the patient is obese. If bile flow is obstructed, fat-soluble vitamins, such as A, D, E, and K, and bile salts may need to be administered.

Medications. A narcotic analgesic may be required for pain relief during an acute attack of cholecystitis. Hydromorphone (Dilaudid), a morphine derivative, is commonly administered in the emergency department as the patient is being evaluated for cholecystitis. Meperidine (Demerol) can also be used as an analgesic.

Oral medications to dissolve gallstones are indicated for patients who cannot tolerate surgery because of comorbid conditions. Ursodiol (Actigall) and chenodiol (Chenix) reduce the cholesterol content of gallstones, leading to their gradual dissolution. Patients with pruritus caused by accumulation of bile salts in the bloodstream may be given cholestyramine (Questran), which binds with bile salts to promote their excretion in the feces. The major adverse effects of medications used to treat biliary disease include diarrhea, abnormal liver function tests, and increased serum cholesterol.

Direct cholelitholysis therapy can also be used for treatment of gallstones. This approach involves the use of a cholesterol-dissolving agent directly infused into the gallbladder by a percutaneous transhepatic biliary catheter; it is indicated for symptomatic, high-risk patients whose gallbladder can be visualized by radiographic study.

> **ALERT!** Rupture of an acutely inflamed gallbladder may result in acute pain that is transient and followed by relief of pain as contents are released from the distended, perforated gallbladder into the abdomen. It is critical to report this finding immediately to avoid sepsis.

CLINICAL CONCEPT

If a narcotic analgesic is needed for pain management in biliary disorders, morphine and codeine are contraindicated because they can cause spasm of the sphincter of Oddi. Dilaudid does not cause spasm of the sphincter of Oddi and is recommended in lieu of morphine or codeine.

Cancer of the Gallbladder and Biliary Tract

Cancers of the gallbladder and biliary tract, termed cholangiocarcinoma, are rare disorders. They usually occur in individuals older than 65 years. The patient usually has cholelithiasis (gallstones) and chronic cholecystitis, which causes intense RUQ pain. Gallbladder cancer often manifests as a palpable mass in the RUQ of the abdomen called **Courvoisier's sign.** Jaundice, anorexia, nausea, and weight loss are common. Enlargement of a left-sided supraclavicular lymph node may be palpable; this is termed **Virchow's node.** Measurement of tumor marker CA 19-9 may be elevated in both cholangiocarcinoma and gallbladder cancer. Carcinoembryonic antigen (CEA) may also be elevated in the blood.

The signs and symptoms occur late in the disease process; frequently, metastasis has occurred by the time the patient is symptomatic. Gallbladder cancers spread by direct extension to the liver and metastasize via the blood and lymph system. Ultrasound and CT scan are commonly used to diagnose gallbladder cancer. However, percutaneous transhepatic cholangiography (PTC) or endoscopic retrograde cholangiopancreatography (ERCP) may be needed to establish the diagnosis of gallbladder cancer. Analysis of bile cytology can be accomplished with these procedures. Magnetic resonance cholangiopancreatography (MRCP) is an alternative, noninvasive way to take images of the bile ducts. At the time of diagnosis, gallbladder cancer usually is often too advanced to treat surgically. Ninety-five percent of patients with primary cancer of the gallbladder die within 1 year. Radical and extensive surgical interventions may be performed, as well as radiation and chemotherapy, but the prognosis is poor, regardless of treatment.

Acute Pancreatitis

Acute pancreatitis can range from mild organ dysfunction to a severe, life-threatening disorder. Normally, the pancreas inhibits digestive enzymes from causing injury and destroying the gland. However, the dysfunctional pancreas undergoes inflammation and cellular injury caused by the leakage of activated pancreatic digestive enzymes into the glandular parenchyma. The enzymatic destruction and autodigestion of the gland can range from mild to severe. Severe forms of the disease include necrotizing and hemorrhagic pancreatitis. Despite the insult to the glandular tissue, it is a reversible disorder with potential for complete resolution.

The incidence of acute pancreatitis in the United States ranges between 110 and 140 persons per 100,000 with an estimated more than 300,000 emergency department visits per year. The median age at onset depends on the etiology: for alcohol-related pancreatitis the median age is 39 years old and for biliary tract–related disease, 69 years old. Acute pancreatitis generally affects males more than females and is more common in African Americans than European Americans. Approximately 80% of patients develop mild to moderately severe disease. However, one-fifth of patients develop severe disease with a mortality rate of approximately 20%.

Etiology

The most common causes of pancreatitis are biliary tract disease and alcohol use disorder. In biliary tract disease, the causative factor is obstruction of the pancreatic duct by a gallstone or other cause, with release of digestive enzymes that back up into the pancreatic gland parenchyma, followed by autodigestion. It has also been theorized that microlithiasis, defined as microscopic-size gallstones, can lodge at the ampulla of Vater, causing obstruction and backup pressure within the pancreas. In alcohol-related pancreatitis, ethanol causes intracellular accumulation of digestive enzymes and their premature activation and release.

Abdominal trauma causes clinical pancreatitis in 5% of cases. Pancreatic injury occurs more often in penetrating injuries, such as from knives and bullets, than in blunt abdominal trauma.

Several infectious diseases may cause pancreatitis, especially in children. Viral causes include mumps virus, coxsackievirus, cytomegalovirus, hepatitis virus, Epstein–Barr virus, echovirus, varicella-zoster virus, measles virus, and rubella virus. Bacterial causes include *Mycoplasma pneumoniae, Salmonella, Campylobacter,* and *Mycobacterium tuberculosis.* Pancreatitis has been associated with AIDS; however, this may be the result of opportunistic infections, neoplasms, lipodystrophy, or drug therapies.

Hypercalcemia from any cause can lead to acute pancreatitis. Such causes may include hyperparathyroidism, excessive doses of vitamin D, familial hypocalciuric hypercalcemia, and total parenteral nutrition. Hypertriglyceridemia can also cause pancreatitis. The risk of acute pancreatitis in patients with serum triglycerides greater than 1,000 mg/dL is about 5%, and for patients with serum triglycerides greater than 2,000 mg/dL, the risk is 10% to 20%. In surgical procedures that cause hypotension, acute pancreatitis can occur because of hypoperfusion and resulting ischemia. Also, after ERCP, hyperamylasemia and abdominal pain caused by pancreatitis is common. Periampullary tumors, masses of the pancreatic head, and cystic lesions of the pancreas can cause obstruction of the pancreatic duct, impeding the flow of pancreatic enzymes, which may lead to inappropriate enzyme activation within the pancreas.

Additional possible causes of pancreatitis include insecticides, methanol, organophosphates, and thiazide diuretics. Up to 500 different medications have pancreatitis as a potential side effect.

 CLINICAL CONCEPT

Patients who engage in heavy drinking are commonly admitted with an acute exacerbation of chronic pancreatitis.

Pathophysiology

Acute pancreatitis is an inflammatory disease of the pancreas that can result from episodes of untreated cholecystitis caused by gallstones. A gallstone can lodge in the common bile duct and obstruct free flow of enzymes from the pancreas. The digestive enzymes then back up and perform autodigestion on the gland parenchyma and destroy the pancreatic cells. Autodigestion leads to severe damage to pancreatic cells, edema, vascular insufficiency, and ischemia of the gland.

Alcohol, drugs, and infectious agents can directly damage the cells of the pancreas. Alcohol and drug metabolites can reach the pancreas and cause premature activation of pancreatic enzymes. Ethanol or toxins can increase the permeability of ductules, allowing enzymes to reach the parenchyma and cause pancreatic damage. Ethanol also increases the protein content of pancreatic juice, decreases bicarbonate levels, and hinders trypsin inhibitor. Without trypsin inhibitor or bicarbonate, acids injure the gland, and protein plugs block pancreatic outflow.

The cause of acute pancreatitis by hypertriglyceridemia is unclear. However, there are two hypotheses. One is that the metabolism of excessive triglycerides by pancreatic lipase to free fatty acids leads to pancreatic cell injury and ischemia. Alternatively, hyperviscosity from excessive triglycerides in pancreatic capillaries leads to ischemia of the pancreas. Specific genetic mutations such as

CFTR and *ApoE* gene mutation are associated with hypertriglyceridemia-associated acute pancreatitis.

Acute pancreatitis is classified as either acute interstitial pancreatitis or acute hemorrhagic pancreatitis. Hemorrhagic pancreatitis can cause retroperitoneal blood accumulation. Chronic pancreatitis is characterized by permanent changes in pancreatic structure and persistent dysfunction even after the precipitating cause has been corrected. Necrotizing pancreatitis, which is the necrosis of cells, edema, and bleeding with loss of gland function, is the most severe condition and is associated with high morbidity and mortality.

After an episode of pancreatitis, both exocrine and endocrine functions of the pancreas can be impaired; with inflammation of the gland, the affected individual can become deficient in digestive enzymes and insulin.

Clinical Presentation

The classic symptom associated with acute pancreatitis is severe abdominal pain, which is characteristically dull, penetrating, and steady. Usually, the pain is sudden in onset and gradually intensifies in severity. Most often it is located in the epigastric region and radiates straight into the back. Nausea, vomiting, and diarrhea occur with accompanying anorexia. Fever, tachycardia, and hypotension commonly accompany the pain. Dyspnea and tachypnea may also occur because of irritation of the diaphragm.

On physical examination, abdominal tenderness, muscular guarding, and distention are observed in most patients; bowel sounds are often diminished or absent. Some patients exhibit jaundice. Patients with severe acute pancreatitis are often pale, diaphoretic, and lethargic. Occasionally, muscular spasms may be noted secondary to hypocalcemia.

Physical examination may also reveal Cullen's sign and Grey Turner sign (see Fig. 32-5). The **Cullen sign** is a dark-blue discoloration around the umbilicus that resembles a bruise resulting from blood in the peritoneal cavity because of hemorrhagic pancreatitis. The **Grey Turner sign** is a dark-blue discoloration resembling bruises along the flanks resulting from retroperitoneal blood dissecting along tissue planes. Erythematous skin nodules may result from subcutaneous fat necrosis; these are typically located on extensor skin surfaces. In addition, polyarthritis is occasionally seen.

Diagnosis

Establishing the severity of acute pancreatitis is critical to predict the patient's course and anticipate complications. Many scoring systems can predict morbidity and mortality. A common scoring system used is the revised Atlanta classification (RAC) (see Box 32-2).

Diagnostic testing involves blood work and noninvasive imaging. Blood work includes complete blood count, blood glucose level, blood urea nitrogen, serum calcium, lactic dehydrogenase, amylase, and lipase.

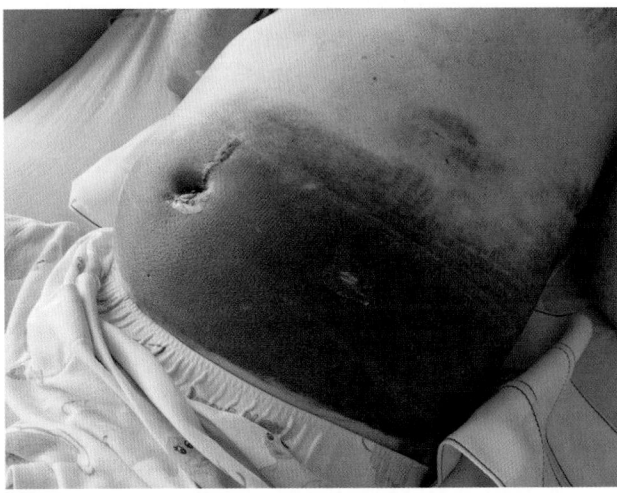

FIGURE 32-5. Cullen sign is a dark blue discoloration resembling a bruise in the periumbilical region of the abdomen. It occurs due to the release of pancreatic enzymes that cause inflammation, fat necrosis, and intra-abdominal bleeding in severe pancreatitis. **Grey Turner sign** is a dark blue discoloration resembling a bruise in the flank regions. It is due to release of pancreatic enzymes that cause inflammation and bleeding within the retroperitoneal region in severe pancreatitis. Both are shown in this photo. *(Source: Barry Slaven/Science Source.)*

BOX 32-2. Revised Atlanta Classification for Diagnosis of Acute Pancreatitis

DIAGNOSIS OF ACUTE PANCREATITIS REQUIRES TWO OUT OF THREE FOLLOWING FEATURES:
1. Abdominal epigastric pain that radiates to the mid-back
2. Elevation of serum amylase or lipase (greater than 3x normal)
3. Imaging study consistent with pancreatic inflammation

From Banks, P. A., Bollen, T. L., Dervenis, C., et al. (2013). Acute Pancreatitis Classification Working Group. Classification of acute pancreatitis–2012: revision of the Atlanta classification and definitions by international consensus. *Gut, 62*(1), 102–111.

The blood level of amylase is 10 to 20 times greater than normal in acute pancreatitis and is also an early response to injury. Serum lipase levels are usually elevated about 72 hours after the onset of symptoms. Noninvasive imaging studies include abdominal and endoscopic ultrasound, CT scan, and MRCP.

The severity of acute pancreatitis is categorized by the revised Atlanta classification according to the presence and duration of organ failure (i.e., respiratory, kidney, or cardiovascular) and the presence of local complications (see Box 32-3). Mild pancreatitis is the most common form of acute pancreatitis and is self-limiting.

Another scoring system is used to predict mortality in patients with pancreatitis. The Bedside Index

BOX 32-3. Revised Atlanta Classification of the Severity of Pancreatitis

Mild acute pancreatitis	No organ failure No local or systemic complications
Moderately severe acute pancreatitis	Organ failure that resolves within 48 hours and/or systemic complications without organ failure
Severe acute pancreatitis	Persistent organ failure >48 hours and/or multiple organ failure

From Banks, P. A., Bollen, T. L., Dervenis, C., et al. (2013). Acute Pancreatitis Classification Working Group. Classification of acute pancreatitis–2012: Revision of the Atlanta classification and definitions by international consensus. *Gut, 62*(1), 102–111.

for Severity in Acute Pancreatitis (BISAP) score was designed as a predictor of mortality based on five variables (see Box 32-4). The lowest score was associated with a less than 1% mortality rate and the highest with a greater than 20% mortality rate.

In addition to scoring systems, individual biomarkers may also have predictive value in acute pancreatitis. C-reactive protein (CRP) is commonly obtained in hospitalized patients. CRP levels of 190 mg/L or greater within the first 48 hours of admission or an absolute increase of greater than 90 mg/L predict severe disease.

CLINICAL CONCEPT

Elevated serum lipase level is a key sign of acute pancreatitis.

Treatment

There is no proven therapy that directly ameliorates pancreatic inflammation. There are two cornerstones in acute pancreatitis management regardless of the etiology: (1) fluid resuscitation to maintain or restore tissue perfusion and (2) nutritional support to counter the catabolic state and decrease the rate of infectious complications. Treatments provide supportive care and minimize pancreatic stimulation. Fluid resuscitation and maintenance of optimal fluid balance are necessary.

It is unnecessary to wait until the pain has resolved before resuming a diet in patients who have acute pancreatitis. In general, patients tolerating oral nutrition should be placed on a low-fat soft or solid diet. If patients are unable to tolerate an oral diet, they should be started on nasoenteral nutrition. The most recent guidelines from the American Gastroenterological Association (AGA) recommend initiating enteral feeding within 24 to 72 hours. Reduced intestinal vascular perfusion in acute pancreatitis can lead to gastrointestinal mucosal damage, peritonitis, sepsis, and organ failure. Early nutrition mitigates these potential adverse effects. Patients who cannot tolerate enteral feeding due to paralytic ileus, obstruction, or other causes should be started on parenteral nutrition within 72 hours.

The patient should receive sufficient analgesic medication for pain control, as abdominal pain may be intense. Dilaudid is commonly prescribed because it does not have gastrointestinal side effects. Neither total parenteral nutrition nor prophylactic antibiotic therapy is indicated in uncomplicated acute pancreatitis.

Hypovolemia can be caused by the exudation of fluid into the inflamed pancreatic retroperitoneal area and by the gastrointestinal fluid losses caused by vomiting and nasogastric suction. This fluid shift should be corrected promptly. Patients who are still hypotensive after adequate volume replacement require placement of central catheters to allow more precise assessment and management of fluid and electrolyte requirements.

Most patients with gallstone pancreatitis can undergo cholecystectomy. Patients with severe gallstone pancreatitis and evidence that gallstones are impacted at the ampulla of Vater in the small intestine

BOX 32-4. Bedside Index for Severity of Acute Pancreatitis (BISAP) Score

PARAMETER	LEVEL	BISAP POINTS
BUN (blood urea nitrogen)	BUN >25 mg/dL	1 point
Impaired mental status	Abnormal mental status evidenced by Glasgow Coma Scale score <15	1 point
Systemic inflammatory response syndrome (SIRS)	Evidence of SIRS	1 point
Age	Older than 60 years	1 point
Pleural effusion	Imaging study shows pleural effusion	1 point
SCORE 0 to 2 points = low mortality risk		
SCORE 3 to 5 points = higher mortality risk		

From Gao, W., Yang, H. X., & Ma, C. E. (2015). The value of BISAP score for predicting mortality and severity in acute pancreatitis: A systematic review and meta-analysis. *PLoS One, 10*(6), e0130412. doi: 10.1371/journal.pone.0130412

require prompt ERCP with sphincterotomy and stone extraction.

The major indication for early surgical intervention is the presence of an acute abdomen. Intestinal perforation or necrosis, which sometimes mimics hemorrhagic acute pancreatitis, can be confirmed and corrected only when a laparotomy is performed.

Alcohol-related acute pancreatitis is a predictor of developing recurrent acute pancreatitis and chronic pancreatitis. The AGA recommends performing a brief alcohol intervention during the hospitalization for alcohol-related acute pancreatitis, and additional educational sessions in 6-month intervals for 2 years after discharge.

Obese patients and those with hypertriglyceridemia should be counseled regarding weight reduction, dietary modifications, and alcohol avoidance. Pharmacological therapies include fibrates, statins, niacin, and omega 3 fatty acids. Patients found to have hypercalcemia during an episode of acute pancreatitis should be evaluated for primary hyperparathyroidism or, less commonly, malignancy and thyrotoxicosis.

Potential Complications of Acute Pancreatitis

Infected pancreatic necrosis should be suspected in patients who have moderate-to-severe acute pancreatitis; who have worsening symptoms after initial improvement; and who develop new fever, marked by leukocytosis, positive blood cultures, or other evidence of sepsis. If necrotic pancreatitis is suspected, an emergency abdominal CT scan with IV contrast enhancements should be performed.

Pancreatic pseudocysts occur in 10% to 20% of cases of acute pancreatitis. A **pseudocyst** is a circumscribed collection of fluid rich in pancreatic enzymes, blood, and necrotic tissue. Diagnosis is made most easily by abdominal ultrasound or CT scan. Small pseudocysts tend to resolve without treatment. Cysts that have been present for more than 6 weeks and are larger than 5 cm in diameter usually require treatment to prevent leakage and cellular injury.

Systemic Complications. The most important systemic complications of acute pancreatitis are cardiovascular, renal, and respiratory failure. Cardiovascular complications include profound hypotension.

Renal failure usually occurs as a result of hypovolemia and decreased renal perfusion. The prevention and treatment of pancreatitis-associated renal failure depend, to a large extent, on correcting fluid and electrolyte abnormalities. Mild and transient respiratory failure can occur as a result of splinting of respiration and atelectasis. In most cases, respiratory failure usually improves as the acute phase of pancreatitis ends. Some patients progress to a more severe form of respiratory failure that resembles adult respiratory distress syndrome (ARDS). This poor prognostic sign is frequently associated with a complicated clinical course or death. Pancreatitis-associated ARDS results from injury to the alveolar membrane or degradation of surfactant by circulating enzymes, which may be released from the inflamed pancreas. Treatment is usually supportive because specific therapy for pancreatitis-associated ARDS has not been defined.

Chronic Pancreatitis

Chronic pancreatitis (CP) is a chronic inflammatory and fibrotic disease of the pancreas with a prevalence of 42 to 73 per 100,000 adults in the United States. Alcohol use disorder is the most common etiology of CP and is diagnosed in 42% to 77% of patients. Like acute pancreatitis, it occurs when digestive enzymes attack the pancreas and nearby tissues, causing episodes of pain.

Chronic pancreatitis often develops in people between the ages of 30 and 40 years. It is three times more common in African Americans than in European Americans. It has a bimodal incidence, with an early onset form at a median age of 19 years and a late-onset form at 56 years. Alcohol-induced, chronic pancreatitis is more common in males, whereas hyperlipidemic-induced disease is more common in females. Hereditary pancreatitis can present in a person younger than 30 years, but it might not be diagnosed for several years.

Etiology

The most common cause of chronic pancreatitis is long-term, heavy alcohol use and can be triggered by one acute attack that damages the pancreatic duct. Other causes of chronic pancreatitis include hereditary disorders, cystic fibrosis, hypercalcemia, hyperlipidemia, drugs, and autoimmune problems, such as Sjögren's syndrome. A diagnosis of hereditary pancreatitis is likely if the person has two or more family members with pancreatitis spanning more than one generation. Up to 50% of individuals with hereditary pancreatitis have mutations of the trypsin inhibitor gene (SPINK1) or the cystic fibrosis transmembrane conductance regulator (CFTR) gene. Chronic pancreatitis has also been associated with primary biliary cholangitis and renal tubular acidosis.

Pathophysiology

Chronic pancreatitis commonly results after several episodes of acute pancreatitis over the lifetime of the affected individual. Cellular injury is apparent with pancreatic fibrotic changes, which involve cellular release of growth factors, cytokines, and chemokines, leading to deposition of extracellular matrix and fibroblast proliferation. The pancreas ceases to function and develops scar tissue that requires patient supplementation of digestive enzymes and insulin.

Clinical Presentation

Most people with chronic pancreatitis experience upper abdominal pain, although some individuals have no pain at all. The pain may spread to the back, feel worse when eating or drinking, and become constant and disabling. In some cases, abdominal pain decreases as the condition worsens, most likely because the pancreas is no longer making digestive enzymes. Other symptoms include nausea, vomiting, weight loss, diarrhea, and steatorrhea. People with chronic pancreatitis often lose weight, even when their appetite and eating habits are normal. The weight loss occurs because the body does not secrete enough pancreatic enzymes to digest food, and malabsorption of nutrients occurs.

Diagnosis

Serum amylase and lipase levels may be slightly elevated in chronic pancreatitis but may be normal if pancreatic tissue is nonfunctional and fibrotic. Laboratory studies to identify causative factors of chronic pancreatitis include serum calcium and triglyceride levels. When common etiologies are not found, testing for genetic conditions such as cystic fibrosis should be done. Fecal studies can reveal steatorrhea, which is a manifestation of advanced chronic pancreatitis. Fecal chymotrypsin and human pancreatic elastase can be useful in confirming advanced chronic pancreatitis with exocrine insufficiency.

Abdominal x-ray may reveal pancreatic calcifications, considered pathognomonic of chronic pancreatitis, which are observed in approximately 30% of cases. A contrast-enhanced computed tomographic (CT) scan is an initial diagnostic test and should be performed for all patients with suspicion of chronic pancreatitis. If CT cannot decipher chronic pancreatitis, ERCP provides the most accurate visualization of the pancreatic ductal system. MRCP provides information on the pancreatic parenchyma and adjacent abdominal viscera. Endoscopic ultrasonography can show characteristic calcifications in the pancreas with chronic inflammation. Biopsy of the pancreas shows fibrotic changes, protein plugs, and calcifications.

Treatment

Treatment for chronic pancreatitis commonly requires hospitalization for pain management, IV hydration, and nutritional support. Nasogastric feedings may be necessary for several weeks if the person continues to lose weight. When a normal diet is resumed, synthetic pancreatic enzymes may be prescribed if the pancreas does not secrete enough of its own. The enzymes should be taken with every meal to help the person digest food and regain some weight. The next step is to plan a diet that is low in fat and that includes small, frequent meals. Drinking plenty of fluids and limiting caffeinated beverages is also important. People with chronic pancreatitis are strongly advised not to smoke or consume alcoholic beverages, even if the pancreatitis is mild or in the early stages.

ERCP drainage procedures can be used to treat pain when medical therapies are unsuccessful. These procedures alleviate pancreatic ductal obstruction from stones, strictures, or both in an effort to reduce intraductal hypertension and thereby pain.

The surgical procedures used include partial resection (Whipple procedure) or distal pancreatectomy. The Whipple procedure, also known as a pancreaticoduodenectomy, is an operation to remove the head of the pancreas, the first part of the small intestine (duodenum), the gallbladder, and the bile duct.

Complications

People with chronic pancreatitis who continue to consume large amounts of alcohol may develop sudden bouts of severe abdominal pain. As with acute pancreatitis, ERCP is used to identify and treat complications associated with chronic pancreatitis, such as gallstones, pseudocysts, and narrowing or obstruction of the ducts. Chronic pancreatitis can also lead to calcification of the pancreas, meaning that the pancreatic tissue hardens from deposits of insoluble calcium salts. Surgery may be necessary to remove part of the pancreas. In cases involving persistent pain, surgery or other procedures are sometimes recommended to block the nerves in the abdominal area that cause pain.

When pancreatic tissue is destroyed in chronic pancreatitis and the insulin-producing cells of the pancreas, called beta cells, have been damaged, diabetes may develop. Persons with a family history of diabetes are more likely to develop the disease. If diabetes occurs, insulin or antidiabetic medications are needed to keep blood glucose at normal levels. A health-care provider works with the patient to develop a regimen of medication, diet, and frequent blood glucose monitoring.

Cancer of the Pancreas

Pancreatic cancer is one of the most lethal cancers and is increasing in incidence in the United States. It occurs in 6% of the population and is the third most common cause of cancer. According to the American Cancer Society, pancreatic cancer affected 62,210 persons in 2022 and 49,830 people died of the cancer. Most patients have no obvious symptoms during disease development and progression to advanced metastasis, whereby tumor cells are highly invasive. Early diagnosis is difficult, which causes this to be one of the deadliest malignant tumors. Most patients eventually relapse; even after a potential radical treatment, the patient's 5-year survival rate is only 2% to 9%. At the time of diagnosis, 52% of all patients have metastatic disease and 26% have regional spread to lymph nodes and vasculature.

Approximately 90% of newly diagnosed patients are older than 55 years, and most are between 70 and 80 years old. The incidence is lower in females than in males globally. In the United States, the incidence in African Americans is higher than that in European Americans, while Asian Americans and Pacific Islanders have the lowest incidence.

Etiology

The cause of pancreatic cancer is unknown; however, risk factors associated with the disease include cigarette smoking, obesity, diabetes mellitus, and chronic pancreatitis. Consumption of nitrites, preservatives found in such processed meats as bacon, has also been associated with a higher risk of pancreatic cancer.

Approximately 5% to 10% of patients with pancreatic carcinoma have some genetic predisposition to developing the disease. Inherited disorders that increase the risk of pancreatic cancer include hereditary pancreatitis, multiple endocrine neoplasia, hereditary nonpolyposis rectal cancer, familial adenomatous polyposis and Gardner syndrome, familial atypical multiple mole melanoma syndrome, Peutz–Jeghers syndrome, ataxia-telangiectasia, Lynch II syndrome, and von Hippel–Lindau syndrome. Several genetic mutations are associated with pancreatic ductal adenocarcinoma: the activated oncogene KRAS and defective tumor suppressor genes *CDKN2A, TP53,* and *SMAD4.* Up to 20% of pancreatic adenocarcinomas are associated with the *BRCA1* and *BRCA2* genes.

Epidemiological studies show a significant increase in the risk of pancreatic cancer in people with diabetes. In type 1 diabetes, the risk increases by 5 to 10 times in patients with a disease duration of more than 10 years. People with diabetes who have been diagnosed with the disease for more than 20 years are at highest risk. However, some researchers have found that the number of microorganisms in the pancreas of patients with pancreatic cancer is 1,000 times that of normal. Smokers have a 74% increased risk of illness, and pancreatic cancer is significantly higher in people who drink more than 30 g of alcohol per day.

Pathophysiology

Cancer of the pancreas can arise from exocrine or endocrine cells. Most pancreatic tumors arise from exocrine cells in the ducts; these are referred to as ductal adenocarcinomas. Tumors arising in small ducts invade nearby glandular tissue, penetrate the covering of the pancreas, and extend into surrounding tissues.

Ductal adenocarcinomas can occur in the head, body, or tail of the pancreas. Tumors of the head of the pancreas quickly spread to obstruct the common bile duct and portal vein. Obstruction of the common bile duct causes bile to back up into the liver. Bile backup leads to bilirubin backup and accumulation in the bloodstream, causing jaundice. Jaundice usually brings the patient to the attention of a health-care provider.

Ductal adenocarcinomas can infiltrate the superior mesenteric artery, the vena cava, and the aorta. Cancer cells that enter the blood vessels can form emboli. Tumors of the body and tail of the pancreas infiltrate the posterior abdominal walls. Lymphatic invasion occurs early and rapidly and involves local and regional lymph nodes. Cancer cells also enter the venous system, causing metastases to the liver. Tumors that metastasize to the peritoneum can obstruct veins and promote development of ascites.

Clinical Presentation

Cancer that arises in the head of the pancreas leads to bile duct obstruction, which causes jaundice (see Fig. 32-6), an early warning sign of pancreatic cancer. The patient with cancer in the head of the pancreas classically presents with painless jaundice, whereas cancer of the body and tail of the pancreas is generally asymptomatic for a lengthy amount of time. Symptoms do not present until late, when there is intraductal destruction and tumor invasion of adjacent tissue.

Often, vague back pain is present. As the disease worsens, there is constant epigastric pain with radiation to the back. Back pain worsens when the patient assumes the supine position; often this causes intense nighttime abdominal pain. Nausea, vomiting, and accompanying anorexia are common.

Cancer of the head of the pancreas can obstruct the common bile duct, which causes backup of bile into the liver. Obstruction of the common bile duct by pancreatic cancer often manifests as Courvoisier's sign. Courvoisier's sign describes an enlarged, palpable gallbladder due to backup of bile and inflammation of the gallbladder and the common bile duct. Bile and bile constituents back up into the common bile duct and back into the liver. Bile constituents accumulate in the liver, which causes high levels of bilirubin to back up into the bloodstream. Bilirubin accumulation in

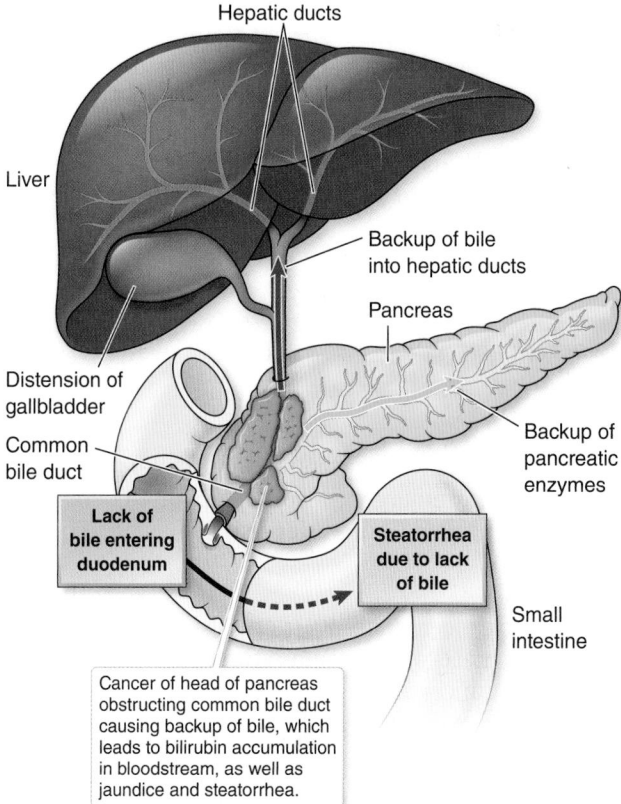

FIGURE 32-6. Cancer of the head of the pancreas.

the bloodstream causes yellowing of the elastin components of the skin and sclera. Bilirubin in the blood is also filtered into the urine, which causes tea-colored urine. Lack of bile causes fat malabsorption and fat accumulation in the stool (steatorrhea). Lack of bile in the intestine causes lack of bilirubin pigment in the stool and, hence, clay-colored stool. Bile backup also causes bile salts to accumulate in the blood that leads to pruritus. Darkening of urine, steatorrhea, and pruritus are often noticed by patients before clinical jaundice occurs. Weight loss occurs because of malabsorption of all nutrients when pancreatic enzymes are no longer produced. Depression is common in patients with pancreatic cancer and may be the most prominent presenting symptom for some individuals.

The onset of diabetes mellitus can be associated with pancreatic cancer. Cancer can invade the beta cells of the pancreas, which secrete insulin. Pancreatic cancer should be considered in a patient older than age 70 years with a new diagnosis of diabetes without any other diabetic risk factors.

> ### CLINICAL CONCEPT
>
> Migratory thrombophlebitis and venous thrombosis also occur with higher frequency in patients with pancreatic cancer and may be the first presentation.

Distant metastases are found in the cervical and other lymph nodes, the lungs, and the brain. In late stages, the patient may present with signs of portal vein hypertension. High pressure within the portal vein causes peritoneal edema that appears as ascites, venous congestion of the liver and spleen demonstrated as hepatomegaly and splenomegaly. Most individuals die of hepatic failure, malnutrition, or systemic disease.

> **ALERT!** The patient with pancreatic cancer classically presents with painless jaundice.

A left supraclavicular lymph node, called Virchow's node, may be enlarged; also a palpable, edematous gallbladder, called Courvoisier's sign, may be found.

Diagnosis

Pancreatic cancer is often a silent disease until its late stages. Laboratory and imaging studies used to diagnose pancreatic cancer are the same as those used for acute and chronic pancreatitis. Jaundice does not become apparent until bilirubin backs up into the bloodstream because of an obstructed common bile duct. The most difficult clinical situation in which to diagnose pancreatic carcinoma is in the patient with underlying chronic pancreatitis. In such cases, the abnormalities seen in imaging studies may not help to differentiate between pancreatic carcinoma and chronic pancreatitis. Abdominal multidetector CT scan is the standard imaging study used in pancreatic cancer and is often used to guide biopsy. ERCP provides the most accurate visualization of the pancreatic ductal system. Transcutaneous or endoscopic ultrasound imaging can also assist in diagnosis. MRCP provides images of the pancreatic parenchyma and adjacent abdominal viscera. Positron emission tomography (PET) can diagnose tumors as it images highly metabolic tissue. Due to the active metabolism of tumor cells, the ability to take up imaging agents is 2 to 10 times that of normal cells, forming an obvious "light spot" on the image. Differential diffusion-weighted imaging (DWI) is a specific MRI technique that can also be used to visualize the cancer.

After visualization of a tumor, biopsy and study of the tissue (termed histopathology) is the gold standard for the diagnosis of pancreatic cancer. Current methods for obtaining histopathology or cell specimens include endoscopic ultrasonography or CT-guided biopsy. Alternatively, cells obtained from ascites fluid can be examined or a laparoscopy can be done to obtain cells from the pancreas.

The carbohydrate antigen 19-9 (CA 19-9 antigen) is a tumor marker found in some cancer patients. It is also normally present within the cells of the biliary tract and can be elevated in acute or chronic biliary disease. However, about 5% to 10% of patients lack the enzyme necessary to produce CA 19-9; in such patients, monitoring the disease with this tumor marker is not possible. CEA is another tumor marker commonly found in gastrointestinal cancers; it is present in 40% to 45% of patients with pancreatic cancer.

Treatment

A laparotomy is performed, particularly if jaundice is present. Laparotomy is used to establish a definitive diagnosis, evaluate the extent of disease, and determine whether palliative bypass surgery is needed. Most individuals require palliative double-bypass of the blocked bile ducts, as well as gastrojejunostomy to prevent duodenal obstruction.

Tumors limited to the pancreas are surgically resectable. Only 15% to 20% of patients with pancreatic cancer are candidates for surgical resection and undergo the Whipple procedure (also called pancreaticoduodenectomy) (see Fig. 32-7). This surgical intervention involves removal of the head of the pancreas as well as a portion of the bile duct, the gallbladder, and the duodenum. Occasionally, a portion of the stomach may also be removed. After removal of these structures, the remaining pancreas, bile duct, and duodenum are sutured back into the intestine.

Staging pancreatic cancer is accomplished using either the Japanese Pancreatic Case Association Criteria or Union Internationale Contre le Cancer (UICC) stage classification (see Box 32-5).

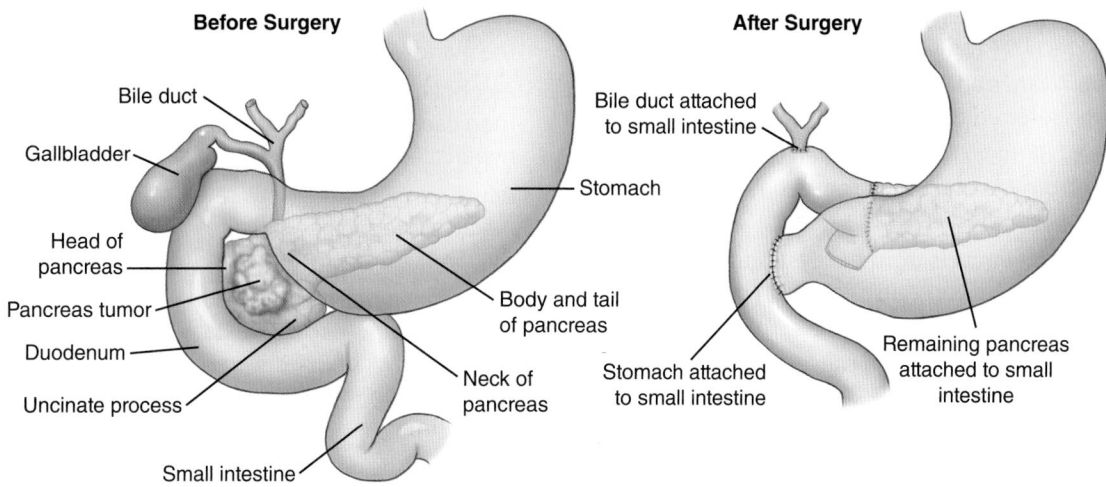

FIGURE 32-7. The Whipple procedure (pancreaticoduodenectomy) is a surgical procedure to remove the head of the pancreas, the first part of the small intestine (duodenum), the gallbladder, and the bile duct.

BOX 32-5. The Japanese Criteria for Staging Pancreatic Cancer

STAGE	DESCRIPTION OF TUMOR AND SPREAD
Stage I	Tumor diameter is less than or equal to 2 cm with no vascular or lymphatic invasion
Stage II	Tumor diameter is greater than 2 cm and less than 4 cm, enveloped cancer infiltration with no vascular invasion or metastasis
Stage III	Tumor diameter is greater than 4 cm with invasion of lymphatics
Stage IV	Tumor diameter is greater than 4 cm with evidence of metastasis

Adapted from Kobari, M., & Matsuno, S. (1998). Staging systems for pancreatic cancer: differences between the Japanese and UICC systems. *J Hepatobiliary Pancreat Surg, 5*(2), 121–127. doi: 10.1007/s005340050021

Surgical resection is commonly followed by chemotherapy. When pancreatic cancer has spread to regional lymph nodes or the mesenteric vasculature, combinations of chemotherapeutic agents are recommended. Chemoradiotherapy may be used in some cases. Patients who have undergone potentially curative treatment for pancreatic cancer should continue to receive ongoing supportive care for symptoms that may result from treatment, including pain, anorexia and weight loss, depression and anxiety, biliary obstruction, pancreatic insufficiency, and venous thromboembolism.

Chapter Summary

- The liver produces and secretes bile for the digestion of fats; the gallbladder stores some of the bile. The liver releases bile into the hepatic duct, which continues on into the common bile duct.

- The gallbladder concentrates and stores bile. It releases the bile into the cystic duct, which then continues into the common bile duct.

- Highly concentrated bile and diminished gallbladder motility can cause bile stasis, which can develop into biliary sludge or cholesterol stones. The process of gallstone formation is called cholelithiasis.

- When cholesterol precipitates out of bile, it becomes a gallstone, also called a calculus.

- Bile stasis, biliary sludge, and gallstones can cause inflammation of the gallbladder and cause cholecystitis.

- Females older than 40 years are frequently affected by cholecystitis caused by cholelithiasis. Symptoms include RUQ abdominal pain, frequent indigestion, nausea, vomiting, eructations, and flatulence.

- The RUQ pain associated with cholecystitis is called Murphy's sign. Pain often radiates to the right scapula.

- Biliary colic is the term used to describe the type of pain that is caused by cholecystitis: a pain that increases to a peak, then wanes and decreases, giving temporary relief. This is referred to as colicky pain.
- The removal of the gallbladder, called laparoscopic cholecystectomy, is one of the most common surgical procedures performed.
- When a gallstone travels from the cystic duct into the common bile duct, it can cause common bile duct obstruction.
- Common bile duct obstruction causes backup of bile into the liver, which causes backup of bilirubin from the liver into the bloodstream. Bilirubin is a yellow compound that attaches to elastin connective tissue. Hyperbilirubinemia causes jaundice, which is yellowing of the skin and sclera.
- When bile is blocked from getting into the intestine, fats are not digested, and steatorrhea (fat in stool) develops. Bile backs up into the liver, hyperbilirubinemia occurs, and bile salts accumulate in the bloodstream. Hyperbilirubinemia causes jaundice, and high bile salts in the blood cause pruritus.
- The pancreas produces digestive enzymes and secretes them into the small intestine through the pancreatic duct for digestion of fats, proteins, and carbohydrates.

- In acute pancreatitis, pancreatic enzymes back up into the gland and cause autodigestion.
- Alcohol use disorder and gallstones are the most common causes of pancreatitis. Hypertriglyceridemia or hypercalcemia can also cause acute pancreatitis.
- Acute pancreatitis causes severe, epigastric pain that radiates into the back.
- Chronic pancreatitis causes gradual deterioration of the pancreas via autodigestion. Episodes of acute pain and symptoms occur. The patient suffers malabsorption from lack of digestive enzymes, diabetes from lack of insulin secretion, and eventual weight loss and malnutrition.
- Cancer of the pancreas often occurs in the head of the pancreas and causes obstruction of the common bile duct. Painless jaundice is commonly the first sign of this condition.
- Cancer of the pancreas requires a surgical procedure called the Whipple procedure.
- Pancreatic cancer has a poor survival rate.

Making the Connections

Signs and Symptoms	Physical Assessment Findings	Diagnostic Testing	Treatment
Cholelithiasis | The formation of gallstones, also called calculi, caused by precipitation of substances contained in bile, mainly cholesterol and bilirubin. Gallstones irritate the inner walls of the gallbladder, causing inflammation; this is referred to as cholecystitis.			
The condition may be asymptomatic during the formation of the gallstones. Once formed, gallstones cause inflammation of the gallbladder, causing RUQ pain, indigestion, flatulence, eructations, nausea, and possibly vomiting. Pain builds up, then decreases, resulting in a biliary colic type of pain.	Murphy's sign: pain upon palpation of the RUQ of the abdomen.	Ultrasonography, CT scans, MRI, and HIDA scans can show gallstones, inflamed gallbladder wall, bile stasis, or sludge. This results in elevated WBC count, ESR, and CRP caused by inflammation. Total serum bilirubin and liver enzymes; aminotransferase, and alkaline phosphatase may be elevated if a gallstone causes obstruction of the common bile duct and backup of bile into the liver.	Laparoscopic surgical removal of gallbladder or open cholecystectomy. Narcotic for pain. If surgery is not an option, medications or lithotripsy can be used to dissolve the stones.

Making the Connections–cont'd

Signs and Symptoms	Physical Assessment Findings	Diagnostic Testing	Treatment
Cholecystitis | Inflammation of the gallbladder; it is generally associated with cholelithiasis, biliary sludge, or bile stasis.			
The condition may be asymptomatic during the formation of the gallstones. Once formed, gallstones cause inflammation of the gallbladder, causing RUQ pain, indigestion, flatulence, eructations, nausea, and possibly vomiting. Pain builds up, then decreases, resulting in a biliary colic type of pain.	Murphy's sign (as above).	Diagnostic criteria for acute cholecystitis (2018 Tokyo Guidelines). Ultrasonography, CT scans, MRI, and HIDA scans can show gallstones, inflamed gallbladder wall, bile stasis, or sludge. This can result in elevated WBC count, ESR, and CRP caused by inflammation. Total serum bilirubin and liver enzymes, aminotransferase, and alkaline phosphatase may be elevated if a gallstone causes obstruction of the common bile duct and backup of bile into the liver.	Laparoscopic surgical removal of gallbladder or open cholecystectomy. Narcotic for pain. If surgery is not an option, medications such as ursodiol or procedures such as lithotripsy can be used to dissolve the stones. Avoid food intake during acute attack, and if bile flow is obstructed, fat-soluble vitamins, such as A, D, E, and K, and bile salts may need to be administered.
Pancreatitis, Acute | A severe, life-threatening disorder associated with activated pancreatic enzymes secreted into the pancreatic tissue and surrounding tissue, causing inflammation and autodigestion.			
Acute abdominal pain, nausea, vomiting. Abrupt onset; may follow a heavy meal or binging on alcohol. Severe epigastric and abdominal pain that radiates straight to the back, which is aggravated when the person is lying supine and is relieved when the person is sitting and leaning forward.	Abdominal distention, hypoactive bowel sounds, tachycardia, hypotension. Cool, clammy skin and fever. Jaundice. Cullen's sign. Grey Turner sign.	Revised Atlanta classification (RAC) for diagnosis of acute pancreatitis. Bedside Index for Severity of Acute Pancreatitis (BISAP). Elevated serum amylase and lipase occurs with pancreatic inflammation. Elevated blood glucose, urea nitrogen, calcium, and triglycerides. Elevated liver enzymes. Elevated bilirubin level. Elevated C-reactive protein (CRP). Urine amylase: elevated levels with pancreatic inflammation. Steatorrhea caused by lack of fat digestion because of decreased lipase in the intestine. ERCP, endoscopic ultrasound, MRCP.	Fluid resuscitation. Nutritional intervention such as oral or enteral feedings. Cholecystectomy may be necessary if gallstones are the cause of pancreatitis. Dilaudid as pain reliever. Alcohol and tobacco abstinence required. Obese patients and those with hypertriglyceridemia should be counseled regarding weight reduction, dietary modifications, and pharmacological therapies that include fibrates, statins, niacin, and omega 3 fatty acids. Persons with hypercalcemia need to have etiology investigated.

Continued

Making the Connections–cont'd

Signs and Symptoms	Physical Assessment Findings	Diagnostic Testing	Treatment
Pancreatitis, Chronic | Characterized by progressive destruction of the pancreas by enzymes. Gradual autodigestion of the pancreas. Gradually fibrotic tissue replaces pancreatic tissue.			
All symptoms associated with acute pancreatitis, although less severe. Episodic abdominal pain, nausea, and vomiting. Episodic epigastric and upper left quadrant pain, anorexia, nausea, vomiting, and flatulence. Steatorrhea: clay-colored stool.	Episodes of abdominal tenderness, vomiting, abdominal distention, lack of bowel sounds, and jaundice. Steatorrhea: clay-colored stool. Dark tea-colored urine.	Elevated serum amylase and lipase occur with pancreatic inflammation. Elevated blood glucose, urea nitrogen, triglycerides, and calcium. Elevated bilirubin level. Elevated liver enzymes. Elevated C-reactive protein (CRP). Urine amylase: elevated levels with pancreatic inflammation. Steatorrhea caused by lack of fat digestion because of decreased lipase in the intestine. ERCP, endoscopic ultrasound, MRCP, and CT scan.	Low-fat diet. Pancreatic enzymes may be needed. Insulin or antidiabetic medications are needed if the pancreas is not able to secrete insulin. Cessation of tobacco use. Alcohol abstinence required; which may require counseling and rehabilitation if alcohol use disorder involved.
Pancreatic Cancer | Neoplastic tumor that develops either in the head of the pancreas (most common) or the body or tail of the gland. Cancer of the head of the pancreas causes obstruction of the common bile duct, which causes backup of bile into the liver and backup of bilirubin into the bloodstream. This causes widespread destruction of the pancreas, with loss of pancreatic enzyme activity and metastasis to the liver.			
When the tumor is in the head of the pancreas, there are early symptoms, whereas if it is in the body or tail, cancer remains silent until there is severe organ involvement. Cancer of the pancreatic head causes obstructive jaundice, steatorrhea, nausea, vomiting, and backup of bile salts, which causes pruritus. Weight loss may be caused by lack of pancreatic enzymes and malabsorption of all nutrients.	Abdominal distention, hypoactive bowel sounds, and jaundice. Steatorrhea. Dark urine. Courvoisier's sign.	Elevated serum amylase and lipase occur with pancreatic inflammation. If pancreas dysfunction occurring, amylase and lipase may not be elevated. Bilirubin and liver enzyme level elevated. Urine amylase: elevated levels with pancreatic inflammation. Steatorrhea caused by lack of fat digestion because of decreased lipase in the intestine. Biomarkers: CEA and CA 19-9 (carbohydrate antigen). ERCP, MRCP, CT scan, and biopsy.	Whipple procedure: surgical excision of cancerous sections of the pancreas. Chemotherapy. Chemoradiotherapy. Pain relief.

Bibliography

Available online at fadavis.com

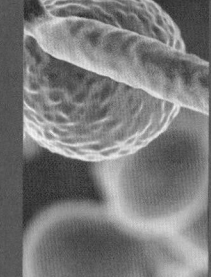

CHAPTER

33

Cerebrovascular Disorders

Learning Objectives

Upon completion of this chapter, the student will be able to:

- Recognize basic anatomical structure and function of the central and peripheral nervous system.
- Identify the circulatory routes from the aorta into the cerebral arteries of the brain.
- Differentiate between the mechanisms of ischemic versus hemorrhagic stroke.

- Describe the signs, symptoms, and clinical manifestations of acute stroke.
- Discuss the assessment and diagnostic tests used to diagnose cerebrovascular disease.
- Explain pharmacological and nonpharmacological modalities used in the treatment of the patient with acute stroke.

Key Terms

Anoxic encephalopathy
Aphasia
Arteriovenous malformation (AVM)
Carotid stenosis
Cerebral infarction
Circle of Willis
Contralateral
Corticobulbar tract
Corticospinal tract

Cushing's triad
Decussation
Expressive aphasia
Glutamate
Hemorrhagic stroke
Intracerebral hemorrhage
Ipsilateral
Ischemic penumbra
Ischemic stroke

Lacunar infarct
Neurological deficit
Receptive aphasia
Spinothalamic tract
Subarachnoid hemorrhage (SAH)
Transient ischemic attack (TIA)
Uncal herniation
Vertebral-basilar insufficiency (VBI)

The nervous system is an intricate web of fibers that enables the human body to interact with the environment. When these fibers are damaged, messages traveling to or from the brain or spinal cord may not reach their target destination. This can lead to numerous complications ranging from an inability to move to a constant struggle with intractable pain. There are various kinds of neurological disorders, and each disorder has an effect on a person's quality of life.

The most common cause of neurological disability is cerebrovascular disease; this involves disorders of the circulatory system of the brain, including cerebral ischemia and cerebral hemorrhage—the most common types of stroke. Both cause brain cell death and permanent neurological impairment.

Epidemiology

Stroke is the fifth leading cause of death in the United States and the leading cause of disability. Commonly, persons who sustain a stroke are left with paralysis of one side of their body; in addition, 20% of individuals who suffer a stroke die within 12 months. In the United States, someone has a stroke every 40 seconds, accounting for 795,000 incidents each year. In 2020, 1 in 6 deaths from cardiovascular disease was due to stroke. Every 3.5 minutes, someone dies of a stroke. The majority of persons who sustain stroke are age 65 years or older, and because of the rising number of older adults in the population, the incidence of stroke is projected to be 1 million persons per year by 2050. The risk of stroke for African Americans is about twice that of European Americans.

Basic Concepts of Cerebrovascular Structure and Function

The overall function of the nervous system is to detect, interpret, and respond to changes in the environment. It is important to review the basic concepts of cerebrovascular and neurological function before stroke can be understood.

Neuroanatomy and Neurophysiology

The nervous system is divided into two regions The central nervous system (CNS) consists of the brain and spinal cord, and the peripheral nervous system consists of cranial and spinal nerves. There are sensory and motor sections located around the midline of the brain; at this area, motor neurons descend down into the spinal cord and sensory neurons arrive up from the spinal cord (see Fig. 33-1).

Movement is dependent on motor neurons that extend from the brain down into the spinal cord. Sensation such as pain, touch, and temperature enter the spinal cord from the periphery and ascend up into the brain. The motor and sensory neurons within the brain are called upper neurons, and the neurons of the spinal cord are lower neurons. The **corticospinal tract** is the major region of upper motor neurons that descend from the brain down into the spinal cord. The **corticobulbar tract** neurons run parallel to the corticospinal tract; they descend from the cortex down into the brainstem where cranial nerves emerge. The **spinothalamic tract** is the major region of sensory neurons that travel from the periphery up into the brain. The corticospinal nerves travel from the brain and cross over at the medulla before reaching the spinal cord. Some of the corticobulbar tract nerves cross contralaterally (to the opposite side) and some remain ipsilateral (same side). At the area referred to as the **decussation** in the medulla, most upper motor neurons cross from one side of the brain to control the opposite side of the body. The spinothalamic tract originates in the spinal cord and crosses at some level within the spinal cord before arriving in the brain. This crossover of neurons causes any type of cerebral injury to manifest sensory and motor deficits on the contralateral side of the body.

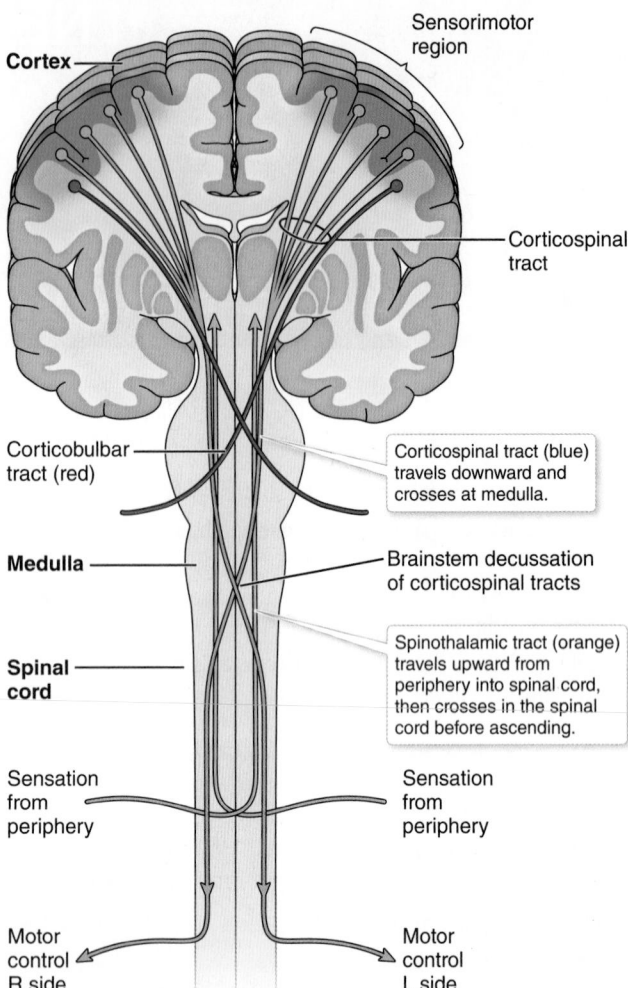

FIGURE 33-1. The sensorimotor region of the brain. Corticospinal tract neurons are motor neurons that travel from the brain into the spinal cord; they cross to the contralateral side of the medulla, an area called the decussation. Spinothalamic neurons are sensory neurons that arise from and travel up the spinal cord before crossing over to the contralateral side before reaching the brain.

The Central Nervous System

The brain can be separated into major regions: cerebrum, cerebellum, midbrain, pons, and medulla (see Fig. 33-2). The midbrain, pons, and medulla together form the brainstem. The cerebrum can be subdivided into lobes.

Cerebrum. The cerebrum makes up most of the brain tissue and is located in the uppermost region of the

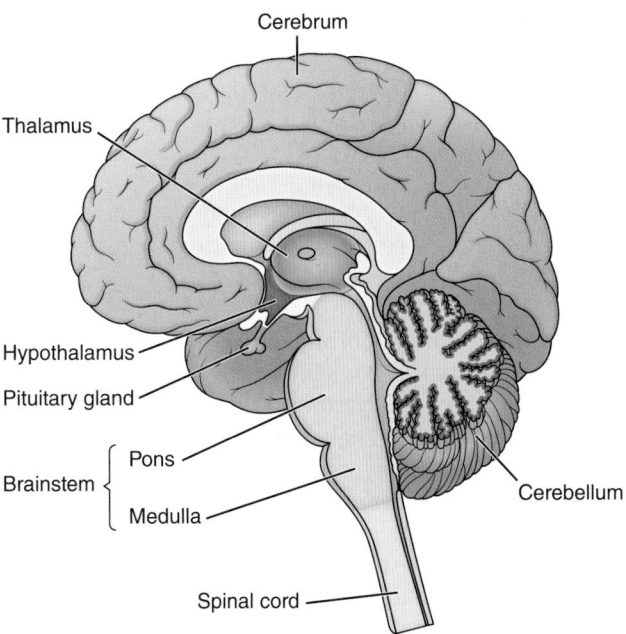

FIGURE 33-2. Major areas of the brain.

brain. It is divided into a right and left hemisphere, which are connected by the corpus callosum. Each hemisphere is also divided into the frontal, parietal, temporal, and occipital lobes. Although each lobe has specific functions, there is some overlapping of responsibilities (see Box 33-1).

Hemispheric Specialization. The location of specific functions within the brain is described as complementary hemispheric specialization (see Fig. 33-3). The cerebral hemisphere associated with language comprehension skills and sequential-analytical processes is referred to as the categorical hemisphere; in most persons, this is the left hemisphere. The other, complementary hemisphere is referred to as the representational hemisphere; in most persons, this is the right hemisphere. It focuses more on recognition of faces, music, and visual-spatial relationships than the other hemisphere.

Speech and Language Center. For most right-handed individuals, the left hemisphere is the categorical hemisphere. The left hemisphere contains areas for language comprehension, speech, and word formation. The ability to speak is controlled by a region called Broca's area, and the ability to comprehend language is controlled by Wernicke's area, which is connected to Broca's area. Dysfunction of Broca's area causes **expressive aphasia;** the affected individual cannot make words, but they do understand what others are saying. Dysfunction of Wernicke's area causes **receptive aphasia.** In receptive aphasia, the affected individual can speak but cannot understand words and uses illogical language.

BOX 33-1. Brain Lobes and Responsibilities

The brain's four lobes each have their own unique responsibilities.

FRONTAL LOBE
- Voluntary movements
- Memory
- Emotion
- Social judgment
- Decision making
- Reasoning
- Aggression

PARIETAL LOBE
- Receiving and interpreting bodily sensations
- Governing of proprioception, the awareness of one's body and body parts in space and in relation to each other

TEMPORAL LOBE
- Hearing
- Smelling
- Learning
- Memory
- Emotional behavior
- Visual recognition

OCCIPITAL LOBE
- Analyzing and interpreting visual information

Adapted from Thompson, G. S. (2015). *Understanding anatomy and physiology: A visual, auditory, interactive approach* (2nd ed.). Philadelphia: F. A. Davis.

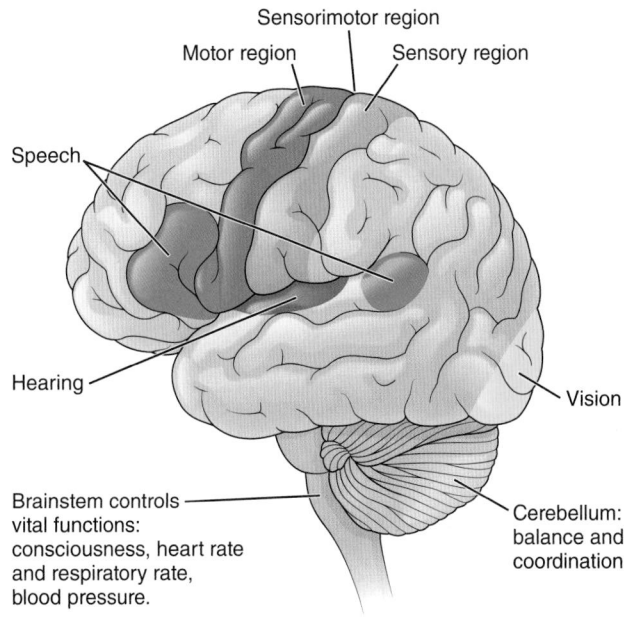

FIGURE 33-3. Functional areas of the brain.

🧬 CLINICAL CONCEPT

Most individuals with damage to the left hemisphere develop **aphasia**, a disorder that makes it difficult to speak or understand language.

Brainstem. The brainstem is divided into three regions: the midbrain, pons, and medulla. These regions allow nerve fibers from the spinal cord to connect with the cerebrum. Cranial nerves originate from the different sections of the brainstem and terminate on various organs. Damage to the brainstem can affect cranial nerve function, which includes changes in pupil size. The midbrain controls auditory and visual responses and modulates movement. The pons connects the cerebellum to the rest of the brain and controls arousal, sleep, and autonomic functions. The medulla oblongata, the "vital sign center," regulates vasomotor tone, cardiac, and respiratory functions.

ALERT! Damage to the brainstem can cause dysfunction of all vital signs and loss of consciousness.

Cerebellum. The cerebellum is located behind the pons and medulla and is responsible for smooth, coordinated movements. It also influences posture and equilibrium. Unlike the cerebrum, damage to one side of the cerebellum affects the ipsilateral (same) side of the body. Injury to the cerebellum leads to a variety of disorders depending on the affected region. Individuals may present with slurred speech and uncoordinated movements that are jerky and slow. Others may present with an ataxic gait (uncoordinated walking). The cerebellum also plays a role in motor learning. When a motor skill is learned, such as riding a bike, the cerebellum stores this information and later provides individuals with the ability to perform the skill without having to relearn it.

The cerebellum is perfused by the branches of the posterior cerebral artery, which derives blood flow from the basilar artery. The vertebral arteries bring blood up to the basilar artery. The vertebral arteries commonly succumb to arteriosclerosis with age. With arteriosclerosis, there is decreased perfusion of the basilar artery and posterior cerebral artery. Decreased blood flow within the posterior cerebral artery causes lack of blood supply to a lobe of cerebellum, thereby causing loss of coordination and ataxia. **Vertebral-basilar insufficiency (VBI)** is the syndrome that occurs when there is decreased vertebral and basilar artery blood flow and consequent decreased blood supply to the cerebellum (see Fig. 33-4).

Cerebrovascular Circulation

Brain cells have a high metabolic demand and require a constant supply of oxygen and nutrients. The cerebral blood supply arises from the vertebral and carotid arteries in the neck. The right and left vertebral arteries branch off the subclavian artery to supply the brain's posterior aspect. The left common carotid artery arises from the aortic arch; the right common carotid artery

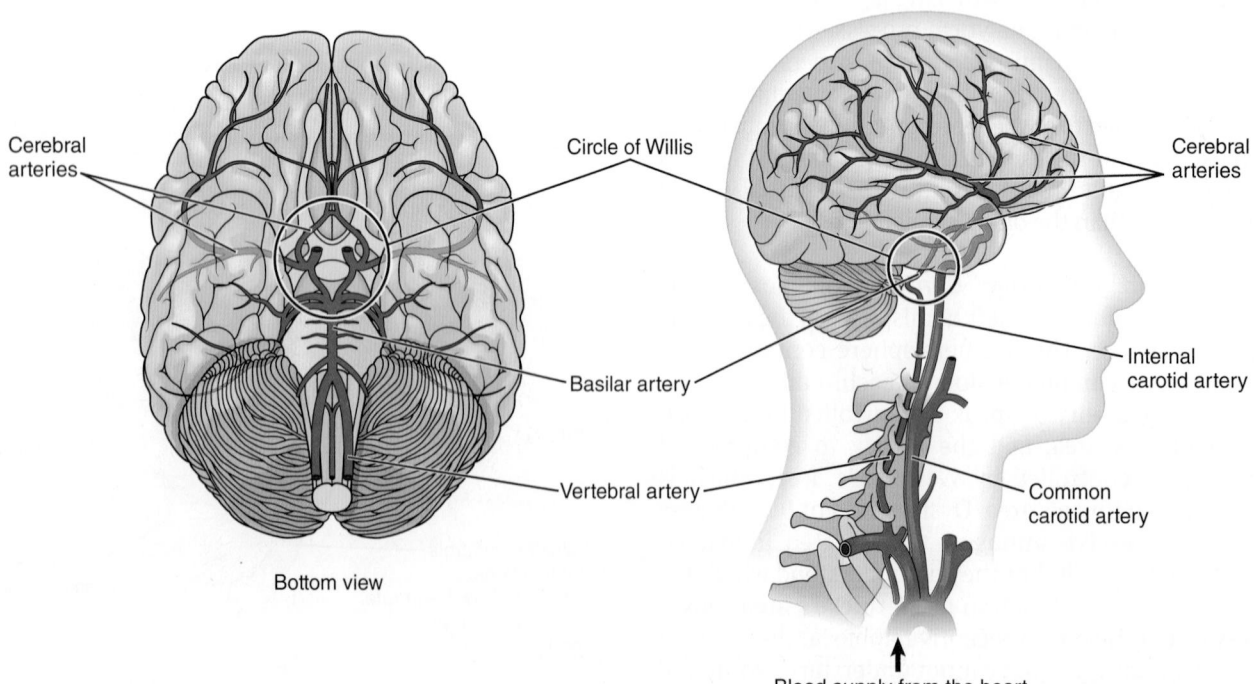

Cerebral arteries

Circle of Willis

Cerebral arteries

Basilar artery

Internal carotid artery

Vertebral artery

Common carotid artery

Bottom view

Blood supply from the heart

FIGURE 33-4. Vertebral-basilar circulation. The vertebral arteries travel up the neck, thread through the vertical bones, and come together at the basilar artery, which flows into the circle of Willis.

arises from the brachiocephalic artery. Both common carotid arteries bifurcate to form the internal and external carotid arteries, and the right and left internal carotid arteries supply the brain's anterior and middle cerebral arteries. The anterior cerebral artery supplies the brain's frontal lobe. The middle cerebral artery supplies the lateral cortex, which comprises 80% of the brain's tissue. The route of the internal carotid artery into the middle cerebral artery is a common route of thrombi that reach the brain. Thrombi often arise from the aorta to the internal carotid artery, which flows into the middle cerebral artery.

The vertebral arteries are located on both posterior sides of the neck. The vertebral arteries unite to form the basilar artery, which bifurcates to form the posterior cerebral arteries. The anastomosis of the posterior cerebral arteries and the terminal branches of the internal carotids form the **circle of Willis.** Located at the base of the brain, the circle of Willis provides collateral circulation in the event that one of the major cerebral vascular routes should occlude (see Fig. 33-5).

> ### 🩺 CLINICAL CONCEPT
>
> The middle cerebral artery supplies a large area of brain tissue; when occluded, it causes deficit of a major region of the brain. Most strokes involve a branch of the middle cerebral artery.

> **ALERT!** The circle of Willis is a frequent site of aneurysm formation. Cerebral aneurysms are weaknesses of the arterial wall that are susceptible to rupture, causing a hemorrhagic stroke.

Cranial Nerves

Cranial nerves arise from the brain and travel to places on the head, face, neck, and shoulders. There are 12 pairs of cranial nerves, numbered from I through XII, and they act as tiny antenna that sense changes in the brain. The majority of the cranial nerves have their origin high in the cortex in the corticobulbar tract, which runs parallel to the corticospinal tract. Some of the cranial nerve tracts cross over to the opposite side of the brain before arising from the brainstem and connecting to their end organ. The terminal portions of the cranial nerves come off the midbrain, pons, and medulla (see Fig. 33-6).

Cranial nerves have either motor or sensory functions; some have both. Cranial nerves are sensitive to changes in circulation of the brain and intracranial pressure. In conditions of stroke, tumor, or brain injury, the cranial nerves can become dysfunctional. When examining a patient, cranial nerve dysfunction commonly indicates that there is a disturbance within the opposite side of the brain. For example, when an individual suffers a stroke in the right cerebral hemisphere, there will be a left-sided facial droop caused by the dysfunction of cranial nerve VII, the facial nerve (see Table 33-1).

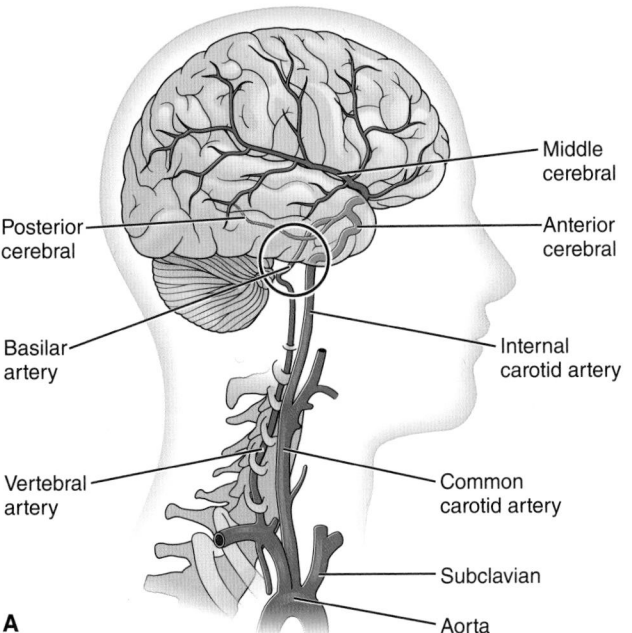

A

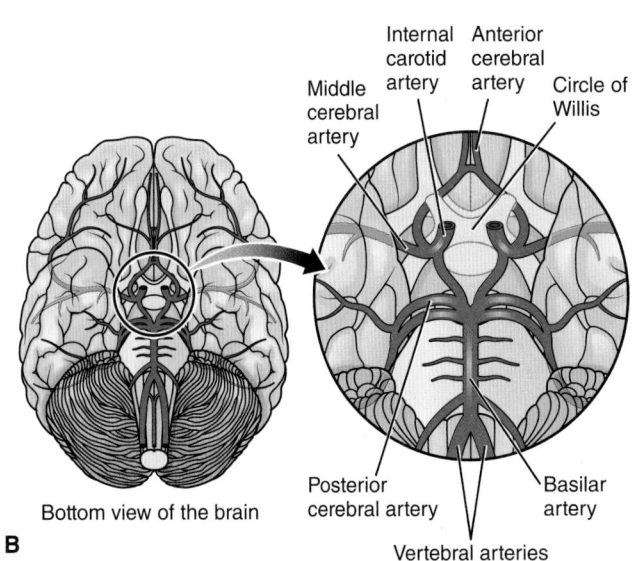

Bottom view of the brain

B

FIGURE 33-5. Circulatory routes from the neck to the brain include the internal carotid and vertebral arteries. **(A)** The common carotid artery divides into the internal carotid artery, which ascends into the circle of Willis. The vertebral arteries ascend up through the vertebrae and come together at the basilar artery, which flows into the circle of Willis. **(B)** The circle of Willis is a network of arteries at the underside of the brain. Major arteries that come off the circle of Willis include the middle cerebral artery, anterior cerebral artery, and posterior cerebral artery.

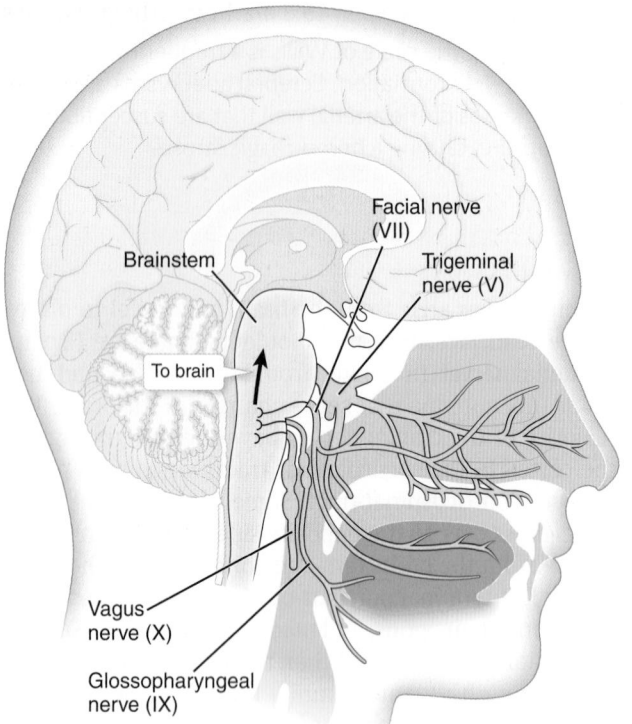

FIGURE 33-6. Some of the cranial nerves have their origin deep in the brain. Many originate high in the cortex within the corticobulbar tract and then some cross over to the contralateral side of the brain and arise off the midbrain, pons, and brainstem. Cranial nerves can act as antennae that can sense changes in intracranial pressure.

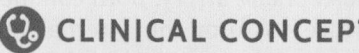 **CLINICAL CONCEPT**

Cranial nerve abnormalities are commonly a sign of increased intracranial pressure or dysfunction of a region of the brain.

Cerebral Metabolism

The brain is the most energy-consuming organ in the body, using 20% of the body's oxygen. Also, brain cells solely use glucose to function. Brain cell metabolism requires a continuous supply of oxygen and glucose. In hypoglycemic conditions, brain cells dysfunction, which can result in loss of consciousness. Lack of cerebral blood flow causes cerebral hypoxia, which causes brain dysfunction. A lack of oxygen for as little as 10 seconds causes a loss of consciousness; a lack of oxygen for 5 to 6 minutes causes brain cells to die. Because brain cells are not capable of anaerobic metabolism, an alteration in oxygen supply can cause irreversible brain damage. Hypoxia or hypoglycemia can have a profound effect on the brain, often causing loss of consciousness and, in some cases, brain death.

TABLE 33-1. Cranial Nerves and Their Functions		
Cranial Nerve	**Type of Neuron**	**Basic Functions**
I Olfactory	Sensory	Smell
II Optic	Sensory	Vision
III Oculomotor	Motor	Extraocular movements (EOMs) and pupil response
IV Trochlear	Motor	EOMs
V Trigeminal	Mixed (motor and sensory)	Facial sensation Masseter muscle control of chewing
VI Abducens	Motor	EOMs
VII Facial	Mixed (motor and sensory)	Facial expressions and taste over anterior two-thirds of tongue
VIII Auditory or Vestibulocochlear	Sensory	Hearing and equilibrium
IX Glossopharyngeal	Mixed (motor and sensory)	Elevation of pharynx in swallowing, taste over posterior one-third of tongue, and salivation
X Vagus	Mixed (motor and sensory)	Gag reflex and parasympathetic control of body
XI Accessory	Motor	Turn the head and shrug
XII Hypoglossal	Motor	Tongue movement

Basic Pathophysiological Concepts of Cerebrovascular Disorders

A stroke is a specific type of brain injury caused by ischemia of brain tissue or hemorrhage of a cerebral blood vessel; it is a clinical syndrome whereby a disruption in cerebral circulation triggers abrupt neurological deficits that are permanent. An **ischemic stroke** is caused by a thrombus or embolus that lodges in a cerebral artery and blocks blood flow to the brain tissue. Ischemia of brain tissue leads to **cerebral infarction,** which is the death of brain cells. A **hemorrhagic stroke** (also called **intracerebral hemorrhage)** is caused by rupture and hemorrhage of a cerebral artery, leading to compression and toxicity of brain cells and loss of cerebral blood flow. Approximately 85% of strokes are due to ischemia, whereas 15% are hemorrhagic strokes (see Fig. 33-7).

Another kind of ischemic injury of the brain is called a **transient ischemic attack (TIA).** Many persons call this a "mini-stroke," which is an inaccurate label. A TIA is a disruption of cerebral circulation with neurological deficits that are reversible and last for less than 24 hours. In a TIA, the body naturally dissolves the clot that caused the ischemia, circulation returns, and there is no permanent neurological injury. However, TIA is often a warning sign of future stroke.

Ischemic Stroke

Ischemic strokes result from an obstruction in cerebral blood flow by a thrombus or embolus. The arterial vessels most commonly involved in ischemic stroke are the internal carotid and middle cerebral arteries. A clot

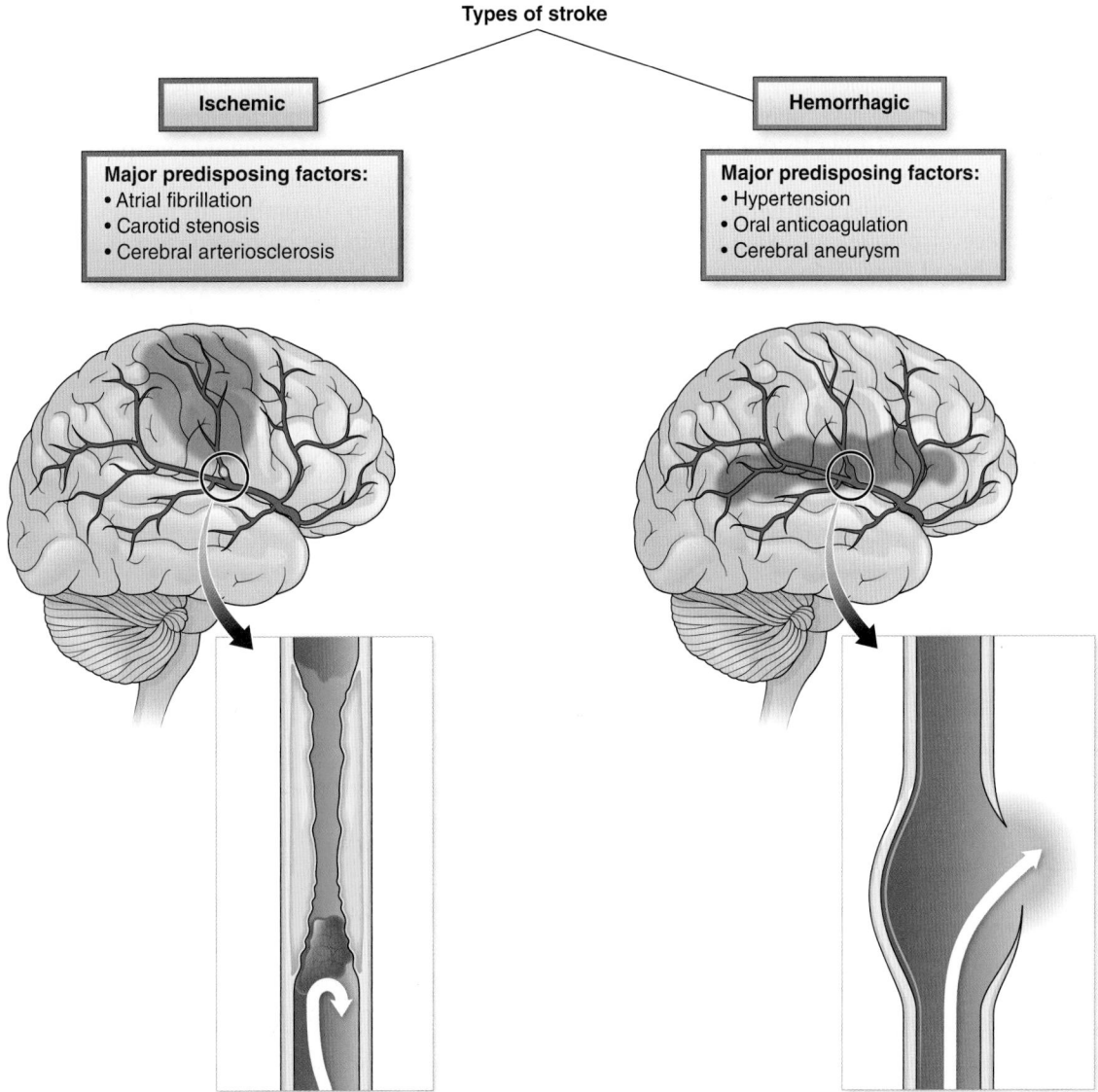

FIGURE 33-7. There are two types of stroke: ischemic and hemorrhagic. An ischemic stroke occurs when an obstruction blocks blood flow to the brain. A hemorrhagic stroke occurs when a vessel wall ruptures and bursts within the brain. Ischemic strokes are more common than hemorrhagic strokes.

commonly travels up the internal carotid artery into the middle cerebral artery and becomes lodged, causing ischemia of brain tissue. Ischemia leads to cerebral infarction: death of brain tissue. The middle cerebral artery is a cerebral artery commonly affected by stroke because it supplies the brain with more than 80% of its blood flow.

A clot or thrombus that causes ischemic stroke commonly arises from one of three mechanisms: arteriosclerosis of a cerebral artery, atrial fibrillation which causes a cardioembolic event, or carotid stenosis that can also cause an embolic event (see Fig. 33-8).

Cerebral Arteriosclerosis

A thrombus is frequently the cause of an ischemic stroke. Thrombi arise from arteriosclerotic plaque; they commonly develop in either the neck or the heart's left atrium and travel up the carotid artery and into the brain. As described in the chapters on cardiovascular disease, endothelial injury usually starts the process of arteriosclerosis. Endothelial injury can be incited by a number of predisposing factors, including free radical injury, hypertension, hyperlipidemia, or high glucose levels in diabetes. As arteriosclerotic plaque builds up, the blood vessel diameter decreases; this, in turn, lessens blood flow to the tissue. Alternatively, arteriosclerotic plaque often breaks and pieces of plaque become emboli. Either as a thrombus or embolus, a piece of plaque can lodge in an arteriole and obstruct blood flow. These mechanisms can occur in cerebrovascular vessels, causing ischemia and infarction of brain tissue.

Atrial Fibrillation

Atrial fibrillation is another cause of ischemic stroke. In left-sided atrial fibrillation, the left atrium is quivering—not contracting sufficiently—and this leads to stasis of blood in the chamber. Stasis of blood increases susceptibility of clot formation in the left atrium. Once formed, clots can travel from the left atrium to the left ventricle and into the aorta. From the aorta, the clot can ascend into the common carotid artery to the internal carotid artery and lodge in a cerebral vessel, most commonly the middle cerebral artery, which leads to brain tissue ischemia (see Fig. 33-9). If ischemia is prolonged, infarction of cerebral tissue and brain cell death occur. Brain cell death leads to loss of neurological functions; this is referred to as a **neurological deficit.** The travel of a clot from the left atrium to the brain is referred to as a cardioembolic event.

Carotid Stenosis

Arteriosclerosis of the carotid artery, called **carotid stenosis,** is also a common cause of ischemic stroke. In arteriosclerosis of the carotid artery, the lumen of the carotid artery narrows from plaque buildup. Normally, the endothelial lining of the carotid artery is smooth and blood cells travel unencumbered. With carotid artery stenosis, the once-smooth endothelial surface becomes irregular because of accumulated plaque. This rough surface promotes platelet adherence and aggregation, which leads to thrombus formation. Once formed, clots can stay in the narrowed carotid artery and cause obstruction of blood up to the brain. Alternatively, a clot

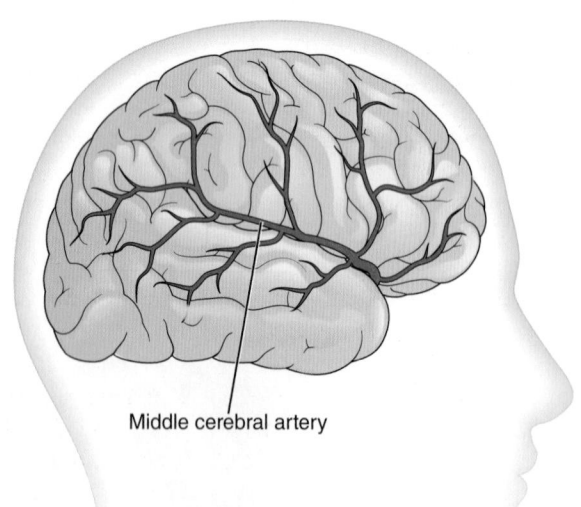

FIGURE 33-8. Parietal view of one hemisphere of the brain. Note the areas that are perfused by the anterior, posterior, and middle cerebral arteries. The major portion of the brain is perfused by the middle cerebral artery, which is involved in most strokes.

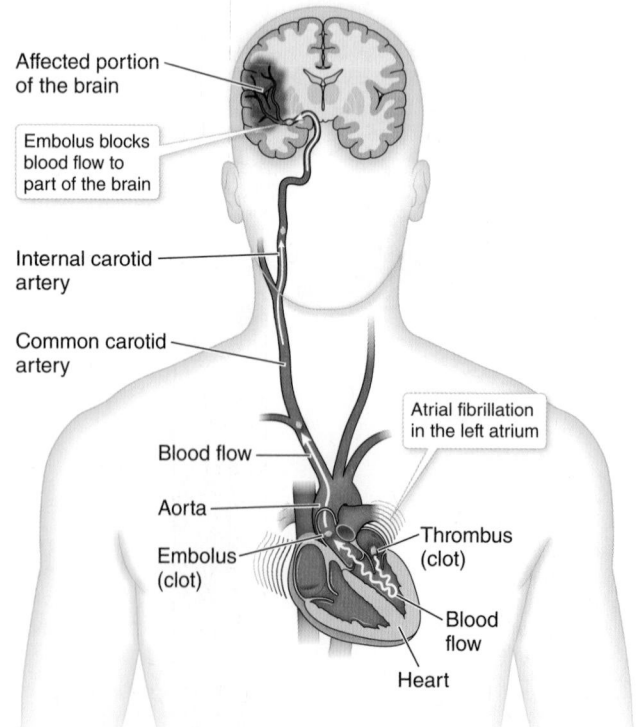

FIGURE 33-9. A thromboembolism can develop in the left atrium with atrial fibrillation. The clot travels from the left atrium to the left ventricle and up through the carotid artery to the middle cerebral artery. It then lodges in the middle cerebral artery and causes ischemia of the brain region.

can dislodge and travel up into a cerebral artery. Either scenario leads to obstructed blood flow to the brain and ischemic stroke (see Fig. 33-10).

> **ALERT!** Left atrial fibrillation and carotid stenosis are the most common causes of ischemic stroke.

Ischemia and Ischemic Penumbra

Cerebral ischemia often occurs gradually and symptoms are progressive. The process of ischemia can appear over several hours and progress to maximal deficit over several days. The core area of tissue ischemia can increase over time. The survival of this area of ischemia is dependent on collateral circulation and the length of time that the tissue is ischemic. Restoration of blood flow to the area is critical and can reverse some of the neurological dysfunction. As time passes, brain cells die, so prompt treatment is mandatory. Failure to restore blood flow results in the tissue becoming infarcted with consequent brain cell death. As the brain cells die, they are replaced by scar tissue called neuroglia (gliosis).

When a cerebral artery is occluded, cerebral perfusion pressure is diminished. Autoregulation of cerebral circulation is nonfunctional and is not able to restore blood flow to the area. Oxygen deprivation allows neurons in the core area of ischemia to progress to irreversible cerebral infarction in minutes. However, brain cells that lie at the perimeter of the stroke region are hypoperfused but are not irreversibly damaged (Fig. 33-11). The perimeter around the core ischemic

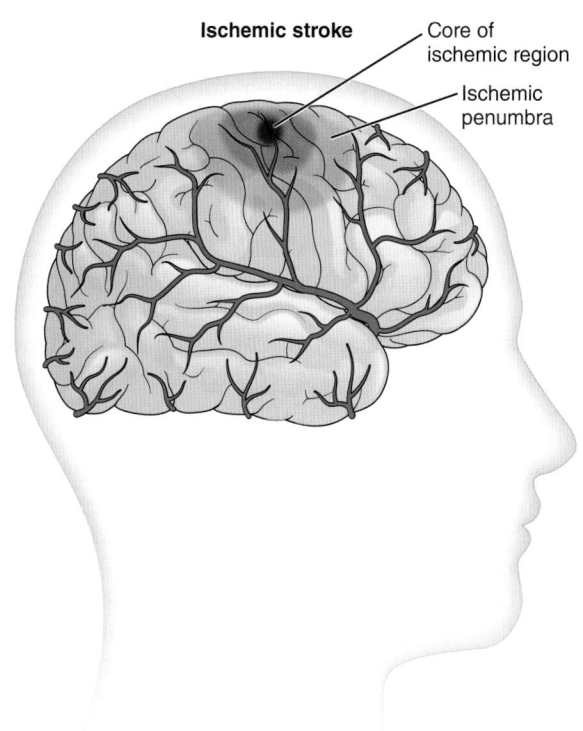

FIGURE 33-11. In ischemic stroke, there is a central core where the clot lodges and damages brain tissue. It is surrounded by the ischemic penumbra, which is brain tissue that is salvageable if reperfused.

area is called the **ischemic penumbra.** The rapid reperfusion of this area is critical because, if left untreated, the penumbra will also succumb to ischemia and infarction. Within the ischemic penumbra and surrounding brain tissue, some cerebral edema occurs, which also contributes to hypoperfusion and further damage of brain cells.

Glutamate Toxicity

Ischemic cellular injury in the brain has reversible and irreversible changes. Early changes involve the failure of cellular ion pumps. Movement of potassium across the cell membrane alters cell membrane action potentials. This causes depolarization of neuronal membranes and increased calcium ion influx. With this depolarization, there is increased release of the excitatory neurotransmitter glutamate into the synaptic space.

Ischemia impairs cellular metabolism and leads to excessive glutamate accumulation in the ischemic penumbra. **Glutamate** opens cation channels and causes an influx of Na+ and Ca++, which are necessary for action potentials to occur. Normally, the signaling for the uptake of Na+ and Ca++ is terminated by the synaptic reuptake of glutamate; increased intracellular levels of Na+ and Ca++ then return to normal. However, if the process is not reversed, persistent elevation of intracellular Ca++ activates degradative enzymes and results in cell death. During a stroke, ischemia impairs the normal mechanism for the removal of glutamate from the synapse. Sustained elevations of extracellular glutamate increase intracellular Ca++, lead to cellular

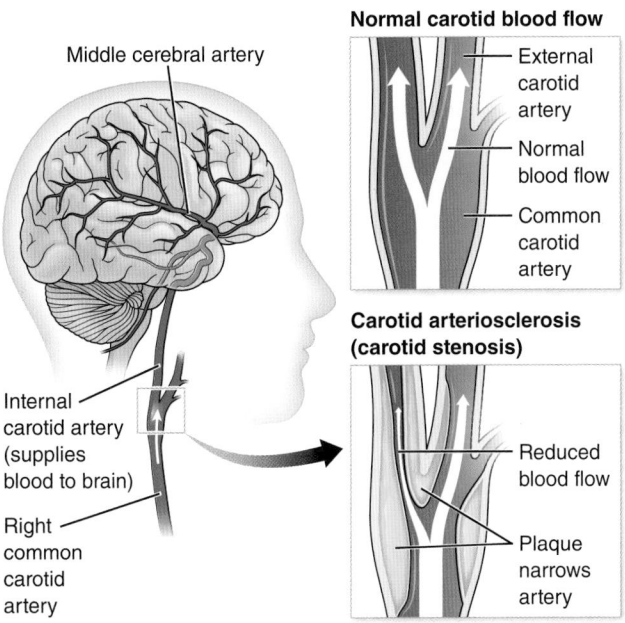

FIGURE 33-10. In carotid stenosis, the carotid artery is narrowed because of buildup of arteriosclerotic plaque. A piece of plaque or a clot can break off and travel up into the middle cerebral artery and cause ischemic stroke.

death, and extend the stroke region (see Fig. 33-12). Progression to cellular death occurs through irreversible neuronal injury. As part of the process, mitochondrial function is impaired. This promotes the release of free radicals that further alter cellular functions and damage cell membranes.

Transient Ischemic Attack

A TIA is similar to ischemic stroke except that it is temporary and resolves. Approximately 50,000 Americans experience TIAs each year. The estimated incidence of TIA is 1.19/1,000 persons. Without treatment, approximately 50% of persons who have experienced a TIA will have a stroke within the following year. TIAs were once considered benign events, but it is now understood that they are true medical emergencies that may signal impending stroke. Therefore, rapid assessment and early intervention are imperative.

In TIAs, individuals present with temporary neurological symptoms that can last for several minutes to hours. TIAs, as the name implies, are transient: neurological deficits that commonly completely resolve within an hour. They are caused by an embolus that suddenly dislodges in an arteriosclerotic arterial vessel and causes arterial occlusion in the brain. This leads to tissue anoxia and clinical presentation similar to stroke. However, in TIAs, the body's fibrinolytic system dissolves the occlusion and the focal deficits disappear in less than 24 hours.

A TIA may be most noticeable to bystanders but not to the person enduring the transient neurological impairment. Confusion, disorientation, inability to communicate, and memory impairment affect the patient. Patients who report to the emergency department with signs of TIA are commonly brought in by another person. Often a TIA is resolved by the time the patient presents to the emergency department. However, an interview of the patient and observer is key to diagnose TIA. TIA requires treatment to decrease risk of stroke in the future.

Small vessels in the brain can become occluded, causing small areas of ischemic brain damage that often cause no major symptoms. Small areas in the brain that endure ischemia from occluded tiny blood vessels are called **lacunar infarcts.** These extremely small infarcts in the brain are often associated with hypertension, smoking, and uncontrolled diabetes.

CLINICAL CONCEPT

To encourage individuals to seek immediate treatment, TIA is sometimes referred to as "brain attack." Laypersons also refer to them as "mini-strokes."

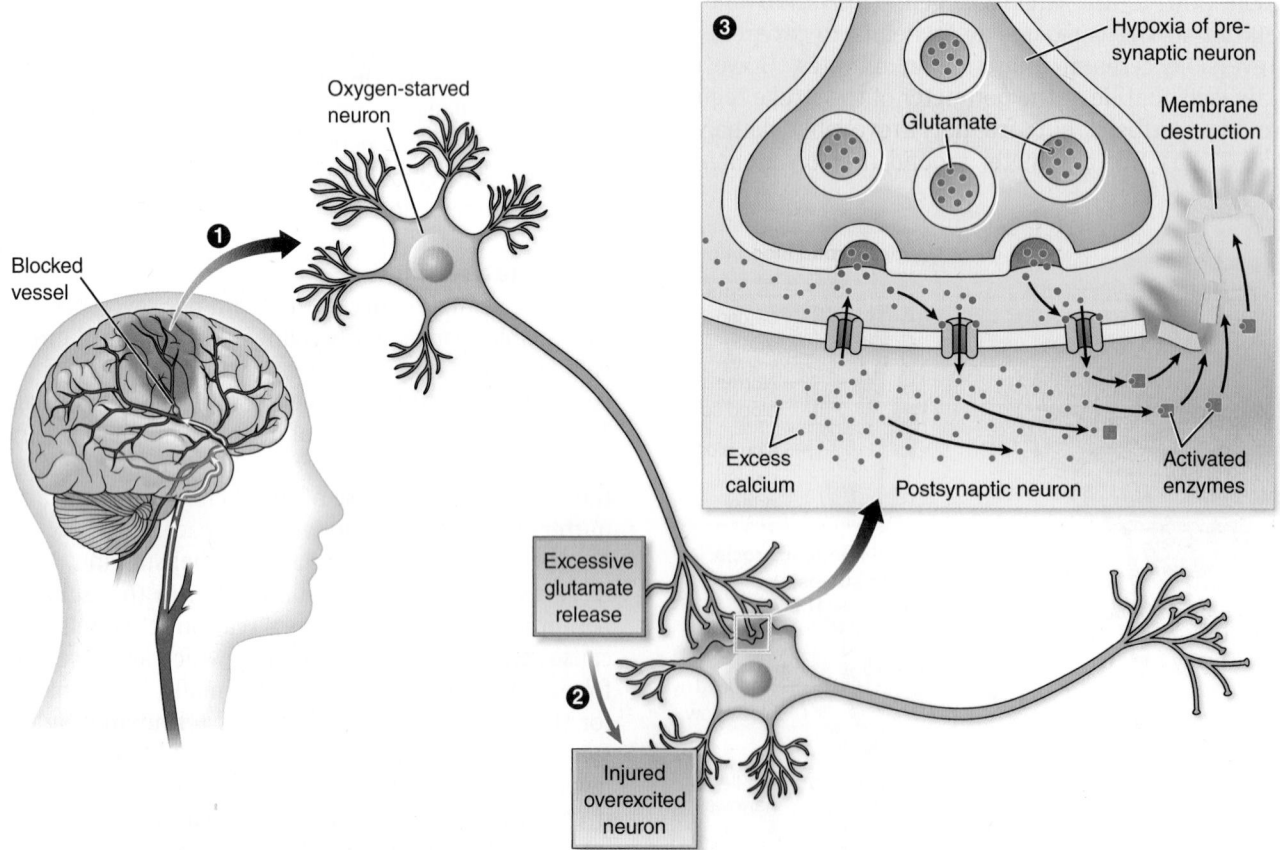

FIGURE 33-12. The effect of glutamate in ischemic stroke. (1) In ischemia, the hypoxic brain cells release excess glutamate. (2) The excess glutamate causes overexcitation of the postsynaptic neurons and triggers an influx of calcium. (3). This influx of calcium causes activation of enzymatic degeneration of brain cells.

Hemorrhagic Stroke

Hemorrhagic stroke occurs when a cerebral artery ruptures and can no longer bring blood to the brain tissue. Hemorrhagic stroke is less common than ischemic stroke; however, it is more severe and causes more brain damage. The cerebral artery is commonly a branch of the middle cerebral artery deep within the brain tissue. A cerebral artery ruptures from excessive pressure and blood leaks into the brain, causing cerebral edema, increased intracranial pressure, and tissue destruction.

Microaneurysms in the walls of cerebral arterial branches are common in older adults. These microaneurysms rupture, causing small bleeds within the brain tissue. Cerebral amyloid angiopathy is another finding in the cerebral arteries of older adults. These cause fragility of vessels, small ruptures, and bleeds. In autopsy studies, cerebral microhemorrhages are detected in 5% to 23% of older individuals. These cerebral microbleeds are asymptomatic and do not appear on imaging studies. Microbleeds have been associated with hypertension, uncontrolled diabetes mellitus, anticoagulant therapy, and cigarette smoking. Hypertension and anticoagulant treatment combined increase the risk of hemorrhagic stroke.

A specific type of cerebral hemorrhage occurs when an arterial branch in the subarachnoid space ruptures; this event, called a **subarachnoid hemorrhage** (SAH), may be the result of head trauma or aneurysm rupture. The most common sites for cerebral aneurysm are in those arteries that make up the circle of Willis within the subarachnoid space (see Fig. 33-13).

After rupture of a cerebral artery, blood flows into the brain tissue, where it becomes compressed and often displaced. This compression leads to tissue ischemia and cerebral edema. Vasospasm of adjacent blood vessels occurs from exposure to blood, which subjects brain tissue to ischemia. In addition, the blood that is released from the ruptured artery is chemically toxic to the brain cells, causing brain cell death. If there is rupture of a large cerebral artery, ischemia, cerebral edema, lack of cerebral circulation, and a significant lack of oxygen delivery to brain tissue lead to a condition called **anoxic encephalopathy,** which causes decreased levels of consciousness. If there is a large region of cerebral edema, swelling brain cells, which are enclosed by the cranial bone, have little room for expansion. Pressure that builds within the skull is directed downward toward the foramen magnum, the area where the spinal cord enters the brainstem. The pressure in the brain can lead to decreased cerebral circulation and **uncal herniation,** which occurs when rising intracranial pressure causes portions of the brain to move from one intracranial compartment to another. It is a neurological emergency because pressure on the brainstem causes life-threatening complications. Signs include decreased level of consciousness and vital sign abnormalities.

 CLINICAL CONCEPT

With increased intracranial pressure, a patient may experience irregular respiratory rate, bradycardia, and hypertension. These changes, collectively known as **Cushing's triad,** are an ominous finding.

A large cerebral hemorrhage causes a hematoma (large clot) that can expand—most significantly in the first 24 hours poststroke. Enlargement of the hematoma is associated with worsening neurological deterioration. Hemorrhagic arteries in the brain can continue bleeding for days, causing destruction of brain tissue. Large hemorrhages cause elevated intracranial pressure and diminished levels of consciousness. They can cause blood to enter the brain's ventricles, which drain the cerebrospinal fluid. Obstruction of the drainage of cerebrospinal fluid can cause hydrocephalus and coma.

The first 24-hour period is critical for neurosurgical intervention to evacuate the hematoma. The slogan "time is brain" applies to hemorrhagic stroke and implies that with each hour that passes, more brain tissue can be affected by the enlarging hematoma.

If the hematoma cannot be evacuated, the clot resolves with time, the body reabsorbs some of the blood, and it becomes smaller. The recruitment of macrophages occurs as part of the inflammatory response. The macrophages phagocytize both the hemorrhagic and ischemic areas. The area is liquefied and a cavity is formed. Astrocytes form scar tissue that fills in the cavity.

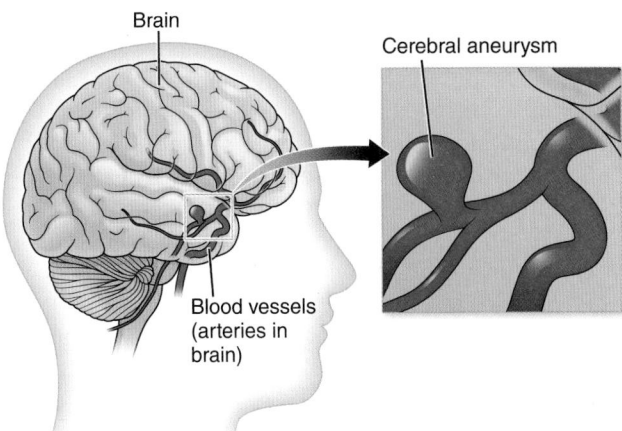

Brain

Cerebral aneurysm

Blood vessels (arteries in brain)

FIGURE 33-13. A cerebral aneurysm is a weakening in the wall of an artery that is susceptible to rupture. If the aneurysm ruptures, it causes a cerebral hemorrhage. Cerebral aneurysms often develop on the circle of Willis in the brain. Because they resemble berries hanging off a tree, they are commonly called "berry aneurysms."

ALERT! A large cerebral hemorrhage can cause cerebral edema that places pressure on the brainstem and causes death.

Assessment of Cerebrovascular Disease

The basic risk factors for stroke are similar to those for cardiovascular disease. These include age greater than 65 years, arteriosclerosis, hyperlipidemia, uncontrolled diabetes mellitus, alcohol use disorder, hypertension, smoking, obesity, and family history. African Americans, Hispanic Americans, and Native Americans have a higher rate of stroke than European Americans. There are some specific risk factors for ischemic stroke versus hemorrhagic stroke. The use of oral contraceptives is a risk factor, specifically for ischemic stroke, because oral contraceptives increase susceptibility to thrombus formation. A thrombus can become lodged in a cerebral artery and cause ischemia. Individuals with sickle cell disease are at increased risk for ischemic stroke because of possible vaso-occlusive crises. These episodes can cause obstruction of cerebral arterioles and cause cerebral ischemia. Carotid arteriosclerosis and atrial fibrillation are also risk factors specifically for ischemic stroke, as discussed previously (see Box 33-2).

The major predisposing factor of hemorrhagic stroke is hypertension. Hypertension can create high pressure against the cerebral arteries that can weaken the vessel walls. An **arteriovenous malformation (AVM)** can also lead to the development of intracerebral bleeding. An AVM is a congenital abnormality that connects an artery with a vein within the brain tissue. AVMs cause weakened areas in vessel walls that are vulnerable to rupture. Other risk factors for hemorrhagic stroke include cerebral aneurysm, amyloid vasculopathy, brain tumor, bleeding disorders, liver disease, anticoagulant medications, thrombolytic medication, CNS infection, and vasculitis. Amyloid vasculopathy is the deposition of abnormal proteins that weaken the integrity of arterial walls in the brain. The etiology of amyloid accumulation is unknown. Liver disease causes decreased coagulation factor synthesis, leading to increased risk for bleeding.

> **ALERT!** It is important to recognize that patients on anticoagulants or antiplatelet medications are at risk for intracranial bleeding, particularly if they sustain head injury or fall.

Signs and Symptoms

Patients who suffer either ischemic or hemorrhagic stroke present with similar signs and symptoms. Because both types of stroke cause damage to the brain, neurological deficits are demonstrated. The area of the brain perfused by the middle cerebral artery is the most common region affected in either type of stroke. The middle cerebral artery supplies the sensory and motor cortex in both hemispheres of the brain. It also supplies the speech center, which is most commonly in the left hemisphere. Therefore, strokes affecting the right hemisphere usually cause sensory and motor neurological deficits. Strokes affecting the left hemisphere commonly cause sensory, motor, and speech deficits.

In either kind of stroke, neurons within the left or right hemisphere become injured and die. Because of the anatomical crossover of nerve tracts at the medulla, patients present with neurological symptoms on the contralateral side of the cerebral hemisphere

---

BOX 33-2. Risk Factors for Stroke

The risk factors for stroke are similar to the risk factors for arteriosclerosis, coronary artery disease, and peripheral arterial disease.

- Hypertension
- Tobacco use
- Diet high in salt, fat, and calories
- Excessive use of alcohol
- Hyperlipidemia
- Heart disorders (particularly disorders that increase formation of clots; myocardial infarction, atrial fibrillation; infective endocarditis)
- Uncontrolled diabetes
- Obesity (particularly abdominal obesity)
- Previous stroke or TIA
- Use of cocaine or amphetamines
- Bleeding disorders (hemorrhagic stroke risk factor)
- Coagulation disorder (ischemic stroke risk factor)
- Vasculitis/amyloid vasculopathy (hemorrhagic stroke)
- Arteriovenous malformation (hemorrhagic stroke risk factor)
- Cerebral aneurysm (hemorrhagic stroke risk factor)
- Sickle cell disease (increases risk of ischemic stroke that mainly affects African Americans; ischemic stroke can occur if sickle cells cause vaso-occlusive crisis in an artery supplying blood flow to the brain)
- Physical inactivity
- Oral contraceptives (estrogenic component of oral contraceptives increase risk of clot formation)
- Family history of stroke
- Age (stroke risk increases with age)
- Race and ethnicity (African Americans, Hispanic Americans, and American Indian/Alaska Natives have a greater chance of having a stroke than do non-Hispanic European Americans or Asian Americans)

Adapted from Giraldo, E. A. (2018). *Overview of stroke*. https://www.merckmanuals.com/professional/neurological-disorders/stroke/overview-of-stroke

that is injured (see Fig. 33-14). Eighty percent of upper motor neurons cross over to the contralateral side of the body. However, 20% of the neurons remain on the ipsilateral side ipsilateral (same) side of the hemisphere. For example, patients who suffer ischemia in the left cerebral hemisphere will exhibit weakness or paralysis on the right side of the body. However, the patient has use of the 20% of ipsilateral neurons on the right side of the body that are retrained during the rehabilitation period (see Fig. 33-15).

Stroke manifestations occur most often as neurological deficits on one side of the body. Common symptoms of stroke include hemiparesis (weakness of extremities on one side of the body) or hemiplegia (paralysis; complete loss of function of extremities on one side of the body), loss of sensation in an extremity on one side of the body, slurred speech, and facial droop with weakness. Some patients have disorientation, confusion, and drowsiness, which can become stupor or coma.

Aphasia, a language disorder whereby individuals are unable to speak or understand the spoken word, is also a common presentation. In the majority of the population, language is a function of the left hemisphere. Two of the areas most critical for language that are usually found in the left hemisphere are Broca's area and Wernicke's area. Ischemic damage to the left hemisphere often results in aphasia. Damage to Broca's area usually causes expressive aphasia, whereas damage to Wernicke's area causes receptive aphasia. In expressive

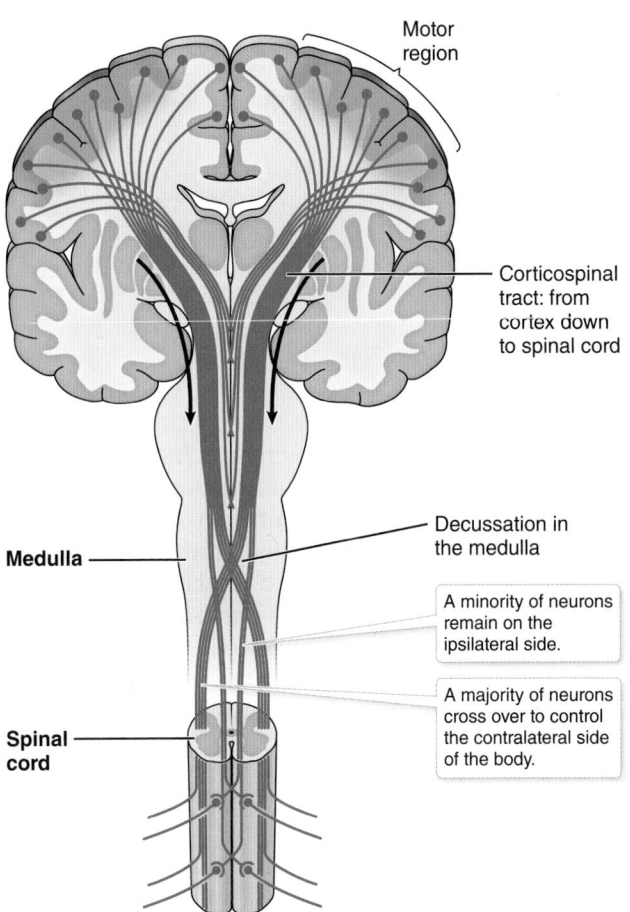

FIGURE 33-15. The neurons of the corticospinal tract are motor neurons. The majority of corticospinal neurons cross at the medulla to the contralateral side of the spinal cord to control the opposite side of the body, but a minority of corticospinal neurons remain ipsilateral to control the same side of the body. The corticospinal tract is also called the pyramidal tract. The region of crossover is called the decussation.

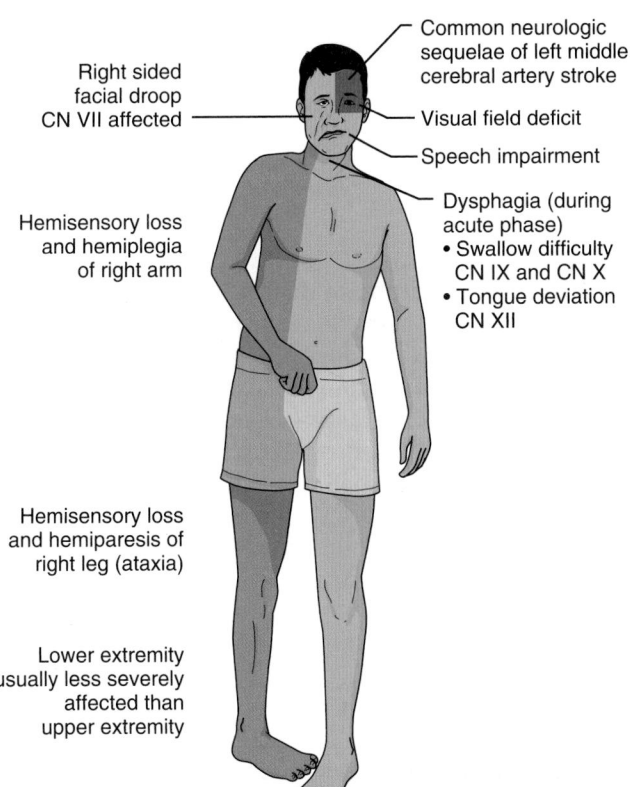

FIGURE 33-14. Neurological deficits resulting from left middle cerebral artery stroke.

aphasia, individuals are unable to form words but can understand others. In receptive aphasia, however, individuals are unable to understand spoken words.

Subarachnoid hemorrhage (SAH), a specific type of cerebral hemorrhage due to trauma or ruptured aneurysm, presents differently from other kinds of hemorrhagic or ischemic stroke. About 80% of patients with SAH report a sudden onset of what they describe as the "worst headache of their life" or "thunderclap" headache. A previous severe headache 2 to 8 weeks before the SAH is a common finding present in up to 40% of patients. Findings accompanying the headache can include vomiting, photophobia, seizures, stiff neck, localized neurological deficits, and decreased level of consciousness.

Vertebral-basilar insufficiency (VBI) is ischemia of the vertebrobasilar circulation. This is most commonly due to arteriosclerotic plaque buildup in the vertebral arteries (see Fig. 33-4). Dizziness, vertigo, headaches, vomiting, diplopia, blindness, ataxia, imbalance, and weakness in both sides of the body are the most common symptoms.

CLINICAL CONCEPT

The American Heart Association and American Stroke Association suggest using the acronym FAST to recognize signs of a stroke:

Facial droop

Arm weakness

Speech difficulty

Time to call 911 and check the time when the symptoms began

Diagnosis

Any patient with a sudden change in neurological function should be assessed for a TIA or stroke. There is no reliable clinical presentation to distinguish between cerebral ischemia or hemorrhage. However, a slow progression of one-sided weakness or sensory loss and slurring of speech are more characteristic of ischemic stroke. Sudden headache, elevated blood pressure, and a depressed level of consciousness are more indicative of a hemorrhagic stroke.

Patient assessment needs to include neurological and cardiovascular examinations. This includes auscultation of carotid arteries for bruits, blood pressure in both arms, and ophthalmoscopic examination of the retina for changes associated with hypertension, such as arteriovenous nicking. Diagnostic testing needs to include electrocardiography, chest x-ray, blood work, and brain imaging studies. This testing should rule out other pathological processes with symptoms that could mimic stroke, such as hypoglycemia, hyperglycemia, vasculitis, migraine, seizure disorders, metabolic encephalopathy, recent head trauma, and tumors.

Computed Tomography

Computed tomography (CT) scans without contrast are preferred during the acute phase of the stroke (see Fig. 33-16). The importance of the CT scan is to rapidly identify or exclude hemorrhage as the etiology of the stroke. Once hemorrhage is eliminated as the etiology of the stroke, thrombolytic therapy is an option for treatment. Thrombolytic therapy acts to dissolve the clot that is causing ischemic stroke. Thrombolytic therapy is contraindicated in hemorrhagic stroke.

ALERT! It is key for a patient with stroke symptoms to obtain a CT scan as soon as possible.

Cerebral ischemia may not be evident during the first 24 hours of the stroke. The use of contrast dye with CT scan, termed *CT angiography,* can allow better visualization of ischemia. CT scans are also helpful in identifying the presence of abscesses, neoplasms, or other conditions that may mimic stroke symptoms.

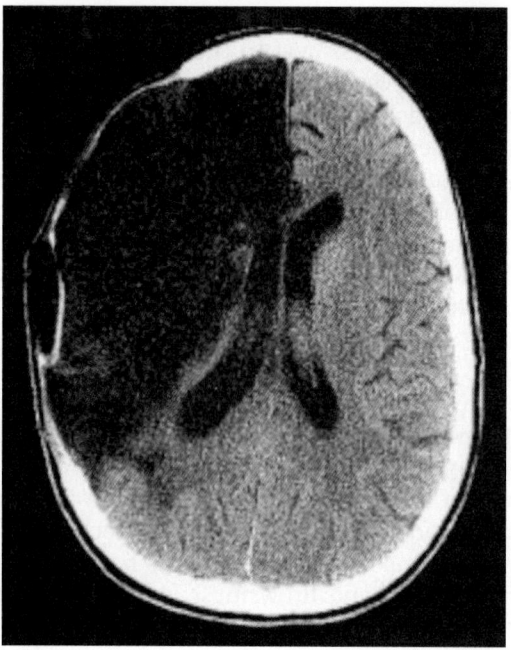

FIGURE 33-16. A CT scan showing stroke. *(From Science Source.)*

Magnetic Resonance Angiography

Magnetic resonance angiography (MRA) can distinguish between cerebral hemorrhage and ischemia. The MRA can be used to determine the presence of a clot or aneurysm. Additional applications of MRA include diagnosing severe carotid artery occlusions.

Transcranial Doppler

Transcranial Doppler is a noninvasive ultrasound procedure that can be used on certain areas of the skull. It is used in critical care to assess intracranial pressure, confirm the lack of cerebral circulation in brain death, detect vasospasm in SAH, and monitor blood flow during thrombolytic treatment and carotid endarterectomy.

National Institutes of Health Stroke Scale

The National Institutes of Health Stroke Scale (NIHSS) was developed as a way to quantify deficits attributed to a stroke and track the progress of treatment. The NIHSS is a graded neurological examination that evaluates visual fields, ataxia, speech, language, cognition, and motor and sensory function (see Table 33-2). Each section has a graded point scale based on level of function. The points are then added for a total score. Essentially, the higher the score, the greater the neurological deficit. A range of scores correlates with the patient's clinical presentation.

When the NIHSS score is used in combination with the size of the damaged area, as measured by the diffusion weighted imaging magnetic resonance imaging (DWI-MRI), it is possible to assess the severity of stroke and identify the patients who have the greatest potential for recovery. The DWI-MRI is an excellent tool that can detect small, evolving ischemic and infarcted areas. In addition to the NIHSS score and size of the ischemic

TABLE 33-2. National Institutes of Health Stroke Scale

Category	Scale	Score
1A. LEVEL OF CONSCIOUSNESS (LOC) (alert, drowsy, etc.)	0 = alert 1 = drowsy 2 = not alert 3 = responds only with reflex motor or autonomic effects or totally unresponsive, flaccid, or areflexic	_____
1B. LOC QUESTIONS (month, age)	0 = answers both correctly 1 = answers one correctly 2 = answers neither correctly	_____
1C. LOC COMMANDS (open/close eyes; make fist/let go)	0 = performs both correctly 1 = performs one correctly 2 = performs neither correctly	_____
2. BEST GAZE (eyes open, patient follows examiner's finger or face)	0 = normal 1 = partial gaze palsy 2 = forced deviation	_____
3. VISUAL (introduce visual stimulus/threat to patient's visual field quadrants)	0 = no visual loss 1 = partial hemianopia 2 = complete hemianopia 3 = bilateral hemianopia	_____
4. FACIAL PALSY (show teeth, raise eyebrows, squeeze eyes shut)	0 = normal 1 = minor paralysis 2 = partial paralysis 3 = complete paralysis	_____
5A. MOTOR ARM, LEFT 5B. MOTOR ARM, RIGHT (elevate arm to 90 degrees if patient is sitting; 45 degrees if patient is supine)	0 = no drift 1 = drift 2 = some effort against gravity 3 = no effort against gravity 4 = no movement	_____ _____
6A. MOTOR LEG, LEFT 6B. MOTOR LEG, RIGHT (elevate leg 30 degrees with patient supine)	0 = no drift 1 = drift 2 = some effort against gravity 3 = no effort against gravity 4 = no movement UN = amputation	_____ _____
7. LIMB ATAXIA (finger–nose; heel down shin)	0 = absent 1 = present in one limb 2 = present in two limbs UN = amputation	_____
8. SENSORY (pinprick to face, arm, trunk, and leg– compare side to side)	0 = normal 1 = mild-to-moderate sensory loss 2 = severe to total sensory loss	_____
9. BEST LANGUAGE (name item, describe a picture, read sentences)	0 = no aphasia 1 = mild-to-moderate aphasia 2 = severe aphasia 3 = mute, global aphasia	_____
10. DYSARTHRIA (evaluate speech clarity by patient repeating listed words)	0 = normal 1 = mild-to-moderate dysarthria 2 = severe dysarthria UN = physical barrier	_____

Continued

TABLE 33-2. National Institutes of Health Stroke Scale—cont'd

Category	Scale	Score
11. EXTINCTION AND INATTENTION (use information from prior testing to identify neglect or double simultaneous stimuli testing)	0 = no abnormality 1 = visual, tactile, auditory, spatial, or personal inattention 2 = profound hemi-inattention or extinction to more than one modality	___
SCORE RANGE	**LEVEL OF NEUROLOGICAL IMPAIRMENT**	
Less than 5	Mild impairment	
Between 5 and 15	Mild to moderate impairment	
Between 15 and 25	Moderately severe impairment	
Greater than 25	Very severe impairment	

Adapted from National Institutes of Health, NIH Stroke Scale. https://www.stroke.nih.gov/documents/NIH_Stroke_Scale_508C.pdf; Adams, H. P., Jr., Davis, P. H., Leira, E. C., et al. (1999). Baseline NIH Stroke Scale score strongly predicts outcome after stroke: A report of the Trial of Org 10172 in Acute Stroke Treatment (TOAST). *Neurology, 53*(1), 126–131.

or infarcted area, the time since the onset of symptoms is considered when assessing a patient. This information is combined into a 7-point scale. The best outcome is associated with scores of 5, 6, and 7, with 87% recovering. Scores of 3 and 4 have a 57% recovery rate. Only 7% of those with scores between 0 and 2 recover.

Treatment

Treatments differ for ischemic stroke and hemorrhagic stroke. Therefore, rapid diagnosis of the type of stroke that is occurring is extremely important for correct treatment initiation. A CT scan should be performed as soon as the patient enters the health-care facility. A DWI-MRI is a superior imaging device for identifying ischemic stroke; however, many medical settings do not have this technology. Once the CT scan or MRI determines whether there is an ischemic or hemorrhagic condition of the brain, rapid delivery of treatment can facilitate recovery.

Treatment begins with stabilization to prevent further brain injury. It is important to maintain a patent airway and to stabilize blood pressure and cardiac rhythm. Regulation of body temperature and blood glucose levels is also important.

🔬 CLINICAL CONCEPT

After stroke, blood pressure should be slowly lowered if hypertension is present. Studies show it is best to keep systolic pressure at 140 mm Hg.

Treatment for Ischemic Stroke

Treatment for acute ischemic stroke utilizes IV thrombolysis, which dissolves the clot that is blocking arterial blood flow and allows for reperfusion to occur. It is important that this thrombolytic therapy be administered within 3 to 4.5 hours of symptom onset, because this provides the best chance for patient recovery and survival. Ideally, thrombolysis within 60 minutes shows the best results. Studies show that for every 15-minute reduction of door-to-IV needle time, there is a 5% lower chance of in-hospital mortality.

Recombinant tissue-type plasminogen activator (rt-PA), often called a "clot-buster," is the thrombolytic agent most often used. IV administration of rt-PA rapidly dissolves the clot that is causing the ischemia of brain tissue. Studies show that if IV rt-PA is administered within the first 3 hours of symptom onset, patients are 30% more likely to have minimal or no disability at 90 days.

ALERT! Not all ischemic stroke patients are candidates for rt-PA. A strict protocol excludes patients who have a specific set of conditions, which includes susceptibility to bleeding. A patient must have no risk or potential for any type of bleeding to receive rt-PA.

Despite following strict protocols, studies show 2% to 7% of individuals develop hemorrhagic bleeds after thrombolytic treatment. It is important to identify the patients who will benefit the most from thrombolytic therapy, as there are specific contraindications to it (see Box 33-3). If a patient receives rt-PA, there is a waiting period of 24 hours before long-term anticoagulant medication can be initiated.

Patients may be treated with aspirin to decrease platelet aggregation and clot formation in the acute phase of ischemic stroke. Some patients are candidates

> ### BOX 33-3. Thrombolytic Contraindications in Ischemic Stroke
>
> Generally, thrombolytic drugs will not be given if the patient has:
> - Recent head injury
> - Bleeding problems
> - Bleeding ulcers
> - Pregnancy
> - Recent surgery
> - Been taking anticoagulant medications
> - Trauma
> - Uncontrolled high blood pressure

for endovascular mechanical thrombectomy, which is surgical removal of a clot from the occluded artery. A catheter called a stent retriever is used to directly break up a clot and allow cerebral blood flow to resume. Thrombectomy is used on selected patients who have persistent vessel occlusion despite treatment with IV rt-PA. Studies have found that mechanical thrombectomy can be implemented within 6 to 24 hours of the time that the patient was last known to be well. Patients need to be eligible according to a strict protocol. The procedure needs to be in a stroke center with expertise in both mechanical thrombectomy and infarct volume determination using MRI or perfusion CT.

After the ischemic stroke, clopidogrel is an antiplatelet medication that may be used. In some patients aspirin and clopidogrel are used in combination in the first 90 days after the ischemic stroke.

During long-term poststroke treatment, rehabilitation is initiated in an attempt to train neurons to develop new pathways for movement of extremities, maintain proper body alignment, and prevent muscle atrophy. During rehabilitation, the neuroplasticity of the brain can allow the patient to recover some motor function. The first 4 weeks after a stroke is a particularly valuable time for the potential to develop new patterns of motor function in the rehabilitation process.

Behavior modifications such as a low-cholesterol diet, smoking cessation, and weight loss are recommended as long-term strategy. Antilipidemic medications such as statin drugs are usually prescribed to keep cholesterol levels low, and blood pressure management is important.

If carotid stenosis is present, to decrease the chance of another ischemic stroke, carotid endarterectomy may be necessary. This surgical procedure opens up the carotid artery and removes obstructive arteriosclerotic plaque in order to restore blood flow to the brain. Alternatively, a carotid stent may be inserted through an endovascular intervention, called angioplasty, which threads a catheter into the carotid artery from a peripheral artery. The stent can keep the carotid artery unobstructed and clots can be prevented from embolizing into the cerebral arteries. Anticoagulants such as warfarin (Coumadin)

may be prescribed for some patients—particularly those with atrial fibrillation. Instead of warfarin, newer agents, such as dabigatran (Pradaxa), rivaroxaban (Xarelto), apixaban (Eliquis), or edoxaban (Savaysa) may be used for long-term prevention of ischemic stroke.

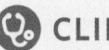 **CLINICAL CONCEPT**

Thrombolytic therapy has shown to be most effective if administered within 60 minutes of the onset of stroke symptoms.

Treatment for Cerebral Hemorrhage

Cerebral hemorrhage commonly occurs rapidly, and treatment involves first establishing hemodynamic stabilization. Reversal of any preexisting anticoagulation is required.

Intubation and blood pressure reduction may be needed early in treatment. Some studies suggest that blood pressure reduction to less than 150 mm Hg systolic can reduce the size of the hematoma formed by the hemorrhage. Intravenous calcium channel antagonists or beta-adrenergic blockers are recommended to reduce blood pressure. Cerebral edema is present in at least half of patients with cerebral hemorrhage and can progress, reaching maximum volume 7 to 12 days after onset. IV mannitol or hypertonic saline may be used if there is significant cerebral edema. These hypertonic fluids can rapidly pull fluid out of the brain cells to decrease cerebral edema. Intracranial pressure monitoring is necessary if these agents are used. Anticonvulsants are recommended if the patient has seizures. The patient's prognosis is dependent on the size of the hemorrhage.

Studies show that up to 20% of patients with an intracerebral hemorrhage have been on anticoagulant therapy. If the patient has been on anticoagulants, reversal of treatment using an antidote or prothrombin complex concentrate (PCC) is recommended. PCC is a combination of coagulation factors II, IX, X, and VII. Fresh-frozen plasma can be used if PCC is not available. If the patient was on warfarin, vitamin K is necessary to reverse the effect. If the patient was on heparin, protamine sulfate is required. For patients on dabigatran, idarucizumab is indicated to reverse treatment. If the patient has received the thrombolytic agent, rt-PA, cryoprecipitate or IV tranexamic acid is indicated. Platelet infusion may be necessary in patients on antiplatelet agents.

Intraventricular hemorrhage occurs in up to 45% of patients with intracerebral hemorrhage. This can cause obstruction of drainage of CSF and hydrocephalus. These patients require external ventricular drain placement (EVD). EVD should be considered in any patient with high intracranial pressure, uncal herniation, transventricular hemorrhage, and Glasgow Coma Scale score of less than 8.

Intracerebral hemorrhage can be surgically treated according to a strict protocol. Various criteria are used to establish that an intracerebral hemorrhage can be surgically treated. Patient age, comorbid conditions, size and location of the hemorrhage, and timing of the hemorrhage are involved in the decision to use surgery. Surgical procedures include craniotomy and hematoma evacuation under direct visual guidance.

If cerebral aneurysm or AVM is present, endovascular therapy using coil embolization or microsurgical clipping is performed. For surgical treatment, the cerebral vessel has to be in a location that is surgically accessible. Evacuation of hematoma is most emergent in cerebellar areas of the brain as they are in close proximity to the brainstem. Pressure on the brainstem can be fatal.

Chapter Summary

- There are two major kinds of stroke: ischemic and hemorrhagic.
- Ischemic stroke is caused by a thrombus or embolus that lodges and obstructs cerebral blood flow.
- Hemorrhagic stroke is caused by rupture and bleeding of a cerebral artery within the brain.
- The cerebral artery most commonly affected by stroke is the middle cerebral artery.
- Ischemic stroke is often caused by an embolus that travels from the common carotid artery into the internal carotid artery to the middle cerebral artery.
- Left atrial fibrillation increases risk for clots that can travel up to the brain from the aorta and cause ischemic stroke.
- Ischemia of the cerebellum can be caused by vertebral-basilar arterial insufficiency.
- Hemorrhagic stroke is often caused by rupture of a cerebral aneurysm or AVM.
- Cerebral aneurysms are most commonly found on the circle of Willis within the subarachnoid space.
- An SAH is a type of cerebral hemorrhage that causes a sudden, severe "thunderclap" headache.
- African Americans, Hispanic Americans, and Native Americans have a higher risk of stroke than European Americans.
- Atrial fibrillation and carotid stenosis are the major predisposing factors for ischemic stroke.
- Hypertension is the major predisposing factor for hemorrhagic stroke.
- The motor neurons that originate in the brain and travel down into the spinal cord are within the corticospinal tract.
- The neurons of the corticospinal tract cross over at the decussation in the medulla.

- Ischemic or hemorrhagic injury of one side of the brain causes symptoms on the contralateral side of the body.
- One-sided weakness, loss of sensation of one extremity, facial droop, and slurring of speech are common signs of stroke.
- A TIA is a strokelike syndrome that lasts minutes to hours and then resolves.
- A TIA is a major risk factor for stroke.
- A CT scan is a diagnostic test that is promptly required to differentiate an ischemic stroke from a hemorrhagic stroke.
- Early treatment can salvage the neurons within the ischemic penumbra in an ischemic stroke.
- rt-PA is a thrombolytic agent that can be used to dissolve the thrombus in some patients with ischemic stroke.
- There are eligibility criteria and a 4.5-hour time frame in which rt-PA can be administered.
- Surgical mechanical thrombectomy is used on eligible patients with ischemic stroke.
- Minimally invasive surgery through craniotomy may be possible in hemorrhagic stroke, depending on location of the bleed.
- Surgical evacuation of the hematoma in hemorrhagic stroke is most urgent in the cerebellar region of the brain due to the proximity to the brainstem.
- In hemorrhagic stroke, uncal herniation can cause pressure on the brainstem, which can be fatal.
- Signs of pressure on the brainstem including hypertension, bradycardia, and decreased level of consciousness are referred to as Cushing's triad.

Making the Connections

Disorder and Pathophysiology

Signs and Symptoms	Physical Assessment Findings	Diagnostic Testing	Treatment

Ischemic Stroke | An area of the brain undergoes ischemia and infarction. Two main etiologies: (1) A thromboembolism commonly causes obstruction of a branch of a cerebral artery. Usually, a piece of arteriosclerotic plaque breaks away from an area of carotid artery stenosis and travels up to a branch of the middle cerebral artery. (2) The left atrium undergoes atrial fibrillation with stasis of blood and clot formation. The clot travels from the left atrium into the left ventricle, into the aorta, and upward into the carotid artery into a cerebral artery. Alternatively, an arteriosclerotic cerebral artery causes tissue ischemia.

Signs and Symptoms	Physical Assessment Findings	Diagnostic Testing	Treatment
Motor and sensory loss is evident on the opposite side of the body than the cerebral hemisphere undergoing the ischemia. Hemiparesis (weakness) or hemiplegia (paralysis) is observed. If the left hemisphere undergoes ischemia, most of those affected will suffer aphasia.	Hemiparesis or hemiplegia of limbs is observed on the opposite side of the cerebral hemisphere affected. Sensation is diminished on one side of the body. Speech problems are evident if the cerebral ischemia is of the left hemisphere.	CT scan without contrast or MRI demonstrates area of injury.	Thrombolytic is administered if the ischemic stroke began less than 4.5 hours ago and the patient is eligible. Aspirin is given with anticoagulants to prevent further damage. Some patients are eligible for surgical thrombectomy.

Lacunar Infarct | Small blood vessel infarction associated with hypertension.

Signs and Symptoms	Physical Assessment Findings	Diagnostic Testing	Treatment
No symptoms or evidence of neurological changes are present.	No symptoms or evidence of neurological changes are evident.	CT scan or MRI demonstrates small area of infarction.	Aspirin or anticoagulant therapy is used to prevent further injury.

Transient Ischemic Attack (TIA) | Ischemia of the brain that is caused by the same etiologies as ischemic stroke: thromboembolism from carotid stenosis or atrial fibrillation. Ischemia of the brain is caused by a thromboembolus that dissolves within 24 hours. The ischemia is reversible after the thrombus dissolves.

Signs and Symptoms	Physical Assessment Findings	Diagnostic Testing	Treatment
Motor and sensory loss is evident on the opposite side of the body than the cerebral hemisphere undergoing the ischemia. Hemiparesis (weakness) or hemiplegia (paralysis) is observed. If the left hemisphere undergoes ischemia, most of those affected will suffer aphasia.	Hemiparesis or hemiplegia of limbs is evident on the opposite side of the cerebral hemisphere affected. Loss of sensation on one side of body. Speech problems are evident if cerebral ischemia is of the left hemisphere. Gradually improving neurological examination. Neurological examination is back to normal within 24 hours, with no remaining neurological deficits.	CT scan or MRI may not be helpful if ischemia area has resolved. Electrocardiogram. Carotid artery CT scan.	Aspirin or anticoagulant therapy is used to prevent recurrence. Carotid stenosis surgery, called endarterectomy, or treatment of atrial fibrillation may be done to prevent recurrence.

Continued

Making the Connections–cont'd

Signs and Symptoms	Physical Assessment Findings	Diagnostic Testing	Treatment
Hemorrhagic Stroke | Cerebral artery rupture occurs, which causes a large amount of blood to compress the brain tissue and cause brain death. Subarachnoid hemorrhage is one type of hemorrhagic stroke.			
Motor and sensory loss is evident on the opposite side of the body than the cerebral hemisphere undergoing the hemorrhage. Hemiparesis (weakness) or hemiplegia (paralysis) is observed. If the left hemisphere undergoes hemorrhage, most affected patients will suffer aphasia. Subarachnoid hemorrhage causes severe headache with changing level of consciousness.	Sudden onset. Elevated blood pressure. Rapid deterioration of cognitive function. Motor and sensory loss on opposite side of the affected cerebral hemisphere. If the left hemisphere undergoes hemorrhage, most of those affected will suffer aphasia.	CT scan or MRI demonstrates specific area of bleeding in the brain. Over the following day, CT scans are done to evaluate bleeding into the brain. CT angiography is most precise.	Supportive care. Reversal of any anticoagulant treatment is necessary. Decrease cerebral edema with IV mannitol or hypertonic saline. Patient may need intubation and mechanical ventilation. Neurosurgery to evacuate the hematoma may be possible in some patients.

Bibliography

Available online at fadavis.com

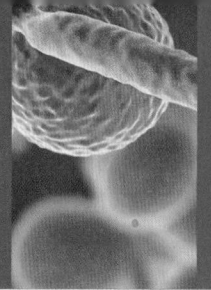

Learning Objectives

After completion of this chapter, the student will be able to:

- Recognize the neurotransmitters that are involved in central and peripheral nervous system transmission of impulses.
- Describe the pathophysiological mechanisms involved in major chronic and degenerative neurological disorders.

- Identify signs and symptoms that are the clinical manifestations of chronic and degenerative neurological disorders.
- Discuss various assessment techniques used to diagnose chronic and degenerative neurological disorders.
- Recognize the different treatment modalities involved in the management of chronic and degenerative neurological disorders.

Key Terms

Acetylcholine
Ataxia
Atonic
Athetosis
Aura
Basal ganglia
Chorea
Diencephalon

Dopamine
Gamma aminobutyric acid (GABA)
Glutamate
Ictal period
Interictal period
Midbrain
Migraine
Myelin

Myoclonus
Postictal period
Seizure
Serotonin
Substantia nigra
Tonic
Unified Parkinson Disease Rating Scale (UPDRS)

Chronic and degenerative neurological disorders have a profound effect on patients and their caregivers. Some chronic neurological conditions, such as migraine headache and epilepsy, can be prevented and treated. In contrast, degenerative neurological disorders, such as Parkinson's disease and amyotrophic lateral sclerosis (ALS), are progressive and slowly debilitating in nature. The patient with a degenerative disorder has difficulty carrying out activities of daily living (ADLs), which impairs the patient's ability to function independently. Degenerative neurological disorders commonly require ongoing physical and occupational therapy to maximize function of the individual.

Epidemiology

Headaches, which are one of the most common disorders treated in the primary care and emergency clinical settings, account for 1% to 4% of all emergency department (ED) visits and are the ninth most common reason for a patient to consult a clinician. Clinicians classify 90% of headaches reported to them as tension headache or migraine headaches. Migraine headaches occur in more than 30 million people per year. Approximately 75% of all persons who experience migraines are female.

Seizure is a common, nonspecific manifestation of neurological injury and disease. It can appear as a temporary absence of attention, uncontrolled contractions of muscle groups, or whole-body convulsion. Epilepsy is a disorder that causes chronic, unprovoked seizures that are often unpredictable. The lifetime likelihood of experiencing at least one epileptic seizure is about 9%, and the lifetime likelihood of receiving a diagnosis of epilepsy is almost 3%. However, the prevalence of active epilepsy is only about 0.8%.

Degenerative neurological diseases are those disorders that diminish neurological impulse transmission in the body. The common result is lack of independent muscle contraction, postural imbalance, and loss of sensation and movement. Some degenerative disorders can also affect cognitive function. Parkinson's disease is one of the most common degenerative neurological disorders, affecting approximately 1% of individuals older than 60 years. It is estimated that 1 million persons are living with Parkinson's disease in the United States, with 60,000 new diagnoses each year. The cause of Parkinson's disease is unknown, but the areas of the brain affected are clearly defined. Multiple sclerosis (MS) is an immune-mediated degenerative neurological disorder. Slowly, motor and sensory nerves are demyelinated, but remissions from the disease can occur. The incidence of MS is increasing worldwide and currently affects 2.8 million persons in 2020. Nearly 1 million persons in the United States are living with MS.

Basic Concepts of Neurological Function

The human nervous system is composed of the central nervous system (CNS) and peripheral nervous system (PNS). The CNS includes the brain and spinal cord, whereas the PNS includes the somatic nerves—motor and sensory types—and the autonomic nervous system (ANS). The CNS is composed of two types of neural cells: neurons and glial cells. Neurons transmit impulses, process information, and connect with other neurons. The nervous system can be likened to electrical circuits that control the body. Between the neurons are synapses—gaps between neurons through which neurotransmitters travel from one neuron to another. Glial cells provide structural support for the neurons and phagocytose foreign matter and cellular debris.

Neurons

The three basic types of neurons are motor neurons, sensory neurons, and interneurons. The neuron has four major anatomical parts: dendrites, cell body, axon, and axon terminals. Incoming signals from other neurons are received through its dendrites. The outgoing signal to other neurons flows along its axon. A neuron may have many thousands of dendrites, but it will have only one axon. The fourth distinct part of a neuron, the axon terminals, are located at the end of the axon. These are the structures that contain chemical mediators called neurotransmitters.

Neurotransmitters

Some neuron-to-neuron connections are electrical synapses where an impulse travels to another neuron. However, at some neural synapses, axon terminals release neurotransmitters through which signals flow (Fig. 34-1). Common neurotransmitters of the nervous system include acetylcholine (Ach), norepinephrine, serotonin, dopamine, gamma aminobutyric acid (GABA), and glutamate.

Acetylcholine is found within the CNS, PNS, and ANS. It can act as either an excitatory or inhibitory neurotransmitter, depending on what neurons secrete it. For example, within the ANS, Ach functions as an inhibitory neurotransmitter to slow the heart rate. However, within the PNS, it behaves as an excitatory neurotransmitter at neuromuscular junctions.

Serotonin, or 5-hydroxytryptamine, is a neurotransmitter chemically derived from tryptophan. It is found primarily in the gastrointestinal tract, platelets, and CNS. In the CNS, it is found primarily in the dorsal raphe

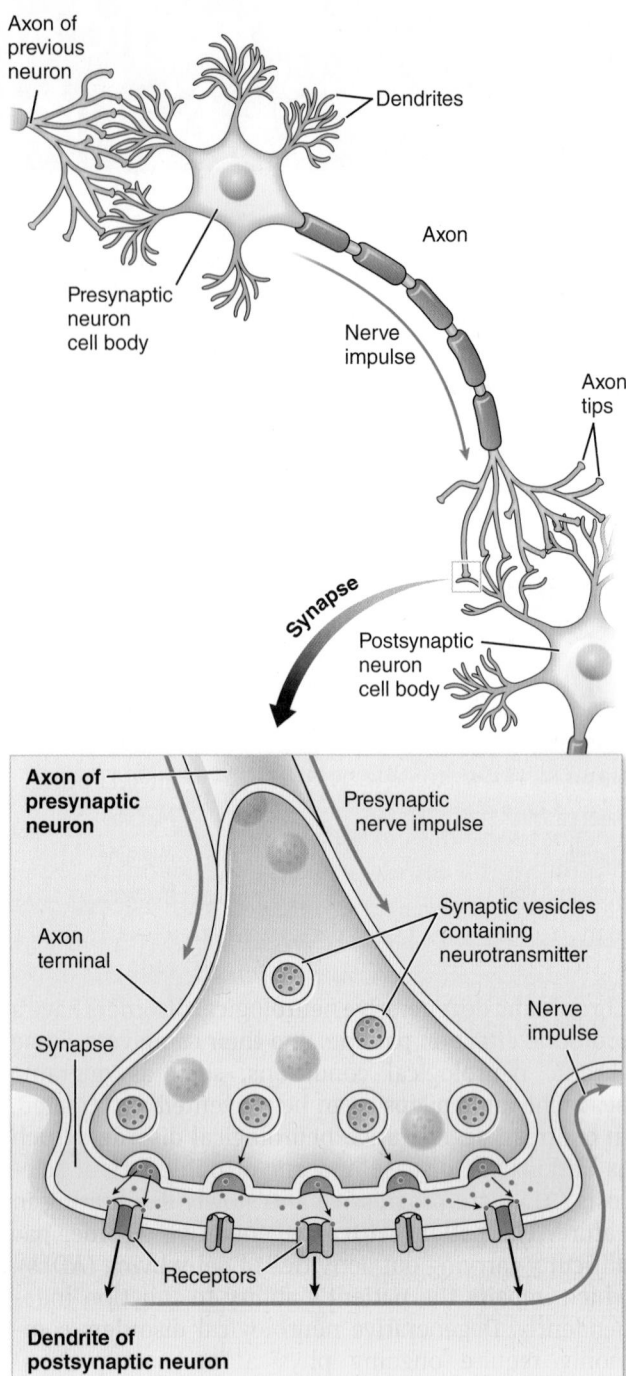

FIGURE 34-1. The neuron and transmission of impulses. **(A)** Neurons transmit impulses to each other in an orderly manner. Dendrites come off the cell body to pick up impulses, and the impulse travels down the axon. **(B)** A synapse is a space between two neurons where neurotransmitters are secreted from a presynaptic neuron to a postsynaptic neuron. Neurotransmitters bind to receptors on the postsynaptic neuron, which stimulates an impulse.

region of the brainstem and is thought to be a contributor to feelings of well-being.

Dopamine has many functions, including roles in:

- Behavior and cognition
- Voluntary movement
- Motivation

- Punishment and reward
- Attention
- Working memory
- Learning

Dopaminergic neurons are mainly located in the substantia nigra of the midbrain's basal ganglia region. Dysfunction of dopaminergic neurotransmission in the CNS has been implicated in a variety of neuropsychiatric disorders, including social phobia, Tourette's syndrome, Parkinson's disease, schizophrenia, neuroleptic malignant syndrome, attention deficit-hyperactivity disorder (ADHD), and substance and alcohol use disorders.

Gamma aminobutyric acid (GABA), the chief inhibitory neurotransmitter in the CNS, typically has a relaxing, antianxiety, and anticonvulsive effect on the brain. It also has an inhibitory effect on muscles, which decreases spasms and allows for muscle tone.

Norepinephrine is an excitatory neurotransmitter in the brain and stress hormone within the endocrine system. Stress activates a region of the brainstem called the locus coeruleus—the origin of most norepinephrine pathways in the brain. Neurons using norepinephrine project from the locus coeruleus to the cerebral cortex, limbic system, and the spinal cord. Another neurotransmitter, **glutamate,** is considered a major mediator of excitatory signals in the CNS and is involved in cognition, memory, and learning. Glutamate is kept within the nerve terminal vesicles; after being released from the neuron, specific transporters must rapidly remove it from the extracellular space, as extracellular accumulation of glutamate causes brain cell injury and cell death.

Nerve Conduction

Neurons conduct impulses called action potentials that begin at the cell body and travel down the axon. This stimulates ions such as sodium (Na+), potassium (K+), and calcium (Ca++) to move across the membrane of the axon. Ions move back and forth across the axon membrane through ion channels that open and close (see Fig. 34-2). When ion channels open, charged particles such as Na+ flood across the membrane at a tremendous rate. When the concentration of ions on the inside of the neuron changes, the electrical property of the membrane changes. The influx of Na+ through ion channels during neurotransmission makes the inside of the neuron more positive. This is called depolarization of the neuron. When depolarization reaches a peak called a threshold, an action potential is generated. After depolarization, potassium channels of the neuronal membrane open, resulting in outward movement of potassium ions during a phase called repolarization. Repolarization refers to the return of the membrane potential to a negative value after the depolarization phase of an action potential.

Typically, the repolarization phase of an action potential results in hyperpolarization, which is attainment of a membrane potential that is more negative

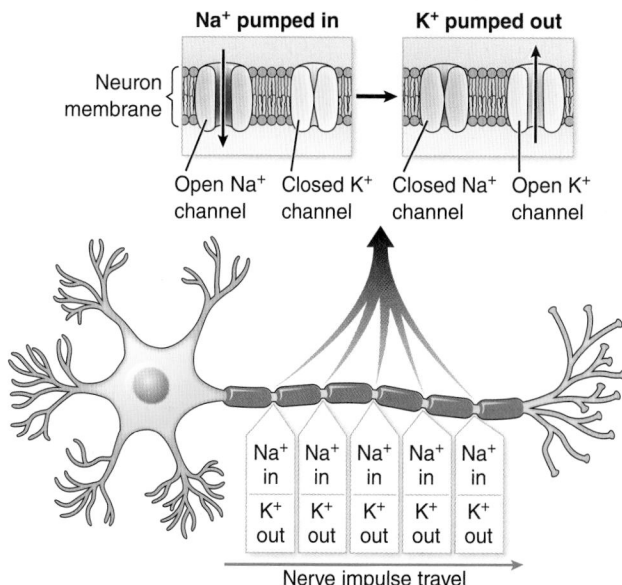

FIGURE 34-2. Ion channels across a neuron membrane. Neurons conduct impulses called action potentials that begin at the cell body and travel down the axon. This stimulates ions, such as sodium (Na+) and potassium (K+), to move across the axon's membrane. Ions move back and forth across the axon membrane through ion channels that open and close.

than the resting potential (see Fig. 34-3). It is important that there is a refractory or resting period between impulses that provides time for the membrane to return to baseline levels. An excitatory phase (depolarization) and an inhibitory phase (repolarization) exist with each action potential—this keeps the impulse moving in a unidirectional manner. Impulses that do not maintain a systematic orderly, excitatory, inhibitory, and resting phase become irregular and chaotic, as occurs in seizure disorders.

Myelin

Myelin is a protective sheath that is formed around axons of some neurons in the nervous system. It acts as an insulator of the electrical signal that is conducted down the axon in neurotransmission and is comparable to the insulation around an electrical wire. The myelin sheath contains a variety of fatty substances called lipids and is considered white matter. In the nervous system, neuron cell bodies are located within the gray matter, whereas axonal tracts and glial cells are within the white matter.

Myelination takes place through glial cells wrapping around the axons in a spiral fashion. Myelin allows for a rapid, efficient conduction of a nerve impulse down its axon. Without an even coating of myelin, nerve impulses can become disrupted and potential for conduction can be lost; nerves can eventually wither away. In disorders that cause degeneration of myelin, some regrowth is possible with time, though eventually myelin cannot regenerate; at this point, whole nerve degeneration occurs, causing complete nerve tract disruption.

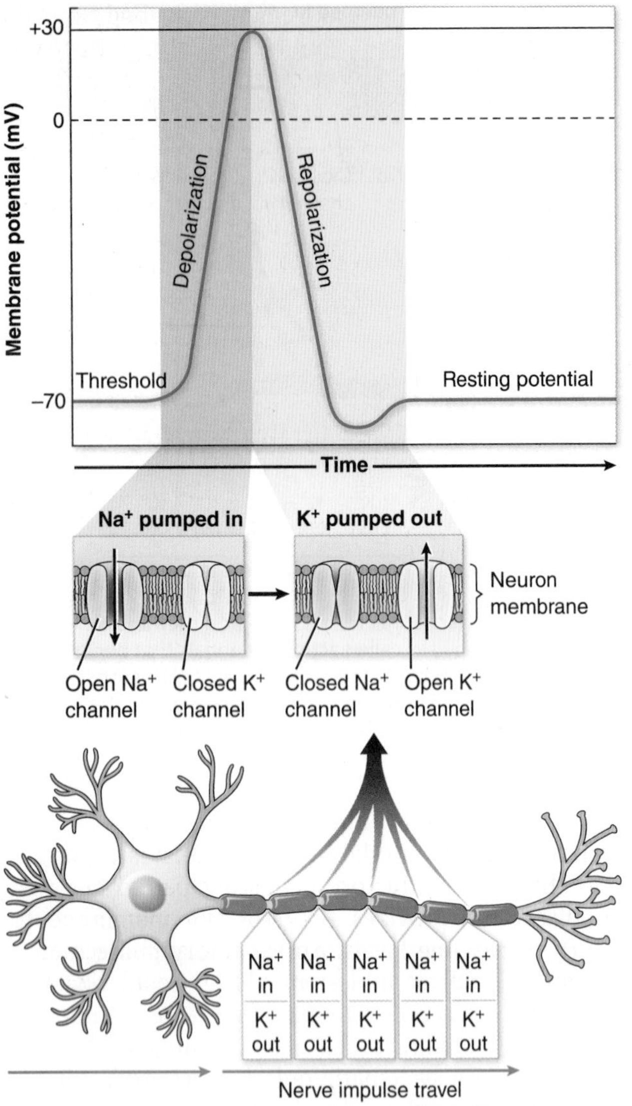

FIGURE 34-3. In neuron transmission, sodium (Na+) ion channels open and Na+ ions enter the cell membrane. The influx of Na+ through ion channels during neurotransmission makes the inside of the neuron more positive. This is called depolarization of the neuron. When this depolarization reaches a peak called a threshold, an action potential is generated. After depolarization, the neuronal membrane opens potassium channels, resulting in outward movement of potassium ions during a phase called repolarization.

Basic Neuroanatomy

Cerebral Cortex

The cerebrum, or cortex, is the largest part of the human brain; it is associated with higher brain functions such as thought and action. The cerebral cortex is divided into four sections, called lobes (see Fig. 34-4):

1. Frontal lobe: associated with reasoning, planning, parts of speech, movement, emotions, and problem-solving
2. Parietal lobe: associated with movement, orientation, recognition, and perception of stimuli
3. Occipital lobe: associated with visual processing

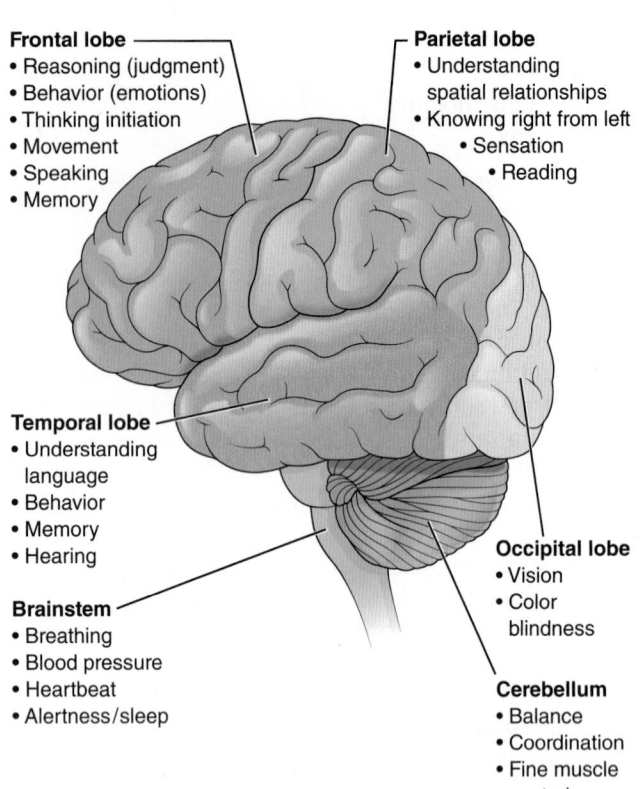

FIGURE 34-4. Brain anatomy and functional areas.

4. Temporal lobe: associated with perception and recognition of auditory stimuli, memory, and speech

Cerebellum

The cerebellum contributes to coordination, precision, and accuracy of movement. It receives input from sensory systems and from other parts of the brain and spinal cord, and integrates these inputs to fine-tune motor activity. Damage to the cerebellum causes lack of coordination, imbalance, and a gait disturbance termed **ataxia**.

Diencephalon

The **diencephalon** is the posterior part of the forebrain that connects the midbrain with the cerebral hemispheres; it consists of the thalamus and hypothalamus (see Fig. 34-5). The diencephalon relays sensory information between brain regions and controls many autonomic functions of the PNS. It also connects structures of the endocrine system with the nervous system and works in conjunction with limbic system structures to generate and manage emotions and memories.

Brainstem

The brainstem is responsible for basic vital life functions such as breathing, heartbeat, and blood pressure. It is made up of the midbrain, pons, and medulla (see Fig. 34-6). The **midbrain** is involved in functions such

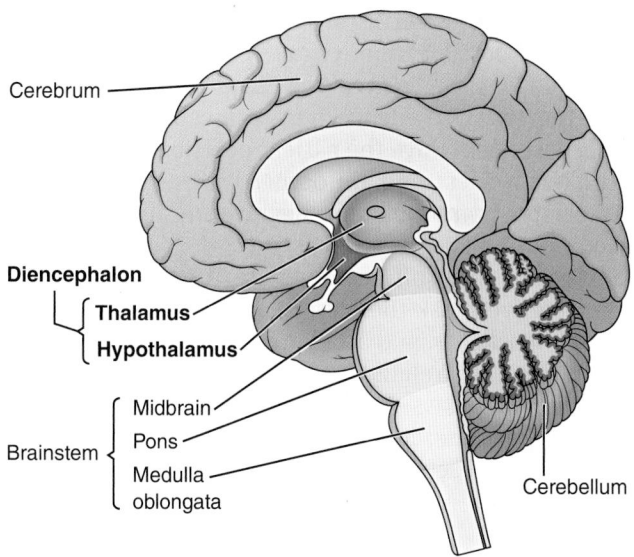

FIGURE 34-5. The diencephalon region of the brain. The diencephalon is located between the cerebral hemispheres and the brainstem. It includes the thalamus and the hypothalamus. Nearly all sensory impulses travel through the thalamus, which sorts out the impulses and directs them to particular areas of the cerebral cortex. The hypothalamus is located in the midline area inferior to the thalamus. It helps to maintain homeostasis by controlling body temperature, water balance, sleep, appetite, and some emotions, such as fear and pleasure. Both the sympathetic and parasympathetic divisions of the ANS are under the control of the hypothalamus, as is the pituitary gland. The hypothalamus influences the heartbeat, the contraction and relaxation of blood vessels, hormone secretion, and other vital body functions.

as vision, hearing, eye movement, and body movement. The anterior part contains the cerebral peduncle, a huge bundle of axons traveling from the cerebral cortex through the brainstem. These fibers, along with other structures, are important for voluntary motor function. The **basal ganglia** is a portion of the midbrain that modulates voluntary motor function and routine behaviors. The **substantia nigra** is a portion of the basal ganglia that synthesizes dopamine.

The pons is involved in motor control and sensory analysis. For example, information from the ear first enters the brain in the pons. It also has parts that are important for level of consciousness and sleep. Some structures within the pons are linked to the cerebellum and are involved in movement and posture.

The medulla oblongata is part of the brainstem between the pons and spinal cord. It is responsible for maintaining vital body functions, such as breathing, sleep–wake cycles, blood pressure, and heart rate.

Basic Pathophysiological Concepts of Neurological Dysfunction

The cellular causes of nervous system disorders commonly involve the sodium and potassium ion channels within the axonal tracts. The generation of an impulse is thwarted in ion channel disorders. In other disorders, the layers of myelin covering the axons are disrupted, which interferes with the smooth travel of impulses.

Ion Channel Disorders

Ion channel disorders, also called channelopathies, are responsible for a growing number of neurological diseases. Most are caused by mutations in ion channel genes or by autoantibodies formed against ion channel proteins. One example is epilepsy, a syndrome of repetitive synchronous firing of neuronal action potentials. Action potentials are normally generated by the opening of sodium channels and the inward movement of sodium ions down the intracellular concentration gradient. Depolarization of the neuronal membrane opens potassium channels, resulting in outward movement of potassium ions, repolarization, closure of the sodium channel, and hyperpolarization. Sodium or potassium channel subunit genes have long been considered candidate disease genes in inherited epilepsy; recently, such mutations have been identified. These mutations appear to alter the normal gating function of these channels, increasing the inherent excitability of neuron membranes in regions where the abnormal channels are expressed. Whereas the specific clinical manifestations of channelopathies are variable, one common feature is that manifestations tend to be intermittent or paroxysmal, as occurs

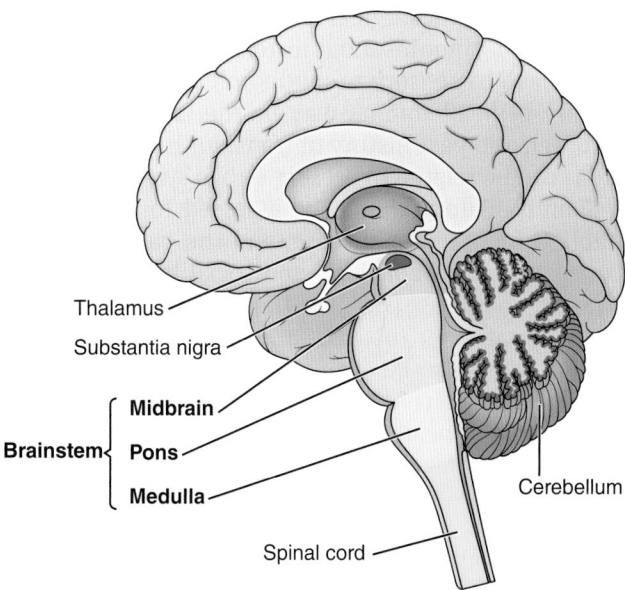

FIGURE 34-6. The components and functions of the brainstem. The brainstem is located in front of the cerebellum. It passes messages back and forth between the brain and other parts of the body. The cerebrum, cerebellum, and spinal cord are all connected to the brainstem, which has three main parts: the midbrain, pons, and medulla oblongata. The brainstem controls vital functions, including breathing, consciousness, cardiac function, involuntary muscle movements, and swallowing.

in epilepsy, migraine headache, dysautonomia, and periodic paralysis.

Myelin and Myelin-Related Disorders

In demyelinating diseases, the myelin sheath around some axons is targeted. The most common demyelinating disease is MS, which is suspected to be an autoimmune disease. Antibodies created by the body attack the myelin on varying sensory and motor axons. After patches of myelin deteriorate, oligodendrocytes repair the damage, but also form scar tissue called gliotic plaques. These hard plaques then begin to interfere with the flow of electrical impulses that move through the axon. Some diseases such as ALS have been found to cause demyelination of motor neurons, and others such as MS have demyelination of both sensory and motor neurons.

Assessment of the Neurological System

The clinician must carefully observe the patient during the history and physical when a neurological disorder is suspected, because neurological symptoms are often subtle.

 CLINICAL CONCEPT

Many neurological disorders are difficult to diagnose upon initial examination, because degenerative neurological diseases are progressive and the full picture of the disorder is not often apparent with early symptoms.

Assess vision, hearing, orientation, and cognitive ability first to ensure that the patient can give an accurate history. If the patient is unconscious, the clinician should make an assessment based on the Glasgow Coma Scale, vital signs, and pupil response. The cause for the loss of consciousness must be sought, primarily through blood tests and imaging studies. (For more on the Glasgow Coma Scale, see Chapter 35.)

 CLINICAL CONCEPT

If the patient is cognitively impaired, obtain the patient's history from the patient's parent, spouse, partner, or guardian, if able.

If the patient is conscious, note speech, demeanor, hygiene, and emotional state. Administration of the Mini-Mental Status Examination (MMSE) may be necessary if cognitive impairment is suspected. The MMSE is a multiple-question test of orientation, cognition, and memory (see Chapter 36 for a discussion of the MMSE). If this is not possible, mini-cognitive assessment through clock drawing can be used (see Chapter 36).

If there is any evidence of trauma, causation must be fully described. Have the patient describe pain, if present. When does the pain occur? Where is it located? Associated symptoms and aggravating and relieving factors should be assessed.

If the patient suffered a seizure, it needs to be fully characterized. Ask the patient about recent falls, dizziness, blackouts, and accidents. Although the patient often does not relate these events to a neurological disorder, they are significant signs. Also ask about loss of consciousness, sudden weakness in an extremity, or slurring of speech.

 CLINICAL CONCEPT

If the patient has been accompanied by someone who observed the incident, make sure to ask this person about loss of consciousness, extremity weakness, and slurring, as these symptoms are best described by a third party and not the patient.

Ask the patient about difficulty with range of motion, numbness, or sensation. Handedness is important in establishing which cerebral hemisphere controls language. In almost all right-handed persons, the left hemisphere is responsible for language. If the patient is taking any medication, it is necessary to evaluate any possible effects on the nervous system. Past medical and surgical history need to be assessed. For example, inquire about history of diabetes because it can lead to sensory or autonomic neuropathy. Past history of head trauma may be the cause of seizure disorder, and past history of transient ischemic attack (TIA) can be related to present stroke symptoms.

Family history should be assessed for any inheritable or contagious disease, and the patient should be asked about behavioral and social habits. Ask the patient about use of over-the-counter medication, alcohol, caffeine, tobacco, and illicit drug use. The patient must also be evaluated to determine whether they can carry out ADLs independently.

Inspect the head for any signs of trauma. Have the patient smile to observe if a facial droop is present. Have the patient close their eyelids tightly as you try to open them. A fundoscopic examination of the retina can reveal if there is excess intracranial pressure. Papilledema—swelling of the optic disc—can occur in stroke, tumor, or other causes of cerebral edema. Have the patient open their mouth and check to see if the uvula and tongue are midline; if they are deviated, there is probable gag dysfunction.

A full neurological examination, which includes sensory, motor, reflex, and balance functions, is needed. The patient should stretch out both arms where hands and fingers can be observed for tremor. Tremor, fasciculations, motor rigidity, or spasm should be noted. It is important to assess the patient's upper and lower motor strength. This can be quickly done by assessing the patient's bilateral grip strength and quadriceps strength against the clinician's resistance. With the patient's eyes closed, sensation to light touch with a cotton ball and pinpoint discrimination with a paper clip can be assessed. Lack of sensation in the feet is significant, particularly if a patient has a history of diabetes mellitus.

Examination of the patient's gait can reveal a lack of neurological integrity. The patient should be able to easily rise from a chair. Assess deep tendon reflexes of the upper and lower extremities, and evaluate the cranial nerves, which can reveal CNS problems. Assess the Babinski reflex, which is tested with stimulation of the sole of the foot. A negative Babinski reflex, in which the toes flex inward with stimulation of the sole of the foot, is normal in adults. A positive Babinski reflex, where the patient's toes flare in response to stimulation of the sole of the foot, indicates an upper motor neuron disorder.

 CLINICAL CONCEPT

An upper motor neuron disorder indicates that the source of the problem is in a neuron in the brain's area of motor control or along its path down into the spinal cord. A lower motor neuron disorder indicates the source of the problem is at the region where motor nerves exit the spinal cord (see Fig. 34-7).

Risk Factors

Risk factors vary across neurological disorders; some disorders have no known risk factors, whereas others have been linked with specific ones. For example, stroke is common in those with cardiovascular risk factors, including hypertension, hyperlipidemia, uncontrolled diabetes, tobacco use, and lack of exercise, but myasthenia gravis (MG), ALS, and MS have no known risk factors. Head injury is a risk factor for intracranial bleeding, which leads to neurological symptoms and places the patient at risk for seizures. Hormonal fluctuations increase susceptibility to migraine headaches. Severe upper respiratory infection can precede meningitis. Some medications can increase the risk of seizure, loss of consciousness, or confusion. Alcohol use disorder and illicit substance use disorder can also increase susceptibility to neurological symptoms such as seizure. Familial or genetic factors are sometimes the only conditions that predispose individuals to neurological disease. This is particularly true of Huntington's disease (HD).

Signs and Symptoms

Signs and symptoms of degenerative neurological disease are often the only clues to diagnosis. Falls, accidents,

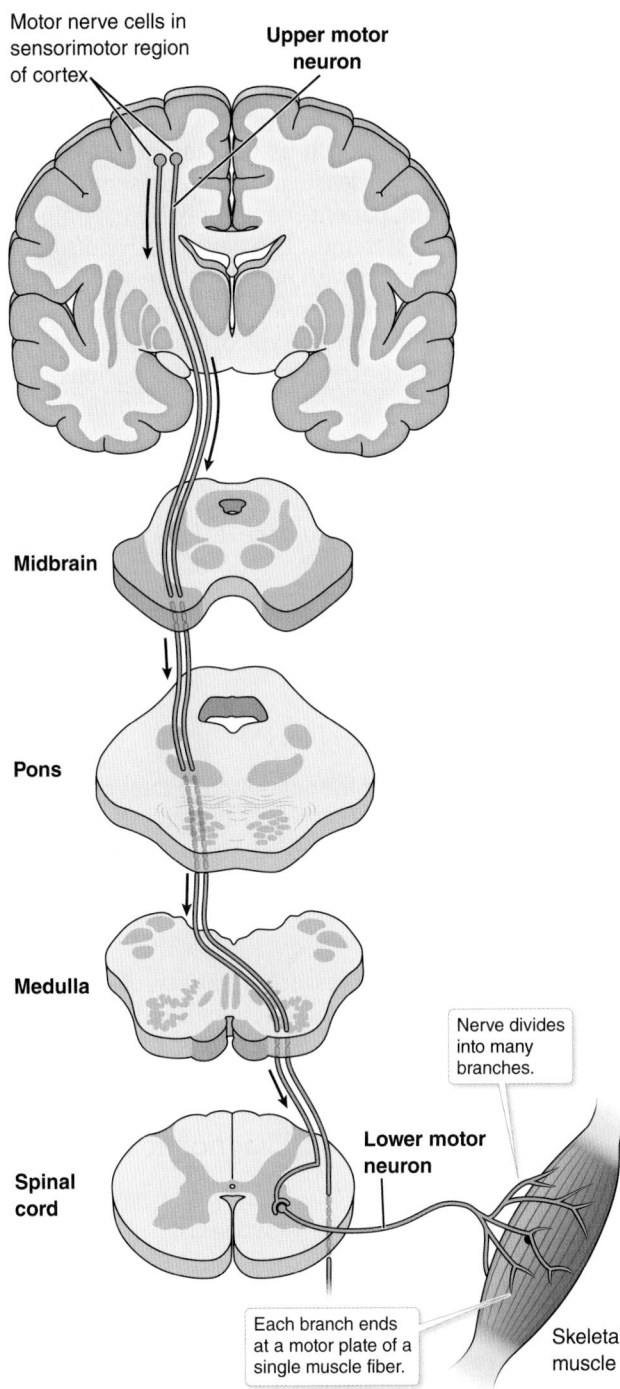

FIGURE 34-7. Upper and lower motor neurons. The upper motor neuron cell bodies are located in the cortex in the brain's area of motor control. The lower motor neuron cell bodies are located in the spinal cord.

and dizziness can be symptoms of neurological disease, which the patient may not think significant, as they often occur in the absence of neurological disease as well. Often a neurological disorder can present with mild and intermittent twitching, subtle weakness, or numbness in one extremity. Stroke often initially presents with numbness or weakness in one extremity, known as hemiparesis. MS can also present with sensory and motor symptoms similar to stroke. With disorders such as MS, the patient commonly presents to the clinician a number of times before the disorder can be diagnosed, as the symptoms are often subtle and confused with other diagnoses. Other neurological disorders may present with obvious gait disorder, rigid muscles, slowed motion, and loss of automatic movements, such as blinking and swinging the arms. Parkinson's disease commonly presents in this manner; in addition, patients commonly have a unique, characteristic resting tremor. The degenerative disorder of MG uniquely presents with ptosis of the eyelids.

Seizures, a symptom of epilepsy, can present in different ways depending on the type of epileptic disorder. A grand mal seizure presents with loss of consciousness and repetitive tonic and clonic muscle contractions; it is unmistakable as a seizure. However, an absence seizure is more difficult to diagnose because it simply presents as an episode of inattention.

Severe headache can also have different associated symptoms depending on the type of headache. For example, nausea and vomiting commonly accompany migraine headaches but not tension headaches.

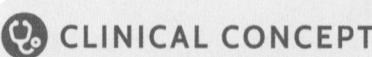

CLINICAL CONCEPT

Papilledema, swelling of the optic disc, indicates elevated intracranial pressure.

Diagnosis

Researchers and clinicians use a variety of diagnostic imaging techniques and chemical and metabolic analyses to detect, manage, and treat neurological disease. Laboratory screening tests of blood, urine, or spinal fluid are used to help diagnose disease and better understand the disease process. Blood tests are also used to monitor levels of therapeutic drugs used to treat epilepsy and other neurological disorders.

Genetic testing of DNA extracted from white blood cells in the blood can help diagnose HD and other genetic diseases. Analysis of the cerebrospinal fluid that surrounds the brain and spinal cord can detect meningitis, acute and chronic inflammation, rare infections, and some cases of MS. Chemical and metabolic testing of the blood can indicate protein disorders, some forms of muscular dystrophy and other muscle disorders, and diabetes. Urinalysis can reveal abnormal substances in the urine or the presence or absence of certain proteins that cause diseases, including the mucopolysaccharidoses.

Genetic testing can help parents with a family history of a neurological disease determine whether they are carrying one of the known genes that cause the disorder or find out if their child is affected. Genetic testing can identify some neurological disorders in utero, such as spina bifida and Down syndrome. Amniocentesis, usually done between 14 and 16 weeks of pregnancy, tests a sample of the amniotic fluid in the womb for genetic defects. Chorionic villus sampling (CVS) is performed by removing and testing a very small sample of the placenta during early pregnancy. Uterine ultrasound is performed using a surface probe with gel. This noninvasive test can suggest the diagnosis of conditions such as chromosomal disorders. For other common diagnostic procedures used in neurological disorders, see Table 34-1.

TABLE 34-1. Diagnostic Procedures Used in Neurological Disorders	
X-ray	X-rays of the patient's chest and skull are often taken as part of a neurological work-up.
Fluoroscopy	Type of x-ray that uses a continuous or pulsed beam of low-dose radiation to produce continuous images of a body part in motion. A contrast medium may be used to highlight the images (e.g., used to evaluate the flow of blood through arteries).
Angiography	Angiogram can detect the degree of narrowing or obstruction of an artery or blood vessel in the brain, head, or neck (e.g., used to diagnose stroke or determine size and location of a brain tumor, aneurysm, or vascular malformation).
Biopsy	Removal and examination of a small piece of tissue from the body under microscope. Muscle or nerve biopsies are used to diagnose neuromuscular disorders.
Brain Scan	Imaging techniques used to diagnose tumors, blood vessel malformations, or hemorrhage in the brain. Types of brain scans include CT, MRI, and PET.
Cerebrospinal Fluid (CSF) Analysis	A lumbar puncture (LP) removes a small amount of the CSF that surrounds and protects the brain and spinal cord. The CSF is analyzed microscopically for bleeding, infection, or proteins associated with neurological conditions and to measure intracranial pressure. The patient is asked to lie on one side, in a ball position with knees close to the chest, while the clinician inserts a needle into the spinal sac in the lower back between two vertebrae to inject anesthesia and then withdraw a sample of CSF. A common after-effect of a lumbar puncture is headache, which can be lessened by having the patient lie flat.

TABLE 34-1. Diagnostic Procedures Used in Neurological Disorders—cont'd

Computed Tomography (CT) scan	Noninvasive, specialized imaging technique that produces clear two-dimensional images of organs, bones, and tissues. It is used to view the brain and spine; can detect bone and vascular irregularities, tumors and cysts, herniated discs, epilepsy, encephalitis, spinal stenosis, blood clot or intracranial bleeding in patients with stroke, brain damage from head injury, and other disorders. An *intrathecal contrast-enhanced CT scan* is used to detect problems with the spine and spinal nerve roots.
Electroencephalography (EEG)	Monitors brain activity through the skull. Can be used to diagnose seizure disorders and many other disorders and confirm brain death.
Electromyography (EMG)	It records the electrical activity from the brain and spinal cord to a peripheral nerve root that controls muscles during contraction and at rest. An EMG is usually done in conjunction with a *nerve conduction velocity* test, which measures electrical energy by assessing the nerve's ability to send a signal.
Electronystagmography	Describes a group of tests used to diagnose involuntary eye movement, dizziness, and balance disorders, as well as evaluate some brain functions. Small electrodes are taped around the eyes to record eye movements. If infrared photography is used in place of electrodes, the patient wears special goggles that help record the information.
Evoked Potentials	Measures the electrical signals to the brain generated by hearing, touch, or sight. Used to assess sensory nerve problems, MS, brain tumor, acoustic neuroma, spinal cord injury, test sight and hearing (in infants and young children), monitor brain activity among coma patients, and confirm brain death.
Magnetic Resonance Imaging (MRI)	Uses computer-generated radio waves and a powerful magnetic field to produce detailed images of body structures, including tissues, organs, bones, and nerves. *Functional MRI (fMRI)* uses the blood's magnetic properties to produce real-time images of blood flow to particular areas of the brain.
Myelography	Involves the injection of a water- or oil-based contrast dye into the spinal canal to enhance x-ray imaging of the spine to diagnose spinal nerve injury, herniated discs, fractures, back or leg pain, and spinal tumors.
Positron Emission Tomography (PET)	Two- and three-dimensional pictures of brain activity by measuring radioactive isotopes that are injected into the bloodstream to detect tumors and diseased tissue, measure cellular or tissue metabolism, show blood flow, evaluate seizure disorders, evaluate memory disorders, and determine brain changes following injury or drug abuse.
Polysomnogram	Measures brain and body activity during sleep.
Single Photon Emission Computed Tomography (SPECT)	Nuclear imaging test involving blood flow to tissue used to evaluate certain brain functions.
Thermography	Uses infrared sensing devices to measure small temperature changes between the two sides of the body or within a specific organ. Thermography may be used to detect vascular disease of the head and neck, soft tissue injury, various neuromusculoskeletal disorders, and the presence or absence of nerve root compression.
Ultrasonography	Uses high-frequency sound waves to obtain images inside the body. Neurosonography analyzes blood flow in the brain and can diagnose stroke, brain tumors, hydrocephalus (buildup of cerebrospinal fluid in the brain), vascular problems, and soft tissue problems. Transcranial Doppler ultrasound is used to view arteries and blood vessels in the neck and determine blood flow and risk of stroke.

Treatment

The type of treatment a patient receives will depend on whether or not they are experiencing a chronic or degenerative neurological disorder. Pain-relieving medications, also known as acute or abortive treatment, are types of drugs taken during migraine headaches and are designed to stop symptoms that have already begun. Alternatively, preventive medications can be taken regularly, often on a daily basis, to reduce the severity or frequency of migraines. Agents used for epilepsy or seizures include anticonvulsants such as valproate, lamotrigine, phenytoin, felbamate, topiramate, and carbamazepine. These are preventive medications meant to decrease susceptibility to seizure.

Treatments for degenerative neurological disorders such as MS and MG are aimed at modulating the autoimmune reaction underlying the disorder. For acute exacerbations, corticosteroids can hasten recovery from a given attack, but these medications cannot be used long term. In addition, plasma exchange can be used short term for severe attacks if steroids are contraindicated or ineffective. In neurological disorders such as ALS, Guillain–Barré syndrome (GBS), and HD, treatment is mainly supportive along with patient education.

Pathophysiology of Selected Chronic Neurological Disorders

Chronic neurological disorders vary in their severity. Migraine headache, a relatively benign form of neurological dysfunction, occurs episodically, and although individual episodes can be debilitating, leaves no residual neurological deficit. Epilepsy, in contrast, is a chronic neurological disorder that has major effects on the patient's life. Unpredictable, sudden episodes of seizure occur, usually with no lasting neurological deficit.

Epilepsy

Epilepsy is a chronic neurological disorder characterized by recurrent seizures. A **seizure** is a sudden, abnormal, disorderly discharge of neurons within the brain that is characterized by a sudden, transient alteration in brain function. A seizure may result in an altered level of consciousness as well as a number of motor, sensory, autonomic, and behavioral manifestations. Seizures have various clinical presentations depending on the specific part of the brain that is affected by the abnormal impulse propagation. A seizure can present as a temporary disruption of the senses, a loss of consciousness, muscle spasms, or repetitive convulsions. Seizures can also occur as a symptom secondary to pathological conditions of the brain, such as tumor, CNS infection, stroke, head injury, metabolic imbalance, substance abuse, and acute alcohol withdrawal (see Box 34-1).

BOX 34-1. Common Etiologies of Seizure

Epilepsy
Brain neoplasms
Cerebrovascular disease
Congenital malformation
Degenerative brain disorders such as Alzheimer's disease
Environmental stimuli, such as blinking lights, loud noises, and certain music and odors
Genetic predisposition
Head trauma
Infections
Metabolic disturbances, such as hypoglycemia, hyponatremia, and respiratory alkalosis
Perinatal injury (hypoxia)
Substance abuse
Withdrawal from alcohol or sedative-hypnotic drugs

Epidemiology

Epilepsy, one of the most common chronic neurological conditions, affects more than 3.4 million people in the United States. It is defined as a brain disorder characterized by a predisposition to seizures. The prevalence of epilepsy in the United States is 1% to 3%. It is most common in infants younger than 1 year of age and in adults older than 65 years. Incidence and prevalence of epilepsy are less common in later childhood and young adulthood. Epilepsy affects both genders and is seen in all racial and ethnic groups.

The annual incidence of seizures is approximately 100 per 100,000 individuals aged older than 60 years. Older adults have an increased risk of stroke and degenerative brain disorders such as Parkinson's disease; they are also more susceptible to metabolic disturbances and comorbid illnesses, which may explain why seizures are more commonly seen in this population.

Etiology

Epilepsy has no identifiable cause in about half of those who have the condition. In the other half, the condition may be traced to various factors (see Box 34-2). Head trauma is the most common cause in young adults, whereas stroke is the most common cause in older adults.

Pathophysiology

Traditionally, the diagnosis of epilepsy requires the occurrence of at least two unprovoked seizures at least 24 hours apart. A seizure results when an abrupt imbalance occurs between the excitatory and inhibitory impulses within a region of cortical neurons in favor of a sudden-onset of hyperexcitability. Epileptogenesis refers to the transformation of a normal neuronal region into one that is chronically hyperexcitable. There is often a delay of months to years between an initial CNS injury, such as head trauma, stroke, or infection, and

BOX 34-2. Causes of Epilepsy

GENETIC INFLUENCE

Some types of epilepsy, which are categorized by type of seizure, run in families, making it likely that there's a genetic influence. Researchers have linked some types of epilepsy to specific genes, though it's estimated that up to 500 genes could be tied to the condition. For most people, genes are only part of the cause, perhaps by making a person more susceptible to environmental conditions that trigger seizures. Some of the genes associated with epilepsy syndromes include 20q13.2, 19q12.1, 10q24, 6q24, and Xq21-24.

HEAD TRAUMA

Severe, penetrating head trauma sustained during a car accident or other traumatic injury can cause epilepsy.

MEDICAL DISORDERS

Dementia is a leading cause of epilepsy among older adults, and disorders such as stroke and heart attack that result in damage to the brain can also cause epilepsy. Included in this are diseases that cause brain lesions, including meningitis, AIDS, and viral encephalitis.

PRENATAL INJURY

Before birth, babies are susceptible to brain damage caused by an infection in the mother, poor nutrition, or oxygen deficiencies. This can lead to cerebral palsy in the child. About 20% of seizures in children are associated with cerebral palsy or other neurological abnormalities.

DEVELOPMENTAL DISORDERS

Epilepsy can sometimes be associated with other developmental disorders such as autism and Down syndrome.

---

the first seizure. The injury appears to initiate a process that lowers the seizure threshold in the affected region; spontaneous seizure activity then becomes a chronic occurrence.

Seizures are described as focal or generalized depending on their involvement of one or both hemispheres of the brain. Focal seizures arise from a neuronal area localized within one cerebral hemisphere and are restricted to that hemisphere. Generalized seizures arise within one hemisphere and rapidly involve neurons distributed across both cerebral hemispheres.

Pathological mechanisms that provoke focal seizures are better understood than mechanisms that provoke generalized seizures. Focal seizure activity can begin in a distinct region of the cerebral cortex, known as a seizure initiation phase, and then spread to neighboring regions in a seizure propagation phase. The initiation phase is characterized by two concurrent events in a section of neurons: high-frequency bursts of action potentials and hypersynchronization. The bursting activity is caused by a relatively long-lasting depolarization of the neuronal membrane that results from an influx of extracellular Ca^{++}. This in turn leads to the opening of voltage-dependent Na^+ channels, influx of Na^+, and generation of repetitive action potentials. This is followed by a hyperpolarization mediated by GABA receptors or K^+ channels, depending on the cell type. The synchronized bursts from a sufficient number of neurons result in a spike discharge that can be seen on electroencephalography (EEG).

Clinical Presentation of Seizures

According to the 2017 International League Against Epilepsy (ILAE), there are three major categories of seizures: generalized onset seizures, focal onset seizures, and unknown onset seizures. Figure 34-8 summarizes the characteristics of each type of seizure and how they relate to formulating a diagnosis.

Seizures may have motor symptoms, nonmotor symptoms, or both. There is specific terminology that describes different kinds of motor symptoms. Motor symptoms that include sustained rhythmical jerking movements are termed *clonic* muscle activity. Muscles may become weak or limp, which are termed **atonic** muscles. Muscles may become tense or rigid, termed **tonic** muscle activity. The affected individual may sustain brief muscle twitching, termed **myoclonus.** Alternatively, the individual may endure repeated flexion and extension of the whole body, called epileptic spasms. Nonmotor symptoms are usually called absence seizures when the patient is unaware of seizure activity. During these episodes the individual has staring spells without movement. Absence seizures can also have brief twitches (myoclonus) that can affect a specific part of the body or just the eyelids.

Before a seizure, an individual may have unique sensations referred to as an **aura.** An aura often manifests as the perception of a strange light, an unpleasant smell, or confusing thoughts or experiences. When occurring, auras allow individuals with epilepsy time to prepare for a seizure, which can help prevent injury to themselves and others. The episode of the seizure is often referred to as the **ictal period,** and the phase after completion of the seizure is referred to as the **postictal period.**

The postictal state, the altered state of consciousness that a person enters after experiencing a seizure, usually lasts between 5 and 30 minutes; however, it can last longer in the case of larger or more severe seizures. The postictal state is characterized by drowsiness, confusion, nausea, hypertension, headache, and other disorienting symptoms. Additionally, emergence from this period is often accompanied by amnesia or other memory defects. During this period, the brain recovers from the trauma of the seizure.

Generalized Onset Seizures. Generalized onset seizures may have motor and/or nonmotor symptoms. Motor symptoms may include clonic, tonic, or myoclonic muscle activity. Alternatively, muscles can become atonic, or the individual may endure repeated flexion and extension of the whole body called epileptic spasms. Nonmotor symptoms are usually called absence seizures

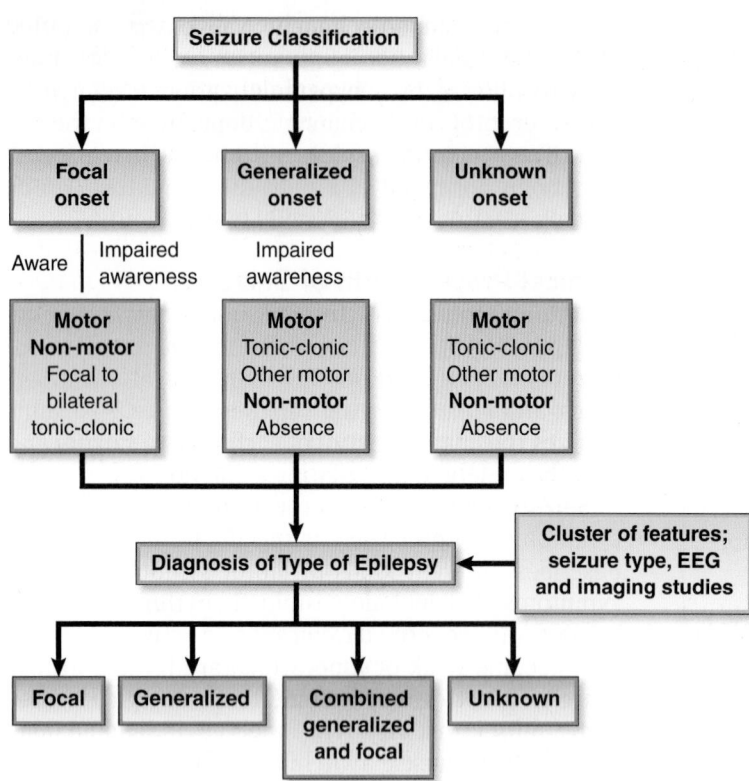

FIGURE 34-8. Type of epilepsy is diagnosed based on classification of the seizure, EEG, and imaging findings. *(Adapted from Fisher, R. S., Cross, J. H., French, J. A., Higurashi, N., Hirsch, E., et al. [2017]. Operational classification of seizure types by the International League Against Epilepsy: Position Paper of the ILAE Commission for Classification and Terminology. Epilepsia, 58(4), 522–530.)*

when the patient is unaware of seizure activity. During these episodes the individual has staring spells without movement. Absence seizures can also have brief twitches (myoclonus) that can affect a specific part of the body or just the eyelids.

Focal Onset Seizures. Focal seizures can cause motor, sensory, autonomic, or psychic symptoms with or without impairment of cognition. For example, a patient having a focal seizure arising from the right primary motor cortex in the area controlling hand movement will experience involuntary movements of the contralateral (left) hand. These movements are typically clonic, repetitive, flexion/extension movements. Because the cortical region controlling the hand is immediately adjacent to the region for facial expression, the seizure may also cause abnormal movements of the face synchronous with movements of the hand. There may also be automatisms, repeated automatic movements, like clapping or rubbing of hands, lip smacking or chewing, or running. Nonmotor symptoms of focal onset seizures include changes in sensation, emotions, thinking or cognition, autonomic functions (such as gastrointestinal sensations, waves of heat or cold, goosebumps, heart racing, etc.), or lack of movement (called behavior arrest). The EEG will show abnormal spike discharges in a very limited region over the related area of cerebral cortex.

Focal seizures are further classified according to patient awareness as either focal onset aware or focal onset impaired awareness seizures. Focal onset aware seizures occur when the affected individual is awake and aware during the seizure. Focal onset impaired

awareness seizures occur when the individual is confused or their awareness is affected in some way during the focal seizure.

Unknown Onset Seizures. An unknown onset seizure is one in which the time of beginning seizure activity is unknown. It may not be witnessed by anyone or occur when the affected person is alone. As more information is obtained, an unknown onset seizure may later be diagnosed as a focal or generalized seizure.

Obtaining History of the Seizure

Obtaining an accurate detailed history of the characteristics of a seizure is critical in establishing an accurate diagnosis. In addition, it is important to ask about the presence of systemic illnesses; history of malignancy; history of head trauma; family history of neurological disorders; and medication, substance, and alcohol use disorder. Seizures need to be described completely. An individual who has observed the patient's seizures is usually the best person to provide an accurate history. Factors preceding the seizure should be described. Precipitating factors or relieving factors regarding the seizure also need to be detailed.

> **CLINICAL CONCEPT**
>
> When a patient first experiences a seizure, the etiological origin is sought. When the patient experiences more than one episode of seizure, however, a diagnosis of epilepsy becomes clearer.

During the history, the patient should be asked to describe auras, loss of consciousness, and any details recalled about the ictal and postictal states. Did the patient note any warning before the seizure? If so, what kind? If an observer was present, ask what happened during the seizure. If the patient has recollection of the seizure, obtain a full description. It is important to ask how the patient felt after the seizure. How long did it take for the patient to get back to normal? How long did the seizure last? How frequently did the seizures occur? Were there any precipitating factors? Relieving factors? Did the patient respond to therapy?

 CLINICAL CONCEPT

If multiple seizures occur in a short time frame, the **interictal period** is the time frame between seizures, when brain activity is more normal.

A complete physical examination should be performed, including a comprehensive neurological assessment and mental status examination. The cranial nerves should be tested completely to obtain clues about intracranial pressure. Physiological illness, metabolic disturbance, head trauma, and substance abuse are often causes for a seizure.

Diagnostic clues about a physical cause of the seizure should be sought during the physical examination. Focal neurological deficits may be present. These are specific neurological impairments due to nerve, spinal cord, or brain dysfunction. One-sided extremity weakness is a common example of a focal neurological deficit. Neurological deficits may be caused by a variety of medical conditions, such as head trauma, tumors, and stroke; various diseases such as meningitis and encephalitis; or as a side effect of medications or abused substances.

 CLINICAL CONCEPT

A quick neurological assessment requires evaluation of vital signs, level of consciousness, pupil reaction, upper and lower extremity strength, and verbal response to a question.

Diagnosis

After the affected individual's seizures are categorized, neurologists can decipher what type of epilepsy is occurring based on seizure category, laboratory studies, EEG, and imaging studies. Laboratory studies are necessary to rule out substance abuse or physiological illness as the cause of a seizure. A complete blood count (CBC), serum chemistry, liver enzymes, and other blood tests pertaining to a suspected clinical illness are necessary. Brain imaging studies, such

as magnetic resonance imaging (MRI) and computed tomography (CT), are helpful, especially if the individual has focal neurological deficits, altered mental status, recent history of head trauma, headache, anticoagulant use, or fever. MRI is the preferred imaging tool, showing epileptogenic lesions in about 20% of people with newly diagnosed epilepsy. Individuals with suspected seizures should have an EEG as part of their diagnostic work-up. Analysis of interictal discharges on the EEG can help to support a diagnosis of epilepsy, help to classify the epilepsy syndrome, and determine the cerebral hemisphere that gives rise to the seizure. Sleep deprivation increases the excitability of the cortical neurons, which decreases the seizure threshold of the brain. Therefore, taking an EEG on an individual who is sleep-deprived will increase the sensitivity of the EEG.

 CLINICAL CONCEPT

The presence of a normal EEG does not rule out a seizure disorder. Approximately 50% of individuals with epilepsy will not show any abnormalities on a single EEG.

Treatment

For nonepileptic seizures, treatment for the underlying condition is necessary. Conditions such as head trauma, stroke, metabolic imbalances, and CNS infection require different treatment modalities and are often reversible.

When there is no identifiable, reversible cause for the seizure, treatment involves the use of antiepileptic drugs. Drug treatment is usually initiated when the individual is experiencing acute or chronic seizures or has clear structural predisposition to seizures. The goal of epilepsy treatment is to prevent further seizures without adverse effects. A wide variety of medications with different mechanisms of action have been successful in enabling many patients to have relatively normal lives with less frequent seizures. The actions of antiepileptic agents commonly modify the activity of ion channels or neurotransmitters in the brain. Antiepileptic agents include phenytoin, valproic acid, carbamazepine, topiramate, zonisamide, ethosuximide, lacosamide, gabapentin, lamotrigine, and benzodiazepines.

A ketogenic diet has been found effective in decreasing epileptic seizures. The diet consists of very low carbohydrate and adequate protein and fat. The low level of carbohydrate causes fat breakdown, increasing fatty acids that transform into ketones. This has proven to be an effective nonpharmacological treatment for children with intractable epilepsy and can be a reasonable option for adults. Research in animal models of epilepsy suggests that the mechanism of action involves alterations in mitochondrial function, effects of ketone bodies on neuronal function and neurotransmitter release, antiepileptic effects of fatty acids, and/or glucose stabilization. Ketone bodies may increase membrane potential hyperpolarization and gamma-aminobutyric acid synthesis, and decrease release of glutamate, norepinephrine, or adenosine.

Studies have shown significant seizure reduction in patients with Dravet and Lennox-Gastaut epilepsy syndromes who are treated with cannabidiol (CBD). The exact mechanism of action is unclear; however, CBD modulates the endocannabinoid receptors that have an anticonvulsant effect. Epidiolex is an FDA-approved form of pure CBD for treatment-resistant epilepsy.

Surgical management may be used for individuals who have seizures that are refractory to medication or for some individuals with a localized focus of their seizures. Electrodes can be placed in the brain via craniotomy. Neurostimulatory pulses can be delivered in a scheduled manner or in response to seizures to counteract seizure activity. There is another option of surgical placement of electrodes for peripheral nerve stimulation. Vagus nerve stimulation has been found to reduce seizure frequency by 50% or more and improve quality of life in one-third of patients. Stereotactic radiosurgery, radiofrequency thermocoagulation, and laser interstitial thermal therapy are surgical techniques that target brain tissue sites involved in seizure activity. These strategies apply irradiation or heat and have been shown to lead to a favorable seizure outcome in 50% to 60% of people with drug-resistant focal epilepsy. Parietal or temporal lobectomies are other surgical procedures that can relieve frequent seizures.

> **ALERT!** During a seizure, the most important goal is to protect the patient from injury. Move objects that could cause injury out of the way. Do not physically restrain the patient and do not put anything in their mouth. Also, because of the risk of postseizure vomiting, after the seizure has ended, place the patient on their left side and turn the head so that any emesis or oral secretions will drain out of the mouth and not be inhaled.

Status Epilepticus

Status epilepticus (SE) is a condition of prolonged seizure activity. In general, a seizure that lasts longer than 5 minutes or having more than 1 seizure within a 5-minute period without returning to a normal level of consciousness between episodes is called status epilepticus. This is a medical emergency that may lead to permanent brain damage or death. In adults, common identifiable causes of SE include trauma, tumor, vascular disease, alcohol withdrawal, and noncompliance with antiseizure medications. Febrile seizures are the most common cause in children. Why some seizures end spontaneously, whereas others become self-sustaining and persist for a prolonged period of time, is not known. Studies are focusing on the neurotransmitter gamma aminobutyric acid type A (GABA$_A$).

Management of any patient presenting with an episode of SE begins with the ABCs (airway, breathing, and circulation). If available, the patient should be placed on a cardiac monitor and pulse oximeter with the application of supplemental oxygen if indicated. Laboratory testing to be considered based on history and physical examination includes blood glucose, electrolytes, magnesium, calcium, phosphorous, complete blood count, serum transaminases, and toxicology screen. If a person has a known diagnosis of epilepsy, levels of the antiseizure medications should be obtained to determine compliance and potentially future alterations in dosing. For those patients who present with fever, cultures of bodily fluids (blood, urine, and cerebrospinal fluid [CSF]) should be considered and antibiotics may be required. Imaging of the head with either axial CT or MRI may be required to identify hemorrhage, ischemia, or a mass. This imaging should not proceed until the patient is stable.

Treatment should be initiated after 5 minutes in cases of convulsive SE, and there is consensus that the first-line treatment is a benzodiazepine (e.g., diazepam, lorazepam, and midazolam). If the seizure does not respond to benzodiazepine administration, other antiseizure medications that are widely used include fosphenytoin, levetiracetam, and valproate. Phenobarbital is also effective but is not usually a first choice owing to the increased risk of sedation.

Refractory SE is defined as seizures lasting longer than 60 minutes despite treatment with a benzodiazepine and an adequate loading dose of a standard intravenous antiseizure medication. SE resistant to standard management continuing for longer than 24 hours has been labeled as superrefractory SE. It is estimated that approximately 15% of all cases of convulsive SE admitted to hospital will fall into this category. Continuous intravenous infusion of antiseizure medications for the treatment of refractory and superrefractory SE is recommended. Pentobarbital has been the agent most widely used. Other agents have included midazolam, propofol, ketamine, high-dose phenobarbital, thiopental, lidocaine, and inhalational anesthetics (e.g., isoflurane).

Sudden Unexpected Death in Epilepsy (SUDEP)

Sudden unexpected death in epilepsy (SUDEP) is premature death in people with epilepsy due to unknown cause. SUDEP is not caused by injury, comorbidities, accidents, or other known factors. Studies suggest that each year, there are about 1.16 cases of SUDEP for every 1,000 people with epilepsy. It is most common in persons with epilepsy 20 to 40 years of age. SUDEP is most commonly unwitnessed and sleep-related. Many individuals with SUDEP are found in prone position with evidence of having had a recent seizure. Studies suggest that SUDEP is preceded by a convulsion followed shortly by apnea and then asystole. Despite its low incidence, SUDEP is the second-greatest neurological cause of potential years of life lost. Frequent convulsions are the major risk factor, particularly if nocturnal. Preventive strategies for SUDEP include reducing the occurrence of generalized tonic-clonic seizures with close attention to compliance with medication or referral for surgical evaluation in persons with lesional epilepsy. Lifestyle measures include detecting cardiorespiratory distress through respiratory and heart rate monitoring devices and preventing airway obstruction through use of safety pillows. Nocturnal nursing care ensures supplemental oxygen, oropharyngeal suction, and patient repositioning from prone to supine. Enhancing serotonergic mechanisms of respiratory regulation using selective serotonin reuptake inhibitors (SSRIs), such as fluoxetine, may be effective. Opiate and adenosine antagonists may also be effective.

Headache

Headaches can be categorized as either a primary or secondary disorder. Primary headaches arise independent of any other medical illness or traumatic cause. Secondary headaches are caused by another primary condition, such as head injury or concussion; vascular problems, such as aneurysms or arteriovenous malformations; medication side effects; sinus disease; and tumors.

Primary Headache

Based on the 2017 International Classification of Headache Disorders (ICHD-3), the most common types of primary headaches are categorized as migraine, tension-type headaches (TTH), and trigeminal autonomic cephalgia (see Box 34-3 for full list).

Tension-Type Headache. TTH, the most common type of primary headache, occurs in as many as 78% of persons. There are three subtypes as described by the International Headache Society:

1. Infrequent episodic TTH, with headache occurring less often than 1 day per month
2. Frequent episodic TTH, with at least 10 headache episodes per month for at least 3 months
3. Chronic TTH, with headaches occurring 15 or more days per month for longer than 3 months

A TTH can last minutes to days. The pain is often described as bilateral with mild to moderate pressure. It does not worsen with physical activity, and there is no associated nausea or vomiting. Some patients may complain of either photophobia (light sensitivity) or phonophobia (sensitivity to sound), but these symptoms are more commonly associated with migraine-type headaches.

Pathophysiology. TTH can be primarily a central neurological disturbance, similar to migraine, or can occur

---

> ### BOX 34-3. International Classification of Headache Disorders-3 (ICHD- 3)
>
> **PART I. PRIMARY HEADACHES**
> 1. Migraine
> 2. Tension-type headache (TTH)
> 3. Trigeminal autonomic cephalgias (TACs)
> 4. Other primary headache disorders
>
> **PART II. SECONDARY HEADACHES**
> 5. Headache attributed to injury/trauma to head or neck
> 6. Headache attributed to cranial or cervical vascular disorder
> 7. Headache attributed to nonvascular intracranial disorder
> 8. Headache attributed to substance or its withdrawal
> 9. Headache attributed to infection
> 10. Headache attributed to disorder of homeostasis
> 11. Headache or facial pain attributed to disorders of the cranium, neck, eyes, ears, nose, sinuses, teeth, mouth, or other facial or cervical structure
> 12. Headache attributed to psychiatric disorder
>
> **PART III. PAINFUL CRANIAL NEUROPATHIES, OTHER FACIAL PAINS, OR OTHER HEADACHES**
> 13. Painful lesions of the cranial nerves and other facial pain
> 14. Other headache disorders

---

as the result of increased cervical and pericranial muscle activity, such as that caused by flexion-extension injury of the neck, poor posture, or anxiety with increased clenching or grinding of the teeth. Electromyographic (EMG) studies have shown muscle contraction in patients with TTH; however, it is unclear if muscle contraction is causative.

Clinical Presentation. The patient often complains of a bandlike pain or diffuse pain over the head. Tight cervical and shoulder muscles commonly accompany headache. Other features of TTH include:

- Stable pattern of headaches over many months or years
- Family history of similar headaches
- Normal physical examination
- Headaches that are consistently triggered by hormonal cycle; specific foods; or specific sensory input of light, odors, or other typical triggers

Diagnosis. The diagnosis of TTH is based on clinical findings. Usually, a TTH does not require laboratory testing or imaging studies if the physical examination is normal.

Treatment. Episodic TTHs are generally treated with simple analgesics such as acetaminophen, aspirin, and other NSAIDs. Medications containing ergotamine, caffeine, barbiturates, and codeine should be avoided. For those individuals with chronic headaches, a prophylactic approach using tricyclic antidepressants and serotonin receptor inhibitors has been used effectively. In conjunction with pharmacological intervention, relaxation therapy, biofeedback, and stress management have been associated with reducing the frequency of headaches.

Migraine Headache.

Migraine headaches are periodic, throbbing headaches that are characterized by altered perceptions, nausea, and severe pain. Approximately 28 million people in the United States suffer from migraine headaches, with a 1-year prevalence of 18.2% among females and 6.5% among males. Seventy-five percent of migraine sufferers are female. The peak prevalence of migraine is between the ages of 25 and 55 years. Individuals with migraine often report it as disabling, as they can have difficulty being productive at home, work, and school.

Pathophysiology.

Knowledge regarding migraine pathophysiology is incomplete, although research into the pathogenesis of migraine headache is ongoing. The current theory proposes four stages of migraine:

1. **Prodrome:** neural hyperexcitability in the brain
2. **Aura:** cortical spreading depression (CSD) occurs
3. **Pain:** trigeminovascular complex activation accounting for the pain
4. **Postdrome:** sensitization of the trigeminovascular complex persists

In the first stage, or prodrome, to the migraine headache, there is a significant hyperexcitability of neurons in the cerebral cortex, most notably the occipital region. Once the nerve cells have reached the threshold of excitability, CSD is initiated. CSD describes a wave of neuronal depolarization that spreads across the cerebrum. This mechanism triggers the aura of migraine and activates trigeminal nerve impulses to the brain. The activation of the trigeminal nerve impulses to the brain by CSD is thought to cause an inflammatory change in the pain-sensitive meninges. Brainstem regions that modulate sensory input to the trigeminal nerves include the locus coeruleus and dorsal raphe nucleus.

In the next stage, a throbbing-type pain begins. Both serotonin and calcitonin gene-related peptides (CGRPs) are thought to play a role in the pain of migraine. During an attack, levels of serotonin are decreased and levels of CGRP are elevated. CGRP is a potent vasodilator of cerebral and dural vessels. The exact role of serotonin in migraine is unclear, though it is known that stimulation of the serotonin receptors can alleviate a migraine. Data also support a role of dopamine; most migraine symptoms can be induced by stimulation of dopamine receptors.

The final postdromal stage of migraine is evident in some patients who present with continued pain on the top of the head, upper trunk, or limb with movement after the headache subsides. These residual pains are believed to be a result of the sensitization of the trigeminal system.

Clinical Presentation.

When a migraine headache is suspected, a complete history and physical examination are necessary to exclude other types of headache. The patient should be asked about events and feelings before the headache. A full description of the headache is necessary to diagnose migraine. Most migraine headaches have a common pattern of presentation described by the sufferer.

The most common presentation of migraine headache is a severe throbbing, one-sided headache that is accompanied by nausea, vomiting, photophobia (sensitivity to light), and phonophobia (sensitivity to sound). However, migraine can also cause bilateral headache. It usually worsens with movements such as climbing stairs, jumping, or leaning over. Migraine headache is usually disabling to the sufferer, and the patient usually needs to lie down. Some migraine headaches may have a preceding aura. The patient should be asked to describe the actions and feelings before a migraine headache to decipher if an aura occurs and assess triggers of the headache (see Box 34-4). It is helpful for individuals to keep a diary of their headaches. This diary should include a description of the symptoms, frequency of the headaches, and any information that could assist in identifying triggers of the migraines. The physical examination is usually normal, yet the patient is incapable of performing tasks or concentrating.

Diagnosis.

The diagnosis of migraine headache is usually based on clinical signs and symptoms. Some

---

BOX 34-4. Migraine Triggers

Migraine headaches may be precipitated by any of the following:

- Emotions such as worry or stress
- Intake of foods containing nitrites, glutamate, aspartate, and tyramine, among other chemicals
- Hormone shifts, as with oral contraceptives and menstruation
- Activities such as excessive exercise
- Lack of sleep or fatigue
- Hunger with an associated drop in blood sugar.

Other triggers of migraine may include medications such as nitroglycerin, histamine, reserpine, withdrawal from corticosteroids, and hydralazine. Some individuals will find that odors such as perfumes, smoke, and other strong odors can trigger their migraine attacks.

Adapted from International Headache Society (HIS) (n.d.). International Headache Classification Disorders-3 (IHCD-3). https://www.ichd-3.org/1-migraine/

clinicians use imaging studies such as CT or MRI to exclude any other cause of headache when diagnosis is questionable. The diagnostic criteria for migraine, which include a normal physical examination and specific signs and symptoms, are listed in Box 34-5.

Treatment. Drugs that are effective in the treatment of migraine headaches include NSAIDs, serotonin receptor agonists (called triptans), and dopamine receptor antagonists. In general, an adequate dose should ideally be administered as soon as possible after onset of the headache. However, migraine therapy is individualized, and there is no one standard approach for all patients (see Box 34-6).

Trigeminal Autonomic Cephalgia. The trigeminal autonomic cephalalgias (TACs) present as an excruciating unilateral headache with prominent cranial parasympathetic autonomic features. This uncommon type of headache affects fewer than 1% of the population. The majority of sufferers are male, and peak age of onset is between ages 25 and 50 years.

TACs activate a trigeminal parasympathetic reflex, with the clinical signs of cranial sympathetic dysfunction. TACs are composed of five diseases: cluster headache, paroxysmal hemicrania, short-lasting unilateral neuralgiform headache attacks with conjunctival injection and tearing (SUNCT), short-lasting unilateral neuralgiform headache attacks with cranial autonomic symptoms (SUNA), and hemicrania continua. The most common kind of headache within this category is a cluster headache.

Pathophysiology. It is theorized that vasodilation is responsible for the pain and the autonomic features of TACs. Similar to the migraine headache, the trigeminovascular system appears to be activated, explaining the patterns of pain. The hypothalamus is postulated to play a prominent role because there are alterations in the circadian rhythms during the cluster period. It is also theorized that the clinical features of TACs can be explained by a lesion involving the cavernous sinus portion of the internal carotid artery. At this site, both the nociceptive and

---

BOX 34-5. ICHD-3 Classification of Migraine Headache

There are various types of migraine headaches—mainly migraine without aura and migraine with aura. During the history, the patient should be asked to describe the whole experience of the disorder, which includes setting, feelings, and actions before the migraine, as well as the type of pain and duration of migraine and associated symptoms.

MIGRAINE WITHOUT AURA

Migraine without aura is the most common type of migraine and is characterized by a headache that lasts from 4 to 72 hours if untreated. It is usually described as a pulsating or pounding pain on one side of the head, usually frontotemporal. The pain is of moderate or severe intensity and is aggravated by physical activity. During the headache, the individual may experience nausea, vomiting, phonophobia, and photophobia.

MIGRAINE WITH AURA

Migraine with aura is characterized by focal neurological symptoms that precede the headache. Aura of migraine can be described by patients as loss of vision or visualization of flickering lights, zig-zag lines, or spots. An aura can include strange tastes in the mouth and odors. Some patients may also have numbness and tingling in the extremities. Those with familial hemiplegic migraine experience severe weakness in one side of the body.

Aura associated with migraine often develops over a period of 5 to 20 minutes and can last up to 1 hour; all symptoms of aura are completely reversible. Headache can either start with aura or follow the aura and is clinically the same as migraine without aura, as previously described.

Some patients with migraine may also experience premonitory symptoms hours to 2 days before a migraine attack. These symptoms include fatigue, loss of concentration, neck stiffness, photophobia and phonophobia, nausea, blurred vision, yawning, or pallor.

CHRONIC MIGRAINE

Headache occurring on 15 or more days/month for more than 3 months, which, on at least 8 days/month, has the features of migraine headache.

COMPLICATIONS OF MIGRAINE

Complications include:
- A migraine lasting more than 72 hours
- Aura symptoms persisting 2 weeks or more without infarction on neuroimaging
- Ischemic brain lesion associated with migraine
- Seizure triggered by migraine with aura

PROBABLE MIGRAINE

Migraine-like attacks missing one of the key features required to fulfill all criteria for a type or subtype of migraine and not fulfilling criteria for another headache disorder.

EPISODIC SYNDROMES ASSOCIATED WITH MIGRAINE

This group of disorders occurs in patients who also have migraine without aura or migraine with aura, or who have an increased likelihood to develop either of these disorders. Additional conditions that may occur in these patients include episodes of motion sickness and periodic sleep disorders, including sleep walking, sleep talking, night terrors, and bruxism.

BOX 34-6. Treatment of Migraine Headaches

In the past, NSAIDs and opiate analgesics have been effectively used in the treatment of migraine. A combination of butalbital, caffeine, and aspirin known as Fiorinal has also been used to effectively treat migraine headache. However, stimulation of serotonin receptors through the use of selective serotonin receptor agonists known as triptans has become the preferred migraine treatment for many sufferers.

Triptans are available in oral, nasal spray, and subcutaneous preparations and as parenteral medication. A triptan transdermal patch has also proven to relieve pain and associated migraine symptoms. Triptans include sumatriptan, rizatriptan, almotriptan, eletriptan, zolmitriptan, and naratriptan. In some cases, coadministration of a long-acting NSAID can reduce rates of headache recurrence. Sumatriptan/naproxen is a combined medication. Ergot alkaloids such as ergotamine and dihydroergotamine are nonselective serotonin receptor agonists that are also effective. Dopamine antagonists such as droperidol are sometimes used to stop migraine headache and accompanying nausea and vomiting.

Transcranial magnetic stimulation (TMS) has been effective for migraine headache in persons older than 18 years old. TMS is a handheld device that releases a pulse of magnetic energy to the occipital region of the head.

PREVENTION

To prevent migraines, patients should be advised to avoid triggers such as lack of sleep, fatigue, stress, vasodilators, oral contraceptives, and dietary components such as wine. Patients who have frequent migraine headaches, such as five or more attacks per month, are candidates for preventive therapy. Preventive drugs should be taken daily and there is usually a 2- to 12-week lag period before an effect is seen. Preventive drugs include beta blockers such as propranolol, tricyclic antidepressants such as amitriptyline, and anticonvulsants such as valproate. *Clostridium botulinum* (Botox) injections into the scalp and temple have also been approved for preventive migraine therapy. Medications that block calcitonin gene-related peptide (CGRP) receptors are the newest preventive medications. These are monoclonal antibodies that target the neuropeptide CGRP, which causes the widespread vasodilation in migraine. The newly approved CGRP antagonists are erenumab, fremanezumab, and galcanezumab.

---

autonomic fibers that innervate the eye are in close proximity to each other.

Clinical Presentation. TACs are often described as attacks of severe, strictly unilateral pain that are orbital, supraorbital, temporal, or in any combination of these sites, lasting from 15 to 180 minutes and occurring from once every other day to eight times a day. The pain is associated with unilateral conjunctival injection (eyes appear "bloodshot"), tearing of the eye, nasal congestion, rhinorrhea (runny nose), forehead and facial sweating, pupil constriction, drooping eyelid and/or eyelid edema, and/or with restlessness or agitation.

Individuals are often unable to sit quietly when experiencing a TAC. This is in sharp contrast to the patient with a migraine headache, who will often withdraw to a dark quiet room.

🩺 CLINICAL CONCEPT

With TAC, the patient describes intense pain, usually around the temple region of the head. Conjunctivitis and rhinorrhea with diaphoresis may be present. Otherwise, the physical examination is normal.

Diagnosis. The diagnosis of TAC is usually based on clinical signs and symptoms. Some clinicians use imaging studies such as CT or MRI to exclude any other cause of headache when diagnosis is questionable.

Treatment. Acute treatment that aims to terminate an attack should be taken at the onset of the attack. Ideally, this approach should work within seconds or minutes; hence, parenteral rather than oral treatments are required. The most established effective acute treatments for cluster attacks are subcutaneous/intranasal triptans and inhaled high-flow 100% oxygen. Subcutaneous sumatriptan is the most effective triptan for cluster headache and can be given up to twice per day. For preventive treatment, verapamil is recommended; however, other agents such as lithium, topiramate, or gabapentin can be substituted, if verapamil is ineffective. A greater occipital nerve block using a local anesthetic and corticosteroid can also be used. A newer treatment found to be effective as a preventive agent is an anti-CGRP monoclonal antibody, galcanezumab, administered once per month. The most effective agent to prevent paroxysmal hemicrania is indomethacin. SUNCT and SUNA can be effectively prevented with lamotrigine.

Secondary Headaches

With secondary headaches, it is important to discern whether the headache is related to another medical condition. Some secondary causes, such as sinusitis, are easily treatable. Trigeminal neuralgia, also called tic douloureaux, is a significant cause of facial pain.

However, the most serious secondary cause of headache is brain tumor.

Sinus Headache. The International Headache Society describes an acute sinus headache as occurring in conjunction with acute sinusitis; fever and rhinorrhea may also be present. The pain is caused by sinus pressure and can worsen when the patient leans over. The facial areas over the frontal and maxillary sinuses may be tender to palpation. Transillumination of the sinuses may show nontransparency. Sinus x-rays may be needed to confirm diagnosis. The usual treatment of sinus headache includes the use of antibiotics and nasal decongestants.

Headache Caused by Brain Tumors. Approximately 50% of individuals with brain tumors will experience a headache. The headaches are usually dull and constant and may or may not have a throbbing quality. The location of the headache is commonly bifrontal, with pain worse on the same side as the tumor. However, generalized head pain has also been reported, perhaps because of an increase in intracranial pressure. Increased intracranial pressure may lead to the classic triad of headache, nausea, and papilledema—swelling of the optic nerve that can be visualized using an ophthalmoscope. It is a key diagnostic finding with increased intracranial pressure. Cranial nerve testing may reveal abnormalities.

> **ALERT!** Patients with the following symptoms need further evaluation to rule out the possibility of a brain tumor:
> - Abnormal neurological examination
> - Change in prior headache patterns
> - Worsening of headache with a change in body position, such as bending over, or with coughing, sneezing, or any maneuver that raises intrathoracic pressure or intracranial pressure
> - Worsening headaches at night that awaken the patient from sleep

Trigeminal Neuralgia (Tic Douloureux). Trigeminal neuralgia (also called tic douloureaux) is caused by irritation of the trigeminal nerve (cranial nerve V). This disorder can be part of another disease such as MS, tumor, tooth disorder, or herpes zoster. It is a chronic pain condition that causes sharp, sporadic, shocklike pain on one side of the face. It most often affects adults older than age 50, particularly females. It is usually triggered by contact with the face, as with shaving, toothbrushing, eating, drinking, talking, or exposure to the wind. A variety of imaging studies such as MRI, CT scan, and x-ray are needed to rule out other causes of trigeminal irritation. However, imaging studies may not reveal any cause for the pain. Carbamazepine (Tegretol), an anticonvulsant, is the treatment of choice. If carbamazepine is not effective, other possible drug choices include phenytoin (Dilantin), gabapentin (Neurontin), lamotrigine (Lamictal), topiramate (Topamax), and valproic acid (Depakene, Depakote). A muscle relaxant such as baclofen (Lioresal) can be tried alone or in combination with an anticonvulsant. Narcotic pain relievers, such as oxycodone, hydrocodone, or morphine (several brand names), may be taken briefly for severe episodes of pain. If pain continues despite medication, some surgical procedures may bring relief.

Pathophysiology of Selected Neurodegenerative Disorders

Common major neurodegenerative disorders include Parkinson's disease, ALS, and MS. They are all slowly progressive diseases that affect motor or sensory nerves, or both.

Parkinson's Disease

Parkinson's disease is a common neurodegenerative disorder affecting approximately 1.5 million people in the United States. The National Parkinson Foundation estimates that 60,000 new cases are diagnosed each year. This slow and progressive disorder is typically diagnosed in the fifth or sixth decade of life. However, approximately 10% of those with Parkinson's disease are younger than 40 years of age; these individuals are classified as having young-onset Parkinson's disease. In rare instances, Parkinson-like symptoms can appear in children and teenagers in a disorder known as juvenile parkinsonism; this disorder has a different clinical course from typical Parkinson's disease and is usually attributed to hereditary causes.

Parkinson's disease affects both males and females equally, and there is no evidence that it is more prevalent in different ethnic groups or in any particular geographic regions. The clinical course of the disorder is highly variable for each individual.

Etiology

Most cases of Parkinson's disease (85% to 90%) are of unknown etiology. Genetics plays a relevant role in the etiology of familial Parkinson's disease, which is responsible for 10% of cases. A mutated protein called leucine-rich repeat kinase 2 (*LRRK2*) is a common cause of familial Parkinson's disease. The *LRRK2* genetic mutation is located at 12p11–p13. Exactly how the protein affects synaptic function remains unclear. Mutations are also found in other genes, including the parkin gene at 6q25–27 and the alpha-synuclein gene at 4q21–23. The parkin gene causes mitochondrial dysfunction, and the alpha-synuclein gene causes an accumulation of an abnormal protein called alpha-synuclein.

In addition to genetics, important risk factors of Parkinson's disease include advancing age, as well as certain viral infections and chemical exposures. Injection of a street drug containing a meperidine analog can produce parkinsonian symptoms. Repeated exposure to other chemicals such as pesticides and repeated head trauma may provide an increased risk as well.

Pathophysiology

Pathologically, Parkinson's disease is mainly associated with progressive loss of dopamine-producing cells in the substantia nigra, which is within the basal ganglia of the midbrain. The basal ganglia modulates movements, such as posture, standing, walking, or writing. In the basal ganglia, Ach and dopamine are the neurotransmitters that modulate the body's movements. Ach stimulates muscle movement, whereas dopamine has an inhibitory effect on movement. The depletion of dopamine in Parkinson's disease creates an imbalance of these two neurotransmitters. The effects of unopposed Ach are apparent in the tremor and abnormal spasmodic, muscle movements. Signs of the disease do not become apparent until 50% to 80% of the substantia nigra is degenerated.

In Parkinson's disease, there is also an accumulation of an abnormal protein called alpha-synuclein found in structures called Lewy bodies in the brainstem, spinal cord, and regions of the cortex. It is still unclear how alpha-synuclein causes the disorder, but the accumulation of this protein is associated with neurodegeneration and cell death.

Pathology can also involve the ANS, which causes nonmotor symptoms such as orthostatic hypotension, sleep disturbances, gastrointestinal disturbances, and impaired thermoregulation.

Clinical Presentation

The triad of bradykinesia, resting tremor, and muscle rigidity are the classic manifestations of Parkinson's disease. The onset is typically slow and insidious, and the resting tremor is often the first symptom. As the disease progresses, bradykinesia, defined as slowed movements, and akinesia, which is the absence of movement, commonly occur as well. Initial manifestations may first appear on one side of the body, but eventually the symptoms involve bilateral, symmetrical areas of the body. As the disease progresses and the substantia nigra deteriorates further, individuals have progressive difficulty with automatic movements. Daily tasks such as walking, dressing, writing, eating, and others become difficult. There is postural imbalance and, at times, difficulty with initiation of movement.

Tremor. The classic tremor of Parkinson's disease is a resting, "pill-rolling" tremor of the hand and finger; this is often the first motor symptom of the disease. The tremor usually presents unilaterally and then becomes bilateral, often spreading to the legs and sometimes the head, jaw, and face. Interestingly, a resting tremor ceases when purposeful movement of the limb occurs.

CLINICAL CONCEPT

With Parkinson's disease, a tremor can appear as though the person is rolling a pill in their hand, which is why the term "pill-rolling" is used to describe the tremor.

Rigidity. Rigidity is often felt by the patient as a tightness or stiffness in the arms, legs, neck, and trunk and presents initially on one side of the body with a gradual progression to both sides. On physical examination, the most notable finding will be the cogwheeling or ratchety movement felt by the examiner when passively moving the affected body part. This cogwheeling movement is caused by cocontraction of agonist and antagonist muscles. Rigidity of muscles is also manifested in facial muscles, causing a facial masking or emotionless stare that typifies the expression often seen in Parkinson's disease. Individuals may also experience decreased blink rates; soft, monotonous, low-volume speech; and difficulty swallowing.

Bradykinesia. Bradykinesia, a state of slowed movements, can inhibit independent functioning. Patients may first see the effect in distal muscles of the arms and legs. Patients may have difficulty initiating gait or rising from a chair. Bradykinetic manifestations of the upper extremities include decreased arm swing, handwriting micrographia, and decreased fine motor function. Patients may also experience akinetic episodes, which they may describe as being "frozen" in place.

Postural Instability. Postural instability caused by the loss of postural reflexes usually manifests at later stages of disease progression. Patients may take very quick and short steps forward, or they may step backward rapidly and uncontrollably. This, coupled with truncal rigidity and decreased ability to make corrective adjustments in balance, increases the risk for falling.

Nonmotor Symptoms. Nonmotor symptoms can be classified into three categories:

1. Nonmotor symptoms with ANS involvement
2. Nonmotor symptoms without ANS involvement
3. Neuropsychiatric symptoms, including cognitive changes

These symptoms can be very disabling, as they often affect socialization, motivation, and quality of life.

A large majority (90%) of individuals with Parkinson's disease experience symptoms attributed to the neurodegenerative effects of the disease on the ANS. These symptoms include constipation, dysphagia, orthostatic hypotension, drooling, sexual dysfunction, abnormal sweating, and thermoregulation, as well as urinary and bladder dysfunction. Nonmotor symptoms without ANS involvement include speech disturbances; seborrheic dermatitis; sleep disorders, including restless leg syndrome, daytime sleepiness, insomnia, and fatigue; and olfactory and visual dysfunction.

Neuropsychiatric symptoms such as depression are commonly associated with Parkinson's disease, with a prevalence as high as 40%. Although depression is often referred to as a nonmotor symptom, the cause of depression may be either endogenous—as a result of the neurodegeneration process related to the disease—or exogenous—resulting from variables such as age of onset, disease severity, and disability.

Cognitive dysfunction in Parkinson's disease can affect as many as 80% of individuals and range from decreased executive functioning ability to severe symptoms of dementia. Other neuropsychiatric symptoms include anxiety and apathy. The neuropsychiatric manifestations of Parkinson's disease are associated with worsening disability, poor quality of life, poorer outcomes, and increased caregiver distress.

Diagnosis

The diagnosis of Parkinson's disease is usually made on the basis of clinical symptomatology. It can be diagnosed by clinical signs with the mnemonic TRAP: **T**remor at rest, **R**igidity, **A**kinesia or bradykinesia, and **P**ostural/gait instability. There are no laboratory tests that identify the disorder; however, recent studies are focusing on the protein alpha-synuclein. Several studies have found a decreased amount of alpha-synuclein in the cerebrospinal fluid of patients with Parkinson's disease. Genetic testing is not generally used routinely, but is used in research studies. Mutations of the *LRRK2* gene are currently under investigation as a diagnostic test. CT scan and MRI reveal normal results, but imaging of the brain dopamine system with positron emission tomography (PET) or single photon emission CT (SPECT) shows reduced uptake of dopaminergic markers. A substantial and sustained response to dopamine medications also helps.

Currently, the Movement Disorder Society suggests using a modified form of **Unified Parkinson Disease Rating Scale (UPDRS)** for assessing PD progression. This is a comprehensive multipage questionnaire completed by the clinician and patient. The patients are assessed based on cognition and mood (Part I: nonmotor), daily living activities (Part II: motor experiences), motor examination (Part III), and complications encountered in motor examinations (Part IV). The responses are scaled, such as 0 = normal, 1 = slight, 2 = mild, 3 = moderate, 4 = severe, accordingly. The maximum total UPDRS score is 199, indicating the worst possible disability from PD.

Treatment

Treatment goals in Parkinson's disease are to relieve symptoms and maximize independence and mobility while preserving the individual's quality of life. The cornerstone of treatment is dopamine replacement therapy. Levodopa (L-DOPA), the metabolic precursor of dopamine, in combination with carbidopa, a peripheral decarboxylase inhibitor, are used together. Carbidopa inhibits peripheral metabolism of levodopa and allows more of the levodopa to act at the brain. Commonly, after years of levodopa, a diminishing response occurs. Dopamine agonists such as pramipexole and ropinirole can be used as adjuncts to levodopa. Monoamine oxidase (MAO)-B inhibitors such as rasagiline and selegiline can provide symptomatic benefit as monotherapy in early disease and as adjuncts to levodopa. The enzyme that shuts down dopamine in the synapse is catechol-O-methyl transferase (COMT). Therefore, COMT inhibitors such as entacapone and tolcapone are used to prolong the effect of dopamine in the synapse.

Anticholinergic medications can be used for the treatment of resting tremor, but they are not particularly effective for bradykinesia, rigidity, gait disturbance, or other features of advanced Parkinson's disease.

> **ALERT!** Anticholinergic medications have many undesirable side effects such as dry mouth, double vision, lack of perspiration and poor heat dissipation, confusion, and lack of concentration ability.

Surgical procedures such as deep brain stimulation (DBS) of the subthalamic nuclei or globus pallidum are effective for a select group of individuals with advanced disease. This therapy consists of placing thin wires containing distal electrodes stereotactically into the brain with the more proximal ends connected to extension cables that tunnel subcutaneously to an impulse generator (IPG). The IPG is placed beneath a patient's skin in the infraclavicular or intra-abdominal region. DBS effectively reduces motor signs of the disease and improves dyskinesia and quality of life.

Stem cell therapy may have the benefit of replacing and repairing damaged dopamine-producing nerve cells within the brain. A common source of mesenchymal stem cells is umbilical cord blood. Studies show that mesenchymal stem cells can differentiate into dopamine neurons that provide benefits following transplantation in animal models of Parkinson's disease.

Exercise therapy is often recommended for individuals and should be used as an adjunct to pharmacological therapies, as it has significant positive effects on functional independence, motor function, ADLs, and quality of life. Physical, occupational, and speech therapy also improve quality of life.

Amyotrophic Lateral Sclerosis

ALS, also referred to as Lou Gehrig's disease, is a progressive neurodegenerative disorder characterized by a loss of upper and lower motor neurons and eventually resulting in respiratory failure. Symptoms include painless muscle weakness and atrophy.

The worldwide incidence of ALS ranges from 0.4 to 2.6 per 100,000 population per year. The prevalence of ALS is 6 per 100,000 individuals. In the United States, it is estimated that 20,000 individuals have ALS, and 6,000 Americans are diagnosed with the disease on an annual basis. In the United States, ALS affects European Americans more than other racial and ethnic groups. It is usually diagnosed between 40 and 70 years of age, with more males affected than females.

Etiology

The etiology of ALS is unknown, but there are some proposed risk factors, including heavy-metal toxic effects, environmental and occupational exposures, cigarette smoking, repeated physical trauma, and participation in heavy physical activity such as professional athletics.

Two classifications of ALS have been described: familial (inherited) ALS and sporadic ALS. Approximately 5% to 10% of all cases of ALS are thought to be familial, with mutations in the superoxide dismutase gene 1 accounting for approximately 20% of familial cases. Mutations in the *TAR* DNA-binding protein gene 43 and *FUS* gene occur in about 4% to 5% of the familial ALS cases (see Box 34-7). Altogether, mutations in specific genes have been identified in about 30% of familial ALS cases.

Pathophysiology

ALS is a rapidly progressive, neurodegenerative disease that destroys the motor neurons that control voluntary muscles. Upper motor neurons, which are motor neurons located in the brain, send messages to lower motor neurons located in the spinal cord, and then to different voluntary muscle groups. In individuals affected by ALS, both the upper and lower motor neurons become sclerotic and die. They can no longer send messages to the muscles. The muscles that are no longer receiving messages from the upper and lower neurons weaken and atrophy. Specific gene mutations, particularly of the *FUS* gene, are under investigation as the instigators of motor neuron death.

Eventually, the damage to the motor neurons becomes so great that the brain is unable to start or adequately control voluntary muscle movement. The affected muscles become progressively weaker until they reach paralysis. Muscles that control the patient's speech, swallowing, and breathing also become impaired. Ultimately, the patient will require artificial ventilation in order to breathe. Because ALS damages only motor neurons, the sensory neurons remain intact—the abilities to see, detect sensation, hear, taste, and smell are not affected. Cognitive ability also remains intact.

Clinical Presentation

There are upper motor neuron (UMN) symptoms due to degeneration of the cortical motor neurons and brainstem. There are lower motor neuron (LMN) symptoms that affect the neurons exiting the spinal cord. Signs of UMN disease include muscle tone increase, slow movement, and hyperreflexia. The presence of the Babinski sign, or upward response of the plantar reflex, is also evidence of UMN dysfunction. Symptoms of ALS may be described as "limb onset" and "bulbar onset." With limb onset, patients may experience clumsiness, gait disturbances, and difficulty with simple actions, such as holding a cup or buttoning a shirt. Patients with bulbar onset may experience challenges with chewing, swallowing, and speaking, such as slurred speech. Patients may also experience muscle cramps, spasms, or twitches. Patients with ALS have no cognitive impairment and are aware of their gradually declining ability to function. Additionally, patients do not always progress on a linear path. Weeks to months may pass with little to no function loss.

Diagnosis

The diagnosis of ALS is usually made on the basis of clinical symptomatology and is a diagnosis of exclusion. There are no laboratory tests that identify the disorder, no biomarkers for the condition, and findings on MRI and CT scan are unremarkable. Laboratory tests are done in patients with ALS to exclude other conditions. These tests include complete blood count, electrolytes, liver and thyroid function tests, creatine kinase, erythrocyte sedimentation rate, antinuclear antibody, rheumatoid factor, vitamin B_{12}, anti-GM1 ganglioside antibody, serum protein electrophoresis with immunofixation, and 24-hour urine protein electrophoresis with immunofixation.

EMG studies may be helpful to rule out muscle or neurological conditions that may mimic ALS. After all other diagnoses have been excluded, the revised El Escorial criteria (2015) requires at least one of the following: the progression of UMN and LMN dysfunction in at least one limb or body region or LMN dysfunction in one region identified by clinical examination and/or

---

BOX 34-7. The *FUS* Gene and ALS

Recently, there has been growing interest in the *FUS* gene (also called *FUS/TLS* for "fused in sarcoma–translated in sarcoma" gene) found on chromosome 16. This gene programs for FUS protein, which is normally found inside the motor neuron cell nucleus, where it serves its primary function as a ribonucleic acid–binding protein. Researchers have found that mutated *FUS* genes direct the manufacture of mutant *FUS* protein that forms characteristic yarnlike cytoplasmic inclusions in spinal motor neurons in both familial and sporadic cases of ALS. Because this has been noted in both types of ALS, there is growing interest regarding the *FUS* gene.

by EMG in two regions (i.e., lumbosacral, bulbar, thoracic, cervical). The EMG findings consist of sharp waves and/or fibrillation and neurogenic potentials.

Genetic testing is recommended if the patient has a family history suggestive of ALS. This should be contemplated if a minimum of one first- or second-degree relative has ALS and/or frontotemporal dementia (FTD). If ALS or FTD is present within three generations, the association should be termed familial ALS.

The Revised Amyotrophic Lateral Sclerosis Functional Rating Scale (ALSFRS-R) can be used to assess progression of the disease. The ALSFRS-R is a 12-item scale with each item scored from 0 (unable) to 4 (normal ability) with a possible total score range of 0 to 48. The higher the score, the better the patient is physically functioning. The items evaluate speech, salivation, swallowing, handwriting, cutting food and handling utensils, dressing and hygiene, turning in bed, walking, climbing stairs, dyspnea, orthopnea, and respiratory insufficiency.

Treatment

There is no cure for ALS. However, the medication riluzole (Rilutek) is believed to reduce the damage to motor neurons by decreasing the release of the excitatory neurotransmitter glutamate. The exact mechanism is not entirely understood. Other treatments for ALS are designed to manage symptoms of the disease and improve the quality of life. Medications to reduce fatigue, relieve muscle cramps, control spasticity, and reduce excessive oral secretions can be beneficial to patients. Gentle, low-impact aerobic activity and range-of-motion and stretching exercises can help prevent painful muscle spasticity and contractures. When respiratory muscles weaken, the use of intermittent positive pressure ventilation may be used to ease the work of breathing during sleep. Decisions regarding patient preference for life-sustaining treatment, such as mechanical ventilation, versus palliative care approaches should be discussed soon after the diagnosis of ALS and should be revisited on several occasions before respiratory failure occurs.

> **ALERT!** Dysphagia resulting from ALS increases the patient's risk for aspiration of food and oral secretions. Dysfunction of the diaphragm muscle causes respiratory failure in ALS.

Multiple Sclerosis

MS is a chronic neurological disorder that affects the brain and spinal cord. It is a demyelinating disorder that results in inflammation and damage to the myelin and other cells within the CNS. This progressive condition eventually results in CNS damage and neurological disability. The disease is characterized by remissions and exacerbations.

The prevalence of MS worldwide is approximately 2.5 million individuals, and 400,000 individuals living in the United States have the disorder. It is most commonly diagnosed among young adults between 18 and 48 years of age, and affects twice as many females as males. MS is more likely to occur among individuals of northern European heritage, although people from African, Asian, and Hispanic ancestry also can develop the disorder. Prevalence is higher at greater distances from the equator and in countries with cooler climates, which has been suggestive of some environmental influences in its pathogenesis.

Etiology

Although the etiology of MS remains unknown, the damage to the myelin of the CNS and peripheral nerves is caused by an autoimmune inflammatory disorder. Several risk factors, including genetic predisposition, viral or other infective process, trauma, or exposure to heavy metals, may trigger the autoimmune response in MS.

Pathophysiology

It is theorized that activated T cells that have been abnormally sensitized to attack myelin cause the damage of MS. T cells damage the CNS myelin; this acts as a stimulant for more T cells to be activated and damage more myelin. Ultimately, demyelination of multiple areas of the CNS results.

The white matter tracts of the CNS are most commonly affected by the demyelination process. However, gray matter tracts can also be involved. Both sensory and motor neurons are affected. There is a predilection for the optic nerves. At times, the inflammatory phase can resolve and areas of demyelination can heal, allowing the disease to go into remission. Alternatively, areas of demyelination can remain damaged and form irreversible fibrotic scar tissue. These fibrotic areas of the myelin disrupt the conduction of impulses traveling throughout the nervous system, and this causes the various sensory and motor symptoms of MS.

Subtypes of Multiple Sclerosis

Multiple sclerosis can be categorized as the following: clinically isolated syndrome (CIS), relapsing-remitting MS (RRMS), secondary progressive MS (SPMS), and primary progressive MS (PPMS). CIS is the initial presentation in 80% of MS cases. CIS encompasses an acute clinical attack affecting one or more CNS sites. Optic neuritis (inflammation of the optic nerve) is a common initial sign of MS. Months to years can pass before CIS can evolve into RRMS. With RRMS, there are episodes when inflammation and demyelination of neurons is actively occurring, then recovery and remission occur. During the relapse, neuron degeneration causes symptoms, then with remission, some repair of myelin can occur. During active episodes, autoreactive lymphocytes cross the blood–brain barrier. This triggers a cascade of inflammation, oxidative damage, mitochondrial injury, and development of the characteristic MS plaque in the brain. Female:male ratio of MS with RRMS is 2:1 and age of onset is around 30 years. Over time, there is accumulation of disability and incomplete recovery from each relapse. Ten to 15 years after the diagnosis of RRMS, up to 80% of people develop SPMS. There is further axonal injury and atrophy in both white and gray brain matter.

Ten to 15% of patients have an initial event and then progressive disability from the outset, usually due to spinal cord disease. This is defined as PPMS. The age of onset is around 40 years, roughly a decade older than for relapse onset MS, and male to female ratio is 1:1. Due to spinal cord dysfunction, patients often have progressive spastic paraparesis and more diffuse brain axonal loss and atrophy.

Clinical Presentation

The most common symptoms of MS are weakness, numbness, tingling sensations, balance problems, blurred vision, and fatigue. The patient suffers both sensory loss and motor impairment. MS follows several different courses that are associated with particular symptoms, patterns of disability, and recommended treatments. About 85% of patients have the most common form of MS, the relapsing-remitting form. This consists of brief episodes, lasting anywhere between several weeks to 3 months, of various symptoms, occurring approximately every 1 to 3 years; these are followed by a complete or almost complete return to normal function. Progressive deterioration without remissions can occur as a form of the disease known as PPMS. PPMS affects about 10% to 15% of individuals with MS.

For patients with relapsing-remitting MS, the most common and early symptoms involve the eyes. Because the optic nerves are heavily myelinated, when those nerves are attacked, patients may experience a temporary distortion or loss of vision in one eye, impairment in color perception, or pain with eye movement. Individuals commonly present with sensory symptoms, such as numbness or paresthesias. Sensory symptoms and debilitating fatigue are often seen at the time of diagnosis. In addition to symptoms related to optic nerve degeneration, signs caused by damage to cerebellar nerves commonly present initially. The cerebellar symptoms include ataxia, tremor, and dysarthria. Uhthoff's phenomenon (transient fluctuation or worsening of MS symptoms with a rise in body temperature) and Lhermitte's sign (an abnormal electric-shock-like sensation down the spine or limbs on neck flexion) are characteristic symptoms of MS.

Severe motor nerve damage typically occurs late in the disease. Motor symptoms include hemiparesis, paraparesis, and quadriparesis. Individuals with MS may have difficulty walking or performing tasks that require coordination. Spinal cord involvement may also lead to urinary and fecal incontinence and sexual dysfunction because the spinal tracts controlling these functions are heavily myelinated.

Individuals with MS are more likely than the general population to experience affective and cognitive symptoms. It is theorized that the neurobiological risk factors associated with MS contribute to the increased risk of depressive disorders and cognitive impairment among these patients. The lifetime risk for major depression in individuals with MS may be as high as 50%. Recent data suggest that 45% to 65% of individuals with MS experience some cognitive impairment. Although MS affects a variety of cognitive domains, recent memory, abstract reasoning, attention, and visual-spatial perception are most often affected. Immediate recall, long-term memory, and language skills seem to be the least disrupted in MS.

Dehydration or malnutrition can result because of swallowing difficulties or an inability to care for oneself. Individuals with MS have dysphagia in later stages of the illness, increasing the risk of aspiration pneumonia. Urinary retention and urinary sphincter dysfunction are common symptoms, placing the individual at a higher risk for urinary tract and kidney infections.

After several decades, approximately 50% of individuals with relapsing-remitting MS go on to develop secondary progressive MS, in which they have continually progressive deterioration and consequent disability.

ALERT! In degenerative neuromuscular disorders, dysphagia occurs because of weakened esophageal muscles, which is why the assessment of the gag reflex is necessary before feeding a patient. The diaphragm can weaken; therefore, assessment of respirations is also necessary.

Diagnosis

MS cannot be diagnosed after only a single symptomatic episode, because symptoms are only clues. Diagnosis requires the appearance of lesions of demyelination detected on imaging studies and patient report of specific neurological deficits. MRI, which shows characteristic MS plaques, is a key clinical tool in terms of diagnosis and therapeutic monitoring. The McDonald criteria, which include specific neurological examination findings; MRI evidence; and patient symptoms are used to diagnose MS. Blood studies are usually normal. The clinician should perform blood work to help exclude conditions such as other autoimmune disorders, infections such as Lyme disease, endocrine abnormalities such as thyroid disease, and vitamin B_{12} deficiency. Cerebrospinal fluid may be evaluated for oligoclonal bands (OCBs) and immunoglobulin G (IgG), as well as for signs of infection. OCBs are found in 90% to 95% of patients with MS, and IgG is found in 70% to 90%. Evoked potentials, which are recordings of the timing of CNS responses to specific stimuli, can be useful neurophysiological studies for evaluation of MS.

Treatment

Because MS is suspected to be an autoimmune disease directed against the CNS, available treatments involve preventing inflammatory cells from traveling across the blood–brain barrier. Immunomodulating agents reduce clinical attacks of new MS lesions, and they may have an effect on disability progression. There are numerous agents currently approved for use in MS. These include interferon beta, glatiramer acetate, natalizumab, fingolimod, alemtuzumab, rituximab, cyclophosphamide, mitoxantrone, and cladribine. The newest disease-modifying agents are monoclonal antibodies that target the specific immune cells that are attacking the neurons in MS. These include ofatumumab, ublituximab, veltuzumab, ocrelizumab, and obinutuzumab. These monoclonal antibodies appear to reduce the accumulation of lesions within the CNS as seen on MRI findings.

Another recently approved treatment, autologous hematopoetic stem cell transplant (AHSCT), is used for highly active, aggressive MS. AHSCT is a multistep procedure that first ablates the patient's immune system to reduce the autoantibodies that are destroying neurons. Then it reconstitutes the immune system with hematopoietic stem cells. Optimal candidates for AHSCT are young, ambulatory, and have inflammatory-active RRMS. Complete suppression of MS disease activity for 4 to 5 years has been documented in 70% to 80% of patients with relapsing–remitting MS who have undergone AHSCT. Neurological improvements have also been demonstrated.

Huntington's Disease

HD is an inherited, progressively degenerative neurological disorder that results in involuntary motor symptoms, cognitive decline, and emotional and behavioral symptoms. It is an autosomal-dominant CNS disorder caused by cellular deterioration in specific areas of the basal ganglia and cortex. Currently, there is no treatment to halt or slow the progression of HD.

Estimates of the international prevalence of HD range from 4 to 8 of every 100,000 individuals. In the United States, it is estimated that 30,000 individuals have HD. Because it is an autosomal-dominant disorder, each child of a parent with HD has a 50% chance of inheriting the gene that causes the illness. Typically, symptoms appear between 30 and 50 years of age and can progress over 10 to 30 years. Duration of illness varies, with a mean of approximately 19 years. Pneumonia and cardiovascular disease are the most common primary causes of death.

Pathophysiology

HD is a genetic disorder caused by a single mutated gene on chromosome 4 that produces an abnormal repetition of the DNA bases cytosine, adenine, and guanine, leading to synthesis of a mutated form of the protein called huntingtin. The mutated protein collects within the cytoplasm of brain cells, but exactly how it causes the disease is unknown. It is linked to neurodegeneration in certain parts of the brain. This degeneration is evident in portions of the basal ganglia, caudate nuclei, and the globus pallidus. These structures, which are found deep within the brain, regulate coordinated movement and emotional expression. HD also affects the cerebral cortex and causes problems with perception, memory, and thinking. It is clear, based on the known pathogenesis of HD, that a neurotoxic mutant HTT protein is principally responsible for the pathological and clinical features of HD.

Clinical Presentation

The early symptoms of HD disease vary greatly from person to person, but there are three common clinical manifestations:

1. Involuntary motor symptoms
2. Emotional and behavioral symptoms
3. Cognitive symptoms

Involuntary Motor Symptoms. The involuntary motor symptoms of HD include two components: dyskinesia, or excess movement, and the loss of voluntary movement. Movements in HD are described as **chorea,** which are brief, irregular, dancelike movements, and **athetosis,** which refers to twisting and writhing movements. Walking may become difficult and include odd postures and leg movements. When chorea is severe, there are thrashing motions referred to as ballismus. As HD progresses, dystonic, rigid postures may develop and eventually worsen, speech becomes slurred, and verbal communication and swallowing become progressively more difficult. In late-stage HD, maintaining adequate caloric and fluid intake becomes challenging because of dysphagia and the high caloric demands caused by worsening chorea movements.

Emotional and Behavioral Symptoms. Approximately 30% of individuals with HD develop a major depressive episode. Additionally, 10% of patients with HD develop episodes of mania in which irritability and elation are prominent. Other common behavioral symptoms of HD include anger and agitation. Delusions and hallucinations are less common but can occur.

Cognitive Symptoms. The early cognitive changes of HD include apathy, impaired mental flexibility, and slowed thought processing. Recognition memory is relatively spared. As HD progresses, the individual might have difficulty remembering new information and making sound decisions and judgments.

Diagnosis

The discovery of the HD gene, at locus 14p16.3, has resulted in the development of a test that is able to detect the majority of individuals who are at risk for developing HD. In order to perform the genetic test, a small sample of blood is tested for the presence or absence of the HD genetic mutation.

Research is emerging to identify a biomarker that accurately predicts onset of HD or disease progression. The mutant HTT (mHTT) protein in the CSF as a biomarker of HD is one such under investigation. The CSF is enriched in the brain-derived proteins that are altered in HD but soluble mHTT is present in extremely low concentrations in CSF, making detection very difficult. Studies show that neurofilament light protein (NfL) and tau are important neuron-specific components of the neuronal cytoskeleton in HD. Similar to mHTT, NfL and tau levels in CSF have been shown to correlate with HD and may reflect useful markers of neurodegeneration. Plasma NfL levels appear to directly correlate with CSF levels, making this a potential peripheral biomarker of neuronal injury and disease progression in HD. Plasma NfL also correlates with rates of brain atrophy and cognitive decline in HD patients and may predict disease onset in HD mutation carriers.

Treatment

Currently, treatment development is emerging that targets the HTT gene DNA, RNA, and protein. Investigations are focusing on the use of the clustered regularly interspaced short palindromic repeats (CRISPR)/ Cas protein 9 (CRISPR/Cas9) system, which is gene editing, but this is still in the early stages of preclinical development. The goal is to selectively inactivate mutant *HTT* genes. Other research that uses human embryonic stem cell–derived neural stem cells (hNSCs) transplanted into the brain of mice with HD has resulted in symptomatic improvement. There is potential for cell-based therapies that offer hope for patients who have HD. Presently, treatment focuses only on supportive care measures for those with HD.

Treatment of chorea with antipsychotic medications such as haloperidol and olanzapine may be symptomatically beneficial. Antidepressant medications have been used for the mood and behavioral symptoms of HD.

Physical and occupational therapies and regular exercise may help the person with HD feel better physically and emotionally. Speech therapy, swallowing interventions, and interventions that promote adequate nutrition and hydration are commonly utilized in the later stages of HD.

Guillain–Barré Syndrome

GBS is an acute peripheral neuropathy that leads to progressive limb weakness over the course of several days up to 4 weeks. Incidence worldwide is 1.3 cases per 100,000, with males affected more frequently than females. There is a slight peak of incidence in adolescence and young adulthood, which may be caused by cytomegalovirus (CMV) infections and *Campylobacter jejuni*. It also occurs more often in older adults and may be a result of decreased immune suppressor mechanisms.

GBS is a postinfectious disease, with most patients having an antecedent infection of either the upper respiratory tract or gastroenteritis. These infections have resolved by the time of onset of the neuropathy. In many cases, the pathogen responsible for the antecedent infection is unidentified. However, the most common pathogens that result in GBS are *C. jejuni,* CMV, Epstein–Barr virus, and *Mycoplasma* pneumonia. The syndrome has also occurred after immunization with various types of vaccines.

Pathophysiology

The proposed pathogenesis for GBS is one in which a previous infection evokes an autoimmune response in the peripheral nerves. Most patients report an infectious illness in the weeks before onset. Many of the identified infectious agents are thought to stimulate the production of antibodies that attack the infectious agent, as well as the body's normal myelin sheaths covering nerve axons. The cause of this cross reaction is unknown. Pathological findings include the infiltration of lymphocytes around spinal nerves exiting the spinal cord, peripheral nerves, and cranial nerves, followed by macrophage attack of myelin. This reaction results in defects in the conduction of electrical nerve impulses, with eventual absence of conduction causing flaccid paralysis of muscles. Recovery can occur with remyelination. However, in some patients, severe inflammation is followed by complete axonal destruction. Acute inflammatory demyelinating polyradiculoneuropathy is the most widely recognized form of GBS in Western countries, but there are subtypes known as acute motor axonal neuropathy (AMAN) and acute motor-sensory axonal neuropathy (AMSAN).

Clinical Presentation

The cardinal clinical presentation of GBS is one of progressive, usually symmetric, muscle weakness accompanied by absent or depressed deep tendon reflexes. Paresthesias and numbness are usually the first symptoms. Symptoms usually manifest quickly over a period of several days and plateau at about 4 weeks. The weakness can vary from mild weakness in the lower limbs, causing difficulty walking, to nearly complete paralysis of all extremities and respiratory muscles, requiring the support of artificial ventilation.

Acute inflammatory demyelinating polyneuropathy (AIDP) involves distal muscle weakness of the lower extremities followed by more proximal muscles, trunk, upper extremities, and cranial nerves. This is a unique clinical presentation that characterizes GBS, and it is often referred to as ascending paralysis. Patients have sensory and motor nerve involvement. Seventy percent of patients with AIDP often experience autonomic dysfunction, most commonly manifested as tachycardia fluctuating with bradycardia, hypertension fluctuating with hypotension, urinary retention, ileus, and loss of sweating. Recovery from AIDP is often steady and occurs within a few weeks or months; however, little improvement can be expected in disabilities that linger beyond 2 years.

AMAN is a motor form of neuropathy in which tendon reflexes are absent, though some patients are hyperreflexic during the early recovery phase. Autonomic dysfunction is rare in this subgroup. AMSAN is similar to AMAN, but very rare. It is associated with severe illness and slow recovery.

Diagnosis

Clinical examination reveals symmetrical ascending muscular weakness, diminished deep tendon reflexes, and variable sensory loss. Laboratory investigations show an increase of proteins without pleocytosis in the CSF. Serum antiganglioside antibodies may also appear in the more atypical forms of GBS. Electromyography and electroneurography are highly useful clinical tools because they reveal the characteristic decrease in the amplitude of muscle action potential, lessening of nerve conduction speed and blockage of the nerve-to-muscle signal transmission. These electrophysiological tests are the most specific and sensitive assessments for the precise diagnosis of GBS. Spinal MRI with intravenous gadolinium (Gd) may also provide a diagnosis by depicting the contrast enhancement in the nerve roots comprising the cauda equina within the first weeks after the symptom onset.

Treatment

There are two facets of treatment for GBS. The first is supportive, because GBS can have life-threatening sequelae. The second goal of treatment is to lessen the nerve damage.

Supportive care is of utmost importance in GBS, as 30% of patients develop neuromuscular respiratory failure requiring mechanical ventilation. Continuous hemodynamic monitoring is also required, especially in patients with autonomic involvement. Prophylaxis for deep vein thrombosis, physical and occupational therapy, and psychological support are also necessary when caring for these patients.

The treatment of GBS is intravenous (IV) administration of immunoglobulins (IVIG) in doses of 1 g/kg/day for 2 days, or 0.4 g/kg/day IVIG for 5 days. A second viable option is plasmapheresis, also known as plasma exchange. If these two therapeutic methods fail to achieve neurological improvement, corticosteroid therapy (IV methylprednisolone) is recommended.

Myasthenia Gravis

MG is a relatively uncommon autoimmune neuromuscular disorder that can occur at any age. It has a prevalence of 100 to 200 per million worldwide, with 10 to 20 new cases per million each year. Prevalence has increased over the past 50 years, likely because of better recognition of the disease, aging of the population, and the longer life span of affected persons.

Pathophysiology

MG is an autoimmune disease caused by the loss of functioning Ach receptors in the neuromuscular junction. Most individuals with MG test positive for Ach receptor antibodies (see Fig. 34-9). Some individuals with the disorder have no detectable levels of antibodies against Ach receptors; this is known as seronegative MG. There is compelling evidence that there is also an antibody-mediated autoimmune component in this form of the disorder, but no tests have been able to detect antibodies in this form.

Normally, in a healthy individual, a nerve impulse releases Ach at the neuromuscular junction, where it travels across to reach Ach receptors concentrated in the folds of the muscle endplate. The muscle contracts when enough of the receptor sites have been activated by the Ach. In MG, there is as much as an 80% reduction in the number of Ach receptor sites because of the deterioration caused by Ach receptor antibodies. The end result of this process is inefficient neuromuscular transmission, which is manifested as muscle weakness and easy fatigability. Commonly, the extraocular muscles, such as those that control eyelids, are first affected in MG and may be the predominant manifestation of the disorder. This is commonly manifested as ptosis of the eyelids. It is unknown why there is a predilection for ocular muscles.

Pathological Autoimmune Mechanism. The mechanism of the body's immunological attack on Ach receptors is not understood. MG can be considered a B-cell– or T-cell–mediated disease. It is known that the antibodies against Ach receptors are IgG immunoglobulins derived from B cells. However, the importance of T cells in the pathogenesis of MG is becoming increasingly apparent. The thymus is the central organ in T-cell–mediated immunity, and thymic abnormalities such as thymic hyperplasia or thymoma are well recognized in myasthenic patients. Approximately 70% of patients with MG have hyperplasia of the thymus gland. It is also likely that genetic factors contribute to the development of the disorder. Patients with MG frequently have other immune-mediated diseases such as rheumatoid arthritis or Graves' disease, as well as a family history of autoimmune disorders.

Clinical Presentation

MG can present in one of two ways: in an ocular form or a generalized form. In the ocular form, the muscle weakness occurs only in the eyelids and extraocular muscles. In the generalized form, the weakness involves a combination of limb, esophageal, and respiratory muscles, as well as involvement of the ocular muscles.

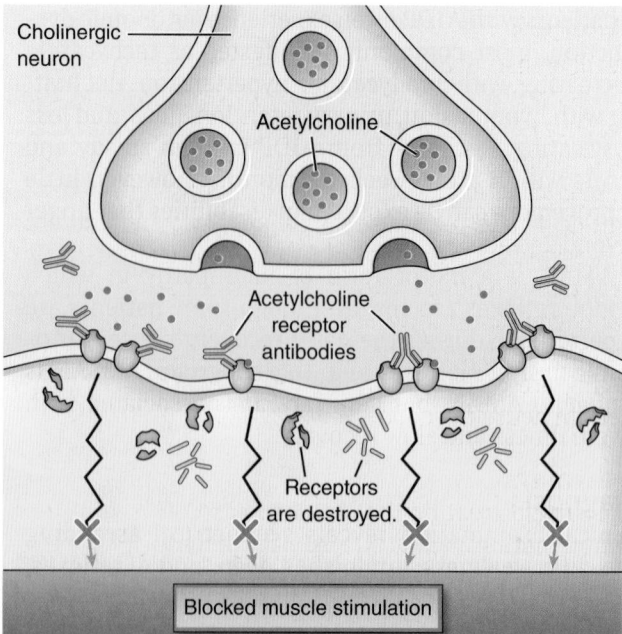

FIGURE 34-9. Myasthenia gravis. MG is a neuromuscular disorder caused by autoantibodies that destroy acetylcholine (Ach) receptors at neuromuscular junctions. As the disease progresses, increasing numbers of Ach receptors are destroyed, which decreases the ability of Ach to stimulate muscle. In MG, there is progressive weakness of the muscle. Fatal consequences can result when respiratory or swallowing muscles are weakened.

Ptosis and diplopia will be the presenting symptoms in as many as half of those diagnosed with MG. In addition, 50% of patients who present with ocular symptoms are likely to develop generalized disease within 2 years. Approximately 15% of patients will develop speech and esophageal symptoms, including dysarthria, dysphagia, and fatigue while chewing. Very few patients will present with only limb weakness.

The cardinal feature of MG is a fluctuating skeletal muscle weakness, often with true muscle fatigue. The fatigue is seen as a worsening of muscle contractile force, not a sense of tiredness in the muscle. This is most notably seen with repetitive motion, such as blinking, walking, or even talking. For example, after only a few minutes of constant talking, the voice can become slurred, with increased difficulty in forming words. After resting, the voice can return to normal. However, this cycle can be repeated if constant talking continues.

Early in the disease, the symptoms of weakness can fluctuate throughout the day. Muscle strength may be best in the morning hours and decrease throughout the day. As the disease progresses, the symptom-free periods shorten and symptoms become constant along a continuum of mild to severe. Factors that worsen myasthenic symptoms include emotional stress, concurrent illness, hypothyroidism or hyperthyroidism, hormonal fluctuations, and increases in body temperature. MG can eventually lead to myasthenic crisis (see Box 34-8).

BOX 34-8. Myasthenic Crisis

Myasthenic crisis is weakness resulting from MG that is severe enough to cause respiratory failure necessitating ventilator support. Precipitating factors include infection, surgery, and tapering of immunosuppression, or it can be a spontaneous event. The patient in crisis experiences severe respiratory muscle weakness that increases risk for aspiration. The individual with an exacerbation of MG symptomatology must be closely monitored in an intensive care unit for respiratory failure. The patient's forced vital capacity and negative inspiratory force are monitored every 2 to 4 hours. Although arterial blood gases can be monitored, they are not a sensitive measure of respiratory muscle weakness.

CLINICAL CONCEPT

It is important to assess respiratory function and gag reflex in patients affected with severe MG because the diaphragm, intercostal muscles, and swallowing muscles can be affected.

ALERT! Aspiration and respiratory failure are major causes of death in severe MG and other neurodegenerative diseases.

Diagnosis

The diagnosis of MG is based on a combination of clinical history of fluctuating muscle weakness and the presence of serum autoantibodies, which are most frequently directed at the acetylcholine receptor (AChR), muscle-specific kinase (MuSK), or lipoprotein-related peptide 4 (LRP4). In some patients, antibodies cannot be detected. In these patients, the diagnosis is based on electrophysiological testing. The presence of an abnormal decrement during low-frequency repetitive nerve stimulation or an increased jitter in single-fiber EMG testing are considered to be indicative of an impairment in neuromuscular transmission.

Treatment

The current treatment of autoimmune MG is based on a combination of lifestyle advice, including exercise, symptomatic treatment, immunosuppressive drugs and interventions, and thymectomy. Acetylcholinesterase (AchE) inhibitors enhance the bioavailability of acetylcholine at the neuron-muscle synapse. Pyridostigmine bromide, an AchE inhibitor, is usually the first-line treatment and may be sufficient as stand-alone treatment in patients with mild or moderate MG. Salbutamol, a selective B_2-adrenergic agonist, is an effective treatment for patients with congenital myasthenic syndrome, including those with AChR deficiency syndromes, or autoimmune MG. Ephedrine is a sympathomimetic agent that mainly affects adrenergic receptors. Its mechanism of action in MG is not well understood. Corticosteroid treatment, usually by means of oral prednisone, is currently the mainstay of immunosuppressive treatment but is associated with many well-known side effects. Nonsteroidal agents such as azathioprine, cyclosporin, mycophenolate, methotrexate, and tacrolimus have been used. However, emerging corticosteroid-sparing treatments with immunomodulators are showing promise. Complement protein inhibitors, eculizumab, ravulizumab, and zilucoplan are potential treatments for the future.

If rapid treatment is warranted, therapeutic options include IV immune globulin, plasmapheresis, or plasma exchange, which removes Ach receptor antibodies from the circulation. Thymectomy is recommended for patients with a thymoma.

Chapter Summary

- The neuron has four major anatomical parts: dendrites, cell body, axon, and axon terminals.

- Incoming signals from other neurons are received through its dendrites. The outgoing signal to other neurons flows along its axon. Some axons are myelinated, covered with a lipid-rich substance that acts as insulation and keeps impulses traveling smoothly in one direction.

- An upper motor neuron disorder indicates that the source of the problem is in the brain's area of motor control, the sensory-motor cortex. A lower motor neuron disorder indicates that the source of the problem is at the region where motor nerves exit the spinal cord.

- A positive Babinski's reflex in an adult indicates upper motor neuron dysfunction.

- Disorders of ion channels are responsible for a growing number of neurological diseases. Most are caused by mutations in ion channel genes or by autoantibodies formed against ion channel proteins.

- If a patient is unconscious, the clinician should make an assessment based on the Glasgow Coma Scale, vital signs, and pupil response.

- Epilepsy is a chronic neurological disorder characterized by recurrent seizures. A seizure is a sudden, abnormal, disorderly discharge of neurons within the brain that is characterized by a sudden, transient alteration in brain function. There are three categories of seizures: generalized onset, focal onset, and unknown onset.

- Before a seizure, an individual may have unique sensations referred to as an aura.

- The most common types of primary headaches are tension-type headaches, migraine headaches, and trigeminal autonomic cephalgia.

- A TTH is the most common type of primary headache, occurring in as many as 78% of persons.

- Migraine headache is a severe, throbbing, one-sided headache that is accompanied by nausea, vomiting, photophobia, and phonophobia. Migraine headache is usually disabling to the sufferer. Some migraine headaches may have a preceding aura.

- Cluster headache is a form of trigeminal autonomic cephalgia that has key identifiable unilateral symptoms: rhinorrhea, tearing of the eye, conjunctival injection, forehead and facial sweating, pupil constriction, drooping eyelid and/or eyelid edema, and/or restlessness or agitation.

- Parkinson's disease is mainly associated with progressive loss of dopamine-producing cells in the substantia nigra, which is within the basal ganglia of the midbrain. The basal ganglia modulates movements, such as posture, standing, walking, or writing.

- Parkinson's disease can be diagnosed by clinical signs with the mnemonic TRAP: **T**remor at rest, **R**igidity, **A**kinesia or bradykinesia, and **P**ostural/gait instability.

- ALS is a progressive neurodegenerative disorder that is characterized by a loss of upper and lower motor neurons.

Swallowing and respiratory function are affected in terminal stages.

- MS is a progressive neurodegenerative disorder of both motor and sensory nerves often characterized by remissions and exacerbations

- HD is a neurodegenerative, genetic disorder caused by a single mutated gene on chromosome 4 that programs the manufacture of an abnormal protein called huntingtin that collects within brain neurons. Clinical manifestations include movement disturbances such as athetosis, chorea, and ballismus.

- In degenerative neuromuscular disorders, dysphagia occurs because of weakened esophageal muscles; because of this, assessment of the gag reflex is necessary before feeding a patient with a degenerative neuromuscular disorder. Involvement of the diaphragm can cause respiratory dysfunction; therefore, respirations should also be assessed.

- GBS is an acute peripheral neuropathy that leads to progressive limb weakness over the course of several days up to 4 weeks. This ascending paralysis often occurs after an infection or vaccine.

- MG is an autoimmune disease caused by autoantibodies that attack Ach receptors in the neuromuscular junction. The first symptom of the disorder is often ptosis. As the day progresses, patient muscle weakness increases.

Making the Connections

Disorder and Pathophysiology

Signs and Symptoms	Physical Assessment Findings	Diagnostic Testing	Treatment
Epilepsy | Abnormal electrical discharge of neurons in the brain, an imbalance of neurotransmitters, or both. Ion channel abnormalities causing hyperexcitability of regions of brain neurons, causing seizures.			
Generalized seizure: loss of consciousness and tonic-clonic contractions of muscle. Postictal memory loss. Absence seizure: loss of attentiveness for period of time. Before a seizure, an individual may have unique sensations referred to as an aura.	Generalized: loss of consciousness, involuntary muscle contractions, autonomic symptoms, postictal vomiting common. Focal: spasms of a specific muscle group with awareness or lack of awareness. Absence: loss of attentiveness.	Most patients have a normal EEG when not having a seizure. EEG is abnormal during seizure. Brain imaging may exhibit the cerebral hemisphere seizure origin. Metabolic panel is used to rule out electrolyte imbalances or toxicities.	Anticonvulsant medications to prevent seizures. Safety measures during seizure activity such as adjusting environment to prevent patient injury. After seizure, patient placed on side to prevent aspiration.
Tension Headache | Pericranial and cervical muscle tension.			
Band of pain around head. Cervicothoracic muscle stiffness.	Normal physical examination.	Diagnosis mainly based on symptoms.	Acetaminophen, aspirin, or NSAIDs.
Migraine Headache | Hyperexcitability of neurons, cortical spreading depression, trigeminal nerve complex activation, dural blood vessel sensitivity. Ion channel abnormalities may be associated.			
Commonly lasts 4 to 72 hours. May or may not be accompanied by an aura. Nausea, vomiting, photophobia, and phonophobia are common.	Normal physical examination.	Normal laboratory tests and imaging studies. Specific criteria for diagnosis of a migraine headache.	NSAIDs to decrease inflammation. Triptans, which are serotonin agonists, are first-choice medications. Propranolol, botulinum toxin treatment, and CGRP antagonists (e.g., erenumab) are preventive medications. Avoidance of triggers.

Making the Connections–cont'd

Signs and Symptoms	Physical Assessment Findings	Diagnostic Testing	Treatment
Trigeminal Autonomic Cephalgia | Main type is called a cluster headache. Activation of the trigeminovascular system, autonomic nerves, and hypothalamus play prominent roles.			
Stabbing, unilateral headache. Nasal discharge, tearing of the eye, pallor, and perspiration over one side of the face.	Rhinorrhea, conjunctival injection, tearing of the eye, sweating, eyelid edema, and pallor over one side of the face. Restlessness and agitation.	Diagnosis mainly based on symptoms.	100% oxygen inhalation, or 6 mg subcutaneous or nasal spray sumatriptan. Short course of oral or IV corticosteroids. Preventive medication includes verapamil, lithium carbonate, methylergonovine, and topiramate. Preventive treatments include anti-CGRP monoclonal antibody, galcanezumab, administered once per month. Indomethacin is used to prevent paroxysmal hemicrania. SUNCT and SUNA can be prevented with lamotrigine.
Parkinson's Disease | Progressive loss of dopamine-producing cells, especially in the substantia nigra of the basal ganglia that modulates movement and posture.			
Clinical signs TRAP: **T**remor at rest, **R**igidity, **A**kinesia or bradykinesia, and **P**ostural/gait instability.	Stiff posture, muscle stiffness, blank expression, gait disturbances, and resting tremor. "Freezing" episodes where individual cannot initiate movement; micrographia, slowed movements, depression, cognitive disturbance. Autonomic disturbances.	Diagnosis mainly based on symptoms. Normal laboratory tests and imaging studies. Genetic susceptibility and current research regarding accumulation of mutated protein in brain. Significant symptom improvement with trial of levodopa indicates Parkinson's disease.	Levodopa–carbidopa medications to replace dopamine in the brain and decrease peripheral effects of dopamine. Dopamine agonists. Catechol-O-methyl transferase inhibitors to decrease breakdown of dopamine. Anticholinergic drugs to balance acetylcholine effects.
ALS | Progressive neurodegenerative disorder characterized by a loss of upper and lower motor neurons.			
Gradual loss of control of muscles.	Muscle weakness and atrophy, dysarthria, dysphagia. Sensation intact.	A diagnosis of exclusion. Laboratory tests to exclude other causes of disorder. EMG muscle studies.	No cure. Riluzole (Rilutek^R). Supportive and palliative care.
MS | Autoimmune, demyelinating disorder that results in inflammation and damage to the myelin and other cells within the CNS, ANS, and PNS.			
Ocular and cerebellar symptoms often are initially present. Vision disturbances and gait and balance problems often are initial symptoms.	Motor and sensory weakness. Visual problems. Incoordination and gait disturbance (ataxia). Uthoff phenomenon, Lhermitte sign.	Condition cannot be diagnosed after only a single symptomatic episode. Cerebrospinal fluid evaluated for oligoclonal bands (OCBs). Symptoms are clues to diagnosis; however, diagnosis requires the appearance of demyelination lesions detected on MRI imaging studies. McDonald criteria are used to diagnose. EMG and evoked potential tests are also used.	Numerous immunomodulators (monoclonal antibodies) and immunosuppressives to decrease autoantibody effects. Corticosteroids to decrease inflammation. Autologous hematopoietic stem cell transplant (AHSCT) possible for highly active, aggressive MS.

Continued

Making the Connections–cont'd

Signs and Symptoms	Physical Assessment Findings	Diagnostic Testing	Treatment
HD | Autosomal-dominant neurological disorder; genetic mutation on chromosome 4 that codes for huntingtin protein; causes progressive lack of muscle control.			
Involuntary motor symptoms, cognitive decline, and emotional/behavioral symptoms.	Motor control deficits. Chorea, athetosis, ballismus, and cognitive impairment.	Presymptomatic blood test for the presence of the mutated HD gene. Biomarkers mHTT, NfL.	Supportive treatment. CRISPR/Cas9 technology may offer treatment in future.
GBS | Postinfectious disease with resulting neuropathy; ascending paralysis, previous infection evokes an autoimmune response in the peripheral nerve; can occur postimmunization also.			
Progressive, usually symmetric, ascending muscle weakness accompanied by absent or depressed deep tendon reflexes, paresthesias, and numbness.	Motor and sensory deficits, distal to proximal, starting in lower limbs and moving upward.	Clinical examination, EMG, spinal MRI.	May require temporary mechanical ventilation, IV immunoglobulin, corticosteroids, or plasmapheresis (plasma exchange).
MG | Autoimmune antibodies directed against muscle acetylcholine receptors.			
Muscle weakness; often manifests as ptosis or easy fatigability.	Muscle weakness; ptosis of eyelids; worsens as day continues.	Serum autoantibodies to AChR, muscle-specific kinase (MuSK), or lipoprotein-related peptide 4 (LRP4) EMG.	Acetylcholinesterase inhibitors such as physostigmine to allow more acetylcholine to remain in the synapse. Salbutamol, ephedrine may be effective. Nonsteroidal agents such as azathioprine, cyclosporin, mycophenolate, methotrexate, and tacrolimus have been used. Corticosteroids and immunosuppressive therapy to decrease effects of autoantibodies. Complement protein inhibitors eculizumab, ravulizumab, and zilucoplan are potential treatments for the future.

Bibliography

Available online at fadavis.com

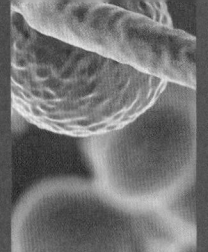
Brain and Spinal Cord Injury

Learning Objectives

Upon completion of this chapter, the student will be able to:

- Identify common risk factors and causes of traumatic brain injury and spinal cord injury.
- Recognize basic pathological mechanisms that occur during traumatic brain injury and spinal cord injury.
- Understand the signs and symptoms of major types of traumatic brain injury and spinal cord injury.

- Describe neurological assessment techniques, laboratory tests, and imaging studies used in the diagnosis of traumatic brain injury and spinal cord injury.
- Discuss basic treatment modalities used in traumatic injury and spinal cord injury.
- Explain the long-term consequences of traumatic brain injury and spinal cord injury.

Key Terms

Acceleration-deceleration
Areflexia
ASIA Impairment Scale
Basilar skull fracture (BSF)
Battle's sign
Cauda equina
Cauda equina syndrome
Cerebral perfusion pressure (CPP)
Concussion
Conus medullaris

Coup-contrecoup injury
Cushing's triad
Cytotoxic cerebral edema
Decerebrate posture
Decorticate posture
Diffuse axonal injury (DAI)
Glasgow Coma Scale (GCS)
Intracranial pressure (ICP)
Monroe–Kellie hypothesis
Neurogenic shock

Paraplegia
Postconcussion syndrome (PCS)
Quadriplegia
Raccoon eyes
Spinal shock
Tetraplegia
Transtentorial herniation
Traumatic brain injury (TBI)
Uncal herniation
Vasogenic cerebral edema

Traumatic brain injury (TBI) is sudden physical damage to the brain. The damage can result from a closed head injury, such as that caused by the head hitting an external unmovable object or surface. This commonly can occur during falls, sports injuries, assaults, and motor vehicle accidents. The damage can also result from a penetrating brain injury, such as that caused by a bullet or knife piercing the skull. Contact sports often cause TBI in the form of **concussion.** TBI can cause a diminished or altered state of consciousness that can result in alteration of cognitive abilities or physical functioning.

Traumatic spinal cord injury (SCI) is damage to the spinal cord that results in loss of mobility or sensation. In most cases, the spinal cord remains intact, but the damage causes loss of nerve function below the area of injury.

Epidemiology

According to the CDC, there were approximately 223,135 TBI-related hospitalizations in 2019 and 64,362 TBI-related deaths in 2020. This represents more than 611 TBI-related hospitalizations and 176 TBI-related deaths per day. However, these estimates do not include the many TBIs that were only treated in the emergency department, primary care, urgent care, or those that went untreated. Individuals aged 75 and older had the highest numbers and rates of TBI-related hospitalizations and deaths. Males were nearly twice as likely to be hospitalized and three times more likely to die of a TBI than females.

The 2022 annual incidence of SCI was approximately 54 cases per one million people in the United States, which is equal to 18,000 new SCI cases each year. New SCI cases do not include those who die at the location of the incident that caused the SCI. As of June 2022, the National Spinal Cord Injury Model Systems Database contained information on 35,953 persons who sustained traumatic SCIs. Each year, males are affected by SCI more than females, and motor vehicle accidents are the leading cause. Falls, violence, and sports injuries are also major causes of SCI. The majority of SCIs occur to persons between the ages of 16 and 30.

Basic Concepts in Neurovascular Physiology

The brain sits inside a rigid protective skull surrounded by meningeal membranes and cerebrospinal fluid (CSF). Broad anatomical regions of the brain have been mapped. However, functions of some regions of the brain still remain unknown.

Cerebral Anatomy and Physiology

The cerebrum of the brain consists of four lobes:

1. Frontal lobes: These are responsible for consciousness, judgment, and emotional responses. These processes comprise executive function, which controls how individuals react to the world.
2. Temporal lobes: These are responsible for hearing ability and memory acquisition. The center for speech is predominantly found in the left cerebral hemisphere.
3. Parietal lobes: These are responsible for sensory discrimination, such as touch perception and manipulation of objects.
4. Occipital lobes: These control vision.

The brainstem contains the vital sign center that controls respirations, heart rate, and blood pressure. It also contains the reticular activating system, which is responsible for the sleep–wake cycle and levels of alertness.

Intracranial Pressure

The bones of the skull form a rigid cranial compartment that contains brain tissue (80%), CSF (10%), and blood volume (10%). The pressure of these three elements must remain balanced to maintain normal **intracranial pressure (ICP)**. ICP—the pressure inside the skull, brain tissue, and CSF—is normally 5 to 15 mm Hg in the resting, supine adult. Changes in ICP occur because of volume changes in the brain tissue, cerebral blood flow, or CSF. To maintain normal ICP, any increase in the volume of any one of the components must be compensated for by a decrease in the volume of another. For example, as a slow-growing brain tumor increases the volume of brain tissue, the CSF production is slowed to compensate and maintain normal ICP. Once the volume of the brain tumor exceeds the volume of the CSF reduction, ICP increases. This concept of maintaining normal pressure within the cranium is known as the **Monroe–Kellie hypothesis** (see Fig. 35-1).

When the compensating mechanisms are totally exhausted, ICP will increase, as demonstrated by the volume–pressure curve in Figure 35-2. The ICP is maintained until a maximum point is reached. At this point, it takes only a small amount of volume increase to cause a large increase in ICP.

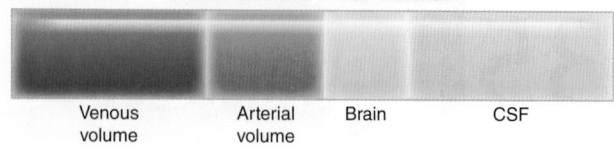

Normal state — ICP normal

Venous volume   Arterial volume   Brain   CSF

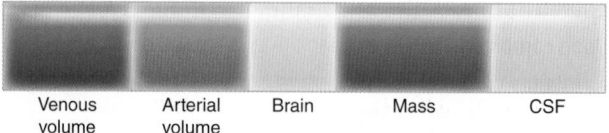

Compensated state — ICP normal

Venous volume   Arterial volume   Brain   Mass   CSF

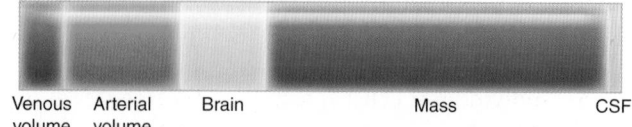

Decompensated state — ICP elevated

Venous volume   Arterial volume   Brain   Mass   CSF

FIGURE 35-1. The Monroe–Kellie hypothesis states that an increase in one compartment of the brain is compensated by a decrease in other compartments of the brain. An example of this is how the growth of a brain mass will cause compensatory decreases in cerebral spinal fluid and venous compartments.

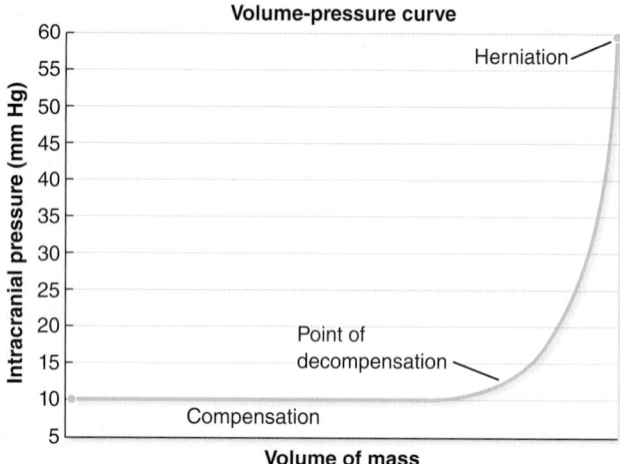

FIGURE 35-2. The volume–pressure curve in ICP. As the volume of an expanding mass in the brain increases, ICP rises until compensatory mechanisms are overcome. The point of decompensation is reached when further expansion of the brain mass causes a steep rise in ICP. The final result is herniation of the brain.

> ### 🩺 CLINICAL CONCEPT
>
> Increased ICP is directly related to increased mortality in patients with TBI.

Level of Consciousness

Consciousness is associated with self-awareness and the ability to interact with the environment; this active process is the result of neuronal activity within the brain. Content of consciousness refers to the cognitive function and is mediated by the cerebral cortex. A declining content of consciousness results in confusional states where a person is unable to maintain a coherent stream of thought or action. There are many causes of confusion, both neurological and nonneurological in origin.

Consciousness itself, however, is not located within specific areas of the brain, and maintaining consciousness depends on interconnected neural pathways within the brain. These include the upper brainstem, the reticular activating system, and their interactions with the cerebral hemispheres. Whenever there is an alteration in the interconnected pathways, there can be a change in the level of consciousness (LOC). The change is measured by patient responses to stimulation or to the environment and includes communication, emotional responses, and appropriate gestures.

An individual's LOC is a measure of their arousability and reaction to the environment. An individual's consciousness can be described on a continuum. Alertness is the highest LOC, where the individual is awake and fully interactive with the environment. Lethargy is a state in which the individual is sleepy but can be aroused easily. An obtunded person is more difficult to arouse. An obtunded or stuporous individual in a lower LOC is difficult to arouse and has little or no interaction with the environment. Coma, where the individual is in a sleeplike state and has no interaction with the environment, is the lowest LOC.

> ### 🩺 CLINICAL CONCEPT
>
> Signs of increasing ICP include decreased LOC, pupillary dilation, headache, vomiting, increased blood pressure, and papilledema.

Basic Pathophysiological Concepts of Brain and Spinal Cord Injury

Although brain injury can occur because of different mechanisms, certain pathophysiological alterations result, regardless of the etiology. These alterations include changes in ICP, cerebral perfusion pressure, and LOC.

Mechanisms of Injury in TBI

TBI is the result of external forces that are transferred directly or indirectly to the brain. Four mechanisms can result in skull or brain injuries:

1. Blunt trauma: This occurs when an object hits the skull forcefully, causing fractures of the skull and damage to the underlying brain. Examples of blunt trauma include being struck in the head with a baseball or being a passenger in a motor vehicle accident whose head hits the dashboard.

2. Acceleration-deceleration: When the skull stops abruptly, as in a motor vehicle accident, the brain continues to move forward, rotating within the skull and causing shearing of brain tissue against the skull's rough interior edges. This movement is referred to as **acceleration-deceleration** and causes stretching and shearing of neural axons, resulting in diffuse axonal injuries. In acceleration-deceleration, the brain bounces off the skull and moves in the opposite direction of the first impact, then strikes the back of the skull and damages the opposite area. This type of injury is also referred to as a **coup-contrecoup injury** (see Fig. 35-3).

> ### 🩺 CLINICAL CONCEPT
>
> Shaken baby syndrome is an example of a coup-contrecoup injury. "Coup" refers to the site of first impact, whereas "contrecoup" refers to the injury site opposite the impact area.

3. Penetrating injury: When a foreign object penetrates the skull and brain, the skull is fractured and brain tissue is injured. The amount of damage depends on the size of the foreign object and its velocity. High-velocity projectiles, such as bullets, produce a cavity along the primary missile tract as the bullet destabilizes brain tissue and converts body fluids to steam, blasting apart a channel and creating extensive brain damage. Penetrating trauma causes an increase in infection as the foreign body disrupts the meningeal layers and carries external debris,

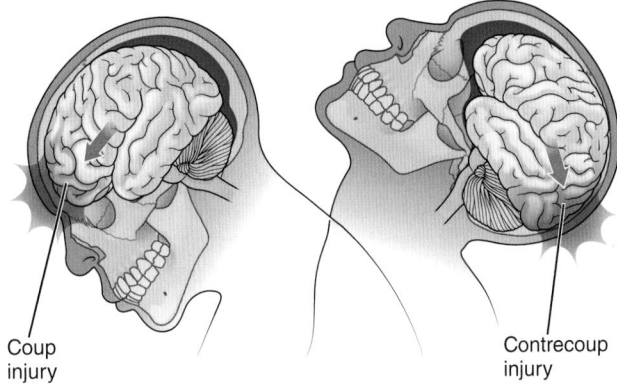

Coup injury   Contrecoup injury

FIGURE 35-3. Acceleration-deceleration injury. This type of traumatic head injury, also called coup-contrecoup injury, occurs as a whiplash accident when the brain bounces back and forth inside the skull. The coup injury happens when the head stops abruptly because of an impact and the brain then crashes into the skull. The contrecoup injury occurs when the brain then bounces inside the skull and impacts the opposite side of the skull.

such as gunpowder and pieces of skull and hair, into the brain. A penetrating injury usually causes a skull fracture, which ruptures the middle meningeal artery and leads to an extensive arterial bleed in the epidural space.

4. Blast injury: The extent of injury caused by explosions depends on the type and amount of explosive material and the distance between the individual and the blast. One blast of an explosive can produce multiple effects on the body. A primary injury results from the detonation of explosives; this produces a pressure wave that is particularly destructive to gas-filled structures of the body, such as the lungs and inner ears. This wave can produce an acceleration-deceleration injury within the skull. A secondary injury is one caused by penetrating and blunt injuries from flying debris and bomb fragments. Tertiary injuries occur when individuals are thrown by the blast, resulting in blunt trauma. Quaternary injuries are related to burns, inhalation of gases, and angina that result from the experience.

Intracranial Hypertension

High ICP, referred to as intracranial hypertension, is an important secondary cause of neurological injury in patients with acute TBI or neurosurgical procedures (see Box 35-1). Elevated ICP can cause damage of brain cells days after the initial traumatic event. ICP can be measured using an intraventricular catheter.

Dynamics of ICP and Cerebral Blood Flow

The pressure of cerebral blood flow in the brain is referred to as **cerebral perfusion pressure (CPP).** Cerebral perfusion pressure depends on mean arterial pressure (MAP) in the body and ICP. The following equation represents the relationship:

$$CPP = MAP - ICP$$
$$MAP = \tfrac{1}{3} \text{ systolic pressure} + \tfrac{2}{3} \text{ diastolic pressure}$$

Through a process called pressure autoregulation, the brain is able to maintain a normal cerebral blood flow (CBF) with a CPP ranging from 50 to 150 mm Hg. When pressure autoregulation is intact, decreasing CPP results in vasodilation of cerebral vessels, which allows CBF to remain unchanged. This response has been called the vasodilatory cascade. Alternatively, an increase in CPP results in vasoconstriction of cerebral vessels and reduction of CBF. When pressure autoregulation is impaired, ICP decreases, and increases with changes in CPP. At CPP values less than 50 mm Hg, the brain may not be able to compensate adequately, and CBF falls. Lack of cerebral blood flow causes inadequate oxygen and glucose for the brain.

Mechanisms That Increase ICP

Mechanisms that increase the volume of one or more of three compartments—circulation, brain tissue, and

---

BOX 35-1. Major Causes of Intracranial Hypertension

Major causes of intracranial hypertension can occur singularly or in combination. In primary causes of increased ICP, normalization of ICP depends on rapidly addressing the underlying brain disorder. In the second group, intracranial hypertension is due to an extracranial or systemic process that is often treatable. The last group is composed of the causes of increased ICP after a neurosurgical procedure.

Intracranial (Primary)
- Brain tumor
- Trauma (epidural and subdural hematoma, cerebral contusions)
- Nontraumatic intracerebral hemorrhage
- Ischemic stroke
- Hydrocephalus
- Idiopathic or benign intracranial hypertension
- Other (e.g., pseudotumor cerebri, pneumocephalus, abscesses, cysts)

Extracranial (Secondary)
- Airway obstruction
- Hypoxia or hypercarbia (hypoventilation)
- Hypertension (pain/cough) or hypotension (hypovolemia/sedation)
- Posture (head rotation)
- Hyperpyrexia
- Seizures
- Drug and metabolic (e.g., tetracycline, rofecoxib, divalproex sodium, lead intoxication)
- Others (e.g., high-altitude cerebral edema, hepatic failure)

Postoperative
- Mass lesion (hematoma)
- Edema
- Increased cerebral blood volume (vasodilation)
- Disturbances of CSF

CSF—will increase ICP (see Fig. 35-1). Cerebral edema is a common cause of increased ICP. Major causes of cerebral edema include trauma, hemorrhage, tumor, inflammation, and ischemia. Trauma causes a shearing stress on the brain that leads to **vasogenic cerebral edema.** In this form of edema, the pores of the brain's capillaries open wide, allowing proteins and fluids to leak from the blood into the tissues.

Cerebral hemorrhage creates another form of cerebral edema. A ruptured cerebral vessel creates a pool of blood that forms a space-occupying lesion within the closed cranium. The collection of blood is toxic to brain cells and places pressure on brain tissue, which rapidly increases ICP.

In the case of a brain tumor, the excess tumor tissue changes the equilibrium of the ICP's components. When the volume of brain tissue increases, CSF and circulation decrease to maintain normal ICP. However, at some point, circulation and CSF cannot sufficiently diminish to counterbalance the brain tissue expansion. This is when ICP increases and symptoms become apparent. A brain tumor also compresses blood flow, which causes venous congestion and increased hydrostatic pressure, resulting in edema. Alternatively, when an inflammatory condition is present in the brain, the permeability of capillary membranes increases and allows fluid to flow out into the tissue, creating edema.

Another kind of edema, **cytotoxic cerebral edema,** forms with cerebral ischemia or hypoxia. If not reversed, it results in brain cell death. Ischemia leads to failure of ion pumps, which leads to cellular swelling. Cellular swelling increases the volume of brain tissue, which increases ICP. Also, when there are low oxygen levels or high carbon dioxide levels in the brain, a reflexive cerebral vasodilation is initiated. This increases the brain's blood volume, leading to increased ICP.

> **ALERT!** Compression of the jugular vein with tracheostomy ties or tight cervical collars reduces blood flow from the brain, resulting in increased venous blood volume within the brain. This can lead to increased ICP. Care must be taken to avoid this in patients with TBI.

Mechanisms That Decrease ICP

Decreasing volume of any one of the three compartments—brain tissue, CSF, or circulation—will decrease the ICP (see Fig. 35-1). For example, externally draining CSF via a catheter placed in the ventricles will lower ICP. Blood volume can also be reduced by lowering blood pressure. Infusing a hypertonic solution such as IV mannitol can rapidly decrease intracellular pressure and lower cerebral edema. A low carbon dioxide level will vasoconstrict cerebral arteries, reducing the volume of blood delivered to the brain. Removing brain tissue, such as occurs in a lobectomy, will likewise decrease volume and ICP.

Another method to decrease ICP is a decompressive craniectomy, in which a section of the skull is removed, creating an opening in the closed space of the skull and allowing expansion of the brain. This allows the ICP to increase without the danger of compressing brain tissue (see Fig. 35-4).

> **ALERT!** All polytrauma patients should be treated as if there is an SCI until proved otherwise. Spinal immobilization is required in all trauma patients.

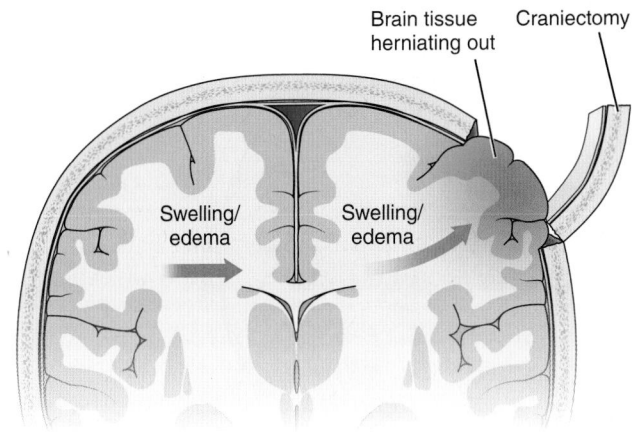

FIGURE 35-4. Open craniectomy allowing brain tissue decompression. Decompressive craniectomy is a neurological procedure in which part of the skull is removed to allow a swelling brain room to expand without being squeezed. It is performed on victims of TBI.

Brain Death

Brain death is the irreversible end of all brain activity (see Box 35-2). Vital centers of the brainstem control heart rate, respiratory rate, blood pressure, and LOC, referred to as brainstem reflexes. When ICP is elevated, the brain tissue is compressed and forced downward in the skull to become herniated or displaced to another region of the brain. The most common type of herniation is a **transtentorial herniation,** also called **uncal herniation.** Part of the temporal lobe (the uncus) is forced through the tentorial notch—the opening in the sheet of tissue between the temporal lobe and cerebellum (see Fig. 35-5). This brain tissue compression results in death to brain tissue. If the herniation compresses vital centers of the brainstem, death ensues.

> ### BOX 35-2. Brain Death
>
> The cardinal findings of brain death are coma, absence of brainstem reflexes, and apnea. Before determination of brain death, patients must have normal temperatures and be free of drugs that depress brain activity, such as barbiturates and alcohol. Only a neurologist or neurosurgeon can determine a patient's brain death. Ancillary tests to confirm brain death include electroencephalogram, cerebral angiogram, and nuclear cerebral flow study. Repeated EEGs will reveal no brain activity for at least 30 minutes. A cerebral angiogram and nuclear cerebral blood flow study that show complete absence of intracranial blood flow can be used to confirm the diagnosis of brain death.

Normal position
of brain tissue

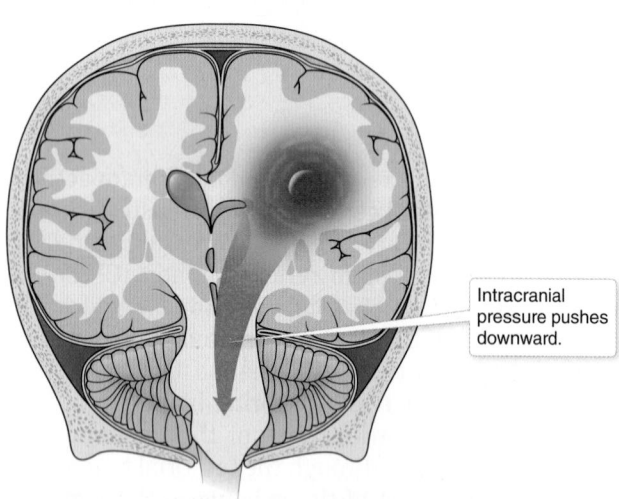

Brainstem: controls
vital functions
(consciousness,
heart rate, BP,
respiratory rate)

Foramen
magnum

Intracranial
pressure pushes
downward.

FIGURE 35-5. Uncal herniation. The skull is a rigid structure that houses the brain and related structures; it cannot accommodate expansion of the tissues and fluid within. Should there be swelling or bleeding within the brain tissue or cranial cavity, ICP pushes brain tissue downward. This is a critical condition because it places pressure on the brainstem, the center of all vital functions.

Neurological Assessment of TBI

Individuals who sustain any type of significant trauma, particularly of the head or spine, should be evaluated to determine the nature and extent of the injury. A thorough history of the events that led to the injury is essential, along with a complete description of the presenting signs and symptoms.

Components of the Assessment

A neurological examination is essential in the trauma setting to evaluate the function of the vital portions of the central nervous system. The severity of brain injury is determined after the patient has been fully resuscitated and any drugs or alcohol have cleared the patient's system, usually at 24 to 48 hours postinjury.

The physical examination should begin with careful observation of the patient and inspection for signs of head trauma (see Table 35-1).

The examination should focus on testing the patient's LOC, mental status, cranial nerves, sensory status, motor status, and deep tendon reflexes. In comatose patients, the examination consists of observing the patient closely and eliciting reflexes to assess the level of cerebral input. The Glasgow Coma Scale is a commonly used system for grading the severity of brain injury and serves to supplement the neurological assessment of patients in the trauma setting.

Other indices of severity of injury are duration of unconsciousness and post-traumatic amnesia (PTA). Patients with severe TBI are generally unconscious at least 24 hours and have PTA that lasts longer than 7 days, usually 1 to 4 weeks. Patients with moderate TBI are unconscious between 1 and 24 hours and have PTA duration of 1 to 7 days. Patients with mild TBI may or may not experience unconsciousness; if they do, it will be for less than an hour. PTA duration for a mild TBI is fewer than 24 hours. Both longer periods of unconsciousness and longer duration of PTA are associated with decreased functional recovery.

Declining Levels of Consciousness

Declining LOC involves reduced responsiveness to stimuli. It exists on a continuum that ranges from drowsiness to stupor, and finally to coma. All levels except coma involve being able to arouse the person to respond; however, each level requires more effort and results in less response.

The difference between consciousness and unconsciousness can be determined by eye opening. People

TABLE 35-1. **Head Trauma Findings**	
Findings that may be present on inspection in direct head trauma.	
Bony-Step Off	Palpable discontinuity in the shape of the skull due to displaced fracture
CSF Rhinorrhea	Exudation of cerebrospinal fluid (clear liquid) from the nose
CSF Otorrhea	Exudation of cerebrospinal fluid (clear liquid) from the ear
Hemotympanum	Dark blood visible behind the tympanic membrane (eardrum)
Battle's Sign	Dark bruising visible in the skin overlying the mastoid process (bony prominence just posterior to the ears)
Raccoon Eyes	Dark bruising visible in the skin around the eyes

who are able to respond to stimulation by opening their eyes are not in a coma. Patients in a vegetative state can open their eyes and are not comatose, though they are not aware of their environment. Individuals who progress up to a minimally responsive state are slowly gaining awareness of their environment.

 CLINICAL CONCEPT

Treat all patients in coma or vegetative state as if they are able to hear their surroundings.

A return of the sleep–wake cycle is the first sign that a patient is slowly improving. The longer the patient is not responsive to stimuli, the poorer the prognosis. Patients who do not open their eyes in response to stimulation after 30 days have a poor prognosis.

The Glasgow Coma Scale

The **Glasgow Coma Scale (GCS)** is used to determine the degree of consciousness impairment associated with head injury and was designed to be used as a noninvasive bedside tool capable of charting a patient's LOC over time (see Box 35-3).

A single GCS score cannot determine the degree of injury after head trauma. However, serial GCS scores are useful when they can be compared over time. An initially low GCS score that stays low or a high GCS that decreases predicts a worse outcome than a persistently high GCS or a low GCS that progressively increases with time.

 CLINICAL CONCEPT

PTA duration is a better predictor of cognitive function 2 years postinjury than is length of coma.

Coma and Posturing

A person in a coma often takes on one of two rigid positions due to increased ICP (see Fig. 35-6). **Decorticate posture** is a position in which a person is stiff with flexed arms, clenched fists, and legs held out straight. The arms are flexed in toward the body, and the wrists and fingers are flexed and held on the chest. This type of posturing results from damage to the corticospinal tract. **Decerebrate posture** is an abnormal position where the arms are held straight out and toes pointed downward. The shoulders and neck are slightly arched as the patient lies supine. Decerebrate posturing results from upper brainstem damage and indicates more extensive brain damage than does decorticate posturing.

Clinical Manifestations of ICP

As ICP increases within the skull, cranial nerves and brain tissue are compressed. Early signs of increasing ICP

BOX 35-3. Glasgow Coma Scale

EYE OPENING RESPONSE
- Spontaneous–open with blinking at baseline: **4 points**
- To verbal stimuli, command, speech: **3 points**
- To pain only (not applied to face): **2 points**
- No response: **1 point**

VERBAL RESPONSE
- Oriented: **5 points**
- Confused conversation, but able to answer questions: **4 points**
- Inappropriate words: **3 points**
- Incomprehensible speech: **2 points**
- No response: **1 point**

MOTOR RESPONSE
- Obeys commands for movement: **6 points**
- Purposeful movement to painful stimulus: **5 points**
- Withdraws in response to pain: **4 points**
- Flexion in response to pain (decorticate posturing): **3 points**
- Extension response in response to pain (decerebrate posturing): **2 points**
- No response: **1 point**

CLASSIFICATION
- Severe head injury: **score of 8 or less**
- Moderate head injury: **score of 9 to 12**
- Mild head injury: **score of 13 to 15**

From Centers for Disease Control and Prevention. (n.d.). Glasgow Coma Scale. http://www.cdc.gov/masstrauma/resources/gcs.pdf; Teasdale, G., & Jennet, B. (1974). Assessment of coma and impaired consciousness. *Lancet, 2*(7872), 81–84; Teasdale, G., & Jennet, B. (1976). Assessment and prognosis of coma after head injury. *Acta Neurochirurgica, 34*(1–4), 45–55.

---

include headache, caused by direct compression of brain tissue; vomiting, caused by compression of the vomiting center in the medulla; and decreasing LOC, caused by compression of the reticular activating system.

Pressure on the third cranial nerve (oculomotor) caused by an uncal herniation will produce an altered response of the pupil to light and alter the pupil's size (see Fig. 35-7). If ICP continues to rise and causes significant pressure on the brainstem, a triad of symptoms called **Cushing's triad** occurs. These late signs consist of hypertension with a widened pulse pressure (difference between systolic and diastolic pressures), slowed heart rate (bradycardia), and slowed respirations (bradypnea).

ALERT! Increased intracranial pressure can displace downward onto the brainstem, which is a life-threatening event. Cushing's triad–bradycardia, bradypnea, and hypertension–is a sign of this disorder and requires immediate action.

Decorticate posturing

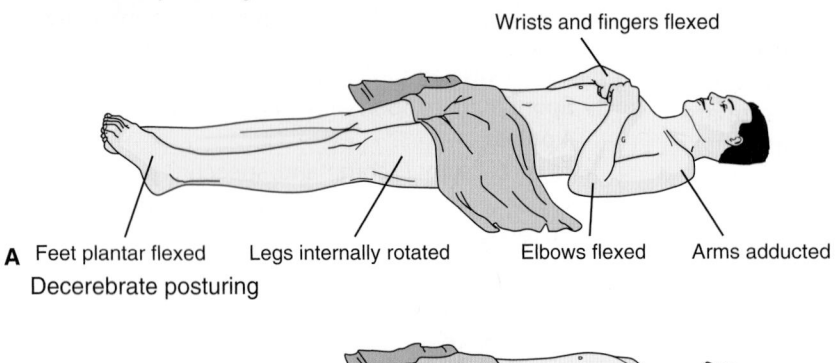

A

Decerebrate posturing

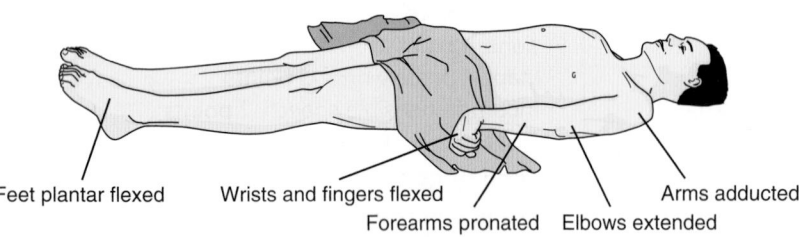

B

FIGURE 35-6. Decorticate and decerebrate posturing in coma. The patient can assume either decorticate (**A**) or decerebrate (**B**) postures depending on what part of the brain is damaged. Decorticate posture results from damage to the corticospinal tract, whereas decerebrate posture results from upper brainstem damage. In both postures, the patient exhibits extended, adducted legs with foot drop: a plantar flexion of the feet. In decorticate posture, the arms and wrists are flexed. In decerebrate posture, the arms are adducted and wrists are pronated.

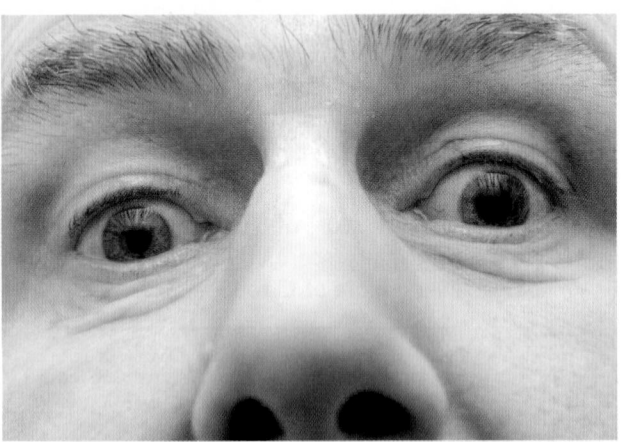

FIGURE 35-7. Pupil size alteration after head injury. *(From SPL/Science Source.)*

Cranial Nerve Testing

The cranial nerves arise in the brain and exit at the brainstem. They are thin, antenna-like nerve tracts that are sensitive to any change in ICP. The cranial nerves should be assessed on both sides, and findings should be symmetric. Asymmetry can indicate upper neuron damage or specific injury to that cranial nerve. Cranial nerves II through XII are evaluated in the neurological examination.

The pupil reaction to light shows whether there is an intact pathway from the retina via the optic nerve (CN II) to the midbrain then back to the pupillary sphincter muscle via the oculomotor nerve (CN III). The presence of asymmetrically responsive pupils may be caused by any defect along this neural pathway or due to brainstem damage.

Extraocular movements (EOMs) are controlled by the oculomotor (CN III), trochlear (CN IV), and abducens (CN VI) nerves. The oculocephalic reflex is also called "doll's eyes movements," where the eyes move in the direction opposite to head movement. The absence of this reflex suggests brainstem dysfunction in the comatose patient but can be normal in the awake/conscious patient. The lack of a corneal reflex on either side in the comatose patient suggests damage to the trigeminal nerve (CN V) or facial nerve (CN VII).

Loss of hearing can suggest damage to the vestibulocochlear nerve (CN VIII). Lack of a gag reflex or asymmetric elevation of the uvula is indicative of damage to either the glossopharyngeal nerve (CN IX) or the vagus nerve (CN X). Significant weakness or asymmetry of the shoulder shrug involves the accessory nerve (CN XI), and deviation of the tongue to one side occurs with damage to the hypoglossal nerve (CN XII).

Sensory Testing

For responsive patients, a sensory examination may be performed. Different kinds of sensations are perceived by the brain via different pathways, and specific patterns of sensory impairment can be a clue to the location or nature of the injury. The skin surface on the four extremities should be systematically tested to determine any pattern of the deficit. Light touch is assessed by applying a very light stimulus, such as a cotton swab. Pain sensation typically is assessed using the sharp end of a paper clip. Joint position sense can be tested when the examiner grasps the sides of a distal phalanx (furthest digit segment) of a finger or toe and slightly displaces the joint up or down. The patient, with eyes closed during this part, is asked to report any perceived change in position.

Motor Testing

The motor examination requires inspection, palpation, and functional testing with tone and strength testing of individual muscle groups. First, the clinician should inspect and palpate to detect visible abnormalities. Muscle twitches, tremors, involuntary movements, or tenderness should be noted. The clinician should assess the patient's injuries and be cautious with manipulation of any extremities to prevent worsening of any injuries.

Before testing strength, have the patient hold their arms outstretched with palms upward for several seconds and observe any abnormal inward rotation or downward drift in their hands from their initial position, known as "pronator drift." This is an indication of corticospinal defect in the cerebral hemisphere on the opposite side.

Muscle tone is judged by palpation of the muscles of the extremities and by passive movements of the joints by the examiner. Any change in resistance to movement should be noted.

Often clinicians complete a rapid motor assessment by asking the patient to grip the clinician's hands with all their strength bilaterally. Then the clinician asks the patient to move each lower leg against the clinician's resistance.

For complete motor assessment, muscle strength should be assessed in the extremities, neck, and trunk. This is accomplished by providing resistance to movement of muscle groups in both directions and assessing any indication of diminished strength. The following scale is used to describe muscle strength, rated on a scale of 0/5 to 5/5 as follows:

- 0/5 – No contraction
- 1/5 – Muscle flicker, but no movement
- 2/5 – Movement possible, but not against gravity
- 3/5 – Movement possible against gravity, but not resistance
- 4/5 – Movement possible against some resistance
- 5/5 – Normal strength

Deep Tendon Reflex Assessment

The deep tendon reflexes are used to test the sensory and motor fibers of spinal nerves. The tendons of specific muscles are tapped using a reflex hammer. A reflex response should be noted immediately following the hammer stimulus. The biceps, triceps, patella, and ankle reflexes are commonly tested. The right- and left-side response should be symmetrical. Reflex responses to stimuli can be rated according to the following scale:

- 0 – Absent reflex
- 1+ – Trace response
- 2+ – Normal response
- 3+ – Brisk response
- 4+ – Nonsustained clonus (repetitive vibratory movements)
- 5 + – Sustained clonus

Evaluating Coordination and Gait

Coordination and gait reflect the function of the cerebellum; therefore, they are tested separately from other sensory and motor testing. If the patient is ambulatory, assess the patient's walking motion. Observe the patient's posture, gait, coordinated automatic movements (swinging arms), and ability to walk in a straight line. The Romberg test is conducted with the patient standing with heels and toes together with eyes closed. The examiner should observe if the patient sways or fails to maintain posture. Rapid repetitive movements can be tested by having the patient place their palms on their thighs and turning the palms upside down rapidly for a few seconds. In the finger-to-nose test, the patient places the tip of a finger on their nose and then touches the examiner's finger, which is placed at arm's length distance away. This motion should be repeated as rapidly as possible, while the examiner changes the finger location. A lower extremity equivalent of this test is the heel-to-shin test. In this test, the patient places one heel on the opposite knee and then moves the heel up and down along the shin. With both the finger-to-nose and heel-to-shin test, each extremity should be tested separately.

Mental Status Examination

A mental status examination is a short test that evaluates the patient's orientation, cognition, language ability, and memory. Day, month, year, and season are commonly asked of the patient. Also some mathematical skills and spatial sense are assessed. This can be accomplished using the mini-mental status examination (MMSE) or mini-cog test. In dementia, a clock-drawing test can be used.

Severity of TBI

TBI is a nonspecific term for an injury to the brain due to various injury mechanisms (i.e., blunt, penetrating, or blast injury). TBI can be classified as mild, moderate, or severe; this classification is based on the GCS score. The term "concussion" indicates mild TBI and is defined as a reversible impairment of neurological function following head injury. Clinical features of concussion include LOC during the traumatic injury, "seeing stars" (visual changes), and other symptoms such as headache, dizziness, nausea, and vomiting. A concussion or mild TBI can result in a transient change in mental status, while a severe TBI can result in extended periods of unconsciousness, and in some cases, can lead to coma or even death. The following is the classification of TBI, based on associated GCS score and mortality rates:

- Mild/minor TBI: GCS 13 to 15; mortality 0.1%
- Moderate TBI: GCS 9 to 12; mortality 10%
- Severe TBI: GCS less than 9; mortality 40%

Individuals with mild TBI can develop postconcussive syndrome (PCS), which includes headaches, lethargy, mental dullness, and other symptoms that can persist for several months after a TBI. Impaired consciousness can occur in response to damage to the brainstem; however, toxicity or metabolic disorders can also cause decreased LOC. These disorders must be investigated with the assessment of head trauma.

Diagnostic Studies

Computed tomography (CT) scan, the test of choice for acute TBI, demonstrates areas of acute bleeding and pressure on the brain's vital structures.

Serial CT scans over a number of days can be used to follow hemorrhage size, mass effect, or CSF volume in more seriously injured patients. CT angiography (CTA) uses a dye to highlight the larger blood vessels of the brain or neck. These pictures are two-dimensional, but advanced technology enables viewing as three-dimensional images so that traumatic aneurysms, vascular dissections, or occlusions can be seen. This is particularly necessary for skull fractures.

Magnetic resonance imaging (MRI) examines the brain's deeper structures. It may be used in mild TBI during the evaluation of persistent symptoms, showing subtle areas of edema or microhemorrhage. MRI is also indicated in patients with more severe TBI to gain a more detailed picture of the brain's deeper structures. The utility of MRI is limited because of its many contraindications, including retained metal fragments and internal pumps or pacemakers. Electroencephalogram (EEG) uses scalp electrodes to monitor the brain's electrical activity. In addition to evaluating seizures, EEG can be used therapeutically to determine the depth of drug-induced coma.

Treatment of TBI

Emergency Treatment for TBI

The ABCs of resuscitation and neurovascular stabilization are priorities in emergency care of head or spinal cord injury. The clinician needs to ensure adequate oxygenation and blood flow to the brain, control of blood pressure, and stabilization of the head and neck. The patient should be stabilized in the supine position with cervical bracing and spinal immobilization on a flat board, after which the patient should be transferred to a trauma care unit. Once the patient is stable, surgery may be necessary to reduce additional damage to the brain tissues. Surgical procedures to remove intracranial blood accumulation between the skull and layers of meninges, such as epidural or subdural hematoma, may be needed. Accumulation of blood can place pressure on the brain. Craniotomy or craniectomy may be necessary to relieve pressure and facilitate removal of a hematoma. If the skull is fractured, stabilizing the cranial bone and removing debris from the brain may be necessary. Adding a shunt or drain can relieve pressure inside the skull and allow excess fluid to drain. Cerebral edema, if present, can be decreased with hypertonic IV fluid such as IV mannitol.

Treatment of Mild TBI

Most patients with mild TBI will improve within 3 to 6 months without any interventions. Patients and families need education regarding expected symptoms and reasonable coping mechanisms. Promotion of adequate sleep can help minimize symptoms. Certain activities, such as working on a computer and intense concentration, can cause fatigue. The person with TBI should reduce these kinds of activities or take frequent rest periods. In addition, alcohol and other drugs can slow recovery and increase the chances of reinjury. Children and teens who may have sustained a concussion during sports should stop playing immediately. They should not return to play until a health-care provider who is experienced in evaluating concussion confirms they are ready. Reinjury during recovery can slow healing and increase the chances of long-term problems. Daily headaches benefit from prophylactic medications, including antidepressants, antiepileptics, and migraine-type medications. Patients should be counseled that overuse, defined as more than six doses per week, of over-the-counter medications such as ibuprofen or naproxen sodium may exacerbate headache by leading to rebound headaches. For the same reason, narcotics should be avoided.

Patients with moderate to severe TBI are admitted to an intensive care unit. Many require short-term mechanical ventilation. There is potential for this level of injury to worsen, resulting in increased ICP. Therefore, frequent neurological assessment of the patient's LOC with pupil size and reactivity is necessary.

After acute treatment is completed, rehabilitation therapies may be necessary. Therapies usually begin during inpatient care and then continue posthospitalization. These include physical therapy, occupational therapy, speech therapy, cognitive therapy, and psychological and vocational counseling.

Pathophysiology of Selected Types of TBI

There are different kinds of TBIs. Head injury can affect either a particular structure within the brain or the entire brain. Symptoms depend on the location as well as the extent of the injury. Treatment varies according to the extent of brain tissue damage. Types of TBI include diffuse axonal injury, concussion, cerebral contusion, intracranial bleeding, and skull fractures.

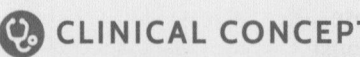

CLINICAL CONCEPT

TBI is commonly due to closed head injury caused by external impact from sudden, violent motion. It can also be caused by penetrating brain injury from gunshot or a sharp laceration wound.

Diffuse Axonal Injury

Diffuse axonal injury (DAI) is one of the most common types of TBI. The damage occurs over a widespread area of brain tissue, mainly white matter, where axons are located. It is the major cause of unconsciousness and persistent coma after head trauma.

Etiology

DAI occurs when the brain moves back and forth in the skull, hitting into the cranial bone, as a result of coup-contrecoup injury or acceleration-deceleration injury. Motor vehicle accidents, sports-related trauma, violence, falls, and child abuse (such as shaken baby syndrome) are common causes of DAI.

Pathophysiology

DAI is characterized by diffuse swelling of neuronal axons, hemorrhage or laceration of the corpus callosum, and hemorrhages in the brainstem. Rapid stretching of axons damages the axonal structure, resulting in a loss of elasticity and impairment of impulse transmission. Calcium entry into damaged axons initiates activation of proteases, which causes further brain cell damage. Swollen, stretched axons may become disconnected. A DAI can also cause swelling in the brain. Swelling causes increased pressure in the brain and can cause decreased blood flow to the brain, along with compression of nerves and tissue.

Clinical Presentation

DAI presents with a wide range of consciousness disorders, varying from full alertness to deep coma. Most patients with DAI fall into the classification of severe TBI and are scored less than 8 points on the GCS, provided that the comatose condition lasts for at least 6 hours after trauma. A person with a mild or moderate DAI who is conscious may show signs of neurological impairment, depending on which area of the brain is affected. Autonomic nervous system dysfunction is often evident and accounts for symptoms such as dizziness, headache, vomiting, palpitations, blood pressure variations, and sweating.

Classification of DAI

As a part of TBI, DAI is divided into mild, moderate, and severe, depending on the score on the GCS. Score between 13 and 15 points indicates mild injury; 9 and 12 points is moderate injury; less than 8 points is severe injury. According to the severity of cellular injury, DAI is classified into three grades: Grade I—DAI with axonal lesions in the cerebral hemispheres; Grade II—DAI with focal axonal lesions in the corpus callosum; Grade III—DAI with focal or multiple axonal lesions in the brainstem. Some researchers suggest extended classification system with additional Grade IV—involvement of the substantia nigra or tegmentum of midbrain lesions. Another classification of DAI is based on the MRI findings: Grade I—lesions in the hemispheric and/or cerebellar white matter; Grade II—lesions in the corpus callosum; and Grade III—lesions in the brainstem in areas typical for DAI.

Diagnosis

DAI is difficult to detect using imaging studies, though MRI is the preferred test for diagnosis. CT scan is less sensitive to DAI, with many patients exhibiting a normal CT scan upon presentation. The degree of microscopic injury is considered to be greater than that seen on diagnostic imaging. DAI is suggested in any patient who demonstrates clinical symptoms disproportionate to CT scan findings.

Potential Biomarkers in TBI

Many research studies have attempted to correlate the neuronal injury in DAI and TBI with specific cellular biomarkers. CT and MRI studies often do not demonstrate the severity of injury of the brain in DAI or mild TBI. Therefore, cellular micromolecules released during neuronal injury in the brain can assist the clinician to make diagnoses, monitor efficacy of treatment, and speculate about prognosis. Many biomarkers hold promise in advancing our understanding of TBI during initial injury through injury resolution. Studies are focusing on the following micromolecules that are evidence of neuronal injury in DAI or TBI: β-amyloid precursor protein (β-APP), neurofilament protein (NF), glial fibrillary acidic protein (GFAP), ubiquitin carboxy-terminal hydrolase L1 (UCH-L1), and S100 β. These are critical biomarkers of neuronal death in TBI and research is still evolving. Eventually, biomarkers that correlate with the severity of neuronal injury may help create clinical guidelines and guide treatment of TBI patients.

Treatment

Immediate treatment involves neurovascular stabilization. Until ruled out, the patient should be treated as if there is a cervical injury. The main contributing factor to secondary injury is the neuroinflammatory process caused by the damaged axons and glial cells that leads to proinflammatory cytokine release and oxidative stress. It is fundamental to initiate treatment with anti-inflammatory and neuroprotective drugs immediately after TBI, if possible within 4 hours postinjury, to achieve optimal outcome. Another factor that worsens the neurological status and outcome is ICP. This requires the use of hyperosmolar agents (mannitol, hypertonic sodium solution) to reduce cerebral edema. There are also selected nonpharmacological therapies to reduce ICP that are employed in the acute trauma phase such as elevating the head in bed to 30 degrees and brief episodes of hyperventilation to maintain PCO_2 within 28 to 33 mm Hg with the aim of reducing cerebral edema. In the long term, effective, individually targeted, continuous multidisciplinary rehabilitation programs should also be employed. If the patient has sustained a mild or moderate DAI, rehabilitation should begin after the patient is stabilized and awake. Rehabilitation includes physical therapy, occupational therapy, and speech therapy.

ALERT! All patients with head injury should be treated as if there is also cervical spine injury until proven otherwise.

Concussion

A concussion, also called mild TBI, is a physiological disruption in brain function caused by traumatic forces that may or may not involve loss of consciousness. It is manifested by temporary memory loss and alteration of mental state. The trauma initiates a cascade of metabolic changes in the brain. Not well investigated in the past, concussion has recently become an area of intense research. Concussion in sports activities, in particular, is the subject of many current research studies.

Most information about concussion comes from studies of injured athletes. In studies of high school athletes, concussion accounts for 8% to 11% of all injuries in football. The incidence rate in ice hockey is estimated at 12% of total injuries. In a survey of competitive college athletes engaged in all sports at a university in Ohio, 32% reported concussive symptoms after a blow to the head. Many cases of concussion go unreported because athletes do not want to suffer ineligibility for sports-related activity. Other individuals do not seek medical care for mild head injury, because they perceive the injury as unimportant. For these reasons, the true incidence of concussion is underestimated. At least a 24-hour reprieve from sports activity is mandatory after a concussion. The CDC has a complete set of treatment recommendations for patients with concussion (see the CDC Heads Up Concussion Action Plan).

Etiology

Concussions result from a blow to the head or severe shaking of the head and neck. Contact sports activities, motor vehicle accidents, and shaken baby syndrome are common causes of concussion.

Simple concussions progressively resolve without complications, a process that can take only a few hours or last up to 10 days. Complex concussions consist of persistent symptoms that recur with exertion and are associated with conditions such as seizure, prolonged loss of consciousness (longer than 1 minute), or prolonged impairment of cognitive function.

A previous concussion is a significant risk factor for sustaining another concussion. Studies show that the risk of sustaining a concussion is four to five times higher in patients who had at least one concussion in the past.

Pathophysiology

Several different theories attempt to explain the pathophysiology of concussion. All theories contain the following basic concepts:

1. Concussion may be caused by a direct blow to the head, face, neck, or elsewhere on the body that involves a traumatic force transmitted to the head.
2. Concussion results in an acute, short-term neurological dysfunction that resolves spontaneously.
3. Concussion results in neuropathological functional changes in the brain but no structural brain injury.
4. Concussion results in symptoms that may or may not involve loss of consciousness.
5. Concussion is typically associated with grossly normal structural neuroimaging studies.
6. Multiple concussions can have a cumulative effect on the brain.

Concussion occurs when traumatic impact causes a sudden strain on the brain tissue from rotational or acceleration-deceleration forces. On a cellular level, the strain on neurons in the brain causes metabolic dysfunction, resulting in diffusion of intracellular potassium ions into the extracellular space. This stimulates release of excitatory amino acids, particularly glutamate. Glutamate accumulation is toxic to neurons and causes a temporary disruption of neuronal cell membranes, overstimulating the neurons and causing the neuronal membranes to open their pores. From the extracellular space, sodium flows into the neuron membrane pores, followed by water. This is followed by temporary neuronal cellular swelling. Cellular ions stabilize, swelling resolves over time, and cellular homeostasis is returned, with no remaining structural changes in the brain.

Clinical Presentation

Concussions are characterized by an alteration in consciousness, such as being dazed, confused, or "seeing stars," or, less commonly, a brief loss of consciousness. Headache, dizziness, confusion, double vision, sensitivity to light and noise, slowed reaction time, and flat affect are common initially. Imbalance and lack of coordination are also present. Both pretraumatic (retrograde) amnesia and post-traumatic (antegrade) amnesia can occur. Usually, the duration of amnesia, or memory loss, is brief, lasting seconds to minutes, depending on the injury.

Vomiting may suggest a significant brain injury with associated elevated ICP. Other signs of increased ICP include worsening headache, increasing disorientation, and changing LOC. If these symptoms are present, the possible causes of increasing ICP include subdural hematomas, epidural hematomas (EDHs), or some other type of intracranial hemorrhage.

Postconcussion syndrome (PCS) is the persistence of symptoms for more than 3 weeks after the initial injury. The symptoms associated with this include headache, dizziness, imbalance, fatigue, irritability, insomnia, and concentration or memory difficulties.

Diagnosis

The initial assessment of an acute concussion should begin with cardiac and pulmonary stabilization: checking the airway, breathing, and circulation (ABCs). Cervical spine injury should be considered, and the unconscious individual should be treated as having a potential cervical spine injury. Those with prolonged loss of consciousness should be transported rapidly to an appropriate medical facility.

For the conscious individual suspected of having sustained a concussion, a thorough neurological examination should be performed, including assessment of orientation to person, place, and time. This should be followed by questions to test recent memory, because these are the most sensitive in diagnosing concussion. The clinician should determine whether amnesia has occurred and attempt to determine length of time of memory dysfunction before (retrograde) and after (anterograde) injury. Even seconds to minutes of memory loss can be predictive of outcome. Recent research has indicated that amnesia may be up to 4 to 10 times more predictive of symptoms and cognitive deficits following concussion than is LOC (less than 1 minute). The ability to perform simple tasks and postural stability should be assessed also.

Because concussion results from a disturbance in brain function rather than structural injury, neuroimaging studies, such as CT and MRI, are not routinely recommended. Neuroimaging studies should be reserved for patients with concussion who have LOC, GCS less than 15 at 2 hours or less than 14 at any time, post-traumatic amnesia, post-traumatic seizure, focal neurological deficit, clinical deterioration of condition, and suspected skull fracture. If neuroimaging studies have to be performed, MRI is preferred to avoid exposure to radiation. MRI is superior to CT in its ability to detect white matter injury and is particularly useful for patients with prolonged or worsening symptoms. CT is the test of choice to evaluate for intracranial hemorrhage and skull fractures.

According to the American Association of Neurology (AAN), concussions can be divided into Grade 1, 2, or 3. In Grade 1, there is no loss of consciousness and mental status changes resolve in less than 15 minutes. In Grade 2, there is no loss of consciousness and mental status changes resolve in longer than 15 minutes. In Grade 3, the patient has a loss of consciousness.

The GCS is not an adequately sensitive instrument for mild traumatic head injury. A few different concussion assessment checklists are available for sports-related injuries. The CDC recommends a concussion assessment toolkit based on the AAN guidelines to aid in the evaluation of a concussion. The tool assesses multiple cognitive, physical, and emotional symptoms initially and at 15 minutes and 30 minutes postinjury. The AAN Acute Concussion Evaluation (ACE) tool can be found at https://www.cdc.gov/headsup/pdfs/providers/ACE_ED-a.pdf.

There are certain "red flags" that require patient evaluation in the emergency department (see Box 35-4). The patient with these signs should have a CT scan to rule out intracranial bleeding or other structural pathology. The Sport Concussion Assessment Tool, 5th edition (SCAT5) is an evaluation tool that can be used on student athletes aged 13 and older. This tool can be found at https://bjsm.

BOX 35-4. Acute Concussion Evaluation Tool "Red Flags"

Patients with a concussion require emergency department evaluation if one or more of the following conditions are present:

- Physical evidence of trauma above the clavicles
- Anticoagulation or coagulopathy
- Alcohol or drug intoxication
- Neurological deficit
- Unequal pupils
- Persistent vomiting
- Seizure or short-term memory deficit
- Drowsiness with difficult arousal
- History of alcohol use disorder
- Headache that worsens
- Slurred speech
- Neck pain
- Weakness or numbness in arms or legs
- Change in state of consciousness
- Increasing confusion or irritability
- Cannot recognize persons or place

---

bmj.com/content/bjsports/early/2017/04/26/bjsports-2017-097506SCAT5.full.pdf.

Another SCAT is available for children younger than age 13.

Any athlete with suspected concussion should be removed from play, medically assessed, and monitored for deterioration. No athlete diagnosed with concussion should be returned to play on the day of injury. If an athlete is suspected of having a concussion and medical personnel are not immediately available, the athlete should be referred to a medical facility for urgent assessment. Athletes with suspected concussion should not drink alcohol, should not use recreational drugs, and should not drive a motor vehicle until cleared to do so by a medical professional. Concussion signs and symptoms evolve over time, and it is important to consider repeat evaluation in the assessment of concussion. Past studies have shown that CT scan is normal in more than 90% of concussion patients. However, if headache does not resolve or the patient becomes disoriented or begins to show decreased LOC, medical evaluation is necessary.

Treatment

Most people recover after a concussion, but how quickly they improve depends on many factors. These factors include severity of the concussion, age, state of health before the concussion, and care after the injury. Rest is the most important treatment measure. Patients with concussions are advised to rest for the first 24 to 48 hours and up to 7 days, with a gradual return to regular activities as appropriate. The clinician should assess the patient for neurological deficits, including inspection of pupils, and assessment of orientation to time, place, and person. Counting backward by sevens or reciting the months in reverse order are common tests of cognition. Clinicians assess grip strength, leg strength, ability to speak clearly, gait, and postural stability. The patient should avoid physically demanding activity and not return to work, school, or sports activity without conferring with a physician. The patient can be given a mild pain reliever such as acetaminophen. NSAIDs and aspirin should be avoided as they can increase bleeding. Nausea, if severe, can be treated with ondansetron.

Concussed individuals should return for further medical care and evaluation 24 to 72 hours after the concussive event if the symptoms worsen. The patient may be released after assessment from hospital or emergency department to the care of a trusted person with instructions to return if the patient displays worsening symptoms such as change in consciousness, convulsions, severe headache, extremity weakness, vomiting, bleeding, or hearing deficits.

The CDC has specific five-step treatment guidelines, called the Head's Up Program, regarding recovery from concussion. These can be found on the CDC website: http://www.cdc.gov/headsup/basics/return_to_sports.html.

 CLINICAL CONCEPT

Approximately 90% of concussion symptoms are transient, and symptoms typically resolve within 10 to 14 days. However, persistent postconcussive syndrome occurs when symptoms such as headache, fatigue, dizziness, poor concentration ability, memory difficulties, and insomnia persist beyond 3 months.

Cerebral Contusion

A cerebral contusion is considered a bruise of the brain tissue that occurs with head trauma. Often a contusion consists of scattered areas of bleeding on the brain's surface, most commonly along the undersurface and the frontal and temporal lobes. Cerebral contusions typically result from coup-contrecoup injury. They may also occur with penetrating TBI.

Etiology

The most common causes of contusion include blows to the head from motor vehicle accidents, gunshots, blunt trauma force, falls, and assault. People at high risk are those with mobility problems, those who are active in high-impact contact sports, and people who are taking anticoagulants.

Pathophysiology

A combination of vascular and tissue damage occurs in cerebral contusion, which commonly results from a coup-contrecoup injury. Most of the force of impact from a small, hard object tends to remain at the injury site, leading to a coup contusion. In contrast, impact from a larger object causes less injury at the impact site, and energy is dissipated at the opposite side of the brain because of head motion, called a contrecoup contusion. Cerebral edema typically develops around cerebral contusions within 48 to 72 hours after injury; it is problematic because the brain is contained within the skull, a bony cranial vault with little room for cellular expansion. The swollen brain tissue may become compressed against the bone, which then leads to brain cell damage. Swollen brain tissue can also increase ICP, which decreases blood flow to brain tissue leading to ischemia, infarction, and necrosis. Also, if cerebral edema is severe, downward pressure may be placed on the brainstem, and herniation of brain tissue is possible, which leads to death. Pressure on the brainstem can compress the oculomotor nerve (CN III), which may be exhibited as a dilated pupil. Pressure on the brainstem also affects vital centers and the reticular activating system, exhibited as changes in vital signs and decreased LOC.

Clinical Presentation

The signs and symptoms of a contusion include severe headache, dizziness, vomiting, increased size of one pupil, and sudden weakness in an arm or leg. The person may seem restless, agitated, or irritable. Often, the person has memory loss. These symptoms can last for several hours to several weeks, depending on the severity of the injury. As the brain tissue swells, the person may feel increasingly drowsy or confused. Vital signs may show decreased heart rate and decreased respirations and hypertension, which are signs of pressure on the brainstem. These changes in vital signs require immediate medical attention. If the person is difficult to awaken or loses consciousness, this is a medical emergency.

Diagnosis

Immediate CT scan is needed when cerebral contusion is suspected. However, the true amount of neuronal damage in the injured region can be underestimated. MRI scans have greater sensitivity for cerebral edema. Skull x-ray is necessary to look for fracture. Skull fracture commonly causes rupture of the middle meningeal artery, which results in an epidural hematoma (EDH). Daily CT scans may be needed in the days following cerebral contusion to assess progression or resolution. Cerebral angiography is often performed to visualize blood vessel damage and possible aneurysms.

Treatment

Cardiopulmonary lifesaving measures are the priority with any head injury. The patient should be assessed for ABCs, as well as treated and stabilized as if they have a cervical spinal injury. In the emergency setting, IV mannitol is frequently used to decrease cerebral edema. Craniectomy may be performed, where a piece of skull is removed to relieve the pressure on the brain cells. If cerebral hematoma is present, evacuation of the blood is performed through a craniotomy.

> **ALERT!** Delayed enlargement of brain contusion or hematoma is the most common cause of clinical deterioration and death. Periodic neurological assessment is essential after head injury.

Intracranial Bleeding

Head trauma can cause three types of intracranial bleeds: Epidural hematoma (EDH), subdural hematoma (SDH), or subarachnoid hemorrhage (SAH). Each condition presents in a distinct manner, and each is treated differently. To understand intracranial bleeding, an understanding of the meningeal layers that protect the brain is necessary (see Fig. 35-8).

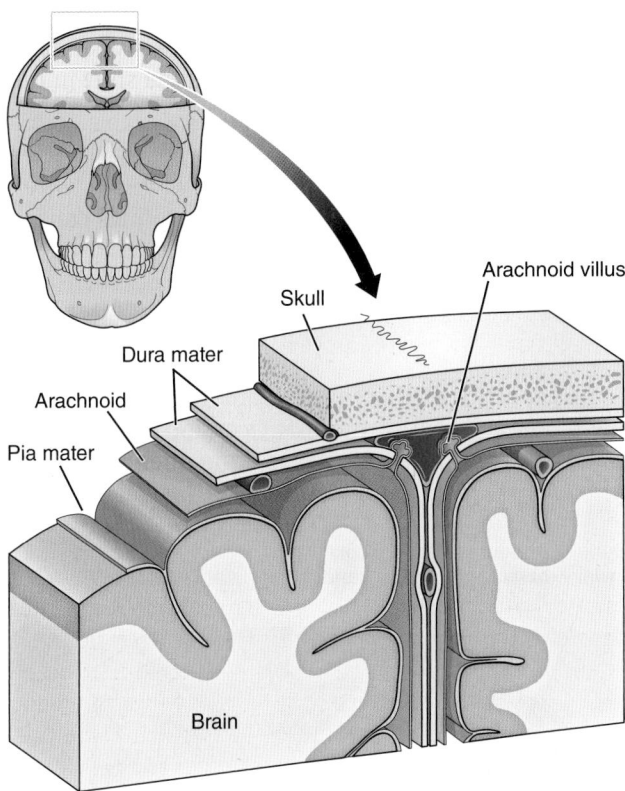

FIGURE 35-8. The meninges. The meninges are layers of membranes that envelop and protect the central nervous system. There are three meningeal membrane layers: the dura mater, arachnoid mater, and pia mater. Between each of the layers is a space. Between the skull bone and dura mater is the epidural space. Beneath the dura mater is the subdural space. Beneath the arachnoid membrane is the subarachnoid space. It is important to note that the middle meningeal artery runs very close to the skull bone above the dura mater. In skull fracture, the middle meningeal artery commonly ruptures and causes an EDH. There is a network of veins within the subdural space, and head trauma often causes rupture of subdural veins, which causes a subdural hematoma. Also, note that the CSF is contained beneath the arachnoid membrane within the subarachnoid space.

Epidural Hematoma

An EDH is a bleed in the space below the skull bone and above the dura mater (see Fig. 35-9). EDH occurs in 1% to 2% of all head trauma cases and in about 10% of patients who present with traumatic coma. Patients younger than 5 years and older than 55 years have an increased mortality rate. Patients younger than 20 years account for 60% of EDHs. EDH is the most serious complication of head injury.

Normally, the middle meningeal artery runs along the skull bone, so close to the bone that it leaves its impression upon the skull. A fracture in the temporal bone of the skull most commonly leads to rupture of the middle meningeal artery, which forms an EDH. Rupture of the artery causes rapid and voluminous arterial bleeding in the epidural space. The bleeding places an increasing amount of pressure on the brain tissue. Brain tissue becomes compressed, and a midline shift in the brain can be visualized on imaging studies within an hour of the injury.

Following injury, there is typically a decreased LOC, then a lucid period, followed by rapid deterioration in physiological status. The patient can be conscious and talking, yet a minute later become apneic, comatose, and minutes from death. Other symptoms include severe headache, vomiting, and seizure. Cushing's triad of hypertension, bradycardia, and bradypnea are indicators of pressure on the brainstem. LOC may be decreased, with decreased or fluctuating GCS. Dilated, sluggish, or fixed pupil(s), bilateral or ipsilateral to injury, suggest increased ICP or herniation. Signs of uncal herniation consist of coma, fixed and dilated pupils, and decerebrate

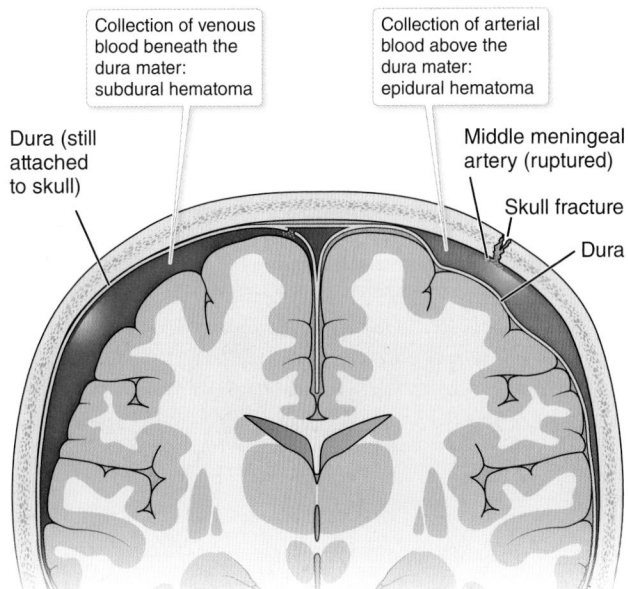

FIGURE 35-9. Epidural and subdural hematoma. An EDH is a collection of arterial blood above the dura mater that is caused by rupture of the middle meningeal artery. This is commonly associated with skull fracture. A subdural hematoma is a collection of venous blood that is beneath the dura mater. Both of these hematomas can place excessive pressure on the brain and cause neurological damage or death.

posturing. Hemiplegia contralateral to the brain injury and a positive Babinski's sign are present.

> **ALERT!** A positive Babinski's sign occurs when stimulation of the sole of the foot causes the toes to flare out. The Babinski's sign is normal in a newborn, but in the adult, it indicates upper neuron cortical dysfunction.

> **ALERT!** Delayed recognition and diagnosis of EDH is a major cause of death.

After severe head trauma, immediate CT scan and skull x-ray are necessary; skull x-ray commonly shows fractures, whereas CT scan will show evidence of bleeding into the epidural space. If bleeding has been prolonged, a midline shift in the brain tissue will be apparent (see Fig. 35-10).

EDH is a neurosurgical emergency requiring a craniotomy and surgical evacuation of the hematoma. The patient requires cardiopulmonary stabilization with airway and blood pressure control, as well as intubation for mechanical ventilation, IV access, oxygen, and cardiac monitoring. Hyperventilating the patient often can decrease ICP. Phenytoin provides prophylaxis against early post-traumatic seizure.

Subdural Hematoma

An SDH results from bleeding that accumulates in the space below the dura mater above the arachnoid membrane. The SDH occurs from tearing of bridging veins located in the subdural space. Acute SDH is the most common type of traumatic intracranial hematoma, occurring in 24% of patients who present in a coma. The bleeding from the subdural veins is slow but can accumulate with time to create substantial ICP that compresses brain tissue. An acute SDH occurs within 72 hours of head injury, whereas a subacute SDH can take several days to accumulate to levels that cause symptoms. Chronic SDH is one that has been present for up to 3 weeks.

Complete neurological examination is necessary. Neurological deficits are commonly not present until there is substantial bleeding into the subdural space. Repeat follow-up neurological examination is required in 2 to 5 days when SDH is suspected. Coagulation profiles are particularly important for patients taking anticoagulants, as well as for patients with alcohol use disorder, who may have coagulation deficiency, placing them at high risk for SDH. CT scan and skull x-ray are therefore necessary. CT scan may or may not show apparent bleeding into the subdural space immediately after injury (see Fig. 35-11). Repeat CT scan is necessary in the next few days when SDH is suspected. If bleeding has been prolonged, a midline shift in the brain tissue will be apparent.

> ### CLINICAL CONCEPT
>
> Alcohol use disorder increases the risk for development of SDH after head trauma.

Large, acute SDHs require craniotomy to evacuate the blood and reduce the ICP. Occasionally, a SDH is small and causes little pressure or no midline shift. In

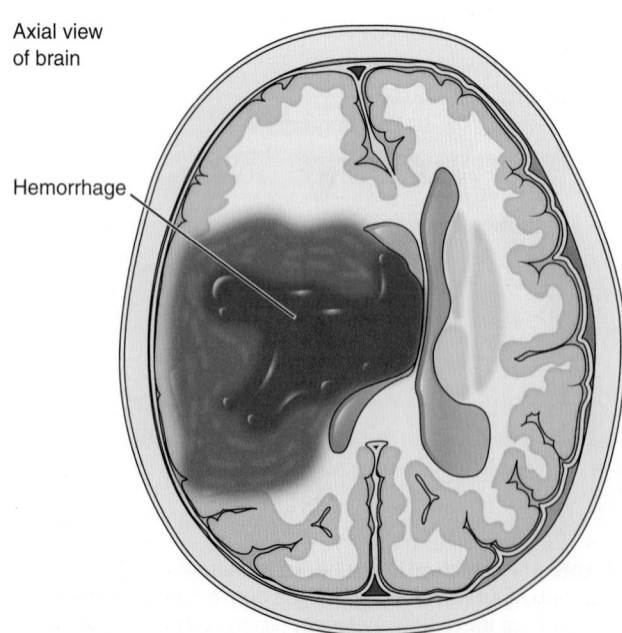

Axial view of brain

Hemorrhage

FIGURE 35-10. In space-occupying lesions, bleeding, and edema of the brain, a midline shift can occur. The pressure of the lesion pushes against the brain tissue.

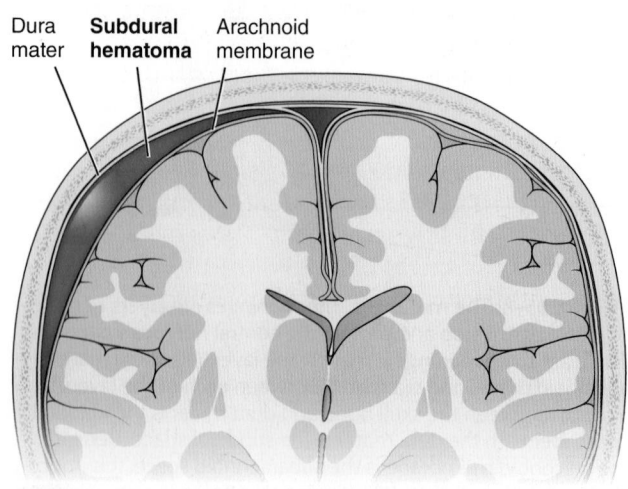

Dura mater   **Subdural hematoma**   Arachnoid membrane

FIGURE 35-11. Subdural hematoma. Head trauma can cause a subdural hematoma, which occurs when veins rupture beneath the dura mater within the subdural space. Blood accumulates beneath the dura mater and above the arachnoid membrane. Accumulation of blood can place pressure on the brain, causing neurological damage.

this case, surgery may be withheld or delayed. A small SDH can slowly be reabsorbed by the brain.

Chronic SDHs result from multiple episodes of minor head trauma in close proximity. Alternatively, small SDHs can fail to be reabsorbed and increase in size as a result of osmotic fluid shifts or membrane formation. Chronic SDHs can be evacuated by craniotomy and catheter placement under the dura mater to drain out the blood.

 CLINICAL CONCEPT

SDH can occur in older adults after minor head trauma, particularly in those who are taking anticoagulants.

Traumatic and Aneurysmal SAH

There are two types of SAH: traumatic and aneurysmal. Traumatic SAH is one of the most common head injuries, accounting for 39% of all closed head injuries. Conversely, aneurysmal SAH is not common; most cases of SAH are due to head trauma. The annual incidence of SAH is 6 to 16 cases per 100,000 population, with approximately 30,000 episodes occurring each year. Approximately 80% of cases of aneurysmal SAH occur in people aged 40 to 65 years, with 15% occurring in people aged 20 to 40 years.

Etiology. Traumatic SAH results from tearing of the cerebral and meningeal vessels within the subarachnoid space of the brain. Causes include rotational-acceleration injury of the brain; stretching of the vertebral artery because of hyperextension of the neck; and sudden trauma to the carotid artery, which raises intra-arterial pressure in the brain. Skull fracture and cerebral contusion are commonly found with traumatic SAH. Post-traumatic cerebral vasospasm also commonly occurs in traumatic SAH. Blood breakdown products within the subarachnoid space are believed to trigger vasospasm of cerebral arteries. Blood from a ruptured cerebral artery is toxic to brain cells.

Cerebral aneurysms usually occur in the terminal portion of the internal carotid artery and the branching sites on the large cerebral arteries in the anterior portion of the circle of Willis. Aneurysms begin as small outpouchings through defects in the muscle layer of an artery wall. They are often called saccular "berry aneurysms" because of their resemblance to a berry on a vine (see Fig. 35-12). These defects are thought to expand as a result of pressure from pulsatile blood flow and blood turbulence, which is greatest at the arterial bifurcations. A mature aneurysm lacks the tunica media, which is replaced by connective tissue. The probability of rupture is related to the tension on the aneurysm wall. Certain conditions increase one's risk for cerebral aneurysms (see Box 35-5).

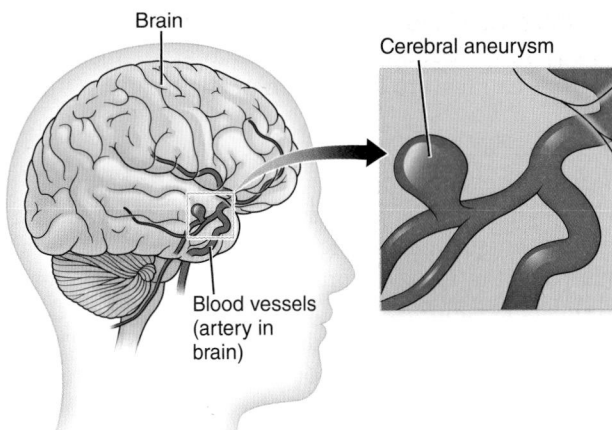

Brain

Cerebral aneurysm

Blood vessels (artery in brain)

FIGURE 35-12. A cerebral aneurysm is a weakening in a cerebral artery wall that bulges out and is susceptible to rupture.

BOX 35-5. Risk Factors for Cerebral Aneurysms

- Aortic coarctation
- Bacterial infections
- Cerebral arteriovenous malformation
- Cerebral atherosclerosis
- Congenital conditions: persistent fetal circulation, hypoplastic/absent arterial circulation
- Ehlers–Danlos syndrome
- Family history of stroke
- Fibromuscular dysplasia
- Fungal infections
- Granulomatous angiitis
- Hypertension
- Klippel-Trenaunay-Weber syndrome
- Long-term analgesic use
- Marfan syndrome
- Metastatic tumors to cerebral arteries: atrial myxoma, choriocarcinoma, undifferentiated carcinoma
- Moyamoya disease
- Osler-Weber-Rendu syndrome
- Persistent headache
- Polycystic kidney disease
- Pregnancy-induced hypertension
- Pseudoxanthoma elasticum
- Systemic lupus erythematosus
- Vascular asymmetry in the circle of Willis

Pathophysiology. Aneurysmal SAH and traumatic SAH have different etiologies, but the pathophysiological mechanisms that cause brain damage are the same. The rupture of a cerebral artery causes a large amount of blood to rapidly fill the subarachnoid space. The blood exerts pressure on the brain, irritates the meninges, and destroys brain cells in its path. If the skull fractures and meningeal layers are torn, this can act as a portal of entry for microorganisms, causing meningitis. SAH can also cause an obstructive hydrocephalus, which is an accumulation of CSF within the brain. The buildup of blood and CSF creates a large amount of ICP that can lead to herniation of the brainstem and death.

Clinical Presentation. In up to 50% of aneurysmal SAH, signs and symptoms precede rupture of the cerebral aneurysm. Leakage of blood from a cerebral aneurysm can cause symptoms. Headache, dizziness, orbital pain, and diplopia can appear 10 to 20 days before rupture. Nuchal rigidity may be present. These symptoms may be ignored or thought to be related to a migraine syndrome. Cranial nerve dysfunction along with memory loss are present in 25% of patients.

 CLINICAL CONCEPT

The rupture of a subarachnoid cerebral aneurysm that results in intracranial bleeding causes an intense "thunderclap" headache. The patient often describes it as the "worst headache of my life." This is a medical emergency because vital signs degenerate rapidly.

The circle of Willis is often the site of a cerebral aneurysm. The cranial nerves exit the brain adjacent to the circle of Willis, and a cerebral aneurysm or leakage of blood from a cerebral aneurysm can compress the cranial nerves. Oculomotor nerve dysfunction with pupil dilation can be exhibited, and vision loss can be caused by compression of the optic nerve. Hemiparesis can result from middle cerebral artery (MCA) aneurysm or ischemia. Patients may also have aphasia, hemineglect, or both.

In the assessment of SAH, clinicians commonly utilize a tool such as the Ottawa Subarachnoid Hemorrhage Rule (OSAH). According to Perry et al. (2017), the OSAH Rule can determine which patients who are neurologically intact but experiencing a new, rapidly peaking headache require investigation. This rule can help standardize which patients with headache do not require investigation to rule out SAH. Careful application of the rule can identify patients who need CT scanning and lumbar puncture to rule out SAH.

Unfortunately, in aneurysmal SAH there are often no outward signs of the impending rupture or hemorrhage, and death occurs within minutes of the event. Patients who suffer the sudden rupture of the aneurysm complain of "the worst headache of my life" just before unconsciousness. The patient is commonly found comatose, and death quickly ensues.

Diagnosis. The diagnosis of SAH can be based on CT scan without contrast, cerebral angiogram, and lumbar puncture. CT scan is followed by lumbar puncture, which demonstrates blood in the CSF. A noncontrast CT followed by CT angiogram of the brain can rule out SAH with greater than 99% sensitivity.

Treatment. Current treatment recommendations involve management in an intensive care unit setting because the patient requires hemodynamic stabilization. Breathing, blood pressure, and heart rate are maintained with consideration of the patient's neurological status. Additional medical management is directed toward the prevention and treatment of complications. Surgical treatment consists of clipping the berry aneurysm. Endovascular treatment is also often done. A catheter can insert thin wire coils into the aneurysm to block it off from blood flow.

Skull Fractures

The skull is prone to fracture in certain regions where the cranial bone has low density. Susceptible areas include the temporal bone, orbital fossa, base of the skull, and foramen magnum. Temporal bone fractures represent 15% to 48% of all skull fractures, whereas basilar skull fractures represent 19% to 21% of all skull fractures.

A **basilar skull fracture (BSF)** is a critical type of skull fracture. Basilar skull fractures are fractures of the occipital part of the skull; an area of bone that is thin and fragile. BSF make are mainly caused by high-velocity blunt trauma and falls from significant heights. BSFs are often associated with other central nervous systems (CNS) pathologies like epidural hematoma due to the weakness of the temporal bone and the close proximity of the middle meningeal artery. At least 50% of BSFs are associated with another CNS injury and about 10% have cervical spine fracture.

Etiology
Skull fracture occurs with a direct blow to the head or traumatic injury of the body, such as a fall, where the head hits an unmovable surface. Risk factors for skull fracture include motor vehicle accidents, contact-sports activities, and falls.

Pathophysiology
Skull fractures are categorized as linear, depressed, or basilar, and may or may not involve injury to the brain tissue. Linear fracture, the most common type of fracture, does not affect brain tissue. Depressed fractures occur when an object fractures the skull with sufficient force to push bone fragments into the brain. Depressed fractures are commonly open fractures that involve underlying brain tissue. The temporal bone is the most commonly fractured bone of the skull. Basilar skull fractures, fractures at the base of the skull, occur in the temporal bone. Fractures that involve the temporal bone continue along the skull base with a pattern that follows the weakest points of the anatomy. The temporal bone encloses vital structures such as the inner ear organs, cranial nerves, meningeal membrane, carotid artery, and jugular vein. Injury to any of these structures can occur with temporal bone fracture. Injury to cranial nerves III, IV, VI, VII, and VIII are possible.

Clinical Presentation

BSFs are critical injuries. They occur most often along the middle fossa and may involve brain injury. Fractures in the middle fossa may produce **Battle's sign,** which is bruising of the mastoid process behind the ear on the affected side. There may also be a CSF leak from the ear (CSF otorrhea) or the nose (CSF rhinorrhea). Fractures in the frontal fossa can result in periorbital ecchymosis, referred to as **raccoon eyes;** edema; and CSF leak from the nose (see Fig. 35-13). Dizziness, hearing loss, nystagmus, and hemotympanum (bulging purple tympanic membrane) may be noted on examination of the individual. It is important to recognize that symptoms of BSF can be delayed by 1 to 2 days post-trauma.

Diagnosis

To diagnose a skull fracture, an x-ray of the head is usually done, followed by a CT scan. MRI or magnetic resonance angiography (MRA) is of value for suspected vascular injury. Anyone with a head injury should have a complete neurological examination. Multidetector CT (MDCT) thin-slice scanning through the face and skull base may aid in the detection of subtle fractures. Pneumocephalus should raise the suspicion for a basilar skull fracture. Further imaging with CT angiography and venography (CTA, CTV) to assess for vascular injury should be considered in the acute setting.

🐾 CLINICAL CONCEPT

After skull fracture, discharge from the nose (rhinorrhea) or ear (otorrhea) should be tested for beta-2-transferrin and glucose, which are diagnostic for CSF. Loss of CSF can cause headache, nausea, vomiting, and dizziness.

Treatment

Treatment for skull fractures involves controlling pain, promoting healing, and preventing complications. The primary concern with skull fracture is potential TBI and epidural hematoma. Most linear skull fractures do not require specific treatment. If there are no complications of brain injury or epidural hematoma, the patient is treated for any external head wound and discharged with instructions to watch for late-developing signs of neurological deficit that may indicate a brain injury.

A linear skull fracture at the base of the skull can cause a tear in the meninges surrounding the brain. CSF, which is a clear or pink-tinged fluid, can leak from the nose or ear. A concern is that the tear in the meninges may provide a path for infection; therefore, an antibiotic may be prescribed. A tear in the meninges can seal by itself in as little as 48 hours, but patients are nonetheless often admitted to the hospital for a brief period for observation.

In a depressed fracture, if bone fragments are dislodged, surgery may be required to align, elevate, or remove fragments. If the bone has not penetrated the meninges and there are no signs of brain injury, a full recovery can be expected. However, concussion symptoms may persist for months. Treatment is often determined by the depth of the depression, whether it is accompanied by an open wound, and the degree of accompanying brain trauma. Deep, open skull fracture is frequently accompanied by brain damage. Surgery is often required to elevate the bone and remove any fragments. Surgery may also be needed to treat bleeding inside the skull. In these cases, mild to severe impairment and disability caused by the brain injury can be expected. If cerebral bleeding or edema is present, the patient often requires a craniotomy or craniectomy, which removes a small section of skull bone to allow expansion of brain tissue.

Spinal Cord Injury

SCI results from compression, stretching, or laceration of the spinal cord following trauma. It can also occur from conditions that impair blood flow to the spinal cord. Injury to the spinal cord leads to temporary or permanent loss of normal sensory, motor, or autonomic function. These deficits are seen immediately following the injury. Further deterioration may occur as edema of the spinal cord develops. Incomplete **quadriplegia** (also called **tetraplegia),** which involves paralysis of all four extremities, is the most common type of SCI. **Paraplegia,** the next most common type of SCI, is the term for paralysis of the lower body. Newer terminology to describe SCI refers to the exact level within the spinal cord where the patient has a deficit. For example, "Complete SCI at C4, Incomplete SCI at L4."

Several factors affect morbidity and mortality following SCI: the patient's age at the time of injury, level of injury within the spinal cord, and the number of muscle groups affected. The degree of muscle

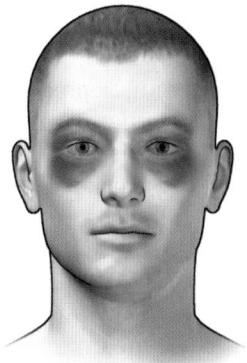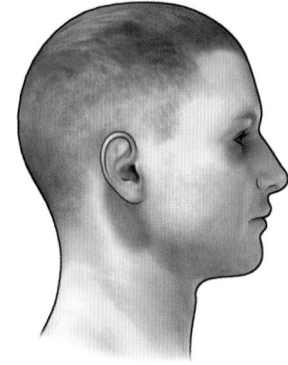

FIGURE 35-13. Signs of basilar skull fracture. Ecchymoses around both eyes ("raccoon eyes") and a bruise behind the ear ("Battle's sign") are key signs of basilar skull fracture.

weakness and sensory loss has the greatest impact on survival and early complication rates. Mortality rates are highest during the first year post-SCI, with 30% of persons rehospitalized during the first year. The most common causes of death in SCI are the complications of pneumonia and septicemia.

Epidemiology

According to the CDC, there are approximately 54 cases of new spinal cord injuries per million, or 17,700 cases in the United States annually. In 2022, there were approximately 36,000 persons who sustained traumatic SCI. Males account for 80% of cases of SCI. Motor vehicle accidents are the leading cause of SCI, followed by falls, acts of violence, and sports injuries.

Basic Concepts in Spinal Cord Anatomy and Physiology

The spinal cord is an extension of the brain that travels through the base of the skull down through the vertebral bones of the back and terminates at the level of the first lumbar vertebra. Like the brain, the spinal cord is surrounded by the meninges, which contain CSF. The end portion of the spinal cord is called the **conus medullaris.** The spinal nerves that continue down from it are referred to as the **cauda equina** (see Fig. 35-14). Vertebrae can be fractured by trauma, but unless the spinal cord within is injured, there will be no motor or sensory deficits.

In the spinal cord, the white matter surrounds the gray matter and contains ascending and descending neural tracts (see Fig. 35-15). The ascending tracts are sensory tracts that carry touch, pressure, vibration, position sense, pain, and temperature information to the brain. The tracts carrying pain and temperature

cross over to the opposite side of the spinal cord, so that when the injury to the spinal cord is incomplete, damage to this tract causes loss of sensation on the opposite side of the body from the initial injury. The descending tracts are motor tracts that carry voluntary and involuntary motor commands down from the brain. Motor tracts from the brain also cross to the opposite side of the spinal cord.

CLINICAL CONCEPT

The symptoms seen in SCI vary based on the neural tract that is injured. Injuries to the descending tracts result in motor deficits, whereas damage to the ascending tracts cause sensory deficits.

Within the gray matter are neuron cell bodies and their dendrites. These are located within three horns of the spinal cord (dorsal horn, ventral horn, and lateral horn) and are surrounded by white matter. The dorsal horn cells are sensory, the ventral horn cells are motor, and the lateral horn contains the cell bodies of the sympathetic and parasympathetic fibers.

The spinal nerves that exit at each level of vertebrae control the sensation and motor response of specific areas of the body. The dermatome map (see Fig. 35-16) illustrates which vertebral-level spinal nerve innervates which area of the body. The functions of the spinal nerves can be classified according to their location in the vertebral column. Cervical nerves in the neck provide movement and feeling in the neck, upper extremities, and upper trunk. The phrenic nerve originates from cervical nerves 3, 4, and 5 to control the diaphragm. The thoracic nerves supply the trunk and abdomen, whereas the lumbar nerves innervate

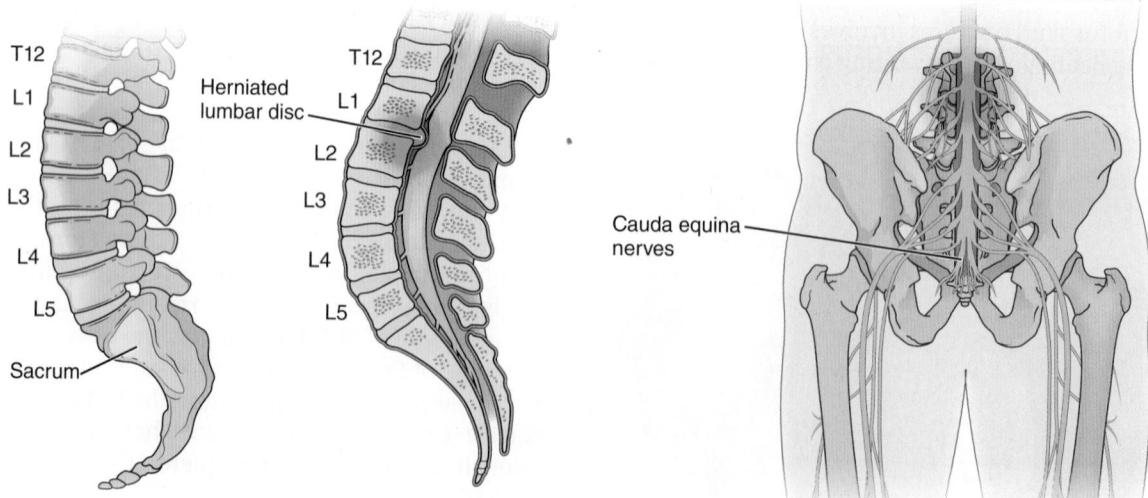

FIGURE 35-14. Cauda equina syndrome. In cauda equina syndrome, a herniated disc compresses the nerves that come off the bottom of the spinal cord, called cauda equina nerves. Symptoms include back pain radiating down the legs, weakness of legs, and bladder or bowel incontinence. This is a medical emergency.

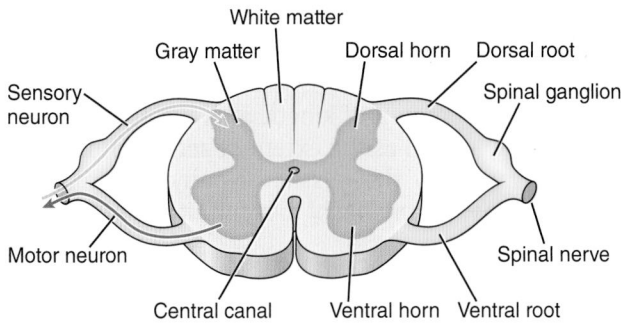

FIGURE 35-15. Cross-section of the spinal cord. Spinal nerves contain sensory and motor components. In the spinal cord, the sensory nerves enter via the dorsal root and then synapse within the spinal cord. The motor nerves exit the spinal cord via the ventral root.

the legs, bladder, and bowel; they are also responsible for sexual function.

Basic Pathophysiological Concepts in SCI

Injury to the spinal cord can be primary or secondary and varies as to the mechanism of injury. A complete SCI indicates that there is no motor or sensory function below the site of injury. Preservation of some function occurs in an incomplete injury.

Primary Injury
Mechanical forces of trauma can damage neurons and their supporting glial cells immediately. Trauma

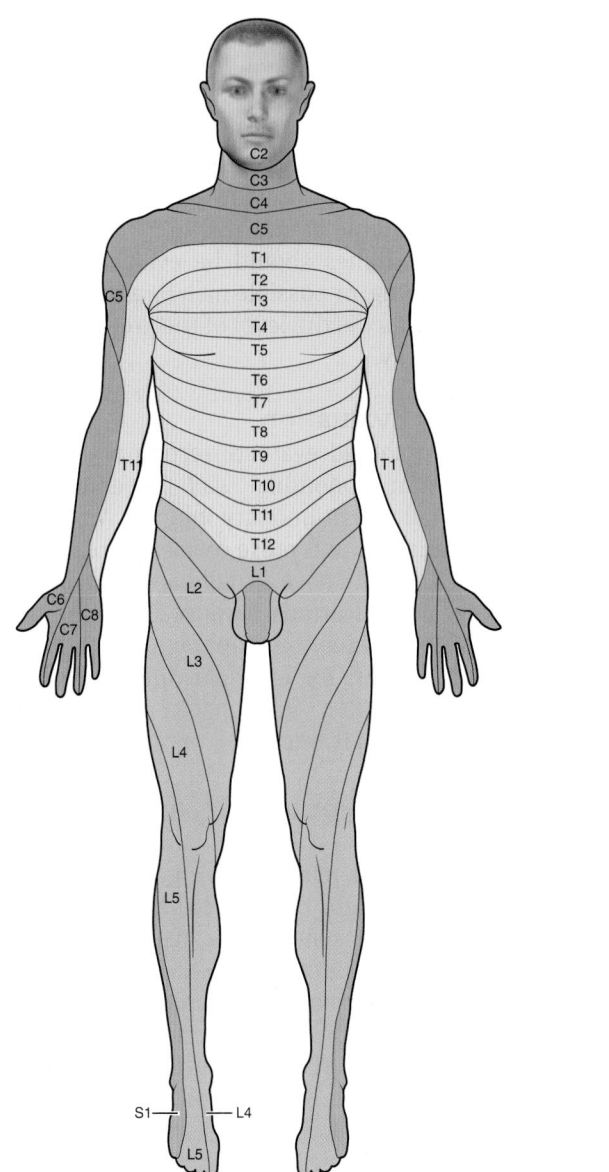
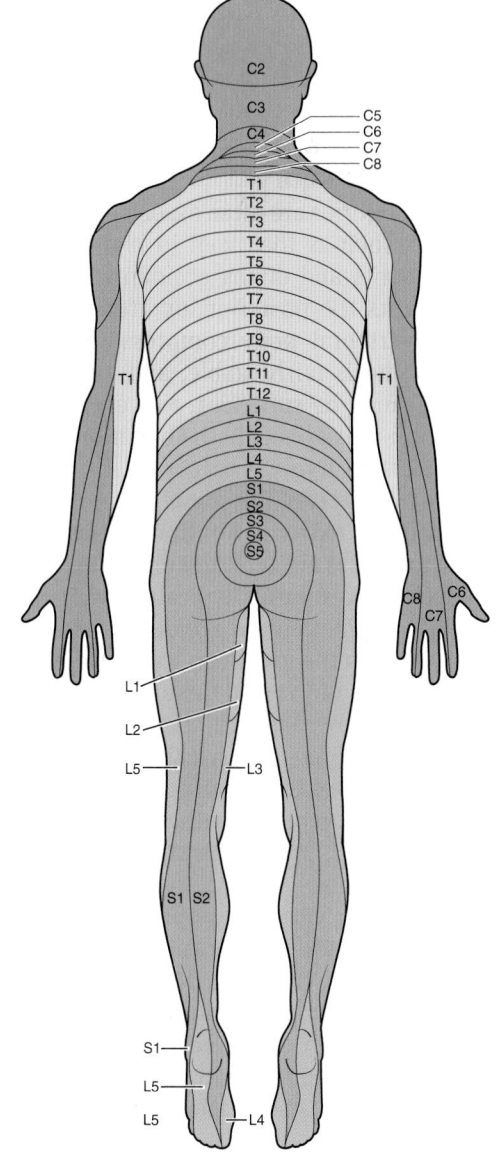

FIGURE 35-16. Dermatome map. A dermatome is an area of skin that is mainly supplied by a single spinal nerve. There are 8 cervical nerves (C1 has no dermatome), 12 thoracic nerves, 5 lumbar nerves, and 5 sacral nerves. Each of these nerves carry sensory stimuli, including pain, from a particular region of skin to the spinal cord and up to the brain. Dermatomes can be used in physical examination of the patient to localize a region of neurological deficit.

can stretch or tear the spinal cord or cut off circulation, which interrupts the function of ascending and descending nerve tracts. The physical damage can result in immediate hemorrhage and neural cell death, which in turn creates an ischemic environment.

Secondary Injury

The ischemia caused by the primary injury initiates multiple secondary processes that worsen the damage over hours to weeks. The ischemia causes a cytotoxic edema similar to that found in TBI. An inflammatory reaction with endothelial injury is activated by the primary injury. Over time, these processes cause a cascade of tissue damage and scarring within the area of injured spinal cord, which inhibits regeneration of neurons.

Disruption of the neural tracts interrupts messages between the brain and the spinal cord below the level of injury. Unstimulated axons atrophy, and a fluid-filled cyst forms within the spinal cord gray and white matter. This cyst occupies several segments above and below the primary injury site. Glial cells proliferate to form scar tissue.

Mechanisms of Injury

Hyperflexion injuries are often associated with sudden deceleration, such as that seen in high-speed motor vehicle accidents and diving accidents. The extreme flexion disrupts the posterior longitudinal ligament, leading to vertebral body compressions. In milder cases, the spine is fairly stable, and external orthosis (bracing) may be sufficient. However, in cases of severe flexion that affects both the anterior and posterior structures, surgery is necessary.

Rotational injuries of the spinal column result from lateral flexion or extreme rotation of the spinal column. These injuries are typically unstable.

Hyperextension injuries typically result from falls or rear-end motor vehicle accidents and are most commonly seen in the lower cervical spine. If hyperextension is followed by forced flexion, often referred to as "whiplash," more severe injuries may result. Initial treatment may require a cervical collar and traction to realign the spine and reduce pressure on the spinal cord. Surgical decompression that relieves the stress on the spinal cord, as well as stabilization, is often required.

Axial loading or vertical compression occurs when overwhelming vertical force is applied to the vertebral body, causing burst fractures. Mechanically, fracture of the vertebral body and disruption of the posterior elements result from compressive forces. Treatment goals include realignment with traction, followed by bracing or surgical stabilization, depending on the degree of instability.

A penetrating injury is one that enters the spinal column and has direct spinal cord contact. Low-velocity stab wounds cause actual spinal cord contact or vascular injury by the instrument or bony fragments, resulting in neurological deficit. Low-impact wounds are likely to cause incomplete injury and subsequently have a more favorable prognosis. In high-velocity mechanisms, such as gunshots, damage is directly related to the amount of kinetic energy applied to the spinal cord, as well as the extent of actual spinal cord trauma caused by the missile or bony compression. Missile injury is more likely to result in complete SCI.

Assessment in SCI

Initially, for trauma patients, a general survey is important. First, the clinician should focus on life-threatening conditions. Assessment of ABCs is a priority. The patient should be treated as if they have a cervical spine injury with cervical bracing while lying flat on a transfer board. The patient should be log-rolled when each spinous process of the entire vertebral column is examined from the occiput to the sacrum. A history should focus on symptoms related to the vertebrae and motor or sensory deficits. The patient should describe the mechanism of injury, which indicates the potential for spinal injury.

The musculoskeletal system should be examined first to identify and provide initial treatment for potentially unstable spinal fractures. The spine and paravertebral tissues should be evaluated for pain, swelling, bruising, or possible malalignment. The skeletal level of injury is the level of the greatest vertebral damage on x-ray.

Pulmonary Evaluation

The clinician should evaluate respiratory rate, chest wall expansion, abdominal wall movement, cough, and chest wall and pulmonary injuries. Arterial blood gas (ABG) analysis and pulse oximetry are important. Injuries at C4 and above usually are associated with respiratory complications because C4 is the phrenic nerve that innervates the diaphragm. With high thoracic cord injuries, for example (injuries that occur from T2 through T4), vital capacity is 30% to 50% of normal, and cough is weak.

Hemorrhage, Hypotension, and Neurogenic Shock

In acute SCI, shock may be neurogenic, hemorrhagic, or both. **Neurogenic shock** occurs when the SCI is above T6 because sympathetic nerves are affected. Sympathetic nervous system (SNS) dysfunction prevents the tachycardia and peripheral vasoconstriction that should normally counteract and characterize hemorrhagic shock. Therefore, it is important for the clinician to suspect hemorrhagic shock even when tachycardia is absent. SCIs at C4 and above affect respiration ability. Injuries at T6 or above can cause SNS dysfunction, causing hypotension and bradycardia.

Sensory Function Testing

In sensory function assessment, the clinician should test light touch, proprioception, vibration, and pain. The clinician can use a pinprick to evaluate pain sensation. The sensory dermatome map is used for this assessment. The patient's intact sensory level is determined by pinprick and light touch of the most caudal (lowest) dermatome. Sensory index scoring is as follows:

- 0: absent
- 1: impaired or hyperesthesia
- 2: intact

 CLINICAL CONCEPT

In sensory index scoring, a score of 0 is given if the patient cannot differentiate between the point of a sharp pin and the dull edge.

Motor Strength Testing
Muscle strength always should be graded according to the maximum strength attained, no matter how briefly that strength is maintained during the examination. The muscles are tested with the patient in the supine position. Muscle strength scoring is from 0/5 to 5/5. Normal muscle strength of 5/5 is muscle activity against resistance (see prior section on neurological assessment).

Motor level is determined by the most caudal muscles that have muscle strength of 3 or above while the segment above is normal (5/5).

Neurological Level and Extent of Injury
Neurological level of injury is the most caudal level at which motor and sensory levels are intact, with motor level assessed 0 to 5 and sensory level defined by a sensory score of 2. There are key muscles that should be tested according to the American Spinal Injury Association (ASIA) assessment tool. A rectal examination is necessary to check motor function or sensation at the anal junction. The presence of either motor or sensory function is considered sacral-sparing. Specific tests that examine the sacral nerve roots are listed on the ASIA assessment tool. The presence of sacral spinal nerve reflexes is a key factor because it is evidence of the integrity of spinal cord long tract fibers. Indication of the presence of sacral fibers is of significance in defining the completeness of the injury and the potential for some motor recovery.

The extent of injury is defined by the **ASIA Impairment Scale** using the following categories:

- A = Complete: No sensory or motor function is preserved in sacral segments S4–S5.
- B = Incomplete: Sensory, but not motor function, is preserved below the neurological level and extends through sacral segments S4–S5.
- C = Incomplete: Motor function is preserved below the neurological level, and most key muscles below the neurological level have a muscle grade lower than 3.

- D = Incomplete: Motor function is preserved below the neurological level, and most key muscles below the neurological level have a muscle grade greater than or equal to 3.
- E = Normal: Sensory and motor functions are normal.

ASIA has established that the neurological level of injury is the most caudal level with normal sensory and motor function. For example, a patient with a C5 injury has, by definition, abnormal motor and sensory function from C6 down. The ASIA classification uses the description of the neurological level of injury in defining the type of SCI, such as "C8 ASIA A with zone of partial preservation of pinprick to T2" (see Table 35-2).

Diagnosis
When SCI is suspected, x-rays are used to demonstrate alignment of the spinal column. In some cases, fractures can be seen. X-rays do not provide information regarding the spinal cord but do show injury or malalignment of the bones that may cause or aggravate injury to the spinal cord. Body size greatly affects the quality of x-ray images. The cervical-thoracic junction is often not well visualized in patients with short or muscular necks.

CT scans can evaluate the spinal anatomy in greater detail than traditional x-rays. Subtle fractures and soft tissue injury are more evident with this imaging technique. Technological advances in CT scanning can show the spinal column in three dimensions. CT scan can also provide information on the integrity of the vertebral and carotid arteries, which sometimes become occluded or dissected after cervical spine injury.

TABLE 35-2. SCI and Loss of Function

Level of Injury	Loss of Function
Between C1 and C3	Unable to breathe without respirator Loss of bowel and bladder control Unable to move arms and legs
Between C4 and C7	Severe weakness in arms with no motor function or sensation in legs Loss of bowel and bladder control
Thoracic spine	Paralysis in legs but arms can still function Truncal instability Loss of bowel and bladder control
Lumbar sacral	Loss of bowel and bladder control Upper body strength and sensation normal Motor weakness or paralysis and sensory loss in hips and legs

Adapted from American Spinal Injury Association (ASIA). (2012). Assessment tool from the American Spinal Injury Association. http://www.asia-spinalinjury.org

MRI can provide detailed pictures of the spinal cord, intervertebral discs, and CSF spaces. Trauma-related pathology seen on MRI includes herniated discs, spinal cord contusions, ligament integrity, and nerve root compression. Patients with cervical or high thoracic SCI should be carefully monitored for respiratory decompensation that may occur when they are placed in the supine position.

Myelography is an alternative for those with contraindications to MRI. It demonstrates obstructed CSF flow around the spinal cord or compression of the spinal cord, but is not able to demonstrate intrinsic spinal cord pathology. The test, which involves the injection of radiopaque dye into the CSF compartment, is performed through a lumbar puncture or a C1–C2 puncture. X-rays or CT scans are then obtained of the spinal anatomy. Myelography involves some risk in the SCI patient that can exacerbate unstable injuries. Other potential complications of myelography include seizures, spinal cord puncture, and spinal headache.

Treatment

When treating a patient with SCI, attending to the ABCs of resuscitation takes precedence. The patient should be stabilized in the supine position with cervical bracing and spinal immobilization on a flat board, after which the patient should be transferred to a trauma care unit. After complete neurological examination, pain relievers can be given, and pneumatic compression stockings are needed to prevent thromboembolism. In addition, the patient needs wound care, warm IV fluid, oxygen, and urinary catheterization.

Urgent surgical decompression of the spinal cord should be performed to preserve intact neurological function. Hypotension is common after SCI due to neurogenic shock. This can lessen circulation to spinal cord neurons. Hemodynamic support with vasopressor medications to avoid hypotension (defined as a systolic blood pressure less than 90 mm Hg) and to augment mean arterial pressure greater than 85 to 90 mm Hg has been recommended by many investigators. Dopamine, norepinephrine, and phenylephrine are vasopressor agents that have been used in various studies. Corticosteroids are a controversial neuroprotective treatment for acute SCI. Most experts do not recommend the use of corticosteroids. However, some studies do show early postinjury administration of methylprednisolone can benefit some patients. Once the possibility of bleeding is excluded, low molecular weight heparin is administered to prevent deep venous thromboembolism.

> **ALERT!** The patient with SCI needs cervical bracing and should be log-rolled during examination or transfer for diagnostic tests.

Selected Pathophysiological Disorders Related to SCI

Trauma to the spinal cord results in loss of function to the area distal to the trauma. However, an insult to one section of the cord leads to the development of **spinal shock,** which eventually resolves during the healing process.

Spinal Shock

Primary injury to the spinal cord results in a state of **areflexia,** which is demonstrated by flaccid muscles, paralysis, absence of sensation at and below the level of injury, and bowel and bladder dysfunction.

Loss of the anal reflex or bulbocavernosus reflex is the hallmark of spinal shock. Autonomic function (vasoconstriction and shivering) is also lost at the level of injury and below. The completeness of the SCI is indeterminable until spinal shock state abates. Return of the anal or bulbocavernosus reflex indicates the resolution of spinal shock, which usually occurs hours to weeks postinjury. The flaccidity of spinal shock is slowly replaced with spasticity and hyperreflexia in most patients.

The patient with spinal shock should first be hemodynamically stabilized with constant monitoring of blood pressure and electrocardiography. Systolic blood pressure should be kept greater than 100 mm Hg and heart rate greater than 60 beats per minute. Motor assessment of the major muscle groups of upper and lower extremities should be tested periodically. It is important to note asymmetrical movement of muscle groups or lack of motor ability. Differences in full strength, antigravity, and no movement should be noted. Periodic testing of the sensation of the extremities is also necessary. In patients with C4 injury or above, respiratory function and ABCs should be monitored. Mechanical ventilation is commonly needed. In patients with respiratory compromise, suctioning and respiratory physiotherapy are necessary. The patient in spinal shock is at high risk for deep venous thromboembolism; pneumatic compression devices can be used on the lower extremities. The patient should be kept in proper body alignment with splinting of extremities and have body position changed periodically, such as raising the head of the bed and going from bed to chair.

> ### 🔍 CLINICAL CONCEPT
>
> The bulbocavernosus reflex is the contraction of the anal sphincter with squeezing of the glans penis or tugging on a Foley catheter. The presence of the reflex indicates intact S1, S2, and S3 nerves. In spinal shock, there is loss of the reflex.

Neurogenic Shock

Although sometimes used interchangeably with spinal shock, neurogenic shock is a distinctly different condition that affects patients with SCI. It manifests in patients with injuries at the sixth thoracic vertebrae or above, resulting in the lack of normal sympathetic outflow from the T1–L2 region of the spinal cord. This means the SNS does not release norepinephrine, which results in a predominant parasympathetic effect, causing bradycardia. Without norepinephrine, blood vessels do not constrict, resulting in peripheral vasodilation. This allows blood to pool in the extremities, decreasing venous return to the heart, and, eventually, reducing cardiac output and systemic blood pressure. The presence of bradycardia with hypotension differentiates neurogenic shock from hypovolemic shock, as with hypovolemic shock, tachycardia occurs in response to hypotension.

The patient with neurogenic shock should be hemodynamically stabilized with constant monitoring of blood pressure and electrocardiography. Measures used in the treatment of spinal shock are also necessary in neurogenic shock.

Complete and Incomplete SCI

SCI is classified by the degree of functional loss. Complete injuries result in the loss of all voluntary motor and sensory function below the level of injury. Accurate functional loss cannot be determined until spinal shock resolves. Individuals with complete or incomplete spinal injury are assessed and monitored, as described in spinal and neurogenic shock. With incomplete SCI, some motor or sensory function below the injury can remain intact. Several types of syndromes are associated with incomplete SCI.

Central Cord Syndrome. Central cord syndrome often occurs after hyperextension of the cervical spine that causes compression of the neurons within the center of the spinal cord. Because of the arrangement of the corticospinal nerve tracts within the spinal cord, there is greater motor dysfunction in the upper extremities than the lower extremities. Sensory and bladder function may or may not be intact. Partial to near-complete recovery can occur in younger, healthy patients. However, recovery is variable for those patients older than 50 years.

Anterior Spinal Artery Syndrome. This syndrome is associated with disruption of blood flow to the anterior two-thirds of the spinal cord, resulting in spinal cord ischemia and infarction. Injuries that cause anterior spinal artery syndrome include acute intervertebral disc herniation, bone fragments impinging on the anterior surface of the spinal cord, or disrupted aortic blood flow. The patient suffers paralysis, loss of sensation, and inability to discriminate pain and temperature. Because circulation remains intact in the dorsal columns of the spinal cord, proprioception, light touch, and vibration sense are undisrupted.

Brown-Séquard Syndrome. This type of incomplete SCI is commonly associated with penetrating injuries that lead to hemisection of the spinal cord, in which there is damage of ascending and descending neural tracts on one side of the spinal cord. The following symptoms can result from damage to the neuron tracts:

- Interruption of the lateral corticospinal tract causes ipsilateral (same side) paralysis and the presence of a Babinski's sign on the side of the lesion.
- Interruption of dorsal spinal cord column results in ipsilateral loss of tactile discrimination, vibratory sensation, and position sense (proprioception).
- Interruption of the lateral spinothalamic tract causes contralateral (opposite side) loss of pain and temperature sensation.

Horner's Syndrome. Horner's syndrome is associated with injuries at or above T1 that disrupt the cervical sympathetic tract of neurons. It is characterized by miosis (constricted pupil), anhidrosis (lack of sweat), and ptosis (drooping eyelid) on the affected side.

Conus Medullaris Syndrome. Conus medullaris syndrome occurs following injury to the lowest portion of the spinal cord (conus medullaris), particularly fractures of L1 and L2. The patient suffers urinary retention, erectile dysfunction, constipation, relaxed anal sphincter, sensory loss in the inguinal area, loss of anal and bulbocavernosus reflexes, and motor weakness. Motor impairment varies but can include paralysis and muscle atrophy caused by spinal cord motor neuron involvement.

Cauda Equina Syndrome. **Cauda equina syndrome** results from compression of the bilateral nerve roots of the lumbosacral region. Motor and sensory losses are variable and depend on which nerve roots are affected. Incontinence is the major sign of this syndrome, which can follow fractures of the lower lumbar spine, sacrum, or acute herniated discs of the lower lumbar region. (See Figure 35-14.)

Complications of SCI

A number of complications can result from SCI. They may be local, affecting the neurological system, or systemic, affecting other body systems.

Local Complications

Syringomyelia. About 3% of people with SCI develop syringomyelia, which is a fluid-filled cyst, termed a syrinx. The cyst forms within the spinal cord and can enlarge over time to cause compression of spinal nerves. Individuals enduring this complication may not experience any symptoms or may have symptoms of weakness of the extremities, pain and stiffness of the back and shoulders, headache, or lack of sensation in the hands. The patient may require a surgical decompression procedure.

Neuropathic Joint Arthropathy (or Charcot Joint Arthropathy). Neuropathic joint arthropathy is the slow destruction of a joint (including those in the hips, knees, ankles, shoulders, elbows, and spine), which can occur years after an SCI. Patients may develop deformed joints and pain below the sensory level of injury and reduced neurological function. Patients may require bracing, medications, and/or spinal fusion surgery.

Spasticity. Spasticity is contraction of muscles that cause rigid joints and deformity. The patient can have difficulty walking (if this occurs in the ankles), inability to use the hands (if this occurs in the fingers), and may experience discomfort. Common spasticity treatments include physical therapy, muscle relaxants, intrathecal drug therapy, botulinum toxin injections, and surgery.

Systemic Complications

Cardiovascular Complications. Hypotension is a common SCI complication, particularly in persons with cervical or thoracic injury. About 60% of people have symptomatic orthostatic hypotension, which causes dizziness, weakness, and a temporary loss of consciousness when going from sitting/lying down to standing. Common treatment includes wearing compression stockings or abdominal binding, and medication therapy.

Autonomic Dysreflexia. The sympathetic and parasympathetic nervous systems can dysfunction after SCI. Autonomic dysreflexia is caused by a complication below the level of injury, such as bowel impaction, bladder distention, or pressure sores. During autonomic dysreflexia, involuntary functions, such as breathing, blood pressure, and heart rate, become unregulated. Long-term preventive health-care measures that include bowel and bladder management are essential to prevent autonomic dysreflexia.

Pulmonary Complications. Cervical and thoracic SCI can weaken the chest, abdominal muscles, and diaphragm, resulting in respiratory infections. Typical infections include the common cold, bronchitis, and pneumonia. Patients may also experience sleep apnea and respiratory failure. Antibiotics or ventilator-assisted respiratory function may be necessary.

Other Systemic Complications

- Secondary immunodeficiency: SCI can diminish strength of the immune system, placing the patient at risk for infections (including pneumonia, urinary tract infections, and wound infections).
- Bladder dysfunction: SCIs at or above L1–L2 cause dysfunction of the bladder muscle, which can cause problems emptying the bladder, urinary incontinence, and frequent urinary tract infections.
- Bowel dysfunction: Many persons with SCI have bowel dysfunction that causes constipation, fecal impaction, and increased risk of infection.
- Pressure injury: Pressure sores can occur in areas of skin over bony prominences. Common areas of skin breakdown include the sacrum, buttocks, outer thighs, feet, and ankles. Wound infections can occur in these areas, which can lead to sepsis.
- Neurogenic heterotopic ossification: Individuals with long-term SCI can have abnormal bone formation, called neurogenic heterotopic ossification, in the connective tissue around joints. It commonly occurs in the large joints of the hips, knees, elbows, and shoulders, causing pain and spasticity.
- Neuropathic pain: Many patients with long-term chronic SCI report neuropathic pain: paresthesias, hyperalgesia, and allodynia. Hyperalgesia is high pain sensitivity to stimuli that are usually not regarded as painful. Allodynia is exaggerated painful stimuli from neural pathways that are used repetitively and are usually not causative of pain. The pain can be above or below the level of SCI. Treatment may include antidepressants, antiepileptic drugs, surgery, acupuncture, transcutaneous neural stimulation, and cognitive-behavioral therapy.

Chapter Summary

- TBI is sudden physical damage to the brain that can result from a closed head injury, such as that caused by the head's impact with an external unmovable object or surface.

- Certain pathophysiological alterations occur with brain injury, such as changes in ICP and LOC.

- The brain has three compartments: CSF, brain tissue, and blood. According to the Monroe–Kellie hypothesis, an increase in one compartment of the brain is compensated for by a decrease in other compartments.

- Four mechanisms can result in skull or brain injuries: blunt trauma, acceleration-deceleration (also called coup-contrecoup), penetrating trauma, and blast injury.

- When ICP increases, the brain tissue is compressed and forced downward in the skull to become herniated or displaced to another region of the brain. The most common type of herniation is a transtentorial (also called uncal) herniation.

- A decrease in the LOC is the earliest sign of neurological decline.

- Pressure on the brainstem will cause Cushing's triad: hypertension, bradycardia. and bradypnea.

- Pressure on the oculomotor nerve (CN III) causes pupils to become fixed and dilated.

- The GCS is used to assess the degree of consciousness impairment associated with head injury. The GCS incorporates both LOC and orientation, and is determined by rating three areas: eye opening, verbal response, and motor response.

- DAI, often caused by the coup-contrecoup mechanism, is characterized by diffuse swelling of neuronal axons, hemorrhage or laceration of the corpus callosum, and hemorrhages in the brainstem. DAI commonly leads to coma.

- A concussion is a physiological disruption in brain function that may or may not involve loss of consciousness. It is manifested by temporary memory loss and alteration of mental state. It leaves no permanent structural damage to the brain.

- A cerebral contusion is considered a bruise of the brain tissue that occurs with head trauma. Cerebral edema with increased ICP occurs, which can cause loss of consciousness.

- An EDH is associated with skull fracture and rupture of the middle meningeal artery. Increased ICP can be caused by the rapid arterial bleeding. Brainstem compression can cause death.

- A subdural hematoma is caused by venous bleeding into the subdural space. This bleed can occur over a period of hours to days.

- A cerebral aneurysm is most commonly found on the circle of Willis. They are often called "berry aneurysms" because they look like berries hanging off a vine.

- An SAH can be caused by trauma or rupture of a cerebral aneurysm.

- Leakage of an SAH can cause neurological deficits over a number of days. Alternatively, an SAH can be a sudden event that leads to bleeding into the subarachnoid space, compression of brain tissue, and uncal herniation, which can cause death.

- Acute SAH can cause thunderclap headache; "worst headache of my life" is the common complaint of the patient.

- Skull fractures are categorized as linear, depressed, or basilar and may or may not involve injury to the brain tissue. Basilar skull fracture is a most critical disorder.

- Periorbital ecchymosis ("raccoon eyes"), Battle's sign (bleeding in the mastoid region), CSF rhinorrhea, and CSF otorrhea are signs of basilar skull fracture.

- The symptoms seen in SCI vary based on the neural tract that is injured. Injuries to the descending tracts result in motor deficits, whereas damage to the ascending tracts causes sensory deficits.

- Primary injury to the spinal cord results in a concussive effect causing a state of areflexia, which is demonstrated by flaccid muscles, paralysis, absence of sensation at and below the level of injury, and bowel and bladder dysfunction.

- The ASIA assessment tool is used to evaluate SCI.

- Within the ASIA classification system, the terms "paraplegia" and "quadriplegia" are not used. Instead, the ASIA classification uses the description of the neurological level of injury in defining the type of SCI.

Making the Connections

Disorder and Pathophysiology

Signs and Symptoms	Physical Assessment Findings	Diagnostic Testing	Treatment

Brain Injury

Diffuse Axonal Injury (DAI) | DAI is characterized by rapid stretching of axons that damages the axonal structure, resulting in a loss of elasticity and impairment of impulse transmission. Swollen, stretched axons may become disconnected. A DAI can also cause swelling in the brain. Swelling causes increased pressure in the brain and can cause decreased blood flow to the brain, along with compression of nerves and tissue.

Signs and Symptoms	Physical Assessment Findings	Diagnostic Testing	Treatment
DAI results in immediate loss of consciousness, and most patients (more than 90%) remain in a persistent comatose state. A person with a mild or moderate DAI who is conscious may show signs of neurological impairment, depending on which area of the brain is most affected.	The patient may be comatose or exhibit specific neurological deficits that are related to the exact area of the brain injury. For example, those with injury in Broca's area of the brain will exhibit difficulty with speech. Others who suffer injury to the cerebral motor cortex will exhibit symptoms related to movement of extremities.	MRI is the preferred test for diagnosis. CT scan is less sensitive to DAI, with many patients exhibiting a normal CT scan upon presentation. The degree of microscopic injury usually is considered to be greater than that seen on diagnostic imaging.	Immediate treatment involves hemostabilization. The patient should be treated as if there is a cervical injury until this is ruled out. Measures should be implemented to reduce swelling of the brain, such as IV mannitol and steroids. Surgery is not an option for those who have sustained a DAI. If the patient has sustained a mild or moderate DAI, the rehabilitation phase will follow once the patient is stabilized and awake. About 90% of survivors with severe DAI are unconscious. The 10% who regain consciousness are often severely impaired.

Concussion | Concussion occurs when rotational or acceleration forces are applied to the brain, resulting in the shear strain of the tissue. On a cellular level, there is a disruption of neuronal membranes, resulting in an efflux of intracellular potassium ions into the extracellular space. This results in release of excitatory amino acids, particularly glutamate. Glutamate accumulation is toxic to neurons and temporarily causes a disturbance of surrounding neurons. Glutamate overstimulates the neurons and temporarily causes the neuronal membranes to open their pores. Sodium flows into the cell pores, followed by water, and temporary cellular swelling occurs. Depending on how much cellular swelling occurs, resolution occurs over time with no remaining structural changes.

Signs and Symptoms	Physical Assessment Findings	Diagnostic Testing	Treatment
Alteration in consciousness, such as being dazed, confused, or "seeing stars," or, less commonly, a brief loss of consciousness. Headache, dizziness, and flat affect are common initially. Pretraumatic (retrograde) amnesia and post-traumatic (antegrade) amnesia can occur. Usually, the duration of amnesia is brief (seconds to minutes), depending on the injury. Vomiting may suggest a significant brain injury with associated elevated ICP. Other signs of increased ICP include worsening headache, increasing disorientation, and changing LOC.	Temporary disorientation. Amnesia for events before and just after the injury. Flat affect. Vomiting. Imbalance caused by dizziness.	Check ABCs. Cervical spine injury should be considered, and the unconscious individual should be treated as having a potential cervical spine injury. Thorough neurological examination should be performed, including assessment of orientation to person, place, and time. The ability to perform simple tasks and postural stability should also be assessed. The CDC recommends a concussion assessment toolkit based on the AAN guidelines to aid in the evaluation of a concussion.	Cognitive and physical rest are recommended. Bedrest, fluids, and a mild pain reliever such as acetaminophen may be prescribed. Ice may be applied to strains or superficial bruises to relieve pain and decrease swelling. No return to play or vigorous activity is recommended while signs or symptoms of a concussion are present. At least 24-hour reprieve. Experts recommend that those who suffer concussion should not return to playing sports on the same day as the injury.

Making the Connections–cont'd

Signs and Symptoms	Physical Assessment Findings	Diagnostic Testing	Treatment
Postconcussion syndrome is the persistence of symptoms for more than 3 weeks after the initial injury; symptoms include headache, dizziness, fatigue, irritability, insomnia, and concentration or memory difficulties.		The tool assesses multiple cognitive, physical, and emotional symptoms initially and at 15 minutes and 30 minutes postinjury; it can be found at http://www.cdc.gov/headsup/index.html. Imaging is not normally required unless one or more of the following conditions are present: • Physical evidence of trauma above the clavicles • Anticoagulation or coagulopathy • Age older than 60 years • Alcohol or drug intoxication • Neurological deficit • Persistent vomiting • Seizure or short-term memory deficit • History of alcohol use disorder A CT scan is normal in more than 90% of concussion patients. However, if headache does not resolve or patient becomes disoriented or begins to show decreased LOC, hospitalization is necessary.	Neurological assessment is required. For concussion care, consult CDC Heads Up program guidelines.

Cerebral Contusion | A combination of vascular and tissue damage leads to cerebral contusion, similar to bruising of the brain. A contusion is often a coup-contrecoup type of injury. Cerebral edema typically develops around cerebral contusions within 48 to 72 hours after injury. Cerebral edema is problematic because the swollen brain tissue may become compressed against the bone, which then leads to brain damage. Also, if cerebral edema is severe, uncal herniation of brain tissue is possible, which can lead to death.

Signs and Symptoms	Physical Assessment Findings	Diagnostic Testing	Treatment
Severe headache, dizziness, vomiting, increased size of one pupil, or sudden weakness in an arm or leg may be present. Individual may seem restless, agitated, or irritable. Often, the person may have memory loss. These symptoms can last for several hours to several weeks, depending on the severity of the injury. As the brain tissue swells, the person may feel increasingly drowsy or confused. If the person is difficult to awaken or loses consciousness, immediate medical attention should be sought.	Neurological examination may show neurological deficits such as weakness in one extremity. Patient may seem irritable or restless. Memory loss is common. These symptoms can last for several hours to several weeks, depending on the severity of the injury. As the brain tissue swells, the person may feel increasingly drowsy or confused.	Immediate CT scan is needed, though the true volume of neuronal damage in the contused tissue can be underestimated. MRI scans have greater sensitivity for cerebral edema. Skull x-ray is necessary to look for skull fracture, which is commonly associated with EDH. Serial CT scans over the days following cerebral contusion are used to assess progression or resolution. Cerebral angiography is often performed to visualize blood vessel damage and possible aneurysms.	Lifesaving measures are the priority with any head injury. The patient should be assessed for airway, breathing, and circulation. The patient needs to be treated and stabilized as if they have a cervical spinal injury. In the emergency setting, IV mannitol is frequently used to decrease cerebral edema. Surgical resection of the contused brain tissue is indicated when the patient has brain swelling that increases the ICP above an acceptable degree.

Continued

Making the Connections—cont'd

Signs and Symptoms	Physical Assessment Findings	Diagnostic Testing	Treatment
			Craniectomy may be performed where a piece of skull is removed to relieve the pressure on the brain cells. If cerebral hematoma is present, evacuation is performed through a craniotomy.

Epidural Hematoma (EDH) | Rupture of the middle meningeal artery into the epidural space; bleeding into the space between the cranial bone and dura mater (layer of meninges) can rapidly place pressure on the brain.

Signs and Symptoms	Physical Assessment Findings	Diagnostic Testing	Treatment
Patient may have no notable symptoms and deny need for medical attention. Possible loss of consciousness, severe headache, vomiting, and seizure may be present. Patients may have dramatically delayed deterioration. The patient can be conscious and talking, yet a minute later be apneic, comatose, and minutes from death.	Decreased LOC, with decreased or fluctuating GCS, may be present. Dilated, sluggish, or fixed pupil(s), bilateral or ipsilateral to injury, suggest increased ICP or herniation. If the ICP rises and causes significant pressure on the brainstem, Cushing's triad occurs: bradycardia, bradypnea, and hypertension. In coma, patients take on decerebrate or decorticate posturing. Positive Babinski's sign is observed whenever the upper motor neurons are involved.	Complete neurological examination is performed, including GCS. Immediate CT scan and skull x-ray are necessary. Skull x-ray commonly shows fractures, whereas the CT scan will show evidence of bleeding into the epidural space. If bleeding has been prolonged, a midline shift in the brain tissue will be apparent. A decrease in LOC is the earliest sign of neurological decline.	This is a neurosurgical emergency requiring a craniotomy and surgical evacuation of the hematoma. The patient requires hemodynamic stabilization with airway and blood pressure control. The patient also needs intubation for mechanical ventilation, IV access, oxygen, and cardiac monitoring. Hyperventilating the patient often can decrease ICP. Phenytoin provides prophylaxis against early post-traumatic seizure.

Subdural Hematoma | A subdural hematoma results from bleeding that accumulates below the dura mater but above the arachnoid membrane. The subdural hematoma occurs from tearing of subdural bridging veins. Venous bleeding is slow but can accumulate with time to create substantial intracranial pressure that compresses brain tissue. An acute subdural hematoma occurs within 72 hours of head injury, whereas a subacute subdural hematoma can take several days to accumulate to levels that cause symptoms. Chronic subdural hematoma is one that has been present for up to 3 weeks.

Signs and Symptoms	Physical Assessment Findings	Diagnostic Testing	Treatment
Patients may have headache, nausea, vomiting, and exhibit neurological deficits such as: • Confused or slurred speech • Difficulty with balance or walking • Lethargy or confusion • Loss of consciousness • Seizure • Slurred speech • Visual disturbances • Weakness of an extremity	Patients may exhibit neurological deficits such as: • Confused or slurred speech • Difficulty with balance or walking • Lethargy or confusion • Loss of consciousness • Seizure • Slurred speech • Visual disturbances • Weakness of an extremity Cushing's triad indicates brainstem dysfunction; bradycardia, bradypnea, and hypertension. Positive Babinski's sign is observed whenever upper motor neurons are involved.	Complete neurological examination is performed, including GCS. Immediate CT scan and skull x-ray are performed. CT scan may or may not show evidence of bleeding into the subdural space. If bleeding has been prolonged, a midline shift in the brain tissue will be apparent. Repeat neurological examination and CT scan in the following days are necessary if subdural hematoma is suspected.	Large acute subdural hematomas require craniotomy to evacuate the lesion and reduce the ICP. Occasionally, a subdural hematoma is small and causes little pressure or midline shift. In this case, surgery may be withheld or delayed. A small subdural hematoma can slowly be reabsorbed by the brain. Chronic subdural hematomas can be evacuated by craniotomy and catheter placement under the dura to drain out the blood.

Making the Connections–cont'd

Signs and Symptoms	Physical Assessment Findings	Diagnostic Testing	Treatment
Subarachnoid Hemorrhage (SAH) | Aneurysmal SAH and traumatic SAH have different etiologies; however, the pathophysiological mechanisms that cause brain damage are the same: the rupture of a cerebral artery causes a large amount of blood to rapidly fill the subarachnoid space. The blood exerts pressure, irritates the meninges, and destroys brain cells in its path. SAH also causes an obstructive hydrocephalus, which is an accumulation of CSF within the brain. The buildup of blood and CSF place a large amount of intracranial pressure that can lead to herniation of the brainstem and death.			
Patients describe the worst headache they have ever experienced. Dizziness, orbital pain, diplopia, nuchal rigidity, memory loss, one-sided body weakness, or difficulty with speech may be observed. Often no outward signs of the impending hemorrhage are evident, and either coma or death occurs within minutes after an aneurysmal SAH.	Oculomotor nerve dysfunction with pupil dilation can be exhibited. The pupil, extraocular movements, or vision can be disturbed by compression of the oculomotor nerve. Vision loss can be caused by compression of the optic nerve. If the brainstem is injured, Cushing's triad—hypertension, bradycardia, and bradypnea—occur. Positive Babinski's sign if upper motor neurons are involved.	Complete neurological examination, including GCS. Immediate CT scan. CTA. Lumbar puncture. OSAH Rule.	The patient requires hemodynamic stabilization. Breathing, blood pressure, and heart rate are maintained with consideration of the patient's neurological status. Surgical treatment consists of clipping the ruptured berry aneurysm or catheter insertion of thin wire coils into the aneurysm to block it off from blood flow. In traumatic SAH, evacuation of blood and prophylactic antibiotics are necessary. Craniotomy or craniectomy may be needed if intracranial bleeding or swelling is a problem.
Skull Fracture | Skull fractures are categorized as linear, depressed, or basilar, and may or may not involve injury to the brain tissue. Linear fracture, the most common type of fracture, does not affect brain tissue. Depressed fractures occur when an object fractures the bone with sufficient force to push fragments into the brain; these are commonly open fractures that involve underlying brain tissue. The temporal bone is the most commonly fractured bone of the skull. Basilar fractures, fractures at the base of the skull, occur in the temporal bone.			
Bruising, headache, edema, rhinorrhea (nasal CSF discharge), or otorrhea (ear CSF discharge) may be present. LOC is variable according to the area of injury.	Basilar skull fractures may produce "Battle's sign," which is bruising of the mastoid process behind the ear on the affected side. There may also be a CSF leak from the ear. Fractures in the frontal fossa can result in periorbital ecchymosis, referred to as "raccoon eyes," edema, and CSF leak from the nose.	Complete neurological examination, including GCS. Skull x-ray. CT scan. MRA if vascular injury is suspected.	Linear fractures need little treatment except pain relief and instructions to check for any late-developing neurological deficits. Depressed fracture may require surgery and prophylactic antibiotics. Craniotomy or craniectomy may be needed if intracranial bleeding or swelling is a problem.
Spinal Cord Injury **Spinal Shock** | A traumatic, concussive effect on the spinal cord causing a state of areflexia. Mechanical forces of trauma can immediately destroy neurons and their supporting cells (glial cells), stretch or shear vasculature, and interrupt descending nerve tracts.			
Flaccid muscles, paralysis, absence of sensation at and below the level of injury, plus bowel and bladder dysfunction. Late-developing muscle spasticity and hyperreflexia.	Demonstrated by flaccid muscles, paralysis, absence of sensation at and below the level of injury, plus bowel and bladder dysfunction.	Blood pressure monitoring. Cardiac monitoring. CT scan. MRI. Deep tendon reflex tests. Bulbocavernosus reflex check.	Hemostabilization and spinal stabilization and immobilization. Oxygen. Maintain systolic blood pressure greater than 100 mm Hg with adequate fluid and vasopressor support.

Continued

Making the Connections–cont'd

Signs and Symptoms	Physical Assessment Findings	Diagnostic Testing	Treatment
In cervical injury, the inspiratory and expiratory muscles are weakened, impairing cough mechanisms. Thoracic injuries from T1 to T12 involve varying degrees of loss of abdominal and intercostal muscles.	Loss of the bulbocavernosus reflex is the hallmark of spinal shock. Loss of shivering and vasoconstriction at the level of injury also occurs. Flaccidity is slowly replaced with spasticity and hyperreflexia.	Motor assessment tests major muscle groups of the upper and lower extremities. Subtle differences can be difficult to determine. Differences in full strength, antigravity, and no movement should be visible. Noticing asymmetrical or absent limb movement is critical. Tests of proprioception, pain, and temperature for all extremities are recommended. If pulmonary function is affected, as in injuries to C4 and above, pulmonary function testing, ABGs, and oxygen saturation are tested.	Maintain heart rate greater than 60 beats per minute with vasopressors and atropine as necessary. Venoembolism prevention. Splinting of extremities to maintain normal alignment. Progressive mobilization: head of bed elevated, out of bed to chair. If pulmonary function involved, mechanical ventilation. Suctioning and chest physiotherapy can clear secretions, resolve atelectasis, and improve oxygenation.

Neurogenic Shock | Mechanical forces of trauma can immediately destroy neurons and their supporting cells, stretch or shear vasculature, and interrupt descending nerve tracts. Injuries at the sixth thoracic vertebrae or above cause lack of normal sympathetic outflow from the T1–L2 region of the spinal cord. Lack of norepinephrine from the SNS results in the parasympathetic system causing bradycardia. Also, blood vessels do not constrict, resulting in peripheral vasodilation. Blood pools in the extremities, decreasing venous return to the heart, which reduces cardiac output and systemic blood pressure.

Signs and Symptoms	Physical Assessment Findings	Diagnostic Testing	Treatment
Flaccid muscles, paralysis, absence of sensation at and below the level of injury, plus bowel and bladder dysfunction. Late-developing muscle spasticity and hyperreflexia. In cervical injury, the inspiratory and expiratory muscles are weakened, impairing breathing and cough mechanisms. Thoracic injuries from T1 to T12 involve varying degrees of loss of abdominal and intercostal muscles.	Bradycardia, hypotension. Flaccid muscles, paralysis, absence of sensation at and below the level of injury, plus bowel and bladder dysfunction. Flaccidity is slowly replaced with spasticity and hyperreflexia.	Blood pressure and cardiac monitoring, along with CT scan, MRI, and testing of deep tendon reflexes. Bulbocavernosus reflex check. Motor assessment tests major muscle groups of the upper and lower extremities. Subtle differences can be difficult to determine. Differences in full strength, antigravity, and no movement should be visible. Noticing asymmetrical or absent limb movement is critical. Tests of proprioception, pain, and temperature for all extremities are recommended. If pulmonary function is affected, as in injuries to C4 and above, pulmonary function testing, ABGs, and oxygen saturation are tested.	Hemostabilization and spinal stabilization and immobilization. Oxygen. Maintain systolic blood pressure greater than 100 mm Hg with adequate fluid and vasopressor support. Maintain heart rate greater than 60 beats per minute with vasopressors and atropine as necessary. Venoembolism prevention. Splinting of extremities to maintain normal alignment. Progressive mobilization: head of bed elevated, out of bed to chair. If pulmonary function involved, mechanical ventilation. Suctioning and chest physiotherapy can clear secretions, resolve atelectasis, and improve oxygenation.

Making the Connections—cont'd

Signs and Symptoms	Physical Assessment Findings	Diagnostic Testing	Treatment
Complete or Incomplete SCI | Same as above; if there is cervical injury at or above C4, the diaphragm is paralyzed, impairing breathing and cough mechanisms. Thoracic injuries from T1 to T12 involve varying degrees of loss of abdominal and intercostal muscles. SCI at T6 or above causes sympathetic nervous system dysfunction.			
Flaccid muscles, paralysis, absence of sensation at and below the level of injury, plus bowel and bladder dysfunction. Late-developing muscle spasticity and hyperreflexia. In cervical injury, the inspiratory and expiratory muscles are weakened, impairing breathing and cough mechanisms. Thoracic injuries from T1 to T12 involve varying degrees of loss of abdominal and intercostal muscles.	Bradycardia, hypotension. Flaccid muscles, paralysis, absence of sensation at and below the level of injury plus bowel and bladder dysfunction. Flaccidity is slowly replaced with spasticity and hyperreflexia.	Blood pressure monitoring. Cardiac monitoring. CT scan. MRI. Deep tendon reflex tests. Bulbocavernosus reflex check. Motor assessment tests major muscle groups of the upper and lower extremities. Subtle differences can be difficult to determine. Differences in full strength, antigravity, and no movement should be visible. Noticing asymmetrical or absent limb movement is critical. Tests of proprioception, pain, and temperature for all extremities are recommended. If pulmonary function is affected, as in injuries to C4 and above, pulmonary function testing, ABGs, and oxygen saturation are tested.	Hemostabilization and spinal stabilization and immobilization. Oxygen. Maintain systolic blood pressure greater than 100 mm Hg with adequate fluid and vasopressor support. Maintain heart rate greater than 60 beats per minute with vasopressors and atropine as necessary. Venoembolism prevention. Splinting of extremities to maintain normal alignment. Progressive mobilization: head of bed elevated, out of bed to chair. If pulmonary function involved, mechanical ventilation. Suctioning and chest physiotherapy can clear secretions, resolve atelectasis, and improve oxygenation.

Bibliography

Available online at fadavis.com

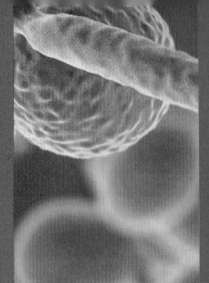

Psychobiology of Behavioral Disorders

Learning Objectives

Upon completion of this chapter, the student will be able to:

- Identify neurotransmitters and areas of the brain involved in behavior and emotional responses.
- Recognize methods of assessment, laboratory testing, and imaging used in the diagnosis of behavioral and emotional disorders.
- Describe signs and symptoms that are characteristic of common behavioral and emotional disorders.
- Recognize the distinguishing characteristics of psychosis as opposed to mood disorder.

- Differentiate between the signs of delirium, depression, and dementia.
- Comprehend dual diagnosis and the treatment required in patients with coexistent mental illness and substance use disorder.
- Discuss nonpharmacological and pharmacological treatment of behavioral and emotional disorders.

Key Terms

Agnosia

Amnesia

Amygdala

Anomia

Apathy

Apraxia

Attention deficit-hyperactivity disorder (ADHD)

Benzodiazepine (BNZ)

Bipolar disorder

Cognitive-behavioral therapy (CBT)

Delirium

Dementia

Gamma aminobutyric acid (GABA)

Generalized anxiety disorder (GAD)

Interpersonal psychotherapy

Kindling theory

Limbic system

Locus coeruleus

Major depressive disorder (MDD)

Mini-Mental Status Examination (MMSE)

Monoamine oxidase inhibitors (MAOIs)

Neocortex

Panic attack

Post-traumatic stress disorder (PTSD)

Psychosis

Selective serotonin reuptake inhibitors (SSRIs)

Serotonin

Serotonin-norepinephrine reuptake inhibitors (SNRIs)

Sundowning

Tardive dyskinesia (TD)

Tricyclic antidepressant (TCAs)

Psychiatry, the study of the mind, attempts to explain human thoughts, emotions, and behaviors. As the scientific knowledge base has expanded over the years, clinical psychiatry has undergone significant changes in theory, practice, and treatment. For example, psychiatric illnesses in the 17th and 18th century were explained in terms of evil spirits, in which persecution and isolation of the patient were customary treatment modalities. In the 19th century, Freud emphasized how the environment and past traumas influenced the individual's psyche. Although this was an advancement in the theory of mental illness, treatment modalities were lacking. Isolation and restraint were customary treatments, and the idea of chemical sedation was first introduced.

The late 20th century introduced psychobiology, a field of neuroscience that analyzes how biological

processes influence mood, cognitive activity, and behavior. The emphasis turned toward neuroanatomy and neurobiology, and psychiatry began to focus on the function of the brain's naturally occurring chemical mediators—the psychoactive neurotransmitters. Since then, research has flourished regarding how specific neurotransmitters from certain areas of the brain influence mental processes such as cognition, mood, memory, perception, fear, addiction, pain, and anger.

In the latter part of the 20th century, psychiatry became increasingly focused on neurotransmitters, particularly how they could be biologically manipulated to treat disorders. Now, in the 21st century, psychiatry is emerging as psychobiology, a neuroscience where diagnosis and treatment of mental illness focus on brain neurochemistry. Our knowledge base in psychobiology is growing because of increasing psychopharmacological investigation and advancements in neuroimaging technology. Twenty-first-century clinical psychiatry is based on an expanding field of psychobiology, an area of study that encompasses neuroanatomy, neurophysiology, and new discoveries in genetics. The field of psychogenomics is creating a novel way of looking at susceptibility to mental illness and addiction. This field of genetic discoveries will likely characterize 21st-century psychiatry.

Epidemiology

Research in psychiatric epidemiology shows that mental disorders are common throughout the United States, affecting tens of millions of people each year, and that only a fraction of those affected receive treatment. Depression is the leading cause of disability worldwide. Approximately 52.9 million adults, or 21% of the U.S. population, experience mental illness each year. Males and females have the same likelihood of developing mental illness over the course of their lifetime, though females report symptoms and seek treatment more often than males. One-half of all chronic mental illness begins by age 14, and three-quarters by age 24. Out of all those affected by mental illness, approximately half do not receive treatment.

Basic Concepts of Psychobiology

Major areas of the brain that are associated with behavior and emotional responses include the hypothalamus, neocortex, and limbic system. The autonomic nervous system (ANS) and endocrine organs also influence our thoughts, behaviors, reactions, and emotions. In turn, our thoughts, behaviors, reactions, and emotions can influence the ANS via a mind–body connection. The study of psychobiology focuses on the unique connection between brain, body function, and behavior.

Neuroanatomy and Psychobiology

The current theory of psychobiology specifically concentrates on the interaction between the limbic system and the neocortex. The **limbic system** refers to a central rim of cortical tissue within the cerebral hemisphere (see Fig. 36-1). It includes specific structures, such as the amygdala and hippocampus, and is surrounded by the **neocortex,** a highly developed area of the cerebrum.

The limbic system is primarily responsible for emotional reactions and participates in mental functions such as learning, motivation, and memory formation. The limbic system includes the hypothalamus,

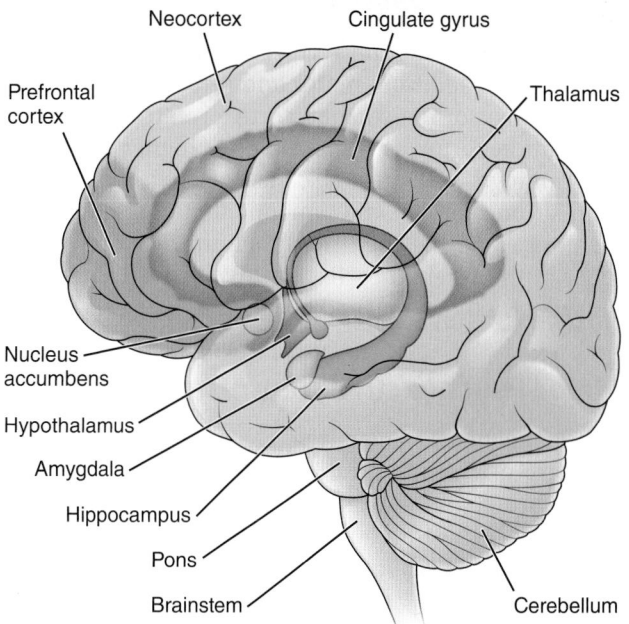

FIGURE 36-1. The limbic system. The limbic system is a complex set of structures that lies on both sides of the thalamus, just under the cerebrum. It includes the hypothalamus, hippocampus, amygdala, and several other nearby areas. It appears to be primarily responsible for our emotional life and the formation of memories.

hippocampus, amygdala, olfactory cortex, septal nuclei, nucleus accumbens, cingulate cortex, basal ganglia, ventral tegmental area, and periaqueductal gray matter. Each area is involved in processing information entering the brain in different ways. The hippocampus plays an important role in the formation, consolidation, and retention of memories, spatial navigation, and the regulation of stress. Stimulation of the **amygdala** evokes fear, anger, and aggression. The hypothalamus is involved in hunger, satiety, sleep onset, and thermoregulation. The olfactory cortex processes the sense of smell. The septal nuclei and nucleus accumbens play a role in reward and reinforcement. The hippocampus is mainly involved in memory. The cingulate cortex is involved in emotion formation and processing, learning, and memory. Areas of the basal ganglia and ventral tegmental area are involved in reward learning, cognition, and inhibition and motivation. The periaqueductal gray matter plays critical roles in autonomic function, motivation, and behavioral responses to threatening stimuli. The limbic system of the brain interacts and projects neuronal pathways into the prefrontal cortex, neocortex, midbrain, brainstem, and the spinal cord.

The neocortex's role is to modify the limbic system responses, which tend to be impulsive and reactive. The neocortex's actions are described as executive decision making, judgment, and insight in response to stressors.

The cerebral cortex is involved in processing and integrating information received from other areas of the brain. In addition, motor and sensory function in certain areas of the cerebral cortex, referred to as the association cortex, is responsible for higher cognitive functioning. This area is concerned with language acquisition, abstract and symbolic thought, long-term memory, and other cognitive functions. The prefrontal lobes of the cerebral cortex are involved with personality, decision making, and insight.

Major Psychoactive Neurotransmitters

The major neurotransmitters released by the brain's neurons are serotonin (5-hydroxytriptamine), norepinephrine, and dopamine. Norepinephrine is present in its highest amounts in the hypothalamus, and then in the medial limbic system areas. About 70% of the norepinephrine is concentrated in axon terminals arising in the medulla and locus ceruleus of the rostral pons. A large amount of serotonin is within axons of other ascending fibers, especially those starting in the reticular formation of the midbrain, and ending in the amygdala, septal nuclei, and lateral areas of the limbic lobe. Neuronal axons of the ventral tegmental parts of the midbrain have large amounts of dopamine. Three pathways in the hippocampal formation are believed to utilize glutamate, aspartate, or both as the major excitatory neurotransmitter.

Serotonin has several actions related to mood and behavior. Decreased serotoninergic activity is associated with depression and is seen in bipolar disorders. Serotonin is also involved in inhibiting the transmission of painful stimuli. A reduction in catecholamines, particularly norepinephrine, is related to depression. The activity of norepinephrine is referred to as noradrenergic activity. Dopamine has been studied because of its role in movement disorders such as Parkinson's disease, but it also plays a major role in behavior and addiction. It is theorized that an excessive level of dopaminergic stimulation is related to the development of schizophrenia. Enhanced dopaminergic activity is also experienced as a positive reward response in a patient with an addiction.

Gamma aminobutyric acid (GABA) is another psychoactive neurotransmitter. Neurons that produce GABA are called GABAergic neurons; these have chiefly inhibitory action at receptors.

Genetics and the Environment

Research studies have been conducted on monozygotic and dizygotic twins regarding mental illness, and researchers commonly conclude that the interaction of genetics and environment is responsible for mental illness. In some disorders, it seems that genetics play a particularly significant role. For example, a patient with depression usually has a family member who also has depression. However, studies show major depressive disorder (MDD) is a polygenic disorder, with multiple loci being identified, each with a small effect. There are 102 gene loci that are associated with the disorder. This suggests that other factors also play a role in mediating the risk for MDD. It is well established that environmental factors, especially stress and exposure to adverse life events, contribute to the risk. Therefore, it is proposed that aside from hereditary genetic DNA variants, epigenetics mediate the depression risk following exposure to an adverse life event. In **attention deficit-hyperactivity disorder (ADHD)**, familial and twin studies have demonstrated a hereditary risk of 60% to 90%. Alternatively, studies show that exposure to environmental toxins, such as nicotine, in utero increases the risk of developing ADHD. Children whose mothers smoked during pregnancy are almost twice as likely to develop ADHD as those whose mothers were nonsmokers. It is theorized that early exposure to nicotine alters neuronal maturation and brain structure in the fetus. However, for most psychiatric disorders, multiple genes are responsible. Schizophrenia has a polygenic architecture in which hundreds or even thousands of variants collectively contribute to risk.

Basic Pathophysiology Concepts of Behavioral Disorders

As brain anatomy and physiology have been studied in relation to behavioral disorders, specific alterations in psychobiology have been identified. Because of breakthroughs in neuroscience and improvements in imaging technology, actual changes of brain structure and function can be visualized in some mental disorders. Imaging studies are used to assist in the diagnosis of patients with certain psychiatric disorders. Psychobiology is an emerging science, and the following theories and research findings are becoming the basis for treatments.

Kindling Theory and Bipolar Disorder

Neurons in the brain become active when stimulated, and the **kindling theory** asserts that if neurons are stimulated too frequently, they become overly sensitive to further stimulation. The theory was originally applied to epilepsy to explain that repeated seizures made the brain sensitive to lower levels of stimulation, and therefore to more seizures. Interestingly, the kindling theory has recently been applied to bipolar disorder. The rapid cycling between the manic and depressive stages that characterizes bipolar disorder stimulates neurons, and the neurons become sensitized so that progressively less stimulation is needed to evoke a response from them. The more frequently the cycling occurs, the more sensitized or vulnerable the brain becomes to repeated episodes. This rapid cycling affects approximately 20% to 30% of patients who are diagnosed with bipolar disorder. Therefore, the kindling theory has been applied to both bipolar disorder and epilepsy. There is a similar hyperexcitability of neurons in both disorders. For this reason, antiepileptic drugs, which decrease neuron excitability, have a mood-stabilizing effect on persons with bipolar disorder.

Alterations in the Prefrontal Cortex

Alterations in dopaminergic and noradrenergic activity in the prefrontal cortex have been linked to several behavioral disorders, including frontotemporal lobe dementia, Parkinson's dementia, and ADHD. Examination with single photon emission computed tomography (SPECT) has demonstrated decreased metabolic activity in the prefrontal area in patients with ADHD. The prefrontal cortex is the area that normally would exert control over the limbic system, and decreased activity in this area is consistent with the loss of executive function and poor impulse control seen in individuals with ADHD. It also provides a rationale for the use of medications that increase dopaminergic and noradrenergic activity in the prefrontal cortex in the treatment of ADHD.

Changes in the prefrontal cortex are also associated with bipolar disorder. Magnetic resonance imaging (MRI) and computed tomography (CT) scans have indicated that the prefrontal cortex is smaller in patients with bipolar disorder than in patients who do not have the condition.

Other Anatomical Alterations

Neuroimaging studies of the brain have demonstrated both cerebral atrophy and enlarged ventricles in patients who have schizophrenia. Additionally, changes have been identified in the white matter of the temporal and occipital lobes of patients with schizophrenia. White matter consists of myelinated neuronal tissue, so changes in white matter have the potential to alter neuronal function and neurotransmitter activity.

Alterations in Brain Physiology and Neurotransmitters

The integrated actions of the cortex and the hypothalamus are responsible for the physiological responses to normal daily life. Under normal circumstances, the ANS and hypothalamus work together to maintain homeostasis. However, in clinical depression or repeated episodes of severe persistent stress, this relationship can be altered.

When a patient experiences the physiological stress response, activation of the hypothalamic–pituitary–adrenal (HPA) axis and the sympathetic nervous system (SNS) are enhanced. The result is that excessive amounts of both cortisol and catecholamines are produced. These increases have specific physiological effects, such as increased heart rate, blood pressure (BP), and elevated blood glucose levels. Behavioral changes and changes in appetite accompany the high levels of cortisol and catecholamines. Over time, elevated cortisol levels can inhibit the serotonergic activity within the brain and lead to depressed mood.

Psychiatric Assessment

Psychiatric assessment involves obtaining information about psychological and physical symptoms, as well as all current medications, supplements, and substance use. Because physical symptoms are associated with behavioral disorders, patients need to be evaluated to rule out medical conditions that may also have similar symptomatology. For example, anxiety includes physiological arousal of the SNS, resulting in restlessness, irritability, trembling, and increased heart rate. Similar symptoms are seen in hyperthyroidism, hypoglycemia, complex partial seizures, and caffeine intoxication. Therefore, medical conditions associated with the behavioral symptoms must be ruled out before a diagnosis of mental illness is made.

Behavioral disorders are complex phenomena, and diagnosis can be challenging. Specific criteria for diagnosing behavioral disorders are contained in the *Diagnostic and Statistical Manual of Mental Disorders,* which is published by the American Psychiatric Association and is currently in its fifth edition (*DSM-5*). Also, screening tools such as the Mini-Mental Status Examination (MMSE), Alcohol Use Disorder Identification Test (AUDIT), Mini-Cog test, Beck Depression Inventory, CAGE questionnaire, and Geriatric Depression Scale are commonly used to assess mental disorders. There are numerous psychological assessment tools for mental health that can assist qualified clinicians to make formal diagnoses; see a collection of tools at https://www.psychologytools.com/download-scales-and-measures/.

Mini-Mental Status Examination

The **Mini-Mental Status Examination (MMSE)**, the most commonly used psychiatric test in clinical practice, is a brief questionnaire used to screen for cognitive impairment or dementia. It is also used to follow the course of cognitive changes in an individual over time, making it an effective way to document an individual's response to treatment. The MMSE includes simple questions and problems in a number of areas: orientation, short-term memory, basic arithmetic, language use, comprehension, and basic motor skills. The test can be administered in 10 minutes or less, and numerical scores can be calculated to show whether the patient's cognition is normal or is slightly, moderately, or severely impaired. Although the MMSE has shown efficacy in the diagnosis of severe dementia in many individuals, the assessment tool has been criticized for its inaccuracy in individuals with less than a high school education and low literacy. Studies have also shown that the MMSE has limited utility for diagnosing minimal cognitive impairment, which occurs in early stages of dementia. Because of the shortcomings of the MMSE, a Modified MMSE known as 3MS has been developed, which has shown greater reliability and sensitivity for testing early dementia and those with low literacy. Some of the questions from the MMSE have been revised in the 3MS.

Mini-Cognitive Examinations

A rapidly administered, mini-cognitive examination can be used in lieu of the comprehensive MMSE or 3MS. The clinician asks the patient to remember three words, such as "bat," "cow," and "tree." Then the clinician asks the patient to perform the clock-drawing test. The clinician supplies a paper for the patient and asks the patient to draw an arbitrary time on the clock, such as 1:50 (see Fig. 36-2). The clock-drawing test requires a number of cognitive, motor, and perceptual functions for successful completion. After the patient completes drawing the clock, the patient is asked what three words were to be remembered before drawing the clock. Remembering the three words and drawing a completely normal clock suggest that a number of functions are intact and contributes to the weight of

evidence that the patient may, for example, be able to continue to live independently. Alternatively, an inability to remember the three words and a grossly abnormal clock are indicators of cognitive impairment warranting further investigation.

Another screening tool that quickly and briefly screens for cognitive impairment is the trail drawing test. The patient is provided a set of consecutive numbers or letters placed on a page in an arbitrary order. The patient is asked to connect the numbers or letters from one to another in proper order. This has been shown to test executive functioning in older individuals. Executive functioning involves cognitive flexibility, concept formation, and self-monitoring. With impaired executive functioning, instrumental activities of daily living (IADLs), such as accounting, shopping, medication management, and driving, may be beyond the person's capacity even though memory impairment is mild. Executive dysfunction is one element in the *DSM-5* criteria for the diagnosis of dementia.

> ### 🩺 CLINICAL CONCEPT
>
> Screening a patient for the IADLs is more sensitive for cognitive impairment than activities of daily living (ADL) screening.

Depression Assessment

Depression is one of the most common psychiatric disorders in both younger and older adults. Persons who are depressed have characteristic symptoms such as feelings of sadness, loneliness, irritability, worthlessness, hopelessness, agitation, and guilt that may be accompanied by an array of physical symptoms. The Beck Depression Inventory and the Geriatric Depression Scale are examples of available screening tools that can be used in the diagnosis of depression. The patient answers questions regarding specific symptoms such as appetite, sleep, concentration ability, and anhedonia. The assessment tool yields a numerical score that indicates mild, moderate, or severe depression.

Psychiatric Treatment

Successful treatment of mental disorders includes education, psychoactive medication, and psychotherapy. Technological interventions are also available when counseling and medication are ineffective.

Psychotherapy

There are different types of psychotherapy, and each focuses on a different aspect of the person's life. Psychodynamic psychotherapy is a therapeutic process

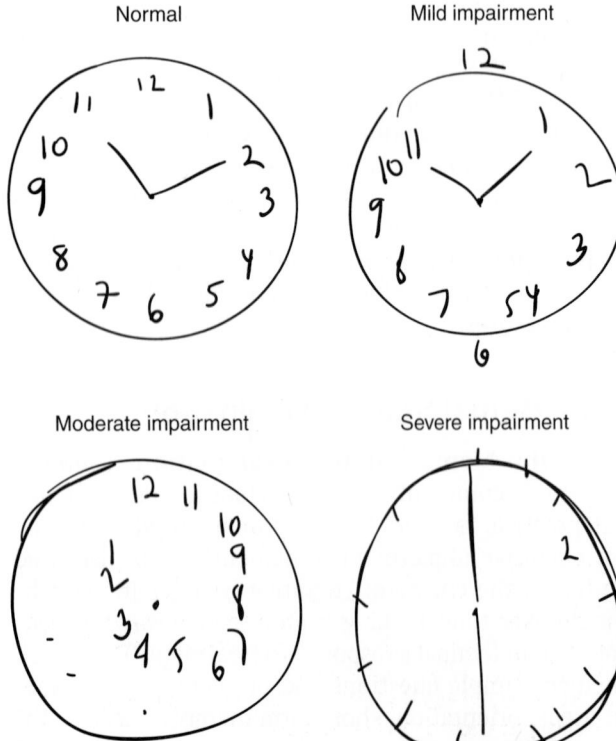

FIGURE 36-2. The clock-drawing test for cognitive status. The patient is asked to draw a clock displaying a specific time, such as 1:50. This simple test has been shown to be more sensitive for early Alzheimer's disease than several other screening tools and can be scored according to standard protocols.

that enables the patient to explore feelings and past traumatic experiences. The therapist investigates the patient's background and childhood to look for patterns or significant events that may play a role in the patient's current difficulties. Psychoanalysis, the type of therapy associated with Sigmund Freud, is a form of psychodynamic therapy.

Cognitive-behavioral therapy (CBT) focuses on specific problems and is commonly used for anxiety and depression. This form of therapy is based on the belief that irrational thinking or faulty perceptions cause psychological dysfunction. A cognitive-behavioral therapist often works with a patient to change thought patterns and problematic behaviors that have been developed through years of reinforcement.

Interpersonal psychotherapy focuses on the patient's interpersonal relationships and skills. It is based on the belief that interpersonal factors strongly contribute to psychological problems, and it aims to change the person's interpersonal behavior by fostering adaptation to current interpersonal roles and situations.

Supportive psychotherapy and education are necessary to assist the patient, family, and others to understand the psychological disorder. Group therapy is a form of supportive psychotherapy where two or more patients work with one or more therapists or counselors. This method is a popular format for support groups, where group members can learn from the experiences of others and offer advice. Group therapy can help patients by providing a peer group of individuals who are currently experiencing the same symptoms or who have recovered from a similar problem. Group members can also provide emotional support and a safe forum to practice new behaviors.

> ### 🧠 CLINICAL CONCEPT
>
> CBT and interpersonal therapy are the most commonly used types of psychotherapy.

Psychoactive Medications

Psychoactive medications, also called psychotropic medications, are substances that cross the blood–brain barrier to affect the brain's neurochemistry and alter mood, thoughts, or perceptions. They act by increasing the synthesis of one or more neurotransmitters or reducing its reuptake from the synapses. Alternatively, they can act by decreasing synthesis of one or more neurotransmitters or antagonizing the neurotransmitter at the receptor (see Fig. 36-3). There are six main categories of psychoactive medications:

1. Antidepressants, which treat disorders such as clinical depression, dysthymia, anxiety, eating disorders, and borderline personality disorder

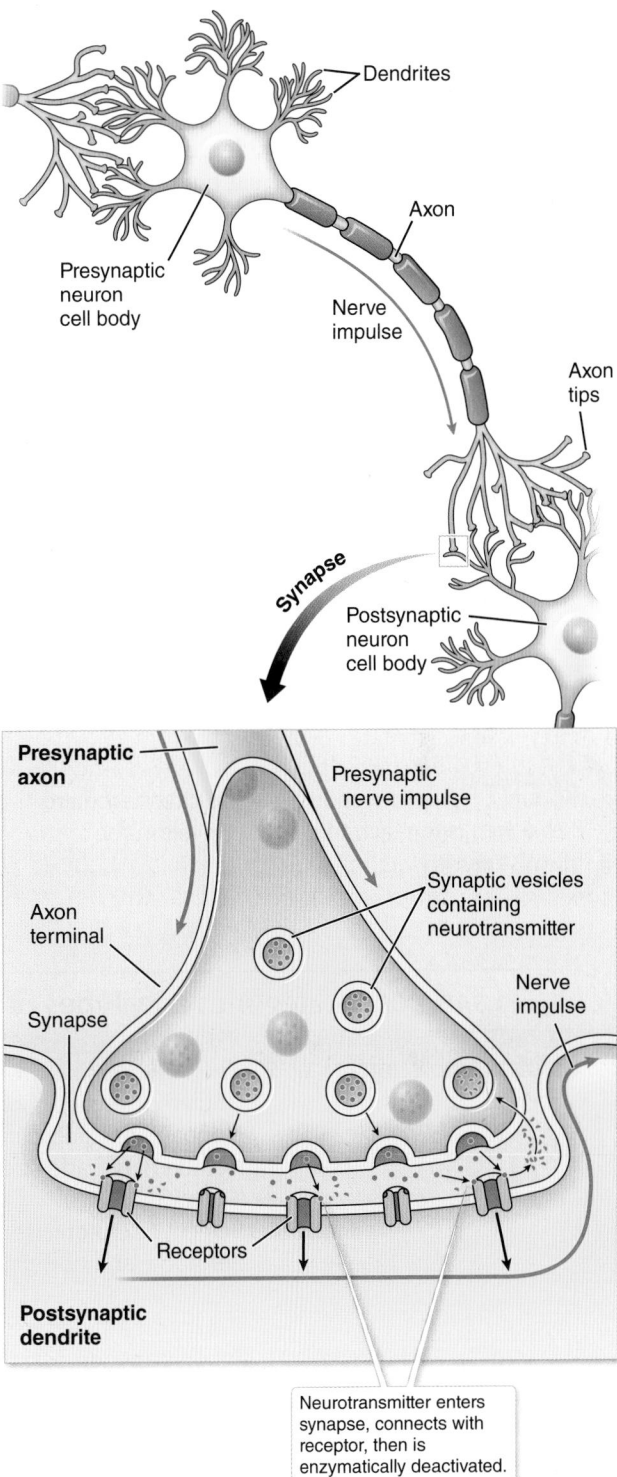

FIGURE 36-3. The process of neurotransmission. The axon of a presynaptic neuron releases chemical neurotransmitters into a synapse. Neurotransmitters include norepinephrine, dopamine, and serotonin. The neurotransmitters stimulate a receptor on the postsynaptic neuron. After the neurotransmitter stimulates the receptor, it may be degraded by enzymes and deactivated. Alternatively, a neurotransmitter can be reabsorbed into the presynaptic neuron for deactivation.

2. Stimulants, which treat disorders such as ADHD and narcolepsy and suppress the appetite
3. Antipsychotics, also referred to as neuroleptics, which treat psychoses such as schizophrenia and augment the effects of antidepressants
4. Mood stabilizers, which treat bipolar disorder and schizoaffective disorder; some anticonvulsant medications are mood stabilizers
5. Anxiolytics, which treat anxiety disorders
6. Depressants, which are used as hypnotics, sedatives, and anesthetics

There are different types of drugs within each category of psychoactive medication (see Table 36-1).

CLINICAL CONCEPT

Treatment that consists of psychoactive medications in conjunction with psychotherapy is most commonly recommended for mental illness.

ALERT! Most psychoactive medications require 3 to 6 weeks to reach therapeutic levels in the bloodstream.

Antidepressants

There are several different types of antidepressant medications, including **selective serotonin reuptake inhibitors (SSRIs), tricyclic antidepressants (TCAs), monoamine oxidase inhibitors (MAOIs), serotonin–norepinephrine reuptake inhibitors (SNRIs),** noradrenergic and specific serotonergic antidepressants (NaSSAs), and dopamine reuptake inhibitors (DRIs).

Selective Serotonin Reuptake Inhibitors. SSRIs are the most widely used medications for the treatment of depression. They are also used for anxiety, insomnia, panic disorder, obsessive-compulsive disorder (OCD), and eating disorders. They inhibit neuronal reuptake of serotonin in the central nervous system (CNS), which increases the concentration of serotonin in the synaptic cleft. This leads to increased serotonergic activity within the brain. It is theorized that serotonin contributes to feelings of well-being, regulation of mood and appetite, memory, and sleep. Decreased serotoninergic neurotransmission has been proposed to play a key role in the etiology of depression.

Like most antidepressants, SSRIs require 3 to 6 weeks to reach a therapeutic blood level and beneficial effect. SSRIs are well tolerated by most patients and have fewer adverse effects than other antidepressants. They do not cause psychological or physiological dependence. SSRIs lack the anticholinergic and

TABLE 36-1. Categories and Types of Therapeutic Psychoactive Medications

Major Therapeutic Classification	Drug Category	Commonly Used Agents
Antidepressants	Dopamine receptor inhibitors (DRIs)	Bupropion
	Monoamine oxidase inhibitors (MAOIs)	Phenelzine
	Noradrenergic and specific serotonergic antidepressants (NaSSAs)	Mirtazapine
	Selective serotonin receptor inhibitors (SSRIs)	Prozac
	Serotonin and norepinephrine receptor inhibitors (SNRIs)	Venlafaxine
	Tetracyclic antidepressants (TeCAs)	Trazodone
	Tricyclic antidepressants (TCAs)	Amitriptyline
Antipsychotics (Neuroleptics)	First generation • Phenothiazines • Butyrophenones • Thioxanthenes Second and third generation	Chlorpromazine Haloperidol Flupentixol Aripiprazole Olanzapine Quetiapine Risperidone Ziprasidone
Anxiolytics Mood stabilizers	Benzodiazepines Anticonvulsants Lithium	Lorazepam Lamictal
Psychostimulants	Amphetamines Methylphenidate Norepinephrine reuptake inhibitors	Adderall Ritalin Duloxetine

cardiovascular side effects typical of the TCAs, but like many psychiatric medications, they have adverse sexual effects, including decreased libido and anorgasmia. SSRIs are a preferable type of antidepressant because they have a low cardiotoxicity and their lethality is low in suicide attempts compared with other drugs.

> **ALERT!** A rare but life-threatening adverse event associated with SSRIs, called serotonin syndrome, is thought to be caused by either too high a dose of the SSRIs or interactions with other drugs, resulting in overactivation of the central serotonin receptors. The clinical presentation of serotonin syndrome includes agitation, confusion, rapid heart rate, loss of muscle coordination, hyperreflexia, diarrhea, high fever, and loss of consciousness.

SSRIs are useful in patients with substance use issues because they do not cause psychological and physiological dependence. Fluoxetine (Prozac) is the prototypical SSRI medication. When discontinuing an SSRI, one should slowly taper the dose downward. There is a "discontinuation syndrome" that causes anxiety, dizziness, sweating, and insomnia if SSRIs are abruptly stopped.

> **ALERT!** Antidepressants may increase suicidal thoughts in children, adolescents, and young adults during the first few months of therapy.

Tricyclic Antidepressants. TCAs were among the first antidepressants to be developed. In the past, TCAs were the first choice for pharmacological treatment of clinical depression. They have been increasingly replaced by the SSRIs and other newer antidepressants. TCAs' beneficial effects occur because they increase norepinephrine and serotonin in the synapse of brain neurons. They are effective for major depression, particularly treatment-resistant depression. They are also prescribed for chronic pain; generalized anxiety; and panic, social anxiety, and obsessive-compulsive and eating disorders. Amitriptyline (Elavil) is the prototypical TCA. Common side effects of TCAs are caused by anticholinergic activity and include dry mouth, blurred vision, tachycardia, constipation, urinary retention, and orthostatic hypotension resulting in dizziness. TCAs also cause sedation and therefore may be given at bedtime to utilize this side effect's benefit for sleep. TCAs are cardiotoxic in overdose and can cause death. Potential adverse reactions include cardiac dysrhythmias, myocardial infarction, and heart block.

> **ALERT!** TCAs cause anticholinergic activity and are contraindicated in patients who have narrow-angle glaucoma or prostatic hypertrophy, orthostatic hypotension, or cardiac arrhythmias. Because of possible cardiovascular effects, TCA overdose can be fatal.

Monoamine Oxidase Inhibitors. MAOIs are another class of medications used for the treatment of major depression. These drugs block the activity of monoamine oxidase, the enzyme that destroys norepinephrine, dopamine, and serotonin. Their effect allows the neurotransmitters, particularly norepinephrine, to remain longer in the synapses of the brain. In addition to depression, MAOIs are used for panic disorder, social phobia, atypical depression, bulimia, **posttraumatic stress disorder (PTSD),** and borderline personality disorder. An example of an MAOI inhibitor is phenelzine (Nardil). The major drawback of MAOIs is their possible fatal dietary and drug interactions, as they cannot be taken with tyramine-containing foods such as dried meats, cheese, and wine. The combination can provoke a malignant hypertensive crisis. MAOIs have potential interactions with many other medications. When changing to another antidepressant medication, there is a 2- to 3-week "washout" period when the patient must slowly taper the dose of MAOI to zero. This period when there is no antidepressant medication is another drawback of MAOIs. Because of the potential side effects, MAOIs are a last choice of antidepressant therapy. Recently, a transdermal form of MAOI has become available without the unsafe side effects.

Serotonin–Norepinephrine Reuptake Inhibitors. SNRIs are another class of drug used in the treatment of major depression and other mood disorders. They are sometimes also used to treat anxiety, OCD, ADHD, chronic neuropathic pain, and fibromyalgia syndrome and for the relief of premenopausal syndrome. SNRIs increase the levels of serotonin and norepinephrine in brain synapses. Venlafaxine (Effexor), duloxetine (Cymbalta), and desvenlafaxine (Pristiq) are the key drugs in this class. As with SSRIs, the abrupt discontinuation of an SNRI usually leads to withdrawal, or discontinuation syndrome, which could include states of anxiety and other symptoms.

 CLINICAL CONCEPT

To discontinue an MAOI or SNRI, the patient should slowly taper the dose under the supervision of a professional.

Noradrenergic and Specific Serotonergic Antidepressants. NaSSAs, also called tetracyclic antidepressants, are a class of psychiatric drugs used primarily as antidepressants. They act by antagonizing norepinephrine and serotonin receptors, which allows the neurotransmitters to remain longer in the synapse. Mirtazapine (Remeron) is the main drug within this class.

Dopamine Reuptake Inhibitors. Low dopamine levels are associated with depression. A DRI increases the amount of dopamine that remains in the neural synapse. DRIs are used for major depressive episodes, particularly treatment-resistant depression. DRIs are also used in the treatment of ADHD, narcolepsy, and obesity. They stimulate the narcoleptic individual to maintain wakefulness and assist in the management of obesity by suppressing appetite. They are also used for social anxiety disorder and other anxiety disorders. The most common DRI used for therapeutic purposes is bupropion (Wellbutrin).

ALERT! High doses of bupropion increase susceptibility to seizure. Antiseizure medications used in conjunction with bupropion can act to decrease susceptibility to seizure and may be used as mood stabilizers.

Mood Stabilizers

Lithium has been a standard medication used for many years to prevent the fluctuating mood swings of depression and mania in bipolar disorder. Anticonvulsant medications, when used in conjunction with antidepressants, can also stabilize mood disorders. Common agents are carbamazepine (Tegretol), divalproex sodium (Depakote), valproic acid (Depakene), and lamotrigine (Lamictal). The exact mechanism of action of lithium and anticonvulsant medications is unknown. However, if lithium is ineffective for a patient, switching to an anticonvulsant is successful in stabilizing mood in many patients.

Psychostimulants

Psychoactive medications that stimulate the central and peripheral nervous system can also be added to a drug regimen if a patient is suffering treatment-resistant depression. Common agents include methylphenidate (Ritalin) and amphetamine/dextroamphetamine (Adderall). The addition of an amphetamine can enhance alertness, endurance, productivity, and motivation. Amphetamines have been used for many years for ADHD and narcolepsy. However, it is important to understand that amphetamines affect the cardiovascular system and increase heart rate and BP. These drugs can cause anxiety and

heart failure in some patients. Often, the side effects of appetite suppression and insomnia are reasons to discontinue stimulant medications.

Benzodiazepines

Benzodiazepines (BNZ) are medications that bind with the GABA receptor to decrease neuronal activity. These medications promote muscle relaxation and a decrease in anxiety. Adverse effects include sedation, physical dependence, fatigue, ataxia, memory difficulties, slurred speech, and weakness. Alprazolam (Xanax), diazepam (Valium), clonazepam (Klonopin), and lorazepam (Ativan) are commonly used BNZs.

ALERT! Because of sedating effects, BNZs can increase the risk of falls in older adults.

ALERT! Used in combination with alcohol, BNZs can create synergistic effects that may cause CNS depression and respiratory arrest in cases of accidental or intentional overdose.

Antipsychotic Medications

Antipsychotic medications block dopamine in the brain, which is theorized as the cause of schizophrenia. These drugs, also called neuroleptics, can inhibit delusions, hallucinations, and disordered thought. They are also used to bolster the antidepressant effects in bipolar disorder. There are three generations of antipsychotic medications: first, second, and third.

First Generation Antipsychotics. Phenothiazines are first generation antipsychotic medications that are used in schizophrenia and are extremely sedating. Chlorpromazine (Thorazine), haloperidol (Haldol), thioridazine (Mellaril), and perphenazine (Trilafon) are prototypical antipsychotic agents that have been widely used in the past. These agents have a wide spectrum of side effects and are used infrequently in clinical settings today. Side effects include weight gain, hyperprolactinemia, decreased white blood cell count, glucose intolerance, restlessness (called akathisia), sexual dysfunction, and involuntary movements called tardive dyskinesia. Hyperprolactinemia can cause breast enlargement and milk discharge (called galactorrhea) in both males and females. **Tardive dyskinesia (TD),** which causes uncontrollable movements of the face, mouth, tongue, and extremities, can occur in long-term users of these medications. At times, patients need an increasing dosage of phenothiazines to prevent breakthrough episodes of psychosis. Patients can experience chemical dependence on these first generation antipsychotic agents.

Second Generation Antipsychotics. Second generation antipsychotic drugs, also called atypical antipsychotic agents, are used for schizophrenia as well. These medications are preferred over first generation antipsychotics because they cause fewer side effects; for example, they do not cause tardive dyskinesia. These medications are commonly used as adjuvant agents in severe mood disorders such as acute mania and bipolar depression. Risperidone (Risperdal), quetiapine (Seroquel), olanzapine (Zyprexa), ziprasidone (Geodon), and lurasidone (Latuda) are second generation antipsychotic agents.

> **ALERT!** TD is a potentially permanent movement disorder resulting from chronic use of dopamine receptor blocking agents. Any antipsychotic agent can cause TD. Switching from a first generation to a second generation antipsychotic with lower dopamine affinity, such as clozapine or quetiapine, may reduce TD. Vesicular monoamine transporter 2 (VMAT2) inhibitors, deutetrabenazine and valbenazine, have been recently approved as treatment for TD.

Third Generation Antipsychotics. Third generation antipsychotic medications include aripiprazole (Abilify). The mechanism of action is similar to other antipsychotic medications, although there are fewer side effects.

Pathophysiology of Selected Psychiatric Disorders

Behavioral disorders and psychiatric illness may affect many areas of the brain and therefore many areas of the individual's functioning. Some disorders may be primarily biological, whereas others may have a greater component of learned behavior. Studies of psychobiological disorders have strongly relied on neuroimaging studies of the brain and psychopharmacological research. A research base regarding the psychobiology of mental illness is emerging, but a great deal of study is still needed.

Anxiety Disorders

Anxiety, a vague sense of dread related to an unspecified danger, is a universal human emotion. During periods of anxiety, physiological stimulation of the SNS causes somatic symptoms such as restlessness and irritability, increased heart rate, hyperventilation, a sense of impending doom, and an inability to process stimuli. Extreme anxiety is called panic; at this level of anxiety, a person is often immobilized and in need of constant monitoring. Anxiety disorders include **generalized anxiety disorder (GAD),** panic attacks, OCD, specific phobias, social anxiety disorder, acute stress disorder, and PTSD.

Generalized Anxiety Disorder

GAD is one of the most common psychiatric disorders and affects 40 million persons in the United States. An estimated 5.7% of U.S. adults experience GAD at some time in their lives. GAD is described as having excessive anxiety and worry (apprehensive expectation), difficulty controlling the worry, and associating the anxiety and worry with three (or more) physical and cognitive symptoms of restlessness, feeling keyed up or on edge, being easily fatigued, difficulty concentrating or mind going blank, irritability, muscle tension, and sleep disturbance. GAD has a prevalence rate of 18% to 23% in adults aged 18 and older in primary care settings within the United States. In family practice settings, the highest number of cases of GAD occurs in persons 36 to 45 years of age, and the lowest rate occurs in persons 60 years and older. According to the CDC, those aged 18 to 29 have highest rates of GAD. In 2019, 9.4% of children aged 3 to 17 years (approximately 5.8 million children) had diagnosed anxiety disorder. According to large population-based surveys, up to 33.7% of the population are affected by an anxiety disorder during their lifetime. There is substantial underrecognition and undertreatment of these disorders. According to the CDC, more than 40% of persons with anxiety disorder are not receiving treatment. Females are almost twice as likely as males to be diagnosed with GAD over their lifetime. Although the prevalence of GAD decreases with age in males, it increases in females.

Etiology. Anxiety is a natural response and a necessary protective mechanism in humans. The emotion of anxiety alerts the individual that there is a threat to safety in the environment. Anxiety is naturally associated with a wide range of physical and affective symptoms, as well as changes in behavior and cognition; however, anxiety can also become a pathological disorder when it is excessive, uncontrollable, and triggered by no specific external stimulus.

Genetic risk factors are under investigation, and researchers have found a genetic predisposition for two types of anxiety disorders: a panic–generalized anxiety–agoraphobia group and a specific phobias group. Important risk factors also include comorbid substance use disorder and family history. Anxiety disorder often co-occurs with major depression, alcohol use disorder and other substance use disorders, and personality disorders. Differential diagnosis from physical conditions—including thyroid, cardiac, and respiratory disorders, and substance intoxication and withdrawal—is imperative. If untreated, anxiety disorders tend to recur chronically.

Pathophysiology. Anxiety is believed to arise from the neurons in the region of the brain called the amygdala. The amygdala analyzes the emotional significance of environmental stimuli and stores emotional memories. Pathways exiting from the amygdala travel to multiple brain structures, including the parabrachial nucleus, resulting in dyspnea and hyperventilation; the dorsomedial nucleus of the vagus nerve, activating the parasympathetic nervous system; and the lateral hypothalamus, resulting in SNS activation. The amygdala also sends neuronal signals to the prefrontal cortex, where cognitive experiences of specific anxiety disorders are integrated.

 CLINICAL CONCEPT

Chest pain and shortness of breath are common symptoms of anxiety disorder that are mistaken for cardiovascular disease.

Clinical Presentation. Patients with GAD are often overwhelmed by worry about their health, family, work, and finances. Worrying is difficult to control, often negatively affecting relationships and social and occupational activities. Patients with GAD commonly present with physical symptoms of dizziness, hyperventilation, insomnia, headaches, muscle aches, fatigue, and gastrointestinal symptoms. It is important to rule out medical disorders and other psychiatric disorders, particularly depression. GAD and depression are often present together. The clinician should also rule out medications or other substances such as caffeine, alcohol, and amphetamines as a source of anxiety.

Diagnosis. It is important for the clinician to be aware of the medical disorders that can cause anxiety (see Box 36-1). Laboratory tests such as complete blood count (CBC), metabolic panel, liver enzymes, serum creatinine, cardiac troponin, and enzymes should be used to rule out medical disorders before diagnosing GAD. It is also prudent to perform an electrocardiogram (ECG) when suspecting GAD.

There is a list of criteria for the diagnosis of GAD (see Box 36-2). A self-report questionnaire is also available to assist clinicians in diagnosing anxiety disorders. The seven-item GAD scale, called GAD-7, is a reliable, valid, and easy-to-use self-report questionnaire for evaluating the presence and severity of GAD.

 CLINICAL CONCEPT

Anxiety and depression are often present together. SSRIs can be used to treat this combination of disorders.

BOX 36-1. Disorders That Present With Anxiety

CARDIOPULMONARY DISORDERS
- Angina pectoris
- Cardiac arrhythmia
- Cardiomyopathy
- Congestive heart failure
- Hypertension or hypotension
- Mitral valve prolapse
- Myocardial infarction
- Syncope

ENDOCRINE DISORDERS
- Hypercortisolism
- Hyperthyroidism
- Hypoglycemia
- Hypoparathyroidism
- Hypothyroidism
- Pheochromocytoma

METABOLIC CONDITIONS
- Hyperkalemia
- Hyperthermia
- Hypocalcemia
- Hypoglycemia
- Hyponatremia

NEUROLOGICAL DISORDERS
- Encephalitis
- Neoplasms
- Parkinson's disease
- Postconcussion syndrome
- Seizure
- Vertigo

NUTRITIONAL STATES
- Anemias
- Caffeine overload
- Folate deficiency
- Pyridoxine deficiency
- Vitamin B$_{12}$ deficiency

PSYCHIATRIC DISORDERS
- Depression
- Panic disorder
- Social anxiety disorder
- Substance-induced anxiety disorder

RESPIRATORY DISORDERS
- Asthma
- Chronic obstructive pulmonary disease
- Hypoxia
- Pneumonia
- Pneumothorax
- Pulmonary edema

Treatment. Psychological treatments, particularly CBT, and pharmacological treatments, particularly SSRIs and SNRIs, are effective, and their combination could be more effective than is treatment with either

BOX 36-2. Diagnostic Criteria for General Anxiety Disorder

A. Excessive anxiety and worry (apprehensive expectation), occurring more days than not for at least 6 months, about a number of events or activities (such as work or school performance).

B. The person finds it difficult to control the worry.

C. The anxiety and worry are associated with three (or more) of the following six symptoms (with at least some symptoms present for more days than not for the past 6 months).
NOTE: Only one item is required in children:
1. Restlessness or feeling keyed up or on edge
2. Being easily fatigued
3. Difficulty concentrating or mind going blank
4. Irritability
5. Muscle tension
6. Sleep disturbance (difficulty falling or staying asleep, or restless, unsatisfying sleep)

D. The anxiety, worry, or physical symptoms cause clinically significant distress or impairment in social, occupational, or other important areas of functioning.

E. The disturbance is not attributable to the physiological effects of a substance (e.g., a drug of abuse, a medication) or another medical condition (e.g., hyperthyroidism).

F. The disturbance is not better explained by another mental condition, for example, anxiety or worry about having panic attacks in panic disorder, negative evaluation in social anxiety disorder (social phobia), contamination or other obsessions in OCD, separation from attachment figures in separation anxiety disorder, reminders of traumatic events in post-traumatic disorder, gaining weight in anorexia nervosa, physical complaints in somatic symptom disorder, perceived appearance flaws in body dysmorphic disorder, having a serious illness in illness anxiety disorder, or the content of delusional beliefs in schizophrenia or delusional disorder.

Reprinted with permission from American Psychiatric Association. (2013). *Diagnostic and statistical manual of mental health disorders* (5th ed.). American Psychiatric Association, Washington, D.C.

individually. CBT is a short-term (e.g., 10 to 20 weeks), goal-oriented, skills-based treatment that reduces anxiety-driven biases to interpret ambiguous stimuli as threatening, replaces avoidant and safety-seeking behaviors with approach and coping behaviors, and reduces excessive autonomic arousal through strategies such as relaxation or breathing retraining.

SSRIs and SNRIs have antianxiety and antidepressant effects. The main difference between treatment of anxiety and depressive disorders is the starting dose. Patients with anxiety tend to be sensitive to most drug side effects, so the recommended starting dose is half that recommended for depression. That dose should be maintained for 1 to 2 weeks and, if tolerated, subsequently doubled. Although the starting dose is lower than that for depression, the therapeutic dose for treatment of anxiety disorders is the same or higher. A common error is failure to titrate the antidepressant dose to reach a therapeutic dose. Underdosing is one of the contributors to the low proportion of guideline-concordant treatment of anxiety in primary care settings.

Often, the patient requires a short course of a benzodiazepine (BNZ) to diminish anxiety symptoms. The use of BNZ is controversial as they can be addictive. BNZs promote binding of GABA, a neuroinhibitory transmitter, to GABA receptors. BNZs have a rapid onset of action, and short- to intermediate-acting agents such as lorazepam (Ativan) are preferred because they are less likely to accumulate and lead to excessive daytime sedation. Long-acting agents, such as diazepam (Valium), alprazolam (Xanax), chlordiazepoxide (Librium), and clorazepate (Tranxene), are not recommended as they can cause drowsiness and sleepiness. BNZs should be avoided in patients who have previously demonstrated addictive behavior. Discontinuation should be carried out gradually over several weeks in all patients who have had 4 or more weeks of treatment to avoid withdrawal symptoms such as agitation, insomnia, irritability, and restlessness.

Other drugs that could be used as adjuncts to treat anxiety disorders are gabapentin and pregabalin. However, these are used mainly for neuropathic pain and seizures and only as off-label agents for GAD. These agents target anxiety symptoms by modulation of GABA biosynthesis and nonsynaptic GABA neurotransmission in the brain. There has been growing concern about the potential for gabapentin and pregabalin abuse. Atypical antipsychotics, such as quetiapine, also have good evidence as adjunctive medications in GAD; however, their metabolic adverse effects may limit their use. Quetiapine inhibits central serotonergic, including $5HT_{2A}$, and dopaminergic, including D_2, receptors. Buspirone, an azapirone, nonbenzodiazepine anxiolytic, is an effective treatment for GAD. Buspirone is an agonist of the serotonin receptor subtype 5-hydroxytryptamine-1A and is a nonaddictive, nonsedating alternative. However, buspirone requires 1 to 3 weeks to reach therapeutic blood levels and has a short half-life, necessitating dosing two to three times per day. Beta blockers, such as propranolol or atenolol, have some evidence of efficacy in acute prevention of performance anxiety (a form of social anxiety disorder), but not in other anxiety disorders.

In individuals who have not fully responded to initial GAD treatment and in whom there are clinically significant mood fluctuations (e.g., hypomania or irritability), studies show augmentation with agents that have mood-stabilizing properties, such as valproate or lamotrigine, can be effective.

Hydroxyzine has shown efficacy in treatment-resistant anxiety. It is usually needed two to four times a day. It is more sedating than BNZs and buspirone, and thus potentially useful for treating insomnia associated with GAD.

Stress management is a necessary skill for those who suffer from chronic anxiety. In addition to pharmacotherapy or CBT, aerobic exercise is recommended for treatment of GAD in patients who are medically capable. In particular, high-intensity exercise appears to be more effective than low-intensity as a complement to first-line therapy for GAD. Relaxation techniques such as mindfulness, deep breathing, yoga, and meditation are commonly taught to those with GAD. Patients are often asked to keep track of their episodes of anxiety with a log. This log can be used in CBT, which can analyze the triggers of anxiety and teach alternative reactions. The patient also needs education about medications and substances that can cause anxiety.

Panic Disorder

Panic disorder is an anxiety disorder characterized by recurrent, unexpected episodes of extreme anxiety. **Panic attacks** are discrete periods of intense apprehension, fear, and terror, with associated physiological symptoms of extreme anxiety. Association with the place of the panic attack can result in a pervasive avoidance of places and situations in which a panic attack could occur.

The lifetime prevalence rate of a panic disorder is reported to be at 3.5% in the community. This is likely a low estimate, however, because many affected individuals do not report these episodes. In clinical settings, the rate is reported to be 10% to 30% in respiratory and neurology clinics and up to 60% in cardiology settings. One-half to one-third of individuals diagnosed with panic attacks in community samples also have agoraphobia, a fear of being outside of the home alone. Panic disorders usually occur in persons of adolescent age through young adulthood up to the mid-30s. Those with first-degree biological relatives with panic disorder are eight times more likely to develop panic attacks.

Etiology. There is a genetic component to panic attacks, and multiple genes are associated with the disorder. The neuroanatomical model for panic disorder focuses on specific areas in the amygdala or hypothalamus that are hyperexcitable and make the individual susceptible to unprovoked panic symptoms. Neurotransmitter-focused studies have mainly implicated alterations in the GABA-benzodiazepine receptor and serotonin receptor systems. Panic attacks often occur at times of significant life stress. Studies have shown that childhood adversity such as a history of physical or sexual abuse increases the risk of panic disorder in adult years.

Pathophysiology. The central and peripheral neurological systems are involved in panic disorder.

Biological theories stress a genetic etiology and argue strongly against the idea that panic is merely a reaction to distressing stimuli. The psychobiology of panic disorder has been extensively investigated in terms of neuroimaging studies and pharmacological evidence.

Sympathetic System Stimulation. Anxiety reactions are associated with increased levels of catecholamines such as epinephrine. The **locus coeruleus** is a part of the brainstem involved in physiological responses to stress and panic attacks. The locus coeruleus includes 50% of all adrenergic neurons in the CNS and sends projections to many parts of the brain, including the hippocampus, amygdala, limbic system, and the cerebral cortex (see Fig. 36-4). Stimulation of the locus coeruleus causes fear and anxiety. Antianxiety medications inhibit firing of neurons in the locus coeruleus and decrease the noradrenergic response.

GABA–BNZ System. The GABA receptor complex is involved in panic attacks. Binding of a BNZ to the GABA receptor results in a slowing of neuronal depolarization and neurotransmitter release. Decreased GABA–BNZ binding seen on SPECT scanning is

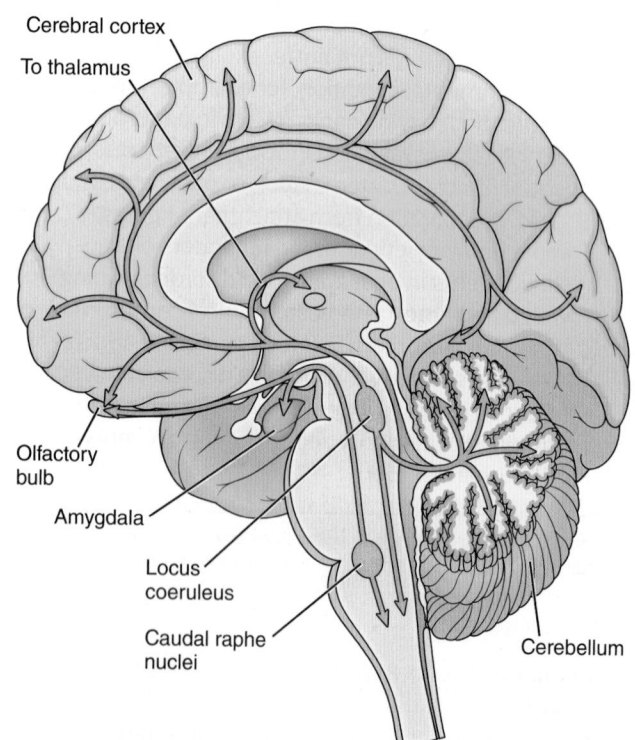

FIGURE 36-4. Locus coeruleus and amygdala. The principal centers for norepinephrine-secreting neurons are the locus coeruleus and the caudal raphe nuclei. The ascending nerves of the locus coeruleus project to the frontal cortex, thalamus, hypothalamus, limbic system, and cerebellum. Nerves projecting from the caudal raphe nuclei ascend to the amygdala and descend to the midbrain. The locus coeruleus is involved in arousal and autonomic activity. The amygdala is involved in memory and emotional reactions.

observed in the hippocampus and prefrontal cortex in patients with panic disorder, whereas decreased BNZ binding in the prefrontal cortex and insula has been seen on positron emission tomography (PET) scans of patients with panic disorder.

Neurocircuitry of Fear. The neurocircuitry of fear model proposes that panic attacks are similar to animal fear and avoidance responses. A panic response is theorized to originate in the amygdala. Input to the amygdala is modulated by the thalamus and prefrontal cortex. Projections from the amygdala extend to various parts of the brain involved in the fear response, such as the locus coeruleus (arousal), brainstem (respiratory activation), HPA axis (stress response), and cortex (cognitive interpretation of the stressor).

Clinical Presentation. Symptoms of a panic attack develop quickly and may include palpitations or increased heart rate, sweating, trembling, shortness of breath, feeling of choking, chest pain, nausea, chills or hot flushes, and paresthesias. In addition, the individual may feel dizzy, detached from oneself, and a sense of unreality. They fear losing control and think that they are dying.

🩺 CLINICAL CONCEPT

Commonly, individuals with panic attacks believe they are having a heart attack and go to an emergency department for treatment.

Diagnosis. The American Psychiatric Association's *Diagnostic and Statistical Manual of Mental Disorders, Fifth Edition (DSM-5)* diagnostic criteria define a panic attack as an abrupt surge of intense fear or discomfort that occurs from a calm or anxious state. The symptoms typically reach a peak within minutes and resolve within an hour. Panic attacks may be triggered or untriggered; however, for a diagnosis of panic disorder, some of the attacks must be untriggered or unexpected. During the attack, an individual manifests at least 4 of the following 13 symptoms:

- Palpitations, pounding heart, or accelerated heart rate
- Sweating
- Trembling or shaking
- Sensations of shortness of breath or smothering
- Feelings of choking
- Chest pain or discomfort
- Nausea or abdominal distress
- Feeling dizzy, unsteady, light-headed, or faint
- Chills or heat sensations
- Paresthesias (numbness or tingling sensations)

- Derealization (feelings of unreality) or depersonalization (being detached from oneself)
- Fear of losing control or "going crazy"
- Fear of dying

Panic disorder is frequently associated with agoraphobic avoidance, substance use, increased utilization of medical services, and reduced quality of life. Individuals with panic disorder appear to have a higher likelihood of suicide attempts compared with the general population.

Although no specific tests exist for panic disorder, several medical conditions can mimic the disorder. A complete history and physical examination and laboratory testing should be carried out before diagnosis of panic disorder. Medical conditions that should be ruled out before diagnosing a panic disorder include:

- Alcohol or drug withdrawal
- Angina
- Aortic dissection
- Cardiac arrhythmias
- Hyperparathyroidism
- Hyperthyroidism
- Hypothyroidism
- Mitral valve prolapse
- Myocardial infarction
- Pheochromocytoma
- Vertigo

There are clinician-administered and patient self-assessment instruments used as diagnostic tools and to monitor response to treatment. The gold standard instrument for the disorder is the Panic Disorder Severity Scale. This is a seven-item scale that covers key clinical aspects of the syndrome (attack frequency, attack intensity, anticipatory anxiety, phobic avoidance, avoidance of internal bodily sensations, relationship impairment, work impairment).

Treatment. Psychotherapy in the form of CBT can be effective when the disabling aspects of anxiety are reduced with pharmacotherapy. Among medications for panic disorder, SSRIs have been the most widely tested in clinical trials and shown to be most efficacious compared with placebo. Patients who have co-occurring depression with anxiety disorder will benefit from SSRIs as monotherapy to treat both the panic disorder and depression. If SSRIs are not effective, SNRIs can be used. Augmentation of SSRIs or SNRIs with a BNZ is effective. BNZs produce a rapid response in reducing anxiety. Long-acting BNZs such as clonazepam are recommended. BNZs should be avoided in persons with history of substance use disorder. Nonbenzodiazepine alternatives include gabapentin, pregabalin, and mirtazapine. In patients who experience treatment-resistant panic disorder, TCAs or MAOIs can be used.

Supportive psychotherapy and education are necessary to assist the patient to understand and confront anticipated anxiety. Different techniques may be used to help the patient learn to control the physiological responses of panic, understand the triggers of the panic disorder, and alleviate stressors.

> **ALERT!** Patients with hypertension who take MAOIs should have their BP periodically monitored because MAOIs can incite a hypertensive emergency. MAOIs should not be used with other drugs that can increase BP.

Obsessive-Compulsive Disorder

OCD is a chronic illness that has a waxing and waning course; it is characterized by persistent and repetitive thoughts, impulses, or images that are intrusive and inappropriate. They may cause marked distress and anxiety. These thoughts are often related to contamination, the order of objects, or sexual imagery. To relieve the anxiety caused by the obsessions, the patient actively engages in compulsive activities, or rituals, to neutralize the thoughts through actions such as hand washing, praying, cleaning, or putting objects in order. In OCD, a progressive deterioration in an individual's occupational and social functioning may occur.

The lifetime prevalence rate of OCD in community studies is 2.5% in adults and 1% to 2% in children. Age of onset is earlier in males (ages 6 to 15 years) than females (ages 20 to 29 years), but OCD can begin at any time. One-third of first episodes occur between the ages of 10 to 15 years, and 75% develop by age 30 years. The onset of OCD is usually gradual and insidious, and the predisposition to develop the condition is genetically linked.

Pathophysiology. The etiology and pathophysiology of OCD are incompletely understood. Evidence from functional brain imaging studies shows hyperactivity in some cortical and subcortical regions of the brain—specifically, the orbital frontal cortex, limbic system, thalamus, and caudate. There are abnormalities in serotonergic, dopaminergic, and glutamatergic neurotransmission in these regions. Twin studies have supported the idea that heredity is involved in OCD, with a genetic influence of 45% to 65% in studies in children and 27% to 47% in adults. Monozygotic twins are concordant for OCD (80% to 87%), compared with 47% to 50% concordance in dizygotic twins. Interestingly, case reports have revealed OCD arising in children and young adults following acute group A streptococcal infections. Fewer reports cite herpes simplex virus as the apparent precipitating infectious event. It has been hypothesized that these infections trigger a CNS autoimmune response that results in neuropsychiatric symptoms.

Clinical Presentation. OCD is characterized by recurrent obsessions and compulsions that are severe enough to cause social and occupational impairment. Obsessional thinking is repetitive, persistent, intrusive, and distressful to the individual. The individual feels that the obsessions are out of their control. A temporary reduction in anxiety results from the completion of a compulsive ritual. If the patient is unable to complete the ritual, anxiety will increase, and physiological symptoms of anxiety will occur.

> **CLINICAL CONCEPT**
>
> Compulsive rituals such as hand washing temporarily relieve the distress of obsessions in patients with OCD.

Diagnosis. There are no specific tests for OCD, but two instruments, the Yale-Brown Obsessive Compulsive Scale and the Obsessive-Compulsive Inventory, may be used in addition to the MMSE.

Treatment. CBT and SSRIs are the recommended first-line treatment for OCD. CBT may be focused on changing the patient's response to anxiety-producing situations.

Post-Traumatic Stress Disorder

PTSD is a specific type of anxiety disorder that develops in response to a highly stressful event in a person's life. Symptoms of PTSD follow life-threatening events in which a person perceives actual or threatened death, serious injury, or a threat to physical integrity. The person may have been the victim of, or a witness to, horrific events. PTSD commonly occurs in soldiers, survivors of rape, Holocaust survivors, prisoners of war, and physically and emotionally abused children.

Epidemiological studies of the U.S. general population estimate that PTSD will affect 15% to 24% of adults at some time in their lives. The incidence of PTSD depends on the type of stressful event studied. For example, the stressful event of sudden and unexpected loss of a loved one—the most common experience that causes PTSD—accounts for 39% of cases in men and 27% of cases in women. In general, women have a greater lifetime prevalence of PTSD than men. Persons of all ages are susceptible to it.

The following are risk factors for PTSD:

- Being female
- Experiencing intense or long-lasting trauma
- Having experienced trauma earlier in life
- Having other mental health problems, such as anxiety or depression
- Lacking a good support system of family and friends
- Having first-degree relatives with mental health problems, including PTSD
- Having first-degree relatives with depression
- Having been abused or neglected as a child

Pathophysiology. The pathophysiology of PTSD remains relatively unclear, with research suggesting the involvement of the HPA axis, ANS, serotonin, and endogenous opioids. It is proposed that individuals with PTSD have higher levels of sympathetic arousal at the time of the trauma than those who do not have PTSD. In persons with PTSD, autonomic responses to both innocuous and harmful stimuli are elevated, but the effects are more noticeable with harmful stimuli.

In the normal response to stress, the body releases catecholamines and cortisol as it attempts to adapt to the stressor. In PTSD, the stress response becomes dysfunctional, resulting in chronic autonomic hyperactivity. Stimulation of the ANS causes the hyperarousal and intrusive thoughts seen in patients with PTSD. The patient experiences an increase in heart rate, respiratory rate, and BP. When an individual experiences prolonged and repeated trauma, the SNS is stimulated and endogenous opioids are released by the body. When any stimulus triggers the past trauma, an analgesic effect caused by endogenous opioids develops in the patient with PTSD. This opioid effect is known as psychic numbing. It is theorized that when the levels of natural opioids dwindle, hyperactivity occurs, similar to opioid withdrawal.

Neuroimaging studies are increasing our knowledge base regarding PTSD. MRI of the brain shows a decrease in volume of the hippocampus in those with combat-related PTSD and survivors of childhood abuse. When veterans with PTSD relive mental experiences of combat, PET imaging demonstrates increased blood flow to the amygdala and anterior cingulate and a decrease in blood to Broca's area. Such neuroimaging patterns are beginning to reveal the brain's activity during nonverbal, emotional reactions in PTSD.

ALERT! PTSD can cause suicidal or homicidal actions by the patient.

Clinical Presentation. Individuals who experience PTSD typically have flashbacks, insomnia, hyperarousal, and hypervigilance. An environmental cue can reactivate the traumatic experience, causing the patient to respond in the same way they would during the original stressful event. Commonly, such behaviors are socially inappropriate and can lead to legal problems and incarceration.

PTSD can have a chronic course leading to impairment in daily functioning and decreased personal well-being. There may be a reduced capacity to master life skills and impairment of role performance. Chronic stress is associated with dysfunction of the nervous system; HPA axis; and cardiovascular, metabolic, and immune systems.

Increased arousal in patients with PTSD may affect ANS functioning, with resultant changes in cardiac function. Individuals with PTSD report a significantly greater number of current and lifetime medical conditions than those without PTSD. Medical conditions include anemia, arthritis, asthma, back pain, diabetes, eczema, peptic ulcer, and kidney and lung disease.

Diagnosis. The essential feature of PTSD is the development of characteristic symptoms following exposure to an extreme traumatic stressor. The person's response to the event must involve intense fear, helplessness, or horror.

CLINICAL CONCEPT

In children, the PTSD response involves disorganized or agitated behavior.

Diagnostic criteria include a strong emotional response that involves fear, helplessness, or horror, as well as impairment in daily functioning and symptoms that begin within 3 months after the trauma. To be diagnosed with PTSD, the individual must demonstrate three types of symptoms:

1. Reliving the trauma
2. Avoidance
3. Hyperarousal

Persons who relive the traumatic event have distressing images, nightmares, or flashbacks. The individual also demonstrates persistent avoidance of situations associated with the trauma and hyperarousal in the form of insomnia, hypervigilance, or difficulty concentrating. The disorder can be acute, with symptoms lasting less than 3 months, or chronic, with symptoms lasting 3 months or more. The full symptom picture causes clinically significant distress or impairment in social, occupational, or other areas of functioning. Delayed onset can occur if symptoms do not erupt until at least 6 months after the traumatic event.

Treatment. Persons with PTSD often self-soothe with alcohol or illicit drugs because the stigma related to mental health problems often prevents them from seeking help. Either disruptions in significant relationships or disproportionate anger may cause an individual to enter treatment for PTSD.

Antidepressants, antipsychotics, BNZ medications, and psychotherapy are used to treat PTSD. The serotonergic system has been implicated in the symptoms of PTSD. Behavioral inhibition and constraint are mediated by serotonergic pathways. The angry and irritable effects seen in patients with PTSD may be related to a deficit in serotonin. This supports the use of the SSRI types of antidepressants in PTSD. Additionally, clonidine or prazosin can be helpful in treating trauma-related nightmares and sleep disruption.

Mood Disorders

Mood disorders are common worldwide and may affect as much as 14% of the world's population. In the United States, more than 20 million people have been diagnosed with a mood disorder. Individuals with mood disorders have an increased risk of self-harm or suicide, as more than 90% of people who die by suicide have been diagnosed with either a mood disorder or substance use disorder.

Family studies indicate that if one parent has a mood disorder, the risk that a child will have the disorder is between 10% and 25%. The risk doubles if both parents have a mood disorder. Genetic factors may explain 50% to 70% of the etiology of mood disorders, as predisposition to the disease is inherited.

Major Depressive Disorder

Major depressive disorder (MDD) has the highest lifetime prevalence of any psychiatric disorder, at 17%. It affects one in every five individuals and is the leading cause of disability worldwide. Females experience MDD twice as frequently as males. This difference in prevalence is thought to be the result of hormonal influences, childbirth, and psychosocial factors. The mean age of onset for MDD is 40 years, with half of all patients diagnosed between 20 and 50 years, although the disorder may be found across the life span. The U.S. Preventive Services Task Force (USPSTF) recommends that primary-care clinicians screen for depression in the general adult population, adolescents aged 12 through 18, and females during the postpartum period.

> **ALERT!** Suicide is the major complication of mood disorders. The lifetime risk of suicide in mood disorders is 10% to 15%, although two-thirds of depressed individuals have suicidal ideation. Females attempt suicide more often than males, but males are more likely to die by suicide because they tend to utilize more lethal means.

Etiology. MDD is considered a multifactorial disease with various causes and triggers such as genetic susceptibility, stress, and other pathological processes. MDD is believed to result from a genetic–biochemical–environmental interaction. Some genetic mutations and polymorphisms affect the response of receptors to certain neurotransmitters, which, in turn, affects the resistance of the brain's chemical balance to stressors. However, it is not yet fully understood which genes or types of genetic changes, alone or in combination, can represent reliable genetic markers of depression.

To date, the greatest contribution to the understanding of the pathogenetic mechanisms of MDD has been made by physiological, biochemical, and pharmacological studies. These studies have allowed the formulation of several theories that attempt to describe the development of MDD on biochemical, cellular, anatomical, and physiological levels. No one theory completely explains the etiology or pathophysiology of MDD. However, there are commonalities in theories. Most theories of the etiology of depression involve an imbalance in monoamine neurotransmitters: 5-hydroxytryptamine (5-HT)/serotonin, norepinephrine, and/or dopamine. Also most theories include the etiological factor of chronic stress, and the subsequent malfunctioning of the hypothalamic–pituitary–adrenal (HPA) axis. The impact of repeated stressful incidents is a common theme in theories of depression. These repeated stressors continuously stimulate the defense and adaptation mechanisms of the individual and eventually lead to their exhaustion.

The functioning of GABA and glutaminergic systems also appears altered in depression. Some studies demonstrate abnormally decreased plasma and CSF levels of GABA and glutamine in patients with MDD. The cholinergic system is also implicated in the pathogenesis of depression because the muscarinic cholinergic system is overactive or hyper-responsive in depression.

Pathophysiology. The underlying pathophysiology of MDD is not clearly understood. Research focuses on disturbances in the neurotransmitters of the CNS: serotonin, norepinephrine, and dopamine. Neuroimaging and pharmacological research have been intricately involved in reaching conclusions about the influence of neurotransmitters in the development of MDD.

The role of CNS serotonergic activity in the pathophysiology of MDD is suggested by the efficacy of SSRIs in treatment. Also, studies show that depressive symptoms can be produced in research subjects when there is tryptophan depletion, which causes a reduction in CNS serotonin levels.

CLINICAL CONCEPT

Many persons suffer from a type of major depression called seasonal affective disorder (SAD). This disorder is most often seen in the winter months and resolves during the spring and summer. Studies show that SAD is mediated by alterations in CNS levels of serotonin and is likely provoked by alterations in circadian rhythm and lack of sunlight exposure.

Neuroimaging studies show that depression is associated with decreased metabolic activity in the neocortex of the brain and increased activity in the limbic system. By using PET images, researchers have found an area of the prefrontal cortex with abnormally diminished activity in patients with depression compared with nondepressed individuals. This region has widespread connections with areas that regulate dopamine, norepinephrine, and serotonin.

Some endocrine changes are also associated with depression. For example, the postpartum period is a time of fluctuating hormone levels when females are vulnerable to depression. Menopause, a time of decreasing estrogen, often triggers depression in females, and low testosterone levels are associated with depression in males.

Clinical Presentation. The most common signs and symptoms of MDD include anhedonia, early morning awakening, low energy and motivation, difficulty concentrating, and social withdrawal. Persons may have feelings of guilt, hopelessness, insomnia or hypersomnia, increased or decreased appetite, or psychomotor agitation or slowing.

In patients suspected of suffering from MDD, a complete assessment is necessary to rule out any medical illnesses with similar symptoms. For example, hypothyroidism can present with depression. Obtaining a list of medications, supplements, and any other substances used is important, because many of these are associated with the side effect of depression. Table 36-2 and Table 36-3 list medical conditions and medications that are linked to depression. Family history is important because there is a significant genetic role in the development of depression.

TABLE 36-3. Common Medications That Can Cause Depression

Classification	Drug
Cardiovascular medications	Clonidine Digitalis Beta adrenergic blockers Reserpine Thiazide diuretics
Cancer agents	Chemotherapeutic agents Corticosteroids Interferon
Endocrine medications	Adrenocorticotropic hormone Corticosteroids Anabolic steroids Oral contraceptives
Gastrointestinal medications	Cimetidine Ranitidine
Drugs with abuse potential	Opioids Alcohol Cocaine Marijuana Sedative-hypnotics

TABLE 36-2. Major Medical Conditions That Commonly Cause Depression

Category	Disorder or Condition
Cancer	Lung cancer Pancreatic cancer
Cardiovascular	Heart failure Myocardial infarction Stroke
Endocrine	Hypothyroidism Hyperthyroidism Addison's disease Cushing's disease
Infectious	AIDS Influenza Hepatitis Infectious mononucleosis Lyme disease
Neurological	Parkinson's disease Multiple sclerosis Alzheimer's disease
Nutritional deficiencies	Iron deficiency Thiamine deficiency Vitamin B_{12} deficiency

CLINICAL CONCEPT

Patients with depression spend more time in bed than patients with diabetes, hypertension, arthritis, or chronic lung disease and have as much functional disability as patients with heart disease.

In addition to the patient's current signs and symptoms, a history of prior episodes and treatment for depression (successes and failures) is an important guide to determine current treatment. Psychosocial history of childhood deprivation; abandonment; and physical, emotional, or sexual abuse are important trauma-related data to be assessed because they are contributing factors for depression. A depressed patient should be clearly questioned about suicidal thoughts and plans.

Diagnosis. Diagnosis is based on having at least five of the following symptoms for a minimum of 2 weeks:

- Sad mood most of the day, nearly every day
- Decreased interest in pleasurable activities (also called anhedonia)
- Weight loss or gain

- Daily insomnia or hypersomnia
- Psychomotor retardation or agitation
- Fatigue or loss of energy
- Feelings of worthlessness
- Inappropriate guilt
- Diminished levels of concentration and decisiveness
- Recurrent suicidal thoughts and plans

These symptoms cause significant distress and occupational and social impairment. Objective assessment tools are also used in the diagnosis of depression, including the Patient Questionnaire-9 (PQ-9), Hamilton Depression Rating Scale, Zung Self-Rating Depression Scale, Raskin Depression Scale, Beck Depression Inventory, Edinburgh Postnatal Depression Scale, and Geriatric Depression Scale. All of these are valid and reliable self-report questionnaires. Primary-care clinicians find the PQ-9 a highly specific assessment tool for depression.

Thyroid testing is recommended in depressed patients to rule out hypothyroidism as a cause of symptoms, because 8% of all patients with depression have a thyroid disorder. The thyrotropin-releasing hormone stimulation test is indicated in patients whose marginally abnormal thyroid test results suggest subclinical hypothyroidism.

Treatment. Depression can be treated with antidepressant medications, psychotherapy, electroconvulsive therapy (ECT), transcranial magnetic stimulation (TMS), and vagus nerve stimulation (VNS). Commonly, individuals are prescribed an antidepressant and are referred for psychotherapy. When prescribing an antidepressant, the clinician often uses a trial-and-error approach because different types of medications are therapeutic for different individuals. Most antidepressant medications require 3 to 6 weeks to reach therapeutic blood levels. This waiting period is extremely difficult for the depressed patient. It is important that the depressed patient has psychotherapeutic support during this waiting period.

The SSRIs are the first-line treatment medications for depression, as well as the most commonly used drugs for depression. Fluoxetine (Prozac) is the prototypical SSRI; other common medications used are venlafaxine (Effexor) and duloxetine (Cymbalta), which are SNRIs that block the reuptake of serotonin and norepinephrine. Bupropion (Wellbutrin), another commonly prescribed antidepressant, is a norepinephrine–dopamine reuptake inhibitor. Since the release of fluoxetine in the mid-1980s, the number of SSRIs and SNRIs has grown substantially. However, their use in children and adolescents is still debated, thus indicating a need for more research into their safety and efficacy. Recent meta-analyses generate many questions about the overall benefits versus costs of using SSRIs to treat major depression in children and adolescents.

TCAs and MAOIs are not first-line medications for MDD; however, they can be used for treatment-resistant depression. Because of the anticholinergic effects of TCAs and the potential side effect of elevated BP with MAOIs, different SSRIs and SNRIs should be tried first. Antipsychotic drugs and anticonvulsant medications are often added to the antidepressant regimen. These medications can amplify the antidepressant effect and stabilize mood. Common antipsychotic medications used include quetiapine (Seroquel) and aripiprazole (Abilify). Anticonvulsants include lamotrigine (Lamictal) and carbamazepine (Tegretol).

Ketamine is a pharmaceutical agent that may also be used in treatment-resistant depression. Treatment-resistant depression is diagnosed when the disorder has not responded to at least two pharmaceutical treatments. Ketamine is an anesthetic drug that acts as an *N*-methyl-D-aspartate receptor (NMDA) antagonist and targets glutamate. Rapid resolution of depression and suicidal ideation after single intravenous infusions of low doses of ketamine has been reported in patients with bipolar depression. Ketamine is available as an intravenous infusion and may require more than one treatment to demonstrate results. Ketamine is also available as a nasal spray (Esketamine). Ketamine can cause side effects that require patient monitoring such as high blood pressure, nausea and vomiting, perceptual disturbances, and feelings of dissociation. It also has addictive properties.

ALERT! Severe adverse events, such as an increased risk of suicidal thoughts and behavior, in adults and youth receiving antidepressants have been reported, leading to the implementation of a boxed warning on the labels of all antidepressants for pediatric use.

ECT, which induces a seizure in a well-anesthetized patient, is highly effective in treating depression. The mechanism of ECT is not fully known, but it is suspected that the induced seizure stimulates available neurotransmitters. ECT can be helpful in up to 70% of patients who fail to respond to antidepressants.

VNS was approved by the U.S. Food and Drug Administration in 2005 for treatment-resistant depression. A VNS system is surgically implanted to deliver electrical pulses to the vagus nerve, with mood elevation as the outcome. The device was first used in treating drug-resistant epilepsy. Elevated mood was observed in some of the treated patients, giving rise to use the device in depressed individuals.

TMS, a noninvasive procedure that delivers magnetic impulses to the cortex, can be used for treatment-resistant depression. It uses a stimulating coil placed directly on the head where magnetic impulses pass unimpeded through the skull. Transsynaptic effects depolarize the neurons, leading to increased secretion of growth factors such as brain-derived neurotropic factor. Some studies show that TMS can initiate neuronal reorganization and neurogenesis. Rapid magnetic pulses over the dorsolateral prefrontal cortex have demonstrated antidepressant effects.

Bipolar Disorder

Bipolar disorder is a mood disorder characterized by cyclical episodes of depression and mania; it includes two subtypes. Bipolar I and bipolar II disorders share similar characteristics, but bipolar I disorder includes an abnormally and pervasive elevated, expansive, or manic mood of at least 1 week; psychotic features; and potential harm to self or others, frequently requiring hospitalization. In bipolar II disorder, the expansive, elated, or irritable mood is manifested as a less elevated mood, also called hypomania. In bipolar II, no psychotic features are noted and depression is the major problem; there is also less impairment in social and occupational functioning compared with patients with bipolar I disorder.

Bipolar disorder typically begins in adolescence or early adulthood. The annual prevalence of bipolar disorder is 4% within the adult population. Bipolar I disorder is equally prevalent in males and females, but females are more likely to experience mood cycles, defined as four or more episodes per year. Manic episodes are more common in males, whereas females are more prone to mixed depression and mania.

A family history of bipolar disorder conveys a greater risk for mood disorder and bipolar disorder. Patients with bipolar disorders frequently have a substance abuse or anxiety disorder. In both MDD and bipolar disorders, males are at greater risk to have a comorbid substance abuse problem.

Pathophysiology. Neuroimaging studies have demonstrated that mood regulation takes place in the prefrontal cortex and the amygdala. In adults with bipolar illness, there is an alteration in connection between the dorsolateral prefrontal cortex and the amygdala, with an increased response by the amygdala to emotional cues. PET and SPECT scans show increased temporal lobe activity and increased amygdala volume. Some structural changes of the brain seem to cause the disorder, and some seem to be caused by the disorder.

Bipolar disorder has a strong genetic predisposition. In a landmark study, researchers found a connection between bipolar illness and a genome that encodes for an enzyme called diacylglycerol kinase (DGKA). DGKA is a crucial part of the lithium-sensitive pathway, and lithium is known as the first-line drug to treat bipolar illness. It is also known that chromosomes 13 and 15 are involved in both schizophrenia and bipolar illness.

Clinical Presentation. A patient with bipolar I disorder may be admitted to an inpatient facility for behavior that is unacceptable in society, because they cannot care for themselves, or are psychotic. A patient in a manic episode of bipolar I disorder has an elevated, expansive, or irritable mood. The person may be euphoric and have pressured speech and flight of ideas. The patient may talk in rhymes, called clang association, and may attempt to entertain others but instead intrude on conversations. Later, the euphoric mood changes to irritability, after which the patient can become demanding, testing rules and limits on behavior. Early in the manic episode, the patient may not sleep and is hyperactive and hyperverbal. The patient may wear colorful clothes, excessive makeup, and flamboyant hairstyles. Sexual interest and behaviors toward others are common during the manic episode. The patient is typically very impulsive and needs monitoring to avoid aggression or unwanted sexual behaviors toward other patients. Patients in a manic episode demonstrate poor judgment, lack of insight, and can be regressed in their behavior. Attention span may be limited. Patients can be preoccupied with religion, politics, finances, sexuality, or persecution. Paranoid or grandiose delusions are common. Patients may also self-medicate with alcohol or drugs to help themselves sleep or to escape their distress.

In lieu of manic episodes, a patient with bipolar I or II disorder may exhibit hypomania. Hypomania is similar to mania except the patient has no psychotic symptoms. The individual may be far more productive or outgoing and sociable than usual. This change in functioning and in mood is not subtle—the change is directly noticeable by others (usually friends or family members) during a hypomanic episode. A hypomanic episode is also not severe enough to cause serious impairment in social or occupational functioning, or to necessitate hospitalization.

A major complication of the mania associated with bipolar I disorder is exhaustion and cardiac collapse caused by lack of rest and sleep. Patients lose weight because they forget to eat as a result of hyperactivity and distractibility. They may also be a danger to themselves or others when they are psychotic, because suicide and homicide are complications of the illness. Social and occupational impairments are complications of not being treated or noncompliance with medications. It can be challenging to help the patient adhere to the treatment regimen because the patient "feels so good" in the manic state and may not want to return to a more euthymic (mood-stable) condition. Ups and downs of mood cycling are more common in bipolar I disorder than bipolar II disorder.

Diagnosis. The diagnosis of a bipolar disorder is based on the clinical presentation. The patient may present in either a manic or depressive phase of the disorder. Notably, the depressive episodes of bipolar disorder are defined by the same criteria as MDD in the

DSM-5, so that distinguishing bipolar from MDD frequently depends on identifying a history of manic or hypomanic symptoms. Past medical and psychiatric histories need to be obtained, including prior medications and treatment success or resistance. A family history of mental illness, particularly bipolar disorder, is a crucial component of the assessment. Routine bloodwork such as CBC and serum chemistry should be done to rule out any concomitant illnesses.

Treatment. Treatment for bipolar disorder includes medications and psychotherapy. Categories of medications used include mood stabilizers such as lithium, anticonvulsants, and atypical antipsychotic medications. Antipsychotics are used to reduce agitation and to promote rest. Mood stabilizers are one of the most common groups of medications used to treat the symptoms of mania and hypomania. Lithium is included in this class of medications, as well as several anticonvulsant drugs such as carbamazepine, valproic acid, and lamotrigine.

Although it is still considered the ideal mood stabilizer, lithium's mechanism of action remains unclear. It has effects on several neurotransmitter systems: serotonin, dopamine, norepinephrine, and acetylcholine.

ALERT! Lithium has a narrow therapeutic/toxic ratio, so plasma concentrations must be monitored closely. The signs and symptoms of lithium toxicity include increased tremors, nausea, vomiting, ataxia, and change in mental status. If untreated, lithium toxicity can lead to coma or death.

Antipsychotics may also be used to treat bipolar disorder. This class of medication is often used to control mania or decrease psychotic symptoms that can be present during the manic phase of the illness. Antianxiety medications can also be used during the manic phase.

ALERT! Antidepressant (SSRI) medications alone are not recommended for the treatment of bipolar disorder I or II, due to the risk of causing a sudden manic or hypomanic episode in the patient. When used, antidepressants should be combined with a mood stabilizer medication to avoid these problems.

Schizophrenia

Schizophrenia is a neurobiological disorder considered a **psychosis,** an abnormal condition of the mind where the affected person loses touch with reality. The person often suffers from delusions and hallucinations. In schizophrenia, patients may express themselves in various ways:

- Neologisms: using words with special meanings to the individual
- Clang associations: rhyming
- Word salad: a collection of random words
- Echolalia: repeating of others' words
- Echopraxia: repeating movements made by another person
- Flight of ideas: varied unconnected thoughts

Individuals often think they are being told to complete certain actions by someone. There is lack of insight and judgment. Often there is bizarre behavior, such as wearing inappropriate clothing or having inappropriate social, sexual, or aggressive interactions.

A delusion is a thought that is not grounded in reality. Three specific delusions are classic positive symptoms of schizophrenia:

1. Thought broadcasting: thinking one's thoughts are broadcasted so that everyone can hear
2. Thought insertion: thinking that others are inserting thoughts into the individual's head
3. Thought withdrawal: thinking that thoughts are being drawn out of the person's head by others

The lifetime prevalence rate of schizophrenia in the United States is approximately 0.5% to 1% of the population. Annual incidence of new cases ranges from 0.5 to 5.0 per 10,000 people per year. Geographical differences exist, as the disorder seems to be more common in urban areas compared with rural areas. Schizophrenia is equally prevalent in both males and females. Peak age of onset for males is age 10 to 25 years; for females, however, the onset peaks between 25 and 35 years. Approximately 90% of patients in treatment for schizophrenia present to mental health providers between the ages of 15 and 55—most experience their first symptoms and episode in their 20s. Onset before age 10 or after age 60 is extremely rare.

First-degree biological relatives of patients with schizophrenia have a 10 times greater risk for developing the disorder. Substance use disorder is a common comorbidity of schizophrenia. This includes alcohol, cannabis, and illicit drugs. Disordered use of such substances results in poorer overall functional ability. In addition, 90% of individuals with schizophrenia are prone to nicotine addiction. Individuals with schizophrenia represent between 15% and 45% of homeless persons; this is attributed to the difficulties these persons have remaining employed and socially functional.

Pathophysiology

The exact cause of schizophrenia is unclear, but a number of theories exist. Many studies using pharmacological agents and neuroimaging have attempted to delineate the cause. There is a genetic component to all forms of schizophrenia, with identical twins having a

50% concordance rate of the illness. The vulnerability-liability theory postulates that genetics lead to vulnerability, but the environment also exerts influence in the cause of schizophrenia. It is also theorized that an individual is at risk for developing schizophrenia if the father is older than age 60 years at the time of birth. This suggests a risk caused by altered sperm development in older males.

The dopamine hypothesis of schizophrenia is derived from the fact that antipsychotic drug treatment is based on antidopaminergic activity. Psychotic symptoms, such as delusions, have been linked to excessive dopamine levels. However, the cause of dopamine excess is unclear. The specific dopamine pathway involved is also unclear, though it is known that dopaminergic neurons project from the midbrain to the limbic system and the cerebral cortex.

Other neurotransmitters are theorized to be involved in schizophrenia. For example, an excess of serotonin has been hypothesized to cause symptoms of schizophrenia. Loss of GABAergic neurons in the hippocampus of some patients with schizophrenia may lead to hyperactivity of serotonin. The serotonin antagonistic activity of clozapine (Clozaril), an atypical antipsychotic drug, in the treatment of chronic schizophrenic patients provides support for this theory. Changes in levels of norepinephrine have been shown to be involved in the symptom of anhedonia experienced by patients with schizophrenia. The neurotransmitter glutamate may also be involved based on the fact that phencyclidine, a glutamate antagonist, causes an acute psychosis similar to schizophrenia.

Neuroimaging studies demonstrate a neuropathological basis for schizophrenia, including a loss of brain volume. CT scans note lateral and third ventricle enlargement, as well as reduction in cortical tissue. Reduced symmetry in the temporal, frontal, and occipital lobes has been noted.

On autopsy of persons with schizophrenia, there appears to be a decrease in the size of a number of brain regions, including the amygdala, hippocampus, parahippocampal gyrus, and prefrontal cortex. MRIs show that the hippocampus in individuals with schizophrenia is smaller than normal and has a disturbance in the transmission of glutamate. Disorganized distribution of neurons within the hippocampus of patients with schizophrenia has also been documented.

The basal ganglia and the cerebellum are also of interest to scientists because of movement disorders that occur in schizophrenia. Some researchers believe that instead of discrete brain areas as the focus of the illness, schizophrenia is a disorder of brain neural circuits that are caused by early developmental lesions.

Immune abnormalities seen in schizophrenia include a decreased T-cell interleukin-2 production, a reduced number of peripheral lymphocytes, abnormal cellular and humoral reactivity to neurons, and the presence of anti–brain cell antibodies.

Clinical Presentation

Early symptoms of schizophrenia may precede diagnosis. For example, an adolescent with schizophrenia may have not had friends, preferring solitary activities, such as watching television or playing on computers, versus group and social activities. The prodromal phase of the illness may begin with vague bodily symptoms and increased emphasis on religious or philosophical ideas; peculiar behavior; changes in affect; and unusual speech, behaviors, and perceptual sensations. The clinical presentation of a patient with schizophrenia varies from someone who is disheveled, aggressive, actively hallucinating, and delusional to someone who is mute and shows lack of spontaneous speech or movement.

Patients with schizophrenia often have a blunted or flattened affect, poverty of speech (alogia), **apathy,** lack of motivation (avolition), decreased spontaneous movements, and inattention to hygiene/grooming. Inattention, poor problem-solving and decision-making skills, and feelings of dysphoria and hopelessness are common. There may be suicidal feelings. Marked dysfunction occurs in the areas of employment, interpersonal relationships, self-care, and quality of life.

Patients frequently claim to hear voices. These voices may be loud or muffled, and there may be more than one voice in a conversation. The patient may also mumble to himself or herself in response. Command hallucinations tell the person to do something, often to hurt self or others, and are dangerous. Visual hallucinations are possible and are experienced as shadows, waves, or spirits. Patients are often paranoid and lack trust in others such as health-care providers.

Violence, suicide, and homicide are complications of untreated schizophrenia. Patients who are untreated may be violent because of impulsivity and delusions of persecution. Emergency management includes use of antianxiety and antipsychotic medications to control aggression. Suicide is a leading cause of premature death in patients with schizophrenia. Suicide attempts are made by 20% to 50% of patients, which is a 20-fold increase compared with the general population.

Diagnosis

Diagnosis is made based on the clinical presentation and exclusion of any organic causes. A complete psychiatric evaluation, history, and physical examination are needed to rule out any physical or drug-induced psychosis. Also important is a complete history of the patient's illness, adherence to treatment, social network, housing, and current medications. Serum laboratory tests should be performed to rule out medical illness.

Treatment

Although antipsychotic medications are the gold standard treatment for patients with schizophrenia, research has found that psychosocial interventions that include psychotherapy can improve clinical outcomes. Hospitalization may be necessary for safety and to stabilize the patient on antipsychotic medications. Outpatient treatment includes intensive partial hospitalization programs, medication evaluations, and support groups. The recovery model of schizophrenia treatment stresses patient responsibility to manage mental illness and build upon patient strengths so that they may live productive lives. Patients need education about their disease and the importance of adherence to the medication regimen.

Schizophrenia is treated medically through use of both traditional antipsychotics and the newer second generation of atypical antipsychotics. Traditional antipsychotics are dopamine receptor antagonists. Because of the possible motor side effects caused by the typical antipsychotics, such as acute dystonia, akathisia, pseudoparkinsonism, and tardive dyskinesia, patients are prescribed the newer second generation antipsychotics. Second generation antipsychotic drugs are serotonin–dopamine receptor antagonists. Remission occurs in approximately 70% of those who adhere to treatment.

Attention Deficit-Hyperactivity Disorder

ADHD is the most common psychiatric condition affecting children in the United States. This disorder has a dramatic impact on the child, family, and community. Approximately 30% of students with ADHD repeat a grade, up to 33% fail to complete high school, and only 5% to 10% complete college. ADHD is also associated with adolescents engaging in antisocial activities in approximately half of the cases. These teens are prone to unintentional injuries compared with those who do not have ADHD.

The prevalence rates for ADHD range from 1.9% to 14.4%. In school-aged children, the prevalence rate has been estimated to be between 3% and 7%. It is estimated that between 50% and 70% of children with ADHD will continue to have symptoms of the disorder as adults.

Several risk factors for ADHD have been identified. ADHD symptoms have been associated with infection such as meningitis and encephalitis, closed head injury, lead poisoning, hypoxia, and maternal substance use during pregnancy. ADHD is more common in low-birth-weight infants. It can occur with other disabling conditions such as sensory impairment and serious psychological and emotional disturbances. It can also occur in the presence of other extrinsic influences, such as poor socioeconomic background and dysfunctional parenting, though it is not a direct result of these environmental or physical conditions. In the past, ADHD was thought to be related to nutritional intake of sugar or artificial additives; however, there is no scientific evidence to support this.

Pathophysiology

There is no clear etiology in ADHD. Biological and environmental factors, such as genetics, perinatal complications, neurological illness, allergies, and environmental toxins, have been correlated with the disorder.

ADHD is a heterogeneous, nonprogressive, neurological condition. Genetic, neurological, and environmental influences play a role in its development. The condition is highly inheritable, with estimates of 60% to 90% across generations. Twin studies confirm a genetic link between identical twins. ADHD is thought to be a polygenic disorder that interferes with encoding and functioning of the neurotransmitters and the corresponding receptors. Investigations focus on genes responsible for dysregulation of dopamine and norepinephrine, their receptors, and their transporters. These two neurotransmitters influence attention, arousal, impulsivity, and mood. The role of neurotransmitter dysregulation in ADHD is supported, in that medications that affect the dopaminergic and noradrenergic systems are successfully used to control ADHD symptoms. The right prefrontal cortex, caudate nucleus, and globus pallidus appear to be smaller, show less blood flow, and display decreased electrical activity in children with ADHD compared with those without it. These areas of the brain are usually rich in dopamine receptors.

Perinatal complications, including antepartum hemorrhage, prolonged labor, and low Apgar scores at 1 minute, are more common among children with ADHD. Those infants with low birth weight and injury to the white matter are at increased risk for developing ADHD. The brains of children with ADHD show prefrontal cortex function abnormalities.

Clinical Presentation

Children with ADHD have very high levels of activity that make them look driven, restless, and never tiring in nature. The child may be unable to comply with school routines because of restlessness, causing them to become disruptive in the classroom. They may make noise, hum, squirm in their chairs, or tap at their desks. ADHD does not have an effect on intellect, but it can interfere with academic performance.

Children with ADHD cannot filter out extraneous stimuli, and distraction takes the form of an inability to concentrate. This makes completion of classwork difficult. At home, children with ADHD have difficulty listening to adults and carrying out multistep instructions. They seem to be in a hurry and rush to complete a task; in addition, they start many activities without completing them. Children with ADHD are impulsive. They may interrupt others and may not have patience to wait their turn, which can result in them becoming disliked by peers. Children with ADHD tend to befriend children who have issues with authority.

Other psychiatric disorders, such as conduct disorder and oppositional defiant disorder, are comorbidities of

ADHD. These disorders occur with high frequency in up to 30% to 50% of children with ADHD. Mood and anxiety disorders are also comorbid conditions and affect the degree of impairment and the course of the disorder. Compared with research control subjects, children with ADHD who are followed in adolescence and adulthood show higher rates of antisocial behavior and substance abuse.

Diagnosis

ADHD is suspected in a child who has academic and behavioral problems in preschool or elementary school. No laboratory tests, neurological assessments, or attention assessments have been established as diagnostic in the clinical assessment of ADHD. However, individuals need to be evaluated to rule out any complicating medical illnesses.

ADHD can be diagnosed in adults. Symptoms include difficulty maintaining attention, as well as hyperactivity and impulsive behavior. Adult ADHD symptoms can lead to a number of problems, including unstable relationships, poor work or school performance, and low self-esteem.

Treatment

Psychostimulant therapy is routinely prescribed to enhance a child's ability to focus on schoolwork and to reduce the child's inattention, impulsivity, and hyperactivity. The medications include methylphenidate (Ritalin) and amphetamine preparations. In persons with ADHD, psychostimulants work in a paradoxical way to increase attention and task-directed behavior while reducing hyperactivity, impulsivity, restlessness, and distractibility. This response is theorized to be the result of the neocortex being stimulated to exert executive control over more impulsive behaviors. There is a risk of substance abuse with the psychostimulants.

Methylphenidate (Ritalin) is the most widely used psychostimulant because of its simplicity of use and safety. Concerta is an extended-release version of methylphenidate. An amphetamine mixture called Adderall has proven effective, but drug abuse has been seen with this prescription medication. Atomoxetine (Strattera), another effective type of medication, is a nonstimulant SNRI that has the advantage of minimal risk of illicit abuse.

Dementia

Dementia is a decline of reasoning, memory, judgment, and other cognitive functions. The decline in cognition impairs the ability to carry out ADLs such as household chores, driving, and handling finances, and personal care such as bathing, dressing, and feeding. Although common in older adults, dementia is not a normal part of aging. It can be caused by reversible or irreversible causes. Dementia is more than age-related forgetfulness; it is a serious illness. Individuals with dementia lose the ability to reason, are unable to solve

problems, and cannot think abstractly. They are disoriented to time and place, and eventually they cannot identify persons.

Approximately 4 to 5 million people in the United States have some degree of dementia, and that number will increase over the next few decades with the aging of the population. Dementia affects about 1% of people aged 60 to 64 years and as many as 30% to 50% of people older than 85 years. It is the leading reason for placing older adults in long-term care facilities.

Three major causes of dementia are Alzheimer's disease, vascular disease, also known as multiinfarct dementia, and Lewy body dementia (LBD). Other causes include Parkinson's disease, metabolic disorders, Creutzfeldt–Jakob disease, and Huntington's disease (see Box 36-3).

Pathophysiology

There are different pathophysiological processes for the major types of dementia: Alzheimer's disease, multiinfarct dementia, and LBD. Alzheimer's disease (AD) is by far the most common cause of dementia and accounts for up to 80% of all dementia diagnoses.

Alzheimer's Disease. AD, a progressive neurological degenerative disease of the brain, is characterized by significant changes in brain tissue. There is an accumulation of neurofibrillary tangles, senile plaques (also called beta-amyloid plaques), and cerebrocortical atrophy of the brain. Healthy neurons have an internal support structure partly made up of structures called microtubules. These microtubules act like tracks, guiding nutrients and molecules from the cell's

---

BOX 36-3. Causes of Dementia

The following conditions can cause cognitive impairment:
- Alcohol use disorder
- AIDS dementia
- Alzheimer's disease
- Brain tumor
- Creutzfeldt-Jakob disease
- Drug reactions
- Huntington's disease
- Infection of brain structures
- Lewy body dementia
- Metabolic disorders
- Normal pressure hydrocephalus
- Nutritional deficiencies
- Parkinson's disease
- Pick disease
- Progressive supranuclear palsy
- Syphilis
- Toxic exposures
- Vascular dementia (also called multiinfarct dementia)

body down to the ends of the axon and back. A special kind of protein, tau, makes the microtubules stable. In AD, tau proteins are changed chemically and become unstable. Tau protein begins to pair with other threads of tau to become neurofibrillary tangles. When this happens, the microtubules disintegrate, collapsing the neuron's transport system, resulting in malfunctions in communication between neurons. Increasing destabilization of neuronal structures leads to death of brain cells. The tangles and plaques eventually build up and take over normal neural tissue in the brain. There is also oxidative damage in areas of the brain; oxidative stress produces reactive oxygen species, also called free radicals, which cause brain cell damage and cellular apoptosis.

AD is also characterized by a deficiency of acetylcholine, which is involved in memory functions. Cholinergic deficiency has been implicated in the cognitive decline and behavioral changes of the disease. Activity of the synthetic enzyme choline acetyltransferase (CAT) is significantly reduced in the cerebral cortex, hippocampus, and amygdala in patients with AD. Loss of cortical CAT and decline in acetylcholine synthesis in biopsy specimens have been found to correlate with cognitive impairment. Because cholinergic dysfunction may contribute to the symptoms of patients with AD, drugs that enhance acetylcholine in the brain constitute a rational basis for symptomatic treatment.

Risk factors for AD include increasing age: after age 65 years, the risk for the disorder doubles every 5 years. Family history increases an individual's chance of acquiring AD. The strongest genetic risk involves the apolipoprotein e4 (*APOE-e4*) gene. Other risk genes have been identified but not conclusively confirmed. Females may be more likely than males to develop AD, in part because they live longer. Some evidence suggests that the same factors that increase risk for heart disease also increase risk for AD: lack of exercise, smoking, hypertension, high cholesterol, and poorly controlled diabetes. Studies have found an association between lifelong involvement in mentally and socially stimulating activities and reduced risk of AD. Factors that may reduce the risk of AD include higher levels of formal education; a stimulating job; mentally challenging leisure activities, such as reading, playing games, or playing a musical instrument; and frequent social interactions.

Vascular Dementia. There are many causes of vascular dementia (also called multiinfarct dementia). Vascular dementia is thought to be an irreversible form of dementia, and its onset is caused by a number of small strokes or, sometimes, one large stroke preceded or followed by other smaller strokes. The main subtypes of vascular dementia are:

- Mild cognitive impairment caused by multiinfarct dementia
- Vascular dementia caused by a strategic single infarct

- Vascular dementia caused by hemorrhagic lesions
- Mixed Alzheimer's and vascular dementia

Vascular lesions can be the result of diffuse cerebrovascular disease or focal lesions—usually both. Mixed dementia is diagnosed when patients have evidence of AD and cerebrovascular disease, either clinically or based on neuroimaging evidence of ischemic lesions. Vascular dementia and AD often coexist.

Risk factors for vascular dementia include hypertension, smoking, hypercholesterolemia, diabetes mellitus, cardiovascular disease, and cerebrovascular disease. Arteriosclerosis and hypertension are the major causes of cerebrovascular disease.

Lewy Body Dementia. LBD is a disease associated with abnormal deposits of a protein called alphasynuclein in the brain. These deposits, called Lewy bodies, interfere with neurotransmission in the brain. The etiology is unknown, but the condition affects 1 million persons per year and can occur as early as age 50. LBD is similar to Parkinson's disease and affects multiple areas of the brain. The disease eventually affects the cerebral cortex, disturbing thoughts, perception, and language; the limbic system and hippocampus, causing emotional, behavioral, and memory problems; and the midbrain, affecting movement. It worsens progressively over a time span that can range from 2 to 20 years.

Clinical Presentation

The onset of dementia can be subtle at first. **Amnesia** is commonly the first symptom experienced, though language, perceptual skills, reasoning, and personality are affected and may be more noticeable initially. This is especially true in individuals whose symptoms begin before age 65 years. Memory loss can begin with **anomia,** which is the forgetting of names of things and people. Despite being reminded, individuals with this condition often repeatedly forget the same information. Usually memory loss involves short-term memory before long-term memory. For example, persons with dementia often have difficulty remembering events from a few minutes ago or last week but can remember events from childhood. Individuals often can remember and reminisce about the most influential time of their life, such as a time when they were successful in their career or a parent of young children.

Early in dementia, individuals can become disoriented and forget their way home or their original destination. They may not remember the day of the week or month. Reality orientation may frustrate the individual.

The individual with dementia may demonstrate poor judgment, lack of ability to reason, and inability to think abstractly. For example, balancing a checkbook and managing finances become difficult tasks. **Apraxia,** which is difficulty in performing familiar tasks, occurs. The individual may forget how to get dressed properly or how to prepare a meal. Often self-hygiene becomes unmanageable. The individual often exhibits **agnosia,** which is forgetting the purpose of familiar items. They might exhibit this behavior in subtle ways, such as placing a toothbrush in a sugar bowl or a wristwatch in the refrigerator.

Often the person with dementia exhibits rapid mood swings or personality changes, such as becoming paranoid, angry, or fearful for no apparent reason. It is important for significant others to realize that cognitive impairment and gradual losses of abilities can be extremely anxiety-provoking for the individual with early dementia. Individuals may express this anxiety in a number of ways, including withdrawing from social situations or becoming impatient and irritable when reminded of their lack of cognitive ability.

Apathy, or loss of initiative to become involved in activities, is common. Individuals with dementia usually do not take part in exercise unless prompted and shown how to perform physical fitness activities. Persons with dementia commonly exhibit insomnia or hypersomnia because of lack of maintaining a proper sleep–wake cycle. **Sundowning,** when the individual shows symptoms of acute confusion, disorientation, hallucinations, and mood swings during late day into night, often occurs. Behavior can become erratic, violent, and difficult to manage. Sedation is frequently employed, which adds to the disruption of circadian rhythms.

With severe dementia, individuals have difficulty recognizing relatives and caregivers. Individuals often also have problems with language. They may experience difficulty finding the proper words, and they often substitute inappropriate words, making sentences incomprehensible. With end stages of dementia, individuals often do not speak or perform activities.

Diagnosis

Individuals suspected of having dementia require a complete history and physical examination. A physical illness should be vigorously sought and ruled out before making the diagnosis of dementia, because many possible physical illnesses can have symptoms that resemble those of dementia. Nutritional deficiencies, metabolic imbalances, drug toxicity, thyroid disease, infection, and heart failure can present with cognitive impairment, confusion, and disorientation in older adults. Often the patient with cognitive impairment is not a reliable historian, and family members need to be interviewed. A complete neurological examination and MMSE should be done. In addition, a depression screening test should be performed, because a "pseudodementia" type syndrome occurs in depression in older adults.

CLINICAL CONCEPT

At times, the MMSE can be an intimidating test for the patient because it highlights the person's cognitive impairment. In these cases, clock drawing can be a quick test of cognitive ability.

Laboratory tests should be performed to diagnose the cause of dementia. These tests should routinely include a CBC, erythrocyte sedimentation rate, glucose level, renal and liver function tests, serological tests for syphilis, vitamin B_{12}, thiamine level and red blood cell (RBC) folate levels, and thyroid function tests. Although not done routinely, blood toxicology tests can detect drug metabolites or heavy metal poisoning.

Neuroimaging studies may include CT and MRI of the brain. The absence of cerebrovascular lesions on CT scanning or MRI is evidence against vascular etiology. The features on CT or MRI that are suggestive of vascular dementia are bilateral multiple infarcts located in the dominant hemisphere and limbic structures, multiple lacunar strokes, or periventricular white matter lesions extending into the deep white matter. PET scans may be useful for differentiating vascular dementia from Alzheimer's disease. Hypoperfusion and hypometabolism can be observed in the frontal lobe, including the cingulate and superior frontal gyri, in patients with vascular dementia; a parietotemporal pattern is observed in patients with Alzheimer's disease. Tests that may be useful for evaluation of stroke and vascular dementia include echocardiography, Holter monitoring, and carotid duplex Doppler scanning.

Specific laboratory tests and neuroimaging studies are available for AD; however, these are not widely available. Most diagnoses of AD are made by clinical examination by a neurologist.

A PET scan is a noninvasive diagnostic imaging study that can visualize beta amyloid deposits in the brain. However, amyloid PET imaging in practice is still limited because it is not covered by most insurance carriers and its cost for most patients is prohibitive. Currently, the majority of patients who undergo amyloid PET imaging do so as participants in clinical trials. A more-invasive but less-costly diagnostic test involves lumbar puncture, which examines CSF for Ab42, hyperphosphorylated tau peptide (p-tau), and total tau protein content. However, most patients are not offered these tests, as they are not widely available.

Genetic testing can be done to check for the *ApoE* gene on chromosome 19, which is associated with AD.

Treatment

When all physical illnesses have been ruled out and dementia is diagnosed, both nonpharmacological and pharmacological treatments can be used. Medications may be needed to control behavior problems caused by a loss of judgment, increased impulsivity, and confusion. Cholinesterase inhibitors, which increase the neurotransmitter acetylcholine in the brain synapses, are used to slow the process of dementia. Another type of drug targets *N*-methyl-D-aspartate (NMDA) receptors to block glutamate, which is hypothesized to cause neural damage in AD. Both of these kinds of medications have shown only modest results. Medications used in dementia include:

- Antipsychotics: haloperidol, risperidone, olanzapine, quetapine
- Mood stabilizers: fluoxetine, imipramine, citalopram
- Serotoninergic drugs: trazodone, buspirone
- Stimulants: methylphenidate

Certain drugs may be used to slow the rate at which symptoms worsen. These drugs include:

- Donepezil (Aricept)
- Rivastigmine (Exelon)
- Galantamine (Reminyl)
- Memantine (Namenda)

Pharmacological approaches involving antipsychotic or sedative medications are often used as first-line treatment in dementia patients. More than 40% of people with dementia in long-term care facilities in the United States are taking antipsychotic drugs. Experts agree that prescription of these medications without attempting nonpharmacological treatment options is of particular concern because of the substantial adverse effects associated with their use. Side effects such as sleepiness, lethargy, falls, and extrapyramidal movement disorders occur with antipsychotic sedating medications.

The newest pharmacological research is focusing on the etiological pathological findings of neurofibrillary tangles (composed of p-tau) and senile plaques (beta amyloid). One type of medication is a monoclonal antibody, aducanumab, which targets abnormal beta amyloid (Ab) and facilitates its removal from the brain. Another approach to decreasing Ab plaque burden in the brain is the inhibition of the enzymes that produce the Ab peptide from its precursor, amyloid precursor protein (APP). Currently, multiple drugs are in development which target b-site APP cleaving enzyme 1 (BACE1), which is thought to be essential for the production of Ab peptides. Verubecestat, elenbecestat, and lanabecestat are BACE inhibitors under development.

Vaccines against the tau protein have shown both safety and efficacy in animal models, and, in one recent small study, an antitau drug demonstrated a good safety profile and even stimulated a positive immune response in human patients. Several other early phase trials of drugs that target the tau protein are currently under way, though results are yet to be published.

CLINICAL CONCEPT

The Beers Criteria is a list of medications that have potentially harmful side effects in older adults. It is a guideline for safe drug use in the older population.

Behavioral and nonpharmacological approaches are key strategies in the care of the dementia patient. Dementia is commonly the reason for the patient's admission to a long-term care facility. For the patient with dementia, a daily routine that remains stable is important. Having the same caregivers for daily care also provides stability. The patient needs familiar items brought from the home environment if transitioning to a long-term care facility. For example, photos can remind the patient of people and places from the individual's past. Likewise, music and artwork that the patient enjoyed provide a sense of constancy.

Reality Orientation. Reality orientation is one of the most widely used management strategies for dealing with people with dementia. It aims to help people with memory loss and disorientation by reminding them of facts about themselves and their environment. It can be used both with individuals and with groups. In either case, people with memory loss are oriented to their environment using a range of materials and activities. This involves consistent use of devices such as signs, labels, calendars, holiday decorations, notices, and other memory aids. Caregivers attempt to bring the patient into the current time. There is debate regarding the efficacy of this approach. Some investigators claim that reality orientation sessions increase people's verbal orientation in comparison with untreated control groups. However, it is also claimed that reality orientation can remind patients of their cognitive deterioration and provoke anxiety.

Validation Therapy. Validation therapy, developed by researcher Naomi Feil, originated because of studies that showed lack of efficacy of reality orientation. Feil suggested that some of the features associated with dementia, such as retreating into the past, are active strategies on the part of the affected individual to avoid stress, boredom, and loneliness. Feil believes that people with dementia can retreat into an inner reality based on feelings rather than intellect, because they find the present reality too painful. Validation therapists therefore attempt to communicate with individuals with dementia by empathizing with the feelings and meanings hidden behind their confused speech and behavior. The caregiver focuses on what is important to the patient and what time period in life was most influential to the patient and uses these memories to motivate the patient. Validation therapists deal with the patient in the time frame that the patient feels comfortable with. If the patient concentrates on past events in life, this is supported. Caregivers assess the patient's reality and work within the patient's world rather than try to reorient the patient to the present. Some investigators assert that validation therapy promotes contentment, results in less negative affect and behavioral disturbance, produces positive effects, and provides the individual with comfort.

Reminiscence Therapy. Reminiscence therapy involves helping a person with dementia to relive past experiences, especially those that might be positive and personally significant, such as family holidays and weddings. This therapy can be used with groups or with individuals. Group sessions tend to use activities such as art and music to provide stimulation.

Reminiscence therapy is seen as a way of increasing levels of well-being and providing pleasure and cognitive stimulation. The therapy also has a great deal of flexibility, as it can be adapted to the individual.

Physical Activity and Nutrition. Often, the patient with dementia lacks the initiative to perform physical activities. Caregivers can assist in that role by taking patients on supervised walks. Exercise enhances patient oxygenation; muscle tone; and cardiovascular, gastrointestinal, and mental health. Physical activity is also important for maintenance of the patient's circadian rhythm. For nonambulatory patients, there are some exercise regimens that can be done in a chair. Persons with dementia also need prompting to eat. Because receiving adequate nutrition can be a problem, meals should be prepared consisting of foods easy for the patient to eat. In severe dementia, the patient needs to be fed.

Delirium

Delirium is defined as a transient, usually reversible, state of cerebral dysfunction. It is manifested by a wide range of neuropsychiatric abnormalities and can be exhibited as a hyperactive or a hypoactive state. For example, drug toxicity often causes impulsive, aggressive delirium behavior, whereas liver failure and renal failure often cause withdrawal and lethargy. Delirium is often mistaken for dementia or depression (see Table 36-4). The clinical hallmarks are decreased attention span and a waxing and waning type of confusion. Hallucinations, delusions, and psychotic behavior are often part of delirium. It is sudden in onset, and there is usually no apparent inciting event. The patient requires thorough assessment and physical examination to diagnose the reason for delirium. Hospitalization, the postoperative state, electrolyte imbalances, and infection are major causes. Early diagnosis and resolution of symptoms are correlated with the most favorable outcomes.

Delirium has been found in 14% to 56% of older hospitalized adults. It is present in 10% to 22% of older patients at the time of admission, with an additional 10% to 30% of cases developing after admission. Prevalence of postoperative delirium following general surgery is 5% to 10%, and as high as 42% following orthopedic surgery. Delirium has been found in 40% of patients admitted to intensive care units, which commonly have no windows and constant fluorescent lighting that can be disorienting to the older patient.

Almost any medical illness, intoxication, or medication can be a risk factor for delirium. Often, delirium is multifactorial in etiology; however, medications are the most common reversible cause. Electrolyte disturbances, metabolic abnormalities, dementia, sleep deprivation, substance abuse, infections, intensive care sensory deprivation, and postoperative states also commonly provoke delirium. Dementia is one of the most consistent risk factors for delirium; underlying dementia is observed in 25% to 50% of patients.

TABLE 36-4. Differences Among Delirium, Dementia, and Depression

Features	Delirium	Dementia	Depression
Onset	Sudden	Gradual	Gradual
Course	Fluctuating	Progressive	Progressive
Duration	Days	Months to years	If untreated, months
Consciousness	Altered level of consciousness	Alert	Alert with possible symptoms of pseudodementia
Attention	Impaired	Normal in early dementia, diminished in late dementia	Alert with possible symptoms of pseudodementia
Psychomotor Effects	Increased or decreased	Normal, except in severe dementia can be agitated or retarded	Agitation or retardation
Reversibility	Fully reversible with treatment	Not reversible	Fully reversible with treatment

The presence of dementia increases the risk of delirium two to three times. For other risk factors, see Box 36-4.

Pathophysiology

The mechanism of delirium is not fully understood, but studies of delirium focus on the effects of the neurotransmitters acetylcholine, dopamine, and serotonin. It is theorized that decreased levels of acetylcholine are part of the pathogenesis of delirium. In the brain, a reciprocal relationship exists between cholinergic and dopaminergic activities. In delirium, an excess of dopaminergic activity occurs. Other causes of delirium involve disruption of cortisol and beta-endorphin circadian rhythms. This mechanism has been suggested as a possible explanation for delirium caused by exogenous glucocorticoids. Recent studies have suggested a role for inflammatory cytokines such as interleukin-1 and interleukin-6 in the pathogenesis of delirium. Following a wide range of infectious, inflammatory, and toxic insults, endogenous pyrogen, such as interleukin-1, is released from the cells. Head trauma

and ischemia, which frequently are associated with delirium, are characterized by brain responses that are mediated by interleukin-1 and interleukin-6. Delirium commonly occurs as a response to infection in older adults. Clinical studies have found that serotonin is increased in patients with septic delirium.

Clinical Presentation

Delirium always should be suspected when a patient exhibits a sudden deterioration in behavior, cognition, or function, especially in patients who are older, demented, or depressed. Delirious patients may have psychotic symptoms such as visual hallucinations or delusions. Some patients with delirium also may become violent, suicidal, or homicidal. Symptoms tend to fluctuate over the course of the day, with some improvement in the daytime and maximum disturbance at night. Reversal of the sleep–wake cycle is common. See Box 36-5 for signs and symptoms of delirium.

In patients with delirium, a careful and complete physical examination, including a mental status examination and neurological examination, is necessary. The clinician should also look for signs of infection. Physical

---

BOX 36-4. Common Risk Factors for Delirium

Delirium is a state of temporary, transient disorientation or psychotic behavior that can be caused by numerous conditions. The following are the most common conditions associated with delirium:

- Alcohol or sedative withdrawal
- Cerebrovascular accidents
- Closed head injury
- Hyperthermia
- Hypoxia
- Malnutrition
- Polypharmacy (particularly in older adults)
- Postictal state
- Sensory deprivation
- Sleep deprivation
- Structural lesions of the brain
- Unfamiliar environment (mainly in hospitalized older adults)
- Use of physical restraints

METABOLIC CAUSES
- Acid–base disturbances
- Fluid and electrolyte abnormalities
- Hepatic failure
- Hypoglycemia
- Renal failure
- Vitamin deficiency states (especially thiamine and cyanocobalamin)

CARDIOVASCULAR CAUSES
- Anemia
- Cardiac dysrhythmias

- Heart failure
- Shock

INFECTIOUS CAUSES
- CNS infections
- HIV-related brain infections
- Pneumonia
- Sepsis
- Urinary tract infections

DRUG- AND ALCOHOL-INDUCED CAUSES
- Illicit drugs, including:
  - Alcohol
  - Cannabis
  - Heroin
  - Lysergic acid diethylamide, also known as LSD
  - Phencyclidine, also known as PCP
  - Substance intoxication
- Medications, including:
  - Anticholinergics
  - Antiparkinson drugs
  - Centrally acting antihypertensives
  - Corticosteroids
  - Histamine-2 blockers
  - Narcotics
  - Sedative hypnotics
- Withdrawal from alcohol, opioids, and benzodiazepines

BOX 36-5. Signs and Symptoms of Delirium

The following conditions frequently occur in delirium:
- Clouding of consciousness
- Difficulty maintaining or shifting attention
- Disorientation
- Dysarthria
- Dysphasia
- Fluctuating levels of consciousness
- Hallucinations
- Illusions
- Tremor

examination is often difficult because patients have difficulty sustaining attention, are disoriented, and have impaired short-term memory and poor insight.

Diagnosis

The diagnosis of delirium is made by the clinical presentation because no laboratory test can diagnose delirium. Obtaining a thorough history is essential. Delirious patients are unreliable historians, so getting a detailed history from family and caregivers is particularly important. A mini-cognitive test can be administered that asks the patient to draw a clock with a specific time as directed by the examiner. The test can also include a test of the patient's short-term memory by asking the patient to remember three words and then, 5 minutes later, asking the patient to recall them. Other diagnostic instruments are the Delirium Symptom Interview and the Confusion Assessment Method (CAM).

To make an accurate diagnosis, knowledge of the patient's baseline mental status is necessary. The CAM for the Intensive Care Unit (CAM-ICU) offers the clinician the opportunity to identify delirium in critical care patients, especially patients on mechanical ventilation. The CAM-ICU makes use of nonverbal assessments to evaluate the important features of delirium. The *DSM-5* lists specific diagnostic criteria for delirium (see Box 36-6).

Treatment

Components of delirium management include non-pharmacological supportive therapy and pharmacological management.

Nonpharmacological Management. Fluid and nutrition should be provided because patients with delirium do not remember to eat or drink. For the patient suspected of having alcohol toxicity or alcohol withdrawal, therapy should include multivitamins, especially thiamine. Environmental modifications that enhance reorientation of the patient should be devised. Memory cues such as a calendar, clocks, and family photos may be helpful. The patient should

be moved near a window for orientation to daylight. The environment should be stable, quiet, and well lit. Family members and staff should explain all procedures, reinforce orientation, and reassure the patient. Sensory deficits should be corrected, if necessary, with eyeglasses and hearing aids. Physical restraints should be avoided. Delirious patients may pull out IV lines, may climb out of bed, and may not be compliant. Perceptual problems lead to agitation, fear, combative behavior, and wandering. Severely delirious patients require constant observation and should never be left alone or unattended. The patient requires one-on-one attention by a health-care provider.

Pharmacological Therapy. Delirium that threatens injury to the patient or others should be treated with medications. The most common medications used are antipsychotic drugs such as haloperidol and benzodiazepines such as lorazepam.

Substance Use Disorder and Addiction

Common substances involved in substance use disorders include alcohol, marijuana, cocaine, opiates, amphetamines, and hallucinogens. Although many individuals use such drugs, not all become addicted. Addiction is a compulsive need for and use of a habit-forming substance, such as heroin, nicotine, and alcohol, and is characterized by tolerance and well-defined physiological symptoms upon withdrawal.

 CLINICAL CONCEPT

A patient experiencing a mental health disorder and substance use disorder simultaneously is said to have a dual diagnosis.

Alcohol, the most commonly used addictive drug, is mainly a CNS depressant. In low doses, alcohol disinhibits the individual, which may lead to out-of-character activities. At higher doses, individuals show irrational thinking, lack of judgment, and absence of motor coordination.

Cannabis is considered the most commonly used psychoactive drug in the world. The drug can be smoked or ingested, and its psychoactive properties are due to the cannabinoid delta-9-tetrahydrocannabinol (THC). The potency of cannabis has increased significantly in the past decade and has led to cannabis-related adverse effects in the U.S. population. Cannabis use disorder is estimated to occur in 10% of regular cannabis users. The disorder is characterized by a persistent cannabis use that results in clinically significant functional impairment. Typical manifestations include impaired school or work function, giving up of previously enjoyed social and recreational activities,

BOX 36-6. Diagnostic Criteria for Delirium

A. A disturbance in attention (i.e., reduced ability to direct, focus, sustain, and shift attention) and awareness (reduced orientation to the environment).

B. The disturbance develops over a short period of time (usually hours to a few days), represents a change from baseline attention and awareness, and tends to fluctuate in severity during the course of a day.

C. An additional disturbance in cognition (e.g., memory deficit, disorientation, language, visuospatial ability, or perception).

D. The disturbances in Criteria A and C are not better explained by another preexisting, established, or evolving neurocognitive disorder and do not occur in the context of a severely reduced level of arousal, such as coma.

E. There is evidence from the history, physical examination, or laboratory findings that the disturbance is a direct physiological consequence of another medical condition, substance intoxication or withdrawal (i.e., due to a drug of abuse or to a medication), or exposure to a toxin, or is due to multiple etiologies.

Specify whether:

Substance intoxication delirium: This diagnosis should be made instead of substance intoxication when the symptoms in Criteria A and C predominate in the clinical picture and when they are sufficiently severe to warrant clinical attention.

Substance withdrawal delirium: This diagnosis should be made instead of substance withdrawal when the symptoms of Criteria A and C predominate in the clinical picture and when they are sufficiently severe to warrant clinical attention.

Medication-induced delirium: This diagnosis applies when the symptoms in Criteria A and C arise as a side effect of a medication taken as prescribed.

Delirium due to another medical condition: There is evidence from the history, physical examination, or laboratory findings that the disturbance is attributable to the physiological consequences of another medical condition.

Delirium due to multiple etiologies: There is evidence from the history, physical examination, or laboratory findings that the delirium has more than one etiology (e.g., more than one etiological medical condition; another medical condition plus substance intoxication or medication side effect).

Specify if:

Acute: lasting a few hours or days

Persistent: lasting weeks or months.

Specify if:

Hyperactive: The individual has a hyperactive level of psychomotor activity that may be accompanied by mood lability, agitation, and/or refusal to cooperate with medical care.

Hypoactive: The individual has a hypoactive level of psychomotor activity that may be accompanied by sluggishness and lethargy that approaches stupor.

Mixed level of activity: The individual has a normal level of psychomotor activity even though attention and awareness are disturbed. Also includes individuals whose activity level rapidly fluctuates.

Reprinted with permission from American Psychiatric Association. (2013). *Diagnostic and statistical manual of mental health disorders* (5th ed.). American Psychiatric Association, Washington, D.C.

and use of cannabis in potentially hazardous situations (e.g., while driving).

Opioid use disorder is considered an epidemic in the United States, with 2.1 million individuals affected. The number of opioid drug overdose deaths increased by nearly 30% from 2019 to 2020 and has quintupled since 1999. Prescription and illicit opioid drugs are both part of this epidemic. Opioid use disorder is defined as a problematic pattern of opioid use that leads to serious impairment or distress. The most commonly prescribed opioids include hydrocodone, oxycodone, oxymorphone, morphine, codeine, and fentanyl. Heroin is the most common illicit opioid. It can be injected, ingested, or inhaled. Heroin use has more than doubled among adults aged 18 to 25 in the past decade. Studies show that in those addicted to heroin, the first opioid drug abused is commonly a prescription opioid. There is a rising trend in the United States in which heroin sold on the street is "cut" with fentanyl, a highly potent opioid. Nearly 75% of the 91,799 drug overdose deaths in 2020 involved an opioid. Over 19% of all opioid overdose deaths in 2020 involved heroin. The sharpest increase involved synthetic opioids, primarily fentanyl and fentanyl analogs. In 2020, more than 56,000 people died from overdoses involving fentanyl.

Opioid use disorder can be mild, moderate, or severe according to specific criteria (see Box 36-7). Signs of opioid intoxication are diminished respiratory rate and constricted pupils. Acute complications include non-cardiogenic pulmonary edema and respiratory failure. Complications of chronic use are primarily infectious and include skin abscess at an injection site, cellulitis, mycotic aneurysms, endocarditis, talcosis, HIV, and hepatitis. Physiological and psychological dependence on heroin occurs. Patients can experience withdrawal when they cannot obtain heroin.

BOX 36-7. Opioid Use Disorder: Symptoms and Severity

To be diagnosed with an opioid use disorder, a person must have a problematic pattern of opioid use leading to clinically significant impairment or distress, as manifested by at least two of the following, occurring with a 12-month period:

An opioid use disorder may be mild, moderate, or severe.

Mild: 2 to 3 symptoms Moderate: 4 to 5 symptoms Severe: 6+ symptoms

Loss of Control

1 Opioids are often taken in larger amounts or over a longer period than was intended.
2 There is a persistent desire or unsuccessful efforts to cut down or control opioid use.
3 A great deal of time is spent in activities necessary to obtain the opioid, use the opioid, or recover from its effects.
4 Craving, or a strong desire or urge to use opioids

Social Problems

5 Recurrent opioid use resulting in a failure to fulfill major role obligations at work, school, or home
6 Continued opioid use despite having persistent or recurrent social or interpersonal problems cause or exacerbated by the effects of opioids.
7 Important social, occupational, or recreational activities are given up or reduced because of opioid use
8 Recurrent opioid use in situations in which it is physically hazardous
9 Continued opioid use despite knowledge of having a persistent or recurrent physical or psychological problem that is likely to have been caused or exacerbated by the substance

Pharmacological Problems

10 **Tolerance,** as defined by either of the following: (a) A need for markedly increased amounts of opioids to achieve intoxication or desired effect; (b) A markedly diminished effect with continued use of the same amount of opioid.
11 **Withdrawal,** as manifested by either of the following: (a) The characteristic opioid withdrawal syndrome (refer to Criteria A and B of the criteria set for opioid withdrawal); (b) Opioids (or a closely related substance) are taken to relieve or avoid withdrawal symptoms.

Reprinted with permission from American Psychiatric Association. (2013). *Diagnostic and statistical manual of mental health disorders* (5th ed.). American Psychiatric Association, Washington, D.C.

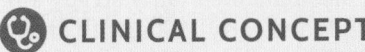

CLINICAL CONCEPT

Substance use disorder occurs when a person needs alcohol or a drug to function normally. Abruptly stopping the substance leads to withdrawal symptoms. Addiction means that a person has a strong urge to use the substance and cannot stop. Tolerance occurs when an individual consistently needs a higher dose of a substance to get the desired effect.

Cocaine may be smoked, inhaled, used topically, or injected. Acute cocaine intoxication causes excitation, and the patient often shows agitation, paranoia, tachycardia, tachypnea, hypertension, and diaphoresis. Complications of acute and chronic use can include myocardial ischemia or infarction, stroke, pulmonary edema, and rhabdomyolysis.

Acute intoxication with amphetamines presents with signs of SNS stimulation such as tachycardia and hypertension. Amphetamines cause anorexia, insomnia, and occasionally seizures.

Different hallucinogens present with a variety of organ system effects. Phencyclidine has been known to cause extreme excitation, muscle rigidity, seizures, rhabdomyolysis, and coma.

Prescription drug abuse is common. Narcotics, stimulants, and sedatives are common prescription drugs of abuse. Deliberate or accidental overdose frequently occurs. Similarly, some over-the-counter medications, such as cough and cold medicines containing dextromethorphan, can also lead to significant CNS effects.

Use of inhalants is underreported and is most common in adolescents. Individuals inhale chemical vapors from a variety of substances, many of which are common household products. The practice of inhaling these substances is called "huffing." The inhalants give the user a euphoric effect, but potential risks include brain damage and death. Some adults also use inhalants, particularly nitrites, and often inhale substances to enhance their sexual experiences. The inhalation of bath salts is becoming a substantial problem among teens. Bath salts give the individual a cocaine-like euphoric feeling. The powders sold as "Ivory Snow," "Bliss," "Vanilla Sky," and other brand names contain the ingredient mephedrone, a stimulant that can cause rapid heart rates, seizures, and hallucinations.

The prevalence of substance use disorders is difficult to estimate because users often do not admit or recognize their habit. Reports indicate that roughly two-thirds of all adults drink alcohol occasionally. Approximately 13% of people in the United States are persons with alcohol use disorder, and one person in five who uses alcohol for recreational purposes becomes dependent for some period of time. Studies performed in urban emergency departments indicate that up to 20% of patients may have problems with alcohol.

Heavy cocaine use has remained fairly steady since its peak in the late 1980s and early 1990s, with an estimated 600,000 to 700,000 regular users. In 2020, more than 19,000 people in the United States died from an overdose involving cocaine. In rural communities, use of methamphetamine, also known as crystal meth, is on the rise. This drug is easily manufactured from a base ingredient found in over-the-counter cold medications. It is most often abused by those 15 to 25 years old.

Pathophysiology

A dopamine reward system in the brain is hypothesized as a reason for substance abuse. A specific allele (A1 allele) of the D2 dopamine receptor (*DRD2*) gene located at 11q23 is associated with addictive behaviors such as alcohol use disorder, substance use disorder, smoking, obesity, and compulsive gambling. Studies show that persons with the A1 allele of the *DRD2* gene have a diminished number of dopamine receptors and a propensity for addictive behaviors. It is hypothesized that in an effort to compensate for deficiencies in the dopaminergic system, substance abusers may seek to stimulate circuits of the brain involved in behavioral reward and reinforcement. Each drug with abuse potential works on the CNS in a slightly different way (see Table 36-5).

Clinical Presentation

Euphoria and sedation are the most common effects of abused drugs. Different kinds of withdrawal symptoms are observed with illicit and prescribed drug abuse.

Alcohol Withdrawal. Many persons with alcohol use disorder experience "the shakes" approximately 12 to 24 hours after their last drink. The shakes are tremors caused by overexcitation of the CNS. These tremors may be accompanied by tachycardia, diaphoresis, anorexia, and insomnia. After 24 to 72 hours, the person with alcohol use disorder may have seizures. Delirium tremens (DT), which begins 3 to 5 days after the last drink, is characterized by disorientation, fever, tremulousness, and visual hallucinations. This medical emergency should be treated on an inpatient basis.

Opioid Withdrawal. Withdrawal symptoms from opioids may begin just a few hours after their last use, although onset of withdrawal may be delayed in patients abusing long-acting opioids. Along with a strong craving for the drug, opioid withdrawal produces yawning, tears, diarrhea, abdominal cramping, piloerection, and rhinorrhea. Symptoms of withdrawal usually peak around 48 hours and again at 72 hours. Withdrawal usually subsides after 1 week, but some heavily dependent users may have mild symptoms for up to 6 months.

Amphetamine Withdrawal. Amphetamine withdrawal is fairly mild. Patients may complain of depression, increased appetite, abdominal cramping, diarrhea, and headache.

Cocaine and Hallucinogen Withdrawal. Cocaine and hallucinogens do not have a typical withdrawal pattern. These drugs are considered psychologically rather than physically addicting.

Benzodiazepine and Other CNS Depressant Withdrawal. Discontinuing prolonged use or abuse of high doses of CNS depressants can lead to serious withdrawal symptoms such as grand mal seizures. BNZs are the drug of choice for withdrawal seizures. When BNZ drugs are discontinued after prolonged use, symptoms such as agitation, restlessness, and insomnia are common.

Diagnosis

Individuals interviewed about substance use commonly underestimate their consumption and deny their substance use disorder. When performing the history, the clinician should question patients about their drug or drugs of choice and the frequency, amount, and method of use. Also, it is important to obtain information about prior detoxifications, concomitant use of other substances, date of first use, and time interval from last use. A short assessment tool for alcohol use is called the CAGE questionnaire. A single positive response to the CAGE questions is considered suggestive of an alcohol problem, and two or more positive responses indicate the presence of such a problem, with a sensitivity and specificity of approximately 90% in most studies.

Several other screening methods exist, with the brief Michigan Alcohol Screening Test the most widely used screen suitable for emergency department use. Another screening tool that is used often is the TWEAK questionnaire (see Box 36-8).

An opioid use disorder can be classified as mild, moderate, or severe. An assessment tool published by the American Psychiatric Association can be used to evaluate an individual's severity of opioid use (see Box 36-7).

The physical examination should be a complete assessment of the patient because individuals with

TABLE 36-5. Substance of Use Disorder and Pathophysiological Mechanism

Drug	Pathophysiological Mechanism
Alcohol	Psychodepressant
Amphetamines	Psychostimulant
Cocaine	Psychostimulant
Heroin (opiates)	Psychodepressant/ psychostimulant
Marijuana (THC)	Psychodepressant

BOX 36-8. The TWEAK Questionnaire

The TWEAK Questionnaire involves the following questions:

T - Tolerance (2 points): How many drinks can you hold? (Five or more indicates tolerance.)

W - Worried (2 points): Have close friends or relatives worried or complained about your drinking in the past year?

E - Eye openers (1 point): Do you sometimes take a drink in the morning when you first get up?

A - Amnesia (1 point): Has a friend or family member ever told you about things you said or did while you were drinking that you could not remember?

K - K/Cut down (1 point): Do you sometimes feel the need to cut down on your drinking?

Scoring: A 7-point scale is used to score the test. The Tolerance question scores 2 points if (a) the patient reports they can hold more than five drinks without falling asleep or passing out or (b) if it is reported that three or more drinks are needed to feel high. A positive response to the Worry question scores 2 points. A positive response to the last three questions scores 1 point each.

From Russell, M. (1994). New assessment tools for drinking in pregnancy: T-ACE, TWEAK, and others. *Alcohol Health and Research World,18*(1), 55–61.

substance use disorders are much less likely than the general population to have regular medical care. In the patient with acute intoxication, a blood and urine toxicology screen for substances and a blood or breath alcohol level is needed. CBC, serum electrolytes, glucose, blood urea nitrogen, liver enzymes, and serum creatinine are necessary. Gastrointestinal bleeding, anemia, bone marrow suppression, and possible infection are concerns. Complications of cocaine intoxication may require a cardiac or CNS evaluation that may include an ECG and brain CT scan.

Treatment

Supervised withdrawal is the primary treatment method in opioid use disorder. Medications used include methadone and buprenorphine, opioid agonists, and alpha-2 adrenergic agonists such as clonidine and lofexidine. The aim of supervised withdrawal is to safely transition the patient to medication-assisted treatment. Supervised withdrawal alone does not generally result in sustained abstinence because it does not address reasons the patient became dependent on opioids. Psychotherapy should be used in conjunction with supervised withdrawal. Complete detoxification from opioids is achieved only in transitioning a patient to the opioid antagonist intramuscular naltrexone; transitioning to either methadone

or buprenorphine will still maintain the patient in a state of physiological dependence on these opioid agonists. Buprenorphine is an opioid partial agonist which can be used for pain relief and opioid addiction. It can diminish the effects of physical dependency to opioids, such as withdrawal symptoms and cravings. It has an increased safety profile and low potential for abuse. Naltrexone is an opioid receptor antagonist used primarily in the management of opioid dependence. The drug works by blocking the euphoric effects of opioids, which lessens the patient's urge to use opioids. This long-acting antagonist is commonly used as part of a rehabilitation program. Opioid-receptor antagonists work by modulating the dopaminergic mesolimbic pathway. This area of the brain is theorized to be the major center of reward associated with drugs involved in addiction. Buprenorphine and naloxone are in a combination medication, Suboxone, which also can be used in a comprehensive rehabilitation regimen.

ALERT! Naloxone is a short-acting opioid receptor antagonist that is used in emergency conditions of overdose.

Disulfiram (Antabuse), a drug used to treat chronic alcohol use disorder, allows only partial metabolism of ethanol. Increased levels of serum acetaldehyde concentrations are generated by this partial metabolism. High acetaldehyde levels in the bloodstream cause an intense "hangover" type reaction, including headache, nausea, myalgias, and postural hypotension. Therefore, if the patient uses alcohol while on disulfiram, they become intensely ill. The discomfort associated with this syndrome is intended to serve as a negative stimulus, but the reaction may be severe enough to cause hypotension and death. Persons must consent to the use of disulfiram in their rehabilitation and should be clinically monitored.

A patient with an alcohol addiction may require vitamin supplementation with thiamine (200 mg), folic acid (1 mg), and a multivitamin. If the patient develops agitation or tremulousness, short-term use of benzodiazepines may be needed.

All patients with a substance use problem require referral to a detoxification clinic for treatment. Substance use disorder is a lifelong disease that can be only controlled, not cured. In the detoxification center, treatment initially consists of managing the varied symptoms of withdrawal, which can range from cravings to hallucinations and seizures. Once physical withdrawal is complete, group and individual counseling begins and continues on an inpatient, outpatient, and group support basis with groups such as Alcoholics Anonymous and Narcotics Anonymous.

Chapter Summary

- Statistics show that approximately 18.5% of the U.S. population suffers from some type of mental illness each year.

- Women and men have the same likelihood of developing mental illness, although women report symptoms and seek treatment more often than men.

- Out of all those affected by mental illness, approximately half do not receive treatment.

- The MMSE is the most commonly used psychiatric test in clinical practice.

- The major neurotransmitters of the brain that are involved in mental illness include serotonin (5-hydroxytryptamine), norepinephrine, dopamine, and GABA.

- A combination of medication and psychotherapy is recommended for most psychiatric disorders.

- Cognitive-behavioral and interpersonal therapy are the most common types of psychotherapeutic treatment.

- Anxiety disorders include GAD, panic attacks, OCD, specific phobias, social anxiety disorder, acute stress disorder, and PTSD.

- MDD is the most common psychiatric disorder in adults and older individuals.

- Bipolar I disorder involves manic episodes, hypomanic, and major depressive episodes.

- Bipolar II disorder involves no mania, at least one hypomanic episode, and at least one major depressive episode.

- Types of antidepressant medications include SSRIs, TCAs, MAOIs, and SNRIs.

- Antidepressant medications require 3 to 6 weeks to reach therapeutic blood levels.

- Many psychoactive medications have anticholinergic side effects, including dry mouth, blurred vision, tachycardia, constipation, urinary retention, and orthostatic hypotension.

- Schizophrenia is a neurobiological disorder considered a psychosis. A psychosis is an abnormal condition of the mind where the affected person loses touch with reality. The person often suffers from delusions and hallucinations.

- Psychotic symptoms, such as delusions, have been linked to excessive dopamine levels.

- ADHD is the most common psychiatric condition affecting children in the United States. The cause is unknown. Treatment includes psychostimulants such as amphetamines.

- The two main causes of dementia are Alzheimer's disease and vascular disease.

- The characteristics of dementia include amnesia, anomia, agnosia, apraxia, aphasia, and apathy.

- Pharmacological approaches involving antipsychotic or sedative medications are often used as first-line treatment in dementia patients. More than 40% of people with dementia in long-term care facilities in the United States are taking antipsychotic drugs.

- Cholinesterase inhibitors, drugs that enhance acetylcholine stimulation in the brain, are used to slow the progression of dementia. Glutamate receptor antagonists are also used to counteract neural damage. Antipsychotic agents are also commonly used in dementia.

- Delirium is a transient, usually reversible, cause of cerebral dysfunction and is manifested by a wide range of neuropsychiatric abnormalities. Delirium is often caused by drug toxicity, metabolic problems, infection, electrolyte disturbances, renal failure, or liver failure. Delirium is often mistaken for dementia or depression.

- Common substances involved in substance use disorders include alcohol, marijuana (cannabis), cocaine, opioids, amphetamines, and hallucinogens.

- Addiction is a compulsive need for and use of a habit-forming substance characterized by tolerance and well-defined physiological symptoms upon withdrawal.

- Drug tolerance occurs when a subject's reaction to a specific drug and concentration of the drug are progressively reduced, requiring an increase in concentration to achieve the desired effect.

- Withdrawal symptoms, specific noxious physiological effects, occur if the individual who is addicted does not maintain regular use of the drug.

- Supervised withdrawal is used for opioid use disorder, using the medications methadone and buprenorphine, which are opioid agonists, as well as alpha-2 adrenergic agonists such as clonidine and lofexidine.

- Nalextrone, an opioid antagonist, is used to counteract the detrimental effects of opioid poisoning or overdose.

- Alcohol is the most commonly used addictive drug. The CAGE questionnaire is a useful tool in the diagnosis of alcohol use disorder.

- Cannabis is considered the most commonly used psychoactive drug in the world.

Making the Connections

Signs and Symptoms	Physical Assessment Findings	Diagnostic Testing	Treatment
GAD | Anxiety is believed to arise from the neurons in the region of the brain called the amygdala. The amygdala analyzes the emotional significance of environmental stimuli and stores emotional memories. Pathways exiting from the amygdala travel to multiple brain structures, including the parabrachial nucleus (resulting in dyspnea and hyperventilation), the dorsomedial nucleus of the vagus nerve (activating the parasympathetic nervous system), and the lateral hypothalamus (resulting in SNS activation). The amygdala also sends neuronal signals to the prefrontal cortex, where cognitive experiences of specific anxiety disorders are integrated.			
Feelings of uncontrollable worry and fear, often accompanied by trembling, hyperventilation, diaphoresis, digestive problems, paresthesias, and palpitations.	Patient may be hyperventilating. Patient may have tachycardia, diaphoresis, and trembling.	Use of GAD assessment tool. Normal CBC, thyroid, cortisol, and serum chemistry laboratory tests. Normal ECG. Normal toxicology screen.	BNZ, which enhances GABA neuron signals in the brain. GABA has an antianxiety effect for use as a short-term medication. SSRI, which has antidepressant and antianxiety effects, for long-term management. Buspirone, another antianxiety agent, is an alternative to SSRIs. CBT. Stress management, education, deep breathing, yoga, and meditation.
Panic Disorder | *Sympathetic System Stimulation:* Intense anxiety reactions are associated with increased levels of catecholamines from the locus coeruleus to the hippocampus, amygdala, limbic system, and the cerebral cortex. *GABA–BNZ System:* Decreased GABA–BNZ binding in the hippocampus and prefrontal cortex. Decreased BNZ binding in the prefrontal cortex and insula. *Neurocircuitry of Fear:* Input to the amygdala is modulated by the thalamus and prefrontal cortex. Projections from the amygdala extend to various parts of the brain involved in the fear response, such as the locus coeruleus (arousal), the brainstem (respiratory activation), the hypothalamus–pituitary–adrenal axis (stress response), and the cortex (cognitive interpretation of the stressor).			
Shortness of breath, palpitations, dizziness, nausea, and feelings of alarm or overwhelming fear.	Hyperventilation, tachycardia, diaphoresis, pallor, and trembling.	Use of GAD assessment tool. Normal CBC, thyroid, cortisol, and serum chemistry laboratory tests. Normal ECG. Normal toxicology screen.	BNZ, which enhances GABA neuron signals in the brain. GABA has an antianxiety effect for use as short-term medication. SSRI, which has antidepressant and antianxiety effects, for long-term management. CBT. Stress management, education, deep breathing, yoga, and meditation.
Obsessive Compulsive Disorder | Hyperactivity in some cortical and subcortical regions of the brain; specifically, the orbital frontal cortex, limbic system, thalamus, and caudate. There are abnormalities in serotonergic, dopaminergic, and glutamatergic neurotransmission in these regions.			
Persistent repetitive thoughts and rituals or actions that are inappropriate and may become disabling.	Normal physical examination.	No specific laboratory tests. Use assessment tool such as Yale-Brown Obsessive Compulsive Scale.	SSRIs keep more serotonin in the synapse of neurons in the brain. Psychotherapy can also be used.

Continued

Making the Connections–cont'd

Signs and Symptoms	Physical Assessment Findings	Diagnostic Testing	Treatment
PTSD | Chronic dysregulation of HPA glands. Enhanced SNS responses. Alterations in the medial prefrontal cortex, hippocampus, and visual association cortex.			
Insomnia and hyperarousal following a life-threatening or traumatic episode. Avoidance of places reminiscent of trauma. Presence of flashbacks or reliving the traumatic experience.	Normal physical examination. If patient is reexperiencing the trauma, patient will have hyperventilation, tachycardia, diaphoresis, and possibly violent, impulsive behavior.	No specific laboratory tests. Use assessment tool PTSD scale.	Clonidine decreases sympathetic neuron activity. Prazosin decreases sympathetic activity. SSRIs prolong serotonin action in the synapses. SNRIs keep serotonin and norepinephrine in the synapse for prolonged time in the brain. Psychotherapy can be used.
MDD | Decreased metabolic activity in the neocortex of the brain and increased activity in the limbic system. Area of the prefrontal cortex with abnormally diminished activity in patients with depression compared with nondepressed individuals. This region has widespread connections with areas that regulate dopamine, norepinephrine, and serotonin.			
Depressed mood, sadness, loss of pleasure, disturbed sleep patterns, disturbed eating pattern for 2 weeks' duration.	Normal physical examination.	Rule out other causes of symptoms. Use an assessment tool such as Zung Self-Rating Depression Scale, Beck Depression Inventory, Raskin Depression Scale, Geriatric Depression Scale, or the Hamilton Rating Scale for Depression. Thyroid-stimulating hormone, cortisol levels are normal. Dexamethasone suppression test.	SSRIs raise serotonin levels in the brain. SNRIs raise both serotonin and norepinephrine levels in the brain. MAOIs prevent breakdown of norepinephrine. TCAs raise norepinephrine levels in the brain. NaSSAs, also called tetracyclic antidepressants, dopamine receptor inhibitors (DRI). Antipsychotic agents can be added to the regimen to boost antidepressant activity. Anticonvulsants can be added that have mood-stabilizing effects. VNS. TMS. Electroconvulsive therapy. Psychotherapy. Ketamine (subanesthetic dose) for treatment-resistant depression.
Bipolar I and II Disorder | Alterations in the prefrontal cortex and the amygdala. Altered temporal lobe activity. Patients with bipolar disorder experience manic, hypomanic, and/or depressive episodes.			
Bipolar I disorder includes manic episodes, hypomanic and major depressive episodes. Bipolar II disorder is marked by lack of mania, at least one hypomanic episode, at least one major depressive episode.	Normal physical examination.	Laboratory tests and toxicology screen normal.	Lithium acts as a mood stabilizer. Anticonvulsant and antipsychotic drugs have mood-stabilizing effects. Antidepressants are often used. Psychotherapy is used.

Making the Connections–cont'd

Signs and Symptoms	Physical Assessment Findings	Diagnostic Testing	Treatment
Schizophrenia | Increased dopaminergic concentrations in the amygdala and the caudate nucleus. Brain atrophy.			
Positive symptoms: delusions, hallucinations, disorganized speech, flight of ideas. Negative symptoms: blunted affect, apathy, lack of motivation, lack of speech or spontaneous movement.	Normal physical examination.	Laboratory tests and toxicology screen normal.	Traditional first generation antipsychotics such as Haldol are antidopaminergic agents. Second generation antipsychotic medications such as clozapine, quetapine, ziprasidone, or olanzapine are antidopaminergic agents. Psychotherapy is used.
ADHD | Alterations in the neurocircuitry in the prefrontal cortex. Neurotransmitter alterations.			
Restless, driven, and never tiring in nature. Easily distracted. Both academic and behavioral difficulties.	Normal physical examination.	Normal laboratory tests and toxicology screen.	Methylphenidate and amphetamine preparations are stimulants that have a paradoxical effect in persons with ADHD. Psychotherapy is used.
Dementia | *Alzheimer's Disease:* Neurofibrillary tangles, beta-amyloid deposition in brain. Cortical atrophy. *Vascular Dementia:* Multiple sites of infarction or single large hemorrhage or ischemia of brain. *Lewy Body Dementia:* Accumulation of alpha-synuclein proteins damaging multiple areas of the brain.			
Anomia, amnesia, agnosia, apraxia, apathy. Aphasia. Cognitive impairment. Disorientation to person, place, or time.	Poor performance on MMSE. Inability to carry out ADLs independently.	MMSE or clock drawing.	Antiacetylcholinesterase drugs, such as rivastigmine, allow more acetylcholine to remain in the synapse. Memantine, an NMDA receptor antagonist, may be used. Antipsychotics decrease dopaminergic transmission. Levodopa and other Parkinson's disease medications may be used for LBD. Attention to nutrition and hydration is needed. Validation therapy, music, art, and reminiscence therapy are utilized.
Delirium | Various causes, such as infection, metabolic imbalances, polypharmacy, or sensory deprivation caused by intensive care unit.			
Sudden onset of disorientation, confusion, hallucinations, or violent behavior.	Physical examination findings depend on cause of delirium.	Rule out infection and metabolic imbalances. Various laboratory tests to rule out medical cause of behavior.	Antipsychotic drug such as Haldol® has antidopaminergic effects. Attention to nutrition and hydration is required. Reality orientation is needed.

Continued

Making the Connections—cont'd

Signs and Symptoms	Physical Assessment Findings	Diagnostic Testing	Treatment
Substance Use Disorder and Addiction | Addiction is a compulsive need for and use of a habit-forming substance characterized by tolerance and by well-defined physiological symptoms upon withdrawal. A dopamine reward system in the brain is hypothesized as a reason for substance use disorder. The A1 allele of the *DRD2* gene is associated with alcohol use disorder, drug use disorder, smoking, obesity, compulsive gambling, and several personality traits.			
CNS stimulation symptoms or depression symptoms, depending on substance used.	Findings depend on which substance is involved.	Toxicology screen.	In a detoxification center, treatment initially consists of managing the varied symptoms of withdrawal, which can range from a craving to hallucinations and seizures. Once physical withdrawal is complete, group and individual counseling begins and continues on an inpatient, outpatient, and group support basis.

Bibliography

Available online at fadavis.com

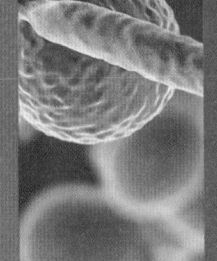

Musculoskeletal Trauma

Learning Objectives

Upon completion of this chapter, the student will be able to:

- Recognize the basic anatomy, histology, and physiological growth and healing processes of bone.
- Identify common types and mechanisms of bone, ligament, tendon, and soft tissue trauma.
- Describe how to perform clinical assessment of the patient with musculoskeletal trauma.

- Identify the factors that can delay healing and potential complications of musculoskeletal trauma.
- Recognize laboratory tests and imaging studies commonly used to diagnose musculoskeletal trauma.
- Discuss treatment modalities used in the management of musculoskeletal trauma.

Key Terms

ABCDEs (of trauma assessment)
Actin
Adhesive capsulitis
Avascular necrosis (AVN)
Basic multicellular unit (BMU)
Bursa
Callus
Cancellous bone
Compartment syndrome
Cortical bone
Crepitus
Delayed union
Diaphysis

Epiphysis
Fat embolism
Kyphosis
Lateral epicondylitis
Malunion
Metaphysis
Myocytes
Myosin
Nonunion
Open reduction and internal fixation (ORIF)
Osteoblasts
Osteoclasts

Osteocytes
Osteoprogenitor cells
Pes cavus
Pes planus
Plantar fasciitis
Rhabdomyolysis
RICE therapy
Sarcomeres
Sequestrum
Temporomandibular joint (TMJ)
Trabecular bone
Valgus
Varus

Trauma causes more than 180,000 deaths per year in the United States. It is the leading cause of death for those aged 1 to 44 years and causes more years of lost productivity before age 65 years than coronary artery disease, cancer, and stroke combined. Musculoskeletal disorders, including those acquired from traumatic events, are commonly managed in the outpatient setting. In the United States, 5.6 million fractures occur per year, corresponding to a 2% incidence. Although most musculoskeletal disorders are not life-threatening, they are a frequent cause of work disability and productivity losses in industrialized countries.

Epidemiology

Motor vehicle–related accidents, work-related injuries, sports activities, and fractures related to osteoporosis are common causes of musculoskeletal trauma. Musculoskeletal injuries occur frequently, result in significant disability, and consume a major portion of health-care resources. According to the Centers for Disease Control and Prevention (CDC), there were 160,000 injury-related deaths in the United States in 2017. Motor vehicle accidents caused more than 40,000 of the injury-related deaths, and falls caused approximately 35,000 deaths. In 2017, falls among older adults cost the U.S. health-care system $30 billion in direct medical costs, and motor vehicle–related deaths and injuries cost more than $90 billion.

Basic Concepts of the Musculoskeletal System

The musculoskeletal system includes the muscles and bones of the skeleton, including the cartilage, ligaments, and tendons. Muscle and bone provide the framework for body shape and work together to accomplish controlled, precise movements. Contracting muscle fibers use the skeleton for stability and leverage to achieve different postures, positions, and movements.

Bones

The 206 bones in the adult body perform the following five main functions:

1. Structural support of the body: The skeletal system provides structural support for the entire body. Individual bones or groups of bones provide a framework for the attachment of soft tissues.
2. Storage of minerals: Bone is composed of 65% calcium hydroxyapatite, a mixture of mainly calcium and phosphorus, and 35% organic matrix, which includes osteoprogenitor cells, osteoblasts, osteocytes, and collagen. Bone stores 99% of the body's calcium, 85% of the body's phosphorus, and 65% of the body's magnesium and sodium.
3. Production of blood cells: Bone marrow produces red blood cells (RBCs), white blood cells (WBCs), and platelets. There are two types of bone marrow: red and yellow. Red bone marrow is hematopoietic; it synthesizes all blood cells. Hematopoietic bone marrow is called myeloid tissue. Yellow marrow is called stromal bone marrow; it produces fats, cartilage, and bone. At birth all bone marrow is red; with age, some red marrow is converted to yellow marrow.
4. Protection of body organs: The skeleton surrounds the soft tissues and organs and helps to protect them from impact injuries.
5. Provide leverage and movement: Many bones function as levers that can change the strength and direction of the forces generated by muscles.

Bone Structure

The skeleton contains two forms of bone: **cortical bone,** which is solid and dense, and trabecular, also called **cancellous bone,** which is nonsolid. **Trabecular bone** is composed of a meshwork that makes the bone porous. The proportion of interior cortical and trabecular bone varies with each bone. The wrist, hip, and vertebrae are composed primarily of trabecular bone.

Microscopic Structure of Bone. The outer layer of bone is called the periosteum. Under the periosteum is a layer of cortical bone that contains units called osteons. Each osteon is composed of concentric layers of cortical bone, termed lamellae, that surround a central canal, termed the Haversian canal. Haversian canals travel longitudinally through bone and contain capillaries, nerves, and lymphatic vessels. Haversian canals are connected to each other via horizontal conduits, called Volkmann canals. These canals transport blood and nutrients to bone cells (osteocytes). Each osteocyte sits in a region called a lacunae. Tiny canals, called canaliculi, travel between the lacunae carrying nutrients to the bone cells (see Fig. 37-1). Within the center of long bones, such as the femur and humerus, is a medullary cavity lined by endosteum, a layer of connective tissue. The medullary cavity is the innermost central cavity that contains the bone marrow (see Fig. 37-2). The endosteum is an active participant in bone growth, repair, and remodeling. Within the endosteum osteoprogenitor cells differentiate into osteoblasts, which then develop into osteocytes. Also, within this layer there are hematopoietic stem cells that further develop and mature into specific blood cells: RBCs, WBCs, and platelets.

Bone Development and Growth

Osteogenesis, or bone growth, begins at about 6 weeks after fertilization, and portions of the skeleton continue to grow until about the age of 25 years. Most

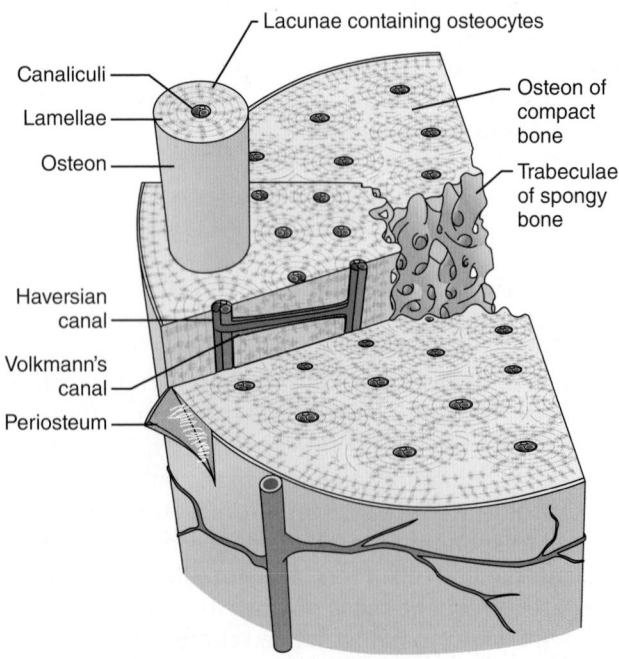

FIGURE 37-1. Microscopic structure of bone.

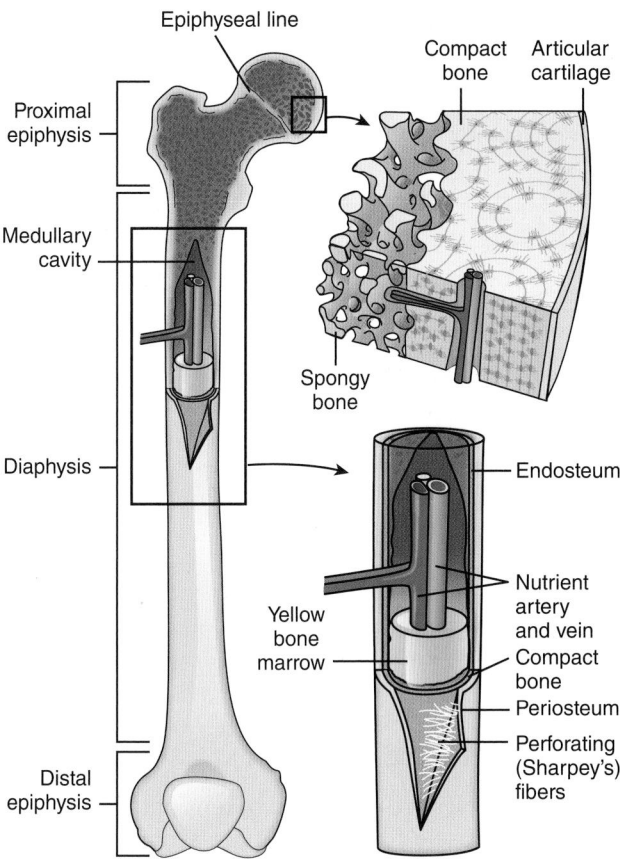

FIGURE 37-2. Anatomical structure of a long bone.

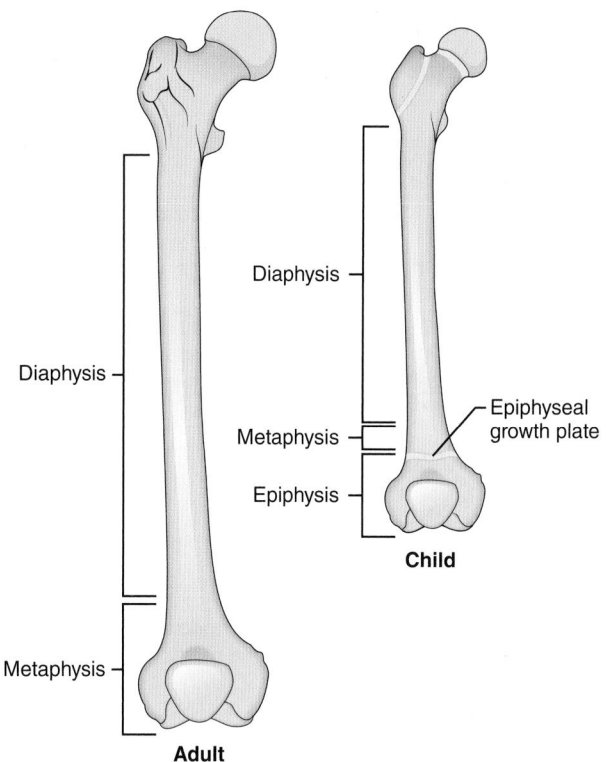

FIGURE 37-3. Epiphysis, metaphysis, and diaphysis of bone.

bones originate as hyaline cartilage; chondrocytes are progenitor cartilage cells. The cartilage is gradually converted to bone through a process called ossification. Bone growth begins at the center of the cartilage. As bones enlarge, bone growth activity shifts to the ends of the bones called **epiphyses,** also called growth plates, which results in an increase in bone length.

The **diaphysis** is the term used to describe the shaft of long bones. It is made primarily of compact cortical bone surrounding a central marrow cavity. The **metaphysis** is the region between the epiphyseal growth plate and the diaphysis portion of bone; it contains mainly trabecular bone (see Fig. 37-3). The metaphysis undergoes extensive remodeling as children grow.

There are different types of bone cells:

- **Osteoblasts:** These bone-forming cells secrete osteoid, which forms the bone matrix. They also begin mineralization and are unable to divide.
- **Osteocytes:** These are mature osteoblasts that maintain metabolism and nutrient and waste exchange; they are unable to divide.
- **Osteoclasts:** These function in resorption and degradation of existing bone, the opposite of osteoblasts.
- **Osteoprogenitor cells:** These are immature cells that differentiate into osteoblasts. These do divide.

Bone Physiology

Osteoblasts and osteoclasts act together and are considered the functional unit of bone called the **basic multicellular unit (BMU)** (also called the bone remodeling unit) (see Fig. 37-4). Bone tissue must be constantly replaced to preserve its strength and integrity. Bone remodeling is organized by two opposite activities: bone formation by osteoblasts, which produce the organic bone matrix, and bone resorption by osteoclasts, which dissolve bone mineral and the extracellular matrix. Bone remodeling is a lifelong process where mature bone tissue is removed from the skeleton and new bone tissue is formed. New bone tissue develops in the process termed modeling, where osteoblastic activity predominates. Once the bone has reached maturity, breakdown and renewal are caused by osteoclasts in a process called remodeling. Osteoclasts adhere to bone and break it down through acidification and proteolytic enzymes. As osteoclasts leave the site, osteoblasts move in to cover the excavation site and begin the process of new bone formation by secreting osteoid, which is eventually mineralized into bone. The processes of bone formation and resorption occur together, and their balance determines the skeletal mass. These processes also control the replacement of bone following injuries that cause fractures and microdamage.

In adults, approximately 1 million BMUs are active at one time, causing the remodeling of 10% of the skeleton annually. Peak bone mass is achieved in early adulthood, between ages 30 and 35 years. Bone mass is influenced by many factors, including nutrition, physical activity,

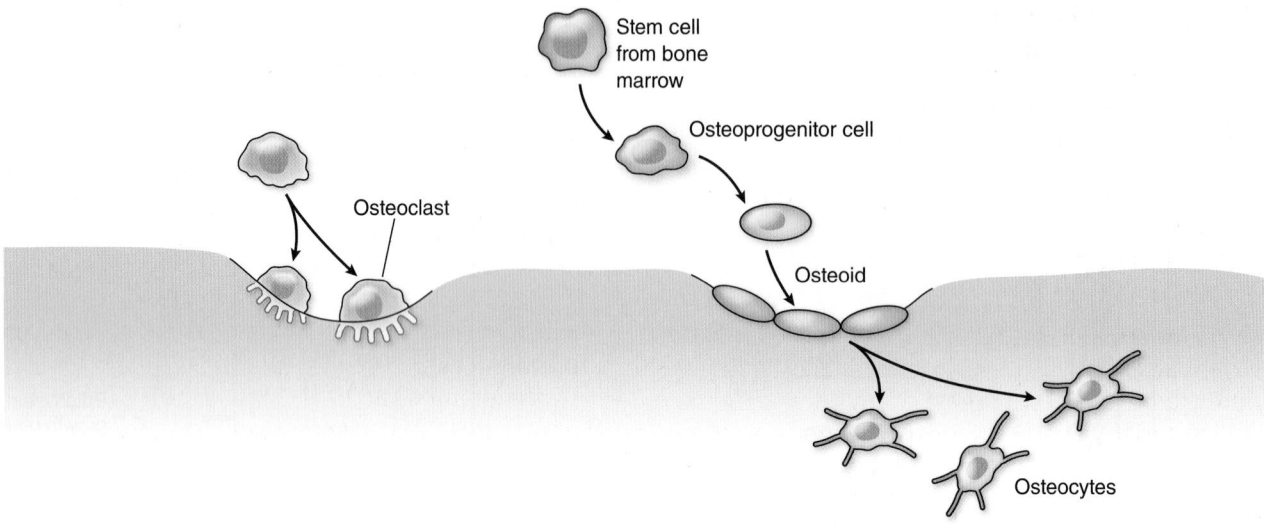

FIGURE 37-4. Bone modeling and remodeling. Bone dynamics encompass continual formation and deterioration (resorption) of bone matrix. The interaction of osteoblasts, osteoclasts, and osteocytes is referred to as a BMU.

age, hormonal status, and vitamin D receptors. Beginning at age 30 or so, the amount of bone resorbed by the osteoclasts exceeds that which is formed by osteoblasts, resulting in a steady decrease in bone mass with age. The propensity for bone loss increases with age.

Bone metabolism is highly dependent on calcium, vitamin D, parathyroid hormone, and calcitonin (see Chapter 38, Figure 38-1). These hormones and nutritional elements are influential in bone growth and maintenance of bone integrity. Calcium absorption from the gastrointestinal (GI) tract is facilitated by vitamin D. Vitamin D activation is dependent on kidney and parathyroid gland function and adequate sunlight. Calcium and vitamin D are key in the maintenance of bone health. Without vitamin D, calcium is not absorbed, and hypocalcemia occurs. Hypocalcemia stimulates the parathyroid gland to secrete parathormone, which activates osteoclasts to break down bone to release calcium. If calcium rises to high levels, calcitonin is stimulated. Calcitonin is a hormone released by the C cells of the thyroid gland that suppresses osteoclastic activity. Calcitonin blocks excess calcium release from bone. It opposes parathyroid gland action and integrates calcium into the bone. Because of the importance of calcium and vitamin D in maintaining bone health, supplements of both are commonly recommended to prevent bone loss. Also, as a person ages, a diet with adequate calcium is very important.

CLINICAL CONCEPT

Adequate intake of calcium and vitamin D, in combination with weight-bearing and physical activity, are essential to stimulate bone growth and maintain adequate bone strength.

Skeletal Muscle

Skeletal muscles are composed of tens of thousands of individual muscle fibers, which are arranged in bundles called fascicles. Each fascicle contains approximately 10 to 30 muscle fibers encased in connective tissue called endomysium. Each muscle fiber is made up of myofibrils that are arranged parallel to each other. Each myofibril consists of **sarcomeres,** the contractile units of skeletal muscle, which consist of thin and thick filaments that slide over one another to cause contraction of the muscle. The thin filaments are made of the protein **actin,** whereas the thick filaments are made of the protein **myosin.** Protein nutrition is important for the development of skeletal muscle.

Skeletal muscle is under voluntary control of the somatic nervous system. Skeletal muscle can become hypertrophied when worked against high resistance. Conversely, muscle can become atrophied if immobile for long periods. Loss of neurological stimulation, nutrients, or blood supply can also cause atrophy.

CLINICAL CONCEPT

Casting or immobilization of a bone for a lengthy period can cause atrophy of surrounding muscle.

Tendons and Ligaments

Tendons and ligaments are made of tough fibrous connective tissue, parallel arrays of collagen fibers that are closely packed together. Tendons attach muscles to bone and transmit load from muscle to bone, resulting in joint motion. Ligaments attach bone to bone and augment mechanical stability of a joint. Common sites of tendons include:

- Rotator cuff of the shoulder
- Insertion of the wrist extensors and flexors at the elbow
- Patellar and popliteal tendons and iliotibial band at the knee
- Posterior tibial tendon in the leg
- Achilles tendon at the heel

Tendons are subject to many types of injuries. There are various forms of overuse tendon injuries, called tendinopathies. These types of injuries generally result in inflammation and degeneration or weakening of the tendons, which may eventually lead to tendon rupture. Rupture of a tendon requires a complex, prolonged healing process and usually requires surgical intervention.

Alternatively, ligaments connect bones to other bones to form a joint. Capsular ligaments that act as mechanical reinforcements are part of the articular capsule that surrounds synovial joints. Extracapsular ligaments join together and provide joint stability. Cruciate ligaments occur in pairs. Ligaments can gradually lengthen when under tension and return to their original shape when the tension is removed. However, when stretched past a certain point or for a prolonged period, they cannot retain their original shape. Like tendons, ligaments can rupture; this also requires surgical intervention. There are many ligaments throughout the body, but some of the most vulnerable ligaments surround the knee, including the cruciate ligaments, collateral ligaments, and patellar ligament.

When injured, most ligaments heal by a process that is similar to scar formation. Unlike healthy ligaments, healed ligaments consist of a hypertrophic mass of type III collagen. This immature collagen is characterized by smaller-diameter fibrils, which result in a mechanically inferior structure compared with normal collagen. A healed ligament often fails to provide adequate joint stability, which can lead to reinjury, a chronically lax joint, or progression to degenerative joint disease. Ligament injuries sometimes require surgical intervention.

Basic Pathophysiological Concepts of Musculoskeletal Trauma

Musculoskeletal trauma can involve bone fracture, soft tissue injury, skeletal muscle injury, and neurovascular damage. Bone and muscle injury can cause immobility, serious complications, and lasting disability if the healing process is hindered. Prolonged immobility can have numerous consequences such as deep venous thromboembolism, pneumonia, and pressure injuries that lead to infection (see Chapter 4 for complications of immobility).

Sprains and Strains

Sprains and strains are common injuries that have similar signs and symptoms but involve different parts of the musculoskeletal system. A sprain is an overstretching of a ligament with a possible tear. A sprain occurs in response to a quick twist or pull of the muscle. It can be caused by a force that displaces a joint from its normal alignment. Sprains most commonly occur around joints. The most common location for a sprain is in the ankle. Inflammation with bruising, swelling, instability, and painful movement are common symptoms experienced after a sprain occurs.

There are three grades of sprains:

- Grade I: mild injuries where there is no tearing of the ligament and no lost joint function, although there may be tenderness and slight swelling.
- Grade II: caused by a partial tear in the ligament, these sprains are characterized by obvious swelling, extensive bruising, pain, difficulty bearing weight, and reduced function of the joint.
- Grade III: caused by complete tearing of the ligament where there is severe pain, loss of joint function, widespread swelling and bruising, and the inability to bear weight; have symptoms similar to those of bone fractures.

A strain is an overstretching of tendons and muscle. Strains often occur in the lower back and in the hamstring muscle and result from overuse of muscles, improper use of the muscles, or as the result of injury in another part of the body when the body compensates for pain by altering the way it moves. Pain, weakness, limited range of motion, and muscle spasms are common symptoms experienced after a strain occurs.

Muscle Contusions

A bruise, or muscle contusion, can result from an injury from a direct blow or an impact, such as a fall. A bruise results when muscle fiber and connective tissue are crushed; torn blood vessels may cause a bluish appearance. Most bruises are minor, but some can cause more extensive damage and complications.

Bone Fractures

Bone is routinely subjected to a variety of loading forces: tension, compression, bending, torsion, and shear. Usually, these forces are within normal physiological parameters. When forces exceed physiological parameters or when a bone abnormality exists, fracture may occur. A fracture is any disruption, complete or incomplete, in the continuity of a bone. There are several common types of fracture (see Table 37-1). Information concerning the mechanism of injury can often help to identify the type of fracture sustained and guide initial treatment until radiological evaluation is obtained.

TABLE 37-1. Types of Fracture

Type	Description	Type	Description
Closed (Complete)	A fracture in which bone fragments separate completely, are not displaced, and remain beneath overlying tissue	Incomplete	A fracture in which the bone fragments are still partially joined

Intervertebral disc

Vertebral compression fractures

Intervertebral disc

Closed fracture

Type	Description	Type	Description
Open (Compound)	A fracture of bone that protrudes to the outside of the body	Compression	A fracture that consists of the crushing of cancellous bone

Vertebral compression fracture

Open or compound fracture

TABLE 37-1. Types of Fracture–cont'd

Type	Description	Type	Description
Transverse	A fracture where parts of the bone are separated but close to each other 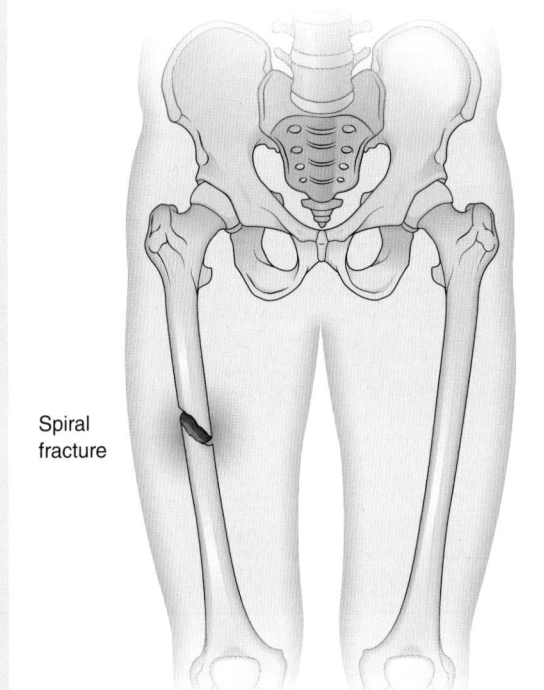 Transverse fracture	Comminuted	A fracture with more than one fracture line and more than two bone fragments that may be shattered or crushed 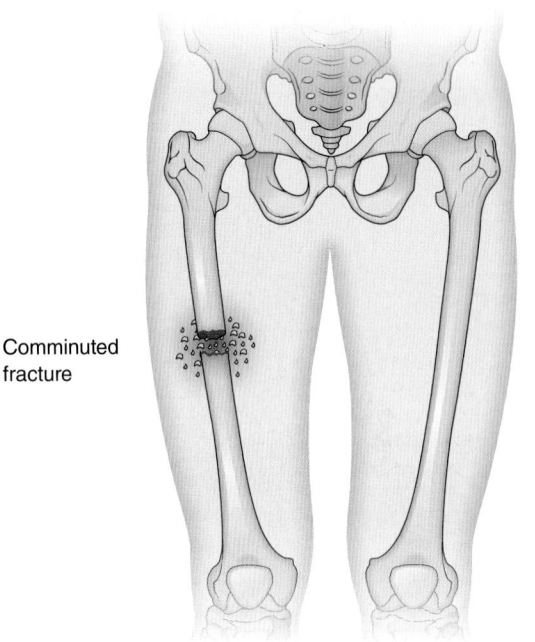 Comminuted fracture
Spiral	A twisting force to the thigh causes a fracture line that encircles the shaft Spiral fracture	Stress fracture	A failure of one cortical surface of the bone, often caused by repetitive activity 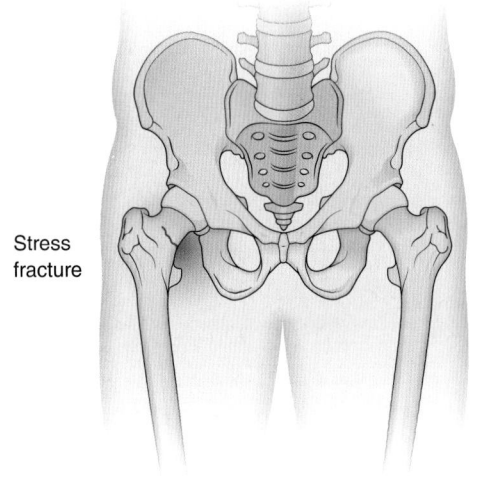 Stress fracture

Continued

TABLE 37-1. Types of Fracture–cont'd

Type	Description	Type	Description
Avulsion	Separation of a small fragment of bone at the site of attachment of a ligament or tendon	Impacted	A fracture in which one part of the fracture is compressed into an adjacent part of the fracture

Avulsion fracture

Impacted fracture

Type	Description
Greenstick	An incomplete break in the bone with the intact side of the cortex flexed (one side is broken and the other is bent); usually seen in children

Greenstick fracture

Soft Tissue Injury

Soft tissue injuries can occur alongside bone fractures, but they can also happen in isolation. The two types of soft tissue, contractile and inert, assist in differentiating the exact site of injury. Contractile tissue includes the structures involved in muscle contraction: the muscle belly, bony insertion, and tendon. Active contraction and passive stretching will elicit pain if the contractile tissue has been injured. In contrast, inert tissue does not take part in muscle contraction but plays a supportive role in muscle functioning. Inert tissue includes the joint capsules, ligaments, bursae, fasciae, dura mater, and nerve roots.

To identify inert tissue injuries, clinicians can use clinical signs and symptoms to isolate the structures involved. Generally, passive stretching provokes pain in an inert tissue injury. However, there may also be swelling and erythema, joint instability, weakness, limited motion, and diminished deep tendon reflexes present.

Neurovascular Injury

When musculoskeletal injury occurs, it is important to identify if there is a concomitant neurovascular injury as well. Damage to the brain, spinal cord, nerve roots, and peripheral nerves can cause irreversible dysfunction if left untreated. Injury to the neurological system can cause a loss or decrease in the level of consciousness (LOC), weakness or paralysis, pain, and paresthesias, as well as other sensory deficits.

When soft tissue and bone are damaged, the integrity of the vascular system may also be compromised, leading to hemorrhage, hematoma formation, and ischemia of tissue and organs. Although it is vital to identify neurovascular injuries during the initial assessment, they may also occur later on in the later stages of healing, which is why it is imperative to routinely assess neurovascular integrity with any type of musculoskeletal injury throughout the course of treatment.

 CLINICAL CONCEPT

Neurovascular integrity should be frequently assessed in an area of musculoskeletal injury. Pulses, sensation, color, and function should be assessed in areas just distal to the injury.

Bone Healing

Fracture healing takes place through five stages:

1. Fracture and inflammatory phase: In the inflammatory phase, bleeding initially occurs between the edges of fractured bone, and a hematoma develops during the first few hours and days. Inflammation in the area causes vascular permeability and the attraction of WBCs. Macrophages, monocytes, lymphocytes, and polymorphonuclear WBCs infiltrate the bone area. This phase peaks approximately 48 hours after the injury and can last up to a week.

2. Granulation tissue formation: In the next phase of healing, fibroblasts are attracted to the area of injury and there is a growth of vascular tissue. Nutrient and oxygen supply during this early process is significant. This stage lasts approximately 2 weeks.

3. Callus formation: During this phase of healing, a **callus** is formed, which consists of osteoblasts and chondroblasts in granulation tissue. These cells synthesize the extracellular organic matrix of woven bone and cartilage, producing newly formed mineralized bone usually after 6 weeks postinjury.

4. Lamellar bone deposition: This fourth phase is a strengthening phase where ossification is beginning. The meshlike callus of woven bone is replaced by sheets (lamellae) of mineralized bone that are organized parallel to the axis of the bone and are mechanically stronger than the bone of a callus. The length of time of this phase depends on the injury; it occurs in the weeks following callus formation.

5. Remodeling: The final phase involves remodeling of the bone at the site of the healing fracture by osteoclasts and osteoblasts. The formation is sculpted and refined by the mechanical stresses imposed on the bone. Adequate strength commonly occurs in 3 to 6 months.

Some factors that influence fracture healing include patient age, medication use, nicotine use, and nutrition (see Box 37-1). Adequate nutrition, especially adequate calcium intake, is needed for bone healing. After bone has healed sufficiently, weight-bearing builds bone strength. Other factors that affect fracture healing include the type of fracture, degree of trauma, systemic and local disease, and infection (see Chapter 9 for factors that affect wound healing).

 CLINICAL CONCEPT

The use of nicotine, corticosteroids, cytotoxic medications, anticoagulants, or immunosuppressive agents during bone's healing process can alter the inflammatory response and inhibit healing.

CLINICAL CONCEPT

After fracture, a bone callus is sufficiently mineralized to show up on x-ray within 6 weeks in adults.

BOX 37-1. Factors That Promote Bone Growth and Healing

- Calcium intake (1,000 to 1,200 mg/day–depends on age)
- Exercise (particularly weight-bearing exercise)
- Vitamins A, B_{12}, C, and K
- Vitamin D (400 to 1,000 units/day)
- Magnesium
- Potassium
- Phosphorus
- Hormones
- Calcitriol synthesized by kidneys
- Growth hormone synthesized by pituitary gland
- Thyroxine synthesized by thyroid
- Sex hormones
- Parathyroid hormone (PTH)
- Calcitonin synthesized by thyroid

Skeletal Muscle Healing

Skeletal muscle is in a constant state of regeneration, which is heightened in response to injury. When muscle fibers are damaged, several mechanisms work simultaneously to regenerate injured tissue. Initially the inflammation reaction attracts WBCs to the area of injury. This stage of healing requires an adequate blood supply of the injured area. If blood supply has been significantly damaged, regeneration cannot take place until new blood vessels penetrate the area.

Regeneration of single muscle fibers or entire muscles can then occur with activation of muscle stem cells, called satellite cells, which migrate to the area of injury. This process usually takes place within 18 hours of the injury. The muscle stem cells differentiate into muscle fiber cells called **myocytes.** Within each myocyte are bundles of myofibrils that are composed of sarcomeres. There are thick and thin filaments within the sarcomeres of myocytes called actin and myosin; these filaments are the structures involved in muscle contraction. Myoblasts that do not form muscle fibers dedifferentiate back into satellite cells and remain adjacent to a muscle.

The extent of injury to nerves and blood vessels has a clear effect on the maintenance of neurovascular control and how quickly the damaged area can obtain nutrients. Muscle histology is also a factor and can change after injury, as fewer numbers of muscle fibers are present, with a subsequent reduction in muscle mass. Repaired muscle is not as strong as it was before injury, although it may be able to contract just as quickly. Muscle may also heal with fibrous scar tissue instead of with new muscle fibers. Scar tissue is a normal part of the healing process for many injuries but can obstruct muscle regeneration and interfere with the normal contraction and elasticity of skeletal muscle.

Trauma Assessment

A comprehensive assessment is necessary for individuals with major musculoskeletal trauma that consists of life-threatening injuries. This assessment involves a primary survey to evaluate immediate life-sustaining needs of the patient followed by a secondary survey after the patient is stabilized hemodynamically. With isolated musculoskeletal injuries, a focused approach is used to evaluate the specific injury, forces involved, and potential sequelae.

The first part of the assessment of patients presenting with major musculoskeletal trauma due to multiple injuries is the primary survey. During this time, life-threatening injuries are identified and resuscitation is begun. The mnemonic **ABCDE** can be used as a memory aid for the order in which problems should be addressed in the primary survey (see Box 37-2). If the patient is unconscious, the Glasgow Coma Scale (GCS) should be used to test eye opening, best motor response, and best verbal response (see Chapter 35, Box 35-3).

After the patient is hemodynamically stable, the secondary survey, focusing on the specific musculoskeletal problems and health history, can occur. The clinician needs to obtain specific information about the musculoskeletal symptomatology. Asking the patient about activities directly before the onset of injury can help to identify the mechanism and loading forces involved. A comprehensive musculoskeletal assessment should move from head to toe to identify all wounds. The number and distribution of involved joints should also be noted. Suspected fractures need immediate immobilization and evaluation with diagnostic tests. Open fractures require irrigation and placement of a sterile dressing while awaiting urgent orthopedic consultation.

Health History

A detailed health history should be obtained for information about the individual's age, gender, ethnicity, occupation, and current and previous health status;

BOX 37-2. ABCDEs of Acute Trauma Assessment

With major trauma, the following lifesaving measures are instituted first:
- **A**irway with cervical spine protection
- **B**reathing and ventilation
- **C**irculation and hemorrhage control
- **D**isability and neurological evaluation
- **E**xposure and environmental control

Source: Initial assessment and treatment with the Airway, Breathing, Circulation, Disability, Exposure (ABCDE) approach. (2012). *Int J Gen Med, 5*, 117–121. Published online Jan 31, 2012. doi: 10.2147/IJGM.S28478

the problem that prompted the need for health care; and related effects or changes in the areas of mobility, strength, and activities of daily living. Past medical and surgical history should be obtained along with medications taken on a regular basis, including over-the-counter supplements and herbal therapies. Past medical and surgical history can influence the treatment currently necessary. Many medications affect musculoskeletal health: long-term use of steroids can lead to osteoporosis and muscle weakness, and anticoagulant drugs may cause bleeding disorders that contribute to such conditions as hemarthrosis. It is also important to obtain information on any past or present allergies; family history; and the patient's usual level of activity, diet, and exercise. Sports activities and other activities that can cause injury are important. The patient should be asked about their use of safety measures, such as sports equipment, helmet, and seat belts. Occupational exposures or hazards should be identified. Travel destinations within the past year can be helpful in evaluating exposure to specific diseases, such as Lyme disease. Exposure to sexually transmitted diseases, as well as past diagnoses or treatment, should be ascertained because some have musculoskeletal manifestations. Other previous therapeutic measures, such as occupational or physical therapy, previous diagnostic tests, joint aspiration, or past injuries related to neurological or vascular problems, should be identified.

Physical Examination

In the physical examination, first note the patient's general appearance, body build, contours, alignment, and symmetry. Also describe the patient's gait, posture, and spinal alignment (see Fig. 37-5).

Guided by the history, the physical examination helps to distinguish between mechanical problems, soft tissue injury or disease, and inflammatory or noninflammatory joint disease or bone fracture. Sensation should be tested using perception of sharp or dull throughout the dermatomes. Pain or paresthesias caused by irritation of a spinal nerve are exhibited in the corresponding area of dermatome (see the dermatome map in Chapter 35, Figure 35-16). Paying special attention to the injured tissue, with a comparison of sensation in a noninjured area, can be helpful in ascertaining whether a sensory deficit exists.

Muscle girth should be measured for symmetry to detect atrophy, which indicates a chronic etiology. Assess deep tendon reflexes and circulatory status. When evaluating an extremity after injury, the unaffected side should be checked first and used as the baseline. For an injured extremity, findings distal and proximal to the site of the injury should be compared. To evaluate peripheral vascular integrity, the color, capillary refill time, temperature, presence of peripheral pulses, degree of sensation of the body part, and a pain evaluation should be documented (see Box 37-3).

Passive and active range of motion (ROM) should be evaluated. Passive ROM requires that the patient keep the muscles relaxed while the examiner moves the joint, whereas active ROM requires that the patient use their muscles for movement. Passive ROM should equal active ROM except when there is paralysis of muscles or a ruptured tendon. As the joint moves through ROM, any stiffness, clicking, or limitation of movement should be noted. **Crepitus,** or joint clicking, may be caused by articular surface abnormalities or joint inflammation, or can be normal. However, when crepitus is present without pain or limited motion, it is generally of no clinical significance.

While putting the muscle through passive ROM, note muscle tone. Muscle should be evaluated for spasticity, hyperreflexia, or fasciculations, with comparison of one side to the other. Muscle strength should be assessed in the injured extremity as well as the normal

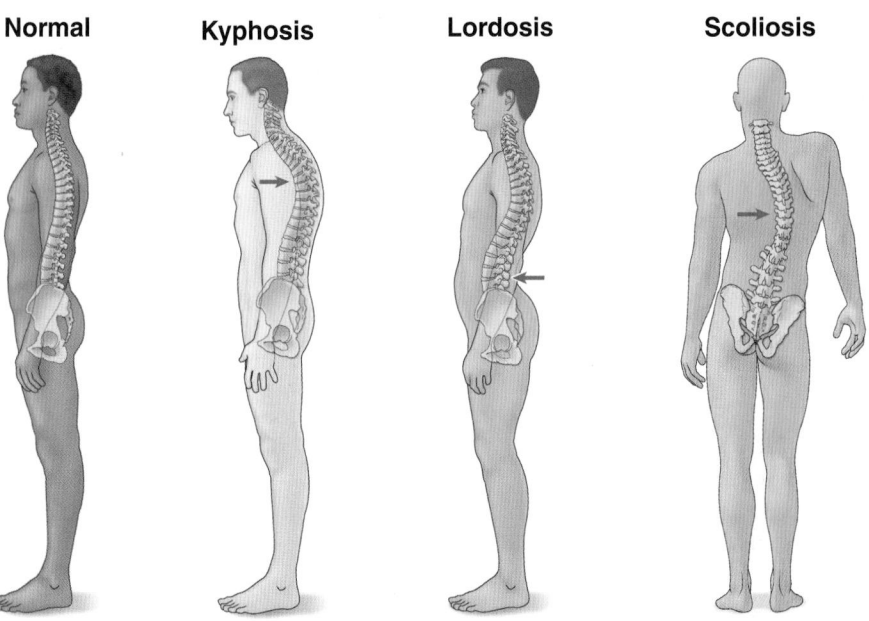

Normal **Kyphosis** **Lordosis** **Scoliosis**

FIGURE 37-5. Types of spine curvature.

BOX 37-3. Assessment of Musculoskeletal Trauma

When performing an assessment on a patient with suspected musculoskeletal trauma, always compare the injured side or extremity to the uninjured side or extremity for symmetry, and make sure to assess for the following:

- Color
- Temperature
- Circulation: capillary refill <3 seconds
- Pulse strength 0/4 to 4/4
- Swelling
- Muscle strength 0/5 to 5/5
- Pain on a scale of 0 to 10, with 0 being no pain and 10 being the worst pain imaginable
- Radiation of pain
- Active and passive ROM
- Sensation 0/3 to 3/3
- Deep tendon reflexes 0/4 to 0/4
- Tenderness
- Paresthesias: feeling of numbness and tingling
- Wounds/wound drainage
- Joint clicking (crepitus)
- Joint instability
- Joint stiffness
- Joint swelling

one. It can be evaluated using the Lovett scale, which is described in Table 37-2.

Signs and Symptoms

The signs and symptoms of traumatic musculoskeletal injury depend on the location, extent of injury, and mechanisms involved. With significant trauma,

TABLE 37-2. Lovett Scale of Muscle Strength

Score	Grade	Description
0	Zero	No palpable contraction of muscle
1	Trace	Palpable contraction of muscle; no joint motion
2	Poor	Complete ROM with gravity eliminated
3	Fair	Complete ROM against gravity; no added resistance
4	Good	Complete ROM against gravity; some added resistance
5	Normal	Complete ROM against gravity with full resistance

soft tissue injury, internal derangement, and fracture, there may be significant bleeding, tissue disruption, swelling, and pain. Constitutional signs, such as fever, weight loss, and malaise, are commonly seen with infection, sepsis, or systemic rheumatic disease. If these conditions involve a joint, the joint may become warm, swollen, and painful. Traumatic joint injuries are usually characterized by stiffness or limitation of movement, swelling or redness, and pain or aching, and may have unilateral or bilateral involvement.

Muscular injuries typically involve limitation of movement, weakness or fatigue, paralysis, tremor, spasm, clumsiness, wasting, aching, and pain. Skeletal injuries are commonly characterized by numbness, tingling or pressure sensation, pain with movement, crepitus, abnormality or change in bone contour, and difficulty with gait or limping. Significant pain on palpation or on weight-bearing suggests a missed or occult injury.

Diagnostic Studies

X-rays are used to identify fractures, dislocations, tissue derangement, or bony abnormalities after a traumatic event. They are useful when there is a loss of joint function, when pain continues despite conservative management, when infection is suspected, or when there is a history of malignancy. Ultrasound studies may be useful in the detection of soft tissue abnormalities, specifically synovial (baker's) cysts, rotator cuff tears, and various tendon injuries. Computed tomography (CT) scan provides an evaluation of the axial skeleton; helical or spiral CT may be used to detect obscured fractures. Magnetic resonance imaging (MRI) is useful when specific disorders are suspected, such as rotator cuff tear, spinal stenosis, avascular necrosis (AVN) of the bone, or mechanical derangement of bones. Bone scintigraphy (nuclear bone scan) is a laboratory test that involves injection of radiopaque dye to visualize bone and surrounding tissue. This is commonly used to detect areas of inflammation, osteomyelitis, or bone tumors. Nerve conduction studies such as electromyography (EMG) may be used when neurological abnormalities or paresthesias are present. A dual energy x-ray absorptiometry (DEXA) scan measures bone density. This specialized dual beam scan visualizes the bone mineral density (BMD) of the hip and lumbar vertebrae and compares that to the BMD of an approximately 25- to 30-year-old adult. This scan is used when osteoporosis is suspected.

ALERT! Before any study using contrast dye, the clinician should ask the patient about kidney function, medication use (particularly metformin), and allergies to dye. Metformin can cause lactic acidosis in patients injected with contrast dye.

Treatment

Patients presenting with acute trauma should be immediately assessed for the ABCDEs and evaluated using advanced trauma support algorithms. Those with fracture, those with injury to the neurological or vascular system, and those with multiple traumatic injuries require emergent consultation and treatment. Because certain musculoskeletal injuries are a risk factor for deep vein thrombosis (DVT) and pulmonary embolism (PE), some patients may need to be placed on anticoagulant therapy.

> **ALERT!** Orthopedic surgery patients are particularly susceptible to DVT and PE. Orthopedic surgery predisposes individuals to DVT because of venous stasis, vessel injury, and hypercoagulability of blood with venous pooling.

Most musculoskeletal injuries are self-limiting, and improvement should be expected over a period of weeks. Activity limitations, if appropriate, should be reserved for the most acute period (2 days or less) to control spasm and edema. In most cases, the goal is to promote a gradual reintroduction of activities, depending on the patient's symptoms. Pharmacological and nonpharmacological therapies should be used for symptom management. Pharmacological agents include NSAIDs or acetaminophen as the first-line choice, topical analgesia, opioids for moderate to severe pain, and skeletal muscle relaxants, which can be given over a 1- to 2-week course to control spasm or tightness.

> ### 🔬 CLINICAL CONCEPT
>
> **RICE therapy** is used for mild to moderately severe injuries:
> - R: rest for initial 24 to 48 hours
> - I: ice application on injured region for 20 minutes of each waking hour during the initial 48 hours after injury
> - C: compression, with brace or splint, if necessary
> - E: elevation above the level of the heart

Other nonpharmacological therapies may include physical therapy, massage, acupuncture, transcutaneous electrical nerve stimulation (TENS), or chiropractic care. Patients who have progressive symptoms or decreased loss of function may need to be referred to a specialist for evaluation of surgical options. Those with ongoing pain symptoms may benefit from a referral to a pain management specialist.

The process of realigning bones and ancillary structures for maximal healing and restoration of proper function is called reduction. There are two kinds of reduction:

1. Closed reduction: A device is worn outside the musculoskeletal area.
2. Open reduction: An incision is commonly necessary for realignment, with surgical insertion of hardware.

External devices used for closed reduction include splints, casts, and traction devices. With open reduction, fixation devices can be inserted inside or outside the body. Internal fixation devices are surgically inserted inside bone. External devices are pieces of hardware that are connected to the internal bone from outside the body. Fixator devices are made of stainless steel or titanium. Commonly, patients undergo **open reduction and internal fixation (ORIF).** Open reduction means that the region of injury was opened for surgical repair. Internal fixation prevents micromotion of bone across fracture lines; this decreases the risk of improper healing (see Fig. 37-6). After reduction, immobilization is needed so that healing takes place with proper skeletal alignment. Also immobilization prevents further injury to soft tissue, nerves, and blood vessels. Splints, casts, slings, and braces support and protect fractures, dislocated joints, and injured soft tissues such as tendons and ligaments. A collar is commonly used for neck injuries. A soft collar can relieve pain by restricting movement of the head and neck. Collars can also take some of the weight of the head off the neck. Stiff collars are generally used to support the neck when there has been a fracture in a cervical vertebra.

Traction can also be used for immobilization. Traction applies tension to correct the alignment of bones

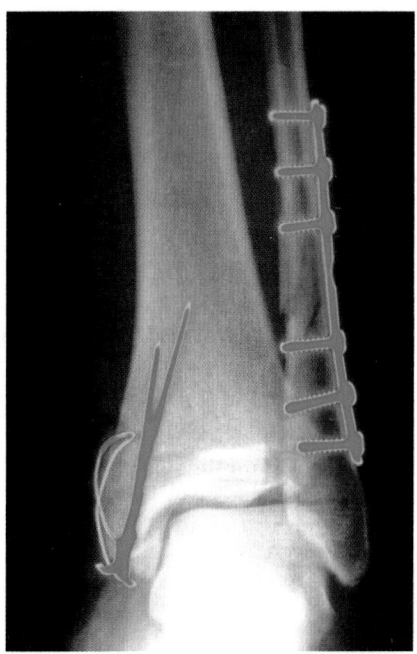

FIGURE 37-6. X-ray showing hardware that reinforces healing of the interior bone. *(From Scott Camazine/Science Source.)*

and hold them in the correct position. For example, if the bone in the thigh breaks, the broken ends may tend to overlap. Use of traction will hold them in the correct position for healing to occur.

Common Complications of Musculoskeletal Trauma

The potential acute complications of bone injury include vascular injury with bleeding, infection, compartment syndrome, thromboembolism, and fat embolism syndrome. If there is extensive muscle injury, rhabdomyolysis can be a significant complication. To prevent neurovascular damage, periodic assessment of the injured area and distal regions is necessary. Compartment syndrome is an uncommon complication but becomes apparent to the patient because of intense pain. As in any breach of skin integrity, infection is a possible complication, particularly in compound fracture. After the acute phase of healing, later musculoskeletal complications include AVN; post-traumatic arthritis; and delayed healing, malunion, or nonunion.

Vascular Injury and Bleeding

Vascular injury of major blood vessels that causes bleeding can occur in musculoskeletal trauma. The vasculature of the extremities is particularly vulnerable to injury because of the close proximity of the blood vessels to the bones. Trauma is the most common cause of hemorrhagic shock. Arterial injuries are particularly prevalent in cases of proximal tibial, supracondylar humeral, distal femoral, and pelvic fracture. Blunt trauma, crush injuries, and high-velocity penetrating injury, such as gunshot, can cause arterial injury and bleeding. Fractures with arterial injury can cause ischemia of the limb, hemorrhage, hypovolemia, and shock. Survival of the limb is correlated with rapid diagnosis and treatment of the vascular damage. Measurements with Doppler or ultrasonography are useful diagnostic tools for rapidly evaluating patients with arterial vascular trauma. Arteriography can demonstrate vascular abnormalities. Bleeding may be apparent, or an expanding hematoma may be visible with poor distal pulse. The clinician needs to be vigilant for signs of limb ischemia, which include pallor, pulselessness, and coolness. If bleeding is severe, the patient will demonstrate decreasing blood pressure and tachycardia. For patients with severe hemorrhage, replacement of blood loss can be accomplished with blood products or crystalloid solutions such as lactated Ringer's solution. Antifibrinolytic medications such as tranexamic acid or aminocaproic acid may be used to facilitate clot formation by blocking breakdown of fibrin. They can be used for patients with severe bleeding—optimally within 3 hours of traumatic injury.

> **ALERT!** To assess neurovascular status, always check pulses and sensation distal to a musculoskeletal injury. Decreased blood flow and neural function can lead to the 5 Ps: pain, pulselessness, pallor, paresthesias, and paralysis.

Compartment Syndrome

Compartment syndrome occurs when tissue pressure exceeds perfusion pressure in a closed anatomical space. Compartments are groups of muscles, nerves, and blood vessels within a space that is contained by a tough fascial membrane. The fascial membrane cannot accommodate swelling or bleeding because it is inflexible (see Fig. 37-7). Swelling or bleeding within a compartment can exert high pressure that causes collapse of arteries and veins and impingement on nerves. The tissue within the compartment receives diminished arterial blood supply, and venous return is reduced with waste buildup. Nerves within the compartment are compressed, which decreases sensation and motor ability of the muscle. The patient complains of pain that is out of proportion to the degree of injury. Progression of compartment syndrome can cause tissue ischemia, necrosis, and functional impairment. This condition can occur in any compartment, such as the hand, forearm, upper arm, abdomen, buttock, or thigh, but it most commonly occurs in the anterior compartment of the leg. The clinician should suspect compartment syndrome when the patient has acute pain, decreased or absent pulse distal to the injured region, sensory loss or paresthesias distal to the injury, and pallor indicating lack of circulation and delayed capillary refill. Irreversible tissue damage can occur within 6 hours of decreased perfusion. Compartment pressures can be objectively measured as greater than 30 mm Hg. Acute compartment syndrome is a medical emergency, and immediate surgical fasciotomy is necessary.

> **ALERT!** An immediate surgical evaluation is required at the first sign of compartment syndrome.

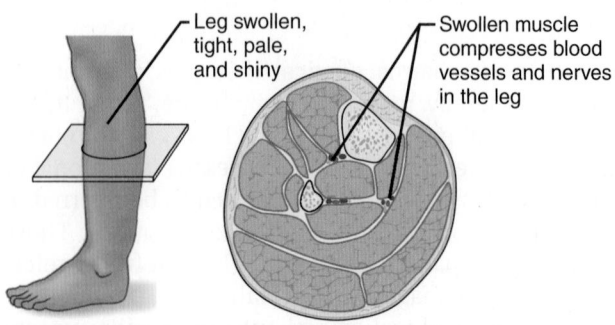

Compartment syndrome:

Leg swollen, tight, pale, and shiny

Swollen muscle compresses blood vessels and nerves in the leg

FIGURE 37-7. Compartment syndrome.

Rhabdomyolysis

Rhabdomyolysis, the breakdown of skeletal muscle tissue, can also occur in compartment syndrome. In rhabdomyolysis, muscle breakdown products, particularly myoglobin, accumulate in the bloodstream. At the kidney, large amounts of myoglobin need to be filtered out of the blood at the nephrons. Myoglobin is toxic to the nephrons and in large quantities will cause nephron tubule dysfunction. Acute renal injury is common with rhabdomyolysis. Clinically, rhabdomyolysis is exhibited by a triad of symptoms: myalgia, weakness, and myoglobinuria, demonstrated by tea-colored urine. However, more than 50% of patients do not complain of muscle pain or weakness, and the initial presenting symptom is dark urine. An elevated creatine kinase (CK) level is the most sensitive laboratory test for evaluating an injury to muscle that has the potential to cause rhabdomyolysis (assuming no concurrent cardiac or brain injury).

Infection

Complications of open wounds and surgical intervention include local infection in the form of cellulitis or osteomyelitis and systemic infection in the form of sepsis. Conditions that heighten susceptibility to infection include diabetes, peripheral vascular disease, and IV drug use. Osteomyelitis should be suspected in cases of poor healing of bone, termed delayed union or nonunion. The most common pathogen involved is *Staphylococcus aureus.* Other pathogens that may cause infection are group A streptococci, anaerobic bacteria, *Pseudomonas aeruginosa, Escherichia coli,* and enterococci. The patient with sepsis will present with fever, chills, and increased pressure in the affected area. The affected area will be warm, edematous, and erythematous, and if infection is advanced, purulent discharge with foul odor will be present. Blood cultures, complete blood count (CBC) with differential, C-reactive protein, and erythrocyte sedimentation rate (ESR) are necessary laboratory tests to monitor the infection. Commonly performed imaging studies are x-ray, MRI scan, technetium-99 bone scintigraphy (nuclear bone scan), and leukocyte scintigraphy. IV antibiotic treatment based on culture and sensitivity is essential during hospitalization followed by oral antibiotics for 5 weeks. Débridement of the wound by removing infected bone and necrotic tissue, also called the **sequestrum,** is necessary for healing to occur. If there is an implant or prosthesis, surgical removal of orthopedic hardware is usually required.

Deep Venous Thrombosis and Pulmonary Embolism

Injury to a vessel wall, venous stasis, and hypercoagulability of blood are the three conditions, known as Virchow's triad, that increase susceptibility to DVT. After musculoskeletal injury, blood vessels are damaged and blood pools within the damaged area. The sequelae of musculoskeletal injury predispose a patient to DVT because of the vessel damage and venous stasis. Within the pooled blood, venous thrombus formation is common. A venous thrombus can detach from anywhere in the venous system and embolize to the pulmonary circulation. Therefore, PE is the dreaded sequela of DVT.

Commonly, a PE will begin as a clot in a leg vein that travels into the inferior vena cava. From the inferior vena cava, the clot reaches the right atrium, right ventricle, and pulmonary arterial circulation. As a PE at that point, it can obstruct blood flow through the lungs and cause hypoxia and possibly death.

Orthopedic surgery carries a high risk of DVT and PE. With any kind of surgery there is vessel damage, and with orthopedic surgery, immobilization is usually needed postoperatively. Therefore, surgical vessel damage and venous stasis caused by immobilization increase the risk of clot formation. Commonly, there are few to no symptoms exhibited by the patient with DVT. The area of DVT may be tender, edematous, and warm, and there can be a palpable ropiness along the course of the involved vein. To diagnose DVT, a D-dimer blood test, prothrombin time, partial thromboplastin time, fibrinogen level, and platelet count should be done.

A patient experiencing a PE may exhibit dyspnea, cyanosis, cough, tachypnea, hemoptysis, chest pain, or tachycardia. Most patients who suffer a PE show no symptoms, and many suffer rapid cardiovascular collapse. A ventilation-perfusion scan, helical CT scan, or CT pulmonary angiogram can demonstrate a PE.

Prevention of DVT and PE is the therapeutic strategy used for patients undergoing orthopedic surgery. Anticoagulation is the recommended pharmacological approach to prevent DVT and PE. If DVT is strongly suspected, the surgical insertion of a Greenfield filter into the inferior vena cava may be recommended. The filter can catch any venous clot that is making its way up to the pulmonary artery. Other therapies for DVT and PE include thrombolysis and pulmonary thrombectomy.

Fat Embolism and Fat Embolism Syndrome

Long-bone and pelvic fractures are associated with fat embolism. A **fat embolism** occurs when fat globules from the marrow of fractured bone enter the circulation. The clinical manifestations may develop 24 to 72 hours after trauma, when fat droplet emboli obstruct the pulmonary microvasculature and other microvascular beds, such as in the brain. Fat embolism syndrome (FES) is the systemic manifestation of fat emboli within the microcirculation that results in a cascade of sequelae. Pulmonary dysfunction occurs as an initial symptom in 75% of patients; in 10% of the cases it progresses to respiratory failure. Symptoms include tachypnea, dyspnea, and cyanosis; hypoxemia may be detected hours before the onset of respiratory complaints. In 86% of patients with FES, emboli travel to the brain and cause cerebral symptoms. These changes range from acute confusion to drowsiness, stupor, or coma. In some patients, a nonpalpable petechial rash on the chest, axillae, conjunctivae, and neck appears within 24 to 36 hours. Serial chest x-rays show bilateral pulmonary infiltrates and nodular "ground glass" opacities, which are fat emboli. CT and MRI scan of the chest and brain can demonstrate fat emboli. Ventilation-perfusion scans can show PE. Transesophageal ultrasound can show fat emboli entering the right atrium from the venous circulation. There is also a specific set of clinical criteria for the diagnosis of FES (see Box 37-4).

Hemodynamic stabilization is the priority in FES. Infusion of fluids—normal saline and lactated Ringer's—are used to flush out emboli. Corticosteroids and albumin infusion are also commonly used. Albumin enhances intravascular fluid volume and binds to fatty acids released from a fat embolism. Early stabilization of long-bone fractures is key to decrease the risk of bone marrow embolization into the venous system. Rigid fixation of long-bone fractures within 24 hours has been shown to reduce the incidence of FES.

BOX 37-4. Clinical Criteria for Diagnosis of Fat Embolism Syndrome

One major criterion, four minor criteria, and the presence of macroglobulinemia are required for the diagnosis.

Major criteria for diagnosing FES are as follows:
- Symptoms and radiological evidence of respiratory insufficiency
- Cerebral sequelae unrelated to head injury or other conditions
- Petechial rash

Minor criteria are as follows:
- Tachycardia (heart rate >10 beats/min)
- Pyrexia (temperature >38.5°C or 101.3°F)
- Retinal changes of fat or petechiae
- Renal dysfunction
- Jaundice
- Acute drop in hemoglobin level
- Sudden thrombocytopenia
- Elevated erythrocyte sedimentation rate
- Fat microglobulinemia

From Gurd, A. R., & Wilson, R. I. (1974). The fat embolism syndrome. *J Bone Joint Surg (British Volume)*, 56B(3), 408–416.

Avascular Necrosis

Avascular necrosis (AVN), deterioration of bone caused by insufficient blood supply, is commonly associated with fractures of the femoral head and neck, scaphoid, talar neck and body, and proximal humerus. The patient with AVN experiences pain and weakness. The examiner will find motor weakness; abnormal gait, if a lower extremity is involved; and lack of rehabilitation progress. An MRI or bone scintigraphy are used to detect AVN. Treatment involves surgical removal of necrotic bone.

Post-Traumatic Arthritis

Post-traumatic arthritis is common in intra-articular fractures, particularly in those fractures that are inadequately reduced. The patient complains of persistent pain and achiness of the involved joint; the examiner will note crepitus in the joint and motor weakness. Diagnostic tests include x-ray and CT scan. Treatment may require arthroscopic débridement, osteotomy, arthroplasty, or arthrodesis. Arthroscopic débridement is the removal of damaged cartilage or bone tissue within a joint. Osteotomy is the removal of pieces of bone. Arthroplasty involves resurfacing or remodeling of a joint. This is most commonly done by replacing a joint with a prosthesis. Arthrodesis is the surgical immobilization of a joint. An example is a spinal fusion, which is a procedure that fuses two vertebrae together when there is instability of the bones causing nerve impingement and pain.

Delayed Healing of Fracture

When a fracture has not healed after the expected period, an assessment of union status should ensue. **Delayed union** is defined as a fracture that is taking more time than normal to heal. **Malunion** is the healing of bone in an unacceptable position. **Nonunion** is the permanent failure of healing of bone. In each of these conditions, the patient experiences persistent pain and dysfunction of the affected limb. The examiner will note motor weakness, abnormal function of the limb, and abnormal gait if it occurs in a lower extremity. The most common cause of delayed healing or nonunion is infection of bone (osteomyelitis) (see earlier discussion of infection). Other causes include malalignment or nonstabilization of bones; poor circulation, nutrition, or oxygenation; or metabolic disease such as diabetes. Healing can also be delayed by corticosteroid or anticoagulant use, smoking, or radiation (see Chapter 9). Diagnosis of delayed healing is made via x-ray, CT scan, and bone scintigraphy. If cellulitis or osteomyelitis is found, IV antibiotics are necessary. Débridement of the dead bone and necrotic tissue is necessary. Treatment also includes stabilization of the fracture and possibly bone grafting. Treatment of malunion involves surgical correction of the anatomical abnormality.

Pathophysiology of Selected Disorders of Musculoskeletal Trauma

Certain musculoskeletal areas of the body are susceptible to specific kinds of injury. The following disorders of musculoskeletal trauma are those seen most commonly in the clinical area.

Strains and Sprains

The paravertebral musculature and muscles of the extremities are commonly affected by strains and sprains. Strains occur when muscles or tendons are pulled, small blood vessels tear, and nerve endings are irritated. Sprains occur when ligaments, the connective tissue linking bones together, are stretched and overextended. Strains and sprains may present with some edema, but usually no deformity is noted.

Cervical Strain

More than 1 million cases of cervical strain injuries caused by motor vehicle accidents occur annually in the United States. Cervical strain is most often caused by an acceleration-deceleration injury, commonly known as whiplash. It is estimated that the annual incidence of symptoms caused by cervical strain is 3.8 cases per 1,000 population.

Etiology and Pathophysiology. Cervical strain is produced by an injury to the muscles and tendons because of excessive forces placed on the cervical spine. Elongation and tearing of muscles or ligaments occur with secondary edema and inflammation. The most common cause of cervical strain is whiplash injury caused by a motor vehicle accident. Repetitive stress injuries to the cervical spine or abnormal posture can also cause cervical strain. Such injuries can result from occupational situations that require odd positioning of the neck.

Clinical Presentation. The clinician should elicit a complete history to evaluate how the cervical injury occurred. The most common symptoms of cervical strain are suboccipital headache and motion-induced neck pain. There is difficulty sleeping because of cervical pain. At the time of the accident, neck pain may be minimal, with an onset of symptoms occurring during the subsequent 12 to 72 hours. Shoulder, scapular, and arm pain may also occur.

> **ALERT!** In the acute phase of neck trauma or multitrauma injury, immobilization of the cervical spine is mandatory until it is certain that there is no spinal cord damage. Acute cervical spinal cord injury involving C1 through C4 can cause respiratory failure.

Less common symptoms of cervical strain include visual disturbances, such as blurred vision and diplopia; tinnitus; dizziness; concussion; and disturbed concentration and memory.

In the physical examination, the clinician must rule out cervical spine fracture, herniated disc, and spinal cord injury. If weakness, numbness, or paresthesias of the arms are present, there may be cervical spinal nerve impingement, also called cervical radiculopathy.

> **CLINICAL CONCEPT**
>
> Cervical radiculopathy is impingement of a cervical spinal nerve; it often occurs because of vertebral bony degeneration and misalignment, disc herniation, and vertebral compression fracture. Neck pain with radiation into the arm, paresthesias, and weakness of the arm are symptoms.

Examination findings include cervical paravertebral muscle spasm and tenderness. There is neck stiffness, and the posture may show a forward tilt of the head, flexed neck, rounded shoulders, and asymmetry of the neck or shoulders. Palpation may reveal muscle spasm tightness, crepitation, swelling, enlargement of joints, and tenderness. Decreased active and passive ROM of the neck is noted. Deep tendon reflexes of the arms should be normal.

> **ALERT!** Injuries of the cervical spine at or above C4 can cause respiratory failure. The fourth cervical spinal nerve is the phrenic nerve, which innervates the diaphragm. Fatal cervical spine fractures occur in upper cervical levels, either at craniocervical junction C1 or C2.

Diagnosis. Cervical spine x-rays may be normal or show straightening of the normal lordotic curve of the neck. An MRI is the best study for evaluating the status of the vertebral bones, discs, and spinal cord.

Treatment. Early treatment with nonopioid analgesics for pain relief, anti-inflammatory agents, and muscle relaxants for spasms are the main medications used for cervical sprain or strain injuries. A soft cervical collar may be recommended for minor neck injuries. A cervical collar can facilitate healing by taking the weight of the head off the neck. A rigid cervical collar or neck brace may be used for more severe cervical injury. In cases of vertebral fracture and spinal cord injury, vertebral fusion surgery may be required. Postsurgery, a halo traction device may be used to stabilize the cervical spine.

Lumbar Strain and Sprain

Low back pain is one of the most common reasons patients seek health care. The most common cause is lumbosacral strain and sprain. The lifetime prevalence of low back pain in the United States is 60% to 80%, and it is the most common cause of work-related disability in persons younger than 45 years. Other more serious causes of low back pain that need to be excluded before diagnosing lumbar strain or sprain are herniated disc, vertebral fracture, and spinal cord injury.

Etiology. Sprains are ligamentous injuries that are caused by a sudden contraction, sudden torsion, severe direct blows, or a forceful straightening from a crouched position. Individuals also commonly sustain a low back strain or sprain while lifting heavy objects. During such activities, tremendous loads are placed on the lumbar spine, which may cause a temporary instability and lead to a subsequent injury to the soft tissue that surrounds the spine. Sprain and strain commonly occur when there is lateral bending with flexion-extension or axial rotation with lateral bending of the lumbar spine.

Pathophysiology. Strains are defined as tears, either partial or complete, of the muscles and tendons. Muscle strains and tears most frequently result from a violent muscular contraction during an excessively forceful muscular stretch. Any posterior spinal muscle and its associated tendon can be involved, although the most susceptible muscles are those that span several joints.

The lumbar spine and the hips are responsible for the trunk's mobility. The L4–L5 and L5–S1 areas bear the highest loads and tend to undergo the most motion. Consequently, these areas are found to sustain the most spinal strain or sprain injuries.

> ### 🔬 CLINICAL CONCEPT
>
> The L4–L5 and L5–S1 segments of the vertebrae are most often involved in lower back strain and sprain. In L4–L5 spinal nerve impingement, the dorsiflexion of the foot is weak. In L5–S1 spinal nerve impingement, the plantar flexion of the foot is weak.

Clinical Presentation. Lumbar strain and sprain can present similarly to more serious conditions such as herniated disc or spinal nerve impingement. The clinician has to evaluate the history and perform a comprehensive motor and neurological assessment of the lower extremities. The physical examination findings often cannot make the clear distinction between muscle and nerve damage. Diagnostic testing also often cannot demonstrate the extent of muscle, ligament,

and soft tissue damage. However, it can make the necessary distinction of nerve versus muscle involvement.

History. During the history of a patient with low back pain, the following key information needs to be elicited:

- The mechanism of injury, with an exact description of the event leading to the pain
- The exact localization and duration of the pain
- Any pain radiation
- Movements that aggravate or minimize the pain

Typical symptoms are sharp pain, tenderness, and spasm over the posterior lumbar paravertebral spinal muscles or at the insertion of the muscle at the iliac crest. ROM, particularly in flexion, is usually painful and decreased.

If the injury is limited to a sprain or strain injury, structural deformities and neurological symptoms are absent. Any neurological problem, such as numbness or weakness of the lower extremity, indicates the possible presence of a herniated disc or spinal nerve root impingement.

> ### 🔬 CLINICAL CONCEPT
>
> Low back pain accompanied by radiating pain down the leg indicates spinal nerve impingement, a syndrome called sciatica.

> **ALERT!** If lumbar pain is accompanied by urinary or fecal incontinence, cauda equina syndrome is probable. Cauda equina syndrome, a medical emergency, occurs when the bundle of nerves at the end of the spinal cord is compressed.

Physical Examination. The clinician should evaluate the patient's back with the patient in a standing position. Assessment should include inspecting the back for obvious deformities or changes in alignment. The patient should be asked to assume changes in position according to full ROM: flexion, extension, lateral flexion, and rotation. The clinician should note restricted ROM. Evaluation of ROM provides clues to muscle spasm and aggravating factors that worsen the patient's pain.

With the patient in the prone position, the clinician should palpate the paravertebral musculature, areas of muscle spasm, and the location of any point tenderness, if present.

Evaluation of the lower extremities should include a motor examination, a sensory evaluation, and reflex testing at the knees and ankles. The patient should be asked to stand on the toes and walk on the heels, if possible. Standing on the toes requires dorsiflexion of the foot and tests the L4–L5 spinal motor nerve, whereas walking on heels requires plantar flexion of the foot and tests the L5–S1 spinal motor nerve. Testing of sensation of the patient's lower extremities according to the sensory dermatomes can assist in diagnosis. Also, the patellar and Achilles reflex need to be assessed.

With the patient in the supine position, the clinician should test for the straight-leg raising sign, also called Lasègue's sign (see Fig. 37-8). The straight-leg raising test helps to evaluate disc involvement, sciatica, or a neurological deficit, as it places strain on the sciatic spinal nerve roots. The supine patient should lie with both legs extended in a relaxed position on a table. The examiner should raise one of the patient's legs to a 30- to 70-degree angle from the table. A patient complaint of pain radiating down the leg is a positive straight-leg raising sign, which indicates sciatica. In addition, the clinician should conduct the Patrick test, also called a FABER (flexion, abduction, and external rotation) test (see Fig. 37-9). The patient should lie supine and flex one leg at the knee. The examiner should abduct and externally rotate the patient's thigh. A positive Patrick sign is the presence of pain with this maneuver and points to a sacroiliac joint inflammation, termed sacroiliitis. This test is negative in lumbosacral sprains and strains.

Diagnosis. Laboratory studies are generally not indicated in the evaluation of lumbosacral spine sprain or

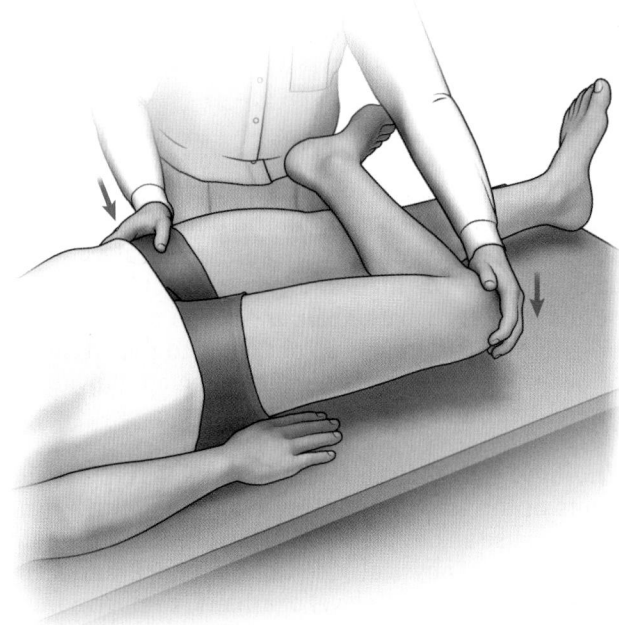

FIGURE 37-9. The Patrick test, also known as the FABER test (flexion, abduction, and external rotation), is performed to evaluate function of the hip joint or the sacroiliac joint. The test is performed by having the tested leg flexed, abducted, and externally rotated. If pain is elicited on the ipsilateral side anteriorly, it is suggestive of a hip joint disorder on the same side. If pain is elicited on the contralateral side posteriorly around the sacroiliac joint, it is suggestive of pathology in that joint.

strain injuries. Anteroposterior and lateral x-rays of the lumbar spine should be routinely obtained to:

- Exclude a fracture, rheumatic disease, or a tumor growth
- Evaluate degenerative joint disease as well as overall spinal alignment

With lumbar strain and sprain, there should be no abnormal finding except soft tissue swelling. If neurological signs are present, a CT scan or MRI should be done to evaluate for disc herniation and involvement of the spinal nerve roots.

Treatment. Cold therapy, initially performed for a short period up to 48 hours, can be applied to the affected area to limit the localized tissue inflammation and edema. The patient should maintain a low level of activity. Activities, particularly those involving lifting and extreme ROM of the spine, should be avoided. The patient should be instructed on how to perform activities without straining the back muscles. Heat therapy can be applied after the acute phase. Anti-inflammatory agents and muscle relaxants are commonly prescribed. Intramuscular (IM) injections of muscle relaxants or NSAIDs at the site of the pain may help control muscle spasms. There should be no manipulation of the affected area during the injury's acute phase. A supportive lumbosacral corset may also be used to help control muscle spasms. The patient

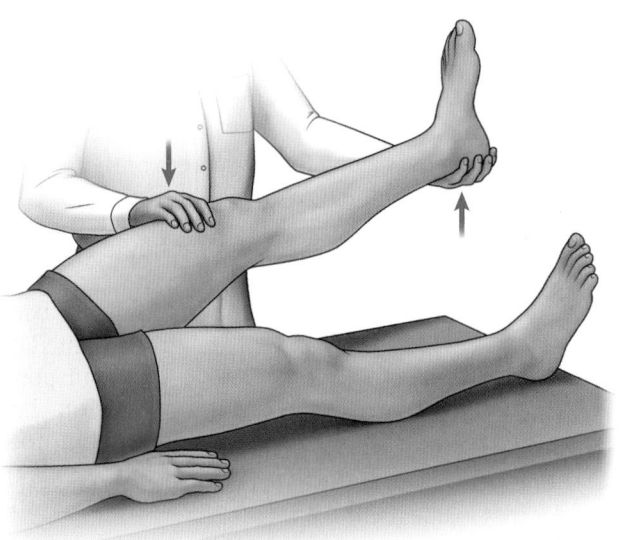

FIGURE 37-8. Straight-leg raising test. The straight-leg test, also called Lasegue's sign, is a test done during the physical examination to determine whether a patient with low back pain has an underlying herniated disc. With the patient lying supine on an examination table, the examiner lifts the patient's leg while the knee is straight.

should be referred to a physical therapist. Abdominal obesity aggravates low back pain; therefore, weight reduction is advised if this is a problem.

Ankle Sprain

Sprained ankles have been estimated to constitute up to 30% of injuries seen in sports medicine clinics. More than 23,000 people per day in the United States, both athletes and nonathletes, require medical care for ankle sprains. The highest incidence of ankle injuries occurs in football, basketball, and soccer players. However, most ankle sprains do not come to the attention of health-care providers because affected individuals often treat themselves.

Etiology. Mechanical forces exceeding the tensile limits of the ankle joint capsule and supportive ligaments cause ankle sprains. Risk factors of ankle sprain include lack of physical conditioning, poor proprioception, obesity, and high level of athletic competition.

Pathophysiology. The most commonly injured site is the lateral ankle complex, which is composed of the anterior talofibular, calcaneofibular, and posterior talofibular ligaments. Approximately 85% of sprains are caused by inversion of the foot during plantar flexion of the ankle; most injuries involve the anterior talofibular ligament. Recurrent ankle sprains are common. The cause is unknown, although it is postulated that the scar tissue of healed ligaments creates a weak, unstable joint.

Clinical Presentation. Individuals with ankle sprain complain of severe pain that worsens with weight-bearing. It is most important to exclude ankle fracture; the ability to walk on the foot usually indicates no fracture. The clinician should palpate the ankle for bony point tenderness, especially over the medial malleolus, lateral malleolus, base of the fifth metatarsal, and midfoot bones. Point bony tenderness at one of these areas, as well as bony deformity or crepitus, suggests the possible presence of a fracture. Sensation of the foot should be normal. Palpation of the dorsalis pedis and posterior tibial arterial pulses are necessary. Active ROM must be assessed, because Achilles tendon ruptures can mimic ankle sprains.

There are three grades in the classification of ankle sprains:

- Grade 1: Injuries cause a stretch of the ligament, mild swelling, little or no functional loss, and no joint instability. The patient is able to fully or partially bear weight.
- Grade 2: Injuries cause a stretch of the ligament with partial tearing, moderate-to-severe swelling, ecchymosis, moderate functional loss, and mild-to-moderate joint instability. Patients usually have difficulty bearing weight.
- Grade 3: Injuries cause complete rupture of the ligament, with severe swelling, ecchymosis, an inability to bear weight, and moderate-to-severe instability of the joint.

Diagnosis. The Ottawa Ankle Rules, a set of conditions that occur in ankle injury, assist in the diagnosis of ankle sprain versus fracture (see Box 37-5). Drawer and talar tilt examination techniques are used to assess ankle instability. X-rays are necessary to rule out fracture; in addition, CT scanning may be needed to exclude stress fractures. Electromyographic examinations of individuals with severe ankle sprains have shown that 80% of these patients have some degree of peroneal nerve injury.

Treatment. RICE therapy is the mainstay of acute treatment; more comprehensively, the combination of protection, relative rest, ice, compression, elevation, and support (PRICES) is used. Anti-inflammatory agents can decrease swelling and pain. A compression dressing or splint can be applied to severe sprains. Physical therapy during the recovery phase is aimed at the patient regaining full ROM, strength, and proprioceptive abilities.

Cumulative Trauma Disorders

Cumulative trauma disorders, also referred to as repetitive strain injuries, are caused by constant stresses exerted on a particular body part. The trauma takes place over months to years.

Stress Fracture

A stress fracture is caused by repetitive stress on bone. Commonly, stress fractures occur on the second and

---

BOX 37-5. **The Ottawa Ankle Rules**

According to the Ottawa Ankle Rules, an ankle x-ray is required only if there is pain in the malleolar zone and any one of the following:

- Bone tenderness along the distal 6 cm of the posterior edge of the tibia or tip of the medial malleolus, OR
- Bone tenderness along the distal 6 cm of the posterior edge of the fibula or tip of the lateral malleolus, OR
- An inability to bear weight both immediately and in the emergency department for four steps

A foot x-ray is required only if there is pain in the midfoot zone and any one of the following:

- Bone tenderness at the base of the fifth metatarsal (for foot injuries), OR
- Bone tenderness at the navicular bone (for foot injuries), OR
- An inability to bear weight both immediately and in the emergency department for four steps

Adapted from Stiell, I. G., McKnight, R. D., Greenberg, G. H., et al. (1994). Implementation of the Ottawa Ankle Rules. *J Am Med Assoc, 271*, 827–832.

third metatarsals, tibia, and fibula. In the majority of cases, no acute traumatic event precedes the symptoms. Recall that the normal physiological function of bone involves constant remodeling, with osteoclasts and osteoblasts performing opposing activities. Stress fractures develop when extensive microdamage occurs before bone can be adequately remodeled. Bones prone to stress fractures are those constantly involved in weight-bearing activity, those involved in high-impact activity, or those that are weakened by osteoporosis.

Risk factors for stress fractures include genetics, female sex, White ethnicity, low body weight, lack of weight-bearing exercise, intrinsic and extrinsic mechanical factors, amenorrhea, oligomenorrhea, inadequate calcium and caloric intake, and disordered eating. A decreased testosterone level in male endurance athletes has also been implicated as a risk factor. Studies show a high incidence of stress fractures in military recruits, distance runners, tennis players, and ballet dancers. The females most at risk for stress fractures are those who restrict their food intake and those who have dysmenorrhea.

The symptom of a stress fracture is localized bone pain that increases with weight-bearing. On physical examination, there is tenderness along an involved bone upon palpation and percussion. X-ray, bone scanning, MRI, and CT scanning are the preferred tests for diagnosis, although it is important to note that stress fractures may not be apparent on x-ray for the first 2 to 4 weeks after injury.

CLINICAL CONCEPT

The triad of disordered eating, amenorrhea, and osteoporosis are conditions that are extremely prevalent in female athletes with low body fat.

Carpal Tunnel Syndrome

Carpal tunnel syndrome (CTS) is a cumulative trauma disorder that causes increased pressure on the median nerve in the wrist. The carpal tunnel, located at the base of the palm, is surrounded by carpal bones and is wrapped by the transverse carpal ligament. The median nerve runs anteriorly from the forearm into the wrist through the carpal tunnel.

The prevalence of CTS in the United States is estimated at 3.7%, and the annual incidence is estimated at 0.4%. Incidence is probably higher because some persons do not seek health care for CTS. CTS is more prevalent in middle-aged persons and predominately in females. It occurs in persons with occupations that require repetitive strain risk, such as assembly packers, waiters, computer keyboard workers, musicians, or craftspeople. Also, compression of the median nerve can occur during pregnancy or because of oral contraceptive–related edema. There is a strong

association between being overweight or obese and the presence of CTS.

Clinical Presentation. Classic CTS is associated with symptoms that affect at least two of the first through third fingers. The index finger, thumb, and middle finger are commonly affected. Wrist pain and radiation of pain proximal to the wrist may also occur. Patients typically complain of an intermittent "pins-and-needles" or paresthesias in the median nerve distribution of the hand. Pain is generally worse at night than during the day. Patients may awaken with a burning pain or tingling that may be relieved with shaking their hands.

Diagnosis. Phalen's sign may be elicited by hyperflexion of the wrist for 60 seconds. The patient with CTS experiences paresthesias in the median nerve distribution of the hand. Tinel's sign occurs by tapping the anterior surface of the wrist over the median nerve. This produces paresthesias in the median distribution of the hand. Hand and arm x-rays may be needed to rule out other problems; EMG is also sometimes used in the diagnosis.

Treatment. To relieve CTS, rest, splinting, pain management, and surgical decompression may be necessary. Early in the course of the syndrome, the neurological findings are reversible. If untreated, CTS can result in thenar atrophy, chronic hand weakness, and numbness in the median nerve distribution of the hand.

Lateral Epicondylitis

Lateral epicondylitis, also called tennis elbow, occurs in up to 50% of tennis players. However, this condition is not limited to tennis players; it is the result of overuse from many activities. Any activity involving wrist extension or supination can be associated with overuse of the muscles originating at the lateral epicondyle (elbow). The typical patient is a man or woman aged 35 to 55 years who either is a recreational athlete or one who engages in rigorous daily activities.

The most important structure involved in epicondylitis is the extensor carpi radialis brevis (ECRB) muscle, which arises from the lateral epicondyle of the humerus. The etiology of lateral epicondylitis involves inflammatory processes of the radial humeral bursa, synovium, periosteum, and the annular ligament. There is also microscopic tearing with formation of scar tissue in the origin of the ECRB. This microtearing can lead to structural failure of the origin of the ECRB muscle. Patients complain of lateral elbow and forearm pain exacerbated by use.

Upon examination, the patient has a point of maximal tenderness just distal to the lateral epicondyle in the area of the ECRB muscle, as well as weak muscle grip with painful movement of the forearm. Wrist extension or supination against resistance with the elbow extended should provoke the patient's symptoms. Another helpful test is the chair-raise test. The patient stands behind a chair and attempts to raise it by putting their hands on the top of the chair back and lifting. In patients with lateral epicondylitis, pain results over the lateral elbow. X-ray, CT scan, and MRI are used to diagnose epicondylitis.

Rest, ice, nonsteroidal analgesics, splinting, steroid injection, and physical therapy are treatment measures for lateral epicondylitis. Approximately 90% to 95% of patients with the disorder recover with conservative measures and do not require surgical intervention. Patients whose condition is unresponsive to 6 months of conservative therapy are candidates for surgery.

Bursitis

Bursae are fluid-filled, saclike structures between skin and bone or between tendons, ligaments, and bone. They act as cushions to lubricate and decrease friction between bone, ligaments, and tendons. Bursitis occurs when the synovial lining produces excessive fluid, leading to localized swelling and pain.

Bursitis accounts for 0.4% of all visits to primary care providers. The incidence of bursitis is higher in athletes, with an incidence of up to 10% in runners. The most common locations of bursitis are the subdeltoid, olecranon, ischial, trochanteric, and prepatellar bursae.

The most common cause of bursitis is repetitive injury or overuse. Repetitive injury within the bursa stimulates the inflammatory cascade, which causes local vasodilation and increased vascular permeability. Bursitis can also be caused by autoimmune disorders, gout or pseudogout, infection, traumatic events, and hemorrhagic disorders. Systemic diseases such as rheumatoid arthritis, ankylosing spondylitis, psoriatic arthritis, scleroderma, systemic lupus erythematosus, pancreatitis, Whipple disease, oxalosis, uremia, hypertrophic pulmonary osteoarthropathy, and idiopathic hypereosinophilic syndrome have also been associated with bursitis.

Clinical Presentation. Patients complain of pain with motion of a joint and discomfort at rest. There is swelling and decreased ROM of the affected joint. The bursa, which is not normally palpable, becomes enlarged, tender, and painful. Pain is aggravated by movement of the joint, tendon, or both.

On physical examination, patients have tenderness at the site of the inflamed bursa. If the bursa is superficial, physical examination findings are significant for localized tenderness, warmth, edema, and erythema of the skin. Decreased active ROM with preserved passive ROM is suggestive of bursitis, but the differential diagnosis includes tendinitis and muscle injury. A decrease in both active and passive ROM is more suggestive of other musculoskeletal disorders. Patients with septic bursitis may have fever, bursal warmth, tenderness, and associated cellulitis.

In chronic bursitis, the affected extremity may show atrophy and weakness. Tendons may also be weakened and tender. Chronic bursitis leads to continual pain and can cause weakening of overlying ligaments and tendons; ultimately, this can result in rupture of the tendons.

Diagnosis and Treatment. Diagnostic tests include x-ray, ESR, and WBC count. Treatment for pain control includes rest, ice, compression, elevation, and medications (RICEM), which include NSAIDs, acetaminophen, and corticosteroid injections. If no response occurs to other treatments, a mix of corticosteroid and local anesthetic can be injected into each tender site.

Temporomandibular Joint Disorder

The **temporomandibular joints (TMJ)** connect the jaw to the skull in front of each ear. The joint allows for side-to-side movement and up-and-down motion, as well as protrusion and retraction of the jaw. An estimated 10 million people have TMJ disorders, and roughly 25% of the population has symptoms at some point in their lives. Adults aged 20 to 40 years are most often affected, with a preponderance of females to males.

The pathophysiology of TMJ disorder mainly occurs because of local repetitive injury. Repetitive and cumulative trauma caused by nocturnal jaw clenching, nocturnal bruxism (teeth grinding), and jaw clenching because of stress play a significant role. Irritation of the mandibular branch of the trigeminal nerve results in pain at the TMJ. Conditions such as rheumatoid arthritis, osteoarthritis, and dental malocclusion can also cause the disorder.

Patients complain of pain over the TMJ area, as well as the preauricular region and masseter muscles. Pain is aggravated by chewing, and there may be clicking of the TMJ. There is also tenderness and swelling of the muscles surrounding the TMJ.

Diagnostic tests include a dental examination to rule out causes of TMJ that result from malocclusion. X-ray, CT, or MRI of the jaw may be necessary. A diagnostic nerve block of the mandibular branch of the trigeminal nerve can also be helpful in diagnosis. If the patient does not experience pain relief with the nerve block, other causes of facial pain are likely.

Treatment includes pain management with anti-inflammatory agents, physical therapy, and possibly acupuncture. TMJ caused by malocclusion may require orthodontic treatment. Signs and symptoms of TMJ disorders improve over time with or without treatment for most patients.

Common Fractures

A fracture is a break of the integrity of bone, which is commonly caused by trauma. Pathological fractures occur when there is weakening of the bone by osteoporosis, infection, degeneration, necrosis, or a space-occupying lesion in the bone.

Hip Fracture

A hip fracture is a fracture of the proximal end of the femur. In older adults, the hip can undergo osteoporotic degeneration, a weakness in the hip that often causes a fall. An estimated 340,000 hip fractures occur each year. Furthermore, 9 of 10 hip fractures occur in patients aged 65 years and older, and 3 of 4 occur in females. European American females are twice as likely to suffer hip fracture compared with African American and Hispanic females. In both males and females, the rate of hip fracture increases with age, doubling each decade after age 50 years. Nearly half of all hip fractures occur in adults older than 80 years.

> **ALERT!** Death after a fall is often caused by the complications that set in after hip fracture and immobility. One out of five older adults with hip fracture dies within a year of the injury because of complications.

CLINICAL CONCEPT

The hip, wrist, and vertebrae are the most commonly fractured bones in older adults with osteoporosis.

Etiology. Osteoporosis is a major cause of hip fracture. Osteoporotic fracture usually occurs in the femoral head or neck, where there is mainly trabecular (nonsolid) bone. Hip fracture caused by osteoporosis often causes a fall in older adult patients. Young adults can sustain hip fracture because of high-energy trauma caused by accidents or athletic activity. Stress fracture of the hip can also occur in an otherwise healthy person.

Pathophysiology. The hip is a ball-and-socket joint: the acetabulum within the pelvic bone serves as the socket and the head of the femur as the ball. This region is composed of trabecular bone, which is a meshwork of nonsolid bone, which is more susceptible to the degenerative changes of osteoporosis than solid, cortical bone.

In older adults, a common pathological process is osteoporotic degeneration of the hip followed by instability of the joint and consequent fall. The hip becomes unable to bear the individual's weight and gives way, causing a traumatic fall. Femoral neck fractures are common in the presence of osteoporosis, whereas femoral head fractures are more common in younger patients as a result of trauma.

Hip fractures involve fracture of any aspect of the proximal femur, from the head to the first 4 to 5 cm of the subtrochanteric area. They can be classified based on their relation to the hip capsule (intracapsular and

extracapsular), location (head, neck, trochanteric, intertrochanteric, and subtrochanteric), and degree of displacement (see Fig. 37-10). Femoral neck fractures often disrupt the blood supply to the head of the femur. Superior femoral head fractures normally are associated with anterior dislocations, whereas inferior femoral head fractures are associated with posterior dislocations. Higher-grade displacement implies worse prognosis. Fractures of the femoral head and neck are intracapsular, whereas those of the trochanteric, intertrochanteric, and subtrochanteric regions are extracapsular. Intracapsular hip fractures frequently have complicated healing. The thick capsule that surrounds these fractures separates them from adjacent soft tissue and capillaries, leading to impaired callus formation. Nonunion necrosis and AVN are frequent complications of these fractures.

Clinical Presentation. The patient usually presents with a history of a fall or extreme trauma. In addition, older adult patients often have a history of osteoporosis and may have a history of vertebral compression or wrist fracture, which are also fractures caused by osteoporosis. Commonly, the patient is a thin, older, European American female. Older patients should be asked about their current medications, as well as comorbid conditions such as hypertension, diabetes mellitus, and cardiovascular disease. Family history of osteoporosis and other disorders should be elicited.

In younger adults, there is usually trauma that has caused other injuries in addition to hip fracture. Up to 70% of patients with femoral head fractures-dislocations have experienced associated injuries, which include injuries to other extremities, intra-abdominal or intrapelvic injuries, neck injuries, and head injuries. The exact events leading to the trauma

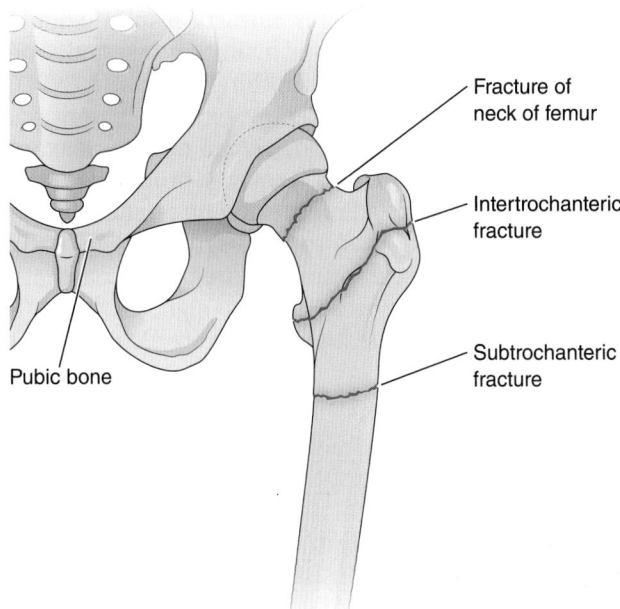

FIGURE 37-10. Sites of hip fracture in the femur.

need to be investigated to evaluate the risk of associated injuries.

Physical Examination. The patient's vital signs and signs of blood loss should be assessed. The hip and femur position should be inspected, which can provide clues to the type of injury endured. In different types of fractures, the lower extremity assumes different characteristic positions. The abduction or adduction of the leg should be noted as well as the internal or external rotation. In the acute phase the affected leg may appear shorter than the other. Pain and tenderness will be apparent with any motion of the leg. In assessing ROM, first test external and internal rotation with the extremity held in extension. If a fracture exists, especially one that is displaced, ROM will be extremely painful; if this happens, movement of the leg should be discontinued. A neurovascular examination distal to the site of fracture is essential. Pulses, reflexes, sensation, and motor ability should be assessed as tolerated by the patient. If the patient is a trauma victim, the pelvis should be assessed for fractures by stressing the pelvis anteriorly to posteriorly through the iliac crests and symphysis pubis, and laterally to medially through the iliac crests.

Diagnosis. All x-ray views of the extremities and pelvic bones should be completed. If radiographic findings are ambiguous, CT scan or MRI should be considered. A view of the contralateral hip for comparison is necessary.

Treatment. The patient who complains of hip pain should be immobilized in the supine position. The clinician should perform the ABCDEs of trauma assessment and immobilize the patient's cervical spine. Orthopedic as well as neurological or cardiovascular consultations should be sought. If fracture or deformity of the femur is obvious, a traction splint should be applied and an IV line for hydration inserted. The patient should be placed on nothing-by-mouth (NPO) status and have supplemental oxygen. Parenteral analgesia is necessary; in addition, a muscle relaxant may be necessary. For open fractures, broad-spectrum antibiotics should be administered and tetanus immunization should be given as necessary. Surgical ORIF or hip replacement is often required. Anticoagulant therapy is necessary because of the high risk for DVT. Calcium and vitamin D supplements are also needed.

Vertebral Compression Fracture

Vertebral compression fractures are pathognomonic of osteoporosis. Osteoporotic vertebral collapse occurs when the body's weight exceeds the bone's ability within the vertebral body to support the load. The interior of the vertebrae consists of trabecular, meshlike bone, which weakens and degenerates in osteoporosis. Consequences include postural changes, particularly kyphosis, loss of height, and pain.

Vertebral compression fractures affect approximately 25% of all postmenopausal females in the United States. Prevalence steadily increases with advancing age, reaching 40% in females 80 years of age. Females diagnosed with a compression fracture of the vertebrae have a 15% higher mortality rate than those who do not experience fractures. Because the older adult age group is the fastest growing segment of the U.S. population, the incidence of vertebral compression fracture will likely increase. More than 700,000 new vertebral compression fractures occur every year, accounting for more than 100,000 hospital admissions and resulting in close to $1.5 billion in annual costs.

Etiology. Vertebral compression fracture often occurs because of a pathological fracture, also called a fragility fracture. A pathological fracture occurs in the vertebrae because of preexisting disease within the bone that undermines the structural integrity. Osteoporosis is the most common cause of vertebral compression fracture. Cancer, such as prostate, breast, or lung cancer, often metastasizes to the vertebral bones and weakens the inner bone tissue. The fracture of vertebrae can also occur because of a localized infection of the bone caused by osteomyelitis, which may occur in people with diabetes and in those who abuse IV drugs. Tuberculosis of bone, called Pott's disease, can also cause vertebral compression fracture. Ischemia of bone can cause osteonecrosis, which can also lead to fracture. Risk factors for osteoporosis and vertebral compression fracture are categorized as modifiable and not modifiable (see Box 37-6).

BOX 37-6. Risk Factors for Vertebral Compression Fracture

NONMODIFIABLE RISK FACTORS
- Osteoporosis
- Advanced age
- Bilateral ovariectomy
- White or Asian race
- Early menopause
- Female gender
- History of fractures in adulthood
- History of fractures in a first-degree relative
- Premenopausal amenorrhea for more than 1 year
- Presence of dementia

MODIFIABLE RISK FACTORS
- Alcohol use
- Dietary calcium or vitamin D deficiency
- Estrogen deficiency
- Frailty
- Insufficient physical activity
- Low body weight
- Presence of osteoporosis
- Prolonged use of glucocorticoids or anticonvulsants
- Tobacco use

Pathophysiology. The vertebrae are composed of trabecular bone, which are horizontal and vertical strands of bone that form a meshwork and appear as scaffolding. Vertebral compression fracture occurs because of the collapse of the internal latticelike meshwork of the vertebral bone. The vertebral bone becomes thinned and flattened. Osteoporosis, the most common cause of vertebral compression fracture, is a reduction in skeletal mass caused by an imbalance between bone resorption and bone formation. Cancer of the prostate, lung, and breast often metastasizes to vertebral bone and the tumor cells weaken the bone's internal strength. Infection of the bone, termed osteomyelitis, can also cause bone degeneration, which weakens bone strength. Ischemia of bone can cause osteonecrosis, which can also lead to compression fracture.

Vertebral compression fractures can result from low-energy trauma, such as falls, as well as high-energy trauma, such as motor vehicle accidents. Pathological fractures, which occur secondary to low-energy trauma, are characteristic of osteoporosis, infection, or metastatic cancer in bone. In pathological fracture, bone can break when under stress such as weight-bearing. Even minor loads can lead to vertebral compression fractures (see Fig. 37-11).

Clinical Presentation. Individuals with a vertebral compression fracture may be asymptomatic or may experience pain in the lower back, upper back, or neck. Some people may also have hip, abdominal, or thigh pain. A hunched-over posture, also called **kyphosis,** is common. There may be numbness, tingling, and weakness of the extremities; such symptoms could indicate compression of the nerves at the fracture site. It is considered a medical emergency if the patient reports incontinence or an inability to urinate, as these symptoms can mean impingement on the spinal cord.

 CLINICAL CONCEPT

Osteoporosis of the cervicothoracic vertebrae causes kyphosis in females.

Diagnosis. Imaging studies such as x-ray can visualize the vertebrae involved in the compression. X-rays demonstrate the wedged appearance of compressed vertebrae; often, more than one vertebra are involved. CT or MRI scans may be necessary, particularly to exclude impingement on spinal nerves.

Treatment. Calcitonin can relieve the pain of vertebral compression. There may also be a need for muscle relaxants and analgesics. External support devices provide postural stability. The surgical procedures vertebroplasty and kyphoplasty are sometimes recommended. These procedures attempt to build up the compressed area of bone with a surgical type of cement. Calcium and vitamin D supplements as well as bisphosphonates may be necessary to treat osteoporosis.

Femur Shaft Fracture

The femur, the strongest bone in the body, is surrounded by sturdy musculature and rich blood supply. The shaft of the femur, also called the diaphysis, requires a significant amount of force to fracture. Because of the abundant blood supply, fracture of the femur causes a large amount of bleeding. In addition, when fractured, the bone is commonly displaced because of the tension of the musculature that surrounds it.

The incidence of femoral fractures is reported as 1 case per 10,000 population per year. In individuals younger than 25 years and those older than 65 years, the rate of femoral fractures is 3 fractures per 10,000 population annually. Femur shaft fractures are most common in males younger than 30 years because of motor vehicle accidents and sports injury.

Etiology. Fracture of the femur shaft occurs because of a large, high-energy force, which may be generated by automobile, motorcycle, or recreational vehicle accidents or gunshot wounds. In these cases, the femoral fracture is often accompanied by other traumatic injuries of the body. The femur is also commonly injured in contact and high-speed sports such as skiing, football, hockey, rodeo, and motor sports. Alternatively, a femoral stress fracture can occur from repetitive forces that overload the bone, causing microfracture. Stress fractures occur most often in repetitive-overload sports such as running, baseball, and basketball. Less commonly, a fracture of the femur occurs because of tumor or metabolic disease within the shaft

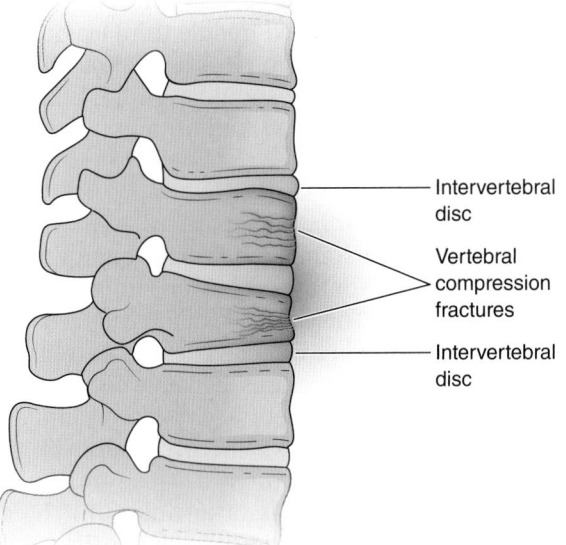

FIGURE 37-11. Vertebral compression fracture. The most common type of fracture in the vertebrae is a compression fracture, commonly in the thoracic spine. The vertebral body is commonly weakened by osteoporosis before a compression fracture occurs.

Intervertebral disc

Vertebral compression fractures

Intervertebral disc

of the bone. The area of the lesion becomes structurally weakened, which leads to fracture.

Pathophysiology. There are several types of femoral shaft fractures (see Table 37-1 for illustrations):

- Transverse: A transverse fracture is a simple break of the bone across the shaft of the femur. The fracture line is perpendicular to the long line of the shaft.
- Spiral: The fracture line encircles the shaft like the stripes on a candy cane. A twisting force to the thigh causes this type of fracture.
- Comminuted: In a comminuted fracture, the bone is broken into a number of pieces, as occurs in a crushing injury.
- Open: In an open fracture, also called a compound fracture, the break of the bones causes angulation sufficient to protrude through the skin, leaving a wound that is open to the environment; open fractures are extremely vulnerable to infection.

Clinical Presentation. The patient will usually report a high-velocity injury, pain, and inability to bear weight on the affected extremity. Patients may be noted to have bruising, shortening of one leg, and a great deal of swelling. On physical examination, femoral fracture and associated injuries must be assessed. A head-to-toe examination is indicated. The pelvis, hips, and knees require palpation, and any lower extremity deformity should be placed in alignment. An assessment of pulses, circulation of the leg, and sensation distal to the injury is essential. Swelling of the thigh, hematoma, and loss of ROM are common. Blood loss can be severe (see "Vascular Injury and Bleeding" above).

Alternatively, stress fractures of the femur are observed with increasing frequency in joggers. The onset of stress fractures is usually gradual, though it may be sudden or severe. Patients may report groin or thigh pain. Symptoms of stress fractures are aggravated by activity and relieved by rest.

Diagnosis. The clinician should order x-rays of the involved leg, with pelvic and knee views as well. Usually, views of the thorax and opposite leg are important to exclude other traumatic injuries. If x-rays are ambiguous, CT scan may reveal a fracture more clearly. Radionuclide scanning may be needed in cases of stress fracture. An arteriogram is often necessary to assure patency of circulation within the leg.

Treatment. Pain management is necessary for these fractures, and surgical reduction and fixation is commonly required. Traction is also often necessary. Open fractures require antibiotics and tetanus toxoid. Frequent monitoring of distal pulses and sensation is necessary to ensure neurovascular integrity.

Clavicle Fracture

Clavicle fractures, the most common of all childhood fractures, account for 5% of all fractures and nearly half of significant injuries to the shoulder girdle. Falls are the most common cause, and the most frequent site of injury is the middle of the clavicle. The annual incidence rate is estimated to be between 30 and 60 cases per 100,000 population. Males are affected twice as often as females, with a high incidence in males younger than 30 years because of sports injuries. A smaller peak of incidence occurs in older patients in whom the injury is sustained during low-energy falls.

Pathophysiology. Clavicular fractures are classified according to where the break occurs. Group I fractures, the most common variety, occur in the middle third of the clavicle. Group II fractures involve the distal or lateral third, and Group III fractures occur in the medial third. Clavicle fractures are often greenstick fractures, which means that they splinter when fractured (see Table 37-1).

The clavicle is vulnerable to fracture because of its protruding, superficial position on the chest. These fractures are common with high-energy force injuries or multiple traumatic injuries. With clavicle injury, other important structures are subject to damage. For example, the subclavian artery and vein are both in close proximity to the middle portion of the clavicle. The brachial plexus also passes behind the clavicle posterior to the subclavian vessels and is at risk with displaced fractures of the middle clavicle. The subclavius muscle lies between the clavicle and brachial plexus—though small, it is believed to prevent more frequent damage to the brachial plexus.

Other areas in close proximity also require thorough examination. Injury to the apices of the lung often occurs with displaced middle third clavicle fractures. There can be rib fractures, scapula fractures, and other fractures about the shoulder girdle; pulmonary contusion; pneumothorax; hemothorax; and closed head injuries.

Clinical Presentation. The patient with clavicular fracture will report some kind of high-energy trauma. Persons often fall onto a shoulder and complain of pain in the region. The clinical examination will reveal a deformed area along the clavicle and extreme tenderness. Often, the fractures become displaced. The clinician needs to complete a physical examination, particularly of the thorax. There can also be damage to the vascular structures in close proximity to the clavicle. Some findings of an injury to the subclavian vessels are hematoma overlying the clavicle, presence of a bruit over the region, diminished or absent pulses in the extremity, first rib fracture, brachial plexus injury, and a wide mediastinum on chest x-ray. The lungs should be auscultated to exclude pneumothorax.

Diagnosis. Chest x-ray is essential in clavicular fracture. X-ray views of the sternoclavicular joint and shoulder girdle should be the focus.

> **ALERT!** Pneumothorax needs to be ruled out with clavicular or rib fractures.

Treatment. Realignment of the clavicle and the use of a sling for 4 to 6 weeks following the injury is the common treatment. During this period, the patient should perform active ROM of the elbow and hand. After 4 to 6 weeks, the patient can begin ROM of the shoulder as tolerated. Use of the sling may be discontinued as pain allows. For more complicated displaced fractures, surgery and fixation may be necessary. The patient may also need treatment for associated injuries.

Distal Radius Fracture

Fractures of the distal radius in the wrist are a very common type of fracture. Peak incidence occurs in persons aged 18 to 25 years, as well as persons older than age 65 years. The mechanism of injury is unique to each group, with high-energy injuries being more common in the younger group and fall injuries being more common in the older group. There are two types:

- Smith fracture: a fracture of the distal radius most commonly caused by falling onto a flexed wrist or a high-energy force to the lower arm. The distal fracture fragment is displaced ventrally (anteriorly).
- Colles fracture: a similar fracture of the distal radius in the forearm caused by falling onto an extended wrist or a high-energy blow to the lower arm; in Colles fracture, there is dorsal (posterior) displacement of the wrist and hand.

Etiology. Motorcycle or motor vehicle accidents, falls from a height, and similar traumatic situations are common causes for a distal radius fracture. Trauma is the leading cause in the 15- to 24-year-old age group. Older patients have much weaker bones and can sustain a fracture of the radius from simply falling on an outstretched hand in a ground-level fall. This type of fracture in an older adult is often caused by osteoporosis. As the population lives longer, the frequency of this type of fracture will increase.

Pathophysiology. A distal radius fracture is caused by a high amount of force placed on the bone, more than the bone can sustain. The Smith and Colles fractures are the most common wrist injuries. If the wrist is flexed during the trauma, the fragmented radius becomes displaced anteriorly, resulting in a Smith fracture. In contrast, if the wrist is extended during the trauma, causing posterior displacement of the fragmented radius, the result is a Colles fracture (see

Fig. 37-12). The event that caused the fracture should be thoroughly investigated. If the fracture is caused by a fall in an older adult, the patient should be questioned about the circumstances surrounding the fall and assessed for the cause. Loss of consciousness, myocardial infarction, transient ischemic attacks, and loss of balance and coordination can be the etiology. These conditions require further investigation and diagnostic testing.

Clinical Presentation. The patient should describe events leading to the fall or trauma. A history of prior fractures should be sought, and the patient should be asked about a history of osteoporosis, which can cause reduction of the wrist to be challenging and may require fixation. Pain is present in the wrist, and there may be some deformity and bruising of the wrist's soft tissues. The wrist bones should be examined along with radial and ulnar circulation, development of the hand, ROM, and sensation in the hand. The opposite wrist and hand should be compared. The median nerve function needs to be periodically monitored from the time of the initial examination through treatment. Extreme tenderness and lack of ROM of the wrist will be noted.

Diagnosis and Treatment. X-rays of the wrist and arm should be done. Most fractures can be treated conservatively with a cast or splint. For example, fractures with no or minimal displacement can be treated in a cast for 6 weeks. If the distal ulna is fractured and unstable, it can be treated in a short arm cast. Fractures in older adults that are compressed

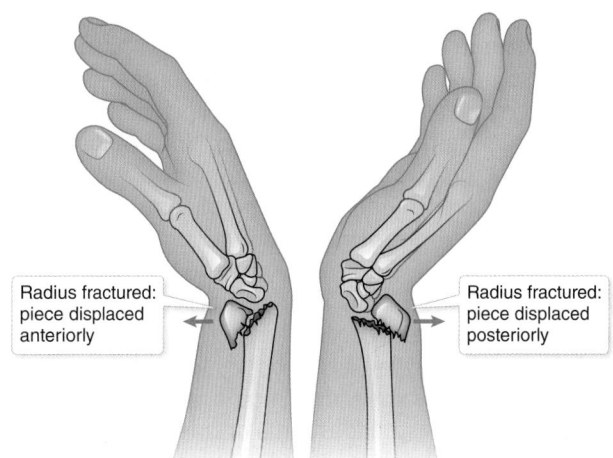

Radius fractured: piece displaced anteriorly

Radius fractured: piece displaced posteriorly

Smith fracture: commonly due to fall onto a flexed hand

Colles fracture: commonly due to fall onto an extended hand

FIGURE 37-12. Radius fractures: Smith vs. Colles fracture. A Colles fracture, also called an extension fracture of the wrist, is a break in the radius with posterior displacement. A Colles fracture commonly occurs when a patient sustains a fall on an extended hand. A Smith fracture, also referred to as a flexion fracture of the wrist, is a break in the radius with anterior displacement. A Smith fracture commonly occurs when a patient sustains a fall on a flexed hand.

dorsally can be minimally painful and may appear to be clinically stable; these fractures may be treated with only a splint. Patients with unstable or weak bones may require surgical reduction and internal or external fixation.

Tibia–Fibula Fracture

Fractures of the tibia are the most common long-bone fractures. The annual incidence of open fractures of long bones is estimated to be 11.5 per 100,000 persons, with 40% occurring in the lower limb. Lower leg fractures include fractures of the tibia and fibula. Of these two bones, the tibia is the weight-bearing bone. Fractures of the tibia generally are associated with fibula fracture, because an interosseous membrane connects the two bones. Tibia–fibula fractures can occur as a result of low-energy injuries, such as falls, as well as athletic injuries or high-energy injuries, such as motor vehicle accidents and gunshot wounds.

Pathophysiology. The shin, or anterior surface of the tibia, has a very thin layer of subcutaneous tissue, and the bone is easily palpable below the surface. As a result of this, many injuries to the lower leg cause open fractures, which are susceptible to infection.

At the lateral malleolus in the ankle region, the fibula is thinly covered by subcutaneous tissue. It is important to note that the common peroneal nerve, which is susceptible to injury from a fibular fracture, crosses over the fibula and is superficial in this region. In addition, the popliteal artery, which runs along the tibia, is susceptible to injury, which is why neurovascular compromise can easily occur in lower limb fracture.

Diagnosis and Treatment. During the history, the patient usually reports a traumatic injury. Associated areas traumatized by the injury also commonly need assessment; treatment should be prioritized. The patient complains of pain, swelling, and inability to bear weight on the leg. The examination commonly shows edema, ecchymosis, and point tenderness. The clinician should perform a neurovascular assessment of the leg; gross deformities should be noted and splinted. Open fractures require emergency orthopedic consultation. Diagnostic testing requires x-ray of the affected leg as well as the opposite leg for comparison. X-rays of the knee, tibia, fibula, and ankle should be viewed. If widespread trauma occurred to the lower body, the hip and pelvis should be x-rayed as well.

In treating fractures of the lower leg, the patient should be immobilized; in addition, the priority is performing the ABCDEs of trauma assessment. Pain management and lower leg immobilization may require a cast or splint; antibiotics are necessary for an open fracture. The clinician should monitor tibial fractures frequently for compartment syndrome. Crutches are necessary for patient ambulation; orthopedic consultation is necessary to determine whether surgical reduction or fixation is necessary.

Foot Fracture

The foot contains 26 bones: the calcaneus, talus, navicular, cuboid, 3 cuneiform bones, 5 metatarsal bones, and 14 phalanges. The most common causes of fracture in the foot include a twisting injury as in athletics, trauma directly to the foot, or cumulative trauma that causes a stress fracture.

Several types of fractures occur to the forefoot bone on the side of the little toe (fifth metatarsal). For example, ballet dancers may break this bone during a misstep or fall from a pointe position. An ankle-twisting injury may tear the tendon that attaches to the fifth metatarsal and pull a small piece of the bone away. A more serious injury in the same area is a Jones fracture, which occurs near the base of the fifth metatarsal bone and disrupts the blood supply to the bone. This injury takes longer to heal and may require surgery.

Stress fractures frequently occur in the bones of the forefoot that extend from the toes to the middle of the foot (see Fig. 37-13). Stress fractures, tiny cracks in the bone surface, can occur with sudden increases

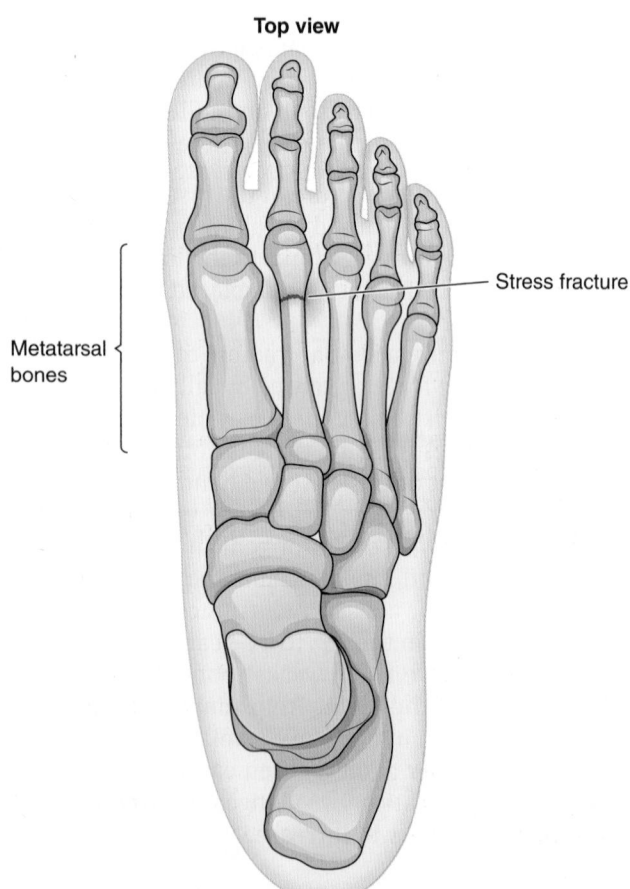

Top view

Stress fracture

Metatarsal bones

FIGURE 37-13. Stress fracture of the foot. A stress fracture is a small crack in a bone that is often caused by overuse injury. Most stress fractures occur in the weight-bearing bones of the foot and lower leg. When muscles are overtired, they are no longer able to lessen the shock of repeated impact to the foot. When this happens, the muscles transfer the stress to the bones, potentially resulting in small cracks or fractures. The most common sites of stress fractures are the second and third metatarsals of the foot.

in training, such as running or walking for longer distances or times, improper training techniques, or changes in training surfaces. Toe, tarsal, and navicular fractures are common sites of stress fractures in athletes.

Dislocation and fracture can occur at the Lisfranc (tarsometatarsal) joint. The Lisfranc joint, found at the base of the second metatarsal, is formed by a six-bone arch that includes the first, second, and third cuneiforms and first, second, and third metatarsals. Calcaneal (heel) fracture can also occur, usually because of a fall from a significant height.

Clinical Presentation. Symptoms of fracture in the foot are pain, deformity, tenderness, and swelling. Bruising and soft tissue injury are common. The patient usually cannot perform ROM or bear weight.

Diagnosis. To diagnose foot fracture, the clinician should grasp the first and second metatarsals and move them alternately through plantar flexion and dorsiflexion. The Ottawa Foot Rules, a tool that predicts significant midfoot fractures, are guidelines used to determine whether x-rays are necessary. If any of the following are present, an x-ray is required:

- Point tenderness over the base of the fifth metatarsal
- Point tenderness over the navicular bone
- Inability to take four steps

Diagnostic testing includes x-ray, MRI, and ultrasound. A CT or bone scan may be required if a foot fracture is not apparent on plain x-ray. A thorough neurovascular examination is necessary when diagnosing foot injury.

Treatment. Elevation of the leg and analgesics may be necessary until the swelling and pain are relieved. In toe fracture, the procedure of "buddy taping" the toes to each other is used to stabilize the fracture.

Other Common Musculoskeletal Injuries

Other kinds of upper extremity musculoskeletal injuries are rotator cuff injury, shoulder dislocation, brachial plexus palsy, and ulnar nerve injury. Meniscal and ligament tears in the knee are common sports injuries. In the foot, a common inflammatory disorder called plantar fasciitis can cause pain.

Rotator Cuff Injury

Rotator cuff injury or strain is an injury to any of the four rotator cuff muscles in the shoulder (see Fig. 37-14). The rotator cuff muscles, a group of muscles that work together to provide stability for the shoulder's glenohumeral joint and control shoulder rotation, include the supraspinatus, infraspinatus, teres minor, and subscapularis. The most commonly

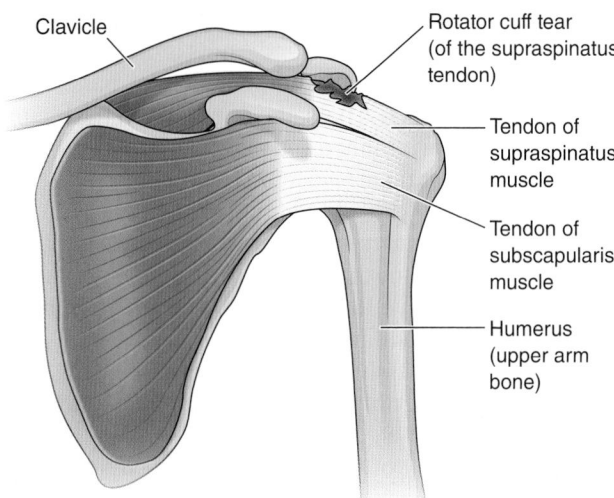

View of left shoulder girdle from the front

FIGURE 37-14. Rotator cuff injury. The rotator cuff is a group of muscles, tendons, and ligaments around the shoulder joint. The four muscles that form the rotator cuff are the supraspinatus, infraspinatus, teres minor, and subscapularis. A rotator cuff injury includes any type of irritation or damage to the rotator cuff muscles or tendons. Causes of rotator cuff injury may include falling, lifting, and repetitive arm activities.

injured muscles are the supraspinatus and infraspinatus. Sports involving constant shoulder rotation, such as baseball pitching or swimming, often cause rotator cuff injury.

There are two major types of rotator cuff injuries:

- Tears of the tendons and muscles
- Tendonitis, which is inflammation of the tendons

Clinical Presentation. The patient's chief symptoms are usually pain, weakness, instability, and limited ROM in the shoulder. Associated symptoms such as swelling, numbness in the arm, uneven rotation, or "popping" of the shoulder may be present. Pain is often felt over the anterolateral part of the shoulder and is exacerbated by overhead activities. Night pain is a frequent symptom, especially when the patient lies on the affected shoulder.

The patient should be asked about aggravating factors and relieving treatments that have been tried and encouraged to describe the events surrounding any shoulder injuries; previous medical treatment, such as physical therapy; previous injections; and any surgical interventions. The clinician should assess the patient's occupation and sporting activities. In older adults, symptoms often are not associated with any specific activity or injury.

The patient requires a thorough physical examination of the shoulder using specific types of maneuvers that assist with diagnosis. Examination should begin with patient observation during the history portion of the evaluation. The clinician needs to carefully inspect the shoulder from the anterior, lateral, and posterior positions. Swelling, atrophy, or asymmetry should be noted. Supraspinatus and infraspinatus muscle atrophy can be observed in rotator cuff tears and in entrapments of the suprascapular nerve. Tenderness is often localized to the greater tuberosity and subacromial bursa. The biceps tendon, which is palpated anteriorly in the bicipital groove, can be inflamed and painful in this condition.

Total active and passive ROM in all planes and scapulohumeral rhythm should be evaluated. Patients with rotator cuff tears tend to have a decrease in glenohumeral joint motion. Decreased active elevation with normal passive ROM is usually observed in rotator cuff tears secondary to pain and weakness. When both active and passive ROM are decreased, this usually suggests onset of frozen shoulder, also known as **adhesive capsulitis.**

Assess internal rotation by having the patient reach around to their back with an extended thumb up the spine. Patients with normal internal rotation reach the T5–T10 level. Note any accompanying pain and specific pain location in ROM testing.

Rotator cuff injuries cause the impingement syndrome. Pain occurs with elevation of the arm, over the head or reaching behind the back. In this position, the rotator cuff tendons are compressed against the anterior acromion process of the scapula.

Strength Testing. The clinician should perform strength testing to isolate the relevant muscles individually. Several maneuvers can be used to assess the strength of the individual muscles (see Box 37-7). The anterior cuff (subscapularis) can be assessed using the lift-off test, which is performed with the arm internally rotated behind the back. Lifting the hand away from the back against resistance tests the strength of the subscapularis muscle. The posterior cuff (infraspinatus and teres minor) is isolated best in 90 degrees of forward flexion with the elbow flexed to 90 degrees, testing external rotation. Significant weakness in external rotation is observed in large rotator cuff tears.

Testing the strength of the supraspinatus muscle can be achieved with the elbow extended, the shoulder in full internal rotation, and the arm in the scapular plane (thumbs-down position). Testing of the scapula rotators (trapezius and serratus anterior) is also important. Serratus anterior weakness can be observed by having the patient lean against a wall. Winging of the scapula as the patient pushes against the wall indicates serratus anterior weakness.

Diagnosis. Diagnostic tests include x-ray, MRI, and ultrasound view of the shoulder. X-ray may not show rotator cuff injury; arthrography may be necessary. It is also important that the clinician exclude all other possible causes of shoulder pain, such as angina pectoris and cervical radiculopathy.

Treatment. A physical therapy rehabilitation program is necessary in rotator cuff injury. Pain and inflammation management are required to allow for an active

---

BOX 37-7. Rotator Cuff Assessment Tests

DROP-ARM TEST
Abduct the patient's shoulder to 90 degrees and ask the patient to lower the arm slowly to the side in the same arc of movement. Severe pain or the patient's inability to return the arm to the side slowly indicates a positive test result, which indicates a rotator cuff tear.

NEER IMPINGEMENT TEST
The patient's arm is maximally elevated through forward flexion by the examiner, causing a jamming of the greater tuberosity against the anteroinferior acromion. Pain elicited with this maneuver indicates a positive test result for impingement.

HAWKINS TEST
The examiner forward flexes the arms to 90 degrees and then forcibly internally rotates the shoulder. This movement pushes the supraspinatus tendon against the anterior surface of the coracoacromial ligament and coracoid process. Pain indicates a positive test result for supraspinatus tendonitis.

APPREHENSION TEST
Abduct the arm 90 degrees and fully externally rotate, while placing anteriorly directed force on the posterior humeral head from behind. The patient becomes apprehensive and resists further motion if chronic anterior instability is present.

RELOCATION TEST
Perform the apprehension test with the patient supine and the shoulder at the edge of the table. In a positive relocation test result indicative of anterior instability, a posteriorly directed force on the proximal humerus causes resolution of the patient's apprehension and usually allows more external rotation of the humerus.

---

rehabilitation program. A combination of rest, icing for 20 minutes three to four times per day, and acetaminophen or an NSAID is advised. The patient should also be advised to sleep with a pillow between the trunk and arm to decrease tension on the supraspinatus tendon and to promote blood flow. Corticosteroids injected directly into the problem region of the shoulder can facilitate the rehabilitation program.

Shoulder Dislocation
The shoulder is the most commonly dislocated joint in the body. Under normal conditions, the glenohumeral ligaments, the joint capsule, and the rotator cuff muscles maintain shoulder stability. However, a high-energy force from a fall or a striking blow may be sufficient to cause shoulder dislocation, most of which occurs anteriorly.

The inferior glenohumeral ligament is commonly injured during an anterior shoulder dislocation. The injury may be a tear of the ligament or capsule off one of its bony attachments, or it may be a stretch injury. Tears in the rotator cuff muscles or injury to the axillary nerve can also cause shoulder weakness and consequent dislocation.

Clinical Presentation. Patients with a dislocated shoulder complain of severe pain; during a traumatic incident, they may feel the shoulder pop out of its socket. Different shoulder positions during the trauma dislocation cause injury to different ligaments, so the clinician should try to determine the shoulder position at the time of the injury. For example, with an anterior dislocation, the patient reports having the arm abducted and externally rotated.

Some persons have very lax joints; these individuals may report feeling like a joint can roll, rather than pop, out of the socket. However, they are sometimes able to readjust their shoulder joint back into place. Some patients feel numbness and tingling down their arm at the time of the dislocation.

 CLINICAL CONCEPT

Patients with previous shoulder dislocations are more apt to redislocate.

In the physical examination, the anteriorly dislocated shoulder is obviously deformed and tender with poor ROM. Posterior shoulder dislocations may not be as obvious because the patient appears to only be guarding the extremity, usually holding the arm against the abdomen.

A detailed neurovascular examination is needed both before and after the shoulder has been reduced, because injury to the axillary nerve during shoulder dislocation has been reported to be as high as 40%.

Diagnosis and Treatment. Diagnostic tests include x-ray, CT scan, and MRI scan. Treatment of an acute shoulder dislocation includes maneuvers to reduce the dislocation of the shoulder joint, most commonly the glenohumeral joint. The patient may require conscious sedation or general anesthesia so that there is relaxation of the shoulder musculature. Once reduction has been accomplished, postreduction x-rays are necessary to confirm a normalized joint.

After reduction of the joint dislocation, the arm should be immobilized in a sling for 1 to 3 weeks. The patient should maintain ROM of the elbow, wrist, and hand, and ROM exercises should be continued when the patient comes out of the sling. Rehabilitative therapy that includes active and passive flexion, extension, abduction, and internal and external rotation begins at about the third week, when the patient comes out of the sling. Patients are encouraged to incrementally achieve 10 degrees of improvement in their ROM per week; rehabilitation should restore full ROM over

6 to 8 weeks. In patients who have recurrent shoulder instability, surgery is considered.

 CLINICAL CONCEPT

Immobilization of the shoulder for a lengthy period can cause adhesive capsulitis (also called frozen shoulder) (see Box 37-8).

BOX 37-8. Frozen Shoulder

Frozen shoulder is an inflammatory disorder of the shoulder that manifests as stiffness and lack of ROM. Most patients with frozen shoulder have had a period of shoulder immobilization for some reason and then have resulting limited active and passive ROM in the shoulder.

Also called adhesive capsulitis, frozen shoulder commonly affects persons aged 40 to 70 years and is estimated to occur in 2% to 5% of the general population. Females tend to be affected more frequently than males. Frozen shoulder is associated with several conditions, including inactivity, trauma, surgery (including but not limited to shoulder surgery), inflammatory disease, hyperthyroidism, ischemic heart disease, and diabetes. Incidence among patients with insulin-dependent diabetes is 36% with bilateral shoulder involvement.

In the history, information should be gathered regarding the onset and duration of symptoms, trauma or surgery, and affected side. The patient usually complains of pain and stiffness in the shoulder with an inability to stretch the arm above head level. The patient should be asked about any existing conditions. Because frozen shoulder is associated with diabetes, hyperthyroidism, ischemic heart disease, and cervical spinal nerve impingement, these disorders should be excluded using screening tests. Any previous treatments that the patient has received for the shoulder should be documented, as should the individual's current medications. Questions should be directed toward any upper extremity neurological complaints. Any history of cervical pain or radiculopathy should be thoroughly evaluated during the clinical examination to exclude a diagnosis of herniated cervical disc.

The patient's posture should be observed while seated. It should also be noted whether the patient is leaning to one side secondary to pain and whether they are holding the neck to one side secondary to spasm or pain. The clinician should try to exclude a cervical condition contributing to the shoulder stiffness.

Diagnostic tests include x-ray, CT scan, and MRI. Treatment involves physical therapy and anti-inflammatory agents, and corticosteroid injection into the shoulder may be necessary. Surgery may be needed if other treatments are unsuccessful.

Brachial Plexus Injury

The brachial plexus is a group of nerves that originate at the cervical spinal cord in the neck and run into the axillary region of the arm with branches into the hand and fingers. Nerves within the plexus control the hand, wrist, elbow, and shoulder. The plexus consists of both motor and sensory nerves originating from the C5–T1 nerve roots (see Fig. 37-15).

A recent study showed that brachial plexus injuries occur in slightly more than 1% of multitrauma victims. Motorcycle accidents carry especially high risks, with the incidence of injury approaching 5%. Head injuries, thoracic injuries, fractures, and dislocations affecting the shoulder girdle and cervical spine are particularly common associated injuries.

Etiology and Pathophysiology. Most injuries of the brachial plexus involve the spinal nerves C7, C8, or T1. Pressure, damage, stretching, and crushing injuries can all damage the brachial plexus. A brachial plexus injury, also referred to as Erb's palsy, occurs because of a violent pull of the entire arm and shoulder from the rest of the body. These injuries usually result from high-speed motor vehicle accidents or high-energy forces in activities such as football or wrestling. A fall from a significant height or penetrating injuries such as gunshot wounds can also result in brachial plexus injury. In addition, a brachial plexus injury can occur at birth because of difficult delivery of the newborn's shoulders.

Minor injury occurs when the brachial plexus nerves are stretched. More significant injuries occur with an avulsion, when the nerve root is torn from the spinal cord. The sensory and motor consequences of brachial plexus injury (nerves C5–T1) affect the arm, hand, and fingers (see Table 37-3).

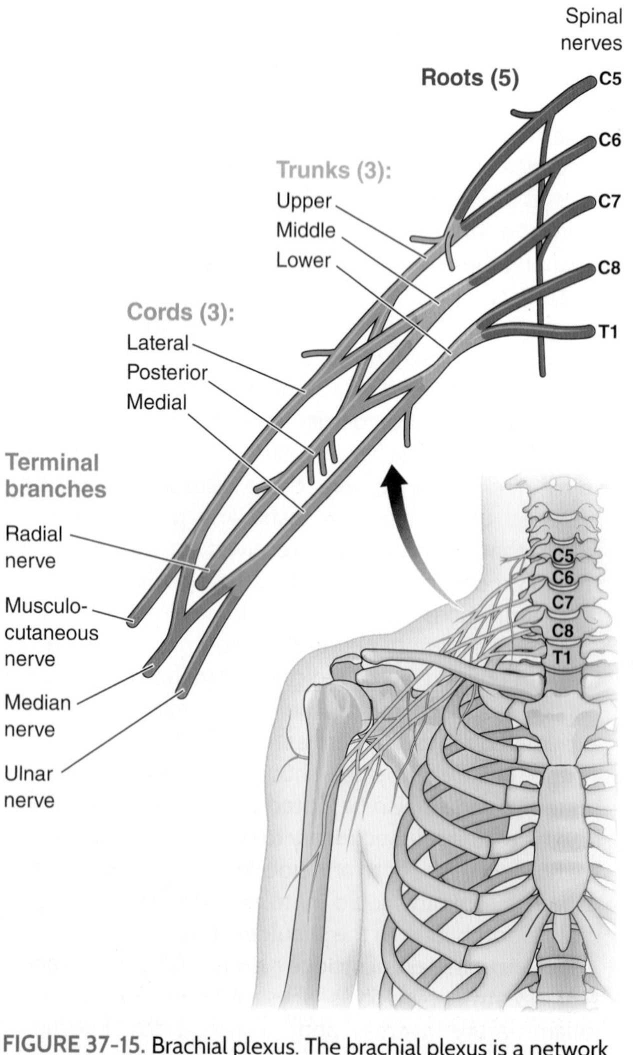

Clinical Presentation. The patient will often report a traumatic event that pulled the arm away from the body with high force. Injuries may also be caused by compression between the clavicle and first rib, penetrating injuries, or direct blows. Recognition may be delayed by other injuries, particularly to the spinal cord and head. The patient complains of feeling a shocklike pain or burning sensation, as well as numbness and weakness down the arm. Signs and symptoms of severe injuries can include an inability to move the shoulder, elbow, or fingers; complete lack of sensation in the arm; and severe pain.

Spinal nerves

Roots (5)
- C5
- C6
- C7
- C8
- T1

Trunks (3):
- Upper
- Middle
- Lower

Cords (3):
- Lateral
- Posterior
- Medial

Terminal branches
- Radial nerve
- Musculo-cutaneous nerve
- Median nerve
- Ulnar nerve

C5
C6
C7
C8
T1

FIGURE 37-15. Brachial plexus. The brachial plexus is a network of nerves that arise from the cervical (C5–C8) and first thoracic spinal nerves. The network consists of the musculocutaneous, radial, ulnar, and median nerves of the arm.

CLINICAL CONCEPT

Horner syndrome, a disorder of the sympathetic nervous system, causes classic symptoms of autonomic dysfunction, including ptosis (lid droop), enophthalmos (sinking of the eye into the orbit), anhidrosis (dry eye), sweating, and miosis (small pupil). Because the chain of sympathetic nerves is in close proximity to the thoracolumbar spinal nerves, T1 within the brachial plexus is often affected in Horner syndrome. T1 controls the intrinsic muscles of the hand, and resultant sensory and motor dysfunction can occur.

There can be swelling in the shoulder region and diminished or absent pulses in the arm. There can also be associated cervical spine, head, and clavicle fractures. It is important for the clinician to examine each cervical nerve root individually for motor and sensory function. Sensory and motor examination according to the sensory and motor dermatomes is important; examination of wrist and finger sensation and motion with respect to the median, ulnar, and radial nerves may help start to locate the lesion within the brachial plexus. Elbow flexion and extension determine radial nerve function, whereas shoulder abduction tests the axillary nerve.

TABLE 37-3. Brachial Plexus Motor Testing

Cervical Root	Clinically Relevant Gross Motor Function
C5	Shoulder abduction, extension, and external rotation; some elbow flexion
C6	Elbow flexion, forearm pronation and supination, some wrist extension
C7	Diffuse loss of function in the extremity without complete paralysis of a specific muscle group, elbow extension, consistently supplies the latissimus dorsi
C8	Finger extensors, finger flexors, wrist flexors, hand intrinsics
T1	Hand intrinsic muscles

anatomical position, it is subject to entrapment and pressure injury.

Etiology and Pathophysiology. The ulnar nerve is the peripheral branch of the medial cord of the brachial plexus, consisting of fibers C8–T1. Proximally, it is located medial to the axillary artery and then to the brachial artery to the middle of the arm. It pierces the intermuscular septum and follows the medial head of the triceps muscle to the groove between the olecranon process and the medial epicondyle. At this location, ulnar injury commonly occurs because of its superficial location. A blow that strikes the ulnar nerve will cause a sharp pain that radiates into the fingers. The area of the ulnar nerve at the elbow is commonly called "the funny bone" (see Fig. 37-16).

Clinical Presentation. In the history, the patient will complain of symptoms from mild, transient paresthesias in the ring and small fingers to contracture

Diagnosis and Treatment. Diagnosis includes clinical examination, x-ray, CT myelogram, MRI, EMG, and nerve conduction studies. The nerves of the brachial plexus can be tested for sensation and motor function to find exactly which brachial nerves are involved in the injury (see Table 37-3 and Table 37-4). Often, brachial plexus injury is a part of multitrauma injuries. Therefore, the ABCDEs of trauma assessment should be followed. After the patient is stabilized, bracing of the arm in the anatomical position is important. Neurological pain often cannot be remedied by traditional analgesics; however, antidepressants and anticonvulsants may ease neurological pain. Transcutaneous nerve stimulation (TNS) and acupuncture have been used for pain control as well. Neurovascular surgery often is necessary; physical therapy and rehabilitation are also required. Prevention of contractures of the arm is a key concern.

Ulnar Nerve Injury

The ulnar nerve, a peripheral branch of the brachial plexus, runs from the axillary region down into the arm and becomes superficial at the elbow's olecranon process. It then continues into the wrist and innervates the ring and small finger. Because of the ulnar nerve's

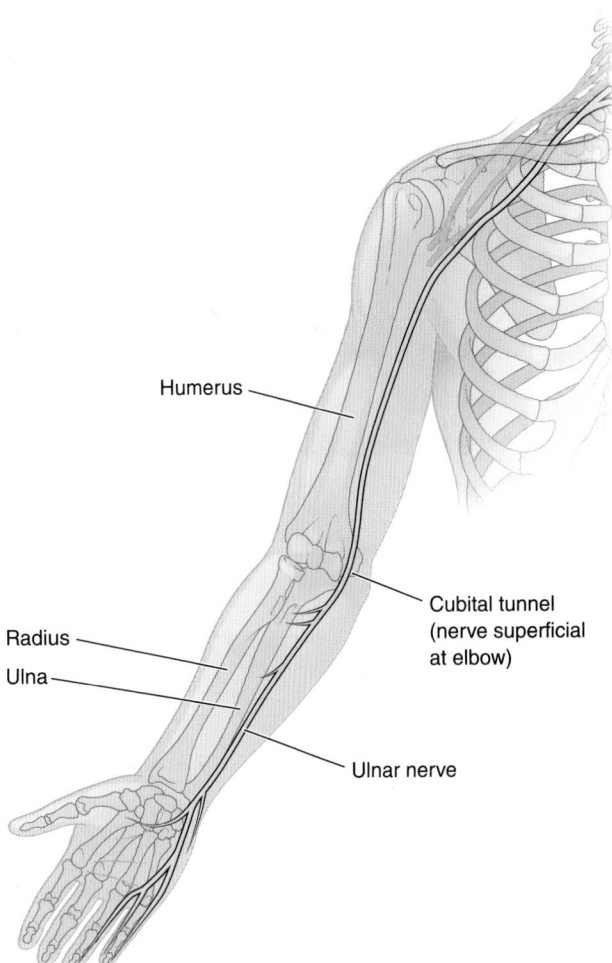

FIGURE 37-16. The distribution of the ulnar nerve. The ulnar nerve originates in the brachial plexus of the axillary region and becomes superficial at the elbow. It continues into the ring finger and little finger of the hand. Common injuries include entrapment of the ulnar nerve or trauma to the ulnar nerve at the elbow. When the ulnar nerve is pinched, the sensation is referred to as "hitting the funny bone."

TABLE 37-4. Brachial Plexus Sensory Testing

Location of Deep Pressure Test	Affected Spinal Nerve	Nerve
Thumb	C6	Median nerve
Middle finger	C7	Median nerve
Little finger	C8	Ulnar nerve

of these digits and severe intrinsic muscle atrophy. The patient usually reports severe pain at the elbow or wrist with radiation into the hand or up into the shoulder and neck. Patients may report difficulty performing rotation, flexion, and extension of the wrist. When the patient rests on the elbows, numbness and paresthesias down the ulnar side of the arm can occur.

The clinician should examine the neck and shoulder and move down the affected extremity to the elbow. The course of the ulnar nerve should be palpated from the axilla to the forearm and wrist. Pain on neck movement could indicate cervical disc disease or a problem with the brachial plexus. Masses on the ulnar side of the arm could indicate a soft tissue tumor or hematoma compressing the ulnar nerve. At the elbow, deformity and mobility should be assessed. Comparison of the opposite arm is necessary.

The strength of the flexor carpi ulnaris and flexor digitorum profundus muscles should be assessed by having the patient flex the wrist and make a fist. Intrinsic muscle function is tested by asking the patient to cross the long finger over the index. Only two muscles can be tested accurately in the hand: the abductor digiti quinti and the first dorsal interosseous. The thumb should be tested in the pinch position for Froment sign (see Fig. 37-17).

In ulnar nerve injury, numbness in the arm usually precedes motor loss. Muscle wasting and contracture of the ring and small digits are indicative of a chronic compressive syndrome.

CLINICAL CONCEPT

A positive Froment sign indicates dysfunction of the ulnar nerve motor fibers.

Diagnosis and Treatment. The clinician should obtain x-rays of the neck, chest, elbow, and wrist. Entrapment of the ulnar nerve may occur at more than one level. MRI may be necessary for visualization of soft tissue lesions. EMG tests and nerve conduction studies are indicated to confirm the area of entrapment and examine the extent of the pathology.

Treatment of ulnar neuropathy at the elbow can include splint devices, physical therapy, rehabilitation, or surgery. NSAIDs may relieve nerve irritation. Surgical intervention is indicated if numbness or paresthesias occur despite other treatment and if motor function problems occur. Vitamin B_6 supplements may improve neurological function.

Plantar Fasciitis

Plantar fasciitis is an inflammatory degenerative disorder of the connective tissue in the sole of the foot. The plantar fascia originates at the calcaneus (heel bone) and attaches to deep ligaments of the metatarsal heads (see Fig. 37-18). The pain may be substantial, resulting in difficulty walking. There are many causes of heel pain, although plantar fasciitis is the most common cause for which medical care is sought. Peak incidence occurs in females aged 40 to 60 years. Females are affected twice as often as males.

Normal

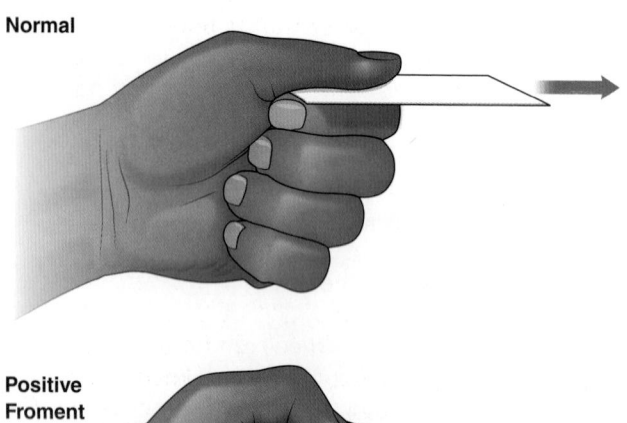

Positive Froment sign

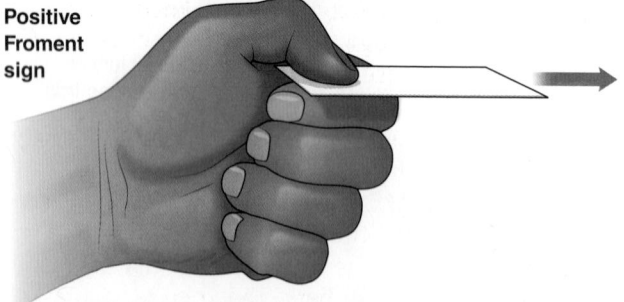

FIGURE 37-17. Froment sign. The Froment test assesses the strength of the adductor pollicis, which is weak with an ulnar nerve palsy. A patient is asked to hold an object, usually a flat object such as a piece of paper, between the thumb and index finger in a pinch grip. The examiner then attempts to pull the object out of the patient's hands. A normal individual will be able to maintain a hold on the object without difficulty. With ulnar nerve palsy, the patient will experience difficulty maintaining a hold and will compensate by flexing the flexor pollicis longus of the thumb to maintain grip pressure, causing a pinching effect.

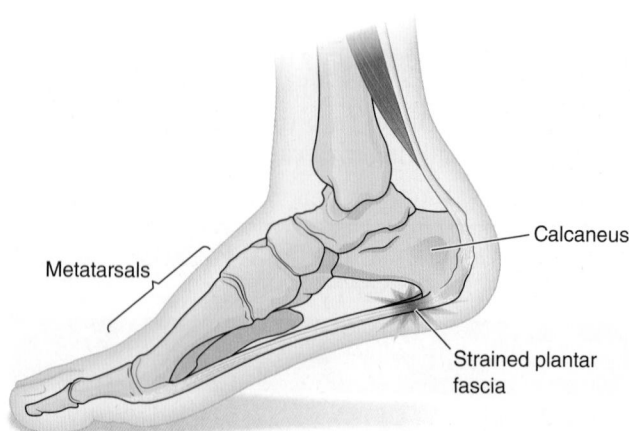

FIGURE 37-18. Plantar fasciitis. Inflammation of the connective tissue that is attached from the metacarpal bones to the calcaneus (heel). It can cause intense pain.

Many individuals mistakenly refer to plantar fasciitis as a heel spur. Although heel spurs can be the cause for the disorder, cumulative trauma is the most common etiology. Approximately 10% of the U.S. population experiences bouts of heel pain, which result in 1 million visits per year to medical professionals for treatment of plantar fasciitis.

Etiology. Most cases of plantar fasciitis are caused by cumulative stress on the foot. Incorrect performance of athletic activities, such as running in nonsupportive shoes, can cause plantar fasciitis. Structural flaws of the leg or foot are also risk factors for the disorder. These anatomical causes include **pes planus** (flat feet), overpronation of the foot, **pes cavus** (high arches of the foot), leg-length discrepancy, excessive lateral tibial torsion, and excessive femoral anteversion. Tightness in the gastrocnemius, soleus muscles, and Achilles tendon is also a risk factor for plantar fasciitis.

Risk factors that increase susceptibility include obesity, occupations requiring prolonged standing and weight-bearing, and heel spurs.

Pathophysiology. The pathophysiology of plantar fasciitis is believed to be secondary to repetitive microtrauma (microtears). The resulting damage at the calcaneal–fascial interface occurs with weight-bearing secondary to repetitive stressing of the arch. Excessive stretching of the plantar fascia can result in microtrauma either along its course or where it inserts onto the medial calcaneal tuberosity. This microtrauma, if repetitive, can result in chronic degeneration of the plantar fascia fibers. The loading of the degenerative and healing tissue at the plantar fascia may cause significant foot pain.

Clinical Presentation. Patients with plantar fasciitis complain of sharp heel pain with the first couple of steps in the morning or after other long periods without weight-bearing. Pain is experienced chronically in the sole of the foot. Patients may report that before the onset of pain, they had increased the amount or intensity of athletic activity, such as running. They may have also started exercising on a different type of surface or may have recently changed footwear.

Plantar fasciitis accounts for about 10% of running-related injuries.

The pain of plantar fasciitis can usually be reproduced by palpating the area of the sole where the plantar fascia inserts into the heel bone. The anteromedial aspect of the plantar fascia is tender. Less frequently, the pain will localize directly below the heel bone or even in the midsection of the plantar arch. In more severe cases, pain may be reproduced by palpation over the proximal portion of the plantar fascia. A tight Achilles tendon is commonly a secondary finding; ankle dorsiflexion may be limited as a result.

Other maneuvers that may reproduce the pain of plantar fasciitis include passive dorsiflexion of the toes, which is sometimes called the windlass test, and having the patient stand on the tiptoes and toe-walk.

Diagnosis and Treatment. The clinical examination is usually enough to diagnose the condition. However, x-rays can be useful to rule out heel spurs, and CT or MRI may be needed to rule out stress fracture. Traditional treatment usually begins with 6 weeks of consistent and daily icing, stretching, NSAID therapy, strapping and taping, and over-the-counter shoe orthotics. Counseling regarding activity modification, as well as choice of shoe gear, is important. After 6 weeks, some cases require additional treatment with a night splint to keep the foot in dorsiflexion, as well as a possible corticosteroid injection, along with the initial regimen for another 6 weeks. Injection therapy, immobilization in a cast or walker boot, and physical therapy are sometimes needed. For severe cases, fasciotomy, a surgical intervention that cuts the connective tissue to release tension, may be required.

Ligament or Meniscus Injury of the Knee

Knee pain occurs in 20% of the general adult population and accounts for almost 3 million outpatient and emergency department visits per year. Overall, 18.1% of U.S. males and 23.5% of U.S. females aged 60 years and older report knee pain for 6 weeks before seeking medical care. Sixty percent of knee injuries are sports-related, although trauma of the knee is the second most common occupation-related injury.

The knee joint, the largest synovial joint of the body, is a combination of two interdependent joints: the tibiofemoral and the patellofemoral joints. The condyle surfaces of the tibia and the femur come together at the knee. Between these surfaces are cartilaginous structures known as the medial and lateral menisci, which act as shock absorbers. The knee must support as much as five times an individual's body weight, and this force is transmitted through the condyles of the femur and the tibia. A fibrous capsule lined with a synovial membrane composes the knee joint with ligaments surrounding the tibia, femur, and patella bones.

Two collateral ligaments and two cruciate ligaments surround the joint capsule. The collateral ligaments are the medial collateral ligament (MCL), which counteracts abductive forces coming from the medial side of the knee, and the lateral collateral ligament (LCL), which limits excessive adductive forces coming from the lateral side of the knee. The anterior cruciate ligament (ACL) and the posterior cruciate ligament (PCL) crisscross the joint and brace the knee against excessive anteroposterior forces. The ACL serves as the primary knee stabilizer, preventing forward displacement of the tibia on the femur. Damage to the ACL causes the most joint instability. Also at the knee, the quadriceps muscle fuses into the patellar ligament, which inserts onto the tibial tubercle.

There are many bursae in the knee that cushion it and alleviate frictional forces between the susceptible structures. In the back of the knee joint, in the popliteal fossa, are vital neurovascular structures, including the popliteal artery (see Fig. 37-19).

Etiology and Pathophysiology. Valgus- or varus-directed forces and anterior- or posterior-directed forces can cause injuries to the knee (see Fig. 37-20 and Box 37-9). Direct blows to one side of the knee provoke injury to the contralateral collateral ligaments and patellar dislocation. Pure **valgus** forces, those occurring on the lateral aspect of the knee, are more common than **varus**-directed contact on the medial side of the knee. The MCL is more prone to injury than the LCL. A combination of valgus or varus stress, whether direct or indirect, delivered to a twisted leg accounts for a wide array of injuries. Vulnerable structures include the collateral and cruciate ligaments, the menisci, and the joint capsule.

> ### 🩺 CLINICAL CONCEPT
>
> The MCL, medial meniscus, and the ACL are the triad of injuries commonly seen in knee trauma.

Clinical Presentation. The patient should be questioned about how the knee injury occurred. The patient

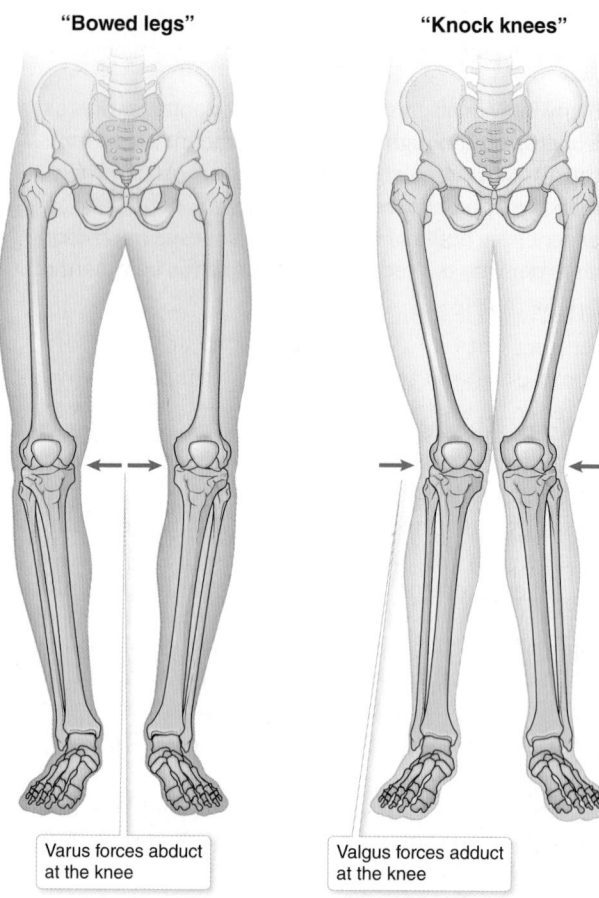

FIGURE 37-20. Valgus vs. varus forces directed at the knee.

Varus forces abduct at the knee

Valgus forces adduct at the knee

should describe the motion of injury and point to the area of pain. The clinician should ask about previous injuries to the knee, and the patient should explain medical problems, past surgeries, and current medications, as well as occupation and recreational activities.

Most patients with ACL damage report a snapping sensation at the time of injury and complain of immediate and profound pain that is exacerbated with motion and weight-bearing. An acute knee injury heralded by a pop or snap, followed by rapidly evolving edema almost always affirms a rupture of the ACL. This injury displaces the tibia backward and pulls apart the PCL. Patellar injury with disruption of normal articulation or fracture may also result.

> ### 🩺 CLINICAL CONCEPT
>
> In cases of trauma, the patient should be completely examined for life-threatening injuries before focusing on the knee injury. The ABCDEs of trauma assessment are applied to the patient. After the patient has been stabilized, the knee can be the area of concentration.

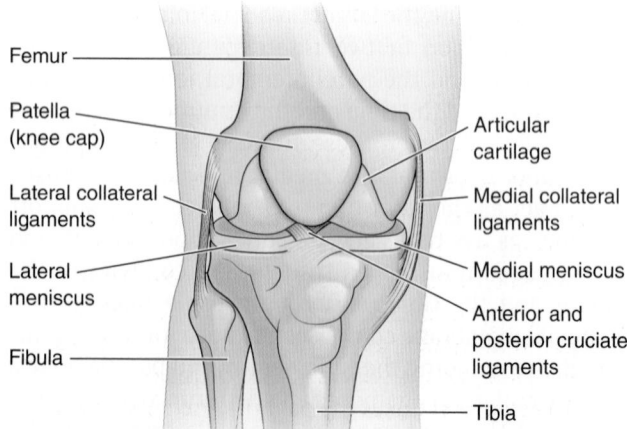

Femur
Patella (knee cap)
Lateral collateral ligaments
Lateral meniscus
Fibula
Articular cartilage
Medial collateral ligaments
Medial meniscus
Anterior and posterior cruciate ligaments
Tibia

FIGURE 37-19. Knee joint. The structures around the knee joint that are most commonly affected by injury include the menisci and ligaments.

Focus the initial examination on inspection, palpation, and neurovascular evaluation of the knee. The clinician should examine the injured knee in

BOX 37-9. Types of Knee Injuries

SPRAINS

Sprains to the knee are characterized by the stretching of the ligaments or the joint capsule, whereas a strain refers to stretching along the course of muscles or tendons. Collateral ligament and cruciate ligament sprains, as well as muscular strains, are common in the knee.

RUPTURE OF THE ACL

Rupture of the ACL is among the most serious of the common knee injuries. ACL tears are associated with anterior blows that hyperextend the knee, as well as strong deceleration forces to the knee. Most patients with ACL damage complain of immediate and profound pain, exacerbated with motion, and inability to bear weight on the knee. Disruption of the ACL may occur alone or with other knee injuries, especially a meniscal injury or MCL tear.

MENISCAL TEAR

Rotational movements may cause a meniscal tear. The medial meniscus is firmly fixated compared with the more mobile lateral meniscus. It is attached to the MCL capsule and has less elasticity than the lateral meniscus, which makes it vulnerable to injury. Menisci do not have pain fibers; the tearing and bleeding into peripheral attachments, as well as the traction on the joint capsule, cause the pain.

comparison with the contralateral knee. Observe the patient in a standing position. When an uninjured patient stands with feet together, the medial aspects of both knees and ankles are normally in contact. The knee should be inspected for edema, ecchymosis, masses, patella location and size, muscle mass, erythema, and evidence of local trauma, such as abrasions, contusions, or lacerations. After a knee injury, onset of edema and pain tends to occur within the first 3 hours after injury. The clinician should verify the knee's mechanical trauma by attempting to perform passive ROM. Also, the clinician should observe if the patient can walk or bear weight on the knee. The posterior aspect of the knee should be palpated for the popliteal pulse, abnormal bulges, popliteal thrombophlebitis, or baker's cysts.

CLINICAL CONCEPT

A baker's cyst, which originates from a herniation of the synovial membrane through the posterior aspect of the joint capsule, tends to be associated with intra-articular disease.

The knee should be palpated in slight flexion. This position can be facilitated by placing a pillow under

the popliteal fossa. Stress testing of the knee should be performed by applying gentle pressure in various valgus, varus, anterior, and posterior directions. In bursitis, there is tenderness, erythema, warmth, and swelling; however, ROM is usually not restricted.

Specific maneuvers that are used in the assessment of the knee are listed in Box 37-10.

BOX 37-10. Knee Assessment Tests

The following are some specific maneuvers used to investigate the individual structures of the knee.

ACL

- Anterior drawer test: The patient assumes a supine position with the injured knee flexed to 90 degrees. The clinician fixes the patient's foot in slight external rotation by sitting on the foot and then placing the thumbs at the tibial tubercle and fingers at the posterior calf. With the patient's hamstring muscles relaxed, the clinician pulls anteriorly and assesses anterior displacement of the tibia (positive anterior drawer sign).
- Lachman test: The test is performed with the patient in a supine position and the injured knee flexed to 30 degrees. The clinician stabilizes the distal femur with one hand, grasps the proximal tibia in the other hand, and then attempts to sublux the tibia anteriorly. Lack of a clear endpoint indicates a positive Lachman test.

MCL

- Valgus stress test: This test is performed with the patient's leg slightly abducted. The clinician places one hand at the lateral aspect of the knee joint and the other hand at the medial aspect of the distal tibia. Next, valgus stress is applied to the knee at both 0 degrees (full extension) and 30 degrees of flexion. With the knee at 0 degrees, the PCL and the articulation of the femoral condyles with the tibial plateau should stabilize the knee; with the knee at 30 degrees of flexion, application of valgus stress assesses the laxity or integrity of the MCL.

MENISCAL STABILITY

- McMurray test: Patients with injury to the menisci usually demonstrate tenderness at the joint line. The McMurray test is performed with the patient lying supine. To assess the medial meniscus, the test is performed with the patient supine and the knee flexed to 90 degrees. The examiner grasps the patient's heel with one hand to hold the tibia in external rotation, placing the thumb at the lateral joint line and the fingers at the medial joint line. The examiner flexes the patient's knee maximally to impinge the posterior horn of the meniscus against the medial femoral condyle. A varus stress is applied as the examiner extends the knee.

Diagnosis. The clinical examination is an important component in the diagnosis. Other studies of importance include x-ray, CT, and MRI scan. Ultrasound can be used to diagnose effusions, tendon ruptures, and popliteal cysts. Arthrocentesis, the examination of the fluid surrounding the knee, may be necessary.

Treatment. Initial treatment of most knee injuries includes RICE therapy. For the first 1 to 3 days, therapeutic measures are used that minimize tissue damage and reduce pain and inflammation. The knee may be splinted to provide support and to prevent further injury. Intra-articular injection of an analgesic or surgical treatment may be required.

In cases of trauma, the ABCDEs should be applied before focusing on the knee. Stabilization of the lower extremity and monitoring the neurovascular status of the limb are essential. If there is resistance to realignment, this should not be attempted. Wounds should be covered with saline-soaked sterile gauze.

Chapter Summary

- Trauma is the leading cause of death for persons aged 1 to 44 years.
- Peak bone mass is achieved in early adulthood, around age 30 to 35 years.
- There is a wide spectrum of types of musculoskeletal trauma, from acute, life-threatening injuries to mild sprains and strains.
- Motor vehicle accidents, sports activities, falls, and osteoporosis are major causes of musculoskeletal trauma.
- Whenever musculoskeletal trauma occurs because of high-energy forces, astute assessment skills are necessary. Associated organ trauma, neurovascular damage, and collateral fractures are common.
- A sprain is an overstretching of tendons and ligaments with possible tear. The most common location for a sprain is in the ankle.
- A strain is an overstretching or contraction of muscle. The most common locations for strain are the lower back and hamstring.
- Cumulative trauma disorders are "wear and tear" injuries caused by constant stresses exerted on a body part. Common cumulative trauma disorders are stress fractures and carpal tunnel syndrome.
- There are many different types of bone fractures, and all require immobilization for healing to occur.
- Fracture healing takes place through five stages: fracture and inflammatory phase, granulation tissue formation, callus formation, lamellar bone deposition, and remodeling.
- Initial treatment of most musculoskeletal injuries includes RICE.
- To assess neurovascular status, always check pulses and sensation distal to a musculoskeletal injury. Signs of neurovascular compromise include the 5 Ps: pain, pallor, paresthesias, pulselessness, and paralysis.
- A compartment consists of bone, muscle, nerves, and blood vessels that are enclosed by a fascial membrane.
- Compartment syndrome occurs when tissue pressure exceeds perfusion pressure in a closed anatomical space. The pressure causes severe impingement on nerves and blood vessels that can lead to muscle and bone ischemia. Intense pain that is out of proportion to the nature of the injury is the major symptom of compartment syndrome.
- Although immobilization is necessary for healing, it increases the risk of complications, such as deep venous thrombosis, contracture, and muscle atrophy.
- Compound or open fractures are vulnerable to infection.
- The history of how the trauma occurred is an important feature of diagnosis. Physical examination findings often reveal deformity, pain, and limited ROM.
- Vertebral compression fracture is pathognomonic of osteoporosis.
- The hip, wrist, and vertebrae are the most commonly fractured bones in older adults with osteoporosis.
- The shoulder is the most commonly dislocated joint of the body.
- Frozen shoulder is indicated when active and passive ROM of the shoulder are decreased.
- Trauma of the knee is the second most common occupation-related injury. The MCL is the most frequently injured ligament in the knee.
- Rupture of the ACL is among the most serious of knee injuries and causes the most joint instability.

Making the Connections

Signs and Symptoms	Physical Assessment Findings	Diagnostic Testing	Treatment
Cervical Strain | Acceleration-deceleration mechanism of injury causing elongation and tearing of cervical muscles or ligaments with subsequent edema, hemorrhage, and inflammation. Commonly occurs in motor vehicle accidents, while lifting heavy objects, and with abnormal postures.			
Suboccipital headache; motion-induced neck pain; shoulder, scapular, or arm pain. Visual disturbances, dizziness, difficulty sleeping. Onset of symptoms usually delayed 12 to 72 hours after incident.	Tenderness along cervical spine, paravertebral muscle spasm, swelling.	X-ray shows soft tissue injury.	Short-term use of soft cervical collar, muscle relaxants, heat application to area, possibly steroid injections. Rigid cervical collar or neck brace for more severe injury. With unstable cervical fracture halo traction is used. Pain management.
Lumbar Strain or Sprain | Active strain and sprain of lumbosacral muscles or ligaments with frequent intervertebral disc herniation, causing impingement on spinal nerves.			
Sharp pain, stiffness, and tenderness in the lumbosacral region, often with pain radiation down into one leg (called radicular pain or sciatica). Numbness and tingling along dermatome into lower extremity. In cauda equina syndrome, bladder and bowel incontinence or saddle paresthesias.	Lumbosacral paravertebral tenderness and swelling. Lack of sensation in dermatome areas of lower extremity. Possibly diminished deep tendon reflexes and weakness in lower extremity. L4–L5 spinal nerve tested with patient's ability to walk on heels. L5–S1 tested with patient's ability to walk on toes.	Inspect ROM. Ask patient to touch toes, dorsiflex and plantarflex foot. Straight-leg raising test. Patrick test. Sensory dermatome testing. Test Patella and Achilles DTRs.	Back support belt, periodic stretching exercises (no prolonged sitting or lying), muscle relaxants, heat application to area, possibly steroid injections. Pain management. Avoidance of heavy lifting, jogging, climbing. Physical therapy, TENS, massage, ultrasound treatments, chiropractic treatments.
Ankle Sprain | Commonly caused by inversion of foot during plantar flexion of ankle; most injuries involve the anterior talofibular ligament.			
Intense pain, swelling of ankle joint, weakness of foot, inability to bear weight, popping sound during injury.	Tenderness, commonly over either malleolus; edema; ecchymosis; and deformity of ankle. Decreased ROM. Check posterior tibial and dorsalis pedis pulses.	Order ankle x-ray based on Ottawa Ankle Rules.	Rest, ice, compression, elevation (RICE); cessation of weight-bearing may be prescribed. Compression dressing, air stirrup splint, or plaster or fiberglass posterior splint for more severe sprains. Pain management. Physical therapy.
Stress Fracture | Repetitive stress on bone; most commonly tibia, fibula, and second and third metatarsals.			
Localized bone pain that increases with weight-bearing.	Tenderness along involved bone.	X-ray, bone scanning, MRI, and CT scanning preferred for diagnosis.	Rest with gradual return to increased activity once pain subsides. Pain management.

Continued

Making the Connections—cont'd

Signs and Symptoms	Physical Assessment Findings	Diagnostic Testing	Treatment
Carpal Tunnel Syndrome | Increased pressure on the median nerve in the carpal tunnel in the wrist. The index finger, thumb, and middle finger are commonly affected.			
Numbness, tingling, pain in the hand and proximally in the forearm along the distribution of the median nerve.	Wrist pain radiation of pain proximal to wrist. Intermittent paresthesias in the median nerve distribution of hand. Pain worse at night.	Clinical examination, including finding paresthesias in the median distribution of the hand after Phalen's sign and Tinel's sign.	Rest, splinting, surgical decompression possible. Pain management.
Lateral Epicondylitis | Repeated extension of the wrist and pronation and supination of the forearm.			
Tenderness of the lateral epicondyle, weak grip strength, painful movement of wrist and forearm.	Tenderness of the lateral epicondyle, weak grip.	X-ray, CT, or MRI.	Rest, ice, nonsteroidal analgesics, splinting, steroid injection, physical therapy. Pain management.
Bursitis | Inflammation of the bursa commonly caused by repetitive. motion injury.			
Pressure and painful motion of joint. Discomfort at rest.	Swelling, warmth, tenderness of joint. Decreased ROM.	ESR, x-ray.	Moist heat, immobilization, intrabursal steroid injections, possibly surgery. Pain management.
TMJ Disorder | Repetitive stress on TMJ caused by jaw malocclusion, anterior disc disorder, abnormal chewing patterns, facial trauma, bruxism.			
Pain over TMJ area, preauricular area, and muscles of mastication, aggravated with chewing or bruxism.	Tenderness, swelling of the masseter, temporalis, medial pterygoid, digastric, and mylohyoid muscles. Clicking of TMJ.	Dental examination to rule out dental etiology.	Physical therapy, patient education, acupuncture possibly. Pain management.
Hip Fracture | Most occur as a fracture through the femoral neck or fracture from greater trochanter to lesser trochanter; intertrochanteric or beneath the trochanters; subtrochanteric. Common sequela of osteoporosis.			
Pain centered in groin, immobility.	An externally rotated and shortened leg. Motion to the extremity will produce severe pain centered around the affected groin. Edema and ecchymosis possible.	X-ray.	Surgical reduction and fixation, hip replacement sometimes required. Anticoagulant therapy caused by high risk for deep venous thrombosis. Hip fracture indicates osteoporosis is likely; therefore, Ca++/vitamin D supplements needed. Pain management.
Vertebral Compression Fracture | A thinning of the vertebral body. A 15% to 20% or more decrease in vertebral body height. Common sequela of osteoporosis.			
Back pain, kyphosis, loss of height. Pain worsened by ambulation.	Tenderness over spine. Pain with ambulation. Kyphosis. Paravertebral muscle spasm.	X-ray and DEXA scan of spine.	Calcitonin, muscle relaxants, analgesics, external support devices, vertebral surgery; vertebroplasty, kyphoplasty. Osteoporosis likely in patient; therefore. Ca++/vitamin D supplements needed.

Making the Connections—cont'd

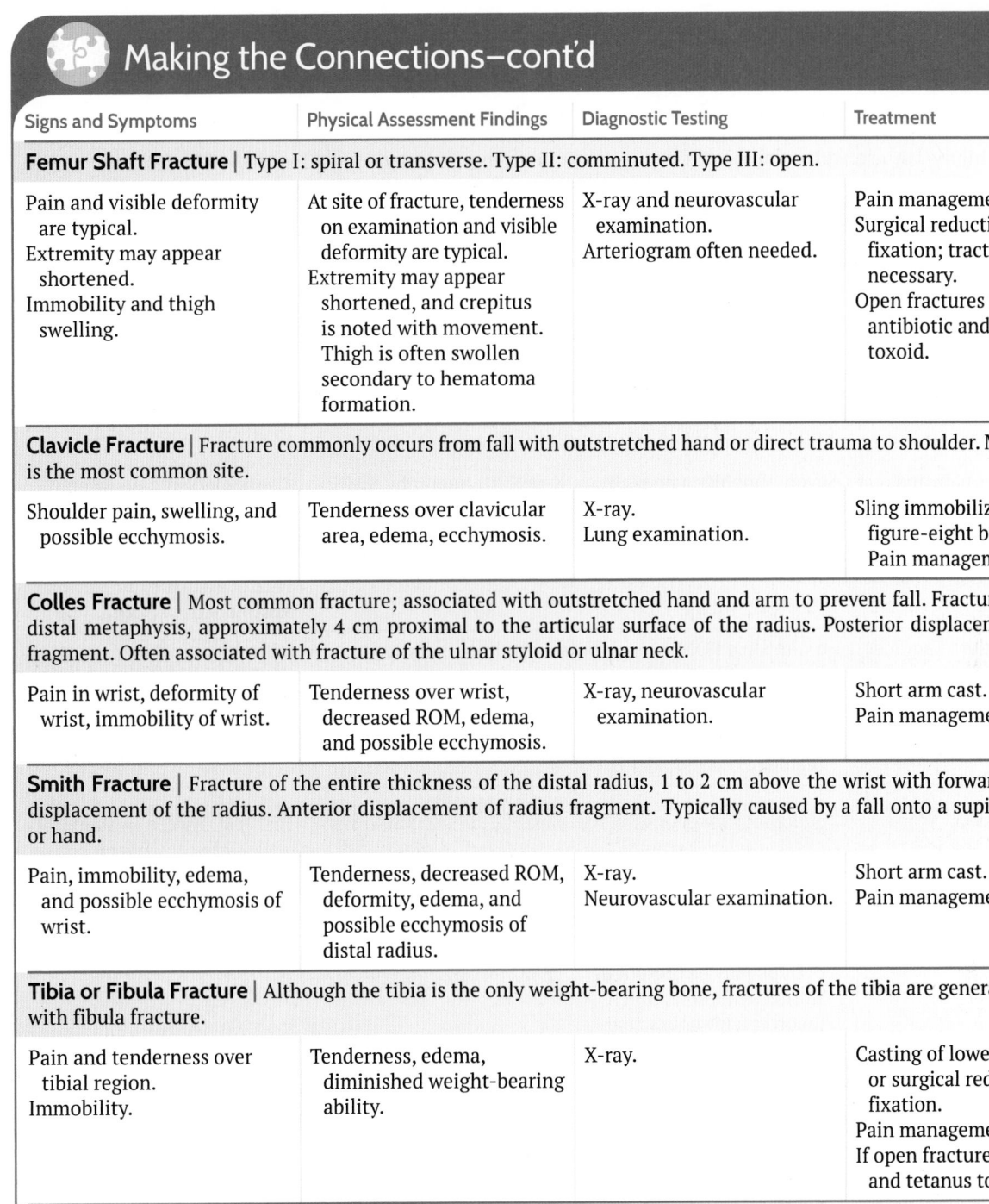

Signs and Symptoms	Physical Assessment Findings	Diagnostic Testing	Treatment
Femur Shaft Fracture | Type I: spiral or transverse. Type II: comminuted. Type III: open.			
Pain and visible deformity are typical. Extremity may appear shortened. Immobility and thigh swelling.	At site of fracture, tenderness on examination and visible deformity are typical. Extremity may appear shortened, and crepitus is noted with movement. Thigh is often swollen secondary to hematoma formation.	X-ray and neurovascular examination. Arteriogram often needed.	Pain management. Surgical reduction and fixation; traction is often necessary. Open fractures require antibiotic and tetanus toxoid.
Clavicle Fracture | Fracture commonly occurs from fall with outstretched hand or direct trauma to shoulder. Middle clavicle is the most common site.			
Shoulder pain, swelling, and possible ecchymosis.	Tenderness over clavicular area, edema, ecchymosis.	X-ray. Lung examination.	Sling immobilization or figure-eight bandaging. Pain management.
Colles Fracture | Most common fracture; associated with outstretched hand and arm to prevent fall. Fracture through the distal metaphysis, approximately 4 cm proximal to the articular surface of the radius. Posterior displacement of radius fragment. Often associated with fracture of the ulnar styloid or ulnar neck.			
Pain in wrist, deformity of wrist, immobility of wrist.	Tenderness over wrist, decreased ROM, edema, and possible ecchymosis.	X-ray, neurovascular examination.	Short arm cast. Pain management.
Smith Fracture | Fracture of the entire thickness of the distal radius, 1 to 2 cm above the wrist with forward and upward displacement of the radius. Anterior displacement of radius fragment. Typically caused by a fall onto a supinated forearm or hand.			
Pain, immobility, edema, and possible ecchymosis of wrist.	Tenderness, decreased ROM, deformity, edema, and possible ecchymosis of distal radius.	X-ray. Neurovascular examination.	Short arm cast. Pain management.
Tibia or Fibula Fracture | Although the tibia is the only weight-bearing bone, fractures of the tibia are generally associated with fibula fracture.			
Pain and tenderness over tibial region. Immobility.	Tenderness, edema, diminished weight-bearing ability.	X-ray.	Casting of lower extremity or surgical reduction and fixation. Pain management. If open fracture, antibiotic and tetanus toxoid.
Foot Fracture | Most common causes of foot fracture include fracture from twisting, trauma directly to the foot, and cumulative trauma.			
Pain, deformity, swelling, difficult weight-bearing on foot.	Tenderness, edema, deformity of foot, diminished weight-bearing.	To facilitate diagnosis, grasp first and second metatarsals and move them alternately through plantar flexion and dorsiflexion. X-ray, MRI, or ultrasound or CT or bone scan if foot fracture occult on plain x-ray. Neurovascular examination.	Nondisplaced fractures are treated with non–weight-bearing short leg cast. ORIF for displaced fractures. Crutch walking. Neurovascular monitoring to prevent compartment syndrome. For toe fracture, common treatment is buddy tape the fractured toe to an adjacent toe and apply a rigid flat-bottom shoe.

Continued

Making the Connections—cont'd

Signs and Symptoms	Physical Assessment Findings	Diagnostic Testing	Treatment
Rotator Cuff Injury | A spectrum of disease, ranging from acute reversible tendonitis to massive tears involving the supraspinatus, infraspinatus, and subscapularis muscles. Caused by a history of repetitive overhead activities.			
Shoulder pain, decreased ROM, shoulder weakness.	Decreased active elevation of arm with passive ROM.	X-ray, MRI, or ultrasound. EMG testing.	Pain management, anti-inflammatory agents, rest, icing. Corticosteroid injections possible. Physical therapy.
Shoulder Dislocation | Anterior dislocation, the most common type of shoulder dislocation, occurs when the humeral head is forced out of the glenohumeral joint, rupturing or detaching the anterior capsule from its attachment to the head of the humerus or from its insertion into the edge of the glenoid fossa.			
Severe shoulder pain and decreased ROM. Obvious shoulder deformity.	Severe shoulder pain with passive ROM. Severely decreased active ROM.	X-ray, arteriography, EMG.	Conscious sedation when reducing shoulder joint. Shoulder immobilization using a sling and swathe. Neurovascular examination. Postreduction x-ray.
Frozen Shoulder | Shoulder has diminished ROM caused by previous immobilization.			
Pain and immobility of the shoulder joint.	Decreased active and passive ROM of the shoulder. Tenderness over the deltoid region of the shoulder.	X-ray, ultrasound, MRI, EMG.	Moist heat, anti-inflammatory agents, pain management. Physical therapy.
Brachial Plexus Injury | High-energy trauma to the upper extremity and neck, causing stretching and injury of the brachial plexus.			
Pain in neck and shoulder, paresthesias, swelling, weakness or heaviness of the extremity.	Tenderness and weakness of arm. Edema of shoulder. Ptosis of eyelid and miosis of pupil may be present in Horner syndrome, which involves a lower brachial plexus lesion.	X-ray, CT scan, myelography, MRI, angiography, sensory nerve action potentials, EMG testing.	Surgery, nerve grafting, physical therapy. Pain management.
Ulnar Nerve Injury | Ulnar nerve entrapment. Pressure or injury to the ulnar nerve along its course may cause paralysis of the muscles. One of the most severe consequences is loss of the intrinsic muscle function in the hand.			
Numbness, motor loss, and possible muscle wasting along course of ulnar nerve.	Motor and sensory losses along course of ulnar nerve.	X-ray of elbow and wrist. MRI or EMG may be necessary. Motor and sensory conduction velocities.	Avoidance of pressure on elbow. Anti-inflammatory agents, oral vitamin B_6. Decompression surgery may be needed.
Plantar Fasciitis | Thickening of plantar fascia caused by overuse and degeneration. Sometimes a calcification at the calcaneus (heel spur) is present.			
Pain, which is intense in morning and lessens with activity.	Anteromedial aspect of plantar fascia is tender. Ankle dorsiflexion is limited secondary to pain. Excessive pronation of foot.	Clinical examination findings, x-ray.	Daily icing, stretching, and NSAID therapy, along with orthotics. Night splints to maintain foot in dorsiflexion during sleep. Corticosteroid injection possible. Plantar fasciotomy may be needed.

Making the Connections—cont'd

Signs and Symptoms	Physical Assessment Findings	Diagnostic Testing	Treatment
Ligamentous or Meniscus Injury of Knee	Knee can suffer acute traumatic injury, infectious injury, chronic overuse injury, or degenerative injury. Knee joint dislocation can occur from high-energy trauma.			
Pain, limited ROM, inability to bear weight, and gait disturbance.	Specific knee maneuvers that stress the joint are used to localize the area of injury. Common maneuvers include the anterior drawer test, Lachman test, and McMurray test.	X-ray, CT scan, MRI, arteriogram, synovial fluid aspiration, and analysis.	RICE, cast, brace, or surgical treatment.

Bibliography

Available online at fadavis.com

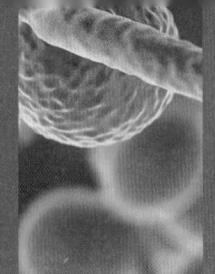

Degenerative Musculoskeletal Disorders

Learning Objectives

Upon completion of this chapter, the student will be able to:

- Identify normal anatomy and physiology of the muscle, bone, and joints.
- Describe the etiologies and pathological mechanisms of degenerative disorders of the musculoskeletal system.
- Identify signs, symptoms, and clinical manifestations of degenerative disorders within the musculoskeletal system.

- Recognize the assessment techniques, laboratory tests, and imaging studies used in the diagnosis of degenerative disorders of the musculoskeletal system.
- Discuss pharmacological and nonpharmacological treatment modalities used in the management of degenerative disorders of the musculoskeletal system.
- Describe the potential complications of degenerative disorders of the musculoskeletal system.

Key Terms

Arthritis
Arthropathy
Bisphosphonates
Bone mineral density (BMD)
Bouchard's nodes
Calcitonin
Calcitriol
Cortical bone
Degenerative disc disease (DDD)
Dual-energy x-ray absorptiometry (DEXA)

Female athlete triad syndrome
FRAX Risk Assessment Score
Heberden's nodes
Lubricin
Osteoarthritis (OA)
Osteocalcin
Osteomalacia
Osteopenia
Osteophyte
Osteoporosis

Parathyroid hormone (PTH)
Radiculopathy
Rickets
Sciatica
Selective estrogen receptor modulator (SERM)
Spinal stenosis
T score
Telopeptides
Trabecular bone

Bone health is a critical component of an individual's overall health and quality of life, and bone disease generates pain, anxiety, depression, and a general decline in a person's well-being. Bone density reaches its peak at approximately age 30 years. After age 30, bone deterioration, known as osteoclastic activity, outpaces bone growth, or osteoblastic activity. **Osteoporosis** occurs with aging when osteoclasts cause an increased rate of bone deterioration. **Osteoarthritis (OA)** is the degeneration of joints caused by aging; the joints of the hands and knees are particularly affected.

Epidemiology

Osteoporosis, the most common degenerative disease of bone, is a disorder of bone demineralization. The disease is more common in females than males, with over 200 million affected annually worldwide. Among females, one in three suffer an osteoporotic fracture sometime in their lifetime, with the most common fracture sites being the wrist, hip, and vertebrae.

Seventy-five percent of females who suffer osteoporotic fracture are older than age 65. With the aging of the population, by the year 2050, it is estimated that the number of females who suffer hip fracture worldwide will increase by 240%. In addition, one in five males suffer from osteoporosis; by 2050, this number is estimated to increase by 300%.

OA, the deterioration of joints that commonly occurs with aging, is the most common cause of disability in the United States, with approximately 20 million adults diagnosed annually. Obesity and aging are factors that are increasing the incidence of OA in the United States. Obesity, which affects more than one in three adults, causes excess weight-bearing for the knee and hip joints. It is estimated that two out of three obese adults in the United States will suffer OA of the knee in their lifetime. By 2030, it is projected that 67 million adults will be suffering from some form of arthritis.

Degenerative disc disease (DDD) is also a very common musculoskeletal problem in the population. The discs between vertebrae become compressed or malaligned, particularly in the lumbar area of the spinal column, causing impingement of spinal nerves. It is the most common cause of back pain in adults throughout the world.

Low back pain is the second most common reason for patient visits to primary-care providers in the United States. Vertebral compression and herniated intervertebral discs can cause intractable pain that requires surgery.

Basic Concepts of Healthy Bone and Joint Function

The major structures of the musculoskeletal system—the bones, muscles, tendons, and ligaments—work together to produce flexible skeletal movement. The skeleton protects the internal organs and tissues and is a storehouse for calcium and phosphorus, which are bound to a matrix made up largely of collagen. In combination, these minerals form calcium hydroxyapatite crystals, $Ca_{10}[PO_4]_6[OH]_2$, the major constituent of bone. In addition to providing mechanical support, bone contains hematopoietic cells. Bone marrow is the birthplace of all blood cells—red blood cells (RBCs), white blood cells (WBCs), and platelets.

There are two basic types of bone: trabecular and cortical. **Cortical bone** is solid bone. **Trabecular bone,** also called cancellous, is nonsolid bone with an interior latticelike composition. It is found in high amounts in the upper femur, vertebrae, and wrist. Osteoporosis affects all bones equally, but the areas of trabecular bone display the degeneration first. Osteoporotic deterioration of the latticework of trabecular bone rapidly weakens the nonsolid structure. The bone often weakens because of weight-bearing, and fracture occurs; this is commonly the patient's initial sign of osteoporosis.

Bone Health

Bone is in a constant state of change. The skeleton is sculpted when new bone is formed by osteoblasts, and bone resorption is activated by osteoclasts. Osteoblasts secrete alkaline phosphatase, which raises the calcium and phosphorus content of bone. Healthy bone production is directly related to bone's calcium content. There are three calcium-regulating hormones: **parathyroid hormone (PTH), calcitriol** (which is a form of vitamin D), and **calcitonin.** The parathyroid glands, found nestled within the thyroid, regulate calcium balance in the body. PTH can activate both bone formation and bone breakdown. PTH stimulates osteoblast formation and maturation while at the same time stimulating osteoclastic activity. The bone remodeling process requires both building up and breaking down of bone. Although PTH stimulates these opposing processes, its net effect favors bone formation: the gain of bone tissue. PTH is secreted when calcium concentration in the blood decreases. PTH stimulates bone to release calcium and

acts at the kidneys to reabsorb calcium into the bloodstream. It has the dual role of regulating blood calcium levels and bone calcium content. PTH also facilitates renal synthesis of a major component of vitamin D. Vitamin D is derived from the kidneys and dietary consumption. Vitamin D is activated by ultraviolet light and then facilitates absorption of calcium from the gastrointestinal tract. Bone is composed of calcium hydroxyapatite ($Ca_{10}[PO_4]_6[OH]_2$): a combination of calcium and phosphorus. Calcitonin is a hormone produced by the thyroid gland, which is stimulated by increased calcium levels in the blood; it enhances calcium entry into bone and inhibits osteoclast activity, which in turn, blocks bone breakdown (see Fig. 38-1).

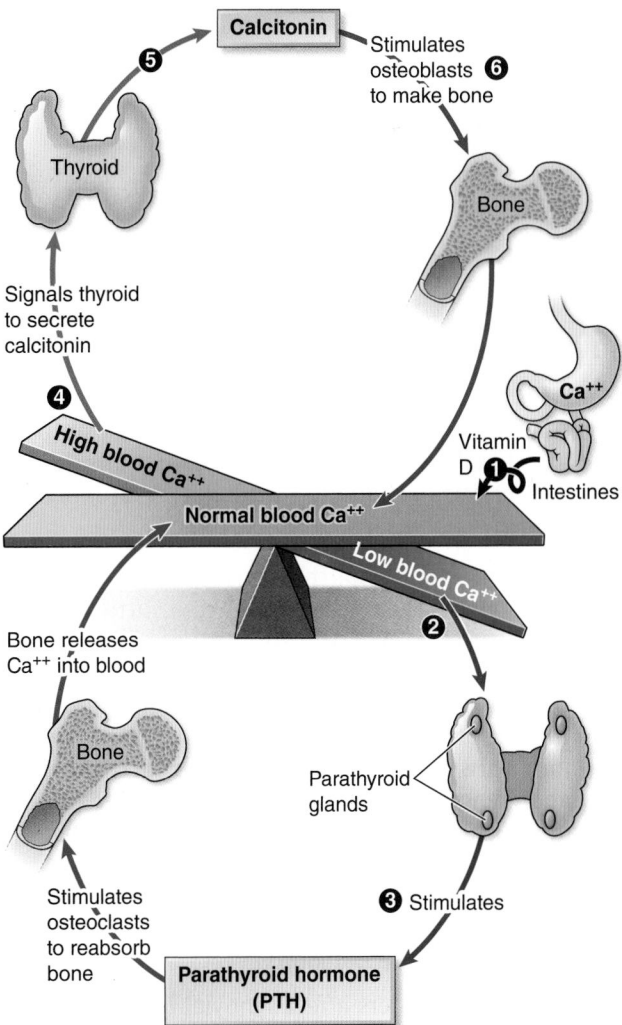

FIGURE 38-1. Calcium balance in the body. (1) Calcium is ingested in the diet, broken down by HCL in the stomach, and absorbed into the bloodstream via the intestine with facilitation by vitamin D. (2) When calcium levels are decreased in the blood, the parathyroid glands are stimulated to release PTH. (3) PTH acts at bone to activate osteoclasts to break down bone and release calcium, which raises the calcium level in the blood. When calcium levels normalize, the parathyroid receives feedback and shuts off. (4) Alternatively, high calcium levels in the blood stimulate the thyroid gland to release calcitonin. (5) Calcitonin activates osteoblasts to build bone.

Sex hormones also have an effect on skeletal health. Estrogen has a suppressive effect on osteoclasts, which in turn, inhibits bone breakdown. During menopause as estrogen levels fall, osteoclastic activity increases. Testosterone stimulates muscle growth, which places stress on the bone, thus increasing bone formation and strength. However, because the body's natural production of sex hormones declines with age, it is crucial that maximum bone health is established in the growth years. To build strength, bone requires the stress of weight-bearing exercise such as walking. The stronger the bones are in young adulthood, the better able they are to deal with changes that occur with aging and other health disorders. There are many different natural, physiological changes of aging that predispose to decreased bone mass (see Box 38-1).

 CLINICAL CONCEPT

Overuse of sunblock and cover-ups that block the sun can inhibit activation of vitamin D.

Joint Health

A joint is the location where two or more bones come together. Joints allow mobility and mechanical support and are classified structurally and functionally. Joints can be classified according to the degree of mobility they allow:

- Synarthrosis: A synarthrosis is a joint where two bones make contact and there is little or no mobility. Most synarthrosis joints are fibrous joints, such as skull sutures.
- Diarthrosis: A diarthrosis is a joint that allows the most movement. Because all diarthrosis joints are synovial joints, the terms "diarthrosis" and "synovial joint" are interchangeable. Examples include the shoulder, elbow, knee, hip, hand, and fingers.
- Amphiarthrosis: An amphiarthrosis is composed of cartilage and permits slight mobility. Examples include the vertebral joints.

Most joint disorders affect synovial joints. A synovial joint is composed of an outer fibrous capsule, which encases interior synovial membranes, articular cartilage, and synovial fluid. The bones come together and move easily because of the smooth surfaces of articular cartilage and lubricating synovial fluid (see Fig. 38-2).

A joint disorder is termed an **arthropathy;** when the disorder involves inflammation of one or more joints, the disorder is called **arthritis.** Arthropathies are called polyarticular when involving many joints and monoarticular when involving only a single joint.

BOX 38-1. Physiological Changes of Aging That Predispose to Osteoporosis

- Predominance of osteoclast-mediated bone resorption over osteoblast-mediated bone formation after age 30
- Predisposition to calcium and vitamin D deficiency
- Less robust vitamin D–enhanced absorption of calcium from the intestine
- Decline in growth hormone levels in both males and females
  - Decline in estrogen in females, allowing osteoclastic activity to outpace osteoblastic activity
  - Decline in testosterone in males
- Shift from osteoblastogenesis to predominant adipogenesis in the bone marrow
- Lactose intolerance (decreased ability to digest dairy products) due to lactase deficiency
- Decreased weight-bearing activity, high-impact, and strength-developing exercise
- Increase in sedentary lifestyle (e.g., due to comorbidities, osteoarthritis, decreased stamina)
- Involuntary loss of muscle mass with age; 5% lost muscle mass per decade after age 30
- Tendency to decrease protein intake with age (e.g., tendency to have less meat in the diet)
- Increased predisposition to comorbidities that can contribute to bone loss and frailty
- Increased intake of medications that may contribute to bone loss (e.g., inhaled or oral corticosteroids)
- Decreased exposure to sunlight (e.g., homebound infirmed older adults, nursing home residents)

Adapted from Demontiero, O., Vidal, C., & Duque, G. (2012). Aging and bone loss: New insights for the clinician. *Therapeutic Ad Musculoskeletal Dis, 4*(2), 61–76; Walston, J. D. (2016). Common clinical sequelae of aging. In L. Goldman & A. I. Schafer (Eds.), *Goldman-Cecil medicine* (25th ed.). Philadelphia, PA: Elsevier Saunders.

Basic Pathophysiological Concepts of Degenerative Musculoskeletal Disorders

Degenerative musculoskeletal disorders include osteoporosis and OA, which are both related to aging of the skeleton. The pathophysiological processes of these two diseases differ and cause a great deal of pain and disability for the adult population.

Degeneration of Bone

Bone is constantly sculpting itself. Bone remodeling is a process that consists of bone resorption by osteoclasts, followed by a period of repair during which new bone tissue is synthesized by osteoblasts. It is an ongoing process of construction and deconstruction in adults, and is the principal metabolic skeletal process. Both

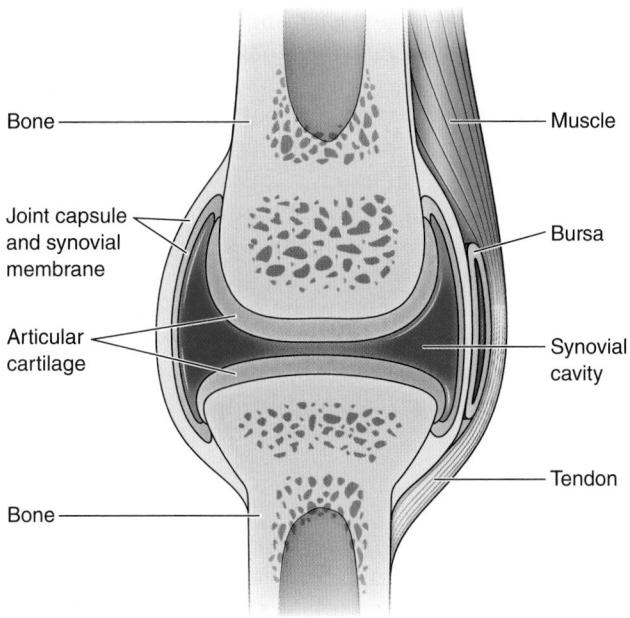

Bone

Joint capsule and synovial membrane

Articular cartilage

Bone

Muscle

Bursa

Synovial cavity

Tendon

FIGURE 38-2. Typical synovial joint.

osteoblasts and osteoclasts perform bone remodeling, which repairs microdamage of the skeletal architecture and extracts calcium from bone to maintain blood calcium levels. Remodeling is stimulated mainly by excessive or accumulated stresses on bone. Weight-bearing stress and a cadre of circulating factors—including estrogens, androgens, calcium, phosphate, vitamin D, PTH, PTH-related peptide, growth factors, interleukins, prostaglandins, and tumor necrosis factor (TNF)—regulate the rate of bone remodeling.

Bones contain a certain percentage of solid, cortical bone and a percentage of meshlike trabecular bone. Bones that contain a large amount of trabecular bone are the wrist, vertebrae, and upper femur (hip). When osteoclastic activity greatly overtakes osteoblastic activity in trabecular bone, the links of bone within the meshwork disintegrate, leaving it vulnerable to fracture. Microscopic cracks in vertebral bone are some of the first fractures noted when osteoclastic activity is unopposed.

> ### 🦴 CLINICAL CONCEPT
> Bones most susceptible to the effects of osteoporosis include those with a high amount of trabecular bone: hips, wrist, and vertebrae.

Bone formation, which occurs throughout life in the remodeling process, requires adequate calcium in the diet. Insufficient calcium in the diet—which is common among middle-aged and older adults—causes inadequate calcium blood levels that stimulate parathyroid gland activity. PTH regulates blood calcium by stimulating bone remodeling, triggering vitamin D

synthesis in the kidney, enhancing gastrointestinal absorption of calcium, and reabsorbing calcium at the kidney. Although all these actions by PTH adjust the blood level of calcium, bone calcium is sacrificed to adjust the blood level. The remodeling of bone is dominated by the osteoclastic activity in calcium deficiency. Although the recommended daily calcium intake for adults is 1,000 to 1,200 mg per day, the average daily intake in the United States is 600 to 800 mg of calcium; this amount is suboptimal and is one of the major reasons for the high number of adults affected by osteoporosis.

Degeneration of Joints

Osteoarthritis (OA) is the most common type of degenerative joint disease, and its pathogenesis has been studied extensively. Interestingly, OA affects certain joints and not others. The joints commonly affected are the cervical and lumbosacral spine, hip, knee, and first metatarsal phalangeal joint. Spared joints include the wrist, elbow, and ankle. According to anthropologists, the joints in the human body were first designed for animals that used four limbs to walk. The center of gravity is widely displaced in a four-legged animal, whereas in a biped, the weight of the body falls mainly on the knees and hips. It is theorized that OA develops in areas that were not designed for walking upright. The knees and the hips take on the majority of the body weight in the upright position; according to darwinian scientists, this is a relatively new change in the evolution of man from ape. According to evolutionists, the human body is still evolving to accommodate this biped position. The upright position itself predisposes to degeneration of the weight-bearing joints.

The mechanics of the knee have been studied extensively. It is estimated that under intense activity, the knee bears five times the body weight. However, studies reveal that ideal body weight is sustainable, whereas obesity causes excessive loading force on the knees. Anatomical studies reveal that abnormal structural changes of the knee and hip are common in the population. Structural changes exist in persons who suffer joint injury; however, physical and mechanical changes also occur in the joints of asymptomatic persons with age.

Articular Cartilage Deterioration

The major change occurring in the joints as a result of aging is articular cartilage loss. Cartilage is a thin slice of flexible tissue on the surfaces of the ends of two opposing joints. In conjunction with synovial fluid, it provides a cushion upon which two joint surfaces move. Cartilage absorbs the impact of forces affecting the bones across a joint. It is made up of chondrocytes (cartilage cells), which synthesize collagen, and aggrecan; this matrix gives cartilage tensile strength. Chondrocytes also produce enzymes that break down the matrix, in concert with cytokines and growth factors that modulate the synthesis of new cartilage. A dynamic equilibrium of cartilage formation and degradation is occurring at all times. Healthy cartilage has slow, consistent synthesis of matrix occurring in synchrony with slow breakdown of matrix. Similar to bone, it is in a constant state of modeling and remodeling. However, with excess weight-bearing or injurious force, cartilage becomes metabolically active and chondrocytes are stimulated to synthesize more degradative enzymes. The matrix starts to break down with unfurling of the collagen matrix and deteriorated aggrecan. With continued excessive force to bear, the cartilage becomes weak and loses its resilient stiffness and cushioning of the joint surface. Chondrocytes continually exposed to excessive force begin to undergo apoptosis, or programmed degeneration. The excessive force placed on a joint caused by obesity activates the degradation process of cartilage. Although weight-bearing incites metabolic changes leading to joint health, excessive weight acts as a pressure force upon joints, particularly the knees and hips. Similarly, the impact of a traumatic force across a joint incites the enzymatic deterioration process of cartilage. Athletes who sustain repeated injury of a joint undergo cartilage loss with each injury. Repetitive knee injuries suffered by athletes are a particularly common precursor to OA of the knee.

With loss of cartilage comes alterations in subchondral bone, the bone just below the cartilage layer. Growth factors, cytokines, osteoclasts, and osteoblasts become activated in the subchondral bone, which thickens and develops microscopic cracks. Shearing of the microvasculature leads to decreased blood flow to subchondral bone.

At the margin of cartilage loss, osteophytes can develop. **Osteophytes** are small bony projections that can impinge on nerves and obstruct blood supply to the joint's components.

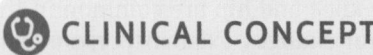

CLINICAL CONCEPT

Osteophyte formation is a hallmark of OA.

Synovial fluid is a lubricating liquid inside a joint that minimizes shearing force between bones in the joint during motion. A synovial membrane exists between the surfaces of the bones in the joint; this is a very thin membrane composed of fat, macrophages, and fibroblasts. The fibroblasts produce **lubricin,** a mucinous glycoprotein that acts as a lubricant for the joint's bone surfaces. In OA, the synovial membrane often becomes inflamed and edematous. Inflammation of the synovial membrane causes a migration of macrophages into the tissue, and the synovium proliferates and secretes enzymes that further degrade the cartilage within the joint. Also, the concentration of lubricin diminishes with synovial inflammation.

The outer joint protectors include the joint capsule, ligaments, tendons, muscles, and sensory nerves. These joint protectors prevent the joint from malalignment. Muscles, ligaments, and tendons contract at different times throughout joint movement and dissipate joint impact. Edematous fluid that accumulates in a joint with OA stretches the joint capsule, making it less effective as a protector. Sensory nerves are stretched, which causes pain.

Assessment

Assessment of the patient with degenerative bone and joint disease requires a complete history and physical examination. The patient should be asked about the present health concern or problem that prompted them to seek health care. The following are important assessment considerations:

1. Onset of the problem and how it developed (sudden or gradual)
2. Location of pain (joints, bone, muscles, soft tissues)
3. Presence of swelling (presently, in the past, or intermittent)
4. Subsequent course (progressive, intermittent, continual, or exacerbations and remissions)
5. Impact on daily life
   - Activities of daily living (ADLs)—dressing, bathing, eating, transfers
   - Household tasks—cooking, cleaning, washing, gardening, etc.
   - Employment—physical or sedentary, any repetitive tasks
   - Recreational/hobbies—outdoor activity, walking, cycling, etc.
6. Previous management and response (how the patient has achieved relief, what aggravates the problem, any consultation with another health-care provider)
7. Current medications or supplements and allergies (e.g., long-term use of corticosteroids or anticonvulsants, which can cause osteoporosis)

After the patient has fully described the present health concern, the clinician should ask questions regarding the following:

8. Past medical and surgical history (any history of fracture or injury, other health problems, hospitalizations, or surgeries)
9. Family history (any history of this disorder or other disorders in the family; it is best to try to ask about past three generations; a genogram may be drawn)

10. Psychosocial history (any present or past use of tobacco, alcohol, marijuana, illicit drugs)
11. Past and present occupation, diet and exercise, sedentary or active lifestyle, recent travel, recreational activities (any occupational exposures, repetitive tasks, heavy lifting, or frequent outdoor activities)
12. Associated complaints (any current problems other than the musculoskeletal complaint—a review of systems may shed light on the present illness)

In the physical examination, the clinician should first describe the patient in terms of posture, any limitation in movement, any visible signs of distress, or bruises or injuries. The area of pain should be examined last. Height, weight, and vital signs should be assessed. If the patient is ambulatory, it is important to ask the patient to "get up and go." The clinician should observe the patient's gait as they arise from a chair and walk approximately 10 feet. Observe if the patient can bear weight on the lower extremities.

The body should be examined in an orderly sequence and should be inspected for erythema, bruising, swelling, and deformity. The joints can be palpated for warmth, tenderness, and crepitus, which may be heard with range of motion (ROM). Muscle tone, ROM, and muscle strength should be assessed. During the examination, the clinician should compare the body for symmetry. In the seated position, examine the head and neck, clavicles, upper thoracic region, shoulders, elbows, forearms, wrists, and hands. With the patient in the seated and standing positions, examine hips, knees, ankles, and feet. The patient should be asked to bend forward and attempt to touch their toes. As the patient bends forward, the paravertebral musculature should be observed from behind for symmetry. In general, upper extremity strength can be assessed by the bilateral hand grip of the patient. The lower extremity strength can be assessed by asking the seated patient to push with lower legs against the resistance of the clinician.

- **Swelling** can be rated as 0 to 3 (0 = none, 1 = mild, 2 = moderate, and 3 = marked). Swelling can be due to inflammation, synovial proliferation, or fluid accumulation. The inspection should also include any bony enlargement, thickening of overlying structures, palpable masses, or atrophy of surrounding tissues.
- **Tenderness** can be rated 0 to 3 (0 = none, 1 = patient says it is tender, 2 = says it is tender and winces, 3 = says it is tender, winces, and withdraws).
- **Muscle strength** can be rated in a range of 0 to 5 (see Table 38-1).
- **ROM:** the clinician should assess the patient's ROM in the area of concern and ascertain which motion aggravates the pain.

TABLE 38-1. Rating Muscle Strength

MUSCLE STRENGTH RANGE: 0 TO 5		
0	None	No visible or palpable contraction
1	Trace	Visible or palpable contraction with no motion
2	Poor	Full ROM without gravity
3	Fair	Full ROM against gravity
4	Good	Full ROM against gravity, moderate resistance
5	Normal	Full ROM against gravity, maximum resistance

Diagnosis

A wide range of diagnostic modalities are used to assess musculoskeletal disorders. Common diagnostic tests are explained here:

- After a complete history and physical, x-rays are a common next diagnostic test. X-rays can delineate bone structures and soft tissues.
- Computed tomography (CT) scan is superior to x-ray for demonstrating complex structure and subtle injuries to tissues.
- Magnetic resonance imaging (MRI) is optimal to evaluate soft tissue, occult fractures, articular cartilage, masses, marrow abnormalities, synovitis, and infectious processes. MRI is the most sensitive modality for detecting fractures and is recommended if there is clinical suspicion for fracture and radiographs are negative.
- Ultrasound may be used to evaluate masses in soft tissues, vasculature, ligaments, tendons, bone, cartilage, effusions, and foreign bodies.
- Bone scans (also called scintigraphy) use intravenously administered radionuclide that binds to hydroxyapatite crystals in bone to detect changes in the skeleton's level of bone formation. Bone scans can detect abnormalities in bone, such as fractures, stress fractures, osteomyelitis, tumors, and osteoblastic metastases, before anatomical changes can be detected on x-ray.
- Single-photon emission CT (SPECT) is used in conjunction with bone scans to provide a three-dimensional image and improve specificity and sensitivity. Bone scan with SPECT can detect vertebral bone lesions and distinguish between aggressive and nonaggressive lesions.
- Dual energy x-ray absorptiometry (DEXA) is a test of bone mineral density (BMD) used to diagnose osteoporosis. The hip and lumbar vertebrae

are specifically visualized, and BMD is measured in terms of a **T score.** The T score indicates the patient's BMD results in comparison to BMD in a healthy 30-year-old young adult. A T score is standard deviation (SD) from the mean. Simple x-rays do not show osteoporosis until the bone is more than 40% deteriorated.

- Specific blood and urine tests can also be used to show evidence of osteoporosis, as well as various types of arthritis and autoimmune disease. Joint synovial fluid can be aspirated and analyzed.

Treatment

Many treatment options are available for musculoskeletal degenerative disorders. Aspirin, NSAIDs, and corticosteroids are major anti-inflammatory agents used to relieve pain and improve mobility. Oral or intra-articular injections of corticosteroids are used. However, long-term use of aspirin, NSAIDs, or corticosteroids have adverse effects. Side effects of aspirin and NSAIDs include gastrointestinal irritation and ulceration. Long-term use of NSAIDs can also cause kidney dysfunction. Corticosteroids have widespread adverse side effects, including osteoporosis, glucose intolerance, hypertension, gastrointestinal ulceration, weight gain, mood changes, cataracts and glaucoma, and immunosuppression if used chronically. Therefore, corticosteroids should only be used for a short period in low doses. COX-2 inhibitors are anti-inflammatory agents that specifically target the prostaglandins that perpetuate pain and inflammation. Newer anti-inflammatory agents, called biological agents, are immunomodulators that target cytokines that cause pain and inflammation. However, immunosuppression can occur with long-term use of these drugs. A wide range of medications is used for osteoporosis, including bisphosphonates, selective estrogen receptor modulators, PTH, and biological agents. However, prevention via the intake of sufficient calcium and vitamin D (Calcitriol) is the most effective treatment. Once fracture occurs, surgical fixation is usually necessary because osteoporotic bone is fragile and cannot heal sufficiently.

Different types of arthritis require different treatment modalities depending on the etiology of the disorder. For example, rheumatoid arthritis (RA) requires medications that oppose the immunological destruction of joints. Immunosuppressant drugs (biological agents) are commonly used in RA (see Chapter 11). OA, in contrast, does not involve the immune system and mainly requires anti-inflammatory medications. Relief of joint pain and inflammation is essential to maintain ROM in all types of arthritis. Surgical treatments can involve fusion of vertebrae, vertebroplasty, joint replacement, and arthroscopy. Physical therapy is commonly needed during rehabilitation.

Pathophysiology of Selected Degenerative Bone and Joint Disorders

The most common degenerative bone disease, osteoporosis, slowly develops without symptoms until late in the disease. The individual is unaware of the bone density breakdown until fracture occurs. OA is also a disease that slowly develops; however, unlike osteoporosis, the development of OA is a painful process. Patients are aware of the joint breakdown because of the tenderness of the joints.

Osteoporosis

Osteoporosis, meaning "porous bone," is a common yet serious disease, characterized by low bone density and structural deterioration of bone tissue. This, in turn, leads to bone fragility and an increased risk of fractures, especially of the trabecular bone in the hips, vertebrae, and wrists. **Osteopenia** is the term used for thinning of the trabecular matrix of the bone before osteoporosis, whereas osteoporosis is the term used when actual breaks in this matrix have occurred.

An estimated 10 million Americans suffer from osteoporosis, and another 34 million are determined to be at risk. It is estimated that one in two females and one in four males older than age 50 years will suffer an osteoporotic fracture in their lifetime.

Osteoporotic hip fractures are specifically linked to an increased risk of mortality. Risk of mortality is 2.8 to 4 times greater among hip fracture patients during the first 3 months after the fracture compared with nonaffected individuals. Nearly one in four hip fracture patients will die within 12 months after the injury from related complications. Immobility and its many detrimental effects are the cause for a decline in health after hip fracture (see Box 38-2).

> ### 🔬 CLINICAL CONCEPT
>
> Only 25% of hip fracture patients will make a full recovery; 40% will require nursing home care, 50% will need a cane or walker, and 24% of those older than age 50 will die within 12 months.

Patho-Pharm Connection

Major Degenerative Musculoskeletal Disorders

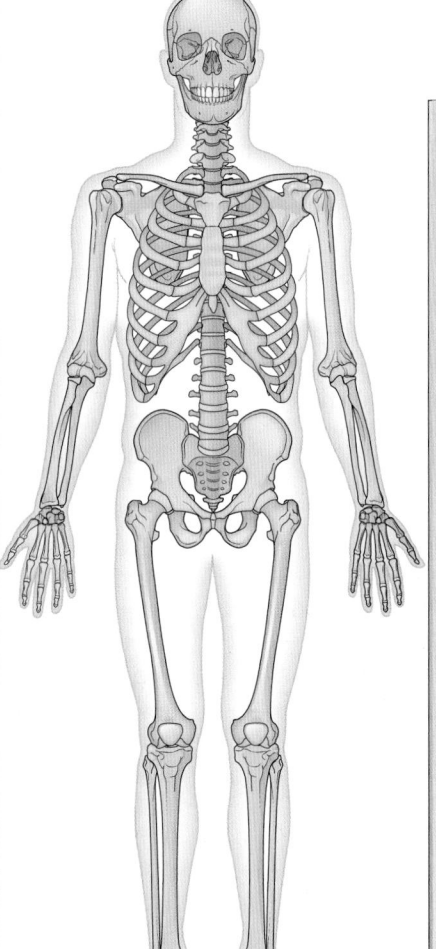

Degenerative Disc Disease

Affects cervical and lumbar vertebrae

NSAIDs: anti-inflammatory agents
(e.g., ibuprofen, naproxen)

Corticosteroid/lidocaine injections:
anti-inflammatory/local anesthetic

Rheumatoid Arthritis

NSAIDs (e.g., ibuprofen)

COX-2 inhibitors (e.g., celecoxib)

DMARDs (disease-modifying
anti-rheumatic drugs)
(e.g., methotrexate, leflunomide,
hydroxychloroquine)

Biologic agents (e.g., abatacept,
adalimumab, anakinra, certolizumab,
etanercept, golimumab, infliximab,
rituximab, sarilumab, tocilizumab)

Targeted DMARDs
(e.g., baricitinib, toafacitinib, upadacitinib)

Osteoarthritis

Affects hands, wrists, knees, hips

NSAIDs: anti-inflammatory agents
(e.g., ibuprofen, naproxen)

COX-2 inhibitor: inhibits prostaglandins
that contribute to inflammation
(e.g., celecoxib)

Topical medications: in the form of
analgesic patches or NSAID creams, rubs,
or sprays that may be applied over the skin
of affected areas to relieve pain

Osteoporosis

Affects hips (upper femur; head and
neck of femur), wrist, and vertebrae

Calcium supplements
Calcitriol (vitamin D)

Bisphosphonates: inhibit
osteoclastic deterioration of bone
(e.g., alendronate, risendronate
ibandronate, zoledronic acid)

**Selective estrogens receptor
modulators (SERMs):** simulate
estrogen receptors on bone
(e.g., raloxifene, bazedoxifene)

Parathyroid hormone analogue:
anabolic building of bone
(e.g., teriparatide, abaloparatide)

Biologic agents
Denosumab: inhibits RANKL protein, which
in turn inhibits osteoclastic activity
Romosozumab: inhibits sclerostin, which
in turn inhibits osteoclastic activity

Calcitonin-Salmon: nasal spray—
mechanism is unclear; may stimulate
calcitonin receptors on osteoblasts or may
inhibit calcitonin receptors on osteoclasts

Gender, genetics, age, and nutritional deficiency of calcium or vitamin D are key elements that can affect an individual's risk of osteoporosis. Lack of weight-bearing exercise, alcohol use, and smoking are also major risk factors (see Box 38-3).

Etiology

Primary osteoporosis generally results from a prolonged negative calcium balance, which can be caused by poor dietary habits, lack of weight-bearing exercise, decline in sex hormones, and lack of daily exposure to natural sunlight.

In the bone remodeling process throughout life, ideally osteoblastic-mediated bone formation and osteoclastic-mediated bone reabsorption would be equal. With age, due to many different factors (see Box 38-1), osteoclastic activity outpaces osteoblastic activity. To enhance skeletal formation, calcium consumed in the diet must first be absorbed from the intestine. Much of the calcium consumed does not make its way to the skeleton; studies indicate that in adults only 30% of calcium intake is actually absorbed. Also some calcium is excreted from the body into the intestine, so the actual net absorption is even lower.

BOX 38-2. Consequences of Immobility

Immobility increases patient susceptibility to:

- Pressure injury, which leads to skin breakdown and, eventually, wound infection
- Slowed bowel peristalsis, which leads to constipation
- Lack of muscle stimulation, which leads to muscle atrophy
- Lack of aerobic exercise, which leads to deconditioning of the cardiovascular system
- Lack of weight-bearing activity, which leads to osteoporosis
- Venous stasis, which predisposes to thromboembolism
- Slowed urinary excretion, urinary stasis, and precipitation of calcium, which leads to kidney stones
- Lack of deep breathing, lack of effective coughing, and stasis of secretions, which leads to pneumonia
- Social isolation and lack of mental stimulation, which leads to depression

BOX 38-3. Risk Factors for Osteoporosis

- Female gender
- Postmenopausal age in female
- Lack of estrogen in female
- Lack of testosterone in male
- Family history
- Females of Asian and European ancestry
- Thin and small-framed females
- Lack of recommended daily intake of calcium and vitamin D
- Lack of weight-bearing exercise
- Excess alcohol consumption
- Excess caffeine consumption
- Smoking
- Long-term use of corticosteroids
- Excess carbonated soft drink consumption
- Gastric bariatric surgery
- Eating disorders such as anorexia
- Hyperthyroidism or excessive intake of thyroid medication
- Hyperparathyroidism
- Anticonvulsant medications

Calcium absorption is facilitated by vitamin D in the intestine. However, as a person ages, vitamin D–enhanced intestinal absorption of calcium is less robust. When calcium absorption is insufficient, blood calcium levels fall, stimulating PTH to reabsorb calcium from bone tissue.

Over time, the combination of these factors causes the inner matrix of bone to thin and eventually break down. The breakdown of bone matrix predisposes to fracture, particularly in areas that contain nonsolid, trabecular bone.

 CLINICAL CONCEPT

Weakening and fracture of bone from osteoporosis commonly affect the areas of predominately trabecular bone first: hip, wrist, and vertebrae. The head and neck of the femur are the primary locations of hip fracture. In vertebral fractures, flattening and compression of vertebral bones occur.

Secondary osteoporosis is caused by disorders that have a direct effect on bone tissue. For example, some hormonal disorders, if not corrected, have a major effect on bone density. Hyperparathyroidism negatively affects serum calcium balance caused by excess secretion of PTH, which reabsorbs calcium from bone to raise the blood levels. This bone resorption from the skeleton leads to weakened bone and increased fracture risk. Hypogonadism in children and young adults causes the loss of the protective effects of estrogen and testosterone, which can result in severe osteoporosis. Exogenous glucocorticoids (corticosteroid medications) taken for prolonged periods can cause deterioration of bone tissue. Malabsorption syndrome, celiac disease, and inflammatory bowel disease diminish both calcium and vitamin D absorption from the intestine and therefore increase susceptibility to osteoporosis.

Pathophysiology

The hallmark of osteoporosis is a reduction in bone density caused by an imbalance between osteoclasts and osteoblasts. Under physiological conditions, bone formation and resorption are in equilibrium. However with age, osteoclastic activity outpaces osteoblastic activity. Early childhood nutrition and physical activity are important to the development of bone strength in an adult. Hereditary factors also play a major role in determining an individual's peak bone strength. Genetics account for up to 80% of the variance in peak bone mass between individuals.

Osteoblasts and activated T cells in the bone marrow produce a cytokine that promotes osteoclast formation—in other words, osteoblastic activity provokes osteoclastic activity to keep cellular activity in balance. Osteoclasts require weeks to resorb bone, whereas osteoblasts need months to produce new bone.

Bone mass peaks by the third decade of life and slowly decreases afterward. After age 30 years, bone resorption exceeds bone formation and leads to osteopenia and, in severe situations, osteoporosis. Females lose 30% to 40% of their cortical bone and 50% of their trabecular bone over their lifetime, as opposed to males, who lose 15% to 20% of their cortical bone and 25% to 30% of trabecular bone. Testosterone endows males with more bone mass, and therefore, males have more bone reserve during old age.

Accelerated bone loss can occur in **female athlete triad syndrome,** a disorder in which a young woman exercises excessively, causing energy deficiency, amenorrhea, and osteoporosis. Disordered eating, such as conscious restriction of food intake, anorexia, or bulimia, can be part of this disorder. Amenorrhea occurs due to suppression of the hypothalamic–pituitary–ovarian axis and low body fat, which leads to low estrogen. Energy deficiency is the main cause of this syndrome. There is an imbalance in the amount of energy consumed and the amount of energy expended during exercise.

Accelerated bone loss can occur in perimenopausal females and older males (see Box 38-1). Loss of gonadal function and aging are the two most important factors contributing to the development of osteoporosis. Studies have shown that bone loss in females accelerates rapidly in the first years after menopause. The lack of the gonadal hormones, estrogen and testosterone, stimulates osteoclast progenitor cells and promotes breakdown of bone. Estrogen deficiency not only accelerates bone loss in postmenopausal females but also plays a role in bone loss in males. Estrogen deficiency sets the stage for intense bone resorption accompanied by inadequate bone formation. T cells and cytokines are activated in the estrogen-deficient environment. In the absence of estrogen, T cells, and cytokines, interleukin-1, interleukin-6, and TNF-alpha significantly promote osteoclast activity. T cells and cytokines also inhibit osteoblast activity and cause premature apoptosis of osteoblasts. Finally, estrogen deficiency sensitizes bone to the bone-deteriorating effects of PTH.

Calcium, vitamin D, and PTH work together to maintain bone homeostasis. Insufficient dietary calcium or impaired intestinal absorption of calcium causes hypocalcemia; this, in turn, stimulates the parathyroid gland to release PTH, which acts on bone tissue to release calcium. This process eventually demineralizes the bone. Other endocrinological conditions, such as Cushing's disease, or medications, such as glucocorticoids, can cause osteoporosis. In Cushing's disease hyperadrenal activity releases an excess of glucocorticoids, which suppress osteoblast function and promote osteoblast apoptosis.

Clinical Presentation

Osteoporosis is known as a silent disease because diagnosis is often not made until after the individual has already suffered an osteoporotic fracture. Weakening of vertebral bodies results in vertebral compression fractures. Osteoporosis reduces vertebral mass by decreasing the strength of the internal latticework of bone. Other common osteoporotic fractures are those of the wrist and hip, with the hip defined as the upper femur head and neck. Osteoporotic fractures of the hip often cause the patient to fall when bones are severely weakened and cannot support the patient's weight. Fragility fractures, which occur without trauma, are characteristic of osteoporosis. Alternatively, osteoporotic fractures can be caused by traumatic falls from a lying, sitting, or standing position or from high-energy trauma, such as a motor vehicle accident. Complaints of back pain that radiate around the trunk are a symptom of vertebral involvement. Increasing deformity, kyphosis, and loss of height are other common symptoms.

Diagnosis

Several diagnostic tests can be utilized to diagnose osteoporosis. **Dual energy x-ray absorptiometry (DEXA)** measures bone density in the lumbar spine and hips, the areas that most commonly suffer osteoporosis. DEXA is precise and allows for monitoring patients who are being treated for osteoporosis over time. Quantitated CT provides a true volumetric measurement of trabecular bone density in the spine. Alternatively, ultrasound densitometry uses sound waves to assess bone mass in a variety of peripheral sites, such as the heel or wrist. **Bone mineral density (BMD)** measurement results are compared with a reference population of young, healthy adults of approximately age 30 years; this is called a T score. The World Health Organization (WHO) has established definitions of osteopenia and osteoporosis based on BMD measurements (see Box 38-4).

The **FRAX Risk Assessment Score** should be included in the total assessment of an individual's risk of osteoporotic fracture. It is a self-assessment tool

---

> ### BOX 38-4. World Health Organization Definitions of Bone Health
>
> According to the WHO, bone health has the following four definitions:
> - **Normal:** BMD is within 1 SD of the mean bone density for young adult females (T score at –1 and above).
> - **Low bone mass (osteopenia):** BMD is between 1 and 2.5 SD below the mean for young adult females (T score between –1 and –2.5).
> - **Osteoporosis:** BMD is 2.5 SD or more below the normal mean for young adult females (T score at or below –2.5).
> - **Severe or "established" osteoporosis:** BMD is 2.5 SD or more below the normal mean for young adult females (T score at or below –2.5) in a patient who has already experienced one or more osteoporotic fractures.
>
> The WHO definition applies to postmenopausal females and males aged 50 years or older.

that uses a range of risk factors to predict a person's risk of fracture. The tool gives a 10-year probability of a fracture in the spine, hip, shoulder, or wrist for people aged between 40 and 90. The National Osteoporosis Foundation recommends using FRAX to calculate fracture risk for patients who have bone density T scores between −1.0 and −2.5 in the spine, femoral neck, or total hip region. Persons with these T scores have decreased bone mass (osteopenia) but have not developed osteoporosis yet. The FRAX assessment includes questions about:

- Age
- Smoking
- Family history of hip fracture
- Prior history of fracture
- Glucocorticoid use (e.g., prednisone)
- Arthritis
- Femoral neck BMD

Taking multiple risk factors into account allows the FRAX formula to make a better estimate of risk for fracture than past methods. The FRAX tool can be obtained as an application for electronic devices from https://www.sheffield.ac.uk/FRAX/index.aspx.

Blood tests that are helpful in the diagnosis of osteoporosis include blood calcium levels, thyroid function tests, PTH levels, estradiol levels in females, testosterone levels in males, and osteocalcin levels. **Osteocalcin** is a major protein found in bone; when blood levels are high, this indicates bone resorption is occurring. There are also biochemical marker tests that measure the rate at which a person is breaking down or resorbing bone. Urine **telopeptides** are bone-specific collagen breakdown products that also indicate bone breakdown.

CLINICAL CONCEPT

The DEXA scan, which measures BMD in the lumbar spine and hip, is the most commonly used diagnostic imaging study that can diagnose osteoporosis.

Treatment

Lifestyle changes that are positive for bone health are the first way an individual can take control. This is especially important for the prevention of osteoporosis, as well as maintenance if a person has been diagnosed with osteopenia. For the individual with diagnosed osteoporosis, supportive devices such as lumbar supports or other types of bracing may be helpful. At least 1,000 mg of calcium and 400 IU of vitamin D supplements are needed daily. Pharmaceutical regimens include the use of antiresorptive agents, anabolic medications, and hormonal therapies. **Bisphosphonates,** such as risedronate, are antiresorptive agents that suppress osteoclast activity. Estrogen-like

drugs, termed **selective estrogen receptor modulators (SERMs),** are also antiresorptive agents. SERMs, such as raloxifene, act like estrogen on bones but do not have other side effects. Estrogen is not used, as it can cause venous thromboembolism and acceleration of estrogen-dependent cancers.

CLINICAL CONCEPT

Bisphosphonates have been associated with atypical bone fractures in females. They must be taken with water, and the patient should be in the sitting or upright position for 30 minutes because they can be extremely irritating to the esophageal and gastric mucosa.

Denosumab, an injectable antiresorptive agent, can be used if other drugs prove ineffective or intolerable. Denosumab is a monoclonal antibody that binds to the osteoclastic protein sclerostin, blocking bone resorption by osteoclasts. It can be used to prevent fracture in individuals with osteoporosis. Calcitonin, which is particularly useful in vertebral compression, can also be used to prevent bone loss and enhance bone formation. Studies show mixed results regarding the efficacy of calcitonin. Teriparatide (TPTD), a medication similar to PTH, and PTH itself are considered anabolic agents, as they stimulate osteoblastic activity and bone formation. Studies show that the treatment sequence of antiresorptive and anabolic medications is important. There is substantial increase in BMD if anabolic medications, such as TPTD or PTH, are used as initial treatment followed by antiresorptive therapy. In contrast, studies indicate that BMD responses to TPTD are lower in patients who are pretreated with antiresorptive therapies.

CLINICAL CONCEPT

Denosumab should not be used in patients with hypocalcemia, as painful muscle spasms can occur. Denosumab has also been associated with osteonecrosis of the jaw. Persons undergoing dental treatment should inform dental health providers if they are currently on this medication.

Surgical treatments, termed vertebroplasty and kyphoplasty, are available for painful spinal compression fractures and are performed if other treatments fail. These are minimally invasive procedures that inject bone cement into the fractured area of the vertebrae. Collapsed vertebrae are reexpanded, which reduces pain and helps the person become more active again.

Osteoarthritis

OA commonly occurs in individuals older than age 40 years. It is the most common form of arthritis and the leading cause of chronic disability in the United States. The disease occurs equally in males and females. Those who have had trauma to joints over the course of their life, such as athletes, are at particular risk. With the combined effects of aging and increasing obesity in the global population, this syndrome is becoming more prevalent, with worldwide estimates suggesting that 250 million people are currently affected. Clinically, the knee is the most common site of osteoarthritis, followed by the hand and hip.

Risk factors for OA include aging, obesity, history of participation in team sports, history of trauma or overuse of a joint, and heavy occupational work. Obesity has become a particularly common risk factor, as excess body weight places excess pressure on the knees and hips. In addition, static or dynamic malalignment of the pelvis, hip, knee, ankle, or foot can contribute to the development of osteoarthritic changes. Muscle weakness, imbalance, and inflexibility can also be risk factors because an individual's risk for injury increases with poor muscle health.

CLINICAL CONCEPT

The increase in obesity has increased the number of orthopedic surgeries related to repair and replacement of weight-bearing joints.

Etiology

OA results from stresses applied to the joints, especially the weight-bearing joints such as the ankle, knee, and hip. Degenerative alterations begin in the articular cartilage as a result of either excessive loading of a healthy joint or relatively normal loading of a previously disturbed joint. It is chronic, with degeneration occurring as a result of the breakdown of chondrocytes and adjacent subchondral bone. The contribution of genetics in OA is estimated to be between 40% and 80%, with a stronger genetic contribution in OA of the hand and hip than the knee. There are some rare monogenetic disorders associated with early onset OA. In contrast, late-onset OA is often multifactorial and caused by many common DNA variants, together with other risk factors.

CLINICAL CONCEPT

Previous joint injury is a major cause of OA. For example, older professional athletes commonly have OA of the knees and hips caused by injury during their career.

Pathophysiology

OA is a slowly progressive, degenerative, and inflammatory disease. Excess pressure on a joint gradually wears away the cartilage surface, exposing the subchondral bone. Inflammation occurs as cytokines, various inflammatory mediators, and metalloproteases are released into the joint and degrade the cartilage. In an effort to repair the cartilage early in the process, chondrocytes synthesize a fluid called proteoglycans. This excess fluid causes swelling of the joint. Proteoglycans and cartilage degeneration can occur for years. As OA progresses, however, the level of proteoglycans decreases, causing the cartilage to lose elasticity and crack. Microscopically, there is loss of cartilage, resulting in the narrowing of the joint space.

In the weight-bearing joints, a greater loss of joint space occurs because of the great pressures these joints endure. Erosion of the damaged cartilage in an osteoarthritic joint progresses until it exposes the underlying bone.

Bone stripped of the protective cartilage comes into contact with the opposing surface. Eventually, the increasing stresses exceed the bone's strength. The subchondral bone becomes exposed and responds, inflammation increases, and the joint eventually becomes thickened and dense at areas of pressure. The traumatized subchondral bone may also undergo cystic degeneration, caused by either osseous necrosis secondary to chronic impaction or to the penetration of synovial fluid.

At the margin of cartilage loss, osteophytes can form. Osteophytes are small bony projections that develop along the rim of bone adjacent to cartilage loss. Osteophytes are an important hallmark of OA. In malaligned joints, osteophytes will grow larger on the side of the joint subjected to the most stress. Osteophytes can impinge on nerves and obstruct blood supply to the joint's components. This nerve impingement will cause pain.

Clinical Presentation

The patient history commonly includes complaints of deep, aching joint pain, occurring especially after exercise or weight-bearing. Symptoms may be relieved with rest. Other symptoms include joint pain during cold weather, stiffness when arising in the morning, crepitus of the joint during motion, joint swelling, altered gait, and limited ROM. The patient may report a burning sensation felt in the associated muscles and tendons or experience muscle spasm and contractions in the tendons with motion. The patient's occupation and recreational activities should be investigated because these activities often increase susceptibility to OA through repetitive use or injury of certain joints. Family history and past medical history are important features of the history. There is a genetic predisposition to arthritis, and certain comorbidities can increase the risk of OA.

Upon physical examination, joint deformity and tenderness may be evident. The involved joints demonstrate decreased ROM. The fingers are often involved in OA, with classic swelling at the distal interphalangeal joint, called **Heberden's nodes.** There is also classic swelling at the proximal interphalangeal joint, called **Bouchard's nodes** (see Fig. 38-3). In OA, regional muscles may atrophy and ligaments may become lax because of decreased movement. Symptoms can be exacerbated by obesity, poor posture, and occupational stress.

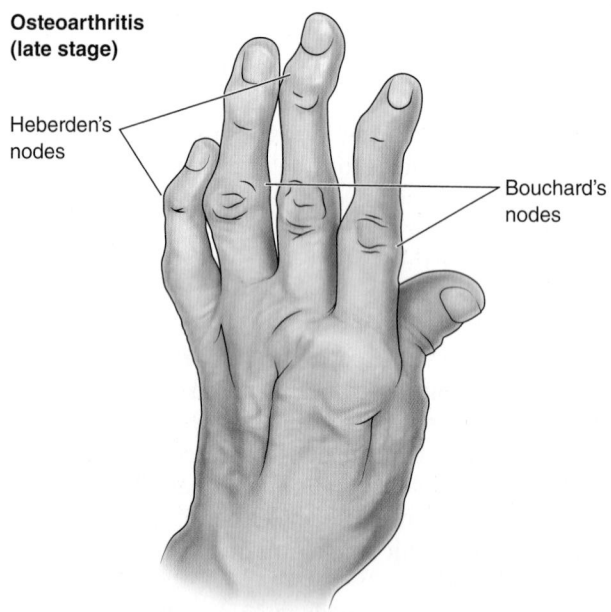

Osteoarthritis (late stage)

Heberden's nodes

Bouchard's nodes

FIGURE 38-3. In OA, the hands can develop two kinds of deformity. Heberden's nodes are swellings in the distal interphalangeal joints. Bouchard's nodes are swellings in the proximal interphalangeal joints.

Also, during the physical examination, it is important for the clinician to differentiate OA from RA. In early RA, the patient's joints may present similarly with swelling, tenderness, and limited ROM. However, RA is an autoimmune disease that is accompanied by systemic symptoms such as fever, elevated WBC count, and other signs of inflammation. The joints are often not affected symmetrically in RA as in OA, and there is greater joint deformity in RA. The hands, especially the metacarpal and phalangeal joints, are particularly affected by RA, and abnormalities are apparent on examination (see Table 38-2).

Diagnosis

No specific laboratory tests can provide a diagnosis of OA, but biochemical markers such as serum osteocalcin and hyaluronic acid levels can reflect the presence of synovitis in earlier stages of the disorder. In turn, the biochemical markers can be a valuable tool in evaluating the effects of specific treatments in the course of OA progression. Clinical examination can often provide a diagnosis with reasonable certainty, with actual confirmation of OA made through x-rays. OA is characterized on x-ray by joint space narrowing and with the presence of osteophyte and subchondral sclerosis. MRI is often indicated only if abnormalities other than OA are expected based on symptomatology and the physical examination.

Treatment

Treatment goals are to relieve pain, maintain mobility, and minimize disability. Treatment includes exercise and lifestyle modification, use of medications, supportive measures to reduce stress on the affected joint, and, in some cases, surgery. Conservative measures such as weight control and a balance of rest

TABLE 38-2. The Differences Between Osteoarthritis and Rheumatoid Arthritis		
	OA	**RA**
Etiology	Degenerative joint disease caused by aging or excessive trauma to a joint	Autoimmune disease; antigen unknown; autoantibodies found in joint space
Incidence	10% of population	1% of population
Joints Most Commonly Affected	Knee, hip, hand, and proximal interphalangeal and distal interphalangeal joints	Hand; metacarpophalangeal joints
Pathophysiology	Joint swelling and osteophyte formation	Joint swelling and deformity, intense inflammation with joint erosion
Symptoms	Joint pain, stiffness, and tenderness worst in morning; better as day progresses	Joint pain, stiffness, tenderness, and systemic symptoms such as fever, myalgias, and fatigue
Major Treatments	Acetaminophen, NSAIDs, COX-2 inhibitors, glucosamine chondroitin, cortisone injections, hyaluronic acid injections, joint replacement	Methotrexate and monoclonal antibody biological agents

with low-impact exercises can be very helpful. Regular exercise, such as daily walking or swimming, is encouraged. These measures alone can relieve joint stress and delay the progression of OA.

Medications include various NSAIDs. These act by inhibiting the formation of prostaglandins, which are key components in inflammation. Ibuprofen is a common drug used for this purpose.

> ALERT! Risks of long-term NSAID use include peptic ulcer with gastrointestinal bleeding and kidney failure.

The use of oral steroids is not recommended for treatment of OA; however, intra-articular injection of glucocorticoids such as hydrocortisone can provide short-term pain relief lasting from a few weeks to a few months. Artificial joint fluid containing hyaluronic acid, such as Synvisc, can also be given via intra-articular injection to provide pain relief for up to 6 months.

Effective treatment also includes reducing stress on the affected joint by supporting or stabilizing it with braces and assistive devices, such as a cane or walker. Other supportive measures include the use of moist heat, massage, and low-intensity exercises that help to regain or maintain motion and flexibility of the joint and ligaments.

Surgery may be necessary when the disease has progressed in severity and other measures have become ineffective. Referral of patients with end-stage OA to a surgeon should be considered if all appropriate conservative options, delivered for 6 months, have been unsuccessful. An osteotomy can be performed to relieve stress on the joint by changing the alignment of bone. This can be done through excision of bone spurs. An osteoplasty, the scraping and removal of deteriorated bone from the joint, can also be performed. Arthrodesis, the surgical fusion of bones, is used primarily in the spine. Lastly, partial or total joint arthroplasty is a common procedure in which the deteriorated bone is removed and replaced with a prosthetic appliance; the knee and hip are the joints most commonly replaced by prostheses. Total joint replacement is recommended if there is marked joint space narrowing and evidence of bone loss. The epidemic of obesity has increased the need for total hip and knee replacements.

Rickets

Rickets is a failure of osteoid calcification due to a genetic, nutritional, or metabolic disorder involving bone development. In children, there is a lack of mineralization in the growth plates of bone. The majority of cases are either due to vitamin D or calcium deficiency. The incidence and prevalence of rickets are difficult to estimate, as different regions of the world vary in their rates. Calcium deficiency continues to be a major cause of rickets in Africa and Asia. Vitamin D–deficiency rickets is increasing in the Americas, Europe, and parts of the Middle East. Vitamin D deficiency is pandemic in Europe, affecting nearly 18% of the population in winter, but with 3 to 71 times higher risk in dark-skinned ethnic minority groups. Public health studies have identified traditional diets low in calcium, dark skin, and cultural full-body clothing as the predominant causes of rickets and osteomalacia in sunny parts of the world such as the Indian subcontinent, the Middle East, and Africa. In high northern or southern latitudes the seasonal lack of the ultraviolet-B (UV-B) spectrum of sunlight causes seasonal vitamin D deficiency (also called "vitamin D winter"). In high-latitude countries, the dark-skinned immigrant and resident population is at greatest risk.

According to the Centers for Disease Control and Prevention, the incidence of rickets in America has been rising in the past few decades. However, there are very few recent studies regarding the actual incidence in the United States. A retrospective study shows there has been a sixfold increase in cases of rickets in children between 1990 and 2000. In 1990, the incidence of rickets was 3.7 per 100,000, and this number rose to 24.1 per 100,000 children in 2000. There is a greater incidence of rickets in impoverished children and higher incidence among African American children in the United States compared with European American children. The incidence has been particularly high in breastfed infants. Vitamin D deficiency in the pregnant and lactating mother predisposes to the development of rickets in the breastfed infant. Rickets is most commonly diagnosed in children by age 2. Reasons for the increasing incidence of rickets in children include lack of sufficient calcium and vitamin D in the diet, excessive sunscreen use in children that blocks sunlight, cultural practices that require totally covering the body, and breastfeeding by females who are deficient in calcium and vitamin D. Currently, there is also a tendency for children to spend more time indoors instead of playing outdoors in the sun.

Etiology

There are several different types of rickets: nutritional, congenital, vitamin D resistant, hypophosphatemic, neoplastic, drug induced, and rickets of prematurity. Nutritional rickets can occur as a consequence of inadequate intake of calcium, vitamin D, phosphate, or a combination of these. Congenital rickets and vitamin D–resistant rickets result from a genetic deficiency in the enzyme that converts calcidiol to calcitriol in the kidney. Inheritance is autosomal recessive, and the gene is located in band 12q13.3. Hypophosphatemic rickets is a metabolic disorder caused by homozygous loss-of-function mutations in the *SLC34A3* gene, which in turn causes the kidneys to fail to reabsorb phosphate. Drug-induced rickets can occur in patients who take anti-convulsant medications, corticosteroids, or certain cholesterol-controlling medication.

Neoplastic rickets is a paraneoplastic syndrome with hypophosphatemia secondary to decreased renal phosphate reabsorption, normal or low serum 1,25-dihydroxyvitamin D concentration, osteomalacia, and myopathy. Several mesenchymal tumors of bone or connective tissue (including nonossifying fibromas, fibroangioma, and giant cell tumors) secrete a phosphaturic substance (parathyroid-like protein) that results in rickets. Rickets can also occur due to suboptimal sunlight exposure, which leads to vitamin D deficiency. Rickets can develop in pediatric patients with malabsorption syndromes or end-stage renal disease. Breastfed infants may also develop rickets, as human milk contains only 20 to 40 IU/L of vitamin D.

Pathophysiology

Rickets is mainly caused by a deficiency of vitamin D, which is required for calcium absorption from the intestine. Cholecalciferol (vitamin D_3) is formed in the skin when exposed to sunlight and is also attained from the diet. After activation by sunlight, cholecalciferol undergoes hydroxylation in the liver and kidney and then becomes the active metabolite calcitriol (chemical name 1,25-dihydroxycholecalciferol). Calcitriol acts at three sites to regulate calcium metabolism: (1) it promotes absorption of calcium and phosphorus from the intestine into the bloodstream; (2) it increases reabsorption of phosphate in the kidney; and (3) it acts on bone to release calcium and phosphate into the bloodstream. Calcitriol also directly facilitates calcification of bone. These actions result in an increase in the concentrations of calcium and phosphorus in the bloodstream, which in turn leads to the calcification of osteoid. Calcification primarily occurs at the growth plates of bones in children. Calcification affects the formation of all osteoid in the skeleton in adults.

In the absence of vitamin D, the body only absorbs 5% to 15% of dietary calcium and 50% to 60% of dietary phosphorus—the major minerals that compose bone. Hypocalcemia causes neuromuscular irritability and bone degeneration. A drop in serum-ionized calcium triggers the parathyroid glands to release PTH, which acts on bone to release calcium. The loss of calcium from bones causes the major pathology in rickets—bone weakness, bone deformity, and susceptibility to fracture.

Clinical Presentation

In the history, malnutrition, intestinal malabsorption, lack of milk products, or lack of sunlight may be reported. The pathological process generally begins in infants between 4 and 12 months of age. A child usually experiences symptoms by age 2 and is brought to the attention of a clinician. Rickets affects bone development in infants because the long bone regions of growth, called the epiphyses, and costochondral junctions, are rapidly expanding at this time. X-rays in children with rickets show irregular, widened growth plates with cupping and fraying of bone. Malformation of these bone regions causes protrusion of the sternum and tibial and femoral bowing. Thoracic asymmetry and widening of the thoracic base is a result of muscle traction on the softened rib cage. Delay in fontanelle closure is also a physical sign of this disease. Tooth development may be affected, resulting in delayed tooth eruption, enamel hypoplasia, and early dental caries. Physical deformities become apparent when rickets is present for months to years. These deformities can include low height and weight for age, enlargement at the ends of bones, craniotabes (softening of cranial bones), and torsional deformities of the extremities. Proximal muscle weakness and delayed gross motor milestones are apparent in infants and toddlers. Carpopedal (wrist) spasms, tetany, seizures, laryngospasms, and hypocalcemic cardiomyopathy can also occur because of the hypocalcemia. Hematological disorders seen in children with rickets include hypochromic anemia and hypoplastic bone marrow. The spleen and liver can become enlarged because they begin to take over hematopoiesis in bone marrow failure.

Diagnosis

A patient presenting with the symptoms of rickets requires laboratory tests that measure serum and ionized calcium levels, serum alkaline phosphatase, serum phosphorus, 25-hydroxyvitamin D, 1,25 hydroxyvitamin D, PTH levels, and urine calcium. Serum calcium, vitamin D, and phosphorus levels will be low. PTH levels and alkaline phosphatase levels will be elevated. X-rays will show the common changes that occur in rickets, such as varus deformity (bowing) of the legs, costochondral swellings called "rachitic rosary," lumbar lordosis, widened wrists and knees, and greenstick fractures. An x-ray of an anterior view of the knee is the best single x-ray for infants and children younger than 3 years. This view can demonstrate the metaphyseal end and epiphysis of the femur and tibia, which have rapid growth at these ages.

Treatment

The best treatment strategy for rickets is to prevent vitamin D deficiency. Poor calcium intake by a pregnant mother predisposes the infant to bone malformations. Prenatal vitamins with vitamin D and calcium are necessary for optimal maternal child health, as well as increased consumption of fortified daily products. Breastfed infants should receive vitamin D supplementation of at least 400 IU/day. For older children, dairy products should be fortified with vitamin D to ensure adequate intake. Children and adolescents should get regular exposure to sunlight and drink at least 500 mL of vitamin D–fortified milk daily.

Vitamin D loading is necessary for those afflicted with rickets. Vitamin D treatment may be administered gradually over several months or in a single-day dose of 15,000 mcg (600,000 U) of vitamin D. Using the gradual method, 125 to 250 mcg (5,000 to 10,000 U) is given daily for 2 to 3 months until healing is established and the alkaline phosphatase concentration normalizes. If the vitamin D dose is administered in a single day, it is usually divided into four or six oral doses. An intramuscular injection is also available. Vitamin D (cholecalciferol) is a fat-soluble vitamin that is well stored in the body and released gradually over many weeks. Studies show that children with rickets require a daily calcium intake of 1,000 mg or 2,000 mg over 24 weeks. Daily UV light exposure of 10 to 30 minutes is also needed for vitamin D metabolism. Darker-skinned children may require a longer period of light exposure. Physical therapy and weight-bearing exercise are important to strengthen bone and muscle tone.

Osteomalacia

Osteomalacia is a disorder of vitamin D deficiency that is similar to rickets, only it occurs in adults. In adults, vitamin D deficiency is not necessarily caused by malnutrition; rather, lack of sufficient exposure to sunlight, renal disorders, cancer, and malabsorption most commonly cause this adult disorder.

The incidence of vitamin D deficiency has largely decreased because of the use of fortified milk and vitamin supplements in the Western world. Despite this, vitamin D–related osteomalacia occurs in certain populations at risk, including the homebound older adults who have little sun exposure, as well as insufficient dietary calcium and vitamin D; patients with malabsorption related to gastrointestinal bypass surgery or celiac disease; and immigrants to cold climates from warm climates, especially females who wear traditional veils or dresses that prevent sun exposure.

Etiology
Osteomalacia can result from low nutritional intake of vitamin D, abnormal vitamin D metabolism, chronic renal failure, tumor-induced osteomalacia, and certain ingested substances such as aluminum or fluoride. Other causes of this condition include cancer, liver disorders, use of anticonvulsant medication, and poor phosphates in the diet.

Pathophysiology
The basic problem in osteomalacia is lack of calcium absorption caused by vitamin D deficiency. Hypocalcemia then stimulates the parathyroid gland to secrete PTH, which causes breakdown of bone in order to raise blood calcium levels. Consequently, individuals suffer bone demineralization. Because bones become weakened, ambulation becomes difficult, and intense bone pain occurs.

Additionally, with the lack of vitamin D and calcium, the parathyroid glands keep secreting PTH in an attempt to raise blood levels of calcium. As a result, the parathyroid glands become overactive. Secondary hyperparathyroidism is thus a feature of osteomalacia. Osteomalacia is often misdiagnosed as fibromyalgia, chronic pain syndrome, or dysthymia (depression).

Clinical Presentation
The patient will often present to the clinician because of lumbar back pain. The patient usually reports that walking—particularly upstairs—is difficult. The clinician should investigate the patient's current medications, medical and surgical history, and family history. Renal failure and intestinal malabsorption may be reported in the history. The patient's diet and lifestyle also should be described. The patient may have malabsorption of calcium, lack of sunlight exposure, or lack of fortified dairy products in the diet. Alternatively, ingestion of aluminum or excess fluoride can cause osteomalacia.

Osteomalacia is a difficult diagnosis that is made mainly via laboratory testing. In a physical examination, the patient with osteomalacia may feel pain when pressure is applied to the sternum or anterior tibia. Symptomatic proximal muscle weakness and diffuse bone pain are also part of the physical findings. With symptomatic proximal muscle weakness, the patient has difficulty rising from a squatting position. The patient may experience diffuse bone pain from stress fractures in the axial skeleton and lower extremities.

Diagnosis
Abnormal blood test results that characterize osteomalacia include low 25-hydroxyvitamin D, elevated PTH level, hypophosphatemia, and elevated alkaline phosphatase. There is usually a normal calcium level until late in the progression of the disease.

Radiological findings for this condition are nonspecific generalized osteopenia noted on x-ray. A DEXA scan can best demonstrate osteopenia. Pseudofracture, also called Looser's zones, can be found along the surfaces and shafts of long bones. A pseudofracture is a band of bone material with decreased density along the surface of bone that gives the appearance of a partial fracture. Subperiosteal resorption, increased cortical thinning, and bone porosity are x-ray findings that occur because of secondary hyperparathyroidism caused by osteomalacia. CT, MRI, or technetium bone scans can confirm the diagnosis. In some cases, a bone biopsy may assist in the diagnosis.

Treatment
In osteomalacia, vitamin D deficiency and low phosphate levels require correction. Initial vitamin D supplements would include 50,000 IU of ergocalciferol (vitamin D_2) until normalized. Maintenance doses

would be 1,000 IU of vitamin D_3 (Calcitriol) daily. If the underlying etiology is tumor-induced osteomalacia, removal of the tumor would reverse this condition. The patient should get adequate sunlight and increase calcium in the diet.

Increased ingestion of foods high in phosphates helps lessen the hypophosphatemia. In addition, phosphate supplements may be needed. Parenteral nutrition may also be necessary in some incidents. Foods such as dairy products, hard cheeses, eggs, bread products that contain baking powder, yeast and beef extracts, herrings, kippers, and sardines can help increase phosphate levels.

Degenerative Disc Disease

DDD is a common cause of pain, motor weakness, and neuropathy. The disorder has effects on the nervous system because anatomically the vertebrae and discs surround the spinal nerves. Motor spinal nerves exit from the spinal cord and travel through narrow openings of the vertebral bone out to the periphery to stimulate muscles of the extremities. Similarly, sensory spinal nerves from the extremities enter the spinal cord through narrow vertebral bone apertures carrying sensory messages from the environment. With age, intervertebral discs and vertebral bone become compressed. The openings in the vertebrae often become so narrow that the bone or discs impinge on the entering and exiting nerves. With impingement on nerves, DDD can cause pain and dysfunction of motor and sensory spinal nerves and impede movement and sensation in the extremities.

The disorder most commonly occurs in the cervical and lumbar regions of the vertebral column. DDD of the lumbar vertebrae is a common cause of low back pain, which is the second most common reason for patient visits to primary health-care providers. DDD of lumbar through sacral vertebrae is commonly referred to as sciatica, as the sciatic nerve is impinged. Seventy percent of cases of low back pain are caused by lumbar strain or sprain, 10% are caused by age-related degenerative changes in the intervertebral discs, 4% are caused by herniated discs, 4% are caused by osteoporotic compression fractures, and 3% are caused by spinal stenosis. All other causes account for less than 1% of cases.

Back pain is the most common cause of work-related disability in persons younger than 45 years in the United States. Back pain is commonly caused by lumbar DDD, and it affects males and females equally. Lumbar DDD onset most often occurs between ages 30 and 50 years. DDD of the cervical spine also commonly occurs but can be silent; it can be observed with MRI in 25% of asymptomatic individuals aged younger than 40 years and 60% of those aged older than 40 years. The true incidence and prevalence of cervical DDD are uncertain; however, 51% of adults experience neck and arm pain at some point in their lifetime.

Etiology

DDD is a disorder of the intervertebral discs—the fibrocartilaginous cushions that are located between the vertebral bones and allow for vertebral flexibility. The discs, which normally act as spongy shock absorbers for the spine, deteriorate, resulting in malalignment of the spinal column. The intervertebral disc is considered the most critical component of the load-bearing structures of the spinal column. DDD causes malalignment of the vertebral bones which, in turn, increases susceptibility to spinal nerve impingement; this is also called **radiculopathy.**

> **CLINICAL CONCEPT**
>
> Cervical and lumbar radiculopathy are the most common types of spinal nerve impingement disorders.

Risk factors include heavy lifting, sudden traumatic twisting of the torso, obesity, family history, aggressive exercise routine, and poor physical conditioning. There is also a genetic predisposition to DDD.

Pathophysiology

DDD most often occurs due to intervertebral disc flattening in the cervical or lumbar region of the vertebral spine. The intervertebral disc consists of a gelatinous center called the nucleus pulposus, which is surrounded by strong cartilage called the annulus fibrosus. With age, discs lose moisture and change from supple structures that are flexible to rigid structures with less elasticity. As discs flatten and collapse, there is consequent malalignment of the vertebral bones. With a herniated disc, the nucleus pulposus is squeezed out of place and bulges through the annulus fibrosus. A herniated disc often causes impingement on a spinal nerve, which can cause motor and sensory problems in the region supplied by that nerve.

Osteophyte formation is a common occurrence in DDD; these bony formations can narrow the spinal canal—a condition called spinal stenosis (see Fig. 38-4). Disc degeneration can also lead to disorders such as spondylolisthesis (forward slippage of the disc and vertebrae) and retrolisthesis (backward slippage of the disc and vertebrae).

Clinical Presentation

The patient with lumbar DDD will commonly present to the clinician because of back pain, weakness, or numbness in a lower extremity. Cervical DDD causes neck pain, weakness, or numbness in an upper

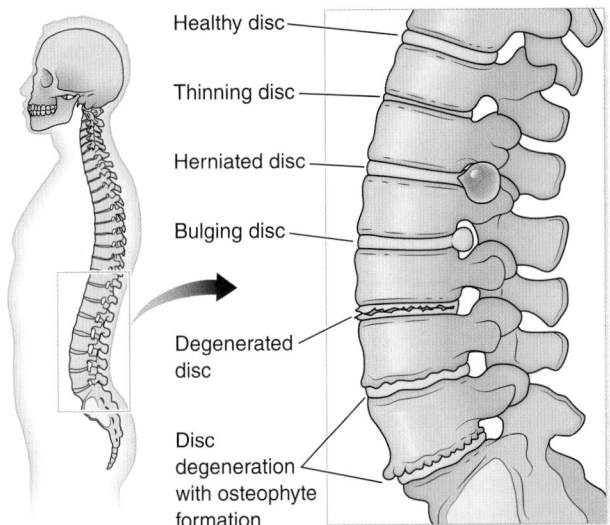

Healthy disc

Thinning disc

Herniated disc

Bulging disc

Degenerated disc

Disc degeneration with osteophyte formation

FIGURE 38-4. Degenerative disc disorders include disc thinning and compression, herniated disc, and osteophyte (bone spur) formation. Any of these problems can cause spinal nerve impingement.

BOX 38-5. Signs and Symptoms of Degenerative Disc Disease

Signs and symptoms of lumbar DDD include:
- Pain in the low back that radiates down the back of the leg (also called sciatica)
- Pain in the buttocks or thighs
- Pain that worsens when sitting, bending, lifting, or twisting
- Pain that is minimized when walking, changing positions, or lying down
- Numbness, tingling, or weakness in the legs
- Foot drop
  Signs and symptoms of cervical DDD include:
- Chronic neck pain that can radiate to the shoulders and down the arms
- Numbness or tingling in the arm or hand
- Weakness of the arm or hand

extremity. The pain is described as radiating down the back of the leg or down the arm. A history of heavy-force trauma, twisting injury, or heavy lifting can provoke the painful event.

The diagnosis of DDD requires a physical examination, with special attention paid to the musculoskeletal and neurological system of the back and extremities. This involves testing muscle strength, deep tendon reflexes, and sensory dermatomes. The dermatomes can give information about which spinal nerve is involved in the disorder. Dermatome maps are helpful in interpreting the level and extent of sensory deficits that are the result of spinal nerve impingement or spinal cord injury.

With a herniated disc, pain is usually intensified with coughing, sneezing, straining, stooping, standing, or jarring motions. Motor weakness, sensory deficit, and decreased deep tendon reflexes can occur in the upper extremities in cervical DDD, whereas motor weakness, sensory deficit, and ambulation problems may occur in lumbar DDD (see Box 38-5).

The most common vertebral discs involved in DDD are the lumbar and sacral: L4, L5, and S1. The lumbar spinal nerves L4–S1 make up the sciatic nerve, which arises from the spinal cord and travels down the lower extremity. When lumbar spinal nerve 4 (L4) is involved, the patella reflex may be diminished. When L5 is affected, dorsiflexion of the foot is difficult. When S1 is affected, the Achilles reflex may be diminished and plantar flexion of the foot may be difficult. The most common sensory deficits from spinal nerve impingement are paresthesias, particularly of the leg and foot. Spinal nerve impingement in the L4 through S1 regions is often referred to as **sciatica.**

During the physical examination, the clinician should perform a straight-leg raising test. During this test, the clinician places the patient in the supine position and raises the patient's leg on the affected side. The maneuver applies traction along the sciatic nerve, exacerbating pain if the nerve is irritated. The test is positive if pain is produced when the leg is raised to 60 degrees or less and dorsiflexion of the foot causes pain in the back.

CLINICAL CONCEPT

Signs of nerve impingement at L4–L5 include weak or absent ability to dorsiflex the foot, sensory loss in the lower leg and foot, and decreased patella reflex. Signs of nerve impingement at L5–S1 include weak or absent ability to plantarflex the foot, sensory loss in the lower leg and foot, and decreased Achilles reflex.

Diagnosis

Tests useful in diagnosing DDD include x-ray, CT, myelography, and MRI. MRI is the preferred imaging procedure as it can demonstrate multiplanar evaluation with good soft tissue contrast, giving more accurate interpretation of disc changes. An MRI can be used to identify the type of degenerative disc changes according to the Pfirrmann classification for disc morphology. The Pfirrmann classification describes the stages of changes in disc degeneration progression from one stage to the next, becoming more progressive in the destruction of disc architecture, in moving from grade I to V. Generally, grades I–III are early disc degeneration and grades IV–V are advanced disc degeneration. Electromyography can also be used to help identify peripheral neuropathies caused by associated nerve root irritation.

Specific laboratory tests can be used as a complement to other forms of testing and screen for causes of spinal pain not related to disc disease or arthritis. These include complete blood count, differential WBC count, serum protein electrophoresis, and erythrocyte sedimentation rate.

Treatment

Treatments for DDD include both conservative and surgical measures; conservative measures are usually tried first. These noninvasive measures include physical therapy, pain management techniques, and alternatives such as chiropractic care. The goal of these measures is to alleviate pain and increase mobility.

Physical Therapy. Physical therapists use a variety of techniques in the treatment of back pain, including the use of heat and cold packs, electrotherapies, massage, biofeedback, traction, and therapeutic exercise. The use of braces limits spinal motion and therefore enhances healing. Bracing is also used for support following specific spinal surgical procedures, such as fusions. Depending on the problem, both rigid and soft braces are available. The goal is to provide support to the spine and rest for the spinal muscles.

Pain Management. Traditional drug therapy for those with DDD may include options such as acetaminophen, NSAIDs, muscle relaxants, narcotics, and antidepressants. Narcotics are prescribed for short-term use because of their addictive potential. Antidepressants have analgesic properties and can also improve sleep.

Interventional pain management techniques use injections to an identified area to reduce pain. Of these techniques, epidural steroid injections are the most common. An anti-inflammatory agent, usually cortisone, is injected in the area surrounding a specific nerve or region of the spinal canal. The cortisone reduces swelling in the area, thus reducing pain. These injections can last for weeks to months, depending on the individual, and can help patients benefit from their therapy programs.

Chiropractic Care. Chiropractic therapy focuses on adjustment and manipulation techniques of the articulating joints and tissues of the spine. The goal of chiropractic manipulation is to take pressure off sensitive neurological tissue, thereby increasing ROM. This, in turn, will restore blood flow and reduce muscle tension.

Surgery. If conservative treatments are not successful, surgery may be recommended. It is often necessary when back or leg pain limits normal activity and when there is weakness or numbness in the legs, making walking or standing difficult. If the lumbosacral spinal nerves are compressed and causing bladder or bowel dysfunction, immediate surgery is necessary.

> **ALERT!** Compressed lumbosacral nerves in DDD, which cause loss of bowel or bladder function, is called cauda equina syndrome (CES). This is a medical emergency (see Box 38-6).

Traditional surgical options for DDD include decompression and stabilization surgery. Decompression surgery involves removal of tissue pressing on a nerve. Decompression surgery can be done through various methods. Mechanical decompression involves water- and air-driven suction cutting probes using CT guidance or fluoroscopic guidance to remove the bulging disc material. Decompression surgery also involves removal of bone termed facetectomy, laminectomy, laminotomy, and foraminotomy. Thermal decompression uses lasers to remove the bulging disc material and relieve nerve impingement. Chemical decompression uses chymopapain, a proteolytic enzyme, or ethanol to decompose the bulging disc tissue.

Minimally invasive techniques in decompression surgery using endoscopic procedures have recently become popular. Endoscopy also allows spine surgeons to navigate to areas that were not accessible previously. Having a magnified endoscopic view of the intervertebral disc and dura, one can safely decompress the neural elements of adhesion from DDD, and provide targeted radiofrequency to specific pain-generating nerves.

Following decompression, the spine may be unstable, thus requiring stabilization surgery or spinal fusion surgery, which joins two or more vertebra into one single stabilized unit. Often, decompression and stabilization surgery are performed at the same time. As with decompression, spinal fusion can be performed anteriorly or posteriorly, depending on the disease specifics. Spinal fusion surgery involves removal of the intervertebral disc material and then filling in this space with bone graft. Bone grafts are usually autografts; in many cases, taken from the patient's pelvic bones. However, allograft or cadaveric bone may be used if the patient has poor bone quality, such as occurs in osteoporosis. Bone graft substitutes, biological substances that can stimulate bone growth, are also available. In some cases, a surgeon may insert sterile spinal hardware, such as rods, screws, or wires, to increase spine stability as the bones fuse.

Spinal Stenosis

Spinal stenosis is an anatomical narrowing of the intervertebral foramina or nerve root canal in the vertebrae that allow spinal nerves to enter and leave

BOX 38-6. Cauda Equina Syndrome

Emerging from the lumbar and sacral nerve roots is the cauda equina. These nerves control sphincter muscles, sexual function, perineal sensation, and sensation and motor function throughout the legs. Damage to this area is known as CES. Causes of CES include fracture or dislocation of the lumbar part of the spine, herniated lumbar discs, spinal stenosis, neoplasms, and inflammatory conditions such as Paget's disease and ankylosing spondylitis. CES causes weakness of the legs, leads to bowel and bladder dysfunction, and requires immediate treatment.

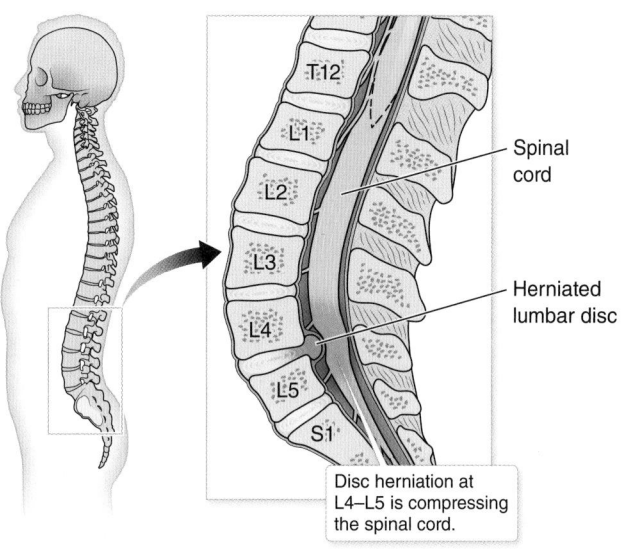

Spinal cord

Herniated lumbar disc

Disc herniation at L4–L5 is compressing the spinal cord.

the spinal cord. The narrowing of the vertebral openings causes nerve impingement and entrapment, termed radiculopathy. The lumbar and cervical regions are most commonly involved.

Approximately 250,000 to 500,000 persons in the United States have symptoms of spinal stenosis. This represents about 1 of every 1,000 persons older than age 65 years. Lumbar spinal stenosis is the leading diagnosis for adults older than 65 years who undergo spine surgery. The incidence of spinal nerve entrapment is reported as 8% to 11%. The lower lumbar nerves that are involved most often include L5 (75%), L4 (15%), L3 (5.3%), and L2 (4%).

Etiology
Narrowing of the bony parts of the spinal column can be congenital, acquired, or both. Some people are born with a small spinal canal, but acquired spinal stenosis can occur from trauma or spinal tumors. Aging is often a factor in the formation of spinal stenosis. The intervertebral discs deteriorate with age, and arthritis of the spine commonly occurs. These changes can narrow the nerve root canals and put pressure on the spinal nerves.

Pathophysiology
Spinal stenosis is the narrowing of the lower vertebrae that causes compression on spinal nerves. The patient often has a history of DDD, and spinal stenosis develops over time. It is usually not related to a traumatic event, but it is related to gradual spinal degeneration; most commonly, narrowing of the space around the spinal cord is caused by bony overgrowth (osteophytes) from OA or DDD as a result of aging. Osteophytes can compress a spinal nerve and cause pain, sensory disturbances, and motor symptoms.

Clinical Presentation
The first step in diagnosing spinal stenosis is conducting a medical history and a physical examination. Symptoms related to spinal stenosis are similar to those of intervertebral disc herniation. Commonly, the compressed nerve causes paresthesias, pain, and weakness of the limbs. Cervical spinal stenosis causes symptoms in the arms, whereas lumbar spinal stenosis causes symptoms in the legs.

Specific signs and symptoms of spinal stenosis include:

- Back pain in lumbar spinal stenosis or neck pain in cervical spinal stenosis
- Numbness, weakness, cramping, or pain in the legs or arms in lumbar spinal stenosis or cervical spinal stenosis, respectively, and foot drop in lumbar spinal stenosis
- Incontinence in severe spinal stenosis caused by impingement of sacral nerves that control bladder and bowel function.

Diagnosis and Treatment

Diagnostic procedures for spinal stenosis include spinal x-ray, MRI, CT, myelogram, and bone scan. In the majority of patients, symptoms of spinal stenosis respond favorably to nonoperative management. Medical management usually begins with rest, NSAIDs, muscle relaxants, and physical therapy. If there is little relief from the NSAIDs, opioid analgesics and steroid injections may be helpful. Epidural steroid injections and nerve blocks may also relieve the discomfort. In addition, alternative therapies such as acupuncture and chiropractic intervention may be utilized. Nonsurgical treatment is used initially unless the symptoms are intolerable and prevent the patient from normal functioning. For example, a decompressive laminectomy may be performed to relieve pressure on the nerve roots and vertebroplasty used to prevent spinal instability. Problems with bowel or bladder function require immediate decompression surgery.

Chapter Summary

- Osteoporosis is a disorder of bone demineralization that occurs with aging. Lack of calcium or vitamin D in the diet, immobility, age, gender, genetics, and certain medications can predispose patients to osteoporosis.

- Osteoporosis often causes hip, wrist, or vertebral compression fractures.

- A DEXA scan is necessary to visualize BMD in order to diagnose osteoporosis.

- Calcium and vitamin D supplements, bisphosphonates, and calcitonin are used to treat osteoporosis.

- OA commonly occurs with aging.

- Obesity, repetitive trauma to a joint, age, and genetic predisposition place a patient at risk for OA.

- OA can appear like RA; however, RA is an autoimmune disease.

- Osteomalacia (also called rickets when occurring in children) is degeneration of bone caused by hyperparathyroidism, or insufficient calcium or vitamin D in the diet.

- Osteophytes are common outgrowths of osteoarthritic bone surfaces that can impinge on nerves and cause pain.

- DDD often causes impingement on spinal nerves. Cervical and lumbosacral intervertebral discs are most often affected.

- A herniated disc often causes impingement on a spinal nerve, also called radiculopathy. Spinal nerve impingement commonly causes weakness or paresthesias of an extremity.

- The most common DDD is sciatica, impingement on the sciatic nerve that causes pain radiating down the leg.

- X-rays are commonly used for diagnosis of degenerative diseases of the musculoskeletal system. However, x-rays are often insufficient, and CT scan, DEXA scan, or MRI are necessary.

- Nonsurgical therapies commonly used in DDD include NSAIDs, epidural steroid or analgesic injections, and muscle relaxants.

- Surgical procedures include decompression and spinal stabilization where herniation of intervertebral disc ablation and vertebral fusion can diminish nerve impingement.

Making the Connections

Signs and Symptoms	Physical Assessment Findings	Diagnostic Testing	Treatment
Osteoporosis | Bone demineralization caused by greater osteoclastic activity compared with osteoblastic activity. Trabecular bone has high susceptibility to fracture, especially the wrist, upper femur (hip), and vertebrae.			
Often no symptoms until vertebral collapse that can cause back pain.	Loss of height. Kyphosis. Fracture (hip, wrist, vertebrae).	DEXA scan; specifically measures bone density in lumbar spine and hip. BMD is 2.5 standard deviations or more below the normal mean for young adult females (T score at or below −2.5).	Weight-bearing exercise to strengthen bone by stimulating osteoblastic activity. Calcium 1,200 mg/daily to strengthen bone. Vitamin D 400 IU/daily to increase calcium absorption. Bisphosphonates to inhibit osteoclastic activity. Raloxifene, an estrogen-like medication that strengthens bone. Teriparatide (or PTH) to strengthen bone. Denosumab, a biological agent. Vertebroplasty or kyphoplasty to fortify osteoporotic bone.
Osteoarthritis (OA) | Slowly progressive, degenerative, and inflammatory disease. Excess pressure on a joint gradually wears away the cartilage surface, exposing the subchondral bone. Inflammation occurs as cytokines, various inflammatory mediators, and metalloproteases are released into the joint and degrade the cartilage. Osteophytes form along the margin of cartilage loss, impinging on nerves and causing pain.			
Pain, stiffness of joints, decreased ROM, and swelling of joints.	Tenderness of joints, decreased ROM, swelling of joints, crepitus heard with joint motion. Heberden's nodes. Bouchard's nodes.	X-ray, CT, MRI.	Moist heat to decrease muscle spasm and pain. NSAIDs to decrease inflammation. Intra-articular injection of glucocorticoid decreases pain and inflammation. Supportive devices such as walker or lumbar brace support. Surgery, including osteotomy, osteoplasty, and arthroplasty, that fortifies joints.
Rickets | A failure of osteoid calcification due to a genetic, nutritional, or metabolic disorder involving bone development. In children there is a lack of mineralization in the growth plates of bone. The majority of cases are either due to vitamin D or calcium deficiency.			
Short stature; lack of bone growth. Deformity of bones caused by hypocalcemia. Muscle cramping caused by hypocalcemia.	Short stature. Deformity of bones. Muscle cramping. Seizures. Tooth hypoplasia.	Serum and ionized calcium, serum alkaline phosphatase, serum phosphorus, 25-hydroxyvitamin D, hydroxyvitamin D, PTH levels, and urine calcium.	Vitamin D (Calcitriol) to increase absorption of calcium from gastrointestinal tract. Calcium supplement in diet to strengthen bone.

Continued

Making the Connections—cont'd

Signs and Symptoms	Physical Assessment Findings	Diagnostic Testing	Treatment
Seizures caused by hypocalcemia. Tooth hypoplasia.		X-rays will show varus deformity (bowing) of the legs, costochondral swellings called "rachitic rosary," lumbar lordosis, widened wrists and knees, and greenstick fractures.	Phosphorus in diet to strengthen bone. Sunlight to activate vitamin D.

Osteomalacia | Lack of calcification of bones caused by deficient vitamin D or calcium in adult.

| Bone pain. | Tenderness of bone.
Difficulty with ambulation. | X-ray, vitamin D level, calcium level, phosphate level. | Vitamin D to increase calcium absorption.
Calcium supplement to strengthen bones.
Phosphorus in diet to strengthen bone.
Sunlight to activate vitamin D. |

Degenerative Disc Disease (DDD) | Intervertebral discs dehydrate and collapse, causing malalignment of the discs and vertebral bones. In a herniated disc, the central nucleus pulposus tissue of the disc is squeezed out of place and bulges through the annulus fibrosus, causing impingement on a spinal nerve. Spinal nerve impingement causes inflammation, pain, paralysis, lack of sensation, and paresthesias in the region supplied by the spinal nerve. Most common discs involved are L4, L5, and S1.

| Pain (cervical or lumbar commonly) with radiation (legs or arms commonly), numbness, paresthesias, difficulty walking if DDD in lower spine. | Tenderness of site of DDD, paraspinal muscle spasm, numbness in arms or legs depending on site of DDD. | X-ray, CT, or MRI can demonstrate disc collapse and vertebral malalignment. Electromyography can show muscle dysfunction. | Heat to reduce pain and muscle spasm.
NSAIDs to decrease inflammation.
Short-term narcotic to relieve pain of spinal nerve impingement.
Muscle relaxants to reduce muscle spasm.
Antidepressants to decrease neuropathic pain.
Intra-articular injection of glucocorticoid diminishes inflammation.
Physical therapy attempts to realign vertebrae, strengthen muscles, and decrease spasm.
Acupuncture is used for pain relief.
Chiropractic treatments are used to realign discs.
Supportive devices, such as walker or cervical collar, are used to decrease impingement on spinal nerves.
Decompression surgery is used to obliterate the disc impingement on the spinal nerves.
Surgical fusion is used to realign discs and vertebrae with supportive hardware. |

Making the Connections–cont'd

Signs and Symptoms	Physical Assessment Findings	Diagnostic Testing	Treatment
Spinal Stenosis	Spinal stenosis is anatomical narrowing of the openings in the vertebrae that allow spinal nerves to enter and leave the spinal cord. The narrowing causes nerve impingement and entrapment. Impingement causes pain, sensory loss, and paralysis.			
Pain (cervical or lumbar commonly) with radiation (legs or arms commonly), numbness, paresthesias, difficulty walking if in lower spine.	Tenderness of site, paraspinal muscle spasm, numbness in arms or legs, depending on site.	X-ray, CT, or MRI can demonstrate narrowing of vertebral openings and impingement on spinal nerves. Electromyography can demonstrate muscle dysfunction.	Heat to relieve pain and muscle spasm. NSAIDs to decrease inflammation. Short-term narcotic to relieve pain. Muscle relaxants to decrease muscle spasm. Intra-articular injection of glucocorticoid to decrease inflammation. Physical therapy attempts to realign vertebrae, strengthen muscles, and decrease spasm. Acupuncture may relieve pain. Chiropractic treatment attempts to realign vertebrae, strengthen muscles, and decrease spasm. Supportive devices, such as a walker or cervical collar, are used to decrease nerve impingement. Decompression surgery is used to eradicate nerve impingement. Surgical fusion is used to eradicate nerve impingement and realign vertebrae with supportive hardware.

Bibliography

Available online at fadavis.com

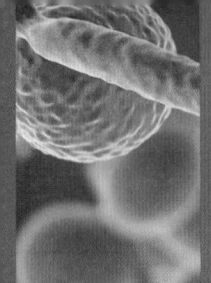

Infectious and Inflammatory Musculoskeletal Disorders

Learning Objectives

Upon completion of this chapter, the student will be able to:

- Identify normal anatomy and physiology of the muscle, bone, and joints within the musculoskeletal system.
- Describe the etiologies and mechanisms of musculoskeletal inflammation and infections.
- Identify signs, symptoms, and clinical manifestations of musculoskeletal inflammation and infection.
- Recognize the assessment techniques, laboratory tests, and imaging studies used in the diagnosis of musculoskeletal inflammation and infection.

- Discuss pharmacological and nonpharmacological treatment modalities used in the management of musculoskeletal inflammation and infection.
- Describe the complications that can develop in musculoskeletal inflammatory and infectious disorders.

Key Terms

Borrelia burgdorferi

Contiguous spread

Erythema migrans (EM)

Gout

Haversian canal

Hematogenous spread

Hyperuricemia

Lamellae

Myositis

Podagra

Pott's disease

Rheumatology

Sacroiliitis

Sequestra

Tophi

Tumor necrosis factor (TNF)

Volkmann canal

Inflammatory disorders of the musculoskeletal system are common in the adult population. The field of **rheumatology** involves the study of inflammatory muscle, bone, and joint disease. Inflammatory joint disease, or arthritis, can be caused by infection, autoimmune disease, or metabolic disorders. Infectious microorganisms commonly cause osteomyelitis and septic arthritis. Autoimmune processes cause disorders such as rheumatoid arthritis (RA), psoriatic arthritis, systemic lupus erythematosus, and ankylosing spondylitis. Inflammatory joint disorders can also be caused by metabolic disorders such as gout. Aging, obesity, and past injury to joints are the most common causes of osteoarthritis (OA). Inflammation of the skeletal muscles is called **myositis,** a disorder that progressively weakens the muscles. Like arthritis, some forms of myositis are caused by an autoimmune reaction. The autoimmune inflammatory joint disease RA is discussed in Chapter 11 and OA is discussed in Chapter 38.

Epidemiology

This chapter focuses on the specific musculoskeletal inflammatory disorders including osteomyelitis, septic arthritis, Lyme disease, gout, types of myositis, ankylosing spondylitis, and TB of bone.

Osteomyelitis is an infection of bone tissue with most cases occurring after trauma to bone or secondary to vascular insufficiency or diabetes mellitus. The incidence of osteomyelitis after open fracture is reported to be 2% to 16%, depending on the severity of trauma and type of treatment administered. The incidence of osteomyelitis in persons with diabetic foot ulcers is 20% to 60%, depending on the severity of the wound. Septic arthritis is the most serious cause of an inflamed, swollen joint. The estimated incidence of septic arthritis in industrialized countries is 6 cases per 100,000 per year. In patients with underlying joint disease or with prosthetic joints, the incidence increases approximately 10-fold, to 70 cases per 100,000 of the population.

Gout is the most common inflammatory arthritis and occurs when hyperuricemia leads to the formation and deposition of monosodium urate crystals in and around the joints. Recent reports of the prevalence and incidence of gout range from a prevalence of <1% to 6.8%. It is most prevalent in older adult males.

Basic Concepts of the Musculoskeletal System Relevant to Inflammation and Infection

The bones and joints are commonly involved in inflammatory or infectious disease. Understanding the normal physiology of these structures is important for the study of musculoskeletal system diseases (see Chapter 37 for musculoskeletal anatomy and physiology).

Bone Structure and Susceptibility to Infection

Bone is normally resistant to infection; however, infection can occur if there is exposure to a pathogenic microorganism, if the microorganism is virulent, and if a large number of organisms are present. Although the musculoskeletal system may be infected by any microorganism, the great majority of infections are bacterial. Bacteria can enter bone when a break in bone integrity is exposed to the environment, as in a compound fracture or surgical fixation of a fracture. Alternatively, bone can be infected via the bloodstream. Bacteria invade the cortex of bone via the **Haversian canal** and **Volkmann canal** systems located beneath the periosteum. Haversian canals contain the blood vessels, nerves, and lymphatic vessels that travel longitudinally within the bone. Volkmann canals also contain blood vessels and travel horizontally between the Haversian canals to connect them.

The functional unit of bone, called an osteon, consists of concentric layers, or **lamellae,** of compact bone that surround a central Haversian canal. Osteoblasts develop into osteocytes, which occupy small spaces within compact bone called lacunae. Osteocytes contact each other via a network of small transverse canals, or canaliculi. This network facilitates the exchange of nutrients and metabolic waste (see Fig. 39-1).

Certain risk factors compromise immunity and make the patient susceptible to bone infection. These risk factors include nutritional deficiency; comorbid diseases such as diabetes; and immunosuppressive medications such as corticosteroids, methotrexate, or biological medications such as tumor necrosis factor inhibitors. In addition, any patient with an implanted synthetic or allograft prosthetic material (such as a hip replacement) has an increased risk for musculoskeletal infection. Studies indicate that all biomaterials

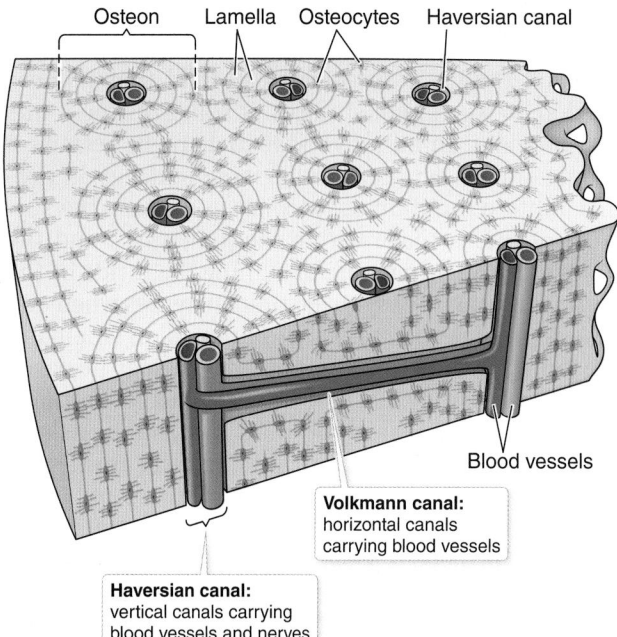

FIGURE 39-1. Haversian and Volkmann canals of compact bone. In compact bone, layers of matrix are arranged in concentric, onionlike rings (called lamellae) around a central canal (called a Haversian or osteonic canal). This basic structural unit is called an osteon (**A**). Transverse passageways, called Volkmann canals, connect the Haversian canals (**B**). These canals transport blood and nutrients from the bone's exterior to the osteocytes locked inside.

commonly used for surgical fixation of bone increase the incidence of *Staphylococcus aureus* infections. Adherence of bacteria to the surface of implants is promoted by the microorganism's outer capsule, a polysaccharide called glycocalyx. This protective capsule acts as a barrier to immune defense mechanisms and antibiotics. In addition, the capsule makes culture of organisms difficult.

Joints

Cartilage provides a smooth, well-lubricated surface for joints and allows movement between bones with low frictional resistance. Normal articular cartilage is durable and elastic, providing a shock absorber for joints. However, articular cartilage does not have a blood supply; it obtains oxygen and nutrients from the surrounding joint fluid. When a joint is bearing weight, the pressure squeezes fluid, including waste products, from the cartilage; when the pressure is relieved, the fluid seeps back in together with oxygen and nutrients. An excessively heavy load on a joint is a common cause of injury. Once injured, cartilage has a limited ability to repair itself. Damaged or abnormal cartilage loses its resistance to wear. The two joint surfaces grind together and shed particles of cartilage, which further contribute to joint surface wear. As the joint mechanics deteriorate, the rate of wear increases. The process may continue until most of the joint cartilage is lost.

Synovial Fluid

Synovial fluid is a viscous, clear fluid that reduces friction between joint surfaces. It stabilizes the joints and provides an adhesive seal that freely permits a sliding motion between cartilaginous surfaces. In normal joints, a thin film of synovial fluid covers the surfaces of the cartilage within the joint space and the synovium, the thin membrane lining the inside of the joint. The volume of synovial fluid increases when disease is present and creates a joint effusion (edema of the joint) that is clinically apparent and may be easily aspirated for study. Because normal articular cartilage has no microvascular supply of its own, it is at risk for ischemia. Chondrocytes or cartilage cells are farther from supporting microvasculature than are any other body cells. Cartilage has limited repair capabilities; damaged cartilage is usually replaced by fibrocartilage scar tissue.

In the synovium, as in all tissues, essential nutrients are delivered and metabolic by-products are cleared by the bloodstream. However, there is limited exchange between the bloodstream and a synovial joint. This limitation hinders the transport of therapeutic agents into inflamed synovial joints. No therapeutic agent is known to be transported into or selectively retained within a joint space. Consequently, intra-articular injection is often needed for medication delivery.

Basic Pathophysiological Concepts of Musculoskeletal Inflammation and Infections

Compared with other cell types in the body, bone is more resistant to infection. However, certain conditions increase the risk. There are various ways in which a microorganism can come in contact with bone. Inflammation of bone due to infection is termed osteomyelitis. Inflammation of musculoskeletal tissue can also occur with traumatic injury or autoimmune disease.

Bone Infection and Inflammation

Inflammation of the musculoskeletal tissues can occur via contiguous or hematogenous spread of infection. **Contiguous spread** is best exemplified by *S. aureus* infection of the musculoskeletal system. *S. aureus* is part of the skin's normal flora but can become pathogenic when it invades interior tissues via contiguous spread. Contiguous spread occurs by invasion of the microorganism via a puncture or wound. *Staphylococcus, Pseudomonas,* and anaerobic bacteria commonly spread to the musculoskeletal system in this manner.

Hematogenous spread occurs when bacteria from tissues within the body spread via the bloodstream to the musculoskeletal system. Pathogens, such as group A streptococci or *Streptococcus pneumoniae* that are usually limited to the oropharynx or lung, can be transported within the bloodstream to musculoskeletal tissues.

The development of osteomyelitis involves five stages:

1. Inflammation: This stage represents initial inflammation with vascular congestion and increased pressure within the interior bone; obstruction to blood flow occurs with intravascular thrombosis.
2. Suppuration: Infectious material within the bones forces its way through the Haversian system and forms an abscess beneath the bone surface.
3. Sequestrum: Increased pressure, vascular obstruction, and thrombi compromise the periosteal and endosteal blood supply, causing bone necrosis in approximately 7 days.
4. Involucrum: This is new bone formation from the stripped surface of periosteum.
5. Resolution or progression to complications: With antibiotics and surgical treatment early in the course of disease, osteomyelitis resolves without any complications. If there is no resolution, complications can arise such as gangrene, necrotic tissue that becomes infected with bacteria, commonly a *Clostridium* species.

Inflammation of musculoskeletal tissue can also occur from autoimmune disease that develops as a result of breakdown in the basic mechanisms regulating the immune system: identifying self versus non-self. For unknown reasons, an immunological reaction develops within the host against its own tissue, with resulting inflammation and injury. The common autoimmune processes include direct T-cell–mediated cellular injury, B-cell antibody-dependent cellular injury, and antigen or antibody immune complex deposition. Autoimmune diseases can be organ specific, such as ankylosing spondylitis, which affects the sacroiliac joints, or systemic, such as systemic lupus erythematosus (SLE), which causes multiorgan dysfunction.

Systemic autoimmune disorders are commonly characterized by exacerbations and remissions. Despite significant research, there is currently no cure for these diseases; the goal of therapy is to lengthen the time between disease exacerbations.

CLINICAL CONCEPT

An exacerbation is a period of worsening disease that can be detected by flare-up of patient symptoms and laboratory changes. A remission is a period of diminished apparent disease when symptoms are decreased and laboratory changes often normalize.

Joint Infection and Inflammation

The infection of a joint can occur in different ways:

- Via injection or during joint movement through direct colonization
- By direct contact with a neighboring infected site
- By hematogenous or lymphogenous spread of a pathogen

Bacterial arthritis can be categorized as acute, chronic, or reactive, which differ in the type of joint infection and their triggering bacteria. Reactive arthritis (ReA) is an autoimmune reaction that develops in one or more joints triggered by a bacterial infection in another part of the body. *Chlamydia,* gonococcus, *Salmonella, Shigella, Yersinia,* and *Campylobacter* infections are the most common triggers of ReA.

 CLINICAL CONCEPT

Chlamydia is the most common cause of ReA in the United States and is usually acquired through sexual contact. Individuals with human leukocyte antigen (HLA) known as HLA-B27 are genetically predisposed to ReA.

The knee joint is the most common site for a joint infection, and the hip is the second most frequent site. The same types of bacteria can infect the hip joint as well as other large joints. Hip joint infections, however, can exist silently with few symptoms for a long period.

An increased rate of infection occurs in a predamaged joint or a joint with a prosthesis. When implanting a prosthesis, the joint is vulnerable to infection because bacteria can enter the joint during surgery. The joint is also vulnerable because the implanted prosthetic material lowers resistance and facilitates infection that enters via the hematogenous route. The prosthetic materials act as binding sites for various bacteria. In addition, the virulence and resistance of the bacteria are involved in the mechanism of infection. Joint infections can also be the starting point of a progressive infection spreading through the contiguous, lymphatic, or hematological route. In general, the detection and treatment of joint infection (also called infectious or septic arthritis) is an acute situation that requires prompt diagnosis and treatment. A delay can allow progression of the infection and cause sepsis.

In contrast to joint infections, inflammatory disorders that occur in joints are termed inflammatory arthritis; these are characterized by pain, swelling, tenderness, and decreased function of the joints. The most common forms are RA, psoriatic arthritis (PsA), SLE (lupus), and ankylosing spondylitis (AS). In these disorders, an autoimmune reaction occurs where antibodies, white blood cells (WBCs), and cytokines attack joint tissue. The etiology of autoimmune disorders is unclear; however, they cause chronic inflammation. Synovitis, cartilage breakdown, bone erosion, and ligament damage can occur. Gout is an inflammatory arthritis caused by a metabolic disorder. Defective purine metabolism causes uric acid crystal accumulation in the blood, joints, and tissues. Swollen, red, exquisitely tender joints characterize the disorder.

Assessment

When assessing the patient with an inflammatory or infectious musculoskeletal disorder, the clinician should evaluate the following:

- Local signs of inflammation, including erythema, tenderness, swelling, and discharge
- Onset, location, and duration of symptoms
- Symmetry or asymmetry of bones, muscle, or joints on opposite sides of the body
- Aggravating factors
- Alleviating factors
- Severity of pain
- Systemic symptoms such as fever, malaise, weakness, or fatigue
- Range of motion (ROM) of affected bones or joints, palpating tender areas last

A comprehensive history and physical examination are necessary with musculoskeletal disorders. It is important to inquire about current medications, medical and surgical history, recent trauma, and family history.

 CLINICAL CONCEPT

The clinician should always examine and compare one area of the body with the opposing area of the body for symmetry. For example, when examining a swollen knee, it should be inspected in comparison to the knee on the opposite leg.

To gather a thorough history, the patient must be interviewed about any risk factors, including occupation or lifestyle factors that can lead to the musculoskeletal infection or inflammatory process. Medical disorders such as diabetes, sickle cell anemia, immune disease, and peripheral arterial disease often set the stage for musculoskeletal infection. The patient should also be questioned about past medical history of systemic disorders or infections such as Lyme disease, tuberculosis (TB), sexually transmitted illnesses (STIs), gout, wound infection, endocarditis, HIV, or autoimmune disorders. If Lyme disease is suspected, the patient should be asked about recent travel, outdoor activities, pets, and if the patient has noticed any rashes. The clinician should inquire about current occupational hazards, any recent trauma, IV drug use, alcohol use, and recent wounds. Past musculoskeletal injuries should be described in full by the patient. Past surgery, particularly orthopedic surgery and prosthetic implantation, should be noted, as these are important risk factors of musculoskeletal infection. In addition, the patient's current medication list should be reviewed because some drugs can change the metabolic profile or decrease immunocompetence.

During the physical examination, the clinician should note the patient's gait and posture, as these can give clues to the location of inflammation or infection and the disability associated with them. Skin rashes should be noted, as these are sometimes related to musculoskeletal disorders. The clinician should ask where exactly pain is located and examine that part of the body last. Examination of the surrounding region for any open wounds, discharge, swelling, or erythema is important. It is critical to evaluate blood flow and sensation in the area around the tender region.

Diagnosis

The patient's complete blood count (CBC) with differential, erythrocyte sedimentation rate (ESR), and C-reactive protein (CRP) are important indicators of inflammation or infection. High WBC count and elevated ESR and CRP are indicative of active inflammation or infection. Analysis of discharge or joint fluid with culture and sensitivity (C&S) can reveal the precise infectious agents in osteomyelitis or septic arthritis. Laboratory tests for autoantibodies are key in autoimmune disorders. The most common imaging study is x-ray. However, computed tomography (CT) scan and magnetic resonance imaging (MRI) can yield more information because they visualize areas with more detail. Ultrasound examination and dual energy x-ray absorptiometry (DEXA) scan can be used to investigate bone density and can show abnormal results in osteomyelitis. Nuclear bone scans are particularly useful in osteomyelitis and can detect infection earlier than other imaging studies. Blood cultures and bone biopsy are often needed in osteomyelitis.

Treatment

Anti-inflammatory and antibiotic agents are commonly used in infectious or inflammatory musculoskeletal disorders. Anti-inflammatory agents, such as cortisone, may be injected directly into a joint. Osteomyelitis often requires high doses of broad-spectrum antibiotics. Septic arthritis often requires intra-articular administration of antibiotic and steroids. In autoimmune disorders, immunosuppressant agents can diminish damage caused by the disease process. Commonly in autoimmune disorders, anti-**tumor necrosis factor (TNF)** inhibitors are used. The inflammatory process in gout requires specific agents that reduce the production of uric acid. Colchicine is a classic drug

used in gout. Surgical débridement of necrotic tissue in osteomyelitis is frequently required. Amputation is a last resort but may be the only way to limit the disease process if gangrene is present.

Pathophysiology of Selected Infectious Musculoskeletal Disorders

Infections of the musculoskeletal system can be caused by pathogens that focus their destruction on bones, muscles, or joints. Alternatively, systemic infectious disease can affect the whole body, leaving the musculoskeletal system damaged along with other organs. Osteomyelitis and septic arthritis are diseases where infection is localized in the bone or joint, whereas systemic infections such as Lyme disease affect the whole body and indirectly cause harm to musculoskeletal and neurological systems.

Osteomyelitis

Osteomyelitis is infection of the bone caused by a microorganism, most commonly a bacteria. Although bone is normally resistant to bacterial colonization, events such as trauma, surgery, presence of foreign bodies, or prostheses may disrupt bony integrity and lead to the onset of bone infection.

The incidence of osteomyelitis in adults and children is 1 in every 5,000 adults. Neonatal incidence is approximately 1 case per 1,000. The incidence of osteomyelitis in diabetic patients is 16%; after a foot wound, the incidence increases to 30% to 40%. Among individuals who have been treated for an episode of acute osteomyelitis, the prevalence of chronic osteomyelitis is about 5% to 25% in the United States. The presence of a prosthesis increases the risk of osteomyelitis. The incidence of prosthetic joint infection among all prosthesis recipients ranges from 2% to 10%.

Etiology
The most common cause of osteomyelitis for all age groups is *S. aureus*. However, sickle cell disease is often associated with osteomyelitis caused by the *Salmonellae* species. Puncture wounds through athletic shoes have been linked to *S. aureus* and *Pseudomonas* infection. Anaerobes of the *Bacteroides* species and *Clostridium* are also significant pathogens, especially in patients with diabetes mellitus.

The three basic categories of osteomyelitis are hematogenous, contiguous, and chronic osteomyelitis. Each type is acquired differently and has distinct characteristics.

Hematogenous Osteomyelitis. Hematogenous osteomyelitis arises from a bacterial source within the bloodstream. The infectious process typically has a rapid onset of symptoms within a few days to a week after infection by a pathogen. More than 85% of hematogenous osteomyelitis occurs in children younger than age 17. In adults, thoracic or lumbar vertebrae are typically involved. Regardless of age, males are affected more often than females.

 CLINICAL CONCEPT

Children are especially at risk for hematogenous osteomyelitis because of the rapid growth and vascularity of immature bone tissue.

Contiguous Osteomyelitis. Contiguous osteomyelitis results from direct bacterial infection of bone or by extension of an adjacent soft tissue infection. Trauma and surgery are the most common causes of direct bacterial infection in younger individuals. In the older adult, pressure injuries or infected joint prostheses are typical sources of infection. Those with peripheral vascular disease (PVD) are especially at risk because of impaired blood flow. Diabetes mellitus also predisposes individuals to osteomyelitis because of impaired blood flow and reduced immunocompetence. Osteomyelitis in diabetes often develops when a localized foot lesion becomes infected.

 CLINICAL CONCEPT

Older adults, especially those with underlying diseases such as diabetes, are at increased risk for contiguous osteomyelitis.

Chronic Osteomyelitis. Osteomyelitis begins as an acute infection; however, when untreated or undertreated, the destructive process may progress to a chronic disease. Chronic osteomyelitis, which is noted primarily in adults, is defined by the length of time of disease, a lack of response to antibiotic therapy, or presence of necrotic bone. Acute osteomyelitis is considered to be chronic when infection persists longer than 6 to 8 weeks or fails to respond to appropriate antibiotic therapy. The key feature of chronic osteomyelitis is the development of necrotic bone tissue that distinctly separates from the surrounding living bone. Necrotic bone lacks blood supply and cannot attain levels of antibiotic; therefore, it is susceptible to gangrene.

Pathophysiology
Healthy adult bones are normally resistant to bacteremia because bones are not highly vascular, so infection is slow to develop. However, in hematogenous osteomyelitis, bone becomes invaded with bacteria that are present within the bloodstream. The bacteria invade, lodge in bones, and often form an abscess. Because the abscess deprives the bone of its blood supply, the bone tissue dies and becomes necrotic. Sections of necrotic bone that separate from viable bone tissue and form devascularized fragments surrounded by exudate are called **sequestrae.**

In adults, the most common region infected in hematogenous spread is vertebral bone and adjoining intervertebral discs. The infection then commonly spreads into the joint space and adjoining vertebral bodies. Vertebral osteomyelitis at any age is most often a secondary complication of a remote infection. In approximately one-half of vertebral osteomyelitis cases, the source of primary infection is the urinary tract or skin, and in one-third, it is endocarditis.

Contiguous osteomyelitis involves direct bacterial invasion through trauma or local extension. Patients with diabetic neuropathy are at higher risk of developing contiguous spread osteomyelitis secondary to infection of diabetic foot wounds. Peripheral vascular disease can also lead to osteomyelitis from a local infection. Diabetes plays an especially important role, as it both perturbs the immune response and compromises the macrovascular and microvascular blood supply.

The invading pathogen provokes an inflammatory response with vascular engorgement, edema, leukocyte accumulation, and formation of exudate. Once the inflammatory process begins, blood vessels thrombose, and exudate extends into the cortex. When the cortex is disrupted, the bone becomes weaker, predisposing the bone to pathological fracture.

Chronic osteomyelitis occurs when an infection has been in the bone for a lengthy duration, from weeks to months. The bone is deteriorated, and there are no viable blood vessels in the necrotic bone. The avascular, anoxic necrotic bone is a breeding ground for bacteria, particularly anaerobic bacteria. *Clostridia* bacterial species are ubiquitous in the environment and proliferate in areas with low oxygen tension. These resilient, spore-forming bacteria produce toxins that break down surrounding tissue and produce gas. *Clostridium perfringens* is a common type of bacteria that thrives on necrotic tissue, secretes toxins, emits gas, and causes gas gangrene. Gangrene requires amputation.

Clinical Presentation
The individual with osteomyelitis will often develop generalized symptoms: chills, fever, and malaise. Localized tenderness, erythema, edema, and pain with movement of the infected extremity are common. Loss of ROM can occur as the infection progresses. Postoperative patients, particularly those who have undergone orthopedic surgery or prosthetic implants, may demonstrate delayed wound healing and cutaneous drainage. Those with coexisting diabetes or peripheral

arterial disease often lack sensation in the affected extremity and therefore experience less pain. With less pain, the patient is less aware of the infection and will present later in its course. The patient may not seek health care until infection becomes severe. This is commonly the case with patients who have diabetes: they often seek health care late when there is no chance of saving the limb and amputation is the only way to limit the infection.

Diagnosis

The patient history can aid in identifying the mechanism of infection and most likely pathogen. The history obtained from the patient with osteomyelitis should identify present or recent infections of the oropharynx, bladder and kidneys, skin and soft tissue, and musculoskeletal system. The patient should be asked about IV catheter use, IV drug abuse, or hemodialysis. Underlying medical conditions such as sickle cell anemia, diabetes mellitus, PVD, alcoholism, AIDS, and other forms of immunosuppression should be addressed. The patient should also be asked about any recent trauma such as fracture, animal bite, gunshot wound, puncture wound, or any recent invasive surgical or diagnostic procedure.

The diagnosis of osteomyelitis is sometimes challenging because laboratory tests and culture may not indicate infection. Laboratory analyses are not diagnostic for osteomyelitis, but do provide helpful information. The CBC may reveal an elevation of WBCs, but the WBC count, as well as other components of the CBC, can be within normal limits. When the WBC count is elevated, there is usually an increased number of neutrophils. The ESR is elevated in nearly 90% of cases. CRP rises earlier than ESR rate, but neither of these laboratory values are specific for a diagnosis of osteomyelitis. Blood cultures are positive in only 50% of patients. It is important to recognize that culture or aspiration of infected tissue fails to identify the pathogen in approximately 25% of cases.

Plain x-rays of the affected area often appear unremarkable until late in the osteomyelitis process or abscess formation occurs. It usually takes at least 2 weeks for plain x-rays to demonstrate osteomyelitis; therefore, they are not a reliable diagnostic study. However, plain x-rays are important to rule out other diagnoses, including fracture and malignancy. Malignancy, in particular, can masquerade as infection and infection can appear as a malignancy.

Enhanced osteoclastic activity can be seen on technetium-99 bone scintigraphy (Tc^{99m}; also called radionuclide bone scan) 10 to 14 days before any abnormality appears on plain x-ray. Radionuclide bone scan is better than plain x-ray but not highly specific for osteomyelitis.

MRI, CT scanning, and ultrasonography can be used to confirm infection. Although ultrasound can exhibit an effusion of a joint, abscess, or soft tissue involvement, it is inaccurate in identifying the bone infection. MRI is the most sensitive of these diagnostic tests and is particularly helpful in exhibiting soft tissue involvement.

White blood cell scans are currently regarded as highly reliable studies. A combined white blood cell and bone marrow scan is the current study of choice for investigating suspected osteomyelitis. In white blood cell scans, the patient's white blood cells are labeled with a radionuclide (such as Tc^{99m}) and then returned to the patient intravenously. Increased white blood cell uptake of the radionuclide substance is seen in areas of bone infection as "hot spots" on the scan. However, normal bone marrow also takes up white blood cells to some degree. To differentiate between bone infection and physiological marrow uptake, the white blood cell scan is combined with a bone marrow scan that uses Tc^{99m}-labeled colloid. The bone marrow scan provides a map of physiological white cell uptake that is then compared with the white blood cell scan. The difference in white blood cell uptake between the two studies indicates a focus of infection (Lee et al., 2016)

Fluorodeoxyglucose positron emission tomography (FDG-PET) provides more anatomical information in osteomyelitis than any conventional imaging technique. The radionuclide binds to hypermetabolic tissues that have high glucose uptake. FDG-PET has been shown to have the highest sensitivity of all radionuclide techniques in the detection of chronic osteomyelitis. However, these types of scans are not widely available (Lee et al., 2016).

Needle aspiration of bone for culture, commonly under CT guidance, often identifies the causative organism. Bone biopsy for culture should be performed in all patients, except those with hematogenous osteomyelitis who have blood cultures that have positively identified the causative organism. It is important to appreciate that cultures may not always be positive, which is termed culture-negative infection. Here, the bone is infected but an organism is unable to be cultured.

Treatment

Antibiotic therapy is initially begun intravenously for 2 to 6 weeks. The gram-positive bacterium *Staphylococcus aureus* is the most frequently isolated etiological agent of osteomyelitis. *Streptococcus pyogenes, Streptococcus pneumoniae,* and *Kingella kingae* are also important causes. Fungal organisms such as *Blastomyces, Coccidioides, Candida,* and *Aspergillus* can also cause osteomyelitis in certain clinical scenarios. Systemic antibacterial or antifungal agents are used to treat the infection depending on the suspected organism. Most often, a broad-spectrum agent is used initially until culture and sensitivity (C&S) reports are obtained. Ideally, specific agents are chosen based on the C&S results. Oral therapy follows IV therapy. Correction of hyperglycemia and amelioration of peripheral vascular disease are critical components of therapy in patients with osteomyelitis related to chronic wounds.

Surgical débridement of necrotic tissue and debris, as well as surgical drainage of an abscess, are commonly necessary. Those with prosthetic joints are often treated with the joint prosthesis in place. However, in prosthetic joint infections, bacterial adherence to prosthetic surfaces forms biofilms, which can lead to increased resistance to the host's immune system and to antimicrobials. Removal of the prosthesis may be necessary.

Infected bone has a decreased oxygen content and low permeability of antibiotics. Hyperbaric oxygen therapy, which is pressurized 100% oxygen delivery, can increase oxygen content of the blood and bone. Increased oxygen content boosts WBC function and intensifies eradication of gram-positive organisms (such as *S. aureus)* and some gram-negative microbes. Hyperbaric oxygen also increases penetration of antibiotics, such as aminoglycosides and cephalosporins, into the infected bone. Hyperbaric oxygen therapy of 100% oxygen at 2 atmospheres of pressure for 2 hours per day for a total of 30 treatments has been effective for those with chronic osteomyelitis.

All patients with osteomyelitis should be reevaluated every 3 months for at least 2 years to monitor for relapses, which can occur years after the initial infection. Complications of osteomyelitis occur as a result of delayed initiation of therapy or failure to respond to therapy. Delayed initiation of therapy most commonly occurs when individuals seek care late in the course of illness or when there is misdiagnosis by the health-care provider. Failure to respond to therapy can result from improper antimicrobial agent selection, dosing, or limited antibiotic penetration. Excessive necrotic tissue, abscess formation, and debris at the infectious site can limit antibiotic tissue penetration, making débridement—surgical removal of necrotic tissue—necessary. Additionally, patients with medical conditions, such as immunosuppression or altered sensory and vascular status, are more prone to complications.

Complications can include pathological fractures, especially in weight-bearing bones weakened by infection of the cortex. Removal of the infected joint prosthesis, with mandatory mobility restrictions, may be required in those who develop osteomyelitis postoperatively. Amputation of a digit or distal extremity has been required with advanced, chronic infection.

Septic Arthritis

Septic arthritis, also known as infectious arthritis or pyogenic arthritis, is a direct invasion of the joint space by pathogenic microorganisms: bacteria, viruses, or fungi. Although any infectious agent may cause septic arthritis, bacteria are most common causes.

Incidence of septic arthritis ranges from 2 to 10 cases per 100,000 in the general population per year. Sexually transmitted infections, caused by gonococcal and non-gonococcal microorganisms, can cause reactive arthritis in joints. It is estimated that 5% of those with chlamydia infection develop reactive arthritis in a joint. The incidence of reactive arthritis caused by gonococcal infection is 2.8 cases per 100,000 persons per year. Septic arthritis associated with prosthetic implants, which occurs in 2% to 10% of prosthetic recipients, is the most common and challenging form of the disorder. Septic arthritis is also becoming increasingly common in older adults and among those who are immunosuppressed. Of all persons with septic arthritis, 45% are older than 65 years. Those with concurrent disease states are most commonly affected. Fifty-six percent of patients with septic arthritis are male.

Risk factors for septic arthritis include age, underlying medical conditions, and penetrating injury of a joint. Neonates and those older than age 60 are at highest risk for septic arthritis. In children, the epiphyseal growth plate of bones—rich in vascularity—is the region where infection commonly occurs.

In adults, underlying medical conditions that increase the risk of septic arthritis include diabetes, RA, SLE, liver disease, chronic renal failure, IV drug use, organ transplantation, malignancy, and AIDS. Joint-specific factors include puncture wounds, recent joint injection or aspiration, and surgery.

Etiology

Pathogenic microorganisms most commonly invade a joint space via the bloodstream because the synovium of the joint is highly vascular and microbes pass from the blood to the synovial space. Less commonly, organisms enter the joint through direct penetration or contiguous spread from infected surrounding tissue. Direct infection can occur from penetrating or blunt trauma to the joint; this may include diagnostic needle aspiration of the joint or treatments with intra-articular injections of corticosteroids. Prosthetic joint infections are caused by intraoperative contamination in 60% to 80% of cases and bacteremia in 20% to 40% of cases.

Bacterial pathogens have been identified as the most common causes of septic arthritis. Bacterial septic arthritis is often classified as nongonococcal or gonococcal. *S. aureus* remains the most common cause for the vast majority of cases of nongonococcal arthritis in adults and children older than 2 years. Other common pathogens include *Streptococcus* groups A and B, *Streptococcus viridans,* and *S. pneumoniae.* Gram-negative enteric bacilli, such as *Escherichia coli, Salmonella, Proteus,* and *Pseudomonas* species, are common causes of septic arthritis in infants, children, and adults, especially those with recent trauma or abdominal infection. Chlamydia and gonorrhea are the most common sexually transmitted diseases that cause reactive arthritis in the joints.

CLINICAL CONCEPT

Viral infections, such as rubella, hepatitis B, parvovirus B19, and lymphocytic choriomeningitis, can directly infect joints or create antibody–antigen complexes that cause inflammation in joints. With viral infection, multiple joints are usually affected without the formation of purulent exudate; this is also true for the causative agent of Lyme disease, *Borrelia burgdorferi.* Mycobacterial or fungal arthritis typically presents as chronic granulomatous arthritis that affects a single joint.

Pathophysiology

In a healthy joint, synovial fluid has some bactericidal capabilities that allow for resistance of infection. Synovial cells that line the joint can phagocytose microorganisms to protect the joint from bacterial invasion. However, chronic conditions such as RA and SLE decrease the immune defenses in the joints. In hematogenous spread, bacteria are transported from an infectious site in the body into the bloodstream to the arterioles of the bone epiphysis and the synovium. Once the microorganism has invaded the joint space, the microvasculature of the synovial membrane becomes infected. In the infectious process, WBCs synthesize cytokines and other inflammatory products. The end result is the deterioration of essential collagen and intra-articular cartilage. The cytokine and inflammatory products cause joint effusion, creating swelling that obstructs the delivery of blood and nutrients to the joint. If the inflammatory process continues, the microorganism may invade the adjacent bone.

Clinical Presentation

Patients with septic arthritis often present with inflammation of the synovium, with an acutely painful, edematous, and erythematous monoarticular joint. Fever and malaise occur early in the infectious process. Those who have underlying chronic illnesses or are immunocompromised may not present with fever. Individuals often seek health care because of joint pain and limited ROM. In adults, the joints most commonly involved include the knee, hip, elbow, shoulder, and joints of the hand. In children, the hip is the most commonly affected joint.

Diagnosis

The history and physical examination for the individual with suspected septic arthritis are similar to that for osteomyelitis. An important focus of the patient history is investigation of underlying medical conditions, such as RA or diabetes, which increase the risk of septic arthritis. The clinician should also investigate any recent problems that may have allowed microorganisms to enter and multiply within the joint structures. The patient should be asked about any recent trauma, invasive procedure,

or prosthetic implant. The patient's occupation and lifestyle factors may be related to risk for septic arthritis. Patients should be asked about recent sexually transmitted infection such as Chlamydia or gonorrhea. For other elements of the history, see the "Osteomyelitis" section.

X-ray has a limited role in the evaluation of septic arthritis. Soft tissue swelling around the joint, although not diagnostic, is the most common initial finding. Late findings include bone destruction. Ultrasonography can confirm the presence of an effusion, but does not provide clues as to the underlying cause. Radionuclide bone scanning is able to localize areas of inflammation through increased dye uptake, but cannot distinguish infectious from noninfectious etiologies. CT scans and MRIs are more sensitive, but also cannot distinguish between infectious and noninfectious etiologies.

A definitive diagnosis of septic arthritis requires the detection and identification of bacteria from the blood or synovial fluid by Gram stain or culture. This often requires aspiration of the joint and analysis of the synovial fluid for crystals or microorganisms. For example, the presence of more than 50,000 WBCs/mm³ with more than 75% polymorphonuclear leukocytes in the synovial fluid is common in septic arthritis caused by bacteria. Gram stain is less than 60% sensitive for detection of bacteria in synovial fluid, so fluid should also be cultured. Three sets of blood cultures should be obtained to rule out bacteremia that can lead to the joint infection. If an STI is suspected, cervical or urethral discharge should be cultured. Elevated ESR and CRP levels are not diagnostic, but can be helpful in monitoring response to therapy.

Treatment

Management of septic arthritis involves drainage of the joint, short-term joint immobilization for pain control, and antibiotic administration. Joint aspiration provides fluid for diagnostic analysis and also decreases the joint swelling to relieve pain and allow circulation into the joint. A few aspiration procedures to decrease swelling may be needed during the first 1 to 2 weeks of therapy. Joint immobilization, without weight-bearing, is important while synovitis resolves. The joint should be maintained in a functionally neutral position, with passive ROM exercises scheduled on a regular basis. Once synovitis resolves, physical therapy is used to promote optimal function of the affected joint.

Prompt administration of antibiotic therapy for bacterial infections should be administered to promote complete recovery. The initial antibiotic therapy should cover *S. aureus* and *Streptococcus* species; *Chlamydia* and *Gonococci* should be covered in the sexually active patient. The antibiotic is usually administered IV initially for 2 to 4 weeks. However, a shorter course of IV therapy, with a switch to oral antibiotics, has also proven efficacious in some cases. Oral antibiotic therapy should not be initiated until there are no systemic symptoms and the joint cultures are negative for pathogens.

For those with a prosthetic joint infection, optimal treatment involves removal of the prosthesis and a 6-week course of antibiotics. Replacement of the prosthesis should involve using an antibiotic-impregnated bone cement and new prosthesis.

 CLINICAL CONCEPT

Joint dysfunction is the major complication of septic arthritis. In adults, the optimal treatment eradicates bacteria from the synovial fluid within 6 days of initiating antibiotic therapy. *S. aureus* infection, a challenging form of septic arthritis, has been linked to chronic complications such as permanent joint damage with limited ROM or chronic pain in approximately one-half of cases. The mortality rate of *S. aureus* is typically 10%, but can approach 50% in the immunosuppressed patient.

Mycobacterium Tuberculosis

Although pulmonary TB is the most common form, *Mycobacterium tuberculosis* can spread to other areas of the body through the bloodstream and can involve multiple organs, particularly the vertebrae. *M. tuberculosis* accounts for 10% to 35% of extrapulmonary TB (EPTB) and most often involves the spine (50%), but may also result in tuberculous arthritis in the hip (15%) or knee (15%) and extraspinal tuberculous osteomyelitis. In 2021, approximately 7,860 cases of TB were reported in the United States—an incidence rate of 2.4 per 100,000 population. TB incidence is higher than expected among Hispanics, African Americans, and Asians, based on the percentage of these ethnic minority groups in the U.S. population (CDC, 2021). There is a high number of TB cases among people experiencing homelessness, people who use illicit IV drugs, immunocompromised persons, and individuals who are incarcerated. In less-developed countries, such as rural China, sub-Saharan Africa, and Central and South America, TB is endemic. Globally, 9.9 million new cases occurred in 2020 and 1.5 million persons died of TB that year.

 CLINICAL CONCEPT

Immunocompromised individuals, especially those with AIDS, are at greatest risk for EPTB, particularly of the bone.

Etiology

M. tuberculosis is an acid-fast, aerobic, slow-growing bacillus. Within the United States, the individual's immunological status is the most important factor in the development of EPTB.

Pathophysiology

Following multiplication of *M. tuberculosis* within the lung, the bacillus may spread throughout the body via the bloodstream. Although any bone can be infected, infection of the vertebrae is most common.

Vertebral TB is also referred to as tuberculous spondylitis, or **Pott's disease.** Pott's disease, a combination of osteomyelitis and arthritis, usually involves more than one vertebra. Compression of spinal nerves that causes pain is common. Thoracic vertebrae are most commonly affected, followed by lumbar and cervical vertebrae. Infection of the vertebral bone most commonly begins in the anteroinferior aspect of the vertebral body with involvement of the intervertebral disc and adjacent vertebrae. Abscesses can develop in the paravertebral muscles, with abscess extension into adjacent tissues. Severe kyphosis (cervicothoracic curvature of the spine) can occur in conjunction with destruction of the vertebrae. TB can cause severe destruction of the vertebrae with resulting spinal nerve impingement. If the spinal nerves are severely affected, paralysis can occur.

Clinical Presentation

The patient most commonly complains of chronic back pain. The reported average duration of symptoms at diagnosis is 4 months. The patient may complain of symptoms of spinal nerve impingement such as weakness and numbness of a lower extremity. Some patients report fever and weight loss. Cervical spine TB is less common but is potentially more serious because severe neurological complications can cause breathing problems. Cervical TB symptoms include neck muscle spasm, hoarseness, and dyspnea.

When examining a patient who may have vertebral TB, the clinician should carefully inspect and palpate the vertebrae, as well as carefully observe the patient's posture and gait. The patient should bend over to touch the toes with the clinician observing from the back of the patient to look for asymmetry of the paravertebral muscles. The patient's vertebrae should be palpated for tenderness, and a comprehensive neurological examination should be done. Neurological deficits may be noted if there is spinal nerve compression. Neurological manifestations can range from single spinal nerve impingement to paralysis of a limb. Clinical manifestations of vertebral TB may vary depending on the site of skeletal involvement, but the typical presentation of tuberculous arthritis includes pain, joint swelling, and decreased ROM.

Diagnosis

Exposure to TB is a key component of the patient history. The classic symptoms of pulmonary TB—cough, night sweats, and weight loss—are often *not* present in skeletal TB. The essential history components for the patient with skeletal TB include known or suspected exposure to *M. tuberculosis*. The patient should be asked about recent travel to or from a region where TB is endemic, such as China or underdeveloped countries. Immunosuppression increases susceptibility to TB infection, so patients should be asked about current medications, medical conditions, surgical history, and HIV status.

Diagnosing EPTB is difficult because classic signs or symptoms of TB may not be present. It is important to note that a purified protein derivative (PPD) skin test may be negative in EPTB because fewer bacteria are necessary to infect nonpulmonary sites. Also, patients who are immunocompromised may not have the ability to mount an immune reaction to the PPD antigen. The PPD test can be negative in immunodeficient individuals due to anergy.

Biopsy of bone tissue is the method of diagnosis in vertebral TB. Chest x-ray reveals pulmonary involvement in less than one-half of patients with EPTB. X-ray findings of the affected vertebral bone include soft tissue swelling and joint space narrowing. Vertebral lesions cause compressive fractures, exhibited as flattening of the vertebral bone. Joint aspiration and fluid analysis contain *Mycobacteria* in nearly 80% of cases.

Advanced infection and destruction of the vertebrae can lead to spinal deformity with instability, vertebral collapse, and spinal nerve compression. Involved joints may result in joint deformity, chronic pain, and limited ROM.

Treatment

The treatment principles of pulmonary TB also apply to EPTB. A detailed discussion of baseline evaluation, antituberculous therapy, and follow-up can be found in Chapter 20. An extended 12-month regimen is often required for individuals with skeletal TB. When neurological impairment or spine instability is present, surgery may be necessary to drain abscesses, débride infected tissue, stabilize the spine, or relieve spinal cord compression.

> ### CLINICAL CONCEPT
> Vertebral TB usually does not present with the classic signs of pulmonary TB. It is important to assess the patient for spinal nerve compression in vertebral TB, as quadriplegia, paraplegia, or cauda equina syndrome can occur.

Lyme Disease

First discovered in Lyme, Connecticut, Lyme disease is caused by the tick-transmitted spirochete *B. burgdorferi*. It is the most common vector-borne disease in the United States.

Lyme disease most often occurs in the late spring and summer months when ticks are most active and human outdoor activity is highest. The disease has been detected more frequently in males than females, with a higher incidence in those 5 to 14 years of age and 50 to 59 years of age. Approximately 20,000 cases are reported annually in the United States. Although most of the states report Lyme disease, more than 95% of cases come from just 12 states: Connecticut, Delaware, Maine, Maryland, Massachusetts, Minnesota, New Hampshire, New Jersey, New York, Pennsylvania, Rhode Island, and Wisconsin. Within these states, incidence can vary from one community to another. In the states where Lyme disease is most common, the average is 34.7 cases per 100,000 persons. However, the incidence is speculated to be much higher because many people do not seek health care and misdiagnosis by health-care providers is common.

> ### CLINICAL CONCEPT
> The greatest risk for Lyme disease is occupational or recreational outdoor exposure in a tick-endemic region. Individuals who live in areas with a high deer population are at increased risk of Lyme disease.

Etiology

Lyme disease bacteria live in mice, squirrels, deer, and other small mammals. In the northeastern and north central United States, the black-legged deer tick (*Ixodes scapularis*) is the most common agent of transmission (see Fig. 39-2). On the West Coast, the western black-legged deer tick (*Ixodes pacificus*) is the agent of transmission.

Ticks feed on infected animals, resulting in transfer of the spirochete *B. burgdorferi* to a tick. The ticks can become attached to grass or foliage in forested areas; individuals or their pets then can contract the tick when walking through the forested areas. The bacteria *B. burgdorferi* is transferred to a human

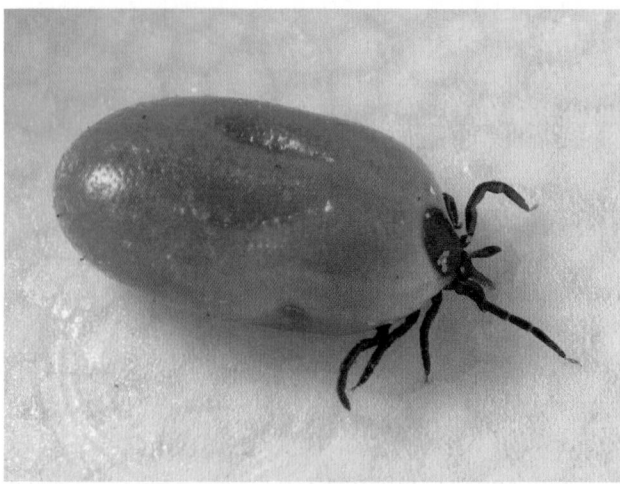

FIGURE 39-2. Deer tick. *(Courtesy of CDC/Gary Alpert–Urban Pests–Integrated Pest Management (IPM).)*

through a tick bite. Human infection may result when a tick is attached for 24 to 48 hours. Adult ticks are less likely to transmit the disease because they are noticed and removed; nymphs (immature ticks), however, can easily go undetected, especially in hairy areas of the body, because they may be only slightly larger than the period at the end of a sentence.

The incubation period is typically 7 to 14 days after tick exposure, but can be between 3 and 31 days. Less than 50% of individuals recall any tick bite.

Pathophysiology

Lyme disease pathophysiology is not completely understood. Spirochete infection causes many of the disease manifestations, but the infected individual's immune response is thought to contribute as well. Before the tick delivers the bacteria, it injects a substance to inhibit the individual's immune response. Once the bacterium is introduced through the tick bite, the spirochete may be eradicated by the individual's defense mechanisms. However, in many cases the bacterium remains viable. The spirochete secretes enzymes that aid in replication of the bacteria; the infection can be picked up by blood or lymph and disseminated throughout the body. This hematogenous dissemination can occur within days to weeks of initial infection. Once the *B. burgdorferi* spread throughout the body, the bacteria tend to be difficult to detect with laboratory tests. The spirochete has been known to infect the skin, heart, joints, eyes, central nervous system (CNS), peripheral nerves, and other parts of the body.

Clinical Presentation

Commonly, the patient presents with a vague combination of arthralgias, myalgias, excessive fatigue, and headache. However, the vague presentation does not give the clinician sufficient clues to suspect Lyme disease. Most patients do not report a tick bite, and the rash is often not present. Uniquely, some patients present with facial nerve palsy (also called Bell's palsy) with no recollection of a tick bite or rash.

There are three stages of Lyme disease:

1. Early localized
2. Early disseminated
3. Late disseminated

Each stage has specific characteristics, but regardless of stage, children may present differently than adults.

Early Localized Disease. Early localized Lyme disease is the most common stage of presentation, occurring 3 to 30 days after a deer tick bite. In 70% to 80% of cases, the individual presents with a localized rash called **erythema migrans (EM),** which often begins as an erythematous macule or papule at the site of the tick bite. The rash enlarges over several days to form a round lesion with a clear area in the middle of the ring, called a "bull's-eye rash" (see Fig. 39-3).

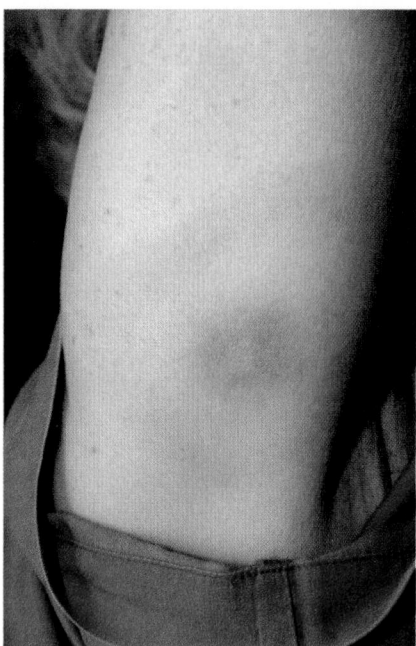

FIGURE 39-3. EM rash of Lyme disease. *(Courtesy of CDC/James Gathany.)*

EM can also present as an oval-shaped lesion, with various shades of red, pink, and purple, which can be mistaken for a spider bite or skin infection. The rash is not painful or pruritic (itchy), and the patient may ignore it. Those infected with early Lyme disease often present with skin rash and vague generalized flu-like symptoms: fever (usually low grade), chills, myalgias, arthralgias, fatigue, and headache. Regional enlargement of lymph nodes (lymphadenopathy) in the area draining the tick bite may be found.

Early Disseminated Disease. Early disseminated Lyme disease occurs from 3 to 12 weeks after the tick bite. The infected individual will usually have one or more EMs and the vague, generalized symptoms as described in early localized disease. *B. burgdorferi* infection can result in lymphocytic meningitis (neck pain and intense headache), cranial neuritis (paralysis of facial nerves), carditis (various degrees of reversible heart block, myocarditis, or pericarditis), and ocular involvement (visual changes or unilateral blindness).

Late Disseminated Disease. When the bacteria are not eradicated, the individual develops late disseminated Lyme disease. This stage occurs months to years following the tick bite. By then, the individual experiences severe joint pain and swelling of large joints, often the knees (in 60% of cases). In a small percentage of patients, CNS involvement can cause subacute encephalopathy, or confusion and difficulty with concentration. If spinal nerves are involved, neural inflammation (polyradiculopathy) can develop with symptoms of shooting pains, numbness, or tingling of the hands or feet.

CLINICAL CONCEPT

More than 50% of individuals who develop Lyme disease do not recall any tick bite.

Diagnosis

The diagnosis of Lyme disease is based on symptoms, physical findings, and a history of exposure to ticks. The clinician who suspects Lyme disease needs to inquire about the patient's occupational or recreational outdoor activities. Particular attention should be given to activities undertaken within the past month. Although the recollection of a tick bite is helpful, it is not essential. The patient should also be asked about any recent rashes

Laboratory tests are commonly falsely negative in patients with early disease, though they are more reliable for the later stages. The Centers for Disease Control and Prevention recommend a two-step process; both tests can be done using the same blood sample. Enzyme-linked immunosorbent assay (ELISA) or immunofluorescent assay (IFA) are the recommended initial laboratory tests. These tests are highly sensitive; the vast majority of those with Lyme disease—and some individuals without the disease—will test positive. Sometimes these tests may provide a result of "indeterminate" or "equivocal," meaning a positive or negative result cannot be determined. For those with positive or indeterminate or equivocal results on ELISA or IFA, Western blot confirmation is the second recommended laboratory test. Western blot is designed to be specific, in that it is only positive if the person is truly infected.

Treatment

For those living in an area endemic with Lyme disease and sustaining a known tick bite, the Infectious Disease Society of America recommends a prophylactic single dose of the antibiotic doxycycline. All others who have removed ticks should be closely monitored for signs and symptoms of Lyme disease for 30 days. If EM or generalized symptoms develop, antibiotic therapy is warranted. The treatment of choice is a 21-day course of doxycycline, although alternative antibiotics have been used. The response to antibiotics can vary widely because there are more than 300 strains of *B. burgdorferi* worldwide and more than 100 strains in the United States alone.

Commonly, Lyme disease is not readily identified in its early stages. However, if antibiotic treatment is begun early, Lyme disease can be cured. Even with antibiotics, a small percentage of infected individuals have symptoms that last months, years, or even a lifetime. Patients report neuropathic pain, difficulty concentrating, arthritis, and altered mobility. The cause of these symptoms, called post-Lyme syndrome, is not known. It is theorized that the individual has an autoimmune response that remains overactive long after the infection has been eradicated.

Common Musculoskeletal Inflammatory Disorders

Common musculoskeletal inflammatory disorders include RA, gout, SLE, scleroderma, PsA, AS, and dermatomyositis. Most of these disorders occur because of autoimmune reactions triggered by unknown factors. For RA, SLE, and scleroderma, see Chapter 11.

Gout

Gout, also termed gouty arthritis, is a disorder of recurrent inflammation triggered by **hyperuricemia,** which is elevated uric acid in the blood and high uric acid crystals in the synovial fluid. Prevalence in the United States has risen over the last 20 years, and the disorder now affects 8.3 million Americans—or 4% of the population. The prevalence of increased uric acid levels (hyperuricemia) also rose, affecting 43.3 million (21%) adults in the United States. It is important to note that not all persons with hyperuricemia develop gout. Experts estimate that only 5% of individuals with hyperuricemia develop the condition. This leads to questions of why only a small portion of those affected with hyperuricemia progress to symptomatic gout. Many factors are thought to predispose individuals to the syndrome (see Box 39-1).

BOX 39-1. Risk Factors for Gout

High alcohol consumption increases the risk of gout because alcohol stimulates hepatic uric acid production and renal uric acid reabsorption. Specific dietary intake may contribute to the development of gout or exacerbations of primary gout. A diet filled with purine-rich foods, such as meat and seafood, has been linked to exacerbations of primary gout.

The use of medications such as niacin, ethambutol, pyrazinamide, cyclosporine, levodopa, diuretics, or salicylates has been implicated in the development of secondary gout and may contribute to exacerbations in those with primary gout. Chemotherapeutic agents used in the treatment of cancer can also trigger attacks of gout. Chemotherapeutic agents cause the death of high numbers of cells, which yields high amounts of cellular DNA; this is made up of purines, which are sources of uric acid. Additionally, trauma or surgery can cause an acute attack of gout. Conditions such as hypertension, diabetes, renal insufficiency, hypertriglyceridemia, hypercholesterolemia, obesity, and early menopause are associated with a higher incidence of gout.

Gout often affects the peripheral joints of males older than 30 years of age. For unknown reasons, certain joints of the body, such as the first metatarsal, are specifically affected. Males are four times more likely to develop gout than females. Females are rarely affected until after menopause, as estrogen is believed to be protective against hyperuricemia. Twenty percent of individuals with gout have a family history of the syndrome. Gout is more prevalent in African American males; this is thought to occur because African American males have a higher incidence of early hypertension and are often treated with diuretics. Hyperuricemia is an adverse effect of thiazide and loop diuretics, which can trigger an episode of gout in predisposed individuals.

Etiology

Gout may be designated as primary or secondary. Primary gout, a metabolic disorder, constitutes 90% of cases. The vast majority of individuals with primary gout have a defect in renal excretion of uric acid, termed underexcretion of uric acid. Genome-wide association studies (GWAS) indicate that genetic variants in *URAT1, OAT4, OAT10,* and *GLUT9* genes, which direct transport of uric acid in the nephrons, cause hyperuricemia. GWAS data have also indicated that genetic variants of a secretory pump, termed ABCG2, in the intestine, cause hyperuricemia. Ten percent of persons with gout are oversecretors of uric acid.

Secondary gout can be attributed to a variety of disorders, including myeloproliferative (abnormal growth of bone marrow cells) or lymphoproliferative disease (abnormal production of WBCs), neoplastic disease, glycogen storage disease, psoriasis, and sarcoidosis. Secondary gout is also associated with obesity, lead intoxication, alcoholism, and use of specific medications. In addition, gout can occur in cancer chemotherapy because of the accelerated breakdown of cells. Increased breakdown of cellular DNA leads to elevated uric acid levels.

Pathophysiology

Uric acid, a weak acid that remains ionized at the body's normal pH, is a by-product of purine metabolism. Ninety-eight percent of extracellular uric acid is in the form of monosodium urate, needlelike crystals that are deposited in connective tissues throughout the body when uric acid levels exceed a concentration of 6.8 mg/dL. Crystallization within synovial fluid results in the acute painful joint inflammation of gouty arthritis. Over time, aggregates of uric acid crystals become deposited in subcutaneous tissue surrounding joints, termed **tophi.** A tophus is a palpable, subdermal, hard nodule commonly visible in the Achilles tendon, joints of the hands, elbows, or pinnae of the ears.

Clinical Presentation

Symptoms of gout occur after 15 to 20 years of constant, asymptomatic levels of hyperuricemia. The classic presentation of acute gout is a sudden onset of inflammation and excruciating pain in one joint—commonly the joint of the great toe. **Podagra,** an acute inflammation of the metatarsophalangeal joint of the great toe, is the most common presentation (see Fig. 39-4). Other joints, including the ankle, knee, wrist, or elbow, may be affected. Symptoms include a warm, tender, swollen, and erythematous joint with possible fever.

Usually, the discomfort of gout begins at night or early in the morning. The affected joint is inflamed, erythematous, and exquisitely sensitive. Symptoms may subside after a few days to weeks without treatment when an interval between attacks occurs, where the individual remains symptom free.

Because chronic gout may involve more than one joint, it can be confused with osteoarthritis and RA. As the disease progresses, asymptomatic intervals shorten, more joints become involved, and attacks last longer. Tophi around joints are pathognomonic of gout (see Fig. 39-5). Extra-articular manifestations can also develop: low-grade fever, nephropathy (kidney disease), and nephrolithiasis (kidney stones).

CLINICAL CONCEPT

The classic presentation of acute gout is a sudden onset of inflammation and excruciating pain in the metatarsophalangeal joint of the great toe, a condition called podagra.

The major complications of gouty arthritis are related to joint and kidney involvement in the disease process. Untreated or undertreated gout can lead to the development of painful, disabling destruction of cartilage and bone. Irreversible joint deformity and loss

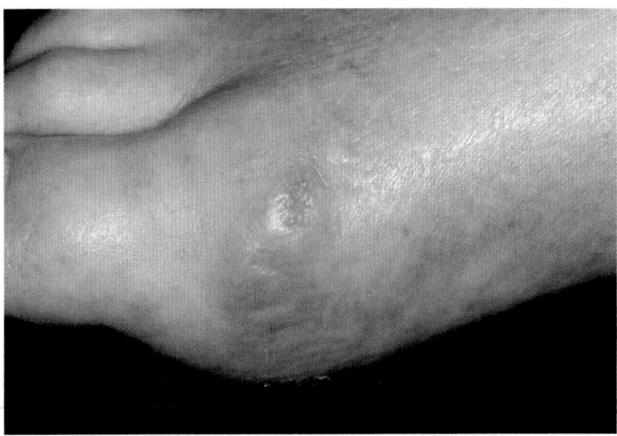

FIGURE 39-4. Podagra of gout. Podagra is an inflamed, reddened area around the joint of the great toe caused by gout, which is an arthritis caused by an excess of uric acid in the bloodstream. Crystals of uric acid collect inside the synovial space within the toe joint, causing inflammation and acute pain. *(From Dr. P. Marazzi/Science Source.)*

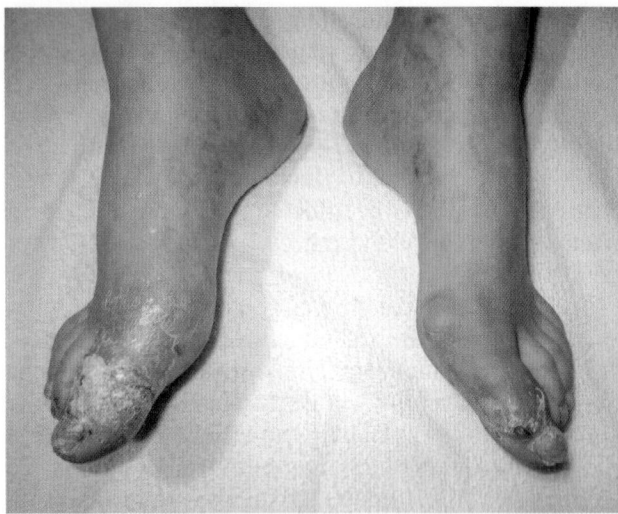

FIGURE 39-5. Tophi of great toe caused by gout. Tophi are swellings that contain uric acid crystals. *(Courtesy of James Heilman, MD.)*

of motion have been reported. Tophi can grow to significant sizes and require surgical removal. Prolonged hyperuricemia can lead to the formation of uric acid renal calculi (kidney stones). Individuals with gout have a 1,000-fold increased incidence of renal calculi; this is especially true when patients excrete more than 1,100 mg of uric acid in a 24-hour urine sample. Forty percent of persons with gout develop kidney stones. Persons with gout can also develop urate nephropathy, in which uric acid crystals are deposited in the tissue of the kidneys and cause renal dysfunction.

Diagnosis

Symptoms and frequency of attacks of gout should be described in the history. The patient should be asked about alcohol consumption, current medication use, and dietary intake of meat. Ingestion of foods rich in purines such as cooked or processed meats of animal origin increases levels of uric acid. Also, alcohol ingestion, either beer or hard liquor, can trigger gout. The patient should also be asked about a history of medical conditions, such as proliferative or neoplastic disease (cancer), psoriasis, sarcoidosis, or other inflammatory disorders. It is important to ask the patient about recent chemotherapeutic treatments, potential lead exposure, recent weight change, trauma, or surgery. Family history of gout is significant, as there is a genetic cause of the disorder.

Diagnostic tests should be aimed at ruling out different diagnoses such as pseudogout, cellulitis, septic arthritis, RA, and bunion bursitis. All these disorders resemble gout but are not related. Laboratory tests should include serum uric acid levels, CBC, ESR, CRP, and rheumatoid factor.

A 24-hour urine uric acid of more than 900 mg suggests overproduction of urate. A serum uric acid level of more than 7 mg/dL in males or 6 mg/dL in females is suggestive of gout, but is not diagnostic. Uric acid

levels should not be relied upon to provide a diagnosis. Although most individuals with gout have elevated uric acid levels intermittently during the course of the disease, hyperuricemia may not be present during an acute attack. Furthermore, having hyperuricemia alone does not mean that an individual will develop gout. In fact, most individuals with elevated serum uric acid do not develop gout.

X-rays often reveal soft tissue inflammation and asymmetric swelling during the acute phase of gout. However, in the early stages, x-rays may be normal. As the disease progresses, subtle changes in bony structures may be noted on x-ray; yet these findings do not typically occur until after at least 1 year of uncontrolled disease. Small punched-out lesions can develop within the periphery of affected joints but may not be detected unless two views of the x-ray are obtained. The classic sign of late-stage gout is the development of multiple large tophi. Joint space narrowing will also be apparent on radiological films.

Ultrasound is recommended, as it can show a specific sign, called a double contour line, over intra-articular cartilage within affected joints. This line on ultrasound is a shadowy line running parallel to the subchondral bone of a joint secondary to deposition of monosodium urate crystals. Aggregates of uric acid microcrystals can be detected as shadows within joints. Bone erosions can be detected as discontinuous regions of bone. CT scan cannot detect early inflammation, but intra-articular tophi can be well visualized. Dual energy CT (DECT) scan is a quick, noninvasive method to visualize uric acid crystals, soft tissue changes, and early erosions at high-resolution before x-ray.

The gold standard of diagnosis is aspiration of joint fluid for culture and urate crystals. The procedure is critical to the diagnosis of gout in order to rule out other inflammatory or infectious joint disorders. The detection of urate crystals, which are needlelike in appearance under the microscope, establishes a positive diagnosis of gouty arthritis. During acute attacks, the synovial fluid may contain a WBC count of 20,000 to 50,000 cells/mm^3, with a predominance of polymorphonuclear neutrophils.

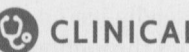 **CLINICAL CONCEPT**

It is important to differentiate gout from pseudogout (see Box 39-2).

Treatment

The management goal for gout is to treat acute attacks and prevent further attacks. It is important to begin administration of medications early in the disease to enhance treatment response. Pain can also be controlled with joint immobilization and decreased weight-bearing.

BOX 39-2. Differentiating Gout From Pseudogout

Pseudogout is a form of arthritis that mimics gout in presentation. The inflammation of pseudogout is caused by the formation of calcium pyrophosphate crystals, which have the microscopic appearance of rod-shaped crystals with blunt ends. Pseudogout is also called calcium pyrophosphate disease.

Although anyone can develop pseudogout, risk greatly increases with advancing age. Older adults are more prone to the disease because they have a higher incidence of preexisting joint disease such as osteoarthritis. Knees are most commonly involved, but ankles, shoulders, elbows, wrists, or hands can be affected. Diagnosis is made with joint aspiration and microscopic evaluation for calcium pyrophosphate crystals.

NSAIDs are first-line agents to counteract the inflammation. Starting doses should be high for the initial 2 to 3 days, with a gradual dose reduction over the next 2 weeks; patients should be asymptomatic for at least 2 days before discontinuation of the NSAID. COX-2 inhibitors such as celecoxib can be alternatively used to reduce inflammation.

 CLINICAL CONCEPT

Only 7% of those with gout remain attack-free for more than 10 years: 78% of those with gout will have a recurrent attack within 2 years; 62% will have one within the first year after diagnosis. Nonpharmacological therapy includes maintaining or obtaining an ideal body weight, avoiding rapid weight loss, limiting overall alcohol and dietary meats (which contain purines that raise uric acid), avoiding binge drinking, drinking a minimum of 2 to 3 liters of fluid per day, and avoiding medications associated with hyperuricemia whenever possible. The medications allopurinol and probenecid are recommended to prevent further attacks of gout. Allopurinol decreases uric acid synthesis, and probenecid increases renal excretion of uric acid. The goal is to keep uric acid levels between 5.5 mg/dL and 6.5 mg/dL.

Once an infectious process is ruled out, oral corticosteroids can be initiated if NSAIDs are ineffective. Moderately high doses are used for 1 to 3 days and tapered over 2 weeks because more abrupt tapering can initiate a rebound flare. Intra-articular injections of corticosteroids can also directly reduce inflammation.

Colchicine is the oldest available agent for the treatment of acute gout. The drug has no analgesic activity but specifically blocks the inflammation caused by uric acid crystals. It is used for sudden attacks of gout. Colchicine is most effective when initiated during the first 12 to 24 hours of an attack. As an alternative, interleukin-1 antagonists, such as anakinra, are recommended for flare-ups. These drugs are particularly useful in resistant cases or in persons who cannot tolerate NSAIDs, corticosteroids, or colchicine.

Allopurinol and probenecid are used for long-term control of serum uric acid levels in gout. Allopurinol is a xanthine oxidase inhibitor that reduces synthesis of uric acid. Probenecid enhances excretion of uric acid. Alternatively, febuxostat, another newer xanthine oxidase inhibitor, can be used. Febuxostat can reduce uric acid to lower levels than allopurinol and is particularly useful in patients with renal insufficiency. However, some studies have shown a higher rate of thromboembolism with use of febuxostat that can cause myocardial infarction or stroke.

Persons treated for gout must also receive education about reducing red meat and organ meats, such as liver or kidney, in their diet. Beer and distilled liquor should also be avoided.

Polymyositis and Dermatomyositis

Polymyositis and dermatomyositis are part of a group of musculoskeletal diseases known as idiopathic inflammatory myopathies. These two conditions are both characterized by inflammation and destruction of muscle fibers. Polymyositis is the inflammation of multiple muscle groups in the body. Dermatomyositis is the inflammation of muscle with involvement of the skin.

Polymyositis and dermatomyositis are rare disorders. The prevalence rate of polymyositis ranges from 6 to 10 cases per 1,000,000 individuals. Polymyositis is a disease of adults older than age 20 years; dermatomyositis occurs more commonly in those younger than age 15 years and those older than age 50 years. African Americans have a higher incidence of polymyositis and dermatomyositis than European Americans, and females are affected by polymyositis nearly twice as often as males.

Etiology

The definitive cause of polymyositis and dermatomyositis is not known, but specific abnormalities within the immune system have been noted. Both polymyositis and dermatomyositis have been linked to the autoimmune disorders RA, SLE, and scleroderma. Dermatomyositis in the adult has also been linked to underlying malignancies. There is also a genetic predisposition, as these disorders are often familial.

Pathophysiology

Although the cause of both disorders is unclear, experts have hypothesized that a viral illness, injury, or microvascular damage leads to the release of muscle proteins that are misidentified as antigens. With both polymyositis and dermatomyositis, autoantigens begin an inflammatory process involving T cells, B cells, interferon gamma, interleukin-2, and TNF-alpha. The WBCs and inflammatory mediators surround muscle fibers and ultimately destroy them. In dermatomyositis, the WBCs and inflammatory mediators also gather around cutaneous blood vessels. This clustering of inflammation around cutaneous vessels causes dermatological changes.

Clinical Presentation

The onset of polymyositis and dermatomyositis is gradual with proximal muscle weakness appearing over a period of weeks to months. The initial signs and symptoms include malaise, fever, myalgias, muscle weakness, muscle pain and tenderness, and lethargy. Fatigue, weakness, fever, and malaise are often mistaken as a viral illness. Polymyositis and dermatomyositis involve striated muscles (voluntary skeletal muscles) simultaneously, resulting in symmetrical muscle weakness. Because early signs and symptoms are vague and generalized, diagnosis may be delayed and often is not made until symmetrically patterned muscle weakness or rash is apparent

Although polymyositis spares the dermis, dermatomyositis is associated with a classic skin rash that involves the eyelids, face, chest, and extensor surfaces of the extremities. The presence of a symmetric purple-red colored macular skin rash and eyelid edema suggests a diagnosis of dermatomyositis.

It is important for the clinician to gather detailed history information. As these disorders are linked to other autoimmune diseases, essential components of the history include a personal or family history of RA, SLE, and scleroderma. Underlying malignancies may also precede the development of polymyositis or dermatomyositis, so the history should focus on previous medical and surgical conditions or potential undiagnosed lung or breast cancer.

Diagnosis

Laboratory tests that indicate inflammation, such as creatinine phosphokinase and ESR, can be elevated 5 to 50 times above the normal range in both polymyositis and dermatomyositis. Other muscle enzymes may be elevated, including lactic dehydrogenase, aspartate aminotransferase, alanine aminotransferase, and aldolase. Additionally, patients may have leukocytosis, a positive rheumatoid factor, or positive antinuclear antibodies. Electromyography studies reveal characteristic muscle changes in nearly all patients with polymyositis or dermatomyositis: muscle membrane irritability and changes of motor unit action potentials.

Muscle biopsy is the most definitive test for polymyositis and dermatomyositis, revealing stages of muscle inflammation. In dermatomyositis, inflammatory cells surrounding blood vessels and atrophy of muscle cells are identified.

Treatment

The goals of treatment are to minimize muscle weakness and improve the ability to maintain activities of daily living (ADLs). Corticosteroids, such as prednisone, and immunosuppressive agents are considered first-line treatment. They are often initially administered at high doses and tapered as symptoms subside and creatinine phosphokinase levels decrease to normal range. In patients who fail to respond or develop intolerable side effects, other agents such as azathioprine, cyclosporine, chlorambucil, methotrexate, and cyclophosphamide have resulted in symptom improvement.

Another key treatment component is individually designed physical therapy to prevent contractures and enhance functional ability. Ideally, physical therapy should be initiated early in the disease course so that mobility and strength may be optimized. Most patients improve with treatment; full recovery is accomplished in approximately 50% of patients.

> ### 🔬 CLINICAL CONCEPT
>
> Most individuals with polymyositis or dermatomyositis respond to immunosuppressive therapy, and 5-year survival rates have been estimated at more than 80%. Specific complications linked to mortality include advanced muscle weakness, pulmonary involvement, cardiac involvement, dysphagia and aspiration pneumonia, associated malignancies, and adverse effects of immunosuppression.

Psoriatic Arthritis

PsA is a chronic inflammatory disease of the joints and connective tissue that is linked to the skin disorder psoriasis (see Chapter 41). In 85% of affected individuals, psoriatic skin disease precedes joint disease. PsA has been linked to other autoimmune disorders, including RA. PsA affects males at a slightly higher rate than females, with the onset of the disease occurring most often between 30 and 50 years of age.

There are five patterns or forms of PsA:

1. Distal interphalangeal (DIP) predominant: known as the "classic" form, DIP occurs in only approximately 5% to 10% of those with PsA
2. Arthritis mutilans: a severe, destructive arthritis that accounts for 5% of those affected by PsA
3. Symmetric arthritis: symmetrical arthritis, which affects fewer than 25% of those with PsA, is similar in appearance and destruction to RA, but has a milder course
4. Asymmetric arthritis: the most common type of PsA, occurring in up to 70% of affected patients
5. Spondylitis: this form, characterized by inflammation of the spinal column, occurs in more than 5% of individuals with PsA

Although patients can initially present with any one of these forms of arthritis, the patterns of PsA can change during the course of the disease, and up to 60% of patients do not have one permanent pattern of the disease course.

Etiology

The exact etiology is unknown, but PsA is believed to be an autoimmune disorder with T-cell–mediated immune response. Like other autoimmune disorders, environmental, genetic, and immunological factors are thought to be key factors in the development of PsA. Environmental factors include infectious agents and physical trauma. There is a genetic component to the disease, with PsA often present in several members of a family.

Pathophysiology

The pathophysiology of PsA is similar to that of other types of inflammatory arthritis. In psoriasis and PsA, T cells infiltrate the skin and joints. The T-cell infiltration sets off a cascade of immune-mediated inflammation. B lymphocytes, also involved in the inflammatory reaction, synthesize immunoglobulins. Immunoglobulins then become deposited in the epidermis and synovial membranes, leading to the classic psoriatic scaly skin lesions and inflammation within joints.

Clinical Presentation

The symptoms of PsA are similar to those of other arthritic diseases such as RA and gout. Patients may differ in their patterns of psoriatic involvement of skin and joints. Depending on the pattern or form of the disease, PsA can develop slowly with mild symptoms or quickly with severe symptoms.

PsA typically presents as pain, swelling, and erythema of the affected joints with accompanying extra-articular symptoms: generalized fatigue, redness, and pain of the eye; plaque psoriasis of the skin; and psoriatic nail changes. The nail changes occur in more than 80% of patients: pitting, ridging, and onycholysis (painless separation of nail from the nailbed).

When differentiating between the forms of PsA, signs and symptoms can vary significantly. DIP-predominant PsA primarily involves the distal joints of the fingers and toes. Those with arthritis mutilans suffer from destruction and erosion of the small joints of the hands, feet, and spine. Symmetric PsA usually affects multiple symmetric pairs of joints and can be disabling. Asymmetric arthritis may present with inflammatory changes in both large and small joints and does not occur in the same joints on both sides of the body. These patients may develop dactylitis (inflammation of all the finger joints), with a "sausagelike" appearance of the fingers or toes. The joints may also be warm and red, with periodic joint pain. Spondylitis (inflammation of the vertebral joints) often develops later in the disease and affects males

and older patients disproportionately. Often, those with spondylitis have **sacroiliitis,** which is inflammation of the sacroiliac joint, along with complaints of pain, stiffness, and difficulty with movement of the cervical, thoracic, or lumbar spine.

Diagnosis

A detailed history should focus on both current and previous skin and nail changes. The patient will often complain of psoriatic skin changes before the development of joint symptoms. Family history of psoriasis should also be investigated.

A definitive diagnosis of PsA cannot be made without evidence of classic psoriatic skin and nail changes. Health-care providers rely on the history and physical examination to diagnose PsA. Although tests are used to rule out other disease processes, there is no specific test to diagnose PsA.

Laboratory tests can be only somewhat helpful in diagnosing the patient with presumed PsA. Although ESR is elevated in only 40% to 60% of patients with PsA, the degree of ESR elevation often correlates with the severity of skin involvement. A high ESR occurs in severe cases of PsA, whereas low elevation of ESR occurs with mild disease. At least 20% of those with PsA will have an elevated serum uric acid level because of rapid skin turnover, breakdown of the skin's nucleic acids, and metabolism of these nucleic acids to uric acid.

In the early stages of PsA, x-rays do not reveal signs of arthritis and are not usually helpful in making a diagnosis. In the later stages, x-rays may show changes that are characteristic of PsA and not found with other types of arthritis. In those with DIP disease or arthritis mutilans, changes on x-ray of the fingers demonstrate a "pencil and cup" phenomenon where the end of the bone gets whittled down to a sharp point.

Treatment

Treatment goals for the individual with PsA are to control the inflammatory process and improve quality of life. NSAIDs and local corticosteroid injection are used in joint disease, as they decrease inflammation, pain, and stiffness. Standard treatment of PsA includes disease-modifying antirheumatic drugs (DMARDs), specifically TNF inhibitors. The TNF inhibitors, adalimumab, golimumab, and certolizumab, have been shown to have similarly significant benefits on arthritis, psoriasis, and radiographic damage. TNF inhibitors relieve more severe symptoms and slow or halt the joint and tissue damage. Another DMARD, ustekinumab, an interleukin inhibitor, has also been proven effective against PsA.

For persons with progressively severe symptoms or treatment resistance, methotrexate (MTX) has been used. MTX is recommended only for severe, disabling cases of PsA that do not respond to other treatment. MTX blunts the immune response and depletes the body of folic acid. Folic acid must be supplemented in patients on MTX. MTX can also cause hepatotoxicity, which can lead to cirrhosis, bone marrow toxicity, and severe anemia.

Topical vitamin D and corticosteroids can be used for mild PsA and for relieving its dermatological effects. Phototherapy using ultraviolet A and B light has also shown efficacy; however, the skin must be examined frequently for cancerous changes.

CLINICAL CONCEPT

Early recognition, diagnosis, and treatment of PsA can help minimize the extensive joint damage that occurs in later stages of the disease. Without adequate treatment, PsA can become disabling. Those with more progressive forms of the disease, such as arthritis mutilans, can suffer from significant impairment early on in the disease process.

Ankylosing Spondylitis

Ankylosing spondylitis (AS) is a systemic rheumatic disease that can affect multiple tissues throughout the body, such as the eyes, heart, lungs, and kidneys. Most commonly, ankylosing spondylitis is known as a form of chronic inflammation of the spine and the sacroiliac joints, which results in pain and stiffness in and around the spine. Other problems that can accompany AS include arthritis of joints in the extremities, iritis (inflammation of the eyes), and pulmonary fibrosis (scarring throughout the lungs).

Within the United States, the prevalence of AS is approximately 0.5% to 1% among European Americans, 3% to 4% in African Americans, and 18% to 50% in Native Americans. It is more common in males than in females, with symptoms commonly beginning in late adolescence or early adulthood. In females, the sacroiliac joint and joints away from the spine are more frequently affected, and the disease often progresses more slowly than in males.

Etiology

The exact etiology of AS remains unknown, though the tendency to develop it is believed to be genetically inherited, as most patients (90% to 95%) with AS are born with HLA-B27 on the surface of their cells. The genes that promote HLA-B27 increase the tendency of developing AS, whereas additional factors—perhaps environmental or infectious—are necessary for disease development.

Pathophysiology

The initial inflammation of AS is thought to occur as a result of an activation of the body's immune system by a bacterial infection, possibly *Klebsiella pneumoniae*, or a combination of infectious pathogens. Once activated, the immune system remains chronically stimulated with resulting tissue inflammation long after the initial bacterial infection has resolved.

The primary site of inflammation for AS is the enthesis (the point where tendons and ligaments join the bone around a joint) around the vertebral joints. For unknown reasons, macrophages and lymphocytes infiltrate and erode the enthesis and periosteum. Fibroblasts then proliferate and synthesize collagen to repair the region. However, collagen is fibrous tissue that eventually undergoes calcification and ossification (hardening). Flexibility is lost with ossification. After time, all the cartilage of the spinal joint is replaced by bony scar tissue and the joints become rigid. Simultaneously, the eroded bone undergoes repair with osteoblast activation and proliferation. The osteoblasts lay down callus (new bone), which is eventually replaced by compact, lamellar (stronger, layered) bone. Because of the bone repair, the shape of the bone's surface changes as the new bone grows outward and forms a new enthesis at the end of a deteriorated ligament. As calcification of the spinal ligaments progresses, intervertebral disc fibers, which are normally spongy and elastic, are replaced with bone as well. As the chronic remodeling occurs, the intervertebral discs, bones, and ligamentous tissue fuse, creating a rigid column of vertebrae.

Clinical Presentation

The symptoms of AS are related to inflammation of the spine, joints, and other organs. Classic signs and symptoms of early disease are low back pain and stiffness beginning in young adults in their early 20s. Pain is commonly centered over the sacrum and may radiate bilaterally to the buttocks, groin, and down the legs. As a result of inflammation, decreased flexion of the lumbar spine is usually the earliest observed sign. The individual has difficulty bending forward to touch their toes. Sacroiliitis is identified by palpation of tender points along the sacroiliac joints. When the disease progresses to involve the cervical spine, flexibility of the neck will also decrease. The extensive spinal changes in severely affected persons can cause kyphosis, inflexible hip, knee, and ankle joints. The individual eventually has difficulty ambulating. Other complications are described in Box 39-3.

Diagnosis

The history for the patient with AS needs to focus on identifying the spinal changes that aid in diagnosis. Family history is important because there is believed to be a genetic predisposition.

In addition to the patient's symptoms and physical examination findings, the diagnosis of AS is based on radiological findings and blood tests. X-rays are the single most important imaging technique to detect, diagnose, and monitor patients with this condition. Early bone and joint changes of calcification and later ossification can be detected on x-rays.

CLINICAL CONCEPT

When AS progresses up the spine, complete fusion of the vertebral bodies results in the x-ray appearance of a "bamboo spine."

ESR and CRP levels are elevated during the acute inflammatory phases of the disease and may be detected in 75% of all patients during their initial presentation. Alkaline phosphatase is elevated in approximately 50% of patients during active ossification (bone hardening). The blood test for genetic marker HLA-B27 is positive in the vast majority of patients.

Treatment

Treatment is targeted at controlling pain and maximizing mobility by reducing inflammation. Treatment plans incorporate physical therapy and home exercise to reduce pain and stiffness, along with medications to decrease inflammation and suppress immunity. NSAIDs such as naproxen and indomethacin are first-line agents used to decrease pain and stiffness of the spine and other joints. When NSAIDs fail to provide adequate symptom control, immunosuppressants are considered. TNF-blocking medications, such as adalimumab, are extremely effective for halting disease progression, decreasing inflammation, and improving spinal mobility. Interleukin-17 (IL-17) inhibitors, such as secukinumab, are also highly effective. MTX has been shown to be somewhat effective, but has a significant potential for hepatotoxicity, which can lead to cirrhosis, bone marrow toxicity, and severe anemia.

Physical therapy is an important part of treatment and can maintain flexibility and pain relief.

Polymyalgia Rheumatica

Polymyalgia rheumatica (PMR) is an inflammatory condition characterized by acute onset of bilateral morning stiffness in the shoulder and upper arms. It occurs less commonly in the neck, pelvic girdle, lower back, and thighs. Range of motion in the shoulders and arms is limited; however, there is no observable inflammation. It most commonly affects older females, rarely develops before age 50 years, and usually occurs after age 60 years. Median age at the time of diagnosis is 72 years. The onset can be abrupt, with patients transitioning from going to bed feeling well to awakening in the morning with pain and stiffness. The average annual incidence in the United States is 52.5 cases per 100,000 persons aged 50 years and older.

Etiology

The etiology of PMR is not known, but individuals with the condition often have elevated IL-2 and IL-6 levels. There is also a prevalence of elevated antibodies to adenovirus and respiratory syncytial virus in individuals with PMR. Occurrence in close family members suggests a genetic role in the pathophysiology of the disease.

Pathophysiology

The pathophysiology of PMR is basically a severe inflammatory reaction with immune components. A proposed theory suggests that in a genetically predisposed patient, an environmental factor—potentially a virus—initiates macrophage activation, resulting in production of cytokines. The production of the cytokines, along with ILs and lymphokines, further stimulates a cascade of immune-mediated inflammation that induces the clinical manifestations characteristic of PMR. There is evidence that the affected muscles are infiltrated with T cells around their respective blood vessels. For reasons not completely understood, patients with PMR are also commonly affected by giant cell arteritis (also called temporal arteritis).

Clinical Presentation

The signs and symptoms of PMR can be nonspecific; however, the abrupt onset of myalgia is a key sign of the disorder. Pain and stiffness are reportedly worse in the morning, lasting at least 1 hour. The shoulder girdle is the first region to become symptomatic in most patients. In the remainder of individuals, the hip or neck is the initial area affected. More rarely, pain occurs in distal joints such as those of the hands and wrists. There may be no remarkable findings on physical examination except muscle tenderness and decreased active ROM caused by pain. Rarely, the affected individual may have systemic symptoms such as low-grade fever, weight loss, malaise, fatigue, and depression.

CLINICAL CONCEPT

Of persons with PMR, 10% to 20% also suffer giant cell arteritis (temporal artery inflammation), which can cause vision loss. Patients should seek immediate treatment if headache, changes in vision, pain over the temporal artery, or high fever occur. In the later stages of PMR, disuse muscle atrophy (atrophy caused by lack of physical activity) with proximal muscle weakness and contractures of the shoulder may lead to limitation of passive and active ROM.

BOX 39-4. Diagnostic Criteria for Polymyalgia Rheumatica

Diagnostic criteria for PMR include:
- Age 50 years or older at onset of symptoms
- Bilateral pain or aching with morning stiffness for at least 1 month, which involves at least two of three areas: neck or torso, shoulders or arms, hips or thighs
- ESR of 40 mm/h or higher
- Prompt improvement of symptoms to steroid treatment

Diagnosis

The diagnosis is based on clinical presentation. Criteria for diagnosis have been suggested (see Box 39-4). Blood tests may assist in ruling out other disease processes, but they are not very helpful in confirming a diagnosis of PMR. X-rays of joints are usually not remarkable. ESR is often elevated but may not be significantly high. There is a rapid positive response to low-dose oral corticosteroids in PMR, which is pathognomonic of the disorder.

The history of the patient with PMR does not usually lead the health-care provider to the diagnosis. Other joint and muscle disorders are first ruled out before PMR is considered. The abrupt onset of symptoms and the manifestation of bilateral muscle and joint involvement are key factors in the diagnosis. Family history is also important because of genetic predisposition.

Treatment

Therapeutic goals are to control painful myalgia, improve muscle stiffness, and resolve constitutional symptoms of the disease. The disorder is best treated with anti-inflammatory medications and nonpharmacological therapy. Oral corticosteroids are the first line of treatment; however, they are needed on a long-term basis, which causes adverse effects (e.g., glucose intolerance, osteoporosis). Corticosteroids can completely resolve symptoms within 72 hours but need to be taken for up to 12 months. NSAIDs have been tried, but they are required in high doses that subject the patient to gastrointestinal and renal side effects. MTX has been ineffective and anti-TNF agents have proven inadequate to treat PMR.

Because of the side effects of corticosteroids, other drugs are tried in PMR. New agents, including IL-6 receptor inhibitors such as tocilizumab, have been found to be effective. These drugs can be taken long term and have a steroid-sparing effect. A bone mineral density study such as a DEXA scan is recommended at the onset of treatment. Because patients require long-term corticosteroids, bisphosphonate therapy, vitamin D, and calcium supplements are recommended to prevent corticosteroid-induced osteoporosis. Physical therapy is recommended, as it can help the patient maintain mobility.

 CLINICAL CONCEPT

The risk of vertebral fractures is five times greater in females with PMR. Therefore, calcium and vitamin D supplementation should be recommended for all patients taking corticosteroid therapy.

Chapter Summary

- The clinician should always examine and compare one area of the body with the opposing area of the body for symmetry when assessing musculoskeletal disorders.
- The great majority of musculoskeletal infections are bacterial, particularly when a break in bone integrity is exposed to the environment, as in a compound fracture or surgical fixation of a fracture.
- *S. aureus* is the most common bacteria that causes osteomyelitis (infection of bone). Individuals with diabetes mellitus are at particularly high risk for osteomyelitis of the lower extremities because of compromised distal blood flow and immunosuppression.
- Treatment of osteomyelitis commonly requires removal of an infected joint prosthesis. It also often requires débridement of sequestra, which is dead bone tissue.
- Complications of osteomyelitis can include pathological fractures, especially in weight-bearing bones weakened by infection of the cortex.

- Conditions in diabetes mellitus, including lack of sensation and decreased circulation in the lower extremities, favor bacterial invasion; gangrene often necessitates amputation of the lower extremities.

- Lyme disease affects persons who live in deer-infested environments. The deer tick carries the bacterium *B. burgdorferi*. Carried by unaffected deer, the tick does not cause pathology until it bites a human and injects the bacteria.

- A classic targetlike rash called EM often heralds the pathophysiology of Lyme disease, which can cause widespread arthralgias, myalgias, and neurological impairment.

- A 3-week course of the tetracycline antibiotic doxycycline is required to treat Lyme disease.

- Septic arthritis is a type of musculoskeletal infection that can arise from *Staphylococcus* that infects a joint. It can also occur in conjunction with a sexually trans-mitted gonorrhea or *Chlamydia* infection.

- Musculoskeletal inflammatory disease occurs most often because of autoimmune disorders, where the body forms autoantibodies for unknown reasons.

- Remissions and exacerbations often describe the pattern of autoimmune musculoskeletal inflammatory diseases.

- Corticosteroids are highly effective treatment in many autoimmune, musculoskeletal inflammatory disorders. However, long-term corticosteroids can cause adverse effects such as glucose intolerance and osteoporosis.

- Many autoimmune musculoskeletal inflammatory disorders are treated effectively with TNF or IL inhibitors.

- In RA, scleroderma, SLE, PsA, polymyositis, and dermatomyositis, antibodies against the body's own joints and muscles cause inflammation.

- Gout is an inflammatory disorder that is associated with elevation in serum uric acid levels. Treatment of gout requires anti-inflammatory agents and medica-tions to reduce uric acid levels. Colchicine is used for acute episodes of gout, followed by allopurinol, which reduces uric acid levels.

- The individual with PsA usually presents with a red, scaly, patchy rash commonly on the extensor surfaces.

- AS is a disorder caused by calcification and ossification of the intervertebral discs, surrounding ligaments, and vertebrae–mainly of the sacroiliac joints. Rigidity and inflexibility of the spine occur.

- PMR is a disorder of inflammation that commonly affects the muscles of the shoulder girdle.

Making the Connections

Signs and Symptoms	Physical Assessment Findings	Diagnostic Testing	Treatment
Osteomyelitis | Acute or chronic microbial invasion of bone and bony structures. Infectious process results in inflammatory destruction that may be localized or spread through other bony tissues. *S. aureus* is the most common bacterial pathogen.			
Generalized symptoms of chills, fever, and malaise are common. Limited ROM. Pain.	Localized symptoms include tenderness, erythema, edema, and pain with movement of the affected extremity.	Radionuclide bone scan demonstrates area of infection. White blood cell radionuclide scan best diagnostic imaging study. Bone biopsy needed for culture of infection.	IV antibiotic therapy for 2 to 6 weeks followed by oral therapy. Débridement of necrotic tissue and debris may be necessary. Hyperbaric oxygen treatment can enhance healing.
Septic Arthritis | Infectious or pyogenic arthritis with direct invasion of the joint space by bacteria, viruses, mycobacteria, or fungi causing effusion. Classified as nongonococcal or gonococcal. Most commonly affects the knee or hip of adults and the hip in children.			
Fever and malaise; acutely painful, edematous, and erythematous joint. Pain will limit the ROM of the joint.	Acutely tender, edematous, and erythematous joint. Fever.	Definitive diagnosis requires detection and identification of microorganism from blood or synovial fluid.	Treatment focuses on drainage of joint, short-term immobilization for pain control, and admin-istration of appropriate antimicrobial agent. Antibiotics are typically administered IV for 2 to 4 weeks, followed by oral therapy. Intra-articular injection of antibiotics may be necessary.

Continued

Making the Connections—cont'd

Signs and Symptoms	Physical Assessment Findings	Diagnostic Testing	Treatment
Mycobacterium tuberculosis | Extrapulmonary invasion of *M. tuberculosis* into bone and bony structures. Most commonly involves the spine in a condition called Pott's disease; less commonly affects the hip or knee.			
Localized pain, joint effusion, and decreased ROM are common complaints.	Localized pain, joint effusion, decreased ROM, and kyphosis. Abscesses can extend into adjacent tissue.	Purified PPD skin test may be negative in those with extrapulmonary TB. Chest x-ray may reveal lung involvement, but bone x-ray findings are usually nonspecific early in the disease process. Excisional biopsy is the preferred method of obtaining tissue for diagnostic evaluation.	Treated with antitubercular drugs for long-term therapy. A multidrug regimen extended to 12 months is recommended.
Lyme Disease | Most common vector-borne disease in the United States. It is caused by a tick-transmitted spirochete, *B. burgdorferi,* which is often carried by deer. Transmitted by the deer tick to the human, it can affect the heart, joints, eyes, and CNS.			
Early localized disease occurs 3 to 30 days after tick bite; symptoms include EM rash, fatigue, fever, chills, myalgias, arthralgias, and headache. Late disseminated disease occurs months to years after tick bite; symptoms can include severe joint pain with edema and chronic cardiac, neurological, musculoskeletal, and CNS effects.	EM "bull's-eye" type rash. Fever, extreme fatigue, joint swelling, Bell's palsy are common.	Diagnosis based on patient's symptoms, physical examination findings, and a history of possible exposure to infected ticks. A two-step laboratory test (ELISA or IFA followed by Western blot) can assist with the diagnosis.	A 21-day course of the antibiotic doxycycline is recommended for those with early localized disease. Early disseminated disease is treated with a longer course of antibiotic. Late disseminated disease warrants IV antibiotic therapy and should be managed by an infectious disease specialist.
Gout | A syndrome characterized by recurrent inflammation as a result of hyperuricemia in blood and body fluids. An inborn error causes overproduction or inadequate renal excretion of uric acid. Uric acid forms an insoluble precipitate that deposits in joints, as well as connective and subcutaneous tissues.			
Pain, swelling, redness, and tenderness of joint; most commonly, the metatarsal-phalangeal joint in the great toe; exquisitely tender.	Sudden onset of a warm, painful, erythematous joint. Podagra, inflammation of the metatarsal-phalangeal joint of the great toe, is the most common presentation.	Serum uric acid level of greater than 7 mg/dL in males or 6 mg/dL in females is suggestive of gout. Radiographic studies often reveal soft tissue edema. Ultrasound and CT scan can show signs of joint contour associated with gout. The gold standard of diagnostics is joint aspiration and fluid analysis for urate crystals.	NSAIDs and colchicine are used for acute attacks. Recurrent attacks are prevented with medications to decrease uric acid production (e.g., xanthine oxidase inhibitor; allopurinol) or increase renal excretion (e.g., probenecid). Other anti-inflammatory medications used include IL-1 antagonists (e.g., anakinra and the newer uric acid inhibitor, febuxostat).

Making the Connections—cont'd

Signs and Symptoms	Physical Assessment Findings	Diagnostic Testing	Treatment
Polymyositis and Dermatomyositis | Autoantigens begin a series of processes that result in the production of several inflammatory cells. Inflammatory cells surround and ultimately destroy individual muscle fibers and small groups of fibers. In dermatomyositis, the inflammatory cells group around blood vessels and cause damage to the cutaneous vasculature as well as muscles.			
Initial symptoms include malaise, fever, lethargy, and muscle swelling, pain, or tenderness.	Muscle weakness in proximal extremities appears over weeks to months. Classic skin changes include a symmetric purple-red macular rash that affects the eyelids, chest, and extensor surfaces of extremities.	Creatine phosphokinase and ESR can be elevated 5 to 50 times above the normal range. Electromyography is abnormal. Muscle biopsy is the most definitive test.	Immunosuppressants play an important role in limiting the disease process. Corticosteroids are considered first-line agents; they are started at high doses until symptoms improve, then gradually tapered. Physical therapy should be initiated early in the disease to optimize strength and mobility.
Psoriatic Arthritis (PsA) | A chronic inflammatory disease of joints and connective tissue that is linked to psoriasis. T lymphocytes infiltrate skin and joints and initiate a cascade of immune-mediated inflammation. Immunoglobulins become deposited in the skin and synovial membranes.			
Pain and swelling of joints are observed on both sides of the body. Spondylitis usually affects the spine and sacroiliac joint.	Red, scaly, silvery plaque rash (psoriasis) and nail pitting are key findings for all forms. Swelling over joints.	A definitive diagnosis requires evidence of classic psoriatic skin and nail changes. In later stages, x-rays may reveal characteristic changes: "pencil and cup" phenomenon.	NSAIDs and corticosteroids are used. DMARDs, mainly anti-TNF agents, such as golimumab. Topical vitamin D and corticosteroids. Phototherapy may be used. MTX if other treatments are ineffective.
Ankylosing Spondylitis | Systemic rheumatic disease that can affect multiple tissues, but commonly results in chronic inflammation of the spine and sacroiliac joints. Collagen calcifies and ossifies, replacing all cartilage of the affected area with bony tissue. Vertebral bodies become fused with bony bridges to adjacent vertebrae. Inflammation can affect many other organ systems, including the lungs, eyes, heart, kidneys, and gastrointestinal system.			
Low back pain (centered over the sacrum) and morning stiffness in young adults. Eyes, heart, lungs, nerves, and gastrointestinal system can be affected.	Limited ROM is common; the thoracic vertebrae develop an inflexible forward curvature. Eyes, heart, lungs, nerves, and gastrointestinal system can be affected.	X-rays are the single most important diagnostic test. A loss of joint space can be detected. More classic signs are the appearance of a "bamboo spine" as the vertebrae fuse. Nonspecific laboratory tests are often elevated: ESR, CRP, and alkaline phosphatase. Genetic marker for HLA-B27 is positive in the vast majority of cases.	Physical therapy and exercise reduce pain and stiffness and improve posture, joint mobility, and lung capacity. NSAIDs; naproxen and indomethacin can be used with corticosteroids used as an adjunct. TNF-blocking medications, such as anakinra, and IL-17 inhibitors, such as secukinumab, are effective.

Continued

Making the Connections—cont'd

Signs and Symptoms	Physical Assessment Findings	Diagnostic Testing	Treatment
Polymyalgia Rheumatica (PMR) | Autoimmune disorder with monocyte activation (potentially by a virus) leading to cytokine production and immune-mediated inflammation. Appears to be related to giant cell arteritis (also called temporal arteritis).			
Abrupt onset of myalgia; pain and stiffness are worse in the morning and last more than 1 hour.	Shoulder swelling, pain, limited ROM of other joints.	A presumed diagnosis is based on clinical presentation. Diagnostic tests are not very helpful.	Oral corticosteroids are used, except there are adverse effects. NSAIDs are often used, especially as corticosteroids are "tapered." IL-6 receptor inhibitors, such as tocilizumab, are effective and corticosteroid-sparing treatment.

Bibliography

Available online at fadavis.com

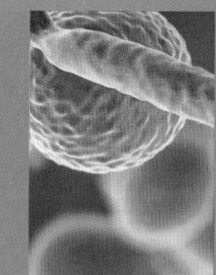

CHAPTER

40

Cancer

Learning Objectives

Upon completion of this chapter, the student will be able to:

- Identify common risk factors and etiologies that can lead to cancer.
- Differentiate among the characteristics of benign versus malignant neoplasia.
- Recognize the pathological mechanisms involved in the development of cancer in the body.
- List assessment techniques, laboratory tests, and imaging studies used to diagnose cancer.

- Recognize the most common types of cancer and their symptoms and clinical manifestations.
- List common complications caused by cancer that can lead to comorbidities.
- Discuss the pharmacological and nonpharmacological treatments used to manage cancer.
- Describe common side effects associated with cancer treatment modalities.

Key Terms

Adenocarcinoma
Adenoma
Alpha-fetoprotein (AFP)
Anaphase
Anaplasia
Apoptosis
Benign
Brachytherapy
Cachexia
Carcinoembryonic antigen (CEA)
Carcinoma

Cell cycle
Cytokinesis
Differentiation
Epi-drugs
Epigenetics
Epimutations
Interphase
Kinases
Leukemia
Lymphoma
Malignant

Melena
Metaphase
Metastasis
Oncogene
Paraneoplastic syndrome
Prophase
Sarcoma
Telophase
TNM system
Tumor suppressor gene
Vascular endothelial growth factor (VEGF)

A cancerous neoplasm, also termed neoplasia, is an abnormal mass of cells that grows in an uncoordinated manner and proliferates independently at a rate greater than normal cells. Cancerous changes in cells result from sporadic (nonhereditary) and inherited genetic alterations that persist and perpetuate the growth of cancer (neoplastic) cells. Sporadic genetic alterations commonly arise from exposure to carcinogens in the environment. For a large number of cancers, there exists a hereditable genetic alteration that originated with either parent of the cancer patient. Other cancers develop because of defective **tumor suppressor genes**—genes that guard against cancer formation. There are also cancers that develop because of mutated proto-oncogenes, which are genes that control normal cell growth and proliferation. Mutated proto-oncogenes become **oncogenes** that allow unrestrained cell division. Cancer can also be caused by dysfunctional DNA repair genes or faulty cellular apoptosis mechanisms. Dysfunctional DNA repair genes do not fix errors of the genome and allow mutations to persist and drive cells to synthesize aberrant proteins. Faulty cellular apoptosis mechanisms do not initiate programmed cellular degeneration, allowing abnormal cells to endure and propagate.

Regardless of the cause, cancer cells look distinctly different from normal cells. Cancer or neoplastic cells are nonuniform in architecture, disorganized, and misshapen. The cells are undifferentiated or anaplastic, which means that they do not resemble their normal counterparts. Cancer cells fail to function like healthy cells and often secrete abnormal proteins, hormones, invasive enzymes, and growth factors. Cancer cells compete with normal cells for space, blood supply, oxygen, and nutrition. They regenerate, multiply rapidly, and may travel to distant sites in the body (termed metastasis), where they take up residence and proliferate further. They possess an unlimited life span, as well as genetic instability, and disregard cell cycle checkpoints and repair mechanisms. In general, cancer can be seen as a parasite that draws what it needs for survival from the human host, gathers strength from its surroundings, constantly regenerates, multiplies exponentially, and leaves its victims debilitated.

Epidemiology

Cancer is the second leading cause of death behind cardiovascular disease. The most significant risk factor for cancer overall is age: two-thirds of all cancers occur in those older than age 65 years. For persons from birth to age 39 years, 1 in 72 males and 1 in 52 females develop cancer; for those ages 40 through 59 years, 1 in 12 males and 1 in 11 females develop cancer; and for those between ages 60 and 79 years, 1 in 3 males and 1 in 5 females develop cancer.

In males, the most common cancer is prostate cancer; in females, breast cancer. When rates for both sexes are combined, however, the most common cancer is lung cancer, which also happens to be the most common cause of cancer death. Cancers of the lung, female breast, prostate, and colon constitute more than 50% of cancer diagnoses and cancer deaths in the United States. Cancer occurs more often in males than in females and, for reasons that are unclear, African American males have the highest incidence and mortality.

Etiology of Cancer

It is estimated that 5% of human cancers are caused by viruses or chronic inflammation, 5% by radiation, and the remaining 90% by chemicals. Of these, an estimated 30% are caused by the use of tobacco products and the rest by chemicals associated with diet, lifestyle, and the environment. All chemical carcinogens or their derivatives contain highly reactive oxygen species (ROS) (also called free radicals), which are electron-deficient compounds that react with electron-rich sites in the cell. The cell's membrane and DNA, in particular, are chemically attractive to ROS. ROS can break down the plasma membrane, which leaves the organelles and nucleus vulnerable

to further injury. DNA alterations lead to subsequent mutated RNA and aberrant protein synthesis. Approximately 6 million chemicals have been identified as carcinogens. Of these, it is estimated that more than 50,000 are used regularly in commerce and industry. However, fewer than 2,000 have been closely examined for their carcinogenic potential. According to the International Agency of Research on Cancer (IARC), the U.S. Environmental Protection Agency (EPA), and the U.S. National Toxicology Program's Report on Carcinogens (RoC), there are more than 100 known human carcinogens (see Box 40-1 for common chemical carcinogens).

Basic Concepts Related to the Understanding of Cancer

There are basic concepts that pertain specifically to the study of cancer. These concepts include:

- The cell cycle
- Immunocompetence as it relates to tumor development
- Tumor classification and staging
- Cancer genetics
- Role of viruses in cancer
- Stages of carcinogenesis
- Metastasis and tumor angiogenesis

BOX 40-1. Selected Agents Classified as Human Carcinogens by the International Agency for Research on Cancer (IARC) and the National Toxicology Program Report on Carcinogens (ROC)

- Acetaldehyde
- Aflatoxin
- Arsenic
- Asbestos
- Benzene
- Benzo(a)pyrene
- 1,3 Butadiene
- Cadmium
- Chromium VI
- Coal tar
- Dioxins
- Estrogens
- Ethanol
- *Helicobacter pylori*
- Ionizing radiation
- Formaldehyde
- Radon
- Vinyl chloride

From Malarkey, D. E., Hoenerhoff, M., & Maronpot, R. R. (n.d.). Carcinogenesis: Mechanisms and manifestations. Retrieved from https://focusontoxpath.com/carcinogenesis-mechanisms-and-manifestations

- Biomarkers of cancer cells
- Nomenclature used in neoplasia
- Paraneoplastic syndromes
- Cancer cachexia

The Cell Cycle

The **cell cycle** is a sequence of growth stages that a cell moves through for mitosis and regeneration. The cell must go through stages G_0, G_1, S, G_2, and M to undergo mitosis (see Fig. 40-1). In stage G_0, the cell is at rest and is not actively engaged in the cell cycle. In stage G_1, cells enter the cell cycle, grow, and prepare for DNA replication. In the S stage, synthesis of DNA occurs; each of the 46 chromosomes is duplicated by the cell. In the G_2 stage, there is checking of the duplicated chromosomes for any errors and needed repairs. During the G_1, S, and G_2 stages, the cell is growing and performing activities necessary for mitosis; this preparatory phase is commonly called the **interphase.** After interphase, the mitosis (M) stage occurs, separated into four phases: **prophase, metaphase, anaphase,** and **telophase.** During prophase, chromosomes condense, the nuclear membrane dissolves, and spindle fibers appear. During metaphase, the 46 chromosomes begin to reorganize as two separate sets of 23 chromosome pairs. During anaphase, the two sets of chromosomes are pulled to opposite poles by the spindle fibers. Lastly, in telophase, two distinct nuclear envelopes form, spindle fibers dissolve, and chromosomes condense within each nucleus. During **cytokinesis,** the cytoplasm splits into two distinct cells, each containing 23 pairs of chromosomes, forming two daughter cells.

Cancer cells are constantly moving through the cell cycle stages. During the cell cycle, there are several checkpoints where DNA replication mechanisms can be stopped if errors have occurred in the synthesis of cell parts before mitosis. Cells can undergo repair, recycling, or apoptosis (programmed degeneration) if errors exist. Commonly, if errors are identified during the G_2 stage in the cell cycle, the cell is signaled to undergo apoptosis. However, cancer cells do not undergo scrutiny at checkpoints, or repair, and do not undergo apoptosis.

There are several cell-cycle checkpoint proteins called **kinases.** These proteins include cyclin-dependent kinase, checkpoint kinase, WEE1 kinase, aurora kinase, and polo-like kinase. In cancer, the genes encoding these proteins are often mutated so these checkpoint kinases do not work, leading to unrestrained cancer cell growth. These deregulated kinase proteins are overexpressed in many malignancies.

Cancer cells disregard the growth inhibitors released by neighboring cells. As the cancer cells proliferate, they accumulate on top, around, and beside each other, take over boundaries of organs, crowd out normal cells, and may even break free and travel to distant body sites. Cancer cells are invasive and

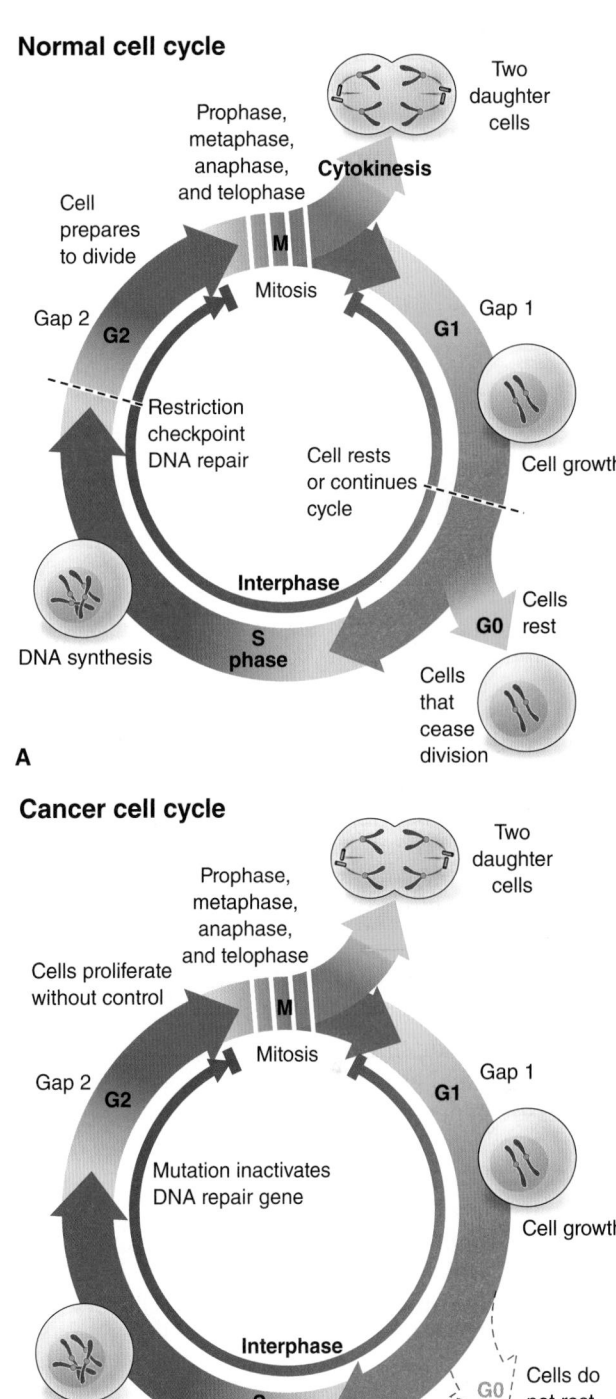

FIGURE 40-1. The normal cell cycle versus the cancer cell cycle. **(A)** Normal cell cycle. The cell cycle is an ordered sequence of events that occurs when cells multiply and regenerate. The specific stages are G_0, G_1, S, G_2, and M. During G_0, the cell is quiescent and at rest. In stage G_1, enzymes called cyclin-dependent kinases activate the cell to enter the cell stage. In the S stage, the cell is synthesizing new DNA in preparation for mitosis. In stage G_2, there is a checkpoint that senses DNA damage and delays the cycle to allow DNA repair before entry into mitosis. In the M stage, mitosis occurs. Mitosis phases include interphase, prophase, metaphase, anaphase, telophase, and finally cytokinesis when daughter cells are formed. After mitosis, the cell enters a resting stage (G_0) and awaits another signal to enter the cycle. **(B)** Cancer cell cycle. Cancer cells go through the cell cycle constantly. There are no restrictive checkpoints or resting phases. They are actively proliferating without control.

equipped with enzymes that break down surrounding membranes.

Immunocompetence as It Relates to Tumor Development

The immune system constantly surveys the body for foreign substances or "nonself" antigens. When a "nonself" antigen is discovered, the immune system initiates an attack to destroy the invading substance. This attack also occurs when the body produces a defective or mutated cell; the body recognizes it as "nonself" and the immune system destroys it. With neoplasm development, once abnormal cells start proliferating, the immune system attacks and destroys these aberrant cells. However, with age, mutated cells can escape immune surveillance, perpetuate themselves, and form tumors. Because immunocompetence declines with aging, older adults are more susceptible to tumor development.

Cancer Genetics

All cancers originate from changes in DNA. Genetic mutations are required for the transformation of a normal cell into a cancer cell. These mutations can be hereditary or sporadic. Hereditary genetic mutations are passed down from parents to offspring. Sporadic genetic mutations are acquired during a person's lifetime due to carcinogen exposure. Types of genes that are involved in the development of cancer include tumor suppressor genes, oncogenes, DNA repair genes, and genes that control apoptosis. Tumor suppressor genes normally function to restrain cell growth. However, these genes can also become defective and lose the ability to inhibit cell growth and division, thus allowing cancer formation. The *TP53* gene, the tumor suppressor gene in cells, controls cellular **apoptosis,** which is the natural death of cells with damaged DNA. Approximately half of all cancers have a defective *TP53* gene. The *TP53* gene, known as the "guardian of the genome," is located at the short arm of chromosome 17 at region 13.1 (17p13.1). With a defective *TP53* gene, cells with damaged DNA are not destroyed; they proliferate unchecked and progress to malignancy.

Proto-oncogenes are genes that stimulate and regulate a cell's movement through the cell cycle, resulting in cellular growth and proliferation. When mutated, proto-oncogenes become oncogenes that stimulate constant, unrelenting cellular proliferation and cell cycling.

DNA repair genes code for proteins that correct errors that arise when cells duplicate their DNA before cell division. DNA repair genes are critical for the maintenance of genome integrity. DNA repair genes are active throughout the cell cycle, particularly during the G_2 stage. Defective DNA repair genes can lead to errors in DNA, which in turn cause subsequent errors in RNA and mutated proteins. Certain forms of cancer involve defects in DNA repair.

Epigenetic changes also contribute to the development of cancer. **Epigenetics** is the study of how behaviors, lifestyle, and environmental factors can influence genes and the way the genes are expressed. Epigenetics is a rapidly expanding field, and the study of epigenetic regulation in cancer is emerging. Epigenetic changes do not change your DNA sequence, but change the way your body reads the DNA sequence. They are reversible changes that work by turning genes either "on" or "off." Epigenetic changes affect gene expression in the following ways (CDC, 2022):

- DNA methylation: A chemical group is added to the DNA, which can turn a gene "on" or "off."
- Histone modification: Histones are proteins that can wrap around genes and turn them on or off.
- Nocoding RNA modification: Not used to make proteins; it influences how ribosomes read the RNA to make proteins.

The environment and human behavior are main causes of epigenetic alterations. Poor diet, lack of exercise, drugs, exposure to environmental chemicals or radiation all have the potential to cause epigenetic mutations (also called **epimutations)** that can lead to cancer. Smoking cigarettes, for example, has been shown to affect DNA methylation patterns across multiple organ systems. The affected genes have been linked to several major diseases including cancer, osteoporosis, chronic obstructive pulmonary disease (COPD), cardiovascular disease, and rheumatoid arthritis. An important fact about epigenetics is that the changes to genes can be passed down from parent to child, called transgenerational inheritance. In other words, some epigenetic effects are inherited. People with certain genetic mutations carry a relatively high risk of developing cancer during their lifetimes, and these mutations can often be passed on to offspring. It is thought that about 1 in 20 to 1 in 10 (5% to 10%) of all cancers are due to inherited mutations (Emory Winship Cancer Institute, 2022). Unlike genetic mutations, epimutations are reversible. The terms epigenetic treatments or **epi-drugs** refer to drugs that reverse abnormal epigenetic modifications in cancer cells. Epi-drugs are not cytotoxic; their goal is to "reprogram" cancer cells. The targets of epigenetic therapy are the enzymes involved in epigenetic modifications (Emory Winship Cancer Institute, 2022).

Cancer is also caused by deregulation of programmed cellular degeneration, also called apoptosis. The balance between cell proliferation and apoptosis is critical in normal tissue homeostasis. Deregulation of apoptosis in normal cells results in many diseases, including cancer. Some genes signal cells to degenerate when damage or aging occurs. If these genes are dysfunctional, normal apoptosis of cells will not occur, allowing abnormal cell accumulation.

Role of Viruses in Cancer

Certain malignancies are associated with cancer-inducing viruses. For any virus to live and propagate, it must insert its genes into the host cell's genome. The host cell then becomes a manufacturer of the virus. In viral-induced cancer, the mechanisms of action differ among viruses, but the mechanisms always involve the activation of growth-promoting pathways or inhibition of tumor suppressors in infected cells. Examples of cancers activated by viruses include cervical cancer, Burkitt's lymphoma, and hepatocellular carcinoma (HCC).

 CLINICAL CONCEPT

Cervical, anorectal, vaginal, vulvar, penile, and oropharyngeal cancers are associated with human papillomavirus (HPV), Burkitt's lymphoma is associated with Epstein-Barr virus (EBV), and hepatocarcinoma is associated with hepatitis B and C viruses.

Stages of Carcinogenesis

Carcinogenesis is a complex, multistep process that can be divided into three major stages: initiation, promotion, and progression (see Fig. 40-2). Initiation involves the alteration, change, or mutation of genes arising spontaneously or induced by exposure to a carcinogenic agent. Genetic alterations can result in dysregulation of biochemical signaling pathways associated with cellular proliferation, apoptosis, or DNA repair function.

The promotion stage is considered to be a relatively lengthy and reversible process in which actively proliferating preneoplastic cells accumulate. Within this period, the process can be altered by chemopreventive agents that affect growth rates.

Progression is the phase between a premalignant lesion and the development of invasive cancer. Progression is the final stage of neoplastic transformation, where genetic and phenotypic changes and cell proliferation occur. This involves a rapid increase in tumor size. The proliferating cells may undergo further mutations with invasive and metastatic potential.

Metastasis and Tumor Angiogenesis

Malignant cancer cells are invasive, penetrative, and destructive to surrounding tissue. They penetrate through basement membranes and metastasize from a primary site to a distant site through lymph or blood. Certain tumors have common sites of metastasis, as shown in Table 40-1.

Tumor cells that metastasize must embed where there are sufficient nutrients, blood supply, and oxygen. For establishment in a target organ, the tumor must develop its own blood vessels and connect to the preexisting blood supply. Cancer cells are suited for this task because they secrete **vascular endothelial growth factor (VEGF),** a substance that gives them the capability to develop new blood vessels.

Biomarkers of Cancer Cells

Biomarker testing is used increasingly as a means of identifying the type of cancer affecting the patient. Biomarkers are specific genes, proteins, enzymes, growth factors, or other substances that are unique to the cancer cells affecting the patient. They identify certain tumor characteristics that can be used to assign specific treatments and can be used to ascribe a prognosis regarding the disease. There are unique patterns of biomarkers that affect how certain cancer treatments work. There are also biomarkers that can help diagnose and monitor cancer during and after treatment. A biomarker test is commonly used

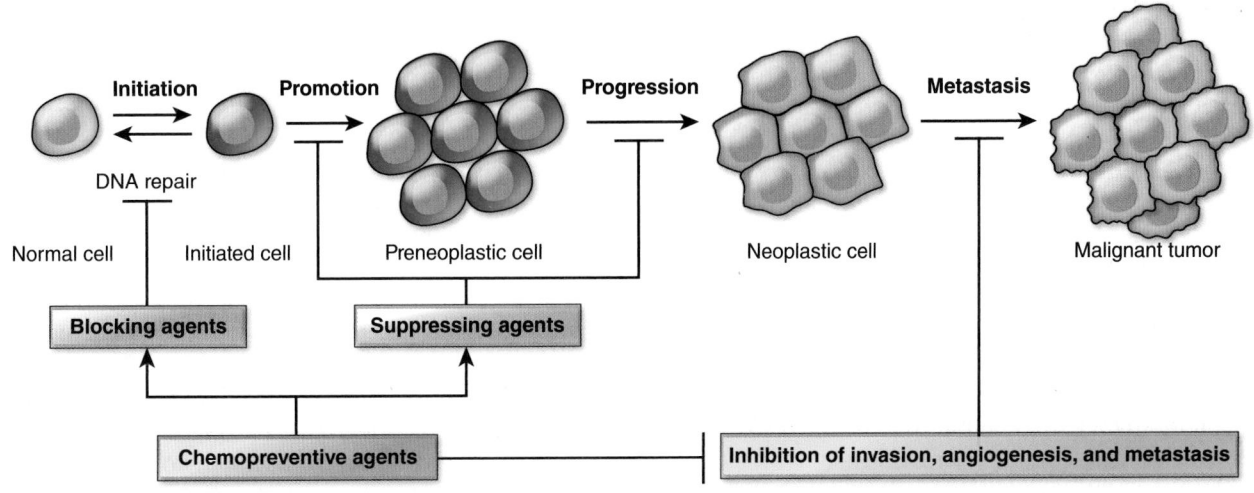

FIGURE 40-2. Stages of carcinogenesis.

TABLE 40-1. Common Metastatic Sites for Tumors

Cancer	Common Site of Metastasis
Lung	Bone, brain
Colon	Liver
Breast	Bone, brain, liver, lung
Prostate	Vertebrae
Melanoma	Brain

along with other diagnostic tests. Biomarker testing for cancer cells may also be called:

- Tumor testing
- Tumor genetic testing
- Genomic testing or genomic profiling
- Molecular testing or molecular profiling
- Tumor subtyping
- Immunophenotyping
- Immunohistochemistry

Biomarkers can be found on a biopsy of the cancer cells or in the blood, urine, stool, or other tissues or bodily fluids depending on the type of cancer. Some cancer treatments referred to as biological therapy, targeted therapies, and immunotherapies may only work for people whose cancers have certain biomarkers. For example, breast cancer cells that are referred to as HER2 positive have a certain surface protein that responds to a specific type of treatment. For examples of other common biomarkers, see Box 40-2.

Biomarkers can be used to:

- Estimate prognosis
- Determine the stage of cancer
- Detect cancer that remains after treatment (residual disease) or that has returned after treatment
- Assess how well a treatment is working
- Monitor whether the treatment has stopped working

Serial measurements, which show how the level of a marker is changing over time, are usually more meaningful than a single measurement. For example, a decrease in the level of a tumor biomarker in the blood may indicate that the cancer is responding to treatment, whereas an increasing or unchanged level may indicate that the cancer is not responding. Circulating tumor biomarkers may also be measured periodically after treatment has ended to check for recurrence (the return of cancer) (National Cancer Institute, 2021).

Nomenclature of Neoplasia

Neoplasia means "new growth," commonly referred to as a tumor. Tumors can be benign and noncancerous or malignant and cancerous. There are terms used to describe benign tumors and malignant cancers according to the type of tissue that is affected.

- **Benign** tumor—abnormal cells that remain localized; a benign tumor does not travel to other sites in the body
- **Malignant** tumor—spreads to other areas of the body
- **Adenoma**—benign tumor occurring in the lining of glandular tissue or organ (an example is a polyp found in the colon)

BOX 40-2. Examples of Biomarkers Used in Cancer Diagnosis and Treatment

BIOMARKER	WHAT IS ANALYZED	HOW USED FOR CANCER
Alpha-fetoprotein (AFP)	Blood	Diagnosis of liver cancer and response to treatment
BCL2 gene rearrangement	Bone marrow, blood, tumor biopsy	Diagnosis of certain lymphomas, leukemias, and choose treatment
CA-125	Blood	Diagnose ovarian cancer and assess treatment response and track recurrence
JAK2 gene mutation	Blood and bone marrow	Diagnosis of certain types of leukemias
CEA	Blood	Colorectal cancer response to treatment and track recurrence
ECFR gene mutation	Tumor biopsy	Determine treatment and prognosis of non–small-cell lung cancer
KRAS gene mutation	Tumor biopsy	Determine treatment and prognosis of non–small-cell lung cancer and colorectal cancer
Nuclear matrix protein 22	Urine	Bladder cancer response to treatment
Thyroglobulin	Blood	Response to treatment and recurrence of thyroid cancer

From National Cancer Institute. (NCI) (2021). Tumor markers in common use. https://www.cancer.gov/about-cancer/diagnosis-staging/diagnosis/tumor-markers-list

- Lipoma—derived from fat cells; among the most common benign tumors
- Hemangioma—benign collection of blood vessels in the skin or internal organ
- Desmoid tumor—although benign, can be highly invasive but does not metastasize
- Nevi—noncancerous moles on the skin that are very common
- Myoma—muscle tumor (a specific kind of benign muscle tumor of the uterus is called a leiomyoma)
- **Carcinoma**—malignant epithelial cells that line inner and outer surfaces
- **Adenocarcinoma**—cancer of the glandular or ductal tissue
- **Sarcoma**—cells undergoing cancerous changes are of mesenchymal origin, such as connective tissue, cartilage, and bone
- Osteoma—benign tumor of bone; however, osteosarcoma is malignant
- Chondroma—benign tumor of cartilage; however, chondrosarcoma is malignant
- **Leukemia**—cancerous changes in the leukocytes
- **Lymphoma**—cancerous lymphocytes in the lymph nodes and lymphoid tissue

Tumor Classification and Staging

The diagnosis of cancer relies heavily on tissue biopsy and analysis. Compared with normal cells, cancer cells are disorganized and nonuniform in architecture. **Differentiation** refers to the extent that neoplastic cells resemble normal cells, both structurally and functionally. Lack of differentiation is called **anaplasia,** a term that indicates total cellular disorganization, abnormal cell appearance, and cell dysfunction. Ordinarily, **benign** tumors are well differentiated and remain localized, cohesive, and well demarcated from surrounding tissue. Benign tumors are not invasive, do not destroy surrounding tissue, and do not break away

or travel from the tumor cell mass. In general, **malignant** tumors range from well differentiated to poorly differentiated, but they are invasive and destructive to surrounding tissue. Malignant, metastatic cells can be highly anaplastic with little resemblance to cells in their site of origin. Malignant cancer cells also lack adhesion to the tumor mass and easily break free to travel to distant sites in a process called **metastasis.** They travel via the lymphatic system or bloodstream. For this reason, often the first metastatic site is a lymph node. For the differences between benign and malignant tumors, see Table 40-2.

After establishing that a tumor is malignant, the tumor is examined and classified by grading and staging. Grading and staging predict the disease course and assist in the formulation of a treatment plan. Malignant tumors can be graded I through III. Grade I indicates that the cells are well differentiated, grade II cells are moderately differentiated, and grade III indicates poorly differentiated or anaplastic. Different classification systems are used to stage tumors. Staging classifies the tumor according to size, invasiveness, and spread. One commonly used classification method is the **TNM system.** T is for tumor size, N is for lymph node involvement, and M is for metastasis to distant organs. For example, if a patient has a 2.5-cm tumor in the right breast, palpable lymph nodes, and a computed tomography (CT) scan indicative of a metastatic lesion in the liver, it would be staged as $T_2N_1M_1$ breast cancer. See Table 40-3 for an example of staging for breast cancer using a TNM classification system.

Paraneoplastic Syndromes

Paraneoplastic syndromes are symptom complexes related to cancer's presence and action on the body. However, these are not symptoms caused by cancer's space-occupying effects, nor are they caused by cancer's metastatic effects. A **paraneoplastic syndrome** is an unexpected pathological disorder provoked by the presence of cancer in the body (see Table 40-4).

TABLE 40-2. Differences Between Benign and Malignant Tumors

Characteristic	Benign Tumors	Malignant Tumors
Differentiation	Well differentiated; resembles tissue of origin	Poorly differentiated (also referred to as anaplasia); does not resemble tissue of origin
Rate of growth	Progressive, slow	Erratic, slow to rapidly proliferative
Life span	Variable	Cells have unlimited life span
Genetics	Genetic stability	Genetic instability, mutations can occur
Local invasion	Cohesive cells, well-demarcated tumor	Invasive and infiltration of the surrounding normal tissue through enzymatic destruction
Metastasis	None	Frequent

TABLE 40-3. TNM Classification System

T (TUMOR)	
T_X	Main tumor cannot be measured
T_0	Main tumor cannot be found
T_{is}	Carcinoma in situ
T_{1-4}	Progressive increase in tumor size or involvement
N (NODES)	
N_X	Cancer in nearby lymph nodes cannot be measured
N_0	No cancer in nearby lymph nodes
N_{1-3}	Increasing involvement of regional lymph nodes
M (METASTASIS)	
M_X	Metastasis cannot be measured
M_0	Cancer has not spread to other parts of the body
M_1	Cancer has spread to other parts of the body

From National Cancer Institute. (2015). Retrieved from http://www.cancer.gov/cancertopics/factsheet/detection/staging

TABLE 40-4. Common Paraneoplastic Syndromes

Cancer	Paraneoplastic Syndrome
Lung	Cushing's syndrome, SIADH, hypercalcemia, myasthenia-like syndrome, acanthosis nigricans, dermatomyositis
Breast	Hypercalcemia, disorders of the CNS and peripheral nervous system, dermatomyositis
Pancreas	Venous thrombosis (Trousseau's syndrome), carcinoid syndrome, Cushing's syndrome
Hepatocellular	Polycythemia, hypoglycemia

A common type of paraneoplastic syndrome involves the secretion of endocrine hormones unrelated to the cancer tumor. For example, a patient suffering from lung cancer often endures excessive secretion of adrenocorticotropic hormone (ACTH) from the tumor. Another common paraneoplastic syndrome is hypercalcemia. For unclear reasons, in many types of cancers, the body produces a parathyroid-like hormone that stimulates bone breakdown and calcium accumulation in the blood. Cancers most often associated with paraneoplastic hypercalcemia are breast, lung, kidney, and ovary. Another inappropriate hormone secreted during lung cancer is antidiuretic hormone (ADH). Syndrome of inappropriate ADH (SIADH) can occur as a paraneoplastic disorder causing edema, hyponatremia, and hypertension. The body can also have an immune reaction to a neoplasm. Commonly, cutaneous signs of a malignancy occur. Paraneoplastic pemphigus is an autoimmune reaction that causes painful ulcerative lesions of the mucous membranes in persons with non-Hodgkin's lymphoma or chronic lymphocytic leukemia. Paget's disease is a breast cancer that is associated with a pruritic, well-demarcated, erythematous, scaly rash on the areola of the breast. Acanthosis nigricans is a hyperpigmented thickening of the skin that develops in axillae, neck, groin, and intertriginous areas. It is commonly associated with adenocarcinoma of the stomach or liver, or leukemia. A paraneoplastic syndrome is peculiar and unrelated to the cancer that has initiated the condition. However, it can be the cause of the first signs and symptoms of illness, and its investigation can lead to a diagnosis of the cancer that initiated it.

Cancer Cachexia

Patients with cancer commonly develop a progressive loss of body fat and lean body mass known as **cachexia.** The patient suffers profound weakness, unintentional weight loss, fatigue, loss of appetite, and anemia. The cause of the cachexia is theorized to originate with cytokines and mediators released by white blood cells (WBCs) that are attacking the tumor. The cytokines and mediators include tumor necrosis factor-alpha (TNF-alpha), interleukin-1, and proteolysis-inducing factor. These mediators induce the breakdown of muscle and fat and give the patient a wasted (cachectic) appearance.

Assessment

In cancer patients, important information is obtained from every portion of the history and physical examination. Because cancer can present in a variety of ways, various chief complaints may bring the cancer patient to the health-care provider. Patients with cancer often present with general complaints of anorexia, excessive fatigue, and weight loss. The clinician should inquire about any tumor or cancer in the past medical and surgical history. Also, the patient should be asked about the existence of any illnesses that predispose individuals to cancer, such as ulcerative colitis, chronic hepatitis, cervical HPV infection, chronic *Helicobacter pylori* gastritis, and breast and skin lesions. Family history may suggest an underlying familial predisposition to cancer. A genogram can map out this family history for a clearer view of susceptibilities. Social history can describe the behaviors, environmental exposures, and lifestyle habits that increase susceptibility to cancer. Behaviors such as smoking, alcohol abuse, unsafe sexual practices, and occupational exposures should be investigated. The review of systems can reveal a spectrum of symptoms that indicate a paraneoplastic syndrome, metastatic disease, or signs of a primary cancer.

Physical Examination

The clinician should perform a thorough physical examination, which may demonstrate findings consistent with a primary cancer, cancer metastasis, or paraneoplastic syndrome. The clinician should carefully palpate the regions of lymph nodes, such as cervical, axillary, epitrochlear, supraclavicular, infraclavicular, and inguinal. The thyroid should also be inspected and palpated. The breast examination on the female is of particular importance, so the clinician should inspect and palpate all areas of the breast and axilla.

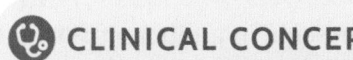

CLINICAL CONCEPT

Virchow's node is the term used for an enlarged, left-sided, supraclavicular lymph node. This can indicate breast, lung, or abdominal cancer.

Auscultation of the heart and lungs is critical, as is palpation of the abdomen. Paraneoplastic syndromes or metastasis of cancer can present with abnormalities of the heart and lungs. For example, an occult lung tumor or metastasis of cancer to the lungs can present as pulmonary crackles, wheezes, or obstructive atelectasis (collapse of alveoli). The abdominal examination should include palpation of the liver, a common site of metastasis. The patient's skin should be thoroughly inspected for suspicious lesions—those that are asymmetric with irregular borders, varied in color, and larger than a pencil eraser in diameter. The patient should be questioned about any changes in moles or bothersome skin lesions. Wounds that are not healing in a timely manner can also be indicative of cancer. Males should have a digital rectal examination (DRE), which allows palpation of the prostate gland; a fecal occult blood test (FOBT) can be done in conjunction. The male testicles should be palpated for masses or lesions. Females require a pelvic examination and FOBT as well. An anal Papanicolaou (Pap) smear is necessary for persons at risk of anorectal cancer.

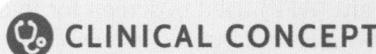

CLINICAL CONCEPT

A hard, nodular prostate gland, which is a sign of prostate cancer, can be palpated through the rectal wall.

Diagnosis

The diagnosis and prevention of cancer rely heavily on specific screening tests that are available for various types of cancer (see Table 40-5). For example, the Pap smear is used in the diagnosis of cervical cancer. The HPV test screens for HPV, which is linked to cervical, anal, and oropharyngeal cancer. Mammograms detect

TABLE 40-5. Effective Cancer Screening Tests

Effective cancer screening tests can find cancer early. Clinicians may recommend certain screening tests based on the patient's specific risk factors.

Screening Test	Recommended
Colonoscopy, sigmoidoscopy, high-sensitivity stool DNA test	Persons age 50 and older
Low-dose helical CT scan (also called spiral CT scan)	Persons with risk factors such as smokers age 40 and older
Mammography	Persons with risk factors and those age 40 and older
Breast MRI	Females who have the *BRCA1* and/or *BRCA2* gene
Pap test and human papillomavirus (HPV) testing	Females at high risk and/or females age 21 and older
Alpha-fetoprotein	Persons at risk for liver cancer
CA-125 test with transvaginal ultrasound	Females at risk of ovarian cancer
Prostate surface antigen (PSA) test and digital rectal examination	Males at risk for prostate cancer
Skin examination	Persons at risk for skin cancer

From National Cancer Institute (2019). Retrieved from https://www.cancer.gov/about-cancer/screening/screening-tests#effective-screening

breast cancer. DREs and blood prostate surface antigen (PSA) tests are used to detect prostate cancer. Magnetic resonance imaging (MRI), CT scans, and bone scans are other techniques that assist in the diagnosis of cancer. Colonoscopy is commonly recommended at age 50, and then every 10 years to screen for colon cancer. Endoscopy may be recommended for persons at risk of gastric cancer. If lesions are found, biopsy can be done with each of these procedures.

Screening for tumor cell markers is clinically important in identifying and tracking progression of cancers before, during, and after treatment. Tumor cell markers are products of cancer cells such as hormones, enzymes, genes, antigens, or antibodies that are found in blood, spinal fluid, or urine. Some of these tumor markers are called *oncofetal antigens* because they are normally found during fetal development. Examples of these antigens are **carcinoembryonic antigen (CEA),** commonly used to monitor cancer treatment, and **alpha-fetoprotein (AFP)** used to screen for liver cancer (see Table 40-6).

Treatment

Cancer treatments vary; however, the standard therapies include surgery, radiation, chemotherapy, and immunotherapy, also called biological cancer therapy. Surgery, used for many types of cancers, has the highest cancer cure rate with solid, well-circumscribed tumors. Surgery is also used to reduce the size of tumors that are impinging on neighboring organs or causing pain. Radiation therapy is used to destroy tumor cells; it is most effective during the S and M stages of the cell cycle.

Chemotherapy that uses cytotoxic drugs destroys cells in the S, M, or G stages of the cell cycle. This type of chemotherapy has a collateral effect on healthy, rapidly multiplying cells such as skin, hair, gastric, and bone marrow cells. The side effects of chemotherapy include dry mouth, anorexia, nausea and vomiting, alopecia (hair loss), and bone marrow suppression.

Immunotherapy, referred to as biological cancer therapy, uses several different mechanisms to enhance the body's immune response against cancer. Treatments promote cytokines' ability to attack cancer, inhibit T-cell deactivation, or use genetically engineered antibodies to target specific antigens or unique receptors on cancer cells, or enzymes produced by cancer cells (see Table 40-7).

Pathophysiology of Selected Types of Cancers

Each type of cancer presents in a different way and requires specific treatments. It is important to understand their different nuances.

Lung Cancer

Lung cancer is a leading cause of cancer-related death in both males and females throughout the world. In fact, 25% of all cancer deaths are the result of lung cancer. In the United States, the disease causes more deaths than colorectal, breast, and prostate cancers combined. In 2022, approximately 237,000 people were diagnosed with lung cancer in the United States. In the same year, there were 130,000 deaths caused by lung cancer. More males are diagnosed with lung cancer than females. However, the rate of new lung cancer cases (incidence) over the past 41 years has dropped 35% for males, whereas it has risen 87% for females. African Americans are more likely to develop and die of lung cancer than persons of any other racial or ethnic group. The age-adjusted lung cancer incidence rate among African American males is approximately 30% higher than for European American males. Close to 70% of patients with lung cancer present with locally advanced or metastatic disease at the time of diagnosis. Early diagnosis is the key to effective treatment.

Cancer of the lung occurs most often in persons older than age 65 years, with an average age of 70 years. Cigarette smoking is responsible for 80% to 90% of lung cancers.

Etiology

The leading cause of lung cancer is cigarette smoking: 85% of patients with lung cancer are current or former smokers. Cigarette smoke contains as many as 1,200 potential carcinogens. Risk increases with

TABLE 40-6. Cancer and Common Tumor Markers	
Cancer	**Specific Tumor Marker**
Colorectal	CEA (carcinoembryonic antigen)
Pancreatic Lung Breast Stomach Thyroid Liver Ovarian	
Breast	CA-15-3 (carcinogenic antigen 15)
Pancreatic	CA-19-9 (carcinogenic antigen 19)
Gallbladder	
Stomach	
Liver	AFP (alpha-fetoprotein)
Testicular	
Ovarian	CA-125 (carcinogenic antigen 125)
Prostate	PSA (prostate surface antigen)

TABLE 40-7. Types of Cancer Immunotherapy

There are several types of cancer immunotherapy currently in use. Each type has a different mechanism and is the optimal treatment for specific kinds of cancer.

Type of Agent	Mechanism of Action	Type of Cancers	Examples of Agents
Immune checkpoint inhibitors (ICIs)	ICIs block inhibitory proteins that suppress T-cell function against cancer cells. By blocking these proteins, there is no inhibition of T cells, which allows T cells to produce a strong antitumor response.	Hepatocellular Head and neck squamous cell Lung cancers Renal/urothelial cell Malignant melanoma	Ipilimumab Pembrolizumab Nivolumab Atezolizumab Durvalumab Avelumab
Adoptive cell transfer	This involves removing a patient's own T cells to genetically engineer the cells to have direct cancer-killing ability. These enhanced cells are then reinfused back to the patient. One example of adoptive cell transfer therapy is the chimeric antigen receptor (CAR) T-cell (CAR-T) therapy.	Leukemia Lymphoma	Tisagenlecleucel Axicabtagene Ciloleucel
Oncolytic viral therapy	Uses either a natural or genetically engineered virus to produce an immune response against cancer cells. The virus targets cancer cells and does not introduce pathogenic infection in normal cells.	Malignant melanoma	Talimogene Laherparepvec
Monoclonal antibody (mAb)	A genetically engineered antibody that is designed to bind to cancer cells. The mAb attaches to a specific receptor on the cancer cell and identifies the cancer cell as a target for the patient's natural immune system. The patient's natural immunoglobulins attack them directly. An mAb can also be used to deliver radiation or chemotherapy directly to cancer cells.	Non-Hodgkin's lymphoma Breast cancer Head and neck cancer Colorectal cancer	Rituximab Trastuzumab Cetuximab
Treatment vaccines	Treatment vaccines expose the patient's own extracted antigen-presenting cells (APCs) to cancer antigens and reinfuse them back to the patient. Then, the APCs activate T cells against the cancer cells. Treatment vaccines do not expose patients to antigens of a new disease.	Prostate cancer	Sipuleucel-T therapy
Cytokines	Cytokines, such as interferons and interleukins, activate the patient's T cells. Therapeutic interleukin promotes T-cell activity and increases immune cytokine production. Interferons have a stimulatory effect on T cells but also directly inhibit tumor cell proliferation.	Metastatic melanoma Renal cell carcinoma Hairy cell leukemia Follicular lymphoma AIDS-related Kaposi's sarcoma	Aldesleukin Recombinant interferon alfa-2b

From National Cancer Institute (2018). Retrieved and adapted from https://www.cancer.gov/about-cancer/treatment/types/immunotherapy

the total number of cigarettes smoked, expressed in cigarette pack-years.

CLINICAL CONCEPT

Smoking history is calculated in pack-years. This is the number of packs of cigarettes smoked multiplied by years smoked. For example, a 60-year-old who smoked two packs of cigarettes per day since age 20 has an $(40 \times 2) = 80$ pack-year smoking history.

Asbestos exposure is another risk factor for lung cancer; if the person is a smoker, there is a synergistic risk of developing lung cancer. Having a first-degree family member (parent, sibling, or child) with lung cancer roughly doubles the risk of developing lung cancer. Having a second-degree relative such as an aunt, uncle, niece, or nephew with lung cancer raises the risk by around 30%. The most important genetic mutations are those involving the *ras* family of oncogenes. The *ras* oncogene family has three members: H-*ras*, K-*ras*, and N-*ras*. These genes are particularly found in cases of non–small-cell lung cancer (NSCLC) in smokers. Other molecular abnormalities found in NSCLC include mutations in the oncogenes *c-myc* and *c-raf* and in the tumor suppressor genes retinoblastoma (*Rb*) and *p53*.

Asbestos can cause a specific type of cancer on the pleural membrane, called mesothelioma. Mesothelioma is a relatively rare cancer with approximately 3,000 new cases diagnosed each year in the United States. It occurs more often in males than in females, and risk increases with age.

CLINICAL CONCEPT

The rate of mesothelioma was highest in the 1970s through 1990s when asbestos was found as the cause for most cases. Workplaces are now restricted from using asbestos, and asbestos is being removed from older construction. Because of this, the incidence of mesothelioma is decreasing.

Other risk factors for lung cancer include radon exposure, arsenic exposure, history of radiation therapy to the chest, pulmonary fibrosis, and history of chronic obstructive pulmonary disease. Radon is a naturally occurring radioactive material in the ground that is prevalent in certain areas of the United States. It releases a gas that increases the risk of lung cancer and is estimated to cause 12% of cases. Also, frequent exposure to cigarette smoke can affect those in the environment. Passive smoke increases a person's risk

of lung cancer by 20% to 30%. Beryllium, nickel, copper, chromium, and cadmium have all been implicated in causing lung cancer. HIV infection has been found to increase risk of lung cancer 2.5-fold. Compared with lung cancer patients in the general population, HIV-infected patients with lung cancer are significantly younger. Most patients with HIV infection and lung cancer present with advanced-stage disease.

Pathophysiology

The pathogenesis of lung cancer involves an overload of carcinogens from smoking and other environmental toxins, plus a genetic predisposition acquired from parents. Smoke and other environmental toxins can paralyze the cilia of the respiratory tract's epithelium. Cilia, which would normally sweep away carcinogens, bacteria, and other foreign substances, become less active, and accumulation of carcinogens occurs.

On a molecular level, a respiratory tract lesion develops and typically undergoes sequential genetic and structural changes from hyperplasia—an increased mass of cells—to dysplasia—a precancerous mass of cells—to an invasive, neoplastic, cancerous mass. There is an activation of oncogenes and a deactivation of tumor suppressor genes that allow the unchecked cell growth and proliferation of cancer. Because there is a lack of cellular apoptosis, the cancer cells multiply rapidly and extensively. The cancer cells also have a capacity for angiogenesis (building of blood vessels) and metastasis. In addition, the cancer causes destructive invasion of surrounding tissue. Lung cancer commonly begins as an area of dysplasia that over time becomes a thickened area of bronchial mucosa. The lesion proliferates and can erode the lining epithelium, grow into the bronchial lumen, or become a mass within the lung tissue. Extension can occur into the pleural surface and then spread to the tracheal, bronchial, or mediastinal lymph nodes.

Lung cancer can develop on bronchial surface epithelium or bronchial mucous glands. It can be divided into two categories: NSCLC, which makes up about 85% to 90% of all lung cancers, and small-cell lung cancer (SCLC). It is important to distinguish between the two: SCLC is a rapidly growing tumor that tends to metastasize quickly, whereas NSCLC develops more subtly over a longer period.

Non–Small-Cell Lung Cancer. The types of NSCLC include adenocarcinoma, squamous cell carcinoma (SCC), and large-cell carcinoma. All have similar treatments but have distinct cellular appearance and clinical characteristics. Adenocarcinoma occurs within bronchial mucosal glands in a peripheral location of the lung. It is the most frequent NSCLC in the United States. Bronchioloalveolar carcinoma is a distinct subtype of adenocarcinoma that arises from alveolar cells and may appear as a solitary peripheral nodule, multiple nodules, or a rapidly progressing pneumonia. SCC accounts for 25% to 30% of all lung cancers. SCC usually occurs in the central parts of the lung as an erosion in a proximal bronchus. Large-cell carcinoma accounts for 10% to 15% of lung cancers, appearing as a large peripheral mass on chest x-ray.

Small-Cell Lung Cancer. SCLC is also divided into several subcategories, which include pure small-cell, mixed small-cell, and combined small-cell carcinoma. SCLC is a more aggressive form of cancer than NSCLC and occurs as a central lesion with enlargement of the hilar and mediastinal lymph nodes, which are centrally located lymph nodes. Commonly, when first presenting to the health-care provider because of pulmonary symptoms, SCLC already has metastasized to other areas of the body. The most common sites of metastasis of lung cancer are the bones, liver, adrenal glands, pericardium, brain, and spinal cord.

Clinical Presentation

The major presenting complaints of lung cancer include cough, hemoptysis (blood in sputum), wheeze, stridor, chest pain, and dyspnea. Patients may complain of weight loss, excessive fatigue, and weakness. Hoarseness may be a sign if the tumor compresses the recurrent laryngeal nerve. A lung tumor can frequently cause an obstructive accumulation of secretions in the bronchioles that appear as pneumonia. The patient may have symptoms of fever and productive cough, which can lead to a misdiagnosis of pneumonia. Lung cancer patients are often asymptomatic, and a tumor may be an incidental finding on a routine chest x-ray. Often, symptoms of a paraneoplastic syndrome may be the first sign of lung cancer (see Box 40-3).

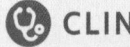 **CLINICAL CONCEPT**

A common paraneoplastic syndrome involves lung tumor secretion of ACTH. Lung tumors can inappropriately secrete ACTH, which chemically resembles melanocyte-stimulating hormone. Melanocytes are often stimulated, giving the patient with lung cancer a tanned appearance.

Over half the patients diagnosed with lung cancer will have metastatic disease at diagnosis. Patients with metastasis may complain of symptoms related to the spread of the cancer, such as bone pain.

Screening for Lung Cancer

Screening of high-risk persons for lung cancer is currently an issue of debate. Currently, most persons with lung cancer present to the health-care provider when they have symptoms that interfere with their daily function, which usually happens at an advanced stage of the disease. Screening the population at risk before symptom occurrence would allow early detection at a treatable and curable stage. However, currently the population at risk is narrowly defined as persons with a history of heavy smoking of more than 30 pack-years, current smokers, or smokers who have quit less than 15 years ago, and between ages 55 and 80 years. The American Cancer Society and U.S. Preventive Services Task Force (USPSTF) recommends lowering the starting age for screening from 55 to 50 years and the smoking history requirements from 30 to 20 pack-years. Currently, only a fraction of the recommended population is screened. The type of screening test that should be recommended is also being debated. Chest x-ray can detect tumors approximately 1 cm in diameter, which already have over 10^9 cells with a disrupted bronchial and vascular epithelia. Studies have also concluded that sputum cytology is insufficiently sensitive or accurate to be included in the routine work-up of any patient suspected of having lung cancer. Many advocate for a low-dose helical (spiral) CT scan of the chest as a screening test. However, cost and accessibility are the problems involved in providing this test for the population at large.

Many investigators are seeking a simple, accurate, reproducible, and inexpensive yearly test as a general screening tool for lung cancer. Several serological biomarkers are under intense study including carcinoembryonic antigen (CEA), serum cytokeratin 19 fragments (CYFRA 21-1), neuron specific enolase (NSE), and squamous cell carcinoma antigen (SCC-Ag).

Diagnosis

Diagnostic tests in lung cancer include chest x-ray, CT or MRI scan, cytological examination of sputum, bronchoscopy, and CT-guided tissue biopsy. Low-dose helical CT scan is particularly useful as a screening tool for persons at high risk for lung cancer. After a biopsy, the tumor cells are classified according to a stage and TNM system.

Biomarkers to Determine Treatment

Patients with either SCLC and NSCLC benefit from using biomarkers in early diagnosis and follow-up of treatment. There are many different biomarkers that can be used for detecting lung cancer, each with different specificity and sensitivity for tumors.

Current national and international guidelines recommend testing for alterations of the oncogenic biomarkers *EGFR, ALK, ROS1, BRAF, RET, MET,* and *HER2,* along with immune biomarkers such as PD-L1 and tumor mutational burden (TMB) to determine the best treatment for lung cancer.

 CLINICAL CONCEPT

Lung cancer stages range from 0 to 4. A small, localized tumor, referred to as in situ, is classified as stage 0. A large tumor is classified as stage 1. When a tumor is classified as stage 2 or 3, there is spread to the lymph nodes. Stage 4 lung cancer indicates that metastasis has occurred.

BOX 40-3. Paraneoplastic Syndromes in Lung Cancer

Lung cancer–SCLC in particular–is the most common cancer associated with paraneoplastic syndromes. Paraneoplastic syndromes are disorders that develop because of hormones, enzymes, cytokines, and other chemical mediators secreted by cancer cells. The following are some of the most common syndromes.

ADRENOCORTICOTROPIC HORMONE SECRETION

Adrenocorticotropic hormone (ACTH) is the most commonly produced hormone in lung cancer patients, particularly those with SCLC. Increased levels of ACTH may be detectable in up to 50% of patients with lung cancer. Because of a chemical similarity between ACTH and melanocyte-stimulating hormone, the lung cancer secretion of ACTH causes stimulation of melanocytes and a darkening of the skin. Cushing's syndrome, caused by excessive ACTH, is sometimes seen as well.

CACHEXIA

Cachexia, which is the wasting of the body's lean body mass, is perhaps the most common manifestation of advanced malignant disease and is responsible for approximately 25% of cancer deaths. TNF-alpha is one of the chemical mediators that cause this complication. TNF-alpha causes anorexia and other metabolic alterations such as weight loss; muscle loss; anemia; and disorders of carbohydrate, lipid, and protein metabolism. Cancer patients exhibit a relative glucose intolerance, insulin resistance, reduced lipogenesis, and decreased muscle protein synthesis.

CLOTTING AND THROMBOSIS

Tumor cells can directly activate the clotting process through two secreted coagulation factors: tissue factor and cancer procoagulant. A variety of hypercoagulable disorders, including Trousseau's syndrome, deep venous thrombosis and thromboembolism, disseminated intravascular coagulation, and others can occur in lung cancer. The incidence of deep venous thromboembolism in cancer sufferers is approximately 40 to 100 per 1,000 persons per year compared with an estimated 1 to 2 cases per 1,000 persons per year in the general population.

HYPERCALCEMIA

Hypercalcemia in lung cancer patients can be caused by cancer metastasis and deterioration of bones or by paraneoplastic syndromes. Cancer tumors can secrete parathyroid hormone peptide, calcitriol, or other cytokines, including osteoclast-activating factors. All these act on bone to release calcium into the bloodstream.

NEUROLOGICAL EFFECTS

Autoantibodies are commonly found in neurological syndromes associated with cancer. SCLC is particularly associated with Lambert-Eaton syndrome, which is a weakening of the limbs caused by autoantibodies found in neuromuscular junctions. Similar to myasthenia gravis, it resolves with cancer treatment.

PANCOAST SYNDROME OR HORNER'S SYNDROME

Pancoast syndrome is a disorder caused by a cancerous tumor in the apical region of the lung. The tumor causes destructive lesions of the thoracic inlet and involvement of the brachial plexus and cervical sympathetic nerves. Severe pain of the shoulder radiating down the arm into the hand and atrophy of hand and arm muscles can occur. A disorder called Horner's syndrome, which is caused by cervical sympathetic nerve dysfunction, can be present. It is characterized by ptosis (drooping of the eyelid), miosis (pupil constriction), hemianhidrosis (lack of sweating), and enophthalmos (sinking in of the eyeball within the orbit).

SYNDROME OF INAPPROPRIATE ANTIDIURETIC HORMONE

Elevated levels of ADH occur in 30% to 70% of lung cancer patients. SCLC can secrete excessive amounts of ADH, which causes excess water reabsorption at the nephron. This is termed syndrome of inappropriate antidiuretic hormone (SIADH). ADH stimulates water reabsorption at the collecting duct of the nephron, creating a high water content of the blood. This excess water causes hypoosmolarity of the bloodstream and dilutes the sodium concentration, called dilutional hyponatremia. The ADH also creates a low water content in the tubule fluid, resulting in highly concentrated urine.

Treatment

Treatment depends on the type and the staging of the lung cancer. The earlier the diagnosis, the more effective the treatment. Lung cancer treatment mainly involves surgery, radiation, and chemotherapy. The key treatment for stages 1 and 2 and localized NSCLC is surgery. A minimally invasive procedure called video-assisted thoracic surgery (VATS) is used, which accesses the chest through small incisions.

Wedge resection is the term used when the patient requires removal of a small section of lung. A segmentectomy is the removal of a segment (part of a lobe) of one lung. A lobectomy–the most common type of

surgery for lung cancer–is the removal of an entire lobe of one lung. A sleeve resection involves removal of a lobe of the lung and part of a bronchus. A pneumonectomy is the removal of an entire lung. Radiation treatment is aimed at destruction of rapidly dividing cells such as cancer cells. Stereotactic body radiotherapy is used to deliver radiation to a specific region of the tumor while limiting injury to the surrounding healthy tissue.

Patients who have inoperable stage 3 lung cancer and metastatic disease receive chemotherapy. Chemotherapy, which usually requires the combination of different agents, is the main form of treatment for those with SCLC. The cornerstone of treatment for any stage of SCLC is etoposide/platinum-based chemotherapy and concomitant radiotherapy to the thorax and mediastinum. Surgical treatment is commonly needed in limited SCLC. Prophylactic radiotherapy to the central nervous system (CNS) is also used because the brain is a common site of metastasis. Immunotherapy has made progress in the treatment of SCLC, and nivolumab, pembrolizumab, atezolizumab, and durvalumab have led to significant improvements in clinical outcomes of SCLC. Future prospects for even better outcomes in SCLC lie in novel ways to integrate immunotherapy and tyrosine kinase inhibitors.

Targeted molecular chemotherapy has been most effective in NSCLC. For example, the growth of adenocarcinoma has been found to require specific growth factors, enzymes, and signaling pathways. Drugs have been developed that target these specific molecular-level cancer mediators. For example, cancer cells have tyrosine kinase receptors that, when stimulated, trigger massive proliferation of the cells. Pharmaceutical agents such as erlotinib, gefitinib, or crizotinib precisely inhibit tyrosine kinase receptors and block the stimulus for cancer growth in NSCLC. Cancer immunotherapy using checkpoint inhibitors such as pembrolizumab, nivolumab, ipilimumab, durvalumab, cemiplimab, avelumab, or atezolizumab have also been effective for the treatment of NSCLC.

Breast Cancer

Breast cancer is the second most common cancer in the United States after lung cancer; one in eight American females will suffer breast cancer in their lifetime. Breast cancer is the leading cause of cancer death in females. In 2019, there were 3.1 million females living with the disease, the average age of whom is 61 years. Breast cancer incidence increases with age. Seventy-nine percent of new cases and 88% of breast cancer deaths occur in females age 50 years and older. In 2019, an estimated 268,000 new cases of invasive breast cancer were diagnosed among females, along with 63,000 cases of in situ (noninvasive) breast cancer. Approximately 2,670 cases of breast cancer were found in males. Approximately 42,000 females and 400 males died from breast cancer in 2019. Breast cancer tends to develop earlier at around age 45 in African American females compared with European American females. African American females have a higher death rate from breast cancer than do European American females. This disparity is attributed to the fact that African American females seek care for breast cancer at later stages in the disease compared with European American females.

About 5% to 10% of breast cancers can be linked to genetic mutations inherited from one's mother or father. Mutations in the *BRCA1* and *BRCA2* genes are the most common. On average, females with a *BRCA1* mutation have up to a 72% lifetime risk of developing breast cancer. For females with a *BRCA2* mutation, the risk is 69%. Breast cancer that is positive for the *BRCA1* or *BRCA2* mutation tends to develop more often in younger females. An increased ovarian cancer risk is also associated with these genetic mutations. Approximately 85% of females with breast cancer do not have the *BRCA* genes—breast cancer develops sporadically. Research into effective diagnostic procedures and treatments has increased the survival rate over the last decade; the 5-year survival rate for females diagnosed with breast cancer is now 89%.

Etiology

Although the specific etiology of breast cancer is unknown, risk factors are clear: prolonged reproductive life, including early menarche and late menopause; age older than 50 years; obesity, caused by increased levels of estrogen in fat deposits; hormone replacement therapy; personal or family history of breast cancer; having no children (nulliparity) or late childbirth after age 30 years; lack of breastfeeding; dense breast tissue; radiation to the chest; and genetic predisposition. The major risk factors for sporadic breast cancer are related to estrogen exposure. Via hormonal action, estrogen can enhance the proliferation of premalignant lesions and cancers with estrogen receptors. However, other mechanisms also play a role, as a significant number of breast cancers are estrogen-receptor negative.

A family history of breast cancer in one first-degree relative, such as a mother or sister, is reported to increase an individual's lifetime risk of breast cancer by 1.8 times. The lifetime risk of breast cancer is up to three times higher if two first-degree relatives are affected by breast cancer, particularly if the relative was diagnosed at an early age (50 years or younger). A family history of ovarian cancer in a first-degree relative, especially if the disease occurred at an early age (younger than 50 years), has been associated with a doubling of breast cancer risk. Females of Ashkenazi Jewish descent have double the risk of breast cancer compared with other ethnic groups.

Approximately 5% to 10% of breast cancers can be attributed to one of two autosomal-dominant genes: *BRCA1* and *BRCA2*. In hereditary cancers, one mutant *BRCA* allele is inherited, and the second allele is affected by a sporadic mutation. The *BRCA1* gene locus is 17q21, and the *BRCA2* gene locus is 13q12.3. Both *BRCA1* and *BRCA2* are defective tumor suppressor genes. The estimates of the risk of breast cancer in females with these mutations vary: by age 70 years, up to 78% of females with *BRCA1* mutations develop breast cancer, and up to 56% of females with the *BRCA2* mutation will develop the disorder.

Aside from *BRCA1* and *BRCA2*, other gene variants are associated with breast cancer. These include *ATM, CHEK2,* and *PALB2, BARD1, RAD51C, RAD51D,* and *TP53*. A recent population study in China showed that non-*BRCA* genes contributed to 38.5% of the mutation carriers, with *PALB2, RAD51D,* and *ATM* being the majority. *PALB2* was found to be particularly important because lifetime risk for breast cancer can reach 58% in those with family history.

 CLINICAL CONCEPT

Genetic testing for *BRCA1* and *BRCA2* can be performed in selected high-risk patients with a strong family history of breast or ovarian carcinoma. Genetic counseling should be available for patients undergoing this test. Many patients with these genetic mutations opt for preventive mastectomy and oophorectomy—surgical removal of the ovaries.

Pathophysiology

Most breast cancers are epithelial cell tumors that develop from cells lining the ducts or lobules of the breast. Less commonly, cancer of the breast arises from nonepithelial cells such as the supporting connective tissue. In most cancers, a triggering factor, which is unclear, causes the breast epithelial cells to proliferate, grow uncontrollably, and invade surrounding tissue.

Normally, estrogen and progesterone act at the breast to stimulate growth and cell proliferation. Estrogen and progesterone receptors are nuclear hormone receptors that promote DNA replication and cell division. In some breast cancers, these estrogen and progesterone receptors are overexpressed; these are called *estrogen receptor-positive* (ER-positive) breast cancers. Another cellular receptor that promotes breast cell growth is human epidermal growth factor receptor 2 (HER2). This cellular receptor is commonly overexpressed in some forms of breast cancer; these cancers are termed HER2 positive.

Categorizing Breast Cancer. Breast cancers can be categorized based on different characteristics, including molecular subtype and histopathology. There are four basic molecular subtypes of breast cancer: luminal A, luminal B, basal (triple negative), and HER2 enriched. Each different subtype behaves differently and requires specific treatments as follows:

- Luminal A: Slow-growing cancers that have a 90% cure rate and are often found on screening mammogram. Treatment usually includes surgery and radiation.
- Luminal B: Aggressive cancers that invade blood vessels and lymph nodes. The tumor is often difficult to surgically remove from surrounding tissue with clear margins. Often a second surgery is necessary.
- Basal (triple negative): very aggressive, rapidly growing cancer that lacks estrogen, progesterone,

and HER2 receptors. These tumors respond to chemotherapy.
- HER2 enriched: These tumors overproduce HER2, which signals breast cancer to grow and spread.

Breast cancers can also be categorized according to the demonstrated changes in the tissue as follows:

- Carcinoma in situ is proliferation of cancer cells within ducts or lobules without invasion of surrounding tissue; designated as ductal carcinoma in situ (DCIS) or lobular carcinoma in situ (LCIS).
- LCIS is a nonpalpable lesion usually discovered via biopsy. LCIS is not malignant, but it indicates an increased risk of future invasive carcinoma in either breast; about 1% to 2% of patients with LCIS develop cancer annually.
- Invasive carcinoma is primarily adenocarcinoma. About 80% of adenocarcinoma is the infiltrating ductal type; most of the remaining cases are the infiltrating lobular type.
- Paget's disease of the nipple is a form of DCIS that extends into the overlying skin of the nipple and areola, manifesting with an inflammatory skin lesion. Characteristic malignant cells called *Paget cells* are present in the breast epidermis. Rare types of breast cancers are termed *medullary, mucinous,* and *tubular carcinomas.*

Breast cancer invades locally and spreads initially through the regional lymph nodes, bloodstream, or both. Metastatic breast cancer may affect almost any organ in the body—most commonly the lungs, liver, bone, brain, and skin. Metastatic breast cancer frequently appears years or decades after initial diagnosis and treatment.

Clinical Presentation

Ninety percent of palpable breast masses are noncancerous; however, all masses require a complete investigation. Most masses that are cancerous are single, nontender, and firm with irregular borders and adherence to the skin or chest wall. The most common place on the breast for a woman to have a tumor is the upper, outer quadrant, where 45% of tumors are found (see Fig. 40-3). By the time a cancer lesion becomes palpable, over half of patients have metastasis to axillary lymph nodes. Other breast changes associated with cancer include nipple discharge, swelling in one breast, nipple or skin retraction, and a specific type of skin appearance called *peau d'orange*—a thickening of skin that resembles an orange peel. Paget's disease of the breast, which involves redness, crusting, pruritus, and tenderness of the nipple, is also characteristic of a cancerous change.

Screening for Breast Cancer

The American Cancer Society recommends that females with an average risk of breast cancer should undergo regular screening mammography starting at age 45 years. Depending on risk, females between

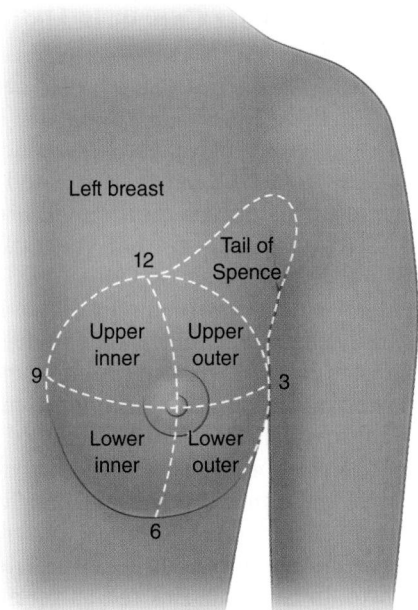

FIGURE 40-3. The breast should be divided into four quadrants when referring to a lesion: upper outer (UO), upper inner (UI), lower outer (LO), and lower inner (LI). Additionally, there is an outer region that includes some of the axilla known as the tail of Spence. Most breast cancer lesions are found in the UO quadrant.

ages 40 and 44, should have the opportunity to begin annual screening; ages 45 to 54 years should be screened annually; and age 55 years and older should transition to biennial screening or have the opportunity to continue screening annually. Females should continue screening mammography as long as their overall health is good and they have a life expectancy of 10 years or more.

Diagnosis

Diagnosis of breast cancer includes a complete history and physical, clinical breast and pelvic examinations, mammogram, breast ultrasound, and biopsy of the lesion. A fine-needle aspiration or excisional biopsy is performed with histology and cytology examination. In some cases, an MRI scan is warranted. The finding of calcifications on a mammogram is associated with breast cancer. In some cases, a ductogram, also called a galactogram, is used to determine the cause of nipple discharge. A fine plastic tube is placed into the opening of the duct in the nipple. A small amount of contrast medium is injected, which outlines the shape of the duct on a mammogram and shows whether a mass is present inside the duct. Scintimammography is a nuclear imaging test that is used when mammography does not show sufficient detail. It is also used to assess high-risk patients, tumor response to chemotherapy, and metastatic involvement of axillary lymph nodes.

Positron emission tomography (PET) scanning is the most sensitive and specific of all the imaging modalities for breast disease. Changes in metabolic activity, vascularization, oxygen consumption, and tumor receptor status can be detected.

Specific tests are performed on biopsy samples of cancer tissue. These tests include the following:

- Estrogen and progesterone receptor test: Measures the amount of estrogen and progesterone receptors in the breast cancer tissue. Breast cancer tissue with more estrogen and progesterone receptors than normal may grow quickly. About 75% of breast cancers are ER positive. About 65% of ER-positive breast cancers are also progesterone receptor positive (PR positive). Cells that have receptors for one or both of these hormones are considered hormone receptor positive. Hormone receptor–positive cancer is also called hormone sensitive because it responds to hormone therapy such as tamoxifen or aromatase inhibitors. Hormone receptor–negative tumors are referred to as hormone insensitive or hormone resistant. Having this information influences the choice of treatment. Treatments that block estrogen and progesterone may stop the cancer from growing.
- HER2/neu test: Measures the number of HER2/neu genes and the amount of HER2/neu protein in a sample of cancerous tissue. Cancerous tissue with a high number of HER2/neu genes or a high amount of HER2/neu protein is aggressive, grows quickly, and is likely to metastasize. This type of breast cancer can be treated with specific biological drugs that target the HER2/neu protein.
- Oncotype Dx assay: Has been used for females with early stage, ER-positive, lymph node–negative breast cancer treated with tamoxifen. This assay analyzes 21 genes (16 cancer genes and 5 reference genes). Using a formula based on the expression of these genes, the likelihood of recurrence of the cancer within 10 years can be predicted.

Diagnostic testing also includes histological examination of lymph nodes. Axillary lymph nodes are particularly significant in breast cancer. The staging of breast cancer is highly reliant on spread to axillary lymph nodes and metastasis. There are five stages of breast cancer that are based on the TNM classification system. As noted earlier, T indicates tumor size, N indicates spread to lymph nodes, and M indicates whether metastasis is present. The TNM results are combined to determine the stage of breast cancer. The five stages are stage 0 (zero), which is noninvasive DCIS, and stages I through IV, which are used for invasive breast cancer.

Treatment

Treatment of breast cancer usually requires surgery, such as lumpectomy or mastectomy, lymph node biopsy, and adjuvant therapy, which includes radiation, hormonal therapy, chemotherapy, and immunological or biological agents. After surgery, adjuvant therapy is aimed at possible micrometastatic disease. It is possible that surgery does not completely destroy all breast cancer cells in the body. Adjuvant chemotherapy targets breast cancer cells that have escaped the breast and regional lymph nodes but have not yet been identified as metastasis.

Adjuvant therapy is used to reduce the risk of future cancer recurrence. It has been estimated to be responsible for 35% to 72% of the reduction in mortality rate. The presence of specific receptors within the cancer lesion is significant in adjuvant treatment. Selective estrogen receptor modulators (SERMs) can inhibit the estrogen receptors of cancerous tissues. Tamoxifen and raloxifene are SERMs that are equally effective in reducing the risk of ER-positive breast cancer in postmenopausal females. Trastuzumab (Herceptin) is an immunotherapeutic agent used to counteract cancers with the HER2 protein. Tyrosine kinase inhibitors target epidermal growth factor receptors that are present in breast cancers. They are commonly combined with other forms of chemotherapy or radiation therapy. Everolimus and lapatinib are examples of tyrosine kinase inhibitors. Aromatase inhibitors such as anastrozole are also used as adjuvant therapy in breast cancer. These agents work by inhibiting aromatase, the enzyme responsible for converting other steroid hormones into estrogen. Bisphosphonates are added to the therapeutic regimen because they may lessen the damage to bone from reduced estrogen. Bisphosphonates such as zoledronic acid inhibit osteoclast function and reduce the resorption of bone.

Drugs called microtubule inhibitors such as eribulin are also used to interfere with the cell cycle of cancer cells. They inhibit the growth phase of microtubules, leading to disruption of mitotic spindles, and, ultimately, apoptotic cell death. Microtubule inhibitors are indicated for breast cancer patients with metastasis who have previously received at least two chemotherapeutic regimens.

Tumor markers, such as CEA, CA15.3 (carcinoma antigen 15-3), and CA27.29 (carcinoma antigen 27-9), can be used for monitoring patients on therapeutic regimens. CA15.3 and CA27.29 levels correlate with the course of disease in 60% to 70% of patients, whereas CEA levels correlate in 40% of patients. After recovery from breast cancer, if a recurrence develops, it is usually within the first 5 years after treatment.

CLINICAL CONCEPT

Individuals with the BRCA1 and BRCA2 genes have an increased risk of breast, ovarian, colon, and pancreatic cancer. Males also have an increased risk of prostate cancer.

Prevention of Breast Cancer in High-Risk Patients

Some females with high risk for breast cancer, such as those with BRCA1 and BRCA2 genetic mutations, opt for risk-reduction therapies. Risk-reduction treatment includes bilateral mastectomy and salpingo-oophorectomy. This option removes all breast tissue and the estrogen stimulus from the ovaries. Risk-reduction mastectomy and oophorectomy have been performed on patients with family history of breast cancer, painful breasts, cancer phobia, and history of breast biopsies (with or without proliferating disease). As a preventive measure, risk-reducing mastectomy remains controversial. Potential benefits include a reduction of risk of breast cancer and increase in psychological peace of mind. It is important for patients to recognize that no mastectomy can remove all breast tissue, and therefore cannot eliminate all risk of breast cancer. In addition, risk reduction mastectomy may cause significant physical morbidity, affect body image, and affect the patient's quality of life.

In patients who have had cancer in one breast, studies show that removing the other breast may reduce the incidence of cancer in that other breast, but there is insufficient evidence that this improves long-term survival. There is the continuing risk of recurrence or metastases from the original cancer.

Alternatively, some patients opt for pharmacological preventive therapy of breast cancer. Prescription of preventive medication depends on the risk of breast cancer according to each patient's medical history. The health-care provider needs to weigh the benefits and risks of preventive pharmacological therapy in each patient. Risk assessment tools such as the Breast Cancer Risk Assessment Tool and the International Breast Cancer Intervention Study Risk Calculator can help identify females at increased risk for breast cancer. The updated USPSTF and American Society of Clinical Oncology guidelines encourage the use of risk-reduction medications in high-risk females. Preventive pharmacological therapies include agents that can block estrogenic stimulus of breast tissue: tamoxifen and raloxifene, which are SERMS; and anastrozole and exemestane, which are aromatase inhibitors.

Ovarian Cancer

Ovarian cancer is the fifth-leading cause of cancer death in females in the United States, with approximately 20,000 females in the United States developing ovarian cancer annually and 13,000 dying from the disease. It affects approximately 12 females per 100,000, per year; there is a 1 in 78 chance that a female will contract ovarian cancer in their lifetime. It is more common in European American females than African American females, and it is more common between ages 55 and 64. Patients with advanced disease at diagnosis have an overall 5-year survival rate of 20% to 30%, but those with an early diagnosis have a 90% to 95% probability of successful treatment. Unfortunately, ovarian cancer commonly remains undiagnosed until its advanced stages because of vague presenting symptoms and a lack of screening tests. Frequently, the cancer has already metastasized upon diagnosis.

Etiology

The etiology of ovarian cancer is unclear. Risk factors include older age, nulligravidity (no history of pregnancy), obesity, smoking, estrogen treatment, infertility, family history of ovarian cancer, and Ashkenazi Jewish descent. Family history is a very important risk factor. From 5% to 10% of cases of ovarian cancer occur in individuals with a family history of the disease. Females who have had breast cancer are at a higher risk of developing ovarian cancer. The use of talcum powder on the vulva and perineum may be associated with increased risk of ovarian cancer. Females who possess the *BRCA1* or *BRCA2* gene, which is a defective tumor suppressor gene, have a high risk of developing ovarian cancer. In families with a history of ovarian or breast cancer, *BRCA* mutations are responsible for about 90% of cases of ovarian cancer. Females with a *BRCA1* genetic mutation have a 35% to 40% risk of developing ovarian cancer, and those with a *BRCA2* genetic mutation have a 10% to 30% risk of developing ovarian cancer. Studies show that advanced ovarian cancer is characterized by a mutated tumor suppressor gene (*TP53*) in almost all tumors. The studies also show that ovarian cancer is linked to mutations in nine other genes, including the neurofibromatosis gene and retinoblastoma gene. There are certain genetic disorders that increase risk of ovarian cancer. These include hereditary nonpolyposis colorectal cancer (Lynch syndrome), Peutz-Jeghers syndrome, MUTYH-associated polyposis, and PTEN hamartoma tumor syndrome.

A person who has been pregnant has a 50% decreased risk for developing ovarian cancer compared with a nulligravida, and those who have engaged in breastfeeding have decreased risk. Females ages 40 to 59 years who have taken oral contraceptives or undergone tubal ligation also have a reduced risk. Oral contraceptive use has been shown to decrease the risk of ovarian cancer in average-risk females by 40% to 50%. The longer the use of oral contraceptives, the greater the reduction of risk.

Pathophysiology

There are three types of ovarian cancer that are classified depending on the area of the tumor's origin in the ovary: epithelial, germ cell, or stromal. Epithelial tumors arise from the surface cells of the ovary and account for more than 90% of cancers. Germ cell tumors arise from tissue that will develop into ova. Stromal tumors arise from tissue that secretes hormones. Germ cell and stromal tumors are less common, accounting for less than 5% of ovarian cancers.

Epithelial ovarian cancer involves the outer epithelial surface cells of the ovary. Ovarian epithelial tumors are cystic lesions with solid components. The surface may be smooth or irregular with cysts that contain straw-colored serous fluid or hemorrhagic fluid. The most common malignant form of epithelial ovarian cancer is termed high-grade serous carcinoma. The majority of high-grade serous ovarian cancers have recently been found to originate in the fallopian tube, not the ovary. Epithelial ovarian cancer spreads initially within the peritoneal cavity. The most aggressive form of ovarian cancer is a germ cell tumor called a dysgerminoma. Metastatic cancerous tissue is often found on the peritoneal surfaces, surface of the liver, outer surface of the small and large bowel and uterus, and para-aortic and pelvic lymph nodes. Outside the peritoneal cavity, the tumors can spread to the pleural cavity, lungs, and inguinal lymph nodes.

Clinical Presentation

Most ovarian cancers cause vague clinical manifestations or no symptoms at all. If the ovarian tumor is sizeable, it can cause lower abdominal pain and abdominal enlargement. The patient may complain of abdominal bloating and difficulty eating because of a feeling of fullness. Nausea, vomiting, and constipation also bring the patient to a health-care provider. Urinary frequency, dysuria (difficulty urinating), back pain, and pelvic pressure are other symptoms. In advanced disease, anorexia, weight loss, progressive weakness, and cachexia are present, as is characteristic of other malignant tumors. Physical examination of patients with ovarian cancer is often normal in the early stages. Later, in advanced disease, there may be ascites and a solid, irregular, fixed pelvic mass or bowel obstruction.

 CLINICAL CONCEPT

In the majority of cases, ovarian cancer is asymptomatic, leading to delayed diagnosis when the disease is at an advanced stage.

Diagnosis

There are no screening modalities for ovarian cancer. However, the CA-125 and transvaginal ultrasound are widely used diagnostic studies. Laparotomy is often the primary procedure used to establish diagnosis and stage of the disease. Cytological analysis of ascites fluid (peritoneal edema fluid), biopsy of the tumor and lymph nodes, and visual inspection of the peritoneum and diaphragm are performed during laparotomy. The staging of disease relies on the acumen of the surgeon performing the laparotomy and the confinement or spread of the tumor. Stage I disease is cancer confined to the ovary or ovaries. Stage II disease is cancer confined to the pelvis. Stage III disease is cancer spread beyond the ovaries and pelvis but confined to the abdomen. Stage IV disease is cancer spread outside the abdomen.

Treatment

Treatment includes surgical resection of the tumor and chemotherapy. Often, the patient requires a total hysterectomy, which includes excision of the unaffected ovary. However, if disease is confined, fertility-sparing surgery can remove only the involved ovary. Surgery plus combination chemotherapy consisting of the platinum-based medication carboplatin and paclitaxel is a common treatment regimen. These agents interfere with mitosis of cancer cells, thereby inhibiting progression of cancer growth. New chemotherapeutic agents under investigation include poly (ADP ribose) polymerase PARP inhibitors. Cancer cells use PARP proteins to regenerate and proliferate. PARP inhibitors olaparib and rucaparib stop the process of regeneration in the cancer cells, prohibiting growth and large tumor formation. If metastatic spread is apparent with surgery, surgical excision of all cancerous tissue is necessary. This may require liver resection, bowel excision, and splenectomy. Chemotherapy can be instilled directly into the peritoneal cavity instead of intravenously, which has shown decreased systemic adverse effects.

A number of different chemotherapeutic agents are being used in platinum-resistant tumors. These alternative agents include tyrosine kinase inhibitors, such as pazopanib, and epithelial growth factor inhibitors, such as pertuzumab. Regardless of the type of chemotherapy used, several cycles of chemotherapy are commonly required. After surgery and chemotherapy, 46% of patients achieve a 5-year survival rate. However, approximately 50% of ovarian cancer patients experience relapse and ultimately die of the disease.

Recurrent ovarian cancer is classified into two categories, depending on the length of time the patient remained disease free after completing platinum chemotherapy: (1) if patient relapse occurs more than 6 months after initial chemotherapy, the cancer is considered platinum sensitive and (2) if the patient experiences earlier relapse, the cancer is considered platinum resistant. Patients with platinum-sensitive disease may exhibit a good response if rechallenged with a platinum-based regimen. However, treatment of platinum-resistant cancers is under investigation. Maintenance therapy to prevent recurrence includes the PARP inhibitor type of chemotherapeutic agents niraparib (Zejula) and rucaparib (Rubraca). A monoclonal antibody medication, bevacizumab (Avastin), has also been effective in the treatment of recurring cancer. A unique therapeutic approach under investigation is called hyperthermic intraperitoneal chemotherapy, which consists of a heated solution of chemotherapeutic agents instilled directly into the peritoneum. Heat has been found to potentiate the effects of chemotherapeutic agents.

Surgical Preventive Treatment

Some patients with high risk for ovarian cancer, such as those with *BRCA1* mutations, choose to undergo risk-reducing surgery. Risk-reduction surgery includes bilateral salpingo-oophorectomy or tubal ligation. Risk-reducing bilateral salpingo-oophorectomy causes postoperative menopausal symptoms including vaginal dryness, hot flashes, and in some patients, decreased sexual function. These prophylactic surgeries have substantially reduced the incidence of cancer in BRCA mutation carriers.

Cervical Cancer

Cervical cancer is the fourth most common cancer in females worldwide (WHO, 2022). Worldwide in 2020, there were 604,000 new cases and 342,000 deaths from cervical cancer. Approximately 90% of cervical cancer cases occur in females of low-income, low-resourced countries. In low-resourced countries, cervical cancer is the second most common type of cancer and third most common cause of cancer death in females. However, in well-resourced, higher-income countries, due to widespread Pap test screening programs and HPV vaccine, there has been a downward trend in the incidence of cervical cancer over the last few decades. Each year in the United States, about 13,000 new cases of cervical cancer are diagnosed and about 4,000 females die of this cancer. Hispanic females have the highest rates of developing cervical cancer, and Black females have the highest rates of dying from cervical cancer in the United States.

Etiology

Females at risk for developing cervical cancer include those who smoke, as well as those with a history of sexually transmitted diseases, HPV infection, two or more lifetime sexual partners, or immunosuppression. HPV infection is the etiological agent in all cervical cancers. It is also an etiological agent in anorectal, penile, vaginal, vulvar, and oropharyngeal cancer.

Cervical cancer most commonly affects females during their 40s and 50s. The most significant predisposing conditions to cervical cancer are long-standing HPV infection and genetics. HPV is a known human carcinogen, and infection occurs in a high percentage of sexually active females. The prevalence of HPV infection in females is highest in those ages 20 to 24 years. However, approximately 90% of HPV infections resolve on their own with no sequelae of cervical cancer. On average, only 5% of HPV infections develop changes consistent with cervical cancer.

There are more than 200 subtypes of HPV; HPV16 and HPV18 are the specific subtypes associated with cervical cancer.

Human leukocyte antigen genes, which code for cellular surface antigens, are also involved in susceptibility to cervical cancer. Females with HLA II- DRB1 and DQB1 alleles who are infected with HPV are highly susceptible to cervical cancer. The chemokine receptor-2 gene on chromosome 3p21 and the *Fas* gene on chromosome 10q24.1 predispose an individual to cervical cancer. It is believed these genes diminish the immune response to HPV. Additionally, HIV infection increases susceptibility to cervical cancer, most likely because of an impaired immune response to HPV infection. Cervical cancer is at least six times more common in HIV-infected individuals, and this increased prevalence has remained essentially unchanged with the use of antiretroviral therapy.

Pathophysiology

In cervical cancer, there are two major kinds of cellular changes: squamous cell carcinoma (SCC), which occurs within epithelial cells, and adenocarcinoma, which involves glandular cells. The earliest preinvasive changes that occur on the cervix are termed squamous intraepithelial lesions. These asymptomatic changes, which are usually diagnosed by Pap smear, are categorized as:

- Low-grade squamous intraepithelial lesions
- High-grade squamous intraepithelial lesions
- Possibly cancerous (malignant)
- Atypical glandular cells of undetermined significance

The intraepithelial lesions are first limited to the cervical epithelium; as invasion occurs, neoplastic cells penetrate the underlying basement membrane. The squamocolumnar junction, an area of rapid cell turnover between the uterus and cervix, is a very common site of cancerous changes.

If a Pap smear shows abnormal cells, a biopsy is done. Dysplasia that is seen on a biopsy of the cervix is called cervical intraepithelial neoplasia (CIN). It is grouped into three categories:

- CIN I: mild dysplasia
- CIN II: moderate to marked dysplasia
- CIN III: severe dysplasia to carcinoma in situ

CIN I and CIN II changes can resolve on their own. CIN III indicates early cancerous changes of the cervix.

Almost 100% of cervical cancer cases test positive for HPV. HPV16 is the most carcinogenic genotype and accounts for approximately 55% to 60% of all cervical cancers. Persistent cervical infection with high-risk HPV types is necessary for the development of cervical cancer and its precursor lesion, CIN III. HPV18 is the next most carcinogenic genotype and accounts for approximately 10% to 15% of cervical cancers. Approximately 10 other HPV genotypes cause the remaining 25% to 35% of cervical cancers. HPV18 causes a greater proportion of glandular cancers, adenocarcinoma, and adenosquamous carcinoma than SCC.

Cervical cancer, both squamous cell carcincoma and adenocarcinoma, tends to grow upward to the endometrial cavity, throughout the vaginal epithelium, and laterally to the pelvic wall. It can also invade the bladder and rectum. The common sites for distant metastasis include lymph nodes, liver, lung, and bones.

Clinical Presentation

Cervical cancer has a long asymptomatic period before the disease becomes clinically evident. Commonly, an abnormal Pap test alerts the individual to a problem. The first symptom of cervical cancer may be abnormal vaginal bleeding, commonly after sexual activity. There also may be vaginal discomfort, discharge, and burning on urination. Cervical cancer can invade the rectum and bladder, leading to constipation, hematuria, and ureteral obstruction. The triad of leg edema, pain, and hydronephrosis (swelling of the kidney) suggests pelvic wall involvement. There are usually no abnormal findings in early-stage cervical cancer on physical examination. As the disease progresses, the cervix may become abnormal in appearance, with an erosion, ulcer, or mass. These abnormalities can extend to the vagina. Rectal examination may reveal an external mass or gross blood from tumor erosion.

Diagnosis

The Pap smear and HPV DNA test performed during pelvic examination are key screening diagnostic studies. Pap smears that suggest invasive disease require further evaluation by colposcopy, colposcopic-directed biopsy, and endocervical curettage. Curettage is the scraping of tissue away from a surface of an organ; in this case, the surface of the cervix. Colposcopy is a direct visualization of the cervix where sites of abnormality can be biopsied. Once the diagnosis of cervical cancer is established, the disease is clinically staged, which involves assessment of any metastasis. A thorough history and physical examination with emphasis on the pelvic examination is necessary. A rectovaginal examination is also important to identify lymph nodes or locally invasive disease. Use of laparoscopy, chest x-ray, gastrointestinal (GI) endoscopy, CT scan, or MRI of the pelvis and abdomen may be needed to establish the degree of metastatic disease. Cervical cancer is staged from stage 0 to stage IV (see Table 40-8).

Treatment

There are different treatment modalities for the stages of disease. Carcinoma in situ (stage 0) is treated with local excisional measures such as cryosurgery, laser ablation, and loop excision. Loop excision uses an electrified wire that cuts around the tumor to remove it.

The treatment of choice for stage IA disease is surgery. Conization, radical hysterectomy, and total hysterectomy are surgical procedures. Conization is a procedure that removes a wedge of tissue from the cervix. If lymph nodes are involved, radiation therapy is needed. Radical hysterectomy with bilateral pelvic lymphadenectomy and combined external beam radiation with brachytherapy is needed for stages II, III, and IVA. **Brachytherapy** involves embedding deposits of radioactive material in the cervical tissue. For

TABLE 40-8. Stages of Cervical Cancer

Stage	Description
Stage 0	Carcinoma in situ. Abnormal cervical cells are localized to the inner surface of the cervix.
Stage I	Cancer is found limited to the cervix. It is divided into stage IA and stage IB, depending on the amount of cancer cells involved. Stage IA and Stage IB can be subdivided into Stage IA1 and IA2 and Stage IB1 and Stage IB2, depending on the size of the tumor.
Stage II	Cancer has spread beyond the cervix but not to the pelvic wall (the tissues that line the part of the body between the hips) or to the lower third of the vagina. Stage II is divided into stages IIA and IIB, based on how far the cancer has spread. Stage IIA and Stage IIB can be subdivided into Stage IIA1 and IIA2 and Stage IIB1 and Stage II 2, depending on the size of the tumor.
Stage III	Cancer has spread to the lower third of the vagina, or to the pelvic wall, or has caused kidney problems. Stage III is divided into stages IIIA and IIIB, based on how far the cancer has spread.
Stage IV	Cancer has spread to the bladder, rectum, or other parts of the body. Stage IV is divided into stages IVA and IVB, based on where the cancer is found.

From National Cancer Institute. (2019.) Stages of cervical cancer. Retrieved from https://www.cancer.gov/types/cervical/patient/cervical-treatment-pdq#_142

stage IVB, individualized therapy is used to provide pain relief. Radiation therapy is used for control of bleeding and pain, whereas systemic chemotherapy is used for metastatic disease. For pelvic recurrence after radiation therapy, modified radical hysterectomy or pelvic exenteration is performed. Pelvic exenteration is a radical surgical treatment that removes all organs—the urinary bladder, urethra, rectum, and anus—from the pelvic cavity.

Prevention of Cervical Cancer

The USPSTF recommends screening for cervical cancer every 3 years with cervical cytology alone (Pap test), every 5 years with high-risk HPV (hrHPV) testing alone, or every 5 years with hrHPV testing in combination with cytology (cotesting) in females 30 to 65 years of age. The USPSTF recommends screening for cervical cancer every 3 years with cervical cytology (Pap test) alone in females 21 to 29 years of age. Cervical cancer is very rare in patients younger than 21 years. A 5-year screening interval for primary hrHPV testing alone or cotesting offers the best balance of benefits and harms for patients ages 21 to 29. According to the USPSTF, evidence from randomized clinical trials and decision modeling studies suggests that screening beyond 65 years of age in females who have had an adequate screening history does not have significant benefit.

The nine-valent HPV vaccine (Gardasil 9 [9vHPV]) is recommended to decrease the risk of HPV-related cancers in males and females ages 9 through 26. This age group is recommended as it is most beneficial to receive HPV vaccine before being sexually active. HPV is the most common sexually transmitted virus; however, not all HPV infection converts to cancer. Adults older than age 26 should consult their health-care provider to decide whether they would benefit from HPV vaccine.

Prostate Cancer

The prostate is a small gland that manufactures and secretes semen, which carries sperm. It uniquely increases in size throughout a male's lifetime. Benign prostatic hyperplasia (BPH), which is an increase in the size of the prostate gland caused by excessive proliferation of cells, is a common condition of middle-aged and older adult males. When examining a male older than age 50 years, it is important to exclude the presence of prostate cancer because both BPH and cancer enlarge the size of the gland and present with similar symptoms.

In the United States, an estimated one in six European American males and one in five African American males will be diagnosed with prostate cancer in their lifetime, with the likelihood increasing with age. Approximately 6 out of 10 males age 65 and older develop prostate cancer. In 2019, approximately 225,000 males were diagnosed with prostate cancer and 31,000 died of the disease. Clinically apparent disease is very rare in males younger than age 50 years; the average age of diagnosis is 66 years. Prostate cancer is the second most common cause of cancer death in males, after lung cancer.

Etiology

The exact etiology of prostate cancer is unknown. However, there are many different risk factors. Having a father or a brother who had prostate cancer doubles one's risk; having both a father and a brother with prostate cancer increases one's risk fivefold. Certain lifestyle factors may also increase the risk of prostate cancer, including consumption of fat, red meat, fried foods, and dairy; high calcium intake; and smoking. African American ethnicity, high alcohol intake, and exposure to Agent Orange and cadmium are also risk factors. Males with the *BRCA1* or *BRCA2* gene or family history of Lynch syndrome are also at increased risk.

Other factors may decrease the risk of prostate cancer, such as a diet rich in plant-based foods and vegetables, especially lycopene-containing foods such as tomatoes. A diet rich in cruciferous vegetables such as broccoli, Brussels sprouts, cabbage, cauliflower, and kale; soybeans; legumes; carotenoids; antioxidants; and fish oil, along with moderate exercise, all decrease the risk of prostate cancer.

Pathophysiology

Prostate cancer mainly develops in the glandular cells of the organ, so it is referred to as an adenocarcinoma. Prostate cancer is initiated by carcinogenic mutations, and its growth is dependent on the male hormone testosterone. Initially, there is an oncogenic or tumor suppressor genetic defect, which causes uncontrolled cellular growth in the gland. As the glandular cells hyperproliferate, further mutations of other genes occur, including the *TP53* gene and *Rb* gene. These changes lead to tumor progression and metastasis. The cancer cells proliferate locally and invasively and often spread to the neck of the bladder, ejaculatory ducts, and seminal vesicles. The cancer metastasizes to bone early in the course of the disease, sometimes before any external symptoms are exhibited. Lung, liver, and adrenal metastases can also occur. In early cancer, the tumor grows slowly but becomes more aggressive as the size of the tumor increases.

Clinical Presentation

Early stage prostate cancer has no symptoms. In more advanced disease, the prostate gland can obstruct urine flow from the bladder. This usually causes urinary symptoms such as decreased force of stream, hesitancy (urine flow stops and starts), and incomplete emptying of the bladder. The patient needs to strain to get urine out and may have frequency of urination. Late-stage symptoms include hematuria, azotemia, anemia, and anorexia. Back pain also is often a late-stage symptom caused by vertebral bone metastasis.

On physical examination, the patient may have no remarkable findings except those on a DRE. The prostate gland can be palpated through the wall of the rectum. The normal prostate, which is a rubbery gland, becomes hard and immovable in cancer. The inguinal lymph nodes may be enlarged, and if vertebral metastasis has occurred, tenderness over the lumbar region is found.

Diagnosis

Diagnosis of prostate cancer involves a DRE, PSA test, and transrectal ultrasound-guided needle biopsy. It is important to keep in mind, however, that PSA screening has low specificity, as most males with elevated PSA do not have prostate cancer, and PSA levels are elevated in both BPH and prostate cancer. The clinician must consider several variables when assessing a patient for risk of prostate cancer: race, age, PSA level, family history of prostate cancer, and findings on DRE.

These variables determine which males require a prostate biopsy. As the PSA level increases, so does the risk of cancer. The American Cancer Society advises that if the PSA level is less than 2.5 ng/mL, retesting of PSA is needed only every 2 years. Males with a PSA level of 2.5 ng/mL or higher should have annual PSA testing. With a PSA level of 4 to 10 ng/mL, the likelihood of finding prostate cancer is about 25%. Most experts do not recommend a biopsy unless the PSA is at least 3 ng/mL or greater. The measurement of bound and free PSA can help to further differentiate mildly elevated PSA levels due to cancer from elevated levels due to BPH. The percentage of free PSA is generally used as an additional factor in making an informed recommendation for or against biopsy in patients with a PSA level of 4 to 10 ng/mL. Free PSA is calculated as a percentage of total PSA; the lower the percentage of free PSA, the higher the likelihood of cancer.

A needle core prostate biopsy under transrectal ultrasound guidance is the most common method of obtaining diagnostic tissue. However, there is increasing use of multiparametric magnetic resonance imaging as well to guide biopsy. The combined images on biopsy is termed targeted fusion biopsy. The problem with needle biopsy is that diseased tissue can be missed. Therefore, a 12-core biopsy is advised, which includes sampling from more areas of the prostate gland. Each core of the biopsy is examined for the presence of cancer. Because prostate biopsy is subject to error, patients with abnormal PSA and negative biopsy are advised to add biomarker testing.

Currently, there are several biomarkers that may be used in addition to the PSA and DRE for diagnosis, treatment, and risk assessment (see Box 40-4).

Classification. Two classification systems are used to determine the pathology and aggressiveness of prostate tumors. The Gleason grading system ranks tumors histologically based on differentiation of tissue. The poorer the differentiation of the cancer cells, the worse the prognosis. The Gleason grading system is based on the two areas of the prostate tissue: the predominantly involved area and a secondary area. Areas of the gland can have different histological patterns. Histological patterns are scored from (1) well differentiated to (5) undifferentiated and summed to give a total score of 2 to 10. Well-differentiated tissue has a favorable prognosis (scores less than 6), whereas areas of less-differentiated tissue are assigned a higher number (7 to 10), which have less favorable prognosis (see Table 40-9).

The TNM (tumor, node, metastasis) staging system gives information about the extent of spread of the prostate cancer. Magnetic resonance imaging is used to detect the cancer as localized to the gland, spread into the capsule of the gland, or extended into lymph nodes or extranodal sites. Radionuclide bone scans (bone scintigraphy) are used to evaluate spread to bone. The most common site for prostate cancer metastasis is the vertebral column (see Table 40-10).

BOX 40-4. Prostate Cancer Biomarkers

BIOMARKER	TYPE OF TEST	DEFINITION
PHI (prostate health index)	Blood	A predictive assay based on the presence of [-2]pro PSA, an inactive precursor of PSA, known to be associated with prostate cancer rather than with benign prostatic hyperplasia.
PCA3 (prostate cancer antigen 3)	Urine	The PCA3 is a urine-based test, collected after DRE with prostatic massage. It measures the noncoding PCA3 gene mRNA, which is overexpressed in cancerous tissue.
ConfirmMDx	Biopsy	This assay measures epigenetic changes (hypermethylation of GSTP1, APC, and RASSF1) present in benign tissue around the tumor, also known as the "halo effect," in order to predict the detection of high-risk disease.
Oncotype Dx	Biopsy	This assay measures the expression of 12 genes involved in different neoplastic pathways. The results are reported as a Genomic Prostate Score (GPS).
Prolaris	Biopsy	Measures the expression of 31 genes known to be contained in aggressive tumors.
Decipher	Biopsy	To assess risk of progression for patients with high-risk features on radical prostatectomy pathology.

Adapted from: Nevo, A., Navaratnam, A., & Andrews, P. (2020). Prostate cancer and the role of biomarkers. *Abdom Radiol (NY), 45*(7), 2120–2132. doi: 10.1007/s00261-019-02305-8

TABLE 40-9. Gleason Grading Scores of Prostate Cancer

Grade Group	Gleason Score	Differentiation/Risk of Tissue
Grade group 1	Gleason score less than or equal to 6	Lowest-risk tissue; favorable prognosis
Grade group 2	Gleason score 3 + 4 = 7	Low- to intermediate-risk tissue
Grade group 3	Gleason score 4 + 3 = 7	Intermediate-risk tissue
Grade group 4	Gleason score 4 + 4 = 8	High-risk tissue
Grade group 5	Gleason scores 9 and 10	Highest-risk tissue; aggressive tumor; poor prognosis

Adapted from Prostate Cancer Foundation (PCF). (2022). Gleason Score and Grade Group. Retrieved from https://www.pcf.org/about-prostate-cancer/diagnosis-staging-prostate-cancer/gleason-score-isup-grade/

According to the National Comprehensive Cancer Network (NCCN) guidelines, additional testing is recommended for patients diagnosed with prostate cancer. Testing for alterations in DNA repair genes (e.g., *BRCA1, BRCA2, ATM, CHEK2*) is suggested for males with very low-risk, low-risk, and intermediate-risk disease if family history is positive for an inherited cancer predisposition syndrome or if the prostate tumor shows intraductal histology.

ALERT! Back pain is often the presenting symptom of late-stage prostate cancer.

Treatment

Treatment options for prostate cancer include active surveillance; watchful waiting; surgical removal of the prostate; and different types of radiation treatment, cryotherapy, brachytherapy (implantation of radiation seeds into the gland), and hormonal therapy. Prostate cancer is appraised as a low-risk or high-risk disease according to the Gleason score, PSA levels, and the patient's age and life expectancy.

For low-risk disease, active surveillance or watchful waiting is increasingly recommended, as prostate cancer is often a slow-growing disease that can be assessed over time. The patient who is a candidate for active surveillance or watchful waiting is usually older than 75 years who has other medical disorders. Active surveillance or watchful waiting is preferable because surgery may pose a greater risk to the patient's health and quality of life, so the clinician monitors the progress of the neoplastic growth using repeat PSA levels every 3 months and biopsy every 12 to 24 months.

For younger persons with localized prostatic adenocarcinoma, treatment depends on an informed patient decision incorporating knowledge about the potential advantages and disadvantages associated with each approach. The basic choices are external beam

TABLE 40-10. TNM Staging System for Prostate Cancer

Tx	Primary tumor cannot be assessed
T0	No evidence of primary tumor
T1	Clinically inapparent tumor, neither palpable nor imaged
T1a	Tumor incidental finding in <5% of resected tissue
T1b	Tumor incidental finding in >5% of resected tissue
T1c	Tumor identified on needle biopsy
T 2	Tumor confined to prostate gland
T 2a	Tumor involves half of one lobe of prostate gland or less
T2b	Tumor involves more than half of one lobe of prostate gland
T2c	Tumor involves both lobes of prostate gland
T3	Tumor extends through prostate capsule
T3a	Extracapsular extension
T3b	Tumor invades seminal vesicles
T4	Tumor invades adjacent anatomical structures such as rectum, bladder, pelvic wall
N1	Positive regional lymph nodes
M1	Distant metastasis evident

Adapted from Cancer Research UK (2022). TNM staging for prostate cancer. Retrieved from: https://www.cancerresearchuk.org/about-cancer/prostate-cancer/stages/tnm-staging.

radiation therapy (RT) with or without brachytherapy, brachytherapy alone, or radical prostatectomy. Ablative techniques such as cryotherapy, high-intensity ultrasound, and photodynamic therapy with an interstitial laser have been advocated, but there are inadequate long-term data to support these as standard approaches.

Active surveillance is not indicated for patients with unfavorable intermediate-risk disease. For high-risk disease, radical prostatectomy, radiation, and hormonal therapy are recommended. There are different types of radiation therapy that attempt to focus directly on the cancer to prevent bladder and colorectal complications. These include proton beam radiation, stereotactically guided radiation, and three-dimensional conforming radiation. Brachytherapy is also used. Testosterone is a major driver of cancer growth; therefore, androgen suppressants are a cornerstone of intervention for advanced disease. In the United States, 5-year survival rates in males with local or regional prostate cancer at diagnosis approach

100%. In males with metastatic disease, however, survival is only 30%. Currently, radical prostatectomy and radiation therapy can result in permanent side effects of erectile dysfunction and urinary incontinence.

Colorectal Cancer

Colorectal cancer is the second leading cause of death resulting from cancer. It is a preventable disease if individuals utilize the recommended screening procedures, which include colonoscopy and FOBT. In 2019, there were 142,500 new cases of colorectal cancer and 53,000 deaths due to colorectal cancer. Males had higher rates of getting and dying from colorectal cancer than females. Although the majority of colorectal cancers are in adults age 50 and older, 17,930 (12%) will be diagnosed in individuals younger than 50 years, the equivalent of 49 new cases per day. Out of an estimated 53,000 people who died from colorectal cancer in 2020, this included 3,640 people younger than age 50. It is estimated that approximately 1 out of 23 males (4.4%) and 1 out of 25 (4.1%) females will be diagnosed with colorectal cancer in their lifetime. The risk of colorectal cancer increases with age; the median age at diagnosis for males is 66, and 69 in females. The incidence and death rate for colorectal cancer is declining for older adults, but for unknown reasons, there is rising incidence in adults younger than age 50. Screening for colorectal cancer has increased over the last decade from 58% to 66%. Decreasing incidence and death rates due to colorectal cancer in older adults is partially attributed to greater colorectal screening rates and removal of polyps during colonoscopy. The relative survival rate for colorectal cancer is 64% at 5 years following diagnosis and 58% at 10 years. The most important predictor of survival is stage at diagnosis. The 5-year survival rate is 90% for those with localized-stage disease but declines to 14% for those diagnosed with metastasis. There is a higher incidence and rate of death (40%) from colon cancer in African Americans than in non-Hispanic European Americans.

 CLINICAL CONCEPT

The American Cancer Society recommends that screening for colorectal cancer should begin at age 45 in the majority of individuals. Screening can be done with high-sensitivity stool-based testing annually, CT colonography (virtual colonoscopy) every 5 years, flexible sigmoidoscopy every 5 years, or colonoscopy every 10 years. Patients and providers may consider the best option. CRC screening recommendations are modified for members of families with hereditary colon cancer syndromes, or patients with inflammatory bowel disease, and in those who have been exposed to abdominal radiation therapy.

Etiology

Current research indicates that environmental and genetic factors have the greatest correlation to colorectal cancer. The majority of colorectal cancers are sporadically occurring tumors; however, there is a striking influence of genetic factors. Colon cancer usually starts as a polyp, a tumorous mass that projects into the intestinal lumen. Familial adenomatous polyposis (FAP) is a well-defined hereditary disorder that predisposes an individual to intestinal polyps; it is an autosomal-dominant condition caused by a mutation of the gene located at chromosome 5q21, also called the adenomatous polyposis coli (*APC*) gene. The *APC* gene is a defective tumor suppressor gene, and it confers an almost 100% likelihood of colon cancer development. In FAP, patients typically develop 500 to 2,500 colonic polyps that cover the mucosal surface of the bowel. Polyps in FAP can become cancerous at an early age—some in childhood. Another similar condition, hereditary nonpolyposis colorectal cancer (HNPCC; also called Lynch syndrome), is an autosomal-dominant familial syndrome characterized by multiple colonic polyps with cancerous potential. There is a smaller number of polyps in HNPCC than in FAP, and HNPCC confers approximately a 40% chance of development of colon cancer.

As many as 10% of patients with colorectal cancer carry one or more pathogenic mutations in cancer-predisposing genes, not including those with FAP or Lynch syndrome. Other genetic mutations associated with colorectal cancer include M-*UTYH*, *BRCA1* and *BRCA2*, *PALB2*, *CDKN2A*, *TP53*, and *CHEK2*.

Other risk factors include inflammatory bowel disease, diabetes mellitus, long-term immunosuppression, high consumption of red meat, high consumption of processed meats, obesity, tobacco use, excessive alcohol use, physical inactivity, insulin resistance, low fiber in the diet, high amount of animal fat in the diet, and diets low in fruits and vegetables. Cancer survivors who received abdominopelvic radiation therapy in childhood or as adults are at significantly increased risk of subsequent gastrointestinal neoplasms, the majority being colorectal cancer. A history of radiation therapy for prostate cancer has been associated with an increased risk of rectal cancer in two large database studies. Patients with cystic fibrosis (CF) and those with hyperpituitarism or acromegaly have an elevated risk of colorectal cancer.

🔾 CLINICAL CONCEPT

Patients with inflammatory bowel diseases such as ulcerative colitis and Crohn's disease have an increased risk of developing colorectal cancer. Although both diseases increase susceptibility, ulcerative colitis seems to be a stronger risk factor. The risk for developing colorectal malignancy increases with the duration of inflammatory bowel disease and the greater extent of colon involvement.

Pathophysiology

Colon cancer most commonly begins as a polyp, which goes through a number of changes to become cancerous (see Fig. 40-4). Polyps with cancerous potential are called *adenomatous polyps*. Approximately 90% of polyps are small—usually smaller than 1 cm in diameter—and have a small potential for malignancy. The remaining 10% of adenomas are larger than 1 cm and approach a 10% chance of containing invasive cancer.

On a molecular level, colon cancer is caused by genetic changes that result in defective tumor suppressor genes, activated oncogenes, or mismatched gene repair. Commonly, an accumulation of multiple genetic mutations results in the progression of normal colonic mucosal cells to benign adenoma to adenomatous polyp to adenocarcinoma. The three types of adenomatous polyps (polyps with cancerous potential)—tubular adenomas, villous adenomas, and tubulovillous adenomas—are characterized as follows:

- Tubular adenomas, also called pedunculated adenomas, have a mass with a stalk coming off the intestinal wall.
- Villous adenomas, also called sessile polyps, have fingerlike projections without stalks that invade the intestinal wall. Villous adenomas are more difficult to remove and have a higher risk of cancerous changes than tubular adenomas.
- Tubulovillous adenomas have characteristics of both tubular and villous adenomas.

Some precancerous lesions are not polyps but flat. A flat area of dysplasia that is confined to the mucosa of the intestinal wall is called carcinoma in situ, which is considered premalignant. When the dysplastic tissue invades the intestinal wall more deeply, it is considered adenocarcinoma.

Clinical Presentation

Colorectal cancer can remain asymptomatic for years. Symptoms develop insidiously and frequently have been present for months before the affected individual seeks medical care. Symptoms include fatigue, weakness,

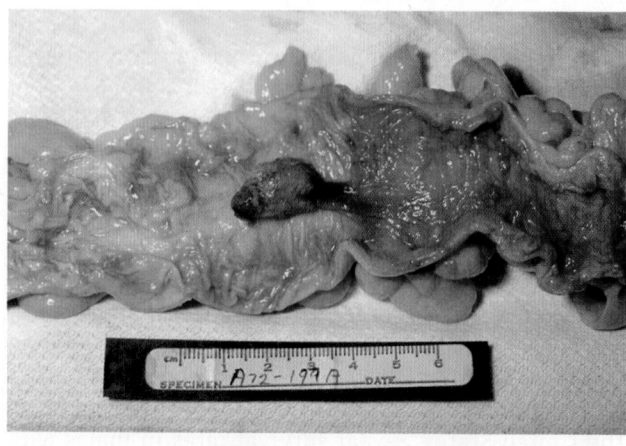

FIGURE 40-4. A colonic polyp. *(Courtesy of CDC/Dr. Edwin P. Ewing, Jr.)*

abdominal cramping, weight loss, iron-deficiency anemia, changes in bowel habits, blood in the stool, diarrhea, and constipation. Lower bowel cancers can present with hematochezia (rectal bleeding) and narrowing of stool caliber. Colon cancer can also cause bowel obstruction.

Iron-deficiency anemia is frequently a sign of slow GI blood loss that occurs in colon cancer. Colon cancer causes a constant microscopic leakage of blood into the intestine. Blood may not be visible in stool but can be occult, causing dark, tarry stools also called **melena**. Blood—an iron source within the body—is slowly depleted. It is paramount to check for GI blood loss in individuals with iron-deficiency anemia. This can be done with performance of an FOBT, stool DNA test, and colonoscopy to ensure that occult colon cancer is not present.

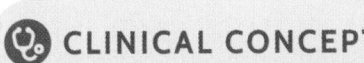 **CLINICAL CONCEPT**

Iron-deficiency anemia can be a key sign of GI blood loss from colon cancer.

All colorectal cancers spread by direct extension into adjacent structures and by metastasis through the lymphatics and bloodstream. Spread commonly occurs to regional lymph nodes, liver, lungs, and bones. The AJCC staging system is a classification system developed by the American Joint Committee on Cancer for describing the extent of disease progression in colon cancer patients. It utilizes in part the TNM scoring system: tumor size, lymph nodes affected, and metastases (see Table 40-11).

Diagnosis

Both diagnostic tests and laboratory tests are used to diagnose colorectal cancer. Diagnostic tests for colorectal cancer include colonoscopy, DRE, FOBT, barium enema, abdominal and pelvic ultrasound, CT scan, MRI, and PET scanning. Capsule endoscopy using an ingestible, camera-equipped capsule is available as a means of virtual colonoscopy. However, this procedure has lower accuracy than colonoscopy. Flexible sigmoidoscopy is performed in some settings for colon cancer screening,

TABLE 40-11. American Joint Committee on Cancer (AJCC) Staging of Colon Cancer

Stage	TNM Designation	Meanings of Different Designations
Stage 0	Tis N0 M0	**Tis:** carcinoma in situ; does not involve muscle layer **N0:** indicates no lymph node involvement **M0:** no metastasis
Stage I	T1, T2, N0, M0	**T1:** tumor involves layer of muscularis mucosa but not muscularis propria, which is deeper **T2:** tumor does involve the muscularis propria **N0:** no lymph node involvement **M0:** no metastasis
Stage IIA	T3, N0, M0	**T3:** tumor invades through the muscularis propria into pericolorectal tissues **N0:** no lymph node involvement **M0:** no metastasis
Stage IIB	T4a, N0, M0	**T4a:** tumor invades through the visceral peritoneum **N0:** no lymph node involvement **M0:** no metastasis
Stage IIC	T4b, N0, M0	**T4b:** tumor directly invades or adheres to adjacent organs or structures **N0:** no lymph node involvement **M0:** no metastasis
Stage IIIA	T1, N2a, M0 T1–2, N1/N1c, M0	**T1:** tumor involves layer of muscularis mucosa but not muscularis propria, which is deeper **T2:** tumor does involve the muscularis propria **N2a:** 4 to 6 regional lymph nodes are positive **M0:** no metastasis **N1:** 1 to 3 regional lymph nodes are positive (tumor in lymph nodes measuring $\geq$0.2 mm), or any number of tumor deposits are present and all identifiable lymph nodes are negative **N1c:** no regional lymph nodes are positive, but there are tumor deposits in the subserosa, mesentery, or nonperitonealized pericolic, or perirectal/mesorectal tissues **M0:** no metastasis

Continued

TABLE 40-11. American Joint Committee on Cancer (AJCC) Staging of Colon Cancer—cont'd

Stage	TNM Designation	Meanings of Different Designations
Stage IIIB	T1–T2, N2b, M0 T2–T3, N2a, M0 T3–T4a, N1/N1c, M0	**T1:** tumor involves layers of muscularis mucosa **T2:** tumor involves layers down to muscularis propria **N2a:** 4 to 6 regional lymph nodes are positive **N2b:** ≥7 regional lymph nodes are positive **T3:** tumor invades through the muscularis propria into pericolorectal tissues **T4:** tumor invades the visceral peritoneum or invades or adheres to adjacent organ or structure **T4a:** tumor invades through the visceral peritoneum (including gross perforation of the bowel through tumor and continuous invasion of tumor through areas of inflammation to the surface of the visceral peritoneum)
Stage IIIC	T3–T4a, N2b, M0 T4a, N2a, M0 T4b, N1–N2, M0	**T3:** tumor invades through the muscularis propria into pericolorectal tissues **T4a:** tumor invades through the visceral peritoneum **N2a:** 4 to 6 regional lymph nodes are positive **N2b:** ≥7 regional lymph nodes are positive **T4b:** tumor directly invades or adheres to adjacent organs or structures
Stage IVA	Any T, Any N, M1a	**T:** can be T1, T2, T3, T4, T4a, T4b **N:** can be N1, N2a, N2b **M1a:** metastasis to one site or organ is identified without peritoneal metastasis
Stage IVB	Any T, Any N, M1b	**T:** can be T1, T2, T3, T4, T4a, T4b **N:** can be N1, N2a, N2b **M1b:** metastasis to two or more sites or organs is identified without peritoneal metastasis
Stage IVC	Any T, Any N, M1c	**T:** can be T1, T2, T3, T4, T4a, T4b **N:** can be N1, N2a, N2b **M1c:** metastasis to the peritoneal surface is identified

T, primary tumor; N, regional lymph nodes; M, distant metastasis.
Reprinted with permission from AJCC. (2017). Colon and rectum. In M. B. Amin, S. B. Edge, F. L. Greene, et al. (Eds.). *AJCC cancer staging manual* (8th ed., pp. 251–274). New York, NY: Springer, 2017. Retrieved and adapted from https://www.cancer.gov/types/colorectal/hp/colon-treatment-pdq#_39

although this procedure cannot examine the entire colon. CT colonography (also called virtual colonoscopy) provides a computer-simulated endoluminal perspective of the air-filled distended colon. The technique uses conventional spiral or helical CT scan or, in the case of magnetic resonance colonography, magnetic resonance images. Colonoscopy is the gold standard for diagnosis of colorectal cancer. During colonoscopy, polypectomy and tissue samples for biopsy can be obtained.

Laboratory tests include complete blood count (CBC), serum iron, serum ferritin, serum carcinoembryonic antigen (CEA), serum carbohydrate antigen (CA)19-9, and liver enzymes. Stool DNA tests (Cologuard) have been developed that detect mutant, fragmented, and methylated DNA from exfoliated colon tumor cells in stool. Genetic testing of blood samples can detect most cases of HNPCC and FAP. The serum CEA and CA 19-9 are tumor markers not used as diagnostic tests, but used for monitoring patients who were treated for colorectal cancer and forecasting prognosis.

Colorectal Cancer Staging
Once the diagnosis of colorectal cancer is established, the local and distant extent of disease needs to be established to determine therapy and prognosis. The tumor, node, metastasis (TNM) staging system of the combined American Joint Committee on Cancer (AJCC)/Union for International Cancer Control (UICC) is the preferred staging system (see Table 40-11).

Treatment
Treatment involves surgical resection of the tumor, which usually requires removal of part of the colon, termed colectomy. Laparoscopic or open surgical procedures are done. The entire peritoneum should be examined, including the liver, pelvis, and diaphragm, for metastasis. Radiation to the pelvis is recommended for patients with cancers of the lower bowel. Chemotherapy is recommended for some patients and has shown modest benefit. Chemotherapy agents include 5-fluorouracil (5FU) with leucovorin, capecitabine, oxaliplatin, and irinotecan in combinations. Biological agents such as bevacizumab (Avastin), cetuximab (Erbitux), and pembrolizumab (Keytruda) are used particularly in metastatic colon cancer. For patients who cannot tolerate surgical resection, radiofrequency ablation, cryotherapy, and hepatic artery infusion of chemotherapeutic agents can be used.

Survival rate is related to the stage of the tumor, lymph nodes involved, and presence of metastasis. Periodic surveillance should take place after surgery. Tests include annual colonoscopy and CEA blood tests every 3 months.

Liver Cancer

Hepatocellular carcinoma (HCC) and cholangiocarcinoma (CC) are the two primary malignancies of the liver. HCC is cancer of the liver cells and CC is cancer of the hepatic bile duct cells. According to the American Cancer Society, approximately 41,260 new cases (28,600 in males and 12,660 in females) were diagnosed in 2022. Approximately 30,520 people (20,420 males and 10,100 females) died of these cancers in 2022. In the United States, the rate of death from liver cancer increased by 43% (from 7.2 to 10.3 deaths per 100,000) between 2000 and 2016. With a 5-year survival of 18%, liver cancer is the second most lethal tumor, after pancreatic cancer. Liver cancer incidence is rising each year—rates have more than tripled since 1980—while the death rates have more than doubled during this time in the United States. It is three times more common in males than females with highest incidence in African American males. The average age at diagnosis is 65 years; 74% of those affected are males.

Liver cancer is more common in countries in sub-Saharan Africa and Southeast Asia than in the United States. This is because hepatitis B and C viral infections are endemic in that part of the world. In many of these countries, liver cancer is the most common type of cancer. More than 800,000 people are diagnosed with this cancer each year throughout the world. Liver cancer is also a leading cause of cancer deaths worldwide, accounting for more than 700,000 deaths each year. On the basis of annual projections, the World Health Organization estimates that more than 1 million patients will die of liver cancer in 2030.

The majority of HCCs occur in patients with underlying liver disease, mostly as a result of hepatitis B or C virus (HBV or HCV) infection or alcohol abuse.

The threat of HCC is expected to increase in coming years due to the increasing numbers of patients who will develop cirrhosis from nonalcoholic fatty liver disease (NAFLD) and nonalcoholic steatohepatitis (NASH). Also the peak in incidence of HCC associated with hepatitis C has not yet occurred. It is estimated that 1.5% of the U.S. population is infected with hepatitis C. Persons born between 1945 and 1965 have a high incidence of hepatitis C, and one-time testing is recommended.

Etiology

Any agent that contributes to chronic, low-grade liver cell damage is a risk factor for liver cancer. The conditions of hepatitis B or C infection, alcoholic liver disease, alpha-antitrypsin deficiency, hemochromatosis, and nonalcoholic forms of cirrhosis predispose individuals to liver cancer. Other risk factors include obesity, diabetes, smoking, long-term androgenic steroid administration, exposure to toxins such as vinyl chloride, or long-term oral contraceptive use. Genetic mutations that predispose to HCC include *TP53, CTNNB1, AXIN1,* and *CDKN2A*. Mutations in the telomerase reverse transcriptase (TERT) promoter genes are the most frequent genetic alterations, accounting for approximately 60% of cases of HCC. These genes unleash uncontrolled cellular proliferation and deactivate tumor suppression.

Pathophysiology

HCC is a primary cancer of the liver and occurs predominantly in patients with underlying chronic liver disease and cirrhosis. It develops when there is a genetic mutation that causes the hepatocytes to proliferate excessively and resist cellular apoptosis. Chronic infections of hepatitis B or C repeatedly provoke the body's own immune system to attack the liver cells. Chronic alcohol abuse repeatedly injures the hepatocytes. A constant cycle of damage followed by cell repair can lead to mistakes during repair, which in turn may lead to carcinogenesis. Dysplastic nodules of cells are the preneoplastic changes seen in HCC. Dysplastic cells arise as a result of environmental assaults (chronic liver damage), genetic mutations, chromosomal rearrangements, and epigenetic changes. These influences lead to uncontrolled cellular proliferation and invasive qualities that transform the cells into carcinoma cells. Cancer cells grow and expand locally, spread within the liver, and then leave the organ to cause distant metastases. In general, cancer presents as a single mass lesion or as diffuse growth.

Clinical Presentation

The symptoms of liver cancer usually occur when the cancer is in an advanced stage. Symptoms include abdominal pain, weight loss, fever, and symptoms associated with cirrhosis, such as ascites, jaundice, or esophageal varices. Esophageal varices are caused by a blockage of the portal vein by a tumor, which causes blood flow to back up into the esophageal veins. On physical examination, the liver is usually enlarged, sometimes tender, and a hepatic artery bruit may be auscultated because of the increased amount of blood flow. In advanced liver cancer, the tumor can spread to nearby tissue or metastasize to distant sites such as the lungs.

Diagnosis

There is no specific diagnostic screening test for liver cancer; however, the AFP blood test is widely used because it is about 60% accurate in detecting liver cancer. If high levels of AFP (greater than 500 ng/mL) are found, this can indicate primary liver cancer, testicular cancer, ovarian cancer, or metastatic cancer in the liver. Imaging procedures to detect liver tumors include ultrasound, CT scan, MRI, and hepatic artery angiography. In patients with high risk for HCC, such as those with hepatitis B, hepatitis C, or cirrhosis, periodic surveillance testing is recommended. This includes ultrasound and AFP levels every 6 months.

The diagnosis of HCC, which can be difficult, often requires the use of one or more imaging modalities. The goal is to detect the tumors when they are 2 cm or smaller in size so that the entire range of treatment options are available. Percutaneous liver biopsy can be diagnostic if the sample is taken from an area of cancer cells localized by ultrasound, CT scan, or laparoscopy. The stages of liver cancer are based on the TNM anatomic system.

Treatment

Treatment of liver cancer includes surgical resection of the tumor, chemotherapy with hepatic transarterial chemoembolization (TACE), brachytherapy, radiofrequency ablation, and liver transplantation. In hepatic transarterial embolization, substances are injected into the hepatic artery to cut off blood supply to the tumor. In chemoembolization, chemotherapy medications are injected directly into the hepatic artery. Radioembolization is also possible; this procedure combines embolization with radiation therapy. This is done by injecting small beads (called microspheres) that have a radioactive isotope (yttrium-90) attached to them into the hepatic artery. In brachytherapy, radioactive seeds are implanted into the liver at the tumor site. Radiofrequency ablation focuses heat to directly destroy tumor cells.

Systemic chemotherapy involves use of molecular targeted therapies or immunotherapy using checkpoint inhibitors. Chemotherapeutic agents can be used in conjunction with other treatment modalities, such as TACE. The agents most studied include sorafenib, lenvatinib, atezolizumab plus bevacizumab, or durvalumab plus tremelimumab.

In the United States, patients with underlying chronic liver disease (cirrhosis, hepatitis C virus infection) are potentially eligible for liver transplant if they fulfill specific criteria (i.e., solitary HCC 5 cm or smaller in diameter or up to three separate lesions, none of which is larger than 3 cm, no evidence of gross vascular invasion, and no regional nodal or distant metastases).

To prevent HCC, the hepatitis B vaccine can prevent infection and subsequently prevent the development of cancer. There is no hepatitis C vaccine; however, there is highly effective treatment. Antiviral therapy for hepatitis C has decreased viral loads to undetectable levels. Different combination therapies have been formulated according to the specific genotype of the virus. Medications can be taken for 12 to 24 weeks for virtual cure of the infection, which then prevents progression to HCC.

Brain Tumors

Brain tumors either originate from the neurons or supportive tissue in the brain, or they may be the metastasis of primary tumors elsewhere in the body. In 2022, malignant primary tumors of the CNS occurred in approximately 25,000 individuals and accounted for an estimated 18,000 deaths in the United States. The rate of new cases of brain and other nervous system cancer was 6.3 per 100,000 per year. The death rate was 4.4 per 100,000 per year. Approximately 0.6% of people will be diagnosed with brain and other nervous system cancer at some point during their lifetime. The peak prevalence of brain tumor is between 55 and 64 years of age, with a slightly higher incidence in males than in females.

Etiology

There is a striking difference in the location of primary brain tumors found in adults versus children. In adults, most brain cancer affects areas superior to the cerebellum and brainstem. In children, most brain tumors occur inferior to the cerebellum. A prior history of irradiation to the head may increase the chance of primary brain tumor. Some inherited diseases, such as neurofibromatosis, tuberous sclerosis, multiple endocrine neoplasia (type 1), Von Hipple–Lindau (VHL) syndrome, Li–Fraumeni syndrome, and retinoblastoma, increase the susceptibility to development of brain tumors. Immunosuppression and infection with HIV increase susceptibility to CNS lymphoma. Metastatic tumors commonly reach the brain via spread through the bloodstream.

 CLINICAL CONCEPT

Lung cancer is the most common tumor that metastasizes to the brain, followed by breast, melanoma, and colon cancer.

Pathophysiology

In general, a benign tumor within an organ has a better prognosis than a malignant tumor. However, benign brain tumors can have similar adverse effects as malignant tumors. Similar to malignant tumors, benign tumors can infiltrate large regions of the brain and cause serious neurological deficits and poor prognosis. Also, whether the brain tumor is benign or malignant, it is difficult to surgically resect large tumors without causing some neurological deficit. In addition, the anatomical site of a brain tumor, whether benign or malignant, can have lethal consequences. Brain tumors increase intracranial pressure (ICP) and place a compressive force on brain tissue. If ICP rises to high levels, it can place pressure on the brainstem, affecting vital functions and potentially leading to fatal consequences. Finally, the pattern of spread of primary brain tumors differs from that of other tumors; even the most highly malignant gliomas rarely metastasize outside the CNS.

The frequency of various tumor types and grades varies by age group. In adolescents and young adults, primary brain tumors are more common than metastatic tumors, and among primary brain tumors, gliomas predominate. In adults older than 30 to 40 years, metastatic brain tumors are prevalent, accounting for more than half of all brain tumors. Glioblastoma and meningiomas are the most common malignant primary brain tumors in adults.

The fifth edition of the World Health Organization (WHO) Classification of Tumors of the Central Nervous System (CNS) (WHO CNS5) has a comprehensive list of tumor classifications with new nomenclature. The WHO CNS5 groups tumors into more biologically and molecularly defined entities with better-characterized natural histories, as well as introducing new tumor types and subtypes (see Box 40-5).

Most Common Primary Brain and CNS Tumors

Gliomas. Gliomas are the most common primary malignancy in the CNS, accounting for approximately 80% of malignant brain and CNS tumors in adults. Gliomas arise from glial cells, which are nonneuronal supportive cells in the CNS. There are three types of gliomas:

- Astrocytoma—composed of astrocytes, which are star-shaped cells often thought of as "nurse" cells for neurons in the brain parenchyma. These cells compose a large portion of the brain parenchyma. There are four grades of astrocytomas; the high-grade tumors are also termed glioblastomas.
- Oligodendroglioma—composed of oligodendrocytes, which are cells in the brain and spinal cord that produce the myelin that protects neurons. Oligodendrogliomas range from less malignant to very malignant.
- Ependymoma—derived from ependymal cells that line the ventricle surfaces of the brain. Ependymomas range from less malignant to very malignant.

Meningiomas. Meningiomas are another type of primary brain tumor in adults. They are the most common primary tumor, accounting for 35% of adult brain tumors. They arise from the dura mater layer of the meningeal membranes. Incidence increases with age and are more common in females, persons with neurofibromatosis type 2, and those who have been exposed to cranial radiation. They are classified from grade 1 (benign) to grade 3 (malignant). Meningiomas are often asymptomatic and are incidentally found on neuroimaging for an unrelated reason. Typically, they can be managed with periodic surveillance or resected surgically.

Schwannomas. Schwannomas are generally benign tumors arising from the Schwann cells of cranial and spinal nerves. The most common is a vestibular schwannoma (also called acoustic neuroma) arising from CN VIII, and accounts for 9% of primary brain tumors. Persons with neurofibromatosis type 1 are predisposed to schwannomas. Persons often present with dizziness, hearing loss, and tinnitus. Small lesions can be managed with periodic surveillance. Larger lesions can be resected surgically.

Craniopharyngioma. Craniopharyngiomas are tumors that develop near or around the pituitary gland. They are benign, slow-growing tumors that have a bimodal incidence; most commonly arise in children or adolescents or older adults. Symptoms are commonly visual problems due to the close proximity of the optic chiasm. Pituitary problems can also develop (see Chapter 24 for more information).

Primary Central Nervous System Lymphoma. Primary CNS lymphoma is a form of non-Hodgkin's lymphoma accounting for less than 3% of primary brain tumors. The incidence of this type of tumor is rising in older adults for unclear reasons. Immunocompromised adults, particularly those with HIV or organ transplant, are at highest risk. It can also occur in immunocompetent older adults with median age of 60 years. It is usually a diffuse large B cell lymphoma that presents as a mass lesion. The patient usually presents with neuropsychiatric symptoms, neurological deficits, and/or seizures. It is treated with glucocorticoids, chemotherapy, and radiation therapy.

BOX 40-5. The Fifth Edition of the World Health Organization (WHO) Classification of Tumors of the Central Nervous System (CNS) (WHO CNS5)

(Only major categories of tumors listed here; for a complete, detailed list, see https://www.ncbi.nlm.nih.gov/pmc/articles/PMC8328013/)
- Gliomas, glioneuronal tumors, and neuronal tumors
- Ependymal tumors
- Choroid plexus tumors
- Embryonal tumors
- Pineal tumors
- Cranial nerve and paraspinal nerve tumors
- Meningiomas
- Mesenchymal, nonmeningothelial tumors
- Melanocytic tumors
- Hematolymphoid tumors
- Histiocytic tumors
- Germ cell tumors
- Tumors of the sellar region
- Metastases to the CNS

Adapted from Louis, D. N., Perry, A., Wesseling, P., et al. (2021). The 2021 WHO classification of tumors of the central nervous system: A summary. *Neuro Oncol, 23*(8), 1231–1251. doi: 10.1093/neuonc/noab106

Medulloblastomas. Medulloblastomas are the most common malignant brain tumor of childhood, accounting for approximately 20% of all primary CNS tumors in children. Medulloblastoma in adults is usually diagnosed between the ages of 20 and 44. Medulloblastomas usually appear as a solid mass in the cerebellum. Medulloblastomas are rapidly growing tumors that can cause headaches, dizziness, imbalance and ataxia, and nausea and vomiting. It is more common in persons with *BRCA1* gene mutations, Corlin syndrome (a type of basal cell carcinoma), and Turcot syndrome (a type of colon cancer). Surgery, chemotherapy, and radiation are treatments.

 CLINICAL CONCEPT

Glioblastoma multiforme (GBM) is the most common and aggressive malignant tumor found in the CNS in adults. Medulloblastomas are the most common malignant tumor found in the CNS in children.

Tumors That Metastasize to the Brain

Brain metastasis is common in adults and arises due to hematogenous spread of another type of cancer. Most frequently, the origin is lung cancer. Most metastatic tumors occur in the gray-white matter junction where there is a large proportion of blood flow. Aside from lung cancer, breast cancer and melanomas have the greatest propensity to metastasize to the brain. Brain metastases are best visualized on MRI and appear as well-circumscribed lesions. Biopsy is rarely necessary as another systemic cancer has usually been diagnosed. Common treatment of brain metastases is radiation therapy. Stereotactic radiation treatments, such as gamma knife, cyberknife, or proton beam, are most commonly used.

 CLINICAL CONCEPT

Brain and spinal cord metastasis from other primary sites of cancer is more common than primary CNS tumors.

Clinical Presentation

Most brain tumors cause symptoms because of the pressure they exert on brain tissue. Increased ICP and cerebral ischemia may cause initial symptoms. Seizure activity may occur due to disruption of neural tissue. A progressive headache (see Box 40-6) is the most common symptom. Progression of a focal neurological deficit, such as weakness of one extremity, sensory loss, and cranial nerve dysfunction, commonly occurs. The patient may report dizziness, unsteadiness, ataxia, apraxia, anosmia, expressive language disorder, drowsiness, and confusion. Cranial nerve disruption often manifests as pupillary changes. Visual

BOX 40-6. Headaches Caused by Brain Tumors

Headaches caused by brain tumors may:
- Be worse when the person wakes up in the morning and clear up in a few hours
- Occur during sleep
- Be accompanied by vomiting, confusion, double vision, weakness, or numbness
- Get worse with coughing or exercise, or with a change in body position

disturbances such as diplopia and visual field deficits, nausea and vomiting, and mental status changes are common. Papilledema, which is swelling of the optic nerve visualized on the retina, may be seen on ophthalmological examination. Cognitive dysfunction, which includes memory problems and mood or personality change, is common among patients with primary and metastatic brain tumors. Most of the neurocognitive deficits associated with brain tumors are subtle. Patients often complain of having low energy, fatigue, an urge to sleep, and loss of interest in everyday activities.

 CLINICAL CONCEPT

Increased intracranial pressure (ICP) can arise either from a large mass or from restriction of cerebrospinal fluid (CSF) outflow, causing hydrocephalus. Symptoms consist of a classic triad of headache, nausea, and papilledema.

Diagnosis

A complete history and physical examination that includes a comprehensive neurological examination are necessary. Examination of the visual fields, retina, and particularly the optic discs should be performed in patients suspected of having increased ICP. Common laboratory testing such as CBC, electrolytes, coagulation studies, and metabolic panel are necessary. The likelihood of brain involvement due to metastasis from a systemic malignancy should be considered. A thorough screening for a systemic malignancy should be done. Chest, abdominal, and/or pelvic CT may be necessary to find the primary site of the cancer.

Gadolinium-enhanced MRI is a preferred modality for diagnosis of brain tumor because of its resolution and enhancement with contrast agents. CT is relied upon primarily in emergency settings for a more detailed view of bony structures and in patients with a contraindication to MRI. Cerebral angiography is often used to visualize the vascular supply of the tumor. Electroencephalography is a useful test in patients with seizures. A PET scan and single photon emission tomography may be used in surgical planning to define the tumor's anatomy. Tissue removed from an accessible tumor biopsy or cerebrospinal fluid analysis is sometimes necessary.

Molecular Biomarkers

The diagnosis and treatment of brain and CNS tumors are increasingly more specific based on molecular biomarkers derived from immunohistochemical analysis of the tumor cells. Biomarkers are continually being discovered that allow for more specific diagnostic, therapeutic, and prognostic information. Biomarkers can be genetic aberrations, proteins, enzymes, or receptors that are unique to the tumor cells (see Box 40-7).

BOX 40-7. Biomarkers Associated With Specific Types of Brain and CNS Tumors

These are examples of molecular biomarkers and genetic aberrations used as diagnostic, therapeutic, and prognostic indicators in different types of brain and CNS tumors.

MOLECULAR BIOMARKER	SPECIFIC TYPE OF BRAIN OR CNS TUMOR
AKT1 mutation	meningioma
ATRX mutation	astrocytomas
APC mutation	medulloblastomas
BRAF mutation	astrocytomas, gangliogliomas, glioblastomas, craniopharyngiomas
BRCA2	medulloblastomas
CDKN2A/B deletion	astrocytomas
CIC mutation	oligodendroglial tumors
EGFR (epidermal growth factor receptor)	glioblastomas
FUBP1 mutation	oligodendroglial tumors
IDH1/IDH2 mutation (isocitrate dehydrogenase)	astrocytomas, oligodendroglial tumors, glioblastomas
MGMT promoter hypermethylation	glioblastomas
NF1 inactivation	neurofibroma
RELA fusion-positive	ependymoma
TERT promoter mutation	astrocytomas, oligodendroglial tumors, glioblastomas, meningiomas
TP53 mutation	astrocytomas, oligodendroglial tumors, glioblastomas
YAP 1 fusion	ependymoma
1p/19q deletion	oligodendroglial tumors

Adapted from Kristensen, B. W., Priesterbach-Ackley, L. P., Petersen, J. K., et al. (2019). Molecular pathology of tumors of the central nervous system. *Ann Oncol, 30*(8), 1265–1278. doi: 10.1093/annonc/mdz164

Grading of Tumors

Brain tumors are a heterogeneous group of malignancies, individually categorized from grade 1 to grade 4 by the WHO. The choice of treatment, particularly the adjuvant radiation and/or chemotherapy, is directly influenced by the WHO tumor grade.

Grade 1 tumors have slow proliferative activity. These tumors can be treated with surgical resection alone. Grade 2 tumors are commonly known as low-grade gliomas. They have comparatively less proliferation rate but can progress to higher-grade tumors. These tumors can be treated with surgery but they often recur. Grade 3 tumors have a high rate of proliferative activity and a high infiltration rate. These tumors are histologically malignant, have an overall survival rate of 2 to 3 years, and can be treated with adjuvant radiation and/or chemotherapy. Grade 4 (life-threatening) tumors have vigorous proliferation activity and can invade nearby tissues. These are cytological malignant tumors with brisk mitotic activity. These tumors require more aggressive treatment with the adjuvant therapy of radiation and chemotherapy.

Treatment

The treatment of brain and CNS tumors varies depending on the location of the tumor, tissue type, and comorbid conditions. The treatment requires care from a multidisciplinary team of health-care providers: neurosurgeon, oncologist, radiologist, and radiation oncologist. Various treatment options are used either to restrict the tumor growth or remove the tumor mass.

The conventional treatment options after the tumor diagnosis include surgery, radiation therapy, and chemotherapy. Surgical resection is preferred, and may provide a complete cure for low-grade tumors. Radiation therapy, including gamma rays, x-rays, and proton rays are used to kill the tumor cells and shrink brain tumors. Stereotactic radiotherapy, also called cyberknife or gamma knife treatment, targets a tumor precisely. A robotic device moves and bends around the patient to deliver radiation doses from thousands of unique beam angles, significantly expanding the possible positions to concentrate radiation to the tumor and minimizing the dose to surrounding healthy tissue. Proton therapy, also called proton beam therapy, is a type of radiation therapy that uses protons rather than x-rays to treat cancer. At high energy, protons can destroy cancer at depths within the body without affecting healthy tissue. They may be used alone or in combination x-ray radiation therapy, surgery, chemotherapy, and/or immunotherapy.

Chemotherapeutic agents act by either disrupting the cell cycle or obstructing the supply of blood to tumor cells. Chemotherapeutic agents used most often to treat brain tumors include temozolomide (Temodar), procarbazine (Matulane), lomustine (Gleostine), and vincristine.

Newer strategies are also in use for the treatment of brain tumors, including targeted drug therapy, electric field treatments and vaccine therapy. Targeted drug therapy includes everolimus and bevacizumab. Everolimus is a protein kinase inhibitor that blocks the enzyme tyrosine kinase active in many types of cancer. Bevacizumab is a monoclonal antibody that inhibits vascular endothelial growth factor (VEGF), thereby restricting circulation of the tumor. In 2015, the first electric field device, Optune, was approved by the U.S. Food and Drug Administration (FDA) as adjuvant therapy for newly diagnosed glioblastoma multiforme.

The newest medications for gliomas are selective cyclin-dependent kinase inhibitors (CDKIs), which block certain steps in the cell cycle of tumor cells. Every cell cycle step is a well-regulated process controlled by cyclin-dependent kinases (CDKs). Currently, brain tumor treatment includes targeting CDKs with drugs such as abemaciclib (Verzenio) and ribociclib (Kisqali).

Because the blood-brain barrier restricts the transport of therapeutic agents to the brain, drug technology is increasingly utilizing nanomedicines as targeted drug delivery. Loading of the chemotherapeutic agents in nano-sized formulation, such as in the liposomes, is in clinical practice. Liposomes have an aqueous inner core enclosed by phospholipid bilayers, and are frequently used as nanocarriers in cancer chemotherapy. Liposomal drug delivery protects chemotherapeutics from degradation, early inactivation, and dilution in the circulation.

Glucocorticoids, which are the mainstay of postoperative management, help decrease tumor-associated vasogenic edema and prevent postoperative and radiation-associated edema. Because long-term use is often necessary, patients should be monitored for potential adverse effects of glucocorticoids. Post treatment anticonvulsant medication may be needed to prevent seizures.

Multidisciplinary treatment is necessary to assist patients with cognitive deficits post-treatment. Cognitive rehabilitation programs that include computer-based attention retraining and compensatory skills training of attention, memory, and executive functioning is used to help patients overcome cognitive deficits. Psychotherapy is recommended for emotional support. Hospice and palliative care should be made available when appropriate throughout treatment. Hospice should be offered if life expectancy is less than 6 months, and to patients who have poor or worsening performance status, are not candidates for surgery or chemotherapy, have deteriorating neurological deficits despite therapy, or have tumor recurrence.

Bone Cancer

Bone cancer is a malignant tumor that develops from the cells of the bone. Primary bone cancer is rare. It accounts for only about 0.5% of all cancers in the United States. In children, however, it accounts for about 5% of all cancers. There are three main types of bone cancer: osteosarcoma, which arises in new tissue in growing bones; chondrosarcoma, which arises in cartilage; and Ewing's sarcoma, which may arise in immature nerve tissue in the bone marrow. Osteosarcoma is the most common of these types, occurring most frequently during adolescence. Often, bone cancer is a metastatic disease from another type of primary tumor in the body. Bone is commonly a metastatic site for breast, lung, prostate, and kidney cancer.

In the United States, the incidence of osteosarcoma is approximately 750 to 900 cases per year. The majority of affected individuals are younger than 20 years old, and the incidence of osteosarcoma is slightly higher in males than in females. Patients with hereditary retinoblastomas have up to 1,000 times greater risk of subsequently developing osteosarcoma. Mutations in the *Rb* gene are also found in 60% to 70% of noninheritable, sporadic osteosarcoma tumors.

Chondrosarcomas, which originate in cartilaginous tissue, have an incidence of 1 per 200,000 population in the United States. Most affected patients are 50 to 70 years old, and the majority are male. Ewing's sarcoma tumors are most common in individuals from birth to the age of 20 years, with approximately 250 cases diagnosed per year in the United States. Males are more frequently affected compared with females. The incidence of these tumors in European Americans is at least nine times higher than it is in African Americans.

Etiology

The cause of primary bone cancer is not clear, but there are several risk factors, including use of high doses of radiation therapy or treatment with some anticancer drugs, hereditary retinoblastoma, bone infarction, chronic osteomyelitis, and a history of Paget's disease, which is a bone-remodeling disorder.

Persons with certain genetic mutations are susceptible to bone cancer. The majority of genetic variants are in the *RB1* (the gene associated with hereditary retinoblastoma) and *TP53* (the gene associated with Li-Fraumeni syndrome [LFS]) genes. Other variants identified include the cancer susceptibility genes *APC*, *PALBB2*, and *MSH2*, as well as *CDKN2A*, *ATRX*, *MEN1*, and *POT1*. Genetic conditions with a known predisposition to osteosarcoma include Rothmund-Thomson syndrome (RTS), RAPADILINO, and Bloom and Werner syndromes.

Pathophysiology

Osteosarcoma, chondrosarcoma, and Ewing's sarcoma affect different age groups and have slightly different pathological mechanisms (described in Clinical Manifestations, following).

Clinical Manifestations

The most common symptom of bone cancer is pain. It commonly starts as a dull ache and progressively worsens. A lump or mass may be felt over the bone.

Fracture can occur if the tumor weakens the integrity of the bone.

Osteosarcoma. Osteosarcoma develops from bone-forming stem or progenitor cells that reside in the skeleton. Areas of rapid bone growth are common sites and may be related to cancer development; however, the etiology is unclear. Osteosarcoma appears most frequently at sites where the greatest increase in bone length and size occurs (e.g., distal femur, proximal tibia, and proximal humerus). There are many chromosomal aberrations associated with osteosarcoma. There is a high frequency of chromosomal deletions in the regions of 3q and 13q (the location of the *RB* gene), 17p (the location of the *TP53* gene), and 18q (the location linked to osteosarcoma arising in the setting of Paget's disease). Combined inactivation of the *RB* and *TP53* pathways is common in osteosarcoma. The genetic region 8q contains the gene *MYC,* which is amplified in up to half of cases of osteosarcoma and may be associated with a poor prognosis. Amplification of *FGFR1* and alterations in the *IGF1R* pathway have also been observed in about 18.5% and 14% of cases, respectively.

The most common site for osteosarcoma is in the bone surrounding the knee (see Fig. 40-5). Osteosarcoma develops in areas of greatest bone growth, such as the distal femur, proximal tibia, and proximal humerus. Patients typically present with pain and swelling in the affected area. A sudden pathological fracture can be the first sign of bone cancer.

Osteosarcomas are classified as stage 1, 2, or 3. Stage 1 osteosarcoma is localized and resectable. Stage 2 is more aggressive, causing more tissue necrosis; it may or may not have metastasized to the lymph nodes and lungs. Stage 3 osteosarcoma has lung metastasis. Osteosarcoma has a 50% to 60% survival rate, and metastasis most commonly occurs to lungs, other bones, and the brain. Surgical amputation of the extremity, most commonly above the knee, is the common treatment.

CLINICAL CONCEPT

Retinoblastoma is associated with later development of osteosarcoma.

Chondrosarcoma. Chondrosarcoma is a very rare disease. Chondrosarcomas are the third most common primary malignancy of bone after Ewing's sarcoma and osteosarcoma. These tumors commonly arise in the central portions of the skeleton, including the pelvis, shoulder, and ribs. They present as painful, progressively enlarging masses. Grade 1 chondrosarcoma grows relatively slowly, has cells with a similar appearance to normal cartilage, and is the least aggressive and invasive. Grades 2 and 3 are increasingly faster-growing cancers, with more varied and abnormal-looking cells, and are much more likely to infiltrate surrounding tissues, lymph nodes, and organs. Grade 4 is the anaplastic and undifferentiated cartilage-derived tumors with the worst prognosis.

The most common sites for chondrosarcoma to grow are the pelvis and shoulder, along with the superior metaphyseal and diaphyseal regions of the arms and legs. However, chondrosarcoma may occur in any bone, and is sometimes found in the skull, particularly at its base. Most tumors are low grade and slow growing, with a 5-year survival rate of up to 90%. Large tumors are more aggressive than small tumors, and metastasis occurs to the lungs and skeleton. Surgical excision and chemotherapy are the treatment modalities used for chondrosarcoma.

Ewing's Sarcoma. Ewing's sarcoma is the second most common primary bone malignancy affecting children and adolescents, after osteosarcoma. Genetic exchange between chromosomes can cause cells to become cancerous. Most cases of Ewing's sarcoma (85%) are the result of a translocation between chromosomes 11 and 22, which fuses the *EWS* gene of chromosome 22 to the *FLI1* gene of chromosome 11. The disease typically involves long bones such as the femur and flat bones of the pelvis. On x-ray, tumors lyse and destroy bone and have a characteristic "onion peel" appearance. Ewing's sarcoma presents as an enlarging, tender, swollen mass and may appear as an infection. Some patients have fever and elevated WBC count and erythrocyte sedimentation rate. It is an

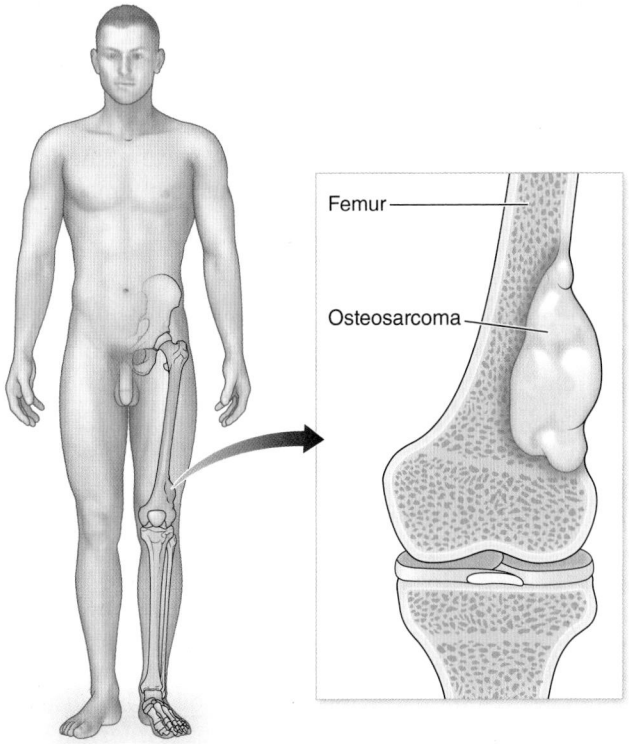

Femur

Osteosarcoma

FIGURE 40-5. Osteosarcoma is cancer of the bone. It is commonly located in the leg, close to the knee.

aggressive disease with a high likelihood of metastasis to the lungs, bones, and bone marrow.

Diagnosis and Treatment

Common laboratory tests used in the diagnosis of bone cancer include CBC, electrolyte level, liver enzymes, platelet count, metabolic panel, renal function tests, and blood levels of lactic dehydrogenase (LDH) and alkaline phosphatase (ALP). The LDH and ALP blood levels are indicative of prognosis. Those with elevated ALP commonly have pulmonary metastasis. Those with elevated LDH have a poorer prognosis than those with normal LDH levels. For each type of bone cancer, an x-ray shows a destructive lesion in bone. CT scan, MRI, and bone scan can delineate the tumor and reveal metastases. Radionuclide bone scanning with technetium-99 (^{99m}Tc)-methylene diphosphonate (MDP/MDI) is important in evaluating for the presence of metastatic or multifocal disease. After the bone scan, an image of abnormal areas should be obtained with CT or MRI. A PET scan can be used to identify other areas in the body where there is active bone cancer. A biopsy of the tumor is needed to examine and grade bone cancer cells. There are four stages and three grades of bone cancer (see Table 40-12). The TNM system is used to stage the cancer, and grade is based on cell differentiation; well-differentiated cancer cells look like bone cells, whereas poorly differentiated cancer looks very abnormal. Well-differentiated tumors have a better prognosis than poorly differentiated. Biopsy of the bone tumor assists in the determination of appropriate treatment.

Treatments for bone cancer depend on the type of cancer. Surgical resection, chemotherapy, radiation, and targeted therapies are used. Chemotherapy is a standard component of most osteosarcoma treatment, both in children and in adults. It has been found that by the time of diagnosis, many cases of osteosarcoma have metastasized; therefore, systemic chemotherapy can be used to reach the distant sites of cancer. Preoperative and postoperative chemotherapy regimens and multimodality treatments are used. There is no worldwide consensus on a standard chemotherapy approach for osteosarcoma. The majority of regimens incorporate doxorubicin and cisplatin with or without high-dose methotrexate (HDMTX) (with leucovorin rescue), called the MAP regimen. For patients who cannot tolerate HDMTX and for institutions that cannot provide pharmacokinetic monitoring for HDMTX, the combination of carboplatin, ifosfamide, and doxorubicin appears to be a reasonable alternative. Most types of osteosarcoma are resistant to radiation.

Patients who present with overtly metastatic osteosarcoma have a poor prognosis; long-term survival rates with standard chemotherapy and surgery range from 10% to 50%. Metastasis to the lungs is the most common site of relapse. This is in contrast to patients with apparently localized disease at presentation, two-thirds of whom will achieve long-term survival with appropriate therapy. Complete resection of all metastatic sites is a prerequisite for long-term survival. Some patients with isolated pulmonary metastases that develop more than 1 year after original treatment will be long-term survivors with just surgical removal of their lung nodules.

In Ewing's sarcoma, metastatic disease is usually present upon diagnosis. Chemotherapy can successfully eradicate the metastatic deposits, and treatment plans all include chemotherapy, usually administered before and following local surgical resection. The combination of vincristine, doxorubicin, cyclophosphamide, and dactinomycin is a common regimen. Adding alternating cycles of ifosfamide and etoposide (I/E) to a vincristine, doxorubicin, and cyclophosphamide (VDC) backbone (VDC/IE) provides further benefit.

For all grades and subtypes of nonmetastatic chondrosarcoma, surgical treatment is necessary. Many types of chondrosarcoma are resistant to radiation and chemotherapy. High doses of radiation are needed in attempts to achieve local control after incomplete resection.

Uterine Cancer

Cancers of the female reproductive system account for almost 15% of all cancers in females. The most common of these malignancies is uterine cancer. Ninety percent of uterine cancer is endometrial cancer and 10% is uterine sarcoma. An estimated 66,000 cases of uterine cancer were diagnosed in 2022 and 12,500 cases were fatal. It is the fourth most common cancer, accounting for 6% of female cancers, following breast, lung, and colorectal cancer. The chance of a female being diagnosed with uterine cancer in their lifetime is 1 in 37. It affects mainly postmenopausal females with the average age of 60 years old. It affects more European American females than African American females; however, more African American females die of it.

Etiology

Premenopausal females are at increased risk for endometrial cancer if they have risk factors such as obesity, nulliparity, anovulatory menstrual cycles, diabetes, tamoxifen treatment, estrogen therapy, and hypertension (see Box 40-8). In addition, these younger females are at higher risk (up to 19% to 25%) for primary ovarian cancer. Females at increased risk of premenopausal endometrial cancer are those with hereditary nonpolyposis colorectal cancer (Lynch syndrome) and Cowden syndrome. These patients are also at increased risk for many other kinds of cancer, including melanoma and cancers of the breast, thyroid, kidney, colon, and rectum. Endometrial cancer can occur because of excess estrogen from various sources, either exogenous or endogenous.

Endogenous estrogen sources include obesity, polycystic ovary syndrome, anovulatory menstrual cycles,

TABLE 40-12. Stages and Grades of Bone Cancer

The stages of bone cancer are designated according to the American Joint Committee on Cancer (AJCC) TNM system. The scale used for grading bone cancer is from 1 to 3. Low-grade cancers (G_1) tend to grow and spread slowly and resemble bone tissue; high-grade (G_3) cancers are rapidly spreading and aggressive and look very different from bone tissue. G_2 cancer indicates it is somewhere between slowly and rapidly spreading. G_X indicates that the cancer grade cannot be determined.

AJCC Stage	Stage Grouping	Stage Description*
IA	T_1 N_0 M_0 G_1 OR G_X	The cancer is 8 cm across (about 3 inches) or smaller (T_1). It has not spread to nearby lymph nodes (N_0) or to distant sites (M_0). The cancer is low grade (G_1), or the grade cannot be determined (G_X).
IB	T_2 N_0 M_0 G_1 OR G_X OR T_3 N_0 M_0 G_1 OR G_X	The cancer is larger than 8 cm (3 inches) across (T_2). It has not spread to nearby lymph nodes (N_0) or to distant sites (M_0). The cancer is low grade (G_1), or the grade cannot be determined (G_X). The cancer is in more than one place on the same bone (T_3). It has not spread to nearby lymph nodes (N_0) or to distant sites (M_0). The cancer is low grade (G_1), or the grade cannot be determined (G_X).
IIA	T_1 N_0 M_0 G_2 OR G_3	The cancer is 8 cm across (about 3 inches) or less (T_1). It has not spread to nearby lymph nodes (N_0) or to distant sites (M_0). The cancer is high grade (G_2 or G_3).
IIB	T_2 N_0 M_0 G_2 OR G_3	The cancer is larger than 8 cm (3 inches) across (T_2). It has not spread to nearby lymph nodes (N_0) or to distant sites (M_0). The cancer is high grade (G_2 or G_3).
III	T_3 N_0 M_0 G_2 OR G_3	The cancer is in more than one place on the same bone (T_3). It has not spread to nearby lymph nodes (N_0) or to distant sites (M_0). The cancer is high grade (G_2 or G_3).
IVA	Any T N_0 M_{1a} Any G	The cancer can be any size and may be in more than one place in the bone (any T) **AND** has not spread to nearby lymph nodes (N_0). It has spread only to the lungs (M_{1a}). The cancer can be any grade (any G).
IVB	Any T N_1 Any M Any G OR Any T Any N M_{1b} Any G	The cancer can be any size and may be in more than one place in the bone (any T) **AND** it has spread to nearby lymph nodes (N_1). It may or may not have spread to distant organs like the lungs or other bones (any M). The cancer can be any grade (any G). The cancer can be any size and may be in more than one place in the bone (any T), and it might or might not have spread to nearby lymph nodes (any N). It has spread to distant sites like other bones, the liver, or brain (M_{1b}). The cancer can be any grade (any G)

From American Cancer Society (2019). Bone cancer stages. Retrieved from https://www.cancer.org/cancer/bone-cancer/detection-diagnosis-staging/staging.html

or estrogen-secreting tumors. Obesity has been associated with an increased risk of endometrial cancer because within adipose tissue, androgenic hormones convert to estrogen compounds. This leads to higher levels of unopposed estrogen in obese females. Nulliparity and infertility are also related to chronic anovulation and unopposed estrogen levels. Frequent alcohol use can elevate estrogen levels. Late menopause and early menarche can be associated with more anovulatory cycles and thus more unopposed estrogen.

BOX 40-8. Risk Factors for Uterine Cancer

Postmenopausal age (usually after age 50)
European ancestry
Metabolic syndrome
Obesity
Unopposed estrogen exposure; estrogen treatment without progesterone
Polycystic ovarian syndrome (PCOS)/chronic anovulation
Early onset menarche
Late onset menopause
Nulliparity
Tamoxifen treatment
Lynch syndrome
Cowden syndrome

Adapted from Passarello, K., Kurian, S., & Villanueva, V. (2019). Endometrial cancer: An overview of pathophysiology, management, and care. *Semin Oncol Nurs, 35*(2), 157–165. doi: 10.1016/j.soncn.2019.02.002

Pathophysiology

Endometrial cancers are divided into two classes, type I and type II, each with differing pathophysiology and prognosis. More than 80% of endometrial cancers are type I and are caused by unopposed estrogen stimulation. Type I is often found in association with endometrial hyperplasia, which is thought to be a precursor. Type I cancers primarily include low-grade endometrioid adenocarcinomas (International Federation of Gynecology and Obstetrics [FIGO]) grades 1 and 2. The FIGO grading system assesses the architectural pattern and nuclear grade. Grade 1 cancers have <5% solid component. They are well differentiated, more closely resemble normal tissue, and typically have a good prognosis. Grade 2 cancers fall in between grade 1 and 3 in resembling normal endometrium. They have 6% to 50% solid component and can be referred to as moderately differentiated. Grade 3 cancers do not resemble healthy endometrial tissue, are considered high grade, and are poorly differentiated. They tend to be more aggressive with a poorer prognosis. They have a greater than 50% solid component. Grade 1 and 2 tumors are generally classified as low grade and fall into the type I classification; grade 3 tumors are classified as high grade and fall into the type II classification.

Type II endometrial cancers are thought to be estrogen independent, occurring in older females, are considered high grade, and have worse prognosis. Type II tumors are considered aggressive and often present at an advanced stage. Type II histologies typically have a poor prognosis and have higher rates of recurrence (approximately 50%), with lower 5-year overall survival (55%).

Endometrial cancer may originate in a small area, such as within an endometrial polyp or in a diffuse multifocal pattern. Early tumor growth is characterized by a spreading pattern. Endometrial cancer growth is characterized by fragility of the tissue and spontaneous uterine bleeding. Later tumor growth is characterized by invasion of the uterine muscle layer and growth toward the cervix.

Clinical Presentation

More than 90% of patients with endometrial cancer will present with abnormal vaginal bleeding. Advanced cases may present with abdominal pain and bloating or other symptoms of metastatic disease. Other presenting symptoms may include purulent genital discharge, unintentional weight loss, and a change in bladder or bowel habits. Fortunately, most cases of endometrial cancer are diagnosed before this clinical presentation because of the recognition of abnormal vaginal bleeding as a possible early symptom of cancer. About 5% of patients may be asymptomatic and diagnosed after abnormal Pap test results.

Diagnosis

Currently, no screening tests for cancer of the uterus are recommended for asymptomatic patients. However, a Pap smear can detect preinvasive cervical cancer at early stages, which can lead to more intense investigation for uterine cancer. Pelvic and transvaginal ultrasound can be used to visualize the uterus, fallopian tubes, and ovaries and pinpoint areas of suspected tumor. An endometrial biopsy can be done through the cervix with a needle or suction. Hysteroscopy with dilation and curettage (D&C) allows for direct visualization of the interior uterus and biopsy of the endometrial tissue. Although no laboratory tests aid in the diagnosis of uterine cancer, a CA-125 blood level is used to monitor the efficacy of treatment of endometrial cancer. Chest imaging should be obtained in all patients to rule out lung metastases before treatment. A CT scan of the chest, abdomen, and pelvis may be helpful in advanced-stage disease.

Treatment

The mainstay of treatment in endometrial cancer is surgery. A total hysterectomy and bilateral salpingo-oophorectomy are indicated with lymph node assessment. This can be accomplished through a minimally invasive laparoscopic procedure if there is nonbulky disease. A thorough survey of the abdomen should be done which includes surfaces of the diaphragm, peritoneum, and serosal surfaces. Omental biopsies and peritoneal washings are often performed for those with high-risk disease. Additionally, radiation has an important role in adjuvant treatment of endometrial cancers, as does chemotherapy. Hormonal therapy also has a role in adjuvant therapy in receptor-positive endometrial cancers. The goal of adjuvant therapy in uterine cancer is to reduce the risk of disease recurrence, and the recommendation for adjuvant therapy is guided by surgical stage, tumor histology, and adverse risk factors. Most endometrial cancers are diagnosed as stage I tumors, low-risk, which are confined to the uterus and histologically grade 1 or 2. Intermediate-risk endometrial cancer is confined to the uterus but invading into the myometrium. This is considered stage IA or IB. Cancer that invades the cervical tissue is considered stage II. High-risk endometrial cancer includes all type II histologies (e.g., serous, clear cell, carcinosarcoma), grade 3 deeply invasive endometrioid carcinoma, and pathological histological stages III and IV. Because of their aggressive nature and possibility for early metastasis, multimodality treatment is typically recommended for high-risk disease.

Most endometrial cancer can be cured with surgery alone, and relatively few patients need adjuvant radiotherapy. Primary radiation therapy is reserved only for patients who are poor surgical candidates or for those with unresectable disease.

Cancer of the Head and Neck

Squamous cell carcinoma (SCC) represents more than 90% of all head and neck cancers. In the United States, SCC of the head and neck comprises about 3% of all malignancies. Over the last few decades, oropharyngeal squamous cell carcinoma in relation to smoking and alcohol use has decreased, due to effective smoking cessation in the population. However, the incidence of oropharyngeal cancer related to oral HPV infection is rapidly rising in incidence. Among those individuals (males and females) with oncogenic oral HPV infections, the lifetime risk of oropharyngeal cancer is 37 per 10,000. Male-to-female incidence rates are greater than three to one.

Upward of 80% of oropharyngeal cancers are attributed to HPV in North America and Europe, with the timing between HPV exposure and progression to carcinogenesis exceeding a decade or more. In 2018, there were 51,540 new cases of oral cavity and pharyngeal cancers in the United States (males: 37,160) and 10,030 people died of these cancers. Over 30,000 cases of oropharyngeal squamous cell carcinoma are projected annually by 2029, of which over 70% will be related to the HPV.

> **CLINICAL CONCEPT**
>
> HPV is the most common sexually transmitted disease globally. It is now becoming the most common cause of oropharyngeal squamous cell carcinoma.

Etiology and Risk Factors

In the past, the most common cause of oropharyngeal cancer was excessive tobacco and alcohol use as they act synergistically to raise risk. However, studies show this cause of oropharyngeal cancer has greatly decreased,

as the rate of smoking among adults has decreased. However, HPV infection is becoming the more common cause of squamous cell oropharyngeal cancer. The subtypes of HPV16 and HPV18 are the etiological agents in most cases. For unclear reasons, the disorder is arising in younger (mean age 57), European American, male adults more than other segments of the population.

Patients who engage in oral sex with multiple partners are at highest risk for HPV-related oropharyngeal cancer. Environmental exposures to paint fumes, plastic by-products, wood dust, asbestos, and gasoline fumes have been implicated as risk factors. Gastroesophageal reflux disease is also a significant risk factor for cancer of the larynx.

Pathophysiology

It is believed that most malignancies in the oropharynx are caused by constant exposure to carcinogens. Long-term exposure to excessive alcohol and tobacco can lead to oropharyngeal cancer. However, long-term HPV infection in the oropharynx is surpassing other causes of oropharyngeal cancer. Over a number of years, HPV is thought to remain dormant in the oropharyngeal region without evidence of lesions. HPV is a small deoxyribonucleic acid (DNA) virus with over 200 subtypes that vary in their cancer risk association. It has long been a known cause of genital warts, termed condyloma acuminata, and cervical cancer. In the past decade, it is increasingly associated with anorectal, penile, vaginal, vulvar, and oropharyngeal cancer. HPV subtype 16 (HPV16) and HPV subtype 18 (HPV18) are the viral genotypes most often associated with oropharyngeal cancers. HPV infects a number of epithelial cell types in the oropharynx; the tonsillar crypts particularly permit direct access for the virus to penetrate the deep cell layer. The tonsillar tissue and base of the tongue are the most common sites of cancer. HPV infections of the oral mucosa are usually cleared by the immune system, but if not, E6 and E7 oncogenes can become activated and cause abnormalities in the cell cycle. In addition, HPV infection over time diminishes the effect of tumor suppressor genes and causes chromosomal instability in the oral mucosal cells. These influences lead to carcinogenesis of the oral mucosa. Mutations at gene *9p21* have been particularly related to oropharyngeal dysplasia. Mutations in the *TP53* and *Rb* genes are also commonly found in oropharyngeal cancer. Cellular changes in oropharyngeal cancers cause squamous cell carcinoma, which can range from well differentiated to poorly differentiated. Poorly differentiated cell changes are found in aggressive tumors with poor prognosis. Thirty percent of cancers are discovered when the lesion is localized and surgically resectable without lymph node infiltration; 60% of cases are found when lymph node infiltration has already occurred. In these lesions, despite spread to the lymph nodes, treatment is usually successful. Less than 10% of patients present with metastatic disease that is incurable.

Clinical Presentation

When gathering history information, it is important for the clinician to question the patient about use of tobacco and alcohol. Tobacco use, particularly chewing tobacco, is highly associated with oropharyngeal cancer. Sexual history is significant and the patient should be asked about past STIs, number of partners, risk of STIs in partners, and sexual practices; particularly oral sex. The patient should be asked about past HPV infection and HPV vaccination. Other disorders in the medical history that can increase risk of oropharyngeal cancer include HIV infection, Epstein–Barr virus (EBV) infection, gastroesophageal reflux, and Fanconi syndrome. Occupational exposures should be noted in the history because certain toxins increase risk. Family history is also important because several genetic mutations are related to oropharyngeal cancers.

When examining the patient, SCCs appear as plaques, nodules, or verrucae (wartlike) lesions. They may be scaly or ulcerated and white, red, or brown. SCCs usually begin as surface lesions with erythema and slight elevation. Early red lesions are asymptomatic and may be either carcinoma in situ or invasive carcinoma. One-third of lesions are white, termed leukoplakia, and only 10% of them are carcinoma in situ or invasive carcinoma.

Head and neck cancers originate in the squamous cells that line the mucosal surfaces, including the oral cavity, pharynx, and larynx. The most common sites for SCC are the tonsils and base of the tongue. Cancer of the larynx can occur and present as hoarseness of the voice. Symptoms such as mild dysphagia, painful swallowing, recurrent throat irritation, or earache occur. In more advanced cases, enlarged cervical lymph nodes are common, and the patient may present with a mass in the neck.

Diagnosis

To diagnose SCC, laryngoscopy and fine-needle aspiration biopsy (FNAB) of the lesion are necessary. Immunohistochemical analysis of the cells for p16 has become a standard approach. p16 is a tumor suppressor protein that plays an important role in cell cycle regulation. Additional testing includes polymerase chain reaction to detect the HPV viral DNA in the cells. CT scans and IV contrast are often used to detect the extent of tumor infiltration into deeper tissues and bone. MRI can be used alternatively with similar accuracy, though ultrasound is less sensitive. PET scanning is being used more frequently in patient work-up. Preoperatively, PET scanning can assess a primary tumor and lymph node and distant metastatic disease.

Treatment

Factors that influence the choice and type of treatment are the site and stage of the primary tumor. The TNM staging system is used for head and neck cancers, similar to the way it is used for other cancers. Surgery, radiation, and chemotherapy are the treatment modalities used. Surgery and radiation therapy are the major treatments for most HPV-induced oropharyngeal cancer. There are high cure rates exceeding 90% for nonsmokers. Recent development of minimally invasive transoral surgical techniques such as transoral laser microsurgery and transoral robotic surgery (TORS) have decreased morbidity and improved functional outcomes compared with traditional open surgical approaches.

 CLINICAL CONCEPT

Currently, there are no effective screening methods available to offer early detection of oropharyngeal cancers. However, the HPV vaccine has the potential to prevent HPV-related oropharyngeal cancers. The Advisory Committee on Immunization Practices recommends the HPV vaccine at age 11 or 12 years in all children (although it can be started at age 9).

Thyroid Cancer

Thyroid nodules are very common, occurring in up to 50% of individuals. Thyroid cancer is found in ~5% of thyroid nodules, so the vast majority are benign. Approximately 44,000 cases of thyroid cancer were diagnosed in 2022 in the United States. Out of that number, there were approximately 2,200 deaths. The incidence of thyroid cancer has tripled in the last 30 years and is a rapidly increasing cancer in the population. However, it is speculated that this may be due to improved diagnostic methods using thyroid ultrasound. On ultrasound, many patients are discovered to have thyroid cysts, growths, and tumors; however, few of these go on to develop carcinomatous changes. Thyroid cancer is three times higher in females than in males and peaks in the third and fourth decades of life. Nearly two-thirds of cases occur in adults younger than age 55 years.

Etiology

The thyroid gland is particularly sensitive to radiation. Radiation exposure of the neck, particularly in childhood, significantly increases the risk for thyroid cancer. Radiation treatments for Wilms tumor, lymphoma, and neuroblastoma also increase risk. Radiation fallout from nuclear power plants or nuclear weapons has been shown to increase risk of thyroid cancer in children. Family history of thyroid cancer increases risk. Genetic disorders that increase risk include familial adenomatous polyposis (FAP), Cowden disease, and familial nonmedullary thyroid carcinoma (FMTC).

Thyroid cancers are commonly categorized as well differentiated versus poorly differentiated; with well differentiated having a good prognosis. Papillary thyroid cancer and follicular thyroid cancer are well-differentiated thyroid cancers accounting for most of thyroid cancer cases.

For papillary carcinoma, hereditary gene variants are seen in chromosomes 9q22.33 and 14q13.3. The B-Raf proto-oncogene (BRAF) is a genetic variant found in many papillary carcinomas. Medullary carcinoma of the thyroid is due to a defect in the *RET* proto-oncogene on chromosome 10 (10 q11.2). Tumors of the thyroid often occur in persons with multiple endocrine neoplasia type 2 (MEN), which is also due to the *RET* gene defect. Oncogenic drivers in follicular thyroid carcinoma are primarily *RAS* single nucleotide alterations (*NRAS, HRAS,* and *KRAS*) and *PAX8/PPARγ* chromosomal rearrangements. Anaplastic thyroid cancer is extremely aggressive, rapid in progression, and commonly lethal. It accounts for 1.7% of all thyroid cancer and 75% of the patients present distant metastasis often in the lungs, bones, and the brain. *BRAF* (20% to 45%), *TP53* (up to 70%), and *RAS* (20% to 40%) mutations are the most frequent alterations in anaplastic cancer. Thyroid nodules are most likely to be malignant in patients older than 60 years and in patients younger than 30 years.

Pathophysiology

Thyroid cancers are categorized as papillary carcinomas, follicular carcinomas, medullary thyroid carcinomas, anaplastic carcinomas, primary thyroid lymphomas, and primary thyroid sarcomas. Among these, 80% of all thyroid cancers are papillary carcinoma. Follicular carcinoma occurs in approximately 10% of cases. Medullary thyroid carcinomas represent 5% to 10% of neoplasms. Anaplastic carcinomas account for 1% to 2% of cases. Primary lymphomas and sarcomas are rare.

Papillary carcinoma, which has the best prognosis, is a slow-growing tumor that arises from the thyroxine (T_4) and thyroglobulin-producing follicular cells of the thyroid. The cells are sensitive to thyroid-stimulating hormone (TSH) and take up iodine. They produce the protein thyroglobulin in response to TSH stimulation. Papillary carcinoma is invasive and grows with fingerlike projections into the gland. Lesions can be unilobular or multilobular. Classic pathological lesions of papillary carcinoma are called psammoma bodies, which are calcifications found in the tumors. Tumors can grow through the thyroid membrane to invade surrounding structures. Growth into the trachea can occur, producing hemoptysis and airway obstruction. The recurrent laryngeal nerves can become involved and cause patients to present with a hoarse, breathy voice and, occasionally, dysphagia. Papillary carcinoma often spreads to the cervical lymph nodes. Clinically evident lymph node metastases are present in approximately one-third of patients at presentation.

Clinical Presentation

Thyroid cancer most commonly manifests as a painless, palpable, solitary thyroid nodule. These nodules are commonly discovered during a routine physical examination of the neck. Rapid growth of a nodule suggests malignancy; malignant thyroid nodules are usually painless. Sudden onset of pain is more strongly associated with benign disease such as thyroiditis than with malignancy. Hoarseness suggests involvement of the vocal cords, and dysphagia may be a sign of impingement on the esophagus. The patient may complain of tightness or a feeling of fullness in the neck and note swollen lymph nodes. Family history of thyroid cancer increases the risk of malignancy. Physical examination should include a thorough head and neck examination, with careful attention to the thyroid gland and cervical soft tissues. Hard, fixed, nontender nodules are more suggestive of malignancy than supple, mobile, tender nodules. Cervical lymphadenopathy can be present.

Diagnosis

History taking, physical examination, laboratory evaluation, ultrasound, radioiodine imaging, and fine needle biopsy (FNB) are most commonly involved in the evaluation of thyroid nodules. Ultrasonography is the first imaging modality usually involved in the evaluation of a thyroid nodule. According to studies, many more thyroid nodules discovered on ultrasound are benign, rather than malignant. Some investigators suggest that currently there is an overdiagnosis of thyroid nodules, causing more biopsies than necessary. It is important to be precise about which nodules should be biopsied. On ultrasound, the characteristics of a nodule that indicate potential malignancy include being solid or predominantly solid, taller in dimension than wide, hypoechogenic, irregular margins, microcalcifications, absent halo, and increased vascularity.

The thyroid can take up radioactive iodine just like it would take up iodine; hence, radioactive isotope I-131 can be used to evaluate thyroid disease. Radioiodine imaging can help determine the functional status of a thyroid nodule. The functionality of the nodule depends on its uptake of radioiodine. Nodules can appear as hyperfunctioning, termed "hot"; intermediate in function or "warm"; or nonfunctioning, termed "cold." Cold nodules consist of tissue that do not take up radioiodine and are nonfunctional. Cancer usually occurs in cold nodules, but carcinoma cannot be excluded on the basis of radioiodine scans. FNB is usually the deciding factor in diagnosis of a cancerous thyroid nodule. CT and MRI can be used to evaluate soft tissue extension of large thyroid masses into the neck, trachea, or esophagus, and to assess metastases to the cervical lymph nodes.

After FNB, molecular analysis of the specimen can identify the presence of gene mutations associated with thyroid carcinoma. Molecular testing quantitatively assesses the proportion of cells carrying common genes mutated in thyroid cancer (e.g., *BRAF, RET*). Molecular testing helps determine which patients need a surgical procedure due to malignancy.

Molecular markers also help guide decisions related to prognosis and the use of a specific targeted therapy for advanced disease.

Treatment

Primary treatment for carcinoma is surgical excision, and total thyroidectomy has been the main treatment modality. Most well-differentiated thyroid cancers are resolved with solely surgical excision. However, some thyroid cancers require follow-up treatment with I-131, which will destroy any remaining thyroid tissue.

In cases of radioiodine-refractory tumors, additional treatment options are considered. These include strict suppression of thyroid-stimulating hormone (also known as thyrotropin, TSH) and external local radiotherapy. Systemic chemotherapy usually does not play a significant role. However, recently, medications such as multikinase or tyrosine kinase inhibitors have been approved for the treatment of radioiodine-refractory thyroid cancer. Although a benefit for overall survival has not been shown yet, these new drugs can slow tumor progression.

After thyroidectomy, thyroid hormone replacement with levothyroxine is needed for life. Thyroglobulin levels are used to monitor recurrences after surgical excision of thyroid cancer.

Kidney Cancer

Cancer of the kidney, or renal cell carcinoma (RCC), is among the 10 most common types of cancer. Among urological tumors, it is third in incidence following prostate and bladder cancer. In the United States, the incidence is 21 per 100,000 males and 11 per 100,000 females, representing the sixth and eighth most common malignancies in males and females, respectively. The peak incidence of diagnosis of RCC is at 64 years of age, and is rare in persons younger than age 45. In the United States, 76,000 new cases were diagnosed in 2021 and approximately 14,000 patients died. African Americans have a 10% to 20% higher incidence compared with European Americans. Most cases of RCC are sporadic, and only 4% are familial. Wilms tumor, also known as nephroblastoma, is a malignant type of kidney cancer that arises in children. It is the most common abdominal malignancy in children. Usually unilateral, most affected children are younger than age 15. The median age for diagnosis is 3.5 years, and 80% to 90% survive Wilms tumor.

Etiology and Risk Factors

The cause of RCC is unknown in most patients; however, there are a number of hereditary and environmental risk factors. Hereditary syndromes that increase risk of RCC include von Hippel Lindau (VHL) syndrome, tuberous sclerosis complex, Cowden disease, hereditary papillary renal carcinoma (HPRC), familial renal oncocytoma associated with Birt–Hogg–Dube syndrome, and hereditary renal carcinoma.

The primary gene implicated in RCC is the VHL gene, known as pVHL, which is a defective tumor suppressor gene. Other risk factors include smoking; obesity; hypertension; end-stage renal disease, diabetes mellitus, systemic lupus erythematosus, immunosuppression for antirejection of a transplanted organ, Hodgkin lymphoma, non-Hodgkin lymphoma, non-melanoma skin cancer, cystic kidney disease; and environmental exposures to asbestos, trichloroethylene, vinyl chloride, cadmium, herbicides, benzene, and other organic solvents. Cigarette smoking is thought to be responsible for one-third of cases and doubles the risk of RCC. Long-term use of NSAIDs is thought to be associated with an increased incidence. In patients undergoing long-term renal dialysis, there is an increased incidence of cystic disease of the kidney, which is a risk factor for renal cell cancer. The etiology of Wilms tumor is unknown. However, a defective tumor suppressor gene on chromosome 11 (11p13) is common. Another genetic defect that predisposes to the tumor is present at 11p15, where there is a duplicated paternal allele. Risk factors include African American ethnicity, family history of Wilms tumor, aniridia (absence of part of the iris in the eye), hemihypertrophy, WAGR syndrome (Wilms tumor, aniridia, genitourinary anomalies, and intellectual disability [previously referred to as mental retardation]), Denys–Dash syndrome, and Beckwith–Weidemann syndrome.

Pathophysiology

RCC encompasses a group of malignancies that originate in the renal cortex, most often in the upper pole of the kidney. The proximal tubule of the nephron is the origin of most RCCs. Most RCCs are clear cell RCC (ccRCC), sometimes referred to as conventional RCC. Papillary RCC (pRCC), the second most common form of RCC, is genetically linked to alterations in chromosomes 7 and 17 and a loss of chromosome Y. Chromophobe RCC (chRCC), the third most common form of RCC, is genetically linked to alterations in chromosomes 1, 2, 6, 10, 13, and 17. RCC is commonly a silent disease found incidentally on an imaging study that was done for another condition. Most renal cancers are discovered at a late stage when metastasis has already occurred. Renal cancer occurs in a sporadic and a hereditary form, and both forms are associated with mutations of the short arm of chromosome 3 (3p), also called the *VHL* gene. A chromosomal translocation between 3p and chromosome 6 or 8 has also been associated with ccRCC. Clear cell RCC presents as a round, well-circumscribed mass with rich vasculature. Each cell has clear cytoplasm that grows along blood vessels in the kidney. With a rich blood supply, the tissue mass can be hemorrhagic. It is common for ccRCC to spread to various locations, such as bone and lungs via the renal vein.

Clinical Presentation

The classic presentation of RCC includes hematuria, flank pain, and palpable abdominal mass. Almost half of RCC cases are asymptomatic and discovered because a renal mass is incidentally detected on x-ray. Other common presenting symptoms include fatigue, weight loss, anemia, and in males, varicocele within the scrotum. Hypercalcemia, liver dysfunction, erythrocytosis, and polyneuromyopathy are paraneoplastic disorders in RCC that occur as a result of tumor secretion of inflammatory cytokines. A paraneoplastic disorder may cause the first presenting symptoms in RCC. Paraneoplastic syndromes may cause high levels of erythropoietin. This leads to polycythemia, high levels of renin causing hypertension, or excess parathyroid peptide leading to hypercalemia. Up to 30% of patients present with metastatic disease in the kidney from bone, lung, and liver cancers. The most common presentation for Wilms tumor is an asymptomatic abdominal mass palpated during physical examination. Careful, light palpation is necessary because vigorous palpation can cause rupture of the tumor.

Diagnosis

Laboratory test abnormalities in RCC include hypoalbuminemia, proteinuria, and hypercalcemia. Ultrasonography of the abdomen can clearly differentiate renal cystic masses from solid masses and may be the initial step in determining whether a renal mass is benign or malignant. Ultrasound can identify the hypervascularity around the periphery of a round mass that is hypoechoic (dense tissue) in RCC. Renal masses must be assessed for enhancement on CT with contrast imaging. MRI is an effective modality used to identify the hypervascularity and abnormal angiogenesis in RCC. A tissue biopsy guided by ultrasound or CT is usually obtained. RCC tumors are staged according to the TNM system. Ultrasound, CT scan, and/or MRI are also used to diagnose Wilms tumor. Nephrectomy and biopsy confirmation of Wilms tumor tissue are essential.

Treatment

Surgical treatment is recommended for localized disease. Partial or total nephrectomy (surgical removal of the kidney) is the major form of treatment. Radiofrequency ablation (application of heat) and cryoablation (application of cold/freezing) are options in patients with stage I RCCs. Partial or total nephrectomy may be performed laparoscopically or as an open procedure. A laparoscopic approach is preferred if feasible because it is associated with less blood loss.

Radiation and targeted cancer therapy are used to treat patients with metastasis. Immune checkpoint inhibitors such as nivolumab or ipilimumab are being used. Multikinase and tyrosine kinase inhibitors (TKIs), such as sunitinib and sorafenib, are also being used to decrease tumor growth. Up to 30% of patients present with metastases, so surgical removal of metastatic tumors is also recommended.

RCC is often a slow-growing disease that occurs in an asymptomatic older patient. Older patients often have other medical disorders that place them at high risk for surgery. For these patients, active surveillance is recommended. In active surveillance, the clinician periodically monitors the progress of the tumor and intercedes when the cancer is causing symptoms. For Wilms tumor, nephrectomy followed by chemotherapy, with or without radiation, constitutes the most common treatment.

Chapter Summary

- Some cancers develop because of defective tumor suppressor genes, which are genes that guard against cancer formation. Other cancers develop because of mutated proto-oncogenes, which are genes that control normal cell growth and proliferation. Mutated proto-oncogenes become oncogenes that allow unrestrained cell division. Alternatively, cancer can result from defective DNA repair genes that do not prevent DNA mutation, or faulty cellular apoptosis mechanisms that do not initiate programmed cellular degeneration.

- The cell cycle is a sequence of stages that a cell moves through for mitosis and regeneration. For cells to undergo mitosis, the cell must go through stages G_0, G_1, G_2, S, and M. At each stage in the cell cycle, normal cells have a checkpoint where they can be repaired or undergo apoptosis if necessary. Cancer cells do not have checkpoints, and they constantly cycle through stages.

- Differentiation refers to the extent to which neoplastic cells resemble normal cells, both structurally and functionally. Lack of differentiation is called anaplasia.

- In general, benign tumors are well differentiated and remain localized, cohesive, and well demarcated from surrounding tissue. Benign tumors are not invasive, do not destroy surrounding tissue, and do not break away or travel from the tumor cell mass.

- In general, malignant tumors range from well differentiated to poorly differentiated, but they are invasive and destructive to surrounding tissue. They also lack adhesion to the tumor mass and easily break free to travel to distant sites in a process called metastasis.

- Staging classifies a cancer tumor according to size, invasiveness, and spread. Staging uses the TNM system: T is for tumor size, N is for lymph node involvement, and M is for metastasis to distant organs.

- A paraneoplastic syndrome is an unexpected pathological disorder provoked by the presence of cancer in the body. A common type of paraneoplastic syndrome involves the secretion of endocrine hormones unrelated to the cancer tumor.

- Tumor cell markers (also called biomarkers) are products of cancer cells, such as hormones, enzymes, genes, antigens, or antibodies, that are found on biopsy, in blood, spinal fluid, or urine. Biomarkers are used to diagnose, treat, and ascribe a prognosis regarding the disease.

- Tumor cells multiply rapidly, constantly progressing through the cell-cycle S and M stages. Radiation has its greatest destructive effect on cells in these two stages. Chemotherapy uses drugs to destroy cells in the S, M, or G stage of the cell cycle. Cancer chemotherapy has a collateral effect on healthy, rapidly multiplying cells such as skin, hair follicles, gastric cells, and bone marrow.

- Most common treatments of cancer include surgery, radiation, chemotherapy, and targeted cancer therapy. Stereotactic radiotherapy, also called cyberknife or gamma knife treatment, targets a tumor precisely. Proton therapy, also called proton beam therapy, is a type of radiation therapy that uses protons rather than x-rays to treat cancer.

- Lung cancer is the leading cause of cancer-related death in both males and females throughout the world.

- Helical CT scan is the best diagnostic test for lung cancer. Currently, there are no screening tests for lung cancer in the population at large.

- Smoking history is calculated in pack-years. This is the number of packs of cigarettes smoked multiplied by years smoked.

- Although it is well known that individuals with the *BRCA1* and *BRCA2* genes have an increased risk of breast cancer, these genes also increase susceptibility to ovarian, colon, and pancreatic cancer, and prostate cancer in males. There are numerous other genes that increase susceptibility to breast cancer: *ATM, CHEK2, PALB2, BARD1, RAD51C, RAD51D,* and *TP53.*

- Some breast cancers overexpress the hormone receptors estrogen/progesterone, and some overexpress the human epidermal growth factor receptor 2 (HER2) receptor. HER2-positive breast cancer is more aggressive than HER2-negative breast cancer. Treatments vary depending on these receptors.

- The oncotype diagnostic assay (oncotype Dx assay) analyzes 21 genes (16 cancer genes and 5 reference genes) and is used in the diagnosis and treatment of breast, prostate, and colon cancer. It is used to customize treatment to the genomic variations caused by specific types of cancer. It is used to predict chemotherapy benefit and predict 10-year risk of recurrence.

- Virchow's node is the term used for an enlarged, left-sided, supraclavicular lymph node. This can indicate breast, lung, or abdominal cancer.

- A Pap smear can detect preinvasive cervical cancer at the earliest stages. HPV can cause cervical, anorectal, vaginal, vulvar, penile, and/or oropharyngeal cancer.

- The liver, brain, and bone are frequent sites of metastasis for other primary cancers.

- For females, nulligravidity (never being pregnant) and nulliparity (never completing pregnancy with live birth) is a risk factor for breast, ovarian, and uterine cancer. Prolonged unopposed estrogen exposure is thought to be related to development of these cancers.

- Early breast cancers are being found using mammography, ultrasonography, and fine needle biopsy.

- Persons should be screened for colorectal cancer beginning at age 45.

- Colorectal cancer should be ruled out in all individuals with iron-deficiency anemia. Melena (black tarry stools) is a key sign of colorectal cancer. A fecal occult blood test (FOBT) can detect melena.

- Beginning at age 45 years, all adults should be screened for colorectal cancer using high-sensitivity stool testing annually, CT colonography every 5 years, flexible sigmoidoscopy every 5 years, or colonoscopy performed every 10 years.

- Brain and spinal cord metastasis from other primary sites of cancer is more common than primary CNS tumors.

- Glioblastoma multiforme is the most common malignant brain tumor in adults.

- Painless hematuria can be a sign of bladder or kidney cancer.

- Prostate cancer screening involves digital rectal examination and prostate surface antigen testing (PSA) annually in males over age 50. A urologist needs to interpret the PSA test to determine which patients require biopsy.

- Prostate cancer commonly spreads to the vertebral bones.

- HPV-induced oropharyngeal cancer is the most common cause of head and neck cancer.

- Hepatitis C is a common cause of HCC. The treatment for hepatitis C virus is 99% effective.

- HCC incidence is expected to increase in the next decade due to cirrhosis associated with NASH and NAFLD.

- Thyroid nodules are found in up to 50% of persons; however, approximately only 5% are carcinomatous.

- Osteosarcoma is the most common type of bone cancer often found in the lower extremity of teens and young adults.

- Renal cell carcinoma is a slow-growing tumor that is commonly diagnosed in a late stage when metastases have occurred.

Making the Connections

Signs and Symptoms	Physical Assessment Findings	Diagnostic Testing	Treatment
Lung Cancer | Small-cell and non–small-cell carcinoma. Begins as cellular dysplasia that develops on bronchial surface epithelium or bronchial mucous glands. Can also develop on the pleura.			
Cough, hemoptysis, wheeze, dyspnea, unintentional weight loss, stridor. Fatigue, weakness, cachexia, hoarseness.	Cachexia, weight loss. Lungs: wheezes, crackles. Hemoptysis. Supraclavicular enlarged lymph node. Tanned skin often occurs because of tumor secretion of ACTH, which stimulates melanocyte-stimulating hormone.	Chest x-ray; helical CT scan or MRI; tumor biopsy, bronchoscopy, bronchial or transbronchial biopsy, node biopsy, and fine needle biopsy by CT guidance.	Surgery to remove tumor and then radiotherapy and chemotherapy to kill any leftover cancer cells.
Breast Cancer | Most are epithelial cell tumors that develop from cells lining the ducts or lobules. A triggering factor, which is unclear, causes the breast epithelial cells to proliferate, grow uncontrollably, and invade surrounding tissue. Some breast cancer is attributed to *BRCA1* or *BRCA2* defective tumor suppressor genes.			
Breast lump or skin changes such as nipple discharge, nipple retraction, swelling of breast, "peau d'orange" skin changes, axillary lymph node enlargement.	Breast lump, which is usually hard, nontender, and immovable. Upper outer quadrant most common region of breast tumor. Possible nipple discharge and skin changes, swelling in one breast, nipple or skin retraction, axillary lymphadenopathy, or peau d'orange skin.	Clinical breast examination and annual or biennial mammogram for females 40 to 49 years of age as decided by physician. Annual mammogram in females 50 to 74 years (American College of Obstetrics and Gynecology). Calcification and densities seen on mammogram indicate breast cancer. Breast ultrasound can be used to examine dense breasts for evidence of cancer. A fine-needle/core needle biopsy; open/excisional biopsy; axillary dissection; and sentinel node biopsy are all performed to stage breast cancer.	Lumpectomy and axillary dissection; sentinel node biopsy and radiation; OR mastectomy; radiation, chemo-hormonal therapy for estrogen receptor–positive tumor; and chemotherapy for HER2-positive cancer.
Ovarian Cancer | Unknown cause of proliferation of ovarian cells; risk increased with *BRCA1* or *BRCA2* gene, nulligravida, infertility, family history, and Ashkenazi Jewish descent.			
Vague abdominal pain, bloating, anorexia, weight loss.	A palpable abdominal mass may be present. May present with no significant findings.	Transvaginal ultrasound, blood CA-125 level, laparotomy, biopsy of ovarian tumor.	Surgery to remove ovary or total hysterectomy is commonly performed, as well as chemotherapy.
Cervical Cancer | Abnormal growth of cervical cells, usually in region between uterus and cervix. HPV is a known cervical carcinogen.			
Abnormal vaginal bleeding.	Abnormal vaginal bleeding. Pelvic examination may show abnormality of cervix.	Pap test, HPV test, colposcopy, rectovaginal examination, CT, MRI, IV pyelogram, and chest x-ray.	Surgery, usually total hysterectomy, brachytherapy, and radiation may be done.

Continued

Making the Connections—cont'd

Signs and Symptoms	Physical Assessment Findings	Diagnostic Testing	Treatment
Prostate Cancer | Cancer that develops in the glandular cells of the prostate. Carcinogenic mutations initiate the cancer, and its growth is dependent on testosterone. Initially, there is an oncogenic or tumor suppressor genetic defect, which causes uncontrolled cellular growth in the gland. These changes lead to tumor progression and metastasis. The cancer cells proliferate and often spread to the neck of the bladder, ejaculatory ducts, and seminal vesicles. The cancer metastasizes to bone early in the course of the disease.			
Asymptomatic in early stages. In advanced disease, prostate gland can obstruct urine flow from the bladder, causing urinary symptoms such as decreased force of stream, incomplete emptying of the bladder, and frequency of urination. Late-stage symptoms include hematuria, azotemia, anemia, anorexia, and back pain.	On physical examination, the patient may have no remarkable findings except those on a DRE. The prostate gland can be palpated through the wall of the rectum. The prostate, which is usually a rubbery gland, becomes hard and immovable in cancer. Inguinal lymph nodes may be enlarged; if vertebral metastasis has occurred, tenderness is found over the lumbar region.	Diagnosis of prostate cancer involves a DRE, PSA test, and biopsy.	Options include active surveillance, watchful waiting, surgical removal of the prostate, radiation, cryotherapy, brachytherapy, and antiandrogen hormonal therapy.
Colorectal Cancer | Most commonly, an adenomatous polyp has cancer potential. Genetic, environmental, and behavioral causes are noted. Genetic conditions called FAP and HNPCC increase susceptibility to cancerous polyp formation. The *APC* gene causes multiple polyp formation, which increases susceptibility to cancer.			
Melena, fatigue, weakness, and changes in bowel habits such as diarrhea or constipation. May be asymptomatic.	Occult blood in the stool appears as black, tarry stool.	Colonoscopy OR flexible sigmoidoscopy shows a polyp, FOBT shows blood. Laboratory tests: iron-deficiency anemia, increase in CEA, increased liver enzymes.	Surgery to remove tumor. Sometimes requires removal of the colon with creation of a stoma and colostomy. Radiation and chemotherapy.
Liver Cancer | Occurs in hepatocytes that undergo chronic inflammation, as in hepatitis B or C or cirrhosis. Cells required to undergo frequent damage repair lose their ability to suppress tumor growth.			
Jaundice, weight loss, abdominal pain, fever, fatigue, weakness.	Abdominal tenderness, unintentional weight loss, jaundice, fever, hepatic bruit, hepatomegaly possible.	Tumor marker AFP; radiological imaging/ ultrasound CT, MRI may show tumor. Liver enzymes abnormal. Possible erythrocytosis, hypoglycemia, hypercalcemia. Liver biopsy or aspiration shows tumor cells.	Liver resection surgery to remove tumor. Chemotherapy to kill all liver cancer cells and any metastasis. Chemoembolization, radiofrequency ablation therapy, proton beam therapy. Hepatitis B vaccine. Hepatitis C treatment.
Brain Tumor | Some tumor growth is related to chromosomal deletions, additions, duplication, and mutations of specific genes. Commonly, a metastatic cancer emerges from another primary cancer.			
Neurological symptoms common, such as one-sided numbness or weakness. Headache, vomiting, seizure, vision disturbances, gait, or cranial nerve problems.	Neurological deficit may be assessed. Seizures, visual disturbance, headaches, vomiting, unstable gait, and cranial nerve dysfunction.	MRI, CT scan, and cerebral angiography can all show a brain tumor.	Surgery to excise or debulk a tumor. Radiation therapy to decrease size of tumor. Chemotherapy to kill cancerous cells.

Making the Connections–cont'd

Signs and Symptoms	Physical Assessment Findings	Diagnostic Testing	Treatment
Bone Cancer | Major types: osteosarcoma, chondrosarcoma, and Ewing's sarcoma. Hereditary retinoblastoma is clearly linked to osteosarcoma. This cancer can often be a metastasis from another primary cancer such as lung, prostate, or breast.			
Pain, swelling, and tenderness of an area of bone. Osteosarcoma occurs around the knee region. Bone tumor can cause a pathological fracture.	Localized pain, swelling, and tenderness are present. Osteosarcoma usually is in distal femur, proximal tibia, and humerus. Chondrosarcoma affects flat bones like shoulder and pelvic girdles. Ewing's sarcoma is seen in diaphyseal regions of long bones and flat bones. Chondroma is tumor of the base of the skull or vertebrae.	x-ray finding, CT scan, or MRI and tumor biopsy.	Treat underlying malignancy with combination of surgery, chemotherapy, and radiation.
Uterine Cancer | Endometrial hyperplasia develops into dysplasia; increased risk because of obesity, nulliparity, anovulatory menstrual cycles, tamoxifen, hormone replacement therapy, polycystic ovary syndrome, alcohol, diabetes, and hypertension; also increased risk in HNPCC.			
Abnormal vaginal bleeding or discharge, bloating, abdominal pain, change in bladder or bowel habits.	May be asymptomatic. Abdominal mass may be palpable.	Hysteroscopy with endometrial biopsy. Transvaginal ultrasound, pelvic x-ray, CT scan, MRI, chest x-ray, CA-125 blood test.	Surgery, chemotherapy, hormonal therapy, and radiation.
Cancer of the Head and Neck | Commonly is an SCC; linked to tobacco and alcohol use; mutations in *TP53* gene, HPV etiology, and gastroesophageal reflux disease.			
Plaques, nodules, verrucae lesions in mouth, under and side of tongue. Leukoplakia.	Plaques, nodules, verrucae lesions in mouth, under and side of tongue. Leukoplakia.	Laryngoscopy. CT scan, MRI, and x-ray. Biopsy.	Surgery, radiation, chemotherapy.
Thyroid Cancer | Unknown cause; papillary carcinoma most common form; increased risk with radiation exposure; genetic syndromes such as FAP, MEN, and the *RET* gene.			
Painless, palpable solitary thyroid nodule. Dysphagia possible.	Painless, palpable solitary thyroid nodule.	Ultrasound, FNAB, radioiodine scanning.	Surgery to remove thyroid. Radioactive iodine treatment. Thyroid hormone replacement treatment.
Kidney Cancer | Unknown cause; increased risk with obesity, smoking, hypertension, cystic kidney disease, environmental toxins, VHL syndrome gene.			
Hematuria, flank pain, weight loss, fatigue.	Abdominal mass, costovertebral angle tenderness, hematuria.	IV pyelogram, CT scan, MRI, ultrasound, biopsy.	Surgery, radiation, immunotherapy.

Bibliography

Available online at fadavis.com

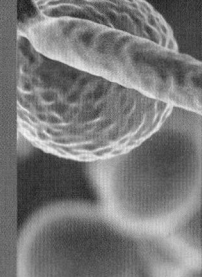

CHAPTER
41

Skin Disorders

Learning Objectives

Upon completion of this chapter, the student will be able to:

- Recognize normal anatomy and physiological mechanisms involved in the function of the integumentary system.
- Describe how the skin can reflect the state of overall health and presence of systemic disease.
- Identify assessment modalities and laboratory tests used in the diagnosis of skin diseases.

- List the risk factors, signs, symptoms, and distinct characteristics of skin cancer.
- Recognize the clinical manifestations of common dermatological disorders.
- Discuss various kinds of nonpharmacological and pharmacological treatments used for skin disorders.

Key Terms

Acne vulgaris
Actinic keratosis
Albinism
Angioedema
Basal cell carcinoma
Bullae
Cimex lectularius
Comedone
Condyloma acuminata
Dermatophytes
Discoid lupus erythematosus (DLE)
Ecchymosis
Eczema (atopic dermatitis)
Erythema multiforme (EM)
Hemangioma
Herald patch

Hidradenitis suppurativa
Hirsutism
Hymenoptera
Kaposi's sarcoma
Lentigos
Lesions
Melasma (chloasma)
Melanoma
Molluscum contagiosum
Nevi
Onycholysis
Onychomycosis
Paronychia
Pediculosis
Pemphigus
Pruritus (itching)

Pulicosis
Rash
Rosacea
Scabies
Stevens–Johnson syndrome (SJS)
Telangiectasias
Tinea
Urticaria
Verrucae
Vesicle
Vitiligo
Wheal
Wood's light
Xerosis

The integumentary system consists of the layers of the skin—the epidermis, dermis, and subcutaneous tissue—that connect the dermis to muscles and accessory structures. The skin, the body's largest and most visible organ, comprises about 16% of body weight and encompasses about 20 square feet. Its thickness varies from 0.5 mm on the eyelids to 4.0 mm on the soles of the feet. The skin contains many tissues, cell types, and specialized structures and mediates many aspects of life. It includes associated tissue such as the hair, nails, and sebaceous and sweat glands. The skin reflects ancestral background and expresses genetic structures, race, age, gender, health, and identity. It also gives evidence of environmental exposure, lifestyle, nutrition, and medication use. The skin is a vital organ that establishes identity and maintains boundaries between the person and the environment.

Epidemiology

Approximately 30% of all Americans have a skin condition, ranging from inflammatory and infectious lesions to skin cancers. With age, skin disorders become more likely. For example, it is estimated that more than 90% of older adults have some form of skin disorder. Persons with skin diseases usually seek help from primary care providers or dermatologists in community-based settings.

 CLINICAL CONCEPT

Approximately half of all primary care visits are for skin conditions.

Basic Concepts and Functions of the Skin and Related Tissue

The skin is accessible and easily biopsied. Health assessments begin with an examination of the skin because the skin provides clinicians with data about health status, age, and systemic disease. Usually, skin examinations focus on the top layer of skin, the epidermis, to determine the skin's health, as well as the person's general health.

The skin performs vital physiological functions that correlate with specific properties of the epidermis, dermis, and subcutaneous tissue. These functions include:

- Temperature control and regulation
- Barrier protection
- Secretion and absorption
- Vitamin D production
- Immunological surveillance

The skin also acts as a mirror for internal disease processes and serves as an indicator of one's general health.

Temperature Control and Regulation

About 80% of heat loss occurs via the skin. The skin plays a major role in temperature regulation, maintaining a constant body temperature of approximately 98.6°F. Extremes of both heat and cold are very dangerous, increasing the risk of organ failure and death.

Temperature sensors in the skin send information about body temperature to the hypothalamus, the temperature-regulating center in the brain. The brain then "feeds" information to the skin's sweat glands and blood vessels. If the message from the hypothalamus is to cool the body, the sweat glands excrete sweat, a mildly salty substance, onto the skin's surface. As the water in the sweat evaporates, the body cools.

In response to hypothalamic stimulation to cool the body, the capillaries—small blood vessels near the surface of the skin—dilate. Heat is lost directly through the skin through radiation and conduction.

If the hypothalamus senses hypothermia, it sends messages to heat the body. The tiny erector muscles of the skin contract, raising small hairs on the skin. This effect traps air and provides insulation that reduces heat loss. Shivering occurs as the body tries to increase its metabolic rate and raise its temperature. Superficial blood vessels also constrict, pulling blood away from the skin's surface and reducing heat loss.

Temperature-regulating systems in the skin can become impaired or overwhelmed by extreme environmental temperature changes. For example, hypothermia occurs after prolonged exposure to frigid water or air. Low environmental temperatures cause severe prolonged constriction of blood vessels that can lead to local ischemia of the skin or frostbite.

Conversely, heat stroke or heat exhaustion can occur because of exposure to high temperatures—those greater than body temperature. Heat stroke occurs because of the widespread vasodilation and loss of fluids that occur in extreme heat. As the body tries to cool itself, severe hypotension or shock can occur. Both extremes of temperature challenge the body's restorative powers; if untreated, they can cause death.

Barrier Protection

The skin forms a natural barrier protecting the body from injury and infection, as well as physical, chemical, and environmental hazards. A flora of harmless bacteria coupled with a thin layer of lipid film formed from sweat and sebaceous secretions covers the skin, repels virulent strains of bacteria, and protects the body from infection. The surface film and the thick surface layer called the stratum corneum stop antigens from entering the body and keep the body waterproof even when it is submerged in water.

Excretion and Absorption

By influencing the composition and volume of sweat, the skin influences total fluid volume and the quantity of excreted waste products, notably uric acid, ammonia, and urea. Of course, the skin plays a minor role in excretion when compared with the kidneys and the lungs. Primarily, it removes water, heat, salt, carbon dioxide, ammonia, and urea from the body. Although the skin is almost waterproof, it plays a role in absorption. Fat-soluble substances, such as vitamins A, D, E, and K, penetrate the skin. Oxygen, carbon dioxide, and other gases also permeate the skin, along with organic solvents such as acetone; carbon tetrachloride; salts of heavy metals like arsenic, lead, and mercury; and the oils of poison ivy and oak. Medication absorption can occur through the skin because of its permeability to fat-soluble substances.

Vitamin D Production

The interaction of ultraviolet (UV) light with the skin is a major factor in vitamin D synthesis. The first step in the production of vitamin D occurs in the skin when the chemical 7-dehydrocholesterol is converted into a precursor of vitamin D, cholecalciferol. Further synthesis occurs in the liver and kidney. Vitamin D regulates calcium and phosphorus metabolism, facilitates calcium absorption from the intestine, and affects bone cell development.

Immunological Surveillance

The skin provides the first barrier in the body's immunological defense. It is a major aspect of the innate immunological response, offering a nonspecific kind of protection against all antigens. Skin surface enzymes, acids, waxy sebum, and other substances act together to repel pathogens that try to enter the body via the skin. Keratinocytes—surface-layer epidermal cells—regulate the immunological response and secrete inflammatory mediators. Langerhans cells detect foreign antigens that have penetrated the epidermis and present antigens to the lymphocytes that take part in the adaptive immunological response.

Mirror for Internal Disease Processes

The skin exhibits the body's internal processes, particularly the body's immunological activity. Urticaria, wheals, blisters, bullae, and various other kinds of inflammatory lesions appear on the skin's surface. These are external signs of the immune response that is actively occurring below the skin's surface.

Some systemic diseases manifest themselves via skin lesions, which are often external signs of disease and can assist in diagnosis. Syphilis is signaled by an asymptomatic rash that resolves; the next lesion, a distinctive chancre, usually appears in the genital area. A herald patch precedes pityriasis rosea. Kaposi's sarcoma (KS) presents as red-purple-brown plaques and nodules, and is an AIDS-defining illness. Clinicians closely examine rashes in school-age children to detect the viral exanthems: rubella, measles, chickenpox, or fifth disease. Rashes on the skin also can indicate drug intolerance, allergic reactions, or communicable diseases.

Indicator of General Health

The skin, the most visible organ, provides information about itself and the rest of the body. For example, changes in the color of the skin and nailbeds reflect circulation and may indicate diseases of the heart, liver, or blood cell synthesis. Persons who lack sufficient oxygen become blue or cyanotic. If bilirubin builds up in the blood, the skin becomes yellow or jaundiced. Erythema, extreme redness of the skin, reflects capillary engorgement, whereas pallor, extreme paleness of the skin, indicates anemia or shock. A bruise, or **ecchymosis,** can exhibit various colors from reddish to brown to yellow-green. A diet with high amounts of beta carotene–containing foods like carrots can turn the skin orange.

Assessment

In a comprehensive assessment, the entire skin surface is examined and any evidence of a skin disorder is documented. Initially, the patient's skin should be viewed from a distance of 4 to 6 feet so the distribution and pattern of lesions can be clearly seen. Abnormal skin is compared with normal skin; specific lesions are visualized and palpated with a gloved hand to determine their color; size; texture; consistency; and the presence of scales, inflammation, or edema. Lesions should be described and measured for documentation. A skin lesion can be marked so that the size of the lesion can be measured and monitored throughout treatment. Sometimes lesions are scraped, biopsied, or cultured. These specimens are visualized, perhaps with the assistance of a UV **Wood's light,** or sent to the laboratory for further analysis.

As part of the integumentary examination, it is important to conduct a complete history that elicits information about:

- Initial appearance of lesions
- Symptoms associated with eruption
- History of allergies
- Medication use
- Exposure to insects, irritants, or UV light
- Other associated systemic symptoms
- Current or previous illnesses
- Presence of photosensitivity
- Remedies the patient has used to treat skin lesions

Persons with histories of skin diseases, hospitalized patients, and nursing home residents should have frequent skin assessments.

 CLINICAL CONCEPT

It is important that the clinician remembers that no two skin disorders look exactly alike; their classic presentations may be distorted by scratching, swelling, infection, or self-treatment. Skin color also affects the appearance of skin diseases.

A common distinction utilized in describing skin lesions is the difference between a rash and a lesion. A **rash** is a temporary eruption of the skin associated with systemic disease, heat, irritation, allergy, or a response to drug therapy. **Lesions** are traumatic or pathological loss of normal skin continuity, structure, or function. A **vesicle** is blister: an area of clear fluid enclosed by thin layer of skin. **Bullae** are large vesicles that appear as thin-skinned bubbles. **Urticaria** is the term for hives, which is a pinpoint, erythematous, pruritic (itchy) rash. **Wheals** are confluent regions of urticaria; erythematous, raised, pruritic lesions.

Clinicians should begin the diagnostic analysis with a graphic description of the presenting skin lesion (see Box 41-1).

 CLINICAL CONCEPT

It is important to mark the borders of skin lesions so that changes can be measured and therapy can be evaluated.

Basic Pathophysiological Concepts of Common Skin Disorders

Skin can be described in terms of color, texture, turgor, tenderness, temperature, moisture, and any secretion that is released. Pathological changes of the skin can affect all these qualities. Also, the intactness of the skin is important for full protection from pathogens. Open skin areas are vulnerable to infection. Skin, nails, and hair can develop primary disorders, or they can display manifestations of an inner pathological process. Sweat glands beneath the skin cool the body, whereas sebaceous glands secrete sebum that protects the skin. However, both sweat and sebaceous glands can dysfunction, which can create problems for the overlying skin.

Disorders of Skin Color

Skin color may reflect systemic disorders or provide clues to the identity of specific lesions. Several disorders significantly affect skin color, including albinism, vitiligo, and melasma.

Albinism, a genetic disorder, deprives skin, hair, and eyes of pigment. It leaves a person with diminished vision and extreme sensitivity to light and UV rays. Individuals with any of the 10 types of albinism have pale or pink skin, yellow hair, and very light or pink eyes. Patients lack the pigment melanin; they should use protection from solar radiation and undergo frequent screening for skin malignancies.

Vitiligo is an acquired skin condition characterized by abnormalities in the production of melanin. It presents as a series of discolored patches on the skin (see Fig. 41-1). Appearing suddenly, these patches present as macules of varying sizes with smooth

---

> ### BOX 41-1. Terms Commonly Used to Describe Skin Lesions
>
> Terms commonly used to describe skin lesions include the following:
>
> - **Atrophy:** thinning and loss of skin layers
> - **Bulla:** large blister (larger than 0.5 cm in diameter)
> - **Crust:** dried yellowish or yellow-brown exudate on the skin
> - **Erythema:** reddened skin; area blanches with pressure
> - **Excoriation:** scratch that breaks the skin's surface
> - **Fissure:** crack in the skin that breaks through keratin
> - **Induration:** hardening or thickening of the skin
> - **Keloid:** irregular, elevated scar tissue formed by excessive collagen growth during wound healing
> - **Lichenification:** hardening or thickening of the skin with markings; lichenification develops from repeated trauma such as scratching
> - **Macule:** defined, flat area of altered pigmentation
> - **Nodule:** solid lump larger than 0.5 cm in diameter
> - **Papule:** raised, well-defined lesion, usually smaller than 0.5 cm in diameter
> - **Plaque:** raised, flat-topped lesion, usually larger than 2 cm in diameter
> - **Purpura:** purplish lesion caused by free red blood cells in the skin; does not blanch on pressure and may be nodular
> - **Pustule:** papule filled with pus
> - **Scale:** fragment of dry skin
> - **Scar:** permanent replacement of normal skin with connective tissue
> - **Telangiectasia:** fine, irregular, red lines produced by dilation of the capillaries
> - **Ulcer:** loss of epidermal and dermal tissue
> - **Vesicle (blister):** blister smaller than 0.5 cm in diameter
> - **Wheals/urticaria:** transient pink, itchy, elevated papules that evolve into irregular red maculopapular patches

---

borders. They commonly appear on the face, neck, axillae, and extremities. The lesions are depigmented, itchy, and easily burned by exposure to the sun or UV rays. The exact cause of vitiligo is unknown, and no treatment has yet been effective. Vitiligo often occurs with hypothyroidism or other autoimmune diseases.

Melasma, also called chloasma, by contrast, is characterized by the appearance of dark macules on the face. More common in brown-skinned females, melasma commonly occurs during pregnancy and in females who use oral contraceptives. Sun damage can also cause this skin discoloration. Blue-eyed and fair-skinned people reveal sun damage more dramatically than dark-skinned people. Large pigmented spots, called age spots or **lentigos,** appear on fair, sun-damaged areas of the

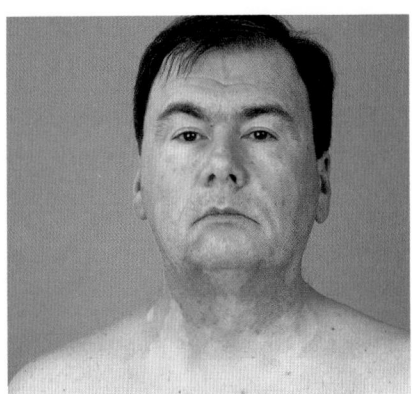

FIGURE 41-1. Vitiligo.

skin, usually on the hands, forearms, and face. As in other disorders of melanin production, preventive measures include limiting sun exposure through the use of sun-screening agents. Skin-bleaching agents applied to darkened areas of the skin can be used for cosmetic purposes.

Associated structures of the skin also demonstrate a change in color with age. Genetically programmed graying of the hair often begins in the 30s at the temples and then extends to the top of the scalp. Over time, hair color becomes progressively lighter, eventually turning white. Body and facial hair also turn gray, but usually more slowly than scalp hair. Although the consistency and distribution of hair are determined genetically, hair thinning and loss also occur with age.

Disorders of Skin Texture

Skin texture provides another manifestation of its health and integrity. The skin and related tissue damaged by repeated infections, overexposure to the sun, trauma, or burns, lose elasticity and functional ability. With age, the skin loses tensile strength and becomes less flexible. Changes in connective tissue reduce the skin's elasticity or turgor. This process of skin aging, called elastosis, is more pronounced in sun-damaged skin.

Some specific diseases—scleroderma and pemphigus, for example—are diagnosed by changes in the skin's texture. Acanthosis nigricans, often associated with diabetes, is characterized by a dark, brownish-black, velvety thickening of the skin.

Dry skin, **xerosis,** is a common dermatological complaint. Dry skin appears to be rough, scaly, and wrinkled. Skin dryness can be caused by dehydration of the stratum corneum, changes in sebaceous gland secretions, decreased sweat, and a flattening of the epidermal ridges, which reduce the ability of fluids to move between the skin's layers.

Dry skin is more easily bruised and irritated. Because pruritus is the major symptom of dry skin, excoriation of the extremities, abdomen, back, and waist are found on examination. Liberal use of moisturizing agents such as emollients, humectants, and occlusives is the major treatment for dry skin. Each of these substances acts differently by replenishing oil on the skin, drawing water from deeper layers of the skin up to the skin's surface, or preventing water loss from the skin. Lotions or creams that contain camphor, menthol, or benzocaine are widely used to decrease pruritus. Temperature control and use of room humidifiers are also helpful.

Pruritus (itching) is a common patient complaint. Sometimes the cause of the itching is localized and associated with a rash or an insect bite. Often persons with severe itching suffer from sleep disturbances. At times, there are no objective data to explain the itching. This manifestation of itching, which is more difficult to diagnose and treat, may be a sign of a systemic illness, such as liver failure, or it may be psychogenic in origin.

Discontinuing drugs known to cause itchy skin or removal of offending agents is usually the first remedy. Treatment addresses the underlying cause of the itching if it can be identified. Local treatment relies on creams, lotions, and antihistamines. Excoriated skin can become infected, so it is important to address pruritus.

Disorders of the Hair

Hair is an extension of the skin that can reflect metabolic changes. For example, hair texture can change with disorders of the thyroid, disruption of sex hormones, nutritional deficiencies, and physiological aging. Hair loss is the most common disorder of the hair and can be congenital, genetic, or acquired. Four types of hair loss account for 95% of visits to dermatologists:

1. Male and female pattern baldness
2. Telogen effluvium
3. Chemical overprocessing
4. Alopecia areata

Male and Female Pattern Baldness
Male pattern baldness, which can begin at any age, is usually genetic and influenced by male hormones. Typically, the hair loss is on the front, sides, and crown of the head. Female pattern baldness is less common and involves a thinning of hair over the entire head. Conversely, **hirsutism,** a type of male pattern hair growth, is often seen in females because of increased androgenic hormones.

Telogen Effluvium
Telogen effluvium, a poorly understood condition, affects the growing or resting cycle of hair follicles. In telogen effluvium, the number of resting follicles increases and the number of growing follicles decreases. The result is a generalized thinning of hair over the entire scalp. This reversible type of hair loss is often associated with chronic stress and nutritional deficiencies.

Chemical Overprocessing

Chemical overprocessing, a common cause of hair loss, follows efforts to change the color, quality, texture, and style of hair by curling, straightening, braiding, rinsing, dying, and tinting. Treatment is aimed at discontinuing the processes that stimulated the hair loss.

Alopecia Areata

Alopecia areata is sudden loss of hair in one area of the scalp. The cause is unknown, and usually the hair grows back in several months. A diagnostic tool for hair loss, the hair pull test, provides clues to the amount of hair that is being shed. Often clinicians biopsy the skin in the thin or bald areas or check for fungal or bacterial infections because some hair loss is caused by scalp ringworm.

Although hair loss secondary to radiation or chemotherapy is not identified as a major type of hair loss, it is common in patients undergoing these treatments. After cessation of treatment, the hair usually returns.

Disorders of the Nails

Nails can be the target of infection or can reflect nutritional status, metabolic changes of the body, or systemic illness. Chronic hypoxia, celiac disease, cirrhosis, malignancies, or inflammatory bowel disease can cause clubbing of the nails, where the nails become convex and fingertips thicken. Clubbed fingernails exhibit Schamroth sign: obliteration of the diamond-shaped space at the proximal end of the nail when the distal phalangeal bones are opposed.

Chronic illness can cause pitting of the nails or depressions called Beau's lines. Pitting is commonly associated with psoriasis, whereas Beau's lines are transverse linear depressions across the nail that can also be caused by trauma or Raynaud's syndrome. Spooning of nails, also called koilonychia, can occur in thyroid or liver disorders, cardiovascular disease, or iron deficiency. Splinter hemorrhages of the nails occur in endocarditis. Yellow nail syndrome, where nails thicken and discolor, occurs in rheumatoid arthritis, immunodeficiency, malignancies, or pulmonary problems. Onycholysis, where the nails separate from the nailbeds, can occur in thyroid or autoimmune disease. An obvious black region under the nail can indicate melanoma beneath the nail or subungual hemorrhage caused by trauma. Persons often show short white lines in the nail, called leukonychia, which may be caused by trauma to the nail. Similar to leukonychia are Muehrcke's lines, which are transverse white lines that span the nail width and are indicative of hypoalbuminemia.

Bacterial or fungal infection is the most common cause of nail disease. When the paronychial fold, a seal between the nail plate and the surrounding tissue, is broken, bacteria and fungi can invade the tissue, producing pain, redness, and swelling called a **paronychia.** An acute paronychia is most often caused by *Staphylococcus*

aureus, and an abscess is commonly present. Chronic paronychias are commonly caused by *Candida* (yeast) infection.

Onychomycosis is the term for a fungal or yeast infection that involves the proximal and lateral nailfolds. *Pseudomonas* bacteria can also infect the space between the nail plate and the nailbed. Like other organisms that invade the paronychial fold, *Pseudomonas* thrive on moisture. Most infectious agents discolor the nails, causing them to darken; the degree of discoloration indicates the depth of the infection (see Fig. 41-2). A bacterial or fungal invasion may be deep enough to cause the nail plate to separate from the nailbed, a process called **onycholysis.**

Disorders of the Sweat Glands

Two common conditions of the sweat glands are hyperhidrosis, which is excessive sweat production, and anhidrosis, which is decreased sweat production.

Hyperhidrosis

Hyperhidrosis may be related to physiological, pathological, or endocrine factors; brain trauma; or drug therapy. Often excessive sweat production is localized to the palms, soles, and axilla. Physiologically, sweat is produced in response to emotions; pain; fear and stress; hot, humid environments; work; and exercise. Pathologically, it is associated with febrile diseases, hyperthyroidism, and diabetes. Trauma to the hypothalamus or its tracts can interfere with heat regulation mechanisms and produce excessive sweating. Sympathomimetic (sympathetic stimulant) drugs and drugs that affect the hypothalamus also lead to sweating.

Anhidrosis

It is not uncommon for newborn and premature infants to exhibit anhidrosis for several weeks after birth. In adults, the causes of diminished sweat

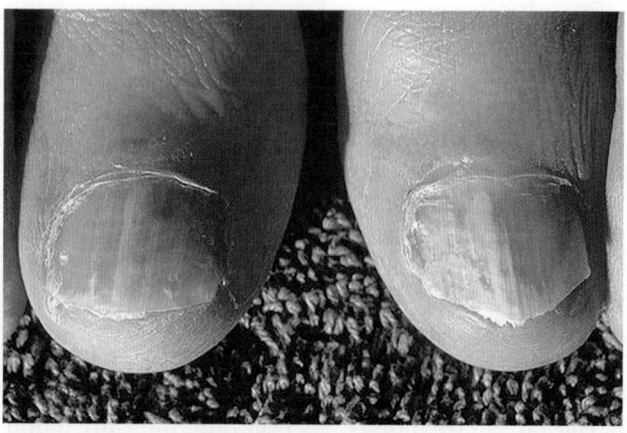

FIGURE 41-2. Finger with onychomycosis infection. *(Courtesy of CDC/Dr. Edwin P. Ewing, Jr.)*

production include head injuries, tumors, occlusion of the sweat ducts, degeneration of peripheral sympathetic fibers as seen in peripheral neuritis, atrophy caused by burns and radiotherapy, and the use of anticholinergic (antiparasympathetic) drugs.

Hidradenitis suppurativa is a disorder of the apocrine sweat glands, which are present in the axilla and groin areas. In this disorder, there is plugging or clogging of the gland openings onto the skin. The glands become obstructed and inflamed, and tender areas of swelling develop under the arm or in the groin. Bacterial infection is common, causing a purulent exudate that drains from the swollen, erythematous, tender glands onto the skin surface. Hidradenitis suppurativa is often a chronic disorder that occurs as remissions and exacerbations. Obesity, stress, and inadequate hygiene will make the glandular swellings worse. Chronic exacerbations can cause glandular swellings to develop fibrotic scar tissue.

CLINICAL CONCEPT

In hydradenitis suppurativa, antibacterial soap should be used to wash the areas daily, and anti-inflammatory agents such as ibuprofen can be used to decrease the swelling and pain. Shaving of the area should be avoided because this can make the lesions worse.

Medical treatment consists of oral antibiotics as well as topical or intralesional injections of antibiotics. Tretinoin (Retin-A) and isotretinoin (Accutane), which are synthetic forms of vitamin A, have also been effective. If medical treatment is ineffective, surgical incision and drainage of the swollen glandular regions is common.

Disorders of the Sebaceous Glands

Acne vulgaris, a common multifactored inflammatory disorder of the sebaceous glands, affects 85% of the population between the ages of 12 and 25 years. Its lesions are inflammatory papules, pustules, nodules, noninflammatory open or closed comedones, and cysts. A **comedone,** the prototypical lesion in acne, is a plug of sebaceous and necrotic cellular material within the opening of a hair follicle. The follicle may be open (blackhead) or almost closed (whitehead). The lesions most commonly appear on exposed areas of the face, chest, and back.

Acne is more common at puberty because hormones stimulate the sebaceous glands. However, it is not unusual for young adults in their late 20s to develop acne. *Propionibacterium acnes* colonize the lesions of acne. Topical agents and oral antibiotics are often required to counteract acne. Tretinoin (Retin-A) and isotretinoin (Accutane), synthetic forms of vitamin A, have been very effective in treating severe acne. However, isotretinoin should be used with caution

in patients, as it can lead to depression and suicidal ideation. It is also contraindicated in pregnancy due to the teratogenic potential.

Acne rosacea, often seen in middle-aged adults, appears as erythematous papules and pustules. Usually these lesions, which are associated with inappropriate vasodilation, appear in the middle third of the face but may extend to the forehead and chin. When the inflammatory process of **rosacea** affects the nose, it produces an unsightly, irreversible swelling and inflammation called rhinophyma. Heat exposure and alcohol consumption accentuate the vasodilation and inflammation of this disease. Although the exact cause of acne rosacea is unknown, it is thought that this inflammation of the sebaceous glands results from infection or from an immune-related response. Sunscreen lotions and protective coverings are recommended. In severe cases, oral antibiotic therapy is used.

Birthmarks and Developmental Conditions Affecting the Skin

Birthmarks are skin lesions that are present at birth or develop in infancy. **Hemangiomas,** benign tumors of blood vessels, are apparent in 30% of newborns, with females more likely to be affected. Port-wine stains are permanent blood vessel abnormalities affecting 0.5% of the population. At birth, these lesions look like pink patches; as the child ages, the birthmark darkens and becomes larger. Strawberry hemangiomas, by contrast, are enlarged blood vessels that grow rapidly after birth and resolve by 6 years of age. Spider veins are enlarged blood vessels that grow with age. A Mongolian spot is a benign darkened area of skin commonly on the back or buttocks.

Treatment

Many persons treat their skin problems with over-the-counter preparations before consulting a health-care provider. Treatments are directed at the etiology of the skin eruption as well as its symptoms. Suspicious lesions are biopsied and may be removed or treated with laser surgery. Inflammatory lesions are treated initially with steroidal creams; if the inflammation is severe, short-term oral steroid therapy is used. Skin infections are treated with topical antibiotic creams. If the infection spreads locally or if the patient develops systemic symptoms of infection, oral or IV antibiotics are used. Treatment of systemic disease, manifested on the skin, is directed to treating the primary disease. When the skin condition is psychogenic in origin, drugs that treat anxiety or depression, as well as psychotherapy, are combined with treatment of the skin lesions.

Of course, preventive treatment of skin disorders is the first step to maintaining healthy skin. Prevention involves protection of the skin and underlying tissues from environmental hazards, UV rays, injuries, sustained pressure, infections, and bites. One of the key preventive treatments of the skin is protection from the sun. Melanoma, basal cell carcinoma, and squamous cell carcinoma (SCC), the three most serious skin conditions, are all associated with sun overexposure.

Selected Precancerous Skin Disorders

There are several different types of precancerous skin lesions. They are common on the sun-exposed areas of the body, particularly the facial areas. Nevi, actinic keratoses, and lentigos are lesions that should be periodically assessed, as these can undergo cancerous changes.

Nevi

Nevi, or moles, are probably the most common benign skin tumors. These lesions, which can be pigmented or depigmented, develop from melanocytes during childhood, usually between 3 and 5 years of age. They present as papules and nodules and vary in size. Atypical or dysplastic nevi are those that are irregular in shape, variegated in color, and have a high susceptibility to cancerous change. These lesions require clinical examination to rule out skin cancer. Persons with a high number of nevi on the body should consult a dermatologist periodically for a whole-body skin assessment.

Actinic Keratoses and Lentigos

Actinic keratosis, a premalignant lesion found on skin that has been damaged by the sun's UV rays, is common in fair-skinned persons. The lesions present as patches of rough, scaly, red plaques. The surrounding tissues are red and may show telangiectasia (branches of delicate capillaries). Lentigos, premalignant skin lesions, usually appear as brown spots on sun-exposed areas. Commonly called solar lentigos, liver spots, or age spots, these lesions are benign, but they bear watching because there is also a lentigo maligna that appears as a freckle on sun-exposed areas. Lentigo maligna are pigmented macules with well-defined borders. Slow-growing, they can reach a size of 5 cm. Over time, the lesions may become raised and wartlike in appearance. Persons with a high number of actinic keratoses or lentigos on the body should consult a dermatologist periodically for a whole-body skin assessment.

> **ALERT!** Any change in size, color, border, or appearance of a nevus can indicate malignant melanoma. A dysplastic nevus can be considered a premalignant stage of melanoma. The actinic keratoses should be examined and biopsied because they can progress to SCC, a metastatic disease. Lentigo maligna can become malignant melanoma.

Most Common Skin Cancers

Skin cancer is by far the most common type of cancer. Malignant melanoma, basal cell carcinoma, and squamous cell carcinoma (SCC) are the three types of skin cancer. These lesions can begin as premalignant dysplasia. Periodic dermatological examination is necessary to identify their occurrence.

Malignant Melanoma

Skin cancer is the most common type of cancer in the United States. **Melanoma** is the most lethal form of skin cancer, killing about one person per hour in the United States. Current estimates are that one in five Americans will develop skin cancer in their lifetime. According the American Cancer Society and the American Society of Clinical Oncologists, an estimated 3.4 million Americans were diagnosed with skin cancer in 2022. Before age 50, skin cancer rates are higher in females compared with males. After age 50, and in general, males have higher rates. European American males have the highest rate of contracting melanoma, with an average age of 61 at diagnosis. Basal cell and squamous cell carcinomas, the two most common forms of skin cancer, are highly treatable if detected early and treated properly. The 5-year survival rate for people whose melanoma is detected early and treated before it spreads to the lymph nodes is 99%. The 5-year survival rate for melanoma that spreads to distant lymph nodes and other organs is 30%.

Etiology

The vast majority of melanomas are caused by sun exposure. Melanoma originates in melanocytes, the cells that produce the pigment melanin, which colors our skin, hair, and eyes. The majority of melanomas are black or brown, but they can also be skin-colored, pink, red, purple, blue, or white. Approximately 30% of melanomas occur in a nevus. Melanoma begins on the surface, but it penetrates deep into the skin, invades the blood and lymphatic vessels, and then metastasizes throughout the body. There are a number of risk factors, but anyone of any skin color can develop melanoma (see Box 41-2).

It is not clear how all melanomas develop, but exposure to UV radiation clearly plays a role, especially in fair-skinned people. A history of sunburns, especially blistering sunburns as a child or teenager, has been shown to increase the risk of developing melanoma. Some inherited traits increase an individual's risk, such as dysplastic nevi (precancerous moles), fair skin, light-colored eyes, freckles, and skin that burns easily or tans poorly. There also is evidence that exposure to UV radiation from indoor tanning equipment increases the risk of melanoma. Genetic studies are finding a number of defective tumor suppressor genes that are linked to malignant melanoma. One such gene is located at 9p21.

BOX 41-2. Risk Factors for Melanoma

Risk factors for melanoma include:
- Fair, sun-sensitive skin that tans poorly or burns easily
- Red or blond hair and blue or green eyes
- Having 50 to 100 or more moles
- Having unusual or irregular-looking moles that are typically larger in size (may be referred to as dysplastic or atypical moles)
- History of sunburns or indoor tanning use
- Close relatives (parents, children, siblings, cousins, aunts, uncles) who have had melanoma
- Immunosuppression caused by disease, organ transplant, or medication
- History of previous melanoma or another skin cancer
- 50 years of age or older

Most melanomas develop in areas that have had exposure to the sun, such as the upper back, torso, lower legs, head, and neck. Other factors associated with increased risk include a family history of melanoma, presence of an atypical nevus (mole), and immunosuppression.

Pathophysiology

Malignant melanomas are cancers of the melanocytes, which have a radial and vertical growth phase. During the radial growth phase, malignant cells grow in a radial, spreading manner in the epidermis. With time, melanomas progress to the vertical growth phase, where malignant cells invade deep into the dermis and are able to metastasize.

The types of melanoma are superficial spreading melanoma, lentigo maligna melanoma, acral lentiginous melanoma, and nodular melanoma. Seventy percent of melanoma is the superficial spreading type. The superficial, lentigo, and acral lentiginous types begin with skin surface growth before deeper penetration and spread. The lesion enlarges, its borders widen irregularly, and the lesion attains various pigments. During this time, the melanoma can be cured by surgical excision. Nodular melanoma is the most aggressive type, with deep penetrative growth and early metastasis. Between 10% and 15% of melanomas are of the nodular type, and another 10% to 15% are of the lentigo maligna type.

A set of predictable stages predisposes individuals to malignant melanoma:

- Benign nevus
- Dysplastic nevus
- Radial growth phase of melanoma
- Vertical growth phase of melanoma
- Metastatic malignant melanoma

Clinical Presentation

Noncancerous moles are generally uniform in color, round to oval in shape, and have a well-defined border. In contrast, melanomas tend to have one or more ABCDE traits:

- A: Asymmetry: one half unlike the other
- B: Border: an irregular, scalloped, or poorly defined border
- C: Color: varied from one area to another; shades of tan, brown, and black; sometimes white, red, or blue
- D: Diameter: usually larger than 6 mm, or the size of a pencil eraser, when diagnosed, but they can be smaller
- E: Evolving: a mole or skin lesion that looks different from the rest or is changing in size, shape, or color

It is important for the clinician to question the patient about their family history of melanoma; approximately 10% of melanoma patients report a family history. Familial pancreatic cancer and astrocytoma are frequently associated with melanoma. In addition, familial atypical mole, or melanoma syndrome, is a disorder that predisposes the patient to multiple dysplastic nevi.

ALERT! A common warning sign of melanoma is change. A change to the shape, color, or diameter of a mole can be a warning sign. Other changes that could indicate melanoma include a mole that becomes painful or begins to bleed or itch.

Diagnosis

The diagnosis of melanoma begins with examination of a suspicious lesion. Careful inspection of the entire skin surface, including the scalp and mucous membranes, is necessary for diagnosis. Palpation of the lymph nodes and abdomen are part of the staging examination for melanoma. Suspicious lesions should be biopsied, evaluated by a specialist, and recorded by chart or photography for follow-up. Computer image analyses are often used to appraise suspicious lesions. If melanoma is diagnosed, chest x-ray, computed tomography (CT) scan, magnetic resonance imaging (MRI) scan of the brain, and ultrasound testing of lymph nodes are necessary to look for any evidence of metastases. Positron emission tomography (PET) scan is also commonly used to look for metastases.

Treatment

Treatment typically begins with complete surgical removal of the melanoma and some healthy skin around the growth. This ensures that all cancerous cells are removed. Treatment for melanoma depends on the stage (see Table 41-1).

To stage melanoma, imaging techniques such as x-ray, ultrasound, CT scan, MRI, PET scan, and radioisotopic bone or organ scan are used. A surgical procedure known as a sentinel lymph node biopsy is also recommended to stage melanoma. In staging melanoma, the thicker the lesion or signs of spread, the worse the prognosis. Stages I and II primary tumors that have not spread have a 98% 5-year survival rate. Stage III melanoma has palpable regional lymph nodes and a 64% 5-year survival rate. Stage IV is distant metastatic disease and has a 23% 5-year survival rate. The distant metastasis of melanoma often occurs in the lungs and brain. If testing indicates that melanoma has metastasized to the lymph nodes or other areas, treatment may include additional surgery to remove the cancer, immunotherapy, radiation therapy, chemotherapy, or a combination of treatments. Various melanoma vaccines are currently under investigation. Melanoma patients have a lifelong risk of developing new melanomas; therefore, follow-up examinations are critical.

Basal Cell Carcinoma

Basal cell carcinoma, the most common form of skin cancer, accounts for more than 90% of all skin cancer in the United States. These cancers rarely metastasize to other parts of the body. They can, however, cause damage by growing deeply and invading surrounding tissue.

Light-colored skin and sun exposure are both important factors in the development of basal cell carcinomas. About 20% of these skin cancers, however, occur in areas that are not sun-exposed, such as the chest, back, arms, legs, and scalp. The face, however, remains the most common location for basal cell lesions. UV radiation from the sun is the main cause of basal cell cancer. Artificial sources of UV radiation, such as tanning beds, can also cause it. Most basal cell cancers appear after age 50 years, but the sun's damaging effects begin at an early age.

A basal cell carcinoma usually begins as a small, dome-shaped bump and is often covered by small, superficial blood vessels called telangiectasias. The texture of the lesion is often shiny and translucent, sometimes referred to as "pearly" (see Fig. 41-3). Basal cell carcinomas grow slowly and deeply, taking months or years to become sizable. Similar to melanoma, a biopsy is necessary for diagnosis. Treatment is also similar to melanoma. However, most cases of basal cell carcinoma can be cured with surgery alone.

Squamous Cell Carcinoma

Of the more than 1 million cases of skin cancer that will be diagnosed in the United States this year, about 20% will be SCC. As with melanoma and basal cell carcinoma, most cases of SCC will be caused by exposure to the sun's harmful UV rays. The risk of developing SCC also increases with age because each exposure to UV rays causes more damage to the skin. As this damage accumulates, the risk of developing SCC grows.

SCC appears as a red, crusted, or scaly patch on the skin; a nonhealing ulcer; or a firm, red nodule. Some SCCs develop from actinic keratoses, which also are caused by exposure to the sun's UV rays. With early detection and proper treatment, SCC is curable. If allowed to progress, however, SCC can invade and destroy much of the tissue surrounding the cancerous tumor, which can be disfiguring. Some SCCs, such as those that develop on a lip or an ear, can be particularly aggressive. If left untreated, aggressive SCCs have a high risk of metastasis to the lymph nodes and other internal organs. Diagnosis must be confirmed

TABLE 41-1. Stages of Melanoma	
Stage	**Description**
Stage 0; in situ	Melanoma that is confined to the epidermis
Stage I–II	Melanoma that is confined to the skin but has increasing thickness; skin may be intact or ulcerated (top layer of skin is absent)
Stage III	Melanoma that has spread to a nearby lymph node and is found in increasing amounts in one or more lymph nodes
Stage IV	Melanoma that has spread to internal organs, beyond the closest lymph nodes to other lymph nodes, or to areas of the skin far from the original tumor

Adapted from the American Cancer Society. (2017). Melanoma skin cancer stages. Retrieved from https://www.cancer.org/cancer/melanoma-skin-cancer/detection-diagnosis-staging/melanoma-skin-cancer-stages.html; AIM at Melanoma Foundation (2014). Stages of melanoma. Retrieved from https://www.aimatmelanoma.org/stages-of-melanoma/; The Skin Cancer Foundation (2019). The stages of melanoma. Retrieved from https://www.skincancer.org/skin-cancer-information/melanoma/the-stages-of-melanoma.

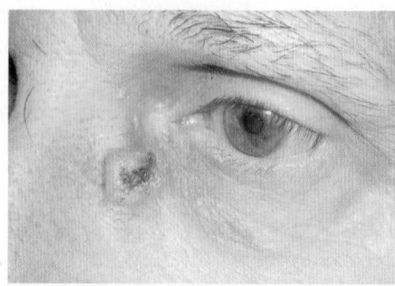

FIGURE 41-3. Basal cell carcinoma.

with a biopsy. Treatment options are similar to those of melanoma. Most patients with localized SCC have cure rates that range from 85% to 95% or greater.

Selected Infectious Disorders Affecting the Skin

Bacteria, viruses, fungi, and parasites can cause skin infection. Some microorganisms are normal inhabitants of the skin, such as *Staphylococcus* and *Candida*. With a breach in skin integrity, these organisms, which normally colonize the skin, can cause infection. The most common parasitic infections are caused by lice and scabies. Because these infections commonly do not require medical attention, their incidence and prevalence statistics are difficult to estimate. For more information about bacterial and viral infections, see Chapter 10.

Diseases Caused by Fungal Infections

Fungi, or mycoses, are saprophytic plantlike organisms present in the environment and part of the normal skin flora. There are two types of fungi: yeast and mold. Yeast, also known as *Candida albicans,* is a single-celled fungus. *Candida* grow in long filaments, called *hyphae.* All fungi grow in warm, dark, moist areas on animals, plants, and in the soil. Children are often infected by fungi present in the soil, on pets, or by contact with an infected child in day care or school. Hygiene plays a protective role in reducing the incidence of fungal infections, especially in children. Superficial fungi, also called **dermatophytes,** such as **tinea** (ringworm), live on the keratinized tissues of skin, hair, and nails and secrete digestive enzymes that cause skin scaling, nail disintegration, and broken hair (see Box 41-3 and Fig. 41-4).

The pruritus associated with tinea lesions and the associated cosmetic changes in the skin, nails, and hair cause persons to seek diagnosis and treatment. Diagnosis of superficial fungal infections is made clinically by a microscopic examination of scrapings

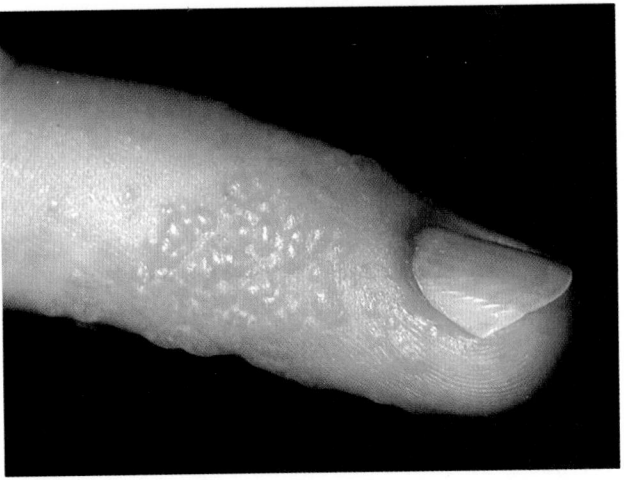

FIGURE 41-4. Tinea. *(Courtesy of CDC.)*

from the lesions or by visualizing the lesions with a Wood's light. When viewed under a Wood's light, fungi take on a fluorescent yellow-green appearance. When fungal infections penetrate the keratinized tissue and invade the skin layers, vesicles, redness, and signs of inflammation appear in the affected areas. Invasive fungi can cause septicemia (bloodstream infection) in an immunocompromised individual.

Treatment of superficial fungal infections is simple and involves the use of topical, and in difficult cases, systemic (oral or IV) antifungal agents. Most topical agents are over-the-counter preparations. Some persons do not tolerate systemic antifungal agents because these drugs interact with other medications. Toxic reactions to antifungal medication, especially liver toxicity, have also been reported.

Diseases Caused by Viruses

Warts, also called **verrucae,** are benign lesions of the skin caused by certain strains of the human papillomavirus (HPV). Transmitted by touch, they are round, rough, gray lesions that can occur anywhere on the body. Plantar warts, usually located at pressure points on the soles of the feet, are also benign lesions. They can be transmitted by skin-to-skin contact or surfaces such as communal showers. Plantar warts can cause callused skin, itching, and discomfort, and may be removed surgically. Genital warts, also called **condyloma acuminata,** are caused by certain strains of HPV that target the mucous membranes of the external genitalia and anus. Eighty percent of sexually active persons become infected with HPV at some point in their lifetime. Spread by vaginal, oral, or anal sexual activity, HPV infection can cause genital warts; cervical, anal, or oropharyngeal cancer; or resolve without consequences. High-risk HPV strains include HPV 16 and 18, which cause about 70% of cervical cancers. Low-risk HPV strains, such as HPV 6 and 11, cause about 90% of genital warts, which rarely develop into cancer.

BOX 41-3. Types of Tinea Infection

Tinea infections (commonly called ringworm) are named for the part of the body they infect:
- **Tinea corpora:** body
- **Tinea cruris:** groin
- **Tinea faciale:** face
- **Tinea capitis:** scalp
- **Tinea pedis:** foot, also called athlete's foot
- **Tinea manus:** hand
- **Tinea unguium:** nail
- **Tinea versicolor:** upper chest, back, or arms

The association among sexual activity, genital warts, and an increased risk of cancer has prompted public health officials to strongly encourage vaccination against HPV before the initiation of sexual activity. The Food and Drug Administration (FDA) has approved an HPV vaccine (Gardasil) for use in individuals ages 9 to 45 years old.

Because HIV infections are transmitted sexually, persons with HIV are at high risk for HPV infection. This increases the risk for cervical, anal, and oropharyngeal cancer in persons with HIV who are co-infected with HPV. In persons with HIV and AIDS, HPV-related genital warts are larger, more numerous, and more uncomfortable than they are in the population that is not HIV-positive. Warts can be removed by freezing, laser treatments, or the application of keratolytics or irritants. Imiquimod (Aldara), podophyllin and podofilox (Condylox), trichloroacetic acid (TCA), or sinecatechins (Veregen) are agents used to treat genital warts.

Another viral disease, **molluscum contagiosum,** causes small bumps to appear on the skin. The bumps are smooth, waxy, and small, about the size of a pinhead, and their central core is filled with a white cheeselike substance. The virus that causes this illness can live in warm water and can be transmitted in spas, baths, and heated swimming pools. In persons with HIV, regardless of their age, the lesions of molluscum contagiosum are more numerous and larger.

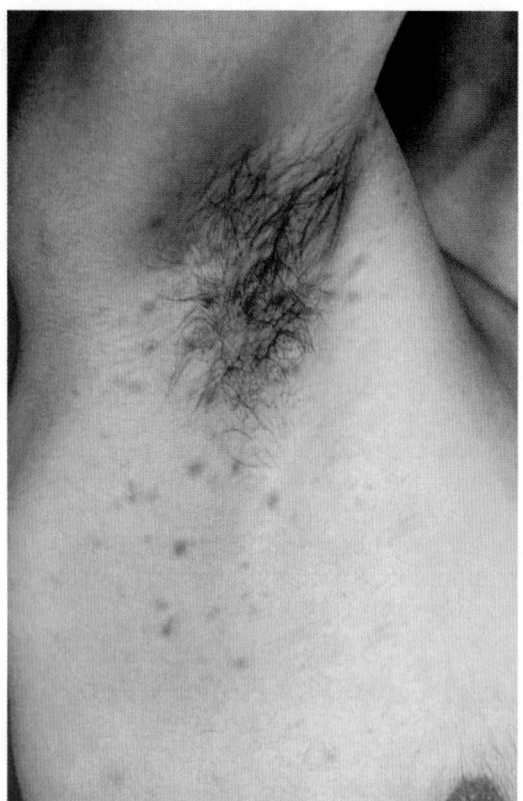

FIGURE 41-5. Scabies. *(Courtesy of CDC/Susan Lindsley.)*

CLINICAL CONCEPT

The vaccine against HPV should be administered to prevent the spread of infection by sexual activity.

Diseases Caused by Arachnid Bites

Arachnids, which include mites, ticks, and spiders, can cause a number of different skin disorders with their bites, ranging from the benign to the serious.

Mite Bites

Mite bites injure the skin and render it susceptible to other infections. **Scabies,** the disease transmitted by mites, is associated with poverty, malnutrition, and sexual promiscuity. Usually scabies is spread by skin-to-skin contact, but it can also be spread via objects, clothing, and bedding because mites can survive for several days without contact with the skin's blood supply.

Activated by warmth, the female mite finds its way to the bottom of the stratum corneum layer of the skin by creating a tunnel or burrow—a narrow, raised, irregular channel. Scabies are often suspected when small papules and visible wavy or linear burrows are present on the interdigital webs of the fingers and toes, folds of the skin, nipples, or genitalia. Because the lesions are itchy, the skin around the burrows is usually excoriated (see Fig. 41-5).

Tick Bites

Ticks are insects that live in grasses and bushes, as well as on forest animals, such as deer. Ticks also commonly bite dogs, humans, and livestock. A female tick punctures the skin, sucks blood, and falls to the ground when engorged. Tick bites produce local damage to the skin, which resembles new moles. In some persons, urticarial wheals appear at the site of puncture. A characteristic "bull's-eye" type of red rash called erythema migrans often develops in bites from ticks carrying the bacterium *Borrelia burgdorferi.* The *Ixodes ricinus* ticks carrying the bacteria can cause Lyme disease after puncturing human skin. Aside from the characteristic rash, some persons develop an isolated cranial nerve VII palsy, termed Bell's palsy. Rare cases of meningitis and myocarditis have also been reported. Although Lyme disease is the most common tick-related illness, other disorders caused by tick bites include ehrlichiosis and anaplasmosis. More formally termed human granulocytic ehrlichiosis (HGE) and human granulocytic anaplasmosis (HGA), these are bacterial infections transmitted by different types of ticks. HGE is caused by the bacterium *Ehrlichia anaplasma* transmitted by the lone star tick *(Amblyomma americanum).* HGA is caused by the bacterium *Anaplasma phagocytophilum,* transmitted by the black-legged deer tick *(Ixodes scapularis).*

Lyme disease, HGE, and HGA can be transmitted after 24 to 48 hours of tick attachment. They have an incubation period of 7 to 14 days and can cause systemic symptoms including fever, chills, headache, myalgias, arthralgias, abdominal pain, and vomiting. It is important to recognize that these symptoms can occur as late as 2 weeks after the original bite. The tick and tick bite are often unnoticed and not readily apparent. Serological testing is commonly done to diagnose tick-borne illnesses, but these can have ambiguous results. Polymerase chain reaction (PCR) is the confirmatory test of choice for these infections. Doxycycline is first-line treatment for all ages for these diseases. In addition to Lyme disease, HGE, and HGA, tick bites can cause Rocky Mountain spotted fever, tularemia, and encephalitis (see Chapter 10 for more information on these diseases).

Spider Bites

Spider bites are common occurrences. They cause pain, redness, itching, swelling, and small puncture wounds. Although most spider bites are benign, the black widow spider and brown recluse spider inject toxic substances into the skin. These spider bites present as target marks, pale areas surrounded by red rings. The person who is bitten experiences local itching, rash, and burning, as well as systemic symptoms, including cramping pain, weakness, fever, sweating, nausea, and vomiting. Severe symptoms include difficulty breathing and increased blood pressure. Children and older adults have more severe symptoms.

Diseases Caused by Insect Bites

Bedbugs

Bedbugs, ***Cimex lectularius,*** are insects associated with a lack of clean mattresses or bedding. They bite children and adults who sleep in unsanitary conditions. Homeless persons are at particular risk of bedbug bites. Although the bite itself is painless, the person awakens to find itchy skin. More careful examination of the skin reveals red wheals arranged in linear patterns (see Fig. 41-6). Because the saliva of bedbugs contains a protein substance, purpuric reactions are not uncommon. Diagnosis of the cause of the skin irritation is made by finding bedbugs in linen or mattresses. Vigorous sanitation of bedding and specific pesticide use are required to kill bedbugs.

Lice

Lice infestation, also called **pediculosis,** is highly contagious. Lice obtain nourishment by attaching themselves to the skin, biting, and sucking blood. They can live on clothing for up to a month. Lice bites produce reddened macules, inflammation, hyperpigmentation, and parallel scratch marks. Although lice bites can cause significant illness—including typhus, relapsing fever, and trench fever—usually, they produce itchy skin and social embarrassment.

Lice bites are more common in children, and lice have an affinity for skin that is covered with hair. When lice penetrate the scalp, the hair becomes dry and lacks luster. Scalp itching is a common symptom. Body lice are associated with poverty, overcrowding, and inadequate hygiene. Some lice infections, called pediculosis pubis, are sexually transmitted. If patients have evidence of pubic lice, they should be screened for other sexually transmitted diseases, and their sexual contacts should be advised and treated.

Diagnosis of lice is made by finding the lice or lice eggs, called nits, in the clothing, bed linen, or the hair of the person who has been bitten (see Fig. 41-7).

Washing the person, their clothing, and the environment is the first step in eradication. Definitive treatment requires the destruction of lice with special soaps, shampoos, and rinses. Fine combs are used to determine whether there are nits in hairy parts of the body. Usually, this process requires repeated applications of soap, shampoo, or rinse. The eradication process may also require shaving the hair.

Mosquitoes

Mosquito bites are commonly encountered during warm months. The mosquito bite produces a localized, itchy wheal. Sweat attracts mosquitoes, which need protein to produce eggs. Mosquitoes bite horses, cattle, small mammals, birds, and people because of their large skin surface and abundant underlying blood supply. In tropical countries, mosquitoes can carry malaria, yellow fever, dengue fever, and encephalitis. Within the past decade, there have been serious outbreaks of mosquito-borne West Nile viral infections in the United States.

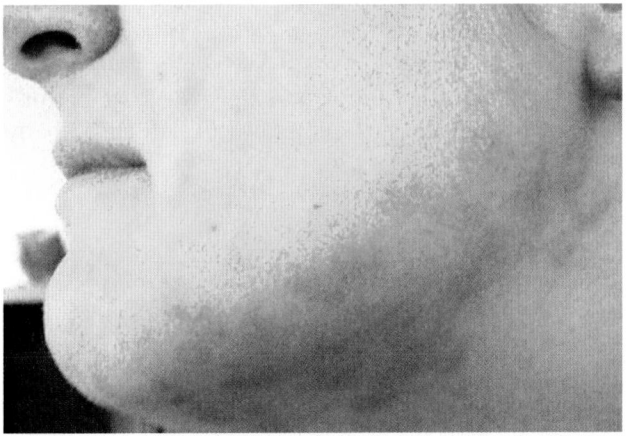

FIGURE 41-6. Bedbug bites. *(Wikipedia: Courtesy of Andy Brookes BSc.)*

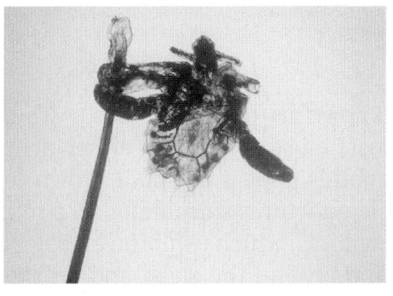

FIGURE 41-7. Head lice. *(Courtesy of Wills Eye Hospital, Philadelphia, PA.)*

Because mosquitoes can cause serious illness, there are public health initiatives related to their eradication: destruction of breeding grounds, emptying of pools of stagnant water, screening of windows and porches, and spraying of wetlands and grassy breeding areas. In areas where mosquitoes are abundant, mosquito netting, protective clothing, insect repellents, and avoidance of tall grassy areas and stagnant water decrease the incidence of exposure and the number of mosquito bites.

Diseases Caused by Hymenoptera Bites

Hymenoptera bites, which include bites from bees, wasps, and fleas, are another common source of skin injury. These bites cause local inflammation, irritation, swelling, and itching. Some Hymenoptera bites trigger the severe allergic reaction termed anaphylaxis. Other reactions result from toxins injected by Hymenoptera that penetrate the skin and cause vesicles and bullae formation. Toxins can produce hematological symptoms in addition to skin lesions.

Bee and Wasp Stings

Bee and wasp stings are immediately painful and swelling and itching persist for about a week. A sting can inject poisonous venom into the skin that can reach the blood supply and cause systemic reactions. Serious, even fatal, allergic or anaphylactic reactions can occur immediately or within 1 hour of the sting.

Treatment requires immediate removal of the stinger if it remains because it is a source of venom, followed by the application of ice to the area. Persons who continue to have symptoms or show any signs of an anaphylactic reaction, such as hives, should receive prompt medical care.

 CLINICAL CONCEPT

Because a sting is a type of puncture wound, some clinicians recommend tetanus immunization.

ALERT! Persons known to be highly allergic to bee stings should carry self-injectable epinephrine to prevent an anaphylactic reaction.

Fleabites

Fleabites, known as **pulicosis,** occur when the flea bites its host, most commonly either a human, cat, or dog. Fleabites appear as small brown lesions and hemorrhagic punctures surrounded by a red, urticarial patch. These bites, which exhibit a zigzag pattern, are usually found around the waist and on the legs. The lesions from the bites are often seen in sets of three (see Fig. 41-8).

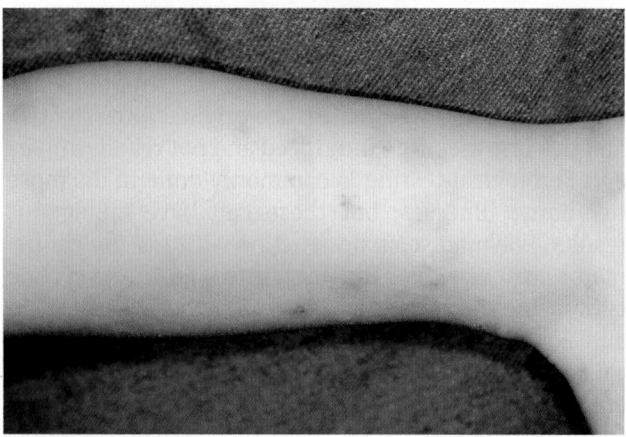

FIGURE 41-8. Fleabites. *(From Scott Camazine/Science Source.)*

Some persons have hypersensitivity responses to fleabites. When disturbed, fleas can jump from one host to another or to rugs, furniture, or bedding and remain in the environment. Pets that go outdoors can transfer fleas to humans. Unsanitary environments are often associated with flea infestation and an increase in bites. Pest control, window screens, removal of garbage and stagnant water, and environmental cleanliness are important modes of preventing fleabites.

Environmental or Physical Injuries Affecting the Skin

Pressure Injuries

Pressure injuries, also called pressure ulcers, decubitus ulcers, and bedsores, are the most common of the skin ulcers. Pressure causes diminished blood flow to the skin, especially skin covering bony prominences, which are particularly vulnerable to pressure. If pressure on the skin is released after several hours, the skin is reddened but not damaged. Sustained pressure produces blisters, followed by reddish-blue discoloration, and finally skin breakdown and tissue ulceration, which create opportunities for infection.

Pressure injuries affect older adults and persons who are immobilized for long periods; they are costly, burdensome illnesses. Persons with diabetes are at special risk for all types of skin ulcers because peripheral nerve damage and lack of circulation accompany the disease.

 CLINICAL CONCEPT

Pressure injuries occur because of sustained pressure on the skin, especially the skin over bony prominences. Change of position and range-of-motion exercises prevent pressure injuries.

Stasis Ulcers

Stasis ulcers are also related to diminished circulation and are usually found in the lower extremities. Venous insufficiency, obesity, pregnancy, family history, old age, and blood clotting disorders are factors associated with the development of stasis ulcers.

The process of developing stasis ulcers is subtle; as the valves in the legs become blocked or incompetent, blood flow back to the heart is compromised. As pressure rises in the veins, fluid seeps from the veins into the surrounding tissues. As a consequence of venous blood pooling and accumulation of wastes, the skin in the area becomes darker, thicker, dryer, and itchy. If untreated, these darkened areas of skin become ulcerated and infected.

Loss of sensation, poor circulation, and itching contribute to the development of these easily infected ulcers. Because blood supply is restricted, infected stasis ulcers are difficult to heal.

Tattooing

Tattooing, the practice of placing permanent color into the skin, has been used for centuries to decorate the skin. If the tattoo artist uses sterile equipment and aseptic techniques, the procedure is relatively safe. Complications, including secondary infections, are unusual. However, if conditions in the tattoo parlor are unsanitary and equipment is unsterile, infections such as hepatitis B or C or HIV can be transmitted.

In July 2006, the Centers for Disease Control and Prevention reported 44 cases in three different states of methicillin-resistant *Staphylococcus aureus* (MRSA) skin infections secondary to receiving tattoos. Usually, complications from tattooing present as toxic reactions or immune responses to the pigment in the dye—especially the pigment in red dye. Some persons respond to tattoos by developing granulomas and contact dermatitis. Others find that they experience an exacerbation of existing skin diseases, such as psoriasis or lupus. Tattoo removal is most commonly performed using lasers that break down the ink in the tattoo.

Pattern Injuries

Pattern injuries are bruises, wounds, or those injuries whose shape suggests the instrument that inflicted them, such as belt buckles, irons, or burning cigarettes. These injuries indicate physical abuse. Usually, the history of the injury is inconsistent with its appearance and severity. Clinicians are required to report evidence that a patient has been abused.

> **ALERT!** Patients with suspected pattern injuries should be screened for other signs of physical abuse, and this should be reported to authorities.

Psychological and Psychiatric Conditions Affecting the Skin

The skin and associated tissues reveal much about the person's emotions and health status. Specialized somatic sensory receptors located in the dermis perceive and transmit sensations of pain, pressure, touch, and temperature to the brain. When the involuntary erector pili muscles that surround the hair follicles contract, hair literally stands on end. This action conveys fright or adaptation to cold.

Pruritus and purpural (bruising) syndromes are common manifestations of psychogenic skin disease. Often, excoriation of the skin from picking, rubbing, scratching, or self-mutilation leads to secondary infections and scarring. A similar manifestation of psychogenic disease is seen in the hair. Trichotillomania is hair loss from repeated urges to pull or twist the hair until it breaks off. Anxiety often reveals itself in obsessive-compulsive behavior, such as pulling, twisting, or removing clumps of hair or biting the fingernails.

The sudden appearance of telogen effluvium and alopecia areata secondary to trauma or surgery can be a psychogenic response to stress. Persons with psychogenic skin disease seek care for symptoms of skin disease, burning, itching, or pain when there is no clinical, physical, or laboratory evidence to explain these symptoms.

Within the past two decades, biomedical science has enhanced clinicians' understanding of psychogenic skin disease. Often, dermatological disorders are manifestations of depression, obsessive-compulsive disorders, anxiety, and pain-prone conditions. Idiopathic pruritus, inflammatory dermatosis, psoriasis, and eczema may also indicate or accompany an underlying emotional disorder.

Self-cutting, self-mutilation, and intentional self-harm are behaviors that may be apparent upon examination of the skin. Self-injury is a relatively common phenomenon in adolescence. Nonsuicidal self-injury disorder (NSSID) is a psychiatric disorder listed in the *DSM-V*. Often, there is no suicidal intent; rather, the action is related to reducing emotional distress, inflicting self-punishment, and/or signaling personal anguish to others. Scars and healed lacerations may be evident on examination of the skin.

Treatment of psychogenic skin disorders is aimed at the skin, hair, or nail symptoms, but it is also directed at uncovering and addressing the underlying causes of the skin manifestations. In addition to therapy for the skin disorder, pharmacological agents for depression, anxiety, and obsessive-compulsive behavior; psychotherapy; and cognitive-behavioral therapy can be effective in persons with NSSID.

Eczema and Other Types of Dermatitis

Inflammation, or dermatitis, characterizes many disorders of the skin, including eczema, contact dermatitis, and seborrheic dermatitis.

Eczema

Eczema, also known as atopic dermatitis, is the most common dermatitis, occurring in two clinical forms: infantile and adult. Vesicle formation, oozing, and crusting with excoriation that begins on the cheeks and spreads to the scalp, arms, trunk, and legs characterize the infantile manifestation of eczema (see Fig. 41-9). This form may become milder as the child ages, sometimes disappearing by age 15 years. However, some persons continue to have eczematous lesions and rhinitis throughout their lives. Adolescents and adults with eczema have dry, lichenified lesions that are either hypopigmented or hyperpigmented; these lesions are usually seen in the antecubital and popliteal areas, spreading to the neck, hands, feet, eyelids, and behind the ears. Because these lesions are itchy, inflammation and infection occur.

Eczema also has a range of clinical presentations: acute, subacute, and chronic. In eczema, there is a recognized interaction among genetic and environmental factors, skin barrier, immune factors, and stress. Persons with eczema often have family histories of asthma or hay fever. The individual has elevated immunoglobulin IgE levels, as it is associated with allergy or type I hypersensitivity reactions. The goal of treatment, usually sought in the acute phase, addresses symptoms such as pruritus, dryness, inflammation, and infection. However, the ultimate therapeutic goal is to keep the eczema in remission. Treatment involves allergen control; good skin care; and avoidance of stress, foods, drinks, and temperature changes that exacerbate the eczema or its symptoms. Topical and occasionally systemic corticosteroids are used. Immune modulators are showing positive results without side effects.

Contact Dermatitis

Contact dermatitis represents delayed hypersensitivity to materials such as metals, chemicals, drugs, and poison ivy. The condition affects the head, neck, trunk, arms, hands, abdomen, groin, and lower extremities. This allergic skin reaction usually occurs days after the skin contact with the allergen. Emollients and topical anti-inflammatory medication are standard therapy.

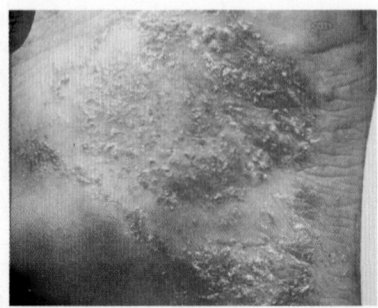

FIGURE 41-9. Eczema.

Seborrheic Dermatitis

Seborrheic dermatitis is an inflammation of the skin caused by excessive secretions of the sebaceous glands. Its lesions are red, usually on the face and scalp, and yield yellow to yellow-brown scales known as dandruff. The lesions appear to be greasy, inflamed, and itchy. Removal of scales by frequent washing of the skin and shampooing of the hair provides some relief from this condition.

Papulosquamous Dermatoses

Papulosquamous dermatoses include psoriasis, pityriasis rosea, and lichen planus. They are distinguished by scaling papules and plaques.

Psoriasis

Psoriasis—a genetic, chronic thickening of the epidermis that presents as overlying silver-white scales covering red, circumscribed, thickened plaques—is a disease of unknown cause found throughout the world. More common in colder climates, the disease affects less than 5% of the American population, although its prevalence increases with age. Psoriasis can be associated with disabling arthritis of the hands and fingers.

Psoriasis is a T-cell–mediated autoimmune response to an unknown antigen. Histories of adults with psoriasis reveal that skin trauma, stress, infection, and the use of medications such as hydroxychloroquine (Plaquenil), angiotensin-converting enzyme inhibitors, and lithium often precede the appearance of psoriasis.

Although the lesions of psoriasis can appear anywhere on the body, they are frequently seen on the extensor surfaces of elbows and knees, as well as on the scalp (see Fig. 41-10). Topical agents and emollients can soften and hydrate the skin. Exposure to sunlight and saltwater baths are known to be helpful. Topical corticosteroids are used with varying results but cannot be used long term. Immunomodulator drugs, also called biological agents or monoclonal antibodies, are a novel category of drugs found to be effective in psoriasis and other autoimmune disorders. These agents act systemically to inhibit inflammatory mediators, tumor necrosis factor alpha (TNF-alpha), and/or interleukins (ILs). There is a growing number of available systemic immunomodulators used to treat autoimmune disorders. Patients using these drugs have an increased risk of infection and need close monitoring during treatment. Testing for tuberculosis is often necessary before initiation of immunomodulators. Treatment varies with the severity of the disease, the age of the patient, and the person's ability to tolerate side effects of systemic drug therapy.

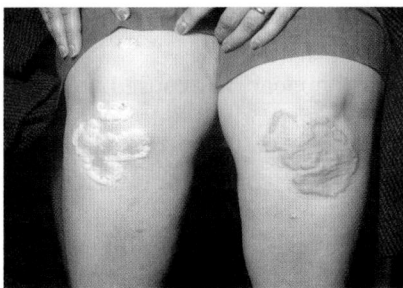

FIGURE 41-10. Psoriasis.

 CLINICAL CONCEPT

Psoriasis lesions bleed when the scales are removed. This diagnostic finding, called Auspitz sign, differentiates psoriasis from other skin disorders.

Pityriasis Rosea

Pityriasis rosea—an oval macular or papular rash surrounded by erythema—appears spontaneously on the skin of young adults. Its cause is unknown, although some infectious agent is suspected because the rash is often found among those who live in close quarters.

The first lesion of pityriasis rosea is a solitary patch, called a **herald patch,** which usually appears on the neck or trunk. As this lesion enlarges and begins to fade, usually between days 2 and 10, successive patches appear on the neck and trunk. When the patches appear on the back, they form a Christmas tree pattern. The patches are itchy, but they clear in 6 to 8 weeks. Treatment is aimed at controlling symptoms and consists of corticosteroids or antihistamines. In some cases, acyclovir can be used to treat symptoms and reduce the length of disease. UV phototherapy can also be considered for severe cases.

Lichen Planus

Lichen planus, from the Greek for tree moss, is a term used to describe flat-topped, small, purple papules with irregular borders, covered with a shiny, white, lacelike pattern. It is a common chronic disease of the skin and mucous membranes, particularly the oral mucosa. The cause is unknown, and pruritus is its main symptom when on the skin. Treatment is aimed at controlling symptoms using topical corticosteroids, or if severe, a short course of oral corticosteroids.

Urticaria and Related Inflammatory Lesions

Acute urticaria is a skin reaction that is commonly caused by an allergy. Severe cases can include angioedema. Urticaria can also occur as a chronic skin reaction because of an unknown allergen.

Urticaria

Urticaria, or hives, are elevated, pink or red, itchy blotches or plaques of varying size. These lesions, also called *wheals,* appear suddenly on the skin or mucous membranes and blanch with pressure (see Fig. 41-11). In about 40% of patients, the appearance of urticaria is accompanied by **angioedema,** the swelling of the eyes, face, lips, and the mucous membranes (see Fig. 41-12). Urticaria may occasionally be associated with acute anaphylactic reactions and laryngeal edema.

The release of histamine from the granules of mast cells is the cause of urticaria. Immunological, nonimmunological, physical, and chemical stimuli can cause mast cell degranulation and release histamine into the skin and the circulating blood. The disease classification of either acute or chronic urticaria depends on the duration of symptoms. If a person has urticaria for longer than 6 weeks, they are considered to have a chronic form of the disease.

Acute urticaria occurs as a discrete, sudden episode, often after the ingestion of medicine, food, or drinks, or following insect stings, viral infections, and exposure to dust mites, pollens, and chemicals.

 CLINICAL CONCEPT

Allergy-prone children, especially those with eczema and rhinitis, are particularly susceptible to acute urticaria, which is associated with the ingestion of food or drink.

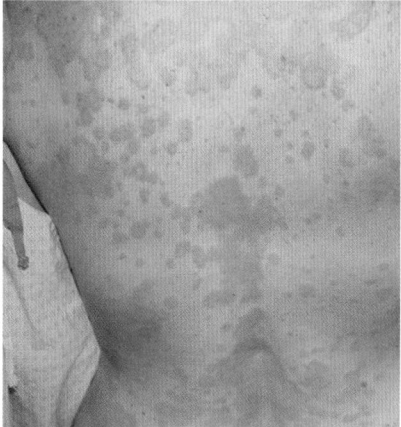

FIGURE 41-11. Urticaria.

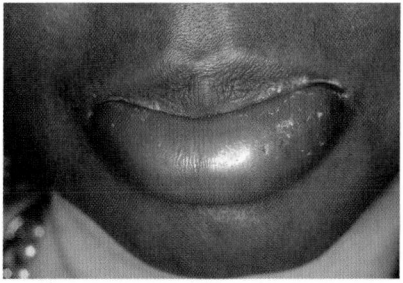

FIGURE 41-12. Angioedema.

Antihistamines are prescribed in acute urticaria. Injectable epinephrine is used if the swelling is severe, if it involves the mucous membranes, or if it is accompanied by the inability to breathe or by the appearance of shocklike symptoms.

History and allergy testing may determine the trigger of urticaria. Avoidance or discontinuation of the offending agents holds the key to prevention. If the patient's history suggests a food or drink allergy, these substances should be eliminated from the diet immediately. Efforts should then be undertaken to discover the chemical or the protein present in the drug, food, or drink that triggered the skin response, because this antigen may be the real allergic trigger. In these cases, eliminating one drug or one food or drink may not stop the attacks.

Chronic urticaria affects adults and is twice as common in females as in males. It appears to be an autoimmune disorder, but extensive laboratory work-ups usually fail to identify a causal agent; avoidance of suspect antigens is not helpful. Approximately half of the persons with chronic urticaria have circulating immunoglobulin G antibodies to a subunit of the immunoglobulin E receptor. These antibodies activate the release of histamine from basophils and mast cells. It may manifest an underlying disease, certain cancers, collagen diseases, or hepatitis B.

Physical urticaria is considered a chronic form of the disease. These intermittent, short-acting manifestations can be induced by rubbing the skin or by exercise, cold, pressure, sunlight, water, vibration, and heat.

Most types of urticaria are treated with antihistamines that block histamine type 1 and type 2. Leukotriene antagonists may also be prescribed. Local therapy, such as oatmeal baths, may also be helpful. Persons with histories of angioedema, extreme swelling of the face and throat, should carry injectable epinephrine with them. Oral corticosteroids and antidepressants are used when urticaria persists.

> **ALERT!** Persons with a history of anaphylaxis or angioedema should carry injectable epinephrine with them.

Disorders Involving the Skin's Blood and Lymphatic Vessels

Vascular lesions are small tumors with chronically dilated blood vessels that arise from the middle to upper dermis. Depending on their size and location, these tumors can be disfiguring.

Senile angiomas are small, asymptomatic, cherry-red, dome-shaped papules that appear on the trunk of older adult individuals. They are a common example of a disorder of the skin's blood vessels.

Telangiectasias appear as a single, dilated capillary. Thought to be genetic, they appear on the face, nose, and other exposed areas likely to be affected by the sun or harsh weather.

Venous lakes appear on exposed areas of the body. They present as small, dark-blue papules that resemble the configuration of a lake.

Cutaneous T-cell lymphoma (CTCL), a rare type of non-Hodgkin's lymphoma, presents as either a low-grade or a high-grade lymphoma, based on how rapidly the disease spreads through the lymph system. Unlike other lymphomas in this class, CTCL affects the skin; in 65% of cases, it is caused by a malignant growth of T cells. The etiology is unknown; diagnosis is made by biopsy. The most common types of CTCL are mycosis fungoides and Sezary syndrome. Nitrogen mustard chemotherapy has been used for more than 50 years for CTCL. A topical formulation, chlormethine gel, is recommended. Other skin-directed therapies include topical corticosteroids, phototherapy, and radiotherapy. Systemic chemotherapy is used in advanced cases of CTCL; bone marrow transplant may also be attempted.

Kaposi's sarcoma (KS) is a cancer that develops within blood and lymphatic vessels. Tumors appear as purple-colored, painless, irregularly shaped lesions on the skin of the face, trunk, and extremities. These blood vessel tumors can also occur within organs such as the lungs and digestive tract. The underlying cause of KS is infection with human herpesvirus 8 (HHV-8). Immunosuppressed individuals are at increased risk for this disorder, particularly those with HIV infection and those who have had organ transplantation. Another type of KS occurs in older males of the Mediterranean and Middle Eastern regions and Africa. It is a slowly progressive cancer that demonstrates similar lesions; however, it is less virulent than HIV-related KS. Diagnosis involves biopsy of the lesion, chest x-ray, upper endoscopy and colonoscopy, and bronchoscopy, depending on the patient's symptoms. Treatment for KS depends on the etiology. HIV-related KS may be treated using different combinations of antiretroviral agents. Transplant-related KS may be treated by changing the immunosuppressive drug regimen. Low-dose radiation, intralesional chemotherapy injections, surgical excision, electrodessication, or cryotherapy of the lesions can be used to manage the disorder.

Autoimmune Skin Disorders

Autoimmune diseases are disorders in which the body reacts against itself. The body forms antibodies that attack part of the body. The autoimmune diseases—scleroderma, systemic lupus erythematosus (SLE), pemphigus, and erythema multiforme (EM)—have specific dermatological manifestations.

Scleroderma

Scleroderma, an autoimmune disease that occurs more often in females than in males, affects the skin's connective tissue and blood vessels. Beginning as a mild inflammation, the lesions of scleroderma develop into patches of yellow, hardened skin. The disease, which may be localized or generalized, alters the skin's appearance and flexibility and restricts movement. As a systemic disease, scleroderma affects internal organs and can cause cardiac problems (for more information, see Chapter 11).

Systemic Lupus Erythematosus

SLE, an inflammatory autoimmune disease, can be limited to the skin or become a diffuse multisystem illness. As a skin disease, **discoid lupus erythematosus (DLE)** is more common in middle-aged females. The lesions of DLE, appearing on exposed areas of the skin, are often seen on the face. Accompanied by photophobia, the classic lesion of DLE presents as a red, plaquelike, asymmetric, butterfly-patterned lesion over the nose and cheeks. Skin biopsies reveal deposits of immunoglobulins, especially IgM, in the lesion and surrounding tissues. Lesions last for months, then resolve or atrophy to return again. Persons with DLE often have random hair loss, telangiectasias over the palms and fingers, urticaria, and Raynaud's phenomenon (for more information, see Chapter 11).

Pemphigus

Pemphigus, a rare, chronic autoimmune disease that is more prevalent between ages 40 and 50 years, causes blisters to form on the epidermis. It is characterized by a painful and pruritic vesiculopustular rash. The etiology is unknown; however, it frequently occurs in persons with a malignancy or chronic illness. In some forms of the disease, blisters penetrate deep into the tissues. Caused by circulating IgA or IgG autoantibodies, the blister formation occurs because the autoantibodies attack the intracellular matrix, causing a separation in the epidermis. In pemphigus vulgaris, the most common form of the disease, blister formation begins on the oral mucosa or the scalp. As the disease progresses, the rash evolves into flaccid, bullous lesions that can rupture, leaving crusty, denuded skin. Corticosteroids and dapsone are used to treat pemphigus.

Erythema Multiforme

Erythema multiforme (EM) is an acute hypersensitivity disorder of the skin and mucous membranes that is associated with allergic or toxic reactions to drugs or microorganisms. Herpes simplex virus (HSV) is the most common microorganism that triggers EM, accounting for more than 50% of cases. *Mycoplasma pneumoniae* is another commonly reported etiology, especially in children. Epstein–Barr, HIV, hepatitis C, and Coxsackie viruses are also known to trigger EM. The medications most often associated with the condition are barbiturates, statins, allopurinol, anticonvulsants, TNF-alpha inhibitors, NSAIDs, tetracyclines, penicillins, nitrofurantoin, phenothiazines, and sulfonamides. EM has also been triggered by other viruses and vaccines.

EM can be a mild or a very serious disease in which immune complex formation and deposits of complement C3, IgM, and fibrinogen develop around superficial dermal vessels, the basement membrane, and keratinocytes. There are no prodromal symptoms of EM, and an initial rash of sharply demarcated, pruritic, red and pink macules appears. These macules evolve into papules and then into large areas of red and pink plaques. The lesions take on a characteristic target appearance with a central, inflamed, red area surrounded by concentric rings of pink, swollen tissue. In the vesiculobullous form of the disease, bullae appear on mucous membranes and as plaques on extensor surfaces of the extremities. When these bullae rupture, they leave erosions and crusts. The mouth, airways, esophagus, urethra, and conjunctiva may be involved.

Underlying infections need to be treated, and the drug or microorganism that triggered the skin's response needs to be identified and eliminated from the patient's system. EM spontaneously resolves in 3 to 5 weeks without complications; however, it can recur. Oral antihistamines and topical and oral steroids may be used to provide symptom relief. In patients with coexisting or recent HSV infection, early treatment with acyclovir or a similar type of drug may lessen the number and duration of cutaneous lesions. Dapsone and Janus kinase (JAK) inhibitors are also used to treat EM.

Stevens–Johnson Syndrome

Stevens–Johnson syndrome (SJS) is a rare but very serious disorder of the skin and mucous membranes usually triggered by an infection or drug. There is a genetic propensity in those with the *HLA-B1502* gene. Other risk factors include HIV infection, past episode of SJS, family history of SJS, and weakened immune system. Infections that can trigger SJS include pneumonia, herpes, HIV, hepatitis A, and bacterial skin infections. Drugs such as allopurinol, anticonvulsants, antipsychotics, NSAIDs, acetaminophen, and antibiotics can also trigger SJS. It begins with flu-like symptoms followed by a painful, red rash that evolves into large blisters and bullae with sloughing of the skin. Symptoms include fever and widespread, red, painful blistering of the skin and mucous membranes of the mouth, eyes, nose, and genital region. Hospitalization is required, as the patient is critically ill and can develop complications. A life-threatening dermatological condition called toxic epidermal necrolysis (TEN) can evolve from SJS. This disorder causes widespread exfoliation.

Respiratory failure, cellulitis, sepsis, and shock can occur. Patients require intensive care with supportive measures such as IV fluids, anti-inflammatory agents, pain medications, and wound care. Treatment includes removal of the offending drug or amelioration of the infection with antibiotics, if infection initiated the syndrome.

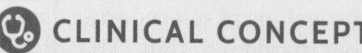 **CLINICAL CONCEPT**

There is a genetic propensity for SJS in persons with the *HLA-B1502* gene. Some drugs should be avoided in this population, as they can trigger SJS.

Chapter Summary

- The surface film and thick surface layer called the stratum corneum stop antigens from entering the body and keep the body waterproof.

- The interaction of UV light with the skin is necessary for vitamin D synthesis.

- A rash is a temporary eruption of the skin associated with childhood diseases, allergies, heat, irritation from clothing, or a response to drug therapy.

- Lesions are traumatic or pathological loss of normal skin continuity, structure, or function.

- Acne is a skin condition caused by *Propionibacterium*.

- Hidradenitis suppurativa is a disorder that causes tender, swollen sweat glands that drain purulent exudate.

- Dysplastic nevi are lesions that are irregular in shape, variegated in color, and have a high susceptibility to cancerous change. These lesions require clinical examination to rule out skin cancer.

- Actinic keratoses, premalignant lesions found on skin that has been damaged by the UV rays of the sun, are common in fair-skinned persons.

- Malignant melanoma tends to have one or more ABCDE traits: **A**symmetry of shape, irregular **B**orders, **C**olor variation, **D**iameter more than 6 mm, and a lesion that is **E**volving.

- Basal cell carcinoma is the most common form of skin cancer and accounts for more than 90% of all cases in the United States. These cancers, often found on the face, rarely metastasize to other parts of the body. They can, however, cause damage by growing deeply and invading surrounding tissue.

- Light-colored skin and sun exposure are both important factors in the development of malignant melanoma, SCC, and basal cell carcinoma.

- Superficial fungi live on the keratinized tissues of skin, hair, and nails. When viewed under a Wood's light, fungi take on a fluorescent yellow-green appearance.

- Warts, termed verrucae, are benign lesions of the skin caused by certain strains of HPV. Plantar warts, also benign and located at pressure points on the soles of the feet, usually cause discomfort and can be removed surgically.

- Genital warts, called condyloma acuminata, are due to specific strains of HPV. Some strains are commonly transmitted during sexual activity and can cause cervical, anal, or oropharyngeal cancer.

- Scabies, caused by mites, can be spread by infected clothing, person-to-person contact, or pet-to-human contact.

- A characteristic "bull's-eye" type of red rash, called erythema migrans, often develops in bites from ticks carrying the microorganism *B. burgdorferi*. These bacteria-carrying ticks can cause Lyme disease after puncturing the skin of humans.

- Other tick-borne illnesses in the United States include ehrichiosis and anaplasmosis.

- Bedbugs, *C. lectularius,* are insects associated with infested mattresses or bedding.

- Head lice infestation, also called pediculosis capitis, is common in schoolchildren as it is extremely contagious.

- Bee and wasp stings are associated with anaphylaxis.

- Fleabites occur when the flea bites its host, most commonly a human, cat, or dog.

- Pressure injuries occur because of sustained pressure on the skin, especially the skin over bony prominences.

- Eczema, the most common dermatitis, is characterized by vesicle formation, oozing, and crusting with excoriation that begins on the cheeks and spreads to the scalp, arms, trunk, and legs.

- Contact dermatitis represents delayed hypersensitivity to materials such as metals, chemicals, drugs, and poison ivy.

- Psoriasis lesions are erythematous lesions with silvery white scales that bleed when removed.

- Pityriasis rosea begins as a solitary patch called a herald patch, which usually appears on the neck or trunk. Successive patches appear on the neck and trunk in a Christmas tree pattern.

- Urticaria (hives) are elevated, pink or red, itchy blotches or plaques of varying size. These lesions can be the first sign of anaphylaxis.

- Urticaria can be accompanied by angioedema, which is swelling of the eyes, face, lips, and mucous membranes.

- Erythema multiforme is an acute inflammatory disorder of the skin and mucous membranes associated with allergic or toxic reactions to drugs or microorganisms.
- Scleroderma and SLE are autoimmune diseases, each with characteristic skin changes. Scleroderma causes the skin surface to become extremely tight and shiny.

- SLE causes a characteristic erythematous "butterfly malar rash" across the cheeks and nose.
- SJS is a severe reaction to drugs or infection that causes flu-like symptoms; a painful, red-purple rash; and large blisters on the skin and mucous membranes. It can lead to sepsis, shock, and multiple organ failure.

Making the Connections

Signs and Symptoms	Physical Assessment Findings	Diagnostic Testing	Treatment
Malignant Melanoma | Arises from the melanocytes. Differ in size and shape and may arise from dysplastic nevi or new molelike growths. Slightly raised and brown or black in color. Can appear anywhere on the body and may be slowly or rapidly growing.			
Patient presents with a lesion that has changed in size, shape, and appearance. Lesion is usually asymptomatic, but occasionally pruritus is observed. Cosmetic concerns about appearance of the lesion are frequent. Skin cancers may appear suddenly or develop over time.	Description and comprehensive skin history reveal sun exposure and change of the lesion's appearance in its symmetry, diameter, color, or border. Melanoma **ABCDE** rules: **A:** Asymmetry **B:** Irregular border **C:** Variable color **D:** Diameter **E:** Evolving The general skin examination shows evidence of sun exposure.	Biopsy, with assessment of spread of disease if the biopsy is positive.	Surgery with a wide excision. Cryosurgery, radiation, and chemotherapy. Yearly skin checkup by a dermatologist. Monthly skin self-assessment by patient. Advice about protection from sun exposure.
Basal Cell Carcinoma | Arises from the nonkeratinizing cells of the basal layer of the epidermis. It is nonmetastasizing.			
Lesion often appears on the face, particularly the nose. Sun-exposed areas are the most common regions of basal cell carcinoma.	Begins as a nodular-cystic, small, pearly, flesh-colored, smooth nodule that enlarges over time.	Biopsy.	Surgery to remove lesion—often needs a very deep excision.
Squamous Cell Carcinoma (SCC) | A more serious epidermal cancer that is aggressive, invasive, and often develops from actinic keratosis.			
Lesion often appears on face or lips, or can be an oral lesion inside the mouth or on the tongue. Sun-exposed areas are the most common regions of SCC.	Presents as red, scaly, slightly elevated lesions with irregular borders.	Biopsy.	Surgery to remove lesion. Radiation or chemotherapy may be necessary.

Bibliography

Available online at fadavis.com

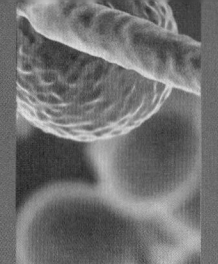

Burns

Learning Objectives

Upon completion of this chapter, the student will be able to:

- Recognize the various etiologies and mechanisms of burn injury.
- Identify the assessment techniques used to evaluate the extent of burn injury.
- Identify the different types of burn injury based on tissue depth and involved total body surface area.
- Describe the localized and systemic responses that occur in burn injury.
- List the most common complications of burn injury.
- Discuss different treatment modalities and pain management used in the care of patients with burns.

Key Terms

Acute radiation syndrome (ARS)

Acute respiratory distress syndrome (ARDS)

Allogeneic skin grafting

Allografts

Autografting

Autologous skin grafting

Burn shock

Carboxyhemoglobin level

Chemical burn

Débridement

Electrical burn

Eschar

Escharotomy

Fasciotomy

Fluid resuscitation

Full-thickness burn

Hypermetabolic state

Inhalational injury

Laser Doppler imaging (LDI)

Lund and Browder method

Major burn

Minor burn

Moderate burn

Myoglobinuria

Partial-thickness burn

Rad

Rems

Rule of nines

Skin grafting

Thermal burn

Total body surface area (TBSA)

Zone of coagulation

Zone of hyperemia

Zone of stasis

Accidental burns, common injuries that can range from mild to life-threatening, are the fourth-leading cause of accidental death after incidents involving falls, motor vehicle accidents, and violence.

Although most acute burn injuries are managed on an outpatient basis, severe burns require hospitalization and surgical intervention. They cause a significant amount of pain, scarring, disfigurement, organ dysfunction, and psychological trauma for those affected.

Burns are categorized according to the source that produces the injury, such as thermal, chemical, electrical, or radiation energy. Regardless of the etiology, a number of factors determine the magnitude and severity of the burn:

- Burn depth
- Percentage of the body surface area injured
- Age of the patient
- Extent of associated systemic involvement

Prognosis after a burn injury has improved over the last four decades because of an increased understanding of the systemic damage produced by burn trauma and the development of interventions that facilitate wound healing and prevent infection. It is necessary to recognize the clinical features of burn injuries to facilitate prompt treatment because the quality of care received within the hours immediately after a burn injury is a major determinant of long-term outcome.

Epidemiology

The National Burn Repository issued a report based on data from 101 hospitals in 37 states regarding burn injuries between 2008 and 2017. During this time, adults ages 20 to 59 made up 55% of burn injury cases, children ages 1 to 15 accounted for 23.5%, and adults over age 60 accounted for 15%. The two most common etiologies were fire/flame and scalds, accounting for 76% of cases reported. Most affected individuals reported burn injuries of less than 10% of **total body surface area (TBSA).** Seventy-four percent of the burn injuries were reported to have occurred in the home. Nearly 95% of cases were due to accidents that caused burn injury, with nearly 13% of these reported as work-related. Just over 2% of cases were suspected abuse and 1% were self-inflicted. Deaths from burn injury increased with burn size. Persons with burns of less than 10% TBSA had a 0.6% mortality rate, whereas persons with burns of 50% TBSA had a 37% mortality rate. Those with more than 90% TBSA had an 84% mortality rate. The most common causes of complications were pneumonia, sepsis, and respiratory failure.

Etiology

Burn trauma can be categorized according to the mechanism of injury, that is, injury from thermal, chemical, electrical, or radiation energy. The etiology is used as a predictor of outcome, but the burn's severity depends on the degree of heat intensity, duration of contact, thickness of skin at the point of contact, percent of body surface area (BSA) affected, and extent of systemic involvement.

Thermal Burns

Thermal burns result after exposure to fire, hot objects, scalding liquids, hot grease, or steam. They comprise over 90% of all burn traumas and produce damage to the skin and underlying tissues after exposure to temperatures greater than 111.2°F (40°C). Thermal burn injuries can range from superficial, affecting only the epidermis, to full thickness, which injure subdermal tissues.

Flame burns caused by house fires or flammable liquids produce direct tissue injury. If clothing composed of synthetic fibers is ignited, a full-thickness burn can result because synthetic fibers melt and increase the depth of injury. Flames can create temperatures of thousands of degrees in a confined space, which increases the occurrence of an associated inhalational injury to the airways of the lungs.

Scald burns are specific types of thermal burns. They occur after exposure to hot liquids, grease, or steam and cause tissue necrosis and cellular death within seconds after exposure to temperatures of 158°F (70°C). Because water has a higher specific gravity and is a better conductor of heat than air, a deeper burn can be produced by hot liquids with lower temperatures of 120°F to 130°F. This has prompted many states to mandate that hot water heaters be set below 140°F, which has decreased the incidence of scald burns from hot bath water. The high heat-carrying capacity of steam can also produce significant inhalational injury.

CLINICAL CONCEPT

Accidental scalding from hot liquid produces a characteristic pattern of splashing. A limb that has a circumferential pattern with a demarcation line from the liquid can indicate that the person may have been deliberately burned. Any suspicious history that does not correlate with the appearance of the burn should alert the clinician that abuse might be involved and should be reported.

Chemical Burns

Chemical burns account for less than 10% of all burn injuries and generally occur after an industrial accident or ingestion of harsh household chemicals, including strong acids, alkalis, and corrosive materials. Chemical burns induce protein coagulation of tissues (protein breakdown) as chemical energy is converted into thermal energy. This produces a characteristic gray coloring of the skin.

The severity of the response, which can be localized or systemic, is proportional to the type, quantity, and concentration of the chemical; duration of contact; and degree of penetration of the tissues. Chemical agents that are common offenders include sulfuric acid, ammonia, lye, and chemical warfare agents. Exposure to the agent must be halted by removing the clothes and vigorously irrigating the area to decontaminate the patient or neutralizing the chemical agent to limit injury.

Electrical Burns

Electrical burns account for less than 10% of all burn trauma and range from mild injury after an electrical shock from a low-voltage household current (110 to 220 volts) to death after exposure to high voltage that exceeds 1,000 volts of energy. The electrical current generates heat when it meets resistance in body tissues and produces damage as the current passes through the body, possibly leaving entrance and exit wounds. The path of electrical energy commonly causes internal organ injury.

The degree of injury depends on the amount of voltage, length of contact, and pathway of current. Most low-voltage household current produces deep burns at the exit and entrance wounds. High-voltage injury is divided into true high-tension and flash injuries produced by a bolt of lightning. Voltage greater than 1,000 produces a high-tension injury that causes extensive tissue, muscle, and bone damage and frequently results in loss of limbs. Lightning strikes—a characteristic flash injury lasting only a few milliseconds—traumatize the victim. Electricity tends to flow along the path of least resistance toward a natural ground. Nerves and muscles produce less resistance and therefore suffer greater damage than tendons, fat, and bones. The pathway of current across the heart is associated with the highest mortality, as the alternating current of the electrical shock disrupts normal cardiac conduction, which can produce cardiac arrest.

 CLINICAL CONCEPT

Electrical injury produces intense tissue damage and cellular death, which can lead to metabolic acidosis. Analysis of arterial blood gases to assess acid–base balance is necessary.

Radiation Burns

The risk of cutaneous injury from radiation burns has increased because of the emerging threat of radiological bioterrorism. Although an emergency response team initially manages this type of disaster, since the September 11, 2001, terrorist attacks against the United States, emphasis has shifted to incorporate the entire hospital in crisis management. Clinicians must be prepared to assess and treat patients who have been exposed to dangerous levels of radiation.

Close proximity to an explosion involving ionizing radioactive material can induce significant harm and produce both thermal burns from the explosion and internal or external radioactive contamination. External contamination from radioactive material is usually limited to the skin or underlying tissue damage by a layer of clothing, although cutaneous burns might not be immediately visible. It is important to obtain the patient's history to determine the degree of exposure. Some patients may report exposure to radiation or contact with an unknown metal object from industrial exposure, although the onset of visible symptoms can appear weeks after exposure. Radioactive exposure is measured in terms of "rads." A **rad** is a radiation dose of energy absorbed by the tissues, similar to a joule of energy. However, the radiation dose of energy does not indicate the biological risk of the exposure, which is measured in **"rems."** For example, one dental x-ray or chest x-ray causes a biological risk of 4 to 15 millirems, which is considered minor.

Injury to the external and underlying tissues from acute radiation exposure is known as cutaneous radiation injury (CRI). Diagnosis of CRI is based on the scope of visible damage, dose of radiation, and depth of penetration. There are four stages:

1. Prodromal stage
2. Latent period
3. Manifest illness stage
4. Third wave of erythema

The prodromal stage can begin within minutes after intense radiation exposure or can emerge over 2 days with exposure to smaller doses of radiation. Radiation doses as low as 200 rads can damage the hair follicles and basal layer of skin and produce early cutaneous symptoms of pruritus, inflammation, and transient erythema, which might not be evident for days to weeks after initial exposure. This is followed by the latent period, which is characterized by a lack of symptoms, although cutaneous and systemic damage is still evolving. As the basal cell layer attempts to repair itself, the body enters the manifest illness stage, and severe skin blistering and erythema are observed. If a significant dose of radiation (exposures greater than 1,000 rads) is encountered, then a third phase of cutaneous symptoms known as the third wave of erythema can occur over months or years postexposure. Exposures greater than 1,000 rads produce late effects with permanent damage to hair follicles, sebaceous and sweat glands, and pigment-producing cells. Skin tissue may become fibrotic, then necrotic, and develop ulcers. Usually pain and pigment changes will occur.

Ingestion, inhalation, or entry of radioactive materials via open wounds can induce internal contamination and produce **acute radiation syndrome (ARS)** if exposure to an excessive dose of penetration radiation occurs over a short period. Initially, the patient may be asymptomatic, but systemic contamination ensues until treatment is initiated to promote elimination of the radioactive material. Doses of 25 rads produce systemic effects such as bone marrow suppression and the consequent deficient synthesis of blood cells. High doses of radiation can produce aplastic bone marrow, which requires blood transfusion to replace the low blood cell production. Patients exposed to the highest levels of radiation experience gastrointestinal (GI) symptoms such as nausea, vomiting, and diarrhea, as well as damage to the central nervous system.

 CLINICAL CONCEPT

Initial treatment of ARS focuses on patient decontamination by removing and bagging clothes and shoes, which usually removes more than 80% of radioactive material.

Gentle irrigation of open wounds helps minimize internal contamination, whereas irrigation of intact skin helps decrease further skin abrasion. Localized injuries are treated symptomatically; the Radiation Emergency Assistance Center should be contacted to guide more intensive treatment.

Basic Pathophysiological Concepts Relating to Burns

Burns cause localized integumentary reactions that can be described in terms of three separate zones on the skin. Burns also cause a systemic reaction, which includes hypovolemia, electrolyte disturbances, acid-base imbalance, and a hypermetabolic state. There are associated injuries to the pulmonary, GI, and renal systems. Persons involved in fire accidents often succumb because of inhalational injury. Burns also impair immunity and increase susceptibility to infection.

Integumentary Responses to Burn Injury

A thermal burn injury produces a localized integumentary response consisting of three zones of injury within the skin and subdermal tissues. The deepest point of injury occurs in the **zone of coagulation.** This is the core of the wound with the greatest degree of irreversible tissue necrosis that occurs from protein coagulation and cellular death. The **zone of stasis,** which surrounds the zone of coagulation, is characterized by decreased tissue perfusion with some vascular damage. However, if intervention is aimed at increasing blood flow to this area, minimizing edema, and preventing infection, tissue damage is potentially reversible. The outer zone, the **zone of hyperemia,** is reddened from vasodilation and increased blood flow but has minimal tissue damage and heals quickly (see Fig. 42-1).

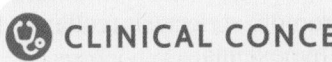

> ### ⊙ CLINICAL CONCEPT
> Normal physiological organ function is disrupted if the thermal injury is greater than 30% of TBSA.

Fluid, Electrolyte, and Acid–Base Imbalance Response to Burn Injury

Cellular damage and cell death release vasoactive substances, including histamine, free radicals, thromboxane, cytokines, and catecholamines, which increase vascular permeability and leakage of albumin and plasma from the blood (extracellular space) into the interstitial space. This shift is greatest during the first 6 to 8 hours after burn injury. As albumin continues to leak out of the bloodstream, colloidal oncotic pressure decreases, which promotes increased fluid loss into the interstitial space. This creates the characteristic severe tissue swelling seen in burned patients. This, coupled with the tremendous evaporative fluid loss from open burn wounds, significantly decreases intravascular and intracellular fluid. If the burn injury encompasses a large surface area, the extensive fluid loss can cause hypovolemic shock. To counteract the loss of albumin and reduced colloid oncotic pressure, intravenous albumin may be infused therapeutically.

Cellular damage from the burn injury causes a large release of intracellular potassium into the extracellular space. This causes hyperkalemia, which increases risk of cardiac arrhythmias.

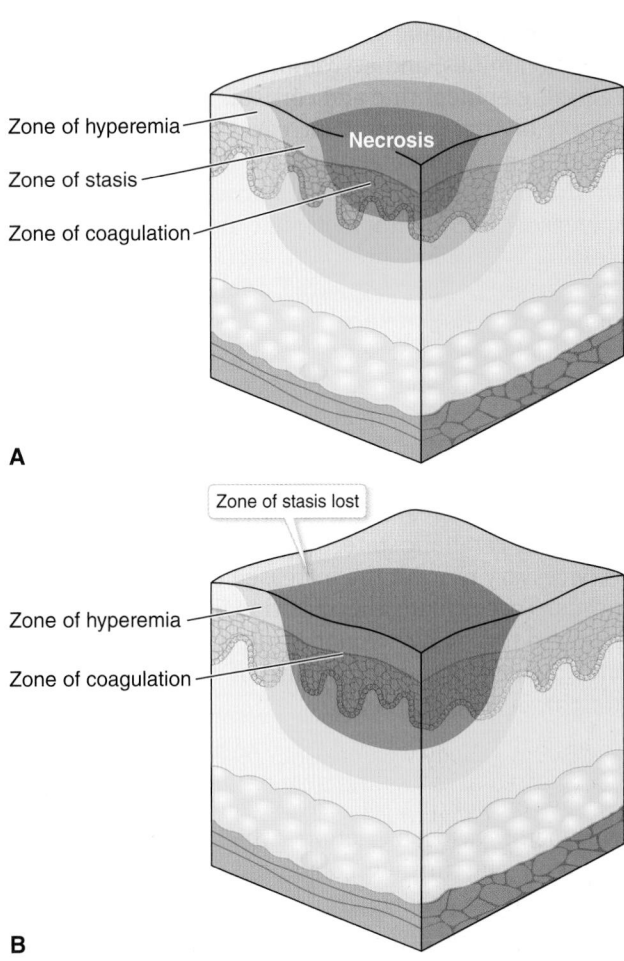

FIGURE 42-1. Zones of injury in burns. **(A)** The central part of a burn, called the *zone of coagulation,* is the worst-affected region. The area surrounding the central burn, called the **zone of stasis,** is characterized by decreased tissue perfusion and can be salvaged with appropriate fluid resuscitation and treatment. **(B)** If treatment is inadequate, the zone of stasis is lost and the central zone of coagulation expands.

In addition to the fluid and electrolyte shifts, acid–base imbalance occurs in extensive burn injury. Severe volume depletion leads to decreased tissue perfusion. Decreased tissue perfusion leads to cellular hypoxia, which triggers anaerobic metabolism. Lactic acid accumulation leads to metabolic acidosis. This is commonly treated with infusion of Ringer's lactate, which can normalize acid–base imbalance.

> **ALERT!** If the patient does not receive adequate fluid resuscitation during the initial resuscitative period of thermal injury, a type of hypovolemic shock termed **burn shock** sets in, which compromises organ perfusion.

Metabolic Changes Due to Burn Injury

A major burn injury triggers the stress response of the body. The body is in an alarm state, with stimulation of the sympathetic nervous system (SNS) releasing catecholamines, and activation of the adrenal glands releasing epinephrine and cortisol. The constant activation of these stimuli increases body metabolism. There is a hypermetabolic state that is proportional to the percentage of TBSA burned. Metabolic rate increases along with metabolic needs of the body. Resting energy requirements increase 50% to 100% compared with an uninjured adult and average 1.3 times the basal metabolic rate. A **hypermetabolic state** heightens energy needs, oxygen consumption, body heat production, and body temperature and causes rapid tissue breakdown. The release of stress hormones activates the mobilization of glycogen, protein, and fat stores, often resulting in a catabolic state, where there is breakdown of lean body mass. To counteract the catabolic state, nutritional supplementation is necessary to meet the increased caloric and protein needs. To calculate the nutritional supplementation required to promote wound healing, the following formula, which is based upon size of the burn and body weight, may be utilized:

$$25 \text{ kcal} \times \text{body weight (kg)} + \% \text{ TBSA}$$

The outpouring of catecholamines also causes peripheral vasoconstriction, which, combined with hypovolemia, further compromises cardiac output. This leads to inadequate organ perfusion and oxygenation. Clinically, hypotension, tachycardia, and decreased urine output will be evident as cardiac output is decreased. If adequate fluid resuscitation is administered during the first 24 hours after burn injury, increased blood pressure is seen as cardiac output is restored to normal.

Pulmonary Responses to Burn Injury

After a severe burn, physiological changes within the pulmonary system are a leading cause of morbidity and mortality. In response to the injury, respiratory rate increases secondary to anxiety or pain, and minute ventilation can increase 2 to 2.5 times the normal rate.

Increased lung capillary permeability and increased pulmonary vascular resistance can affect adequate tissue oxygenation. The pulmonary complications that develop after a major burn are airway edema of the upper respiratory tract and inhalational injury to the lungs. Systemic toxicity can occur from inhalation of toxins such as carbon monoxide. **Acute respiratory distress syndrome (ARDS)** can also be a life-threatening sequela due to capillary permeability after a pulmonary burn injury.

Airway Edema of the Upper Respiratory Tract

Exposure to intense heat and flames produces mucosal damage, erythema, and edema of the upper airway. Edema of the upper airway tissues progresses rapidly, so if the patient manifests signs such as stridor, which is indicative of upper airway edema, the patient should be intubated immediately to prevent total airway obstruction.

Inhalational Injury

Inhalational injury should be suspected in people trapped in an enclosed space and exposed to smoke, noxious fumes, and steam inhalation. It should also be suspected in individuals who lose consciousness because the protective reflex of the vocal cords that limits injury to the lungs is lost, resulting in damage to the lower airway. Depending on the type of burning material, injury of the respiratory tract mucosa from the oropharynx to the alveoli can occur. Damage includes loss of bronchial cilia, decreased alveolar surfactant, interstitial edema, and release of inflammatory substances that increase pulmonary vascular resistance and narrow small airways. All of these factors impair the diffusion of oxygen from the alveoli into the pulmonary capillaries and create a mismatch of ventilation and perfusion, as well as the potential for hypoxemia. It is also important to realize that overhydration from excessive fluid resuscitation can cause accumulation of fluid in the interstitial space, because increased capillary permeability allows the shifts of fluid from the intravascular to the interstitial space. This can cause chest wall edema, which will decrease total lung compliance, promote atelectasis (collapse of alveoli), and perpetuate hypoxemia.

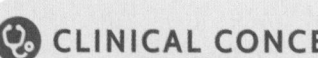

CLINICAL CONCEPT

The risk of inhalational injury and carbon monoxide (CO) poisoning is increased if the patient is burned in an enclosed space.

CO is contained in the smoke and fumes of a fire. In the body, CO binds to hemoglobin and pushes oxygen off, which leads to hypoxia. The initial chest x-ray may be normal, and the patient may be asymptomatic for up to 24 hours before respiratory distress develops. If the patient is demonstrating signs or symptoms indicative of respiratory distress such as stridor, hoarseness, use of accessory muscles, and increased work of breathing, the patient should be intubated immediately to prevent total airway obstruction.

Gastrointestinal Responses to Burn Injury

Patients with burns greater than 35% of TBSA have decreased circulating blood flow to the GI tract due to hypovolemia and the stimulation of the SNS. Hypovolemia and the extensive catecholamine release of the SNS cause both decreased GI circulation and activity. This can impair GI motility, interfere with absorption of nutrients, and lead to paralytic ileus. Hypovolemia and reduced cardiac output can promote ischemia and sloughing of the gastric mucosa. Interventions to increase perfusion to the GI tract include adequate fluid resuscitation and the use of positive inotropic medications such as dopamine to support blood pressure. Additionally, the combination of early enteral feedings and the use of proton pump inhibitors (PPIs) or H_2 blockers is needed to prevent damage to the gastric mucosa. PPIs are recommended for prophylactic acid suppression. This has virtually eliminated the development of Curling's ulcer, a gastric stress ulcer that occurred in severely burned patients years ago, before the availability of PPIs.

 CLINICAL CONCEPT

A Curling's ulcer is a gastric ulcer that develops in individuals who are severely burned due to the extensive stress response. PPIs are commonly administered early in treatment to prevent this disorder.

Effects of Burn Injury on Immunity

A thermal injury causes massive impairment of the immune system; therefore, any prior immunological abnormality has a profound impact on morbidity and mortality. Serum levels of immunoglobulins and complement activation are reduced, and the production and function of white blood cells, such as neutrophils, monocytes, and macrophages, are suppressed. Decreased interleukins-1 and interleukins-2, decreased T-helper cells, and overstimulation of suppressor T cells impair the cellular immune response. An increased risk of infection is promoted by loss of the skin barrier, by excessive nutritional needs induced by the hypermetabolic state, and by increased release of mediators at the wound site that causes suppression of the immune response.

Additionally, an open burn wound provides excellent conditions to support bacterial growth: dead cell debris provides nutrients for the bacteria, and burns reduce blood flow and inflammatory response to invasion of organisms. Thus, aggressive early surgical **débridement** is advocated to improve blood flow to the burned area. This stimulates tissue regeneration and restores phagocytic activity to fight invading organisms while decreasing the risk of opportunistic infection. Opportunistic infections can lead to rejection of skin grafts and delayed wound closure; despite improvement in antimicrobial therapy, sepsis continues to be a leading cause of death in patients with burns.

Renal Responses to Burn Injury

After the initial burn injury, reduced blood flow to the kidneys is proportional to the degree of hypovolemia.

There is also vasoconstriction of the renal arterial circulation due to the stimulation of the SNS. Diminished renal blood flow activates the renin–angiotensin–aldosterone system and stimulates the release of antidiuretic hormone, which causes retention of sodium and water, as well as major loss of potassium, calcium, and magnesium. If fluid resuscitation is inadequate to restore intravascular volume, renal ischemia can develop and lead to acute kidney injury. Laboratory findings include elevated serum creatinine and decreased creatinine clearance. Intervention is aimed at restoring intravascular volume and avoidance of nephrotoxic medications such as aminoglycoside antibiotics and vancomycin. In addition, an electrical burn injury causes significant muscle breakdown and release of myoglobin into the bloodstream. Because of the large size of myoglobin, mechanical obstruction of the renal tubules can develop and lead to acute tubular necrosis and renal failure if fluid resuscitation is inadequate. Therefore, it is recommended to maintain urine output at 50 to 100 mL per hour until laboratory studies indicate that myoglobin levels are normal.

Assessment

Initially after a burn injury, the patient's airway, breathing, and circulation needs should be assessed. Clinicians need to establish hemodynamic stability and oxygenation of the patient and then survey the body for the extent of the burn injury. During assessment of a patient with burns, determining the size and depth of the burn is important because it:

- Provides information about the severity of the injury
- Guides fluid resuscitation
- Determines the need for surgical intervention
- Acts as a strong predictor of mortality

The depth of the burn injury also affects long-term cosmetic appearance and degree of functional impairment. The traditional classification of burns as first, second, third, and fourth degree has been replaced by categories that describe the depth of destruction of the cellular layers of the skin: superficial, partial thickness, and full thickness.

Superficial Burns

Superficial burns, formerly known as first-degree burns, damage only the epidermal layer. They result from severe sunburn, hot liquid splash, or a brief flash burn. The skin is dry, as blistering does not occur, but vasodilation produces a characteristic redness of the skin. Although initially painful, these burns usually heal in less than a week without long-term scarring. It is not necessary to calculate the percentage of BSA affected for a superficial burn.

Partial-Thickness Burns

Partial-thickness burns, formerly known as second-degree burns, can be either superficial partial thickness or deep partial thickness, depending on the degree of tissue necrosis of the dermal layer. Superficial partial-thickness burns char the epidermis and papillary dermal layer, with resultant edema and formation of epidermal blisters. Burned skin is wet, raw, and pink or cherry red in color that blanches with pressure. These burns are quite painful and usually result from hot liquid scalding or direct skin contact with chemicals, flash, or open flame. Although superficial partial-thickness burns can spontaneously heal within 3 to 6 weeks without surgical intervention, some degree of scarring and change in skin pigmentation is possible. However, if the potential for infection is a concern, excision and skin grafting may be necessary.

A deep partial-thickness burn injury extends from the epidermis through the papillary and reticular layers of the dermis. The appearance of the skin is similar to a superficial partial-thickness burn, although skin color may be more mottled depending on the degree of blood flow to the area. The patient may or may not describe pain depending on the viability of nerve tissue. Blisters are commonly present and should not be opened because preventing infection is key in deep partial-thickness burns.

Full-Thickness Burns

Full-thickness burns, formerly known as third-degree burns, damage the epidermis, dermis, hair follicles, and all underlying structures. Pain is rare because of the destruction of nerve endings. The skin's appearance is white, brown, black, or red, and the surrounding tissue is very edematous. These burns are caused by prolonged exposure to intense heat, open flames, electrical currents, or chemical agents. In children or older adults, a hot liquid scald can produce a full-thickness burn.

Diagnosis

Diagnosis of a burn requires assessment of the extent and depth of the burn injury; this also determines the appropriate treatment. The extent of injury is expressed as a percentage of TBSA burned and must be established before developing a plan of care.

There are various methods for determining the extent of the burn wound, including the rule of nines, the Lund and Browder method, and the American Burn Association (ABA) Classification of Burn Injury.

> ### 🩺 CLINICAL CONCEPT
>
> The diagnosis of burns entails the thickness of involved body layers and percentage of BSA.

Rule of Nines

The **rule of nines** is a rapid method used during the prehospital and emergent phase of care. The body is divided into regions that present 9%, or multiples of nine, with the exception of the perineum, which is 1% of BSA. The face and back of the head are 4.5% each, so the entire head is 9%. The anterior and posterior portion of the arm is 9%, and the total for each leg is 18%.

The rule of nines is fairly accurate for adults; however, for children it must be modified because of the differences in BSA between an adult and child. For example, a child's head comprises 18% of their TBSA, because a child's head is large in proportion to the child's body, whereas in the mature adult, the head comprises only 9% of the TBSA. The patient's total area of burn is estimated by adding the percentages of surface area burned (see Fig. 42-2).

> ### 🩺 CLINICAL CONCEPT
>
> In adults, the rule of nines is most commonly used to estimate TBSA involved in a burn.

Lund and Browder Method

The **Lund and Browder method** of assessing burns is a more accurate estimation of affected body surface.

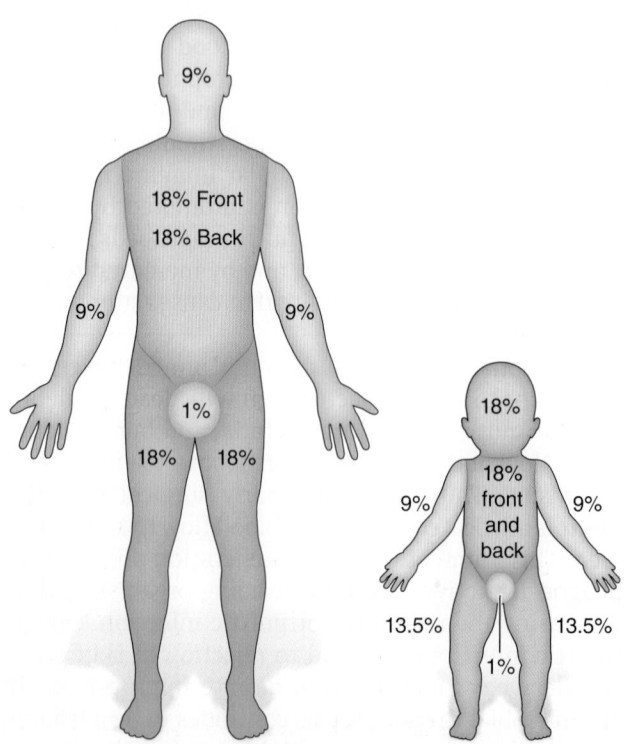

FIGURE 42-2. Rule of nines. The rule of nines is a standardized method used to quickly assess how much body surface area has been burned on a patient. This rule is only applied to partial-thickness (second-degree) and full-thickness (third-degree) burns. The diagrams depict BSA percentages for adults (**A**) and infants of 1 year or younger (**B**).

It divides the body into smaller sections of TBSA and evaluates the percentages of these areas. Again, the patient's total area of burn is estimated by adding the percentages of surface area burned (see Fig 42-3).

American Burn Association Classification of Burn Injury

The ABA Classification of Burn Injury uses both the extent and the depth of burns to classify burns as minor, moderate, or major. The ABA uses the rule of nines to determine TBSA as a basis for their classification.

A **minor burn** injury is described as:

- A partial-thickness burn of less than 15% TBSA in adults and less than 10% TBSA in children
- A full-thickness burn of less than 2% TBSA not involving special care areas, such as the eyes, ears, face, hands, feet, perineum, or joints

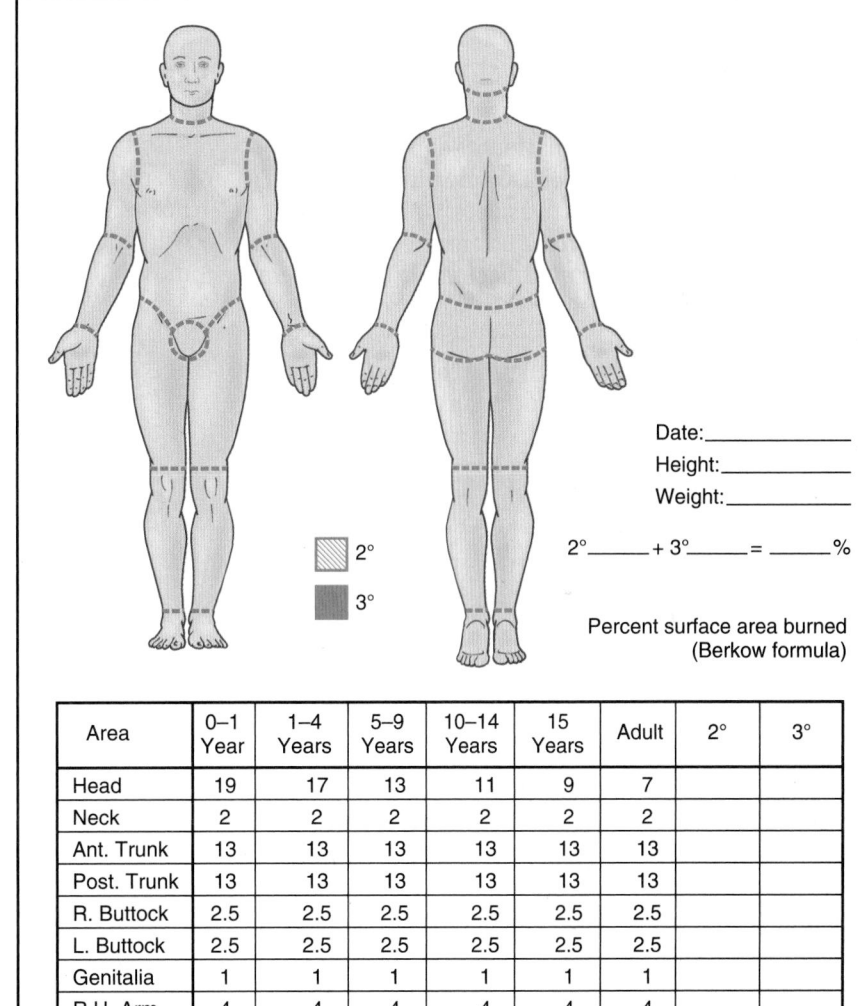

Date:_____
Height:_____
Weight:_____

2°_____ + 3°_____ = _____%

Percent surface area burned
(Berkow formula)

Area	0–1 Year	1–4 Years	5–9 Years	10–14 Years	15 Years	Adult	2°	3°
Head	19	17	13	11	9	7		
Neck	2	2	2	2	2	2		
Ant. Trunk	13	13	13	13	13	13		
Post. Trunk	13	13	13	13	13	13		
R. Buttock	2.5	2.5	2.5	2.5	2.5	2.5		
L. Buttock	2.5	2.5	2.5	2.5	2.5	2.5		
Genitalia	1	1	1	1	1	1		
R.U. Arm	4	4	4	4	4	4		
L.U. Arm	4	4	4	4	4	4		
R.L. Arm	3	3	3	3	3	3		
L.L. Arm	3	3	3	3	3	3		
R. Hand	2.5	2.5	2.5	2.5	2.5	2.5		
L. Hand	2.5	2.5	2.5	2.5	2.5	2.5		
R. Thigh	5.5	6.5	8	8.5	9	9.5		
L. Thigh	5.5	6.5	8	8.5	9	9.5		
R. Leg	5	5	5.5	6	6.5	7		
L. Leg	5	5	5.5	6	6.5	7		
R. Foot	3.5	3.5	3.5	3.5	3.5	3.5		
L. Foot	3.5	3.5	3.5	3.5	3.5	3.5		
Total								

FIGURE 42-3. The Lund and Browder classification. The Lund and Browder classification is a method for estimating the extent of burns on persons of different ages. It is particularly useful in assessing burns in children. In children, the head has a larger surface area and the lower limbs have a smaller surface area than in adults.

A **moderate burn** injury, or uncomplicated burn, is described as:

- A partial-thickness burn of 15% to 25% TBSA in adults or 10% to 20% in children
- A full-thickness burn of less than 10% TBSA not involving special care areas

A **major burn** injury is described as:

- A partial-thickness burn exceeding 25% TBSA in adults or 20% in children
- All full-thickness burns exceeding 10% TBSA
- All burns involving the eyes, ears, face, hands, feet, perineum, and/or joints
- All burns involving inhalation injury, electrical injury, concurrent trauma, and patients at high risk

Laser Doppler Imaging

In addition to clinical estimation of depth and extent of skin injury in burns, **laser Doppler imaging (LDI)** can be used. LDI is a noninvasive, painless scanning procedure that is done 36 to 72 hours after burn injury. Burn depth can be estimated accurately using measurements of skin perfusion with LDI. It can be used to determine which patients require surgical intervention versus conservative medical treatment based on burn depth. Deep burns require surgery, and superficial burns can be treated conservatively, as spontaneous reepithelialization can be expected to occur.

Significant Laboratory Parameters in Burn Injury

There are some basic laboratory tests to perform when treating a patient with burn injury. Upon admission, baseline laboratory results should be obtained, which include a complete blood count (CBC), electrolyte level, urinalysis, arterial blood gas, and a **carboxyhemoglobin level** if the burn injury occurred in a closed space and inhalation injury is suspected. A CBC is monitored routinely to assess the degree of hemoconcentration and the elevation of white blood cells if infection is present. Electrolytes are monitored to evaluate sodium concentration, which decreases secondary to fluid shifts and potassium levels, which are initially elevated as a result of fluid shifts into the extracellular space. Potassium levels return to normal as the burn shock resolves. Creatinine phosphokinase (CPK) is measured in electrical burns to indicate the severity of muscle damage. Renal function tests, including blood urea nitrogen (BUN) and serum creatinine, are routinely measured; elevation of BUN indicates dehydration, and elevation of creatinine indicates renal insufficiency. A urinalysis is used to monitor the adequacy of renal perfusion and the patient's nutritional status. **Myoglobinuria,** or dark brown urine, signals development of tubular necrosis. The breakdown of plasma proteins and dehydration are indicated through spilling protein in the urine

(proteinuria) as nitrogen is excreted in large amounts in catabolic states. Arterial blood gases indicate the presence of hypoxia, as well as acid–base disturbances.

 CLINICAL CONCEPT

In severe burns, muscle breakdown causes myoglobinuria. Myoglobinuria causes acute tubular necrosis, which leads to acute kidney injury.

Treatment

Treatment of burns varies from outpatient application of topical antiseptics to the multidisciplinary team approach of a specialized burn center. Individuals who sustain minor burns can follow the American Burn Association's (2020) first aid treatment guidelines (see Box 42.1). Individuals who sustain a major burn injury will require the intensive care of a burn center. However, most burns are minor and are treated in the emergency department. Burn care occurs in three phases:

1. Emergent phase
2. Acute phase
3. Rehabilitation phase

BOX 42-1. Burn First Aid: Initial Treatment

- Stop the burning process: Apply cool (NOT COLD, NOT ICE) water for at least 5 minutes by running water over the burn, and applying a clean, wet towel.
- Do NOT use butter or ointments on the burn wounds as this may hinder healing
- If possible, remove jewelry, rings, and constrictive clothing. However, if clothing is adherent to burn area, do not remove.
- Protect the burn from constrictive pressure and friction and cover with a clean, dry cotton dressing.
- Relieve pain and swelling with ibuprofen or acetaminophen.
- If blisters are present, leave intact–do not break.
- Seek medical attention if there is a persistent fever not relieved by medication, redness that may extend beyond the border of the burn, or pain is not controlled by ibuprofen or acetaminophen.
- Drink plenty of fluids (electrolyte-containing solutions such as Gatorade) if the person appears to be dehydrated.
- Burned extremities should be elevated above the level of the heart to facilitate circulation.
- Do not delay seeking medical attention if the burn is larger than the size of the victim's hand.

Adapted from American Burn Association (ABA). 2020. Burn first aid. Retrieved from https://ameriburn.org/wp-content/uploads/2020/03/first-aid-fact-sheet.pdf

Emergent Phase

The emergent phase begins with the onset of the injury and continues until completion of fluid resuscitation. During this phase, the estimation of the extent of the burn, first aid measures, and fluid resuscitation are accomplished. The goal is to prevent shock and respiratory distress and to assess and treat additional injuries. The initial focus of care addresses the ABC-DEF (airway, breathing, circulation, disability, exposure, and fluid resuscitation) of trauma care because the systemic injuries, if present, pose a threat to life.

Thermal Burns

All prehospital interventions are aimed at eliminating the heat source, stabilizing the patient's condition, identifying the type of burn, preventing heat loss, and preparing to transport. At the scene of thermal burn injury, the flames must be extinguished so the rescuers can ensure both their own and the victim's safety. The burn wound is then irrigated with cool water to halt the burning process; this gives immediate relief from the pain and limits edema and tissue damage. Restrictive clothing and items such as rings or belts should be removed if in the burned area.

> **ALERT!** It is important never to use ice on a large burn area because it may induce blood vessel constriction, worsen tissue damage, and cause hypothermia.

The next step is to quickly assess the airway and initiate oxygen therapy based on the type and location of injury. Maintain a patent airway, or intubate if the patient is demonstrating signs and symptoms of respiratory compromise. If no respiratory distress is present, 100% oxygen should be administered by face mask and the patient's head elevated 30 degrees. If the burn injury occurred as the result of an explosion or in an enclosed space, there is a higher likelihood of inhalation injury; supplemental oxygen is the treatment of choice to reverse the systemic effects of CO poisoning. No fluids are given by mouth because of a potential for vomiting and aspiration related to stress. A large-bore IV line will be started, preferably in a non-burned area, to initiate fluid resuscitation and prevent burn shock in patients with a TBSA greater than 20%. **Fluid resuscitation** is initiated using crystalloid and colloid solutions, which are similar to the composition of blood. The goal is to provide adequate fluid volume that supports perfusion of organs and maintains acid–base balance. Ringer's lactate is a commonly used intravenous fluid that is effective for fluid resuscitation and treatment of metabolic acidosis, which commonly occurs in large burn injuries. Fluid resuscitation needs to be precisely balanced between providing adequate circulation and preventing overload that can lead to pulmonary edema. Fluid resuscitation should be approximately 0.5 mL/kg/hr in adults. A cardiac monitor should be connected to the patient to evaluate for hemodynamic stability including the presence of dysrhythmias. Hyperkalemia is a common complication of cell injury, which increases risk of rhythm disturbances and cardiac arrest. Vital signs should be monitored to assess the circulatory system, as well as the patient's response to fluid resuscitation. Burned extremities are elevated above the level of the heart to facilitate circulation.

> **CLINICAL CONCEPT**
>
> In patients with a burn of more than 20% of TBSA, IV lactated Ringer's solution is commonly administered.

Chemical Burns

When the injury is related to chemical exposure, brush off the dry chemical agent, remove all clothing, and irrigate with copious amounts of water immediately for approximately 20 minutes to interrupt the chemical's contact with the skin. There may be chemicals that require specialized treatment; if the information is not readily available onsite, call the Poison Control Center for information.

> **CLINICAL CONCEPT**
>
> Health-care providers must wear chemical-resistant clothing and protective equipment before initiating treatment for chemical burns.

> **ALERT!** Acid or alkali contamination of the eyes is the most detrimental type of chemical burn and requires immediate and copious irrigation.

Electrical Burns

For electrical burns, first ensure the source of electrical current has been disconnected. Assess the patient for responsiveness and initiate cardiopulmonary resuscitation (CPR) if indicated.

All patients injured with an electrical burn, including those injured by lightning, have an increased risk for trauma and fractures caused by intense muscle contraction from the electrical current, from a fall, or from the hazardous flash of the electricity. The major concern is the increased risk for cervical spine injury. So, it is imperative that the patient not be moved until the cervical spine has been immobilized with the application of a semirigid collar. This places the cervical spine in a neutral position and reduces the risk of spinal cord compression.

Radiation Burns

For radiation burns resulting from an industrial accident, trained personnel will render the contaminated areas safe for entry. Interventions are focused on shielding, distance, and limiting the time of exposure. Specific conditions exist for a patient to be transferred to a specialized burn center (see Box 42-2).

Acute Phase

The acute phase begins 48 to 72 hours after the burn injury; it includes the start of diuresis (loss of water from the body) and ends with closure of the burn wound. Continued assessment of respiratory and circulatory status related to edema and fluid shifts, nutritional support, infection prevention, and burn wound care are priorities during this phase. Hydrotherapy, excision, and early **skin grafting** (surgical implantation of new skin) of full-thickness wounds are performed as

---

BOX 42-2. Burn Center Referral Criteria

A burn center may treat adults, children, or both. Burn injuries that should be referred to a burn center include the following:

1. Partial-thickness burns of more than 10% of the total body surface area (TBSA).
2. Burns that involve the face, hands, feet, genitalia, perineum, or major joints.
3. Third-degree (full-thickness) burns in any age group.
4. Electrical burns, including lightning injury.
5. Chemical burns.
6. Inhalation injury.
7. Burn injury in patients with preexisting medical disorders that could complicate management, prolong recovery, or affect mortality.
8. Any patient with burns and concomitant trauma (such as fractures) in which the burn injury poses the greatest risk of morbidity or mortality. In such cases, if the trauma poses the greater immediate risk, the patient's condition may be stabilized initially in a trauma center before transfer to a burn center. Clinician judgment will be necessary in such situations and should be in concert with the regional medical control plan and triage protocols.
9. Burned children in hospitals without qualified personnel or equipment for the care of children.
10. Burn injury in patients who will require special social, emotional, or rehabilitative intervention.

From Anonymous (2007). Guidelines for the operation of burn centers. *J Burn Care Res, 28*(1), 134–141.

---

soon as possible after the injury. Infection is combated through application of topical antimicrobial agents to the burn surface areas in addition to daily wound cleansing. Enteral (tube feedings) or total parenteral nutrition feedings will be initiated as necessary to meet the caloric needs for healing and the hypermetabolic state of the patient with burns. Pain management continues to be a priority in the plan of care for the patient with burns, especially before procedures such as dressing changes and wound débridement.

During this time frame, there is a shift of fluids from the interstitial to the intravascular space, and diuresis begins as capillaries regain integrity. There must be continued caution with fluid administration because of the fluid loss from large burn wounds. In older adult patients and in patients with inadequate cardiac or renal function, fluid overload occurs with the resulting signs and symptoms of congestive heart failure (CHF). Early detection and intervention with vasoactive medications, diuretics, and fluid restriction may prevent CHF and pulmonary edema.

The patient with burns is at high risk for sepsis related to the immunosuppression that accompanies extensive burn injuries. Monitoring of the patient's temperature is important for early detection of bacteremia or septicemia. It is not uncommon for patients to have a low-grade fever for several weeks after the burn injury. In order to reduce the metabolic stress and oxygen requirements of the tissue, the patient may be given acetaminophen and a cooling blanket to maintain a temperature of 99°F to 101°F (37.2°C to 38.3°C).

 CLINICAL CONCEPT

The burn wound is an excellent site for bacterial growth such as *Escherichia coli*, the primary source being the patient's own intestinal tract; it is also an excellent site for fungi such as *Candida albicans* to grow.

Tissue specimens are obtained routinely for culture and sensitivity to monitor for colonization by microbes. Antibiotics are not prescribed routinely unless a specific organism has been identified because of the risk of promoting resistant organisms. The exception to this is preoperatively and postoperatively, the patient is given systemic antibiotics because of the increased risk of exposure to the surface bacteria during the débridement.

ALERT! Infection is the major cause of death in the patient who survives a major burn.

The environment is a secondary source of microbes. So when providing wound care, use clean technique when caring directly for burn wounds. Burn wounds are cleansed daily, at a minimum, and by a variety of methods, including immersion in a hydrotherapy tub. Treatments can be metabolically and psychologically stressful for the patient, so paying attention to the patient's physiological and emotional comfort will enhance their ability to participate.

 CLINICAL CONCEPT

Acticoat antimicrobial barrier dressing is a new silver-coated dressing approved for burn wound and donor site treatment. This particular dressing may be left in place for up to 7 days and is remoistened every 3 to 4 hours with sterile water.

The conditions of the wounds are carefully documented, with special attention given to color, odor, exudates, and any signs of reepithelialization. Débridement removes contaminated and necrotic tissue, also called **eschar.** Débridement enhances healing and prepares a site for grafting.

Natural débridement occurs when the dead tissue separates from the underlying tissue spontaneously. The body's natural enzymes cause this separation of burned tissue from the underlying viable tissue. Mechanical débridement involves scissors and forceps to remove the eschar, usually done with the dressing changes. Dressings themselves may be used as a débriding agent, as in the instance of wet-to-dry dressings that remove tissue as the dressing is removed. However, this method of wet to dry can be extremely painful for the patient and cause damage to granulation tissue.

Surgical interventions include escharotomy, surgical débridement, and autografting. **Escharotomy** is a surgical procedure to prevent circumferential constriction of a limb or the chest. Surgical débridement is an operative procedure as opposed to natural débridement. It consists of removing tissue to the level of the viable tissue at the fascia level, also called **fasciotomy.** This procedure is reserved for patients with full-thickness burns because it removes potentially viable fat and lymph tissues.

Skin Grafting

Autografting is a procedure performed in the operating room to provide early burn wound coverage. In this procedure, healthy skin is removed from nonburned areas of the patient, known as donor sites, and transferred to burned areas. This procedure is termed **autologous skin grafting;** the current gold standard in the surgical treatment of burn injury. However, if large areas of burn regions require grafting, the amount of the patient's own skin may be limited.

Allogeneic skin grafting using deceased donor skin grafts **(allografts)** can be used on a patient's burned regions; however, tissue matching is necessary with this procedure. It is not yet possible to completely inhibit the patient's immune reaction against allografted skin. Immunosuppressive drugs are needed to counteract tissue rejection, which in turn leads to immunocompromise of the patient and risk of infection. Despite intensive research efforts, no skin substitute has yet succeeded in sufficiently replacing the function of the patient's original skin.

Over the years, tissue engineering has been able to provide a wide range of industrially manufactured skin substitutes. Dermal skin substitutes include decellularized dermis derived from human or animal sources, artificially constructed scaffolds comprised of highly purified biomaterials, and entirely synthetic polymers. These are currently showing various rates of success.

In the near future, three-dimensional (3D) bioprinting is a potential approach for skin tissue engineering. Bioprinting, involving computer-controlled deposition of scaffolds and cells in a plethora of shapes and patterns, can offer the potential to fully replicate native human skin. As described in literature, multilayered approaches using fibroblast, keratinocytes, and collagen have been used to bioprint human skin.

In patients with large burn areas, it may be necessary to use biosynthetic dressings to provide temporary coverage until skin grafting is possible. These dressings contain animal-derived components and synthetic polymers and should be applied as early as possible. The coverage of the wound decreases pain, promotes healing, and reduces the incidence of infection.

Most skin graft sites are covered with an occlusive dressing to immobilize the graft. Depending on the graft's site, occupational therapy may construct a splint to assist in preventing the graft from dislodging. The occlusive dressing will be left in place for 2 to 5 days after surgery. Great care is taken in positioning and turning the patient to prevent dislodging of the graft or placing pressure on the graft site. The donor site will be painful if not covered because it is a partial-thickness wound. The site must be observed for excess drainage and signs of infection. It is usually covered with a moist gauze dressing and heals within 7 to 14 days.

Rehabilitation Phase

The rehabilitation phase may extend for years after the injury and actually begins during the emergent phase with the application of splints and the initiation of physical therapy. Active and passive range-of-motion exercises are initiated as soon as possible to prevent the development of contractures (inflexible contracted musculature). Scar tissue formation can be modified with pressure dressings, such as Ace wraps over the burn dressings, especially when the patients are ambulating. As the burn wounds are grafted, specialized tubular support bandages are applied to supply an equal amount of pressure to the wounds to prevent or decrease the amount of scar formation.

Pain Management in Burn Injuries

Pain management is one of the most difficult challenges of burn care. Not only does the burn injury produce severe pain, but wound care modalities also induce a significant amount of discomfort above the baseline pain experienced at rest. Yet despite these complications, pain must be treated aggressively to keep it controlled.

In burn care, there are different types of pain depending on the extent and depth of the burn area. A partial-thickness burn causes constant pain when exposed to air because the nerve endings are exposed. Full-thickness burns are not painful in the areas of the deep burn because the nerve endings are damaged, but they are painful at the edges of the burn.

Pain management is initiated during the emergent phase. The patient's degree of pain must be routinely assessed and medicated appropriately to manage the intensity. Any manipulation of the burned area or dressing is very painful, as the removal of bandages commonly causes some denuding of the superficial surfaces of wounds. IV opioids, such as oxycodone or morphine, and fentanyl are commonly necessary 20 minutes before dressing changes. Sedation may also be needed. Oral, intramuscular, and subcutaneous routes are avoided until the patient is hemodynamically stable and has full tissue perfusion. Dressings are changed on a schedule that is dependent on the topical agent used. The staff members performing the dressing change wear gowns, gloves, and hair and eye protection for their protection, as well as the patient's protection. Dressings are usually cut, removed, and disposed of according to the procedure established for contaminated materials. If the dressing adheres to a burn wound, it may be moistened with saline or soaked off in a hydrotherapy tub.

Depending on the severity of the burn, patients can be involved in the initial débridement and cleansing of their wounds. This gives the patient some control over this painful procedure. However, patients with extensive burns cannot perform self-care. Patient-controlled analgesia using IV opioid agents enhances the patient's ability to cope with the pain because the patient has control of the medication.

 CLINICAL CONCEPT

Premedication with analgesics is necessary before dressing changes in severe burn injuries. Opioid agents are usually required to relieve the pain.

Common Complications of Burn Injury

Infection and Sepsis

Infection is the most common complication after burn injury, causing death in 60% of burn victims.

After burn injury, the major barrier to environmental pathogens, the skin, is lost. There is also immunosuppression with deficient T cells and macrophage-mediated defenses. Because circulation is diminished in the burn region, there is a deficient number of white blood cells reaching the area of injury. Significant inflammatory mediators are unable to protect the body. Major pathogens that infect burn wounds include bacteria and fungi. *Staphylococcus aureus,* particularly methicillin-resistant *S. aureus* (MRSA), is a common cause of invasive wound infection. *Pseudomonas aeruginosa,* Enterococcus, *E. coli, Klebsiella pneumoniae,* and *Acinetobacter baumannii* are also common bacterial pathogens. *Candida* is the most common fungal organism. Antibiotic-resistant strains often arise that challenge effective eradication of infection. Prolonged hospitalization is one of the strongest risk factors for the development of infection, as there is potential exposure to other colonized or infected patients and to environmental contamination. According to the ABA, the various types of burn wound infections include wound colonization, wound infection, invasive infection, cellulitis, necrotizing infection/fasciitis, and sepsis. Wound colonization is characterized by the presence of low concentrations of bacteria (fewer than 10^5 organisms) on the surface without invasion. Wound infection consists of more than 10^5 organisms that cause systemic signs and symptoms. Invasive infection involves more than 10^5 organisms in deeper tissue such as muscle or bone. Cellulitis is characterized as erythema, induration, warmth, and tenderness in the tissue surrounding the burn wound. Necrotizing fasciitis is a deep aggressive infection of muscle and bone with destruction of tissue. Sepsis is extensive infection in the bloodstream. Several criteria are used to diagnose sepsis. A diagnosis requires the presence of infection, which can be proven or suspected, and two or more of a list of criteria (see Chapter 46). Significant findings that indicate sepsis include hypotension (systolic blood pressure less than 90 mm Hg or a decrease of more than 40 mm Hg in the patient's normal systolic blood pressure) and serum lactate level greater than 1 mmol/L.

Topical antimicrobials for the prevention and treatment of burn wound infection include mafenide acetate, silver sulfadiazine, silver nitrate solution, and silver-impregnated dressings. The topical agent is applied in a thin layer to the burn wound and then covered with gauze dressings. Fingers and toes are each wrapped separately to promote mobility and ability to heal. Facial burns may be left open to air, but are observed closely to prevent drying that may cause conversion to a deeper burn. Circumferential burns are dressed from the distal portion to the proximal portion, with attention paid to the joints to allow for motion.

When an infection is identified, antimicrobial therapy should be directed at the pathogen recovered on culture. In the setting of invasive infection or evidence of sepsis, empiric therapy should be initiated. Surgical wound care should be directed at thoroughly removing devitalized tissue and debris. A broad-spectrum surgical antimicrobial topical scrub, such as chlorhexidine gluconate, should be used along with preemptive analgesia and sedation to permit adequate wound care.

Acute Respiratory Distress Syndrome

ARDS is a leading cause of death in severe burn injuries. It can evolve into multiple organ failure (MOF), which has an 80% mortality rate. ARDS can occur when there is a large area of burn injury, direct lung injury, inhalation injury, or sepsis. The risk of ARDS increases when the burn is greater than 40% TBSA or the full-thickness burn is greater than 20%. During ARDS, there is capillary hyperpermeability within the lungs that causes fluid to leak into the alveoli. Oxygenation and gas exchange are obstructed, causing hypoxemia. Patients develop respiratory distress with tachypnea, nasal flaring, use of accessory muscles, cough, hypotension, tachycardia, and fever. The patient requires deep sedation and mechanical ventilation and careful fluid management. Extracorporeal membrane oxygenation (ECMO) and vasoconstrictors may be necessary.

Compartment Syndrome

Full-thickness circumferential and near-circumferential skin burns result in the formation of tough, inelastic, dead, burned tissue called eschar. Eschar can cause burn-induced compartment syndrome, which is a buildup of pressure within an area of the body so restrictive that it suppresses circulation to the region. This is caused by the accumulation of extracellular and extravascular fluid within confined anatomic spaces of the extremities or other parts of the body. The excessive fluid causes collapse of blood vessels within the region, which can lead to ischemia and infarction of tissue. Eschar around the torso can cause chest wall restriction and hinder ventilation. Abdominal compartment syndrome can cause hypoperfusion of organs within the abdomen and torso. Circumferential burns involving the neck may cause airway obstruction and restricted venous return. Treatment consists of surgical escharotomy or fasciotomy, which is the excision of the restrictive eschar tissue. This releases tissue restriction and allows for circulation.

> **ALERT!** Compartment syndrome occurs when there is an increase in pressure in a limited space, causing restriction or decreased circulation to muscles and nerves. Early manifestations include pain and decreased peripheral pulses. Later signs include numbness, tingling, and severe pain.

Contractures

Deep dermal and full-thickness burns heal with formation of fibrotic tissue that causes scarring. Epithelial replacement is not possible if skin is burned below a certain level called the stratum reticulare. In areas of deep skin loss, healing occurs by a concentric reduction in the size of the wound with proliferation of fibroblasts, myoblasts, and collagen. This process pulls edges of wounds together, forming constricted regions of tissue called contractures. Contractures often form around joints, which pull the two bones close together so the joint cannot fully open. After healing is complete, surgical reduction of the fibrous tissue and surgical reconstruction using skin grafts can reverse some contractures. Some contractures require several surgeries to achieve a gradual release. Orthopedic surgery and physical therapy may also be needed.

Hypertrophic Scarring

Hypertrophic scars, also called keloids, can occur as burns heal in some patients. This hyperplastic growth of skin forms hyperemic, raised areas of firm skin. Compression dressings and garments can be worn to prevent development of hypertrophic scars. Silicone gel sheets worn over the wound 24 hours a day have been effective. Pressure therapy diminishes the number of myofibroblasts, erythema, thickness, and firmness of hypertrophic scarring and accelerates its maturation. Pressure and silicone gel dressings may exert effects by increasing the temperature of the scar, thereby enhancing the activity of collagenase, which breaks down fibrous tissue. Cosmetic surgery can also reduce hypertrophic scars.

Chapter Summary

- Burns are the fourth-leading cause of accidental death in the United States and can result in injuries that are mild to life threatening.

- Burns are categorized as thermal, chemical, electrical, or radiation injuries.

- The severity of a burn depends on the degree of heat intensity, duration of contact, and thickness of skin at the point of contact.

- Inhalation injury and CO poisoning occur when individuals suffer burns in a closed space. The patient requires measurement of the CO level.

- Ingestion, inhalation, or entry of radioactive materials via open wounds can induce internal contamination and produce ARS.

- High doses of radiation can produce bone marrow suppression or aplastic bone marrow, which requires blood transfusion to replace the low blood cell production. Patients exposed to the highest levels of radiation experience GI symptoms (nausea, vomiting, and diarrhea) and damage to the central nervous system.

- Treatment of ARS focuses on patient decontamination by removing and bagging clothes and shoes, which usually removes more than 80% of radioactive material.
- Electrical shock can cause cardiac conduction abnormalities, including cardiac arrest.
- Thermal injury causes three zones of tissue damage: zone of coagulation, zone of stasis, and zone of hyperemia.
- The traditional degree classification of first-, second-, third-, and fourth-degree burns has been replaced by categories that describe the depth of destruction of the cellular layers of the skin, termed superficial, partial thickness, and full thickness.
- A common method of assessing the extent of burn injury involves the rule of nines, in which the body is divided into regions that present 9%, or multiples of nine.
- The Lund and Browder method is another assessment technique used to evaluate the extent of patient burns.
- Normal physiological organ function is disrupted if thermal injury is greater than 30% of TBSA.
- The ABA Classification of Burn Injury uses both the extent and the depth of burns to classify burns as minor, moderate, or major.

- The focus of care in burns involves the ABCDEF (airway, breathing, circulation, disability, exposure, and fluid resuscitation) aspects of trauma care.
- A tetanus booster is recommended with burn injuries of partial or full thickness.
- Débridement is the removal of dead, necrotic, or infected tissue to improve the healing potential of the remaining viable tissue. Débridement causes pain, and premedication with opioid medication is necessary.
- Aside from localized destruction of tissue, an extensive burn injury can cause pulmonary, renal, and GI complications.
- Myoglobinuria can cause acute tubular necrosis, which leads to acute renal failure.
- Burns cause a hypermetabolic state and fluid shifts that require IV fluids.
- Contractures can occur if the patient with burns remains immobile; active and passive range-of-motion exercises are required.
- Compartment syndrome can occur if there is excess swelling or fluid accumulation within the musculoskeletal compartments.
- Infection is the major cause of death in the patient who survives a major burn.
- Silver nitrate and other antimicrobial agents are often used to prevent infection in burns.

Making the Connections

Signs and Symptoms	Physical Assessment Findings	Diagnostic Testing	Treatment
Superficial Burns | Injury is limited to the outermost layer of the skin (epidermis). Tissue damage is minimal; the protective barrier is not impaired. Overexposure to the sun is the most common cause of injury.			
Painful erythema of the skin. Extremely tender to the touch.	Skin is tender and appears pink, red, and dry. Blisters common. Peeling skin. No break in the epidermal layer of the skin.	None.	Treatment limited to analgesics and moisturizers. The area heals within 3 to 5 days, with no scarring.
Superficial Partial-Thickness Burns | The injury involves the epidermis and limited dermis. The protective barrier is impaired, causing heat and fluid loss. Scalds or brief contact with hot objects is the usual cause of injury.			
Painful redness of the skin and exposure of dermal tissue beneath the epidermis. Blisters.	Skin is bright red, pearl-pink, painful, wet, or blistered. Dermis is exposed. Extremely tender.	Depending on how much BSA is involved, CBC, electrolytes, urinalysis, arterial blood gas, CPK, and carboxyhemoglobin level may be needed. If infection occurs, one may need to culture the exudate.	Topical agents used on the wound area. Débridement. Skin grafting may be needed. Burn heals in 10 days to 2 weeks. Monitor for infection. Tetanus booster. Depending on how much of the body is involved, IV fluids may be needed. Antibiotic treatment may be needed. Pain control.

Making the Connections–cont'd

Signs and Symptoms	Physical Assessment Findings	Diagnostic Testing	Treatment
Deep Partial-Thickness Burns | Injury involves the epidermis and most of the dermis. Wound is not painful, as the nerve endings are destroyed.			
Deep area of exposed tissue. The area appears dry, pale, or whitish-yellow in color. May be nontender if nerves are destroyed.	Deep area of exposed tissue. The area appears dry, pale, or whitish-yellow in color. May be nontender if nerves are destroyed.	Depending on how much surface area is involved, CBC, electrolytes, urinalysis, BUN, serum creatinine, arterial blood gas, CPK, and carboxyhemoglobin level may be needed. Increased risk for infection. If infection occurs, may need to culture the exudate.	Topical agents on wound area. Healing occurs within 3 to 5 weeks. Débridement. Skin grafting may be necessary for injuries within the deeper layers of the dermis. Pain control. Tetanus booster. IV fluids or enteral feedings may be needed, depending on surface area involved. Antibiotic treatment may be needed.
Full-Thickness Burns | Injury involves the entire epidermis, dermis, and underlying subcutaneous tissues. Common causes are direct contact with flames, hot liquids, or steam. Fluid and heat loss are related to the loss of the protective layer.			
Acutely, the layers beneath the epidermis and dermis are totally exposed. Red, raw-appearing wound. No pain sensed.	Skin exhibits a dry, leathery, and white or yellow color that does not blanch with pressure, which indicates it is avascular. Nontender because nerves are destroyed.	CBC, electrolytes, urinalysis, BUN, serum creatinine, arterial blood gas, CPK, and carboxyhemoglobin level. There is an increased risk for infection. Culture of exudate may be needed.	Tetanus booster. Topical agents and wound dressing. Burns heal within weeks to months. Wounds usually require surgical intervention. Débridement and skin grafting. Depending on percentage of body surface involved, IV fluids or enteral feedings may be needed. Antibiotic agents may be needed. Pain control.

Bibliography

Available online at fadavis.com

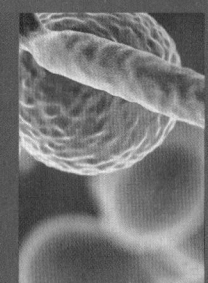

CHAPTER

43

Eye Disorders

Learning Objectives

Upon completion of this chapter, the student will be able to:

- Describe normal anatomy and physiology of the eye.
- Recognize etiologies and pathological mechanisms of common disorders that affect the eye.
- List assessment techniques and imaging modalities used in the diagnosis of eye disorders.

- Describe common signs, symptoms, and clinical manifestations of disorders of the eye.
- Discuss treatment modalities used to correct vision and manage common disorders of the eye.

Key Terms

Accommodation	Glaucoma	Optic disc
Amblyopia	Hordeolum	Papilledema
Aqueous humor	Hyperopia	Pinguecula
Astigmatism	Keratoconjunctivitis	Pterygium
Canal of Schlemm	Lacrimal apparatus	Red reflex
Cataracts	LASIK	Refraction
Ciliary muscle	Lens	Retinal detachment
Conjunctivitis	Macula	Retinoblastoma
Cornea	Miosis	Strabismus
Drusen	Mydriasis	Trachoma
Extraocular movements (EOMs)	Myopia	Vision acuity
Fovea	Optic cup	Vitreous humor

More than 12 million people in the United States are visually impaired; with the aging of the population, this number is estimated to double by the year 2030. Visual impairment may be caused by a number of eye diseases, including age-related macular degeneration (AMD), diabetic retinopathy, glaucoma, and cataracts. The increasing incidence of diabetes is one of the major reasons for the rise in visual impairment in the population. Per some estimates, less than two-thirds of people with diabetes obtain regular visual examinations. Persons with vision loss are more likely to report depression, falls, cognitive decline, and premature death.

To understand the definition of visual impairment, it is necessary to know how vision is measured. **Vision acuity** is measured using an eye chart, and results are

recorded as a pair of numbers. Normal sight is scored as a ratio of 20/20; the numerator indicates that the object to be visualized is at a distance of 20 feet, whereas the denominator indicates how far away the object seems to the patient. Someone with a visual acuity of 20/20 can see letters at a distance of 20 feet away as if they are 20 feet away. Someone with a visual acuity of 20/60 sees letters at 20 feet as if they are 60 feet away. The higher the denominator of visual acuity, the worse the individual's vision. According to U.S. law, if a person's best eye has an acuity of 20/200 or worse and/or if their peripheral vision is less than 20 degrees, then that person is legally blind.

Having good vision is important to safety, independent living, and self-confidence. By comprehending the various eye disorders, clinicians should be able to recognize the signs of impending eye problems and chronic eye conditions to adequately assist patients with visual disturbances.

Epidemiology

According to the World Health Organization (WHO), 1.3 billion people live with some form of visual impairment and 36 million are blind. About 90% of the world's visually impaired live in underdeveloped countries. About 82% of all people who are blind and 65% of those with moderate to severe vision impairment are older than age 50. Globally, uncorrected refractive errors and cataracts are the main causes of visual impairment. In underdeveloped regions of the world, *Chlamydia trachomatis* eye infection is a major cause of blindness. Globally, approximately 80% of vision impairment is preventable and curable. The WHO is currently leading a global action plan to incorporate universal eye health-care services into international health-care delivery systems.

According to U.S. census data, blindness or low vision affects approximately 3% of Americans older than 40 years. The specific causes of visual impairment, and especially blindness, vary greatly by race/ethnicity. An estimated 1 million Americans were legally blind in 2015, and by 2050, this number is projected to grow to 2 million. It is expected that 8 million Americans will have vision impairment by 2050. Those over age 80 will be most affected as age-related macular degeneration (AMD) and cataracts are the main causes of vision impairment.

Basic Concepts of the Structure and Function of the Eye

The eye is a sensory organ with a complex structure and function. It allows us to constantly interpret our environment by bringing images to the brain. It is not until a part of the eye malfunctions that we understand the significance of this sensory organ.

Structure of the Eye

The eye consists of the eyeball, or globe, that sits in the orbit of the skull (see Fig. 43-1). The eyeball is a fluid- and gel-filled sphere. There are three chambers: the anterior located in forefront, the posterior located in the middle, and the vitreous located throughout the back of the eye. The anterior chamber sits between the cornea and the iris (see Fig. 43-2). The watery fluid that circulates within the anterior chamber of the eye is the **aqueous humor.** The posterior chamber is between the iris and lens. The vitreous chamber is between the lens and the retina. The eye has three main layers: sclera, choroid, and retina.

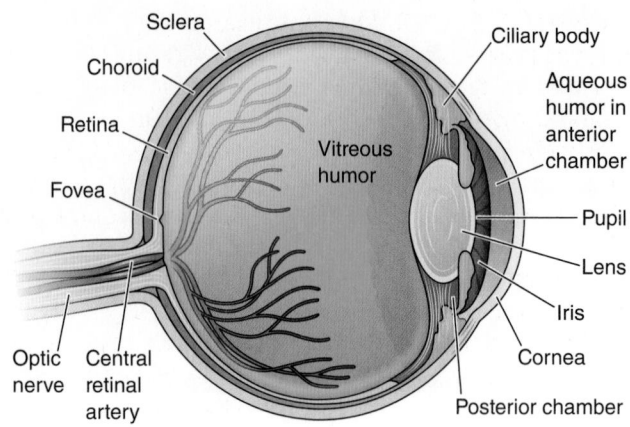

FIGURE 43-1. Cross-section of the eye.

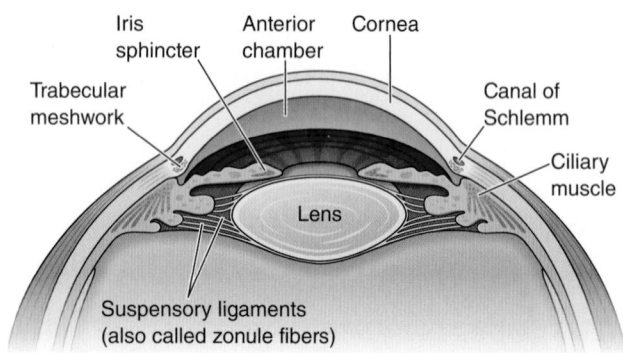

FIGURE 43-2. Close-up view of the anterior chamber and lens.

The sclera is the white outermost layer of the eye. Within the sclera is the **cornea,** the transparent section through which light enters the eye. The choroid is the thin vascular layer between the sclera and the retina. The iris, the colored part of the eye, is located in the choroid layer. The pupil is an opening in the center of the iris. The pupil can dilate, referred to as **mydriasis,** and it can constrict, referred to as **miosis.** Light waves enter the eye through the pupil and are transmitted via the retina and optic nerve to the brain for interpretation. The light waves are focused by the **lens,** which is suspended by zonule fibers attached to the ciliary body. The lens can change shape by the ciliary muscle actions, which cause contraction or relaxation of the zonule fibers. The lens changes shape in order to form a sharp image on the retina—a process called **accommodation.** The body of the eyeball behind the lens is a clear, gel-like substance called **vitreous humor. Refraction** of light occurs as rays travel from the pupil through the aqueous and vitreous humors to the retina, the innermost layer of the eye.

The retina is the sensory portion of the eye that changes light waves into neuroimpulses that travel via the optic nerve to the brain for interpretation (see Fig. 43-3). On funduscopic examination, the optic nerve is visualized as a bright, yellow, round structure located medially on the retina. It consists of a lighter-colored **optic cup** in the center, surrounded by the darker yellow **optic disc.** Blood vessels, both arterial and venous, lead out of the optic disc and perfuse the retina. Approximately two-and-a-half disc diameters to the left of the optic disc is the **macula,** a slightly oval-shaped, blood vessel–free, dark-red area. The central region of the macula is called the **fovea,** which is responsible for sharp central vision.

Attached to each eyeball are four rectus muscles and two oblique muscles that are innervated by cranial nerves (CNs) III, IV, and VI (see Fig. 43-4). Normally, the eyeballs move symmetrically with six possible positions of gaze, also called the six cardinal fields of gaze (see Fig. 43-5). CNs III, IV, and VI control **extraocular movements (EOMs).**

The conjunctiva is a mucous membrane with two parts. The palpebral portion of the conjunctiva is a pink membrane that lines the eyelid, whereas the

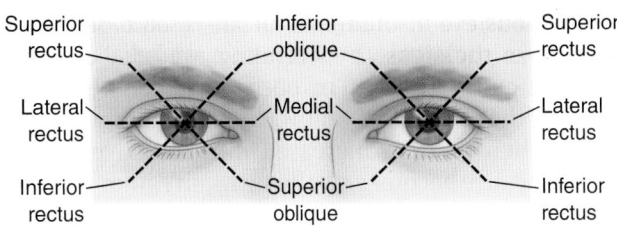

FIGURE 43-5. Six cardinal fields of gaze.

bulbar conjunctiva is colorless and covers the eyeball except for the cornea.

Protecting the anterior portion of the eye are the eyelids, which consist of smooth and striated muscles covered by thin skin. The lateral portion of the eyelids contains eyelashes; they protect the eye from dust and other small particles. Other accessory structures that protect the eye include the brows, lashes, meibomian glands, and lacrimal apparatus. The meibomian glands are located at the rim of the eyelids. They are sebaceous glands that secrete an oily substance. The **lacrimal apparatus** consists of the lacrimal gland, lacrimal sac, and duct (see Fig. 43-6). The lacrimal gland produces tears and is located in the upper lateral region of the orbit under the brow. Tears pass over the eye surface to the lacrimal puncta, tiny openings found at the medial corner of the eyelids. From there, tears collect in the lacrimal sac and then flow into the nasolacrimal duct, which empties into the nose.

Function of the Eye

In order to visualize an object, light rays must pass through the cornea, anterior chamber, pupil, lens, and posterior chamber to the retina. The pupil dilates and constricts in response to light, which allows the appropriate amount of light into the retina. The retina is the gateway where nerve impulses enter the optic nerve to travel to the brain. Blood vessels, the optic nerve, and the macula can be seen on the retina with an ophthalmoscope. The retina is the only place in the body where active blood vessels are directly

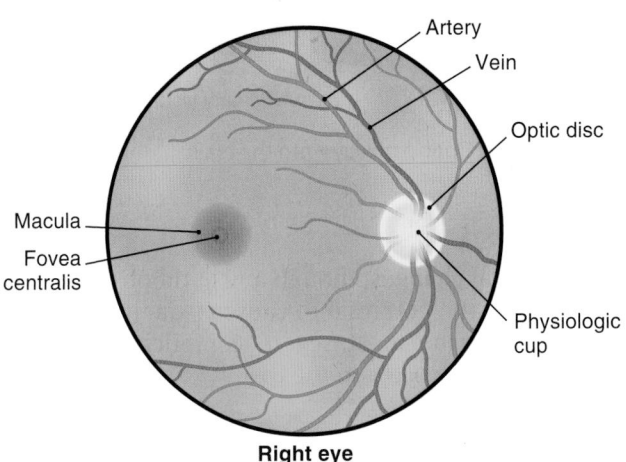

Right eye

FIGURE 43-3. Normal retina.

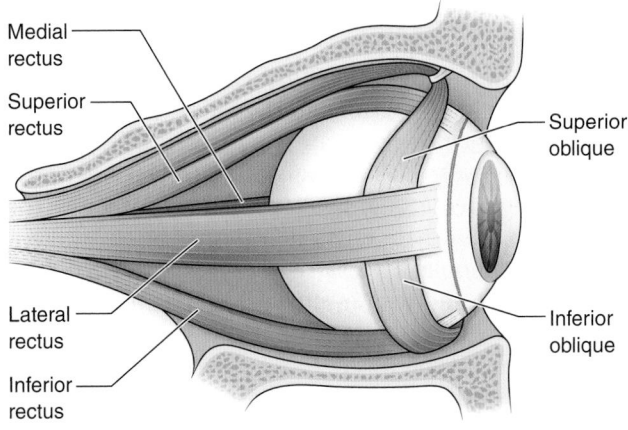

FIGURE 43-4. Extraocular muscles.

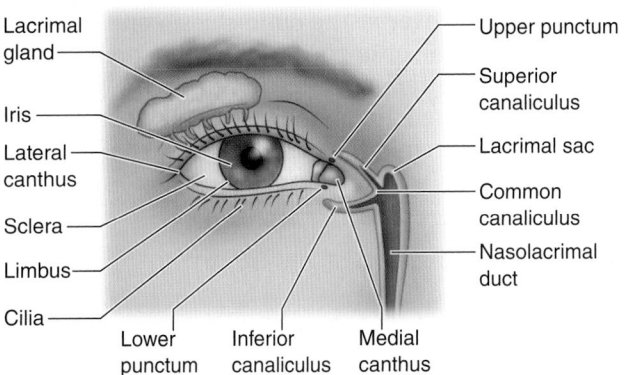

FIGURE 43-6. Lacrimal apparatus.

visible. Therefore, changes in blood vessels associated with arteriosclerosis, hypertension, and diabetes can be seen on the retina. The optic nerve can be visualized on the retina as a yellow, circular, clearly defined disc. When there is increased intracranial pressure, the optic disc becomes swollen with irregular borders, a condition termed **papilledema.**

The lens focuses the light rays on the retina. The ciliary muscle is attached to zonule fibers that are attached to the lens. The **ciliary muscle** is a smooth muscle controlled by the autonomic nervous system that changes the shape of the lens for accommodation—near versus far vision. Sympathetic nervous system stimulation causes relaxation of the ciliary muscle, which places high stress on the zonule fibers attached to the lens that flattens its shape. Conversely, parasympathetic nervous system stimulation causes ciliary muscle contraction, which allows the zonule fibers to relax; in response, the lens bulges. The change of the lens's shape changes how light converges on the retina.

The ciliary muscle also regulates the flow of aqueous fluid through the **canal of Schlemm**—an important structure that regulates intraocular pressure (IOP) (see Fig. 43-2). Sympathetic stimulation causes relaxation of the ciliary muscle, which blocks drainage of the canal of Schlemm. Consequently, aqueous fluid can accumulate within the eye. Parasympathetic stimulation causes contraction of the ciliary muscle, which opens the way for the canal of Schlemm to drain.

> ### 🩺 CLINICAL CONCEPT
>
> Sympathetic or anticholinergic drug action on the ciliary muscle blocks the canal of Schlemm, causing accumulation of aqueous fluid, thereby increasing IOP; high IOP can trigger or worsen glaucoma.

The retina contains specialized nerve cells called rods and cones, also called photoreceptor cells, that further focus images, allow visualization of color, and carry impulses to the optic disc. Nerve fibers from the optic disc form the optic nerve, which sends impulses to the optic tracts, optic radiations, and visual cortex of the brain. Nerve fibers from the nasal portion of each eye cross over at the optic chiasm and travel to the contralateral, or opposite, side of the brain. Nerve fibers from the temporal portion of each eye do not cross over and remain on the ipsilateral, or same, side of the visual (occipital) cortex (see Fig. 43-7).

Basic Pathophysiological Concepts of the Structure and Function of the Eye

The basic pathophysiological processes that occur in the eye are caused by infection and inflammation or

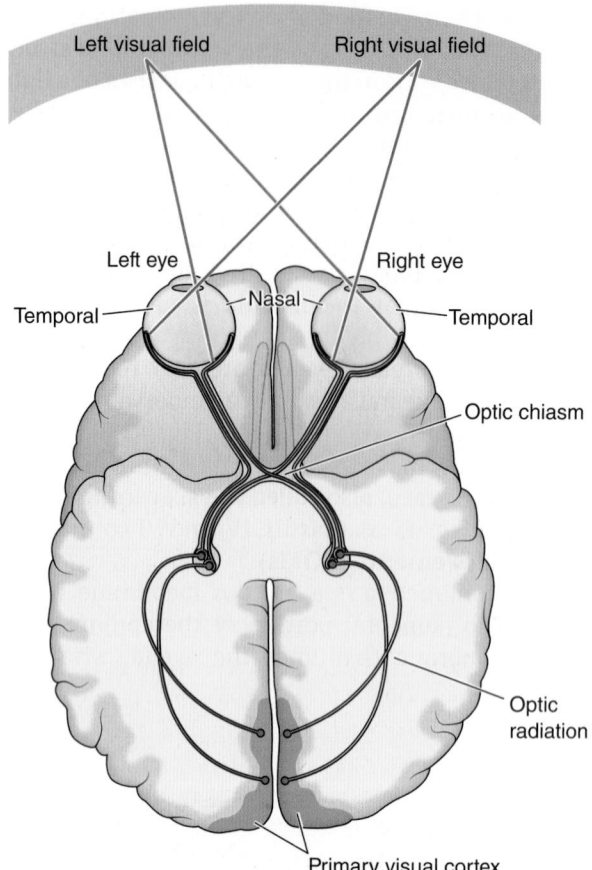

FIGURE 43-7. Optic pathways into the brain.

by structural changes, though any pathophysiological process has the potential to cause visual impairment. Blindness is the most severe complication of any dysfunctional process in the eye.

Infection and Inflammation of the Eye and Surrounding Area

Infection and inflammation can occur in various parts of the eye and surrounding structures. Accurate diagnosis of the cause of the infection or inflammation is crucial in order to choose the correct treatment.

Blepharitis

Inflammation of the eyelids, called blepharitis, is also referred to as granulated eyelids. Symptoms of blepharitis include red, watery eyes; dry, gritty sensation of the eyes; burning sensation in the eye; itchy eyelids; erythematous, swollen eyelids; flaking of the skin around the eyes; crusted eyelashes upon awakening; photophobia; excessive tearing; abnormal eyelash growth; and loss of eyelashes. The eyelids may also appear greasy and crusted with scales that cling to the lashes. Acne rosacea and seborrheic dermatitis are skin disorders associated with blepharitis of the eyelids. Blepharitis can be difficult to treat. Good eye hygiene is key to effectively treating this eye infection.

Stye

A stye, also known as a **hordeolum,** is a bacterial infection that develops near the root of an eyelash and appears on the outside of the eye (see Fig. 43-8). Pain, swelling, and redness of the conjunctiva and eyelid are symptoms. *Staphylococcus aureus* is the most common pathogenic etiology. Physical examination of a stye reveals swelling, erythema, and tenderness to touch. Treatment includes antibiotics and warm compresses with diluted boric acid solution.

Chalazion

A chalazion is a blockage in one of the small meibomian oil glands at the margin of the eyelid (see Fig. 43-9). Symptoms include eyelid tenderness, increased tearing, painful swelling on the eyelid, and sensitivity to light. Warm compresses, steroid injection, and surgical excision are the treatments.

Conjunctivitis

Conjunctivitis occurs when the conjunctiva of the eye becomes infected or inflamed. The conjunctiva becomes red and swollen (see Fig. 43-10), and the eye feels itchy to the affected individual. There may be a purulent or watery discharge from the eye. There are viral, bacterial, and allergic causes of conjunctivitis. Bacterial or viral conjunctivitis, commonly called pinkeye, is highly contagious. Persons can spread the bacteria or virus by touching the eye and then touching the hands of another individual. Contaminated objects or bedding can transmit the microorganism as well. Patients should avoid touching their eyes and

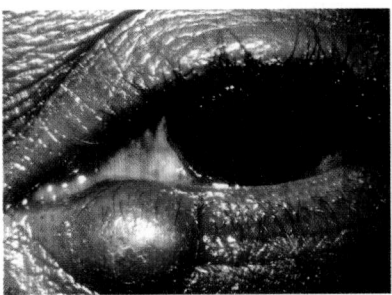

FIGURE 43-8. Stye (hordeolum). *(Courtesy of Wills Eye Hospital, Philadelphia, PA.)*

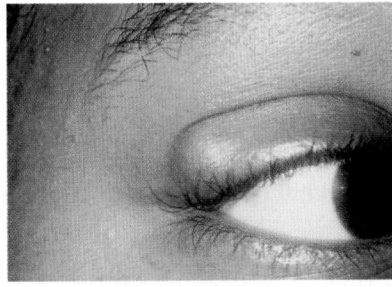

FIGURE 43-9. Chalazion. *(Courtesy of Wills Eye Hospital, Philadelphia, PA.)*

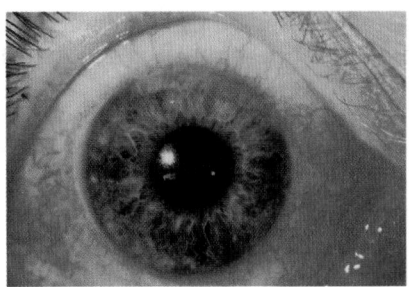

FIGURE 43-10. Conjunctivitis. *(Courtesy of Wills Eye Hospital, Philadelphia, PA.)*

wash hands thoroughly, as infectious conjunctivitis is easily spread.

> ### 🔬 CLINICAL CONCEPT
>
> The microorganisms that most often cause conjunctivitis include streptococcus, staphylococcus, *Haemophilus aegyptius, Chlamydia,* adenovirus, herpes simplex, varicella zoster, enteroviruses, and Coxsackievirus. Swabs for bacterial or viral culture are sometimes necessary. Patients are treated with antibiotic ointment, and antihistamines are useful in allergic conjunctivitis. In herpes simplex or varicella zoster conjunctivitis, acyclovir is necessary.

Keratitis

Inflammation of the cornea, called keratitis, is commonly caused by herpes simplex virus type 1. The virus infects the ophthalmic division of the trigeminal nerve (CN V). Other viruses that cause keratitis include varicella zoster and the adenoviruses. Keratitis can also be caused by misuse of contact lenses, trauma to the eye, occupational toxin exposures, tanning booths, and hypersensitivity reactions. More rarely, keratitis is caused by other infections, such as bacteria, parasites, and fungi.

The inflammation or infection of keratitis affects the outer layer of the cornea, but it can go deeper into the cornea, increasing the risk of impaired vision. The term **keratoconjunctivitis,** meaning corneal and conjunctiva inflammation, is often used. The patient has eye pain, redness, photophobia, and a feeling that a foreign body is irritating the eye. Infectious or inflammatory keratitis can leave a scarred cornea than can interfere with vision. Fluorescein staining of the cornea is necessary to diagnose keratitis. Antibiotics may be needed with bacterial keratoconjunctivitis. Acyclovir is the treatment for herpes simplex or varicella zoster. Corticosteroids should not be used for viral keratitis, as they will worsen the disease. Corneal transplant can be done in severe cases.

Acanthamoeba keratitis can occur if contact lenses are contaminated with ameba: a protozoan organism that is ubiquitous in the soil. This can occur from swimming, showering, or washing with ameba-infested water while wearing contact lenses. Immunosuppressed persons are particularly susceptible. It is usually a localized infection that can lead to corneal scarring, uveitis, scleritis, and cataract. Although rare, acanthamoeba keratitis can lead to granulomatous ameba encephalitis.

Keratoconjunctivitis sicca, commonly called dry eye, occurs when tear production is inadequate. It is seen in many autoimmune disorders. Sarcoidosis, Sjögren's syndrome, and lesions affecting CN V or VII can also cause dry eye. A number of systemic medications can cause this condition, including antihistamines, anticholinergics, and psychotropic drugs. It is treated with artificial tears.

Dacryocystitis

Dacryocystitis, an inflammation of the lacrimal sac, is often caused by an obstruction of the nasolacrimal duct. Incomplete canalization of the nasolacrimal duct or infection is the cause. The most common organisms include *Staphylococcus aureus, Haemophilus influenzae,* beta-hemolytic streptococci, and pneumococci. Newborns frequently have dacryocystitis caused by obstruction of the nasolacrimal duct.

When dacryocystitis infection is present, the area around the lacrimal sac is painful, red, and swollen. The eye becomes red and watery and oozes purulent exudate. Slight pressure applied to the lacrimal sac may push exudate through the opening at the inner corner of the eye, near the nose. Fever is also common.

Dacryocystitis is typically diagnosed by physical examination. Additionally, blood cultures may be necessary. Standard treatment consists of antibiotics and warm compresses. However, if conservative measures are ineffective, this condition is treated surgically.

Scleritis

Scleritis, or inflammation of the sclera, causes severe eye pain that may radiate to the eyebrow, temple, or jaw. Other symptoms include photophobia; tearing without discharge; eye tenderness; and purplish-red, edematous, and engorged blood vessels. Inflammation of the sclera is usually associated with autoimmune diseases such as rheumatoid arthritis and systemic lupus erythematosus. Sometimes the cause is unknown. Treatment involves corticosteroid drops and oral NSAIDs.

Subconjunctival Hemorrhage

Blood vessels can become apparent in the sclera in a subconjunctival hemorrhage (see Fig. 43-11). A subconjunctival hemorrhage occurs when a small blood vessel breaks open and bleeds near the surface of the white of the eye. Alternatively, pinpoint subconjunctival hemorrhage is exhibited by red blood vessels in the sclera; sometimes this is referred to as "injected sclera" or "bloodshot eyes." Sudden increases in pressure, such as violent sneezing or coughing, can cause

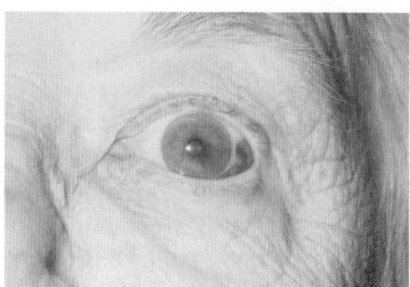

FIGURE 43-11. Subconjunctival hemorrhage. *(Courtesy of Wills Eye Hospital, Philadelphia, PA.)*

a subconjunctival hemorrhage. The hemorrhage may also occur in persons with high blood pressure or those who take blood thinners. A bright red patch appears on the white of the eye, but it does not cause pain or discharge. Vision does not change. No treatment is needed; eventually, the body absorbs the blood.

Uveitis

Uveitis is inflammation of the uveal tract, which includes the iris, choroid, and ciliary body. Common causes include infection or autoimmune disorders, such as rheumatoid arthritis or ankylosing spondylitis; inflammatory disorders, such as Crohn's disease or ulcerative colitis; infections, such as syphilis, toxoplasmosis, and tuberculosis; and eye injury. Symptoms, which can develop quickly, include eye redness and irritation, blurred vision, eye pain, photophobia, and floaters. Uveitis is diagnosed with a thorough examination of the eye with a slit lamp microscope and ophthalmoscopy. Treatment of active inflammation usually involves topical cycloplegic agents (e.g., atropine or cyclopentolate) and topical corticosteroids (e.g., prednisolone ophthalmic). Immunomodulator (e.g., adalimumab) or immunosuppressive agents (e.g., azathioprine) may be necessary for patients with autoimmune uveitis. An intravitreal dexamethasone or fluocinolone implant has been effective for some patients. Some patients may require surgery.

CLINICAL CONCEPT

Keratoconjunctivitis sicca, scleritis, and uveitis can occur in rheumatoid arthritis or other autoimmune diseases.

Structural Disorders of the Eye

A corneal abrasion is the most common type of eye injury. This usually benign condition heals within 24 hours. Other structural eye disorders include entropion and ectropion, which are abnormalities of the eyelids that can cause irritation of the eye. These benign conditions can be surgically treated. A more serious condition is exophthalmos, an eye condition that occurs in hyperthyroidism. The eye bulges and the cornea can dry out, causing irritation or injury. Pterygium and pinguecula are benign growths on the eye that usually do not affect vision.

Corneal Abrasion

Corneal abrasion, the most common type of structural eye trauma, is damage to the epithelial surface of the cornea, usually caused by a foreign body that comes into contact with the eye. It can also be caused by either physical or chemical trauma. Contact lens wearers are more vulnerable to corneal abrasions because foreign bodies may become trapped between the cornea and the contact lens, causing scratching of the corneal membrane. Also, persons who play sports are more prone to corneal abrasions because of the increased risk of foreign bodies entering the eyes.

Often, persons with a corneal abrasion present with the following: foreign body sensation of the eye, gritty eye sensation, unilateral eye watering pain, photophobia, and mild erythema of the conjunctiva. Minor corneal abrasions may be asymptomatic. In cases of a significant abrasion, slit lamp examination reveals a defect in the corneal epithelium. This defect can be confirmed by placing a drop of fluorescein dye in the eye. The fluorescein dye flows into the defect and glows under the light of a Wood's lamp (see Fig. 43-12).

Treatment includes topical antibiotic ointments to prevent bacterial growth. Untreated corneal abrasions are susceptible to infections that may cause corneal ulcerations and blindness.

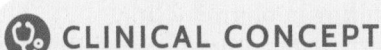

CLINICAL CONCEPT

Most cases of corneal abrasion heal within 24 hours.

Entropion and Ectropion

Entropion and ectropion are benign conditions of the eye. Entropion occurs when the eyelid turns inward and irritates the eye, whereas ectropion occurs when the eyelid turns outward, revealing the pink conjunctival membrane. Both of these conditions can cause eye irritation, excessive tearing, and corneal dryness. Artificial tears and surgery are the treatments.

Exophthalmos

Exophthalmos, also called proptosis, is a bulging of the eye out of the orbit; hyperthyroidism or ocular tumor are the most common causes. In autoimmune hyperthyroidism, also called Graves' disease, exophthalmos often occurs; termed thyroid eye disease (TED). It occurs most frequently in middle-aged females with hyperthyroidism. Inflammatory changes around the eye include lymphocytic infiltration and cytokine activation. Dryness and irritation of the eyes can occur. The cornea becomes inflamed because of the friction that occurs when the patient blinks. Some patients may experience compression of the optic nerve or ophthalmic artery, which can eventually affect the patient's vision, leading to blindness. The cause of the exophthalmos needs to be treated. Corticosteroid drops, artificial tears, and ophthalmic lubricants can be used to relieve symptoms. Targeted immunomodulator agents are available to counteract the inflammatory changes that cause exophthalmos in TED. Teprotumumab, a monoclonal antibody, has been recently approved by the U.S. Food and Drug Administration (FDA) as treatment.

Enophthalmos

Enophthalmos is the recession of the eyeball within the orbit. It may be a congenital anomaly or occur as a result of trauma, collapse of the facial sinuses, Horner's syndrome, or other disorders. Treatment is aimed at the disorder's etiology; surgery may be necessary.

Benign Growths

A **pinguecula** is a benign, yellowish growth that forms on the conjunctiva (see Fig. 43-13a). A **pterygium** is another benign growth that resembles a pinguecula; however, it encroaches on the corneal surface (see Fig. 43-13b). Exposure to ultraviolet light is thought to cause these abnormalities. These remain on the eye unless surgically removed; however, neither requires treatment unless they interfere with vision.

Types of Visual Impairment

Types of visual impairment include myopia (nearsightedness), hyperopia (farsightedness), presbyopia,

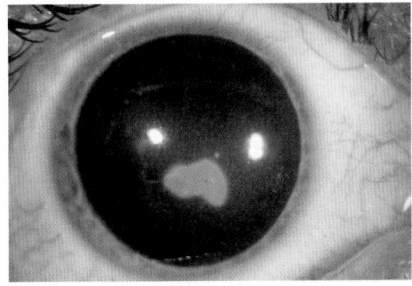

FIGURE 43-12. Corneal abrasion with fluorescein dye. *(Courtesy of Wills Eye Hospital, Philadelphia, PA.)*

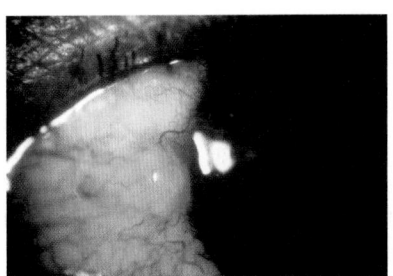

FIGURE 43-13a. Pinguecula. *(Courtesy of Wills Eye Hospital, Philadelphia, PA.)*

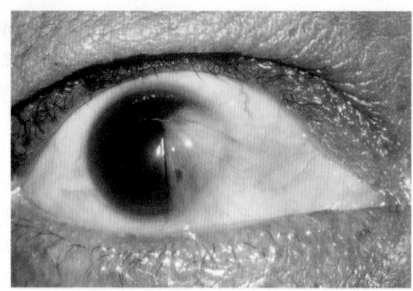

FIGURE 43-13b. Pterygium. *(Courtesy of Wills Eye Hospital, Philadelphia, PA.)*

astigmatism, amblyopia, and color blindness. Perfectly shaped eyeballs promote optimal vision; however, individuals with myopia or hyperopia have different-shaped eyeballs. Their anteroposterior width is either too short or too long. This causes an imperfect focus of light waves through the lens on to the retina.

Myopia

Normally, light enters the eye via the pupil and passes through the lens, which causes bending of the light. The lens is important because it projects an image on the retina. **Myopia,** or nearsightedness, occurs when the eyeball is elongated and visual images are focused in front of the retina (see Fig. 43-14). Individuals with myopia see better when objects are close, which allows the lens to focus light waves onto the retina. Hence, in myopia the farther away an object moves, the blurrier it becomes.

Myopia is very common, affecting approximately one-third of Americans, with aging adults being most affected. Symptoms include blurry distal vision, headache, squinting, and eyestrain. Visual acuity examinations are used to diagnosis myopia. Treatment includes corrective lenses via eyeglasses or contact lenses, or refractive surgery. There are various types of refractive surgery; laser-assisted in situ keratomileusis **(LASIK)** surgery is used most often. Refractive surgery reshapes the cornea itself. Decreasing the curvature of the cornea

by removing tissue from the center corrects for myopia. If left untreated, myopia may worsen with age.

Hyperopia

Hyperopia, or farsightedness, occurs when visual objects are focused behind the retina because of a shorter anteroposterior width of the eyeball. The lens cannot focus the light rays onto the retina. Individuals with hyperopia see better when objects are farther away. The closer an object moves, the blurrier it becomes. Treatment includes corrective lenses or refractive surgery. Refractive surgery, most commonly LASIK surgery, changes the shape of the cornea to correct how light rays focus on the retina. Increasing the curvature of the cornea by removing tissue from the periphery corrects for hyperopia. If untreated, hyperopia tends to worsen with age.

Presbyopia

Presbyopia, a common disorder in aging adults caused by the decreased elasticity of the lens with age, is a vision defect exhibited as a gradually diminished ability to focus on close objects. This begins around the age of 40 years, which is why some individuals start to require reading glasses at this age.

As with hyperopia, individuals need to have objects held at a distance to see clearly. Individuals may first notice that the ability to read small print is more difficult. Treatment for presbyopia includes corrective lenses such as contacts and glasses with bifocals.

Astigmatism

In normal vision, light rays focus directly on the retina. With **astigmatism,** the rays are diffusely spread about the retinal area, resulting in blurred vision.

The cause of astigmatism is the shape of either the lens or the cornea. The eyeball is often referred to as having a football shape rather than its normal spherical shape. These changes in shape distort the light rays entering the eye so that the rays do not center on the retina.

Although some individuals may be asymptomatic, people with astigmatism may experience blurred vision, headaches, and eyestrain. Keratoscope and videokeratoscope are ophthalmic devices to measure and assess the curvature of the cornea to diagnose astigmatism. Treatment for astigmatism includes use of corrective lenses or refractive surgery such as LASIK.

Amblyopia

Amblyopia, also known as lazy eye, affects just 2% to 3% of the population. In this condition, central vision fails to develop properly, usually in one eye, which is called amblyopic. **Strabismus,** commonly called crossed eyes, is a related condition where the visual axes of the eyes are not parallel and the eyes appear to be looking in different directions (see Fig. 43-15). Strabismus often causes amblyopia.

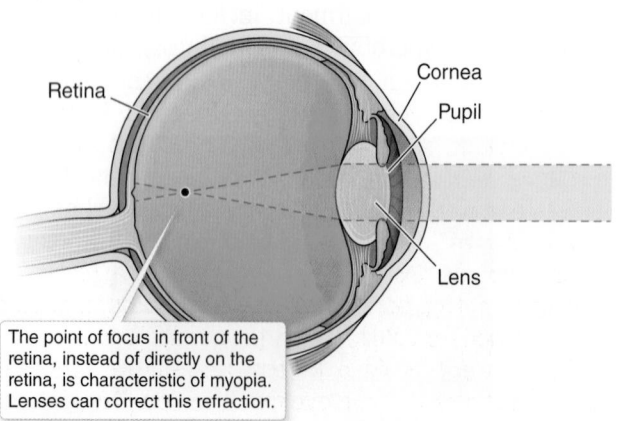

The point of focus in front of the retina, instead of directly on the retina, is characteristic of myopia. Lenses can correct this refraction.

FIGURE 43-14. Refraction of light in myopia.

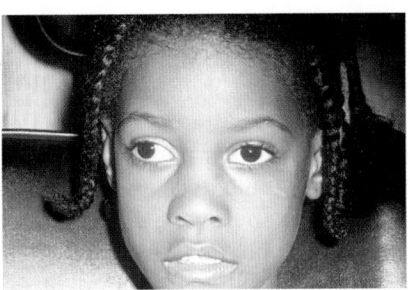

FIGURE 43-15. Strabismus. *(Courtesy of Wills Eye Hospital, Philadelphia, PA.)*

Amblyopia generally develops in children before the age of 6 years; parents, caregivers, or health-care professionals often notice the symptoms. These symptoms include eyestrain, poor visual acuity, squinting, or completely closing one eye to see.

Trauma to the eye at any age can cause amblyopia or strabismus. When amblyopia occurs in a child, the visual cortex of the brain will neglect to interpret images from the amblyopic eye as the child grows. It is important to correct amblyopia as early as possible, before the brain learns to entirely ignore vision in the affected eye.

Promoting use of the amblyopic eye by hindering the visual input from the better eye is the treatment strategy used for amblyopia. This can be accomplished with patching, atropine 1% ophthalmic drops, or optical penalization. If patching technique is not used, alternatively, atropine can be administered into the nonamblyopic eye. Atropine 1% ophthalmic drops block parasympathetic innervation to the ciliary muscle and pupil, causing temporary paralysis of accommodation (cycloplegia) and dilation of the pupil. This results in blurring in the nonamblyopic eye and inability to focus at near distance, thus stimulating the preferential near fixation of the amblyopic eye and subsequent visual improvement. Optical penalization is a method in which a Bangerter filter is applied to the eyeglass lens over the nonamblyopic eye. This translucent filter blurs the vision in the nonamblyopic eye to stimulate the vision in the amblyopic eye.

> **ALERT!** Untreated amblyopia may lead to functional blindness in the affected eye. Although the amblyopic eye has the capability to see, the brain "turns off" this eye because vision is very blurred and the brain elects to see only with the stronger eye.

Color Blindness

Color blindness is a condition that impairs an individual's ability to distinguish certain colors. It occurs in about 8% to 12% of males and in about 0.5% of females. Red/green color blindness, in which the individual has problems distinguishing between reds and greens, is the most common type. The red and green objects in the environment appear gray in color. The disorder is a dysfunction of the rods and cones within the retina. Rods and cones are photoreceptor cells in the retina; rods allow us to see clearly in low light, and cones allow us to make color distinctions. Color blindness is normally diagnosed through clinical testing using the Ishihara color chart. There is no treatment for color blindness, and most persons compensate well for their defect.

The gene for color blindness is carried on the X chromosome and is inherited from the mother. Since color blindness is an X chromosome trait, males have a higher incidence than females. X chromosome traits are dominant over Y chromosome traits in the male.

> **CLINICAL CONCEPT**
>
> The color-blind individual cannot decipher words or numbers on the Ishihara color chart.

Blindness

A person with vision that cannot be corrected to better than 20/200 in the best eye, or who has 20 degrees (diameter) or less of visual field remaining, is considered to be "legally blind."

Assessment of the Eye

Assessment of the eye and vision is part of every comprehensive physical examination. Examination of the pupil and EOMs are key features of the neurological examination. Examination of the eyes and eyelids yields results about the optic, oculomotor, trochlear, abducens, and facial CNs. It is also important to assess the eyelids and orbital region for infection, inflammation, and structural disorders. If the eyes are not accurately evaluated, vision can be permanently affected.

Physical Examination

The structures around the eye, including the eyelashes, eyebrows, and eyelids, should be carefully inspected. The clinician should note any apparent inflammation; swelling; seborrheic debris along lashes and brows; or entropion, ectropion, or ptosis of the eyelids. The patient's eyes should be inspected for exophthalmos, enophthalmos, lesions, deformities, and asymmetry. The conjunctiva, sclera, cornea, iris, and pupil should be examined for color, discharge, and lesions.

Visual acuity should be assessed before proceeding with the rest of the eye examination. The patient should use their corrective lenses and be positioned 20 feet from a Snellen chart (see Fig. 43-16). A patient

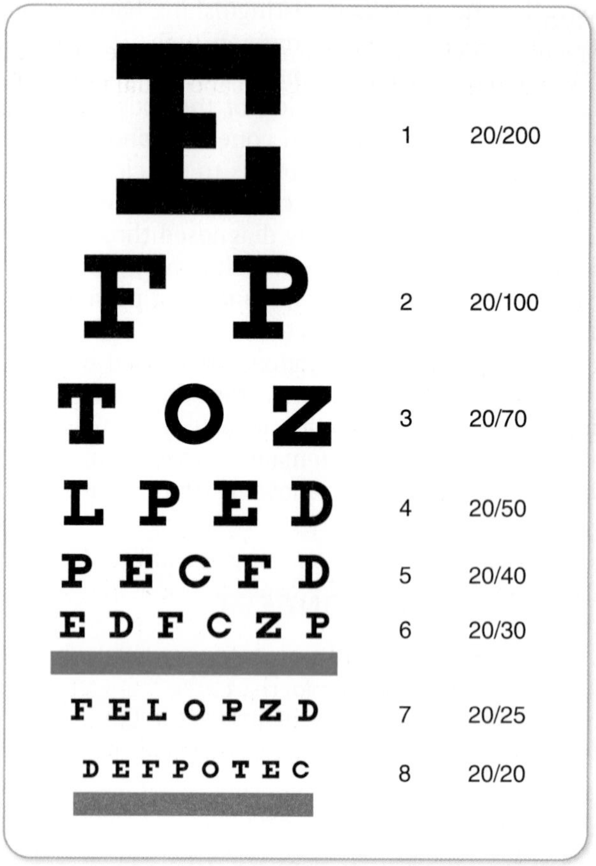

E	1	20/200
F P	2	20/100
T O Z	3	20/70
L P E D	4	20/50
P E C F D	5	20/40
E D F C Z P	6	20/30
F E L O P Z D	7	20/25
D E F P O T E C	8	20/20

FIGURE 43-16. Snellen chart.

should cover one eye and read the letters of each row, beginning at the top. The smallest row that can be read accurately indicates the visual acuity in that eye. Alternatively, the patient's vision can be tested with a Rosenbaum chart, which has lines of numbers. The patient holds this pocket-sized chart at approximately 14 inches from the face. The first line consists of one very large number. Subsequent rows have more lines of numbers that decrease in size. Each eye should be tested one at a time. The smallest row that can be read accurately indicates the visual acuity in that eye.

The clinician should shine a penlight on the pupil of each eye; both pupils should be equally round and reactive to light. A light reflex in one eye should occur consensually in the other eye. To assess the eye's ability to accommodate, observe the patient's pupils as you bring your finger toward the patient's nose. The pupils should constrict as the eyes follow your finger toward the nose. The term PERRLA indicates that the "**P**upils are **E**qually **R**ound and **R**eactive to **L**ight and **A**ccommodation."

The clinician should observe the six cardinal fields of gaze to assess the EOMs (see Fig 43-5). During this examination, the conjugate movement of the eyes should be observed, demonstrating function of the extraocular muscles. The extraocular muscles are the medial, inferior, and superior rectus muscles, as well as the superior and inferior oblique and the levator palpebrae muscles. The extraocular muscles are controlled by the oculomotor nerve (CN III), trochlear nerve (CN IV), and abducens nerve (CN VI). The clinician needs to assess the six cardinal fields of gaze to evaluate the extraocular muscles and CN III, IV, and VI. The clinician should form an "H" or "star" with the index finger in the air as the patient uses only their eyes without moving the head. At the end of EOM assessment, the clinician should bring their finger toward the patient's nose to test convergence of the eyes.

The corneal reflection can be used to assess functional symmetry of extraocular muscles. A penlight can be used to shine a light directly in front of the patient; the reflection of this light on the cornea should appear on both eyes at symmetrical locations. Asymmetry suggests extraocular muscle pathology.

The patient's peripheral vision can be assessed with the clinician standing approximately 2 feet from the patient. The patient should look straight into the clinician's eyes. The clinician then has to bring their own hands around to the sides of the patient. The clinician should slowly move their hands in an arc from back to front toward the front of the patient. Without head movement, the patient needs to report when the hands come into view peripherally. When the clinician's hands are approximately halfway around the patient, they should report peripheral visualization of the clinician's hands.

For a complete examination of the eye, the clinician should complete a funduscopic examination of the patient's retina. This examination requires an ophthalmoscope that shines a bright beam of light through the patient's pupil. For easier inspection, a clinician will often dilate the patient's pupils with administration of an optic mydriatic agent. The patient needs to focus on an object in the distance without changing position of the eyes or head throughout the examination. The clinician needs to shine the ophthalmoscope light on the eye from a distance and observe the pupil's red reflex. The **red reflex** is the reflection of the retina that can be seen when shining light directly on the eye from a distance. It is best seen in a darkened room. After capturing the red reflex, the clinician needs to slowly advance toward the patient; finally, when head to head, the clinician looks into the patient's pupil for a blood vessel. This blood vessel should be followed medially to the optic disc, where its borders and color can be visualized. The disc should have a clear and distinct border, and the optic cup diameter should be less than one-third the disc diameter. The retinal vessels should be examined for color, continuity, and lesions. The retina is the only place on the body where active, live blood vessels can be seen directly. Blood vessels should have clear, smooth borders. The ratio of artery-to-vein diameter should be approximately 2:3. Specific changes of the blood vessels can indicate hypertension, arteriosclerosis, and diabetes mellitus (DM). The ophthalmoscope should be moved laterally on the retina for observation of the macula: a red area without any blood vessels. The macula is an area of central vision that can undergo degeneration with age. The fovea is the central region of the macula.

Diagnosis

Tonometry
A tonometer, a handheld device that measures the pressure within the eye, is similar in shape to a pencil. Once placed on the numbed exterior eye, it can instantly record eye pressure. More often, a tonometer within a slit lamp apparatus shoots a small puff of air into the eye and measures IOP, which is a test to screen for glaucoma.

Slit Lamp Examination
The slit lamp, an instrument with a high-intensity light source, shines a thin beam of light into the eye. A microscope is also contained within the instrument. The slit lamp examination provides a three-dimensional, magnified view of the eye structures in detail. The instrument facilitates an examination of the eye's anterior structures, which include the sclera, conjunctiva, iris, lens, and cornea. The instrument facilitates diagnosis of a variety of eye conditions.

Other Diagnostic Procedures
Other diagnostic procedures used in ophthalmology include x-ray and contrast-media procedures such as orbital venography and angiography. Other imaging techniques include computed tomography (CT) scan, ultrasonography, and magnetic resonance imaging (MRI). For more specific diagnostic methods, see the section "Selected Disorders of Vision."

Treatment

Corrective lenses are the major form of treatment for vision impairment. Alternatively, some patients can be treated with LASIK surgery in lieu of their use of lenses. Many different classes of ophthalmic medications are used in the treatment of various eye disorders. For specific medications, see the section "Selected Disorders of Vision."

Laser coagulation is used in diabetic retinopathy. Many different surgical procedures are also used in ophthalmology.

Corrective Lenses

Corrective lenses are used to treat myopia (nearsightedness), hyperopia (farsightedness), or astigmatism (abnormal shape of the eyeball). Lenses are pieces of transparent material (glass or plastic) that are shaped to bend light rays.

Myopia Correction
Myopic individuals have impaired distance vision. In myopia, the eyeball is elongated and visual images fall in front of the retina. Concave lenses used in myopia spread the light out before it reaches the lens of the eye, allowing the image to fall directly on the retina (see Fig. 43-17).

Hyperopia Correction
Hyperopic individuals cannot see objects in close range, such as reading material. The eyeball is shortened and visual images fall behind the retina. Convex lenses used in hyperopia focus the light on the lens of the eye, causing the image to land directly on the retina (see Fig. 43-18).

Astigmatism Correction
Astigmatism is the result of an irregularly shaped cornea or lens. The eye is shaped like a football instead of a baseball. The eye's shape in astigmatism makes the light rays focus on two spots instead of one on the retina. The cornea has a steep, flat curve that can be corrected with lenses. A cylindrical curve in the corrective lens compensates for the eye's abnormal shape.

LASIK and PRK Surgery

LASIK, commonly referred to as laser eye surgery, is a procedure that can correct myopia, hyperopia, and

Myopia

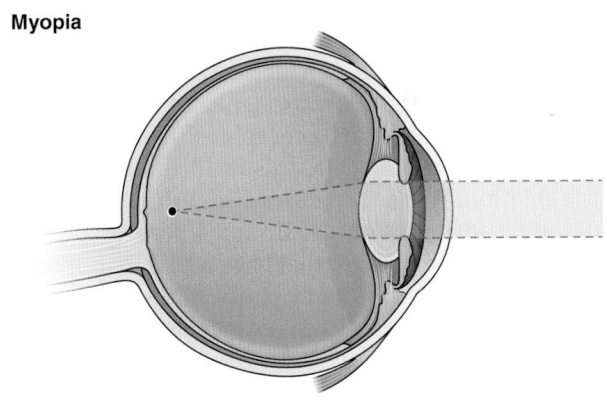

Myopia corrected

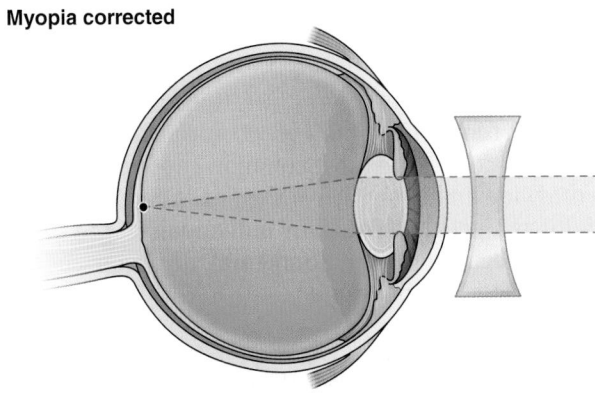

FIGURE 43-17. How corrective lenses change light refraction in myopia.

Hyperopia

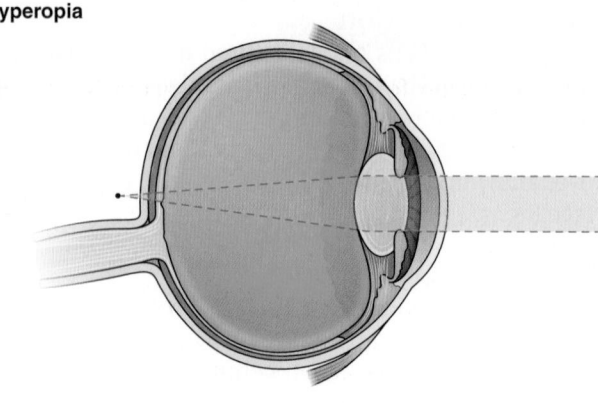

Hyperopia corrected

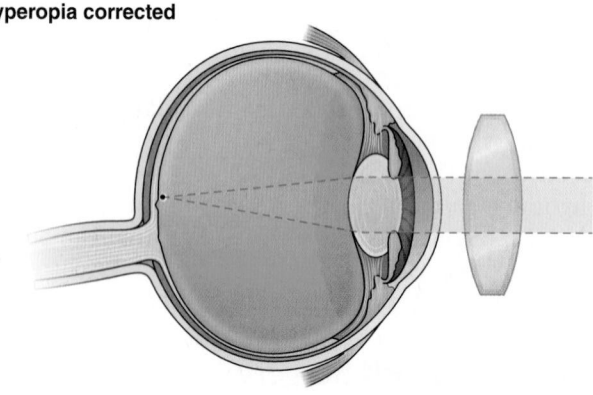

FIGURE 43-18. How corrective lenses change light refraction in hyperopia.

astigmatism. LASIK is performed by using a laser to reshape the cornea to enhance vision. This relatively safe procedure has a low incidence of complications. Other surgical corrective procedures include photorefractive keratectomy (PRK), also called advanced surface ablation. These procedures also reshape the cornea to correct vision. Both LASIK and PRK are advanced technological procedures that have replaced past use of radial keratotomy; for many patients, they offer alternatives to wearing corrective eyeglasses or contact lenses.

Selected Eye Infections and Inflammatory Disorders

Various bacterial and viral infectious and inflammatory disorders affect the eye. *C. trachomatis*, a bacterial infection, is the most common cause of blindness worldwide and is highly contagious. Allergic conjunctivitis is a problem for many individuals in the United States because of environmental antigens such as pollen, dust, or pollutants.

Bacterial and Viral Conjunctivitis

The term *conjunctivitis,* often referred to as pinkeye, describes any inflammatory process that involves the

bulbar conjunctiva, which covers the sclera, and the palpebral conjunctiva, which lines the eyelids. The bulbar conjunctiva is a colorless membrane, whereas the palpebral conjunctiva is a deep pink mucous membrane that keeps the eye moist and protected.

Conjunctivitis is one of the most common nontraumatic eye complaints that presents to the emergency department (ED) or primary-care clinician. Three percent of all ED visits are ocular related, and conjunctivitis is responsible for approximately 30% of all eye complaints. Two percent of all visits to primary-care clinicians are for eye conditions, with 54% of these being either conjunctivitis or corneal abrasion. Bacterial conjunctivitis is more common in children, and viral conjunctivitis is more common in adults.

> **ALERT!** Contact lenses, particularly the extended-wear type, can increase risk of pseudomonal keratitis that can present with symptoms similar to those of conjunctivitis. Keratitis is a more serious condition than conjunctivitis, as perforation of the cornea can occur. Keratitis requires prompt treatment.

Etiology

Bacteria, viruses, parasites, fungi, chemicals, and environmental allergens are the possible etiologies of conjunctivitis. Viral conjunctivitis represents up to 50% of all acute conjunctivitis in primary care. A foreign body in the eye and the use of contact lenses both increase an individual's risk of bacterial or viral conjunctivitis. Exposure to others with conjunctivitis is the most significant risk factor, and the common mode of transmission is from hand to eye.

Pathophysiology

In conjunctivitis, both the palpebral and bulbar conjunctiva undergo inflammation because of a pathogen, allergen, or toxin. *Streptococcus, Staphylococcus,* and *H. influenzae* (biogroup aegypticus) are the most common bacterial organisms that cause conjunctivitis. Viral conjunctivitis is more common than bacterial conjunctivitis, with adenovirus being the most common etiological agent. Adenovirus conjunctivitis, usually accompanied by rhinitis or upper respiratory infection, is relatively benign and self-limited.

Herpes viral infection of the conjunctiva is a more problematic disorder than adenovirus. Herpes viruses remain dormant in the body and can become active at unpredictable times of life. The types of herpes viruses that can affect the eye are herpes zoster and herpes simplex I or II.

Herpes zoster conjunctivitis, also called herpes zoster ophthalmicus, not only affects the conjunctiva but can also cause keratitis, or corneal inflammation. Herpes zoster infection is actually a reactivation of latent varicella zoster. When an individual contracts varicella zoster, the virus becomes dormant and remains in the body; it reactivates as herpes zoster, commonly called shingles. This disorder usually presents as painful blisters on the skin that follow a linear path of a nerve. When this virus is activated along the trigeminal nerve, blisters along the ophthalmic branch affect the cornea. Complications can occur in the form of keratitis, erosion of the cornea, corneal ulceration with keratoconjunctivitis, and bacterial superinfection. Without treatment, corneal scarring can occur.

Herpes simplex virus I or II can also cause conjunctivitis. These viruses, which commonly cause either oral or genital lesions, can infect the eye as well. Similar to herpes zoster infection, herpes simplex causes blisters of the skin along a nerve's path. If the virus infects the trigeminal nerve, the virus can travel on the ophthalmic division of the nerve, which leads to the cornea. Corneal ulceration, keratitis, and keratoconjunctivitis can occur.

Clinical Presentation
Bacterial conjunctivitis produces a mucopurulent exudate, whereas viral infection causes a watery discharge of the eye. In both bacterial and viral conjunctivitis, the patient has a sensation that a foreign body is in the eye; a red, teary eye; or photophobia. The eye may be "glued" shut because of discharge and is usually itchy and edematous with pinpoint subconjunctival hemorrhages. The patient rubs the eyes and blinks frequently, trying to resolve the discomfort with no result. Visual acuity is only slightly affected. Herpes zoster ophthalmic infection causes blistering and erythema along the path of the trigeminal nerve into the eye.

Diagnosis
The diagnosis of conjunctivitis is usually based on the clinical symptoms. Culture of exudate is done with severe infections. Slit lamp examination is necessary if corneal involvement is present.

Treatment
A broad-spectrum, topical, ocular antibiotic is commonly prescribed for bacterial infection. Oral and topical antiviral preparations are used to treat herpes conjunctivitis. In both bacterial and viral conjunctivitis, patients should be discouraged from touching their eyes and should limit direct contact with others until treatment is under way. All bed linens should be thoroughly laundered in hot water. Frequent hand washing is essential.

 CLINICAL CONCEPT

Topical corticosteroid drops can provide relief in bacterial infection; however, corticosteroids will worsen a herpes zoster infection.

Allergic Conjunctivitis

Often mistaken for infectious conjunctivitis, allergic conjunctivitis is extremely common. Airborne antigens, such as pollen, pet dander, dust mites, cockroach debris, cigarette smoke, weeds, and grass, are the most frequent cause of allergic conjunctivitis. Seasonal conjunctivitis occurs during specific times of the year. In spring, trees are the usual stimulus of allergic response. In summer, grasses provoke allergy; in fall, weeds often trigger allergy. People with seasonal conjunctivitis also have allergic rhinitis. In addition, conjunctivitis can occur in atopic individuals—persons with asthma or eczema.

The palpebral conjunctiva becomes inflamed and swollen with a cobblestone appearance. Individuals have tearing and redness of the eye with intense itching. Diagnosis is made from the clinical examination and history. Symptoms are alleviated by the avoidance of allergens; cold compresses, topical vasoconstrictors, and antihistamines can reduce the symptoms. Topical NSAIDs are also used for immune-mediated forms of conjunctivitis. Corticosteroids provide relief, but long-term use can lead to complications such as glaucoma, cataracts, and secondary infection.

Chlamydia trachomatis
C. trachomatis, a bacterial organism, is the leading cause of eye infection worldwide. The most common cause of blindness in underdeveloped countries, it causes an infection called chronic keratoconjunctivitis, commonly referred to as **trachoma.** In keratoconjunctivitis, both the conjunctiva and cornea undergo inflammation.

Trachoma is endemic in parts of Africa, Asia, the Middle East, Latin America, the Pacific Islands, and aboriginal communities in Australia. In 2016, it was estimated that 190 million people live in regions where trachoma is a common public health problem, with 1.9 million suffering blindness or visual impairment. Those most commonly affected are children under 5 years of age. In 1998, the WHO organized an Alliance for the Global Elimination of Blinding Trachoma with the goal of controlling spread of the disease by 2020. By 2021, 69,266 people received surgical treatment for advanced stage of the disease, and 64.6 million people were treated with antibiotics. Global antibiotic coverage in 2021 was 44%. However, the goal of elimination of trachoma has not yet been reached; therefore, the WHO program has been extended to 2030.

C. trachomatis is the most common sexually transmitted infection (STI) in the United States. According to the Centers for Disease Control and Prevention (CDC), in 2015 the rate of *Chlamydia* infection was approximately 646 per 100,000 females in the United States. Therefore, pregnant patients are screened for *Chlamydia* infection and other STIs prior to giving birth. Both *Chlamydia* and gonorrhea can cause eye infection in the newborn during delivery, referred to as as ophthalmia neonatorum (ON). *Chlamydia* is responsible for up to 40% of ON and gonorrhea for less than 1% of ON. To prevent ON, 0.5% topical erythromycin is applied to both eyes of the newborn shortly after birth.

Etiology

Trachoma, a severe eye infection caused by *C. trachomatis* serotypes A, B, Ba, and C, occurs mostly in rural settings where sanitation is poor. Although trachoma is rare in the United States, certain populations living in crowded or low-income areas or with inadequate hygiene are at high risk for this eye disorder. Trachoma is spread through direct contact with the secretions from an infected eye, nose, or throat, or by contact with contaminated objects, such as towels or clothes. Flies can also spread the bacteria. Disease transmission occurs primarily between children and the people who care for them. Repeated episodes of reinfection within a family are common.

Pathophysiology

Active trachoma is characterized by a mucopurulent keratoconjunctivitis that affects mainly the conjunctival surface of the upper eyelid and cornea. There is intense conjunctival inflammation, which leads to conjunctival fibrosis and scarring. Also, there are obvious corneal abrasions, corneal scarring, and opacification. Ultimately, these conditions lead to blindness. Infection concurrently occurs in extraocular mucous membranes, commonly the nasopharynx, leading to a nasal discharge. These nasal secretions commonly cause the spread of infection.

Clinical Presentation

When taking the patient's history, the clinician should include questions regarding recent travel to regions of the world where trachoma is endemic. The patient's current living situation should be investigated because crowded, unsanitary living conditions increase susceptibility. In addition to questions about the discomfort experienced in the eyes, the patient should be asked about family infection. Symptoms of trachoma begin 5 to 12 days after being exposed to the bacteria. Symptoms include cloudy cornea, discharge from the eye, swelling of preauricular lymph nodes, swollen eyelids, and entropion formation. The patient's eyelashes are turned inward (trichiasis). The patient endures eye discomfort and tends to rub the eyes, which allows secretions to spread to others from the hand.

Diagnosis

The patient is often diagnosed based on the clinical manifestations in endemic regions. The best laboratory technique to confirm diagnosis of *C. trachomatis* infection is the nucleic acid amplification test referred to as the polymerase chain reaction. This test amplifies the DNA of the pathogen, which, in turn, identifies the specific organism.

Treatment

The key to treating trachoma is the SAFE strategy developed by the WHO:

S – surgery (for turned-in lashes)
A – antibiotics
F – facial cleanliness
E – environmental improvement

Two antibiotics are used for trachoma control: oral azithromycin and tetracycline eye ointment. Oral antibiotics are necessary because infection occurs in the nasopharynx as well as the eyes. If a topical eye antibiotic is used alone, patients can reinfect themselves from their nasal secretions. Mass antibiotic programs in regions where trachoma is endemic are most effective. Annual treatment programs are recommended for at least 3 years or until prevalence of disease declines to less than 5%.

The promotion of sanitation, improved hygiene, and clean water is key to diminishing contagion. Regions affected by *C. trachomatis* infection require safe drinking water and sanitary disposal of human feces. Improvements in personal and community hygiene are associated with significant reduction in the prevalence of the disease.

Selected Disorders of Vision

Glaucoma, diabetic retinopathy, age-related macular degeneration (AMD), papilledema, and cataracts are among the most common eye disorders that can cause blindness. Each disorder has a distinct pathophysiology and characteristic signs and symptoms. Structural eye disorders such as vitreous hemorrhage and retinal detachment cause unique visual symptoms and can also cause blindness without treatment. Optic neuritis, retinitis pigmentosa, retinoblastoma, and melanoma of the eye are less common disorders, but can also cause blindness if untreated.

Glaucoma

Glaucoma—one of the leading preventable causes of blindness in the world—is caused by elevated IOP, which leads to pressure on the optic nerve with consequent nerve damage and blindness (see Fig. 43-19). There are two main types of the disorder: primary open-angle glaucoma (POAG) and primary angle closure glaucoma (PACG). Open-angle glaucoma is usually silent and slowly progressive, whereas angle closure glaucoma occurs suddenly and is an emergency situation. With appropriate screening and treatment, glaucoma usually can be identified and its progress arrested before significant effects on vision occur.

Ninety percent of glaucoma patients have POAG and 10% have PACG. POAG affects more than 2 million

Healthy eye

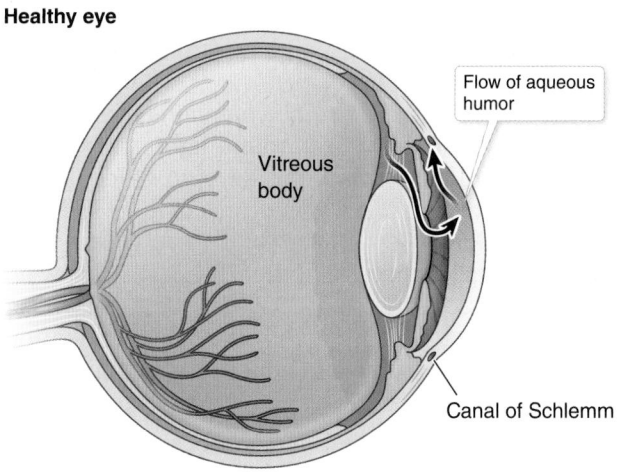

Flow of aqueous humor

Vitreous body

Canal of Schlemm

Glaucoma

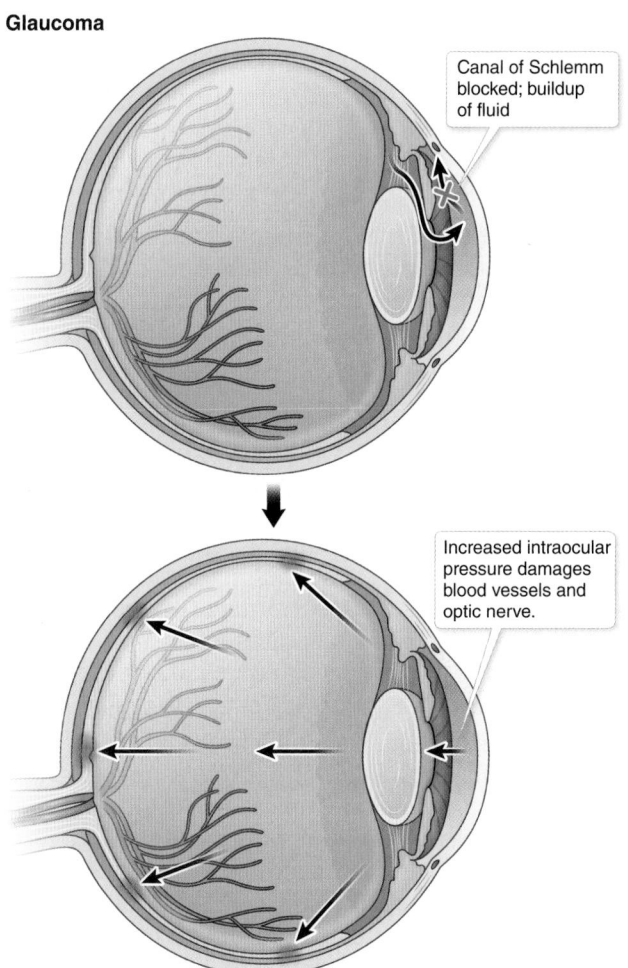

Canal of Schlemm blocked; buildup of fluid

Increased intraocular pressure damages blood vessels and optic nerve.

FIGURE 43-19. Structures involved in glaucoma.

individuals in the United States. With the aging of the U.S. population, this number will increase to more than 3 million by 2020. It is estimated that 1% to 2% of people older than 40 years of age have POAG, with 25% of cases undetected. Glaucoma has been called the "silent thief of sight" because the loss of vision is gradual over a prolonged time, and symptoms occur only when the disease is quite advanced.

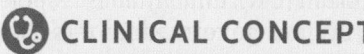

PACG is an acute emergency, and its outcome is dependent on duration from onset to treatment. For unknown reasons, PACG is common in persons of Asian descent, which includes Chinese, Inuit, Southeast Asian, and Asian Indian. PACG occurs in 1 of 1,000 European Americans, but about 1 in 100 Asian Americans. In addition, Asian Americans with PACG are difficult to treat because medical management often fails. Despite treatment, they often suffer a progressive increase in IOP and deterioration in visual acuity. PACG predominately affects females because of their shallower anterior chamber. Older adult patients in their sixth and seventh decades of life are at greatest risk.

Etiology

The cause of glaucoma is unknown; however, there are many known risk factors. For example, age older than 40 years is a risk factor for the development of open-angle glaucoma, with up to 15% of people affected by age 70. As previously noted, ethnicity is a risk factor. Other risk factors include genetic predisposition; myopia; and a history of migraine headaches, cardiovascular disease, diabetes, systemic hypertension, and systemic hypotension.

Specific drugs, such as sympathomimetics, anticholinergics, selective serotonin receptor inhibitor antidepressants, sulfonamides, cocaine, and botulinum toxin, can precipitate PACG. Dim light and rapid correction of hyperglycemia can also trigger it. Studies have identified PACG associated with carotid artery–cavernous sinus fistula, trauma, prone surgical positioning, and giant cell arteritis. Hyperopia (farsightedness) is also a risk factor.

Pathophysiology

POAG and PACG have different disease mechanisms. Although they are triggered by different etiological factors, they basically require treatment that decreases IOP.

Primary Open-Angle Glaucoma. The pathophysiology of glaucoma is not completely understood. There are known structural changes that occur in glaucoma; however, there are many different theories about the cause of retinal cell and optic nerve damage. Significant structural changes found in the eyes involve the ciliary muscle, trabecular meshwork, and canal of Schlemm. The ciliary muscle is attached to a trabecular meshwork that allows free flow of aqueous fluid from the anterior chamber to posterior chamber of the eye. When the ciliary muscle contracts, it allows the drainage of aqueous fluid through the canal of Schlemm; however, with muscle relaxation, the canal is obstructed. The ciliary muscle is innervated by both the sympathetic and parasympathetic nervous system. Stimulation of parasympathetic nerves contract the ciliary muscle, allowing ocular fluid drainage. Stimulation of sympathetic nerves relaxes the ciliary muscle and causes obstruction of ocular fluid drainage.

🧫 CLINICAL CONCEPT

Drugs or conditions that enhance anticholinergic activity have the same effect as sympathetic nerve activation—both cause relaxation of the ciliary muscle and obstruction of fluid drainage. This is particularly important for clinicians to recognize when prescribing drugs with anticholinergic effects. For example, many antidepressants have anticholinergic side effects, so glaucoma can be initiated or worsened by antidepressants.

When ocular fluid drainage is obstructed, the high level of fluid raises IOP and places pressure on the junction of the optic nerve and the retina at the back of the eye. The optic cup in the center of the optic disc enlarges under high IOP. Until recently, it was believed that elevated IOP was responsible for optic nerve damage in glaucoma. However, studies show that only 30% to 50% of all glaucoma patients have elevated IOP; up to 50% do not have high IOP. So, elevated IOP is now believed to be an important—but not the only—factor responsible for optic nerve damage. Other mechanisms of glaucoma are under investigation. Regardless of the mechanisms involved, the outcome of glaucoma is the death of retinal and optic nerve cells, leading to irreversible visual field loss.

Primary Angle Closure Glaucoma. PACG can occur in people who were born with a narrow angle between the iris and the cornea. This type of glaucoma is more common in people who are hyperopic. In PACG, the ciliary muscle is relaxed and the canal of Schlemm is obstructed. Relaxation may occur because of sympathetic or anticholinergic activity or other etiology. With ciliary muscle relaxation, drainage of aqueous fluid is obstructed, resulting in a sudden increase of IOP within the eyes. Consequently, there is a sudden loss of peripheral or central vision.

Clinical Presentation

When gathering information for the history, the clinician should focus on age, use of lenses, past eye problems, family history of glaucoma, ethnicity, and medications. The use of anticholinergic medications is a common trigger of glaucoma. It is important for the clinician to recognize that many medications—including antidepressants, antipsychotics, antihistamines, specific anticholinergic bronchodilators, and muscle relaxants, as well as gastrointestinal and some cardiac drugs—have anticholinergic side effects.

The patient with glaucoma complains of eye pain, eye redness, nausea, halos around lights, and vision loss. In PACG, these symptoms develop suddenly and rapidly, whereas in POAG symptoms may be silent or develop gradually.

On physical examination, the patient may show no signs of illness. Redness of the eye and blood vessels in the sclera may be apparent. Funduscopic examination is necessary. The clinician should inspect the retina, particularly the optic nerve.

ALERT! Anticholinergic drugs and drugs with anticholinergic side effects are contraindicated in glaucoma.

Diagnosis

An examination of the optic nerve is essential to look for an increase in the cup-to-disc ratio. The optic cup is the portion of the optic disc not occupied by nerve fibers. Located in the center of the optic disc, the optic cup-to-disc ratio is normally 0.3 or lower. With glaucoma, there is a progressive increase in optic nerve damage, which increases the optic cup area. Patients with glaucoma have an increased cup-to-disc ratio from 0.7 to 1.0. The greater the optic nerve damage, the greater the vision loss. The patient should be referred to an ophthalmologist for slit lamp examination. Computerized optic nerve imaging is needed if there is any suspicion of damage to the optic nerve.

Treatment

The treatment of glaucoma is aimed at reducing IOP by improving aqueous fluid outflow, reducing the production of aqueous fluid, or both. Treatments available for glaucoma include topical eye medication, oral medications, laser procedures, and incisional surgery. Major drug classes for medical treatment of POAG include the following: alpha-2 agonists, beta blockers, carbonic anhydrase inhibitors, cholinergic agents, and prostaglandin analogs. Traditional surgical procedures to correct glaucoma have included trabeculotomy and glaucoma drainage device implantation to reduce IOP. Micro-invasive surgeries are the newest techniques in glaucoma treatment. These surgeries increase the trabecular outflow using micro-stent insertion or redirection of drainage of aqueous fluid. If glaucoma is left untreated, blindness will occur.

Papilledema

Papilledema is a swelling of the optic nerve caused by an increase in intracranial pressure. Patients with papilledema may report headache, intermittent diplopia (double vision), vomiting and nausea, and tinnitus. Papilledema is a critical sign of intracranial hypertension, a potentially life-threatening situation. On funduscopic examination, the borders of the optic disc are unclear and undefined (see Fig. 43-20). Treatment focuses on the underlying pathological process that caused the elevated intracranial pressure, such as a brain tumor. Untreated papilledema eventually may lead to permanent blindness.

> **ALERT!** Papilledema is indicative of increased intracranial pressure, which requires immediate medical intervention.

Diabetic Retinopathy

Diabetic retinopathy is a change in the retina that occurs in individuals with type 1 or type 2 diabetes. Before the diagnosis of either type of diabetes, vascular changes occur that are caused by periodic high blood glucose levels. Retinopathy, one of these vascular changes, is often present upon the diagnosis of diabetes.

It is estimated that 30.3 million people in the United States are living with diabetes, accounting for 9.4% of the population. In 2015, 25% of adults over age 65 had diabetes, with this number expected to more than double by 2050. It is theorized that 35% of adults with diabetes in the United States have some degree of diabetic retinopathy at diagnosis. With the epidemic of diabetes worldwide, there will be an increase in diabetic retinopathy in the future.

 CLINICAL CONCEPT

Diabetic retinopathy is the most frequent cause of blindness among adults aged 20 to 74 years.

Etiology

There are various risk factors for diabetes (see Chapter 25). High glucose levels and genetic susceptibility are the major risk factors for vascular changes that lead to diabetic retinopathy. It is theorized that before the initial diagnosis of DM, there are intermittent periods of high glucose levels that are asymptomatic, unmonitored, and untreated. During these times, retinal damage probably begins. After diagnosis, if the patient has poor blood glucose regulation, retinal blood vessel changes continue to worsen.

Pathophysiology

There are two forms of diabetic retinopathy: nonproliferative and proliferative. Early in diabetes, nonproliferative retinopathy occurs. On funduscopic examination, tiny aneurysms and hemorrhages are seen. Areas of ischemia of the retina, microinfarcts, and areas of nerve damage called "cotton wool spots" are also seen.

Later in the course of diabetes, proliferative retinopathy occurs. In this stage, diabetes stimulates vasoactive growth factors that cause neovascularization. This is called a proliferative retinopathy because the retina has many more blood vessels than normal. The new blood vessels grow throughout the retina and are seen on funduscopic examination. The new blood vessels have very weak walls, which leads to aneurysms and hemorrhages. Also, new blood vessels grow into the vitreous of the eyeball, which can lead to bleeding behind the vitreous and retinal detachment.

The exact pathophysiological mechanism of retinal vessel aneurysms and hemorrhages in nonproliferative diabetic retinopathy is incompletely understood, but there are many theories. Platelet and red blood cell abnormalities, such as increased erythrocyte aggregation, increased platelet aggregation, and increased platelet adhesion, are seen in diabetes. These changes predispose the patient to sluggish circulation, endothelial damage, and capillary occlusion within the retinal blood vessels. This leads to retinal ischemia, which, in turn, contributes to the development of diabetic retinopathy.

Another theory involves the high glucose levels that occur in DM. Increased levels of blood glucose are thought to cause endothelial injury throughout the body, including the retinal blood vessels. This renders the blood vessel walls susceptible to arteriosclerosis, aneurysm, and rupture.

Other researchers assert that high blood glucose levels stimulate a process called the aldose reductase pathway in certain tissues, which converts sugars into sorbitol. The walls of retinal blood vessels are directly damaged by this increased level of sorbitol, eventually leading to weakness and aneurysms.

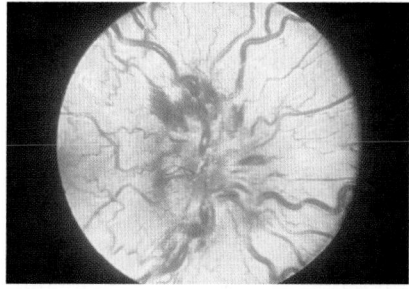

FIGURE 43-20. Papilledema. *(Courtesy of Wills Eye Hospital, Philadelphia, PA.)*

 CLINICAL CONCEPT

When an individual is diagnosed with diabetes, a funduscopic examination should be done to rule out diabetic retinopathy.

Clinical Presentation

The patient history should contain information about the duration of diabetes and daily glucose control. The history should document the patient's current medications and last ophthalmic examination. The history should also contain current medical or surgical disorders such as cardiovascular or peripheral vascular disease. Details about the patient's vision are necessary, so a vision test should be done. Initially, diabetic retinopathy may be asymptomatic or cause only mild vision problems. As the condition progresses, symptoms may include floaters, blurred vision, poor night vision, and vision loss. It usually affects both eyes. Proliferation of new blood vessels is indicative of a poor prognosis.

Diagnosis

In diabetic retinopathy, the retina often shows lesions such as microaneurysms, hemorrhages, hard exudates (lipid residues), cotton wool spots (areas of nerve destruction), and proliferation of fragile, new blood vessels (see Fig. 43-21). A thorough slit lamp examination by an ophthalmologist is needed.

Treatment

Blood glucose control with maintenance of HgbA1c in the 6% to 7% range is necessary to slow the progression of retinal changes. Laser photocoagulation is used to destroy new, fragile vessels and to stop hemorrhages. Drug therapy includes intravitreal injections of ovine hyaluronidase (e.g., Vitrase), antivascular endothelial growth factor (VEGF) inhibitors (e.g., aflibercept and ranibizumab), and intravitreal corticosteroids. Treatment of diabetic retinopathy can decrease the risk of vision loss by over half.

Cataracts

Cataracts, a major cause of blindness worldwide, cause visual impairment because of excessive growth of the epithelial layers of the eye lens (see Fig. 43-22). The lens becomes thickened, with less transparency and flexibility. They commonly affect older adults because lens thickening is a physiological change associated with advancing age. Approximately 20.5 million (17.2%) Americans older than 40 years have a

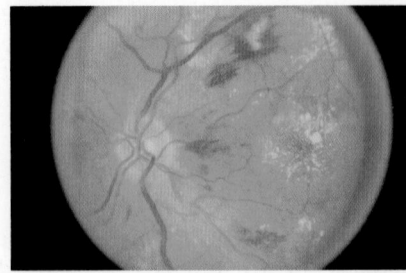

FIGURE 43-21. Diabetic retinopathy. *(Courtesy of Wills Eye Hospital, Philadelphia, PA.)*

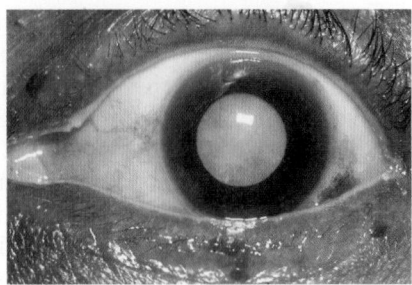

FIGURE 43-22. Cataract. *(Courtesy of Wills Eye Hospital, Philadelphia, PA.)*

cataract in either eye. With the rising number of older adults in the population, this number is expected to increase to 30.1 million people by 2020.

There are different types of cataracts; this section discusses senile and congenital cataracts.

Etiology

Risk factors for senile cataract development include advancing age, cigarette smoking, obesity, diabetes, kidney disorders, musculoskeletal disorders, trauma, long-term steroid use, and exposure to ultraviolet light. In addition to steroids, other drugs associated with increased risk of cataract development include alfuzosin and tamsulosin, which are used to treat benign prostatic hyperplasia.

Congenital cataracts develop in the fetus because of infection contracted during pregnancy. Infections such as rubella, syphilis, toxoplasmosis, and cytomegalovirus are associated with congenital cataract. Other causes of congenital cataract include Down syndrome, Marfan syndrome, and Alport syndrome, as well as many other genetic disorders.

Pathophysiology

Multiple mechanisms contribute to the progressive loss of transparency of the lens in senile cataract formation. As a consequence of normal aging, the lenses in the eyes develop excessive layers of epithelium. The epithelial cells lose the ability to degenerate as new layers of cells proliferate and accumulate. The increased thickness of the lens makes it less able to accommodate. Also, the water solubility of the lens diminishes, making it more inflexible. Protein fibers are normally arranged in a precise manner that makes the lens clear and allows light to pass through without interference. With aging, accumulated damage of the protein fibers of the lenses by free radicals occurs. Protein fibers degenerate and begin to clump together, and clouding of small areas of the lens occurs. As the cataract continues to develop, the clouding becomes denser and involves a greater part of the lens.

Clinical Presentation

A patient with a cataract often presents with a history of gradual loss of vision. Individuals with the condition develop blurry vision and have cloudiness in the lens of the eye. Many people see halos at night around bright objects or they become more sensitive to glare. The patient's eyes have an opacity covering the center of their eyes. The red reflex, which is a reflection of the retina seen on funduscopic examination, is duller than normal in the presence of a cataract.

The progression of cataracts frequently creates changes in the lens that result in myopia. Presbyopia can be counteracted by the myopic effect of cataracts. Patients often report an improvement in their near vision and less need for reading glasses as they experience this phenomenon of second sight. However, this is temporary because the lens increases in excessive thickness with time, which undermines this effect.

A complete ocular examination must be performed, beginning with visual acuity for both near and far distances. When the patient complains of glare, visual acuity should be tested in a brightly lit room. The patient's extraocular muscles should be assessed in all directions of gaze, and it is important to rule out any other causes for the patient's visual symptoms.

Diagnosis
A full ophthalmic examination, which includes dilated eye examination, visual acuity, and tonometry, is recommended. Ocular imaging studies such as ultrasound, CT scan, and MRI are often needed for an adequate view of the back of the eye. If macular involvement or glaucoma is suspected, specialized tests are done as well.

Treatment
Patients may need lenses to improve visual acuity and can be prescribed antiglare sunglasses or magnifying lenses. When cataracts interfere with activities of daily living, surgical intervention is needed. Treatment involves surgical removal of the cataract and replacement with an artificial clear lens called an intraocular lens. Manual small incision cataract surgery (MSICS) is the newest technique used. If cataracts go untreated, the individual will have worsening of vision and possible blindness.

Age-Related Macular Degeneration

AMD is a deterioration of the macula, the specific area on the retina that provides central vision and allows for perception of fine details. As the macula degenerates, central vision deteriorates and the patient develops a blind spot in the center of the visual field. AMD usually produces a slow, painless loss of vision.

AMD is the most common cause of vision loss in the United States in those 50 years or older, and its prevalence increases with age. It occurs in approximately 10% of the population aged 65 to 74 years and in 25% of the population older than age 74. As the population of individuals older than 85 years is projected to increase by the year 2020, the prevalence of AMD is expected to increase from 1.75 million individuals to 2.95 million individuals.

Etiology
AMD is caused by a combination of genetic, behavioral, and environmental factors. Advanced age and family history are nonmodifiable risk factors associated with AMD. Genetic mutations on chromosomes 1, 6, and 10 are associated with the disorder. Genetic factors contribute to approximately 50% of the sibling risk of developing AMD. Smoking, hypertension, obesity, and dietary fat intake are the modifiable risk factors.

Pathophysiology
AMD involves two layers of the eye: the retina, which contains the nerves, and the choroid, which contains the blood supply. There are two types of AMD: nonexudative, also called "dry" macular degeneration, and exudative, also called "wet" macular degeneration. The pathophysiological mechanism of each type is different. More than 90% of patients diagnosed with AMD have the nonexudative type.

 CLINICAL CONCEPT

Nonexudative AMD can progress over the course of decades, whereas exudative AMD can result in vision loss within months.

The pathophysiology of both types involves the retinal pigmented epithelium (RPE), a metabolically active layer of cells that supports the retina's function. RPE cells normally phagocytose degenerated retinal cells and continually recycle and process the cellular materials. The RPE cells normally transport the cellular debris to the vessels of the choroid layer. The debris can then be removed from the region. However, as the RPE cells age, they become less able to process accumulated cellular debris. Changes in the permeability of the choroid membrane with age lead to deposition of material between the RPE and choroid. The deposited material is called **drusen**. The capillaries of the choroid also become less able to absorb extracellular material; this also contributes to drusen formation. Drusen appear as yellow-white accumulations of material in the macula region of the retina.

In the nonexudative (dry) form, drusen accumulate between the retina and the choroid layers of the eye; this can separate the layers, leading to retinal detachment. In the wet form, which is more severe, blood vessels grow from the choroid layer to behind the retina and separate the layers, also leading to retinal detachment.

Clinical Presentation
Patients with AMD usually report a family history of decreased vision late in life, including difficulty with night vision or low light conditions. Commonly, patients with AMD report fluctuations in vision, with

some poor vision days and other days when it appears improved. Patients also report difficulty with reading and seeing faces. Central vision is affected with peripheral vision intact. Areas of yellow-white drusen in the macula region are visible upon funduscopic examination.

Diagnosis

AMD is usually diagnosed by using an Amsler grid to measure central vision. Individuals with macular degeneration will notice black spots in their central vision when looking through the Amsler grid; slit lamp examination is also necessary. Fluorescein angiography is a procedure that can highlight the retinal epithelium.

Treatment

To prevent AMD, consumption of antioxidants, including vitamins A, C, D, and E; zinc; and lutein, is highly recommended, as is a supplement consisting of folic acid, pyridoxine, and vitamin B_{12}. A low-fat diet and smoking cessation, if applicable, are also preventive strategies. Wraparound sunglasses are recommended to diminish glare. Statin medications have been shown to reduce drusen in nonexudative AMD. Laser therapy has shown mixed results. Intravitreous injection of VEGF inhibitors, such as ranibizumab or bevacizumab, has shown successful results in exudative AMD. Aflibercept is a recent FDA-approved VEGF blocker. Photodynamic therapy, which involves injection of photosensitizing dye followed by laser therapy, has shown mixed results. Surgical procedures have also shown mixed results.

Vitreous Floaters

The gel-like vitreous humor makes up the majority of the eyeball. It is an extracellular matrix composed primarily of water, collagens, and hyaluronic acid that extends from behind the lens to the rear wall of the eye. Small amounts of liquefaction of the vitreous gel occur as a normal physiological change of aging. It occurs most commonly in persons with myopia. With gel liquefaction, there is weakened attachment of the vitreous layer to the retina, which is the most common cause of primary vitreous floaters. Vitreous floaters are caused by pieces of the vitreous that pull away from the retinal layer and cast a shadow on the retina. They appear as dark linear, circular, or nodular patterns of debris in the visual field that move with eye and head movements. Vitreous floaters are usually benign and resolve with time. However, in some persons, they can interfere with quality of life. In recent years, neodymium-doped yttrium-aluminum-garnet (YAG) laser vitreolysis has been used as a noninvasive therapeutic technique to eliminate floaters. However, studies show conflicting results regarding efficacy and potential complications that have prevented the widespread adoption of the technique.

Retinal Detachment

Retinal detachment occurs when the retina is pulled away from its normal position in the back of the eye. It can occur at any age, but it is more common in people older than 40 years of age. It affects males more than females and European Americans more than African Americans. It occurs in 1 in 10,000 persons annually.

Etiology

The vitreous gel of the eyeball liquefies with age. As it liquefies, it places traction on the retinal layer, which lies beneath and pulls away, causing a tear. Risk factors for retinal detachment include myopia, prior intraocular surgery, aphakia (absence of the lens), some inflammatory conditions, and genetic susceptibility. Prior intraocular surgery for cataract removal, inflammation caused by cytomegalovirus, and Marfan syndrome are conditions that also increase the risk of retinal detachment.

Retinal detachment is also more likely to occur in people who have had a retinal detachment in the other eye, a positive family history of retinal detachment, and a history of eye injury. In young children and teenagers, eye trauma can cause this condition.

Pathophysiology

The retina is a highly organized layer of neurons in the back of the eye that converts photon energy into neural impulses that are directed into the optic nerve. Retinal detachment occurs when the inner layers of the retina break away from the retinal epithelial cells and choroid layer. Full thickness detachment of the retina is also called rhegmatogenous retinal detachment. This is often caused by fluid accumulation in between the layers from liquefied vitreous, inflammatory conditions of the choroid layer, hypertensive retinopathy, proliferative diabetic retinopathy, sickle cell disease, or penetrating trauma. After retinal detachment occurs, nutrition and circulation to the photoreceptor cells is impaired. The impaired photoreceptor cells undergo apoptosis and degeneration; pigment cells and fibroblasts then abnormally proliferate, leading to irreversible vision impairment. If not treated quickly, the rate of blindness is nearly 100%.

Clinical Presentation

Initial symptoms commonly include the sensation of photopsia, which is a sudden flash of light, accompanied by floaters and disrupted vision. Floaters are described as debris or cobwebs that move in and out of the visual field. Some patients report a shower of black spots in their visual field. Over time, the individual may report a shadow in the peripheral visual field, which may spread rapidly to involve the entire visual field in a matter of days. Vision loss may be described as filmy, cloudy, irregular, or curtainlike. Mono-ocular visual field loss often is reported and requires emergency ophthalmological evaluation.

Diagnosis and Treatment

Ophthalmoscopic examination is used to diagnose retinal detachment. Treatment depends on the type, location, and size of the detachment. Retinal tears are usually treated with laser surgery or cryotherapy (referred to as cryoretinopexy) to reseal the retina to the back wall of the eye. Once the retinal break is sealed, retinal cells reabsorb the fluid and heal the tear within 24 to 48 hours. Patients with severe retinal detachment may require vitrectomy, which involves surgical lacerations through the sclera to drain fluid. Retinal detachments do not improve without treatment.

> **ALERT!** Prompt treatment and repair of retinal detachment are necessary to prevent permanent vision loss.

Retinoblastoma

Retinoblastoma is a malignant tumor of the retina caused by a genetic mutation that generally affects children younger than the age of 6 years. Incidence is 1 in every 15,000 to 20,000 live births. In 60% of cases, the disease is unilateral, and the median age at diagnosis is 2 years. Retinoblastoma is bilateral in about 40% of cases. Survival rates are between 86% and 92%, although many individuals suffer another cancer later in life.

Etiology

The etiology of retinoblastoma is a mutation in the gene located at 13q14, referred to as the *Rb* gene. At the time of initial examination, the clinician should obtain a careful family history and ask specific questions about the occurrence of retinoblastoma, eye problems, or malignancy in any family members. Approximately 5% of patients who develop this disease have a positive family history.

Pathophysiology

Retinoblastoma is a cancerous development in the optic nerve. The tumor arises in the retina and can invade the brain. The tumor cells have an immature appearance and are referred to as retinoblasts. Often the tumor presents as a white mass when seen with the ophthalmoscope.

Clinical Presentation

Signs and symptoms of retinoblastoma include white spots in the pupil, strabismus, redness of the eye, eye pain, and poor vision. Often the abnormality is discovered while viewing photographs of the child. Instead of the typical "red reflex" from the camera flash, the pupil may appear white or distorted. During the examination with the ophthalmoscope, the clinician can see that the red reflex is absent.

Diagnosis and Treatment

An examination of the retina under general anesthesia leads to a diagnosis of the eye tumor. If the cancer is in one eye and the tumor is large, treatment is usually removal of the eyeball, a procedure known as enucleation. If the cancer is in one eye and it is expected that vision can be saved, treatment may include radiation therapy, cryotherapy, and chemotherapy. If the cancer is in both eyes, treatment may include the enucleation of the eye with the most cancer and radiation therapy to the other eye, or chemotherapy followed by local treatment. Combination chemotherapy is demonstrating successful results. Enucleation surgery is done when vision cannot be saved.

The prognosis and treatment options depend on the stage of the cancer and the likelihood of restoring vision in one or both eyes. Without treatment, the cancer will spread through the optic nerve to the brain and cause death in 98% of patients. As previously indicated, treatment often means blindness—including the loss of one or both eyes; patients who survive treatment of retinoblastoma are at risk for second nonocular cancers—notably osteosarcoma later in life.

Chapter Summary

- Vision is measured using an eye chart, and the results are recorded as a pair of numbers called visual acuity. Normal sight is scored as a ratio of 20/20. The numerator indicates that the object to be visualized is at a distance of 20 feet. The denominator indicates how far away the object seems to the patient.

- The leading cause of blindness among European Americans is AMD; among African Americans, cataract and glaucoma account for more than 60% of cases of blindness. Trachoma, an infection caused by *Chlamydia*, is a leading cause of blindness in areas with fewer socioeconomic resources.

- According to the American Medical Association, vision that is worse than 20/200 in the better eye with correction is considered blindness.

- The WHO has specific parameters that categorize vision impairment and blindness. The different types of visual impairment include myopia, hyperopia, presbyopia,

- astigmatism, amblyopia, and color blindness. Different lenses are used to correct vision.
- LASIK, commonly referred to as laser eye surgery, is a procedure that can correct myopia, hyperopia, and astigmatism.
- Infection of the eyelid, termed a stye or hordeolum, is most often caused by *S. aureus*.
- Conjunctivitis, which is inflammation of the conjunctiva, is a common disorder; it is bacterial, viral, or allergic in origin.
- Corneal abrasion, the most common type of structural eye trauma, is damage to the epithelial surface of the cornea, usually caused by a foreign body that comes into contact with the eye. Diagnosis requires fluorescein dye instillation in the eye and inspection with a blue cobalt light, which highlights the area of trauma.
- Diabetic retinopathy is the most frequent cause of blindness among adults aged 20 to 74 years.
- Glaucoma is one of the leading preventable causes of blindness in the world. It is caused by elevated IOP, which leads to pressure on the optic nerve with consequent nerve damage and blindness.
- Papilledema is the swelling of the optic disc caused by increased intracranial pressure.

- A cataract is clouding of the lens of the eye caused by overgrowth of the lens. Cataracts commonly affect older adults because lens thickening is a physiological change associated with advancing age.
- AMD is a deterioration of the macula, a specific area on the retina that provides central vision. As the macula degenerates, central vision deteriorates and the patient develops a blind spot in the center of their visual field. It is the most common cause of vision loss in the United States in those 50 years or older, and its prevalence increases with age.
- Floaters in the visual field commonly occur with age due to small areas of liquefaction of the vitreous gel that pulls away from its attachment to the retina.
- Retinal detachment can occur in older adults as a large section of the vitreous layer pulls away from the retina, leaving a tear. Often this requires emergency surgery.
- Retinoblastoma, cancer of the optic nerve that occurs most often in young children, causes an absent red reflex in the affected eye and a white mass visible on fundoscopy. This often requires enucleation of the eye.

Making the Connections

Signs and Symptoms	Physical Assessment Findings	Diagnostic Testing	Treatment
Bacterial and Viral Conjunctivitis Infection or allergy that causes inflammation of the palpebral portion of the conjunctiva. Exudative discharge may be present in bacterial infection.			
Mild foreign body in the eye and photophobia. Visual acuity slightly affected.	Red, swollen conjunctiva. Bacterial conjunctivitis yields mucopurulent exudates, whereas viral infection and allergy cause a watery discharge.	Culture of exudate if present.	Topical antibiotic. Anti-inflammatory topical drops prevent contagion with bacterial infection.
C. trachomatis A bacterial infection that causes mucopurulent keratoconjunctivitis. There is intense conjunctival inflammation, which leads to conjunctival fibrosis, scarring, corneal abrasions, corneal scarring, and opacification. Ultimately, these conditions lead to blindness.			
Symptoms include discharge from the eye, swelling of preauricular lymph nodes, and swollen eyelids. The eye appears "glued shut." The patient endures eye discomfort and tends to rub the eyes, which allows secretions to spread to others from the hand.	Patient's eyes demonstrate cloudy corneas, discharge from the eyes, swelling of preauricular lymph nodes, swollen eyelids, and entropion formation.	Nucleic acid amplification test, referred to as the polymerase chain reaction. This test amplifies the DNA of the pathogen, which in turn identifies the specific organism.	The key to treating trachoma is the SAFE strategy developed by the WHO: S – surgery A – antibiotics F – facial cleanliness E – environmental improvement Two antibiotics: oral azithromycin and tetracycline eye ointment.

Making the Connections–cont'd

Signs and Symptoms	Physical Assessment Findings	Diagnostic Testing	Treatment
Allergic Conjunctivitis | Inflammation of both the palpebral and bulbar conjunctiva inflammation because of an allergen irritant such as pollen or animal dander.			
The patient has a sensation that a foreign body is in the eye; a red, teary eye; and photophobia. The eye is usually itchy and edematous. Visual acuity is slightly affected.	Redness and tearing of the eye, swelling of the eyelid and surrounding tissue. Watery, nonpurulent discharge from the eye. Pinpoint subconjunctival hemorrhages.	The diagnosis of conjunctivitis is usually based on the clinical symptoms. Culture of exudate is done with severe infections. Slit lamp examination is necessary if corneal involvement is present.	Avoidance of allergen. Antihistamine eye drops.
Glaucoma | Two kinds of disease: POAG and PCAG. POAG has gradual onset; PCAG has sudden onset. Both are caused by an obstructed canal of Schlemm, which normally drains aqueous humor. Obstruction causes accumulation of aqueous humor leading to high IOP and optic nerve damage.			
Painful, red eye; blurry vision. Halos around lights. Vision loss.	Optic cup-to-disc ratio greater than 0.3 due to high IOP.	Ophthalmoscopic slit lamp examination Tonometry.	Treatments available for glaucoma include topical eye medication, oral medications, laser procedures, and incisional surgery. Several different kinds of minimally invasive surgical procedures can reduce intraocular pressure. Major drug classes for medical treatment include alpha-2 agonists, beta blockers, carbonic anhydrase inhibitors, cholinergic agents, and prostaglandin analogs.
Papilledema | Swelling of the optic disc, which is a sign of pressure on the optic nerve and a sign of increased intracranial pressure.			
Headaches, which are worse upon awakening and exacerbated by coughing, holding breath, or other maneuvers that increase intracranial pressure. Nausea and vomiting. Changes in vision, such as temporary and transient blurring, graying, flickering of light, and double vision.	Swelling of optic disc; has become blurred with non-discrete borders.	Dilated visual examination of eye with ophthalmoscope.	Treatment of underlying condition causing high intracranial pressure.
Diabetic Retinopathy | Proliferation of new blood vessels in the retina. Blood vessels are fragile; can cause blindness.			
Floaters, blurred vision, poor night vision, and vision loss. Usually affects both eyes.	Visualization of the retina through funduscopic examination shows lesions such as hemorrhages, microaneurysms, hard exudates, dilatation and beading of retinal veins, cotton wool spots, and proliferation of fragile, new blood vessels.	Funduscopic examination and diagnostic tests related to diabetes such as fasting serum glucose or HgbA1c.	Blood glucose control to slow progression of retinal changes. Laser photocoagulation of blood vessels. Drug therapy includes intravitreal injections of ovine hyaluronidase (e.g., Vitrase), anti-VEGF inhibitors (e.g., aflibercept and ranibizumab), and intravitreal corticosteroids.

Continued

Making the Connections–cont'd

Signs and Symptoms	Physical Assessment Findings	Diagnostic Testing	Treatment
Cataract | Excess protein layers and irregular clumping of proteinaceous substances within the lens. May be a change of physiological aging.			
Blurry vision and cloudiness in lens of eye. Halos at night around bright objects such as light sources. Sensitivity to glare.	Cloudy lens of the eye. Red reflex duller than normal.	Visual acuity test. Slit lamp and tonometry; an instrument within the slit lamp measures IOP (pressure inside the eye).	Antiglare sunglasses. Surgical removal of cataract.
Age-Related Macular Degeneration | RPE cells of the macula region of the retina age and become less able to process accumulated cellular debris. The RPE cells normally transport cellular debris to choroid blood vessels, which remove the debris from area. Changes in the permeability of the choroid membrane lead to deposition of cell debris between the RPE and choroid. The deposited material is called drusen.			
Patients with AMD report fluctuations in vision, with some poor vision days and other days when it appears improved. Patients also report difficulty with reading and seeing faces. Central vision is affected with peripheral vision intact.	Areas of yellow-white drusen in the macula region are visible upon funduscopic examination.	Amsler grid to measure central vision; individuals notice black spots in their central vision when looking through the Amsler grid. Slit lamp examination is necessary. Fluorescein angiography is a procedure that can highlight the retinal epithelium.	Consumption of antioxidants, including vitamins A, C, D, and E; zinc; and lutein, is recommended, as is a supplement consisting of folic acid, pyridoxine, and vitamin B_{12}. A low-fat diet and smoking cessation are preventive strategies. Wraparound sunglasses are recommended to diminish glare. Intravitreous injection of VEGF inhibitors. Photodynamic therapy, which involves injection of photosensitizing dye, followed by laser therapy.
Retinal Detachment | Retina peels away from its underlying layer of support tissue. Initial detachment may be localized, but without rapid treatment, entire retina may detach, leading to vision loss and blindness.			
Symptoms include a sudden or gradual increase in either the number of floaters or light flashes. Appearance of a curtain over field of vision.	Abnormal retina; holes or peeling away of retina from vitreous apparent on ophthalmoscopic examination.	Slit lamp ophthalmoscopic examination.	Emergency laser photocoagulation.

Making the Connections–cont'd

Signs and Symptoms	Physical Assessment Findings	Diagnostic Testing	Treatment
Retinoblastoma | A cancerous development of the optic nerve. The tumor arises in the retina and can invade the brain. The cells of the tumor have an immature appearance and are referred to as retinoblasts.			
Strabismus, redness of the eye, pain, and poor vision.	White spots are seen in the pupil; strabismus of eye and redness of the eye are apparent. Absence of "red reflex" of the pupil during the examination with the ophthalmoscope.	An examination of the retina under general anesthesia leads to diagnosis of the eye tumor.	If the cancer is in one eye and it is expected that vision can be saved, treatment may include radiation therapy, cryotherapy, and chemotherapy. If the cancer is in both eyes, treatment may include the enucleation of the eye with the most cancer and radiation therapy to the other eye, or chemotherapy followed by local treatment. Combination chemotherapy is demonstrating suppression of the cancer. Enucleation surgery of both eyes is done when vision cannot be saved.

Bibliography

Available online at fadavis.com

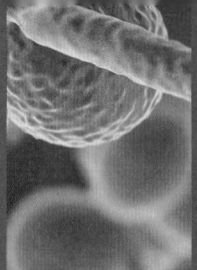

Ear Disorders

Learning Objectives

Upon completion of this chapter, the student will be able to:

- Describe the normal anatomy and physiology of the ear.
- Recognize etiologies and mechanisms of common disorders that affect the ear.
- List assessment techniques, audiometric, and imaging modalities used in the diagnosis of ear disorders.

- Describe common signs, symptoms, and clinical manifestations of disorders of the ear.
- Discuss treatment modalities used to manage common disorders of the ear.

Key Terms

Bony labyrinth
Central hearing impairment
Cerumen
Cholesteatoma
Cochlea
Conductive hearing loss (CHL)
Decibels (dB)
Endolymph
Eustachian tube
Labyrinthitis

Membranous labyrinth
Ménière's disease
Myringotomy tubes
Organ of Corti
Ossicles
Otosclerosis
Perilymph
Pneumatic otoscope
Presbycusis
Semicircular canals

Sensorineural hearing loss (SNHL)
Tinnitus
Tympanic membrane
Tympanostomy
Tympanotomy
Umbo
Vertigo
Vestibular caloric reflex
Vestibular schwannoma

The ears are a pair of organs made up of the external, middle, and inner ear compartments. The functions of the external and middle ear are to collect, amplify, and transmit sound. The inner ear consists of sensory organs that are stimulated by sound waves, which travel through a delicate, integrated circuit of structures and are transformed into neural impulses sent to the brain via the auditory nerve. The inner ear is also stimulated by the position and movement of the head and is thus involved in the maintenance of balance and equilibrium.

Epidemiology

Hearing loss affects approximately 5 to 10 of every 1,000 children in the United States; roughly 1 to 3 children of every 1,000 are born with profound hearing loss, and 3 to 5 children of every 1,000 are born with mild to moderate hearing loss. The incidence of hearing loss increases with age: approximately 17% of adults ages 20 to 69 years suffer hearing loss from excessive noise, and 50% of adults older than age 75 years suffer hearing loss of old age, called

presbycusis. Data from the U.S. census show that almost 3% of the population in the workforce reports having some hearing loss.

Basic Concepts Related to Ear Anatomy and Function

The human ear consists of three separate compartments: the external, middle, and inner ear. The external ear is made up of structures that gather sound and deliver it to a delicate tympanic membrane, which changes sound waves into vibrations. The middle ear takes the vibrations and amplifies them via a triad of delicate bones. The delicate bone vibrations then cause movement of fluid and fine hair cells within the inner ear. Within the inner ear, signals are sent to the auditory nerve, which then takes its impulses to the auditory cortex (see Figure 44-1).

The External Ear

The external ear, which is shaped like a funnel, conducts sound waves through the ear canal to the **tympanic**

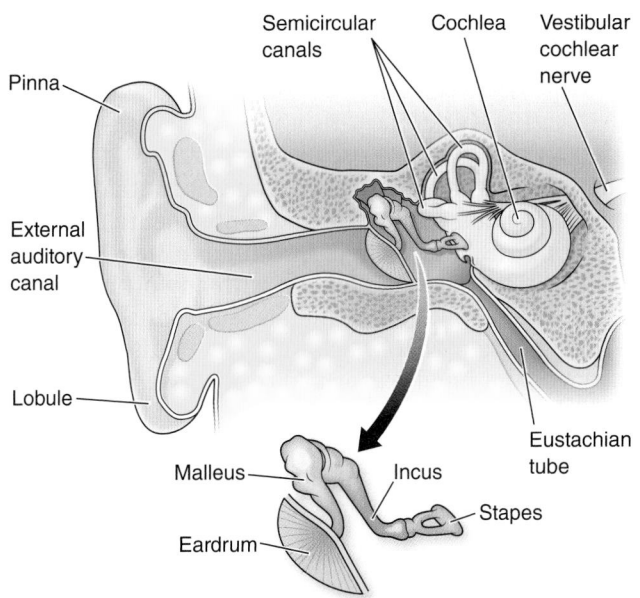

Semicircular canals   Cochlea   Vestibular cochlear nerve

Pinna

External auditory canal

Lobule

Malleus   Incus

Eardrum   Stapes

Eustachian tube

FIGURE 44-1. Anatomy of the ear.

membrane, commonly known as the eardrum. The lining of the ear canal consists of a thin layer of epidermis with fine hairs, sebaceous glands, and glands that produce **cerumen,** or earwax. The function of the external ear is altered when there is blockage, inflammation, or drainage within the canal or disruption of the tympanic membrane.

The Middle Ear

The middle ear is the air-filled space between the tympanic membrane and the inner ear. The middle ear contains three tiny bones called the auditory **ossicles.** These ossicles, which hang from the roof of the middle ear, are the connection between the tympanic membrane and the oval window, which is an opening into the vestibule of the inner ear. The first of the three bones is called the malleus, or the "hammer." The handle of the malleus is called the **umbo.** It connects to the upper portion of the tympanic membrane and can be seen through the membrane. The head of the malleus attaches to the incus, also known as the "anvil," which attaches to the stapes, a stirrup-shaped bone. The stapes, in turn, attaches and is sealed into the oval window by the annular ligament. Sound waves cause vibrations of the tympanic membrane, which moves the ossicles and, in turn, vibrates the oval window and fluid in the inner ear. The two tissue-covered openings—the oval and the round windows—located in the medial wall of the middle ear are responsible for transmission of sound from the middle ear to the inner ear. Vibrations are amplified as they travel from the ossicles in the middle ear to the membrane of the oval window in the inner ear.

The middle ear is connected to the nasopharynx by means of the **eustachian tube.** The eustachian

tube usually remains closed except during yawning or swallowing, which allows equalization of the air pressure between the middle ear and the outside atmosphere. This mechanism of equalizing pressure prevents rupture of the tympanic membrane when there is a sudden pressure change, such as during airplane travel.

CLINICAL CONCEPT

In children, the eustachian tube lies horizontally across from the pharynx, allowing infections to spread easily from the throat to the ear. With maturation, the eustachian tube lengthens and assumes a more vertical orientation, which decreases travel of infection to the ear from the throat.

The Inner Ear

The inner ear is the most complex portion of the ear, containing structures important for both balance and hearing. These structures include the labyrinth, cochlea, and spiral organ of Corti. Balance depends on vision, vestibular function from the ear, and proprioception (neurological position sense).

Balance

The vestibular system of the inner ear regulates movement and balance. It contains a system of communication channels called the labyrinth. There are two parts to the labyrinth: an outer bony wall called a **bony labyrinth** that encases a thin-walled **membranous labyrinth** that floats inside. Within the labyrinth are the **semicircular canals,** which sense head movement, and the utricle and saccule, which sense head position (see Fig. 44-2).

Two separate fluids are found in the inner ear. The periotic fluid, also known as **perilymph,** separates the two labyrinths from each other. The second fluid is otic fluid, also known as **endolymph,** which fills the membranous labyrinth. Perilymph has a composition similar to cerebrospinal fluid, whereas endolymph is comparable to intracellular fluid because of its potassium content.

During physical movement of the head, the flow of the endolymph fluctuates. This movement is sensed by the vestibulocochlear nerve, also called cranial nerve (CN) VIII. Coordinated responses of this nerve provide a sense of balance and stability of movement.

Hearing

The **cochlea** is a snail-shaped bony tubule; the center of this tubule contains the cochlear duct. The cochlea is divided into three parts by the cochlear duct and the spiral lamina, which is a thin, shelflike extension. The three chambers of the cochlea are the scala

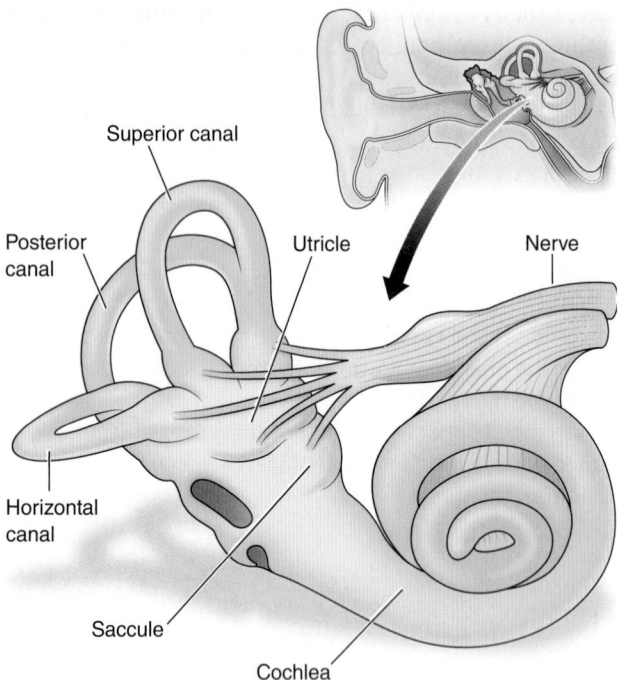

FIGURE 44-2. Inner ear anatomy, demonstrating the relationships of the cochlea, utricle, saccule, and semicircular canals.

Labels: Superior canal · Posterior canal · Utricle · Nerve · Horizontal canal · Saccule · Cochlea

vestibuli, scala tympani, and scala media. Contained within the cochlear duct is the **organ of Corti,** the spiral-shaped receptor organ of hearing. The organ of Corti is made up of supporting cells and many long rows of cochlear hair cells: one row of inner hair cells and three outer rows, all resting on the basilar membrane in the scala media. Afferent sensory nerve fibers from the cochlear nerve are wrapped at the base of the cochlear hair cells. The stapes delivers sound waves to the oval window, which are then transmitted to the scala vestibuli and the scala tympani where the perilymph is located. The transmission of sound occurs when the trapped cilia of the hair cells in the organ of Corti are bent by the movement of the basilar membrane.

Level of hearing is measured in terms of **decibels (dB),** a logarithmic unit that describes loudness of sound, with 0 being the threshold for sound perception of people with normal hearing. A soft whisper is approximately 0 to 20 dB. Normal conversation is approximately 60 dB. Sounds louder than 85 dB can cause hearing loss.

🩺 CLINICAL CONCEPT

Audiometric tests, or hearing tests, evaluate the ability to hear sounds based on both frequency and loudness. The results are utilized to determine whether the individual can hear normal levels of speech.

Basic Pathophysiological Concepts of Common Ear Disorders

Common pathophysiological conditions that affect the ear include conductive and sensorineural hearing loss, tinnitus, and vertigo. **Conductive hearing loss (CHL)** is caused by a problem with any of the structures of the outer and middle ear. **Sensorineural hearing loss (SNHL)** is caused by any disorder that damages the inner ear or auditory nerve. Tinnitus is a ringing or humming heard in the ear in the absence of outside sound. **Vertigo,** the feeling of spinning and imbalance, is the result of labyrinthitis.

Hearing Loss

Hearing loss is marked by the inability to either detect or understand sound. It affects over 30 million people in the United States, including people of all ages and walks of life. Hearing loss can be described as mild, moderate, severe, or profound. These categories are based on the range of sounds that cannot be heard in terms of dB hearing levels.

- Mild hearing loss: The individual cannot hear sounds softer than 26 to 40 dB. Symptoms of mild hearing loss include difficulty following conversations if people are not close to the patient or are in a noisy environment and complaints that others are whispering or mumbling.
- Moderate hearing loss: The individual cannot hear sounds that are softer than 41 to 55 dB. A patient experiencing moderate hearing loss would experience difficulty hearing clearly with background noise and will generally need to wear hearing aids to hear normal conversation clearly.
- Severe hearing loss: The individual cannot hear sounds softer than 60 to 90 dB. This type of hearing loss will generally cause the patient to be unable to hear normal conversational speech. Without the significant assistance of hearing aids, someone with severe hearing loss may not be able to follow even loud conversations.
- Profound hearing loss: The individual cannot hear sounds that are softer than 90 dB. They typically can only hear extremely loud sounds and have difficulty hearing or following conversations. New types of digital hearing aids for profound losses can help. Additional assistance, such as lip reading or sign language training, would also be indicated for patients with profound hearing loss.

Hearing loss may be congenital and present in infancy or acquired in later life. It can be described as genetic, acquired, sudden, progressive, unilateral, bilateral, partial, complete, reversible, or irreversible.

Most types of hearing loss fit into the categories of conductive, sensorineural, or mixed deficiencies (see Box 44-1).

Conductive Hearing Loss

CHL is related to disorders of sound transmission from the outer or middle ear to the receptors in the middle ear. One of the most common causes of CHL is impacted cerumen (earwax). Other possible causes include impaction of foreign bodies, trauma, otitis media (OM), and otosclerosis, which is the hardening of the ossicles.

Sensorineural Hearing Loss

SNHL occurs because of disorders of the inner ear, auditory nerve, or auditory pathways within the brain (see Box 44-1). It is commonly caused by loss of hair cells from the organ of Corti within the inner ear, but it can also occur because of damage to CN VIII or, more rarely, the auditory cortex of the brain, which is located within the temporal lobe. When there is damage to this area of the brain, sounds may be heard but not understood. This type of SNHL is referred to as **central hearing impairment**.

> **ALERT!** Excessive levels of aminoglycoside antibiotics, such as azithromycin, erythromycin, gentamicin, tobramycin, and amikacin, can cause dysfunction of CN VIII. Patients on high doses of these antibiotics are at risk for permanent damage to their hearing and balance. Many other drugs can be ototoxic as well (see Box 44-2).

SNHL may also be caused by genetic disorders or infections while the fetus is in utero. Trauma, tumors, vascular disorders, infection, Ménière's disease, acoustic neuroma, and multiple sclerosis also can cause SNHL. Viral infections that can cause SNHL in the fetus during pregnancy include rubella and cytomegalovirus. Measles, mumps, and meningitis are childhood infections that can also cause it. Genetic disorders that cause SNHL include Waardenburg syndrome, Branchio-oto-renal syndrome, Stickler syndrome, neurofibromatosis type II, Alport syndrome, Treacher Collins syndrome, Usher's syndrome, Down syndrome, and Pendred syndrome. Hearing loss can occur because of exposure to excessively loud noises for a prolonged period. Noise exposure can diminish the individual's ability to hear high-frequency sounds. Eventually, this loss can progress to more severe loss, including the inability to hear the sound frequencies of normal speech. Noise injury commonly occurs in the workplace but may also occur with recreational and social exposure to loud noises (see Box 44-3). This includes the use of personal music devices and attendance at concerts with excessively loud sound systems.

BOX 44-1. Common Causes of Hearing Loss

CONDUCTIVE HEARING LOSS
- Malformation of outer ear, ear canal, or middle ear structure
- Fluid in the middle ear from colds
- Ear infection (otitis media–an infection of the middle ear in which an accumulation of fluid may interfere with the movement of the eardrum and ossicles)
- Allergies
- Poor eustachian tube function
- Perforated eardrum
- Benign tumors
- Impacted cerumen
- Infection in the ear canal
- Foreign object in the ear
- Otosclerosis (a hereditary disorder in which a bony growth forms around a small bone in the middle ear, preventing it from vibrating when stimulated by sound)

SENSORINEURAL HEARING LOSS
- Exposure to loud noise (preventable but not reversible)
- Aging (presbycusis)
- Head trauma
- Infection (e.g., measles, mumps, meningitis)
- Viruses in pregnancy (e.g., rubella or cytomegalovirus can cause SNHL in fetus)
- Autoimmune inner ear disease
- Genetic disorders
- Malformation of the inner ear
- Ménière's disease
- Otosclerosis
- Tumors

BOX 44-2. Common Ototoxic Drugs

- NSAIDs, including aspirin, ibuprofen, and naproxen
- Certain antibiotics, (e.g., aminoglycosides)
- Certain cancer medications
- Diuretics (e.g., furosemide [Lasix])
- Quinine-based medications
- Certain anticonvulsants
- Tricyclic antidepressants
- Antianxiety medications
- Antimalarial medications (e.g., quinine)
- Blood pressure-controlling medications
- Allergy medications
- Chemotherapy drugs (e.g., cisplatin)

BOX 44-3. Occupations and Activities With High Risk of Noise Injury

- Agriculture
- Forestry
- Fishing
- Hunting
- Construction
- Manufacturing
- Mining
- Engineering
- Music industry (musicians, DJs, concert/event organizers, staff, and security)
- Military

 CLINICAL CONCEPT

Noise levels of greater than 85 dB are associated with injury to the cochlea.

Mixed Hearing Loss

Individuals can suffer both SNHL and CHL concurrently, a combination referred to as mixed hearing loss. Causes of mixed hearing loss include barotrauma (pressure changes), otosclerosis, cholesteatoma, and temporal bone fractures.

Tinnitus

Tinnitus is the perception of abnormal sounds in the head or the ear, often described as ringing in the ears. Some patients describe the noise they hear as buzzing, ringing, humming, or hissing in nature. Tinnitus can be continuous or intermittent; unilateral or bilateral; and high, medium, or low pitch. It can occur because of CN VIII disorders, injury from prolonged noise exposure, infection, or medications such as aminoglycosides and aspirin (see Box 44-2). Tinnitus due to excessive aspirin use is termed salicylism.

To resolve tinnitus, it is first necessary to find its cause. Sometimes there are triggers such as red wine, caffeine, or the food additive monosodium glutamate (MSG). Ménière's disease is a common cause of tinnitus that can be treated with medication or surgery.

Vertigo

Patients with vertigo have the sensation that the room is spinning around them, when in fact there is no movement. Additionally, patients report an exaggerated sense of motion with any self-initiated movement. Episodes of vertigo usually last minutes to hours and are often associated with severe nausea and vomiting. This may be because of Ménière's disease or alterations in the labyrinth of the inner ear. It is important to distinguish vertigo from dizziness. A patient who is dizzy reports incoordination and a feeling that they are going to "black out" or fall. Nausea and vomiting do not necessarily accompany dizziness as they do with vertigo.

Assessment

As with any patient assessment, history taking is important when examining for hearing and balance-related disorders. Assess for history of head trauma, exposure to loud noise, and history of ototoxic drug use (see Box 44-2). Ask the patient to fully explain associated symptoms.

If the patient is a child, ask about family history, genetic disorders, congenital infection, OM, history of meningitis, and speech problems. For example, Alport syndrome is a genetic disorder that causes renal failure and sensorineural hearing loss. Patients should also be assessed for thyroid disease as hearing loss, loss of balance, and tinnitus have been associated with congenital and acquired hypothyroidism. Pendred syndrome is a genetic disorder that can cause enlargement of the thyroid (goiter) and progressive loss of hearing.

Health-care providers should understand that normal speech volume is between 50 and 60 dB and that children with hearing loss in this range cannot develop normal speech. Speech problems may be the first manifestation of hearing impairment in children.

 CLINICAL CONCEPT

The American Academy of Pediatrics recommends hearing screening in all infants by the age of 1 month. If a newborn fails the initial test, a thorough audiological evaluation should be performed by the age of 3 months, with appropriate intervention by the age of 6 months.

In the physical examination of the outer ear, there should be no discharge or tenderness of the auricle. A painful outer ear is often present in otitis externa (OE). During a general physical examination, a whisper test can be used to get a general sense of the patient's hearing ability. The patient closes their eyes; then the clinician whispers into the patient's ear. The patient is asked which ear is able to hear the whisper.

Assessment of balance can be done with the Romberg test. The clinician performs this test by asking the patient to stand upright with feet together and then close their eyes. If the patient is unable to maintain this position with eyes closed and begins to sway or fall, the test is considered to be positive. A positive test can be indicative of cerebellar dysfunction, impaired vestibular function caused by damage to CN VIII, or damage to the membranous labyrinth.

Physical examination also includes use of the otoscope, which enables direct view of the patient's tympanic membrane (see Fig. 43-3). A number of key features are visible on the normal tympanic membrane, including the umbo, pars flaccida, and cone of light. Cerumen impaction, foreign body, erythema of the ear canal and membrane, or fluid located behind the tympanic membrane can be seen with an otoscope.

A puff of air propelled against the tympanic membrane from a **pneumatic otoscope** can demonstrate movement of the tympanic membrane. A healthy tympanic membrane is slightly movable when air pressure is propelled against it. In middle ear infection, the tympanic membrane will be immobile and bulging without demonstration of the key features. Pneumatic otoscopy should be performed to detect current or chronic infections, perforation or scarring of the tympanic membrane, cholesteatoma, or fluid behind the tympanic membrane.

Diagnosis

Genetic testing may be useful to determine the etiology of hearing impairment. Many genetic syndromes can trigger hearing loss. Blood tests to search for evidence of thyroid and renal disease are also suggested. Thyroid function, blood urea nitrogen (BUN), serum creatinine levels, and urinalysis should be done.

A specific blood test can identify the presence of connexin-26, a marker for genetic deafness. The test indicates the presence of the *DFNB1* gene, which codes for GJB2, a protein that regulates the composition of the fluid in the cochlea known as endolymph. More than 150 distinct mutations of this gene can cause hearing impairment.

Magnetic resonance imaging (MRI) and computed tomography (CT) scan can uncover abnormalities such as head trauma, tumors, or malformation of the cochlea or the auditory nerve. Other specific tests for hearing loss include audio brainstem response, otoacoustic emissions (OAEs), and audiometry.

Audiometry is performed by placing headsets over the patient's ears and instructing them to raise the corresponding hand when a sound is heard. Pure tone sounds can be presented so that specific volumes at specific frequencies can be documented. CHL and SNHL can be differentiated, and speech recognition can also be tested. Audio brainstem response testing is similar to electroencephalography. When a hearing ear is given a stimulus, the resulting electrographic activity can be followed from the ear to central areas of the brain. In OAE, certain sounds are generated by the inner ear that can be recorded. These sounds are present in normal functioning ears and likely reflect the presence and function of structures responsible for hearing. The sounds may be spontaneous or evoked. How they are produced is unclear.

Treatment

Treatment of ear disorders involves removal of anything that blocks the ear canal, such as impacted cerumen or a foreign body. Antibiotics may be prescribed for some middle ear infections. Children with persistent chronic or recurrent OM with resultant effusions may benefit from the placement of **myringotomy tubes.** These tubes are inserted into the tympanic membrane to allow drainage of discharge from the middle-ear space. If otitis results in the destruction or fixation of the ossicles, surgery on the ossicles may improve hearing function. Hearing aids can be used to increase the sound that is transmitted to the affected ear. Bone-anchored hearing aids may be useful in some patients. Cholesteatoma and vestibular schwannoma, also called acoustic neuroma, are tumors that can be eradicated surgically. In addition, SNHL can be treated with cochlear implantation. A cochlear implant is a surgically implanted device that uses electric stimulation to allow the person to hear. The device captures sound waves and transmits them to a receiver implanted in the cochlea, which in turn sends impulses to the auditory nerve.

Pathophysiology of Selected Disorders of the Ear

Various disorders can interfere with the ear's function. External ear infection, cerumen impaction, middle ear infection, and tumor of CN VIII are the most common disorders.

Disorders of the External Ear

This section discusses the disorders of the auricle and the ear canal. The auricle is easily inspected, and the ear canal requires use of an otoscope.

Cerumen Impaction

The most common cause of reversible hearing loss is impacted cerumen (ear wax). Cerumen can build up

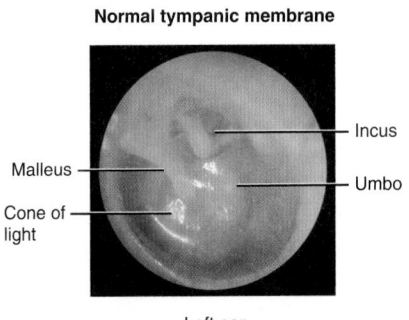

Normal tympanic membrane

Malleus — Incus
— Umbo
Cone of light

Left ear

FIGURE 44-3. Tympanic membrane.

and narrow—or even occlude—the canal despite the ear's ability to self-clean. This condition is usually asymptomatic until complete occlusion of the ear canal occurs. The complaints patients report most often include hearing loss, tinnitus, a feeling of fullness of the ear, or coughing.

Most often, cerumen is removed by irrigation with warm tap water and a bulb syringe. Some health-care providers may choose to use a wire loop or blunt curette to remove excess cerumen. It is best to use warm water as an irrigant to avoid disruption of equilibrium that may occur with cold water because of stimulation of the **vestibular caloric reflex.** The vestibular caloric reflex occurs when the ear's vestibular system is disrupted by cold water placed in the ear canal. Nystagmus, a horizontal movement of the eyes, is a sign of the vestibular caloric reflex.

Otitis Externa

Otitis externa (OE), also called swimmer's ear, is identified by mild to severe inflammation of the external ear. This condition can vary from mild pain when the external ear is manipulated to severe erythematous or tender cellulitis of the external ear. The most common causes are associated with infectious agents, external irritants, and allergic responses. A predisposing factor is water in the ear canal after swimming or bathing, as excess moisture in the canal creates an environment conducive to microbial growth. Common etiological organisms include the bacterial organisms *Pseudomonas* and *Staphylococcus aureus* and the fungal organisms *Aspergillus* and *Candida.*

Clinical Presentation. OE is diagnosed most frequently during the summer months and is usually identified by redness, itching, tenderness, and narrowing of the ear canal because of inflammation. Swelling of the auricle and external canal makes moving the external ear extremely painful. A clear to purulent drainage may be observed depending on the inflammation's severity. There may be temporary CHL secondary to the canal's inflammation.

Diagnosis and Treatment. Diagnosis of OE is usually based on clinical examination. A culture of the discharge can identify the pathogen responsible for the infection. Treatment options usually include an antibiotic or antifungal agent specific to the causative agent in conjunction with a corticosteroid to aid in decreasing the inflammation. Treatment of OE can also include a topical solution of 2% acetic acid, which is antibacterial, and alcohol, which promotes drying.

Instruct the patient to avoid exposing the ear to water until the condition has cleared and to use earplugs while swimming once the infection has resolved. Preventive measures include draining water out of the ears after swimming by tipping the head to the side, drying the ears thoroughly after swimming, and wearing earplugs when swimming.

Disorders of the Middle Ear

Disorders of the middle ear occur within the area behind the tympanic membrane. Often, upper respiratory infections of the pharynx will cause middle ear infections because of the eustachian tube's involvement.

Otitis Media

Otitis media (OM) is the most common disorder to affect the middle ear. This infection results from fluid accumulation in the middle ear. Even though OM can occur at any age, it is seen most commonly in children; peak incidence is usually between the ages of 6 and 24 months.

Etiology. The most common causative bacteria of OM in children are *Streptococcus pneumoniae, Haemophilus influenzae,* and *Moraxella catarrhalis.* More than one bacterium may be responsible for acute OM, and a resistant strain of one of the bacteria listed may be the reason that there is an increase of failed treatment attempts.

OM is most often diagnosed in the winter months secondary to the increase in respiratory tract infections. Infants and toddlers are at highest risk because of their frequent supine position and the anatomical location of their eustachian tube, which is on the same horizontal plane as the middle ear.

Risk factors for OM include male sex, bottle feedings, pacifier usage, day-care attendance, exposure to tobacco smoke, family history of OM, allergic rhinitis, and immune deficiencies.

Pathophysiology. Anatomically, the mucosa of the nasopharynx continues into the eustachian tube of the throat and then into the middle ear. Bacteria of the nasopharynx easily enter the eustachian tube and the middle ear. Infants and children are at highest risk for OM because their eustachian tubes are shorter, wider, and more horizontal in relation to the middle ear, which develops inflammation; an effusion accumulates behind the tympanic membrane. OM can be seen as acute, recurrent, or with an effusion. Effusion related to OM can be serous (clear, watery), mucoid (thick and mucus-like), or purulent (puslike) fluid (see Box 44-4).

Clinical Presentation. Frequent complaints associated with OM include earache, fever, and hearing loss. In infants and toddlers, nonspecific symptoms may include ear tugging, poor feeding, night waking, and irritability. Older children and adults may have rhinorrhea, vomiting, and diarrhea. Pain will increase as an effusion accumulates behind the tympanic membrane. Tympanic membrane rupture is possible when there is too much pressure behind the membrane. Rupture can occur suddenly, resulting in decreased pain and discharge from the ear.

Diagnosis. Diagnosis of OM is made by reviewing the signs and symptoms, as well as performing an otoscopic

---

BOX 44-4. Otitis Media With Effusion

Otitis media (OM) with effusion occurs when there is an intact tympanic membrane with an accumulation of fluid in the middle ear, without signs and symptoms of an infection. People with OM with effusion do not have a fever or other manifestations of an OM infection. Many cases resolve spontaneously in about 3 months. Management includes observation, antibiotics, and corticosteroids. A hearing evaluation may be required if the effusion persists longer than 6 months. A hearing loss of 20 dB or greater may require tympanostomy with tube placement.

BOX 44-5. Complications of Otitis Media

Complications of otitis media (OM) include hearing loss; middle ear problems; and infection of the mastoid process, temporal bone, or the intracranial structures. Hearing loss associated with OM is usually temporary, conductive, and resolves as the effusion resolves. Permanent hearing loss is often related to damage to the tympanic membrane or structure of the middle ear. Tinnitus is another potential complication related to chronic OM.

Adhesive OM is a chronic inflammatory condition characterized by occlusion of the eustachian tube and adhesions in the middle ear because of abnormal healing of an infected middle ear. Often the result of poorly treated or chronic OM, it causes irreversible immobilization of the ossicles, causing conductive hearing loss (CHL). Cholesteatoma, another problem associated with OM, is a mass with white keratin debris that may erode the surrounding tissue and the temporal bone, causing intracranial complications. This condition may be linked to a genetic predisposition or be secondary to chronic OM.

Severe OM can lead to an infection that can extend into the intracranial cavity as well as mastoiditis, which is inflammation of the bone posterior to the auricle.

---

examination, which is usually conducted with a pneumatic otoscope to test the tympanic membrane's mobility. Upon physical examination, the tympanic membrane will be reddened.

A puff of air from a pneumatic otoscope will demonstrate decreased movement of the tympanic membrane. In severe cases of OM, the tympanic membrane will be nonmobile and bulging outward.

Treatment. Treatment for OM varies depending on the individual. Children at high risk, usually those younger than 2 years of age, should be given antibiotics judiciously. Older children who do not present with a fever usually do not require antibiotic therapy, but they do require follow-up in 1 to 3 days. All individuals with acute OM should have supportive therapy, such as analgesics, antipyretics, and localized heat, whether or not antibiotics are prescribed.

When accumulation of fluid is excessive, a tympanotomy may be necessary. A **tympanotomy** is an incision in the tympanic membrane to promote drainage that has accumulated behind it. This procedure also helps to relieve pain, prevent further hearing loss, and prevent spontaneous rupture of the tympanic membrane, which can lead to scarring. A tube is often inserted into the tympanic membrane to maintain an opening for release of discharge in the procedure referred to as a **tympanostomy.** If OM goes untreated or is poorly treated, complications can develop (see Box 44-5).

Tympanic Membrane Perforation

Perforation or rupture of the tympanic membrane can occur as a complication of middle ear infection or be caused by trauma. Common causes of traumatic tympanic membrane perforation include rapid change in ear pressure (e.g., occurring when flying and scuba diving), head trauma, thermal or chemical burns, and direct penetrating trauma. Severe infection can cause tympanic membrane perforation from buildup of fluid. Symptoms of perforation include a buzzing sound in the ear, earache, and hearing loss. Most small ruptures heal spontaneously within 4 weeks. Ear drops should

be avoided. Systemic antibiotics may be prescribed. Cauterization of the edges of the tympanic membrane and patching can be performed. Patches infused with gelatin sponge, basic fibroblast growth factor, and sea buckthorn oil have shown the ability to facilitate the healing of TM perforation Alternatively, surgical tympanoplasty can be done. If untreated, tympanic membrane perforation increases the risk of middle ear infection, cholesteatoma (a keratinized mass), and mastoiditis.

Cholesteatoma

Cholesteatoma is a mass of skin cells that accumulates behind the tympanic membrane or within the mastoid bone. The mass expands and can erode the tympanic membrane, ossicles, and mastoid bone. Persons with cholesteatoma often have a history of middle ear infections. The mass can grow gradually many years after middle ear infection. Commonly asymptomatic, it can present with infection of the middle ear with foul-smelling, bloody discharge and/or hearing loss. If not removed, the mass can expand, erode the middle ear, and cause mastoiditis and meningitis. Surgery is necessary to remove the mass through the ear canal or through postauricular incision by exposing the mastoid bone. Antibiotics are also given.

Otosclerosis

Otosclerosis is caused by a callus that forms on one of the ossicles: the stapes bone. The stapes bone normally receives vibrations from the tympanic membrane and transmits the vibration to the other ossicles. The callused stapes cannot vibrate, and sound transmission is inhibited. The hearing loss is progressive and usually occurs initially in a single ear. The other ear may be involved in the same process sometime later. An audiogram indicates a conductive hearing loss. A special type of testing, stapedial reflex testing, indicates limited or no movement of the bones of hearing. A stapedectomy is a surgical procedure that involves either a total or partial removal of the stapes bone. A prosthesis is then used to restore function. It commonly takes about 4 weeks for the ear to heal and hearing to improve. It is important not to undergo any heavy or strenuous activity during the healing time.

Disorders of the Inner Ear and Auditory Nerve

Labyrinthitis

Labyrinthitis is inflammation of the labyrinth of the inner ear. It occurs as a sudden episode of vertigo that may last several days, and is often associated with hearing loss and tinnitus. It may occur in conjunction with a bacterial or viral infection or an autoimmune disorder. Symptoms of labyrinthitis occur when infectious microorganisms or inflammatory mediators invade the membranous labyrinth and damage the vestibular and auditory end organs. Symptoms often resolve as the infection is treated with antibiotics and antihistamines. Meclizine (Antivert), an antihistamine, is commonly used to reduce the sensation of vertigo produced by the vestibular system of the inner ear.

Ménière's Disease

Ménière's disease, a disorder of the inner ear, was named for the French physician who first described the condition's symptoms. The symptoms are the result of changes in the fluid volume of both the bony and membranous labyrinth of the inner ear. In Ménière's disease, there is an increase in the endolymph that fills the membranous labyrinth, resulting in distention of this portion of the inner ear. Over time, this disorder is associated with progressive hearing loss and tinnitus. Although head trauma is one of the major causes of this disorder, there is frequently no known etiology. Ménière's disease most commonly affects persons ages 40 to 50 years old.

The clinical presentation for Ménière's disease includes episodic vertigo associated with fluctuating SNHL, tinnitus, and a feeling of pressure within the ear. Because there is no specific diagnostic test for this disorder, it is diagnosed by the clinical symptoms. However, a complete history and physical examination must be performed to rule out other causes. Treatment includes a low-salt diet, diuretics, antiemetics,

and anti-inflammatory medications. Transtympanic administration of aminoglycosides is sometimes effective for treatment-resistant Ménière's disease. A Meniett device is also used for treatment-resistant disease. The device delivers pulses of pressure to the inner ear via a tympanostomy tube. Some patients have symptomatic relief when the device is used on a daily basis. The precise mechanism that provides relief is unclear.

A destructive surgical procedure may be necessary in treatment-resistant Ménière's disease. Because a high volume of endolymph in the inner ear sends abnormal signals to the auditory nerve, destruction of these structures may be the last resort to relieve symptoms. Destruction of the inner ear structures, the auditory nerve, or both prevents abnormal signals from reaching the brain. As long as the opposite inner ear and vestibular apparatus function normally, the brain eventually will compensate for the loss of one labyrinth over the following weeks to months.

Vestibular Schwannomas

Vestibular schwannomas, also called acoustic neuromas, are benign tumors that develop from the Schwann cells that surround CN VIII. About 5% are associated with a genetic disorder called neurofibromatosis. The clinical incidence is about 10 to 15 individuals per million people per year. It is most often diagnosed in adults ranging in age from 46 to 58 years.

The symptoms result from compression of CN VIII; these symptoms include tinnitus and decreased hearing with loss of speech discrimination in the affected ear. There is also a persistent loss of balance. The definitive diagnosis is made with an MRI. If symptoms interfere with activities of daily living, it can be removed with microsurgical techniques or with gamma knife radiosurgery.

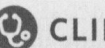 **CLINICAL CONCEPT**

Removal of the schwannoma may not be necessary unless the symptoms increase in severity.

Hearing Loss in Older Adults

Older adults may suffer from **presbycusis,** or degenerative changes that diminish hearing. The changes begin around age 50 years and may remain undetectable for a decade or so. The symptoms are caused by gradual loss of hair cells in the cochlea. In older adult patients, it is important to assess ability to hear both high- and low-frequency sounds. High-frequency sounds are lost first, with a frequent complaint of being unable to hear in a crowded room. Common symptoms of high-frequency hearing loss include:

- Trouble hearing consonants
- Frequently asking others to speak more slowly or clearly
- Difficulty understanding words, especially in crowds or noisy environments

Patients with low-frequency hearing loss have difficulty hearing sounds such as:

- A rumble of thunder
- A car motor running

- Bass music
- Some male voices
- Phone conversations
- Vowels (they're generally spoken at a lower pitch than consonants)

Patients with hearing loss can consult an audiologist, who can prescribe the patient the correct type of hearing aid. There are also over-the-counter hearing aids available as an alternative to prescription hearing aids. Most hearing aids amplify sounds using computer/digital technology.

Chapter Summary

- The functions of the external and middle ear include collecting, amplifying, and transmitting sound.
- The inner ear consists of sensory organs that are stimulated by sound waves. Sound waves are transmitted through a delicate integrated circuit of structures and transformed into neural impulses sent to the brain via the auditory nerve, also called CN VIII.
- The inner ear is also stimulated by position and movement of the head, which is involved in the maintenance of balance and equilibrium.
- Level of hearing is measured in terms of dB. A soft whisper is approximately 0 to 20 dB. Normal conversation is approximately 60 dB. Sounds louder than 85 dB can cause noise trauma and hearing loss.
- CHL is related to disorders of sound transmission from the external or middle ear to the receptors in the middle ear. CHL is commonly caused by OM or cerumen impaction.
- SNHL occurs because of disorders of the inner ear, auditory nerve, or auditory pathways within the brain. SNHL is commonly caused by loss of hair cells from the organ of Corti within the inner ear.
- Tinnitus is the perception of abnormal sounds in the head or the ear, often described as ringing in the ears. Some patients describe the noise they hear as buzzing, ringing, humming, or hissing in nature.
- Vertigo is the sensation that the room is spinning around you.
- Newborns should undergo a hearing screening examination before 3 months of age, and if hearing loss is present, intervention before 6 months of age.
- Excessive levels of aminoglycoside antibiotics can cause dysfunction of CN VIII.
- A specific blood test can identify the presence of connexin-26, a biomarker for genetic deafness. The test indicates the presence of the *DFNB1* gene, which codes for GJB2; this protein regulates the composition of endolymph.

- OE is inflammation of the external ear. The most common causes are infectious agents, external irritants, and allergic responses. Predisposing factors include water in the ear canal after swimming. Common etiological organisms include *Pseudomonas*, *S. aureus*, and *Candida*.
- OM, the most common disorder to affect the middle ear, is an infection that results from fluid accumulation in the middle ear. Even though OM can occur at any age, it is most commonly seen in children.
- Tympanic membrane perforation can occur with trauma or pressure changes. It increases risk of infection and requires patching of the tympanic membrane.
- Labyrinthitis is a sudden episode of vertigo that may last several days; it is often associated with hearing loss and tinnitus.
- Ménière's disease is caused by an increase in the endolymph that fills the membranous labyrinth, resulting in distention of this portion of the inner ear. This disorder is associated with progressive hearing loss, vertigo, and tinnitus.
- Cholesteatoma is a rare growth of skin cells that accumulates behind the tympanic membrane that can erode through bone and cause hearing loss.
- Otosclerosis is the callused fixation of the stapes, which then inhibits it from vibration, which inhibits vibration of the cochlea, causing hearing loss.
- Vestibular schwannomas, also called acoustic neuromas, are benign tumors that develop from the Schwann cells that surround CN VIII. CN VIII becomes compressed and dysfunctional.
- Older adults may suffer from presbycusis, or degenerative changes that diminish hearing. The changes begin around age 50 and may remain undetectable for a decade or so. The symptoms are caused by gradual loss of hair cells in the cochlea.

Making the Connections

Signs and Symptoms	Physical Assessment Findings	Diagnostic Testing	Treatment
Cerumen Impaction | Earwax within the ear canal that impairs sound conduction from the external ear to the inner ear.			
Hearing difficulty. Sense of "fullness" or itching in the ear.	Hearing impairment. Yellow-brown colored earwax buildup in the ear canal seen with otoscope.	None.	Removal of impacted cerumen using irrigation technique or curette.
Otitis Externa | Infection of the auricle and ear canal. Common microorganisms include *Pseudomonas, Staphylococcus,* and *Candida.*			
Pain and tenderness of the auricle, fullness and itching of the ear canal. Discharge from ear canal common. Hearing difficulty.	Tenderness, erythema, and edema of the auricle and ear canal. Purulent or serous discharge from the ear canal.	None.	Antibiotic and steroid treatment. Earplugs when in water.
Otitis Media | Infection of the middle ear region. Discharge accumulation in middle ear. Common microorganisms include *S. pneumonia* and *H. influenza.*			
Earache. Hearing difficulty, sense of fullness. Fever, nausea, and vomiting possible. Children are extremely irritable, tug at ear, do not feed, and may have vomiting.	Bulging, red tympanic membrane. Erythema and edema of the ear canal. Hearing impairment. Often pharyngeal erythema, edema, and rhinorrhea present.	Pneumatic otoscope will demonstrate decreased movement of the tympanic membrane. Throat culture may be needed.	Antibiotic treatment. Antipyretics and analgesic may be needed. Tympanostomy may be necessary in chronic OM.
Labyrinthitis | Inflammation of the membranous labyrinth of the inner ear.			
Dizziness. Loss of balance. Hearing difficulty and tinnitus possible.	Hearing loss. Romberg test may be positive.	None.	Antibiotic and meclizine.
Ménière's Disease | Increased volume of endolymph in inner ear.			
Tinnitus, hearing loss, and vertigo.	Hearing loss. Romberg test: may be positive.	None.	Low-salt diet, diuretics, and steroids. Aminoglycosides may relieve symptoms. Meniett device or destructive surgery may be necessary.
Vestibular Schwannoma | Tumor of the auditory nerve that compresses the nerve and causes hearing impairment.			
Hearing loss, tinnitus, and loss of balance.	Hearing loss. Romberg test may be positive.	MRI.	Surgery.

Bibliography

Available online at fadavis.com

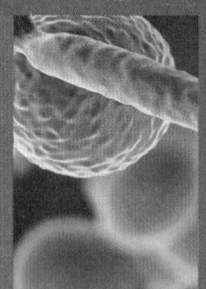

CHAPTER

45

Physiological Changes of Aging

Learning Objectives

Upon completion of this chapter, the student should be able to:

- Discuss current theories of aging, loss of physiological reserve during the aging process, and immunosenescence.
- Identify changes that occur in each organ system within the body during the aging process.
- Recognize the older patient's susceptibility to disorders due to the physiological changes of aging.

- Explain how the older adult commonly presents with atypical clinical manifestations of disease.
- Describe the geriatric syndromes that most commonly occur in older adults.
- Discuss how polypharmacy often occurs due to treatment of multiple disorders in older adults.

Key Terms

Apoptosis
Cataract
Dementia
Diverticulosis
Gastric atrophy
Immunosenescence
Insulin resistance
Lactose intolerance
Life expectancy (LE)

Maximum life span (MLS)
Multicausality
Orthostatic hypotension
Osteopenia
Osteoporosis
Pernicious anemia
Physiological reserve
Polypharmacy
Presbycusis

Presbyesophagus
Presbyopia
Reactive oxygen species
Senescence
Telomerase
Telomere
Type 2 diabetes mellitus (T2DM)

Approximately 52 million persons in the United States are older than age 65 (16% of the total population), and that number is climbing. In fact, the number of older adults is increasing by 2.6% every year, more than double the rate of general population growth. The number of Americans age 65 and older is projected to nearly double to 95 million by 2060, and the 65-and-older age group's share of the total population will rise from 16% to 23%. People age 85 years and older are the fastest-growing segment of the older population. This growth in one segment of the population is unprecedented in the United States.

In 2019, roughly one-quarter of adults age 65 to 74 and nearly half of adults age 75 and older reported having a disability, including cognitive, visual, auditory, ambulatory, self-care, and independent living difficulties. A very small number of older Americans live in nursing homes. Of those age 65 years and older,

1.5 million are in nursing homes, which represents 3.4% of the older adult population; 2% live in assisted living facilities.

The United States is not the only country with an increasing population of older adults. Japan has the largest older adult population, with 27.9% of all Japanese being older than age 60. Although the developed countries have the largest proportion of adults older than age 65, all countries in every stage of development are experiencing rapid growth in their older populations.

Older adult individuals are categorized in three basic groups according to age:

- Young-old: individuals between 65 and 74 years of age
- Middle-old: individuals between 75 and 84 years of age
- Old-old: individuals older than age 85 years

According to the World Health Organization (WHO), older adults can be further categorized based on age: oldest-old include those age 95+, centenarians are age 100+, and supercentenarians are age 110+ (WHO, 2019).

Maximum Life Span Versus Life Expectancy

Study of the aging process involves the concepts of maximum life span and life expectancy. The **maximum life span (MLS)** is the maximum potential years of survival for a species. The MLS for humans has changed over the past century and is now approximately 125 years. This is to say that barring accident, illness, or other biological catastrophe, the human body can function for about 125 years. MLS is contrasted to the concept of **life expectancy (LE),** the expected number of years an organism may live from a particular point in time. According to the Centers for Disease Control (CDC, 2017), in the United States, the average life span for females is 85 years and for males is 83 years.

Although MLS may remain constant for long periods, LE fluctuates based on the ability of the environment to support life. Major improvements in LE have been noted in response to public works initiatives, such as improved food and water supplies and waste disposal. The LE for Americans has nearly doubled since 1900, reflecting the aforementioned improvements in public works, as well as enhanced healthcare quality and quantity. It may be helpful to think of MLS in terms of successful aging and LE in regard to usual aging. Because of research in regenerative medicine and advancing biotechnology, the United States is gaining 1 year of longevity every 6 years.

Basic Concepts of Physiological Aging

Many different disciplines are involved in the study of how and why we age. Although each discipline may research specific phenomena, there are some that are shared by all. When studying why we age, a comprehensive view of all theories is necessary because aging is thought to be a complex and multifactorial process.

Senescence

Senescence refers to a cell's progressive loss of ability to replicate over time. The changes in the human body that take place throughout adulthood are toward decrements in function. This makes the human organism more vulnerable to challenges from disease, injury, or environmental factors. In gerontology and geriatrics, senescence refers to the biological, intrinsic phenomena of aging, including the characteristic patterns of change that are specific to a species and lead to a gradual loss of function of body systems. Senescent changes are universal and easily recognized within a species based on physical appearance and behavior.

Loss of Physiological Reserve

As organisms age, the ability to repair damage and adapt to physiological stressors decreases. This decreased ability is referred to as loss of **physiological reserve.** In humans, physiological reserve is correlated with an individual's functional status. Loss of physiological reserve is part of the reason that older adults are more susceptible to infectious disease than younger adults and may have poorer outcomes from surgery and its complications. Although older adults may be able to function adequately in daily life, they are less resilient to stress compared with younger adults. For example, a urinary tract infection (UTI) is usually a minor inconvenience that is easily resolved for a young adult. In older adults, however, UTIs can lead to urosepsis, a severe body-wide infection. Similarly, in a young adult, influenza is a disorder that resolves within a week, whereas in the older adult, it often leads to pneumonia.

Multicausality

Physiological and pathophysiological changes that occur with aging have many etiologies. Both internal processes and influences from the environment cause senescent cell changes; this combination of factors is referred to as **multicausality.** Biological, epidemiological, and demographic data have generated a number of theories that attempt to identify a process to explain aging. However, in recent years, the search for a single cause of aging, such as a single gene or the decline of a key body system, has been replaced by the view of aging as an extremely complex, multifactorial process. Several processes may interact simultaneously to cause aging.

Theories of Aging

Most researchers believe that different theories of aging are not mutually exclusive and may adequately describe features of the normal aging process in combination.

Programmed Aging of the Cell. The programmed aging of the cell theory asserts that cells have a programmed schedule for aging and degeneration. According to the programmed theory, aging depends on biological clocks regulating the timetable of the life span through the stages of growth, development, maturity, and old age. This regulation would depend on genes sequentially switching on and off signals to the nervous, endocrine, and immune systems responsible for maintenance of homeostasis and for activation of defense responses. For example, the female ovary has a programmed time span of function. In most females, at age 55 years or so, the ovary undergoes **apoptosis,** a programmed degeneration of function. The question asked by many gerontologists is: Like the ovary, do all cells replicate a finite number of times before they die? Some scientists are studying the telomeres of chromosomes to answer this question (see Box 45-1).

Telomere Shortening Theory. A **telomere** is a region of repetitive nucleotide sequences at the end of a chromosome. It has been observed that with each mitotic division of a cell, the telomere regions of its chromosomes shorten. This observation has led to the question: As human telomeres shorten, do cells eventually reach their replicative limit and progress into senescence or old age? The telomere shortening theory focuses on the enzyme telomerase, which allows for replacement of telomeres, which are otherwise shortened when a cell divides via mitosis. It is known that embryonic stem cells express **telomerase,** which allows them to divide repeatedly. With the presence of telomerase, a dividing cell can replace the lost bit of DNA at the end of the chromosome and then divide in uninhibited fashion. Although this unbounded growth property is an exciting finding, caution is warranted regarding this property, as this exact same uninhibited growth enables cancerous growth. Currently, the question is: If telomerase is used to block chromosomal shortening, will this in turn prevent aging of the cell?

Damage-Based Theory of Aging. The damage-based theory of aging asserts that cellular damage occurs over time because of accumulation of toxic by-products of metabolism, ineffective protein synthesis and secretion, or inefficient cellular repair systems. Damage to the genome and cellular organelles leads to cell death.

BOX 45-1. Genetics of Healthy Aging (GEHA) Study

The Genetics of Healthy Aging (GEHA) Study, conducted by 25 partners (24 from Europe plus the Beijing Genomics Institute from China), has identified a number of genes involved in healthy aging and longevity. It is believed that these genes allow individuals to survive to advanced old age in good cognitive and physical function and in the absence of major age-related diseases. Genes related to healthy aging were found by studying selected individuals who survive over the age of 90 years. The study of 2,118 subjects focused on 90-year-old and older White sibling pairs. The analyses demonstrated four regions that show linkage to longevity: chromosome 14q11.2, chromosome 17q12-q22, chromosome 19p13.3-p13.11, and chromosome 19q13.11-q13.32. Although these genes have been identified, it remains difficult to differentiate the effect of the shared environment and that of genetics in the sibling subjects of the study.

Cumulative damage to DNA occurs with age and eventually causes errors in metabolism and protein synthesis. Inaccurate transcription processes yield abnormal RNA, which in turn leads to inappropriate proteins translated by the ribosomes. Proteins needed for structural repair of cells and such processes as hormone synthesis and neurotransmitter generation are all dysfunctional. Damage to mitochondria diminishes the ability of cells to generate energy. Also dysfunctional metabolic processes in the mitochondria yield free radicals. Free radicals then cause additional cell injury. In aged cells, protein synthesis and secretion are disrupted. There is an accumulation of proteins that are not secreted and then interfere with cell function. Damage to lysosomes causes inability of the cell to enzymatically break down wastes. Nonsecreted proteins and waste products accumulate, which interferes with cellular processes.

Free Radical Accumulation Theory. Free radicals are highly reactive chemical compounds; sometimes they are referred to as **reactive oxygen species,** because they contain a free electron on an oxygen atom that endows the free radical with chemical instability and a strong affinity to bind to other molecules. Free radicals are referred to as oxidizing agents because they react with other compounds and cause damage. Free radicals target cellular structures, especially DNA, proteins, and the fatty acids in the cell membrane. For example, cigarette smoke contains free radicals that cause cell damage.

Free radicals cause cross-linkages and biochemical bonds to form between cell proteins and other molecules. The bonds make proteins less flexible, particularly those in muscle and collagen. For example, with free radical damage, muscles lose contractility, skin loses elasticity, and cartilage becomes rigid. Free radicals also injure the endothelial membranes of the arteries and create conditions that are conducive to the formation of arteriosclerotic plaque. Free radicals cause cell damage that produces some of the characteristic changes of aging. With cumulative free radical effects, cells and tissues are irreparably damaged and organs eventually are unable to function properly.

Immunosenescence. **Immunosenescence** refers to the weakening of both the innate and adaptive immune systems with increasing age. Natural killer cells, part of the innate system, become more numerous with increased age but less functional. T lymphocytes, major participants within the adaptive system, are similarly affected, with a decreased ability to recognize and attack the antigens.

New T lymphocytes are essentially not produced in older adults, severely impairing the older adult's ability to combat previously unencountered antigens. B lymphocytes continue to be produced but become less effective in producing antibodies to pathogens. In the population of T and B cells, there is a smaller pool of "naïve" cells that can be programmed for a specific antigen. Cytokine secretion, particularly of tumor necrosis factor, also declines in old age, with concomitant degeneration of the entire process of inflammation. There is a diminished inflammation reaction with decreased external signs and symptoms. With infection, white blood cell (WBC) numbers do not rise to the same level as in younger adults and fever is commonly absent. This is problematic because healthcare providers rely on diagnostic clues such as high WBC levels and fever as signs of infection.

Other factors that diminish an individual's ability to mount a fever include poorer thermoregulation by the central nervous system (CNS), less responsiveness of the hypothalamus, decreased production of endogenous pyrogens (fever-producing substances), decreased ability to produce and conserve body heat, and less vasodilation and subcutaneous fat.

Immunizations may be less effective in the older adult because the immune system does not respond as vigorously as a younger adult to a newly introduced vaccine. Antibody levels do not rise as robustly as in the younger person. This may be particularly true with immunization for influenza, when unique strains of the virus are present each season.

CLINICAL CONCEPT

Signs of infection are blunted in the older adult; there is decreased rise in WBCs, reduced ability to mount a fever, and less sensation of pain. Behavioral changes, such as confusion and disorientation, may be the only symptoms expressed during infection.

ALERT! Recommended immunizations for the older adult include yearly flu vaccine, one-time pneumovax after age 65 years, and varicella zoster (shingles) vaccine.

Life-Prolonging Calorie-Restricted Diets. It has been recognized for quite some time that limiting daily calories to as little as 60% of normal extends the life span of mice up to 40%. In laboratory experiments, calorie-restricted (CR) older adult mice are similar to young mice physiologically in many ways. The CR mice maintain youthful appearances and activity levels longer than non-CR mice and show delays in age-related diseases. The learning ability of CR older mice is more like that of younger adult mice. Reduced calorie intake in mice is associated with reduced free radical activity, less biological waste accumulation, and fewer numbers of damaged mitochondria.

Detractors of CR diets assert that the quality of the diets consumed by the low-body-mass-index individuals are difficult to assess and may lack nutrients important to longevity. Calorie restriction in mice has been reported to hinder their ability to fight infection. Also, CR diets cannot support the caloric demands of exercise in athletics. CR diets increase morbidity and mortality in children and adolescents and should not be emulated by the young. Even though there has been research on CR for more than 70 years, the mechanism by which it works is still not well understood. Currently, CR diets are being studied in monkeys. An ongoing study on rhesus macaques funded by the National Institute on Aging was started in 1989. Results to date have also found a trend toward a reduced overall death rate; however, the results are not of statistical significance (see Box 45-2).

Functional Consequences of Physiological Aging

All systems of the human body are affected by aging. The nature and extent of the changes vary from system to system, as well as from person to person. Lifestyle and environment play a large part in the human aging process.

BOX 45-2. Calorie Restriction and Aging

A small research study investigated the effects of a calorie-restricted (CR) diet with 10% to 25% lower calorie intake than the average "Western" diet. There was a CR group of subjects and a control group of subjects on a typical Western diet. The age range of the control and CR group was 35 to 82 years. Mean body mass index (BMI) was 19.6 in the CR group; the matched control group BMI was 25.9, comparable to the BMI for middle-aged people in the United States. Adjusting for age, the average total cholesterol and low-density lipoprotein (bad) cholesterol levels in the CR group were below those seen in the majority of control subjects. The average high-density lipoprotein (good) cholesterol levels were in the 85th to 90th percentile range for normal middle-aged American males. The CR group also fared much better than the control group in terms of average blood pressure (100/60 vs. 130/80 mm Hg), fasting glucose, fasting insulin (65% reduction), BMI, body fat percentage, and C-reactive protein. The CR group had triglyceride levels as low as the lowest 5% of Americans in their 20s. Systolic and diastolic blood pressure levels in the CR group were about 100/60 mm Hg, a level more typical of 10-year-olds. Fasting plasma insulin concentration was 65% lower. Fasting plasma glucose concentration was also lower.

Cardiovascular System

Changes in the cardiovascular system may represent the most widely varied manifestations of aging and pathology found in humans. In addition, cardiopathology represents the single largest cause of death in the United States, as well as a major source of morbidity, and advanced age is the greatest risk to cardiovascular health. One out of four adult deaths are caused by heart disease each year in the United States; one-half of these deaths are in persons older than 65 years.

Atherosclerosis, the development of cholesterol-laden plaques within the endothelial lining of arteries and increased connective tissue in the walls of the vessels, is common in younger and older adults. Although atherosclerosis is considered a disease, because of the universal presence in humans and animals, it may be more correct to attribute it to aging.

Vascular aging is a process characterized primarily by endothelial senescence. Senescence refers to the limited number of cell divisions one cell can undergo due to genetic and morphological changes. There is a reduction in the bioavailability of nitric oxide (NO) in the endothelium as aging progresses. The lowered levels of NO impair vasodilation in the coronary vasculature and increase endothelial sensitivity to cellular apoptotic signals. This leads to overall decline in endothelial function and potential angiogenesis.

The elastic blood vessels—particularly the aorta, carotid, subclavian, and renal arteries—become stiffer with age. Free radical damage of cell membranes causes protein cross-linking that diminishes elasticity and decreases vasodilation. The heart itself also undergoes changes with age—mainly increased amounts of fibrous and calcified tissues that infiltrate muscle and conductive tissue. The heart of an older adult is less compliant and has some degree of diastolic dysfunction because the chambers cannot expand as widely as in youth. On the other hand, systolic function—contraction of the left ventricle of the heart—is preserved, although systolic blood pressure increases with advanced age.

There is connective tissue infiltration of the conductive tissues in the heart and amyloid deposition in the ventricular endomyocardium with aging. This connective tissue and amyloid deposition interfere with normal cardiac conduction. Cardiac conduction system remodeling commonly occurs around the seventh decade of life. These changes lead to increased incidence of dysfunction of the sinoatrial (SA) and atrioventricular (AV) node and the His-Purkinje system. This often results in episodes of bradycardia, dizziness, syncope, and fatigue. It is also common for older adults to develop the electrophysiological pathologies of atrioventricular and bundle-branch block and atrial fibrillation.

Changes in the conductive tissue cause increased refractory periods for the heart muscle and decreased responsiveness to sympathetic nervous system stimulation. These factors lead to markedly smaller increases in heart rate in the face of stress or exercise. Maximum achievable heart rate decreases linearly with age and may be calculated with the formula 220 − age = maximal heart rate (beats per minute).

Baroreceptors in the arterial walls, which sense changes in blood pressure, are slower to respond. There is less ability to raise blood pressure with position changes, causing increased susceptibility to **orthostatic hypotension.** The heart's reaction to sympathetic nervous system stimulation is blunted, and the increase in heart rate in response to lower blood pressure is limited.

With advancing age, the valves of the heart can undergo pathological changes that lead to valvular stenosis or regurgitation. Calcium commonly accumulates on mitral and aortic valves, leading to valvular stiffness that can progress into valve stenosis. Myxomatous degeneration can affect the mitral valve leaflets, leading to mitral regurgitation. These valvular changes cause pressure changes within the heart chambers and systemic effects.

These "normal" age-related cardiovascular changes serve as the foundation that supports decreased plasticity and limited ability for tissue remodeling during pathophysiological states such as myocardial ischemia and heart failure.

 CLINICAL CONCEPT

It is important to observe for the signs of orthostatic hypotension when changing the position of an older adult from lying to sitting or sitting to standing. The older patient requires a few minutes to adjust to the new position before attempting to walk.

ALERT! Antihypertensive medications can increase susceptibility to orthostatic hypotension. Orthostatic hypotension is a common cause of falls in the older adult.

Respiratory System

The main function of the respiratory system is to provide the cells with adequate oxygenation. The aerobic capacity for older adults decreases about 10% per decade, with peak performance in the early to mid-20s. Males have a slightly greater loss of capacity than females. The changes are related to normal aging and are not indicative of damage from smoking or poor fitness levels. Older adults do not respond as briskly to hypoxia or hypercapnia as younger adults. The usual response of increased respiratory rate, depth, and inspiratory pressure to changing partial pressures of oxygen or carbon dioxide are blunted, although the mechanism is poorly understood. Older adults with serious respiratory conditions such as pneumonia may not exhibit the "early warning signs" of tachypnea and dyspnea, thus delaying diagnosis. Older individuals cannot mount the same maximum heart rate in reaction to hypoxia. Furthermore, aging is accompanied by earlier transition from aerobic to anaerobic metabolism in the body cells, further decreasing respiratory adaptation to exercise.

The elasticity of the thoracic rib cage and lung tissue decreases with age, which causes the resistance to expansion of the chest to increase. In addition, strength of the respiratory muscles decreases, which creates less vital capacity and tidal volume. Residual volume in the lungs, however, increases by as much as 50% from young adulthood. The alveoli lose surface area, and less oxygen is diffused into the pulmonary capillaries. The diameter of the bronchioles and smaller airways also decrease with advancing age. These changes may be caused in part by exposure to atmospheric air, with its many damaging pollutants and free radicals. Remember the theory that aging is related to accumulation of free radical damage from the environment, and the lungs are in constant contact with the inspired air.

The rib cage and vertebrae undergo changes with age that affect respiratory function. Specifically, the costal cartilage becomes calcified, thereby increasing the stiffness of the chest wall. Kyphosis, related to both osteopenia in the vertebrae and collapse of the intervertebral discs, leads to an increased anteroposterior diameter, or barrel chest. The diaphragm becomes less important in ventilation and the abdominal muscles take on a greater role, resulting in an increased effort in both inspiration and expiration. Accordingly, pulmonary function tests are adjusted based on age.

CLINICAL CONCEPT

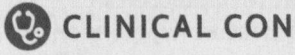

The cough reflex in the older adult is weaker than in the younger adult, which increases stasis of secretions in the lungs. Stasis of secretions increases susceptibility to pneumonia.

Renal System

The renal function in an 85-year-old person is only about 50% of that of a 30-year-old person, which is attributed to loss of nephrons and decreased activity of the nephron tubules. Blood flow to the kidney decreases as a result of atrophy of the arterial blood vessels, particularly in the renal cortex. In addition, the proximal tubules of nephrons decrease in number and length. Although these changes start around age 40 years, they do not become significant until an individual reaches old age. At that time, there will be noticeable decreases in the ability to respond to a fluid overload and to concentrate urine. The older adult will usually demonstrate a lower creatinine clearance than a young adult, indicating less filtration ability of the kidney. The older person will typically excrete lower levels of glucose, acid, and potassium, and the specific gravity of the urine will be lower. The response of the nephrons to antidiuretic hormone is less than in younger adults, and so the ability to concentrate urine is diminished. The kidney in the older adult will not respond to atrial natriuretic peptide as briskly as in the younger adult. This causes less excretion of water from the bloodstream as well. In addition, excretion of hydrogen ions to maintain acid–base balance will not occur as rapidly as the individual ages. The serum creatinine level and the blood urea nitrogen rise in healthy older adults, with a concomitant decrease in glomerular filtration rate (GFR). The older kidney, in contrast to the kidneys in younger adults, excretes more fluid and electrolytes at night than in the daytime. More urine is formed at night, potentially interrupting sleep patterns.

> **ALERT!** Serum creatinine should be checked before administering medications that are excreted by the kidney. Less filtration ability of the kidneys increases susceptibility to medication toxicity.

The ability to respond to a fluid overload by increasing urine production is also decreased in older adults. Because filtration ability of the kidney diminishes with age, impaired excretion of drugs and their metabolites occurs. Drugs and their metabolites can accumulate in the bloodstream, making older adults extremely susceptible to drug toxicity and other adverse medication effects. Often, older adults are on five or more medications, a phenomenon called **polypharmacy.** Drug–drug interactions, which are difficult to predict, often affect the older adult. Because of the adverse effects seen with polypharmacy, some clinicians are attempting deprescribing. Deprescribing is the process of trial drug withdrawal or dose reduction of medications considered inappropriate for the older adult. Research is under way that studies the benefits versus the harm of this practice.

CLINICAL CONCEPT

Dosages of prescribed medication should start low and be increased slowly in the older adult.

Another consequence of reduced renal filtration is an increased probability of hyperkalemia, particularly when certain cardiac or analgesic drugs are used. Hyperkalemia can lead to cardiac dysrhythmias and cardiac arrest.

In the older adult, nephrons are less efficient at reabsorbing water back into the bloodstream and concentrating urine. This increases the older adult's susceptibility to dehydration, a problem that is further complicated by a diminished thirst response; therefore, the older adult will not feel thirsty even when significantly dehydrated.

Genitourinary System

In older adult females, menopause causes some significant changes in the genitourinary system. Genitourinary syndrome of menopause (GSM) is recognized as a combination of gynecological and urological changes that occur due to decline in estrogen levels. These changes include:

- Vulvovaginal atrophy, where the vaginal tissue becomes thinner and vaginal muscle weakens.
- Vulvovaginal dryness, itching, soreness, and dyspareunia are common complaints of older adult females after menopause.
- Decline in estrogen levels also weakens the pelvic musculature, bladder, and urethra.
- Weakening of the bladder musculature can cause stress incontinence, which is leakage of urine when coughing or laughing.
- Changes in vaginal flora, the natural bacterial inhabitants within the vagina, are due to changes in the vaginal glycogen content and pH with menopause, allowing uropathogens to colonize the vagina and increasing susceptibility to UTI.

In older males, one of the most prominent genitourinary changes is enlargement of the prostate gland, termed benign prostatic hyperplasia (BPH). This increase in cellularity of the prostate may constrict the urethra and cause urinary symptoms. The most common urinary symptoms include weakening of the urinary stream, frequency of urination, incomplete emptying of the bladder, and hesitancy (a noncontinuous urine flow). Often, older males require treatment for BPH. Some medications can decrease the urethral constriction, or surgical intervention may be necessary.

Testicular changes are also associated with aging in males. Serum testosterone level decreases, as do sperm volume and motility. There are also more abnormal sperm produced in the older adult male.

Gastrointestinal System

Changes in the digestive system in older adults may have major influences on their quality of life. Motility of the gastrointestinal (GI) tract slows and becomes less coordinated with increasing age because the nerves that supply the system change in function. The autonomic nerves in the entire GI tract decline, beginning in middle age and continuing throughout old age. The denervation is most severe in the distal portion of the tract. The lack of neural strength in the wall of the large bowel and rectum causes decreased peristalsis and constipation.

There is diminished function of the taste and olfactory senses, which in turn changes release of saliva and other digestive enzymes. Also, most older adults experience loosening of the teeth (because of osteopenia in the mandible and maxilla), loss of dentin, gingival recession, and narrowing of the root canal. The muscles involved in swallowing become weaker with age and may not work in concert, increasing susceptibility to dysphagia. The lack of synchronization may be related to loss of cholinergic neurons in the esophagus. **Presbyesophagus** is the term used for age-related changes in the esophagus. In presbyesophagus, there is some loss of strength of the lower esophageal sphincter (LES). With less strength of the LES, acid refluxes up from the stomach into the esophagus. This causes esophagitis and increases susceptibility to gastroesophageal reflux disease.

The stomach lining atrophies with age and produces less intrinsic factor (IF). Lack of IF causes decreased absorption of vitamin B_{12}, which causes decreased red blood cell production in the bone marrow, a condition called **pernicious anemia.** If untreated, pernicious anemia can lead to neurological consequences. Lack of vitamin B_{12} can cause gait disturbance and paresthesias in the lower extremity. Severe vitamin B_{12} deficiency can cause dementia-like symptoms.

Older adults produce less hydrochloric acid (HCl) because the gastric mucosa degenerates, termed **gastric atrophy.** Diminished HCl leads to less absorption of calcium and iron. Lack of calcium increases bone breakdown, and lack of iron can cause reduced hemoglobin synthesis, which leads to decreased red blood cell production. In other words, iron deficiency leads to anemia.

The intestinal wall has decreased muscle and increased collagen and fibrous tissue, whereas the interior lining has villi that become somewhat flattened. The change in the villi makes less surface area available for transport of nutrients into the bloodstream.

The microbes that normally inhabit the intestines change in their proportion to each other, with an increase of enterobacteria in comparison to other bacteria. There is decreased immunity of the GI tract in older adults, which may be related to the change in composition of the intestinal flora. The change in flora predisposes the older adult to GI infections, particularly *Clostridium difficile*. There is also a diminished amount of the enzyme lactase in the intestine. Lactase breaks down lactose; with lack of lactase, **lactose intolerance** occurs; this causes indigestion, gas accumulation, and diarrhea.

Constipation occurs because of the loss of innervation of the intestinal wall, particularly in the colon and rectum. Loss of innervation decreases the motility of the intestinal tract. In addition, the muscle layer of the intestine becomes weaker with age, predisposing individuals to the formation of weakenings in the wall, called diverticula. Diverticula are tiny sacs that develop along the intestinal wall and fill with intestinal contents. The syndrome is called diverticulosis. These diverticula can become inflamed, in which case diverticulitis develops, causing pain in the left-lower quadrant of the abdomen.

Endocrine System

Two endocrine hormones, insulin and thyroxine, undergo changes with advancing age. The pancreatic beta cells that secrete insulin become less active as a normal part of aging, and this is coupled with the body's overall increased **insulin resistance.** Older adults are less physically active than their younger counterparts and have a higher percentage of body fat; both of these factors increase insulin resistance. Older adults also secrete less insulin in response to a glucose load, which is manifested by higher postprandial (after-meal) blood glucose levels. These changes predispose the older adult to glucose intolerance and diabetes.

The thyroid gland shrinks with increasing age, and the hormone thyroxine does not convert to triiodothyronine to the same extent in older adults that it does in younger adults. This makes the older adult susceptible to hypothyroidism. In the older adult, autoimmune hypothyroidism is particularly prevalent. As a result of thyroid changes, the basal metabolism rate is lower, and fewer calories are required to maintain body weight.

During aging, there is also a decline in growth hormone synthesis by the pituitary, which in turn causes a reduction in insulin-like growth factor-1 (IGF-1) production by the liver and other organs. IGFs are peptides that increase anabolic activity in cells. Bone development and mineralization, as well as muscle mass gain, are examples of anabolism. With the reduction of ICFs, there is more catabolic activity in the older adult's body than anabolic activity. Catabolic activity is the breakdown of the elements in the body such as bone and muscle breakdown. The metabolic imbalance in favor of catabolism in older adults leads to reduced protein synthesis, sarcopenia (muscle breakdown), greater osteoclastic versus osteoblastic activity, decreased skeletal muscle strength, decreased neuronal plasticity, reduced energy, and less resilience.

In older adults, there is also decreased peripheral estradiol and testosterone synthesis. This causes increased release of luteinizing hormone (LH) and follicle-stimulating hormone (FSH). In females, there is the degeneration of ovarian function leading to dramatically decreased estrogen levels, which causes menopause. There is a consequent decrease in cardioprotective high-density lipoprotein (HDL), increase in low-density lipoprotein (LDL), and total cholesterol increase. This increases risk of coronary heart disease, myocardial infarction, and stroke in postmenopausal females. The estrogen changes also result in rapid loss of skeletal mass, vasomotor instability, vaginal mucosal atrophy, psychological symptoms, and atrophy of estrogen responsive tissue. In males, there is some drop in testosterone synthesis. This is more marked for free testosterone than for total testosterone, due to an age-associated increase of sex hormone-binding globulin levels. Some males are thought to have the disorder termed low T, or low testosterone. Low testosterone leads to erectile dysfunction, low energy, decreased libido, decreased muscle and bone mass, increased fat mass, and depression. Also, the adrenocortical cells that produce the major sex steroid precursor dehydroepiandrosterone (DHEA) and DHEA sulphate (DHEAS) decrease in activity, often mirrored by a gradual increase in cortisol release. High levels of cortisol are associated with increased catabolism, leading to loss of muscle mass, anorexia, weight loss, and reduced energy expenditure. There is growing evidence supporting the view that chronic cortisol excess may lead to hippocampal atrophy and cognitive impairment during aging. The alterations in cortisol circadian amplitude and phase could be involved in the etiology of sleep disorders in older adults. In both males and females, greater cortisol levels are strongly associated with a greater risk of clinical fractures and increased central fat distribution.

Integumentary System

The most commonly visible characteristics of aging are seen in the integumentary system. The skin is affected by environmental free radicals and sun exposure, which cause cross-linkages in proteins, leading to decreased elasticity. Replacement of epidermal cells slows dramatically with age, and the typical "thin" skin of older adults reflects this slow replacement. Skin breakdown can occur easily. Discoloration of the skin is related to decreased function of melanocytes, and the dryness of older skin is a result of fewer sebaceous glands. The decrease in subdermal fat not only exacerbates the wrinkled appearance of the skin but also removes an important layer of protection involved in older adults' inability to conserve body heat. The loss of sweat glands, hair follicles, and sensory end organs in the skin is related to difficulties in thermoregulation.

The small blood vessels in the skin become more fragile with age so they are more likely to rupture, producing purpura and other lesions. Fewer mast cells and fibroblasts are found in the skin of older adults. The junction between the dermis and epidermis is flattened, creating a more tenuous bond between the two layers, as well as fewer nutrients being passed into the epidermis. This may explain the propensity for older adults to experience injuries to the skin.

Immunosenescence causes decreased immune surveillance of the skin. This immunocompromise and lifetime accumulated exposure to the sun increase growth of skin nodules and nevi with cancer potential. A complete physical examination of the body for cancerous skin lesions annually is necessary.

 CLINICAL CONCEPT

The older adult's skin is delicate and can be sheared off easily. The loss of subdermal fat contributes to the fragility of the skin, increasing susceptibility to pressure injuries.

Musculoskeletal System

Human aging is also marked by changes in muscle mass, strength, and oxygen uptake. Much of the lean muscle mass is replaced by intramuscular fat and connective tissue. For example, the area of lean muscle mass in a cross-section of the human thigh decreases dramatically from age 30 years to age 80 years. Older adults who maintain higher levels of physical activity lose less muscle mass. The loss of muscle mass is accompanied by diminished strength and aerobic capacity of the remaining muscle. These losses appear related to decreased myosin heavy chain and mitochondrial proteins in skeletal muscle. Although muscle protein may be increased with aerobic exercise, once muscle mass is lost, it cannot be regenerated. So an older adult cannot increase the amount of muscle present, but can increase the strength of the remaining muscle.

Both males and females experience age-related loss of bone, particularly in the trabecular (nonsolid) bones of the body, vertebrae, hip, and wrist. Osteoblasts are the cells that build bone, whereas osteoclasts are cells that deteriorate bone. In females, natural estrogen keeps osteoblasts viable; however, after the dramatic decrease of estrogen in menopause, bone resorption caused by osteoclasts outpaces bone formation. With age, decreased bone mineral density (BMD) becomes more common. Osteopenia and osteoporosis are frequently diagnosed in the older adult, particularly females. **Osteopenia** is a decrease in BMD that is a precursor to osteoporosis. Osteoporosis is low BMD that increases susceptibility to fracture. Bone mineral density is measured by a dual energy x-ray absorptiometry (DEXA) scan of the hip and lumbar spine. A DEXA scan compares the patient's BMD to that of a 30-year-old person. **Osteoporosis** is diagnosed if the patient's BMD is 2.5 standard deviations less than the BMD of a 30-year-old.

Nervous System

Older adults are frequently characterized as forgetful, senile, confused, or childish, leading one to expect major changes in the aging nervous system.

Although it is true that there is a small decrease in brain weight—6% to 11%—in some healthy older adults, there is tremendous individual variation in this. Furthermore, it is offset by the large numbers of neurons that compensate for each other. There are changes in the actions of neurotransmitters, as well as in the balance among them. Serotonin, norepinephrine, dopamine, β-endorphins, glutamate, and gamma-aminobutyric acid (GABA) all show decreases in either production or reception with increased age. Behaviors related to sleep pattern and mild memory loss may be related to changes in neurotransmitters. In the peripheral nervous system, loss of myelin accompanies increased age and is likely related to the decrease in nerve conduction velocity. These changes take place at different rates and in different areas of the nervous system.

Neurological health also involves proper nutrition and vitamin absorption. Pernicious anemia, caused by lack of gastric IF, is common in the older adult. Gastric atrophy also causes decreased secretion of HCl in the stomach. Diminished IF and HCl lead to decreased absorption of vitamin B_{12}. Low vitamin B_{12} levels have neurological consequences. In untreated vitamin B_{12} deficiency, there is demyelination of the dorsal columns of the spinal cord, termed subacute combined degeneration (SCD). SCD causes gait instability and paresthesias in the lower extremities. Vitamin B_{12} supplements may be necessary. Intranasal or injectable vitamin B_{12} may be required because some older patients with decreased IF and HCl cannot absorb B_{12} via the intestinal mucosa.

One of the important sequelae of changes in the nervous system is that older adults have pain thresholds that are higher than those found in younger adults. The higher threshold is consistent for many stimuli such as mechanical and thermal injury, although there is some evidence that older adults experience greater levels of visceral pain. Higher pain thresholds may interfere with protective actions, such as pulling away from the source of pain, and may be related to poorer tissue repair. However, length of the stimulus is an important variable to consider, as older adults experience a lowered pain threshold if the stimulus is present over a long period, such as occurs in chronic pain.

 CLINICAL CONCEPT

Older adults may not be aware of an injury because they have less pain sensitivity than younger adults.

Plasticity persists in the nervous system well into old age. The decrements in neurotransmitters and neurons can be delayed, inhibited, or reversed. The current popular notion of "use it or lose it" has a physiological basis. Studies with rats and mice have demonstrated that interesting and enriched environments can increase the levels of neurotransmitters present, as well as functional performance.

The sense organs also undergo age-related changes. The aging eye contains fewer rods and cones than in the younger adult's eye, with concomitant losses in color vision, visual acuity, need for increased contrast, and need for increased ambient lighting. Furthermore, the lens becomes more opaque and stiffer, causing blurring of vision, increased glare, and decreased ability to accommodate. These combined defects are known as **presbyopia,** literally meaning "old vision." **Cataracts** are also common among older adults. Cataracts form because the lens naturally develops thickened layers with age. A cataract can be seen as an opacity over the pupil and iris.

Hearing is also affected by normal aging, with losses in the ability to detect both low- and high-frequency sounds. The result is that the older adult is not able to interpret some speech sounds. Deterioration of the organ of Corti, ganglia, hair cells, and basement membranes are all implicated in **presbycusis,** age-related hearing loss.

Older adults also have less ability to taste salt, sweet, bitter, and sour, which is likely related to a time lag in the turnover of taste buds, rather than a decrease in the total number.

Thermoregulation

Thermoregulation is a function of both the autonomic nervous system and behavioral adaptation. Older adults tend to have lower basal temperatures and often do not produce fevers in response to even overwhelming infection. Fever in older adults is defined as a rise of 2°F (1.1°C) over baseline, or repeated findings of oral temperature of 99°F (37.2°C) or higher, or rectal temperature of 99.5°F (37.5°C) or higher. Even with these lowered criteria, only about 55% of older adults in nursing homes with infections ever demonstrate any fever. The reasons for this are a combination of the fewer antigen-specific antibodies that are produced by older adults, poorer thermoregulation by the CNS, less responsiveness of the hypothalamus, and a decreased production of endogenous pyrogens. Changes in the body, including less subcutaneous fat and less vasodilation, render the body less able to produce and conserve body heat. These changes also lead to lack of fever and increased likelihood of hypothermia. In addition, older adults may be less able to recognize loss of body heat and take the appropriate actions, such as adding more clothing.

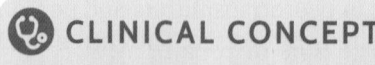

CLINICAL CONCEPT

Older adults are prone to hypothermia and hyperthermia.

Common Age-Related Disorders and Issues

Older adults have increased rates of disease and disability. Most disease is not a consequence of normal aging, but rather of lifestyle choices, injury, and genetics. In addition, most older adults have more than one existing disease, greatly complicating both diagnosis and treatment of new conditions. Furthermore, the many physiological changes of aging lead to unusual presentations of disease. Disease then often causes subtle changes in the older adult's behavior. Frequently, a change in mental status will be the first indication of a pathological process, particularly an infectious one.

CLINICAL CONCEPT

Disease in the older adult, particularly infection, often presents with mental status or behavioral changes, such as confusion and irritability.

It is critically important to remember that treatment goals may be different for older adults. Comorbidities and frailty may dictate less aggressive goals and treatment guidelines.

CLINICAL CONCEPT

Quality of life and functional independence, rather than cure, are the treatment goals for older adults.

Chronic Pain

Chronic pain is too often a factor in the lives of older adults. Common types of pain include joint pain, neuralgias, and cancer pain. Undermedication of pain is common because many older adults assume that pain is a part of aging, whereas health-care providers are concerned about addiction. Overall, slightly more than 3% of patients treated with opioids for chronic pain will demonstrate addiction or substance abuse, but among patients with no prior history of abuse or addiction, that number drops to 0.19%. Chronic pain has serious health consequences for older adults, including loss of functional ability, depression, and structural brain changes. The gray matter in the posterior parietal cortex and white matter in the middle cingulated region are most affected, with subsequent deficits evident in attention and mental flexibility.

Chronic Renal Failure

Chronic renal failure (CRF) is caused by irreversible damage to the kidney and is more common in older adults than in younger adults. Adults older than 65 years are the fastest-growing patient population that requires dialysis; it is estimated that 60% of persons aged 65 years and older have renal impairment, compared with 7% in adults ages 40 to 65 years.

Atherosclerosis and diabetes are the most common causes of CRF in older adults. Most older adults who require assisted living support because of frailty have advanced kidney disease (stage 3 or greater), but very few have been diagnosed with renal impairment. Calculating the patient's estimated GFR is important before administering medications that are metabolized by the kidney.

> **CLINICAL CONCEPT**
>
> As a person ages, GFR decreases by approximately 1 mL/min after age 60. A simple way of estimating the approximate GFR of a patient is by calculating 140 – patient's age.

The definitive treatment for CRF is renal replacement therapy, either through dialysis or through renal transplant. For more information regarding CRF, see Chapter 22.

Dementias

Dementia is defined as a syndrome of loss of cognitive function and memory that is progressive and impedes the functions of daily living, although level of consciousness is not affected until late in the disease process. There are many different causes of dementia, with Alzheimer's disease (AD) being the most common etiology, followed by vascular dementia, Lewy body dementia (LBD), frontotemporal dementia (FTD), and dementias related to specific diseases such as Parkinson's disease or AIDS. It is important to note that people can have more than one etiology for dementia, such as comorbid vascular dementia and AD. Each dementia has different early behavioral manifestations, risk factors, and disease courses.

Alzheimer's Disease

AD is discussed in further detail in Chapter 36, but a few points are important to cover in this chapter. It is absolutely critical to remember that cognitive impairment is not a part of normal aging and must be thoroughly investigated when symptoms first appear. Only 6% to 7% of older adults have illnesses that cause dementia, although the percentage increases to nearly 38% in those age 90 years and older. The average time

from diagnosis of dementia to death from dementia is 7 to 10 years, depending on the type.

The etiology of AD is unknown; however, the pathophysiological processes are the subject of recent research. Genetic mutations within chromosomes 21, 14, 19, and 1 are seen in AD. The *APOE4* gene on chromosome 19 increases susceptibility to AD. Neuron degeneration, accumulation of proteins called beta-amyloid plaques, and lack of acetylcholine occur in the brain in AD. These abnormalities are seen most in the hippocampus and medial temporal lobe, which control memory, thinking, and decision making.

AD is mainly diagnosed by symptoms and clinical examination. Imaging studies such as computed tomography (CT), magnetic resonance imaging (MRI), and positron emission tomography (PET) scans are also used to diagnose AD. Imaging studies show beta-amyloid plaques and reduced size of certain areas of the brain in AD. Cerebrospinal fluid analysis shows abnormal amounts of beta-amyloid and tau proteins. Treatment involves medications, such as acetylcholinesterase inhibitors that can slow the development of AD, and psychosocial support.

> **ALERT!** Cognitive changes are never normal in the older adult and must always be thoroughly assessed.

Vascular Dementia

Vascular dementia, formerly called multiinfarct dementia, is similar to stroke in that a blood vessel is damaged and the tissues beyond it receive no oxygenation. Unlike stroke, however, there are no physical deficits, and cognitive deficits may not be apparent until several infarcts have occurred. The prevalence of vascular dementia is unknown because many cases are unreported; however, it is estimated that 40% of persons with dementia have vascular dementia.

Chronic hypertension and diabetes mellitus, particularly when poorly controlled, put an older adult at higher risk for developing vascular dementia because of the level of damage caused to the microvasculature. The degree of cognitive impairment and behavioral manifestations is dependent on the area of the brain that is affected by ischemia, and because of this, symptoms are quite varied. Imaging studies such as CT, MRI, and PET scans are used to diagnose vascular dementia. Acetylcholinesterase inhibitors, antiplatelet medications, antihypertensives, and antilipidemia medications are used to manage the cognitive decline in vascular dementia.

Lewy Body Dementia

LBD occurs in 10% to 20% of persons with dementia. Incidence and prevalence are difficult to estimate because diagnosis is difficult. It may share etiological factors with Parkinson's disease, in that both demonstrate abnormalities in the substantia nigra, which is part of the basal ganglia in the midbrain. Lewy bodies are abnormal protein clusters that accumulate in the synapses of the basal ganglia, and the number of them does not coincide with the severity of symptoms.

Pathophysiology. In LBD, there are inclusion bodies called Lewy bodies seen inside the cells of many sections of the brain, including the substantia nigra, locus ceruleus, dorsal raphe, and cranial nerve X. The primary constituent in Lewy bodies is alpha-synuclein, a protein with unknown activity. In LBD, acetylcholine is also diminished. Certain regions of the brain with LBD have been studied under single-photon emission computerized tomography (SPECT) to show different areas of perfusion. In LBD, hypoperfusion of the parietal and occipital regions is seen in patients who have visual hallucinations. Hyperperfusion occurs in the frontal cortex, which is thought to be related to delusional behaviors.

Clinical Presentation. A key feature of LBD, and one that differentiates it from other dementias, is fluctuation of symptoms. An older adult with LBD may be quite demented on 1 day, but significantly less so on the next day, although the average level of cognitive impairment is progressive. LBD causes visual hallucinations; delusions; and vivid, frightening dreams. Parkinsonian-like motor symptoms can occur where the patient suffers resting tremor, impaired balance, slowed movements, uncontrollable muscle jerks, and freezing episodes when they cannot move.

Diagnosis and Treatment. Clinical examination of the patient will exhibit signs of dementia, and SPECT shows decreased perfusion in the occipital region of the brain. Acetylcholinesterase inhibitors, antipsychotic drugs, antidepressants, and levodopa/carbidopa may all help control symptoms. Clonazepam and melatonin are helpful for sleep.

Frontotemporal Dementia

FTD, also known as Pick's disease, is a less common type of dementia than AD or vascular dementia. The incidence of FTD is unknown; however, it is thought to be the cause of 10% of cases of dementia. Most patients are affected after age 50 years, with a peak incidence at 64 years old.

Etiology. The etiology of FTD is unknown. There is a strong genetic risk factor; as many as 50% of persons with FTD have a family history of the disease. Mutations are found at 17q21-22, which is the gene that controls the production of the tau protein; tau proteins build up in the brain in FTD. Other genetic mutations on chromosome 17 cause decreased production of the progranulin protein and excess production of the ubiquitin protein.

Pathophysiology. Cerebral atrophy is evident in the frontal or temporal lobe of one or both hemispheres of the brain in FTD. Commonly, there is loss within the brain's language area. Some patients will show motor neuron atrophy.

Clinical Presentation. Persons with FTD demonstrate loss of social skills, the hallmark of this disease. Persons with FTD also become increasingly antisocial and disinhibited, oftentimes using crude language and sexual acting out, as well as being unconcerned about the needs of others. Furthermore, patients with FTD may manifest compulsive oral behaviors, such as overeating, sucking on objects, or eating nonfoods. These behaviors may be extremely upsetting to family members, who may need reassurance that the behaviors are symptoms of the disease. This may be difficult for families to understand, as patients with FTD do not have memory losses or difficulties speaking—symptoms that most people connect with diagnoses of dementia. Additionally, FTD seems to have a strong genetic link within some families, and family members may worry that they, too, will develop the disease. It is important to remind families that the mechanisms of developing FTD are still being investigated and having a relative with FTD does not guarantee that others in the same family will develop it.

Diagnosis and Treatment. MRI and PET scanning of the brain demonstrate cerebral atrophy and hypometabolism in specific areas of the frontal and temporal lobes. Language and neuropsychological tests are commonly administered. Unfortunately, there are few treatment options for FTD, and most are used to control problematic behavior. Antidepressants are commonly prescribed. Trazodone is given to induce sleep.

Type 2 Diabetes Mellitus

Nearly 40% of adults aged 65 years and older meet the diagnostic criteria for **type 2 diabetes mellitus (T2DM)**. Older adults are at increased risk for developing T2DM because of increased cellular resistance to endogenous insulin and pancreatic beta cell dysfunction. Even without diagnosed T2DM, older adults tend to have postprandial glucose levels that are above 200 mg/dL, a condition known as isolated postchallenge hyperglycemia. An elevated glucose level is a risk factor for depression, cognitive impairment, urinary incontinence, falls, persistent pain, and gastroparesis. Older adults, as with all adults, are also at risk of both microvascular and macrovascular complications from DM. The management of blood glucose in older adults, however, is more challenging than with other population groups because of comorbidities, aging changes, and potential injury from falls brought on by hypoglycemia.

Damage from persistent hyperglycemia is more appropriately controlled by attending to other cardiovascular risk factors, such as smoking cessation, weight control, lipid management, and blood pressure control. Glycemic control remains important but will not yield microvascular benefits nearly as quickly as controlling blood pressure and lipids. Taking the older adult's life expectancy into consideration, a more modest HgbA1c goal of 8%, an average blood glucose level of 183 mg/dL, is often targeted for frail older adults, whereas healthy older adults have the same target of lower than 7%, as do younger adults.

Furthermore, many older adults have impaired renal function, and medications such as metformin and angiotensin-converting enzyme (ACE) inhibitors may be contraindicated. Because of alterations in medication metabolism among older adults, it is important to be particularly alert for changes in peak action times of insulins. It may be wise to consider insulin with a very predictable peak of action, such as lispro, over regular insulin or aspart, which have a wider variation in peak and duration of action. For more information about T2DM, see Chapter 25.

 CLINICAL CONCEPT

When working with older patients who have T2DM, it is important to monitor blood pressure and lipid levels with the same vigilance as glucose levels.

Geriatric Syndromes

Geriatric syndromes are health conditions that are common among older adults and have many causative factors. Urinary incontinence, falls, pressure wounds, delirium, and functional decline are some common examples of geriatric syndromes. Frail older adults are more likely to have geriatric syndromes, which lead to increased frailty.

Frailty in an older adult is described as a constellation of symptoms that include weakness, weight loss, decreased balance and physical activity, slowness, social withdrawal, cognitive impairments, and fatigue. The frail older adult has increased vulnerability to stressors and is less able to maintain or regain homeostasis after physiological or psychosocial threat. For example, a frail older adult with coronary artery disease could not endure angioplasty or coronary bypass surgery; therefore, long-acting nitrate medications are used instead.

The factors that lead to frailty include many of the normal changes of aging, plus diseases that are common to older adults. Specifically, changes in the musculoskeletal, neurological, and immune systems, as well as molecular and genetic changes, predispose some older adults to a heightened vulnerability to stressors. Surgery, either emergent or elective, may be the event that precipitates a cascade of events that lead to

greater neuromuscular instability, then to a fall, then to new injuries. Subclinical problems that may have been just beneath the surface of the older adult's functional status begin to appear.

It is extremely difficult to treat geriatric syndromes because of the many contributing factors, but it is important to foster maintenance of function and independence.

Heart Failure

Heart failure (HF) occurs most commonly in older adults because of age-related changes in the cardiovascular system, as well as the high survivorship of ischemic heart disease in the United States. Almost 10% of all older adults have HF, and among all patients with HF, 70% are older than 80 years. With the predicted increase in the population of older adults in the future, HF will become a very prevalent disease.

There are 2 main types of HF: systolic HF and diastolic HF. Older adults are much more likely to have diastolic HF—a stiff left ventricle with decreased compliance and impaired relaxation. As a group, it is common for the older HF patient to receive substandard treatment compared with younger adults. For more information, see Chapter 17.

Hypertension

Not many years ago, isolated systolic hypertension was considered a normal aspect of aging, and older adults were not offered treatment. Some believed that if high blood pressure was treated in older adults, dementia would ensue because blood would not effectively circulate in the brain. Now, although age-related changes clearly may predispose older adults to increased blood pressure, it is recognized that hypertension among older adults is a disease and must be treated, just as hypertension in a middle-aged adult must be treated. Sixty-four percent of male adults older than 65 years have hypertension, and almost 70% of females older than 65 years have the disorder. African Americans have a higher prevalence of hypertension than European American adults. Recently, the American Heart Association/ American College of Cardiology have recommended different blood pressure guidelines and medical management for the older adult (see Chapter 15).

Blood vessels become stiffer with advancing age and contain atherosclerotic plaques. These changes narrow the diameter of blood vessels and increase peripheral vascular resistance. This is most noticeable in the systolic blood pressure of older adults. The older adult's body becomes adjusted to a higher systolic blood pressure for adequate cerebral perfusion. Commonly, 120 mm Hg systolic is too low for the older adult and leaves the person susceptible to orthostatic hypotension.

Also, a significant decrease in GFR is common in the older adult, and this condition has important indications for choice of antihypertensive therapy. The patient's GFR should be calculated before administering medications.

Diuretic antihypertensive therapy commonly causes electrolyte disturbances in older adults. Diuretic therapy also causes frequent urination, which may be problematic in older adults. Calcium channel blockers have been shown to cause ankle edema and reflux esophagitis in some older adults. ACE inhibitors sometimes worsen symptoms of dementia. Different medications have different side effects, particularly in the older adult, who is routinely on six or seven medications, which is why older adults on blood pressure medications require periodic assessment and need careful monitoring. Patient education regarding weight loss, exercise, and a low-sodium diet is an important component of treatment.

Infections

Older adults have alterations in their immune systems that make them more susceptible to infections. Both innate and adaptive immunity decrease in strength and efficiency. The older adult is immunocompromised and less able to fight infection compared with the younger adult. Because the older adult cannot mount a strong immunological response, they do not demonstrate the symptoms that are normally associated with infection. Older adults do not run high fevers and often do not demonstrate a high WBC count with infection. Also, pain sensitivity is decreased in the older adult, and signs of inflammation are blunted. Uniquely, the older adult with an infection may show changes in behavior or disorientation as the only symptom of infection.

Many older adults have significant levels of bacteria in their urine all the time, referred to as asymptomatic bacteriuria (ASB). In fact, older adults who have indwelling catheters have a 100% rate of bacteriuria, yet many of these individuals are without symptoms. Older adults do not demonstrate the typical symptoms of UTI, which include dysuria, frequency, and urgency. Routine urinalysis may show bacteria; however, this is difficult to interpret, as ASB is common in older adults, and urinalysis cannot distinguish between ASB and a true UTI. ASB in the older adult does not require treatment. The clinician has to decide whether to use antibiotic treatment based on the patient's history, vital signs, and changes in behavior.

Pneumonia is also a common infection in the older adult; its prevalence is caused by a combination of age-related changes in the lungs, immune system, and GI system. The thoracic cage becomes stiffer, which decreases the expansion and therefore the capacity for deep breathing. The cough and gag reflexes in the older adult weaken, which increases susceptibility to aspiration. In addition, stasis of pulmonary secretions is common because of the sedentary behavior common in older adults. Older adults who are immobile or on bedrest are particularly susceptible to pneumonia. Pneumonia frequently occurs after an upper respiratory infection or influenza in the older adult. For this reason, an annual flu vaccine and pneumococcal vaccine are recommended for older adults. The pneumococcal vaccine is recommended after age 65 and every 5 to 10 years after the initial immunization. The initial immunization consists of two doses of different types of pneumococcal vaccine: PCV 13 (pneumococcal conjugate vaccine 13 [Prevnar 13]), followed a year later by PPSV23 (pneumococcal polysaccharide vaccine 23 [Pneumovax]).

Altered Medication Effectiveness

Changes that occur in the kidney, liver, intestine, muscle, and subcutaneous fat of older adults have important implications for the pharmacokinetics and dynamics of medications. Absorption, distribution, metabolism, and excretion may all be affected by changes related to aging. Intramuscular injections may be absorbed faster because of the decreased muscle mass, but that is offset by decreased peripheral blood flow that may decrease absorption. Because older adults generally have more overall body fat in comparison to lean muscle, fat-soluble medications such as diazepam will remain in the body longer, leading to a possible overdose if adjustments in timing and dose are not made. Water-soluble medications such as gentamicin, in contrast, will be metabolized more quickly because of the relative lack of free water. The loss of lean muscle mass means that older adults have less protein in their bodies, so the amount of free drug will circulate in higher quantities. Clinicians who work with older adults should become familiar with the most current Beers criteria for potentially inappropriate medication use in older adults.

The liver becomes less effective with increased age, which particularly affects medication metabolism. With age, there is less blood flow to the liver and diminished detoxification capacity. Standard liver function tests such as aspartate transaminase (AST) and alanine transaminase (ALT) often do not accurately reflect pharmacokinetics. The kidney also becomes less effective in excreting drug metabolites. The combination of the decreased functioning of these two organs means that older adults are at risk for accidental overdose.

Conversely, immunosuppression in older adults dictates that antimicrobials be used in doses large enough to be effective, while also carefully monitoring for adverse drug effects. Macrolides such as azithromycin do not concentrate well in older adults, but the acidic anti-infectives such as penicillin, ceftriaxone, sulfonamides, and clindamycin may reach concentrations higher than in younger adults. When possible, culture and sensitivity (C&S) testing should be done to ensure that infections are completely treated.

Polypharmacy and Older Adults

Polypharmacy, defined as regular use of five medications or more, is common in older adults and increases the risk of adverse medical outcomes. Multiple medications may be indicated in patients with more than one chronic health disorder such as heart disease, arthritis, cancer, or diabetes mellitus. In these cases, polypharmacy may be appropriate. However, inappropriate polypharmacy—the use of excessive or unnecessary medications—increases the risk of adverse drug effects, including falls and cognitive impairment, harmful drug interactions, and drug–disease interactions, in which a medication prescribed to treat one condition worsens another or causes a new one. According to a report by the Centers for Disease Control and Prevention (2019), 83% of U.S. adults in their 60s and 70s had used at least one prescription drug in the previous 30 days and about one-third used five or more prescription drugs. The most commonly used drugs were cholesterol, high blood pressure, and diabetes medications.

Older adults with multiple subspecialist physicians and no primary care physician are particularly vulnerable to polypharmacy. A primary care clinician that oversees the comprehensive health management plan and therapeutic goals is needed. Older adults with chronic mental health conditions are at high risk for polypharmacy. These patients are often prescribed psychotropic medications with adverse effects, and more medications may be added to mitigate side effects. Adults residing in long-term care facilities are at high risk of polypharmacy. They are commonly frailer than community-dwelling populations and have multiple medical issues and cognitive impairment. They often cannot share in the decision-making process of prescribing by the clinician. Some cannot communicate their needs or side effects. Up to 91% of patients in long-term care take at least five medications daily.

The American Geriatric Society Beers Criteria® (2019) is an up-to-date compendium of medications to avoid or consider with caution because they often present an unfavorable balance of benefits and harms for older adults. First created by Mark Beers, MD, in 1991, the AGS Beers Criteria is based on an extensive review of more than 1,400 studies. It includes five lists of nearly 100 medications or medication classes to avoid or use with caution in older adults.

A deprescribing strategy is increasingly being utilized by clinicians to eliminate the harmful effects of polypharmacy. The U.S. Deprescribing Research Network, funded by the National Institute on Aging (NIA), is attempting to build an interdisciplinary community of researchers including physicians, pharmacists, nurses, and older adults and their care partners who are interested in improving research in the relatively new field of deprescribing. Its goal is to develop and share resources and support innovative pilot studies to improve the quality of care and health outcomes for older adults. Also, the American Board of Internal Medicine Foundation's Choose Wisely campaign is advocated by the American Geriatric Society, American Psychiatric Association, and the American Society of Health-System Pharmacists. This campaign asks clinicians to conduct comprehensive drug regimen review with patients. The clinician should be aware of all the prescription medications, over-the-counter drugs, and supplements that the patient is taking. They are also asking clinicians to refrain from prescribing drugs with an indefinite time frame. Clinicians should also refrain from continually renewing prescriptions without reassessing the patient. It is recommended that specific therapy goals be examined at every patient visit—disease control (primary/secondary prevention, symptom control/management) vs. acute symptom management. The clinicians should question the utility of adding new medications and deprescribe when appropriate.

An assessment tool called the Beers, STOPP (Screening Tool of Older People's Prescriptions), and START (Screening Tool to Alert to Right Treatment) has been developed to facilitate the detection of potentially inappropriate prescribing in the process of regular medication review in older adults. This tool allows for comparison of a patient's medication list to a set of potentially inappropriate medications and to check for medication duplication, drug–disease interactions, and medication adjustments required for certain disease states such as renal impairment. The STOPP and START criteria are used together to identify medications that may be inappropriate (STOPP) and alternative medications that can be started to safely treat a disease (START). The new paradigm shift of restrained prescribing and deprescribing is evolving in health care. STOPP/START criteria are being incorporated in electronic medical record software algorithms that can be implemented into clinical decision support systems to facilitate their application. Early research has shown that the use of STOPP/START criteria in patient care can lead to a reduction of polypharmacy, inappropriate prescribing, and adverse drug reactions.

Chapter Summary

- Population studies show that the average life span for females in the United States is approximately 85 years; for males, it is 83 years.

- People age 85 years and older are the fastest-growing segment of older Americans.

- Older adult individuals are categorized in three different groups according to age: young-old, individuals aged between 65 and 74 years; middle-old, individuals aged between 75 and 84 years; and old-old, individuals older than age 85 years.

- With age, the ability to repair damage and adapt to physiological stressors decreases. This decreased ability is referred to as loss of physiological reserve.

- Although older adults may be able to function adequately in daily life, they are less resilient to stress compared with younger adults.

- In the telomere shortening theory of aging, telomeres– the end segments of chromosomes–diminish each time the cell divides in mitosis. Telomerase is an enzyme under intense study because it prevents the shortening of telomeres, thereby counteracting aging.

- The damage-based theory of aging asserts that cellular damage occurs over time because of accumulation of toxic by-products of metabolism, ineffective protein synthesis and secretion, and inefficient cellular repair systems.

- Limiting total calories to as few as 60% of the recommended daily allowance extends the life span of mice up to 40%. In laboratory experiments, calorie-restricted older adult mice are physiologically similar to young mice in many ways.

- Cardiovascular changes in the older adult include development of atherosclerosis, stiffening of the elastic blood vessels, development of diastolic dysfunction in the heart, and connective tissue infiltration of the conductive tissues in the heart.

- Respiratory changes in the older adult include a less elastic thoracic cage, which limits lung expansion with inhalation, as well as diminished cough reflex, which increases stasis of secretions in the lungs.

- Renal changes in the older adult include decreased ability of the kidney to filter wastes from the blood and a decreased GFR, which lends to medication toxicity.

- GI changes in the older adult include decreased peristaltic activity, which increases susceptibility to constipation; atrophy of the stomach lining and intestinal villi; and decreased strength of the LES, allowing acid reflux.

- Endocrine changes include some decreased pancreatic efficiency in secretion of insulin, increased cellular insulin resistance, decreased thyroid hormone synthesis, reduced growth hormone that contributes to a catabolic state, dramatic estrogen decline in females due to menopause, and some testosterone decrease in males.

- Integumentary changes in the older adult include the loss of sweat glands, hair follicles, and sensory end organs, which can lead to difficulties in thermoregulation. Skin also becomes less elastic and thinner, increasing susceptibility to breakdown.

- Musculoskeletal changes in the older adult include an increased susceptibility to osteoporosis because osteoclastic activity begins to outpace osteoblastic activity. Lean muscle mass diminishes and body fat increases.

- Nervous system changes in the older adult include an increased pain threshold, which can interfere with protective actions, as well as increased problems with sight, hearing, and taste.

- A majority of older adults with infections demonstrate no fever, and older adults are more susceptible to hypothermia and hyperthermia than younger adults.

- Cognitive changes are never normal in the older adult and must always be thoroughly assessed. Vascular dementia, AD, and FTD are common causes of cognitive impairment.

- Geriatric syndromes are health conditions common among older adults. These conditions have many causative factors. Urinary incontinence, falls, pressure wounds, delirium, and functional decline are common examples of geriatric syndromes.

- Frailty in an older adult is described as a constellation of symptoms that includes weakness, weight loss, decreased balance and physical activity, slowness, social withdrawal, cognitive impairments, and fatigue. The frail older adult has increased vulnerability to stressors and is less able to maintain or regain homeostasis after physiological or psychosocial threat.
- Clinicians who work with older adults should become familiar with the Beers criteria for potentially inappropriate medication use in older adults.

- Polypharmacy affects older adults and can contribute to adverse drug effects, drug–drug interactions, falls, and cognitive impairment.
- An evolving paradigm encourages clinicians to conduct drug regimen reviews, critique medication lists, and consider deprescribing medications in older adults.

Basic Functional Changes of Body Systems With Aging

INTEGUMENTARY SYSTEM
- Decreased skin elasticity.
- Replacement of epidermal cells slows, causing typical "thin" skin of older adults and predisposition to skin breakdown.
- Dryness of skin due to fewer sebaceous glands.
- Decrease in subdermal fat causes wrinkles and inability to conserve body heat.
- The loss of sweat glands, hair follicles, and sensory end organs in the skin is related to difficulties in thermoregulation.
- The small blood vessels in the skin become more fragile and susceptible to rupture, producing purpura and other lesions.
- Immunosenescence and lifetime accumulation of sun exposure cause decreased surveillance of skin and enhanced risk of skin lesions with cancerous potential.

RESPIRATORY SYSTEM
- Aerobic capacity decreases; slowed responses to hypoxia or hypercapnia.
- Stasis of pulmonary secretions and decreased strength of cough increase susceptibility to pneumonia.
- Older adults with respiratory infections may not exhibit the early warning signs of fever, tachypnea, and dyspnea.
- Older individuals cannot mount the same maximum heart rate in reaction to hypoxia.
- Decreased elasticity of the thoracic cage and strength of the respiratory muscles decrease, leading to less vital capacity and tidal volume.
- Residual volume in the lungs increases; alveoli lose surface area, and less oxygen is diffused into the pulmonary capillaries. The diameter of the bronchioles and smaller airways also decreases.
- Kyphosis due to osteopenia in the vertebrae and collapse of the intervertebral discs lead to an increased anteroposterior diameter, or barrel chest.
- Abdominal muscles rather than the diaphragm are used more in breathing, resulting in an increased effort needed in both inspiration and expiration.

CARDIOVASCULAR SYSTEM
- Atherosclerosis of endothelial lining and increased connective tissue in the muscle walls of the arteries lead to decreased elasticity of blood vessels, which contributes to higher blood pressure.
- The heart accumulates fibrous tissue in muscle and conductive tissue. The heart is less compliant, and chambers cannot expand as wide as in youth; this leads to decreased cardiac output.
- There is connective tissue infiltration of the conductive tissues, which increases the risk of arrhythmias.
- Valvular accumulation of calcium and myxomatous changes cause valvular dysfunction.
- Changes in the conductive tissue cause decreased responsiveness to the sympathetic nervous system, leading to smaller increases in heart rate with stress or exercise.
- Baroreceptor reflex in the arterial walls is slower to respond to a drop in blood pressure.
- There is less ability to raise blood pressure with position changes, causing increased susceptibility to orthostatic hypotension.

IMMUNE SYSTEM
- Immunosenescence; weakening of both the innate and adaptive immune systems; natural killer cells and T lymphocytes have decreased ability to recognize and attack the antigens.
- New T lymphocytes are essentially not produced in older adults, severely impairing the older adult's ability to combat previously unencountered antigens.
- B lymphocytes become less effective in producing antibodies.
- Cytokine secretion also declines with concomitant decline in strength of inflammatory reaction.
- Older adults have decreased external signs and symptoms of inflammation or infection.
- With infection, WBC numbers do not rise to high levels and fever reaction is blunted. Immunizations are less effective as the immune system does not respond as vigorously as a younger adult.
- Antibody levels do not rise as robustly as in a younger person.

Continued

Basic Functional Changes of Body Systems With Aging—cont'd

GASTROINTESTINAL SYSTEM

- Motility of the gastrointestinal (GI) tract slows due to decline in function of autonomic nerves, which causes decreased peristalsis and constipation.
- Diminished function of the taste and olfactory senses, loosening of the teeth due to osteopenia in the mandible and maxilla, loss of dentin, gingival recession.
- The muscles involved in swallowing become weaker, called presbyesophagus.
- Some loss of strength of the lower esophageal sphincter (LES) allows acid reflux into the esophagus, leading to esophagitis and gastroesophageal reflux disease (GERD).
- Stomach lining atrophies with age, and produces less intrinsic factor (IF) and less HCL.
- Lack of IF causes decreased absorption of vitamin B_{12}, which can lead to pernicious anemia.
- Diminished HCl leads to less absorption of calcium and iron. Lack of calcium absorption increases bone breakdown, and lack of iron can cause iron-deficiency anemia.
- Intestinal lining villi flatten, leading to less surface available for transport of nutrients into the bloodstream.
- Diminished enzyme lactase in the intestine causes lactose intolerance.
- The muscle layer of the intestine becomes weaker, predisposing to formation of diverticula, which lead to diverticulosis and diverticulitis.

ENDOCRINE SYSTEM

- Pancreatic beta cells secrete less insulin in response to glucose load.
- Body cells develop increased insulin resistance.
- Higher percentage of body fat (versus muscle) increases insulin resistance, which predisposes to glucose intolerance and diabetes.
- The thyroid gland shrinks; hormone thyroxine does not convert to triiodothyronine to the same extent as in younger adults.
- The basal metabolic rate is lower, and fewer calories are required to maintain body weight.
- Decline in growth hormone synthesis by the pituitary; the body has less anabolic activity versus enhanced catabolic state, causing decreased bone and muscle strength.
- Decreased estrogen levels in females due to ovarian degeneration and some decrease in testosterone in males.
- Adrenocortical cells produce decreased sex steroid precursor dehydroepiandrosterone (DHEA), which causes increased cortisol release. Higher cortisol leads to catabolic state of body; bone and muscle breakdown, fat redistribution to central region, sleep disorders, hippocampal atrophy leading to some cognitive impairment.

GENITOURINARY SYSTEM

- In older adult females, menopause causes changes in the genitourinary system due to decline in estrogen levels, resulting in vulvovaginal atrophy, dryness, itching, soreness, and dyspareunia; and weakening of pelvic musculature, bladder, and urethra can cause stress incontinence, which is leakage of urine when coughing or laughing.
- Changes in vaginal flora, the natural bacterial inhabitants within the vagina, allow uropathogens to colonize and increase susceptibility to UTI.
- Enlargement of the prostate gland in males, termed benign prostatic hyperplasia (BPH), may constrict the urethra and cause urinary symptoms: weakening of the urinary stream, frequency of urination, incomplete emptying of the bladder, and hesitancy (a noncontinuous urine flow).
- Serum testosterone level decreases, which decreases sperm volume, motility, and more abnormal sperm produced.

RENAL SYSTEM

- Loss of nephrons, decreased activity of the nephron tubules, and decrease in blood flow to the kidney all decrease filtration ability of kidney (decreased GFR), less ability to respond to a fluid overload and to concentrate urine, and lower creatinine clearance.
- Less ability to maintain acid-base balance and K+excretion; serum creatinine level, and BUN rise.
- Decreased GFR increases susceptibility to medication toxicity. Often, older adults are on five or more medications, called polypharmacy.
- Drug–drug interactions can affect the older adult.
- The response of the nephrons to antidiuretic hormone is less so the ability to concentrate urine is diminished.
- Increased susceptibility to dehydration and fluid overload.

MUSCULOSKELETAL SYSTEM

- Much of the lean muscle mass is replaced by intramuscular fat and connective tissue with diminished strength and aerobic capacity of the remaining muscle.
- Age-related loss of bone, particularly in the trabecular (nonsolid) bones of the body, vertebrae, hip, and wrist.
- Osteoclastic activity is greater than osteoblastic activity, resulting in decreased bone mineral density (BMD).
- In females, dramatic decrease of estrogen in menopause leads to bone resorption outpacing bone formation.
- Osteoporosis is low BMD that increases susceptibility to fracture.
- Bone mineral density is measured by a DEXA of the hip and lumbar spine.
- Osteoporosis is diagnosed if the patient's BMD is 2.5 standard deviations less than BMD of a 30-year-old.

Basic Functional Changes of Body Systems With Aging–cont'd

NEUROLOGICAL SYSTEM

- Neurotransmitters serotonin, norepinephrine, dopamine, β-endorphins, glutamate, and gamma-aminobutyric acid (GABA) all show decreases in either production or reception with increased age.
- Decreased need for sleep and mild memory loss may be related to changes in neurotransmitters.
- In the peripheral nervous system, loss of myelin is related to the decrease in nerve conduction velocity.
- Pernicious anemia, caused by lack of gastric IF, is common in the older adult. Low vitamin B_{12} levels have neurological consequences: demyelination of the dorsal columns of the spinal cord, termed subacute combined degeneration (SCD), causes gait instability and paresthesias in the lower extremities.

- Pain thresholds are higher in older adults than those of younger adults.
- The aging eye contains fewer rods and cones than in the younger adult's eye, with concomitant losses in visual acuity.
- The lens becomes more opaque and stiffer, causing blurring of vision, increased glare, and decreased ability to accommodate.
- These combined defects are known as presbyopia.
- Cataracts form because the lens naturally develops thickened layers with age.
- Hearing is also affected by normal aging, with losses in the ability to detect both low- and high-frequency sounds, called presbycusis, or age-related hearing loss.

Bibliography

Available online at fadavis.com

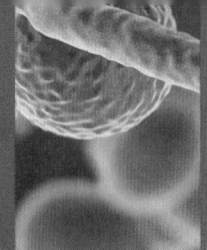

SIRS, Sepsis, Shock, MODS, and Death

Learning Objectives

After completion of this chapter, the student will be able to:

- Describe the pathological mechanisms of systemic inflammatory response syndrome (SIRS), sepsis, shock, and multiple organ dysfunction syndrome (MODS).
- Identify clinical manifestations of SIRS, sepsis, shock, and MODS.
- Compare and contrast the causes and pathological mechanisms of different types of shock, such as septic, hypovolemic, cardiogenic, neurogenic, and anaphylactic.

- Distinguish between the pathological mechanisms occurring in the three different stages of shock.
- Explain the various conditions involved in MODS, including acute respiratory distress syndrome (ARDS), disseminated intravascular coagulation (DIC), abdominal compartment syndrome (ACS), and acute kidney injury (AKI).
- Discuss various treatment modalities used in sepsis, shock, and MODS.

Key Terms

Abdominal compartment syndrome (ACS)
Acute kidney injury (AKI)
Acute lung injury (ALI)
Acute respiratory distress syndrome (ARDS)
Anaphylactic shock
Brain death
Compensatory anti-inflammatory response syndrome (CARS)

Disseminated intravascular coagulation (DIC)
Intra-abdominal hypertension (IAH)
Intra-abdominal pressure (IAP)
Microthrombi
Multiple organ dysfunction syndrome (MODS)
Sepsis
Septic shock

Septicemia
Shock
Systemic inflammatory response syndrome (SIRS)
Ventilation-perfusion mismatch

Patients who are suffering severe illnesses, such as shock, **systemic inflammatory response syndrome (SIRS), sepsis,** and **multiple organ dysfunction syndrome (MODS),** are commonly treated in intensive care settings. Patients with these disorders require minute-to-minute monitoring of vital signs and organ function. Through the use of advanced technology, health-care providers can continuously monitor many of the critical parameters and laboratory values that influence the patient's condition. As technology has progressed, so has our knowledge of the cellular basis of disease. There is more information about inflammation and infection on a molecular basis than ever before, and this allows for specific targets of treatment. Pharmacological agents can aim directly at the biochemical, molecular, and genetic components of disease. These discoveries are reshaping our understanding of the biology of the very ill patient and introducing new treatment modalities. Critical illness can lead to recovery or multiple system failure; often, there is a sequential decline in body function before death. Clinicians can recognize these early signs and symptoms of lethal conditions and stave off death.

Epidemiology

Shock, as defined by sustained hypoperfusion as evidenced by prolonged hypotension (sustained systolic blood pressure less than 90 mm Hg), is experienced by critically ill patients treated in intensive care, emergency, or prehospital settings. It is difficult to estimate the incidence of shock as there are various causes of this sudden, emergent disorder. In an Australian study in 2022, the population-wide incidence of shock was 76 per 100,000 person-years and was more common in males, older patients, rural settings, and those with a lower socioeconomic status. Shock in the prehospital setting was a relatively common clinical problem that the emergency medical system (EMS) manages, complicating nearly 6.8 per 1,000 EMS cases. The overall prognosis for patients with shock in the prehospital setting was poor, with 30-day mortality of approximately 33%.

It is estimated that more than 750,000 people develop sepsis annually in the United States. The disease is often fatal, with an overall mortality rate of

30%. Mortality rates range from 20% to 52% in severe sepsis and 82% for patients with septic shock. In MODS, there is a 20% increase in mortality with each additional organ dysfunction. In the presence of **acute kidney injury (AKI),** the mortality rate increases to 70%.

SIRS occurs in 82% of hospitalized children, with 23% experiencing sepsis, 4% severe sepsis, and 2% septic shock. In children, this widespread inflammatory disorder is termed multisystem inflammatory syndrome in children (MIS-C) or pediatric MIS (P-MIS). Eighteen percent of children with sepsis develop MODS, which increases the mortality rate.

Etiology and Pathophysiology of Shock

Shock is the inability of the heart and lungs to satisfy the metabolic and oxygen requirements of the peripheral tissues. Shock can be thought of as severe hypotension. However, it is important to understand that blood pressure does not define shock. Although a decrease in blood pressure is commonplace in shock, it is not always present—at least not at first. Similarly, heart rate is commonly elevated in shock, but not always.

> **ALERT!** Shock most commonly occurs when blood pressure falls below a systolic measurement of 90 mm Hg or drops 40 mm Hg below the patient's normal blood pressure.

For example, a hypertensive patient with usual blood pressure measurements of 150/90 mm Hg can go into shock with a blood pressure that seems normal, such as 100/70 mm Hg. In a person with chronic hypertension, this low blood pressure may be insufficient to deliver blood to the peripheral and cerebral arterial vessels. In chronic hypertension, the body commonly adjusts to a high blood pressure so that high pressure becomes necessary for arterial perfusion throughout the body. In this way, a patient with chronic hypertension can have inadequate cerebral perfusion and lose consciousness with a blood pressure of 100/70 mm Hg.

Similarly, tachycardia is not always found in a patient with shock. For example, a patient with complete heart block may have a pulse of 25 beats per minute, which does not provide adequate cardiac output to meet the needs of the periphery. This patient is in shock without compensatory tachycardia because the heart is dysfunctional and not capable of a rate

increase. Mental changes, acidosis, renal failure, and death will follow if the heart rate is not raised.

Shock is classified into five broad categories based on etiology:

- Cardiogenic shock caused by cardiac failure
- Hypovolemic shock caused by lack of sufficient fluids or hemorrhage of the body
- Septic shock caused by microbial invasion of the bloodstream
- Anaphylactic shock, a state of severe allergic reaction
- Neurogenic shock, most commonly due to brain or spinal cord injury

It is important to realize that all five categories of shock converge onto the same pathophysiological pathway of cellular hypoxia, which triggers anaerobic metabolism and lactic acidosis (see Fig. 46-1).

Once shock has occurred, prompt reversal of the situation is necessary. This requires treating the cause, as well as the signs and symptoms.

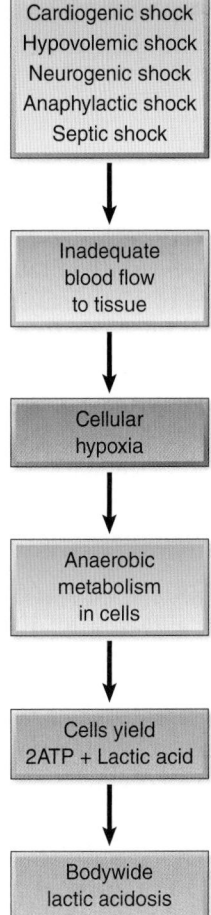

FIGURE 46-1. Mechanism of shock. All types of shock lead to inadequate blood flow to the tissues and cause widespread cellular hypoxia. In hypoxia, anaerobic metabolism occurs in cells. Each cell yields 2 ATP and lactic acid, resulting in widespread lactic acidosis.

> ### CLINICAL CONCEPT
>
> Shock needs to be reversed quickly, or else inadequate organ perfusion and ischemia occur, causing widespread anaerobic metabolism, which leads to lactic acidosis.

Stages of Shock

Shock has three stages: initial, progressive, and irreversible. There are specific pathophysiological changes and patient symptoms in each stage.

Initial Stage

In the initial stage of shock, when there is a sudden drop in tissue perfusion, the SNS and renin–angiotensin–aldosterone system (RAAS) are triggered. The SNS stimulates tachycardia as a compensatory mechanism. The RAAS system increases blood volume and stimulates peripheral vasoconstriction in efforts to bring up blood pressure. However, in shock, these compensatory mechanisms cannot normalize blood pressure, and medical intervention is necessary. The patient is anxious and pale, and their extremities are cold and clammy.

Progressive Stage

If shock is not corrected promptly, a progressive stage ensues in which the lungs, kidneys, gut, pancreas, and liver suffer decreased perfusion. All available blood is conserved for the heart and brain. The patient may begin to show signs of MODS. Commonly, if the kidneys suffer ischemia for 20 to 30 minutes, they begin to fail. The kidneys cannot filter wastes from the blood; therefore, waste products accumulate. The liver and GI system also suffer ischemia. The GI system undergoes ileus, a state where peristalsis ceases. The liver becomes dysfunctional and cannot clear the blood of waste products, so these accumulate in the bloodstream.

Irreversible Stage

Failure to terminate shock during the progressive stage produces the irreversible stage of shock. In this stage, perfusion of the heart and brain begins to decrease. Myocardial and cerebral ischemia occur. If ischemia is prolonged, myocardial infarction (MI) or cerebral infarction (stroke) can occur.

During this stage, there is widespread cellular hypoxia with extensive anaerobic metabolism occurring throughout the body. Anaerobic metabolism utilizes glucose to produce a small amount of energy (2 adenosine triphosphate [ATP]) and lactic acid. Energy stores are rapidly depleted and not replenished. Cellular ATP is insufficient, and the mitochondria do not receive adequate oxygen to make more ATP. Lactic acid builds up in the bloodstream and the cells' ATP pump fails. Sodium and water enter the cell, and potassium exits the cell. The organelles within the cell begin to fail. As cells die, lysosomes break open and release digestive enzymes that break down cellular debris. This is the final step in a downward spiral.

Inflammatory Response in Shock

The release of the necrotic contents of the cellular matrix and membrane is a powerful stimulant of the immune system. The resulting chemotaxis increases the influx of neutrophils, macrophages, and killer T cells. Their action increases the local demand for oxygen and energy that cannot be fulfilled.

The intestine, the home of many bacteria, is always in a state of hypoxia when the body is in shock. The normal intestinal barrier to microbes and their toxins breaks down. The release of microbes and their toxins into the general circulation results in SIRS that causes injury to organs distant from the original insult.

Shock, of any cause, initiates SIRS with the production of cytokines, bradykinin, and histamine. These chemicals have a profound influence on all organs, including the capillary endothelial cells. WBCs adhere to the endothelium, and their output of cytokines causes endothelial injury and dysfunction. Increased capillary permeability causes the accumulation of interstitial edema. Clearly, SIRS plays a large role in MODS seen following shock.

Lactic Acidosis in Shock

Lactic acid production is a result of anaerobic metabolism. Because of hypoperfusion, the liver is unable to convert the lactic acid back to sugar compounds. Renal hypoperfusion causes decreased filtration of the blood and excretion of wastes, which diminishes elimination of lactic acid. As long as a state of shock persists, lactic acidosis will persist and worsen. This lactic acidosis adversely affects cardiac, respiratory, neurological, and brain function. As the lactic acidosis worsens, neurological activity, oxygen and carbon dioxide transport, and cellular enzyme activity become increasingly impaired. Impaired mentation with eventual loss of consciousness, as well as impaired cardiac efficiency and arrhythmias, follow. Cardiac output diminishes despite the powerful stimulus of endogenous catecholamines.

Gastrointestinal Consequences of Shock

In shock, there is severe vasoconstriction of the splanchnic arteries that perfuse the intestine. If hypoxia of the abdominal organs persists they do not function and the following occur:

- Toxins and microbes that normally inhabit the bowel lumen enter the circulation and generate a powerful systemic inflammatory response.
- The pancreas is unable to make sufficient quantities of insulin.
- Secretion of incretins—intestinal hormones such as gastric inhibitory polypeptide (GIP) and

glucagonlike peptide (GLP-1) that increase cellular sensitivity to insulin—are reduced.

- Endothelium of the capillaries of the abdominal organs becomes markedly more permeable. Intestinal edema ensues with loss of intravascular and extracellular fluid into the bowel wall, bowel lumen, and mesentery. This phenomenon is commonly referred to as *intestinal third space fluid loss*, which can sequester many liters of fluid.

Hormone Release During Shock

Epinephrine and cortisol are secreted in large quantities during the stress of shock. Both hormones inhibit the effects of insulin. Glycogen stores in the liver are broken down and converted to glucose. Glucose uptake in the periphery is blocked by the effects of high cortisol and epinephrine levels and by reduced levels of incretins and insulin. The ensuing hyperglycemia

reduces the immune system's ability to resist infection by interfering with the neutrophils' ability to phagocytose and kill microbes.

Activity of the Coagulation System in Shock

In shock, the blood is susceptible to hypercoagulability. Extensive secretion of thromboxane A2 and thromboplastin by the endothelium promotes activation of the coagulation cascade. Inhibition of activated protein C (aPC), a natural anticoagulant that inhibits prothrombin activation, further aggravates the situation. Wide-scale activation of the coagulation system forms many microthrombi, which quickly overwhelm the fibrinolytic system. Clots can lodge in capillaries, blocking blood flow and causing tissue ischemia. Prolonged ischemia causes tissue hypoxia, which leads to cell death, and consequently cellular necrosis (see Fig. 46-2).

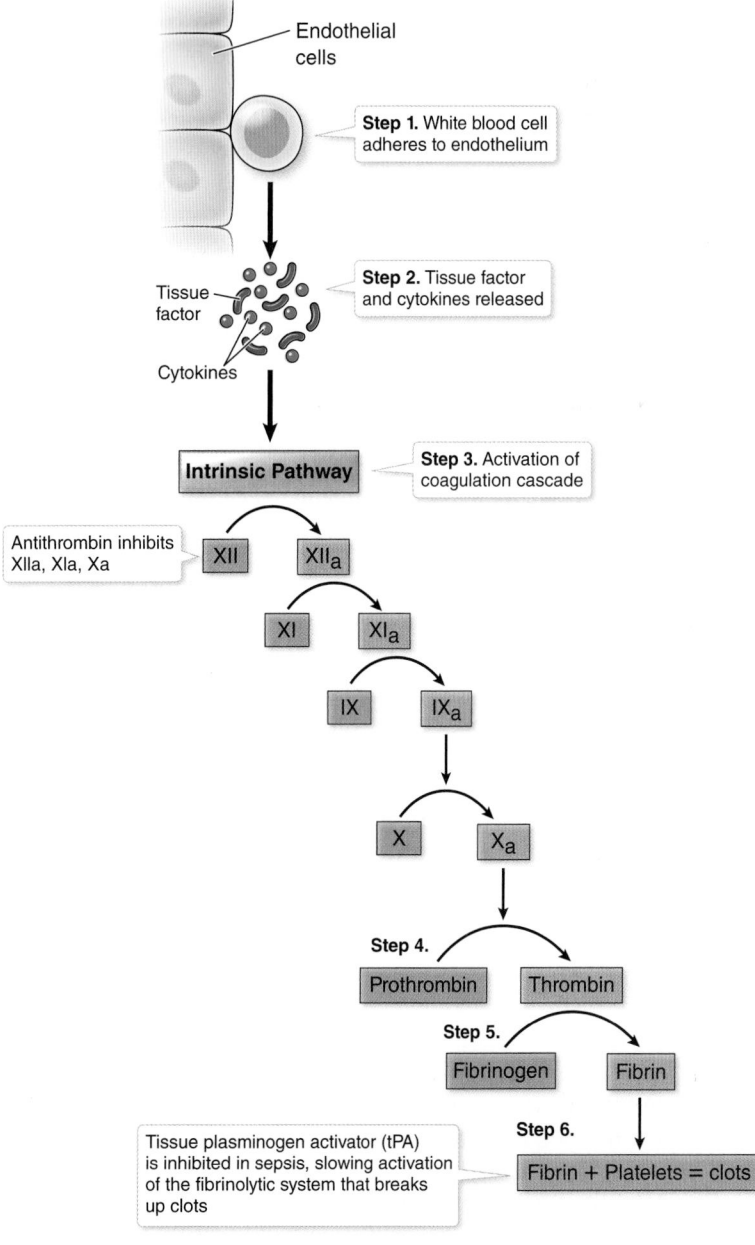

FIGURE 46-2. Microthrombi formation in sepsis. In sepsis, WBCs adhere to the endothelial cells and release cytokines, which damage the endothelial cells. When endothelial cells are damaged, tissue factor (thromboplastin) is activated, which stimulates the coagulation cascade. In the last steps of the coagulation cascade, prothrombin is converted to thrombin, which in turn converts fibrinogen to fibrin. Antithrombin is inhibited by sepsis, and clots form without inhibition. Fibrin binds with platelets to form small clots. Any time clots are formed in the body, the process of fibrinolysis by tissue plasminogen activator should occur. Sepsis, however, inhibits formation of tissue plasminogen activator.

Prevention Versus Treatment of Shock

Clearly, prevention of shock is better than the perfect treatment. Unfortunately, shock often cannot be prevented, and it is important to initiate appropriate therapy without delay. It has been shown that prompt treatment of acute MI prevents cardiogenic shock. Likewise, large-volume fluid infusion in the bleeding patient before shock appears is more effective than after shock occurs. The prevention of sepsis by strict adherence to hand washing and instrumentation protocols has been shown to significantly reduce sepsis in the ICU setting.

The treatment of shock is very complicated and depends on its etiology. Treatment often requires the expertise of several specialists, including an intensivist, surgeon, cardiologist, infectious disease specialist, pulmonologist, and nephrologist.

Specific Types of Shock

There are different types of shock based on the etiology of the condition. Cardiogenic shock is caused by failure of the heart. Hypovolemic shock is caused by a large depletion of blood or fluids from the body. Anaphylactic shock is triggered by a severe allergic reaction. Most often, neurogenic shock occurs because of spinal cord or brain injury. Both anaphylactic and neurogenic shock involve widespread vasodilation, which causes extensive hypoperfusion of tissues.

Cardiogenic Shock

Cardiogenic shock is defined as severe hypotension—lower than 90 mm Hg systolic for 30 minutes, despite adequate fluid status. Cardiogenic shock causes a significant decrease in aortic perfusion, which leads to a loss of circulation in the systemic arteries. The low circulation leads to low urine output, peripheral cyanosis, and altered mental status. The most common cause of cardiogenic shock is severe, acute MI. A severe, acute MI can cause an extensive loss of myocardial muscle and lead to heart failure. Cardiac tamponade, a state where the heart is restricted from pumping blood to the periphery, can also induce a state of shock. In addition, severe tachyarrhythmias and bradyarrhythmias can cause shock. In the very rapid rate of tachyarrhythmias, the heart's ventricles cannot fill with adequate blood volume. Cardiac output is low, and a reduced amount of blood is pumped forward with each contraction. In bradyarrhythmias, the heart is beating at a very slow rate, which causes low cardiac output that cannot supply the tissues with adequate circulation.

Shock Caused by Acute Myocardial Infarction. Cardiogenic shock develops in about 10% to 15% of patients with acute MI who arrive alive at a hospital. In the past, it was thought that cardiogenic shock would occur if an MI destroyed 40% or more of the ventricle. Cardiogenic shock was common with anterior or anterior lateral infarctions. It was thought that the destruction of such a significant amount of myocardium could explain the symptoms of cardiogenic shock on a purely mechanical basis. However, cardiogenic shock can be seen after infarctions that involve less than 40% of the myocardial muscle. Complications of an MI—such as acute mitral valve regurgitation as a result of the necrosis and rupture of the papillary muscles, acute rupture of the ventricular septum, or cardiac tamponade from cardiac perforation—can cause cardiogenic shock. In addition, elements of SIRS play an important role in the development of cardiogenic shock. Elevated temperature, elevated levels of WBCs, and release of inflammatory mediators commonly accompany MIs. Inflammation increases the body's need for oxygen and nutrients, and the heart works harder to supply the body with sufficient blood. This extra work increases the heart's muscle damage.

In cardiogenic shock, the heart is unable to meet the circulation needs of the peripheral tissues. Systemic arterial blood flow decreases. This low arterial blood flow is sensed by the arterial baroreceptors, which in turn stimulate the SNS. The SNS stimulates the peripheral arteries to vasoconstrict. At the same time, the kidney senses low circulation and releases renin, which sets off the RAAS. The RAAS causes release of angiotensin II, which further vasoconstricts the arteries. It also triggers release of aldosterone, which increases sodium and water reabsorption into the bloodstream and increases blood volume. The resistance against the heart is increased because of peripheral artery vasoconstriction. The blood volume is enhanced. Together, the increased arterial resistance and enhanced blood volume intensify the workload of the failing heart, which causes widening of the infarction area; as a result, more cardiac muscle dies.

Shock Caused by Cardiac Tamponade. Cardiac tamponade occurs when there is an increased amount of fluid in the pericardial sac that surrounds the heart, also referred to as pericardial effusion. The fluid within the pericardial sac compresses the heart and restricts the heart's ability to fill with blood. There are various causes of cardiac tamponade, including bleeding into the pericardium caused by trauma, ascending aortic dissection, cardiac perforation following MI, and postoperative bleeding following open heart surgery. Additionally, cardiac tamponade can occur from the accumulation of fluid in the pericardium due to various etiologies, including uremic pericarditis, pericarditis due to autoimmune or infectious disease, radiation treatment, or metastatic cancer.

Normally, the pericardial space contains a very small amount (20 to 50 mL) of clear serous fluid, which does not cause any restriction on the heart. In cardiac tamponade, there is an excess of fluid in the pericardial sac and the atria cannot fill because of the external compression. The reduced filling of the atria causes low blood volume in the ventricles. Cardiac output drops, and the heart compensates by increasing the heart rate.

A sign of cardiac tamponade is pulsus paradoxus, which is exhibited by the jugular veins. Under normal conditions, during inspiration the thoracic cage expands and the jugular venous pressure decreases. However, in pulsus paradoxus, there is an increase in jugular venous pressure during inspiration. The heart is compressed in tamponade; with inhalation, there is further pressure placed around the heart. The pressure on the right atrium causes backflow of pressure into the superior vena cava, which in turn causes backflow of blood into the jugular veins. Consequently, the patient exhibits jugular venous distention with inhalation.

 CLINICAL CONCEPT

Beck's triad is a key sign of cardiac tamponade: distant heart sounds, low blood pressure, and high jugular venous pressure.

In the case of bleeding into the pericardium, the increase in pericardial pressure compressing the heart is very rapid. Small amounts of fresh blood (100 to 200 mL) can cause significant signs of tamponade, as there is no time to allow for the stretching of the pericardium. Death ensues quickly unless the pericardium is decompressed. This requires emergently opening the chest and making an incision into the pericardial membrane to let the blood escape. Such drastic actions are commonly unsuccessful in saving the patient.

In the case of an inflammatory pericarditis, the fluid accumulation is much slower (over weeks) and the pericardium can stretch out to relieve pressure. By the time tamponade occurs, 1 liter of fluid or more has accumulated, and the pericardium is very large and tautly filled. These patients present with a history of a chronic underlying disease, such as renal insufficiency, lupus erythematosus or other autoimmune disorder, tuberculosis, chest wall radiation therapy, or cancer. The presence of chest pain is variable. Tachycardia and hypotension are always present, as are the signs of catecholamine secretion, including cyanosis, tremor, anxiety, and diaphoresis.

Hypovolemic Shock

In hypovolemic shock, the amount of blood in the body's vasculature is reduced. The low blood volume causes low blood pressure. Commonly, hypovolemic shock is caused by extensive loss of blood, as occurs in hemorrhage. Hypovolemic shock can also be caused by loss of extracellular fluid volume through diarrhea (especially in children), vomiting, ascites, or severe burns. Less commonly but significant, loss of adequate venous return can cause hypovolemic shock. Lack of venous return to the heart lowers blood volume in all

the heart's chambers; therefore, less blood is pumped out of the ventricles and into the arterial circulation.

Hypovolemic shock creates conditions that reduce coronary artery blood flow. With severely diminished blood pressure, the aorta suffers low volume; the coronary arteries that come off the aorta will then demonstrate low blood volume. Low coronary artery blood flow can cause myocardial ischemia or infarction.

Compensatory Mechanisms in Hypovolemia. In hypovolemic shock, reduced blood pressure triggers two major compensatory mechanisms. There is a stimulation of the arterial baroreceptors, which are sensors of blood pressure in the walls of the arteries. There is also a trigger of the RAAS. In hypovolemic shock, arterial baroreceptors sense low blood volume, which then stimulates the SNS. The sympathetic stimulus causes peripheral arterial vasoconstriction, which raises blood pressure and directs blood from the periphery to the coronary and cerebral circulations. The sympathetic stimulus also increases the heart rate, which results in tachycardia.

As hypovolemic shock continues, the kidneys sense a drop in circulation and release renin. Renin stimulates the liver to release angiotensinogen, which becomes angiotensin I. Angiotensin I is transformed into angiotensin II by angiotensin-converting enzyme (ACE). Angiotensin II directly stimulates peripheral arterial vasoconstriction and triggers the adrenal gland to release aldosterone. Under the influence of aldosterone, the kidneys increase water and salt reabsorption to restore intravascular fluid volume. Therefore, the body compensates for hypovolemic shock by vasoconstricting all the peripheral arteries, bringing more volume of water into the blood and increasing heart rate.

Hypovolemic Shock Caused by Loss of Blood or Fluids. A normal person can lose up to 20% of their blood volume (approximately 1 liter) without exhibiting any sign of hypovolemic shock. In healthy young individuals, the blood loss can even be greater because the intensity of vasoconstriction and the efficiency of cardiac performance can dramatically hide the signs of shock. The normal blood pressure can fool the caregiver into believing that the patient is stable. However, shock is present and is demonstrated by the signs of inadequate tissue perfusion: cyanosis, tachycardia, reduced urine output, confusion or agitation, poor skin turgor, and thirst. These signs may be missed; only after exhaustion of the ATP that is allowing constriction of the vascular smooth musculature does the blood pressure fall. In these cases, the drop in blood pressure is sudden and death follows quickly if the blood volume is not restored immediately.

Hypovolemic Shock Caused by Diminished Venous Return. Hypovolemic shock can be caused by the lack of venous return to the heart. For example, victims of disasters who are pinned under fallen structures often suffer lack of venous return from the lower extremities up to the heart. The low pressure on the venous side of the circulation leads to inadequate filling volumes in the heart's ventricles and a drop in cardiac output. Consequently, there is a drop in tissue perfusion. The tissues resort to anaerobic metabolism. Production of lactic acid results, and metabolic acidosis ensues. If the situation is not reversed, depletion of ATP occurs, lysosomes break open, and cellular death follows. Cell death releases a host of chemotactic elements and activates the immune system sharply. The SIRS that follows cellular injury is intense and can lead to MODS.

> **ALERT!** Hypovolemic shock induces renal tubular dysfunction and eventual renal tubular necrosis if not reversed. This renal tubular necrosis can be permanent.

Hypovolemic Shock and Coronary Ischemia. Hypovolemic shock can unmask preexisting coronary artery disease. When there is a drop in blood pressure, aortic pressure is reduced. With reduced aortic pressure, there is diminished coronary artery blood flow. If the coronary arteries are already compromised by arteriosclerosis, low aortic blood volume will further diminish low coronary artery perfusion. In addition, in hypovolemic shock, the heart is stimulated by the SNS to increase cardiac contractility and heart rate. Higher heart rate and contractility require more coronary artery blood flow in the heart muscle. Thus, the drop in coronary artery perfusion by hypovolemic shock is accompanied by an increased demand for more coronary artery blood. This lack of sufficient coronary blood flow can precipitate an acute MI. The MI complicates the picture enormously because some heart muscle dies, heart failure begins, and cardiogenic shock ensues. Cardiogenic shock combined with hypovolemic shock has a very high mortality rate.

Anaphylactic Shock

Anaphylactic shock, also known as anaphylaxis, is the extreme manifestation of an allergic reaction. It is unknown why anaphylaxis occurs; it can occur at any time in a person's life, and it is known that prior exposure to an allergen prepares the immune system for repeat exposure. Immunoglobulin E develops memory for a specific antigen, which makes it ready to attack when reexposure occurs. However, the attack on the antigen creates a body-wide reaction. Only a miniscule amount of antigen is necessary, and IgE stimulates the eosinophils, basophils, and mast cells to degranulate, which releases large amounts of histamine, bradykinin, complement, and prostaglandins. Massive vasodilation with increased capillary permeability throughout

the body leads to a hypoperfusion of tissues and hypotension. Shock and bronchospasm occur. Bronchospasm, increased respiratory secretions, and edema of the airways cause respiratory distress. Stridor and wheezing are heard, and laryngospasm can be fatal. The same responses in the skin cause erythema and edema of the dermis (hives and angioedema). Hives may begin as a pinpoint rash but can transform into large areas of red wheals. Angioedema is severe facial swelling, particularly of the eyelids, lips, and tongue. If untreated, this reaction is often fatal.

Almost anything can cause anaphylaxis. Frequent substances include penicillin and other medications, food allergies (shellfish and peanuts are common), iodinated radiological contrast media, Hymenoptera (wasp and red ant) bites, and bee stings.

Neurogenic Shock

Neurogenic shock can occur when the SNS is disrupted by spinal cord injury, brain injury, or during anesthesia. The underlying cause of neurogenic shock is widespread vasodilation that reduces venous return to the heart; this reduces the volume of blood that can be pumped out of the ventricles. Low blood volume causes widespread hypotension. If the spinal cord injury is in the upper thoracic area or higher, there is lack of sympathetic tone; unopposed parasympathetic nervous system (PSNS) discharge then takes over. Parasympathetic stimulation causes bradycardia, and cardiac output becomes very low. Unless corrected, widespread hypoperfusion causes extensive tissue ischemia, which leads to cell death.

> **CLINICAL CONCEPT**
>
> Tachycardia is the expected compensatory response in shock. However, bradycardia occurs in neurogenic shock because of the shutdown of the SNS and unopposed influence of the PSNS.

Other Critical Systemic Illnesses

Infection, burn, trauma, hemorrhage, and major surgery can trigger SIRS, sepsis, septic shock, MODS, and shock. MODS is the cause of death in 50% to 80% of intensive care patients. It is commonly a terminal stage of a deteriorating process triggered by an insult to the body.

Systemic Inflammatory Response Syndrome

SIRS is an overwhelming inflammatory reaction of the body initiated by a severe insult to the body. It is an intense immunological and cytokine response in the body. The precise reason for SIRS is not entirely understood, but it has the potential to do significant damage to body tissues and organs. There are specific criteria for a diagnosis of SIRS (see Box 46-1).

During SIRS, the cardiac, hepatic, respiratory, digestive, and renal systems attempt to compensate for an insult to the body. There is also a large sympathetic nervous system (SNS) and endocrine reaction similar to the alarm stage in the stress response. Heart rate, cardiac output, and respiratory rate increase. Gastrointestinal (GI) activity and urine output are reduced. There are increased levels of catecholamines, glucocorticoids, mineralocorticoids, antidiuretic hormone (ADH), and angiotensin II.

Systemic infection, also referred to as sepsis, often follows SIRS. Following the intense SIRS reaction, there is a period where the immune system is markedly less active (see Fig. 46-3). This period of reduced immunity and increased susceptibility to infection is called the **compensatory anti-inflammatory response syndrome (CARS).** Even if the initial, precipitating insult is not infectious, the intense inflammatory response to the insult is followed by a period of immunological suppression, during which the patient is highly susceptible to health-care–associated infection (HAI). The immune response of the patient is muted, and the source of infection is not obvious. Frequently, the infection is caused by common skin or bowel microbes that normally are not pathogenic.

The majority of patients who manifest a SIRS reaction recover. However, for some, the nature of the initial insult is so severe that prompt recovery does not occur. Preexisting conditions such as cardiac disease, chronic obstructive pulmonary disease (COPD), and renal disease can render the patient unable to withstand the metabolic demands of SIRS. These patients are likely to develop early MODS or die.

An example of the progression of SIRS, CARS, sepsis, septic shock, and MODS can be seen in the following patient scenario: A patient in status asthmaticus

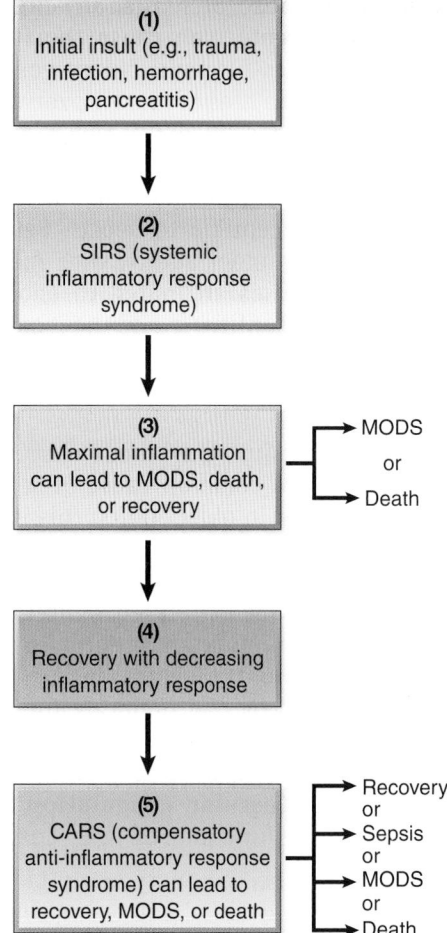

FIGURE 46-3. Mechanism of SIRS. An initial insult leads to SIRS followed by maximal inflammation, which can lead to MODS, death, or recovery with CARS, during which there is decreased immunity. CARS can lead to MODS, death, or full recovery.

(unrelenting asthma) is admitted to the emergency department for life-threatening hypoxemia and severe pulmonary atelectasis. The patient is promptly treated with endotracheal intubation to stabilize ventilation. However, despite the stabilization, the patient develops SIRS in response to the overwhelming stress on the body. CARS, which is a period of low immunity and high susceptibility to infection, follows. During this period, the patient is particularly susceptible to HAIs such as methicillin- or vancomycin-resistant *Staphylococcus aureus,* which often causes pneumonia in intubated patients. The infection starts in the lungs but overwhelms the immunosuppressed patient and leads to infection of the bloodstream (septicemia), also called sepsis. Sepsis often progresses to septic shock. During the period of shock, MODS can develop and lead to death.

Sepsis

Sepsis, also called **septicemia,** is a body-wide infection that overwhelms the immune system and causes severe multiorgan compromise. Although bacteria are

---

the most common cause of sepsis, any organism—viral, fungal, or parasite—can cause the infection. Bacterial sepsis is the active multiplication of bacteria in the bloodstream that results in an overwhelming infection; the term *bloodstream infection* is also commonly used.

Immunosuppressed persons, older adults, and infants are most susceptible to sepsis. Sepsis disproportionally affects older adults, with more than 60% of sepsis diagnoses attributed to adults aged 65 years and older. Identifying and diagnosing sepsis in older adults is highly challenging because older adults often do not present with typical signs and symptoms. Infection usually begins in one organ system and then spreads into the bloodstream, causing sepsis. For example, a common cause of sepsis is a urinary tract infection in older adults; this is termed urosepsis. Pneumonia, abdominal infections, and postoperative infections can also lead to sepsis. Sepsis is sometimes described as SIRS with an infectious origin. There are some important criteria for suspecting sepsis (see Box 46-2). Severe sepsis is defined as sepsis complicated by end-organ dysfunction, as demonstrated by altered mental status, an episode of hypotension, renal insufficiency, or evidence of **disseminated intravascular coagulation (DIC)**—overactivity and dysfunction of the coagulation system.

Septic Shock

Septic shock is defined as a state of severe sepsis with persistent, life-threatening hypotension that is refractory to fluid replacement and vasopressors. Widespread vasodilation occurs in the body during septic shock, and IV fluids and vasoconstrictor medications cannot elevate the blood pressure. The presence of septic shock indicates an infection of great severity, which is the result of a highly virulent microbe. Certain pathogens, such as some *Clostridia, S. aureus, Streptococci A, Yersinia pestis,* and *Meningococci,* can produce potent toxins that rapidly cause septic shock. Infection with one of these pathogens may be overwhelming, and mortality is considerable.

BOX 46-2. Important Criteria to Suspect Sepsis

With sepsis infection, at least one of the following manifestations of inadequate organ function/perfusion is occurring:

- Alteration in mental state
- Hypoxemia
- Elevated plasma lactate level
- Oliguria
- Systolic hypotension <100 mm Hg

 CLINICAL CONCEPT

In septic shock, microbial exotoxins or endotoxins stimulate potent widespread vasodilation. Increased fluids and vasoconstrictors often cannot raise blood pressure.

Septic shock most often develops in people who are immunocompromised. This group includes older adults; infants; postoperative patients; and patients with diabetes, pulmonary disease, renal insufficiency, and cancer, especially if the cancer is advanced or the patient is receiving chemotherapy. Other predisposing factors are chronic corticosteroid therapy, transplants, HIV infection, trauma, and being in an intensive care unit (ICU). Patients who have long-term indwelling catheters, endotracheal tubes, or IV lines are also at risk. These patients can develop sepsis with microbes that are not usually pathogenic or that cause milder infections in people with normal immune systems. At times, the etiology of septic shock is not readily apparent.

 CLINICAL CONCEPT

Blood cultures are positive for bacteria or microbes less than 50% of the time.

Toxins and inflammatory mediators such as interleukins (ILs), nitric oxide (NO), thromboxane A2, prostacyclin, and tumor necrosis factor-alpha (TNF-alpha), cause widespread arterial vasodilation. Capillary permeability is greatly increased with plasma entering the tissues.

Inflammatory mediators also activate the coagulation pathway, which leads to the formation of small blood clots called **microthrombi.** Sepsis also causes injury to the capillary bed endothelium, which stimulates the coagulation cascade and thrombus formation. In addition, some bacterial toxins inhibit the activity of protein C, which is a naturally occurring anticoagulant, as another factor that raises the risk of hypercoagulability. However, conversely, other toxins can activate the fibrinolytic system by activating plasminogen, causing a risk of bleeding. Both clotting and bleeding episodes are possible consequences of sepsis, which is known as DIC.

An outpouring of epinephrine and cortisol accompanies sepsis, which severely reduces insulin sensitivity and incites glycogenolysis (breakdown of glycogen). Blood sugar becomes elevated and difficult to control with insulin. The hyperglycemia impairs the white blood cells' (WBCs') ability to lyse and digest the offending microbes by phagocytosis. The mortality of patients with severe sepsis and hyperglycemia is elevated, and control of glucose levels plays an important part in the treatment of severe sepsis. In uncontrolled diabetes, the high blood glucose potentiates a bacterial infection, as the microorganisms are continually fed by the glucose.

The vasodilation and intravascular fluid loss cause increased cardiac activity. This is a hypermetabolic state, and fever usually develops. The widespread vasodilation, inflammation, and microthrombi can lead to extensive tissue hypoperfusion with ischemia, leading to MODS. The patient may appear pink, and the skin may be warm despite the onset of shock. This stage is called "warm shock."

> **ALERT!** Septic shock is a medical emergency and has a high death rate of up to 60%.

Multiple Organ Dysfunction Syndrome

MODS is a clinical syndrome characterized by progressive and potentially reversible dysfunction in two or more organs or organ systems that is induced by a variety of acute insults, commonly sepsis. It is the leading cause of death in the ICU. There is a common continuum in the critically ill patient that begins with infection, which leads to sepsis, septic shock, and MODS. The exact pathophysiology of MODS in patients with sepsis is not fully understood. However, there are some theories and proposed mechanisms.

Hypoxia–Microvascular Theory
This theory proposes that sepsis or severe inflammatory reactions can initiate MODS, as these conditions cause endothelial dysfunction and microvascular abnormalities. Inflammatory mediators, free radicals, lytic enzymes, and vasoactive substances lead to microcirculatory injury. Erythrocytes cannot navigate through the disrupted microvasculature of different organs, which ultimately leads to cellular hypoxia.

Gut Theory
During severe sepsis, blood flow to the GI system decreases, causing mucosal ischemia and liver dysfunction. Mucosal ischemia leads to increased permeability of the GI wall. The mucosal permeability allows normal bacterial flora of the GI tract to escape into the bloodstream. These bacteria provoke a large immune reaction, resulting in tissue injury throughout the body.

Endotoxin Theory
It is believed that gram-negative bacteria are largely responsible for septic shock and MODS. These bacteria release endotoxins that stimulate a widespread

inflammatory reaction involving ILs, TNF, thromboxane A2, prostacyclin, and NO. These inflammatory actions take place in multiple organ systems.

The pathophysiology of MODS is most likely caused by a combination of the theoretical mechanisms. In MODS, it is common to see respiratory failure occur early in the course of illness, followed by liver failure, GI bleeding, and renal failure. There are four clinical phases of MODS (see Box 46-3).

 CLINICAL CONCEPT

Mortality of MODS increases by about 20% for each additional organ involved. If AKI is involved, the mortality increases to 70%.

Assessment of the Critically Ill Patient

A complete history and physical examination are necessary in the critically ill patient. Often, the patient is unable to give a history; instead, family members or significant others can supply important information. The clinician needs to be aware that critically ill patients demonstrate distinctive signs and symptoms in the different stages of the illness. To establish the level of risk to the patient, the clinician uses various assessment tools.

History

A thorough history is important when dealing with a critically ill patient. Often, the etiology of the critical illness is not readily apparent. For example, hypovolemic shock can occur without obvious blood or fluid loss.

BOX 46-3. Four Clinical Phases of MODS

There are four clinical phases of MODS:
- **Stage 1:** The patient has increased volume requirements and mild respiratory alkalosis, which is accompanied by oliguria, hyperglycemia, and increased insulin requirements.
- **Stage 2:** The patient is tachypneic, hypocapnic, and hypoxemic. There is moderate liver dysfunction and possible hematological abnormalities.
- **Stage 3:** The patient develops shock with azotemia and acid-base disturbances. There are significant coagulation abnormalities.
- **Stage 4:** The patient is vasopressor-dependent and oliguric or anuric. Ischemic colitis and lactic acidosis follow.

Septic shock often develops without fever or positive blood culture. Previous medical history plays a pivotal role. Patients who have recently had chemotherapy or who have a major immunodeficiency disease such as AIDS or leukemia have a much worse prognosis than previously healthy patients. Age is important, with higher mortality in older patients.

Signs and Symptoms

Most critically ill patients develop common signs of generalized systemic inflammation, such as fever, increased pulse, rapid respirations, and hypotension. Tachycardia persists despite the correction of fluid deficits. Tachypnea is present despite the correction of acidosis. Abnormal temperature readings (hyper- or hypothermia) may be present. Leukocytosis or leukopenia may also be present. Multiple investigations to demonstrate a source of infection are often negative. Blood cultures may be positive or negative in sepsis and septic shock.

Sepsis may not be immediately apparent to the clinician. There is no single "gold standard" diagnostic test for sepsis. Various clinical criteria are used to make the diagnosis. Many different assessment tools that use clinical criteria in a scoring system have been developed to assist the clinician in making a diagnosis of sepsis. Commonly, assessment is based on the Systemic Inflammatory Response Syndrome (SIRS) Criteria, Sequential [Sepsis-related] Organ Failure Assessment (SOFA) score, the Logistic Organ Dysfunction System (LODS) score, or the quick SOFA (qSOFA) score. The SIRS Criteria, SOFA, and LODS assessment tools have been critiqued as complex and difficult to administer in non-ICU settings.

The qSOFA score is the simplest screening tool for early recognition of organ dysfunction because of infection (sepsis). It consists of the following three criteria:

- Altered mental status
- Respiratory rate of more than 22 breaths/minute
- Systolic blood pressure of less than 100 mm Hg

When two of these three SOFA criteria are met, organ dysfunction should be suspected.

Shock, no matter what the cause, is the body's inability to supply adequate oxygen and nutrition to vital organs. The following signs and symptoms of inadequate perfusion are some of the parameters clinicians use to diagnose shock:

- Tachycardia or bradycardia
- Tachypnea
- Cyanosis
- Metabolic acidosis
- Changes in mentation or consciousness
- Low urine output
- Electrocardiographic changes
- Cardiac output, either reduced or increased
- Central venous pressure, either high or low
- Total peripheral resistance, either markedly increased or reduced
- Blood pressure is usually low, but not necessarily

The parameters vary depending on the etiology of shock (see Table 46-1).

MODS can result from such disorders as MI, major trauma, burns, hemorrhage, infection, pancreatitis, or major surgery. The SIRS that follows these events can lead immediately to MODS, or there can be a delay of several days to a week between SIRS and the onset of MODS. In that case, there is usually a "second hit" in

TABLE 46-1. Parameters of Shock

	Hypovolemic	Cardiac	Septic	Anaphylactic	Neurogenic
Blood Pressure	↓	↓	↓	↓	↓
Respiratory Rate	↑	↑	↑	↑	↑
Heart Rate	↑	↑ or ↓	↑	↑	↑ or ↓
Temperature	↔	↔	↑ or ↓	↔	↔
Skin Color	Pale	Cyanotic	Flushed or cyanotic	Flushed or hives	Variable
Mental Status	Anxious, thirsty	Anxious	Confused or obtunded	Anxious	Anxious or obtunded to comatose
Cardiac Output	↓	↓	↑ or ↓	↓	↓
Urine Output	↓	↓	↓	↓	↓
Acidosis	Present	Present	Present	Present	Present
Central Venous Pressure	↓	↑	↓ or ↔	↓	↓

the form of infection during the period of CARS. Major infection during this period of immunocompromise can manifest subtly without the usual signs of fever, tachycardia, or tachypnea. Alteration of mental status in this setting is ominous.

Diagnosis

In an effort to predict a level of risk of the critically ill patient, several scoring models have been developed. The APACHE II (Acute Physiology and Chronic Health Evaluation system) scoring model is an example (see Table 46-2). It assesses the probability of survival of an ICU patient based on standard physiological parameters, standard blood tests, Glasgow Coma Scale (GCS) score (see Table 46-3), and medical history in the first 24 hours after admission. There are several easily linked online sites and downloadable programs for personal data assistants where the data are easily entered and the calculations automatic. The scores correlate to the statistically expected mortality.

The Simplified Acute Physiology Score (SAPS II), Sepsis-related Organ Function Assessment score (SOFA), and the Multiple Organ Dysfunction Score are similar assessment tools. In all these scoring systems, the higher the score, the higher the probability of mortality. Although it is useful to have the information afforded by the scoring systems to determine the chances of survival from critical illness, it cannot dictate care.

All these scoring systems correlate statistically with mortality in the ICU, but they refer to the ICU population as a group. The APACHE and other scores represent a level of risk for the group of patients with a particular score, but do not accurately predict outcome for the individual patient with that score. The score is useful when discussing possible outcomes and probabilities of cure or death with family members. The scoring systems are also useful in evaluating the quality of care in an ICU based on the observed mortality versus the expected mortality.

Biomarkers in Critical Illness

Lactate is a commonly used biomarker to identify sepsis. Lactate rises in the bloodstream when organs are undergoing ischemia and consequent anaerobic metabolism, which yields lactic acid. Other biomarkers in sepsis include markers of proinflammatory cytokines and chemokines; C-reactive protein and procalcitonin. Combinations of pro- and anti-inflammatory biomarkers in a multimarker panel may help identify patients who are developing severe sepsis before organ dysfunction has advanced too far.

DIC is diagnosed using a scoring system proposed by the International Society on Thrombosis and Hemostasis, which includes platelet count, prothrombin time, fibrinogen level, and a marker of fibrin formation. The most commonly utilized fibrin-related marker has been the assay for D-dimer.

Treatment of the Critically Ill Patient

There is no single universal treatment for shock. Different types of shock require distinctive treatment modalities. Therefore, treatment relies on the accurate diagnosis of the type of shock that is occurring.

Treatment of Cardiogenic Shock

Cardiogenic shock is most commonly caused by extensive MI. The left ventricle is often involved, which weakens the forward pumping of blood into the aorta and systemic arterial circulation. The treatment goal of MI is reduction of the heart's oxygen needs, support of cardiac output, and revascularization of the myocardium. Beta blockers, given early, reduce the heart's work and oxygen consumption. If there is profound cardiogenic shock, beta blockers may be contraindicated. Aspirin inhibits platelet activation and reduces extension of the infarction. It may also play a role as an anti-inflammatory agent. Dobutamine and dopamine increase cardiac output, but the increase in contractility and heart rate from these drugs increases cardiac work and oxygen demands, which may not be desirable.

Early reperfusion of the myocardium after MI can reduce extension of the infarcted muscle tissue. Revascularization procedures include thrombolytic medications, angioplasty, stenting, or coronary artery bypass. If successful, these procedures are all able to bring blood flow back into the heart muscle and significantly reduce the incidence of cardiogenic shock after an MI.

Acute mitral valve regurgitation, cardiac tamponade, and acute ventral septal defect are surgical emergencies that can occur after MI and have a high mortality.

Acute mitral valve regurgitation requires surgical repair or implantation of a new mitral valve. Acute ventricular septal defect or perforation requires surgical repair. In cardiac tamponade, the heart is constricted by fluid in the pericardial sac surrounding the heart. It is necessary to relieve pericardial pressure, which can be accomplished with a surgical procedure called subxiphoid percutaneous pericardiocentesis. In the procedure, the clinician uses a large-bore needle that is inserted through the chest under the sternum into the pericardial sac (using ultrasound guidance). This incision into the pericardial sac relieves the constriction around the heart.

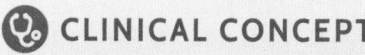

CLINICAL CONCEPT

Cardiogenic shock caused by cardiac tamponade, acute mitral insufficiency, acute ventricular septal defect, or acute ventricular perforation requires emergency surgery.

TABLE 46-2. APACHE II Score

Use the value for each parameter that is the most abnormal during the first 24 hours after admission to the ICU.

Physiological Variable	Point Score								
	+4	+3	+2	+1	0	+1	+2	+3	+4
Temperature rectal (°C)	≥41°C	39°C–40.9°C	–	38°C–38.9°C	36°C–37.9°C	34°C–35.9°C	32°C–33.9°C	30°C–31.9°C	<30°C
Heart rate	≥179	140–179	110–139	–	70–109	–	55–69	40–54	<40
Mean arterial pressure (mm Hg)	≥159	130–159	110–129	–	70–109	–	50–69	–	<50
Respiratory rate, nonventilated	≥49	35–49	–	25–34	12–24	10–11	6–9	–	<6
Arterial pH	≥7.69	7.60–7.69	–	7.50–7.59	7.33–7.49	–	7.25–7.32	7.15–7.24	<7.15
Oxygenation if FIO_2 ≥0.5, use A-aDO_2	≥500	351–499	–	200–350	<200	–	–	–	–
Oxygenation if FIO_2 <50%, use PO_2	–	–	–	–	>70	61–70	–	55–60	<55
Serum sodium	≥180	160–179	155–159	150–154	130–149	–	120–129	111–119	<111
Serum potassium	≥7.0	6–6.9	–	5.5–5.9	3.5–5.4	3–3.4	2.5–2.9	–	<2.5
Creatinine (mg/dL) – *double point score for acute renal failure*	≥3.5	2–3.4	1.5–1.9	–	0.6–1.4	–	<0.6	–	–
Hematocrit	≥59.9	–	50–59.9	46–49.9	30–45.9	–	20–29.9	–	<20
WBC (10^3 cells/mm³)	≥39	–	20–38.9	15–19.9	3–14.9	–	1–2.9	–	<1

AGE

0 points if younger than 44 years
2 points if between 45 and 54 years
3 points if between 55 and 64 years
5 points if between 65 and 74 years
6 points if older than 74 years

HISTORY OF ORGAN DYSFUNCTION OR IMMUNOCOMPROMISE

5 points if yes and emergency postoperative or nonresponsive
2 points if yes and elective postoperative
0 points if no

NEUROLOGICAL EVALUATION

Score = 15 − actual GCS

ICU MORTALITY AS PREDICTED BY APACHE II SCORES

APACHE II score = Physiological Variable Points + Age Points + History of Organ Dysfunction or Immunocompromise Points + Neurological Evaluation Points

TABLE 46-2. APACHE II Score–cont'd

Score	Mortality
0–4	4%
5–9	8%
10–14	15%
15–19	25%
20–24	40%
25–29	55%
30–34	75%
>34	85% or higher

Source: Knaus, W. A., Draper, E. A., & Wagner, D. P. (1985). APACHE II: A severity of disease classification system. *Crit Care Med, 13*(10), 818–829.

TABLE 46-3. Glasgow Coma Scale

Areas of Response	Points
EYES OPENING	
Eyes open spontaneously	4
Eyes open in response to voice	3
Eyes open in response to pain	2
No eye-opening response	1
BEST VERBAL RESPONSE	
Oriented (e.g., to person, place, time)	5
Confused, speaks but is disoriented	4
Inappropriate but comprehensible words	3
Incomprehensible sounds but no words are spoken	2
None	1
BEST MOTOR RESPONSE	
Obeys command to move	6
Localized painful stimulus	5
Withdrawals from painful stimulus	4
Flexion, abnormal decorticate posturing	3
Extension, abnormal decerebrate posturing	2
No movement or posturing	1
TOTAL POSSIBLE POINTS	3–15
MAJOR HEAD INJURY	≤8
MODERATE HEAD INJURY	9–12
MINOR HEAD INJURY	13–15

Mechanical Circulatory Support Devices

An intra-aortic balloon pump (IABP) device can provide lifesaving treatment in cardiogenic shock or severe heart failure. The procedure, called IABP counterpulsation, enhances coronary blood flow, reduces afterload, and decreases the work of the left ventricle. A balloon on a catheter is inserted into the aorta and inflates when the heart relaxes. This inflated balloon creates pressure within the aorta so that the coronary arteries (which arise off the aorta) receive blood flow. The inflated balloon also allows more blood to fill the left ventricle during relaxation by blocking exit of blood into the aorta. When the left ventricle contracts, the balloon in the aorta deflates, and the blood from the left ventricle is ejected into the aorta and then on to the systemic arteries (see Box 46-4).

Despite the use of IABP counterpulsation therapy in patients with cardiogenic shock or severe heart failure, the prognosis of these patients has remained poor. A recent study showed that follow-up of cardiogenic shock patients treated with IABP had a more than 66% mortality rate despite revascularization treatment.

BOX 46-4. Intra-Aortic Balloon Counterpulsation

An IABP is a useful device for cardiogenic shock. This catheter, which has an inflatable balloon on the tip, is inserted into the femoral artery and threaded up the aorta. During diastole of the heart, the balloon is inflated and pressure is created by the open balloon in the aorta. This increased pressure in the aorta increases blood flow into the coronary arteries. During systole of the heart, the balloon is deflated, and there is a suction effect that assists in the drive to push blood forward into the arterial circulation.

Newer percutaneous left- and right-ventricular mechanical circulatory support (MCS) devices are changing the management of cardiogenic shock and severe heart failure. A common type of mechanical circulatory support device is a left ventricular assist device (LVAD), which is a type of mechanical pump that enhances the function of the patient's left ventricle. The LVAD receives blood from the left ventricle and ejects it into the aorta through a tube, decreasing the work of the patient's left ventricle. There are different types of these devices, but they mainly consist of a pumping unit, computerized controller, and battery power source. A cable from the device is placed through the skin of the abdomen and connects to a controller on an external belt (see Fig. 46-4). Often, these patients are on a waiting list for heart transplant and the LVAD is a temporary treatment until they receive a donor heart; this is termed *bridge therapy to transplant*. However, some patients are now deciding to forgo transplant in favor of sustaining life using the LVAD.

Treatment of Hypovolemic Shock

The treatment of hypovolemic shock requires rapid, adequate replacement of the fluid loss. At the same time, every effort should be made to stop the fluid loss, which is not always immediately apparent.

If fluids are replaced before hypotension occurs, shock may be avoided. The initial type of fluids administered is controversial, but most practitioners agree that 1 to 2 liters of normal saline, 5% dextrose in normal saline, or Ringer's lactate solution should be given immediately. These solutions are volume expanders and have a similar ratio of solute and solvent as blood. Persistent bleeding will require blood transfusions, so the patient needs to be tested for blood type and crossmatched with donor blood before transfusion. Some patients can receive type O negative blood to replace blood loss. Fresh frozen plasma infusion is another alternative. Hypertonic IV solution such as 3% sodium chloride may be appropriate in some cases. Some practitioners advocate using mostly crystalloid solutions for hypovolemic shock, such as Ringer's lactate, with transfusions used sparingly. Others recommend the use of colloid solutions such as DextranR, instead of crystalloids. All practitioners agree on the need for rapid fluid resuscitation. However, there is controversy about how much is appropriate. The amount of resuscitation should be gauged by urine output because this is a true measure of tissue perfusion. Ideal urinary output is greater than 30 to 50 mL per hour. Urinary output less than 30 to 50 mL per hour indicates additional infusion of fluids is necessary.

Treatment of Sepsis and Septic Shock

The treatment of septic shock is clearly very complex and may involve multiple specialists, including an infectious disease specialist, a pulmonologist, a surgeon, an intensivist, a cardiologist, and a nephrologist. It requires the use of broad-spectrum antibiotics, support of cardiac output, use of vasoconstrictors, respiratory support, and sometimes surgery to treat the source of infection. Renal failure is frequent, and dialysis may be necessary. Respiratory failure is also frequent, requiring intubation with mechanical ventilator support. Septic shock may be resistant to vasoconstrictors. Angiotensin II is a medication recommended for any type of vasodilatory shock condition. Angiotensin II vasoconstricts the arterial bed and stimulates aldosterone, which increases sodium

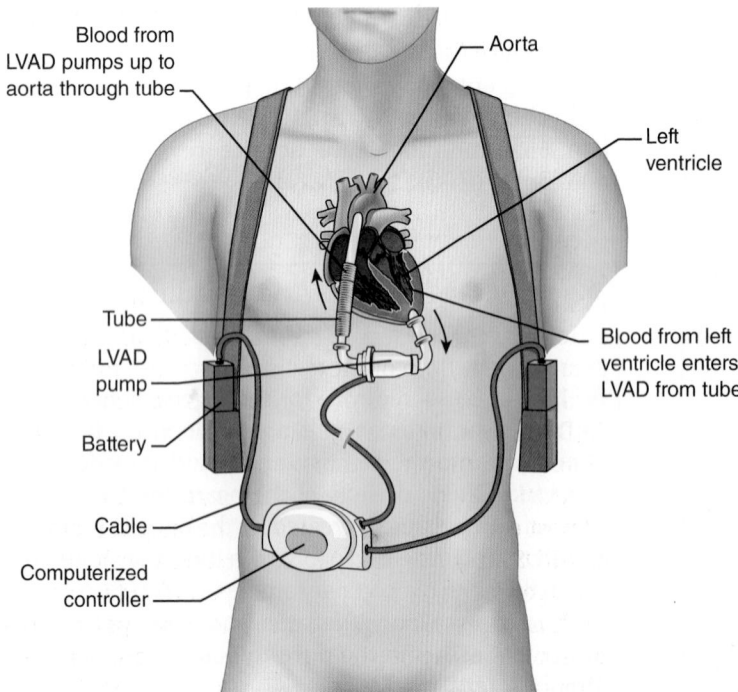

Blood from LVAD pumps up to aorta through tube

Aorta

Left ventricle

Tube

LVAD pump

Battery

Blood from left ventricle enters LVAD from tube

Cable

Computerized controller

FIGURE 46-4. Left ventricular assist device (LVAD).

and water reabsorption into the bloodstream, raising blood pressure.

Control of hyperglycemia with continuous IV insulin and hourly blood sugar determinations reduces mortality. Hypoglycemia must be avoided. The administration of glucocorticoids is controversial. There appears to be a subgroup of patients with inadequate cortisol secretion that may benefit from it. In general, the administration of glucocorticoids to septic patients increases overall mortality. DIC and acute respiratory distress syndrome (ARDS) are commonly triggered by septic shock, and treatment of these disorders may be required. Colloidal volume expanders, such as normal saline with 5% albumin, may also be necessary. Despite the amount of high-tech equipment found in modern ICUs and the advances in the pharmacological treatment of septic shock, mortality remains very high.

> ### 🩺 CLINICAL CONCEPT
>
> Septic shock is associated with a significant increase in capillary permeability. This means that a large portion of the fluids used in resuscitation end up in the subcutaneous tissues, making the patient seem very bloated. This is referred to as third spacing of fluids: a hallmark of septic shock.

The Sepsis Six

Early appropriate management of sepsis saves lives. Once sepsis is suspected, the key immediate interventions that increase survival are described in a care bundle termed the sepsis six. The sepsis six need to be delivered within 1 hour to control the source of infection, restore circulation, and promote oxygen delivery. The sepsis six consists of three diagnostic and three therapeutic steps (UK Sepsis Trust, 2020). In one study, the effective delivery of the sepsis six reduced the relative risk of death by 46.6% (Daniels et al., 2011) (see Table 46-4).

TABLE 46-4. The Sepsis Six

DELIVERY OF THE SEPSIS SIX WITHIN 1 HOUR SAVES LIVES	
Administer oxygen to keep SaO$_2$ >94%	Administer a fluid challenge
Take blood cultures	Measure blood lactate
Administer IV antibiotics	Measure urine output

Published by: UK Sepsis Trust (2020). Clinical resources. https://sepsistrust.org/ professional-resources/clinical/
Copied and adapted from: Bleakley, G., & Cole, M. (2020). Recognition and management of sepsis: the nurse's role. *Brit J Nursing (Mark Allen Publishing)*, 29(21), 1248–1251. https://doi.org/10.12968/bjon.2020.29.21.1248

Treatment of Anaphylactic Shock

Anaphylactic shock is treated with intramuscular or IV epinephrine, antihistamines, and glucocorticoids. IV saline administration is necessary because anaphylaxis causes a large shift of fluid from the bloodstream into the tissues. Intubation may be necessary if bronchoconstriction is severe. The antigen that triggered the severe allergic reaction should be identified. Patients need to carry epinephrine (EpiPen) with them at all times after experiencing anaphylaxis.

Treatment of Neurogenic Shock

The treatment for neurogenic shock consists of IV vasoconstrictors and fluid administration. Some vasodilatory shock conditions, such as neurogenic shock, are resistant to vasoconstrictors. Angiotensin II is recommended for any type of vasodilatory shock condition. Angiotensin II vasoconstricts the arterial bed and stimulates aldosterone, which increases sodium and water reabsorption into the bloodstream, raising blood pressure. Atropine, an anticholinergic agent, may be needed to counteract the parasympathetic-driven bradycardia. The treatment of the underlying central nervous system injury is essential. In cases of spinal injury, stabilization of the injury is key.

Pathophysiology of Selected Types of Organ Dysfunction

In critically ill patients, organ failure can occur. ARDS, renal failure, and DIC are the major disorders involved in MODS that can be lethal. Each organ system failure will present with different signs and symptoms and require different management.

Acute Respiratory Distress Syndrome

Acute respiratory distress syndrome (ARDS) is caused by widespread injury of the alveoli that often occurs in the presence of shock or MODS. This acute condition is characterized by bilateral pulmonary infiltrates and severe hypoxemia. It is important to differentiate ARDS from pulmonary edema caused by heart failure. Both of these disorders cause pulmonary infiltrates; however, in ARDS, there is no heart failure. ARDS is sometimes referred to as the most severe form of **acute lung injury (ALI)**.

ARDS may occur in people of any age; however, it is most common in older adults. The annual incidence of ARDS in the United States increases with advancing age, ranging from 16 cases per 100,000 persons in those ages 15 to 19 years to 306 cases per 100,000 persons in those between the ages of 75 and 84 years. There is a 22% to 44% risk of mortality in ARDS.

Etiology

The most common risk factor for ARDS is sepsis. Other risk factors include lung injury (most commonly, aspiration of gastric contents), systemic illnesses, and traumatic injuries; however, approximately 20% of patients with ARDS have no identified risk factor. Advanced age, cigarette smoking, and alcohol use increase susceptibility. Many conditions can increase the risk of developing ARDS (see Box 46-5).

Pathophysiology

ARDS can result from different mechanisms:

1. Direct lung injury and local inflammation, such as from pneumonitis, aspiration, heat, or chemical inhalation injuries
2. Indirect lung injury from an intense inflammatory reaction elsewhere in the body with systemic inflammatory mediators such as cytokines and microbial toxins damaging the lung

Any injury to the lungs is followed by the secretion of cytokines, superoxidases, and other deleterious substances by the pulmonary macrophages and the neutrophils that rush to the site of injury by chemotaxis. The capillaries of the lungs are particularly rich in neutrophils; migration of these neutrophils occurs quickly after the onset of any pulmonary injury. The presence of inflammatory substances increases the permeability of the alveolar capillaries, and fluid from the bloodstream infiltrates the lung tissue.

Both type I and type II alveolar epithelial cells are injured in ARDS. The loss of type I cells increases alveolar epithelial permeability, leading to increased fluid in the alveoli. Injury of type II cells reduces the production of surfactant. Surfactant is a lubricating substance that lines the alveoli to keep them from completely collapsing. Loss of surfactant decreases pulmonary compliance and causes alveolar collapse.

The increased fluid in the alveoli impedes the diffusion of oxygen into the bloodstream. The combination of alveolar collapse and reduced diffusion of oxygen decreases the arterial partial pressure of oxygen (PaO_2) in the bloodstream. Alveolar carbon dioxide diffusion is much less affected because CO_2 is 20 times more soluble in water than oxygen. The lack of oxygen cannot be overcome by hyperventilating or by administering a high oxygen concentration.

ARDS is also associated with pulmonary artery vasoconstriction, which raises pressure in the pulmonary arterial vessels—a condition called pulmonary hypertension. This constriction of pulmonary arterioles causes a ventilation-perfusion mismatch in the lungs. In **ventilation-perfusion mismatch,** some areas of the lung are ventilated and some areas are not ventilated. Similarly, some areas of the lung have circulation and some areas do not have circulation. There is no uniform transfer of oxygen from the lungs into the bloodstream.

After the acute phase of ARDS, resolution of the disorder can occur, or fibrosis of areas of the lung may develop. In pulmonary fibrosis, the interstitial spaces become filled with collagen and cannot transfer oxygen into the bloodstream. This causes a high mortality rate.

Clinical Presentation

ARDS presents with acute dyspnea and hypoxemia within hours to days of an inciting event, such as trauma, sepsis, drug overdose, massive transfusion, acute pancreatitis, or aspiration. In many cases, the inciting event is obvious; in others, such as drug overdose, it may be difficult to identify.

Patients who develop ARDS are critically ill, often with multisystem organ failure, and they may not be capable of providing a history. In this situation, a history should be sought from family or significant others. The clinician should inquire about recent infection, trauma, drug use, recent surgery, and pancreatitis because these are key preceding conditions. Typically, the illness develops within 12 to 48 hours after an inciting event; although in rare instances, it may take up to a few days.

Signs and Symptoms. Patients are typically short of breath at rest. They breathe rapidly, feel anxious, and need increasingly high concentrations of inspired oxygen. Despite the increase in oxygen administration, the patient's condition does not improve.

In the physical examination, there is tachypnea, tachycardia, and the need for high concentrations of oxygen to maintain oxygen saturation. The patient may be febrile or hypothermic. Older adult patients are often hypothermic. If ARDS is occurring in the presence of sepsis, hypotension, peripheral vasoconstriction with cold extremities, and cyanosis of the lips and fingertips may be apparent. Auscultation of the lungs may reveal bilateral crackles.

BOX 46-5. Major Risk Factors for ARDS

The major risk factors for ARDS include:
- Aspiration
- Bacteremia
- Burns
- Drug overdose
- Fat embolism
- Fractures, particularly multiple fractures and long bone fractures
- Massive transfusion
- Near-drowning
- Pancreatitis
- Pneumonia
- Postperfusion injury after cardiopulmonary bypass
- Sepsis
- Trauma, with or without pulmonary contusion

Manifestations of the underlying etiology may be present, such as acute abdominal findings in the case of ARDS caused by pancreatitis. If sepsis is the cause of ARDS, the clinician should try to identify the cause of infection.

 CLINICAL CONCEPT

In cases of ARDS caused by sepsis, acute abdomen, surgical wounds, intravascular lines, and pressure injuries are commonly the source of infection.

ARDS should be differentiated from pulmonary edema caused by heart failure because the pulmonary findings are similar in both disorders. However, the disorders have different etiologies and require different treatments. The clinician needs to examine the patient to rule out signs of heart failure, which include jugular venous distention, hepatosplenomegaly, ankle edema, and ascites.

Diagnosis

Chest x-ray is the first diagnostic procedure used in ARDS. ARDS is defined by the acute onset of bilateral pulmonary infiltrates, which are evident on chest x-ray. Computed tomography scan can be used if x-ray is not sufficient. It can be difficult to differentiate between pulmonary edema caused by heart failure and ARDS.

An echocardiogram is often done to exclude the possibility of heart dysfunction. The echocardiogram can show left ventricular ejection fraction and valvular dysfunction. Another way to differentiate ARDS from cardiogenic pulmonary edema is to obtain a B type natriuretic peptide (BNP) level. BNP levels are elevated in heart failure. A BNP level of lower than 100 pg/mL in a patient with bilateral pulmonary infiltrates and hypoxemia favors the diagnosis of ARDS rather than heart failure. BNP levels are commonly 400 pg/mL or greater in heart failure.

Another diagnostic procedure that can differentiate ARDS from heart failure is hemodynamic monitoring, also called the Swan–Ganz procedure, with a pulmonary artery catheter. Pressure measurements can be taken in the right side of the heart with this specialized catheter. Heart failure can be excluded based on these measurements.

In ARDS, there is severe hypoxemia apparent in arterial blood gases (ABGs). A low Po_2 will be demonstrated on ABGs. The severity of hypoxemia necessary to make the diagnosis of ARDS is defined by the ratio of the Pao_2 to the fraction of oxygen in the inspired air (Fio_2). ARDS is defined by a Pao_2/Fio_2 ratio of less than or equal to 200. In addition to hypoxemia, ABGs often initially show a respiratory alkalosis caused by hyperventilation. Hyperventilation diminishes carbon dioxide in the lungs, which in turn decreases H^+ concentration in the blood and creates alkalotic (high pH) blood. However, if ARDS occurs because of sepsis, a metabolic acidosis with or without respiratory compensation may be present. In ARDS, as the condition worsens, the respiratory rate decreases; carbon dioxide is retained in the lungs and rises to high levels, which results in H^+ accumulation in the bloodstream, creating respiratory acidosis.

In septic patients, leukopenia (low WBC count) or leukocytosis (high WBC count) may be noted. Thrombocytopenia (low platelet count) may be observed in the presence of DIC. Acute tubular necrosis often develops in the course of ARDS, probably from ischemia to the kidneys. Serum creatinine should be closely monitored, and liver function abnormalities may be noted. Multiple cytokines, such as IL-1, IL-6, and IL-8, are elevated in the serum of patients with ARDS.

Treatment

Treatment in ARDS is mechanical ventilation using low tidal volumes (6 mL/kg based upon ideal body weight). The patient requires different modes of supportive care, including careful use of sedatives and neuromuscular blockade to facilitate mechanical ventilation. These agents place the patient in a state referred to as a medically induced coma. The sedatives and neuromuscular blocking agents inhibit the patient's natural respirations so they do not interfere with the mechanical ventilation. This blockade of the patient's respirations is reversible and alleviates the work of the lungs as ARDS resolves. The patient needs careful hemodynamic monitoring, nutritional support, control of blood glucose, and prophylaxis against deep vein thrombosis and GI bleeding.

Because infection is often the cause of ARDS, early administration of broad-spectrum antibiotic therapy is essential, as is meticulous patient assessment for sources of infection. Removal of intravascular lines, drainage of infected fluid collections, surgical débridement, or resection of an infected site may be necessary.

Some experts advise glucocorticoid administration be used early in the course of ARDS but should not be used in later stages. Inhaled NO has been shown to improve oxygenation; however, NO has not been shown to reduce mortality. Inhaled prostacyclin (iloprost) is another medication that can improve oxygenation, but it has not been found to reduce mortality rates. Some studies suggest a potential role for antibody to TNF and recombinant IL-1 receptor antagonists. More research is necessary before these agents become standard therapies for ARDS.

Interestingly, the prone position has been found to be beneficial in some patients with ARDS. When the patient is placed in the prone position, the posterior area of the lungs endures less pleural pressure and atelectasis. Also less ventilation-perfusion mismatching is found in patients in the prone position and oxygenation is improved. However, the prone position is not recommended for all patients, as some are affected negatively. Complications such as airway obstruction and endotracheal tube dislodgement, hypotension and arrhythmias, loss of venous access, facial and airway edema, and a greater need for paralysis or sedation have all been associated with prone positioning.

Extracorporeal membrane oxygenation (ECMO) is another treatment strategy for acute cardiac and/or respiratory failure in adult patients who are not responsive to conventional treatment. Patients are placed on ECMO temporarily while medications and other treatments are used in the attempt to reverse ARDS. ECMO is a form of cardiopulmonary life support, where blood is drained from the vascular system, circulated outside the body by a mechanical pump, and then reinfused into the circulation. While outside the body, hemoglobin becomes fully saturated with oxygen by an oxygenator and CO_2 is removed by the machine. ECMO currently comes in two varieties: venoarterial (VA) ECMO and venovenous (VV) ECMO. VA ECMO takes deoxygenated blood from a central vein or the right atrium, pumps it into the oxygenator, and then returns the oxygenated blood under pressure to the arterial side of the circulation (typically to the aorta) (see Fig. 46-5). VV ECMO takes blood from a large vein and returns oxygenated blood back to a large vein. Ideal patients for ECMO have potential for resolution of their cardiac or respiratory failure. Patients with MODS are not candidates for this kind of treatment. Both VV ECMO and VA ECMO can be used as a rescue therapy in acute respiratory failure to maintain life while awaiting improvement of the underlying disease. ECMO can be used while the lungs recover or as a temporary solution until a transplant is found in case of end-stage lung disease.

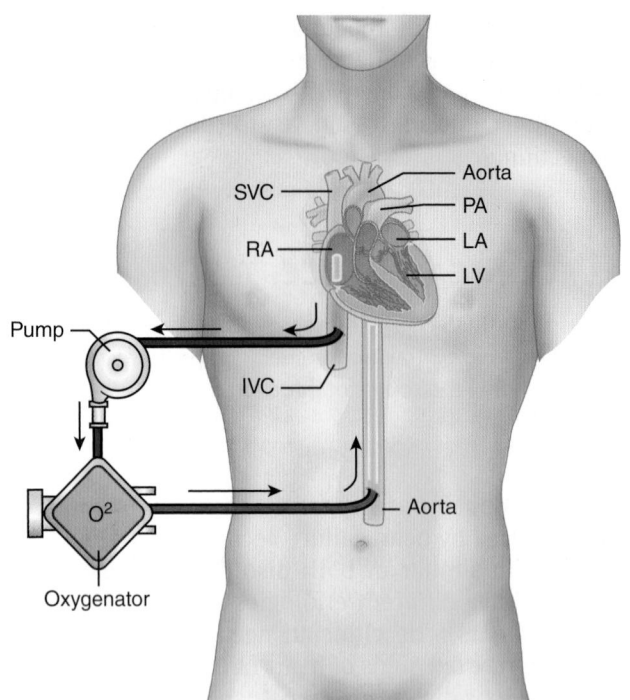

FIGURE 46-5. Venoarterial ECMO in ARDS. Blood is drained from the right atrium and pumped into an oxygenator. Blood is then returned to the aorta. [*RA*, right atrium; *LA*, left atrium; *PA*, pulmonary artery; *SVC*, superior vena cava; *IVC*, inferior vena cava.]

 CLINICAL CONCEPT

In patients with critical illness, family and friends are under stress and likely have many questions and concerns. It is important to communicate with the family and significant others. Clinicians and caregivers should assume that even though sedated, the patient may be capable of hearing and understanding all conversations in the room and may experience pain. Therefore, all conversation at the bedside should be appropriate and all procedures should be performed with local anesthesia and pain medication.

Acute Kidney Injury

In the setting of shock, sepsis, SIRS, or MODS, AKI frequently occurs. Thirty percent of patients in intensive care develop AKI, and there is a high mortality rate in these patients compared with those without AKI. AKI has also been referred to as acute renal failure (ARF) in the past.

Etiology

The most common causes of renal injury are renal ischemia and renal toxicity, also called nephrotoxicity. Renal ischemia occurs because of reduced renal perfusion, which in turn causes ischemic injury of the nephron tubules. This is usually caused by large blood loss from the body or large water deficit in the blood. When the kidney suffers ischemia or injury that causes nephron tubule damage, this is often referred to as acute tubular necrosis (ATN). Renal toxicity commonly occurs because of the toxic effects of drugs such as antibiotics, aspirin, NSAIDs, chemotherapeutic agents, ACE inhibitors, illicit drugs, and iodinated IV contrast dye used in diagnostic tests. Many other drugs are also nephrotoxic.

A combination of ischemic injury and medication nephrotoxicity is often seen in the patient with sepsis. The septic patient often receives combinations of potentially nephrotoxic antibiotics with other drugs or iodinated contrast dye needed for diagnosis. Newer types of contrast dyes are noniodinated, nonallergenic, and nonnephrotoxic.

Pathophysiology

The kidney is responsible for the elimination of nitrogenous waste, nonnitrogenous waste, and nonvolatile acids, as well as the maintenance of electrolyte and water balance. In sepsis, shock, and MODS caused by hypotension, the kidney has to conserve water and maximally concentrate urine. In the adult, the daily average amount of waste the kidney excretes is about 600 mOsm of solutes. In order to excrete this amount, the urine output has to be at least 400 mL/day. Oliguria is defined as a urine output of less than 400 mL/day, whereas anuria is defined as a urine output of 100 mL/day or less. In patients with preexisting renal disease, the added stress of sepsis or MODS can precipitate complete ARF.

In MODS and sepsis, renal ischemia can occur because of several distinct mechanisms:

- Hypotension reduces glomerular perfusion directly.
- The hormonal responses to shock, epinephrine, norepinephrine, vasopressin, and angiotensin II depress glomerular perfusion by vasoconstriction.
- Microthrombi associated with the procoagulant state of shock block the glomerular capillaries.

The nephron tubules are exquisitely sensitive to hypoperfusion. The glomerular capillaries cannot endure extreme drops in blood pressure. Shock for only 15 minutes causes dysfunction of the nephron tubules; longer periods cause tubular necrosis. When there is tubular dysfunction, the tubular cells are unable to concentrate urine. Nephron tubule dysfunction also causes diminished excretion of potassium and less reabsorption of sodium. Hyperkalemia and hyponatremia often occur in AKI. In tubular necrosis, the epithelial cells that line the nephron tubules slough off and clog the tubules. No urine can be excreted from these clogged nephrons; oliguria or anuria exists. Nitrogenous wastes such as blood urea nitrogen (BUN) and creatinine accumulate in the bloodstream as nephron tubules continue to dysfunction. High serum creatinine and BUN are signs of kidney injury.

Clinical Presentation

An accurate history is crucial for diagnosing AKI. People with the following comorbid conditions are at an increased risk for developing it:

- Hypertension
- Chronic heart failure
- Diabetes
- Multiple myeloma
- Chronic infection
- Myeloproliferative disorder (excessive growth of bone marrow cells)
- Connective tissue disorders
- Autoimmune diseases

When the patient has a critical illness such as sepsis or MODS, it is important to review the patient's medications because these can be nephrotoxic. Also, it is important to note if any iodinated dye has been used in diagnostic procedures. Blood loss or transfusions can also cause AKI. The patient's urine output may indicate oliguria or anuria. The patient's mental status may be stuporous because of the accumulation of nitrogenous wastes—a syndrome called uremic encephalopathy.

Diagnosis

Serum creatinine and BUN are elevated in renal injury. Findings of granular brown casts are highly suggestive of tubular necrosis. Casts are cellular debris that come from the nephron tubules and appear in urine. Reddish brown or cola-colored urine suggests the presence of myoglobin or hemoglobin, especially in the setting of a positive dipstick for heme and no red blood cells (RBCs) on the microscopic examination. The urine dipstick test may reveal significant proteinuria as a result of tubular injury.

Treatment

The development of AKI in ICU patients considerably increases the risk of death. Because renal failure can be treated by dialysis, it is rare today for a patient to die of renal failure itself; however, the presence of renal failure does increase the overall mortality.

Abdominal Compartment Syndrome and Intra-Abdominal Hypertension

In **abdominal compartment syndrome (ACS),** the pressure within the abdominal cavity increases to a point that exceeds the perfusion pressure of the capillaries. This causes ischemia and necrosis of the tissues supplied by the abdominal arterial vessels and capillaries.

The abdominal compartment is contained by the retroperitoneum posteriorly and a fibromuscular wall anteriorly and laterally. The retroperitoneum is not distensible, and the fibromuscular wall is only somewhat distensible. The normal **intra-abdominal pressure (IAP)** is usually 0 to 5 mm Hg, and when it increases above 8 mm Hg, **intra-abdominal hypertension (IAH)** exists. IAH causes decreased perfusion of the GI organs. This lack of GI perfusion can lead to ischemia and tissue necrosis, at which time it is called ACS. ACS affects the intra-abdominal viscera such as the intestine, liver, and pancreas, as well as the retroperitoneal viscera (kidneys).

Etiology

The cause of acute ACS is increased capillary permeability of the intestinal vasculature associated with SIRS. Circulating cytokines increase endothelial permeability, and protein-rich fluid escapes into the bowel walls and lumen, the mesenteric walls, and the peritoneal cavity. The fluid in the peritoneal cavity is an example of third-space edema. Peristalsis ceases, and the edematous bowel becomes distended with gas. This accumulation of fluid and gas causes a rapid increase of intra-abdominal volume that exceeds the abdominal wall's ability to distend.

Pathophysiology

As IAP increases, it exceeds the pressure in the inferior vena cava; as a result, the vessel collapses. The venous return to the heart drops, as does cardiac output. The decrease in cardiac output exacerbates the hypoperfusion in all tissues, including the intra-abdominal organs; this reinforces the mechanism by which the IAH was initiated. This positive feedback loop, if unchecked, can lead to death. Increased IAP has multiple adverse consequences:

- Compression of the inferior vena cava reduces cardiac output.
- Renal perfusion is reduced, increasing the likelihood of ATN.
- The barrier breaks down between the bowel wall and the bowel contents with its myriad pathogenic microbes and their toxins. There is diffusion of microbes and toxins into the bloodstream. This phenomenon then leads to sepsis, shock, and MODS.
- The increased IAP pushes up the diaphragm. This compresses the bases of the lungs and causes decreased ventilation.
- The increased intrathoracic pressure is transmitted upward via the jugular veins. There is jugular venous distention and increase in the pressure of the cerebral vasculature; this leads to an increase in intracranial pressure, which causes decreased level of consciousness.

 CLINICAL CONCEPT

In SIRS, IAP can rise to levels that compress the inferior vena cava, restrict venous return to the heart, and cause death.

Clinical Presentation

The patient usually experiences abdominal pain in ACS; the patient feels weak, and systemic blood pressure decreases, causing the patient to lose consciousness. Difficulty breathing or decreased urine output may be the first signs of IAH. Furthermore, patients who develop ACS may be unable to communicate because they are often intubated and critically ill.

Signs and symptoms of ACS and IAH can include the following:

- Increased abdominal girth
- Difficulty breathing
- Decreased urine output
- Syncope
- Melena
- Nausea and vomiting

ACS may be obscured in patients with critical injuries. Many disease processes can contribute to ACS. IAH should be considered in the following patients:

- Intubated patients who are difficult to ventilate
- Patients who have GI bleeding or pancreatitis and are not responding to IV fluids, blood products, and vasopressor medications
- Patients who have severe burns or sepsis with decreasing urine output and are not responding to IV fluids and vasopressors
- Any patient with contradictory Swan–Ganz readings

Diagnosis

One must distinguish between increased IAP, which can be treated conservatively, and full-blown ACS, which is a surgical emergency. Monitoring of IAP is appropriate in patients at risk of IAH. In order to evaluate the abdominal perfusion pressure (APP), subtract IAP from mean arterial pressure (MAP).

APP = MAP – IAP

ACS is present when APP is low, MAP is low, and IAP is high. Normal IAP is approximately 5 to 7 mm Hg. An IAP in excess of 15 mm Hg is associated with significant end-organ dysfunction and failure.

CLINICAL CONCEPT

In order to measure IAP, you need to monitor the pressure in the urinary bladder. Specialized Foley catheters can automatically transduce this value to a patient monitor.

Treatment

In patients at risk for IAH, hourly determination of IAP is appropriate. A trend of increasing IAP requires intervention before ACS develops. Conservative treatment for increasing IAP includes:

- Restriction of fluid resuscitation
- Removing any object that may press on the patient's abdomen, such as an abdominal binder
- Aggressive pain management to relax the abdominal musculature
- Colloid infusions such as albumin to increase intravascular oncotic pressure
- Nasogastric tube suction to remove air and fluid from the stomach and small intestines
- Hemodialysis or hemofiltration to remove excess edema fluid
- Rectal tube to evacuate colonic gas
- Catecholamine support of cardiac output to improve perfusion of the intra-abdominal organs

CLINICAL CONCEPT

The goal in measuring and treating IAP is to keep APP greater than 60 mm Hg.

Hepatic Failure

In conditions of sepsis, MODS, and IAH, liver function is at risk; all of these conditions can decrease the blood supply to the liver. The liver receives about two-thirds of its blood supply from the portal vein and about one-third from the hepatic artery.

Etiology

Arterial blood supply to the liver is reduced whenever there is decreased cardiac output and splanchnic vasoconstriction, as occurs in MODS. The venous perfusion of the liver is compromised when IAH reduces portal vein blood flow. Decreased arterial or venous blood flow to the liver will result in ischemia of hepatocytes and liver dysfunction.

Liver damage can also result from total parenteral nutrition (TPN), the IV infusion of a high-protein, carbohydrate, fat, and electrolyte solution. TPN is used when a patient is NPO (*non per os;* not allowed oral feedings) for an extended period. Although it can support the patient nutritionally for a lengthy time, TPN has possible hepatic complications.

Pathophysiology

In sepsis, shock, and MODS, hepatic arterial flow is diminished in order to conserve blood supply for the heart and brain. Also, splanchnic blood supply to the intestine decreases, which leads to intestinal ischemia. In intestinal ischemia, there is translocation of bacteria from the gut lumen into the portal vein. This portal vein bacteremia leads to direct bacterial infection of the liver. Bacterial toxins poison the mitochondria of hepatocytes, and ATP production in the liver is markedly reduced. This reduced energy then impairs the liver's role of processing wastes.

In addition, TPN treatment can cause liver injury. When a patient is treated with TPN, fatty infiltration of the liver can occur from the administration of too many calories or the administration of too many carbohydrates. This fatty infiltration is a precursor of cirrhosis, which further depresses liver function.

Clinical Presentation

Jaundice, abdominal distention, and decreased level of consciousness will occur with liver failure (for more information, see Chapter 31).

Diagnosis and Treatment

Most patients with acute liver failure tend to develop some degree of circulatory dysfunction. The patient needs IV fluids, airway support, and possibly intubation. Monitoring of metabolic parameters such as liver enzymes, coagulation, and bilirubin is necessary. Maintenance of nutrition and prompt recognition of GI bleeding are crucial.

Disseminated Intravascular Coagulation

DIC is the impairment of the coagulation cascade, which causes episodes of bleeding alternating with bouts of clotting. DIC is exhibited when the entire complex regulatory feedback mechanism of coagulation goes awry.

Etiology

DIC is frequently part of sepsis and MODS. It is known to occur in gram-negative sepsis, major incompatibility transfusion reactions, after placement of peritoneovenous shunts, and amniotic fluid emboli.

Pathophysiology

In DIC, there is major, widespread intravascular clotting and clotting factor depletion. There is also widespread activation of the fibrinolytic (clot-dissolving) mechanisms. Transient episodes of excessive clotting are interspersed with episodes of extreme fibrinolysis, which causes bleeding. Uncontrolled bleeding from all orifices, any wounds, and any IV sites is possible. This characterizes DIC, a syndrome with prohibitively high mortality. Brain injuries with significant, permanent neurological damage frequently occur because of the widespread coagulation of intracerebral vessels.

Clinical Presentation

Mottling and coolness of extremities and decreased peripheral pulses are common early signs of DIC. Bleeding from at least three unrelated sites—such as gingiva, nose, and IV sites—is also found with DIC. The condition often presents with petechiae and ecchymosis, along with blood loss from IV lines and catheters. In postoperative DIC, bleeding can occur from surgical sites externally and internally. Patients with pulmonary involvement can present with dyspnea, hemoptysis, and cough. Comorbid liver disease or hemolytic reactions can lead to jaundice. Neurological changes such as coma are also possible.

CLINICAL CONCEPT

In patients enduring major surgery under general anesthesia, the most common presentation of a transfusion reaction is DIC. The patient will suddenly start to bleed profusely from all cut surfaces and puncture sites.

Diagnosis

Patients with DIC can present with a wide range of abnormalities in their laboratory values. Typically, prolonged coagulation times, thrombocytopenia, high levels of fibrin degradation products, elevated D-dimer, and schistocytes (misshapen RBCs) on peripheral smears are suggestive findings. Laboratory tests need to be frequently done because of the rapidly changing conditions of clotting and bleeding in DIC.

Treatment

Treatment of DIC is controversial and is under current investigation. Hemorrhage caused by DIC requires rapid treatment; initially, treatment of hemorrhage usually occurs with crystalloid solutions, which have the same solute/solvent concentration as normal blood.

 CLINICAL CONCEPT

Ringer's lactate is an example of a crystalloid solution that can temporarily replace lost blood. After the patient's blood type is determined, transfusions of typed RBCs are administered. It is important to recognize that transfusions of RBCs and crystalloid solutions are devoid of clotting factors. Therefore, after the patient is stabilized with crystalloid solutions and receives transfusions of RBCs, a substance containing coagulation factors should be administered. Fresh frozen plasma contains coagulation factors and should be part of the treatment plan in DIC.

The rapid administration of multiple transfusions introduces large amounts of citrate into the bloodstream. This chemical is used as an anticoagulant in banked blood because it binds calcium, an element necessary in almost every step of the coagulation cascade. With multiple transfusions, there is a decrease in the amount of calcium in the blood. Decreased calcium can worsen hemorrhage and reduce cardiac contractility. Therefore, every treatment plan for severe hemorrhage needs to include calcium administration.

 CLINICAL CONCEPT

Blood transfusions contain citrate, which binds calcium. Therefore, treatment with multiple blood transfusions requires calcium supplementation.

The administration of crystalloids, packed RBCs, and fresh frozen plasma in large quantities drops the core body temperature. The coagulation pathways, which are temperature dependent, are impaired in hypothermia. Blood warmers are commercially available and should be used when large amounts of IV fluids are rapidly administered.

 CLINICAL CONCEPT

Multiple transfusions can cause a drop in patient core temperature; therefore, blood warmers are necessary.

Concepts Related to Death

Because of the advances in technology and the emergence of critical care medicine, the concept of what defines death has been debated for almost 50 years. Death was initially defined as the cessation of respiration and circulation. However, because of increased knowledge in the area of neurology, mechanical ventilation, and cardiovascular support, death is currently defined by brain death. Certain neurological criteria must be met in order for a patient to be classified with brain death.

Determination of Death

The gold standard for the determination of **brain death** is the neurological examination. However, before this examination, other morbid conditions must first be ruled out. These include severe electrolyte, acid–base, and endocrine abnormalities; core temperature lower than 89.6°F (32°C); hypotension; and possibility for drug intoxication, poisoning, or neuromuscular blockade. The neurological examination of patients with locked-in syndrome, which is stroke involving the brainstem, hypothermia, or drug intoxication, could mimic that of brain death and lead to misdiagnosis.

Determining Brain Death

The clinical neurological examination assesses the patient for coma, absence of brainstem reflexes, and apnea. A positive examination for the evaluation of brain death includes:

- Presence of coma
- Absence of motor responses
- Absence of pupillary responses to light and pupils at midposition with respect to dilation (4 to 6 mm)
- Absence of corneal reflexes
- Absence of caloric responses (absence of vestibulo-ocular/oculocephalic reflexes)
- Absence of gag reflex
- Absence of coughing in response to tracheal suctioning
- Absence of sucking and rooting reflexes
- Absence of respiratory drive at a $PaCO_2$ that is 60 mm Hg or 20 mm Hg above normal baseline values

Two examinations should be performed; the interval between the two is determined by the patient's age. The recommended intervals are 48 hours for term to 2-month-old newborns, 24 hours for infants older than 2 months to younger than 1 year, and 12 hours for children older than 1 year to younger than 18 years. The interval is optional for adults older than 18 years.

Assessment of Coma and Brainstem Reflexes.
During the neurological examination, presence of coma is determined first, followed by the depth of coma, which is established by the presence or absence of motor response to painful stimulus. The patient's reaction to pain can be determined by pressing on a supraorbital nerve, pinching the sternum, or pressing on the nailbed of a finger. The GCS can be used to establish depth of coma; it is based on certain criteria such as eye opening, motor response, and verbal output (see Table 46-4).

After coma and depth of coma are established, the examination proceeds to evaluate for the presence or absence of brainstem reflexes. Absence of brainstem reflexes includes round or oval pupils in midposition and dilated 4 to 6 mm with no response to bright light. Rapid turning of the head normally elicits eye movements called oculocephalic movements. Oculocephalic movements are absent in brain death. This is confirmed by a procedure called cold caloric stimulation, which is done by irrigating the ear canal with ice water after tilting the head to 30 degrees. If the brainstem is intact, the eyes will deviate toward the cold stimulus. In the coma patient, no neck or eye deviation toward the cold stimulus should be noted. Corneal reflex is evaluated by touching the edge of the cornea with a cotton swab, which causes sudden blinking in the patient with intact brainstem. In the coma patient, there is no blinking in response to this stimulus. Bronchial suctioning is the best stimulus for a cough reflex, and no coughing occurs in the coma patient.

The procedure to determine the lack of independent respiratory drive in coma patients is called apneic diffusion oxygenation. In healthy persons, stimulation of the respiratory center in the brainstem occurs when pressure of CO_2 in blood (PCO_2) reaches 60 mm Hg (in patients with COPD, the value is greater). During the procedure, the mechanical ventilator is turned off and preoxygenation is given through an oxygen catheter in the trachea to eliminate stores of respiratory nitrogen. The PCO_2 will increase at a rate of approximately 3 mm Hg per minute; there will be no spontaneous respirations in a patient with brain death.

Confirmatory Tests for Brain Death.
Confirmatory tests are optional in patients who are older than 1 year of age. For term infants to those up to 2 months of age, two confirmatory tests are needed. From 2 months to 1 year, one confirmatory test is required. Confirmatory tests include:

- Cerebral angiography: performed by an injection of dye in the aortic arch in order to visualize anterior and posterior cerebral circulation of the brain. A positive examination indicating brain death would be lack of flow at the foramen magnum in posterior circulation and lack of flow at the petrous portion of the carotid artery in the anterior circulation.
- Electroencephalography: readings are obtained for at least 30 minutes. A minimum of eight scalp electrodes must be used with a distance of 10 cm between each. In the patient who is brain dead, electrical activity is absent at levels higher than 2 μV per millimeter.
- Transcranial Doppler ultrasonography: a diagnostic test in which a portable 2-Hz pulsed-wave instrument evaluates the middle cerebral and vertebral arteries. The probe may be placed at the temporal bone above the zygomatic arch or the vertebrobasilar arteries through the suboccipital window. In the patient who is brain dead, transcranial Doppler ultrasonography would reveal a lack of diastolic flow and small systolic peaks in early systole.
- Nuclear imaging: in this test, technetium is injected within 30 minutes and x-ray images are obtained immediately, between 30 and 60 minutes, and at 2 hours. Determination of brain death is made if there is no uptake of the technetium.

Postmortem Changes

After death, postmortem changes progress along an approximate timeline. Putrefaction and autolysis are the two processes that start to alter the body immediately after death. Putrefaction involves the action of bacteria on the body's tissues. There is discoloration of the body, gas production with associated bloating, and a foul odor. Autolysis is the breakdown of the body's cells. Upon cell death, lysosomes open within the cell and release the lysozymes that digest dead tissue. In most circumstances, autolysis and putrefaction occur together. In warm climatic conditions, they can result in rapid degradation of the tissues.

Some of the more well-known postmortem changes, such as rigor mortis, livor mortis, and algor mortis, occur in a progressive manner. However, climate, cause of death, and environmental conditions affect their development.

Postmortem changes include:

- Rigor mortis: the postmortem stiffening of the body's muscles. Some muscles may be contracted and remain in position. In most cases, rigor mortis begins within 1 to 2 hours after death; it begins to pass after 24 hours.
- Livor mortis: a purple-red discoloration that appears on dependent portions of the body after the heart stops. It results from the settling of the blood because of gravity.
- Tardieu spots: petechiae and small hemorrhages that occur in dependent areas of the body because of rupture of degenerating blood vessels.

- Algor mortis: the cooling process of the body after death. Cooling takes place only if the environmental temperature is cooler than body temperature at the time of death.

- Purge fluid: exudative fluid from cellular decomposition released from the oral and nasal passages as well as other body cavities.

Chapter Summary

- Shock is classified into five broad categories: cardiac, hypovolemic, septic, anaphylactic, and neurogenic. The hypoperfusion in septic, anaphylactic, and neurogenic shock is due to widespread arterial vasodilation throughout the body. It is important to realize that all five categories of shock cause the same pathophysiological pathway of cellular hypoxia, cellular metabolic exhaustion and dysfunction, and death.

- Shock has three stages. In the initial stage, there is a rapid drop in tissue perfusion. If this is not corrected promptly, a progressive stage of shock ensues in which the lungs, kidneys, gut, pancreas, and eventually the protected areas of the heart and brain suffer cellular injury and no longer function properly. Failure to terminate shock during the progressive stage produces the irreversible stage of shock.

- SIRS is the term used to describe a severe physiological response to inflammation. This inflammation can occur from any source, whether infectious or noninfectious.

- CARS is a sequela to SIRS when the body is highly immunocompromised and susceptible to infection.

- Sepsis is diagnosed when a patient meets SIRS criteria and has a documented or suspected source of infection. The infection can be caused by bacteria, fungi, viruses, or parasites. Common diagnostic procedures include blood culture, urine culture, sputum culture, imaging showing pneumonia or a perforated viscus, and the existence of WBCs in normally sterile fluid. Sepsis is the most common cause of death.

- Severe sepsis is diagnosed when a patient meets sepsis criteria and has signs of end-organ damage or hypoperfusion. Signs of end-organ damage include ARDS, GI ischemia causing ileus, renal insufficiency causing decreased urine output, liver dysfunction causing increased total bilirubin, and DIC.

- Septic shock is diagnosed when a patient meets severe sepsis criteria and has sepsis-induced vascular instability demonstrated by hypotension that is refractory to fluid resuscitation. Widespread vasodilation is the cause of hypotension in septic shock. *Hypotension* is defined as a systolic blood pressure lower than 90 mm Hg, an MAP lower than 60 mm Hg, or a decrease in systolic blood pressure greater than 40 mm Hg.

- MODS is a state of progressive dysfunction of two or more major organ systems in a critically ill patient who cannot maintain homeostasis without medical intervention. In the presence of MODS, there is a 20% increase in mortality with each additional organ dysfunction. In the presence of ARF, the mortality rate increases to 70%.

- During MODS, respiratory failure is referred to as ARDS or ALI. Because of alveolar injury, the lungs become inflamed, edematous, less compliant, and less able to oxygenate the blood.

- AKI is most commonly caused by hypoperfusion of the kidney or by nephrotoxicity of medications necessary to treat sepsis, including aminoglycosides, vancomycin, and iodinated IV radiological contrast media.

- IAH causes decreased perfusion of the GI organs, which can lead to ischemia and tissue necrosis, also called ACS. The intra-abdominal viscera, such as the intestine, liver, pancreas, and retroperitoneal viscera (kidneys), all sustain decreased perfusion in ACS.

- Arterial blood supply to the liver is reduced whenever there is decreased cardiac output and splanchnic vasoconstriction, as occurs in MODS and shock. The venous perfusion of the liver is compromised when IAH reduces portal vein blood flow. Decreased arterial or venous blood flow to the liver will result in ischemia of hepatocytes and liver dysfunction. Liver damage can also result from TPN—the IV infusion of a high-protein, carbohydrate, fat, and electrolyte solution.

- DIC is the impairment of the coagulation cascade, which causes episodes of bleeding alternating with bouts of clotting.

- Death is defined by brain death. Certain neurological criteria must be met in order for a patient to be classified with brain death. The gold standard for the determination of brain death is the neurological examination.

- Postmortem changes occur in a progressive manner: rigor mortis, livor mortis, and algor mortis.

Making the Connections

Signs and Symptoms	Physical Assessment Findings	Diagnostic Testing	Treatment

Systemic Inflammatory Response Syndrome (SIRS) | Overwhelming inflammatory reaction of the body initiated by a severe insult, such as major trauma, burns, hemorrhage, infection, or major surgery. The inflammation reaction, coagulation system, and immune system work in an exaggerated mode to synergistically defend the body. Compensatory anti-inflammatory response syndrome (CARS) is a sequela to SIRS. In CARS, there is immunosuppression and high susceptibility to infection.

Signs and Symptoms	Physical Assessment Findings	Diagnostic Testing	Treatment
Dependent on the source of SIRS reaction: pain, tenderness, cough, shortness of breath (SOB), fatigue, headache, neck stiffness, dysuria, abdominal pain, flank pain, fever, and chills are all possible.	To establish the presence of SIRS, any two of the following criteria should be present: • Heart rate: >90/min. • Respiratory rate: >20/min (or need for mechanical ventilation). • Temperature: 38°C or <36°C.	Chest x-ray. ABGs. Blood lactate. WBC with differential showing leukocytosis or leukopenia. Urinalysis. Gram stain of blood, sputum, purulence, and urine (perhaps cerebrospinal fluid [CSF]). Culture and sensitivity of blood, sputum, purulence, and urine (perhaps CSF). Ultrasonography or CT. Electrolytes, BUN, creatinine, glucose, coagulation, platelet count, partial thromboplastin time (PTT), international normalized ratio (INR). Liver function testing, including bilirubin, ALT, AST, and alkaline phosphatase. Measurement and continued assessment of IAP and APP. Blood glucose monitoring.	***Respiratory, if not intubated*** Assess airway. Administer O_2 by mask or nasal cannula. ***Respiratory, if ventilated*** Administer O_2 at lowest level to maintain Po_2 greater than 60. ***Circulatory*** Administer fluids, vasopressors, or blood as appropriate to keep mean arterial pressure greater than 65 mm Hg and central venous pressure between 8 and 12 cm H_2O. ***Renal*** Administer sufficient fluids to keep urine output at 0.5 mL/kg/hr or greater. If infection is present, broad-spectrum antibiotics are used unless Gram stains allow identification of the specific organism. Drainage of abscess or wounds, if present. Treatment of organ dysfunction is based on symptomology and is given as needed. May include: • Dialysis or hemofiltration • Continuous insulin drip • Mechanical ventilation • Platelet transfusions • Fresh frozen plasma

Sepsis | An infection that begins locally, and through hematogenous spread, it becomes a body-wide infection that overwhelms the immune system and causes severe multiorgan compromise.

Signs and Symptoms	Physical Assessment Findings	Diagnostic Testing	Treatment
Alteration in mental state. Fever or hypothermia. Other symptoms depend on the source of sepsis: pain, tenderness, cough, SOB, fatigue, dizziness, headache, neck stiffness, dysuria, abdominal pain, flank pain, fever, and chills are all possible.	Alteration in mental state: Heart rate: >90/min. Respiratory rate: >20/min (may need mechanical ventilation). Temperature: >38°C or <36°C. Hypotension or normal blood pressure.	Chest x-ray may show pneumonia. ABGs showing hypoxemia. Blood lactate elevated. WBC with differential showing leukocytosis or leukopenia. Urinalysis may show bacteria. Low urine output.	***Respiratory, if not intubated*** Assess airway. Administer O_2 by mask or nasal cannula. ***Respiratory, if ventilated*** Maintain tidal volume (TV) at 6 mL/kg of body weight (BW). Assess for the need for positive end expiratory pressure (PEEP).

Continued

Making the Connections—cont'd

Signs and Symptoms	Physical Assessment Findings	Diagnostic Testing	Treatment
		Gram stain of blood, sputum, purulence, and urine (perhaps CSF). Culture and sensitivity of blood, urine, sputum, and purulence (perhaps CSF). Ultrasonography or CT may show source of infection. Electrolytes, BUN, creatinine, glucose, coagulation, platelet count, PTT, INR.	Maintain F_{IO_2} at lowest level to maintain P_{O_2} greater than 60 mm Hg. **_Circulatory_** Administer fluids, vasopressors, blood as appropriate to keep: MAP >65 mm Hg. Central venous pressure (CVP) between 8 and 12 cm H_2O. Hemoglobin levels adequate. **_Renal_** Administer sufficient fluids to keep urine output ≥0.5 mL/kg/hr. If infection, broad-spectrum antibiotics unless Gram stains allow identification of specific organism. Drainage of wounds or abscesses, if present.

Septic Shock | Septicemia with vasomotor instability; widespread capillary permeability and hypotension. Widespread arterial vasodilation throughout the body causes shock.

Signs and Symptoms	Physical Assessment Findings	Diagnostic Testing	Treatment
Alteration in mental state. Fever or hypothermia. Other symptoms depend on the source of sepsis: pain, tenderness, cough, SOB, fatigue, dizziness, headache, neck stiffness, dysuria, abdominal pain, flank pain, fever, and chills are all possible.	Alteration in mental state: Heart rate: >90/min. Respiratory rate: >20/min (may need mechanical ventilation). Temperature: >38°C or <36°C. Hypotension <90 systolic or 40 mm Hg below patient's normal blood pressure.	Chest x-ray may show pneumonia. ABGs show hypoxemia. Blood lactate elevated. WBC with differential showing leukocytosis or leukopenia. Urinalysis may show bacteria. Low urine output. Gram stain of blood, sputum, purulence, and urine (perhaps CSF). Culture and sensitivity of blood, sputum, purulence, and urine (perhaps CSF). Ultrasonography or CT may show source of infection. Electrolytes, BUN, creatinine, glucose, coagulation, platelet count, PTT, INR.	**_Respiratory, if not intubated_** Assess airway. Administer O_2 by mask or nasal cannula. **_Respiratory, if ventilated_** Maintain administered O_2 at lowest level to maintain P_{O_2} >60. **_Circulatory_** Administer fluids, vasopressors, blood as appropriate to keep MAP >65 mm Hg and CVP between 8 and 12 cm H_2O. Hemoglobin levels adequate. **_Renal_** Administer sufficient fluids to keep urine output ≥0.5 mL/kg/hr. If infection, broad-spectrum antibiotics unless Gram stains allow identification of specific organism. Drainage of wounds or abscesses, if present.

Making the Connections—cont'd

Signs and Symptoms	Physical Assessment Findings	Diagnostic Testing	Treatment
Multiple Organ Dysfunction Syndrome (MODS) | State of progressive dysfunction of two or more major organ systems in a critically ill patient who cannot maintain homeostasis without medical intervention. It can result from such disorders as MI, major trauma, burns, hemorrhage, infection, pancreatitis, or major surgery.			
Alteration in mental state. Fever or hypothermia. Variable symptoms depending on the organ that is failing: pain, tenderness, cough, SOB, fatigue, dizziness, headache, neck stiffness, dysuria, abdominal pain, flank pain, and chills are all possible.	Alteration in mental state: Heart rate: >90/min. Respiratory rate: >20/min (may need mechanical ventilation). Temperature: >38°C or <36°C. Hypotension <90 systolic or 40 mm Hg below patient's normal blood pressure.	Chest x-ray may show pulmonary infiltrates. ABGs show hypoxemia. Blood lactate elevated. WBC with differential may show leukocytosis or leukopenia. Electrolytes, BUN, creatinine, glucose, coagulation, platelet count, PTT, INR. Urinalysis may show bacteria. Low urine output. Gram stain of blood, sputum, purulence, and urine (perhaps CSF). Culture and sensitivity of blood, urine, sputum, and purulence (perhaps CSF). Ultrasonography or CT may show source of infection.	***Respiratory, if intubated*** Assess airway. Administer O_2 by mask or nasal cannula. ***Respiratory, if ventilated*** Maintain administered O_2 at lowest level to maintain Po_2 >60. ***Circulatory*** Administer fluids, vasopressors, blood as appropriate to keep: MAP >65 mm Hg. CVP between 8 and 12 cm H_2O. ***Renal*** Administer sufficient fluids to keep urine output ≥0.5 mL/kg/hr. If infection, broad-spectrum antibiotics unless Gram stains allow identification of specific organism. Drainage of wounds or abscesses, if present.
Acute Respiratory Distress Syndrome (ARDS) | Acute failure of the lungs caused by widespread injury of the alveoli that often occurs in the presence of shock or MODS. Alveoli become filled with fluid from the bloodstream. Condition causes pulmonary infiltrates and inability of lungs to oxygenate blood. Sometimes referred to as the most severe form of ALI.			
Respiratory distress. Possible alteration in mental state.	Possible alteration in mental state. Heart rate: >90/min. Respiratory rate: >20/min (need for mechanical ventilation). Hypotension <90 systolic or 40 mm Hg below patient's normal blood pressure.	Chest x-ray shows pulmonary infiltrates. ABGs show hypoxemia. WBC with differential may show leukocytosis or leukopenia. Electrolytes, BUN, creatinine, glucose, coagulation, platelet count, PTT, INR. Low urine output.	***Respiratory, if not intubated*** Assess airway. Administer O_2 by mask or nasal cannula. ***Respiratory, if ventilated*** Maintain administered O_2 at lowest level to maintain Po_2 >60. ECMO may be used. ***Circulatory*** Administer fluids, vasopressors, blood as appropriate to keep: MAP >65 mm Hg. CVP between 8 and 12 cm H_2O. ***Renal*** Administer sufficient fluids to keep urine output ≥0.5 mL/kg/hr.

Continued

Making the Connections—cont'd

Signs and Symptoms	Physical Assessment Findings	Diagnostic Testing	Treatment
Abdominal Compartment Syndrome (ACS) | Pressure within the abdominal cavity increases to the point that it exceeds the perfusion pressure of the capillaries, causing ischemia and necrosis of the tissues supplied by the abdominal arterial vessels and capillaries. This is called IAH.			
Increase in abdominal girth. Difficulty breathing. Decreased urine output. Syncope. Melena. Nausea and vomiting.	Increase in abdominal girth. Difficulty breathing. Decreased urine output. Syncope. Melena. Nausea and vomiting. Hypotension.	Monitoring of IAP via bladder. APP calculated by APP = MAP − IAP. Compartment syndrome present when APP remains low with refractory acidosis and hypotension despite appropriate conservative intervention. Abdominal x-ray or CT scan or ultrasound. WBC with differential may show leukocytosis or leukopenia. ABGs show respiratory acidosis. Liver function tests. Serum electrolytes, BUN, glucose, coagulation, platelet count, PTT, INR.	Restriction of fluid. Removing any object that may press on the patient's abdomen such as an abdominal binder. Pain management. Colloid infusions such as albumin to increase intravascular oncotic pressure. Nasogastric tube suction to remove air and fluid from the stomach and small intestines. Hemodialysis or hemofiltration to remove excess edema fluid. Rectal tube to evacuate colonic gas.

Bibliography

Available online at fadavis.com

Index

Page numbers followed by "*f*" denote figures, "*t*" denote tables, and "*b*" denote boxes.